Concussion and Traumatic Encephalopathy

Causes, Diagnosis, and Management

Concussion and Traumatic Encephalopathy

Causes, Diagnosis, and Management

Edited by
Jeff Victoroff
Department of Neurology, University of Southern California, Torrance, CA, USA
Erin D. Bigler
Psychology Department and Neuroscience Center, Brigham Young University, Provo, UT, USA

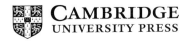

CAMBRIDGE
UNIVERSITY PRESS

University Printing House, Cambridge CB2 8BS, United Kingdom

One Liberty Plaza, 20th Floor, New York, NY 10006, USA

477 Williamstown Road, Port Melbourne, VIC 3207, Australia

314–321, 3rd Floor, Plot 3, Splendor Forum, Jasola District Centre, New Delhi – 110025, India

79 Anson Road, #06-04/06, Singapore 079906

Cambridge University Press is part of the University of Cambridge.

It furthers the University's mission by disseminating knowledge in the pursuit of education, learning, and research at the highest international levels of excellence.

www.cambridge.org
Information on this title: www.cambridge.org/9781107073951
DOI: 10.1017/9781139696432

First published 2019

Printed in the United Kingdom by TJ International Ltd. Padstow Cornwall

A catalogue record for this publication is available from the British Library

Library of Congress Cataloging-in-Publication Data
Names: Victoroff, Jeffrey Ivan, editor. | Bigler, Erin D., 1949– editor.
Title: Concussion and traumatic encephalopathy : causes, diagnosis and management / edited by Jeff Victoroff, Erin Bigler.
Description: Cambridge, United Kingdom ; New York, NY : Cambridge University Press, 2018. | Includes bibliographical references and index.
Identifiers: LCCN 2018000027 (print) | LCCN 2018000312 (ebook) | ISBN 9781107073951 (ebook) | ISBN 9781107073951 (hardback : alk. paper)
Subjects: | MESH: Brain Concussion | Chronic Traumatic Encephalopathy
Classification: LCC RC394.C7 (ebook) | LCC RC394.C7 (print) | NLM WL 354 | DDC 617.4/81044–dc23
LC record available at https://lccn.loc.gov/2018000027

ISBN 978-1-107-07395-1 Hardback

To the young, who – wide of eye and pure of heart – count on us to know the good.

Contents

The color plates are found between pages 682 and 683.

Guiding Apophthegm

Samuel Clemens, Jeff Victoroff and Erin D. Bigler

When in doubt, tell the truth.

Contributors

Amar Agha, M.D., FRCPI
Professor, Division of Neuroendocrinology
Consultant Endocrinologist
Beaumont Hospital and the Royal College of Surgeons
    in Ireland Medical School
Dublin, Ireland

Patrick S.F. Bellgowan, Ph.D.
Program Director, Repair and Plasticity
The National Institutes of Health/The National Institute
    of Neurological Disorders and Stroke
Bethesda, MD, U.S.

Erin D. Bigler, Ph.D.
Professor of Psychology and Neuroscience
Department of Psychology
Founding Director, Magnetic Resonance Imaging (MRI)
    Research Facility
Brigham Young University
Provo, UT, U.S.

Kaj Blennow, M.D., Ph.D.
Professor of Clinical Neurochemistry
Head of Clinical Neurochemistry Laboratory
Department of Psychiatry and Neurochemistry
Institute of Neuroscience and Physiology
Sahlgrenska Academy at the University of Gothenburg
Gothenburg, Sweden

Mark P. Burns, Ph.D.
Associate Professor of Neuroscience
Founding Director, Laboratory for Brain Injury and Dementia
Georgetown University
Washington, D.C., U.S.

Adam Darby, M.D.
UCLA Steve Tisch BrainSPORT Fellow
Department of Neurology
David Geffen School of Medicine at the University of
    California, Los Angeles
Los Angeles, CA, U.S.

Jeffrey Englander, M.D.
Director Brain Injury Rehabilitation (Retired)
Santa Clara Valley Medical Center
San Jose, CA, U.S.

Benton Giap, M.D.
Chair, Department of Physical Medicine and
    Rehabilitation
Santa Clara Valley Medical Center
San Jose, CA, U.S.

Christopher C. Giza, M.D.
Professor of Pediatric Neurology and Neurosurgery
Director, UCLA Steve Tisch BrainSPORT Program
Medical Director for TBI, Operation MEND-Wounded
    Warrior Project
UCLA Brain Research Center
Interdepartmental Programs for Neuroscience and
    Biomedical Engineering
Mattel Children's Hospital – UCLA
David Geffen School of Medicine at UCLA
Los Angeles, CA, U.S.

Nigel Glynn M.D., MRCPI
Consultant Endocrinologist
Saint Bartholomew's Hospital
London, U.K.

Kevin Guskiewicz, Ph.D., A.T.C.
Kenan Distinguished Professor
Departments of Exercise and Sport Science, Orthopaedics,
    UNC Injury Prevention Research Center, and Doctoral
    Program in Human Movement Science
Co-Director, Matthew Gfeller Sport-Related Traumatic
    Brain Injury Research Center
Director, Center for the Study of Retired Athletes
Dean – College of Arts and Sciences
University of North Carolina at Chapel Hill;
Chapel Hill, NC, U.S.

Robin A. Hurley, M.D., F.A.N.P.A.
Professor, Psychiatry and Behavioral Medicine
Wake Forest School of Medicine, Winston-Salem, NC
Adjunct Professor Psychiatry and Behavioral Sciences
Baylor College of Medicine
Associate Chief of Staff for Research and Academic Affairs
Salisbury VA Medical Center, Salisbury, NC
Associate Director, Education
VA Mid-Atlantic Health Care Network; Veterans Integrated
    Service Network 6

Mental Illness Research, Education and Clinical Center
Durham, NC, U.S.

Colleen E. Jackson, Ph.D.
Assistant Professor, Department of Psychiatry
Boston University School of Medicine
Geriatric Research, Education, and Clinical Center
Translational Research Center for TBI and Stress
    Disorders (TRACTS)
VA Boston Healthcare System
Boston, MA, U.S.

Brian Johnson, Ph.D., M.S., R.T.(MR)(N)
Postdoctoral Fellow
Penn State Center for Sports Concussion Research and Service
Departments of Kinesiology and Bioengineering
The Pennsylvania State University,
University Park, PA, U.S.

Barry D. Jordan, M.D., M.P.H.
Associate Professor Clinical Neurology
Weill Medical College of Cornell University
Assistant Medical Director, Burke Rehabilitation Hospital
Chief Medical Officer, New York State Athletic Commission
White Plains, NY, U.S.

Ricardo E. Jorge, M.D.
Professor, Menninger Department of Psychiatry and
    Behavioral Sciences
Beth K. and Stuart C. Yudofsky Division of Neuropsychiatry
Baylor College of Medicine
Houston, TX, U.S.

Giuseppe Lazzarino, Ph.D.
Professor of Biochemistry
Department of Biology, Geology and Environmental Sciences
Division of Biochemistry and Molecular Biology
University of Catania
Catania, Sicily, Italy

Helen Lee Lin, Ph.D.
Department of Psychiatry and Behavioral Sciences
Baylor College of Medicine
Houston, TX, U.S.

Michael F. Martelli, Ph.D., DAAPM
Director, Health and Rehabilitation Neuropsychology
Concussion Care Center of Virginia, Ltd. and Tree of Life
    Services
Glen Allen, VA, U.S.
Medical College of Virginia
Virginia Commonwealth University School of Medicine
Richmond, VA, U.S.

Andrew R. Mayer, Ph.D.
Associate Professor of Translational Neuroscience,
    Department of Psychology
The Mind Research Network/Lovelace Biomedical and
    Environmental Research

Adjunct Assistant Professor, Department of Neurology
University of New Mexico
Albuquerque, NM, U.S.

Curtis McKnight, M.D.
Assistant Professor
Department of Psychiatry
Creighton University School of Medicine
St. Joseph's Hospital and Medical Center
Phoenix, AZ, U.S.

Jon Pertab, Ph.D.
Department of Psychology
Intermountain Medical Center and Riverton Hospital
Salt Lake City, UT, U.S.

Stefano Signoretti, M.D., Ph.D.
Depatment of Neurosciences – Head and Neck Surgery
Division of Neurosurgery
San Camillo Hospital
Rome, Italy

Semyon Slobounov, Ph.D.
Professor of Kinesiology
College of Health and Human Development,
    Penn State University
Professor of Neurosurgery and Orthopaedics
Hershey College of Medicine, Penn State University
Director of Penn State Center for Sports Concussion
    Research and Service
Department of Kinesiology and Neurosurgery
Penn State Center for Sports Concussion
University Park, PA, U.S.

Katherine H. Taber, Ph.D., FANPA
Professor, Edward Via College of Osteopathic Medicine
Blacksburg, VA, U.S.
Assistant Director, Education
VA Mid-Atlantic Health Care Network
Veterans Integrated Service Network 6
Mental Illness Research, Education and Clinical Center
Durham, NC, U.S.
Research Health Scientist
Salisbury VAMC Research and Education Service
Salisbury, NC, U.S.

Barbara Tavazzi, Ph.D.
Institute of Biochemistry and Clinical Biochemistry
Catholic University of Rome
Rome, Italy

Elizabeth Teel, M.S.
Doctoral Candidate
School of Medicine, Department of Allied Health
Human Movement Science Curriculum
Matthew Gfeller Sports-Related Traumatic Brain Injury
    Research Center
University of North Carolina at Chapel Hill
Chapel Hill, NC, U.S.

Roberto Vagnozzi, M.D., Ph.D.
Associate Professor of Neurosurgery
Division of Neurotraumatology nad Neuroradiology
Department of Biomedicine and Prevention, Section of
    Neurosurgery
University of Rome, Tor Vergata
Rome, Italy

Jennifer J. Vasterling, Ph.D.
Professor, Department of Psychiatry
Boston University School of Medicine
Chief of Psychology, VA Boston Healthcare System
President of the Society for Clinical Neuropsychology
    (Division 40 of the American Psychological Association)
Boston, MA, U.S.

Jeff Victoroff, M.D.
Associate Professor of Clinical Neurology and Psychiatry
Keck School of Medicine
University of Southern California, Los Angeles, CA, U.S.

Sonia Villapol, Ph.D.
Assistant Professor
Department of Neuroscience
Laboratory for Brain Injury and Dementia
Georgetown University Medical Center
Washington, D.C., U.S.

Ashley L. Ware
Clinical Psychology Graduate Student
Department of Physical Medicine and Rehabilitation
Baylor College of Medicine
Houston, TX, U.S.

Patricia M. Washington, Ph.D.
Postdoctoral Research Scientist
Columbia University Medical Center
New York, NY, U.S.

Elisabeth A. Wilde, Ph.D.
Associate Professor
Departments of Physical Medicine and Rehabilitation,
    Neurology, and Radiology
Director of Research for Physical Medicine and Rehabilitation
Baylor College of Medicine
Health Research Scientist, Michael E. DeBakey VA
    Medical Center
Houston, TX, U.S.

Rebecca L. Wilken
Graduate Student, Department of Biology
American University
Washington, D.C., U.S.

Nathan D. Zasler, M.D., FAAPM&R, FAADEP, DAAPM, CBIST
Professor, affiliate, Department of Physical Medicine and
    Rehabilitation
Virginia Commonwealth University
Richmond, VA, U.S.
Clinical Associate Professor, Department of Physical Medicine
    and Rehabilitation
University of Virginia, Charlottesville
Charlottesville, VA, U.S.
CEO and Medical Director, Concussion Care Centre of
    Virginia, Ltd.
CEO and Medical Director, Tree of Life Services, Inc.
Vice-Chairperson, International Brain Injury Association

Henrik Zetterberg, M.D., Ph.D.
Professor; Chief Physician
Department of Psychiatry and Neurochemistry
Institute of Neuroscience and Physiology
Sahlgrenska Academy at the University of Gothenburg
Gothenburg, Sweden
UCL Institute of Neurology
Queen Square, London, U.K.

Preface

Jeff Victoroff

Traumatic brain injury (TBI) is the leading cause of death and disability in people younger than age 45 in the United States … most TBIs are mild.

Nguyen et al., 2016, p. 774 [1]

Typical, clinically attended concussive brain injuries often lead to persistent deleterious brain change. Contrary to the guesses of writers from previous centuries, according to the best analysis of the best empirical evidence, more than 40% of survivors of such concussions still suffer from and/or exhibit neurobehavioral deficits at one year or more post-injury. That fact has global implications for human health.

It is not clear at what moment in history that fact became apparent to the scholarly community. It is not clear to whom credit belongs for that startling observation. In fact, rather than a eureka moment followed by proclamation and universal acclaim, the discovery that typical concussions commonly lead to lasting cerebral dysfunction was initially received with blinking dubiety and even stiff-necked resistance. Thankfully (if somewhat belatedly), the world's neurological community has shaken off the dogged dogma of the 20th century and attended with steadily improving observations and steadily increasing alarm to the empirical evidence that concussions are highly heterogeneous and not reliably benign. That is a paradigm shift.

A concussion is a rattling blow or earthquake-like shaking. To discuss such a blow and its possible effects, one is obliged to specify what is concussed. Sometimes, it is the brain. Sometimes, the blow causes injury. When that occurs, the logical specifier is *concussive brain injury* (CBI). The subject of this book, therefore, is CBI.

CBI is not "mild traumatic brain injury (mTBI)." CBI is not mild anything. It means what it says – comprising the spectrum of brain injuries attributable to inopportune visitation by an abrupt external force that, usually, strikes the hair of the head and causes harm. CBI is the most common type of mammalian TBI. Most mammalian CBIs pass without notice or report, which limits our knowledge to a subset. Those are the typical, clinically attended CBIs that account for about 90% of human emergency room visits after head trauma. Athletic trainers, combat medics, and primary care providers also attend such injuries. Confessing from the outset that one can say little

about the huge domain of unreported CBI, one does one's best with the limited available data. The editors of this book feel animated by the thrill of discovery, humbled by the enormity of the problem, and passionate about figuring things out based on first principles. We pledge to do our best.

Many millions of youth in the current generation will suffer CBIs. However, they will be members of the first generation in history to grow up in the new era – an era of scientific revolution about the real effects of blows to the head. This volume is intended to be the first comprehensive textbook of the new era.

Despite centuries of study, some of the most basic questions about CBI remain as opaque as sacred mysteries. What exactly happens in the head? Is that the same from brain to brain? What proportion of concussion survivors suffer brain changes for what time duration, and why them? What does "recovery" mean? Does adaptation to injury carry a hidden cost? Can one CBI cause permanent harm? Is that commonplace or rare? Do one or more CBIs accelerate brain aging, or trigger conventional neurodegeneration, or cause a unique post-concussive dementia? In every concussion survivor or just a few? And what on earth can we do to mitigate the harm of this globally endemic disorder?

Readers are in for a feast. Although our ignorance remains profound and our capacity to intervene remains primitive, a cornucopia of new data and revised conceptualization has grandly enriched the scholarly banquet in just the last ten years. A host of heroic efforts by devoted clinicians and scholars deserves credit for overthrowing the more egregious fallacies of the 20th century. Neuroscientists have graduated from the old "cascade" hypothesis, replacing that thin-slice pathophysiology with a meatier framework that recognizes the interdigitation of force, genetics, and pre-morbid status in a dramatic brain-wide post-concussive melee between scores of degenerative and regenerative factors. Neuroimagers have soundly trounced the "Three-Month Myth," according to which a previous generation of scholars imagined concussion to be self-limited in the overwhelming majority of cases. Neurologists, physiatrists, and psychiatrists have flung aside the straightjacket of clinical homogenization, recognizing that concussion does not do any one thing, or any five things, but has as many presentations and courses as there are genomes. Neuropsychologists, having discovered that paper-and-pencil tests from the 1960s are invalid and insensitive to the effects of CBI, are boldly reinventing their field, dismissing the localizationist fallacy and seeking concordance with the revelations of functional neuroimaging. Neuropathologists have courageously bucked resistance to follow the trail of breadcrumbs back from degenerate brains to repetitive CBIs. Public policy is finally beginning to be informed by concussion science. This textbook – perhaps better called a brief collaborative essay – summarizes the state of the art and attempts, in so far as possible, to anticipate the trajectory of discovery.

What's New?

In-depth epidemiological analysis suggests a much higher incidence of clinically significant CBI than was previously appreciated (see Chapter 2). Critical investigation exposes the dubious validity of much animal research (Chapter 4). Systematic review reveals a much higher than previously recognized rate of persistent post-concussive distress and dysfunction. Moreover, for the first time, biomarkers support the conclusion that prolonged post-concussive psychiatric symptoms must be associated with organic brain damage (Chapters 5 and 10). We need, and do not have, a neuroimaging marker of CBI. That may change shortly, as we adopt machines that permit us to watch a single protein fold (Chapter 6). Recent data show why outcome research will remain mired in fallacy pending adoption of genetic, epistatic, and epigenetic stratification, and why treatments will remain randomly effective pending the discovery of biomarkers with individual predictive validity (Chapter 7). Intriguing evidence suggests that smoked marijuana is the most effective treatment for post-concussive irritability and aggression. The U.S. federal government, however, willfully blocks the urgently needed research (Chapter 10). Neuroscientific advances have overthrown dated theories of aging-related brain change and informed a dramatically new approach to studying the late effects of CBIs, mandating a profound rethinking of "traumatic encephalopathy" (Chapters 11, 13, and 14). As of 2018, for the first time in history, the U.S. Food and Drug Administration has approved a biomarker panel for computed tomography (CT)-positive traumatic brain injury. It is absolutely not a concussion test (Chapter 17). Although research has been heartbreakingly slow to discover efficacious interventions, management of concussed people is beginning to rest on science (Chapters 20, 23, 24–27). Some concussions trigger legal disputes. It is hard for an honest doctor to serve justice in an adversarial system: shadows haunt the cavern where paid experts covene. But federal Rule of Evidence 706 is quietly swinging a light at the edge of that dark place (Chapter 28).

Many survivors of typical, clinically attended concussions feel fine after a week – especially in cases of sport-related concussion. Yet a large proportion of concussion survivors continue to suffer or display neurobehavioral problems for many months or years. Why? In so far as the present parlous state of the science permits, this slender volume has the answer. Readers will be provided with abundant evidence – much of it very recent – that supports what is arguably the first major reconceptualization of concussion in more than a century.

For instance, previous generations conceived of concussion as a transient event and took "recovery" for granted. How would one ever know? Subjective recovery is, of course, highly desirable. So is functional recovery. Neither of these, however, is either reliably measurable or a marker for normalization of brain function. Nor is return of neurofilament light levels to baseline [2]. Nor is the statement, "I'm fine." At the time of this writing, true and complete brain recovery after a typical clinically attended CBI has yet to be demonstrated. Instead of attempting to assess brain recovery – meaning restoration to pre-morbid status with no risk of late effects – most of the old literature discussed results from superficial desktop behavioral assessments or from insensitive bioassays – such as autopsy. Science long ago transcended the assumption of neuropathological omniscience. Although subjecting fragments of dead tissue to chemical manipulations and looking at them was an exciting innovation 125 years ago, the resulting *a posteriori* inferences about the orchestrated dynamic interactions of the ~16 billion adult cortical neurons of at least 17 types [3] are speculative, not probative. One *hopes* that human brains (or some) have the capacity to fully recover after CBI. But, surprising as it may seem, in regard to authentic recovery with no late effects, the jury is out. That recent realization has made CBI a legitimate suspect in the premature aging of tens of millions of brains and galvanized the international quest for better answers.

Although some critical questions remain intractable to the best science, others have recently yielded to the muscular levers of scholarship and technology. Readers will learn, for example:

- why there is a striking mismatch between subjective recovery and biological recovery
- why outcomes vary
- why conventional neuropsychological testing fails to detect indisputable brain dysfunction
- why, despite the supposed protective effects of estrogen, menstruating women are at greater risk for lasting harm
- why "post-concussion syndrome" has been abandoned as a clinical entity
- why determining the late effects of concussion has frustrated neuroscience for more than a century – and how that problem may soon be solved
- why *chronic traumatic encephalopathy* is an extremely common human condition, although a recent academic shanghaiing of that phrase focused attention on a narrowly characterized, dubiously unitary subset of cases
- what evidence-based practices are most likely to help a concussed person in the emergency room – and after.

This is a story about knights, and a few knaves, and a fight to bring scientific rigor to a field long beclouded by lore and sacred cows. The editors submit this text to readers with high hopes and earnest caveats. Textbooks usually explain and support the status quo. In good conscience, we cannot. Dr. Bigler and I, by evolutionary convergence or serendipity, arrived at pretty much the same conclusion at the same time: the barrier to understanding the immense spectrum of human consequences of CBI was not merely the antiquated 20th-century prejudice that dismissed patients with long-term complaints, not only the frugality of funding agencies and the resulting poverty of data, but something deeper: a systematic misunderstanding of health and neurobehavioral dysfunction that seems to have arrested the development of this field for about two generations. We felt compelled to start fresh – to unfetter the narrative from the tyranny of dated terms of art and seek a straightforward, logical, semantically coherent, scientifically muscular conceptual framework loyal to the commands of the data.

We know our earnest wish to just make sense may trigger cognitive dissonance in some readers. Students may become disoriented. Professors whom we call friends may regret their hearty lunches. And, in the end, overthrowing the illogic of 20th-century neurological nosology may prove impossible – leaving our account a historical outlier. Nonetheless, we both feel ethically compelled to do our darndest, informed by our rustic faith in first principles. The stakes are enormous. We dearly hope that – after an awkward period of outrage and adjustment – the result is human benefit.

References

1. Nguyen R, Fiest KM, McChesney J, Kwon C-S, Jette N, Frolkis AD, et al. The international incidence of traumatic brain injury: a systematic review and meta-analysis. *Can J Neurol Sci* 2016; **43**: 774–785.

2. Shahim P, Zetterberg H, Tegner Y, Blennow B. Serum neurofilament light as a biomarker for mild traumatic brain injury in contact sports. *Neurology* 2017; **88**: 1788–1794.

3. Jiang X, Shen S, Cadwell CR, Berens P, Sinz F, Ecker AS, et al. Principles of connectivity among morphologically defined cell types in adult neocortex. *Science* 2015; **350** (6264): aac9462.

Acknowledgments

First and foremost, I thank my patients who survived concussive brain injuries (CBIs). They shared their life stories, thoughts, and feelings. It was not my professors, not my textbooks, not the grand libraries whose stacks I've haunted that alerted me to the gravity of CBI as a human problem. In fact, those didactic sources delayed insight, because, until very recently, the most ravenous scholar would starve looking for impartial and open-minded academic accounts explaining concussion. There are many reasons we can now share the revelations of the last decade or so. In my own case, the first glimmerings of awareness came in the clinic. Repeated, artless, forthright stories of long-term problems after so-called "mild" injuries finally rang a bell in my own head. I am embarrassed that it took so long before I reached astonishment at the mismatch between textbook minimization of the problem and the troubling human truth. The candor and eloquence of concussion survivors set off the alarm that propelled me from complacence to passionate commitment.

Second, I cherish the collaboration, counsel, support, and friendship of Erin D. Bigler. Readers already know Erin is a towering figure – a neuropsychologist whose empirical and theoretical contributions to the understanding of CBI are legendary. His brilliance, depth of thought, work ethic, and innumerable accomplishments are widely familiar and authentically awe-inspiring. None of that explains our friendship. Those who have been privileged to know him know his most precious quality: Erin is a good man. Outsiders might imagine medicine and psychology to attract thoughtful, wise, and compassionate people. They do. But there is a high ceiling and a low floor. In more than 30 years in academic neurobehavioral practice I have never encountered another professor whose gift of virtue – wholehearted devotion to doing what is right – matches Dr. Bigler's.

Third, I must express the deepest regard for our co-authors. If they did not know what they were getting into from the outset of our collaborative essay project, they gradually came to realize that the editors were shooting for the moon. Erin and I, by evolutionary convergence or serendipity, arrived at pretty much the same conclusion at the same time: the problem with truly understanding the human consequences of CBI transcended the combined effects of low-quality research and puritanical suspicion of patients with persistent distress. The problem seems to have been a widespread failure of imagination, such that symptoms that could not be explained by then-available technology were reflexively attributed to psychogenic illness. Asking our co-authors to rethink the problem from first principles was an outrageous imposition. Academics get no credit for book chapters. Our co-authors, therefore, not only volunteered to beautifully summarize their expert knowledge, but to question the very roots of that knowledge – *pro bono*. They more than ably rose to that challenge, transcending the duties of scholarship and, when required, braving the risk of criticism for daring to doubt the received wisdom. We are most warmly appreciative of their special effort.

Fourth, I must somehow credit the giants upon whose shoulders we humbly stand, without writing a list as long and considerate of history as the *Mahābhārata*. Two inspirations from the mid 20th century were the neurologist Cyril Courville and the psychologist Hans-Lukas Teuber. Both cried out like voices in the wilderness, urging deeper thought about traumatic brain injuries. More recent figures, sure to become historical, are neurologist Barry D. Jordan (one of our co-authors) and neuropathologist Bennet Ifeakandu Omalu – both heroes for following the data in the face of contention. Journalist Alan Schwarz (a finalist for the Pulitzer Prize in public service) deserves credit for exposing the despicable behavior of the National Football League on the front page of the *New York Times* – an initiative that hugely raised public consciousness of the dangers of repetitive concussions. In the same vein, Peter Landesman is owed credit for multiplying global awareness of the problem, writing and directing the 2015 film *Concussion*. A team of prolific and indefatigable scholars at Boston University will go down in history for taking the sport-related concussions ball and running with it – energetically exploring the hypothesis that repetitive CBIs sometimes cause a special and tragic spectrum of brain changes. Just two members of that deep team are neuropsychologist Robert Stern and neuropathologist Ann McKee. Kevin Guskiewicz, another of our co-authors, is a sports medicine scientist who, for more than two decades, has played a keystone role in advancing the understanding of sport-related CBI. Yet another of our co-authors, Christopher C. Giza, along with his colleague David A. Hovda, revolutionized the understanding of why trauma can become a crisis for a neuron. That work, synthesized with complementary findings regarding inflammation, molecular genetics, protein conformation, and the connectome, buttresses almost every effort to find an effective early intervention.

These and many other bold individuals have literally fought to get out the truth in the face of tremendous disciplinary and institutional resistance. Not everyone wants it to be known that typical concussions commonly lead to long-term (and possibly permanent) brain damage. This brief collaborative essay may conceivably be regarded as the introduction of a paradigm shift. At the least, it is a heartfelt plea for a long-overdue revolution. It is past time to overthrow the untenable assumptions and insupportable prejudices of 20th-century concussion writing in favor of science, untrammeled by dogma. Our new conceptualization hardly arose *de novo* like an island from a volcano. It is merely the inevitable accretion and synthesis of thousands of novel, careful, open-minded empirical investigations. The original investigators are the soul of today's revolution. The list, really, goes back to Hippocrates – and will hopefully go forward to include a few of our readers.

Finally, we gratefully honor the contributions of Kaylee L. Valverde, Susan Wheatley, and JoAnn Petrie, Ph.D. Erin and I are old guys. We are eager to keep up with neurobiology and imaging technologies, but our understanding of clerical technology peaked with the IBM Selectric. To make this book happen, we turned to experts. These authorities mastered EndNote and other digital magic that has (according to early reports) facilitated coherent scientific documentation. Their energetic and thoughtful support enabled us to deliver a text enhanced with citations and figures that credit our sources and offer our readers direct access to data that will hopefully benefit humanity for generations to come.

Jeff Victoroff

The first acknowledgment goes to patients and research participants who have sustained a concussive brain injury (CBI). They are the inspiration behind all of my research and clinical work with traumatic brain injury (TBI). It was 1975 when I conducted my first neuropsychological exam of a pre-teen with a history of concussion, who was experiencing persisting symptoms. Understanding concussion from a mid-20th-century perspective emphasized its benign nature and inconsequentiality. So why was this child still having problems? Computed axial tomograms or CAT scans – the original acronym – had just been introduced as an initial triage assessment for "closed head injury," as it was referred to then. By today's standards the original CAT scans were laboriously slow and the images based on enormous voxel sizes, as large as a cubic centimeter. Nonetheless it was incredibly exciting to be able to visualize the brain in the living patient, regardless of how crude the image might be.

As reflected in the medical records, the first child I saw had been hit by a car while riding his bike, experienced a brief loss of consciousness as witnessed by family members, but this child had a negative CAT scan and routine skull films when evaluated in the emergency department. Note this was before the universal adoption of the Glasgow Coma Scale (GCS) rating system, so there was no GCS recorded. The child was observed overnight and then discharged. I did not see the child until several months post-injury when there were issues of poor concentration, attention, and memory, particularly notable in terms of diminished academic performance at school, along with what the parents reported as moodiness, poor impulse control, and impulsivity. None of these symptoms/problems had been observed before the injury, but he was also a pre-teen and pubescent. Neuropsychological tests reflected relatively intact cognitive performance and, given the conventional clinical wisdom of the day, as already stated, it was just assumed that over time things would be OK.

While true that the majority of cases of CBI do seem to run a "benign" course, the fact that I was seeing cases with persisting symptoms/problems, as above, was troubling. Animal models of CBI were being developed showing more definitive neuropathology – the brain was being injured, detectable at the microscopic level, even with so-called "mild" injury, but not necessarily at the behavioral level. Then in the 1980s, magnetic resonance imaging (MRI) rapidly ascended as the neuroimaging choice for examining the chronic effects of TBI. I remember a CBI case that had a negative CT scan yet when the original proton density MRI sequence was run, this patient's scan showed multiple scattered "hypointense" foci. As we now know, these abnormalities reflect petechial hemorrhages from shear injury, eventually shown to be hemosiderin deposition.

This was a remarkable discovery, because now there was something "objective" to relate to the symptoms/complaints of the CBI patient. Neuroimaging techniques and technologies to investigate CBI improved steadily and dramatically during the end of the 20th and beginning of the 21st century.

In 1975 I also started teaching psychology and neuroscience courses. On all of my syllabi I had Albert Einstein's famous quote of "looking deep into nature, and then you will understand everything better." But in the 1980s I also started including the following statement, credited to Jeremiah Ostriker, a physicist who championed the theory of dark matter: "In young scientific fields if you say all the accepted positions are wrong, you'll seldom be wrong." Now this was a hard, physical science professor speaking about physics and astronomy, referring to them as still being "young." The first international societies involving neuroscience and neuropsychology were being established at about this same time frame – early 1970s. So, if one rejects the prevailing theory, especially in "young" fields – using Ostriker's axiom – one would likely not be wrong.

With the rapidly improving new advances in neuroimaging we now had hard evidence that, at least some individuals who sustained CBI had demonstrable, underlying evidence of physical neuropathology. This began the quest for examining neuroimaging correlates of CBI and listening to what patients were saying about symptoms/problems they were experiencing.

It also became evident to me that, while neuroimaging technology was improving at an incredibly rapid pace, neuropsychology was not. Neuroscience likewise was exponentially adding new discoveries, especially in the interface of cognitive neuroscience with neuroimaging. One of the neuroscience textbooks I used was titled *The Neuron: Cell and Molecular Biology*. In the preface to the third edition, I.B. Levitan and L.K. Kaczmarek

Acknowledgments xxi

lament the fact that statements in the first two editions were "completely inaccurate." They go on to explain:

It is not that we are acknowledging any major errors of scientific fact in the past editions (although time will certainly show that some of what we now believe about the functioning of the brain is wrong). Rather, the arrival of a new millennium has made nonsense of most of the statements that began "Earlier in this century" [1, p. vii].

All of this became my mantra for exploring CBI. Look deep into nature, reject prevailing theories because they are likely incorrect, embrace new technology and insights that will guide discovery, and establish an improved scientific foundation for the effects of CBI. These views have guided not only my research and clinical work, but also the vision of this book.

I still have my notes from those beginning lectures involved in teaching clinical neuropsychology. What is troubling is that the core aspects of traditional assessment in neuropsychology have not changed in 50 years – the training lecture I gave in 1975 could be given today, basically unaltered. Yes, we have the fourth or fifth edition of a particular test now, but the foundations of that test have not changed. In this 21st-century, information explosion world we now live in, the neuropsychology of concussion has been stagnant, mostly tied to traditional clinical assessment measures that have not advanced the field. Past neuropsychological approaches to understanding CBI have been mostly frozen by its restricted use of conventional techniques. As such, this book rejects many past and prevailing thoughts about CBI that have come out of neuropsychology. It does so because to move a field beyond conventional thought means that those concepts need to be challenged. What is written about in this text provides numerous opportunities for establishing new, testable hypotheses about CBI. We may be entirely wrong about some of what we say about CBI – if so, demonstrate it with the appropriate research study and design, and prove us wrong.

I thank Dr. Victoroff for approaching me to collaborate with him on this project. We had kindred ideas about CBI that we have brought out in this text.

I always acknowledge the support of my wife, Jan, who has tolerated all of my time devoted to academics, research, writing, and clinical work for almost half a century. Many of the images and illustrations in the textbook are with the assistance of my lab director, Tracy Abildskov. His dedication to brain research and neuroimaging is acknowledged, as are the writing and research support from Jo Ann Petrie, Ph.D., and the secretarial assistance of Susan Wheatley, Kaylee L. Valverde, and Adelaine Sowards.

Erin D. Bigler

Reference

1. Levitan IB, Kaczmarek LK. *The Neuron: Cell and Molecular Biology,* 3rd edn. Oxford: Oxford University Press, 2002.

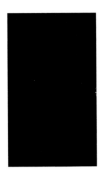

Introduction

Jeff Victoroff

> There is still controversy in the literature whether a single episode of mild traumatic brain injury (MTBI) results in short-term functional and/or structural deficits as well as any induced long-term residual effects.
>
> Zhang et al., 2010[1]

Salve, Elephant!

Zhang et al.[1], in the opening quotation, might be credited with the most politic of understatements. The controversy regarding the effects of concussive brain injury (CBI) is antique, intractable, and intemperate. Of course, controversy is common in medicine. Human biology is only slowly yielding to post-Enlightenment empiricism. As a result, some people perhaps know a bit more than others, but no one knows how things really work. Uncertainty combined with the emotional impact of human malady and professional competitiveness is bound to generate contention.

Yet the degree of agonism dividing the traumatic brain injury (TBI) community is extraordinary. New initiates to the study of CBI may encounter virtually opposite opinions, both pronounced with sober confidence by eminent authorities. Medical students raise eyebrows when instructors with diametrically opposing views take turns at the podium. Young neuropsychology interns learn to couch the impressions in their draft reports to suit the biases of each supervisor. Patients and families of victims are at a loss regarding whom to trust. Fair or not, young contributors quickly acquire labels, like team jerseys, identifying them as champions of one side or the other.

It is important, at the outset, to welcome the elephant in the room. Experts reading this chapter know exactly what the author means. Attend any TBI conference, especially one that focuses on concussion or so-called "mild traumatic brain injury" (mTBI). The tension is palpable. Eager young scholars juggling poster tubes and paper coffee cups display arousal and hope. Published authorities display tighter smiles. The hail fellow well met theater observed between scholarly opponents at most professional gatherings is, in this case, either over-acted or eschewed. The players know each other. The hierarchy is rigid. The lines are drawn in blood.

In a nutshell, some published authorities assert the following as if they were facts:

1. the cerebral consequences of a CBI are reasonably well known, and

2. a single CBI infrequently causes persistent human distress due to brain change.

Other authorities – and the editors of this slender introductory text – disagree.

Figures 1 and 2 illustrate several facets of the burning and seemingly entwined issues that drive the contributors to this textbook: concussion and traumatic encephalopathy. Figure 1 is one of innumerable graphs depicting the change in the prevalence of post-concussive symptoms after a CBI [2]. Note that: (1) the highest level of subjective distress typically occurs just after the injury; (2) fewer victims report distress as times goes on; and yet (3) the curve does not reach zero. It appears asymptotic because about 25% of victims in this study reported persistent symptoms. Figure 2 is a fairly recent

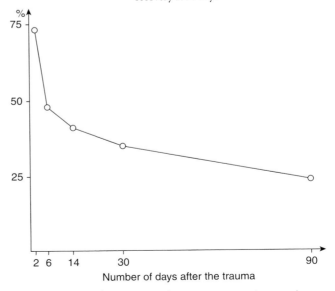

Fig. 1 Percentage of patients reporting one or more post-concussive symptoms on various occasions during the observation period.

Source: Lidvall et al., 1974 [2] Fig. V.1

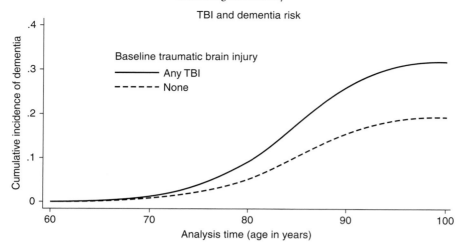

Age at dementia diagnosis in veterans with and without traumatic brain injury (TBI), accounting for mortality

Fig. 2
The cumulative incidence of dementia is shown for veterans with TBI at baseline (solid line) and without TBI at baseline (dashed line), accounting for the competing risk of mortality. Age is used as the time scale to indicate age at dementia diagnosis.

Source: Barnes et al., 2014 [3] http://n.neurology. org/content/83/4/312.short

depiction of the association between prior TBI (mostly concussion) and dementia[3]. Note that: (1) in late middle age, veterans with a history of any TBI begin to deviate in regard to the incidence of dementia from those without a history of TBI; and (2) again, cumulative incidence increases over time.

Students of CBI must account for the findings reported in Figures 1 and 2. Of course, one explanation might be faulty research. Perhaps these findings and all of the similar peer-reviewed findings cannot be reproduced and should be roughly dismissed as statistical flukes or methodological errors. However, for the sake of argument, what if these observations are true? What process might explain both curves?

Assuming for the moment that Figure 1 displays authentically observed data, and that the study is representative, it implies that persistent post-concussive symptoms are common. It does not explain why. In the forthcoming chapters, the reader will have the opportunity to consider many theoretical explanations that have been advanced to account for the commonplace report of persistent post-concussive symptoms – from permanent organic brain injury to self-conscious malingering. Science has yet to prove the cause of persistent post-concussive symptoms – or, more accurately, to measure the relative contribution of multiple potential causes in any individual case. For the time being, however, we will hopefully all accept one compelling conclusion from Figure 1: people's responses to a CBI vary.

Now assume for the moment that Figure 2 also displays observed and representative data. If so, it appears that people who have suffered a TBI (in most cases; a CBI, in most cases, many years prior to the study) have an increased risk of developing dementia at an early-than-usual age. That is, despite the somewhat reassuring downslope of the curve in Figure 1, suggesting that most victims do not complain for very long periods of time, one is confronted with the worrisome upslope of the curve in Figure 2, suggesting that at least some, if not *all*, victims remain at risk of neurological disorder even if decades have passed since their CBI. (This raises the question of whether anybody ever recovers from a concussion – a question to which we will return.)

What process accounts for both curves? The correct answer is "nobody knows." This is perhaps a slightly atypical admission

Table 1 Barriers to knowledge about concussive brain injury

I. Insufficient empirical investigation
II. Lack of a meaningful outcome measure
III. Misplaced faith in a dated conceptual trichotomy
IV. Misplaced faith in flawed modes of inquiry
A. Misplaced faith in authority
B. Misplaced faith in consensus
C. Misplaced faith in cognitive testing
V. Bias, temperament, and conflicts of interest

in the introduction to a medical textbook – to acknowledge our collective and embarrassing ignorance. Yet the only intellectually honest position in CBI studies is to note the giant gaps in empirical investigation that currently divide us from better understanding. In a nutshell, virtually no research has answered the question, "How can we characterize the spectrum of long-term – perhaps lifelong – neurobiological consequences expected after a human concussion?" The word *spectrum* is key. There is no single and identical effect from any two concussions. Resistance to that fact is one of the barriers to knowledge we must overcome.

That having been said, the insight of science is gradually detecting some light at the end of our tunnels. Over about the last decade or so, new empirical findings have discredited the old "we know what happens in concussion and there is little to worry about" mantra. This textbook will show that science supports three dramatically different conclusions:

1. The pathophysiology of concussion is highly variable and poorly understood.
2. The long-term consequences of concussion are highly variable and largely unknown.
3. There are lots of reasons to worry.

Knowledge Versus Opinion

At the risk of getting sucked into the muskeg of epistemology, multiple factors block the route to knowledge. (Table 1 offers a partial list.) A brief examination of these factors may be enlightening, although, admittedly, some factors are better supported by verifiable evidence than others, and some might provoke disciplinary defensiveness.

I. Insufficient Empirical Investigation

An interesting meeting was held in Bethesda, Maryland in July of 2013. The meeting, hosted in part by the National Institute of Neurological Disorders and Stroke, was titled, Brain Trauma-Related Neurodegeneration workshop [4]. The purported goal was to survey "experts" regarding the best research approach to determine whether and in what way concussions may increase the risk of later neurodegeneration. At the opening of that meeting the present author delivered a brief address titled The Hans-Lukas Teuber Memorial Research Presentation. The thrust of those remarks was simple: the National Institutes had been down this road almost 50 years before. They had convened a remarkably similar meeting in year 1968. The title of that one: *Late Effects of Head Injury* [5]. One of their own, a nominal neuropsychologist but actual polymath named Hans-Lukas Teuber, said,

> It is my firm belief, after struggling with these problems for a good many years, that these difficulties can be overcome if we take the following steps: First, we should abandon the distinctions between broader and narrower definitions of the posttraumatic syndrome … Second, I propose we suspend our belief in the separateness of neurological and behavioral signs and symptoms … Finally … If one wants to advance the understanding of head injuries and their consequences, one had better study reasonably large groups of cases for which the initial trauma is fairly well demonstrated and constitutes the *sole* criterion for inclusion … Over the long run, clinicopathological correlations will make sense.
>
> Teuber, 1969 [6], pp. 13–14

In other words, Teuber exhorted his peers,

> Stop fooling around with short-term, small-scale studies that never consider the ultimate impact of TBI on the patient. Abandon the pretense that some symptoms are *neurological* and some are *psychological*. It's high time to perform large-scale, prospective, long-term studies of TBI, considering cognitive, non-cognitive, and somatic changes [6].

Sounds reasonable.

The Institutes declined to follow Dr. Teuber's advice. If they had done so, we would now have almost 50 years of data tracking the effect of concussion on the human brain. TBI does not seem to have been a priority. One reason may have been the misunderstanding, prevalent in the 20th century, that CBIs were benign. Whatever the cause, investigators of CBI are perhaps 50 years behind investigators of vascular disease, infectious disease, and cancer.

In fairness, consider the education of the participants at that long-ago meeting: Most had been taught that concussions are trivial. Despite Koch and Filehne's 1874 report about the impact of repetitive concussions [7], despite the eye-opening

data published by Michael Osnato and Vincent Gilberti in 1927 demonstrating that even mild TBIs may cause a lasting "traumatic encephalitis" [8], and Martland's paper [9] of the next year (1928) about the chronic encephalopathy of boxers titled "Punch drunk," despite Courville's passionate, scholarly, and courageous book *Commotio Cerebri* [10], published in 1953, explaining why minor head injuries can have a major life impact, the typical medical student from the 1960s and 1970s graduated with the belief that concussions generate temporary and innocuous effects.

That belief is mistaken. Both animal and human research strongly confirm the many historic warnings: some victims of concussion suffer lasting harm (see Chapter 2). We are gradually coming to appreciate that, as a result, concussion creates an immense burden on human well-being and social function. TBI is mostly concussion. TBI is the most important cause of disability for people under age 45 [11] Moreover, unlike illnesses that are becoming less common due to therapeutic advances, TBI is a growing epidemic:

> According to WHO [World Health Organization], because incidence is increasing swiftly in low-income and middle-income countries (mostly owing to road traffic accidents), TBI is predicted to become the third leading cause of global mortality and disability by 2020. Furthermore, evidence suggests that TBI is a risk factor for dementia, substance abuse, and other psychiatric disorders. However, few improvements in clinical outcomes for patients with TBI have been achieved over the past two decades, and no effective therapy for TBI has been approved by any regulatory agency [12].

Two thousand years of study. No effective therapy. Despite the magnitude and severity of the problem, despite the pitiful progress in finding solutions, the effort to understand concussion has been inadequately researched.

It is important to make a distinction: one question is whether the most promising research has been performed. A different question is whether TBI research is underfunded. That is, perhaps research funding has been more than adequate but the selection of projects has been unwise. That difficult issue will be addressed periodically throughout this volume; but again, there are two possibilities. One: some of the choice of projects has been unavoidably limited due to the lack of technological capabilities. For instance, at one point in history, structural magnetic resonance imaging (MRI) with a few pulse sequences was the state of the art. Scholars using structural MRI cannot be criticized for failing to detect subtle or long-term brain changes that are apparent with more advanced methods. Similarly, normal rodent brains fail to exhibit a progressive deposition of several aging-related and apparently toxic proteins associated with neurodegeneration. Until transgenic animals could be developed, even a high-quality long-term prospective study of the impact of concussion on rats could not have revealed, for example, increased tau.

However, some of the disappointing choice in research projects is due to a blinders-on mentality, insensitive to the early evidence that concussion can produce long-term changes in brain and behavior. Discounting that evidence (and judging it a waste of money to keep following the patient), many clinical investigators abandon their prospective longitudinal studies at three months.

The second problem, related to the suboptimal choice of research projects, has been the inadequacy of research funding. Every disease has its advocates. Many advocates bemoan what they perceive as inadequate funding. This sometimes bears the taint of special pleading. The question is: does objective evidence exist of disproportionately low funding for TBI research?

> So here we have a disease that results in 80,000 new disabilities annually and the spending on research is a drop in the bucket.
>
> Geoffrey T. Manley, 2011 [13]

> If you think research is expensive, try disease.
>
> Mary Lasker, 1901–1994 [14]

There are many ways to measure research funding for a disease, e.g.:

- total funding for the disease
- funding per patient based on population prevalence
- funding per patient based on annual incidence
- funding relative to the impact of the disease on function
- funding relative to the impact of the disease on economics
- cost of research per life-year gained
- cost of research per quality-adjusted life-year gained.

Some data are available regarding TBI research funding. The best way to summarize the story: things have been dark for a long time, but there are glimmers of light at the end of the tunnel.

Confining our attention to the United States, a review of the most recent "Estimates of Funding for Various Research, Condition, and Disease Categories" [15] reveals that total actual spending on behalf of TBI in 2016 was $105 million. Estimated (enacted) spending for 2018 is $84 million. The respective 2016/2018 figures for HIV/AIDs research: $3.0 billion and $2.47 billion; for diabetes: $1.1 billion and $951 million. Thus, in 2016, compared with TBI, the National Institutes of Health (NIH) invested about ten times as much in diabetes research and 29 times as much in HIV/AIDs research.

In terms of research investment per affected patient, this calculation depends on whether one looks at disease prevalence (total population affected) or incidence (annual rate of new cases). Figure 3 compares the incidence of TBI in the United States with several other conditions. It is self-evident that TBI occurs with much higher frequency than other disorders that receive a good deal of media attention.

However, *incidence* data do not offer a good perspective on the proportion of affected people in the United States. Research investment relative to *prevalence* is theoretically a superior measure, although then we are stuck with attempting to estimate prevalence. Unfortunately, the TBI prevalence figures offered by the Centers for Disease Control and Prevention (CDC) fail to consider the less-than "disabling" effects of concussion – for instance, the many patients who return to work but work inefficiently with greater effort while experiencing irritability, headaches, and divorce – and fail to take into account the suspected contribution of concussion to later dementia. In other words, the CDC prevalence data only consider the small subset of patients regarded as "disabled" due to TBI. In 1999, the CDC's National Center for Injury Prevention and Control estimated that 5.3 million U.S. citizens (2%) were "living with disability as a result of a traumatic brain injury" [17]. A more recent estimate suggests the number is 3.17–3.32 million [18]. The validity of these numbers is highly dubious. As the CDC put it:

> These estimates likely underestimate the prevalence of TBI-related disability as they do not include persons with TBI who were treated and released from emergency departments or other health-care settings, those who

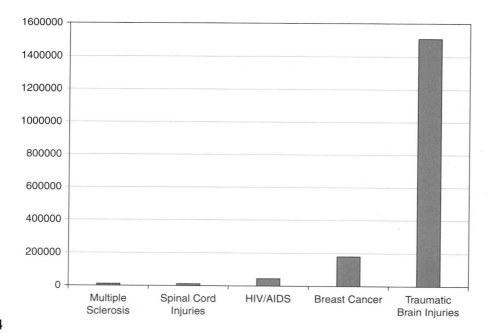

Fig. 3 Comparison of traumatic brain injury with other leading injuries or diseases in the United States. The cost of traumatic brain injury in the United States is estimated to be $48.3 billion annually. Hospitalization accounts for $31.7 billion and fatal brain injuries cost the United States $16.6 billion each year. Even with these staggering statistics, the United States spends less than $50 million annually on research into prevention and cure. Why?

Source: Zitnay, 2005 [16, p. 131]. Reprinted by permission from Springer

were treated in a DoD [Department of Defense] or VA [Veterans Administration] facility, or who did not seek treatment [19].

That major caveat aside, using the 2008 prevalence estimate of 3.2 million, the annual research investment per TBI patient in 2013 was $27.50. The estimated U.S. prevalence of HIV/AIDs in 2009 was 1,148,200 [20]. Ideally, in order to compare with TBI, rather than the number of diagnosed patients, one would compare research investment per disabled patient (since only a subset of HIV-infected persons are disabled [21]). However, making the simplest calculation, $252 was spent per HIV/AIDs patient – almost ten times the level of investment made per patient with TBI.

The third approach is to consider the impact or disease burden per patient. Limited data are available employing this method. However, Gillum et al. [22] performed a novel analysis of NIH funding levels by disease burden. The authors did not specifically tease out "Injuries – TBI" from the broader CDC category, "Injuries." Nonetheless, as illustrated in Figure 4, it is

again apparent that research investment is much higher than expected in HIV/AIDs (and, to a lesser degree, breast cancer and diabetes) and much lower than expected for injuries.

Finally, with regard to how research investments compare with the cost of a disease to society, a conclusion depends very much on the accuracy of the cost estimate. According to the CDC, "The estimated economic cost of TBI in 2010, including direct and indirect medical costs, is estimated to be approximately $76.5 billion" [23]. My guess about the credibility of this official figure: the number is inflated with regard to concussion, since much of the cost of TBI medical care goes for hospitalization after severe injury; and the number is deflated with regard to concussion given that typical estimates of injury impact fail to consider subtle and long-term brain changes. Bearing those caveats in mind, the United States spends one-tenth of a penny on research for every dollar TBI costs our nation every year. I am not an economist. No gold standard exists for the "right" amount of spending per dollar of cost of an illness to society. Yet (gut instinct), spending 1/1000 of the cost of a disease trying to fight it seems suggestive of inadequate funding.

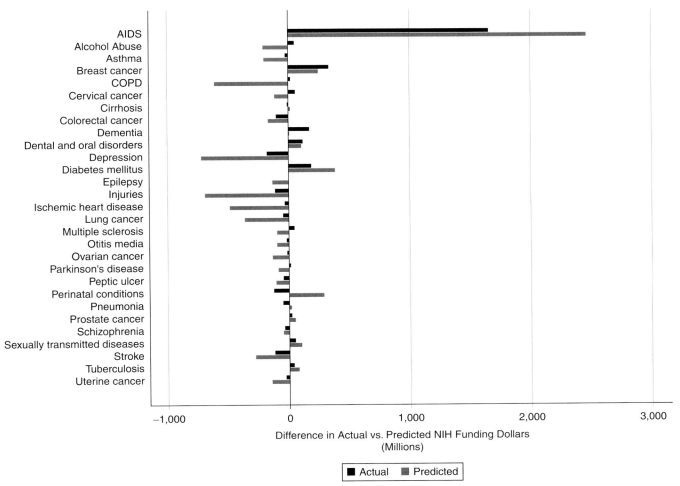

Ten-year comparison of differences between actual and expected disease-specific National Institutes of Health (NIH) funding relative to U.S. burden of disease in disability-adjusted life years (DALYs)

Fig. 4 A comparison of differences between actual and expected funding values as predicted by DALY burden alone in 1996 (light gray) and 2006 (dark gray). Negative values reflect actual funding dollars less than expected and positive values represent actual funding dollars more than expected.

In summary, hope of progress in knowledge about concussion has suffered from: (1) failure to fund research commensurate with the threat to human health; (2) delay in development of technology to objectively assess injury – especially the embarrassing fact that there exists no biologically meaningful outcome measure (see below); and (3) the low priority of research regarding the long-term impact of concussion. The United States – with the most extravagant medical research on Earth – spends a miserly pittance and gets what it pays for.

Thankfully, there are changes in the wind.

It would be unfair and inaccurate for 21st-century scholars to claim that they have been the midwives of a research renaissance. The launch of modern attention to TBI might be dated to 1974, when the NIH began phase I of the Vietnam Head Injury Study – even before computed tomography (CT) scanners were widely available. Phase II began in 1981, by which time MRI scanners had gained a commercial footing [24]. The 1989 U.S. Federal Interagency Head Injury Task Force report set off a sincere effort to determine the incidence of TBIs [25]. In 1992, the U.S. Congress established the Defense and Veterans Brain Injury Program (later renamed the Defense and Veterans Brain Injury Program Centers, DVBIC) – a somewhat disruptive innovation since it bridged the previously disjointed medical operations of the Department of Defense and the Veterans Administration (VA) [26]. Six lead centers went into operation across the nation. Of course, the size of the investment was small and the focus of these early initiatives was on moderate to severe TBI. For instance, the 1996 Traumatic Brain Injury Act authorized just $3 million per year for the CDC and $5 million per year for the Health Resources and Services Administration (HRSA) [27]. And the CDC's 1999 report to Congress on TBI [28] virtually ignored CBI (mTBI).

However, with the new millennium came a gradual escalation in attention to concussion. In 1999 a concussion clinic was established at U.S. Marine Corps Base Camp Pendleton in California. The next year President Clinton signed the TBI Act Amendments of 2000 [29]. For historians of concussion, this was a watershed moment: Section 1302 of those Amendments expanded the study of TBI to include victims of "mild brain injury." Research funding remained very limited; public awareness remained vanishingly low. But mild injury finally appeared on the U.S. federal agenda.

Three social factors have prodded a reassessment of the urgency of funding since that watershed moment at the outset of the 21st century. One is the significant increase in the global incidence of concussion (and global burden of brain injury) due in small part to increased survival after violence and in large part to the enhanced availability of motor vehicles without a safety culture in developing and middle-income countries. Another recent factor increasing the pressure for research has been the high incidence of concussions among warfighters in Iraq and Afghanistan. A third factor is increased awareness that contact sports may cause permanent brain damage. And technical factors have contributed as well. For one, transgenic rodents have been developed that better express human-like neurodegenerative changes. Another factor is that advances in human neuroimaging such as diffusion tensor imaging (DTI)

Table 2 Milestone 21st-century traumatic brain injury (TBI) research initiatives

- 2002: Common Data Element project
- 2003: International Mission on Prognosis Analysis of Clinical Trials in Traumatic Brain Injury (IMPACT)
- 2007: Defense Centers of Excellence for Psychological Health and Traumatic Brain Injury (PH/TBI)
- 2008: Veterans Administration/Department of Defense Evidence Based Workgroup on mTBI/concussion
- 2009: Defense and Veterans Brain Injury Program Centers explored development with NATO of international standards for concussion/mild TBI
- 2011: The International Initiative for Traumatic Brain Injury Research (InTBIR)
- 2012/2013: Head Health Initiative
- 2013: The White House Brain Research through Advancing Innovative Neurotechnologies (BRAIN) Initiative
- 2013: Transforming Research and Clinical Knowledge in Traumatic Brain Injury (TRACK-TBI) pilot study
- 2014: Department of Defense (DoD)/National Collegiate Athletic Association (NCAA) concussion project
- 2015: DoD and Department of Veterans Affairs (DVA) Chronic Effects of Neurotrauma Consortium (CENC)
- 2018: National Football League (NFL) funding pledged for furtherance of the TRACK-TBI study, the DoD/NCAA study, and a National Institute of Aging (NIA) study

and functional MRI (fMRI) have improved detection of injuries. This enables studies that would have been fruitless using the previous generation of imaging devices. Together, all these factors have inspired, if not a renaissance, at least several tentatively promising initiatives. Table 2 is a partial list of recent programs that raise hope of better research funding, research progress, or both. (Sincere apologies to the rest of the world. U.S. progress is emphasized simply because the story is more familiar to this author.) Note, however, that for all the expressions of concern and all the new money, concussions remained trivialized by many.

Forward March

The first step in this forward march: a major impediment to comparing trials of TBI outcome or treatment efficacy has always been the lack of a consensus regarding the best way to measure cognitive, behavioral, and functional outcomes, since results cannot be compared unless metrics are shared. This pressing need drove the National Institute of Neurological Disorders and Stroke (NINDS) Office of Clinical Research to initiate the Common Data Elements (CDE) project. The initial contract was signed in May of 2002 and renewed in 2012 (KAI Research Inc. contract no. N01-NS-7-2372) [30]. Future NINDS-funded research will require the use of the CDEs, or at a minimum be CDE-compatible. Candidly, it is hard to predict the impact of the CDEs. Although the broad aims of the initiative are indisputably vital, the mission statement suggests that we may see a somewhat more pedestrian result: "The primary goal of the NINDS in developing CDEs for clinical research in neurology is to reduce the effort required to train coordinators and create the data collection forms in future studies" [31].

The next big step: in 2003 the U.S. CDC issued its second report to Congress on TBI. The pendulum had swung. For the first time – as mandated by Clinton's 2000 TBI Amendments – concussion was the primary focus. Hence the title: *Report to Congress on Mild Traumatic Brain Injury in the United States: Steps to Prevent a Serious Public Health Problem* [32]. The Introduction of that report warns: "Mild traumatic brain injury or MTBI – also called concussion, minor head injury, minor brain injury, minor head trauma, or minor TBI – is one of the most common neurologic disorders." This report was perhaps something of a wake-up call. Although the risk of lasting dysfunction after a single CBI was far from resolved, policy makers and doctors were put on notice that there might be a risk, and we'd better find out. That very year, the NIH-NINDS funded a multinational, multidisciplinary initiative called the International Mission on Prognosis Analysis of Clinical Trials in Traumatic Brain Injury (IMPACT) [33]. The IMPACT study group has collaborating institutes in Antwerp, Edinburgh, Richmond, VA, and Rotterdam. Having obtained access to 11 large data sets from clinical trials, the consortium has been working for more than a decade to improve the design of trials in TBI [34].

The United States and NATO began fighting various conflicts in the Middle East with the invasion of Afghanistan in 2001. That year, the Army cared for 3393 cases of mTBI [35]. TBI soon gained a reputation as the signature injury of the war. By 2007 – a year in which the Army cared for 11,461 mTBI cases – it had become clear that the available knowledge and resources about moderate to severe TBI were not addressing the military's needs because (1) many soldiers suffered from concussion and (2) many soldiers suffered from post-traumatic stress, with or without concomitant TBI. Based on about 300 recommendations from expert panels, in late 2007, the Deputy Assistant Secretary of Defense for Force Health Protection and Readiness established a new umbrella entity, originally called the Post Traumatic Stress Disorder and Traumatic Brain Injury Research Program. In January 2008 the program came under the auspices of the Congressionally Directed Medical Research Programs and the new name became the Defense Centers of Excellence for Psychological Health and Traumatic Brain Injury [36]. At the time of this writing, the Defense Centers of Excellence oversee three subsidiary programs: the DVBIC, the Deployment Health Clinical Center, and the National Center for Telehealth and Technology, sharing the mission of "advancing excellence in psychological health and traumatic brain injury prevention and care." The law provided for $151 million for post-traumatic stress disorder (PTSD) research and $150 million for TBI research – a gratifying infusion of resources. However, it is challenging to pluck, from public records, an estimate of spending specifically designated for concussion/mTBI.

Further modest steps on the march occurred in 2008, when (1) the Traumatic Brain Injury Act of 2008 [37] reauthorized funding for the CDC and HRSA, and (2) the DVBIC convened a summer consensus conference on management of concussion in the deployed setting. Soon thereafter, the DVBIC released its clinical practice guideline for mTBI in non-deployed settings [38]. The upshot of that meeting was a 16-page report that distilled the military's judgment at that time: "Almost all people recover completely following a concussion" ([38], p. 9).

In 2009 the effort to improve and standardize the clinical approach to concussion became international, when the U.S. DVBIC explored development with NATO of international standards for concussion/mTBI. The same year, the Minneapolis Veterans Affairs Medical Center also prepared for the VA a "systematic review of the evidence" regarding TBI [39]. On the one hand, it was a sign of progress that that report included a discussion of concussion/mTBI. On the other hand – as Chapter 2 of the present text explains – that 2009 VA review failed to assay the literature. No responsible reviewer could read the published evidence and claim, "approximately 90% of mTBI cases follow a predictable course of recovery and do not experience long-term residual symptoms requiring treatment" ([39],p. 6). Chapters 2, 5, 7, and 10 will provide actual data from systematic reviews and let the reader judge. Equally problematic was the VA's claim that "Psychological factors (e.g., depression, anxiety, or PTSD), compensation and litigation, and negative expectations and beliefs are the strongest risk factors" for post-concussive symptoms" (p. 6). Again, Chapters 2, 5, 7, and 10 of the present text demonstrate that other factors are more important.

In April of 2013, President Obama announced the launch of the White House Brain Research through Advancing Innovative Neurotechnologies (BRAIN) initiative [40]. The BRAIN initiative quickly received pledges of $300 million from public and private sources, and comprises a collaboration between five agencies: NIH, National Science Foundation, the Defense Advance Research Projects Agency, the Food and Drug Administration, and the Intelligence Advanced Research Projects Activity. Although TBI is only one of the disorders that this initiative will tackle – and although it remains to be seen what attention will be paid to concussion – there is at least some hope that, over the 12-year anticipated lifespan of the project, advances will occur that enhance knowledge regarding the biology, prevention, and treatment of CBI.

Gratifyingly, in the intervening years multiple new research initiatives have begun. For instance, as shown in Table 2, the Transforming Research and Clinical Knowledge in Traumatic Brain Injury (TRACK-TBI) pilot study that began in 2013 has become an NIH-funded multicenter longitudinal project. In 2014 the DoD began collaborating with the National Collegiate Athletic Association (NCAA) to study thousands of young athletes. In 2015, another component of the DoD and Department of Veterans Affairs joined forces in the Chronic Effects of Neurotrauma Consortium (CENC). The longitudinal designs make all these programs especially promising.

Perhaps the most dramatic recent research developments (indeed, something of a passion play) pertain to the interjection of corporate funding. This has, of course, prompted justifiable concerns about corporate motives.

Early in 2013, after the suicide of linebacker Junior Seau, the National Football League (NFL) pledged to support medical research at NIH with $30 million over five years. But in 2015 the League called an extraordinary and unseemly halt when some support was designated for the highly productive Boston University research team. The NFL literally refused to pay its pledge because the Boston scholars had expressed concerns about the League's ethical behavior [41]. In 2016 the NFL revised its pledge to provide $40 million for medical research, ostensibly to be managed by the Foundation for the National Institutes of Health [42]. Yet a congressional committee found that year that the NFL was improperly steering the money toward a league-connected doctor. The League trimmed its promise to $30 million – but only $12 million was actually provided. The League simply let its contract with NIH lapse in July of 2017, holding on to $18 million.

That broken promise prompted a sharp rebuke from members of the House Committee on Energy and Commerce. Under congressional pressure, in early 2018 the NFL again promised to make good on its gift, pledging $7.65 million to the multicenter NIH/TRACK-TBI project, $7.65 million to the DoD/NCAA longitudinal project, and $2.25 million to the National Institute of Aging [43]. That modest support is welcome. History will judge whether the NFL's principal motive has been compassion, image management, or corporate research and development [44].

These signs are heartening, if somewhat mixed. The new initiatives reflect both increased concern about what concussion does to the human brain and residual loyalty to the belief that the answer is: not much. Yet the field is moving. Readers of this text, in fact, may be witnesses to a historical change in attitudes. Such changes come slowly. Like women's suffrage, school integration, reproductive rights, and many other examples, time is required for large groups to shift their allegiance from one stance to another. That seems to be happening in the domain of concussion. A decade ago, those who were concerned that concussion often causes lasting brain dysfunction were an outsider minority. The tide is turning. The subgroup of victims of concussion with persistent symptoms finally have reason to hope that their distress will not forever be dismissed as psychological frailty or venal self-interest.

What Needs to be Done Right Now?

The present author is not a neurobiologist nor a health care economist (and certainly not a seer). He cannot predict how many dollars of research funding, spent in what way, would prove, after several decades, to have been the wisest investment. He can only express a personal opinion about the most pressing research priorities, and a guess about cost-efficiency. Still, in the course of preparing this collaborative essay, both the editors and authors repeatedly encountered the same knowledge gaps. We do not understand the pathophysiology of CBI beyond the limited domains of inquiry that have been studied (primarily, cerebral blood flow and metabolic changes, readily assayed chemical changes, and currently familiar light microscopic changes) nor beyond the early stage of the process. We do not know the natural history of CBI in any species. We do not understand why outcomes from seemingly identical injuries vary greatly. We have virtually no disease-modifying therapies. And – potentially a matter of urgency given the global aging of the human species – we are only beginning to understand the relationship between CBI and neurodegeneration and how to intervene so that a teenaged CBI victim has a reduced risk from that lifetime sword of Damocles. Filling those knowledge gaps is probably necessary to reduce the accelerating harm that CBI is doing to societies.

Basic Research

Two methodological issues deserve attention. First, as laboratory rodents age, they exhibit little of the deposition of pathological proteins most associated with human neurodegeneration: β-amyloid, hyperphosphorylated tau, and α-synuclein. Transgenic animals have helped overcome this barrier. Such animals have been widely used for more than a decade in basic Alzheimer's disease (AD) and Parkinson's disease research [45–51]. One especially useful model is the 3xTg-AD mouse, which expresses both amyloid precursor protein and tau. And since APOE genotype moderates the human brain's response to injury, the availability of APOE-ε4 transgenic rodents can facilitate modeling of gene–environment interaction [52]. In fact, since 1999 several TBI studies have employed transgenic animals capable of modeling neurodegeneration in TBI research – including a 3xTg-AD experiment [53–55]. If the goal is to determine the relationship between CBI and brain aging or neurodegeneration, the time has perhaps come to say, "Please employ appropriate transgenic models. Do not sacrifice the wrong animal to little purpose."

A second methodological issue: controversy exists about the ideal apparatus for experimental TBI. This issue will be further discussed in Chapters 1 and 2. By far the most popular laboratory tactic has been the fluid percussion injury model, in which a piece of a rodent's skull is removed so that the concussive blow is applied directly to the brain or dura. Yet observers of TBI for almost 1000 years have pointed out that the essence of this injury is force transmitted through – and presumably diffused by – the skull. At the risk of alienating superb local colleagues whose fluid percussion injury work has provided exceptional insights, the present author would ask for experimentalists to review the validity of conclusions made regarding creatures with skulls based on studying creatures without skulls.

Despite literally thousands of publications reporting experimental concussion, primarily using rodents as subjects, it is astonishing that so few laboratories follow their subjects for more than a month. Perhaps this disabling research weakness derives from the old assumption that the effects of CBI are transient. Now that most biologists are aware of evidence suggesting a risk of lasting or permanent brain damage, we need skillful investigators to discover the natural history of CBI. That means subjecting animals to graded injuries and assessing outcomes throughout the remainder of their lives. Without such longitudinal information, it is impossible to determine: (1) the spectrum (which seems to be broad) of natural histories after a given impact; (2) how single or repetitive CBIs interact with aging and environment to effect neurodegeneration; or (3) what interventions, if any, mitigate that effect. The author strongly urges neurobiologists to consider under what circumstances short-term outcome studies justify animal sacrifice. Yes, housing and studying rodents for two to four years is expensive. Yet the most compelling CBI question for human societies seems to be: what are the long-term effects? The importance of answering this question requires a new focus on life course outcome studies.

Translational Research: The Hope for Biomarkers

The most compelling single research gap, in the opinion of many TBI authorities, is that no biomarker exists for TBI. Unless injuries are visible on scalp examination or with neuroimaging, we cannot even conclude whether the head was struck. A biomarker could "mark" many aspects of a particular case of CBI, from confirming that a force impacted the patient's brain to determining the occurrence and amount of neuronal death to predicting functional outcome. Forensic stakeholders are naturally eager for a marker of severity. Table 3 lists several candidates [56–62].

With regard to biomarkers, readers must be wary. For instance, in February of 2018 the U.S. Food and Drug Administration (FDA) announced with considerable fanfare its approval of a two-element commercial blood test for "concussion" [63]. It is nothing of the sort. The approved test analyzes blood levels of ubiquitin carboxy-terminal hydrolase-L1 (UCH-L1) and glial fibrillary acidic protein drawn shortly after a traumatic exposure. Research (not yet published as this volume goes to press) purportedly found that elevations of these markers were 99.5% sensitive for CT scan positivity – that is, visible "lesions." If replicated, that would make the test truly valuable for detecting the 1% of patients most likely to have such imaging findings – an advance in emergency assessment protocols that might spare many patients' exposure to radiation. Yet a typical clinically attended CBI, by definition, shows no gross bleeding on CT. Typical CBIs, in fact, rarely trigger these biomarker elevations, making the test virtually useless for the diagnosis of concussion.

Yet is it realistic to expect a single measure of harm in a neurological condition that reportedly up- and down-regulates ~1000 genes in a matter of minutes? One can certainly settle on arbitrary operational differentiations. For example, some authorities have urged a dichotomy between "uncomplicated" concussion (with a normal CT scan) and "complicated" concussion (with CT abnormalities). Yet the phrase "CT abnormalities" includes such a wide range of radiological findings (e.g., atrophy, ventriculomegaly, calcification, hemorrhage, dysgenesis) that it hardly distinguishes any physiopathological subtype. There might be a little practical value in discriminating between concussions with and without intracranial bleeding. But – apart from providing attorneys with a simplistic classification – it is not clear how patients benefit from testing whether one aspect of their unique and complex findings fits some such arbitrary metric of "severity." Clinicians could surely eschew this kind of actuarial rhetoric, as we do with pneumonia, and just describe what's wrong. The Glasgow Coma Scale was not intended to measure injury severity but to assist clinicians in tracking changes in consciousness. One would rather know what happened to the patient, her vital signs, what she can do now, and whether she might profit from a neurosurgical intervention than know some intern's one-word title for the severity of her injury.

Indeed, can one ordinally rank the severity of ten injuries if each injury alters neurobiology in many ways, resulting in complex and individually unique profiles, such that if we assay five, or ten, or 100 chemicals or cognitive functions, every patient's brain exhibits its private Himalaya of peaks and valleys? The brain does more than one thing. It is not a liver, kidney, or thyroid. We seem unlikely to find any single clinically meaningful cerebral equivalent of a thyroid-stimulating hormone level. Moreover, new facets of basic cell biology are still being (and will forever be) unearthed. To what degree is the harmful effect of CBI due to entatic heme ligation changes in cytochrome c due to dissociation of the Met80 ligand from this "respiratory" protein, converting it to an apoptosis-enabling peroxidase? If a scholar cannot answer that question, why would he or she claim to understand concussion? Basic research suggests that we are just beginning to discover the vast number of neurobiological changes common at various time points after a CBI.

Table 3 Candidate blood biomarkers for concussive brain injury

Neuronal/axonal markers

Neuron-specific enolase (NSE)

Ubiquitin c-terminal hydrolase (UCH-L1)

Alphall-spectrin breakdown products (SBDPs)

Hyperphosphorylated neurofilaments-heavy (NF-H)

Serum neurofilament-light protein (NF-L)

Glial markers

S100 beta (S100β)

Glial fibrillary acidic protein (GFAP)

Myelin basic protein (MBP)

Growth factors

Brain-derived neurotrophic factor (BDNF)

Nerve growth factor (NGF)

Transforming growth factor-beta (TGF-β)

Inflammatory markers

Interleukins (IL-) 1, 6, 8, 10, 12

Interferon-gamma(IFN-γ)

Tumor necrosis factor(TNF)-α

Kallikrein-6 (Klk6)

Soluble Fas (sFAS); soluble vascular adhesion molecule (sVCAM-1); soluble intracellular adhesion molecule (sICAM-1)

Genomic biomarkers

APOE-ε4

Val^{158}Met polymorphism in COMT gene

5HT transporter 5-HTTLPR gene polymorphisms

Others

Heart-fatty acidic binding protein (H-FABP)

Creatine kinase BB

Soluble cellular prion protein (PrPC)

Cortisol

Cleaved tau

Micro-RNAs (e.g., microRNA let-7i)

Note that Table 3 excludes cerebrospinal fluid markers as well as a host of alternatives, including structural and functional neuroimaging markers (e.g., diffusion tensor imaging, or proton magnetic resonance spectroscopy), electrophysiological markers (e.g., event-related potentials, eye movement analysis, and postural stability measures).

Given this conundrum, no single biomarker is likely to satisfy. The biotech companies currently racing for the golden apple will not find it.

Instead, one anticipates the discovery of multiple markers that assay various aspects of injury that may be somewhat dissociable in duration and degree, for instance, CBF changes, metabolic changes, transmission dysfunction, mitochondrial dysfunction, generation of reactive oxygen species, axonal dysfunction and connectivity changes, circuit compromise, inflammation, apoptosis, reactive gliosis, and cell death, all predicting any number of dissociable clinical outcome variables from somatic distress to cognitive deficits to psychiatric problems to late degenerative change. As Kobeissy et al. put the issue, "Many studies suggest that because of the brain's complexity and the heterogeneous nature of brain injury, the measurement of a single biomarker cannot be used to assess TBI evaluation such as diagnosis, prognosis, and management" ([55],p. S103).

So yes, we need biomarkers. Several are promising. But it remains to be seen whether any single chemical measure will reveal the health of a brain better than any single chemical test would reveal the health of an ocean.

Clinical Research to Determine the Risk Factors of Worse Outcome and Traumatic Encephalopathy, and the Modifiable Factors That Protect the Brain

We really must determine the outcomes of CBI. Whether or not one embraces the current concepts of *post-concussive syndrome* or *traumatic encephalopathy*, we need to know who is at the highest risk for distressing or disabling outcomes that persist and for later neurodegeneration. We really need to know who among our children may be at elevated risk. Let's say our research firmly established that a girl who suffered a single concussion playing soccer at age 11 would then have a 17% higher risk of lifetime depression and 1.4 times the normal risk of being demented when she reached age 75. However, if she developed hypertension and it was not properly treated, she'd have a 40% higher risk of depression and 2.8 times the risk of dementia. And if her genotype included one or two APOEε4 alleles, suffering that CBI would make her 16% less likely to graduate from college, 24% more likely to attempt suicide, 42% more likely to divorce, and have 4.7 times the risk of early-onset dementia. On the other hand, if she takes five days of cognitive rest immediately after her injury, or if she exercises in middle age, or if she takes fish oil after menopause, her dementia risk falls significantly toward normal. Might she, her parents, or her pediatrician want to know these things? Might that knowledge influence some life choices, either on the day of soccer sign-ups or later?

These figures are plucked from the air. The author has no way to know if they are too high or too low, or if these putative risk and protective factors will turn out to be important. Nobody does.

The self-evident first step is to launch a multicenter, population-based, prospective long-term longitudinal study. In other words: get to know a large number of young people before CBI. Follow them for the rest of their lives. Determine whether experiencing one or more CBIs has any effect, and whether some people are more vulnerable than others, and whether life choices such as education, the Mediterranean diet, or aerobic exercise might mitigate their risk. This is the one research design that offers a reasonable hope of answering our many questions about cause and effect, and mediating and moderating factors, in scientifically rigorous way.

The Framingham Heart Study [64] – the world's great wellspring of discovery about the natural history of cardiovascular disease, a joint project of the National Heart, Lung, and Blood Institute and Boston University that began in 1948 – was a superb model. Hans-Lukas Teuber urged NINDS to launch a Framingham-like CBI project in 1968 [6]. The present author publicly implored NIH to do the same in 2013. Instead, they cut funding for the Framingham by 40%.

Although no authentic population-based prospective longitudinal study has yet to be funded, at least three exceptionally promising large-scale long-term initiatives are finally under way. One is called "A National Study on the Effects of Concussion in Collegiate Athletes and US Military Service Academy Members: The NCAA–DoD Concussion Assessment, Research and Education (CARE) Consortium" [65]. The second is the NINDS-funded multicenter TRACK-TBI study [66]. Both of these studies include an element of longitudinal follow-up. The third study is called the "Chronic Effects of Neurotrauma Consortium (CENC) multi-centre observational study" [67]. Although this last study is limited to military subjects and will be skewed by a focus on blast injuries, it is the sole prospective longitudinal initiative. The availability of substantial pre-morbid health data makes this 25-year project unique: the investigators will be able to assess injury-related change. All three studies will hopefully yield significant, even fundamental, advances.

In the meantime, even though cross-sectional studies are infuriatingly feebler, a well-designed study of older adults would be a low-risk, high-pay-off investment. Say we recruit 5000 65-year-olds with an unambiguous medical record of CBI and 5000 without. One might compare the two cohorts in any number of ways: neuropsychological testing, psychiatric assessment, neuroimaging, other biomarkers. In fact, we are rapidly approaching the point of having simple tests that detect early-warning signs of neurodegeneration. A big enough sample would allow us control for all manner of potential confounding variables, from contentment on the job to APOE genotype to waist size. Compared with the small-scale preliminary work that's been funded to date, even a study as cheap and dirty as this would be absolutely revelatory.

For these reasons, forgive the redundancy, but the present author must implore those with the resources to step forward. CBI has no angel. It needs one quite desperately. Pending the arrival of our angel – the funder who will some day appear on a spirited Palomino to actualize the first and only high-quality long-term prospective longitudinal studies of concussion employing valid biomarkers in human history – every authority is free to guess what that research will reveal. To guess at the unknown is an irresistible human need. But we uncompromisingly eschew the popular practice of publishing guesses masquerading as knowledge.

II. Lack of a Meaningful Outcome Measure

If a tree falls in the forest …

If a 17-year-old boy named Frederick suffers a CBI, experiences a week of headache and subjective fatigue, and feels fine for the next 60 years, what was the outcome of his concussion? What if he performs just as well on every test of function before and after the concussion, but imaging shows persistent abnormalities in connectivity and reduced cerebral efficiency? What if, due to his CBI, when his wife dies 53 years later, the patient has an 18% increased risk of depression? What if he is asymptomatic and undetectably affected, but has acquired a 6% increase in the risk of dementia at age 77?

As illustrated by Figures 1 and 2, our knowledge about the outcome of concussion tails off after three months, but some evidence suggests a lifelong impact in at least some cases. In essence, due to the scarcity and poor quality of long-term longitudinal studies, we do not know the natural history of CBI (or, more accurately, the spectrum of natural histories). That has led to guessing – and the ongoing crisis of opposing opinions.

What is the "outcome" of a concussion? The very word *outcome* connotes that a cause is followed by an effect. For instance, the outcome from infantile meningitis may be permanent disability, frequent seizures, and early death. The outcome of contracting Ebola virus is usually death. But what of malaria? Survivors are far more common than non-survivors. Survivors vary greatly in their lifetime disease course. For some, the event was a fever dream that thankfully vanished into history. For others, the event was the onset of a chronic and debilitating condition, attended by anxiety about the risk of symptom recrudescence at random times. Contracting malaria may qualify as a *cause* of illness, but who can say when to measure its *effect*? At one year? At 50 years? Who can say how to measure its outcome? Total body burden of *Plasmodium falciparum* protozoans? An average of the patient's perpetually fluctuating level of disability? A subjective measure of distress? A count of lifetime days off work? What if the patient's bouts of illness end at age 45 but the protozoans remain lurking in her blood? Has she "recovered"? What if the patient is completely unaffected (a carrier) but infects her children? Is she sick? Does she have a disorder?

This is the conundrum that undermines the rhetoric in conventional discussions of concussion outcome. The word *recovery* is bandied about as if we knew what that is. Taking young Fred's case: if his concussion obliges his brain to expend more metabolic energy to accomplish the same tasks, or somewhat increases lifetime production of free radicals or toxic proteins, reduces his future chances of well-being, it would seem incorrect to say that he has "recovered" when he feels great and does well on the tests that are currently popular among neuropsychologists. Yet a great deal of literature trumpets the conclusion that CBIs are mostly benign, based on that premise.

Recent research has demonstrated that victims of CBI may: (1) feel well, even when they are not performing well; (2) perform well, even when their brains are struggling to cope (a struggle that perhaps increases the risk of neurodegeneration); and (3) feel and perform well, even though they have acquired frailty that lowers the threshold for many later problems. However, no biomarker exists that detects the severity of a concussion in the acute stage, measures the degree of dysfunction in the chronic stage, or predicts the risk of sequelae over a lifetime.

As a result, it is not clear how best to characterize the "outcome" of a CBI. It may be a very long time before technology reveals the full spectrum of effects and degrees to which they impact health and well-being in different individuals. And, depending on one's conceptualization of "disease," different post-concussive changes may or may not qualify [68–72]. Let us surmise that Fred feels fine two years after his concussion but his brain is less efficient and he has acquired an increased risk of neurodegeneration 50 years later. Whether he is "ill" or "well" may be as much a matter of rhetoric as of science. Even if it were possible to catalog every neurobiological change in Fred's brain, two doctors might label his health status differently. For the sake of simplicity, dodging an interminable debate about the meaning of "disease," perhaps we can agree that if CBI causes a deleterious change, or generates a risk of a deleterious change, that is undesirable.

III. Misplaced Faith in a Dated Conceptual Trichotomy

I therefore put forward the thesis that at the bottom of every case of hysteria there are one or more occurrences of premature sexual experience.

Freud, 1896 [73]

A popular classification divides the sources of symptoms as follows:

1. sickness (so-called "organic" illness)
2. imagining sickness ("psychological" illness)
3. pretending sickness ("malingering" or "factitious disorder").

Any reviewer of the CBI literature will come upon innumerable repetitions of this *sick, imagination, pretense* trichotomy. A common claim is that the initial symptoms of concussion, such as confusion, headache, dizziness, and nausea, are *organic* effects of head trauma; but symptoms lasting more than an arbitrary period of time (one week; one month; three months) are either due to an unconscious *psychological reaction* to trauma – referred to as hysterical, or conversion, or somatoform, or psychosomatic problems – or due to a patient seeking gain – referred to as *malingering*

This dated trichotomy is a hold-over from psychiatry before neuropsychiatry. Even as late as 2000, the American Psychiatric Association's *Diagnostic and Statistical Manual of Mental Disorders* (DSM) – in a striking exception to its purportedly atheoretical stance and exhibition of loyalty to largely discredited psychodynamic theory – claimed that the symptoms of "conversion disorder" are related to "psychological factors" "because the initiation or exacerbation of the symptom or deficit is preceded by conflicts or other stressors" and that those symptoms "are not intentionally produced or feigned, as in Factitious disorder or Malingering" ([74], p. 492). "Conflicts"? A more recent draft of the DSM eschews attribution of illness to "conflicts" but perpetuates the dualist notion that one can draw a line between physiological and non-physiological symptoms: "Medical unexplained symptoms do remain a key feature in conversion disorder … because it is possible to demonstrate definitively that the symptoms are not consistent with medical pathophysiology" ([75], p. 310). What physiological changes are medical? The conceptual frailty of this diagnosis is expressed in the 2013 diagnostic criteria: "Clinical findings provide evidence of incompatibility between the symptom and *recognized* [emphasis added] neurological or medical conditions" ([75], p. 318).

In other words, brain changes that are easy to classify as due to external force, such as immediately altered regional cerebral blood flow related to the neurometabolic cascade, are "recognized" as medical problems while the altered regional cerebral blood flow associated with persistent anxiety or perception of weakness or diminished hope is not "recognized" as a medical problem. That begins to sound like a distinction without a difference.

This antiquated three-way classification is about a century past its expiration date. Candid analysts of this ancient trichotomy will readily acknowledge the two reasons it is no longer acceptable. First, an organic/psychological dichotomy does not seem consistent with what we know about brains. Second, a dichotomy between imaginary and intentional complaints does not seem consistent with what we know about brains and is not clinically diagnosable.

IIIA. An Organic/Psychological Dichotomy Does Not Seem Consistent With What We Know About Brains

What happens in CBI? Say a truck is heading toward you. First, even before impact, the brain changes because of the physiological acute stress/anxiety response that we've known about at least since Cannon's 1915 observations [76,77]. Modern research has identified many acute stress-related neurobiological changes beyond amine transmitter and adrenal steroid hormone effects, including oxidative threat, altered gene expression, and inflammation [78–82]. Some recent evidence suggests that acute cognitive dysfunction after human mTBI – the "where am I?" patient in the emergency department – may be more stress-related than concussion-related, which raises questions about whether disorientation is a trustworthy sign of concussive injury or might just as likely indicate fear [83]. Interestingly, rodent research hints that stress immediately *before* injury may reduce the brain's capacity to remodel *after* injury [84]. In other words, even if the oncoming truck misses you by a centimeter, the traumatic experience can still leave you disoriented and still harm your brain; and if you do get hit, your acute stress may impair your chance of later cerebral healing.

Next, if the truck actually knocks you down and external force strikes your head, the brain changes because of the physiological neurometabolic cascade and a multiplicity of other biological changes caused by diffusion of force through the cerebrum [85–87]. Moreover, strong evidence exists that

CBI (so-called "mild" TBI) may cause either persistent change or late change because of the physiological sequelae of the neurometabolic cascade [3, 8, 88–90].

Next, depending on one's predispositions and reaction to the trauma of CBI, emotional responses such as anxiety or depression (the subjective feelings of brain happenings) may be associated with lasting deleterious changes including frank atrophy, cognitive decline, and accelerated brain aging – especially impacting the hippocampus, amygdala, dorsomedial prefrontal cortex, and anterior cingulate gyrus [91–99]. As a result of above interactive physical/emotional process, one may experience a panoply of psychosocial sequelae beyond anxiety or depression, including cognitive impairment, altered body image, reduced self-confidence, altered job performance, altered family role, perceived limited opportunity, or foreshortened future. All are indisputably mediated by brain change. The net impact on life will vary; that is, even when identical forces strike similar heads one expects individual differences in outcome. Evidence suggests that many facets of the brain's multi-phase, multi-faceted, intercalated response to the injury – from receptor-binding dynamics to mitochondrial respiratory chain enzyme expression to inflammatory cytokine generation – are moderated by gene–environment interactions [100–104].

IIIB. Which One of These Changes is Not Organic?

To find a defender of the old psychological/organic dichotomy, one must reach back in history to the claims of Descartes – who imagined mind and brain to be independent. Even that unsung neuropathologist, Dr. Freud, rejected this conceptually problematic splitting. Long-lasting memory loss, concentration difficulty, fatigue, or irritability due to emotion-associated brain degeneration is perhaps a novel concept. It may lead some clinicians to perceive a mismatch between symptoms and known disease. Their failure to recognize the patient's problem may jibe with the criteria for so-called conversion disorder ("Clinical findings provide evidence of incompatibility between the symptom and *recognized* neurological or medical conditions"). It does not alter the problem's organicity.

Setting aside the fact that all mentation is organic, there is a more practical problem complicating diagnosis of "psychological" symptoms: doctoring is imperfect. Doctors often misdiagnose patients with conventional diseases as being hysterical. Gould and colleagues, for example, reported that 25–50% of patients diagnosed as hysterics were subsequently discovered to have disease that accounted for their symptoms [105]. "A diagnosis of hysteria must be made with great caution as it so often proves incorrect" ([105], (p. 593). Therefore, two dissociable issues deserve consideration. First, since all mental activity is mediated by the brain, all "psychological" symptoms are organic. Second, from a pragmatic point of view, clinicians often lack the capacity to accurately diagnose traditionally classified organic disorders.

Some may ask, "But surely there is a difference between the effects of a subdural hematoma on memory and the effects of depression due to suffering a subdural hematoma on memory?" That sounds reasonable. Yet one suspects that it will be many years before we have better grasped the complex feedforward/feedback dynamics of pre-morbid condition, injury, mentation, and brain change. Today one can refer to multiple neuroimaging studies showing that so-called conversion patients exhibit altered brain function [106–111]. This is straightforward evidence (if any were needed) of the self-evident fact that the brain mediates such symptoms. Of course, it fails to distinguish brain-shaking-related temporal lobe dysfunction from sadness-related temporal lobe dysfunction. And perhaps some day researchers will successfully investigate the precise degree to which the biology of mental processes interacted with the biology of brain shaking in a given concussion (the neuropsychiatric perspective). They might then search for a biological marker of a boundary between those changes that proceeded in the brain without interacting with mental predispositions, thoughts, or emotions (which assumes separation of brain from mind) and those that involved such interactions (which accepts that brain and mind have something to do with one another). That would be quite a technical and taxonomical challenge. Moreover, functional neuroimaging studies suggest that so-called conversion patients have replicable abnormalities of function (e.g., [112]). Feeling sick without pathognomonic objective signs of that sickness (so-called somatoform illness) may involve different brain changes from feeling sick with those signs, but both are due to altered brain function.

Some day, we might discover a neurobiological boundary between brain change that does or does not involve mind. At that point, clinicians may use a biological marker to diagnose brain dysfunction that would have occurred even if the patient had no mind to react, and we can label that oddity "absolutely organic," versus brain dysfunction due to the more common (perhaps universal) interaction of physical brain trauma with genes and environment and mind. For the foreseeable future, all four types of brain disturbances listed above are organic changes caused by CBI.

IIIB1. A Dichotomy Between Imaginary and Intentional Complaints Does Not Seem Consistent With What We Know About Brains

> amid his exaggerations, there is a kernel of truth? … we must not forget that in certain real diseases, mental states including the need to exaggerate or misleads, can be a marker of the primary disease.
>
> Charcot, 1877 [113]

Consider Louise, a healthy, 33-year-old mother of two concussed in a motor vehicle collision. She is angry at the driver of the other car. She is impoverished and hoping for compensation. She has read about CBI and expects that she might suffer memory loss. She complains of memory loss. Why? Who among us – the emergency department physician, the primary care doctor, the consulting neurologist, the neuropsychologist, knows what proportion of her complaint is due to: (1) the acute and chronic effects of external force physically impacting memory circuitry; (2) acute and chronic stress (anxiety and/or depression) physically impacting memory circuitry; (3) "psychological" changes that do not impact

memory circuitry – for instance, a natural wish for sympathy, a lowered threshold to adopt the sick identity, or a sense of a diminished future; (4) expectation; or (5) willful, deliberate, self-conscious, immoral faking?

When people announce health complaints that doctors cannot readily explain with their current knowledge of clinical/pathological correlation, we face three problems. First: there seems to be variability in the degree to which symptoms are consciously versus unconsciously generated. Second: no method exists to measure that degree. Third: our knowledge of clinical/pathological correlation may be faulty. As a result, patient expectation of symptoms is not the only danger of preconceived notions. A doctor's education leads him to expect what he's been told to expect about the effects of concussion. A patient who presents differently becomes the object of suspicion.

So how will the doctor sort patients who *imagine* they have headache or irritability or concentration difficulty after CBI from and those who *pretend*? A century ago it was common to classify symptoms of unknown cause as either hysteria (allegedly unconscious) or malingering (allegedly conscious) [107,113–116]. Lipman (1962) [117] proposed a more nuanced classification of symptom exaggeration: *invention* (when an asymptomatic patient pretends to have symptoms), *perseveration* (when a patient who previously had symptoms alleges they have continued), *exaggeration* (when a symptomatic patient alleges worse symptoms than he feels), and *transference* (when a symptomatic patient deliberately attributes his genuine symptoms to the wrong cause). But that scheme still assumes that both the patient and the clever examiner can distinguish what is driven by consciousness from what is driven by unconsciousness.

That core concept lost credibility as psychologists acknowledged, beginning in the early 1980s, both the conceptual shakiness of a strict division between conscious and unconscious and the impracticality of measuring degree of intentionality (see below). For several decades, a better-accepted model has been that degree of intentionality seems to lie on a continuum of sorts, as proposed by Travin and Potter in 1984 [118] and supported by Rogers (1988) [119] (also see Nies and Sweet, 1994 [120]).

Human thoughts and actions cannot be readily dichotomized as conscious and voluntary versus unconscious and involuntary because there exist varying degrees of both awareness and self-perceived willful intention [121–123]. Several clinical syndromes are illustrative. Patients diagnosed with "psychogenic" seizures very frequently have authentic electrophysiological fits; they are widely considered to exhibit an impossible-to-dichotomize spectrum of intentionality [124–126]. Ganser's syndrome (the syndrome of approximate answers) seems to fall somewhere between conscious/voluntary and unconscious/involuntary [127,128]. Observations on hypnosis offer complementary insights: despite the general consensus that response to hypnotic suggestion is unconscious and that amnesia of hypnotized subjects is genuine, subjects resist acting contrary to their own interests [129] and subjects sometimes have trouble even determining whether they are acting under their own volition. For instance, suggestible but non-hypnotized patients who are primed to produce symptoms usually believe that their behaviors are involuntary [130–132].

IIIB2. A Dichotomy Between Imaginary and Intentional Complaints is Not Clinically Diagnosable

Finally, who can tell the faker from the honest patient? Many of us believe ourselves to be reasonably adept at detecting dissimulation. That is self-delusion. Effective misrepresentation, dissimulation, and outright lying are signal accomplishments of the evolved human brain. This talent plays an important role in pursuing social advantage and success. Even the DSM-5 admits, "the definitive absence of feigning may not be reliably discerned" ([75], p. 320).

As a result of this new candor, there are widespread doubts about the practicality of applying the theoretical trichotomy. Jonas and Pope advised in 1985, "an appropriate strategy might be to set aside the slippery question of what is conscious and what is voluntary, and concentrate on the objective features of patients displaying factitious signs or symptoms" [133]. Kanaan and Wessely put it: "Today many see FD [factitious disorder] and conversion disorder (as hysteria is now known) not as separate categories, but as neighbors on a spectrum of simulated disorder, with clinical distinction usually impossible to make" ([134], p. 47). Friedman echoed this conclusion, "There is, as yet, no reliable way to prove the psychiatric origins for the problem" ([135], p. 307). Prudent clinicians will accept their limits in this regard.

IV. Misplaced Faith in Flawed Modes of Inquiry

IV.A. Misplaced Faith in Authority

WHO is an exemplary center of excellence. Its very existence raises hope for global peace and cooperation. It is a trusted, authoritative voice on matters of life and death. WHO published a paper in 2004 titled "Prognosis for mild traumatic brain injury: Results of the WHO Collaborating Centre Task Force on mild traumatic brain injury [136]. The authors describe having conducted a "systematic search of the literature on MTBI in order to produce a best-evidence synthesis." With regard to the impact of CBI on children: "Twenty-eight longitudinal, 1 cross-sectional study and 1 case series … examined outcome and prognostic factors of MTBI in children" ([136], p. 85). The authors concluded, "There was consistent and methodologically sound evidence that children's prognosis after mild traumatic brain injury is good, with quick resolution of symptoms and little evidence of residual cognitive, behavioural or academic deficits" [136].

This might be taken (and has been cited) as persuasive reassurance. But is the conclusion justified by the review? A brief scrutiny of the "Twenty-eight longitudinal" papers reveals the following: among those 28, only three studies (Bijur et al., 1990 [137]; 1996 [138]; Wrightson et al., 1995 [139]) followed up beyond two years. Neither of Bijur's papers is actually a longitudinal study; they are both case–control studies,

with occurrence of mTBI not even based on medical evidence but on parents' recollection. And, although Wrightson et al.'s study is not strictly speaking longitudinal, since it identified subjects retrospectively, at least the authors had both medical records of the injury and formal testing of the outcomes vs. a comparison group [139]. This minimal standard of design is not present in most of the longitudinal studies cited by WHO.

The authors of the 2004 WHO paper state, "Two phase II cohort studies indicate that post-concussion symptoms in children appear to be largely resolved within 2–3 months of the injury" ([136], p. 85). (They refer to Farmer et al., 1987 [140] and Ponsford et al., 1999 [141].) Setting aside the insensitivity of the follow-up assessments to lingering dysfunction, such a very short follow-up interval can only report the child's status at two to three months. The conclusion that observation can end so soon since obvious problems "largely resolved" presupposes a monophasic illness with no late effects. That may in fact turn out to be one of the courses of CBI. However, it deserves consideration whether the four-year-old who is judged to be fully recovered after nine weeks might go on to drop out of high school, develop social phobia at age 33, or develop dementia five years earlier than expected. The conventional focus in "longitudinal" studies on short-term outcomes may be misleading.

The WHO paper seems to oversimplify some reports. The authors cite the one-year study by Greenspan and MacKenzie [142] as concluding, "mTBI not associated with poor outcome." In fact, Greenspan and MacKenzie wrote: "head-injured children exhibited a greater number of behavioral problems 1 year after head injury when compared with a randomly selected sample of children, ages 6 to 16 years ." Furthermore, the WHO authors did not weight the quality of their sources. The sole long-term longitudinal study they cite with well-documented assessments at injury and follow-up was Wrightson et al. [139]. This study – perhaps the one most worthy of citation – actually reported that mTBI children were cognitively impaired at 6.5 years.

These critiques are by no means a critique of the WHO's landmark effort. The authors themselves bemoaned the lack of quality evidence. In fact, many members of the 2004 WHO team reunited a decade later as the International Collaboration on Mild Traumatic Brain Injury Prognosis. In early 2014 they published a suite of 13 papers in the *Archives of Physical Medicine and Rehabilitation* – an incomparable and humbling summary of the state of the art that will be gratefully cited in this text and many others for the foreseeable future [143]. My comments are only to offer a caution: renowned experts and centers cannot, by virtue of their authority, be assumed to generate trustworthy conclusions about CBI.

IV.B. Misplaced Faith in Consensus

> Consensus means that everyone agrees to say collectively what no one believes individually.
>
> Abba Eban

Consensus is a mode of collective decision making that has been credited to the Society of Friends, or Quakers, more than 300 years ago. Its virtue, proven in many experiments, is that groups sometimes outperform their most proficient group member [144]. Moreover, under the right circumstances, group decisions are "counterintuitively robust" against social influence on individuals[145]. The U.S. NIH ran a Consensus Development Program [146] from 1977 to 2013, assembling groups of experts to propose practice parameters in the face of inconsistent data. The program ended only because, by 2013, other organizations such as the Institute of Medicine and Cochrane Collaboration had assumed this role.

Still, not every medical scholar was enthused about this development. In 1981 Drummond Rennie, then editor of the *New England Journal of Medicine,* commented in that journal that consensus statements about uncertain medical matters are interim approaches in the absence of a proper clinical trial that, unfortunately may "represent the lowest common denominator of a debate" ([147], p. 666). Rennie expressed concern that: "The statements may be taken to embalm a set of truths … This spurious stamp of approval would be very hard for the individual physician to resist." He pointed out that the bland final publications cover up the messy but informative sausage making of passionate debates. He concluded: "This feeling of received truth that is conveyed by consensus statements reminds us that most explorations of nature would have been stillborn if the scientists or navigators or climbers had heeded the advice of consensus panels" ([147], p. 666).

Rennie's concerns mesh with subsequent research. One drawback of consensus meetings is the risk that certain members will dominate the process. For instance, extraverts tend to become group leaders [148], and, as Kameda (1996) found, "The empirical and theoretical results … indicate that … group decisions can … be biased to a certain individual's or faction's advantage through tactical manipulations of consensus procedures"([149], p. 137). One method to reduce this threat is anonymity. In the Delphi approach to consensus, for instance, opinions are submitted by mail without personal identifiers. Yet most consensus meetings are face to face. As Jones and Hunter cautioned, "In open committees individuals are often not ready to retreat from long held and publicly stated opinions, even when these have been proved false" ([150], p. 376).

A different drawback is the simple fact that few consensus recommendations are followed. The process does not usually affect physician behavior and may merely represent "a dialogue among researchers … not a guide to action" [151]. The result of such studies has been a caveat. "The existence of consensus does not mean that the 'correct' answer has been found – there is the danger of deriving collective ignorance rather than wisdom" [150].

Many publications about CBI report the results of conferences at which assemblies of individuals, typically with varying training, expertise, cognitive style, and personalities, have gathered and undertaken the task of finding and publishing shared beliefs – that is, consensus conferences. Perhaps the best-known example is the periodic conclave of the Concussion in Sports Group (CISG). To date the CISG has published four summary and agreement statements. The first followed a 2001 conference in Vienna. Ten participants were given a mandate to describe the agreements reached by the whole [152]. This state-of-the-art document began by proposing a new definition of concussion. Interestingly, this novelty was framed as an effort to supersede a previous consensus: "Over 35 years ago, the Committee on Head Injury Nomenclature of the Congress of Neurological Surgeons proposed a 'consensus' definition of concussion … This definition was recognized as having a number of limitations"([152], p. 6). The CSIG authors acknowledged the major mystery we face: "It is clear that the variations in clinical outcome from the same impact force require a more sophisticated approach to the understanding of this phenomenon than is currently available" ([152], p. 7), as well as the laudable caveat: "the authors acknowledge that the science of concussion is at the early stages" ([152], p. 9). One firm prescription: to better detect whether a CBI victim has declined in cognitive function, pre-injury "baseline testing is recommended" ([152], p. 8).

The second draft of a CISG consensus followed a 2004 meeting in Prague [153]. This draft introduced the Sport Concussion Assessment Tool, a very good checklist to guide clinicians through acute assessment. The authors noted that most concussions resolve in seven to ten days – they called this "Simple concussion" – yet acknowledged that some athletes suffer persistent symptoms – they called this "Complex concussion," and did not question the validity of those long-lasting problems. The authors reiterated their recommendation for pre-participation baseline cognitive testing.

The third CISG consensus statement followed a 2008 meeting in Zurich [154]. Attentive readers noticed a subtle change in tone. The previous definitions of concussions simply stated that resolution typically followed a sequential course. Added in 2009: "In a *small percentage of cases* [emphasis added], however, post-concussive symptoms may be prolonged." The emphasis on the smallness of that percentage was enhanced in the next paragraph:

> There was unanimous agreement to abandon the Simple versus Complex terminology that had been proposed in the Prague agreement … The panel, however, unanimously retained the concept that most (80–90%) concussions resolve in a short period (7–10 days).
>
> [154], p. 756

The authors correctly state that they "retained" the notion from 2005 that most concussions resolve in seven to ten days. But in 2009 they replaced "most" with a number: 80–90%. This represents a newly specific position – that persistent symptoms occur in as few as 10%. The authors supplemented their reassurance about the benignity of CBI: "the majority of injuries will recover spontaneously over several days" ([154], p. 758).

Another change appears in the recommendations for baseline testing. In 2002 and 2005, this was unequivocally recommended, even though it creates an obvious burden on schools and other athletic organizations. In the 2009 paper, the authors were more forgiving: "Although formal baseline NP [neuropsychological] screening may be beyond the resources of many sports or individuals, it is recommended that in all organized high-risk sports *consideration* [emphasis added] be given to having this cognitive evaluation regardless of the age or level of performance" (p. 760). Moreover, in this third iteration, the CISG for the first time approved same-day return-to-play (RTP) after concussion: "some professional American football players are able to return to play more quickly, with even same day RTP supported by National Football League studies" (p. 758). Some readers were astonished that a consensus panel that included some brain experts would sanction the risky protocol of same-day RTP – especially the deference to NFL studies with self-serving conclusions. Of interest, the CISG felt compelled for the first time to issue a disclaimer: "The panel chairperson (WM) did not identify with any advocacy position" (p. 761). Readers might understandably wonder whether, as of 2009, the CISG had indeed begun advocating for a position, tilting their rhetoric to imply that concussions cause little harm.

At the time of this writing, the most recent CISG draft was published in 2013 after a 2012 meeting in Zurich [155]. The definition of concussion was revised: the authors now refer to "brain 'shaking' resulting in clinical symptoms ... that are not necessarily related to a pathological injury" (p. 1). This is the first explicit statement by the CISG of the position that one should not assume that post-concussive symptoms are organic sequelae due to concussive injury. (The present author agrees.) However, after a decade of urging pre-season cognitive testing of athletes the authors withdrew their recommendation for such burdensome baseline testing, due to "insufficient evidence."

The striking change is rhetorical. A new section appears in this fourth draft titled, "Difficult or persistently symptomatic concussion patient." Regarding the "difficult patient," the CSIG states: "Persistent symptoms (> 10 days) are generally reported in 10–15% of concussions. In general, symptoms are not specific to concussion" ([155], p. e3). Every English-speaking physician knows what "difficult patient" connotes: a person whose complaints are judged to be out of proportion to the illness, or who requires more time and attention than the doctor wishes to offer, or who is litigious, or who is judged (by a non-psychiatrist) to be mentally ill [156–158]. "Patient psychiatric pathology is the conventional explanation for why patients are deemed 'difficult'" [159]. A substantial literature addresses doctors' stressful encounters with such patients, with titles such as "Personality disorders: Understanding and managing the difficult patient in neurology practice" [160]; "The difficult patient: Borderline personality disorder in the obstetrical and gynecological patient" [161]; or, in an amicable belch of dehumanization, "Taming the difficult patient" [162]. In short, labeling a person a "difficult patient" is a way to assign blame for the clinician's distress.

It is not clear whether the use of this loaded terminology constitutes evidence that the CISG is biased in favor of the "concussions do little harm" position. However, another revision in the manuscript seems to imply as much. The authors opined, "It was further agreed that CTE was not related to concussions alone or simply exposure to contact sports." Neuropathologists are slowly making strides toward understanding dementia after

TBI. Due to the lack of prospective longitudinal research, it is not yet possible to determine the contribution of one or more sports-related concussions to such cases of dementia, popularly referred to as chronic traumatic encephalopathy. Given the absence of pertinent knowledge, it seems imprudent for a group to declare that they know the answer.

The Wisdom of Crowds?

In 1907, Francis Galton asked nearly 800 people at a fair to estimate the weight of an ox. The average of those estimates was within one pound of the correct weight. This is an example of the wisdom of crowds – the phenomenon in which individual judgments about a fact, averaged together, often yield a better estimate than any individual could produce [163,164]. One might conclude that consensus judgments about CBI are useful.

The limitation of crowd wisdom, however, is that success depends on the participants having some knowledge. Fifty neurologists, working as a collective mind, might or might not guess the weight of an ox, but they could probably estimate the adult IQ of a developmentally disabled toddler or the remaining months of life of a patient with amyotrophic lateral sclerosis. None of them knows the answer, but all of them have pertinent knowledge. In contrast, this group should not be polled to determine the likely height of the first alien to arrive on Earth. They lack field experience in exobiology.

Similarly, there are limitations to the application of consensus meetings to advancing knowledge about CBI. Even assuming that the average participant in such a meeting is a renowned TBI authority, he or she can only estimate unknown facts about which some information is known. Consensus groups such as the CSIG deserve great credit for many thoughtful judgments derived from the hard work of collective thinking. The collective experience of such experts in devising a form likely to collect important information in the acute setting, or judging the efficacy of inpatient rehabilitation, is invaluable. However, hardly anything is known about the spectrum and sequence of brain changes that occur over the 70 years after a single concussion and the genetic and environmental variables that mediate or moderate those changes. Consensus groups cannot "agree" to know about an unknown.

The literature on consensus as a decision-making process, combined with the example of the CISG consensus documents, raises some red flags about trusting groups to decide medical truth:

- Consensus is in the eye of the beholder. Just as the CISG derogated the consensus of the Committee on Head Injury Nomenclature of the Congress of Neurological Surgeons, groups of people sharing strong opinions may trumpet their internal self-agreement as "consensus," and dismiss the opinions of equally capable groups.
- Consensus is an effort to objectify the subjective. The worth of the product depends on many imponderables, including selection and self-selection for group membership, the personality and assertiveness of leaders, shared bias, and group dynamics.
- Consensus about unknowable facts has no value.

IV.C. Misplaced Faith in Cognitive Testing

Two questions would be helpful to settle. One, is there a subgroup of CBI survivors who have persistently reduced cognitive test scores? And if that is so, is that because of the CBI or something else – such as a non-specific emotional response to trauma? Two, whether or not scholars agree about the existence of an unfortunate subgroup with persistently low cognitive test scores, are such scores a good way to assess brain function? Impartial answers to these two questions would be extremely valuable for understanding the spectrum of effects of CBI on humans. Impartial answers, however, are hard to find.

IV.C.1. Is There a Subgroup of CBI Survivors who Have Persistently Reduced Cognitive Test Scores? And if That is So, is That Because of the CBI or Something Else?

A debate has roiled the neuropsychology community for more than a decade. It concerns the simple question: does CBI cause some victims to suffer cognitive impairment lasting more than three months? The adversarial positions might be stated as follows: some neuropsychologists believe that cognitive impairment more than three months after CBI is uncommon. When it does occur, it is due to factors other than brain injury, such as pre-morbid psychiatric problems, desire for compensation leading to faking bad on tests, psychological expectation, or some other behavioral confounder. Other neuropsychologists believe that a subset of CBI survivors have persistently compromised neural function due to traumatic brain change.

This seemingly straightforward question is ripe with nuance. For one thing, the adversaries are not comparing apples with apples. If *cognitive impairment* is an apple, *compromised function*, a broader concept, is an orange. Thus, it is within the realm of possibility that both opinions have merit. For instance, perhaps commonly tested cognitive troubles such as difficulty remembering three words are more likely to recover, while less commonly tested troubles such as multitasking ability are more likely to persist. If so, studies that emphasize traditional domains of cognition might fail to detect important and lasting problems. Alternatively, perhaps cognitive troubles such as difficulty remembering three words tend to recover more quickly while other distressing dysfunctions such as fatigue or irritability or changes in emotional reactivity tend to persist. These questions will be addressed more fully in Chapters 5 and 7.

Another nuance is the definition of *cognitive impairment*. No direct measure of cognitive impairment exists – for instance, the equivalent of a thermometer to measure temperature. All we have are some popular psychological tests and the examiner's instinct. Some of these tests require paper and pencil. Some require a computer. None, not even IQ, are judged to be comprehensive measures of the manifold animal function *mental processing*. Instead, psychologists often propose that a given test provides information about a "domain" – a type of thought in a taxonomy of cognitive function [165,166]. Hence, *cognitive impairment* is not like hearing impairment – a problem that could be mapped along a logarithmic decibel scale – but refers to the presence of trouble with one or many functions, each of which deserves its own measurement.

The validity of so-called "cognitive domains" is worth an essay in itself. Suffice it to say that psychologists do not use this term to refer to brain regions, circuits, nuclei, or a type of neural processing. The phrase is used to distinguish abstract categories of behavior that either seem to hang together *a priori* (for instance, reading and writing both seem to pertain to a "language" domain), or are statistically linked because scores on one test tend to go up and down with scores on another. For instance, factor analysis might reveal that people who have trouble arranging blocks to make a pattern also tend to have trouble quickly substituting symbols for numbers. It is even possible that ablation of one brain part tends to impact scores on both tests. On the basis of such evidence these two tests might be judged to belong to the same "domain," and in fact, many psychologists state that scores on these two tests live in a mental domain they call "performance" – according to a principle of classification that is obviously vague. Despite factor analytic links, little evidence exists that the six "performance" tests on a typical adult IQ battery engage a distinct place, circuit, or neurobiologically distinct type of cerebral processing.

In the same way, ability to figure out that the examiner changed the rules for sorting cards without telling you (the Wisconsin Card Sorting Test) [167] and ability to quickly list a bunch of words starting with "F" (the Controlled Oral Word Association Test) [168] are assigned to a domain called "executive functions." That lumping of disparate behaviors into unitary categories raises the question of whether a domain is anything but a best effort to devise a plausible-sounding unifying theme for abstract constructs that require diffuse and multifocal brain operations that may differ between individuals.

Second, to answer whether CBI causes anything requires a sincere effort to dodge the *post hoc ergo propter hoc* (this followed that so it was caused by that) fallacy. Just because an event commonly follows CBI – for instance, a CBI victim is more likely to receive an emergency department bill than a non-victim – does not mean that cerebral injury per se caused the bill. Therefore, even if scholars agreed that some CBI survivors have reduced cognitive test scores many months after CBI, it would not be proof that CBI *caused* the reduction in test scores.

Causality aside, an impressive effort has been made attempting to determine whether CBI is associated with cognitive impairment lasting more than three months. Earnest teams of psychologists have exchanged remarkable manuscripts arguing for and against the hypothesis that CBI is sometimes associated with lasting cognitive problems [169–185]. A student of acquired brain injury could hardly do better than to read this collection of manuscripts. Setting aside the partisan tone, this is a rich vein of knowledge and thought. Both sides in this famous debate cite multiple provocative empirical observations. Both sides raise vital questions deserving a career's worth of impartial study. The author cannot score this fight blow by blow because his goal is to figure out the science, not to elevate the sweaty arm of a winner. He will focus on providing the reader with a brief summary of the facts and ideas in play.

The modern discussion arguably commenced with an excellent 1995 paper by Dikmen et al. titled "Neuropsychological outcome at 1-year post head injury" [169]. Dikmen et al.'s innovative method was to conduct cognitive testing on 436 victims of TBI and compare those results with findings from 121 patients who suffered trauma other than head injury (orthopedic). The virtue of this approach, at least in theory, is that it controls for the non-specific effects of a traumatic experience, allowing investigators to sort problems specifically attributable to brain trauma from those expected after trauma of any kind. A practical stumbling block to this method is how to match the traumatic severity of a CBI with, for instance, a foot injury. The study reports that the subgroup of 161 head-injured subjects who followed commands within an hour (the "mild" group) "is roughly comparable in median to the trauma controls ([169], p. 82). The authors concluded that significant cognitive impairment one year after mild head injury is unlikely. Yet an equally important finding was the wide range of variability of responses, inspiring the authors' reasonable inference: "high variability … may be viewed as a reflection of the resiliency of brain functions … in some individuals "(p. 87).

That is, people vary. Attempts to lump TBI survivors together, as if the brain's response to a given amount of external force were predictable, ignore the simple truth of biological variation. (Chapter 4 will demonstrate the same observation in rodents. Rats that exhibit longer-lived deficits after mechanically identical injuries should probably not be accused of symptom exaggeration due to expectation, faking bad, frail personalities, or litigiousness.)

Meta-Analysis

Despite multiple studies of varying size and quality, uncertainty has persisted regarding whether or not CBI is associated with lasting cognitive harm. In an effort to overcome that uncertainty, research teams began to publish meta-analyses. This approach combines results of multiple studies in the hope of gaining statistical power, hence, more confidence in the validity of conclusions. In 1997, Binder et al. combined results of eight publications testing 11 samples at least three months post-injury (totals: 314 mild head trauma (MHT); 302 healthy comparisons). One statistical test suggested that MHT impacts cognition beyond 3 months, but only a little (effect size 0.12); another mathematical approach suggested no effect. The authors argued, "the average effect of MHT on neuropsychological performance is undetectable" ([171], p. 428). The authors added a cryptic and provocative comment: "the occurrence of closed-head injury is not random" (p. 430). What they meant is that it's hard to figure out whether CBI hurts the brain because people with pre-existing problems are prone to suffer concussions. Before pointing out some limitations of this 1997 paper, one should credit the authors with a historic attempt to figure out whether CBI can cause lasting cognitive impairment. Taken at face value, this study says no.

Readers familiar with experimental design, however, would immediately ask:

- How were the eight studies selected?
- How high was their quality?
- If an atypical subgroup exists with persistent cognitive impairments, would this approach detect it?

- Were the tests sensitive to the multiplicity of cognitive problems observed after CBI?
- Are scores on cognitive tests what really matter?

Two years later, in 1999, Erin Bigler delivered his Distinguished Neuropsychologist Award Lecture [172]. He did not directly rebut the 1997 claim that cognitive trouble is undetectable more than three months after CBI. In fact, most of his address focused on more severe injuries. Yet Bigler touched upon critical issues relevant to any study of CBI outcome:

1. Cognitive testing does not detect every brain change.
2. "If valid neuropsychological evaluation and testing supports residual deficits, trust that those deficits are organically based" ([172], p. 123). Note: this statement is not radical. Bigler clarified in a later publication that by "organically based" he simply meant that – as readers hopefully agree – psychological symptoms are mediated by organic brain change. For example, Chen et al. reported, "athletes with concussion with depression symptoms showed reduced activation in the dorsolateral prefrontal cortex and striatum and attenuated deactivation in medial frontal and temporal regions" ([186], p. 81). Whether to attribute these organic changes to direct or indirect results of organic brain injury is a different question.
3. Neuroimaging helps, but many CBI patents have normal structural MRI scans. Changes seen on structural MRIs are, in any case, just the tip of the iceberg since more sensitive imaging methods reveal previously unsuspected tissue changes.
4. Bigler predicted, "neurobehavioral probes on line with neuroimaging will likely replace many of the current methods of neuropsychological assessment" ([172], p. 124) (a prediction that seems to be approaching fruition).
5. Bigler urged readers to remember: people vary. "[B]rain–behavior relationships will, in large part, be unique for each individual" (p. 123). For this reason, it would not be wise to generalize about the spectrum of effects of TBI on humans based on an average.

There was a pause, perhaps a collective sucking in of breath. Then Bigler's adversaries responded. In 2003 Lees-Haley et al. published a direct and surprisingly emotional rebuttal to Bigler's five points. Among other critiques, they accused him of a "pervasive tendency to suggest physiological origins" ([174], p. 585). They dismissed his plea to acknowledge individual variation, oddly accusing him of "a preference for relying on individual anecdotal evidence" (p. 587). In regard to Bigler's reporting that sensitive imaging methods reveal unsuspected brain changes, they responded: "We argue that making a reasonable difference in the life of an individual is what defines the significance of brain tissue pathology, not the sheer ability of experts to detect change through neuroradiological imaging or other methods" (p. 588). The present author agrees with this final point. Until sufficient clinical imaging correlations studies are done, until it is known whether these newly detectable phenomena represent brain dysfunction, one should not assume that all post-concussive brain change is deleterious.

Bigler responded. His far-ranging 2003 reply to Lees-Haley et al.'s critique included his clarification of his assertion that post-TBI symptoms are organic: "there are also neurobiological explanations that are part of the so-called psychological features that accompany the trauma of being in an accident, development of chronic pain and stress-mediated disorders" ([173], p. 596). This is hardly a novel idea. Bigler cited William James's seminal 1890 statement: "The causes of our mental structure are doubtless natural, and connected, like all our other peculiarities, with those of our nervous structure" ([187], p. 688). He is merely asking his critics to admit the minimum starting point for modern scientific discussion: Descartes is dead; behavior arises from tissue.

Bigler also implores his critics to accept the straightforward facts that: (1) a continuum exists between the mildest and the most severe possible TBI; (2) different assessment methods will exhibit different degrees of sensitivity to TBI brain changes; and (3) "Short of postmortem histological examination, most pathology cannot be observed in TBI, particularly mild TBI with any type of *in vivo* imaging" ([173], p. 598). In regard to Lees-Haley et al.'s very good point that one should not equate subtle brain change seen on modern imaging with clinically problematic brain damage, Bigler explained his conceptual position. To paraphrase: patients with normal imaging and normal neuropsychological testing may nonetheless be both symptomatic and have demonstrable brain lesions. This leads to a reasonable inference that the brain lesions have something to do with the symptoms, especially since this inference is consistent with the experimental literature that finds permanent changes in the structural and functional organization of the brain after a single concussive head injury. In other words, it remains to be seen whether changes visualized, for instance, with DTI or fMRI have reliable behavioral correlates.

The CISG made a similar point in 2002: "the predictive value of various MRI abnormalities that may be incidentally discovered is not established at the present time" ([152], p. 8). Unfortunately, their use of the qualifier "incidental" suggests premature closure on the question of clinical significance. To date it has not been determined which visible changes are best characterized as incidental, markers of clinically significant brain dysfunction, or harbingers of early death due to neurodegeneration. That is an empirical question begging for an answer.

More data were published by Frencham et al., in 2005 [178]. This meta-analysis merged results from 17 studies published from 1995 to 2004 with the eight older studies cited by Binder et al. in 1997 [171], yielding data on what might be called the "Frencham 25": 25 publications regarding 634 cases of mTBI and 485 comparison subjects. Among the 17 new studies, Frencham et al. found five papers discussing post-acute cognitive testing (meaning three or more months after injury). The authors conducted meta-analysis as if these five studies were comparable, yet the actual timing of testing varied greatly among the five ("3 months," "within 5 years," "6.4 years (average)," "within 8 years," "within 3 years"). Speed of information processing was significantly worse among concussed subjects (effect size 0.47). However, the authors combined these new post-acute studies with Binder's post-acute studies, mixing all types of cognitive testing and generating an effect size for cognition of 0.11, a non-significant result. Again, readers might be impressed by the mirage of concordance across these non-comparable studies, but aggrieved when they discover the assumptions used to analyze them.

In a 2009 publication, Pertab et al. re-examined Frencham's 25 studies [179]. This group focused on the 18 studies that seemed most worthy of inclusion. The authors noted the wide variation in definitions of mTBI among these studies (from "he stopped what he was doing" to "post traumatic amnesia of < 48 h") and the wide variety of mechanisms of injury. Overall effects size for long-term cognitive problems – lumping together all tests – was negligible: –0.08 to –0.09. However, the effect of concussion on verbal paired memory testing was a highly significant –0.81. Pertab et al. also cautioned that assuming the CBI victims form a homogeneous, normally distributed sample could lead to error: "Clinically relevant information from samples that fall on a bimodal distribution … may not be detected with standard meta-analytic techniques" ([179], p. 504). (These authors drew hypothetical curves illustrating that risk.) Pertab et al. were also candid in acknowledging that low test scores do not necessarily mean primary brain damage; many factors other than the mechanics of injury might influence performance in a neuropsychology laboratory. They listed:

- pre-morbid medical, emotional, and personality factors
- litigation and compensation seeking
- demographics (age, education, socioeconomic status, etc.)
- pain and other physical residua.

To summarize Pertab et al.'s contributions:

1. The average of results from injuries defined in different ways may be an uninterpretable average of results from different brain disorders.

2. Lumping together all kinds of test results can obscure the presence of significantly impaired aspects of cognition.

3. Lumping together CBIs with different mechanisms (for instance, a three-foot fall and an 80-kph motor vehicle accident) may obscure the presence of a minority who suffered a neurobiologically different trauma.

4. Lumping together patients with and without persistent symptoms does not permit us to characterize the natural history of CBI followed by persistent symptoms. In essence, judging that no CBI victims suffer long-term problems because the average of all victims on all tests is OK denies the biological fact of individual variation. It is almost akin to stating, "West Africans, on average, are healthy. Therefore, let's not talk about an Ebola problem."

By 2009 mainstream thought about concussion had shifted. More and more neuropsychologists were asking questions about the value of their own product, cognitive test results. As Ruff and Jamora put it that year, "poor postconcussive outcomes cannot be determined by … only focusing on cognitive test findings. Rather a far more sophisticated follow-up protocol warranted" ([182], p. 35).

Rohling et al. countered. In a 2011 publication, they reexamined the "Frencham 25" [176]. Again, their mathematics showed that the effect size on overall cognitive dysfunction after three months was negligible: –0.07. The authors also employed the Q statistic. This is a way to quantify the homogeneity of a sample. Based on these Qs, Rohling et al. asserted that the samples were homogeneous and there was no evidence of an impaired subgroup. Then, in 2012, Rohling et al. published a feisty critique of the notion that meta-analysis might hide a miserable minority with long-term problems [177]. For the sake of argument, this strong paper proposes that 17% of mTBI victims are persistently impaired, then asks whether such a subgroup would be hidden in the meta-analytic process. Assuming that their calculation from their previous paper was correct (that is, that the overall effect size is a tiny –0.07), they show that the only way for such a result to be found in the presence of an impaired subgroup is if that miserable subgroup falls entirely *within the distribution* for normal control subjects. In fact (under their assumptions), to fall outside that normal curve the impaired CBI victims would have to be doing worse than people with moderate mental retardation. Rohling et al. also added to the list of factors that could lower test scores even without brain damage, including (1) *diagnostic threat* (that is, simply being reminded of a TBI can lower scores), and (2) the evidence that people with pre-existing cognitive impairment are more likely to suffer a TBI. If so, observers who attribute impairments they detect after a CBI may be putting the cart before the horse: those cognitive problems may not only have predated the concussion but played a role in causing it. (This recalls Binder et al.'s 1997 comment that TBI "is not random," [171] and highlights the legitimate possibility that some people may be TBI-prone.)

Just two more papers in this campaign of scholarly skirmishes will be mentioned. Bigler et al. published a paper in 2013 that addressed the now-notorious Frencham 25 [184]. They tabulated key information about all 25 studies, permitting readers to judge the methodological flaws for themselves. The authors recited, again, the assumptions made by the meta-analysts (such as assuming that neurological injuries fitting many different definitions are the same injury) and their possible violations of research standards. In particular, they showed how many (if not most) of the original 25 studies fail in formal ratings of research quality. The authors argued that if one confines one's attention to the five highest-quality studies, the effect size became a meaningful 0.56.

Perhaps more importantly, Bigler et al. proposed a simple paradigm shift. They point out what is now old news: cognitive tests are not sensitive to all the brain changes that might impact a person after a concussion, because: (1) they fail to detect many subtle cognitive problems; (2) they fail to detect clinically disabling non-cognitive behavior problems; and (3) the results do not correlate, in any reliable way, with brain change. For example, millisecond scale delays in processing may not measurably degrade performance in a neuropsychology lab, but may nonetheless symptomatically impair complex cognitive functions. New neuroimaging and electrophysiological tests reveal brain abnormalities when neuropsychological testing does not. fMRI studies of concussion, for example, have revealed abnormalities of brain function during memory tasks that were missed in cognitive testing: "TBI-induced differences in working memory functional activity were observed even though differences in behavioral performance between MTBI patients and controls were absent"[188]. In addition, expert psychiatric examination reveals non-cognitive distress – often due to both pre-injury and injury-related factors – that may elude traditional test batteries. Quoting Johnson et al. (2011): "'Neuropsychological testing and conventional neuroimaging techniques are not sufficiently sensitive to detect' ([189], p. 511) neurological changes" (p. 27).

Larrabee et al. responded [185]. In their 2013 manuscript they defended their method of measuring homogeneity. They offered justifiable critiques of several of the sources cited by Bigler et al. They repeated the observation that people with pre-morbid behavior problems are both more likely to have concussion and more likely to complain after concussion. And they reiterated their sensible criteria for future acceptable studies:

1. prospective and longitudinal
2. inclusion of non-head trauma (e.g., orthopedic) comparison subjects to control for non-specific effects of trauma, and
3. controlling for possible psychological confounding factors such as expectancy, diagnostic threat, pain, litigation, malingering, everyday life stress.

Yet the objections to concerns about long-term neurobiological change are simply illogical – compatible with neither the (admittedly limited and technically suboptimal) experimental literature nor with the longitudinal results of neuroimaging.

No one can doubt that a substantial proportion of concussion survivors experience prolonged and even lifelong distress after a single CBI. True, as stated in the preface, little can be said about medically invisible concussions. However, as demonstrated in Chapter 5 of this volume, more than 40% of survivors of typical clinically attended CBI still express or exhibit neurobehavioral problems at or beyond one year post-injury. The question is why outcomes vary so much. The answer is offered in Chapter 7.

Bigler seems to be correct in stating, "it is an untenable and non-supportable position that neuron-based symptoms and deficits do not persist in some individuals who experience mTBI" ([184], p. 206) (although one must be cautious about calling a visualizable brain change a *lesion* until better clinico-imaging studies testing for deleterious effects are done).

When Larrabee et al. write, "The concerns of Bigler et al. (2013) regarding the existence of a neurological etiology for the persisting complaints of some people with history of mTBI are misplaced" ([185], p. 231), they reveal two dated biases. First, they appear to believe that neuropsychological testing is sensitive to brain change. That error was perhaps inspired by the origin story of Western neuropsychology: paper-and-pencil tests without biological validity were promoted as windows into the brain when that infant profession sought respectability and a protected stream of income by controlling certification. Subsequent investigation via test–pathological and test–imaging correlations has demonstrated that conventional tests are neither sensitive to nor specific for traumatic brain change.

Second, in arguing that the "real" cause of persistent dysfunction is "psychological" (often derogated as reflecting "premorbid personality traits"), they perpetuate Cartesian dualism. In essence, they claim that behavioral changes following traumatic brain change are not due to brain change. (It is unclear what other corticated organ might mediate those changes; perhaps the kidney?) As this volume will explain, to debate whether a post-concussive behavior change is "caused" by the concussive blow, versus an emotional reaction to trauma related to a fragile disposition, is to misunderstand the nature of disease. The mechanical effect of a rattling blow is not a disease. The disease is the net effect of a dynamic interaction between that force and all that a concussion survivor ever was or could be. Post-concussive behavior change is entirely mediated by post-concussive neurobiological change.

Thankfully, more than half a century later, with impressive pace and grace, neuropsychology is shaking off its old biases. Today's neuropsychological renaissance has become an indispensable contributor to the enterprise of neuroscience.

As mentioned above, the TBI research community lacks funding for the prospective long-term longitudinal studies that will answer many questions. We do not know the best way to detect and monitor what happens to brains after CBI. However, given the evidence that animals suffer lasting brain and behavioral damage (see Chapter 4), and that persistent abnormal function is readily detected in the brains of many CBI survivors (see Chapters 6, 12, 16, 22) and that even mild TBI victims die young [190], one must be open to the possibility that a concussive blow sets off a long-term neurobiological melee, with deleterious effects in a large proportion of victims.

IV.C.2. Are Cognitive Tests a Good Way to Assess Brain Function?

> Clearly the neuropsychological technique is several steps removed from directly measuring brain function …
> Bigler et al., 2013 ([184], p. 202)

The scientist placed the flea under a bright light. "Jump, flea, jump!" he exhorted. The flea jumped 20 cm. The scientist removed three legs from the flea. "Jump, flea, jump!" The flea jumped 5 cm. The scientist removed the other three legs. "Jump, flea, jump!" The flea was still. "In the flea," reported the scientist, "hearing is mediated by the legs."

Cognitive psychologists have unique abilities. They can quantify many so-called "domains" of behavior, including general knowledge, memory, numeracy, response bias, even sadness and aspects of personality. They do this far better than neurologists, psychiatrists, physiatrists, neurosurgeons, or radiologists. They do this – for the time being – better than any imaging machine. The present author's concern about unwarranted faith in cognitive testing is not a critique of the vital, essential, invaluable contributions of neuropsychologists. It is a comment about the inescapable gap between observations of overt behavior and knowledge of intracranial happenings.

Blood pressure, for instance, is a key physiological function. Among other jobs, it keeps us from falling down. One might measure blood pressure via: (1) a tube in the aorta, (2) a cuff around the arm; (3) feeling the wrist, (4) watching for facial pallor, (5) asking "are you lightheaded?", or (6) observing overt behavior. Has your patient collapsed to the ground, seemingly in a faint, or not? Apart from a direct intravascular measurement, the other methods involve inference. Hearing the patient's response to a query about lightheadedness or observing whether the patient has collapsed to the ground enables inferences about biology from behavior. That is the guiding genius of neuropsychology: inferring brain function from overt behaviors, i.e., quiz taking.

And indeed educated guesswork about happenings in the head based on quizzes can be informative. For more than a hundred years, asking questions and listening for answers was the best way to infer many things about brains. Few would dispute the signal contributions of Broca or Wernicke or Jackson or Harlow. In part this reflects theory of mind: primates have evolved remarkable sensitivity to one another's behaviors and often make good guesses about others' mentations. Although humans are poor lie detectors and highly prone to bias, a neutral observer's reports combined with psychometrically vetted measures often provide helpful insights into what a patient can and cannot do. Over time, largely based on large lesion studies, neuropsychology developed a huge literature demonstrating inconsistent correlations between answers to paper-and-pencil quizzes and the integrity of the brain. In the cases of ablations of a few specific swaths of neocortex, quizzes sometimes provided hints regarding localization. As Rey (1941) [191] described the goals of psychological testing after head trauma:

> The main features of a psychological examination for trauma cases are that it (1) points out existing abnormalities and deficiencies, (2) provides a systematic search for suspected contradictions and inconsistencies, and (3) allows for the differential diagnosis of acquired deficiencies (as a result of the accident) and constitutional deficiencies (existing before the accident) (p. 215).

However, one must be honest about the difference between responses to questions and assays of brain. Figure 5a is the stimulus Rey proposed for the Rey–Osterrieth Complex Figure Test. Figure 5b is an example of an abnormal response. What is wrong with this picture? What troubles this patient? How does that problem impact his or her subjective well-being? Where is the lesion? What is its volume in cubic millimeters? What is its impact on each of the 17 types of neocortical neurons? What is its effect on their axolemmas, and its relationship with microvascular tight junctions, and its reflection of atypical protein folding or clearance, and its interaction with the complement system, and its likelihood of accelerating the onset of dementia by five years? What treatment is most likely to help?

At least three problems limit the accuracy of inference from imperfect scores on cognitive tests. First, wrong responses to tests devised for administration in the odd ecology of an office are inferred to be relevant to day-to-day life. However, virtually no one makes designs with blocks, lists words starting with the letter F, or draws pictures from memory in the course of normal social and occupational functioning. Studies can report statistical *associations* between test scores and naturalistic activities,

Rey–Osterrieth stimulus

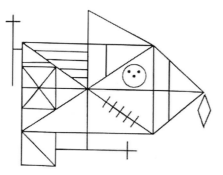

Fig. 5a

Typically, test subjects are first asked to copy this picture free-hand. In the *immediate recall* condition, the subject is asked to draw the same figure from memory. In the *delayed recall* condition, the subject is asked to draw the figure about 20–30 minutes after exposure.

Source: http://editthis.info/psy3242/Rey-Osterrieth_complex_figure. Reproduced with permission from Editions Médicine and Hygiène (Geneva)

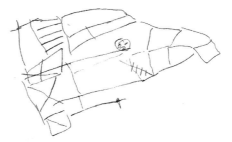

Fig. 5b Example of an abnormal Rey–Osterrieth copy.

Source: Ha et al., 2012 [192] . Reproduced with permission from Dr Sung-Bom Pyun

but these are not tests of vital human functions. Second, as Hughlings Jackson (1875) admonished, the behavior observed after taking out a piece of brain does not tell us what that piece of brain ordinarily does [193]. The *Swiss Watch Fallacy of Behavioral Neurology* is the presumption that each brain part has an identifiable behavioral role. Yet 19th-century inferences from lesion studies (e.g., the dominant inferior posterior frontal gyrus mediates productive language) are routinely exposed as simplistic when functional neuroimaging reveals the multiplicity of regions, nuclei, and circuits that really mediate a given function. Third, when cognitive testers cite putative associations between scores and the integrity of brain parts, they are assuming that all human brains work pretty much the same way. Even identical twins have strikingly different brains. One rarely sees a neuropsychology report in which the inferences have been modified to acknowledge pre-morbid neurobiological variation due to gene-epigene–environment interactions and the uniqueness of every individual's brain-behavior relationships.

Consider a very popular cognitive test: a psychologist names three readily visualizable objects and asks the patient to repeat the names immediately, and again after a delay: "Say 'apple, table, penny." That little cognitive test can potentially be remarkably revealing. Evidence exists that the patient's score is associated with dominant-hemisphere integrity and forgetting even one word may be a sign of dementia. Some evidence suggests that benefiting from cues, or not, adds neuroanatomical specificity. However, imperfect responses on delayed verbal recall can have many causes. If the patient says, "apple, table, ... uhh ... ," one has not measured a specific biological function. That result cannot be decoded to identify a focal nervous system problem. It is not measuring lobar function, regional cerebral metabolism, network connectivity, electrophysiological activity, transmitter release and binding, gene expression, or molecular and submolecular nanosecond-scale events in neuronal compartments. It is not even an observation of physiological change linked to a biological function critical for survival, the way detecting a paling face is reasonably linked to dropping blood pressure. It is perhaps more akin to judging blood pressure by observing whether the patient is upright and chatting

or prone and unresponsive: plausible explanations for the data are protean. Table 4 illustrates this difference. On the left one sees how a behavioral test generates inferences about biology. On the right one sees how a brain test does the same.

Some quiz administrators may debate the implications of Table 4, correctly stating that psychologists also obtain a life history and history of present illness, which could narrow the neuropsychologist's differential diagnosis, or that eight or 18 hours more testing might slightly enhance predictive validity for intracerebral status. Yet would this patient be significantly closer to a tissue diagnosis, prognosis, and treatment plan? Desktop cognitive probes can be tremendously helpful at measuring aspects of behavior that have been assigned to popular constructs such as "working memory" or "executive functions." However, as more fully explained in a forthcoming chapter titled *Concussion and the 21st-Century Renaissance of Neuropsychology* (Chapter 9), results from paper-and-pencil tests cannot reliably localize brain damage, identify the cause, size, or type of a brain lesion, or guide effective medical intervention.

Considered broadly, the concept of neuropsychology has tremendous promise. As scholars continue to investigate how nervous tissue mediates thoughts and emotions, and rigorously test hypothesizes regarding the sensitivity and specificity of given behavioral observations, human suffering should indeed be mitigated. Fortunately, one 20th-century model of neuropsychology – administering desktop tests of unknown validity and guessing about brain function – is rapidly being superseded by a far more sophisticated approach that acknowledges the fallacy of localizationism and embraces the rather thrilling (but still methodologically fraught) prospect of non-invasive imaging of network activity in real time. This slender volume must not be taken as criticizing the discipline, neuropsychology! The editors share both profound respect for the pioneers and wonderment at the pace of discovery since functional imaging has revolutionized behavioral neurology and come closer to cutting the mythic cornerstone of genuine *neuro*psychology: test-brain function correlation.

V. Bias, Temperament, and Conflicts of Interest

The Author's Bias

The author knew a young lady reasonably well. Call her Julienne. She was highly intelligent, personable, independent, fit, French,

Table 4 Behavior testing versus brain testing

	Behavior test	Brain test
Chief complaint	"He talks different"	"He talks different"
Test	Repeat three words after a 120-second delay	Magnetic resonance imaging (MRI) of brain
Results	Speech was somewhat slow. The patient mispronounced one; recalled two out of three	 On T2-weighted coronal MR, an inhomogeneous 4.1 × 3.3-cm mass is visible in the left medial temporal lobe, with many 2–5-mm hyperintense circles around hypointense centers, suggesting luminal areas consistent with feeding arteries and draining veins
Impression	Neuropsychological test report The patient has difficulty repeating three words after a delay. Therefore, he has difficulty with speech or language. Or maybe memory. Or maybe hearing. An ENT consult was requested. No tongue laceration was found. The vocal cords are intact and mobile. There is no evidence of recurrent laryngeal nerve palsy. He does not meet the criteria for spasmodic dysphonia. Audiometry was conducted and ruled out hearing loss in the periphery or the VIIIth-nerve nucleus. Thus, we were able to narrow the problem down to dysfunction somewhere in the brain, perhaps some part of the temporal lobe, or parietal lobe, or frontal lobe, or the white-matter connections between these lobes. Or maybe the cerebellum [184,185] Or maybe the basal ganglia [186]. The dysfunction is either cortical or subcortical – or perhaps both. If it is somewhere in the cerebrum, it is more likely to be on the motor dominant side – unless it's in the cerebellum, in which case it's more likely to be on the non-dominant side. But not always. The lesion is small, medium, or large – that is, if it's a lesion. The underlying problem could be infection, tumor, stroke, or demyelinating disease … or perhaps something else. Or the patient could be feigning. Or this might be conversion. Or this might be due to an attention problem. Intoxication is another possibility Thank you for this interesting consult Addendum Or perhaps he's depressed	Radiology report Probable left medial temporal lobe arteriovenous malformation. Possible left inferior parietal lobe edema. No active hemorrhage. Consider digital subtraction angiography

and (a cheering trait among the habitués of Harvard Square) non-neurotic. She suffered a concussion in a Cambridge bicycle collision. Six months later, her neuropsychological test scores returned to baseline. She was back earning high grades in graduate school, praise at her laboratory job, and the gratitude of the undergraduates she patiently tutored in neurobiology. Three years later, to my surprise, she said, "I'm not right." She described being able to do things, but needing to expend more mental effort. She was able to satisfy the expectations of her mentors and students, but felt sure that, absent her injury, she would have done somewhat more and somewhat better. And her fiancé complained that she had become irritable. The author was finishing his neurology training. Her story did not comport with the model of concussion taught at Harvard Medical School. Distinguished attending neurologists (in fairness, none of whom studied TBI) shrugged. I ran into an old Midwestern mentor at an academy meeting – Joe Foley, a proud and irrepressible Irishman, pioneering scholar, and uncompromising advocate of straight talk. Joe said, "Don't doubt her. I've seen it. Some day we'll understand."

A few years later a book was published titled *Mild Head Injury* [197]. Its concluding chapter was an essay titled "Neurosurgeon as victim" – a candid depiction of neurosurgeon Lawrence F. Marshall's own experience as a CBI patient [198]. He begins, "This 42-year-old moderately coordinated neurosurgeon was in Vail, Colorado." After his skiing-related concussion, he was distractible and forgetful. "These symptoms persisted, but they improved gradually over a period of approximately 18 months." His final self-report: "Function as judged by others remains good, but is not optimal" ([198], p. 277).

These two CBI victims seem to be reporting similar experiences. They got hit. They got better. They went on about their lives uncomplaining and functioning at a high level. Yet they were different. Something was lost. Whatever the brain's astonishing plasticity and self-healing capacities, it never fully recovered.

I cared for TBI patients for decades. I encountered many more people with hard-to-describe, non-disabling but nonetheless disconcerting long-term sequelae of minor head traumas. Thinking back, however, it was Julienne whose "I'm not right" first challenged me to reconsider the received wisdom of the time. Julienne's experience and Dr. Marshall's moving memoir are just anecdotes. They prove nothing. I still do not know why outcomes after CBI are so variable. However, as I have worked on this textbook, as I have pondered the issue of scholarly bias, I must confess that personal contact with such survivors of CBI has influenced my conclusions.

I must also confess to irrational intellectual instincts. Thousands of thoughtful hypotheses are circulating. Many are supported by data. One finds oneself intrigued by a subset of hypotheses that seem to be, for imperfectly justifiable reasons, promising.

Outcomes vary. That is a fact we must address. As of 2018, the present author very tentatively speculates that the astonishing variance in long-term outcomes – demographics, pre-morbid neuropsychiatric status, hydration, hormonal status, litigation status, and impact physics being equal –may be partly conditioned by the individual, collective, and epistatic consequences of – and interdigitating physiological vagaries due to – variations in a suite of four genetically influenced features of the injury response:

(1) stress-related prion-like inter-cellular spread of proneness to make atypically folded proteins and their toxic oligomers;

(2) stress-related immune dysregulation, in part due to damage-associated molecular patterns (DAMPS), triggering both transient activation and lasting priming of microglia, and, in some cases more than others, chronic inflammation;

(3) capacity for clearance of atypically folded or oxidized proteins and inopportune aggregates via *autophagic-* (lysosomal and/or chaperone-), *ubiquitin/proteasomal-*, *extra-cellular protease-*, *circulatory-* (via the blood brain barrier), and *glymphatic-*mediated systems; and

(4) gene-environment-interaction-dependent capacity for post-traumatic plasticity and neurogenesis.

This personal hypothesis is not suggested as a solution to a puzzle, but as an example of the way that neuroscience, having debunked the dogma of typical prompt recovery, *must* divine and test a plausibly dispositive hypothesis explaining the variance. My theory, I would quietly propose, is biologically possible, empirically falsifiable, potentially relevant to drug discovery, and perhaps worthy of discussion.

Anger at Maximizers

Fakers are infuriating. By this, I am not referring to the traumatized person who either semi-consciously exaggerates his symptoms in a bid for help or who unconsciously expresses psychic distress as perception of physical symptoms. I'm referring to the unreconstructed willful liar who feels fine and claims otherwise – most often to gain material resources. That person violates the most sacred principle of the social contract: reciprocal altruism. Unfortunately, cultures that nurture rapacious and unscrupulous trial attorneys are enabling, even encouraging, such egregious behavior. Some data suggest that post-concussive complaints may be significantly less common in less litigious societies (e.g., [199]). Malingerers are an awful drain on the overburdened health care system, and a challenge to one's faith in the innocence of the symptomatic.

Clinicians, perhaps especially in the developed West, periodically meet fakers. The problem is detection. In the case of pain, we must give the patient the benefit of the doubt because no objective measures exist to rebut a claim of "seven out of ten." However, in the case of concussion, one occasionally meets a person whose tale of woe is so absurd, so alien from what little we know about the spectrum of plausible outcomes, as to raise hackles.

"I was minding my own business lying in the gutter when, bam, this lady drove over my head with her baby carriage. The blindness ain't the worst of it, doc. It's the constant flashbacks and the burning earlobes."

Outrage at fakers is probably universal. The threshold for suspicion is not. Doctors fall at different places on an empathy–suspicion scale. Why are some clinicians more likely to empathize with complaints of distress than others? Why are some clinicians more suspicious of malingering than others? This is not intended as a moral lesson. This is merely a summary of some social psychological observations.

Multiple studies report that doctors are more likely to doubt an organic basis for symptoms if (1) the doctor judges that a mismatch exists between claimed disability and the doctor's personal opinion about disability and if (2) the patient creates a lot of work for the clinician [134,135]. Such observations, however, do not identify a psychological difference between clinicians who are more open-minded or more closed-minded to the possibility that the patient's distress is "authentic."

One theme in the study of medical compassion has been robustly supported: those with power are less empathic.

Although humans and other social animals are generally sensitive to one another's distress (e.g., mirror neurons), those with elevated social power are inferior both at detecting and feeling concern about others' suffering. Experiments show that, when confronted with another's distress, persons with more power and money both experience less compassion and exhibit less autonomic reactivity [200,201]. Theories to account for this difference include: (1) a predisposition to positive emotions among the powerful; (2) inattention to the less powerful; and (3) low motivation for empathy because the powerful have little motivation to affiliate with the weak [202–206]. Yet power ownership is an inadequate explanation for differences on the empathy–suspicion scale. In the West, and in many other parts of the world, most doctors have power. They tend to be economically and socially advantaged. What, then, might account for variations in response to patients with persistent symptoms after concussion?

Princeton historian of medicine Keith Wailoo, in his 2014 book *Pain: A Political History* [207], reviews the escalating tension between progressives and conservatives in regard to trusting patients' complaints. The 1960s in the West could be characterized as an era of enlightening interest in human distress, with the rise of an understanding that pain is something real, terrible, and compensable. The 1980s could be characterized as an era of backlash, as conservatives urged crackdowns on the disability culture. More broadly speaking, the author's research reveals systematic bias. Progressives are more likely to accept and empathize with medical complaints of distress. Conservatives are more likely to suspect fraud, ulterior motives, entitlement, and seeking of welfare. The roots of this difference have been attributed to a different valuation of moral rules. Progressives tend to judge what is right based on assessments of fairness, avoidance of doing harm, and care for others. Conservatives share these values. Yet they tend to place more emphasis on ingroup loyalty, respect for authority, and defense of purity [208,209].

These observations are confirmed by psychological research. In studies of personality and morality, conservatives shine in conscientiousness and politeness. However, they resist change, justify inequity, promote authoritarianism, and their moral traditionalism is negatively associated with openness, intellect and compassion (e.g., [210]). A recent survey reports a phenomenon that is conceivably related: in 2014 a RAND Corporation survey found that adults with less education and those who voted for the Republican (conservative) candidate in the 2012 election were approximately twice as comfortable with their sons playing football as adults who were highly educated or who voted for the Democratic (progressive) candidate [211]. One must resist the temptation to generalize from these data. It is surely premature, simplistic, and impolitic to suggest that denial of the possibility of lasting harm from concussion is the special provenance of those with low intellect, low education, and conservatism. At the same time, it would be naïve to ignore social psychological factors that bias belief in cases of scientific uncertainty. In the interest of better understanding barriers to prevention of injury, it may be valuable to consider how attitudes of clinicians, parents, employers, coaches, and

team owners influence both the risk of exposure to CBI and the openness to considering that exposure risky.

Thus, based on the preliminary evidence, I tentatively propose the hypothesis that one factor distinguishing doctors who are open-minded about the authenticity of complaints of lasting distress caused by concussion from those whose are suspicious – or distinguishing doctors who open-mindedly consider the possibility of CBI causing long-term neurobehavioral dysfunction from those who have foreclosed consideration (having decided that such symptoms are psychosomatic) – may be the social psychological dimensions of progressiveness/empathy versus conservatism/authoritarianism. I fully acknowledge that only careful empirical work can test that hypothesis.

Tolerance of Minimizers

Just as unscrupulous lawyers promote the exaggeration of symptoms after head injury, athletes who need to prove their invulnerability and the unscrupulous hangers-on who benefit from denying the athlete's injury facilitate minimization. The Public Broadcasting Service documentary *League of Denial* [212] and the Alexandrian library of written evidence that the producers of that documentary made public strongly suggests that the NFL spent one or more decades willfully suppressing dissemination of evidence that concussions sometimes cause lasting neurological harm. Multiple studies have detected unwillingness of athletes to confess to having experienced concussion or being troubled by lasting symptoms. This makes it difficult to interpret efforts to measure the impact of past concussions on present mental status.

For example, a paper published in 2014 bears the title "Relationship between concussion history and neurocognitive test performance in National Football League draft picks" [213] The subjects were not exactly draft picks. They were potential drafts picks trying to get picked. Subjects were selected as follows:

> Every year in March, approximately 330 potential NFL draft picks are invited to an annual Scouting Combine in Indianapolis, operated by the National Invitational Camp. In attendance are NFL player personnel specialists, coaches, and team medical staff. The athletes are assessed across medical, behavioral, radiographic, and cognitive domains.
> ([213], p. 935).

In other words, young men who have probably spent at least a decade hoping and dreaming to be picked by the NFL are assembled and asked, "Are you healthy or not? How many concussions have you suffered so far?" Just 3.7% reported having had two concussions; 1.4% admitted to having suffered three or more concussions. The 219 subjects in the final sample underwent two neuropsychological test batteries. The authors report, "Concussion history had no relationship to neurocognitive performance on either the Wonderlic or ImPACT" (p. 934).

Consider the research design. Young men who surely perceive being picked by the NFL as a catapult to success, happiness, and unimaginable wealth are asked to admit how unhealthy they are. Could there exist on Earth a cohort more strongly disincentivized to acknowledge a history of head injuries? This manuscript may be the poster child for neglecting to control for conflicts of interest. One could equally perform the converse study and arrive at a different conclusion by telling a bunch of unemployed 22-year-olds: "If you admit to having experienced multiple concussions, you are likely to get $10 million. If you deny having experienced multiple concussions, you will probably get zero." Pride, perceived invulnerability, and secondary gain are weighty influences. So long as athletes are feted, admired, and enriched on the basis of their alleged excellent health, it will be unreasonable to expect candor.

Many stakeholders profit from propelling young people into contact sports. Parents, coaches, trainers, college administrators, team owners, and team physicians each face the temptation to avert their gaze from the evidence of risk. They cavalierly embrace the phrase "return to play" when the accurate descriptor is "return to risk." Many stakeholders profit from dismissing complaints of lasting distress. Defense attorneys, defense experts, insurers, employers, and others have a clear interest in minimizing the risk of lasting harm. Of course, plaintiffs, personal injury attorneys, plaintiff's experts, and so forth have the opposite incentives. The U.S. tort system notoriously promotes adversarial advocacy of medically opposite conclusions. Despite the obvious drawbacks of this system, one hardly expects prompt reform such that experts serve only the court and profit only by impartiality.

In short, human nature will always be a factor in beliefs about concussion. Those of different temperaments and worldviews, those with different incentives and stakes, are likely to differ in regard to those beliefs. The present author will not claim immunity. The best one can hope for is a ferocious commitment to transparency, and steadfast open-mindedness to the supremacy of science over intuition.

The division remains. As Kay et al., put it:

> "Believers" and "nonbelievers" in the possible presence of brain damage in persons who become severely functionally disabled after minor head injuries usually mean different things by postconcussion syndrome. Believers suggest that subtle but permanent brain damage can be present and drive the symptoms in postconcussion syndrome; nonbelievers deny the presence of brain injury and emphasize the neurotic or stress-related aspects of symptomatology in postconcussion syndrome. The tendency for these points of view to polarize professionals has contributed to false dichotomies, usually framed as the false question, Is this functional disability the result of emotional factors or actual brain damage?
>
> ([214], p. 372)

Believers in the possibility of lasting cerebral harm must admit that normalization of desktop test results naturally raises doubt about such harm. Non-believers must be open to considering such findings as those of McMahon et al. (2014) [215]: Among 375 mTBI patients prospectively followed for a year:

> At both 6 and 12 months after mTBI, 82% … reported at least one PCS [post-concussive symptom] symptom. Further, 44.5 and 40.3% of patients had significantly

reduced Satisfaction With Life scores at 6 and 12 months, respectively … 22.4% of the mTBI subjects available for follow-up were still below full functional status at 1 year after injury. The term "mild" continues to be a misnomer for this patient population".

([215], p. 26)

For all the humble caveats that science must confess, the present author takes a single granite stand: the 20th century paradigm of "concussion" is dead. CBIs are never the same as one another and are frequently life changing. He commences this brief collaborative essay with three empirical conclusions our text will prove worthy of happy consensus:

1. Clinically syndromic? Nonsense!
2. Biologically transient? Nonsense!
3. Biographically trivial? Nonsense!

But the consensus that supersedes all others should be this: we do not know enough. We must know more.

Commencement

This introduction, like college, merely acquaints one with the mysteries. On commencement day we go to work to overcome our fledgling limits and mitigate our ignorance. Since the NIH declines to fund the necessary research, it is unclear how quickly progress will be made toward a more definitive and widely accepted understanding of CBI. Yet momentum is gathering. We hope the little book you are holding is a small step in the forward march.

References

1. Zhang K, Johnson, B, Pennell D, Ray W, Sebastianelli W, Slobounov S. Are functional deficits in concussed individuals consistent with white matter structural alterations: Combined FMRI and DTI study. *Exp Brain Res* 2010;20:57–70.

2. Lidvall HF, Linderoth B, Norlin B. Causes of the post-concussional syndrome. *Acta Neurol Scand Suppl* 1974;56:3–144.

3. Barnes DE, Kaup A, Kirby KA, Byers, AL, Diaz-Arrastia R, Yaffe K. Traumatic brain injury and risk of dementia in older veterans. *Neurology* 2014;83:312–319.

4. National Institute of Health. National Institute of Neurological Disorders and Stroke. *Report on the brain trauma-related neurodegeneration: Strategies to define, detect, and predict workshop.* July 22–23, 2013. Available at www.ninds.nih.gov/news_and_events/proceedings/TBI-related_neurodegeneration_workshop_report.htm.

5. Walker AE, Caveness WF, Critchley M, editors. *Late effects of head injury.* Springfield, IL: Charles C. Thomas, 1969.

6. Teuber H-L. Neglected aspects of the posttraumatic syndrome. In Walker AE, Caveness WF, Critchley M, editors. *Late effects of head injury.* Springfield, IL: Charles C. Thomas, 1969, pp. 13–34.

7. Koch W, Filehne W. Beiträge zur experimentellen Chirurgie. Über die Commotio cerebri. *Arch Klin Chir* 1874;17:190–231.

8. Osnato M, Giliberti V. Postconcussion neurosis-traumatic encephalitis: A conception of postconcussion phenomena. *Arch Neurol Psychiatr* 1927;18:181–214.

9. Martland HS. Punch drunk. *JAMA* 1928;91:1103–1107.

10. Courville CB. *Commotio cerebri: Cerebral concussion and the postconcussion syndrome in their medical and legal aspect.* Los Angeles: San Lucas Press, 1953.

11. European Commission. *The international initiative for traumatic brain injury research* (InTBIR). 2014. Available at http://ec.europa.eu/research/health/medical-research/brain-research/international-initiative_en.html.

12. The changing landscape of traumatic brain injury research. *Lancet Neurol* 2012;8:651.

13. Kazakoff L. NFL player's suicide opens discussion on traumatic brain injury. 2011. Available at http://blog.sfgate.com/opinionshop/2011/03/24/nfl-players-suicide-opens-discussion-on-traumatic-brain-injury/.

14. The Lasker Legacy. Lasker Foundation, 2014. Available at www.laskerfoundation.org/about/legacy.htm.

15. National Institute of Health. Estimates of funding for various research, condition, and disease categories (RCDC) March 7, 2017. Available at www.report.nih.gov/categorical_spending.aspx.

16. Zitnay GA. Lessons from national and international TBI societies and funds like NBIRTT. *Acta Neurochir* 2005;[Suppl]93:131–133.

17. Centers for Disease Control and Prevention. CDC estimates of traumatic brain injury-related disability. *Traumatic brain injury in the United States: A report to Congress 2014.* Available at www.cdc.gov/NCIPC/pub-res/tbi_congress/04_estimates_goals.htm.

18. Zaloshnja E, Miller T, Langlois JA, Selassie AW. Prevalence of long-term disability from traumatic brain injury in the civilian population of the United States, 2005. *J Head Trauma Rehab* 2008;21:394–400.

19. The CDC, NIH, DoD, and VA Leadership Panel. *Report to Congress on traumatic brain injury in the United States: Understanding the public health problem among current and former military personnel.* Centers for Disease Control and Prevention (CDC), the National Institutes of Health (NIH), the Department of Defense (DoD), and the Department of Veterans Affairs (VA). 2013.

20. Centers for Disease Control and Prevention. *Diagnoses of HIV infection in the United States and dependent areas,* 2011. HIV surveillance report, volume 23. Available at www.cdc.gov/hiv/library/reports/surveillance/2011/surveillance_Report_vol_23.html.

21. O'Brien KK, Solomon P, Bayoumi AM. Measuring disability experienced by adults living with HIV: Assessing construct validity of the HIV Disability Questionnaire using confirmatory factor analysis. *BMJ Open* 2014;4:e005456.

22. Gillum LA, Gouveia C, Dorsey ER, Pletcher M, Mathers CD, McCulloch CE, Johnston SC. NIH disease funding levels and burden of disease. *PLoS One* 2011;6:e16837.

23. Centers for Disease Control and Prevention. Injury prevention and control: Traumatic brain injury. Severe traumatic brain injury. 2014. Available at www.cdc.gov/TraumaticBrainInjury/severe.html.

24. Raymont V, Salazar AM, Krueger F, Grafman J. "Studying injured minds": The Vietnam head injury study and 40 years of brain injury research. *Front Neurol* 2011;2:1–13.

25. U.S. Interagency Head Injury Task Force. *Interagency head injury task force report.* Bethesda, MD: National Institute of Neurological and Communicative Disorders and Stroke, National Institutes of Health, 1989.

26. Defense Centers of Excellence for Psychological Health and Traumatic Brain Injury (DCoE). Defense and Veterans Brain Injury Center, 2012. Available at www.dcoe.mil/content/Navigation/Documents/About%20DVBIC.pdf.

27. Public Law 104–166. 104th Congress. An act to amend the Public Health Service Act to provide for the conduct of expanded studies and the establishment of innovative programs with respect to traumatic brain injury, and for other purposes. Available at www.gpo.gov/fdsys/pkg/PLAW-104publ166/html/PLAW-104publ166.htm.

28. Centers for Disease Control and Prevention, National Center for Injury Prevention and Control. *Traumatic brain injury in the United States: A report to Congress.* Atlanta, GA: Division of Acute Care, Rehabilitation Research, and Disability Prevention; National Center for Injury Prevention and Control; Centers for Disease Control and Prevention, 1999.

29. Public Law 106–310. 106th Congress. An act to amend the Public Health Service Act with respect to children's health. Available at www.gpo.gov/fdsys/pkg/PLAW-106publ310/content-detail.html.

30. Grinnon T, Grinnon ST, Miller K, Marler JR, Lu Y, Stout A, Odenkirchen J et al. NINDS Common Data Element project – approach and methods. *Clin Trials* 2012;9:322–329.

31. National Institute of Neurological Disorders and Stroke (NINDS). Mission statement. Available at http://nindscommondataelements.wordpress.com/mission-statement/.

32. National Center for Injury Prevention and Control. *Report to Congress on mild traumatic brain injury in the United States: Steps to prevent a serious public health problem.* Atlanta, GA: Centers for Disease Control and Prevention, 2003.

33. International Mission on Prognosis Analysis of Clinical Trials in Traumatic Brain Injury (IMPACT) 2014. Available at www.tbi-impact.org/?p=home/news.

34. Maas AIR, Menon DK. Traumatic brain injury: Rethinking ideas and approaches. *Lancet Neurol* 2012;11:12–13.

35. Knuth T, Letarte PB, Ling G, Moores LE, Rhee P, Tauber D, Trask A. *Guidelines for field management of combat-related head trauma.* New York: Brain Trauma Foundation, 2005.

36. Defense Centers of Excellence for Psychological Health and Traumatic Brain Injury (DCoE). 2014. Available at www.dcoe.mil/.

37. Public Law 110–206 110th Congress. An Act to provide for the expansion and improvement of traumatic brain injury programs.

38. Management of Concussion/mTBI Working Group. VA/DoD clinical practice guideline for management of concussion/mild traumatic brain injury. *J Rehabil Res Dev* 2009;46:CP1–68.

39. Carlson K, Kehle S, Meis L, Greer N, MacDonald R, Rutks I. The assessment and treatment of individuals with history of traumatic brain injury and post-traumatic stress disorder: A systematic review of the evidence, 2009. Available at www.hsrd.research.va.gov/publications/esp/tbiptsd.cfm.

40. Underwood E. NFL kicks off brain-injury research effort. *Science* 2013;339:1367.

41. Wamsley L. NFL, NIH end partnership for concussion research with $16m unspent. National Public Radio July 29th, 2017. Available at: www.npr.org/sections/thetwo-way/2017/07/29/540238260/nfl-ends-partnership-with-nih-for-concussion-research-with-16m-unspent.

42. Peliserro T. NFL says it will commit $100 million in concussion initiative. *USA Today* September 14, 2016. Available at: www.usatoday.com/story/sports/nfl/2016/09/14/nfl-player-safety-concussions/90346224/.

43. Jones M. NFL commits another $16.43 million for concussion research. USA Today. January 5, 2018. Available at: www.usatoday.com/story/sports/nfl/2018/01/05/nfl-commits-another-16-43-million-concussion-research/10074 05001/.

44. Brain Research through Advancing Innovative Neurotechnologies (BRAIN) Working Group Report to the Advisory Committee to the Director, NIH. Brain 2025: A scientific vision. June 5, 2014. Available at www.braininitiative.nih.gov/pdf/BRAIN2025_508C.pdf.

45. Fernagut PO, Chesselet MF. Alpha-synuclein and transgenic mouse models. *Neurobiol Dis* 2004;17:123–130.

46. Götz J, Deters N, Doldissen A, Bokhari L, Ke Y, Wiesner A, et al. A decade of tau transgenic animal models and beyond. *Brain Pathol* 2007;17:91–103.

47. Brion JP, Ando K, Heraud C, Leroy K. Modulation of tau pathology in tau transgenic models. *Biochem Soc Trans* 2010;38: 996–1000.

48. Crews L, Rockenstein E, Masliah E. APP transgenic modeling of Alzheimer's disease: Mechanisms of neurodegeneration and aberrant neurogenesis. *Brain Struct Funct* 2010;214:111–126.

49. Magen I, Chesselet MF. Mouse models of cognitive deficits due to alpha-synuclein pathology. *J Parkinsons Dis* 2011;1:217–227.

50. Lalonde R, Fukuchi K, Strazielle C. APP transgenic mice for modelling behavioural and psychological symptoms of dementia (BPSD). *Neurosci Biobehav Rev* 2012;36:1357–1375.

51. Lalonde R, Fukuchi K, Strazielle C. Neurologic and motor dysfunctions in APP transgenic mice. *Rev Neurosci* 2012;23:363–379.

52. Youmans KL, Tai LM, Nwabuisi-Heath E, Jungbauer L, Kanekiyo T, Gan M, et al. Model of Alzheimer disease: APOE4-specific changes in Aβ accumulation in a new transgenic mouse model of Alzheimer disease. Accumulation in a new transgenic mouse APOE4-specific changes in Ab. *J Biol Chem* 2012;287:41774–41786.

53. Nakagawa Y, Nakamura M, McIntosh TK, Rodriguez A, Berlin JA, Smith DH, et al. Traumatic brain injury in young, amyloid-beta peptide overexpressing transgenic mice induces marked ipsilateral hippocampal atrophy and diminished Abeta deposition during aging. *J Comp Neurol* 1999;411:390–398.

54. Tran HT, Sanchez L, Brody DL. Inhibition of JNK by a peptide inhibitor reduces traumatic brain injury-induced tauopathy in transgenic mice. *J Neuropathol Exp Neurol* 2012;71:116–129.

55. Tajiri N, Kellogg SL, Shimizu T, Arendash GW, Borlongan CV. Traumatic brain injury precipitates cognitive impairment and extracellular Aβ aggregation in Alzheimer's disease transgenic mice. *PLoS One* 2013;8:e78851.

56. Pineda JA, Lewis SB, Valadka AB, Papa L, Hannay HJ, Heaton SC, et al. Clinical significance of αII-Spectrin breakdown products in cerebrospinal fluid after severe traumatic brain injury. *J Neurotrauma* 2007;24:354–366.

57. Manley GT, Diaz-Arrastia R, Brophy M, Engel D, Goodman C, Gwinn, K, et al. Common data elements for traumatic brain injury: Recommendations from the Biospecimens and Biomarkers Working Group. *Arch Phys Med Rehabil* 2010;91: 1667–1672.

58. Kobeissy FH, Guingab-Cagmat JD, Razafsha M, O'Steen L, Zhang Z, Hayes RL et al. Leveraging biomarker platforms and systems biology for rehabilomics and biologics effectiveness research. *PM&R* 2011;3:S139–S147.

59. Berger RP, Beers SR, Papa L, Bell M. Common data elements for pediatric traumatic brain injury: Recommendations from the biospecimens and biomarkers workgroup. *J Neurotrauma* 2010;29:672–677.

60. Crawford F, Crynen G, Reed J, Mouzon B, Bishop A, Katz B, et al. Identification of plasma biomarkers of tbi outcome using proteomic approaches in an APOE mouse model. *J Neurotrauma* 2012;29:246–260.

61. Zurek J, Fedora M. The usefulness of S100B, NSE, GFAP, NF-H, secretagogin and Hsp70 as a predictive biomarker of outcome in children with traumatic brain injury. *Acta Neurochir* 2012;154:93–103.

62. Guingab-Cagmat JD, Cagmat EB, Hayes EB, Anagli J. Integration of proteomics, bioinformatics, and systems biology in traumatic brain injury biomarker discovery. *Front Neurol* 2013;12:1–12.

63. U.S. Food and Drug Administration. FDA authorizes marketing of first blood test to aid in the evaluation of concussion in adults. July 14, 2018. Available at: www.fda.gov/NewsEvents/Newsroom/PressAnnouncements/ucm596531.htm.

64. Framingham Heart Study. 2014. Available at www.framinghamheartstudy.org/.

65. Broglio SP, McCrea M, McAllister T, Harezlak J, Katz B, Hack D, et al. A national study on the effects of concussion in collegiate athletes and US Military Service Academy members: The NCAA–DoD Concussion Assessment, Research and Education (CARE) Consortium structure and methods. *Sports Med* 2017;47:1437–1451.

66. Track-TBI. Transforming Research and Clinical Knowledge in Traumatic Brain Injury. International Traumatic Brain Injury Research Initiative. Available at https://tracktbi.ucsf.edu/.

67. Walker WC, Carne W, Franke LM, Nolen T, Dikmen SD, Cifu DX, et al. The Chronic Effects of Neurotrauma Consortium (CENC) multi-centre observational study: Description of study and characteristics of early participants. *Brain Injury* 2016;30:1469–1480.

68. Kelman S. The social nature of the definition problem in health. *Int J Health Serv* 1975;5:625–642.

69. Merskey H. Variable meanings for the definition of disease. *J Med Philos* 1986;11:215–232.

70. Brown P. Naming and framing: The social construction of diagnosis and illness. *J Health Soc Behav* 1995;Extra Issue:34–52.

71. Nordby H. The analytic–synthetic distinction and conceptual analyses of basic health concepts. *Med Health Care Philos* 2006;9:169–180.

72. Ereshefsky M. Defining 'health' and 'disease.' *Stud Histor Philos Biol Biomed Sci* 2009;40:221–227.

73. Freud S. The aetiology of hysteria. In *The standard edition of the complete psychological works of Sigmund Freud,* volume III (1893–1899): *Early psycho-analytic publications.* London: Hogarth Press, 1962, pp. 187–221.

74. American Psychiatric Association. *Diagnostic and statistical manual of mental disorders, fourth edition (DSM-IV).* Washington, DC: American Psychiatric Press, 2000, pp. 492, 498.

75. American Psychiatric Association. *Diagnostic and statistical manual of mental disorders, fifth edition (DSM-5).* Washington, DC: American Psychiatric Press, 2013.

76. Cannon WB. *Bodily changes in pain, hunger, fear and rage: An account of recent researches into the function of emotional excitement.* New York: D. Appleton, 1915.

77. Selye H. *Stress in health and disease.* Boston: Butterworths, 1976.

78. von Richthofen S, Lang UE, Hellweg R. Effects of different kinds of acute stress on nerve growth factor content in rat brain. *Brain Res* 2003;987:207–213.

79. Garcia-Bueno B, Madrigal JL, Lizasoain I, Moro MA, Lorenzo P, Leza JC. The anti-inflammatory prostaglandin 15d-PGJ2 decreases oxidative/nitrosative mediators in brain after acute stress in rats. *Psychopharmacol* 2005;180:513–522.

80. Shi SS, Shao SH, Yuan BP, Pan F, Li ZL. Acute stress and chronic stress change brain-derived neurotrophic factor (BDNF) and tyrosine kinase-coupled receptor (TrkB) expression in both young and aged rat hippocampus. *Yonsei Med J* 2010;51:661–671.

81. Sugama S, Takenouchi T, Sekiyama K, Kitani H, Hashimoto M. Immunological responses of astroglia in the rat brain under acute stress: Interleukin 1 beta co-localized in astroglia. *Neurosci* 2011;192:429–437.

82. Chen L, Lui S, Wu QZ, Zhang W, Zhou D, Chen HF, et al. Impact of acute stress on human brain microstructure: An MR diffusion study of earthquake survivors. *Hum Brain Map* 2013;34:367–373.

83. Norris JN, Sams R, Lundblad P, Frantz E, Harris E. Blast-related mild traumatic brain injury in the acute phase: Acute stress reactions partially mediate the relationship between loss of consciousness and symptoms. *Brain Inj* 2014;28:1052–1062.

84. Kutsuna N, Yamashita A, Eriguchi T, Oshima H, Suma T, Sakatani K, et al. Acute stress exposure preceding transient global brain ischemia exacerbates the decrease in cortical remodeling potential in the rat retrosplenial cortex. *Neurosci Res* 2014;78:65–71.

85. Giza CC, Hovda DA. The neurometabolic cascade of concussion. *J Athl Training* 2001;36:228–235.

86. Shaw NA. The neurophysiology of concussion. *Progr Neurobiol* 2002;67:281–344.

87. De Fazio M, Rammo R, O'Phelan K, Ross Bullock MR. Alterations in cerebral oxidative metabolism following traumatic brain injury. *Neurocrit Care* 2011;14:91–96.

88. Kiraly MA, Kiraly SJ. Traumatic brain injury and delayed sequelae: A review – traumatic brain injury and mild traumatic brain injury (concussion) are precursors to later-onset brain disorders, including early-onset dementia. *Sci World J* 2007;7:1768–1776.

89. Smith, DH, Johnson VE, Stewart W. Chronic neuropathologies of single and repetitive TBI: Substrates of dementia? *Nat Rev Neurol* 2013;9:211–221.

90. Victoroff J. Traumatic encephalopathy: Review and provisional research diagnostic criteria. *NeuroRehabil* 2013;32:211–224.

91. Sapolsky RM. Why stress is bad for your brain. *Science* 1996;273:749–750.

92. Radley JJ, Sisti HM, Hao J, Rocher AB, McCall T, Hof PR, et al. Chronic behavioral stress induces apical dendritic reorganization in pyramidal neurons of the medial prefrontal cortex. *Neurosci* 2004;125:1–6.

93. Bremner JD. Stress and brain atrophy. *CNS Neurol Disord Drug Targets* 2006;5:503–512.

94. Frodl TS, Koutsouleris N, Bottlender R, Born C, Jäger M, Scupin I, et al. Depression-related variation in brain morphology over 3 years: Effects of stress? *Arch Gen Psychiatry* 2008;65:1156–1165.

95. Hedges DW, Thatcher GW, Bennett PJ, Sood S, Paulson D, Creem-Regehr S, et al. Brain integrity and cerebral atrophy in Vietnam combat veterans with and without posttraumatic stress disorder. *Neurocase* 2007;13:402–410.

96. Lee KW, Kim JB, Seo JS, Kim TK, Im JY, Baek IS, et al. Behavioral stress accelerates plaque pathogenesis in the brain of Tg2576 mice via generation of metabolic oxidative stress. *J Neurochem* 2009;108:165–175.

97. Tavanti M, Battaglini M, Borgogni F, Bossini L, Calossi S, Marino D, et al. Evidence of diffuse damage in frontal and occipital cortex in the brain of patients with post-traumatic stress disorder. *Neurol Sci* 2012;33:59–68.

98. Cardenas VA, Samuelson K, Lenoci M, Studholme C, Neylan TC, Marmar CR, et al. Changes in brain anatomy during the course of posttraumatic stress disorder. *Psychiatry Res* 2011;193:93–100.

99. Shucard JL, Cox J, Shucard DW, Fetter H, Chung C, Ramasamy D, et al. Symptoms of posttraumatic stress disorder and exposure to traumatic stressors are related to brain structural volumes and behavioral measures of affective stimulus processing in police officers. *Psychiatry Res* 2012;204:25–31.

100. Ohira H, Matsunaga M, Isowa T, Nomura M, Ichikawa N, Kimura K, et al. Polymorphism of the serotonin transporter gene modulates brain and physiological responses to acute stress in Japanese men. *Stress* 2009;12:533–543.

101. McAllister TW. Genetic factors modulating outcome after neurotrauma. *PM&R* 2010;2 (Suppl 2):S241–S252.

102. Weaver SM, Chau A, Portelli JN, Grafman J. Genetic polymorphisms influence recovery from traumatic brain injury. *Neuroscientist* 2012;18:631–644.

103. Graham DP, Helmer DA, Harding MJ, Kosten TR, Petersen NJ, Nielsen DA. Serotonin transporter genotype and mild traumatic brain injury independently influence resilience and perception of limitations in veterans. *J Psychiatr Res* 2013; 4: 835–842.

104. Smyth K, Sandhu SS, Crawford S, Dewey D, Parboosingh J, Barlow KM. The role of serotonin receptor alleles and environmental stressors in the development of post-concussive symptoms after pediatric mild traumatic brain injury. *Dev Med Child Neurol* 2014;56:73–77.

105. Gould R, Miller B, Goldberg MA, Benson DF. The validity of hysterical signs and symptoms. *J Nerv Mental Dis* 1986; 174: 593–597.

106. Black DN, Seritan AL, Taber KH, Hurley RA. Conversion hysteria: Lessons from functional imaging. *J Neuropsychiatr Clin Neurosci* 2004;16:245–251.

107. Vuilleumier P. Hysterical conversion and brain function. In Laureys S, editor. *Progress in Brain Research* 2005;150:309–329.

108. Aybek S, Kanaan RA, David AS. The neuropsychiatry of conversion disorder. *Curr Opin Psychiatry* 2008;21:275–280.

109. Voon V, Gallea C, Hattori N, Bruno M, Ekanayake V, Hallett M. The involuntary nature of conversion disorder. *Neurology* 2010;74:223–228.

110. Bryant RA. The neural circuitry of conversion disorder and its recovery. *J Abn Psychol* 2012;121:289–296.

111. Carson AJ, Brown R, David AS, Duncan R, Edwards MJ, Goldstein LH, et al. On behalf of UK-FNS. Functional (conversion) neurological symptoms: Research since the millennium. *J Neurol Neurosurg Psychiatry* 2012;83:842–850.

112. Sierra M, Berrios GE. Towards a neuropsychiatry of conversive hysteria. *Cogn Neuropsychiatry* 1999;4:267–287.

113. Charcot JM. *Oeuvres complètes*, volume 1. Paris: Bureaux du Progrès Médical, 1872. [In English: Charcot JM. *Lectures on diseases of the nervous system*. Sigerson G, trans. London: New Sydenham Society, 1877.]

114. Lazare A. Conversion symptoms. *NEJM* 1981 305:745–748.

115. Goetz CG. J-M Charcot and simulated neurologic disease. *Neurology* 2007;69:103–109.

116. Nicholson TRJ, Stone J, Kanaan RAA. Conversion disorder: A problematic diagnosis. *Neurol Neurosurg Psychiatry* 2011;82:1267–1273.

117. Lipman FD. Malingering in personal injury cases. *Temple Law Q* 1962;35:141–162.

118. Travin S, Potter B. Malingering and malingering-like behavior. Some clinical and conceptual issues. *Psychiatr Quart* 1984;56:189–197.

119. Rogers R. *Clinical assessment of malingering and deception*. New York: Guilford Press, 1988.

120. Nies KJ, Sweet JJ. Neuropsychological assessment and malingering: A critical review of past and present strategies. *Arch Clin Neuropsychol* 1994;9:501–552.

121. Eisendrath SJ. Factitious illness: A clarification. *Psychosomatics* 1984;25:110–117.

122. Eisendrath SJ. Factitious disorders in civil litigation: Twenty cases illustrating the spectrum of abnormal illness-affirming behavior. *J Am Acad Psychiatry Law* 2002;30:391–399.

123. Pilowsky I. A general classification of abnormal illness behaviours. *Br J Med Psychol* 1978;51:131–137.

124. Trimble MR. Pseudoseizures. *Neurologic Clin* 1986;4:53–548.

125. Devinsky O, Gordon E. Epileptic seizures progressing into nonepileptic conversion seizures. *Neurology* 1998;51:1293–1296.

126. Andrade C, Singh NM, Bhakta SG. Simultaneous true seizures and pseudoseizures. *J Cin Psychiatry* 2006:674:673.

127. Deibler MW, Hacker C, Rough J, Darby J, Lamdan RM. Ganser's syndrome in a man with AIDS. *Psychosomatics* 2003;44:342–345.

128. Dwyer J, Reid S. Ganser's syndrome. *Lancet* 2004;364:471–473.

129. Bowers KS. On being unconsciously influenced and informed. In Bowers KS, Meichenbaum D, editors. *The unconscious reconsidered*. New York: John Wiley, 1994.

130. Hilgard ER. *Divided consciousness: Multiple controls in human thought and action*. New York: John Wiley, 1986.

131. Lynn SJ, Rhue JW, Weekes JR. Hypnotic involuntariness: A social cognitive analysis. *Psychol Rev* 1990; 97: 169–184.

132. Spanos NP, deGros M. Structure of communication and reports of involuntariness by hypnotic and nonhypnotic subjects. *Percept Motor Skills* 1983;57:1179–1186.

133. Jonas JM, Pope, Jr. HG. The dissimulating disorders: A single diagnostic entity? *Compr Psychiatr* 1985;26:58–62.

134. Kanaan RAA, Wessely SC. Factitious disorders in neurology: An analysis of reported cases. *Psychosomatics* 2010;51:47–54.

135. Friedman JH. What do neurologists think about conversion disorder? *Nat Rev Neurol* 2011;7:306–307.

136. Carroll LJ, Cassidy JD, Peloso PM, Borg J, von Holst H, Holm L, et al. Prognosis for mild traumatic brain injury: Results of the WHO Collaborating Centre Task Force on mild traumatic brain injury. *J Rehabil Med* 2004; Suppl. 43:84–105.

137. Bijur PE, Haslum M, Golding J. Cognitive and behavioral sequelae of mild head injury in children. *Pediatrics* 1990;86:337–344.

138. Bijur PE, Haslum M, Golding J. Cognitive outcomes of multiple mild head injuries in children. *J Dev Behav Pediatr* 1996;17:143–148.

139. Wrightson P, McGinn V, Gronwall D. Mild head injury in preschool children: Evidence that it can be associated with a persisting cognitive defect. *J Neurol Neurosurg Psychiatry* 1995;59:375–380.

140. Farmer MY, Singer HS, Mellits ED, Hall D, Charney E. Neurobehavioral sequelae of minor head injuries in children. *Pediatr Neurosci* 1987;13:304–308.

141. Ponsford J, Willmott C, Rothwell A, Cameron P, Ayton G, Nelms R, et al. Cognitive and behavioral outcome following mild traumatic head injury in children. *J Head Trauma Rehabil* 1999;14:360–372.

142. Greenspan AI, MacKenzie EJ. Functional outcome after pediatric head injury. *Pediatrics* 1994;94:425–432.

143. Graves DE, Cassidy JD, editors. Results of the International Collaboration on Mild traumatic brain injury Prognosis (ICoMP). *Arch Phys Med Rehabil* 2014;95(3, Suppl):A1–A6, S95–S302.

144. Michaelsen LK, Watson WE, Black RH. A realistic test of individual versus group consensus decision making. *J Appl Psychol* 1989;74:834–839.

145. Davis JH, Kameda T, Parks C, Stasson M, Zimmerman S. Some social mechanics of group decision making: The distribution of opinion, polling sequence, and implications for consensus. *J Personal Soc Psychol* 1989; 57:1000–1012.

146. National Institutes of Health. Retirement of the National Institutes of Health Consensus Development Program 2014. Available at http://consensus.nih.gov/.

147. Rennie D. Consensus statements. *NEJM* 1981;304:665–666.

148. Sager KL, Gastil J. The origins and consequences of consensus decision making: A test of the social consensus model. *Southern Commun J* 2006;71:1–24.

149. Kameda T. Procedural influence in consensus information: Evaluating group decision making from a social choice perspective. In Witte EH, Davis JH, editors. *Understanding group behavior: vol. 1: Consensual action by small groups*. Hillside, NJ: Lawrence Erlbaum, 1996, pp. 137–161.

150. Jones J, Hunter D. Consensus methods for medical and health services research. *BMJ* 1995;311:376–380.

151. Greer AL. The two cultures of public health. *JAMA* 1987;258:2739–2740.

152. Aubry M, Cantu R, Dvorak J, Graf-Baumann T, Johnston K, Kelly J, et al. Concussion in Sport Group. Summary and agreement statement of the First International Conference on Concussion in Sport, Vienna 2001. *Br J Sports Med* 2002;36:6–10.

153. McCrory P, Johnston K, Meeuwisse W, Aubry M, Cantu R, Dvorak J, et al. Summary and agreement statement of the 2nd International Conference on Concussion in Sport, Prague 2004. *Br J Sports Med* 2005;39:196–204.

154. McCrory P, Meeuwisse W, Johnston K, Dvorak J, Aubry M, Molloy M, et al. Consensus statement on concussion in sport – The 3rd International Conference on Concussion in Sport held in Zurich, November 2008. *J Clin Neurosci* 2009;16:755–763.

155. McCrory P, Meeuwisse W, Aubry M, Cantu B, Dvorak J, Echemendia R, et al. Consensus statement on Concussion in Sport – The 4th International Conference on Concussion in Sport held in Zurich, November 2012. *Phys Ther Sport* 2013;14:e1–e13.

156. Hinchey SA, Jackson JL. A cohort study assessing difficult patient encounters in a walk-in primary care clinic: Predictors and outcomes. *J Gen Intern Med* 2011;26:588–594.

157. An PG, Manwell LB, Williams ES, Laiteerapong N, Brown RL, Rabatin JS, et al. Does a higher frequency of difficult patient encounters lead to lower quality care? *J Fam Pract* 2013;62:24–29.

158. Goode RL. Complications of patient selection: Recognizing the difficult patient. *Facial Plast Surg Clin North Am* 2013;21:579–584.

159. Fiester A. The "difficult" patient reconceived: An expanded moral mandate for clinical ethics. *Am J Bioeth* 2012;12:2–7.

160. Ferrando SJ, Okoli U. Personality disorders: Understanding and managing the difficult patient in neurology practice. *Semin Neurol* 2009;29:266–271.

161. Ricke AK, Lee MJ, Chambers JE. The difficult patient: Borderline personality disorder in the obstetrical and gynecological patient. *Obstet Gynecol Surv* 2012;67:495–502.

162. Weiss GG. Taming the difficult patient. *Med Econ* 2002;79:100, 105, 109.

163. Surowiecki J. *The wisdom of crowds: Why the many are smarter than the few and how collective wisdom shapes business, economies, societies, and nations.* London: Little, Brown, 2004.

164. Mannes AE, Soll JB, Larrick RP. The wisdom of select crowds. *J Personal Soc Psychol* 2014:107:276–299.

165. Bloom BS. *Taxonomy of educational objectives, Handbook I. The cognitive domain.* New York: David McKay, 1956.

166. Lezak MD, Howieson DB, Bigler ED, Tranel D. *Neuropsychological assessment,* 5th edition. Oxford: Oxford University Press, 2012.

167. Heaton RK. *A manual for the Wisconsin card sorting test.* Odessa, FL: Psychological Assessment Resources, 1980.

168. Benton AL, Hamsher de SK, Sivan AB. *Multilingual aplasia examination,* 2nd edition. Iowa City, IA: AJA Associates, 1983.

169. Dikmen SS, Machamer J, Winn HR, Temkin NR. Neuropyschological outcome at 1 year post head injury. *Neuropsychology* 1995;9:80–90.

170. Binder LM, Rohling ML. Money matters: A meta-analytic review of financial incentives on recovery after closed-head injury. *Am J Psychiatry* 1996;153:7–10.

171. Binder LM, Rohling ML, Larrabee GJ. A review of mild head trauma. Part I: Meta-analytic review of neuropsychological studies. *J Clin Exp Neuropsychol* 1997;19:421–431.

172. Bigler ED. Distinguished Neuropsychologist Award Lecture 1999. The lesion(s) in traumatic brain injury: Implications for clinical neuropsychology. *Arch Clin Neuropsychol* 2001;16:95–131.

173. Bigler ED. Neurobiology and neuropathology underlie the neuropsychological deficits associated with traumatic brain injury. *Arch Clin Neuropsychol* 2003;18:595–621; discussion 623–627.

174. Lees-Haley PR, Green P, Rohling ML, Fox DD, Allen LM 3rd. The lesion(s) in traumatic brain injury: Implications for clinical neuropsychology. *Arch Clin Neuropsychol* 2003;18:585–594.

175. Rohling ML, Meyers JE, Millis SR. Neuropsychological impairment following traumatic brain injury: A dose–response analysis. *Clin Neuropsychol* 2003;17:289–302.

176. Rohling ML, Binder LM, Demakis GJ, Larrabee GJ, Ploetz DM, Langhinrichsen-Rohling J. A meta-analysis of neuropsychological outcome after mild traumatic brain injury: Re-analyses and reconsiderations of Binder et al. (1997), Frencham et al. (2005), and Pertab et al. (2009). *Clin Neuropsychol* 2011;25:608–623.

177. Rohling ML, Larrabee GJ, Millis R. The "Miserable Minority" following mild traumatic brain injury: Who are they and do meta-analyses hide them? *Clin Neuropsychol* 2012;26:197–213.

178. Frencham KAR, Fox AM, Maybery MT. Neuropsychological studies of mild traumatic brain injury: A meta-analytic review of research since 1995. *J Clin Exper Neuropsychol* 2005;27:334–351.

179. Pertab JL, James KM, Bigler ED. Limitations of mild traumatic brain injury meta-analyses. *Brain Inj* 2009;23:498–508.

180. Ruff RM. Two decades of advances in understanding of mild traumatic brain injury. *J Head Trauma Rehab* 2005;20:5–18.

181. Ruff RM. Mild traumatic brain injury and neural recovery: Rethinking the debate. *NeuroRehab* 2011;28:167–180.

182. Ruff RM, Jamora CW. Myths and mild traumatic brain injury. *Psychol Injury Law* 2009:2: 34–42.

183. Jamora CW, Young A, Ruff RM. Comparison of subjective cognitive complaints with neuropsychological tests in individuals with mild vs more severe traumatic brain injuries. *Brain Inj* 2012;26: 36–47.

184. Bigler ED, Farrer TJ, Pertab JL, James K, Petrie JA, Hedges DW. Reaffirmed limitations of meta-analytic methods in the study of mild traumatic brain injury: A response to Rohling et al. *Clin Neuropsychol* 2013;27:176–214.

185. Larrabee GJ, Binder LM, Rohling ML, Ploetz DM. Meta-analytic methods and the importance of non-TBI factors related to outcome in mild traumatic brain injury: Response to Bigler et al. (2013). *Clin Neuropsychol* 2013;27:215–237.

186. Chen JK, Johnston KM, Petrides M, Ptito A. Neural substrates of symptoms of depression following concussion in male athletes with persisting postconcussion symptoms. *Arch Gen Psychiatr* 2008; 65:81–89.

187. James W. *The principles of psychology* (special ed., vol. II). New York: Henry Holt, 1890.

188. Chen C-J, Wu C-H, Liao Y-P, Hsu H-L, Tseng Y-C, Liu H-L, et al. Working memory in patients with mild traumatic brain injury: Functional MR imaging analysis. *Radiology* 2012;264:844–851.

189. Johnson B, Zhang K, Gay M, Horovitz S, Hallett M, Sebastianelli W, et al. Alteration of brain default network in subacute phase of injury in concussed individuals: Resting-state fMRI study. *NeuroImage* 2011; 59:511–518.

190. McMillan TM, Teasdale GM, Weir CJ, Stewart E. Death after head injury: The 13 year outcome of a case control study. *J Neurol Neurosurg Psychiatry* 2011;82:931–935.

191. Rey A. L'examen psychologique dans les cas d'encéphalopathie traumatique. (Les problèmes.) [The psychological examination

in cases of traumatic encephalopathy (Problems).] *Arch Psychol* 1941;28: 215–285.

192. Ha J-W, Pyun S-B, Hwang YM, Sim H. Lateralization of cognitive functions in aphasia after right brain damage. *Yonsei Med J* 2012;53:486–494.

193. Jackson JH. *On the localisation of movements in the brain.* London: J. & A. Churchill, 1875.

194. Booth JR, Wood L, Lu D, Houk JC, Bitan T. The role of the basal ganglia and cerebellum in language processing. *Brain Res* 2007;1133:136–144.

195. Mariën P, Ackermann H, Adamaszek M, Barwood CH, Beaton A, Desmond J et al. Consensus paper: Language and the cerebellum: An ongoing enigma. *Cerebellum* 2014;13:386–410.

196. Crosson B, Benefield H, Cato MA, Sadek JR, Moore AB, Wierenga CE, et al. Left and right basal ganglia and frontal activity during language generation: Contributions to lexical, semantic, and phonological processes. *J Int Neuropsychol Soc* 2003;9:1061–1077.

197. Levin HS, Eisenberg HM, editors. *Mild head injury.* Oxford: Oxford University Press, 1989.

198. Marshall LF, Ruff RM. Neurosurgeon as victim – a candid depiction of neurosurgeon. In Levin HS, Eisenberg HM, editors. *Mild head injury.* Oxford: Oxford University Press, 1989, pp. 276–280.

199. Mickeviciene D, Schrader H, Obelieniene D, et al. A controlled prospective inception cohort study on the post-concussion syndrome outside the medicolegal context. *Eur J Neurol* 2004;11:411–419.

200. van Kleef GA, Oveis C, van der Löwe I, LuoKogan A, Goetz J, Keltner D. Power, distress, and compassion: Turning a blind eye to the suffering of others. *Psychol Sci* 2008;19:1315–1322.

201. Stellar JE, Manzo VM, Kraus MW, Keltner D. Class and compassion: Socioeconomic factors predict responses to suffering. *Emotion* 2012;12:449–459.

202. Fiske ST. Controlling other people: The impact of power on stereotyping. *Am Psychol* 1993;48:621–628.

203. Anderson C, Berdahl JL. The experience of power: Examining the effects of power on approach and inhibition tendencies. *J Personal Soc Psychol* 2002;83: 1362–1377.

204. De Dreu CKW, Van Kleef GA. The influence of power on the information search, impression formation, and demands in negotiation. *J Exp Soc Psychol* 2004;40:303–319.

205. Galinsky AD, Magee JC, Inesi ME, Gruenfeld DH. Power and perspectives not taken. *Psychol Sci* 2006;17:1068–1074.

206. Piff PK, Kraus MW, Côté S, Cheng BH, Keltner D. Having less, giving more: The influence of social class on prosocial behavior. *J Personal Soc Psychol* 2010;99:771–784.

207. Wailoo K. *Pain: A political history.* Baltimore, MD: Johns Hopkins University Press, 2014.

208. McAdams DP, Albaugh M, Farber E, Daniels J, Logan RL, Olson B. Family metaphors and moral intuitions: How conservatives and liberals narrate their lives. *J Personal Soc Psychol* 2008;95:978–990.

209. Graham J, Haidt J, Nosek BA. Liberals and conservatives rely on different sets of moral foundations. *J Personal Soc Psychol* 2009;96:1029–1046.

210. Hirsh JB, DeYoung CG, Xu X, Peterson JB. Compassionate liberals and polite conservatives: Associations of agreeableness with political ideology and moral values. *Personal Soc Psychol Bull* 2010;36:655–664.

211. Carman KG, Pollard M. 2014. Adults are concerned about sons playing football, especially the more highly educated and Obama 2012 voters. Available at www.rand.org/blog/2014/11/adults-are-concerned-about-sons-playing-football-especially .html.

212. Public Broadcasting Service. Frontline. *League of denial: The NFL's concussion crisis.* October 8 2013. www.pbs.org/wgbh/pages/frontline/league-of-denial/ (2013) and www.pbs.org/wgbh/pages/frontline/league-of-denial/.

213. Solomon GS, Kuhnz A. Relationship between concussion history and neurocognitive test performance in National Football League draft picks. *Am J Sports Med* 2014;42:934–939.

214. Kay T, Newman B, Cavallo M, Ezrachi O, Resnick M. Toward a neuropsychological model of functional disability after mild traumatic brain injury. *Neuropsychology* 1992;6:371–384.

215. McMahon PJ, Hricik A, Yue JK, Puccio AM, Inoue T, Lingsma HF, et al. Symptomatology and functional outcome in mild traumatic brain injury: Results from the prospective TRACK-TBI study. *J Neurotrauma* 2014;31:26–33.

Chapter

1

What Is a Concussive Brain Injury?

Jeff Victoroff and Erin D. Bigler

Ὁκόσοισιν ἂν ὁ ἐγκέφαλος σεισθῇ ὑπό τινος προφάσιος, ἀνάγκη ἀφώνους γίνεσθαι παραχρῆμα

In cases of concussion of the brain from any cause, the patients of necessity lose at once the power of speech.

Anonymous, attributed to Hippocrates [1]

A concussion is a rattling blow – an earthquake-like shaking or a tempest-like buffeting. Dropping a shoe on the floor, swinging an automobile door shut, or perturbing the air by exploding gunpowder are examples.

This chapter would be complete, albeit brief, if it ended thus. However, some readers might balk at embracing this definition of concussion without a little more background. The remainder of this chapter is intended to offer that background. The term *concussion* comes heavily weighted with the baggage of history. Like the shell of the hermit crab, its essence has been hidden by successive accretions. Yet there is a core concept, readily interrogable from what Courville called the "cloud of witnesses" [2]. The goal is not to perpetuate some hoary standard, but to extract a scientifically coherent essence from the testimony of those witnesses.

The first point is that *concussion* is not originally or exclusively a medical term. It originally referred to a simple mechanical phenomenon. A historical review makes it clear that the term has only lately and very inconsistently been employed in reference to a medical problem. To state that a patient "suffered a concussion" is semantically equivalent to saying, "I'm sorry, we did everything we could, but she succumbed to suction." "Doctor, come quick! He seems to be going into compression!" A disease defined by reference to a simple mechanical force is, shall we say, underspecified.

Employing *concussion* in medicine was in fact originally idiosyncratic (albeit expressive). Yet once English-speaking physicians adopted the word, they used it in its simple original sense: a physical blow that causes shaking, whether the result is pulmonary distress, strong hydraulic forces in blood vessels, a jolt to the spine, the eye, the knee, the heart, or the head: "the subject of concussion or commotion … has been a matter of careful study … All the parts of the body may be the subject of such action: Bones, muscles, nerves, viscera; and some assert that the blood itself may be the subject of concussion" [3]; also see[4, 5].

Using the unqualified term *concussion* to refer to a medical problem is inherently problematic. Properly used, the term does not denote the *consequences* of a physical event, but the event itself. By the 18th century, *concussion* began to be used primarily for head and spine injuries. Yet a century of tradition has endowed *concussion* with ambiguous implications, including a blow to the head, the typical clinical symptoms after that blow, or the biological changes contingent upon that blow. By 1950, favoring just one of its hotly debated connotations, some neurologists oddly yoked *concussion* to the connotations "minor," "transient," and "non-structural." None of these qualifiers is supported by linguistics or science. It seems better to say what we mean: that concussive force sometimes hurts the brain, resulting in a concussive brain injury (CBI).

Of course, language is organic and dynamic. Some will rightly argue that a word means what they say it means, if they can convince others to use it in that way. It is in fact true that a popular movement might strive to redefine *concussion* not in accordance with its original essential meaning but instead as "a head injury that does no harm." Equally, one might use *concussion* for "a challenging position for physical intimacy," or "a rare, high-proof, single-malt Scotch whisky." But as Galileo Galilei said in 1612: "Names and attributes must accommodate themselves to the essence of things, not the essence to the names; because first there were the things, and then the names."

We propose that fidelity to the original meaning of concussion may be edifying, clarifying, and a source of relief from untoward contention. A conservative use of language preserves the original meaning of concussion as a mechanical event. Such a mechanical event sometimes causes a medical problem. Therefore – respecting that some authorities will continue to use *concussion* to refer to a neurological disorder with a widely debated slew of operational definitions – we suggest the proper use would be: "This patient's head was apparently impacted by a *concussive force*. As a result, we are concerned that he has experienced a *concussive brain injury* (CBI)."

This language resolves a host of semantic pitfalls. CBI is a *type* of brain injury – the type that results from the rapid transfer of external force (with or without contact, since head acceleration by itself transmits force to the brain). CBI does not mean a uniform suite of symptoms; two millennia of observations have established that the clinical presentation of CBI varies. CBI does not mean a uniform *duration* of distress; it is abundantly clear that the time its effects persist varies as well. CBI does not mean a uniform *amount* of injury; despite the popular conflation of concussion with mildness, a century of debate has failed to establish a biologically meaningful definition of "mild," and no *a priori* reason exists to assume that concussive force always has minor effects. CBI is just the self-explanatory phrase that refers to the most common type of mammalian traumatic brain injury (TBI) – injury due to an abrupt external force that shakes the brain.

Erichsen's use was typical: "Concussion or stunning appears to be a shock communicated to the nervous system from the application of some external violence as will produce commotion of the substance of the brain" ([6], p. 249). Ingvar summarized this original definition neatly in 1923 [7]:

> Commotion is produced by blows against the skull or in the spinal region. Such a blow must mean a concussion of the parts that are hit, as the blow will transmit its energy to the body exposed to it. In principle, the same effect will be produced by a blow from a heavy object as by the intense atmospheric disturbances that follow an explosion ("*vent de l'obus*").
>
> ([7], p. 271)

According to the pithily titled Demographics and Clinical Assessment Working Group of the International and Interagency Initiative toward Common Data Elements for Research on Traumatic Brain Injury and Psychological Health, "TBI is defined as an alteration in brain function, or other evidence of brain pathology, caused by an external force" [8]. We accept this definition. In this chapter, we will do our best to characterize the concussive element of TBI. That is, the empirical evidence appears to support a modest paradigm shift. That shift comprises three elements:

1. Concussion is a mechanical event. It may or may not produce a brain injury. The word does not mean an *amount* of injury, a *duration* of effect, or a *group of symptoms*.
2. CBI is neither physically nor symptomatically homogeneous. It is heterogeneous, not only due to variation in brain changes in the moments after impact, but also due to the interactions between thousands of physiological changes and a lifetime of bio-psychological individuality.
3. It is misleading to characterize CBI as a focal traumatic event comparable to a broken arm. It is a dazzlingly complex, remarkably diverse, and often long-lived cerebral process. It is something special, for trauma to brains alone perturbs the tissue of identity.

Little has been gained by attempting to equate a mechanism of brain damage (shaking due to external force transmitted through the skull) with a particular degree of harm (mildness). It seems wiser to acknowledge that *severity* and *mechanism of injury* are two different things. For instance, pneumonia is a type of lung problem, but one never assumes that *pneumonia* means "a little bit of lung infection." We propose that clinical brain science may possibly accelerate if we recognize this difference. Brains can be hurt in a variety of ways. Sometimes they are starved of oxygen. Sometimes they are afflicted by demyelination. Sometimes they are rattled or shaken or tossed about within the skull. The *type* of injury does not tell us the *amount* of injury. It seems better to acknowledge the wide spectrum of harm caused by a rapid, brain-rattling transfer of external force, without artificially limiting our attention to a neurobiologically indefinable subspecies some wish to call "mild."

To foreshadow the coming argument, ponder for a moment the logical integrity of the usual approaches to defining concussion. Among innumerable explicit and implicit published definitions, one encounters those based entirely on symptoms, on observed pathology (or the lack thereof), on presumed pathophysiology, on imaging results, and on a virtually infinite combination of these factors. Yet CBI cannot be defined reliably by clinical symptoms, because those symptoms vary greatly. For example, CBI might be defined in terms of severity or duration, but every attempt to do so represents the imposition of arbitrary delimiters (such as equation of concussion with mild TBI (mTBI)) that have not been shown to have the slightest pathophysiological validity. CBI cannot be defined reliably by observed pathology, because the pathological changes are variable, and what is "observed" is entirely dependent on the technology used by the observer. CBI might theoretically be defined in terms of today's knowledge of its pathophysiology; yet this would seem imprudent. That the definition would change tomorrow. CBI cannot be defined reliably by reference to any biomarker or neuroimaging result (or by the embarrassingly indefensible criterion "absence of a visible change on conventional neuroimaging") because the technology regarded as *conventional* today will keep changing forever. Some define concussive injury as a "brain effect," but this begs the question of whether concussion is a disorder. A butterfly exerting external force on the great toe may produce a "brain effect." The word *injury* seems a better descriptor of a medical problem.

Although CBI may have focal effects (for instance, bruising or hematoma underlying or opposite the point of impact), concussive injury is rarely just a focal problem. Historically, the adjective most commonly employed to describe its effects was "general." For almost a century, that somewhat ambiguous term has been replaced by *diffuse*. For instance, an American-style football player takes a hit. Even when there are focal cerebral effects (such as contusion underlying the point of impact and contrecoup effects), what observers see – his staggering and imbalance, slowed speech, disorientation, memory loss, often abnormal eye movements – strongly suggests a diffuse (aka, "general") dysfunction of the central nervous system. Evidence suggests differential vulnerability by region, cell type, and subcellular element (Ingvar showed this in 1923) [7]. Thus, *multifocal* effects are also expected. For these reasons, we recommend defining concussive injury in a way that captures the essence of this very important concept without resorting to the arbitrary and the temporarily popular. "The focal, multifocal, and diffuse element of a TBI due to the rapid transfer of energy exerted by an external force transmitted through the skull" says what we know and leaves the door open for further discovery.

Medical science has wrestled since its dawn with the inseparable twin problems of defining (or classifying) disorders and employing that definition in the practical business of diagnosis. Note that *defining* a disorder and *diagnosing* a disorder are two different projects. For example, it is one job to define tuberculosis as "a multifaceted illness due to infection by the tubercle bacillus." It is quite another job to figure out who, among the 12 coughing patients in the waiting room, has that problem. Since the time of Osler, Western medicine has trusted the positivist approach in which clinicians use all available information to determine whether this one patient can be diagnosed with a particular disorder [9–12]. Two approaches cover a plurality of disorders:

1. Defining the disorder in terms of its *cause* permits diagnosis by testing for a biomarker consistent with that cause. For example, we define meningococcal meningitis, trisomy 21, or mercury poisoning by reference to the bacterium, the extra chromosome, or the toxin, and we diagnose by checking for those markers. The more sensitive and specific the biomarker, the greater our confidence.

2. Defining the disorder in terms of *symptoms* requires diagnosis by using some agreed-upon rule. For example, the American Psychiatric Association tells us (paraphrasing), "it's depression if it looks like this, but it's schizophrenia if it looks like that." Although such operationally defined disorders may or may not be biologically valid, written algorithms at last facilitate inter-observer reliability.

However, what if the symptoms vary and there is no biomarker?

The definition of CBI has long been regarded as problematic. It is readily defined in terms of mechanical etiology (injury to the brain due to force impacting the head and transmitted through the skull), but to define it as "head injury" would be a rhetorical circularity that fails to gratify the need to distinguish between the manifold ways a head might be traumatized (for instance, by an icepick, a laser, a fist, or a blast wave). Across medical history, the understanding of CBI has been delayed by the striking diversity of meanings attached to the term "concussion" or to its synonym *commotio cerebri*. The same term has been used to refer to an etiology, a purportedly unitary clinical syndrome, a speculative pathological change, a presumed *lack* of pathological change, a process (e.g., shaking), and – especially among a notorious cohort of early-20th-century writers – a purportedly typical outcome (e.g., transient neurological symptoms, no structural brain change, and complete recovery).

One seeks a definition of concussion that captures its essence and hopefully remains viable for a millennium or two. This requires two efforts. First, teasing out, from a vast and fascinating scientific tapestry, the logical common thread, expressed with words that are likely to retain their meaning. We hope that "force," "injury," "diffuse," and "brain," for instance, have sufficient durability. As much as one might yearn for a neat, readily identifiable combination of cause, symptoms, signs, biomarkers, and pathology (and as certain as it is that august expert panels will continue to publish "consensus" definitions that are merely operational), we submit that further narrowing

the definition of concussion beyond *the element of a TBI due to an external force* would be bowing to one competing school of thought or other without a rationale that survives logical inspection. Second, defining concussion requires openness to neuroscience. The superannuated debate about the meaning of "concussion" comes down to a matter of belief. Some believe – on the basis of knowledge and instinct – that CBI commonly leads to long-lived or permanent organic brain dysfunction. Others believe this is rare. Unfortunately, neuroscience has yet to discover a biomarker that permits us to determine which victims are affected, and to what degree. This perpetuates loyalty to strong opinions about the frequency of persistent harm.

So consider our present conundrum. We are well aware that: (1) more people have CBIs than report them; (2) some of those who report CBIs will overstate and others understate their symptoms – including cohorts of those who misattribute their troubles to CBI, exaggerators, malingerers, compensation seekers, those with lasting brain change directly caused by concussive force, and those with lasting brain change caused indirectly by the interaction of physical force with psychosocial circumstances; (3) neuropsychological testing is insensitive to some brain changes; (4) neuroimaging is not a definitive measure of CBI-related changes. In round numbers: (1) 1% of people aged 15–24 visit U.S. emergency rooms (ERs) for TBI each year – and about 95% of those are CBIs; (2) there are ~ 45 million 15–24-year-olds in the United States. Therefore 450,000 young people show up in the ER each year, of whom about 427,500 have concussions. Since about 90% of ER visits for TBI are "mild," Figure 1.1 permits one to estimate the rates of ER-attended CBI by age group.

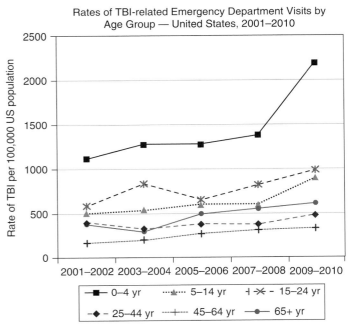

Rates of TBI-related Emergency Department Visits by Age Group — United States, 2001–2010

Fig. 1.1 Rates of traumatic brain injury (TBI)-related emergency department visits by age group.

Source: Centers for Disease Control and Prevention. CDC 2016. ww.cdc.gov/ traumaticbraininjury/data/rates_ed_byage.html [13]

Seventy years after their brain injuries, how many of those 427,500 U.S. adults will be different than they would have been, absent their concussions? 392? 392,000? In the absence of both a logically coherent definition and of sensitive and specific tests for subtle biological change (not to mention a profound resistance to funding the required research), a valid quantitative answer is anyone's guess. Yet the trend of discovery strongly supports the first instinct: many suffer lasting harm.

Part I: A Brief History of the Idea of Concussion

Many of our ancestors, when no fracture was discoverable in the cranium of a person laboring under such symptoms as have been mentioned [disturbance or abolition of the offices of sense and motion, etc.] in consequence of violence offered to the head, contented themselves with calling the case a concussion; and although they had no very precise idea annexed to the term, yet they seldom went farther for a solution; like teeth and worms in infants, or like nerves in women, it satisfied ignorant inquirers.

Percivall Pott, 1768 ([14], p. 231)

What (if Anything) did Hippocrates Think About Concussion?

First, one may never know Hippocrates of Cos's (c. 460 BC – c. 370 BC) thinking on any medical subject. History has only provided us with the collection of documents referred to as the *Hippocratic Corpus*. The authors of this collection, like the authors of the Old Testament, have yet to be identified, and probably contributed their fragments mostly between 400 and 200 BC. Although one supposes the famed Greek healer to have been literate, to date, no evidence has emerged demonstrating that Hippocrates ever wrote anything [15, 16].

Second, of course there is no Greek word, "concussion." The reason that Hippocrates' name is associated in various quasi-historical accounts of brain concussion with the word "concussion" is that his 19th-century translator – who happened to be a physician – elected to use that word.

The first widely available English translation of selected fragments of the *Hippocratic Corpus* was performed by the Scottish physician, Francis Adams, and published by the Sydenham Society in 1849. The book, called *Aphorisms*, Section VII, No. 58, states: "Ὁκόσοισιν ἂν ὁ ἐγκέφαλος σεισθῇ ὑπό τινος προφάσιος, ἀνάγκη ἀφώνους γίνεσθαι παραχρῆμα." Dr. Adams's translation: "In cases of concussion of the brain produced by any cause, the patients necessarily lose their speech." Dr. Adams notes: "the term here used (σεισθῇ)(*seisphe*) implies that the concussion was supposed to be violent" [17].

Given the interest in tracing the roots of the modern concept of so-called "concussion," it may be useful to consider what condition the anonymous author was referring to. The connotations of *seisphe* are clear: this term derives from the verb *sei'o* (σει'ω), "to shake, move to and fro," e.g., *seio egkhos melien* (σειω εΥχος μελιην), "to shake the poised spear." Since

Poseidon was called the Earth Shaker, one divine epithet was *seisi-khphon* (σεισι-χΦων), or "earth-shaker." As one might anticipate of a land with a notorious geological predisposition, the phrase *khphonos seismos* (χΦονος σεισμος) meant earthquake and the term *seismatias* (σεισματιας) means "of earthquakes" [18]. Hence the many English cognates, including *seismic* and *seismology*. An accurate translation of the Hippocratic idea might be "an earthquake-like shaking of the head" or perhaps simply "*headquake*."

It seems irresistible to speculate about what spectrum of problems the Coan and/or Cnidian Schools of Greek medicine meant when they employed the term *seisphe*. If a patient suffered a headquake, did that imply a mode of transmission of force (e.g., a direct blow to the head versus force transmitted indirectly, via the spine)? Did it imply a degree of severity? Did it exclude head injuries of any kind, for instance, those with skull fractures, brain penetration, or causing immediate death? Did Hippocratics distinguish between the expected symptoms or consequences of headquake (e.g., recovery or death) compared with those of other species of head trauma?

One possible way to address these questions is to compare the use of *seisphe* with the terminology in the Hippocratic text titled *On Wounds in the Head* [19]. Here, the Adams translation repeatedly refers to "fracture" and "contusion." The first word is accurately translated from some variant of *regma* (ρηγμα) (e.g., ii, l. 12, *regnutai* (ρηγνυται), meaning breaking or fracture). The second word is usually some variant of *phlao* (φλαω), to crush or pound. Yet the author of *On Wounds in the Head* was probably not referring to contusion of the brain, but instead to contusion of the skull, as implied by the passage, "The bone may be contused and keep its place, and the contusion may not be complicated by fracture" ([19], V., l. 24–27).

One quickly appreciates that, throughout *On Wounds in the Head*, the major diagnostic and therapeutic concern is the condition of the skull. Since the anonymous author of this text commences his work by offering incorrect information about the anatomy of the skull ([20], p. 5), barely mentions the brain, and appears unaware that *head* injury only impacts animal behavior because of *brain* injury, to further pursue the Hippocratic understanding of what moderns call "brain concussion" is to plunge merrily into a blind tunnel. All we have is a circular observation: the 19th-century Scottish physician Adams intuited that the meaning of *concussion* he had learned in his medical training was about the same as what the anonymous Hippocratic author meant by an *earthquake-like shaking of the head*. Dr. Adams thus substituted a British medical term of art, already heavy with connotative baggage, for a Greek idea. Some recent commentators on CBI, apparently relying on Adams's translation of *seisphe* as "concussion," discuss the Hippocratic idea as if it equals something mild and transient. This imposes a narrow, troubled modern medical concept on the original, more interesting text.

The Hippocratic connotation of an earthquake-like shaking is preserved in virtually every Indo-European word for CBI that has been translated as "concussion." For instance, the English word *concussion*, first used in the 14th century, derives from the Latin *concutio*, a cognate of one of various combinations of the prefix *con* ("with") and *quatere* ("to shake") – itself derived from the Proto-Indo European *kweh,t*, or *kwʰt*, a root word meaning "to shake." *Concutio* is the Latin first-person present tense verb meaning, "I shake, agitate." Interestingly, this verb can also mean "I alarm, terrify," connoting emotional shock. Many writers associated concussion with psychic or nervous shock, increasingly so in the early 20th century. (This raises the question of so-called functional versus so-called organic disorders, to which we must return.) Similarly, early French neurological authorities equated concussion with *ébranlement*, which means *shaking* (e.g., [21, 22]).

How, then, did Dr. Adams hit upon the English word *concussion* when he translated the Greek term for earthquake-like shaking? The answer involves a mysterious priest, an idle printer, and the Abbott of Winchester. At some unknown time prior to 1483, an anonymous French priest translated Virgil's *Aeneid* from Latin to French, creating what Salverda de Grave calls the oldest known version of Virgil in "the vulgar tongue." Seven years later (1490), printer William Caxton happened upon this book in his library:

I, sittyng in my studye where as laye many dyuerse
paunflettis an bookys, happened that to my hande came
a lytyl booke in frenshe, whiche late was translated oute
of latyn by some noble clerke of framzce, whiche booke is
named Eneydos …

[23]

According to the *Oxford English Dictionary* [24], the earliest known use of "concussion" in English occurred in Caxton's translation of that French translation of Virgil, from the Latin. Caxton employed the word for a French term describing a tempest-like buffeting: The goddess Juno, seemingly out-of-sorts, called upon the wind deity to assail Aeneas and his little ship with a torment in the air (Figure 1.2).

Concussion is therefore a simple word with a clear derivation. It does not refer to human heads. It does not denote or connote an amount, degree, or duration of force, or even an injury – let alone a particular severity of injury. It refers to *type* of mechanical occurrence – an earthquake-like shaking or tempest-like buffeting. It only acquired its present association with medicine in general and head trauma, in particular, by virtue of Dr. Adams's lyrical 19th-century word choice.

How *concussion* was later redefined to imply something mild – at least in some people's minds – is a captivating tale. It is not a typical history of science story in which punctuated

progress is fueled by heady discoveries. It is more a story of intellectual war, arguably populated by truth seekers and minimizers. To dismiss concussion as something *mild* is to deny both the origin of the concept and the evidences of science.

We submit that the ancient Greek concept of headquake retains value. Without imposing any later notions, one can readily visualize headquake and conceive of this as a physically forceful commotion of the cranium and its contents with varying consequences. The meaning of that commotion can hardly be limited to a degree of severity such as mild, moderate, or severe, any more than the meaning of the term *earthquake* could be rationally confined to "a little shaking." *The fact that a brain was concussed does not mean it was concussed mildly.* Such a commotion can hardly be claimed to exclude skull fracture, or bleeding, or penetrating injury, or death any more than an earthquake can be presumed to exclude an Earth fissure and the leveling of a metropolis. It would seem self-evident that a commotion of the head may produce both a typical suite of symptoms (e.g., headache, dizziness, altered consciousness) and a broad spectrum of outcomes (e.g., from momentary dazing to death), just as an earthquake may have both typical effects (e.g., swaying buildings, falling crockery) and a broad spectrum of outcomes (e.g., from the momentary fright of a lone shepherd (and his more sensitive sheep) to the collapse of a major metropolis.

As reasonable and potentially valuable as the concept of headquake might be, a brief review of the subsequent history of the medical use of concussion and its synonyms reveals the emergence of problematic trends. First, across the centuries, certain authorities took liberties with the core concept of a generalized commotion of the head and brain and appended their favorite arbitrary clinical delimiters – mostly in the direction of narrowing the definition so that it only described a *typical* clinical presentation, rather than the spectrum of changes actually observed. The motivation seems to have been to provide physicians with pragmatic operational strategies to determine that a concussive TBI occurred in the recent past (e.g., "Since she had a head injury and was unconscious for only a week and seems well today, I declare that a concussion occurred"). Unfortunately, this well-meant proclamation of an operational definition would only be valid if a unitary suite of symptoms reliably followed commotion of the head. As we shall see, it does not.

The second problematic historical trend has been an attempt to delimit the use of the term concussion by reference to a presumed pathological process or outcome – for instance, confining its use to those head commotions that cause neurological symptoms but not death. Such an approach would only be valid if one ignores the immense spectrum of outcomes from generalized head/brain commotion and elects to focus on the subset of patients who exhibit a subset of those outcomes. The third problematic historical trend has been an illogical approach to categorization. For instance, a few early physicians distinguished between *concussion* and *skull fracture*, while during another era physicians distinguished between *concussion* versus *compression* versus *contusion*. Such a categorical approach would only be valid if these events were mutually exclusive. Common sense, and subsequent empirical science, shows that they are not.

How Iuno, for tempesshe thooste of Eneas whiche wolde haue goon in to ytalye / prayd the goddys of wyndes / that eueryche by hym selfe sholde make concussyon and tormente in the ayer.

Fig. 1.2 Culley and Furnivall's English translation of Caxton's French translation of Virgil's (Latin) *Aeneid,* Adapted from Culley and Furnivall, 1490 [23].

Through it all, the essence of concussion has waved its hand like a drowning man above the waves of rhetorical sophistry, logical fallacy, and flawed empiricism in hopes of salvation. That essence may or may not satisfy, but it alone persists: virtually every historical authority discusses CBI as a general brain injury due to external force.

Beyond the Hippocratics

A dazzling number of books and manuscripts pertain to CBI. If one grants that *The Edwin Smith Surgical Papyrus* touches upon concussion, we have access to medical views on this extremely common human problem extending back 3500 years [25]. It transcends the most euphoric ambitions of this chapter to discuss every definition of CBI. Some authorities proposed an explicit definition (i.e. "I define concussion as …"); others implied a definition by use (e.g., "This is an exemplary case of concussion because …"). Some of the best minds in Western science have wrestled with the mysteries and tragedies of CBI. Historically minded readers will find a wealth of informative citations in the bibliography of this chapter and may revel in reviewing the original texts. Yet the authors of the present text realize that savoring the history of science is a matter of personal taste. We have sought a balance between the epic and the haiku versions. For the sake of concision, the present chapter will merely offer some key examples that sparked and still inflame the debate.

Even prior to Hippocrates (and probably predating the dawn of humanity), the typical causes and effects of CBI were known. Case 1 of the surgical treatise called *The Edwin Smith Surgical Papyrus* (c. 1500 BCE) provides "instructions" regarding head wounds that do not fracture the skull [25] (Figure 1.3). Of interest: the Egyptian word for brain might best be translated as "skull offal," or the unpalatable refuse of the cranium [26] (Figure 1.4). (It is perhaps slightly disconcerting, at least to those born since Willis assigned imagination to the brain in 1664, to consider the Egyptian perspective – that the stuff of tripe and gizzards fills the space in our otherwise perfectly digestible heads.)

Unfortunately, the authors of that early work focused entirely on signs and rarely mention symptoms, leaving doubt about the relationship between their case report and typical CBI. A better example appears in Homer's *Iliad*, when a javelin delivers a glancing blow to Hector's helmet.

> Swift at his word his ponderous javelin fled;
> No miss'd its aim, but whence the plumage danced

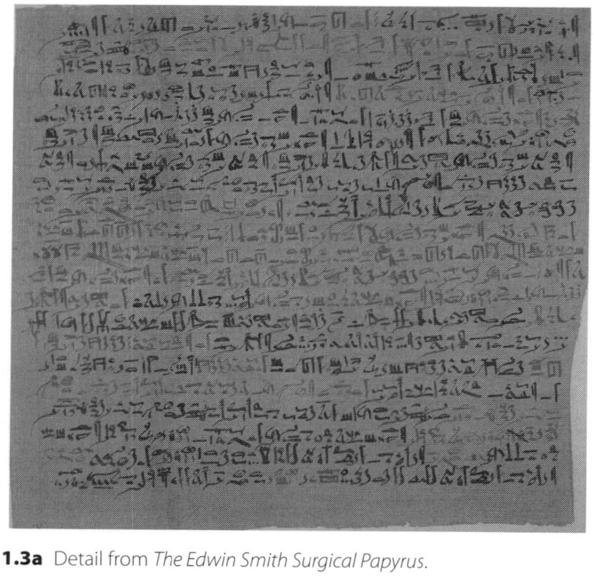

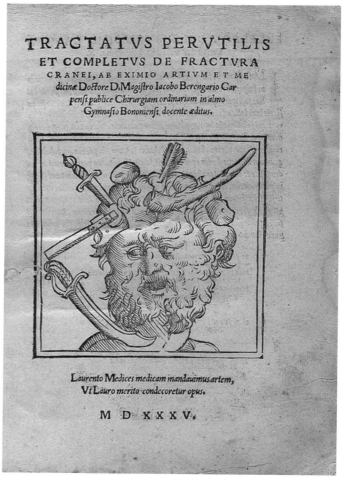

Fig. 1.4 Title page of 1535 edition of da Carpi's text depicting several common forms of concussive brain injury.

Source: da Carpi, 1535 [34]. Complutense University of Madrid

Fig. 1.3a Detail from *The Edwin Smith Surgical Papyrus*.

Source: Used with the permission of the Rare Book Room, New York Academy of Medicine https://ceb.nlm.nih.gov/proj/ttp/smith_home.html

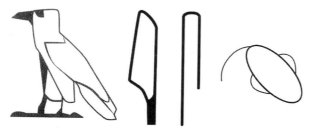

Fig. 1.3b Egyptian hieroglyph for brain, as found in *The Edwin Smith Surgical Papyrus*.

Source: *Edwin Smith Surgical Papryus*, Oriental Institute Publications 3, edited by James Henry Breasted, 1991 reprint of 1930, on p. 511

Razed the smooth cone, and thence obliquely glanced,
Safe in his helm (the gift of Phoebus' hands)
Without a word the Trojan hero stands;
But yet so stunn'd that, staggering on the plain,
His arm and knee his sinking bulk sustain;
O'er his dim sight the misty vapours rise,
And a short distance shades his swimming eyes.

(translation Pope; Book II, ln. p. 335 [27])

Homer poetically crystallizes the clinical essence, documenting the cause (an external force presumably diffused by the helmet), the signs (apparent disequilibrium and motor impact yielding a near fall as well as perhaps abnormal extraocular movements), and the symptoms (altered but not lost consciousness, impaired vision). A medical student offering such detail would deserve praise.

The medical literature in the years between the *Hippocratic Corpus* and the Industrial Revolution (roughly 200 BCE to 1780 CE) is littered with accounts that refer to *commotio cerebri* and pertain to concussion. (One hesitates to call them "definitions of concussion," since that English word first came into use about 1400.) Aulus Cornelius Celsus (c. 25 BC – 50) [28, 29] was an early deviant from the Greek concept of a generalized head shake, limiting the definition of *commotio* to injuries in which the skull is fractured (in exact contradistinction to some modern claims that it's only a concussion if the skull is not fractured). Galen (130–200 CE) updated the Greek concept, clarifying that it's the *brain* injury that matters, and that, as common sense would dictate, the brain can be "shocked" whether or not the skin is broken or the skull is fractured. Rhazes (c. 850–923 CE) was perhaps the first to opine that the symptoms of *commotio* are typically transient (although he hardly limited this disorder to temporary harm) [2, 20, 30]. Lafranchi (1280 CE) agreed that *commotio* sometimes produces a transient disorder, and agreed with Galen that *commotio* and fracture of the skull may occur independently [31–33].

Jacobo Baragazzi was an Italian anatomist. He is better known by the alias he adopted: Berengario da Carpi. He was renowned for his royal connections and his miscreant ways (Putti said "Avarice and cupidity arouse in the spirit of this great man stronger passions than glory or virtue" ([34], p xii)). Yet he possibly deserves credit for a major improvement upon the Greek concept of concussion, drawing attention to the fact that the skull was not the problem; it is the brain. On March 28, 1517, Lorenzo de Medici was wounded with an occipital fracture. "da Carpi" was called to the grandee's bedside in Ancona. He failed to repair the problem. But two months later he rushed into print his thoughts about head injury:

Let us begin therefore with the sign of cranial lesion … redness of the eyes, bilious vomiting, loss of speech, falling to the earth at the time of the heavy blow, and stupor of mind. These signs occur without fracture of the bone. Nevertheless, they can occur due to the motion or concussion of the brain.

[34] (Figure 1.4)

"da Carpi's" concept remained almost entirely undisputed over the next 300 years.

Other 16th-century writers expanded lyrically on the subjective symptoms. In his autobiography (~1568), the notorious artist and rapscallion Benvenuto Cellini (1500–1571) delivered an elaborate, if romanticized, description of his own concussion on escape from prison using linens:

On the descent, whether it was that I thought I had really come to earth and relaxed my grasp to jump, or whether my hands were so tired that they could not keep their hold, at any rate I fell, struck my head in falling, and lay stunned for more than an hour and a half, so far as I could judge. It was just upon daybreak, when the fresh breeze which blows an hour before the sun revived me; yet I did not immediately recover my senses, for I thought my head had been cut off and fancied that I was in purgatory. With time, little by little, my faculties returned.

(transl. Symonds, 1910, Part I, Book 109, [35])

This account meshes well both with the equally poetic account of his own equestrian concussion written by Michel de Montaigne in 1580 [36], and with the contemporaneous description of concussion advanced by Coiter (1573) [37] as a clinical syndrome involving memory loss, loss of speech, poor judgment, and difficulty understanding.

Yet the most authoritative (and hair-raising) Renaissance account of concussion was perhaps that of Ambroise Paré, the French royal barber surgeon. Chapter 9 of his *Oeuvres* is titled "Of the moving, or Concussion, of the Braine" [38] (Figure 5).

you must note that, though the head be armed with a helmet, yet by the violence of a blow, the Veines, and Arteries may be broken, not only those that pass through the sutures, but also those which are dispersed between the two tables in the Diploe … that so the braine might move freely … and this is the true reasons of that vomiting, which is caused and usually follows upon fractures of the scull and concussions of the Braine.

[39]

The progress of empiricism is evident in these words. Setting aside Paré's speculations about pathophysiology, his text is among the first to clarify that concussion and skull fracture, although separable problems, produce similar clinical troubles. He goes on to report his intimate experiences with concussion among his royal patients:

King Henry of happy memory … desirous to honour the marriages of his daughter and sister, with the famous and noble exercise of Tilting … with a blunt lance received so great a stroke … the visor of his helmet flew up, and the truncheon of the broken Lance, hit him above the left eye-brow … the bones being not touched or broken; but the braine was so moved and shaken, that he dyed the eleventh day after the hurt.

What shall I say of the great and very memorable wound of *Francis* of *Loraine* the Duke of *Guise*? He in the fight of the City of *Bologne* had his head so thrust thorough with a lance, that the point entering under his right eye by his nose, came out at his necke betweene his eare and the vertebra, the head of Iron being broken and left in by the violence of the stroke,

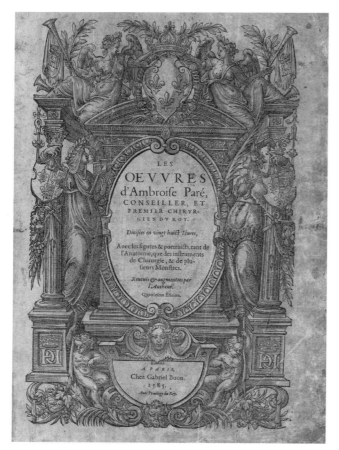

Fig. 1.5a Title page, 1585 edition of Ambroise Paré's text.

Source: Paré, 1585 [38]. Courtesy US National Library of Medicine

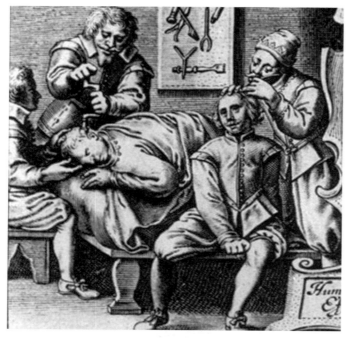

Fig. 1.5b An illustration by Thomas Cecill for Johnson's English translation of Paré, 1634.

Source: Paré, 1634, transl. Johnson [39]. Complutense University of Madrid

which stuck there so firmly, that it could not be drawn or plucked forth, without a paire of Smiths pincers. But although the strength & violence of the blow was so great, that it could not be without a fracture of the bones, a tearing and breaking of the Nerves, Veines, Arteries and other parts; yet the generous Prince by favour of God recovered.

([39], Chapter IX, transl. Johnson, 1634)

Paré clearly regarded the concussive injury as just one element of a head trauma in which an external force produces generalized shaking of and damage to the brain, with or without skull fracture, the outcomes of which span the range from rapid recovery to rapid death. Cases of intermediate severity simply left the victim disabled with a post-concussion syndrome. For example, the case described by Flemish scientist Tertius Damianus, in 1541 (cited in Schenck (alias von Grafenburg), 1584, as cited in Luzzatti and Whitaker 1995–1996 ([40], p. 160):

> In France I saw a man, already adult, who knew not only the common tongue and dialect but also spoke Latin fluently; he was very well educated, and played the bagpipes. [Following an accident], he had lost consciousness, and when he regained his senses he had lost all his knowledge, almost as if he had drunk fully of Lethe's waters of oblivion.

So a concussion means a rattling blow. In medicine, a concussion meant a rattling blow to some part of the body. And in neurology, a concussion meant an injury to the brain due to such a concussive force, leading to a broad spectrum of consequences. What happened? How did we get from this straightforward use of concussion to the current proliferation of meanings, such that some doctors use concussion for a potentially disabling trauma, and other for something mild, transient, and non-structural? Language is plastic. It conforms to the mold of many minds. It's intriguing to trace the devolution of this medical term over the subsequent three and a half centuries, tracking the bloom of confusion.

1600–1700

It was about 50 years after Paré when the meaning of concussion began to be muddled. Of course, most authorities preserved its original meaning. Some focused on the typical symptoms. Fewer looked in the head for the causes. For instance, Fabricius ab Aquapendente (1604) [41] reported that percussion of the head causes lethargy, vertigo, and speechlessness. Wilhelm Fabry (1606) [42], an early observer of the post-concussion state, discussed the idiocy that sometimes follows CBI. Peter Paaw (1616) [43] (also see p[32]) stated that "cerebral commotion, perturbation, and also concussion" might cause death without fracture. Horst (1625) [44] was another to report a fatal case of concussion. Read (1687) [45] gave detailed clinical descriptions of vertigo, tinnitus, visual change, and giddiness – hardly different from Homer's. Bonet's massive *Sepulchretum, sive Anatomia practica* [46], first published in 1679, reported the results of some 3000 autopsies, organized from head to toe (Figure 1.6.)

This anatomist merely repeated the conviction that concussion does its damage by shaking of the brain within the skull.

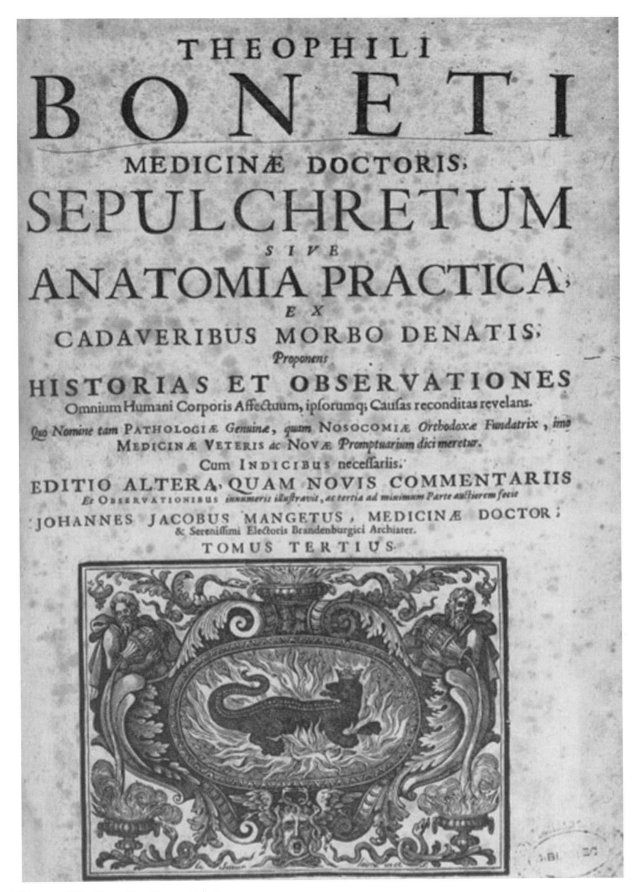

Fig. 1.6 Title page, 1679 edition of Bonet's compendium.

Source: Bonet, 1679 [46]. Complutense University of Madrid

Yet for all these consistent (and redundant) reports, little progress was made in finding the brain damage that underlies all concussive injuries. Pigray (1609/1642) [47] was the exception, the first to cut the brain and report petechial hemorrhages after concussion: tiny specks of bleeding, especially in the white matter. Such simple anatomical observations could have lain to rest the claim that concussion left no mark on the brain. However, rigorous observation was uncommon, and a few bold innovators tested receptiveness of alternative definitions of the much-abused word. For instance, in 1659 Guy de Chauliac inexplicably confined the term concussion to TBI with good outcome [48]. In 1665, Marchetti applied the term to head injuries producing temporary symptoms [49]. In 1674, Boirel opined that concussive injuries were transient disorders, slight shakes associated with no pathological changes, too minor to perturb blood flow, while (in his opinion) skull fractures invariably did so [50].

1700–1800: Running in Place

In the 18th century, CBI was widely observed, frequently discussed, and poorly understood. As in the previous century, the word *concussion* applied to blows to the head transmitting a shaking force through the skull to the brain, with skull fracture or without; with lacerated, bloody brains or brains that seemed untouched; resulting in brief symptoms, or lasting symptoms, or death [51–53]. This was the era when Littré (1705/1730) [54] (Figure 1.7) published his infamous case of a "young and strong criminal" who, fearing the rack, killed himself by backing up 15 steps and running headlong into the wall of his cell:

Un Criminel jeune & fort, qui devoit éttre roué, voulant prévenir fon jugement, prit fa fecouffe de 15 pieds dans le cachot où il étoit enfermee, & la tête baiffée, les main derriere le dos, alla donner de la tête contre le mur oppofe en courant de toute fa force.

([54], p. 54)

Without belaboring the debate: Littré's autopsy of the head showed no obvious injury, leading him to pronounce that concussion may kill without leaving the slightest gross structural damage. However, as many observers have pointed out, the young fellow may simple have broken his neck.

Authorities gained that position by professing reverence for older authorities – chiefly Hippocrates, Celsus, and Galen – and published as news observations made a millennium past. In 1710 [55], François Pourfour du Petit (not to be confused with Jean Louis Petit) described "A medley of wounds … which include piercings and abrasions from swords and sticks, concussions from falling objects, and damage from deeply penetrating bullets." His main contribution was a repetition of the ancient Hippocratic observation of crossed laterality: "limbs and other moving parts of the body are set in motion by animal spirits supplied from that side of the brain which is opposite to that of the parts moved" ([55], p. 166). Rouhault (1720) [56] (also see Courville (1953) [2] and Morgagni (1761) [57] and (1769) [58]) were two of many to echo the old finding that concussions cause intracranial bleeding.

A related 18th-century rediscovery was that trauma to one side of the head harmed the other side: the contrecoup

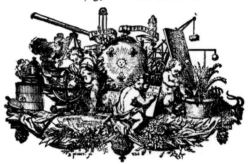

HISTOIRE
DE
L'ACADEMIE
ROYALE
DES SCIENCES.
Année MDCCIV.

Avec les Memoires de Mathematique & de Phyfique,
pour la même Année.
Tirés des Regiftres de cette Academie.

A PARIS,
Chez JEAN BOUDOT, Imprimeur Ordinaire du Roy, & de l'Academie Royale des Sciences, ruë S. Jacques au Soleil d'or, proche la Fontaine S. Severin.
M. DCCVI.
AVEC PRIVILEGE DU ROY.

Fig. 1.7 Title page of the 1730 publication containing Littré's case of 1705. Source: L'Académie Royale des Sciences, 1730 [54]. Complutense University of Madrid

phenomenon. Celsus had discussed this somewhat sooner – at the time when Christ was reportedly living. "It may even happen that the blow may have been upon one part of the head and the fracture at another" (cited by "da Carpi" (1517) [34]). Le Dran (1749) [59] offered a mechanical explanation for this counterintuitive happening: "If the head strikes itself … there always results a commotion of the brain …, because the brain is first directed toward the hard body [skull] and [then] repulsed by it." A more original discovery, noted both by Heister (1719 and 1743 [60]; also see Mettler and Mettler (1945) [20]) and by Jean Louis Petit (1774) [61] was that a blunt or broadly diffused injury that did not fracture the skull could actually do more damage to the brain than a focal injury that broke the skull [61–64]. This notion of diffusion – of potential involvement of the whole brain by a focal impact – was a helpful explanation for link between a loss of consciousness and a fall, since brains mediate not just awareness but also anti-gravity muscle tone. London surgeon William Beckett (1739) [65], for instance, wrote:

To explain the cause of the person's falling to the ground immediately on the reception of the blow, we ought to observe, that the blow caused violent commotio of the whole brain, and so consequently put the spirits into great confusion and disorder, which making irregular incursions into several parts of the body, without direction of the will, could not be confined to the nerves, whose office it was to distribute them to the muscles that keep the body in erect posture; for which reason the machine must unavoidably fall to the ground.

Heister and Petit's comment that the skull moderates the mechanics of the distribution of the impact force is potentially important to interpreting experimental concussion: many laboratories still employ the lateral fluid percussion model, which involves a craniectomy followed by a direct bang to the dura. This skull-less model may not validly reproduce CBI, in which skull injury not only disperses but also absorbs forces that might otherwise cause brain injury. Le Dran made this very point as early as 1749 ([59]; translated by Courville [2]), lamenting, "When the head is struck with violence by a hard body, it is a pity that the skull is able to very strongly resist without breaking." (This, by the way, is one reason modern American football helmets are so effective at defending brains from fractures yet so disappointing at preventing concussions: the human skull evolved to absorb the force of blows, like the crumple zone of an automobile. Interfere with that useful fracture and you may enhance the force of CBI.)

The actual pathophysiological effect of concussions on brains remained unknown. And, as in the 17th century, a handful of 18th-century writers (e.g., Kirkland, 1792 [66]) adopted the linguistic oddity of referring to concussions as mild or reversible. Yet Pott (1768) [14] was clear that concussions varied in severity, having seen cases of temporary nuisance and fatal intracranial bleeding. Perhaps his most telling remark was to point out the fact that the use of the word *concussion* had become corrupt, and his emphasis that the physical effects remained utterly mysterious:

Many of our ancestors, when no fracture was discoverable in the cranium of a person laboring under such symptoms as have been mentioned … in consequence of violence offered to the head, contented themselves with calling the case a concussion; and although they had no very precise idea annexed to the term, yet they seldom went farther for a solution; like teeth and worms in infants, or like nerves in women, it satisfied ignorant inquirers.

([14], p. 231)

The main dispute was about the reason that concussion rendered victims unconscious. Was it the bleeding of the brain, or, conversely, a sudden lack of blood flow? Was it the shaking itself, the pressure in the spinal fluid, or the tiny hemorrhages seen after shaking? Heister (1743) [60] favored the bleeding hypothesis: "Concussion of the Brain from a Fall or a Blow, without receiving any external hurt," the patient will "lie senseless, as if he were in a profound Sleep; Reason in this case will easily inform us, that there is an Extravasation of Blood in the Cavity of the Cranium." Manne (1729) championed the theory that concussion caused its evil by stopping the flow of blood [67]. Le Dran (1749) [59] and Petit (1774) [53] argued

that, since unconsciousness followed whether or not there was a skull fracture and whether or not there was bleeding in the brain, the underlying problem was brain shaking. Morgagni (1761 [57]/1769 [58]) was clear that the vessels of the brain "may be ruptur'd by concuffions" (p. 46). But which vessels? Dease (1776) [68] came closest at divining the truth: as Pigray had seen a century before, the real problem was that shaking caused bleeding in *small vessels*.

Such systematic observations were rare. Dissections were mostly superficial; experiments almost unknown. Like their forebears, 18th-century anatomists hoped that cutting up bodies and glancing about would suffice to reveal cause of disease. The microscope, widely available at the time, was not applied. In despair of uncovering the mechanism of head injury, on April 10, 1766 the French Academy offered a prize for whoever first explained contrecoup [63]. Benjamin Bell summarized the state of the art as of 1788:

Every affection of the head attended with stupefaction, when it appears as the immediate consequence of external violence, and when no mark of injury is discovered, is in general supposed to proceed from commotion or concussion of the brain; by which is meant such a derangement of this organ as obstructs its natural and usual functions, without producing such obvious effects on it, as to render it incapable of having its real nature ascertained by dissection.

([69], p. 132) (Figure 1.8)

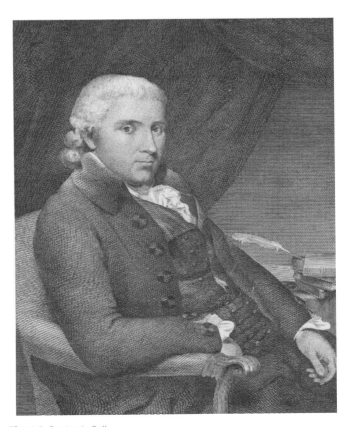

Fig. 1.8 Benjamin Bell.
Source: William and I. Walker; after Sir Henry Raeburn. Benjamin Bell, 1749–1806. Surgeon. National Galleries of Scotland. Purchased 1950

1800–1900: A Certain Undefinable Something, or Cause of Evil

A man receives a blow on the head, by which he is only stunned for a longer or shorter period. What is said to have happened? Concussion of the brain. A man dies instantaneously, or lingers some time after an injury to the head; there are no marks of external violence. Again, what is said to have happened? Concussion of the brain.

(Hewett, 1858 [70])

Leaping to the dénouement: most work on concussion in the 1800s was a perseverative – more publications of cases dressed up by guesswork about biological processes. However, by the tail end of the 19th century, three innovations changed the story of CBI forever. Two shed light. The third slung mud:

1. Neuroscience at last employed the experimental method, concussing the heads of unfortunate animals and looking for change.
2. The microscope, long available, was finally focused on thin slices of brains.
3. The tenebrous concept of hysterical neurosis became a topic of hyperventilating declarations.

As they had during the preceding 200 years, 19th-century neurologists defined concussion as a blow to the head that shakes the brain, causing a wide range of effects [71, 72]. Many more cases were published citing concussion without depressed skull fracture or brain bleeding as the cause of death (often called "pure" or "uncomplicated" concussion) [22, 70, 73–82].

And yet, as implied by Hewett's quote (above) there were minor cases as well. John Erichsen (1853) [6] may have been the first to suggest a sensible reconciliation of the extreme view that concussions are benign with the global observation that they were not: he submitted that concussion has both *typical* outcomes (i.e., resolution after several days) and *atypical* outcomes with persistent or permanent symptoms – perhaps history's first expression of the concept some now call "the miserable minority." Concussion could occur as an isolated insult, or, as Hunter explained in 1835, occur in combination with compression, wounds, and inflammation [83]. Bryant [1888] [84] poignantly captured this diversity of effects, alerting students that, however doctors chose to divvy up injuries with diagnostic terms, concussion was at the root of all brain trauma:

students are taught to think that scalp wounds, fractures of the skull, hemorrhage beneath the bone, concussion and compression of the brain, and inflammation of the brain are separate and independent affections … Yet in all these different classes of cases there is one common injury, one common source of danger, present or remote – viz., the condition of the brain which is associated with the injury, and which has been brought about by the "stunning" force.

British surgeon John Hunter (1835) [83] agreed: the concussive element of a brain injury is the most important, even when the doctor is distracted by skull fracture or bleeding: "When there is depression of bone or extravasation, the symptoms of concussion are lost, though it may be at the bottom of all" ([83], p. 488). As Ommaya (1966) [85] commented, "This statement brings out very clearly the important fact that *the basic problem of head injuries is concussion* [emphasis added]". Moreover, some authorities were aware of long-lasting, disabling post-concussion changes. "In some cases the symptoms of concussion are but slight," wrote Erichsen in 1853 [6], "but major events follow."

This consensus, however, failed to answer the question: *how does shaking hurt the brain?* As Duplay (1882) [80] worded it, "To what anatomical condition does this set of symptoms correspond?" (p. 254). Dissections continued to reveal the same confounding diversity of results: gross bleeding and laceration, tiny specks of blood, or nothing at all. Abernethy (1811) [86] discussed this spectrum of pathology: "I know from examination, that the substance of the brain is sometimes lacerated and disorganized in violent concussions. I have, however, examined other cases of fatal concussions, without observing any such lesion of the substance of the brain" (p. 56). So did Guthrie and Bryant and others. The relevance of the skull was abandoned as a host of empirical observations confirmed Dr. Bell's prescient instinct that the symptoms and outcomes of concussion were associated with damaged nervous tissue. Yet, at mid-century, the real cause of underlying brain damage was still no more sophisticated than "shaking." Hunter [83], for example, attributed bad outcome to "displacement or alteration of the texture of some parts of the brain" (p. 487). Guthrie (1842) [71] was even less specific:

By the term concussion of the Brain, a certain undefinable something, or cause of evil which cannot be demonstrated, is understood to have taken place; … The term concussion is very aptly and forcibly illustrated by the homely but striking expression of our sister country, when a man has been killed by a fall on the head, "that the life has been shook out of him".

([71], p. 7)

Still, dissectors routinely confirmed Pigray's discovery (at some point prior to publication in 1615) [47] of tiny specks of bleeding, "petechial hemorrhages." In 1829, Chassaignac reported examined a sailor's brain after a fatal case of "pure concussion." Chassaignac published that case in 1842. According to one English translation from the French, he described the brain as exhibiting "very minute, miliary, sanguineous extravasations." He is quoted as having opined that "such miliary effusions, insufficient to produce the symptoms of compression [increased intracranial pressure], might give rise to those of concussion; and that such appearances were very likely to be overlooked in autopsies" [87]. Bright (1831) [88], Holmes (1876) [89], and Duret (1878) [90] all found the same. The tininess of these specks, the absence of other changes, and the growing awareness of the little things revealed by microscopy inspired multiple authorities to speculate, in essence: concussion physically damages the brain, but that damage is often too small to see. As Duplay (1882) [80] put it: "The lesions are rather overlooked or escape our means of detection." In fact, as early as 1828, Brodie [74] wrote:

the brain and its coverings appear to be perfect in all their parts; so that the most accurate anatomist can discover nothing different from the natural appearance of these organs … We are not however justified in the conclusion that there is therefore in reality no organic injury … if we consider that the ultimate structure of the brain is on so minute a scale that our senses are incapable of detecting it, it is evident that there may be changes and alterations of structure, which our senses are incapable of detecting also.

Erichsen (1853) [6], Duplay (1882) [80], Obersteiner (1879) [91], and Kocher (1892 [92], 1896 [93]) all echoed that wisdom, predicting the discovery of cellular and even molecular impact of concussive force. The problem was proving it.

Experimental Concussion

At the same time, enthusiasm grew for testing theories about disease by experiments. Jean-Pierre Gama, a former battlefield surgeon, published his *Treatise of Head Injuries and of Encephalitis in which Many Questions Concerning the Functions of the Nervous System are Discussed* in 1830 [63, 94]. He placed slender wires in a glass vessel, filled it with warm isinglass, and allowed it to cool. The result was a gelatinous mass approximating the elasticity of the brain. Percussion made the wires vibrate visibly – thought to be confirmation of the ancient theory that concussion shakes the brain. Gama concluded: "fibres as delicate as those of which the organ of mind is composed are liable to break as a result of violence to the head." One hundred years later, Gama's guess was shown to be correct. Alquié, on the other hand, filled vessels with gelatin, struck them, yet failed to see a shift of the components, concluding that the theory of disturbance of the molecules must be abandoned [95]. This primitive experiment aside, Alquié's conclusions were quite modern. Lane (1896) [77] summarized Alquié's position: "From concussion one or many functions of the head, or parts dependent on it, may be impaired or annulled, and this disturbance may be brief or long lasting" (p. 226).

Most experimentalists, however, turned to vivisection. Dogs, cats, and rabbits were favorite involuntary contributors to that new work. Thus, Fano "instituted experiments, which consisted in suddenly killing dogs by a blow on the head" [78, 80, 87]. He found hemorrhages in six of eight cases and concluded (rather preposterously based on his sample size) "that the morbid condition, designated by the name of concussion of the brain, is a pure creation of the mind" ([78], pp. 366–367). Duret (1878) [90] better limned the typical clinical picture of concussion by sudden injections of fluid into the skull. "The dog was killed immediately afterward, and at autopsy was found an enormous dilatation of the aqueduct of Sylvius" [73, 80]. These results prompted Duret to surmise that "at the moment of a fall on the head, or a blow to the skull, a wave of liquid forms about the cerebral hemispheres and in the ventricles, which distributes the shock to all points throughout the central nervous system" (translation, Goodwin (1989) [96]). Duret's 1878 report inspired Duplay's supremely confident conclusion four years later (1882) [80]: "We can, then, no longer deny the displacement and exaggerated tension of the cerebro-spinal fluid" as the underlying cause of concussive symptoms. "[T]here would seem to exist no possible objection

to this doctrine of the mechanism of cerebral concussion." And yet, for all his presumption about this incorrect mechanism, Duplay, in the end, was exactly right: "The persistent troubles of intelligence, motion and sensibility are due to some material destruction of the parts."

Other investigators were more careful in their observations and more circumspect in their reportage. Famously, in 1874 Koch and Filehne [97] published the results of moderated repeated blows: "The skulls of dogs were hammered with a percussion hammer, weighing from 250 to 500 grammes, until unconsciousness and the other symptoms of cerebral concussions were present" [98], p. 165). The dogs became befuddled but lived. Upon sacrifice, dissection revealed no large-scale anatomical lesions, yet the impact on function was glaringly apparent. This seems to have been the first experimental demonstration that repetitive moderate concussions cause both lasting disability and brain degeneration. Despite this evidence, both effects are debated to this day.

The Arrival of the Microscope: Long Delayed but Brilliantly Disruptive

As noted previously, beginning about 1674 a growing chorus of authorities – including Boirel (1674) [50], Bohn (1694; see Duplay [80]); Heister (1743) [60]; La Faye (1761) [99], Brodie (1828) [74], Baudens (1836) [100], Erichsen (1853) [6], Obersteiner (1879) [91], and Kocher (1901) [101] – all opined that the reason brains sometimes looked intact after concussive injury, even fatal injury, was simply because the damage is *too tiny to see*. What delayed the use of a microscope? Zacharias Jansen had built his 9-power compound microscope in the 1590s! Anton van Leeuwenhoek's vast improvement was good for 270-power. Carefully sketching what he saw, Robert Hooke published his *Micrographia* in 1665 [102] (Figure 1.9).

Since this thrilling device was being widely used to explore the little things in nature starting in the 1660s, why were neurologists still speculating about microscopic brain damage 200 years later, rather than simply looking?

The answer is: neurons are hard to see. Brain scholars slowly gained facility with fixing, cutting, and staining brain slices in the mid 19th century. Ehrenberg first saw cortical fibers in 1833 [103]. Using the much-improved achromatic microscope, Baillarger described the layers of the cortex in 1840 [104] and Berlin noted the remarkable orderliness of neurons, like soldiers on parade, in 1858 (cited in [105]). Meynert vowed to "raise psychiatry to a scientific discipline by means of anatomical fundamentals" (cited in [106]), employing his Zeiss microscope to count the layers of the cortex and follow white-matter tracts [107]. It was also in 1872 that Ukrainian neurologist Vladamir Betz, through laborious experimentation, finally devised a method of hardening and slicing up the brain that permitted a stunningly better view of the pyramidal neuron in gorgeous carmine red [108–111] (Figure 1.10).

Just a year later (1873) [112], Golgi hit upon his silver staining method, unveiling the fine structure of a neuron and its intriguing arboreal projections in basic black (Figure 1.11).

45

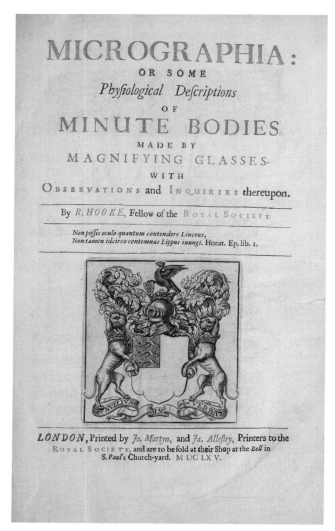

Fig. 1.9 Title page, Hooke's *Micrographia*.
Source: Hooke, 1665 [102]. By permission of Llyfrgell Genedlaethol Cymru / National Library of Wales

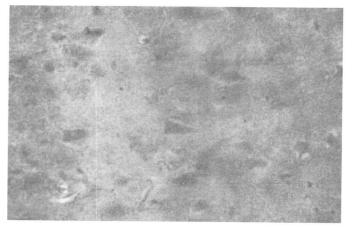

Fig. 1.10 A modern photomicrograph of one of Betz's original slides. [A black and white version of this figure will appear in some formats. For the color version, please refer to the plate section.]
Source: Kushchayev et al., 2011 [105]. By permission of Oxford University Press

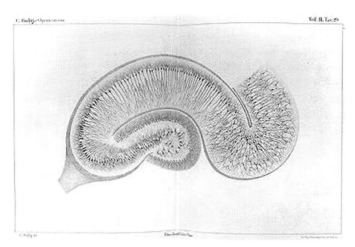

Fig. 1.11 Golgi's free-hand drawing of the hippocampus.
Source: Golgi C. *Opera Omnia Vol II* 1883–1902 [113]

This was a highly disruptive technology. Until then, anatomists held sway, perhaps nursing the understandable pride that only they could uncover the mysteries of disease. Betz boldly took them to task, admonishing that people with microscopes were about to rattle their husky laurels:

> Anatomy should not be considered a completed descriptive or the only applied scientific discipline having the honor to serve medical practice; it is a thing described by a well-known speech of Hamlet to Horatio: "There are more things in heaven and earth, Horatio, Than are dreamt in your philosophy".
>
> [111]

The dam was breached and a flood of information about the tiny changes wrought by brain injury flooded into the literature. Candidly, these discoveries have yet to be granted their due, as a vocal clique continues to resist the fact that CBI lastingly changes the structure of the brain. Yet by the turn of the 20th century it became harder and harder to trumpet that view, as the microscopic findings poured in. Witkowski (1877) [114] may have been the first. To test the theory that concussive injury does its damage by producing anemia of the brain, he first extracted the hearts from his subjects. "[H]e used frogs which he stunned by hitting their heads against a table. After a few time this produced permanent changes such as unsteadiness weakness, and lack of will power" [115], p. 183). (The method used to measure frog will power was not described.) Microscopic examination showed the usual petechial hemorrhages (showing that anemia was not the way concussion hurts brains), but Witkowski could see little more because he had no stains. The German experimentalist Schmaus led the way in that domain in 1890:

> He tied animals to a board and struck repeated heavy blows on the board. Afterward he was able to show widespread degenerations in the nervous system.
>
> (Ingvar 1923 [7], p. 269)

Two years later Alexander Miles asked, "What is the ultimate cause of the symptoms in so-called cases of concussion of the brain?" [76]. He knew that Duret had forcefully injected fluid in 1877, but he doubted that that was a good way to imitate a blow to the skull: "however similar the results in the two cases may be, I cannot admit that the means of producing these are so nearly comparable as M. Duret would appear to indicate" ([76], p. 167). For that reason, Miles resorted to simplicity, pounding on the skulls of human cadavers with wooden mallets and the heads of living rabbits with "the knob of a Kaffir stick"(the fearsome Zulu knobkerrie war-club). Under the microscope, in addition to the well-known petechial hemorrhages he found "collections of colloid bodies, patches of military sclerosis, and chromatolysis and vacuolation of nerve cells." That is, not only cellular but *subcellular* changes were observed (Figure 1.12).

Scagliosi (1898) [116] and Luzenberger (1898) [117] reported similar findings after repeated blows to animals' heads. MacPherson [81] found the same in two cases of fatal human concussion. For example, a 17-year-old boy was struck with a rock by another lad, developing a headache and then becoming "maniacal." He died. Post-mortem examination:

> revealed a fissure fracture a little to the left of the occipital protuberance. There was no depression, no meningitis, and no effusion; nor was there laceration of the brain, or hemorrhage into any part … This, then, is an uncomplicated case of cerebral concussion, which corresponds to Duret's description of fatal concussion.
>
> ([81], p. 1129)

Tillman (1899) [118] discussed a fascinating clue that helps explain why CBI produces behavioral problems such as memory loss and irritability: concussive force is undemocratic, selectively harming some types of neurons while sparing others. The same year Rosenblath [119] had the unusual opportunity of examining the brain of a 17-year-old tightrope walker who had lived for eight months after his concussion. That means the brain reflected the long-term effects of CBI. His key finding was widespread degeneration of the white matter. This not only confirmed Tillman's guess that some brain parts suffer much more than others when the brain is shaken, but also the keen naked-eye finding of 200 years before: tiny post-concussion hemorrhages reliably assail the white matter (especially in the corpus callosum).

And, in a little-cited but thoughtful paper by Skae (1894) [120], the author expressed the core principle of modern neuropsychiatry: all behavioral problems are mediated by brain changes. Dr. Skae examined 70 brains of insane persons from the Stirling District Asylum: 56 (80%) showed nuclear vacuolization. The very same microscopic change, nuclear vacuolization, had been described by Miles and MacPherson in concussion and by Bevan Lewis in epilepsy. As Skae saw it, they had collectively discovered the common underlying brain change in three types of neurobehavioral distress! Moreover, Skae could explain cases of recovery. In a prescient insight, he guessed that the brain tries to *repair itself* after concussion, and he thought he saw the proof: "The discharge of oil from the nuclei, and its presence in spider cells … are obviously an attempt at repair" ([120], p. 1076).

Of course, these were mostly conclusions from fatal concussions. Common sense would predict a spectrum of pathological injury. From the assault of a feather to an anvil, one expects to find some threshold before which the result is life, beyond which is death. Bryant (1888) [84] was one of several authorities who indeed predicted that the brain changes differ in concussions that are more or less severe.

> [A]ny force of a diffused nature, directly or indirectly applied, and whether causing a fracture of the cranium or not, more likely brings about some structural change in the cerebral tissue … when the vibrations are feeble, the injury to the brain structure resulting therefrom is but slight; when they are severe, the mischief may be great.

Yet how could one show that "feeble vibrations" caused "slight" injury to the brain structure? One perhaps required a laboratory apparatus more subtle than a war hammer.

The Traumatic Impact of Traumatic Neurosis

Hysteria (from the Greek for uterus) was hardly new in the 19th century. Doctors had long since agreed that uteri have morbid effects on the brains of women. Bright (1831) [88] exemplified the manly insight of his time:

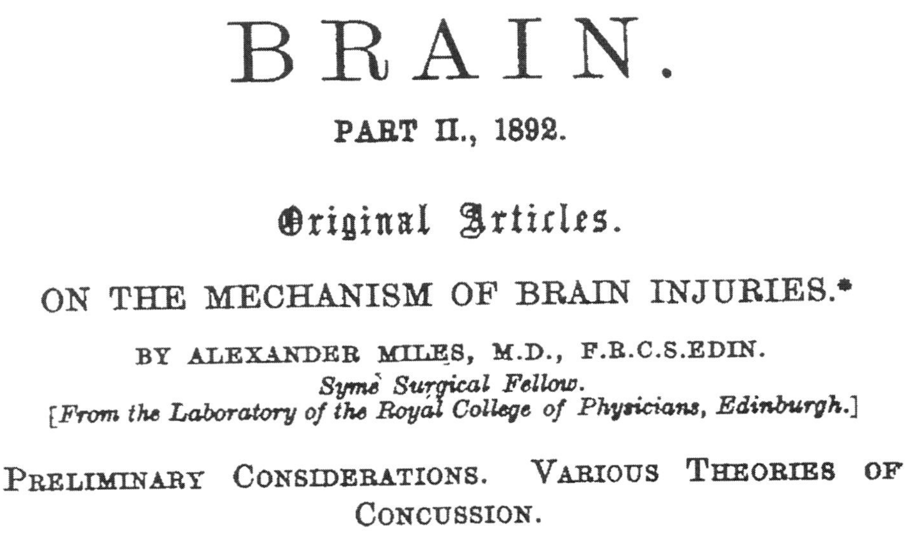

Fig. 1.12 Alexander Miles's report on the pathophysiology of concussion, 1892.

Source: Miles, 1892 [76]. By permission of Oxford University Press

BRAIN.

PART II., 1892.

Original Articles.

ON THE MECHANISM OF BRAIN INJURIES.*

BY ALEXANDER MILES, M.D., F.R.C.S.EDIN.
Syme Surgical Fellow.
[*From the Laboratory of the Royal College of Physicians, Edinburgh.*]

PRELIMINARY CONSIDERATIONS. VARIOUS THEORIES OF CONCUSSION.

Mrs. M., at the age of 74, became the subject of most decided and violent nymphomania ... as rendered it necessary on several occasions to subject her to personal restraint ... the case is interesting as showing a state of the uterus, which was no doubt chiefly instrumental in determining the character of the mental disease ... and no one who is accustomed to hear a description of the varied sufferings of women ... will for a moment feel surprised at any list of ailments, which may accompany its morbid actions.

([88], pp. 465–466)

How, exactly, did Dr. Bright and his worthy colleagues think the uterus drove women insane? "With regard to the actual condition of the nervous system, we know nothing but from the symptoms."

Surely some doctors of that era despaired at the absurdity of this theory. However, the clinical issue is important and unresolved: why do some people complain of symptoms for which we seem to lack an organic explanation or feel tempted to infer a psychic one? This chapter is not the place to attempt a resolution. Chapters 5, 7, and 10 will address the issue in more depth. Yet, about 1880, the history of medical thinking about CBI became irretrievably mixed up with psychiatric growth pangs. Three factors conspired:

1. the rise of the railroads
2. the innovation of workers' compensation
3. the debates of psychodynamic theorists.

Railroads flourished in the mid 19th century. In the United States, the golden spike connected the Central and Union Pacific Railroads into the first transcontinental railroad in 1869. By that time, in both Europe and the Americas, one downside of this modern convenience was becoming apparent. Trains crashed. Railway workers were especially prone to catastrophic trauma. In 1899, President Harrison stated,

> It is a reproach to our civilization that any class of American workmen, should in the pursuit of a necessary and useful vocation, be subjected to a peril of life and limb as great as that of a soldier in time of war [121].

Injuries among survivors were diverse. Many involved the brain, although the most common complaint was "railway spine."

The problem was that some patients had indisputably broken parts while others did not. Savory (1870) [122] described the syndrome:

> After a collision, different persons are found in different degrees of collapse without perhaps any visible injury of local lesions. The condition is referred to as concussion, not of the nerve-centres only, but of the whole system – to shock of both "body and mind".

([122], p. 771)

Owners or insurers of railroads were obliged to compensate identifiable injuries. Owners or insurers understandably questioned the syndrome – in those lacking gross bodily derangements – as likely simulation. Doctors faced the difficult task of sorting out how much of a patient's post-traumatic distress was due to crushed tissue and how much due to the

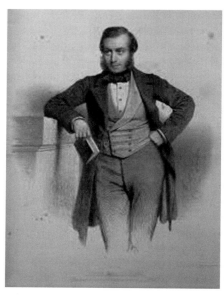

Fig. 1.13 Sir John Eric Erichsen (1818–1896).
Source: Lithograph by C. Baugniet, 1853. Wellcome Collection

residua of terror. (Indeed, medical science has yet to divine a meaningful discriminatory algorithm for so-called organic versus so-called psychological trauma.) Litigation exploded, courts were obliged to arbitrate, and professional expert witnesses found gainful employment. Among these was John Erichsen (Figure 1.13).

In 1866 Erichsen published his book *On Railway and Other Injuries of the Nervous System* [4], distinguishing between concussion of the spine, concussion of the brain, and hysteria (although his sexist thoughts may draw a smile today; see below). On both sides of the Atlantic, a somewhat impolitic debate broke out between those who attributed the physical and mental distress of survivors of railway collisions to organic disease of the nervous system (e.g., Erichsen, 1866 [4], 1883 [5]; Putnam, 1883 [123]; Walton, 1883 [124]; Friedmann, 1892 [125]) and those who largely dismissed this syndrome as hysteria, neurosis, or malingering (e.g., Hodges, 1881 [126]; Page, 1883 [127]; Charcot, 1889 [128]; Gray, 1893 [129]; also see [130–133]). Many authorities point to this era as the first time when large numbers of people were exposed to a new concept – one that remains a source of contention: post-traumatic stress disorder (PTSD).

Regarding workers' compensation: modernity was born in Prussia. Otto von Bismarck, competing with Marxists for popularity and witnessing good workers waving farewell as they steamed west to the American dream, sought worker loyalty. He recognized that German workers despaired of receiving aid should they become hurt on the job. "The real grievance of the worker is the insecurity of his existence." At his insistence, in 1884, the Reichstag passed his "Worker's Accident Insurance" program – a mandate to rescue injured laborers from abject poverty and offer hope via rehabilitation [134]. Very soon thereafter, in 1893, the U.S. Department of Labor delivered its report titled *Compulsory Insurance in Germany* [135]– apparently intending to shame Congress into action. By 1911, impatient with Washington's inertia, the states began passing their own workers' compensation laws.

So as the 19th century drew to its roaring conclusion, courts and agencies played a new role in concussive injury. They dispensed proportional liability. And yet two barriers blocked the way, and still block the way, to devising the best and fairest interventions for victims of concussions. One: the ancient, hopeless debate about where to draw the line between bodily and psychological trauma. Two: the pitiful reality of malingering. Unfortunately, both the flowering of litigation for neurological injuries and the evolution of workers' rights had a perverse effect: if you offer money for exhibiting signs of disability, some people who are healthy, or little harmed, will exhibit what they think are signs of disability. In Harvard neurologist Massaquoi's pithy epigram, "truth bends in proximity to money"(personal communication). How then were doctors at the cusp of the new century to accurately diagnose CBI versus psychic pain versus unreconstructed sociopathy?

Psychiatry might have helped, had it not been splintering into a rivalry between scientists and non-scientists. Charcot insisted that medical complaints without obvious causes are "hysteria." Oppenheim insisted that an injury such as concussion that does not leave gross anatomical wounds might nonetheless damage the brain. (As we will see, this was just the tip of an iceberg. The Charcot versus Oppenheim debate reached its full fury during the first third of the 20th century.) "Hysteria" was not a general term in those early days. It meant something specific, antique, and misogynistic. Here is Erichsen (1866) [4] on railway spine, exhorting readers to use the term properly:

Hysteria … is a disease of women rather than of men, of the younger rather than the middle-aged and old, of people of an excitable, imaginative, or emotional disposition rather than of hard-headed, active, practical men of business. … Does this in any way resemble what we see in "concussion of the spine"? … is it reasonable to say that such a man has suddenly become "hysterical," like a love-sick girl? Or is this term not rather employed merely to cloak a want of precise knowledge …?

([4], p. 93)

Yes to that. A want of precise knowledge beclouded the issue of CBI at the end of the 19th century, as it does today. Lane (1894 [3], p. 48) summarized that century's conclusion about concussion:

It is caused by some external violence which communicates vibration, oscillation, or minute movement to the anatomic elements of the parts acted upon. In the causation, all observers agree; but what occurs in the constituent elements of the parts affected can not be said to be as yet satisfactorily settled.

Clarity at the Very Cusp of the New Century

Now well supplied with microscopes, stains, animal models, and a relatively clear concept of concussion, between 1890 and 1905 neuroscientists began building on this robust experimental foundation. The most enticing target for researchers was to find out whether the brain changes seen after lethal concussion also occurred in the much commoner, milder cases.

Recall that, prior to 1895, few animal experimenters or human dissectors were examining brains of CBI survivors. They simply waited for, or caused, the death of their subjects. They then documented the immediate acute effects of lethal concussions. This produced what is probably the single greatest gap in our knowledge of CBI: what happens to survivors? Do their brains get better? Worse? Both? (The latter, we know now, is correct.) This remains a knotty research task today. To view microscopic changes one must dissect the brain. But to view the changes of *non-lethal* concussion requires caring for the hammered dogs, rabbits, and guinea pigs for weeks or months before cutting their brains – or chancing upon a human who survives concussion only to die later and be quickly collected by a hovering pathologist. Given that stumbling block, how could anyone figure out what goes on in the heads of those who are walking and talking one year, or 50 years, after a CBI? How can we explain why some feel fine, some don't, some carry on with little trouble, and others become disabled?

At the very cusp of the century, an open-minded cohort of new investigators sought that answer. Bikeles (1895) [136], Luzenberger (1897 [137], 1898 [117]), Kirchgasser (1898) [138], Jakob (1912) [139], Tscherbak (1898) [140], Cornil (1921) [141] and others subjected animals to "mild to moderate" experimental concussions. They employed creative methods to rattle the brain without fracturing the skull, including strapping the subject to a plank and hitting the plank [142], applying a vibrating device [143] or decapitating a living mouse and promptly spinning its head at 4000 revolutions per minute [7]. Unlike their predecessors, they allowed the subject to live on for weeks or months before sacrifice. "These authors have studied chiefly the changes that exist some time after the traumatism," as Ingvar summarized. "They have then been able to show degenerative processes affecting cells, nerve fibers and glia" ([7], p. 269).

Similar changes were soon observed in humans. Mott (1917) [144] cut the brains of two soldiers who had died of "shell shock" with no external injuries. In both cases, microscopic examination revealed widespread chromatolysis and white-matter hemorrhages. Tanzi and Lugaro (1914) [145] summarized cases of people who lived on after concussions with persistent mental problems they called "dementia traumatica": "One must admit that following trauma there may be localized gross lesions or mild diffuse lesions following which a chronic process of gliosis and degeneration of nerve cells take place" (Osnato and Giliberti, 1927 [146], p. 187).

The clinical definition of concussion remained the same at the turn of the century. Walter B. Cannon (1901) [147], like his forebears, considered concussion a perturbation of the brain caused by external force that can produce a wide spectrum of effects. He was aware that some writers were troubled by the idea that a concussive injury had such widely varying effects. Moreover, some doctors seem eager to narrow the definition of a disease to match their personal practice experience, or to divide one disease into subtypes they perceived to be different. Hutchinson (1867) [72], for instance, had proposed limiting the use of *concussion* to the "pure" cases and wanted all concussions with bleeding to be considered "not concussion." Cannon, in contrast, urged fidelity to the term's straightforward, artless

49

meaning – a blow with varying effects. To those who wished to define away cases with bleeding from the domain of concussion, he diplomatically proposed that CBI without severe hemorrhage or brain laceration might be called "simple concussion." More importantly, Cannon may have been the first English writer to fully appreciate the implications of the new microscopic findings: concussion might cause neurodegeneration. That is, you may survive your CBI. You may live on. But you could be affected later in life: "progress of the developing necrosis may be slow and diffusion occur gradually" ([72], p. 199).

Advances were also made integrating neurology with psychiatry. Very similar injuries seemed to yield very dissimilar outcomes. No one knew why, but psychological factors seemed plausible. Laudably, some neuropsychiatrists of that era dismissed the growing organic/psychological dichotomy and instead acknowledged the inevitability of interaction and overlap between a traumatic blow to the head, changes in the brain, and effects on the emotions. Thus we have Obersteiner's sensible comment in 1896: "In the majority of apparently truly organic nervous diseases there is also a functional, psychical factor" [148]. Meyer (1904) [149] was more specific. He listed the two effects of "concussion and actual direct traumatisms":

1. "the direct focal and the more diffuse destruction of the nerve tissue …
2. the distinctly diffuse commotions in which the general reaction and the psychic elements predominate, including the remote reactive results of exaggerations of vasomotor and emotional responsiveness".

([149], p. 374)

In other words, early neuropsychiatrists said: (1) the rattling blow of concussion can change emotions; and (2) the mentally upsetting experience of that injury can change emotions. Meyer expressed the resulting dilemma, "how difficult it is to say what symptoms are to be accounted for by the trauma and what others by the mental shock and the effects of the consequences" ([149], p. 424). That thorny problem has yet to be resolved, but at the least, the neuropsychiatric approach began to appear in the medical literature: if you change the brain, you change the mind.

Thus, at the outset of the 20th century, an evolved and persuasive scientific narrative was widely embraced: a person suffers a head injury. Concussive force causes microscopic brain damage (and sometimes other troubles such as skull fracture or brain bleeding). Those brain changes tend to alter emotions and behavior, whether for a minutes or years. At the same time, the stressful life experience of personal injury also alter emotions and behavior. The combination of these factors explains the clinical spectrum doctors had seen since before Hippocrates – from complete recovery, to long-term disability, to death.

It was a brief, gratifying moment of clarity. What followed was a shame.

1900–1925: The Decline and Fall of a Coherent Idea

As we come into the first part of the 20th century the clinical syndrome of concussion as we understand it today was well established. The complaints of later symptoms,

however, were generally regarded as either neurotic or malingering, especially when litigation was involved.

(Wrightson, 2000 [150])

the major part of the literature dealing with such head injuries in which no evidence of fracture can be found, is of an essentially polemic nature, and practically useless.

(Mettler and Mettler, 1945 [20], p. 5)

In 1956, neuropathologist Sabrina Strich publicly lamented the inconsistent concept and superficial investigation of concussion. "[E]xperimenters have been mainly interested in concussion which is supposed to be either fatal or reversible, and not in mechanisms of brain injury which may leave neurological sequelae" [151]. In other words, the word *concussion* had assumed an incoherent identity. The puzzling notion that concussion either leads to complete recovery or immediate death seems as reasonable as a claim that bacterial meningitis either leads to complete recovery or death; it does not seem concordant either with scientific discovery or common sense.

No writers questioned that malingering occurs. No writers questioned that psychic distress may occur absent TBI. The unresolved questions were: (1) which of the structural brain changes seen after concussion are the most important for producing symptoms? (2) how long do organically mediated symptoms persist after concussion? and (3) is persistence common or rare? For historians of science, another question may be equally worthy of investigation: why did neurology deviate from a relatively well-established understanding of concussion in the 1920s? How did this new idea of concussion gain currency – that concussion either killed or had no effect – ignoring the wide range of outcomes that would have been apparent to many hominid observers for perhaps a million years? What happened between 1900 – when concussive injury was well known to produce a spectrum of clinical and pathological effects, including long-term behavioral change and microscopic brain lesions – and mid-century? Why did the concept of concussion become so beclouded? The story is fascinating, and a bit tragic. To preview: three remarkable changes occurred in Northwestern Europe and the United States early in the first half of the 20th century:

1. There was a rapid increase in CBIs.
2. For the first time in history, people were offered money for being (or for seeming to be) disabled.
3. Psychological explanations for physical distress blossomed in popularity.

The sum of these factors, we think, led to unfortunate consequences.

Factor 1: A Rapid Increase in CBIs

The question whether post-concussive symptoms were due to brain pathology or emotional frailty took on added urgency because of two historic developments. One: in 1901 early adopters could buy a three-horsepower Oldsmobile for $650. Mr. Ford invited risk takers to try his Model T in 1908. At that point, automobiles began their ascendancy over railways as a leading generator of TBI. Two: in the summer

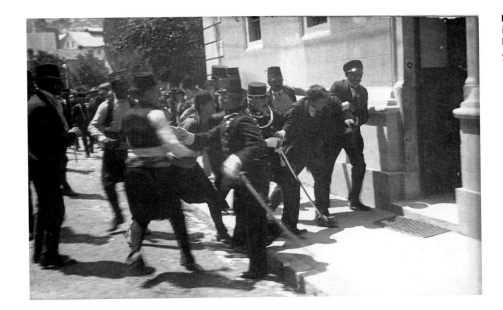

Fig. 1.14 The arrest of Gavrilo Princip immediately after the assassination of Archduke Franz Ferdinand and his wife Sophie.[1]

Source: Popperfoto/Getty Images

of 1914, 19-year-old extremist Gavrilo Princip shot Franz Ferdinand and his wife Sophie in Sarajevo. (It was actually the second assassination attempt on the Archduke that day) (Figure 1.14).

Global havoc and World War I ensued. Thus, in a matter of a few years, railways, autos, 7.92-mm Mauser Gewehr 98 rifles, and other weapons simultaneously added dramatically to the incidence of Western CBI. The widespread exposure to high explosives precipitated a tendentious debate about whether "shell shock" is an organic disorder due to brain commotion, or a mere "functional" disorder – nigh unto reprobate character.

While prehistoric hominids clearly targeted one another's heads, and so did knights and warriors for at least 3000 years, the era from 1900 to 1918 in the Western hemisphere possibly represented the most rapid escalation in closed head injuries to occur on Earth. By 1907 railways became the number one cause of violent death in the United States, reportedly generating more than 12,000 fatal accidents [152]. The automobile, lacking the slightest bow to safe design, supplied physicians with an immense number of cases. And World War I, as just one small element of its unspeakable tragedy, was a manufactory of traumatic exposure. As Walter Schaller had warned in 1918 [153]:

> Industrial insurance and compensation is in effect in many of the states and will ultimately extend to all of them. The war psychoneuroses known as shell shock, which are essentially a group under this heading, must receive attention and disposition in increasing numbers.
>
> ([153], p. 339; Figure 1.15)

The result: larger absolute numbers of CBI patients to deal with – probably more than could be comfortably accommodated by the conventionally trained practitioners of the era.

Factor 2: The Expansion of Payments for Disability

Three forms of compensatory payments marked a dramatic change in the relationship between medicine, economics, and jurisprudence. First came personal injury torts. Such claims were sparsely sprinkled through English common law, and personal injury lawsuits in the United States were rare prior to 1870. In fact, one of the first on record was *Farwell* v. *Boston and Worcester Railroad* (1842) [154, 155]. Thereafter, the rapid growth of the railroads and the expansion of personal injury litigation occurred in parallel. Second, already mentioned, was the German innovation of workers' compensation. Although the U.S. federal government balked at such a progressive idea, the states were less resistant. Wisconsin was the first to pass a law in 1911 and 45 other states followed suit within ten years [134]. Third, in 1917, just as the United States entered World War I, Congress established a novel system of veterans' benefits, including disability compensation administered by what was then called the "Veterans Bureau."

These three initiatives together empowered a volcanic new socioeconomic force. True, some 17th-century pirate captains devised a unique employee loyalty system of monetary compensation for misplaced eyes and limbs. But otherwise, this was a startling change: by 1920, almost for the first time in human history, a person could obtain money for being hurt. Human nature drives the pursuit of advantages. For people with certain temperaments, cheating is a sensible tactic to gain advantages. Personal injury litigation plus workers' compensation laws plus veterans' benefits massively incentivized malingering.

Malingering in the early 20th century not only provoked moral outrage but also represented an authentic threat to the economy. Yet how could the doctor tell who was feigning? Who could read the mind? Humans are known to be energetic, obsessive, but very fallible mind readers. That fact notwithstanding, doctors are routinely asked to determine the "real"

---

[1]   Although often reproduced and titled "Gavrilo Princip captured in Sarjevo in 1914," some scholars believe that this photograph depicts the arrest of Ferdinand Behr, a bystander.

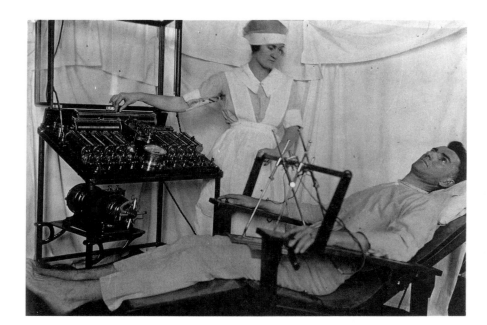

Fig. 1.15 Treating shell shock with Bergonic's electric chair.
Source: Science Photo Library

motives behind a complaint. Understanding that motivation is private and immeasurable, Schaller tried his earnest best to figure out the rate of malingering among 50 carefully studied patients. His conclusion in 1918 may be as close as we can get to the truth: "Although the question of simulation deals particularly with diagnosis, it may be here stated that we have found frank simulation a rare condition, although exaggeration not infrequent" ([153], p. 340).

Factor 3: The Popularity of Psychological Explanations

Dr. Freud, a promising young Viennese neuropathologist, failed to find the mind by peering through his compound achromatic microscope. His reaction was to abdicate his scientific career. He turned to publishing convoluted theories framed as certainties, founding a colorful belief system about the mind. In 1900–1920, his nascent psychoanalytic/psychosexual dynamic movement crept from the intellectual fringe into the mainstream of Western psychiatry [156].

Why would anyone pay attention to such a screed? Despite centuries of clarity regarding the fact that behavior is mediated by the brain, a fervor perpetuated the general public's faith in Descartes's false dichotomy, which fantastically attributed an independent, brain-free existence to the mind (or "soul"). Darwin's discoveries threatened the cozy fantasy of human exceptionalism. Neurobehavioral research was inching close to the third rail, since the findings that all behavior is mediated by the brain were unsettling to those with faith in the spirit. Freud's psychosexual theories found immediate and widespread favor, perhaps in part because they were rather risqué, perhaps because they buttressed the folk belief that physical and mental phenomena must be utterly distinct.

For whatever reason, the burgeoning excitement about psychodynamics had a sorry side-effect on medical diagnosis. It gave physicians a ready answer when they could not figure out the biological problem: it was not biological! (Symonds's

1926 case, discussed below, is illustrative.) When the doctor could not see the cause, he could confidently assign the label "hysterical neurosis." This became a convenient dodge to cover one's ignorance, stigmatize those with emotional distress, and dismiss fears that concussive injuries might be lasting. Schaller (1918) [153] called the syndrome "neurosis following general shock commotion" (p. 338). Many, such as Dercum (1916), believed that pre-morbid psychological frailty was the problem: "It is undoubtedly true that it takes a neurotic disposition to produce a case of traumatic neurosis" [157]. There is a germ of truth here, very worthy of attention. Of course emotions play a role in the response to injury! However, the position of the hysteria extremists may have delayed the rapprochement between neurology and psychiatry for about 50 years.

These three historical factors (increased head injuries, payments for disability, and the popularity of "hysteria") explain a great deal. Set aside the abundant evidence that concussions cause physical brain damage; such subtleties were for professors. When confronted with an employee or citizen or veteran with no obvious physical wound – especially a person who might qualify for monetary compensation – employers, railway or automobile companies, insurers, and the Veterans Bureau all had a strong motivation to find no brain damage. If they could convince the triers of fact that the patient was faking, their problem vanished. Even if some brain damage had indisputably occurred, liable parties had two defensive weapons ready at hand:

1. Declare that the plaintiff has a psychological problem.
2. Declare that the brain injury is "mild."

The British War Office adopted the first defense.

It was 1922. The ghastly, fruitless war was over. Many British soldiers had survived head injuries either from bullets or shrapnel. Others had survived nearby explosions. These two groups got different receptions.

The first group, victims of bullets, was easy to deal with within the framework of surgery and medicine, since a gunshot wound to the head was visible. If the bullet did not penetrate but only grazed the helmet or the bare head, concussion was common. Jefferson (1919) [158] described gunshot wounds of the scalp that rattled the brain. He divided these into "general intracranial upset of a concussional type," which produced symptoms such as headache and vomiting, versus *local* contusions, which produce focal signs. He supported the view that the concussive force causes diffuse brain damage, but that focal injuries can occur as well: "We shall see, in fact, the special signs of a local contusion lifting their heads above the general ruck of signs of the coincident concussion." His language is helpful: "*coincident*." If one strikes the head, Jefferson implies, one expects two simultaneous events. There is a *concussive brain injury*, which is the diffuse effect of any blow transmitted through the skull, and there is sometimes also a *contusion brain injury*, which is a local effect proximate to the point of contact.

So gunshot wounds provoked little debate. Blast exposures did.

Some French neurologists referred to this problem as the wind of explosion ("*vent de l'obus*"), some British authorities as the "zone of brisance" [7, 159]. Whatever the name, the effects of blasts, or "shell shock," were disputed fiercely. After all, a great deal was at stake. Should the soldier be judged disabled, relieved of duty, and compensated for decades with costly veterans' benefits, or should he be sent back to the front line? Like victims of railway accidents who complained of symptoms but had no broken bones, soldiers were highly suspect if they were exposed to a blast, crawled back to the trench with all four limbs attached, then had the bad form to complain of headaches and dizziness.

Confronted with crowds of veterans requesting help, wishing to make decisions based on authoritative advice, the British War Office took the predictable step: they convened a committee. This is the product of that effort:

There was no evidence of organic injury of the nervous system … The loss of memory so common in "shell shock" is ascribed to repressed experience … Painful mental experiences, such as have been referred to, are many cases said to be "converted" and take the form of one or other of the well-recognised hysterical manifestations … Authorities agreed that, in the majority of cases of war neurosis, there already existed a congenital or acquired predisposition to pathological reaction in the individual concerned, and that his constitutional characteristic was of vast importance. … The explosion of a shell … may or may not be the final factor causing the breakdown.

(Army, 1922 [160], pp. 95–97)

These simplistic, one-sided, unscientific conclusions remain a popular response to CBI survivors who dare to complain: blame the victim. Call him hysterical, neurotic, a malingerer, or all three.

The other approach to head injury victims with persistent distress was to minimize. "Sorry about your concussion; thank goodness it was mild." Yet, in the course of diagnosis or litigation, how would one establish that a brain injury was "mild"? Up until about 1925, there did not exist any scale or measure for the severity of concussions. In fact, since all the research

showed a continuum in the amount of brain damage, where would one draw a line between levels of severity? And why bother? A likely explanation will be revealed shortly.

The Fallacy of Benignity

On May 5th, 1924, British surgeon and social psychologist Wilfred Batten Lewis Trotter delivered an address before the Medical Society of London titled "Certain minor injuries of the brain" [162]. *The Lancet* published his remarks.

I may say at once that I use the term concussion, as I think it should only be used in the strict classical sense, to indicate an essentially transient state due to head injury which is of instantaneous onset, manifests widespread symptoms of a purely paralytic kind, does not as such comprise any evidence of structural cerebral injury, and is always followed by amnesia for the actual moment of the accident.

([162], p. 935)

Readers of this chapter, knowing the classical literature, know that Trotter did not. Roughly 300 years of medical history and thousands of medical books employed *concussion* in a consistent way: to refer to a rattling blow to some body part. About 200 years of neurological history employed concussion in a consistent way: to refer to an external force, an impact transmitted through the skull to shake the brain. Trotter hardly uses *concussion* in the "strict classical sense"; quite to the contrary. With rare exceptions such as Boirel back in 1674 [50], no physician regarded concussion as mild, transient, or reversible.

Setting aside Trotter's apparent ignorance of the history of concussion and of multiple contemporaneous neuropathological reports (as revealed by his claim that concussion does not produce structural injury), setting aside his odd claim that the symptoms are confined to the motor system, by what logic and for what benefit does he abandon the essential idea of concussion as

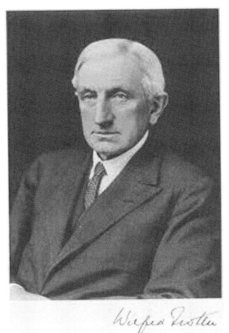

Fig. 1.16 Wilfred Batten Lewis Trotter.

Source: Biographical memoirs of fellows of the Royal Society, Wilfred Batten Lewis Trotter, 1872–1939, TR Elliott Scanned images copyright © 2017, Royal Society. [161] Scanned images copyright © 2017, Royal Society

a blow? He throws in with a handful of etymological revisionists who proposed using the perfectly good English word *concussion* not for a type of injurious event but for a *group of symptoms*. Phelps had cautioned against such deviance in 1892:

> brain injury produces structural change with the same certainty that it occasions palpable symptoms. If the terms concussion and compression be used to indicate a group of symptoms … it is objectionable, both on the score of propriety and as being likely to lead to erroneous diagnosis.
>
> ([163], p. 78)

Trotter declined to take heed. In consequence, he seriously misrepresented the meaning of *concussion* and inexplicably urged doctors to restrict the use of this term for a blow to a small subset of cases – excluding all victims who have skull fracture or hemorrhage, excluding all victims with persistent symptoms. He defined their concussions out of existence.

Trotter himself could not sustain his position. He expressed keen interest in those suffering persistent post-concussive symptoms. In fact, he argued strongly that headache commonly persists long after concussion! He also devised rather fantastic approaches to treatment. As Russell (1932, p. 600) explains:

> If the patient returns at an interval after the injury complaining of severe post-concussional symptoms, the treatment advised by Trotter is of great value and often leads to a complete cure. Rest in the Fowler position both day and night, combined with the use of dehydrating measures such as the regular administration of strong solution of magnesium sulphate, either orally or by the rectum, is the basis of this treatment.
>
> [164]

We agree that such a treatment would surely make a patient express his relief and promptly exit the hospital – if not in that order. Trotter, in addition to innovating bizarre therapies, perhaps deserves the distinction of being one of the first professional concussion deniers: persons who make money by misrepresenting the long-term effects of CBI. In fairness, even though Trotter is a famous advocate of the "Concussions are always benign!" camp, he was clearly aware of the overriding concern: "This tendency of lesions that elsewhere would be trivial and passing to *persist and cause grave symptoms* [emphasis added] is altogether peculiar to the brain" ([165], p. 355).

But the damage was done. After Trotter, the meaning of *concussion* in Western neurology was as fixed and consistent as the visage of Morpheus.

Attorneys and the Invention of Mild Traumatic Brain Injury

Thus, by 1925, American and British neurology was as divided on the concept of *concussion* as psychiatry was regarding Freud's concept of psychosexual dynamics. A contagious sentiment arose such that the previous empathy and curiosity about the long-term effects of concussion were gradually replaced by a dogmatic certainty about "psychical" (emotional) causality. In fact, mapping the history of that troubled era, there is a reasonably neat parallel between the timing of the English-speaking world's transient infatuation with Dr. Freud and the era when many neurologists dismissed concussive complaints as "hysterical."

At this juncture, the movement began to classify head injuries as mild, moderate, or severe.

Why? One factor is surely an apparent human enthusiasm for categorization. We are not content with either an evocative description or even a quantitative measure. For instance, we are not content to say, "That was a bad storm" or even "The wind speed averaged 100 kph"; we must resort to "category 4." We are not content to say an earthquake was a "whopper" or "a 2-meter lateral tectonic plates shift"; we need to say "Richter scale 6.0." From clothing sizes to the turbulence of river rapids, that is our way. Yet, in matters of human distress, is it valid? Why was there not an equally robust and contentious fight about classifying the severity of stroke? Of multiple sclerosis? Of Guillain–Barré, or motor neuron disease, or peripheral neuropathy? Throughout medicine, innumerable disorders present across a wide range of severity. Yet one does not read 100 pulmonologists' competing opinion papers about the definition of mild, moderate, and severe pneumonia. Why, in about 1925, did Western neurologists leap into the role of concussion severity umpires?

Consider the forces in play: tens of thousands of CBI victims were complaining. Only a few had "objective" evidence of injury such as a depressed skull fracture. Many wanted cash. Many exaggerated, some imagined, and a few feigned their distress. No test could tell whose brain had been damaged, or to what extent (our ongoing conundrum). If every complainer were awarded a munificent disability payment, it would bankrupt the fragile system of social supports and threaten the apex of the Industrial Revolution. Indeed, many concussive injuries produced little evidence of lasting harm, so it truly made sense to try to trim the mountain of litigation down to the molehill of legitimate and compensable injuries. Courts, in the interest of justice, urgently needed a way to quantify the harm [166]. As a result, there was tremendous pressure to classify the severity of CBI, so that "mild" injuries could be treated proportionately.

The Reason Why

Although it is perilous to claim one can decrypt the runes of history, we tentatively conclude that a rough weave of factors explains the absurdly inconsistent use of *concussion* in 20th-century medicine. It seems to have more to do with money than with science. Between 1880 and 1925:

1. There was an astonishing increase in concussive brain injuries, which meant a marked increase in patients complaining of symptoms without objective evidence.
2. A new theory in psychiatry encouraged doctors to consider complaints without objective evidence hysterical. (Hysteria about hysteria perhaps reached the apotheosis

of patient derogation with Romanis' and Mitchener's 1930 textbook [167]. They labeled symptoms that persisted for more than two weeks after a concussion "traumatic neurasthenia": "He cannot work, or says he cannot, and becomes dirty, immoral, irritable, and nervous.")

3. A novel and costly social support system evolved that offered money for disability. This incentivized malingering. The malingering of a few made every CBI victim the object of suspicion.

4. Litigants pressed doctors to rank the "severity" of concussions. Yet no one could find a scientific dividing line between mild, moderate, and severe.

5. As a result, arbitrary dividing lines and operational definitions of "mild" were called into being without the benefit of science.

In summary, a never-before-seen combination of historic factors converted the doctor–patient relationship into a cat-and-mouse game, obliging the put-upon neurologist to sit in judgment of the imponderable to declare, "This is mild, this is moderate, this is severe," and – superhumanly – to sit in judgment of the unknowable and declare, "This is organic, this is psychological, and this is fraud."

Modern readers know that such clinical judgments are fraught with subjectivity and simplistic to the point of inanity. In fact, in 1926, Sir Charles Symonds published a paper in *The Lancet* titled "Functional or organic?" [168]. He explained why this dichotomy would prove fallacious: "The one speaks of a lesion of the brain, the other of an attitude of mind. But are these two views really incompatible?" He gives the example of a man who had been referred to him because the patient was allegedly "worrying himself into a state of neurasthenia." Symonds quickly recognized that the man actually suffered from post-influenza encephalitis lethargica.

> Such cases, in which we have every reason to suppose that the neurotic symptoms are due to inflammatory lesions of the nerve-cells, compel us to remember that *behind all disturbance of function there must be some physical change* [emphasis added]. Herein also may be found some justification for the practitioner who maintained that some wise man would some day discover a lesion of the brain to account for such symptoms.
>
> [168]

Unfortunately, that wise man (or woman) has yet to publish his results. Absent such proof, Symonds failed to persuade his colleagues that cases of so-called hysteria were always cases of brain change.

Progress

In 1927, Osnato and Giliberti published the first sophisticated, large-scale study of post-concussive symptoms [146]. Their paper began with that same burning question, "Psychogenic or organic?" Previous investigators rarely followed patients beyond the acute phase. Osnato and Giliberti, in contrast, examined 100 concussion survivors weeks or months after their injuries.

In 51 of those cases there was no skull fracture, and in 32 there was not even a scalp wound. That relatively modest degree of severity makes their paper very important; it was the first real survey of long-term symptoms after slight or "mild" CBI. They found persistent headache in 69%, dizziness in 51%, sleep disturbance in 38%, irritability or moodiness in 23%, restlessness in 22%, and hypersensitivity to noise in 16%. Perhaps most strikingly, they found microscopic evidence of chromatolytic changes they interpreted as degenerative.

Their conclusion can only be interpreted as a direct correction of Dr. Trotter:

> Anatomic and clinical investigations seem to show definitely that our conception of concussion of the brain must be modified. It is no longer possible to say that "concussion is an essentially transient state which does not comprise any evidence of structural cerebral injury." Not only is there actual cerebral injury in cases of concussion but in a few instances complete resolution does not occur, and there is a strong likelihood that secondary degenerative changes develop.
>
> ([146], p. 211)

A year later (1928) [169] Armour courteously stated that he "agreed" with Trotter – although, in fact, he rejected both of Trotter's key claims:

> Two exceptions may be taken to this classical definition of concussion: Is it possible to affirm that the state is essentially transient, unless we limit the expression strictly to the unconsciousness and the immediate paralytic phenomena associated with it? Is it correct to affirm that concussion of the brain does not as such comprise evidence of structural cerebral injury?
>
> [169]

Despite the hardships of the Great Depression, scholars continued laboring to detect those structural changes.

1930 and Beyond

The debate about the meaning of *concussion* persisted. Strauss and Savitsky (1934) [170], in their massive review, soundly rejected Trotter and his followers and repeatedly referred to concussion as an organic brain injury with persistent sequelae. They urged that the term "post-traumatic neurosis" in cases of head injury be abandoned, since neuroscience had discovered abundant evidence of organic brain pathology, even after the lightest concussions. Hall and MacKay (1934) [171] authored a direct rebuttal to Strauss and Savitsky, arguing:

> The neuroses following injury to the head do not differ materially from those after injury to other parts of the body, where no injury to the central nervous system can be in question. Consequently, it seems unwarranted to abandon the concept of neurosis following head trauma.
>
> [171]

This opinion was popular. For example, Colin Russel (not to be confused with Ritchie Russell), formerly President of the

American Neurological Association, published a paper in 1939 on war neurosis. He admitted that "Sir Frederick Mott described minute petechial intracerebral hemorrhages" in the brain of a shell-shocked soldiers, but declared "such cases must be extraordinarily rare" and concluded, "It is now well recognized that there is no difference in the clinical manifestations of these two conditions of shell shock and hysteria" [172].

To be sure, more balanced views were expressed. Munro (1939) [173] cautioned against the capricious assumption that post-traumatic distress was a neurosis motivated by desire for compensation:

> it is neither fair nor correct to conclude … that all patients who have head injuries in the past, and who, at some later date, complain of disabling symptoms that cannot be shown by ordinary tests to be due to objective changes, should be classified with this unsavory minority.
>
> ([174], p. 587)

Meanwhile, neuropathologists continued to discover reasons for concern. In 1930, Minkowski (cited in Russell, 1932 [164]) confirmed earlier reports that concussion caused microscopic breakdown of neurons. Rand and Courville, in a series of reports published between 1931 and 1947 [175–178], reported the most meticulous microscopic examination that had ever been done on the brains of victims of fatal concussion. Their observations help to explain why microscopic examination may never yield a complete answer to what happens in the aftermath of a headquake: "Perhaps the most disturbing feature in efforts to evaluate the nature of cell change is the occurrence of multiple processes acting on a single cell" ([178], p. 98) (this, as it turns out, is exactly what is happening). Yet, from the perspective of an effort to understand the long-term risk of the more common, less severe, everyday concussions, Rand's and Courville's most disturbing findings were hints of progressive brain degeneration: "Not only do death and injury of nerve cells occur as an immediate effect of the injury, but, in addition, progressive changes may take place in nerve cells as a result of processes which are initiated by the injury and which continue for a variable time thereafter." How often does that occur in so-called "mild" head injury? We need to know.

Symonds also published a series of papers on concussion. In 1937, responding to the popular diagnosis of "traumatic neurasthenia," he urged his audience to realize that people with persistent complaints after concussion are not all of a sort: patients so labeled after head injury fall into three groups:

(1) The group in which the situation arising out of the accident (including the compensation situation) leads to the development of hysterical or anxiety states …

(2) The group of patients who are really suffering from post-traumatic dementia …

(3) The group of patients whose constitution before the accident has been of the depressive or anxious type. In this group the injury to the brain precipitates or releases … neurasthenia which is traumatic in a physical, rather than a psychogenic, sense.

[179]

His attention to human individuality, in our opinion, was a major advance. It may be self-evident to the reader that some victims of CBI (or alleged CBI) will give honest reports and others will not. Yet few prior authorities took interest in the fact that there is a broad spectrum of reactions and an extremely important interaction between injury and persona. Symonds in fact concluded that lecture with his memorable maxim: "it is not only the kind of injury that matters, but the kind of head."

This concept is both critical to understanding the interaction between pre-morbid psychological status and reaction to trauma, and hopelessly simplistic. Of course, one can generalize, like Munro (1943) [173]:

> The impact of even a minor craniocerebral injury on the personality of a workman who is constitutionally unable to hold a job or who is so emotionally unstable that his family life is continually disrupted, will be decidedly different from that of the same injury on the personality of an emotionally stable, intellectually competent, adequate individual.
>
> ([173], p. 545)

In point of fact, it is intellectually lazy to conclude that pre-morbid emotional frailty *causes* post-concussive complaints, given the evidence that concussion damages brains, and that even people with neurosis suffer concussions. As Munro himself put it: "This is perhaps an oversimplification of an extraordinarily complex question." The same year (1943) [180], Goldstein offered a piece of common sense: "the evaluation of some symptoms as neurotic or organic does not exclude the possibility that the individual is suffering from organic damage in addition to neurotic reactions or vice versa" ([180], p. 329). He agreed that personality and life circumstances are factors that influence a victim's reaction to a concussion, but he pointed out that this goes both ways. Victims *inflate* or *deflate* their symptoms: "the civilian in peacetime is likely to exaggerate. The soldier dissimulates; he is anxious to lessen his subjective disturbances; he is eager to return to service." Not always. But men in groups often develop machismo loyalty that drives denial of personal distress. The same, by the way, tends to explain the denial of concussions by athletes – one reason that the sports neurology opinion (embracing the doctrine of benignity) tends to be at variance with the non-sports evidence [181].

The Great Divide

We then arrive at some remarkable proclamations of Denny-Brown and Russell. On the eve of U.S. entry into World War II, at a time when American servicemen were expected to sustain many TBIs and the best clinical management remained highly debatable, these giants of 20th-century neurology tried to bring their pioneering laboratory observations to bear on these fractious debates. Yet a careful review of their substantial 1941 *Brain* paper, "Experimental cerebral concussion" [182] reveals that these authors employed six meanings of concussion:

1. "a brief loss of consciousness directly following a blow on the head" (p. 101)

2. "an immediate traumatic paralysis of reflex function, which occurs in the absence of visible lesions in the nervous system" (p. 141)

3. "Concussion … is defined in relationship to immediate loss of consciousness resulting from trauma to the head, with retrograde amnesia" (p. 155).

4. "Concussion is synonymous with traumatic paralysis, of whatever type" (p. 155).

5. "It is concluded that concussion is a generalized reversible "molecular reaction" induced by physical stress" (p. 156).

6. "traumatic paralysis of neural function in the absence of lesions" (p. 159).

Beyond their difficulty defining their subject, this renowned team took some unusual positions regarding experimental evidence – others' and their own. They admitted that when they hammered on cats, dogs, and monkeys, they produced petechial hemorrhages, especially in the white matter. However, they dismissed these brain changes as epiphenomenal, irrelevant to the real effects of concussion ([182], p. 147). Moreover, in something of a historical enigma, they stated that death from experimental concussion "can readily be obtained by repetition of moderately severe blows," yet "No lesions were found in brain or cervical cord even on microscopical section" ([182], p. 107).

No microscopic lesions? Others had detected microscopic lesions since 1890. Odd.

In 1945 [183], Denny-Brown wrote, "It is therefore pertinent to inquire whether any of the phenomena of concussion can be associated with a persistent, structural disorder"(p. 296). This had already been the focus of research for half a century. Curiously, rather than reading and synthesizing that literature, Denny-Brown and Russell mistook it. For instance, even though they had read Mott (1917) [144], Marinesco (1918) [184], Carver and Dinsley (1919) [185], Mairet and Durante (1919) [186], Zuckerman (1941) [187], and others, they forcefully rejected the idea that blast injury concusses the brain. How could they arrive at a conclusion so at odds with the evidence? This is how Denny-Brown dealt with the repeatedly published reports of petechial hemorrhages in the brain after exposure to blast: "The oft cited cases of Mott do not withstand analysis, for the most convincing had been buried by an explosion, and the petechial hemorrhages found in the brain may have been due to CO [carbon monoxide] poisoning from the fumes of explosion" ([183], p. 316). Having thus dismissed the published microscopic findings as mere artifacts of poison gas, Denny-Brown concluded, "No convincing evidence is found to support the hypothesis that explosive blast can produce a cerebral lesion comparable to concussion" ([183], p. 320). As a result of this pair's decisive pronouncements, wounded warriors of World War II, Korea, and Vietnam were enrolled in a veterans' health care system that essentially denied their brain damage over the next 50 years.

Denny-Brown even wrote: "Concussion is not associated with any cerebral lesions recognizable by the naked eye, or by the microscope with any staining process at present available" [183]. This at a time when both cellular and subcellular changes after experimental concussion had been documented, using various stains, for more than 50 years. In fact, Tedeschi (1945) [188] published high-resolution photomicrographs that same year, stating: "concussion may be due to neuronal injury detectable with present histologic methods" (p. 352).

In fairness, despite having failed to see what their peers had seen, Denny-Brown and Russell did predict other avenues of research that would prove helpful. In addition to calling for studies of the effects of CBI on cerebral metabolism, Denny-Brown pointed to the fact that "Its effect on synaptic transmission and the delayed development of a cycle of histological changes are at present complete enigmas which invite investigation" ([183], p. 320) Yet the damage to a biological understanding of concussion was done. Denny-Brown, preaching from his bully pulpit as a Harvard Professor and President of the American Neurological Association, lending gravitas to the fondest hopes of insurance companies, was a hard voice to dismiss.

Neurology embarked on a detour. Eden and Turner (1941) [189], Walker et al. (1945) [190], Merritt (1943; cited in Courville, 1953) [2], Tönnis and Loew (1953) [191], and others began to proclaim that concussion is a temporary, fully reversible problem defined by a group of typical symptoms. The divisive *doctrine of benignity* cadre was at odds with their peers, the contemporaneous clinicians and experimentalists who countered that CBI could obviously lead to brain damage and death [192–195]. Attempting to reconcile the Trotter/Denny-Brown fallacy of benignity with the hard-to-ignore fact that many patients exhibit death or evidence of lasting harm, a few writers tried to revive the old notion of *uncomplicated* versus *complicated* concussion (e.g., Groat et al., 1945 [196]; Meerloo, 1949 [197]). Others, confirming the well-established observation that many concussions are "combined with traumatic interstitial hemorrhage, contusion, or laceration of the brain" [198], tried to revive the discrimination of "pure concussion" from concussions accompanied by other pathological changes (e.g., Windle, 1944 [199], p. 561). Moreover, while Denny-Brown had declared there was no concussion unless the patient lost consciousness, several of his most distinguished contemporaries firmly disagreed based on their experience with patients who were barely dazed but nonetheless exhibited symptoms and signs best explained by brain damage (see Goldstein, 1943 [180]; Miller Fisher, 1966 [200]). In other words, Denny-Brown's and Russell's proclamation was confronted by a host of conscientious objectors who recognized both less and more clinically severe cases as diffuse traumatic brain injuries due to external force.

Science notwithstanding, Western neurology has yet to recover from the curious emanations of Trotter and Denny-Brown and Russell. Their scientifically indefensible doctrine of benignity seems to have had the principal impact of restraining costs and empathy. Armed by these "authorities," insurance companies, employers, the Veterans Bureau, and perhaps many skeptical (or less than empathic) physicians felt authorized to classify hordes of concussed persons with a psychiatric label. To this day, there are neurologists who either try to define concussion as a group of symptoms, or who cling tooth and nail to the notion that CBI is invariably mild, transient, and reversible – and that patients with long-term complaints were fakers or fantasists.

In spite of Trotter's and Denny-Brown's and Russell's idiosyncratic opinions, in spite of the escalation of economic pressures from tort and disability claims, physicians are a reasonably educated bunch. Given the wealth of published evidence that CBI was often serious and sometimes fatal, as well as the superfluity of reports that concussion could cause structural brain injury and long-term disability, it may seem inexplicable that so many physicians bought the "concussion is benign and complainers are imagining their distress" fairytale. Why did so many follow sheepishly at Trotter's heels? (Social psychologists may detect an irony: Trotter's other career led him to author *Instincts of the Herd in Peace and War* (1916) [201]. He pioneered the evocative phrase, "herd instinct.")

There was dissent. Kurt Goldstein, rather than simply championing the empirical facts regarding post-concussive damage, adopted a different focus: the conceptual fallacy of the popular distinction between organic and psychic. Like most neurologists since Willis in the 17th century, Goldstein understood that mind is the result of brain. Therefore, what could it possibly mean to attribute some symptoms to tissue and others to … well, some abstraction called the psyche? In a flurry of seminal publications from his 1931 German-language paper [202], his 1942 textbook [203], and his 1943 English-language papers [180], he asked his peers to reconsider "so-called war neuroses," gently chiding, "According to the organismic point of view the 'psychologic' and the 'physical' do not represent separate occurrences within the organism; the apparent dichotomy is due merely to different ways of investigation." Nonetheless, the Denny-Brown/Trotter doctrine not only held sway during much of the 20th century, but soothes its adherents to this day.

California neurologist Cyril Brian Courville didn't buy it (Figure 1.17).

He was outraged at the treatment that his concussed patients received in court. This seems to have been a major motivation for his definitive, eloquent work, *Commotio Cerebri* (1953) [2]. Courville prefaces his text by telling the story of a woman who had suffered for two years after a concussion. He quotes the defense attorney, "You can see for yourself how little this injury has affected the plaintiff. There she sits, looking as well as you or I!"

Courville was angered by this perverse sophistry:

A series of such experiences gradually led the writer to the conclusion that, by and large the individual who suffered from simple concussion too often gets short shrift when it comes to compensation or award. On numerous occasions … the writer has left the courtroom convinced that … neither the essential nature of concussion nor the mechanism of the resultant symptoms was appreciated. All too often it was presumed that these symptoms were simply a "nervous reaction" to the injury, an inherent defect to be blamed on the patient rather than regarded as a direct consequence of the injury.

([2], pp. ix–x)

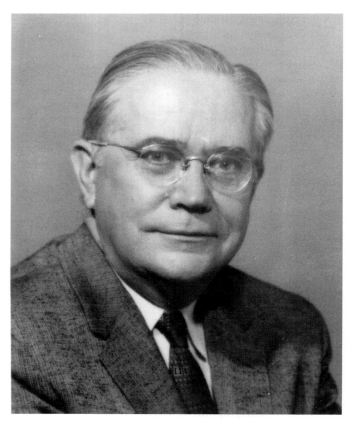

Fig. 1.17 Cyril Brian Courville 1900–1968.
Source: Loma Linda University Photo Archive

Hoping to wrest the train of brain science back on track, Courville composed one of the most astute distillations of *concussion* we have:

It thus seems clear that as a consequence of cerebral commotion two types of lesions may be found: the first a *general effect*; the second consisting of *multiple focal effects* characterized by areas of cell loss … Recognition of these processes helps in the understanding of both the acute and chronic psychic manifestations which follow cerebral concussion.

([2], p. 79)

Part II: A Brief Introduction to What Concussive Brain Injury Does to the Brain

If we are to retain the term "concussion", we feel that it cannot be limited to the effects of the mildest blows since severe blows also concuss. We know that there are serious and even fatal injuries that have been labelled concussion, and rightly so, because there could have been no denial of a concussive element. However, there are descriptions of concussion that stress the importance of a benign clinical outcome.

(Saucier, 1955 [204])

After clinical resolution of signs and symptoms of mild traumatic brain injury (MTBI) it is still not clear if there are residual abnormalities of structural or functional brain networks.

(Johnson et al., 2012 [205], p. 5)

In the parallel universe of the laboratory, many 20th- and early 21st-century neurobiologists gracefully demurred from the hysteria regarding mildness, reversibility, and hysteria to focus, instead, on the empirical question, what brain changes are detectable after CBI? A substantive review would require a detour from the intent of this chapter and can be assembled from the whole of this textbook. This brief introduction is merely a random rag ripped from the emerging tapestry of CBI pathophysiology.

The impact of concussive injuries has primarily been investigated with rodent models. Typical strategies include the hinge-drop model, the closed-skull weight drop, the closed-skull controlled cortical impact, the exposed dura controlled cortical impact, the exposed dura lateral fluid percussion method, and various approximations of blast injury.

At this point, it might do to review the biological definition of CBI. CBI refers to the deleterious effects of an external force applied abruptly to the mobile skull. "Abrupt" is important. The experiments we will review, and the human experiences they are intended to mimic, involve the rapid visitation of damaging force to the head. Winds can waft at 5 knots. That is not a buffeting tempest. Lava can flow at 5 meters per month. This is not a rattling eruption. The visitation of force that causes concussive injury is rapid. The Mafia's head-in-a-vise method of information gathering is not concussive. In animal models, the typical pace of visitation is 4–5 meters per second. No lower limit has been established – again due to a paucity of research. One might speculate, however, that below perhaps 10–100 cm/s the character of the impact shifts from an abrupt blow to a sluggish thump, producing different brain changes.

Second, the head moves. One error of early experiments was fixing the rodent's head in place before delivering the falling ball bearing. This does not replicate natural CBI. Evidence strongly suggests that a fixed, immobile head responds very differently. Obviously, the skull–brain biomechanics are profoundly different: when the knocked head moves, it both absorbs and uses some of the transferred energy in kinesis and enables a sloshing about of brain matter against the bony inner table, possibly with mechanical resonance. That is a completely different scenario from the constrained single slosh of brain if the player's head is pinned to the ground when the baseball arrives.

Thus, concussive force is a quick event. Concussive injury is not. The biological effects comprise both simultaneous and sequential interdigitating structural, ultrastructural, metabolic, oxidative, neurochemical, molecular, inflammatory, genetic, vascular (including the production of edema and compromise of the blood–brain barrier), and neurodegenerative changes of varying degree, duration, and timing. As Giza and Hovda (2001) admonished [206], whatever statements one

makes about "the pathophysiology of concussion" require qualification. No two mammals and no two brain injuries are identical. Both the occurrence and the time course of the many sub-elements of the concussional process vary. There are, nonetheless, five consistent findings worth noting: axonal jeopardy, metabolic change, inflammation, gene expression, and neurodegeneration.

Shear, Stretch, and Axonal Jeopardy

The distribution of microscopic lesions in the brains of patients with head injuries, mild or severe, could now be mapped out. It may eventually be possible to correlate the site and extent of tears with the various post-traumatic syndromes and post-traumatic dementia, and also with the type and direction of the mechanical forces involved.

(Anonymous, 1968 [207])

Magnetic resonance imaging (MRI) studies of human volunteers reveal that the maximum brain deformation after CBI occurs within "a few milliseconds" of impact [208]. Would that that were the end of the story. The second half of the 20th century saw a good deal of earnest scholarship devoted to characterizing those milliseconds, and what comes next. In 1943, Oxford physicist A.H.S. Holbourn proposed that, "when the head receives a blow, the behaviour of the skull and brain … is determined by … Newton's laws of motion" [209]. He opined that it is reasonable to suppose that the brain behaves like the substances whose properties have so far been studied, and therefore that it is injured when the blow is over. The brain is injured, he averred, "when its constituent particles are pulled so far apart that they do not join up again properly … the amount of pulling apart of the constituent particles is proportional to the shear-strain." The author likened the effect to a misaligned pack of cards.

A bundle of spaghetti *al dente* might provide a better analogy. Both white-matter tracts (bundles of axons) and the axolemma (the axon membrane sheathing bundles of neurofibrils – a silken pellicle, nanometers thick) are organized in tidy sheaves of parallel threads. Holbourn's theory of shear injury would help explain the disproportionate damage to white matter in CBI: twist a bundle of half-cooked spaghetti. Many strands will stretch. Keep twisting. Some of those semolina cylinders will break. Twist a bundle of axons and some will stretch or break as well. Two years later, Holbourn (1945) illustrated the mechanical reason why rotational acceleration would be more likely to harm brains in this way than linear acceleration. As he pictured the problem, "The brain moves relative to the skull and is therefore distorted and injured" ([210], p. 726) (Figure 1.18).

The same year (1945) [188], Tedeschi reported the effects of "repeated impacts of minimal intensity" impacting mice. These studies built upon the 1874 observations of Koch and Filehne [97] showing the fatal effects of repeated minor injuries – a finding that now helps explain the persistent or progressive traumatic encephalopathy of athletes who suffer multiple concussions. Confirming Holbourn's theory, Tedeschi

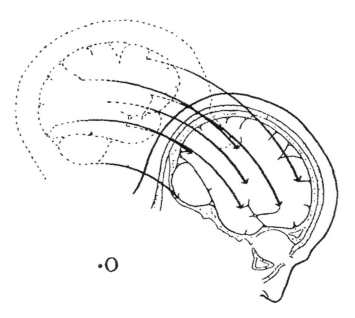

Fig. 1.18 Rotational acceleration in concussive brain injury produces shear forces.

Source: Holbourn, 1945 [210] with permission from Elsevier

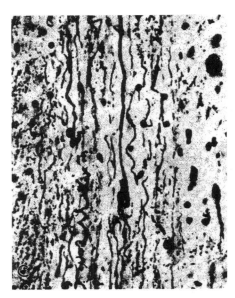

Fig. 1.19 Swelling and twisting in a frontothalamic axon bundle after repetitive experimental concussive brain injury.

Source: Tedeschi, 1945 [188] with permission from Wolters Kluwer Health

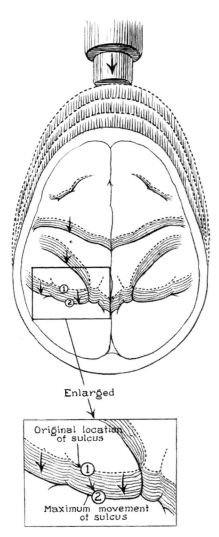

Fig. 1.20 View through Pudenz's and Shelden's lucite calvarium.

Source: Pudenz and Shelden, 1946 [211] with permission from the American Association of Neurological Surgeons

Enlarged

Original location of sulcus

Maximum movement of sulcus

published photomicrographs showing axonal damage and fragmentation of myelin sheaths (Figure 1.19).

One year later, Pudenz and Shelden replaced the skull-caps of macaques with transparent lucite calvaria (1946) [211] (Figure 1.20). A compressed air gun delivered calibrated blows to the head. The relative movements of the brain and skull were recorded with high-speed cinematography at 2000–3000 frames per second. As other investigators had previously shown, if the head was fixed little "convolutional glide" occurred; the freely moving head exhibited far more displacement. The authors documented an association between the degree of rotational movement and the distribution of lesions: frontal and temporal movement was constrained by their fossae. "This restraining effect of the anterior fossa on the frontal lobes must lead to strains within the cerebral tissue" ([211], p. 502). And indeed this is where shear changes were most often found.

About 15 years passed, however, before scientists visualized microscopic evidence of the shear injuries Holbourn had predicted in humans. Sabrina Strich happened upon five patients similar to Rosenblath's unfortunate tightrope walker (that is, people who had been concussed but lived on for months before autopsy. None had a fractured skull). Her microscope permitted her to see the damage that she called "unsuspected from naked-eye appearances." In 1956 [151] she reported, "The most striking finding is a diffuse and often severe degeneration of the white matter throughout the cerebral hemispheres." Like anatomists since the early Renaissance, she found damage to the thick white-matter bundle of the corpus callosum. She pursued her hunch, going on to cut the brains of 43 people who had lived up to two years after their brain injuries. Twenty of those brains showed the same change: degeneration of the white matter with clear

White-matter tract showing Strich's "blobs" (retraction bulbs of Cajal) consistent with shearing of axons

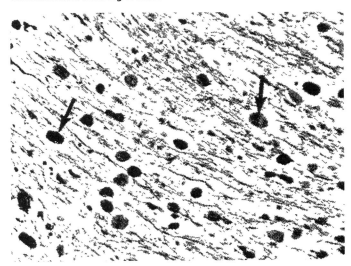

Fig. 1.21 A bundle of the internal capsule of the third case (survival for 24 days). (Holmes silver impregnation ×235). The large blobs are the retraction balls (arrows to two) which form at the ends of severed nerve fibers. Fragmented and degenerating axons can also be seen.

Source: Strich, 1961 [115] with permission from Elsevier

The spectrum of axon damage after concussion

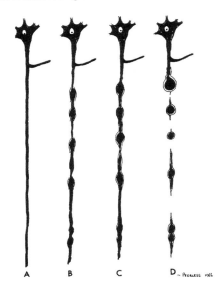

Fig. 1.22 A represents a normal neuron with a collateral branch arising near the cell body. B and C represent the axonal reaction to increasing stretch, while in D, where rupture has occurred, a retraction ball has formed on the proximal end and aggregates of axonal material lie along the course of the axon.

Source: Peerless and Rewcastle, 1967 [212] with permission from the Canadian Medical Association

signs that the axons had been rent asunder. To explain this, she cited Holbourn (with whom she had personal communications) and supported his theory that shear strain might explain this white-matter damage. It was 1961 [115] when Strich published her famous paper in *The Lancet* titled "Shearing of nerve fibres as a cause of brain damage …" As Strich explained: "When a nerve –fibre … is cut, axoplasm flows out of both cut ends and is visible as a large blob." Strich's blobs are called *retraction bulbs of Cajal*. They were abundant and easily recognizable in her subjects, indicating that axons had been transected, spilling their contents like milk from a straw (Figure 1.21).

Yet Strich recognized that the real problem was seeing the microscopic damage in less severe cases, since most concussions do not cause death or months of coma. Her best guess virtually summarized the subsequent 30 years of progress:

Only severe examples of the condition are reported here, but there is every reason to suppose that lesser degrees occur in patients with trauma to the head whether the skull is fractured or not. It also seems possible that if nerve fibres are stretched rather than torn, the lesions may be reversible at some stage, and may play a part in the production of the signs of concussion.

([115], p. 448)

Six years later, Peerless and Rewcastle (1967) [212] found the very same axon damage in 37 patients. They inferred that the degree of concussive force determined the degree of axon damage: mild force led to stretching; severe force led to transection, which generated "blobs" of spilled axoplasm that were still obvious "months and even years after the injury" ([212], p. 581). Figure 1.22 illustrates their conclusion. These authorities went

so far as to declare that microscopic shear injuries in the white matter "represent the basic pathology of all head injury."

How were neurologists, by 1960 well trained to talk about *concussion* as if it were something mild and transient, to absorb these scientific observations? Peerless and Rewcastle memorably counseled:

It is likely that the axonal changes are the basic lesion in all head injury. Contusions, lacerations and surface clots should be considered epiphenomena. The most common clinical syndrome of head injury, concussion, is still often defined as transient loss of consciousness without structural damage, and with no sequelae. It is conceivable that in such cases the axons of neurons may be stretched and distorted by the concussive blow, producing dysfunction but not permanent damage. Between these two extremes there may be all degrees of axonal injury.

[212]

All degrees. A continuum, from least to worst. In other words, if it were not self-evident from the variety of patients visiting any ER, by 1970 it had become clear that categorizing brain injuries as *mild* or *severe* was about as sensible as classifying the sky's infinitely variable clouds as *little* or *big*. (The problem of defining mildness will be addressed in a moment.)

Advances in technology have facilitated a slightly more sophisticated understanding of axonal jeopardy after concussion. Experimental CBI reveals not just the structural changes but the neurophysiologic and chemical changes that show why the structural changes harm mental function. When axons are twisted or stretched, their membranes, too, are physically stretched or twisted. Disruption of the axolemma permits flux of multiple ions through transiently unregulated ion channels and membrane defects that tend to spew neurotransmitters indiscriminately into synaptic clefts. A common effect is that excitatory amino acids (especially glutamate) bind to multiple post-synaptic receptors (especially the N-methyl-D-aspartate (NMDA) receptor). The result is to swing wide the cattle gate that blocks calcium channels. If the only result were depolarization, all might be well. However, excess calcium perturbs the permeability of the inner mitochondrial membrane. Once this happens, the mitochondrial respiratory chain becomes a train wreck of derailed protein complexes and the cell suffers decoupling of oxidative phosphorylation – in other words, that critical little organelle no longer efficiently burns oxygen. Two problems ensue: the mitochondrion begins spitting out reactive oxygen species (ROS) beyond the cell's capacity to scavenge and neutralize them, and the wreck of the respiratory "train" provokes a potentially fatal cellular energy crisis. The ROS, among other mischief, attack and oxidize lipids, yet another threat to membrane integrity. Moreover, the toxic dose of intracellular calcium causes phosphorylation of neurofilaments. They react by compacting. (This conceivably foretells the later appearance of neurofibrillary tangles festooned with hyperphosphorylated tau.) Microtubules lose their neat parallel geometry. It is as if the poles and platforms of a building scaffold simultaneously collapsed. Without that healthy microtubule scaffold to climb, organelles normally transported down the axon tube bunch up, leading to swelling of the axon and, potentially, axotomy (e.g., [213, 214]). All this begins within seconds and typically progresses over 24–48 h.

One ancient question has therefore been answered: whether or not some CBI-related damage is "reversible" – in some cases and to some degree – "structural" damage is *expected* after concussion. The question is – structures viewed at what microscopic resolution? It is possible (though yet to be confirmed) that at some unknown threshold of "mildness," CBI destroys only ultrastructural elements without destroying organelles, or destroys organelles without killing whole cells. Theoretically, "mildness" might some day be defined as a degree of structural plus functional harm verifiably short of triggering apoptosis in even a single cell. Sadly, given the tenor of the times, it may be decades before any international consensus is reached on the biological meaning of "mild."

Injury is not equal throughout the brain. Multiple studies suggest the selective neuronal vulnerability in the ipsilateral cortex, the bilateral thalami, and the bilateral hippocampi, with larger neurons, and especially CA3 neurons, perhaps exhibiting extraordinary injury-proneness (e.g., [215]). This differential vulnerability accounts for the awkward choice between the definitional terms *diffuse* and *multifocal*. Moreover, it is *axonal* damage, rather then *cell body* damage, that seems to predominate after milder brain injuries – a recent finding that may explain the historical delay in recognition of structural brain damage after concussion [216]. Although the traumatic renting of the axolemma, accompanied by calcium

influx, may be resolved in a matter of hours, microtubule breakdown reportedly occurs between six and 24 h post-injury and axonal disconnection due to swelling may persist in humans for weeks [217, 218]. Moreover, in a rodent model, even when cognition has "recovered," based on simple tests, CBI produces "axonal degeneration and sustained perturbation of axonal function" [219]. This is a critical discovery. We will return to the dissociation of cognitive recovery from biological recovery shortly.

Note that the phrase *diffuse axonal injury* (DAI) is a neuropathological condition usually associated with severe TBI. DAI tends to exhibit a stereotypical distribution of petechial hemorrhages in certain axon bundles. Kasahara et al. (2012) [220] rightly cautioned against assuming that the same process accounts for DAI and the more recently discovered multifocal axonal dysfunctional often observed after CBI, or so-called mTBI. The innovation of diffusion tensor imaging (DTI) has allowed visualization of multifocal axonal change in even the mildest of injuries. In adult humans diagnosed with "mTBI," although there is great interindividual variability, the most commonly affected axons seem to be those in the anterior corona radiata, the genu of the corpus callosum, the cingulum, and the internal capsule [221–226]. Whether or not the multifocal axonal changes detected after mild injury are part of a spectrum that includes the pathological condition DAI remains to be seen.

DTI has recently advanced the visualization of axonal jeopardy after CBI: axonal abnormalities are detected by comparing the normally directional diffusion of water as it is neatly constrained to move parallel to axons versus the more chaotic diffusion of water seen after injury. (Figure 1.23b).

The most common current measure of that altered diffusion is called fractional anisotropy (FA) – a measure of the way that the ideal spherical shape of the diffusion pattern of water that one would expect in cerebrospinal fluid is altered by restricted diffusion in axons. Virtually every study comparing groups of concussed persons with normal controls reports the emergence of altered FA within days of injury. However, as Lipton et al.

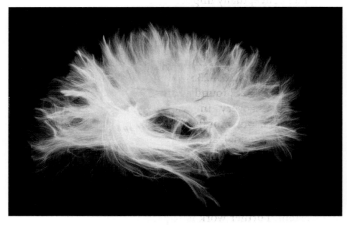

Fig. 1.23a Sagittal view of the corpus callosum white-matter tracts on diffusion tensor imaging. [A black and white version of this figure will appear in some formats. For the color version, please refer to the plate section.]
Source: Shenton et al., 2012 [227]. Reprinted by permission from Springer

Fiber tractography of commonly damaged tracts in mild traumatic brain injury

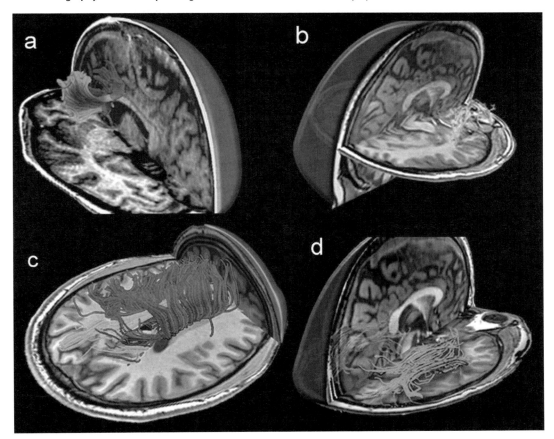

Fig. 1.23b (a) Anterior corona radiata and the genu of corpus callosum; (b) uncinate fasciculus; (c) cingulum bundle in green and the body of corpus callosum in red; (d) inferior longitudinal fasciculus. [A black and white version of this figure will appear in some formats. For the color version, please refer to the plate section.]

Source: Niogi and Mukherjee, 2010 [228] with permission from Lippincott Williams & Wilkins, Inc./Wolters Kluwer

(2012) [225], cautioned, this axonal damage should not be regarded as either "diffuse" or consistent; there is substantial variation in the multifocal distribution of this problem between patients. The changes can persist: Niogi et al. [222] reported that adults with persistent symptoms after "mTBI" exhibited abnormal FA up to 65 months post-injury. Of interest: even "non-concussed" persons exposed to the brain-rattling effects of contact sports exhibit abnormal mean diffusivity [229] (Figure 1.24).

What's conceptually important is the overwhelming empirical evidence that the problem may or may not go away, or may do so in some cases but not in others. In Shenton et al.'s excellent review [227], she cites multiple studies reporting chronic axonal changes after mTBI up to 5.7 years post-injury (e.g., [221–223, 225, 226, 230–233]).

Mayer et al. [226] found a similar patter in children: "Little evidence of recovery in white-matter abnormalities was observed over a four-month interval in returning patients, indicating that physiological recovery may lag behind subjective reports of normality." Yet chronic changes were not detected in every study [234]. Despite what seems to be growing evidence, both Shenton et al. [227], and Slobounov et al. [235] prudently conclude that the results of DTI in chronic mTBI are inconsistent. Further work is required to sort out whether the observed changes (or those visible with alternate new forms of axon imaging) sensitively and specifically detect persistent microstructural damage.

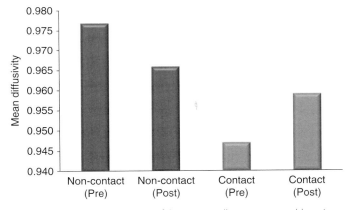

Fig. 1.24 Mean diffusivity values of the corpus callosum among athletes in contact versus non-contact sports, pre- and post season.
Source: McAllister et al., 2014 [229] with permission from Wolters Kluwer Health

The "Neurometabolic Cascade" Hypothesis

The "neurometabolic cascade" hypothesis was a popular conceptualization of a chain reaction of deleterious change, focusing on a few of the thousands of biological occurrences observed in the early phase of the mammalian brain's reaction to TBI. Physical commotion literally stretches or twists neural cell body membranes (and axons) to the point of failing at their duties. Within 60 seconds, ionic flux and neurotransmission, normally tightly regulated by the healthy membrane, both become pathologically dysfunctional. This permits excessive influx of ionic calcium, which in turn provokes multiple molecular and genetic changes, including serious mitochondrial dysfunction and activation of pro-apoptotic enzymes. This is an inopportune moment for mitochondrial unproductiveness that may result in an energy crisis, since the Na$^+$/K$^+$ ATP-dependent membrane pumps need more than usual energy to restore ionic balance. The desperate cell resorts to hyperglycolysis, attempting to produce the needed adenosine triphosphate (ATP). But hyperglycolysis in the face of limited mitochondrial oxido-reductive capacity causes a build-up of toxic lactate and other atypical products. Decoupling of glucose consumption from oxygen consumption

results, among other things, in the production of ROS (a possible contributor to late degenerative effects). These further damage membranes via lipid peroxidation and perhaps play a role in the depletion of nicotinic acid coenzymes. Due to rapid incitement of gene expression (see below), a battle for the life of the cell is waged between the forces of pro- and anti-apoptotic enzymes. The result: a crisis of insatiable energy demand combines with the toxic effects of calcium, ROS, and pro-apoptotic enzymes to damage or kill the neuron via the multifaceted insults of membrane disintegration and apoptosis, or nuclear-mediated self-destruction [213, 214, 236–241]. Figure 1.25 illustrates several features of this putative cascade.

"Neurometabolic cascade" following experimental concussion: a transient energy crisis

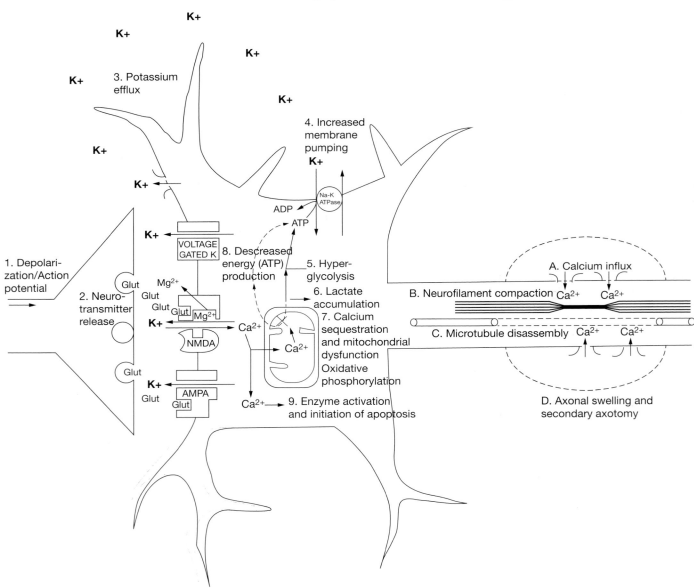

Fig. 1.25 (1) Non-specific depolarization and initiation of action potentials. (2) Release of excitatory neurotransmitters. (3) Massive efflux of potassium. (4) Increased activity of membrane ionic pumps to restore homeostasis. (5) Hyperglycolysis to generate more adenosine triphosphate (ATP). (6) Lactate accumulation. (7) Calcium influx and sequestration in mitochondria leading to impaired oxidative metabolism. (8) Decreased energy (ATP) production. (9) Calpain activation and initiation of apoptosis. A: Axolemmal disruption and calcium influx. B: Neurofilament compaction via phosphorylation or sidearm cleavage. C: Microtubule disassembly and accumulation of axonally transported organelles. D: Axonal swelling and eventual axotomy.

Source: Giza and Hovda, 2001 [236]. Reproduced with permission from Giza CC, Hovda DA.

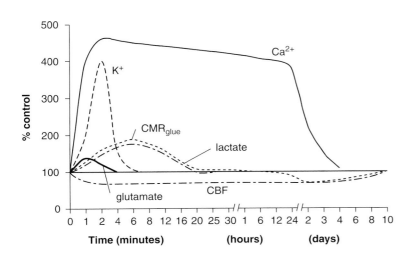

Fig. 1.26 "Neurometabolic cascade" following experimental concussion: a few days of ionic and metabolic perturbation. K+: ionic potassium; Ca²+: ionic calcium; CMRgluc: regional metabolic rate of oxidative glucose metabolism; CBF: cerebral blood flow.

Source: Giza and Hovda, 2000 [242]

At a more global level, the concussed brain exhibits somewhat predictable swings in cerebral blood flow, glucose metabolism, ionic transport, and neurotransmission. Figure 1.26 depicts elements of this broader view of ostensibly transient change.

Declines in neurotransmission are observed through the brain, especially adrenergic, cholinergic, and GABAergic signaling. The pace of recovery varies. Note that the switch to producing ATP via glycolysis causes a seemingly paradoxical but transient (minutes to hours) increase in the brain's metabolic rate of glucose consumption. This contrasts with what happens over the subsequent days: a depression of cerebral glucose metabolism of as much as 50% that lasts about ten days, and a depression in cerebral blood flow that may persist even longer, especially in the hippocampus [216, 217].

It is somewhat difficult to visualize the three-dimensional diffusion or propagation of these manifold facets of injury through the brain, and even more difficult to visualize the dynamics of the fourth dimension of time. It is likely that every lobe, architectonic region, and cell exhibits somewhat different changes following somewhat different temporal trajectories. Some writers suggest maximum damage in the immediate vicinity of the skull impact, with somewhat distance-dependent and tissue vulnerability-dependent damage further away, in part due to the immediate force and in part due to the release of neurotoxic chemicals (e.g., excitatory amino acids and ROS) from the first-hit cells. Yet this proximity-dependent narrative fails to acknowledge the evidence that the initial hit may initiate multiple diffuse or multifocal brain changes poorly linked to local chemical spread, such as diffuse alterations in axonal function, vascular function, inflammation, and gene expression.

One such diffuse effect is the unresolved impact of excess release of excitatory amino acids, especially glutamate. For decades it was thought that excess glutamate pried open calcium channels, permitting toxic calcium influx and all its disadvantageous sequelae. Multiple clinical trials attempted to capitalize on this hypothesis, "protecting" recently injured persons with glutamate antagonists. They failed. The repeated failure of this clinical approach inspired a closer look. In 2004 Biegon et al. [243] published the results of experiments reporting

that, yes, a very brief period of glutamate excess follows TBI. However, for at least the subsequent week, the more serious problem was a trauma-induced insensitivity of the principal glutamate receptor complex, NMDA. Other studies possibly explain what happens: NMDA receptors are linked to calcium channels by two pairs of subunits called NR1 (faster ion flow) and NR2 (slower ion flow). Rodent studies have found that only the NR2 subunits are down-regulated for the week after injury [216]. Flying in the face of conventional wisdom, Biegon and colleagues treated their animals with glutamate *agonists*. It seemed to work. Future investigations will better characterize the role of excitatory amino acids in concussion.

If these are the diffuse and multifocal biological changes of concussive injury, what is a "subconcussive" injury? Those who believe it is reasonable to define concussion clinically might declare, "subconcussion may be operationally defined as concussion so mild that there are no subjective symptoms." Is it mildness, per se, that determines awareness of injury, or perhaps whether or not that particular injury happens to impact the circuitry of consciousness? We agree completely that concussion sometimes occurs without subjective symptoms. However, if concussion is a biological problem, *subconcussion* has no apparent meaning. Concussion's multifaceted neurobiological changes may well occur with or without awareness of injury. Pending further discovery, no scientifically justifiable red line has been found that splits the diffuse and multifocal effects of brain commotion at a point between shaken a little and shaken a little more.

What do the neurometabolic changes of concussion have to do with other types of TBI? Yes, some evidence suggests that skull fracture – like the collapsing crumple zone of a motor vehicle – may sometimes reduce the impact of external force. Yet no logic and no evidence support the contention that skull fracture, massive intracerebral hemorrhage, or impaling on a lance saves the brain from concussive effects. If concussion is a biological problem, it is irrational to diagnose "not concussion" when concussive injury is accompanied by these frequent co-occurrences. As Hunter (1835) [83] suggested and Ommaya (1965) [85] declared, concussion is the core element that underlies virtually every TBI. If the injury involved force impacting the skull, the brain invariably suffers some element of concussive change. The concussive element may be larger or smaller. For instance, Heister (1743) [60] remarked that the concussional element of the brain injury would actually be greater from a blunt impact than from a sharp weapon. Similarly, it has been observed since the 19th century that penetrating gunshot wounds sometime generate minimal concussive changes (and may leave awareness intact), since the impact on the skull produces relatively minor diffuse effects (e.g., [244]). Hence, a fencing foil, an ice pick, or a nail gun will probably produce less concussive injury. Blast injuries certainly transmit external force through the skull to the brain, although physiological peculiarities such as the under-pressure wave require a cautious approach to equating blast with concussive injury [245]. Lightning strike can also cause diffuse brain injury due to external force, and – since this is not a purely concussive effect – represents a legitimate challenge to our definition. Still, one expects almost every externally applied force that harms the brain to involve an element of concussion. Thus, to differing degrees in different cells at different moments post-impact, one expects every TBI to provoke changes such as those depicted in Blennow et al.'s colorful schematic (Figure 1.27).

Perhaps the most controversial question is whether, in some or perhaps many "mild" TBIs, all of these physiological changes might be fully reversible. Rowbotham (1942), for example, declared, "Today it is a firmly accepted belief that the brain can receive a purely non-structural physiological injury sufficient to produce a diffuse neuronal paralysis" ([247], p. 41). More than 75 years later, many authorities still subscribe to that view, whether it is true, or because, like Denny-Brown and Russell, we are hobbled by our technique. Obviously one can experimentally administer lighter and lighter blows until none of these changes are detectable. What remains debatable is whether, when this cascade occurs, any brain survives completely intact, every single neuron happily restored to its exact pre-morbid condition, or the brain as a whole is as plastic and resilient as ever due to true recovery, adaptation, or compensation. That question begs an answer.

Inflammation

In 1968 [248], Oppenheimer published photomicrographs that depicted clusters of microglia in the corpus callosum of a concussed brain (Figure 1.28).

The reader will recall that, for at least 500 years prior to that publication, brain injury scholars had noted the

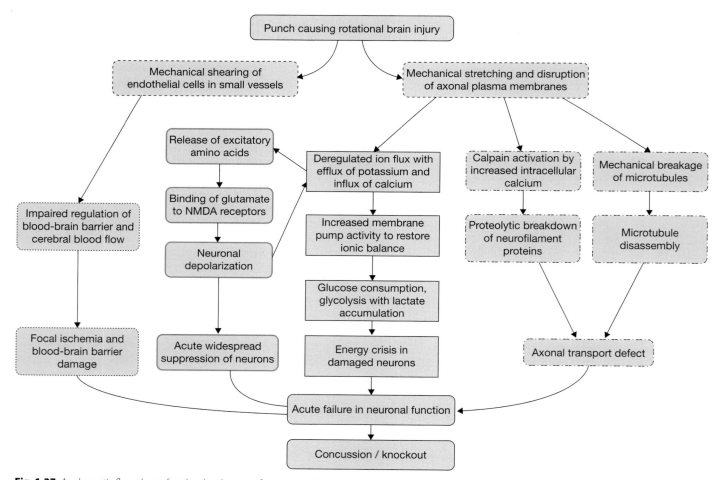

Fig. 1.27 A schematic flow chart of molecular changes after rotational head injury that leads to concussion and knockout with loss of consciousness. Source: Blennow et al., 2012 [246] with permission from Elsevier

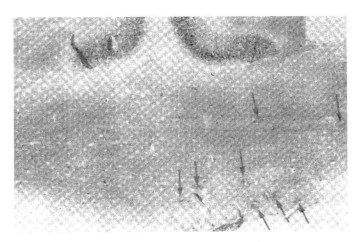

Fig. 1.28 Corpus callosum two weeks after a minor head injury. Arrows indicate the position of microglial clusters.
Source: Oppenheimer, 1968 [248] with permission from BMJ Publishing Group Ltd

vulnerability of the corpus callosum. They were not aware that this is a unique and massive bundle of myelinated axons – hence, likely to show the axonal injuries described and mechanistically explained above. Nor did they know, even though Celsus described inflammation 2000 years ago, that this routinely occurs in brains after a rattling blow. For some analysts, Oppenheimer's finding was a watershed moment. No longer were the persistent structural effects of CBI limited to petechial hemorrhages and shear lesions. The dawning realization that the inflammatory cascade plays an important role in concussion pathophysiology hinted that we were only at the beginning of a historic era of discovery, and that so-called mild TBI is associated with multiple individualized structural and functional changes, including those previously identified with non-brain disease. Shortly after Oppenheimer's publication, an anonymous editorial in the *British Medical Journal* (1969) [249] lyrically summarized the inescapable conclusion:

> It is disturbing to reflect that so valuable an organ as the human brain can, with sudden changes of acceleration, be made to resemble a quivering blancmange … As Oppenheimer says, the demonstration of lesions other than petechial haemorrhages in cases which were clinically labelled "concussion" is of interest, for permanent damage can clearly be inflicted on the brain by apparently minor injuries, and repeated blows (as in the case of the boxer) could lead to a cumulative loss of nervous tissue.
>
> [249]

Several years later, in 1974 [250], Clark published a replication and expansion. He strictly limited his study to 12 TBI survivors – that is, patients who were not killed by their brain injuries but who lived on from 23 h to 277 days. Eleven of the 12 revealed microglial clusters in the corpus callosum (as well as other axonal regions) like those reported by Oppenheimer.

In spite of these early reports, for many years the inflammatory element of CBI received less attention than the axonal and metabolic changes. In part this was an artifact of the slow development of affordable assays permitting accurate measurement of the vast array of inflammatory changes that occur in animals – and perhaps the slow expansion of digital libraries. For instance, in 1996 Engel et al. [251] reported delayed activation of microglia in 17 cases of severe TBI. These authors, apparently unaware of their predecessors, stated, "about microglial reaction in closed traumatic brain injury … no data are available." This minor error aside, the subdiscipline of neuroinflammation has subsequently grown and flourished. So has the evidence that inflammatory response to concussion is common, lasting, and highly variable. It transcends the ambitions of this chapter to review the inflammatory cascade in CBI, or to attempt to sort out findings from: (1) different time intervals after injury in (2) different severities of injuries, involving features of the inflammatory cascade that are (3) beneficial or harmful. Suffice it to say that TBI triggers a complex suite of interactive processes involving pro- and anti-inflammatory cytokines, chemokines, adhesion molecules, complement factors, reactive oxygen and nitrogen species, proteases, infiltrating lymphocytes, and activated microglia [252–256].

Recruitment of central and peripheral inflammatory cells seems to have both neuroprotective effects and secondary neuronal injury effects. One mechanism appears to be an interaction between inflammation and ROS. Another mechanism may be inflammatory suppression of reparative neurogenesis. Some evidence suggests different inflammatory responses in mild versus more severe TBI, and in repetitive versus single concussions [257–259]. Moreover, some evidence implicates inflammatory processes in the dysfunction of the brain long after concussion. At the risk of sooth-saying, neuroinflammation and alterations in immunomodulation may turn out to play critical roles in initiating persistent or progressive neurodegeneration and neurobehavioral dysfunction – or chronic traumatic encephalopathy [260–266]. Figure 1.29 schematically illustrates a hypothesis of the dynamics of the inflammatory response to brain trauma. Table 1.1 lists a few of the inflammatory makers now readily assayed, for instance, in population-based studies of cerebral small-vessel disease [267]. However, at this early stage in the study of CBI-related inflammation, it is entirely unclear how to interpret these markers – for instance, which biomarkers at what serum concentrations in what combinations among people with what genotypes might signal healthful resilience in the face of CBI versus threat to neuronal survival [268].

Advances in neuroimaging have made it possible to assay post-traumatic inflammation *in vivo*. For instance, translocator protein (TSPO) is a five-transmembrane protein spanning the outer mitochondrial membrane. It is increased after experimental TBI, an observation that has been attributed to the expression of activated microglia during neuroinflammation and reactive gliosis. In a sophisticated study published in 2015 [269], nine former National Football League (NFL) players who had been exposed to multiple concussions were compared with matched controls. (For those who are not familiar with this organization, the NFL is a minor league player in the important human domain of competitive team sports. The sport it profits from is violent and obscure, attracting a tiny proportion of human sportsmen compared with, for instance, *fútbol*. It is nonetheless well funded and popular in a certain segment of Western society.) Positron emission tomography scanning was

Proposed dynamics of the central inflammatory response to traumatic brain injury (TBI)

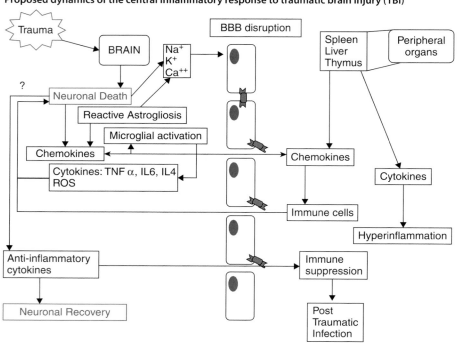

Fig. 1.29 Possible mechanism and the interactions between brain and systemic immunity after TBI. Blood–brain barrier (BBB) disruption allows peripheral immune cell infiltration into the brain. Interaction between brain and peripheral immune organs can cause either hyperinflammation or immune suppression. Anti-inflammatory cytokines may eventually lead to neuronal recovery. IL6: interleukin-6; ROS: reactive oxygen species; TNFα: tumor necrosis factor-alpha.

Source: Das et al., 2012 [261]. Das et al., 2012. Reproduced under the terms of the Creative Commons Attribution licence, CC-BY 2.0

Table 1.1 A subset of putative biomarkers of brain inflammation

- Interleukin-6
- C-reactive protein
- Tumor necrosis factor-α
- Tumor necrosis factor receptor 2
- Fibrinogen
- Osteoprotegrin
- Monocyte chemotactic protein-1
- CD40 ligand
- Intercellular adhesion molecule 1
- P-selectin
- Homocysteine
- Lp-PLA$_2$ activity
- Lp-PLA$_2$ mass
- Vascular endothelial growth factor
- Myeloperoxidase

Source: Shoamenesh et al., 2015 [267]

conducted using ^{11}C DPA-713, a ligand that targets and permits assay of TSPO. The assays were corrected for the effect of the rs6971 allelic polymorphism on binding. (This polymorphism is a potential confound since it affects binding affinity [270].) Structural imaging was also performed with MRI, and cognition assessed with special attention to verbal learning and memory. A history of NFL play was associated with increased TSPO binding in the supramarginal gyrus and right amygdala, while atrophy was apparent in the right hippocampus, and verbal learning (presumably mediated in the same region) was inconsistently impaired. Since the study was conducted years after exposure to CBI, the findings seem to support the hypothesis

that CBI (perhaps especially when repetitive) is associated with very long-term persistence of neuroinflammation that is associated, in turn, with both cell loss and cognitive impairment. While a single study cannot be regarded as definitive, this report suggests the possibility that the inflammatory component of TBI is both pathophysiologically important and, conceivably, a worthwhile target for interventions. Yet the evidence of mixed beneficial/detrimental effects of inflammatory cascades raises a red flag: the guess that anti-inflammatory treatments will help may be exactly wrong. Such treatments may interfere with aspects of the brain's evolved reparative capacity [266, 271, 272].

This commentary is merely a preface. The CBI–inflammation story is unfolding apace and will be discussed further in Chapters 4, 5, and 7.

Gene Expression

Two normal males, aged 24 and 39, each donated his brain to an international consortium called the Allen Human Brain Atlas project. Nine hundred brain regions comprising 170 structures underwent microarray analysis. The goal was to complete a form: for each regional tissue sample or cell type, list the RNA transcripts that comprise its transcriptome [273]. The authors identified 29,412 unique transcripts, a figure that exceeds recent estimates of the total number of human genes. This important advance is part of the revolutionary reconceptualization of brain anatomy and physiology. Initially such data will inform the understanding of species-specific neurobiology. But very soon it will permit precision medicine that accommodates individuality. The relevance to this chapter: CBI provokes changes in gene expression. The immensity of the numbers involved is staggering.

(To detour momentarily: this is one of the cognitive threats that tend to arrest conservative thinkers. They may decline to acknowledge that concussions cause permanent brain damage because they were trained to think of brains like kidneys or hearts: useful organs with finite and definable traits that do pretty much the same things in different people. Organismic heterogeneity differentiating members of the same species is not a focus of medical training. At present, it is not clear in how many millions of ways any two brains differ. Indeed, Holbourn's contention notwithstanding, it has yet to be determined whether mammalian brain function complies with Newtonian physics. Only time will tell whether brains are quanta-free zones. But it is clear, from the numbers alone, that two concussions can differ in a million ways.)

Two approaches have been employed to investigate gene expression after CBI or TBI for more than a decade. Experimental injury can be inflicted on animals, or even on parts of animals. Alternatively, human survivors of brain injury can later donate tissue. In both cases the procedure is the same: mRNA is extracted from the tissue or cell of interest. Reverse transcription produces the corresponding cDNA. Basepairs engineered to fluoresce with cyanine dyes are inserted. This product is then introduced to a glass chip spotted with cDNA arrays from gene libraries. The dye makes the hybridization readily visible, and the location and degree of hybridization tell us the type and amount of mRNA expression in the sample. That reveals which genes are expressed. Next, algorithms test connectivity between genes, which permits pathway analysis – resulting in a graph showing the network relationships between gene/gene products [274].

Most of the animal studies have subjected rodents to lateral fluid percussion injury. Some doubt exists that this is a good model for concussion: the skull is removed, so that transmission of forces is different than if that brain were snug in its usual bony cage as in a typical human injury. Obviously, the concentration of force at a single point is different from the typical blunt trauma. Perhaps most damning, the pharmacological findings that have emerged suggesting efficacious interventions have yet to work in the clinic. Nonetheless, fluid percussion remains globally popular. Typical gene expression studies report complex pathways of up- and down-regulated genes, many pertinent to inflammatory (cytokine and chemokine) factors and growth factors [275]. One study used the apparatus illustrated in Figure 1.30 to produce a mild injury, then analyzed the rapid versus delayed gene expression with a whole-genome microarray [276].

One hour after this traumatic injury, 32 genes were differentially up-regulated and 35 down-regulated (Figure 1.31). More and more genes were affected over the first day. By 48 h after injury, a total of 279 genes had been significantly up- or down-regulated. Some of the same genes that were up-regulated in the minutes after the trauma were profoundly down-regulated a few hours later. Based on animal studies such as this, about 7–9% of genes that have been assayed in experimental TBI exhibit differential expression in injured versus control animals [277]. However, we are far from knowing whether these changes in gene expression represent pathology, an evolved adaptation favoring brain self-repair, or both. In either case, the implications of such rapid swings may be that any good target for pharmacological intervention may be moving. The pathway analysis from this study is depicted in Figure 1.31. This diagram

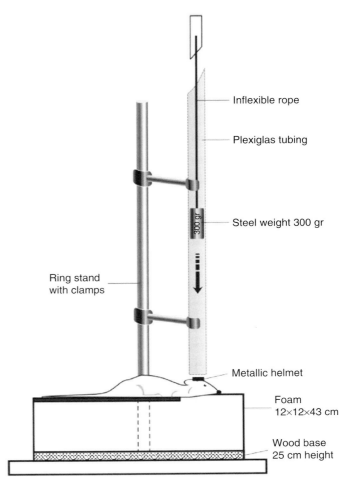

Fig. 1.30 A device for imposing experimental "mild" concussive injury. Source: Colak et al., 2012 [276] with permission from Elsevier

is not offered for close study, but merely as a springboard for the imagination: the complexity of CBI is literally dazzling. Apart from clarifying aspects of basic science, the practical value of such studies may be in determining the activity and interactions of genes involved in neuroprotection, inflammation, and neural recovery with a view toward identifying potentially modifiable processes. Yet perhaps the chief virtue of such figures is to inspire humility. No one understands concussion. No one. But a larger number of scholars, representing a broader spectrum of complementary disciplines than ever in history, is trying.

Another approach is to impose mechanical stress on isolated *in vitro* tissue – for instance, hippocampal slice cultures grown on a deformable silicone membrane. In one study [278], such tissue was exposed to varying levels of stretch, from 10% (judged as mild) to 50% (judged as severe). Again, microarray analysis identified genes that were differentially expressed after injury. In the "mild" protocol, 210 genes were significantly up-regulated and 789 genes were down-regulated. That is, *999 genes were shown to have exhibited altered expression after a mild stretch.* Gene ontology was determined by analyzing the microarray data to determine which of the genes that were differentially expressed belong to which ontological category based on previously published reports. In the case of "mild" stretch, all

Localization and interaction of genes that were differentially expressed
following mild experimental traumatic brain injury

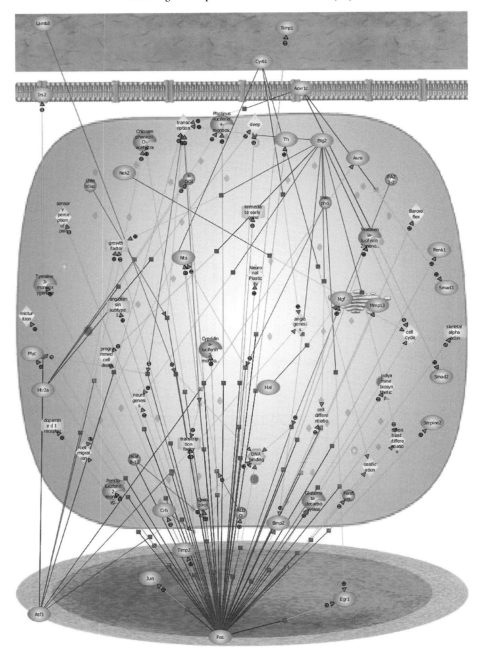

Fig. 1.31 "One hour after trauma (first experimental group), 35 genes were down-regulated, and 32 genes were up-regulated … We observed that most of the genes with altered expression levels after trauma normally function in cell signalling pathways, cell proliferation, cell differentiation and the regulation of transcription … The expression levels of Bdnf, C1ql2, Cbnl, Cd47, Mmp9, Sdc1, Slc27a2, and Tnnt3 were higher in the first hour of trauma than either the control group or at other experimental time points … In contrast, the expression levels of Dmkn, F2rl2, Hal, Htr2a, Pilra, and Slc22a25 were decreased in the first hour of trauma, increasing gradually after 1-h." The classification of affected genes is color-coded. The authors state: "For interpretation of the references to color in this figure, the reader is referred to the web version of the article." [A black and white version of this figure will appear in some formats. For the color version, please refer to the plate section.]

Source: Colak et al., 2012 [276] with permission from Elsevier

the differentially expressed genes belonged to the "biological process" category, inferred to be involved in the integrity of cellular architecture. Figure 1.32 displays a pathway analysis after a 10% stretch injury. As one might have predicted from the previous section on inflammation, one important finding was that pro-inflammatory cytokines play a central role in the molecular interplay; interleukin-1β in particular seems to exhibit many interactions with other genes. Perhaps crucially, the authors commented: "The majority of these expression changes were only found following 10% stretch, indicating that these hippocampal cell cultures have activated protective and repair mechanisms" ([278], p. 355).

These findings support one of the paradigm shifts proposed in this textbook: the "neurometabolic cascade"/energetic crisis conceptualization that has dominated the last two decades of concussion science was a vital advance. It summarized several important facets of short-term negative effects. But it was misleading. Abrupt external rattling force does not provoke a chain reaction of harm. It provokes a thrilling competition among innumerable forces over cellular welfare.

The apparent function of those genes varied widely, but many of the largest effects seemed to be a fortuitous combination: suppressed expression of pro-apoptotic enzymes and boosted expression of anti-apoptotic enzymes, suggesting

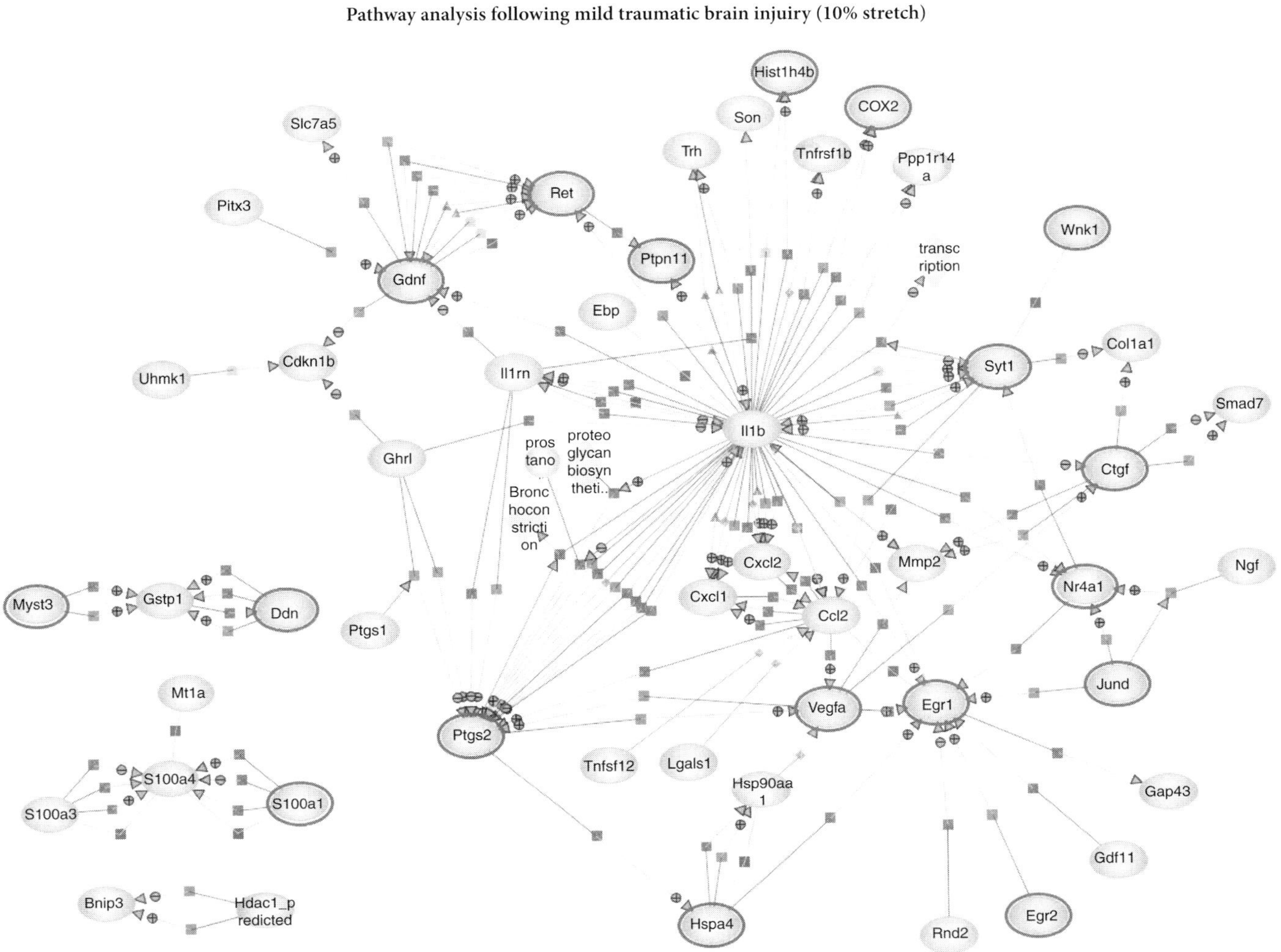

Pathway analysis following mild traumatic brain injury (10% stretch)

Fig. 1.32 "Most of the genes expressed following 10% stretch are involved in signal transducer activity, regulation of transcription, and cell communication … Additionally, we have found that following 10% stretch, certain genes involved in the apoptotic process, such as Vdac1 (voltage-dependent anion-selective channel protein 1), Sh3glb1 (SH3-domain GRB2-like endophilin B1), Phlda1 (leckstrin homology-like domain, family A, member 1), Rock1 (Rho-associated coiled-coil containing protein kinase 1), and Eif4g2-predicted (eukaryotic translation initiation factor 4 gamma, 2) were downregulated. Further, an upregulation was seen in genes involved in the anti-apoptotic process, such as Ccl2 (chemokine [C-C motif] ligand 2), Vegfa (vascular endothelial growth factor A), BIRC3 (baculoviral IAP repeat-containing 3), Tsc22d3 (TSC22 domain family, member 3), Bnip3 (BCL2=adenovirus E1B 19-kDa interacting protein 3), and Nr4a1 (nuclear receptor subfamily 4, group A, member 1)." [A black and white version of this figure will appear in some formats. For the color version, please refer to the plate section.]

Source: Di Pietro et al., 2010 [278]. Reproduced with permission from Mary Ann Liebert, Inc.

that neurons evolved to rescue themselves. In fact, a more recent study by the same group [279] proposed a fascinating hypothesis: might the gene expression changes after CBI represent hibernation? They realized that, after a 10% stretch to hippocampal slice cultures, there was not only (1) a protective combination of down-regulation of pro- and up-regulation of anti-apoptotic genes, but simultaneously (2) down-regulation of transcriptional and translational genes (putting protein synthesis on hold), and (3) down-regulation of genes coding for the mitochondrial electron transport chain complexes I, II, and IV (putting oxidative phosphorylation on hold)! This elegant suite of changes mimics the energy-saving changes in gene expression seen in hibernating animals. Brains, if not people, know to rest after injury.

Altered expression of multiple genes seems to be true for humans as well: Michael et al. [277] employed microarray analysis on tissue from five patients after brain injuries. Four of the five patients had suffered contusions; the fifth had an infarct. A total of 104 or 1200 genes on the microarray were differentially expressed in the "brain injury" group (8.7%). Perhaps the most important finding was individual variation: "of the 95 genes expressed differentially in at least one patient, 25 genes were differentially expressed in more than one patient and 6 genes were differentially expressed in 3 patients" ([277], p. 286). The genes whose expression is altered span an array of functions, including energy metabolism, transcriptional regulation, and signal transduction. Figure 1.33 illustrates the proportions of differentially expressed genes by functional category.

In brief, experimental TBI has unveiled an entirely new level of analysis of the happenings in brains after a buffeting blow. Unstated in this literature is the fact that thousands of

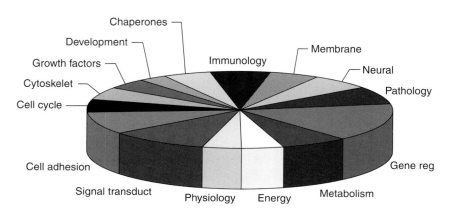

Fig. 1.33 Functional distribution of genes differentially expressed in brain-injured humans.

Source: Michael et al., 2005 [277] with permission from Elsevier

the expressed genes exhibit known variants – haplotypes or allelic polymorphisms. Thus, what we see in these pictures is not what we get. Even if every concussed human brain reliably up- and down-regulates precisely the same 999 genes, imagine the biological permutations and combinations once one adds polymorphic variation!

Altered Protein Degradation, Toxic Accumulation, and Neurodegeneration

Figure 1.34 displays the way that CBI (of unclear severity and multiplicity, but in most cases, "mild") apparently influenced the course of brain aging in a cohort of American-style football players [280]. A single study is hardly definitive. The methodology – for instance, ascertainment of the injuries and behavioral complaints – was suboptimal. Yet this study deserves credit for attending to a nuance: CBI is never the last and only factor influencing brain aging or neurodegeneration. A virtually infinite number of environmental experiences and gene × environment interactions intervene. The authors acknowledged that depression, traumatic stress, and cerebrovascular disease are three such factors. Admitting the infant stage of empirical data collection, admitting the likelihood that some aspect of these curves may later be proven inaccurate, this graphic display should raise eyebrows. What is happening in the brains of our loved ones who survived CBI?

Although Cushing (1917) [281] and, more explicitly, Osnato and Giliberti (1927) [146] proposed that concussion may precipitate neurodegeneration – and in spite of clinical reports since that of Martland (1928) [282] that multiple concussions may cause permanent brain damage – it is only since about 1990 that neurobiologists have escalated their attack on this question. Two putative associations have inspired this renewed interest. First, some evidence suggests that TBI may be the most important environmental risk factor for Alzheimer's disease (e.g., [283]). Second, media attention to the problem of dementia pugilistica among those who earlier pursued contact sports has increased. Some neuropathologists, reviving Parker's terminology (1934) [284], have labeled this second variety of post-concussive neurodegeneration "chronic traumatic encephalopathy." Victoroff's review of every case published between 1928 and 2010 reported considerable clinical diversity, with the majority of post-concussive dementia

cases being progressive and a minority static [285]. The observation of phenomenological diversity raises the question of terminology. The author tentatively proposed the possibility that traumatic encephalopathy with an apparently static and persistent course possibly exhibits somewhat different neurobiological features compared with traumatic encephalopathy with an apparently *progressive* course [284]. Stern et al. [286] proposed distinguishing traumatic encephalopathy with behavioral changes from traumatic encephalopathy with cognitive changes. It remains to be seen whether any categorical pathophysiological difference justifies either distinction.

Be that as it may, abundant evidence has emerged that experimental and clinical concussion are associated with changes in the expression of many potentially toxic proteins typically associated with neurodegenerative disease, including Aβ42, hyperphosphorylated tau, and α-synuclein (e.g., [287, 288]). (Of possible interest: Kang and Lin reported [289] a hazard ratio of 1.97 for the subsequent development of multiple sclerosis among hospital-treated TBI patients. It is premature to evaluate the evidence of this and other possible late sequelae.)

In a recent publication, Ling et al. [290] did their best to weave the threads we've discussed into a somewhat coherent tapestry. As illustrated in Figure 1.35, after a CBI, axonal, vascular, and inflammatory factors conspire. Although the resulting picture will surely be revised, it seems to be a reasonable synthesis of the state of the art. Of course, viewing this landscape of internal melee, two questions immediately come to mind: One: what is the minimal perturbation of the brain that provokes this chain reaction? Two: how often, and under what circumstances, does the chain lead to dementia? Three later chapters in this brief text will attempt to sort that out – in so far as the state of the art allows. A theme the editors cannot resist emphasizing, even at the risk of redundancy: unless and until proper studies determine the late effects of a typical, medically attended CBI, the global health care community has literally no way to accurately estimate the impact of concussion on human well-being. And unless and until we can better guess the magnitude of that total impact, we cannot fairly judge whether the net effects of concussion are merely tragic or catastrophic.

Perhaps the most volcanic question – a question for which the National Institutes of Health decline to fund research – is: can a single CBI deleteriously alter the course of brain aging? If so, do there exist modifiable factors for which intervention might

Additive effects of traumatic brain injury and other risk factors on dementia incidence

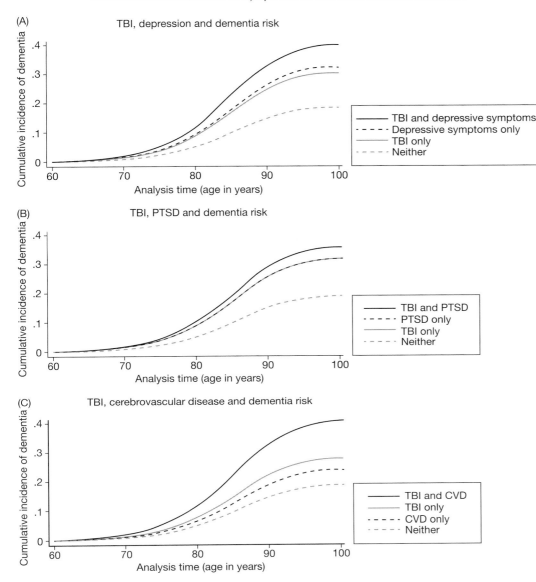

Fig. 1.34 "The additive association between traumatic brain injury (TBI) and other dementia risk factors is illustrated by showing the cumulative incidence of dementia with age as the time scale for veterans with TBI only (gray solid line), other risk factor only (black dashed line), both risk factors (black solid line), or neither risk factor (gray dashed line). Other risk factors examined include depression (A), posttraumatic stress disorder (PTSD) (B), and cerebrovascular disease (CVD) (C)."

Source: Barnes et al., 2014 [280] with permission from the American Academy of Neurology; Wolters Kluwer

mitigate that threat during the 5–75 years after the brain-rattling impact? One study that might trigger concern: Beauchamp et al. [291] reported that children who suffer "mild TBI" exhibit brain atrophy, especially in the hippocampus, ten years later. With a bare minimum of 1.7 million concussions per year in the United States alone (which we will demonstrate in Chapter 2 to probably be an indefensible underestimate), with a rapidly aging global population, we opine that it is a matter of considerable urgency to figure out the proportion of CBI survivors likely to suffer late effects. That number is needed to guide governments and polities. Consider, for a moment, the potential immensity of the stakes. There exists a global net human cerebral potential. There exists a collective human well-being. Is discovering an effective post-concussive intervention a priority for brain health of the order of magnitude of fighting a Zika epidemic? Or, instead, of the order of magnitude of fighting maternal and infant undernutrition, cerebrovascular disease, or air pollution – all suspected of massive and tragic influence on our planet-wide metrics? We need to know.

Setting aside the growing suspicion that one or more concussions may either cause, or lower the threshold for, disabling neurodegeneration, what has empirical science suggested as the explanation for persistent or lifelong clinical distress in some concussed persons? Perhaps even more interestingly, whether or not a patient is aware of brain dysfunction, whether or not a neuropsychologist can detect brain dysfunction, might brain dysfunction nonetheless persist? Laboratory investigations can provide valuable hints, but rodents are shy about enumerating their subjective symptoms, and hard to engage in cognitive tasks during imaging. Better information about the biological basis of persistent post-concussive dysfunction may be inferable from human neuroimaging studies such as those employing proton magnetic resonance spectroscopy (^{1}H MRS), DTI, and functional MRI (fMRI). As Bigler

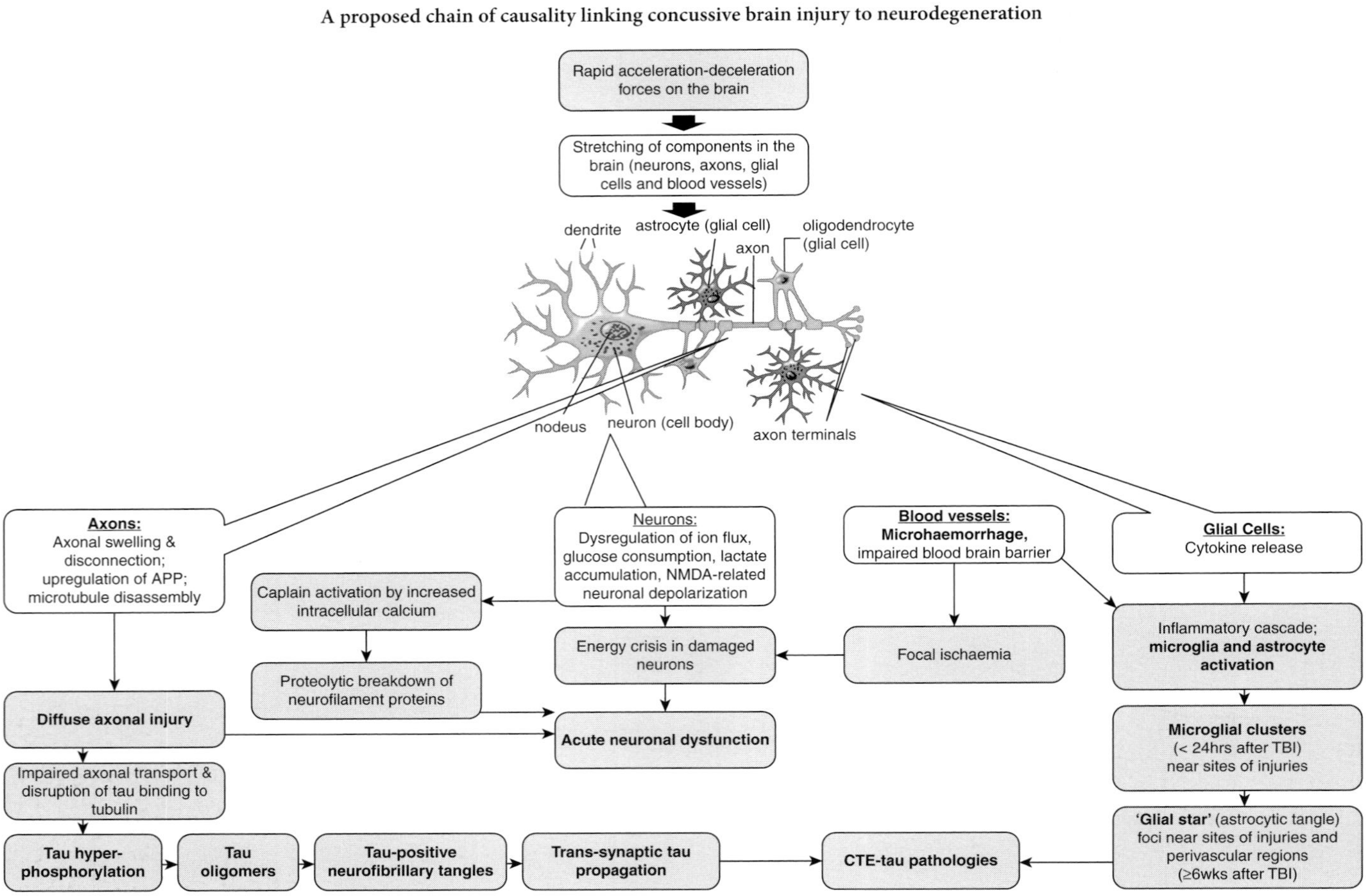

A proposed chain of causality linking concussive brain injury to neurodegeneration

Fig. 1.35 Schematic illustration of the proposed cascade of events triggered by acute traumatic brain injuries (TBIs) and its possible mechanistic links with the development of chronic traumatic encephalopathy (CTE) pathology. APP: amyloid precursor protein; NMDA: N-methyl-d-aspartate. [A black and white version of this figure will appear in some formats. For the color version, please refer to the plate section.]

Source: Ling et al., 2015 [290] with permission from Elsevier

et al. [292] put it, "The entire field of mTBI investigations has changed with the introduction of advanced neuroimaging methods concomitant with an improved understanding of mTBI neuropathology and the opportunity to use neuroimaging and electrophysiological biomarkers." DTI findings have been mentioned above. We will briefly comment on the potential of ¹H MRS and fMRI. All three approaches will receive more rigorous attention in later chapters. Despite the glint of gold in the recent imaging literature, however, two caveats perhaps deserve mention. One: no single method is likely to capture every subtle injury. Dean et al.'s recent caveat [293] gives pause to the optimism of an ideal imaging method: "some individuals may demonstrate a greater difference in one specific modality (e.g., DTI) whilst another may exhibit more of a difference in another modality (e.g., MRS)" (p. 58). Two: the pace of discovery in biomedical imaging is fantastic. Principles of inquiry are all one can take from this discussion. The technology will change in a heartbeat.

Proton Magnetic Resonance Spectroscopy

¹H MRS permits *in vivo* assay of multiple neurochemical compounds, but most attention has been paid to *N*-acetyl aspartate (NAA), creatine (Cr), and choline (Cho). The bio-utility of

NAA remains a bit mysterious. It seems to participate in multiple processes, including myelination, osmolality regulation, and energy production. Evidence suggests that NAA levels may reflect neuronal health – although it is not clear whether the levels better track harm or recovery. Multiple neurological disorders such as stroke and cancer exhibit decreased NAA levels. Although that observation previously led to the presumption that NAA decline is a biomarker for "cell death," that is probably not the case: since 2000 it has been reported that a decrease in NAA levels occurs in TBI in both experimental animals and humans, that the decrease is proportional to the severity of the injury, that, in mild injury, decreased NAA may occur *without* cell death, and that – generally speaking – NAA recovers after mild injury but not after severe injury [294, 295]. NAA apparently tracks neuronal health for two reasons: first, in TBI of almost any severity, membrane permeability is increased. This permits an outflow of NAA to the extracellular space. Second, producing this molecule requires acetyl-coenzyme (CoA). But a neuron suffering the energy crisis described above needs to devote its precious supply of acetyl-CoA to the first-order task of helping to restore its ATP. The result: the more severe the injury, the less acetyl-CoA is available for NAA. That hypothetically makes a decrease in NAA a useful marker for energy depletion – or neuronal "fatigue" (if not exhaustion) – but not necessarily cell death [214].

Cho is considered a marker of cell membrane turnover. Some studies have reported increases after injury (perhaps reflecting lipid peroxidation and recovery); others have reported no change. The level of this compound often serves as a comparator. For instance, a low NAA level compared with a normal or elevated Cho level suggests injury. With regard to Cr: this metabolite is important in the Cr/phosphocreatine shuttle – a system that facilitates rapid transfer of a high-energy phosphate group from the mitochondria for converting ADP to adenosine triphosphate. Its level is also thought to reflect glial function. Although its level is regarded as relatively resistant to the effects of injury, considerable disparity appears in the TBI literature with studies reporting decreased, increased, or no change in this metabolite [214, 296, 297]. If Cr levels are resistant to CBI while NAA levels are sensitive to such injuries, then Cr can be used to normalize NAA findings and a fall in the ratio of NAA to Cr might help quantify neuronal energy jeopardy. If, on the other hand, brain injury changes Cr concentration (and especially if the direction of change is variable), then that ratio cannot be interpreted. It remains to be seen: (1) what absolute or relative levels of these three metabolites reflect what physiological changes; (2) whether the commonly reported ratios detect or predict lasting cerebral harm; and (3) to what degree individual variation (for instance, in the mechanism of concussion, the time after impact, or the demographics and genetics of the patient) complicates interpretation of those ratios. However, most studies regard a decreased NAA/Cr ratio or NAA/Cho ratio as evidence of neurons in trouble. These findings have raised hope that *in vivo* NAA-related assays might serve as a valid measure of injury severity, and perhaps even a marker to monitor the efficacy of treatment or the degree of recovery.

Which brings us to the data regarding ^{1}H MRS in humans after CBI. Vagnozzi et al. [298], for example, scanned 40 athletes who had survived CBI at 3, 15, 22, and 30 days post-injury. As shown in Figure 1.36, the nadir of the ratio between NAA- and Cr-containing compounds was observed on day 3. By self-report, the athletes tended to recover symptomatically by day 15, but the NAA/Cr levels only recovered in all subjects by day 30. This provides further evidence that symptoms, signs, or neuropsychological test results do not accurately reflect brain health. In a subgroup of six doubly concussed athletes, all professing that they no longer had symptoms, restoration of normal NAA occurred at 75–120 days. This evidence supports the virtually universally acknowledged fact, empirically described since Koch and Filehne hammered luckless dogs in 1874 [97], that a second impact during the period of metabolic vulnerability causes a brain injury far more disabling than would otherwise be expected for a blow of that force. As Vagnozzi et al. caution, given both wide variability in the persistence of this biomarker of brain injury and the disconnect between subjective complaints and objective evidence of brain dysfunction, it is impossible to state when a person might "recover" from a concussion [298].

The question remains whether the brain effects of CBI that mediate the persistent or permanent symptoms seen in a subset

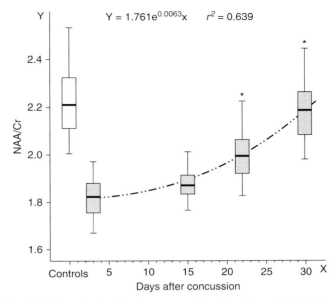

Recovery of *N*-acetylaspartate/creatine-containing compounds in brains of athletes who survived concussive brain injury

$Y = 1.761e^{0.0063}x \qquad r^2 = 0.639$

Fig. 1.36 A box plot showing the recovery of the *N*-acetylaspartate (NAA)/creatine (Cr)-containing compounds ratio occurring in 40 athletes following concussion and reporting the equation and the best fit curve to the data (indicated by a dash-dotted line). Each box is the mean value determined in 30 healthy controls and 40 concussed athletes. Confidence intervals (95%) are represented by vertical bars. *$P < 0.01$ with respect to 3 days.
Source: Vagnozzi et al., 2010 [298], p. 3238 by permission of Oxford University Press

of cases can be detected with this technology. In one study [299], 20 "mTBI" patients and matched controls were scanned to determine whole-brain NAA. The duration of time elapsed from injury to scan ranged from 1.2 months to 31.5 years. In addition to showing that NAA levels were lower among the concussed patients, the study also reported that NAA levels were low up to eight years post-injury and that global atrophy increased over time among the injured. The authors inferred "that the eventual pathologic outcome of mild TBI is loss of cortical neurons" ([299], p. 911).

In another study, Dean et al. [300] reported a reduced Cr/Cho level among 16 "mTBI" patients compared with controls. The metabolite abnormality persisted beyond 12 months. However, that reduced ratio was not confined to those with brain injury: reduced Cr/Cho was found in subjects who complained of post-concussive-type symptoms, *whether or not they had had brain injuries.*

Again, the evidence is ineluctable that post-concussive complaints are associated with altered brain function. The only question is the degree to which causality is rightly attributed to the impact.

Yet the jury is out on the validity of metabolites or metabolite ratios as markers of brain damage. In a seemingly paradoxical finding, for example, Johnson et al. reported that the greater the number of concussions a college athlete had experienced, the *higher* were his NAA/Cho and NAA/Cr levels [301]. The authors speculated that, rather than marking cell death or even energy jeopardy, NAA increase after CBI may be a marker of the mobilization of adaptive and reparative processes.

Functional MRI Studies

It is still early days in the interpretation of fMRI results. Present methods do not measure neuronal activity, but merely infer it from changes in blood oxygenation. The normal "resting state," normal patterns of connectivity, or normal patterns of response to tasks have not been defined in ways that permit robustly reliable comparison across centers. External confirmation of validity – for instance, clinico-imaging-pathological correlation showing that a given complex temporo-spatial pattern of relative hyper- and hypo-activations sensitively and specifically identifies a neurobiological change – is just beginning. Moreover, reports are inconsistent regarding whether a CBI-damaged brain is more likely to exhibit *reduced* activity while performing a task [302–304] – perhaps because it fails to recruit needed cerebral resources – or *increased* activity [305–325] – perhaps because it needs to burn more energy to accomplish the same work [308]. It has become apparent, nonetheless, that fMRI findings contribute to the growing body of evidence that many concussions that superficially seem transient are not. Numerous studies of concussed individuals in the "chronic" phase (setting aside, for a moment, the question of clinical "recovery") report patterns of hyper- and/or hypo-activation persisting as long as 3.6 years [302, 303, 307, 309–314].

The fMRI literature, combined with the renaissance of attention to late-onset neurodegenerative effects, has played havoc with the 20th- century conceptualization of "recovery" after concussion. A few decades ago, one might have been content to opine, "He looks fine, he feels fine, he tests fine – he's fine." Our new information is a reminder of books and their covers: as in the case of latent syphilis, a body can be diseased for decades while all stand by unaware. It was no surprise when studies showed persistent activation abnormalities in symptomatic concussed athletes many months after CBI. Nor was it surprising to learn that athletes who developed post-concussive depression still showed reduced activation in the dorsolateral prefrontal cortex and striatum on average six to seven months later [315] or that soldiers exposed to mild blast injuries exhibit abnormal cerebral function on average 964 days after the event [307].

Yet two other findings are perhaps even more informative regarding the utility of fMRI. First, CBI survivors with completely normal neuropsychological test scores exhibit abnormal patterns of brain activation when performing cognitive tasks [306, 316–318]. This finding might be interpreted as adaptive recovery – except for the fact that, based on some fMRI studies and subjective reports, even if the patient's cognitive performance normalizes, he or she may struggle harder to do the same brain work [308]. Inefficient, effortful processing may be among the largest hidden costs of CBI [319, 320].

Second, and more compelling still, is the finding that *abnormalities of brain function persist in asymptomatic CBI survivors, sometimes long after the patient has "recovered."*

"Recovery" has often been defined as the resolution of subjective symptoms and objective signs. As neuropsychologists devised increasingly sensitive tests, it became apparent that many concussed patients who look and feel neurologically fine are nonetheless somewhat cognitively inferior to their baselines [321]. This discovery informed the first dissociation: between the patient's complaints and the evidence of lasting brain damage. fMRI has pushed the issue further. What is one to say about a patient who has no complaints, a normal neurological examination, and no apparent neuropsychological impairment, when his neuroimaging reveals persistent alterations in processing?

A number of fMRI studies in concussion or so-called mTBI inspire that question. Both resting studies and activation studies, in which the brain is scanned while performing a task, report similar conclusions. McAllister et al. [305, 309], Slobounov et al. [235], and Mayer et al. [322], for instance, have all published studies in which concussed patients display normal neuropsychological function as compared with controls, yet, in the course of performing a cognitive task, exhibit significantly abnormal (in the conventional sense of different from those of normal controls) patterns of cerebral activation at one year after injury [309].

In a related study, Slobounov et al. [323] followed more than 300 men participating in college contact sports for 12 months. Some suffered single CBIs. Although all concussed subjects were asymptomatic by day ten and had returned to baseline on neuropsychological tests, those who exhibited more than 20% suppression of electroencephalogram alpha power in the acute phase continued to exhibit electroencephalogram and balance abnormalities a year later. This seems consistent with the evidence previously presented that neuropsychological testing is often insensitive to the effects of concussion. Mild blast injury is also associated with long-term imaging abnormalities: Scheibel et al. [307] instructed 15 subjects with mild injuries to watch a screen and rapidly identify the stimulus. Compared with normal controls, CBI subjects exhibited significant differences in activation in multiple brain regions (Figure 1.37). Perhaps even more worrisome: Abbas et al. [324] reported that asymptomatic American high school football players *began* their season with different functional connectivity compared with their healthy peers – suggesting that, with or without histories of concussion, children who play contact sports have altered brains. The players also displayed exacerbation of that difference as the season progressed.

These research protocols are not readily comparable. The findings in terms of localization and degree of activation are different between studies. Yet long-lived brain change after CBI was demonstrated using every approach.

In fairness, the deep meaning of the findings illustrated in Figure 1.37 (and many similar studies) is unclear. Although the pattern of activity is *different* from normal, only replication of a given protocol with an increased and better control for potential confounds will confirm validity. Even then, it will be uncertain to what degree we are visualizing a healthful, adaptive response – reorganizing the cortex to do tasks equally well in a new way – versus a devolution to an inferior processing system, possibly associated with an increased risk of dementia.

We are probably decades from understanding the pictures we take of these buffeted brains. Until there exist normed

Altered cerebral activation in survivors of mild traumatic brain injury (TBI) due to blast at 964 days (M) after injury

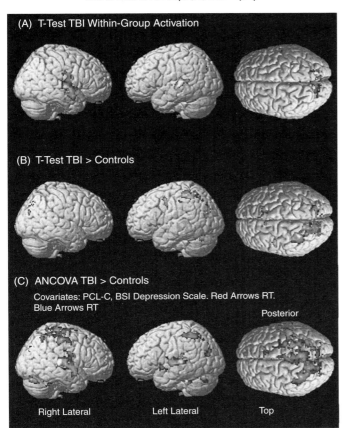

Fig. 1.37 Brain surface images displaying cortical areas with significant t-test and analysis of covariance (ANCOVA) results: (A) significant activation in subjects with TBI; (B) areas where the TBI group had greater activation than the control group; and (C) areas where the TBI group had greater activation than the control group after controlling for blue arrows reaction time (RT), red arrows RT, and scores on the Brief Symptom Inventory (BSI) Depression Scale and Post-traumatic Stress Disorder Checklist (PCL-C). [A black and white version of this figure will appear in some formats. For the color version, please refer to the plate section.]

Source: Scheibel et al., 2012 [307, p. 96] by permission of Cambridge University Press

and validated biomarkers for the many, many ways brains are affected by CBI, and very long-term follow-up reveals their predictive validity for neurodegeneration, we will be gazing at colorful maps and speculating about the location of the dragons. Yet one conclusion seems utterly inescapable: long after CBI, many brains are different. Long after the development of post-concussive symptoms, many brains are different. We propose this is *res judicata*. The questions are: why, and in what way?

If a Tree Falls in a Forest …

Advances in neuroimaging are accelerating the understanding of concussion and so-called mTBI. Other chapters in this textbook provide vastly more sophisticated, nuanced, and informative accounts of these advances. Our purpose here is only to support a point relevant to the question, "what is a concussion?" As we noted at the outset, the question comes down to: is it more reasonable to define and diagnose a medical disorder in

terms of its typical clinical presentation, or in terms of an essential biological problem? Moreover, one is obliged to ask: what is the best way to distinguish between a "change" that is part of the normal physiological accommodation of new circumstances, and a "disorder?" This amounts to a philosophical question about the very concept of disease. In the simplest case, *disease* is a biological problem that causes a decline in ease – either a subjective sense of being unwell or subnormal function in performing the operations of life. If a concussed patient both feels well and performs normally in every respect, is that person's functional organic change a disorder? It is premature to declare that the persistent alterations observed with fMRI identify an essential biological problem. It is open to debate whether functional changes that (as yet) have no certain neuropathological correlates represent "damage" (but see [325]). Perhaps the conceptual key is to distinguish between complete and incomplete adaptation: if the brain rewires itself to do its old job with suave aplomb, it recovered. But if the brain has been obliged either to work harder in its old way, or to invent less energy-efficient work-arounds to keep up with its expected work output, or has been derailed on to a faster track of brain aging, it has not.

Philosophy of disease aside, these findings strongly support a new conclusion that demands consideration and arguably mandates rejection of the "typical clinical" approach to diagnosis: even without clinical symptoms, even without clinical signs, even without neuropsychological deficits, the concussed brain is likely to exhibit long-term changes. As Slobounov et al. (235) unassumingly summarized the robust conclusion from new imaging studies: "There is growing evidence that atypical evolution of mild TBI may be more prevalent due to the fact that physical, neurocognitive, emotional symptoms and underlying neural alterations persist months or even years post-injury."

The Imponderability of Mildness

Why, then, do we still see the phrase "mild traumatic brain injury," even in medical journals? What value, if any, does the phrase "mild traumatic brain injury" have? This irresolvable conceptual conundrum, to which we will return periodically in this text, involves a lesser and a greater problem. The lesser problem is the question of *when* to measure brain injury severity. It is well known that bleeding in the head can be delayed. It is therefore imprudent to classify severity early in the clinical course – for instance, according to the patient's alertness at the moment of registration to the ER. Such a policy would lead to labeling many injuries *mild* that are associated with death within 24 h. It might conceivably be more sensible to classify CBI/TBI severity based on outcome a year later. That might far better characterize the likely impact on quality of life over the ensuing decade or two – if only one could define mild.

However, evidence suggests that CBIs are sometimes associated with deposition of pathological proteins and neurodegeneration, followed by behavioral change, including dementia ~10–70 years after the injury. Therefore, if we embrace a consensus to classify injury severity at 365 days, we will invariably classify some cases as "mild" that, upon longer-term follow-up, are associated with catastrophic cognitive collapse. This might or might not be regarded as accurate severity classification.

The greater problem, by far, is the imponderability of mildness. Assume universal agreement on the lesser issue, with a worldwide consensus to classify severity of brain injury at 365 days after impact. What gold standard specifies the boundary between mild and not mild?

- loss of up to 14 neurons from the medial temporal allocortex but not 15?
- a 5.5% decline in hippocampal efficiency for incorporation of cytosolic AMPA receptors into the post-synaptic membrane in response to an episode of spatial learning, but not a 5.75% decline?
- a decline in NAA levels by 1 s D from lab's standardized age- and sex- and body mass index-adjusted population mean that normalizes within 96 h but not 97 h?
- permanent loss of ultrastructural elements (e.g., microtubules) without permanent loss of microstructural elements (e.g., organelles, especially mitochondria) or of whole cells?

Reflection makes the challenge of a meaningful nomination apparent. As Signoretti et al. eloquently summarized the state of play as of 2011:

> The label "mild" in mTBI does not reflect the severity of the underlying metabolic and physiologic processes, if not even the potential clinical manifestations … The overall doubt that might be generated from the combination of these studies on gene expression with the biochemical works previously cited is that, apparently, not much rationale is left to justify the adjective "mild" when dealing with a concussive injury.
>
> ([214], p. s365)

In point of fact, no biologically meaningful threshold exists. One is thus obliged to nominate some arbitrary, clinical, operational threshold for the upper limit of mildness.

For this reason, we submit that the time has come to reject, dismiss, and abandon the terminology "mild traumatic brain injury." "Mild" tells us nothing important. Despite the wishes of attorneys, epidemiologists, insurance adjusters, and irredeemable pigeon holers, we do not see a compelling reason to refine or perfect a definition of mTBI or to define an immutable boundary between mild and not mild. A far more meaningful distinction, in terms of both biology and human well-being, is between recoverable and not. That is, what matters far more than any arbitrary red-line severity marker is whether a CBI survivor truly, completely, lastingly gets back to his or her baseline. Is this episode more like a transient upper respiratory tract infection followed by both complete restoration of health and enhanced immunity? Or more like a subtle episode of meningitis followed by a subtle brain change? *Did the injury cause, provoke, or trigger a lasting deleterious change in the quality of the person's life?*

Imagining "Recovery"

Recovery is another problematic and borderline ineffable notion. In an effort to classify degree of recovery, many clinicians employ global outcome measures such as the Glasgow Outcome Scale (GOS) [326]. The GOS discriminates between *mild disability* (able to return to work or school) *moderate disability* (able to live independently), and *severe disability* (unable to live independently). Although these global clinical differences correlate rather poorly with biological measures, they rhetorically capture one's instinctive impression of different degrees of disease. This satisfies attorneys. Scientists demur. One problem is that the GOS and other such operational estimates of severity tend to be oblivious to decline from previous level of function. Consider three cases of GOS-mild:

1. a ditch digger who returns to work
2. a ditch digger who returns to work but now regularly beats his wife and children
3. an astrophysicist who returns to work as a ditch digger.

Do these three GOS-mild cases suggest that "mild" is a specific degree of change, or that this rating is satisfactorily informative? It quickly becomes apparent that more nuance is required but hard to operationalize.

The slowly clearing picture of the pathophysiology of concussion provokes another question: does anyone ever recover? Just a generation ago, this question would have seemed absurd. Yet the strong evidence of both inapparent lasting brain dysfunction and later magnification of the risk for neurodegeneration inspires a thought: if a boy sustains a concussion and he acts and feels fine for the next 70 years, yet he's suffered an inscrutable biological change that increases his risk of developing dementia 6 months sooner by 5%, has he "recovered"?

We tentatively propose a practical way to determine the answer to that quasi-metaphysical question: if a CBI survivor never feels, or displays on testing, any adaptive disadvantage – if his or her brain's new way of operating (whether or not it is "inefficient") in no way obliges behavioral adjustments to deal with a higher metabolic cost for the same neural operations, in no way lessens the person's quality of life, functions, or longevity – then a range of post-concussional states may be akin to varying renal function that remains well within the healthy range. By way of comparison (depending on one's laboratory standards): following acute renal failure, many patients are asymptomatic, but their metabolic health varies. A creatinine of 1.8 mg/dL may be in the normal range but is associated with a risk of later kidney dysfunction; a creatinine of 1.5 mg/dL may not be optimum, but has much lower known deleterious associations in the short or long term; and a creatinine of 1.2 mg/dL suggests full recovery. In the same way, there exists a spectrum of brain health among "asymptomatic" CBI survivors. Some have authentically recovered, have returned in every respect to baseline function, and will never exhibit a change in the vulnerability to degeneration. In other cases, perhaps their brain struggles more to accomplish the same tasks (whether or not they are aware of that struggle), or pays a price in cognitive fatigue, or exhibits a subtle impairment of multitasking facility under stress, or exhibits an escalated risk to health in the senium. That CBI is a lasting disorder. Clinical neurology has barely begun to discuss the validity of such distinctions.

Apart from the thought-provoking observation that symptoms do not necessarily track "recovery" in concussion, the question remains why many persons report symptomatic improvement in less than one month, and others, more than 40%, develop persistent or permanent distress [327–330].[2] Some writers have opined that there is no miserable minority [331–333]. They opine that if you pool large numbers of mTBI cases in a meta-analysis, the *average* resolution of symptoms is short and therefore *lasting problems are rare*. The illogic of this argument is self-evident. It equates to declaring, "The *average* gross national product (GNP) of Earth's nations is ~$367 billion. Therefore nations with markedly different GNPs – such as the United States, China, Japan, Germany, France, the United Kingdom, Italy, Brazil, Spain, and Canada – are unlikely to exist." Bigler et al. [292] deserve credit for a scholarly *tour de force* in which they marshaled the evidence and dismantled that argument: the articles that claim that concussive problems infrequently persist are rife with clinical assumptions and statistical errors.

> In conclusion we show methodological violations … that limit Rohling et al.'s [333] critique where their findings merely perpetuate type-II statistical errors. As already stated, it is an untenable and non-supportable position that neuron-based symptoms and deficits do not persist in some individuals who experience mTBI".
>
> ([292], p. 31)

Still, it is a matter of some urgency to need to understand why some victims of concussion seem to exhibit lasting problems, while others do not. At this moment in the history of medicine, one can only speculate about the answers that account for the largest amount of the variance.

One factor may be biological severity. Given the multi-faceted neurobiological correlates of concussive injury, it seems invariable that some victims will suffer more cell loss than others. Yet severity may be moderated in any number of ways. For example, some brains – whether based on age, gender, ethnicity, or innate neurobiological factors – are probably more vulnerable to concussive apoptotic cell loss than others suffering similar injuries. Even if cell loss is identical, some brains perhaps exhibit greater or lesser resilience and adaptive capacity. Di Pietro et al.'s observation that 999 enzymes are up- or down-regulated in concussion offers a possible genetic explanation for clinical variation: presumably some of the genes for pro- and anti-apoptotic enzymes exhibit variants such as allelic polymorphisms [278]. If so, the miserable minority may be explained, in part, by genetic variation in either the allelic type or the expression of these genes. Psychological factors also deserve attention. Many opinions and some evidence suggest that persons with pre-morbid psychiatric distress are more prone to persistent post-concussive symptoms [173].

This prompts a question too monumental for the present essay: what is the relationship between CBI and neuropsychiatric disorders such as depression or PTSD? Shenton et al. [227] expressed a concern that the answer has been unscientifically polarized.

> We would argue that the controversy between mTBI being psychogenic versus physiogenic in origin is not productive because the psychogenic view does not carefully consider the limitations of conventional neuroimaging techniques in detecting subtle brain injuries in mTBI, and the physiogenic view does not carefully consider the fact that PTSD and depression, and other co-morbid conditions, may be present in those suffering from mTBI ([227], p. 139).

A related concept may also deserve consideration: drawing a line between mental and neurological problems is another pre-Enlightenment holdover of the Cartesian false dichotomy. As the renowned behavioral neurologist D. Frank Benson put it, "There may be mindless brains, but there are no brainless minds" (personal communication). All the symptoms of depression and PTSD are mediated by brain change, especially in the circuitry of emotional regulation. All the symptoms of concussion are mediated by brain change, which seems to include changes in the circuitry of emotional regulation. A clinical overlap is inevitable.

We do not propose a definitive response to the "why a miserable minority?" question. We do, however, urge a more vigorous pursuit of an answer (see Chapter 7). Although premature neurodegeneration may harm CBI survivors after a delay, during the months and years following a brain-shaking event it is the more than 40% with persistent dysfunction whose lives, families, friends, and wider social networks are most impacted by concussion (see Chapter 5). Any acute intervention that would reduce the chance of chronicity would be precious.

Diagnostic Semantics

How then, is a clinician to diagnose a typical medically attended CBI? This is a legitimate pragmatic concern. Any agreed clinical criteria, like the atheoretical, non-biological algorithms employed by psychiatrists, could probably be refined to the point where two clinicians will reliably attach the same name to a comparable history and presentation. Even without our being able to assay the pathophysiology, that approach has the practical virtue of classifying the patient as someone who might benefit from neurological attention. Yet, until there is a valid biomarker, employing operational diagnostic criteria to generate a term of art will always leave validity in doubt. One simple solution is to acknowledge doubt, say what we know, and leave it at that. The authors of this chapter (and editors of this volume) implore clinicians to follow a simple rule: be informative.

If, for example, Alejandra comes in telling a story of falling off a newly built wall while commuting to her job in southern Arizona, striking her head, and regaining alertness on the

---

2   Some 20th-century sources opined that only 15% of concussion survivors, or even fewer, exhibited persistent clinically significant dysfunction. Considering CBI as a whole – including the vast majority of cases that are invisible to clinical medicine – no credible estimate of the proportion with either persistent or late effects will be available for the foreseeable future. Considering the subject of this book, typical medically attended CBI, a systematic review offered in Chapter 5 of this volume determined that more than 40% of survivors experience or exhibit persistent dysfunction at and beyond one year post-injury.

U.S. side over three minutes, one can be reasonably sure that her brain sustained a rattling blow. Unless and until definitive biomarkers are discovered, the prudent, scientifically justifiable diagnosis would be "probable abrupt brain rattling" or "probable CBI," which means the same thing. A computed tomography (CT) change compatible with subdural hematoma would not change that diagnosis. Nothing about an intracranial hemorrhage, or a depressed skull fracture, or a sprinkling of shrapnel, or a week of coma, would reduce the likelihood that Alejandra's brain exhibits the thousands of biological changes typical of brain-rattling CBI. It would, however, enhance diagnostic specificity and sometimes alter treatment.

The question is what to write under "impression." Assume Alejandra were lucky enough to have undergone emergency imaging. (A later chapter in this text will discuss the evidence for and against routine CT scanning.) Assume the CT shows a crescentic, homogeneously hyperdense extra-axial fluid collection spreading over the right frontoparietal convexity with a maximum width of 1.2 cm on the axial scan. A doctor who wrote "complicated mild traumatic brain injury" might cheer an attorney. But that clinician, or any clinician who uses terms such as *mild*, *moderate*, *severe*, or *complicated*, has recorded virtually nothing of medical value. Such antique phraseology has no predictive validity, offers no guide to treatment, and obfuscates when it should reveal. In contrast, a doctor might record what he or she knows: "probable abrupt brain rattling with CT imaging consistent with right frontoparietal convexity subdural hematoma with a maximum width of 1.2 cm."[3]

Clinical presentation also matters – although less than was previously thought. The duration of loss of consciousness, Glasgow Coma Scale score, or estimated duration of post-traumatic amnesia (almost never measured with replicable accuracy) might somewhat enhance the specificity of the acute diagnosis. That is, even though the GCS has almost no predictive validity, expert sequential monitoring can be life saving in the acute setting. Again, one strives to inform. A GCS score divorced from a temporal context is less useful than a simple account of the course. The doctor who records "GCS 13" has done far less clinical good than a doctor who records "She came in very confused but an hour later she's less confused." Our dead simple proposal for diagnostic semantics derives from this book's guiding apophthegm: when in doubt, tell the truth.

Part III: Efforts to Define Concussion by Means of "Consensus"

A good deal of awkwardness of expression is encountered in discussing concussion. This stems from the usage of the term "concussion" to characterize both the mechanical incident which produces injury and the state of the injured individual for some indefinite interval afterwards.

Groat and Simmons, 1950 [194, p. 150]

With the preceding history as a springboard, professional groups entered the fray in the 1960s and cobbled together "consensus" definitions of concussion. Since each organization has its own agenda, none of these actually represents an agreement of a representative group of neurologists, neurosurgeons, physiatrists, psychiatrists, neuropsychologists, and neurobiologists studying concussion. The motivations of the leadership of each self-selected committee probably varied. In some cases, the goal seems to have been an earnest effort to review the evidence and develop a useful definition. In other cases, one might be forgiven for concluding that the leaders had another goal: to resolve the ongoing debate between those who considered concussion a mechanism of injury and those who considered it a synonym for mTBI in favor of the latter opinion by means of "expert" fiat. Motivations aside, the question is whether any of these "consensus" definitions are compatible with logic and science.

Before examining these efforts individually, it deserves mention that the number of possible outcomes from such an effort is dazzlingly large. To illustrate how differing opinions about plausible defining factors yield a multiplicity of competing definitions, just consider the issue of consciousness. Different writers (1) specify that consciousness is lost; (2) specify that consciousness is altered; or (3) do not specify the effect of concussion on consciousness. Within the first two groups, different writers (a) specify that the change of consciousness is appreciated subjectively; or (b) specify that that change is observed objectively; or (c) specify that that change is both subjective and objective; or (d) do not specify whether that change is subjective or objective. Setting aside the factor of duration of loss or change in consciousness (which allows for an infinitude of definitions), these alternatives yield 13 potential statements regarding the contribution of consciousness to the definition of *concussion*.

Now consider the fact that, by the mid 20th century, the factors that had been earnestly proposed as definitively distinguishing concussion from non-concussion had grown to about 25. Table 1.2 lists those factors.

The math is trivial: note that, if each of the 25 proposed defining traits were regarded as dichotomous (a grand oversimplification), and the thorny issue of duration is excluded (since inclusion of this issue automatically provides for an infinitude of definitions), the combinations of clinical criteria available to a committee that proposed to generate a consensus definition of concussion would be 2^{25}, or 33,554,432. (Since many variables are ordinal or continuous, rather than dichotomous, the real number is infinite.) This observation perhaps helps to explain both the reportedly fractious ambience of "consensus" meetings and the delay in achieving the laudable goal of international transdisciplinary agreement.

In 1966, the Committee on Head Injury Nomenclature of the Congress of Neurological Surgeons defined concussion as "a clinical syndrome characterized by immediate and transient

---

[3] The authors predict that, within a decade, there will have been sufficient progress in imaging-pathological correlation to permit acute scanning to enhance outcome prediction. For instance, one might soon diagnose "probable CBI with an estimated mean 12–17% stretch of fibers in the uncinate fasciculus per diffusion kurtosis imaging."

Table 1.2 Factors previously employed as defining traits of concussion

1. **Tissue affected** (e.g., whole body, part of body, skull, nervous system, brain)

2. **Mechanical cause** (e.g., unspecified impact, blow, fall, projectile, "outside force")

3. **Immediate _loss_ of consciousness** (e.g., subjective loss of consciousness vs. objectively observed loss of consciousness vs. loss of consciousness not specified in regard to subjectivity vs. objectivity)

4. **Immediate _change_ in level of consciousness** (e.g., subjective change in consciousness vs. objectively observed change in consciousness vs. change in consciousness not specified)

5. **Duration of loss or change in consciousness** (e.g., "transient," "fleeting," "less than five minutes," "less than 24 h")

6. **Effect on memory for the event** (i.e., subjective, objective, or unspecified amnesia for the moment of impact vs. subjective, objective, or unspecified amnesia for the precipitant of the impact, such as fall)

7. **Effect on memories preceding the event** (i.e., subjective, objective, or unspecified _occurrence_ of retrograde amnesia; subjective, objective, or unspecified _duration_ of retrograde amnesia)

8. **Effect on memories following the event** (i.e., subjective, objective, or unspecified _occurrence_ of anterograde amnesia; subjective, objective, or unspecified _duration_ of anterograde amnesia)

9. **Immediate effect on cognitive functions other than consciousness or memory** with or without specification of duration (e.g., loss of speech; for example: _Hippocratic Corpus_)

10. **Immediate effect on motor functions** with or without specification, whether the change was subjective, objective, or not specified, and with or without specification of duration (e.g., "paralysis," "weakness," "fall")

11. **Immediate effect on equilibrium** with or without specification whether the change was subjective, objective, or not specified, and with or without specification of duration (e.g., "dizziness," "disequilibrium," "imbalance," "incoordination")

12. **Immediate effect on gait** with or without specification, whether the change was subjective, objective, or not specified, and with or without specification of duration (e.g., "tipping," "stumbling," "staggering")

13. **Expected to impact autonomic functions** (e.g., nausea, sweating, blood pressure)

14. **Confined to some lower level of severity** (e.g., not worse than "mild head injury," "mild traumatic brain injury")

15. **Explicitly excludes some upper level of severity** (e.g., excludes "grave" injuries, or injuries producing immediate death)

16. **Confined to injuries with purportedly complete recovery** (vs. includes the possibility of a subset with persistent symptoms)

17. **Maximum duration of sequelae specified or not** (e.g., "no more than three months")

18. **Presumed gross pathology specified or not** (e.g., "rupture of a cerebral vein or nerve")

19. **Presumed pathophysiology specified or not** (e.g., humors)

20. **Confined to head or brain injury _absent_ any localizing neurological signs**

21. **Confined to head or brain injury _absent_ any pathological changes visible on gross examination of the brain**

22. **Confined to head or brain injury _absent_ skull fracture**

23. **Confined to head or brain injury _absent_ brain contusion**

24. **Confined to head or brain injury _absent_ brain hemorrhage**

25. **Confined to head or brain injury _absent_ lesions visible on computed tomography scanning**

impairment of neural function, such as alteration of consciousness, disturbance of vision, equilibrium, etc. due to mechanical forces" [334]. A clinical definition such as this based on typical observations is entirely acceptable as an arbitrary operational delineation of a narrow symptom complex. However, it is inherently false if it is used to diagnose a biological problem. Tuberculosis is not invariably a wasting syndrome with frequent cough. Conditions that clinically conform to a "cold" are not invariably self-limited upper respiratory infections due to rhinovirus. Concussion – if regarded as a biological problem – exhibits variation in clinical presentation and outcome. Many cases of mild closed head injury involving general brain commotion due to external force have persistent effects and therefore would be called "not-concussion" by this committee. A minor additional criticism: blast can apparently produce concussive injury. Blast injury is not due to a "mechanical force" and is also excluded by this committee's definition.

In 1997, the Quality Standards Subcommittee of the American Academy of Neurology published a practice parameter for the management of concussion in sports [335]. Their definition: "Concussion is a trauma-induced alteration in mental status that may or may not involve loss of consciousness." Nine "frequently observed" features were appended. This operational clinical definition is less specific than most – making it prone to low levels of interrater reliability. The phrase "may or may not" was surely intended to alert clinicians that the old Denny-Brown and Russell (1941) [182] exclusion of TBIs without complete loss of consciousness should be rejected in favor of C. Miller Fisher's 1966 [336] more liberal allowance for concussion with mere dazing. However, for definitional purposes, the American Academy of Neurology definition comes down to _trauma-induced alteration in mental status_. (One might give the authors the benefit of the doubt that they had intended to include mention of the head; as written, their definition applies to mosquito bites of the great toe.) The American Academy of Neurology definition excludes the possibility that, depending on its intracerebral dispersion, force may provoke a variety of biological changes without necessarily altering mental status. More importantly, this definition includes any type of TBI – e.g., gunshot wound or epidural hemorrhage – without specifying what element of the injury is the concussive element.

In 2001 [337], the first of a series of meeting was held by the self-appointed Concussion in Sport Group (CISG), consisting of attendees at a Vienna meeting organized by the International Ice Hockey Federation, the Fédération Internationale de Football Association (FIFA) Medical Assessment and Research Centre, and the International Olympic Committee Medical Commission. This group stated, "Concussion is defined as a complex pathophysiological process affecting the brain, induced by traumatic biomechanical forces" ([337], p. 6). The group goes on to characterize "typical" features, such as rapid onset of short-lived impairment that resolves spontaneously. However, the definition includes several components that have yet to be proved correct. For instance, it is stated that the brain changes "largely reflect a functional disturbance rather than structural injury." Given the indisputable evidence of immediate physical membrane damage and rapid ultrastructural disruption, it would seem better to state that the frequency, degree, and duration of structural injury have yet to be determined. The definition also declares the existence of "a graded set of clinical syndromes." Yet, to date, none of the proposed grading scales have been shown to discriminate distinct biological processes. Moreover, the concept of a unitary syndrome may be inaccurate, especially as regards the persistent symptoms. McAllister [338] commented, "it is not clear that postconcussive symptoms constitute a syndrome per se. Instead, it may be the case that the various symptoms that commonly co-occur after TBI are relatively independent consequences of a single neurological event." Furthermore, the CISG's definition predicts resolution of symptoms according to "a sequential course." Little evidence supports this contention. Patients vary significantly in the pace at which different symptoms resolve or fail to resolve. As Alves et al. [339] put it, "there is considerable variation between patients in the nature and duration of specific complaints and in findings of neuropsychological deficits after head injury. The expectation that recovery follows a singular course is questionable at best"(p. 25). The group yoked their definition to then-current technology, declaring that concussion is typically associated with "grossly normal structural neuroimaging." Depending on one's interpretation of the phrase "structural neuroimaging," as noted above, one already frequently observes axonal abnormalities after concussion using DTI – and one expects the very rapid advances in medical imaging to reveal more and more. The group also agreed that, "neuropsychological testing is one of the cornerstones of concussion evaluation and contributes significantly to both understanding of the injury and management of the individual." We agree. This strong support for the virtues of neuropsychological testing was an important advance. However, it is vital to note that neuropsychological testing is insensitive to some well-documented persistent brain changes after concussion.

Critiques aside, this definition acknowledges that concussion is a biological problem rather than a symptom cluster – a

major advance over mid-20th-century claims that concussion equals mild injury.

Another major consensus effort was documented in the National Athletic Trainers' Association position statement on management of sport-related concussion [340]. In a section titled "Defining and Recognizing Concussion," the authors state:

> Cerebral concussion … can best be classified as a mild diffuse injury and is often referred to as mild TBI (MTBI). The injury involves an acceleration–deceleration mechanism in which a blow to the head or the head striking an object results in 1 or more of the following conditions: headache, nausea, vomiting, dizziness, balance problems, feeling "slowed down," fatigue, trouble sleeping, drowsiness, sensitivity to light or noise, LOC [loss of consciousness], blurred vision, difficulty remembering, or difficulty concentrating.
>
> ([340], p. 283)

The authors of this 2004 paper cited the American Academy of Neurology's 1997 practice parameter [335] as their source. They further claimed that universal agreement exists regarding several features of concussion: (1) "Concussion may be caused by … an 'impulsive' force transmitted to the head"; (2) "Concussion may cause an immediate and short-lived impairment of neurologic function"; (3) "Concussion may cause neuropathological changes"; however, the acute clinical symptoms largely reflect a functional disturbance rather than a structural injury"; (4) "Concussion … may or may not involve LOC [loss of consciousness]. Resolution of the clinical and cognitive symptoms typically follows a sequential course"; and, (5) "Concussion is most often associated with normal results on conventional neuroimaging studies" ([340], p. 284).

This very well-written declaration ably describes typical concussions. However, it exhibits four problematic features. First, the authors literally equated concussion with something mild. By focusing on the typical clinical syndrome rather than the spectrum, it may mislead readers into underestimating the potential severity of concussion. Second, the claim that acute symptoms are largely functional is inconsistent with the established expectation of acute (if possibly reversible) structural changes. Third, the presumption of a "sequential" course of recovery is ambiguous and debatable. Recovery might better be described as highly variable in character, pace, and completeness. Fourth, imaging methods increasingly regarded as "conventional" routinely show changes, even after mild concussive injury.

In 2006, the American College of Sports Medicine published a consensus statement in which the authors declared, "Concussion or mild traumatic brain injury (MTBI) is a pathophysiological process affecting the brain induced by direct or indirect biomechanical forces" ([341], p. 395). Like other committees, this one described what they called "common features": (1) "Rapid onset of usually short-lived neurological impairment, which typically resolves spontaneously"; (2) "Acute clinical symptoms that usually reflect a functional disturbance rather than structural injury"; (3) A range of clinical symptoms that may or may not involve loss of consciousness (LOC)"; and (4) "Neuroimaging studies that are typically normal." This statement mimics previous consensus statements and shares their failings.

Meanwhile, the CISG has continued to meet periodically. They published revised discussions of sports concussion after meetings in Prague (opinionpublished in 2005) [342], Zurich (opinions published in 2009) [343], again in Zurich (opinions published in 2013) [344], and Berlin (opinions published in 2017) [345].

After the 2004 Prague meeting, the same small group of individuals who had composed the 2001 Vienna statement assembled to write a revision [344]. That small group opined, "No significant breakthroughs in scientifically validated information on concussion had occurred between the two conferences" ([344], p. 3). In the publication that followed, it is stated, "No changes were made to the definition by the Prague Group beyond noting that in some cases post-concussive symptoms may be prolonged or persistent" ([342], p. 196). We defer to the hard-working neurobiology community to judge whether significant breakthroughs were published between 2001 and 2004. We credit the Prague statement for its acknowledgment of the miserable minority. Otherwise, the Prague statement simply reiterates the flawed Vienna statement.

The 2004 Prague meeting was also associated with a momentary detour: a controversial rule was adopted to the effect that "simple" concussion means head injury with symptoms lasting less than ten days, while "complex" concussion refers to cases in which symptoms last more then ten days and/or in which the loss of consciousness is "prolonged" and/or when there are concussive convulsions, and/or when there is "prolonged" cognitive impairment, and/or when there is a history of multiple concussions. Fortunately, this arbitrary and operationally highly ambiguous consensus was promptly abandoned at the 3rd International Conference held in 2008, after study showed that simple/complex distinction lacked predictive validity [343, 347].

The third CISG consensus statement followed a 2008 Zurich meeting and was published in 2009 [343]. In an advance, this meeting "was designed as a formal consensus meeting following the organisational guidelines set forth by the US National Institutes of Health" (p. i81). The previous definition of concussion was preserved. The fourth meeting was again held in Zurich [344]. That publication includes several minor revisions in the definition. Perhaps most importantly from the point of view of clinical diagnosis is the recognition that, "in some cases, symptoms and signs may evolve over a number of minutes to hours." Apart from this very helpful acknowledgment of the diverse presentations of concussion, the new definition preserves the problems of the old: it presumes "graded symptoms" without specifying a coherent grading system. It presumes resolution in a "sequential course" without evidence of a consistent sequence. It denies that microscopic injuries are expected and it repeats the increasingly untenable claim of "No abnormality on standard structural neuroimaging studies" ([344], pp. i76–i77). As Slobounov et al. [235] expressed the dogged problem:

there is still a lack in belief among neuropsychological and clinical researchers that concussion results in long lasting structural injury to the neuron. This idea is reflected in the sentiment of nearly every consensus statement on concussion … and is frequently repeated in these statements.

Times are changing. The much-cited CISG consensus statements aside, a rapid increase in and broadening of the disciplinary base of concussion scholarship has been associated with definitions that perhaps seems less specific, but in fact are more valuable, since they restrict their rhetoric to what is scientifically defensible.

For instance, the U.S. Centers for Disease Control and Prevention state, "A concussion is a type of traumatic brain injury, or TBI, caused by a bump, blow, or jolt to the head that can change the way your brain normally works" [348]. The Brain Injury Association of America [349] expanded on this definition: "Concussions are a type of traumatic brain injury (TBI) caused by a blow or jolt to the head. The injury can range from mild to severe and can disrupt the way the brain normally works." We applaud this simple recital of more or less universally accepted facts. It specifies that concussion is a type of brain injury, not an amount of brain injury. It unequivocally acknowledges the broad spectrum of severity. Rather than dismissing structural injury or guessing at the proportion of cases that are "reversible," it prudently adopts the indisputable concept of brain disruption. We respectfully credit the Brain Injury Association of America for its clear voice among the cloud of witnesses.

In spite of the growing knowledge about the pathophysiology of concussion, and in spite of the growing heft of the body of evidence that concussion often results in lasting harm, there remains certain lore. Most laypersons and many professionals feel more comfortable with the notion that concussion is interchangeable with mTBI. Bodin et al. describe the state of the art: "As a diagnosis, concussion is often used interchangeably with terms such as mild traumatic brain injury (mTBI), minor closed head injury, and mild closed head injury" [350]. Again, language is dynamic. If this use of the term concussion remains sufficiently popular, it may be as hard to shake as any traditional name. Like *phthisis*, it provides a ready term of art for a somewhat mysterious clinical syndrome. Like *cold*, it repurposes a word with another clear meaning as a colloquialism for a reasonably identifiable cluster of symptoms. Laypersons and physicians need not consider that a biological process is involved. Retaining the colloquial use of *concussion* might serve some purpose.

That is, unless one wants to understand the disorder. In that case, a definition shackled to the typical clinical picture will always be misleading. *Phthsis* applies equally well to a number of wasting syndromes. So if physicians are content to diagnose the same condition in persons with tuberculosis, amyotrophic lateral sclerosis, and starvation, there is a virtue to retaining phthisis. *Cold* accurately describes the clinical state resulting from typical rhinovirus infection, some allergic reactions, and early legionnaire's disease. If *concussion* is a synonym for minor closed head injury, it applies equally well to milder presentations of subdural hematoma, epidural hematoma, sub-arachnoid hemorrhage, and scalping.

We reject this quirk of 20th-century medical rhetoric. Concussion is an extremely important type of brain trauma. To repeat Ommaya's [85] resonant dictum, *the basic problem of head injuries is concussion.* Effective prevention, diagnosis, acute therapy, and rehabilitation require knowledge of a patho-physiological sequence. The basic science of concussion cannot be a mix of studies of head injuries with completely different biologies that happen to present with mildness. Fortunately, basic science, reasonably aloof from these rhetorical squabbles, is displaying increasing promise for discovering acute interventions that may interrupt the pathophysiological cas-cade of concussion.

Let's say, at some future time, we have discovered safe and effective therapies for the concussive element of brain injury (meaning the diffuse and multifocal processes briefly described above). Consider a case: a young person is kicked in the head with a football cleat. There is a depressed fracture, a tear in the dura, and a small epidural hemorrhage, leading to coma. Unless those injuries defended the brain from the diffuse and multifocal effects of external force, the patient also has concus-sive damage. If *concussion* is used for *mild*, we will not provide that young person with the known effective anti-concussive therapies, since, after all, her injury fails to meet the definition.

The medical community seems doomed to continue to use problematic phrases such as "mild traumatic brain injury." In part because of the self-evident subjectivity of the term *mild*, it has been very difficult to develop agreed responses to these injuries. For example, Peloso et al. [351] identified 41 mTBI guidelines (of which only three were somewhat evidence-based), hardly any of which employed the same diagnostic criteria. To assure that two doctors can communicate, a purely rhetorical definition requires arbitrary, non-biological operationalization. Hence we have, for instance, the World Health Organization definition of mTBI:

> MTBI is an acute brain injury resulting from mechanical energy to the head from external physical forces.
> Operational criteria for clinical identification include (1) 1 or more of the following: confusion or disorientation, LOC [loss of consciousness] for 30 min or less, posttraumatic amnesia for less than 24 h, and/or other transient neurological abnormalities such as focal signs, seizure, and intracranial lesion not requiring surgery; (2) Glasgow Coma Scale score of 13–15 after 30 min post injury or later upon presentation for healthcare.
>
> [352]

The details amassed in this definition will somewhat enhance interrater reliability. Yet no amount of detail renders such a def-inition specific for any biological process. As Signoretti et al. have written:

> The label "mild" in mTBI does not reflect the severity of the underlying metabolic and physiologic processes, if not even the potential clinical manifestations. The word "mild" implies a general absence of overt structural brain damage.

> However, long beyond the typically reported recovery interval of 1 week to 3 months, at least 15% of persons with a history of mTBI continue to see their primary care physician because of persistent problems.
>
> ([214], pp. S359–S360)

This scientific perspective exposes a root dilemma: Once one defines a medical condition in terms of a clinical presenta-tion, one side steps the question of pathophysiology. Once one dismisses pathophysiology as irrelevant to the definition and diagnosis of a medical problem, one has no target for the scien-tific pursuit of rational therapy.

Conclusion

Understanding concussion is the key to understanding TBI. Evidence suggests that, with a few exceptions, every TBI involves an element of concussive injury, or "headquake." Investigating the thousands of pathophysiological processes underlying and sustaining the effects of typical CBI is the shortest path to discovering effective therapy. And discovering what mitigates the deleterious effects of this core concussive element means enhanced therapy for essentially every survivor of TBI.

We gulp at the slope of the mountain we have chosen to climb. Exhorting one's colleagues to throw off the trammels of tradition is perilous work with unpredictable results. But we can no longer remain silent, appeasing the status quo. We respectfully reject the mythology that concussion is a transient symptom cluster after a trivial blow. We believe that it is more reasonable to define CBI as a protean biological problem with multi-determined effects. We believe that, rather than voting in closed committees for arbitrary definitions tied to "typical" clin-ical observations, the neuroscientific community should make a concentrated effort to understand the pathophysiological basis of this biological problem across its vast spectrum of severity and biological heterogeneity. We believe that no two humans have ever suffered identical CBIs, and that precision medicine will be required to make sense of the astonishing variation in outcomes.

The ultimate question is how to reduce the toll of CBI. It is the brain that is at stake. It is that Egyptian offal that mediates every love and hate, every act of mercy and iniquity, every thought, idea, and dream. Pending the singularity, let's not call it refuse. Let's protect it and help it fix itself. We believe that concussed patients will better be served if students of CBI investigate interventions relevant to its biology, in hot pursuit of something scientifically promising to interdict these short- and long-term threats to the seat of human identity.

References

1. Hippocrates. On wounds in the head. In *Hippocrates, Vol. III* (translated by Withington ET). Cambridge, MA: Harvard University Press, 1931, pp. 7–51.
2. Courville CB. *Commotio cerebri: Cerebral concussion and the postconcussion syndrome in their medical and legal aspects.* Los Angeles, CA: San Lucas Press, 1953.
3. Lane LC. Concussion of the brain. *JAMA* 1894;48–52.
4. Erichsen JE. *On railway and other injuries of the nervous system.* London: Walton and Maberly, 1866.

5. Erichsen JE. *On concussion of the spine: Nervous shock and other obscure injuries to the nervous system in their clinical and medico-legal aspects.* New York: W. Wood, 1883.

6. Erichsen JE. *The science and art of surgery: Being a treatise on surgical injuries, diseases, and operations.* London: Walton & Maberly, 1853.

7. Ingvar S. Centrifugation of the nervous system: An investigation of cellular changes in commotion. *Arch Neurol Psychiatry* 1923;10:267–287.

8. Menon DK, Schwab K, Wright DW, Maas AI. Position statement: Definition of traumatic brain injury. *Arch Phys Med Rehabil* 2010;91:1637–1640.

9. Laor N, Agassi J. *Diagnosis: Philosophical and medical perspectives (episteme).* Dordrecht: Springer, 1990.

10. Thagard P. *How scientists explain disease.* Princeton, NJ: Princeton University Press, 2000.

11. Murphy D. Concepts of disease and health. In *Standford encyclopedia of philosophy*, 2008. Available at http://plato.standford.edu/entries/health-disease/.

12. Rajkomar A, Dhaliwal G. Improving diagnostic reasoning to improve patient safety. *Permanente J* 2011;15:68–73.

13. Centers for Disease Control and Prevention. Rates of TBI-related emergency department visits by age group – United States, 2001–2010. Available at www.cdc.gov/traumaticbraininjury/data/rates_ed_byage.html.

14. Pott P. *Observations on the nature and consequences of those injuries to which the head is liable from external violence.* London: L. Hawes, W. Clarke, and R. Collins, 1768.

15. Singer C, Underwood EA. *Short history of medicine.* New York: Oxford University Press, 1962.

16. Finger S. *Origins of neuroscience: A history of explorations into brain function.* New York, NY: Oxford University Press, 1994.

17. Hippocrates. *The genuine works of Hippocrates, translated by Francis Adams.* London: Sydenham Society, 1849.

18. Liddell HG, Scott R. *An intermediate Greek-English lexicon, founded upon the seventh edition of Liddell and Scott's Greek-English lexicon.* Oxford: 1889.

19. Hippocrates. *On wounds in the head.* Withington ET, editor. Boston, MA: Harvard University Press, 1928.

20. Mettler FA, Mettler CC. Historic development of knowledge relating to cranial trauma. In: Browder J, Rabiner AM, Mettler FA, editors. *Trauma of the central nervous system: Proceedings of the Association, December 17 and 18, 1943.* Baltimore, MD: Williams & Wilkins, 1943 (pp. 1–47).

21. Boyer A. *Traité des maladies chirurgicales, et des opérations qui leur conviennent, vol. 5, 3rd edition.* Paris: Migneret, 1822.

22. Dupuytren G. *Leçons orales de clinique chirurgicale faites a l'Hôtel-Dieu de Paris, vol. V, 2nd edition.* Paris: Germer-Bailliere, 1839.

23. Culley MT, Furnivall FJ. *Caxton's eneydos, 1490; English from the French Liuee des Eneydes, 1483.* London: Kegan Paul, Trench, Trubner, Humphrey Milford, Oxford University Press, 1890.

24. *Oxford English dictionary.* Available at www.oed.com.

25. Breasted JH (transl). *The Edwin Smith surgical papyrus.* Chicago, IL: University of Chicago Press, 1930.

26. Wickens, AP. *A history of the brain from Stone Age surgery to modern neuroscience.* London: Psychology Press, 2015.

27. Homer. *The Iliad.* The Project Gutenberg ebook of The Iliad of Homer by Homer. Available at www.gutenberg.org/files/6130/6130-pdf.

28. Ballance CA. *The Thomas Vicary lecture: A glimpse into the history of the surgery of the brain.* London: MacMillan, 1922.

29. Celsus. *De medicina (translated by Spencer WG).* Cambridge, MA: Harvard University Press, 1938, pp. 475–518.

30. Halstead ME. Historical perspectives on concussion. In: Apps JN, Walter KD, editors. *Pediatric and adolescent concussion.* New York, NY: Springer, 2012, pp. 1–9.

31. Lafranchi G. *Chirurgia magna et parva.* Venice, 1498.

32. Courville CB. The ancestry of neuropathology: Hippocrates and "de vulneribus capitis." *Bull Los Angeles Neurol Soc* 1946;11:1–19.

33. Henry LC. *Microstructural and metabolic changes in the brains of concussed athletes.* Montreal: Département de Psychologie, Université de Montréal, 2011.

34. da Carpi B. *On fracture of the skull or cranium, 1517; translated by Lind, LR.* Philadelphia, PA: The American Philosophical Society, 1990.

35. Symonds JA. *The autobiography of Benvenuto Cellini.* New York, NY: P.F. Collier & Son, 1910.

36. Feinsod M, Langer KG. The philosopher's swoon – the concussion of Michel de Montaigne: A historical vignette. *World Neurosurg* 2012;78:371–374.

37. Coiter V. *Externarum et internarum principalium humani coproris partiumtabulae atque anatomicae exercitationes observationesqe variae.* Norbergae: T. Gerlatzeni, 1573.

38. Paré A. *Les oeuvres d'Ambroise Paré. Conseiller, et premier chirurgien du roy.* Paris: Chez Gabriel Buon, 1585.

39. Paré A. *On the moving of concussion of the brain.* Johnson T, transl. London: Th. Cotes & R. Young, 1634.

40. Luzzatti C, Whitaker H. Johannes Schenck and Johannes Jakob Wepfer: Clinical and anatomical observations in the prehistory of neurolinguistics and neuropsychology. *Neuroling* 1995–1996;9:157–164.

41. Aquapendente FA. Frankfurt, Germany: N. Hoffmanni; 1604. *In Opera omnia anatomica et physiologica.* Leipzig: 1687.

42. Fabry W. *Observationum et curationum chirurgicum.* Basel: 1606, 1611, 1614, 1619.

43. Paaw P. *Amsteldamensis succenturiatus anatomicus continens commentary in hippocretem de capitis vulbneribus.* Lugduni Batavorum: Ioducum & Colster, 1616.

44. Horst G. *Observationum medicalium singularium.* Ulm: J. Saurii, 1625.

45. Read A. *Chirurgorum comes: Or the whole practice of chirurgery.* London: E. Jones for C. Wilkinson, 1687.

46. Bonet T. *Sepulchretum, sive anatomia practica ex cadaverbius morbobdenatis.* Geneva: L. Chouet, 1679.

47. Pigray P. *Epitome des preceptes de medecine et chirurgie: avec ample déclaration des remèdes propres aux maladies.* Paris: P. Mettayer, 1609. Rouen: Chez Jean Manneville, 1642.

48. Chauliac G de. *La grande chirurgie.* Joubert RL, editor. Lyon: J. Ollier, 1659.

49. Marchetti P. *Observationum medico-chirurgicarum rariorum sylloge.* Amsterdam: P. Le Grand, 1665.

50. Boirel A. *Traité de playes de la tête.* Alençon: M. de la Moire et père Malassis, 1674.

51. Wiseman R. *Eight chirurgical treatises*, 6th edition. London: J. Walthoe et al., 1734.

52. Turner D. *The art of surgery*, 5th edition. London: C. Rivington & J. Clarke, 1736.

53. Petit JL. *Des plaies de la tete: Un traité des maladies chirurgicales et des opérations qui leur conviennent.* Paris: Didot le Jeune, 1774, pp. 43–60.

54. Littré A. *Histoire de l'Académie Royale des Sciences.* Paris: Gabriel Martin, Jena-Baptists Coignard fils, Hippolyte Guerin, 1730.

55. Best AE. Pourfour du Petit's experiments on the origin of the sympathetic nerve. *Med Hist* 1969;13:154–174.

56. Rouhault PS. *Traité des playes de tête.* Turin: 1720.

57. Morgagni JB. *De sedibus et causis morborum per anatomen indagatis.* Venetis: Typographia Remondiniana, 1761.

58. Morgagni JB. *The seats and causes of diseases investigated by anatomy, in five books, containing a great variety of dissections, with remarks; translated by Benjamin Alexander.* London: A. Millarj, T. Cadeli, Johnson and Payne, 1769.

59. Le Dran HF. *The operations in surgery of Mons. Le Dran.* Gataker T, translator. London: printed for C. Hitch in Paternoster Row, and R. Dodsley in Pall Mall, 1749.

60. Heister L. *A general system of surgery in three parts (translated into English from Latin by anonymous).* London: W. Innys, C. Davis, J. Clark, R. Manby, J. Whiston, 1743.

61. Petit JL. *Des plaies de la tete: Un traité des maladies chirurgicales et des opérations qui leur conviennent.* Paris: Didot le Jeune, 1774, pp. 43–60.

62. Frowein RA, Firsching R. Classification of head injury. In: Braakman R, editor. *Handbook of clinical neurology,* vol. 13. Amsterdam: Elsevier, 1990, pp. 101–122.

63. Feinsod MA. Flask full of jelly: The first in vitro model of concussive head injury – 1830. *Neurosurg* 2002;50:386–391.

64. Henry LC. *Microstructural and metabolic changes in the brains of concussed athletes.* Montreal: Département de Psychologie, Faculté des Arts et Sciences, Université de Montréal, 2011.

65. Beckett W. *Practical surgery, illustrated and improved.* London: 1739.

66. Kirkland T. *A commentary on apoplectic and paralytic affections and on diseases connected with the subject.* London: William Dawson, 1792.

67. Manne LF. *Observation de chirurgie, au sujet d'une playe à la tête fracas, et une pièce d'os implantée dans le cerveau pendant un mois sans aucune symptome; accompagnée d'une dissertation au sujet des playes de tête avec fracture; suivie des lettres des scavans (Chicoyneau, de la Peyronie, Petit, et Morand) qui ont été consulté à ce sujet par l'auteur.* Avignon: 1729.

68. Dease W. *Observations on wounds of the head.* London: G. Robinson, 1776.

69. Bell B. *A system of surgery,* 3rd edition. Edinburgh: J. & J. Robinson, 1788.

70. Hewett P. Lecture on the anatomy, injuries, and diseases of the head, lecture VI: Concussion of the brain. *Med Times Gaz* 1858:235–237, 287–289.

71. Guthrie GJ. *On injuries of the head affecting the brain.* London: John Churchill, 1842.

72. Hutchinson J. Three lectures on the compression of the brain. *Clin Lect Rep London Hosp* 1867;4:10–55.

73. Delpeche JM. *Précis élémentaire des maladies réputées chirurgicales.* Paris: Méquignon-Marvis, 1816.

74. Brodie BC. Injuries of the brain. *Med-Surg Trans* 1828;14:337.

75. Dupuytren G. Traité théorique et pratique des blessures par armes de guerre; Brussels, 1835 cited by Tonnis and Loew's Einteilung der gedeckten Hirnschadigungen. *Arztl Prax* 1953;36:13–14.

76. Miles A. On the mechanism of brain injuries. *Brain* 1892;15:153–189.

77. Lane LC. *The surgery of the head and neck.* Washington, DC: Levi Cooper Lane, 1896.

78. Fano S. Mémoire sur la commotion du cerveau. *Mem Soc Chir Paris* 1853;3:163–199.

79. Savory WS. Severe concussion of the brain, followed by singular mental phenomena, recovery: Reports of medical and surgical practice in the hospitals of Great Britain. *Br Med J* 1869;376.

80. Duplay M. Concussion of the brain. *Med Surg Reporter* 1882;46:253–256.

81. MacPherson J. Vacuolation of nerve-cell nuclei in the cortex in two cases of cerebral concussion. *Lancet* 1892;1127–1129.

82. Walton GL, Brooks WA. Observations on brain surgery suggested by a case of multiple cerebral hemorrhage. *Boston Med Surg J* 1897;36:301–305.

83. Palmer JF, editor. *Collected works of Hunter, Vol. I: Articles on injuries of the head and fractures of the skull.* London, UK: Richard Taylor, 1835.

84. Bryant T. Cranial and intracranial injuries: Hunterian lecture. *Lancet* 1888;2:405–408, 507–508.

85. Ommaya AK. Trauma to the nervous system: Hunterian lecture delivered at the Royal College of Surgeons of UK on 29 July 1965. *Ann R Coll Surg Engl* 1966;39:317–347.

86. Abernethy J. *Surgical observations on injuries of the head: And on miscellaneous subjects.* Philadelphia, PA: Thomas Dobson, 1811.

87. Anonymous. On concussion of the brain by M Fano, with a report by M. Chassaignac. *Br Foreign Medico-Chirurg Rev* 1854;13:469–470. Citing Chassaignac M. *Mem Soc Chir Paris* 1852–1853; book 3, sections 2 and 3:121–376.

88. Bright R. *Reports of medical cases selected with a view of illustrating the symptoms and cure of diseases by reference to morbid anatomy: Diseases of the brain and nervous system.* London: Longman, 1831.

89. Holmes T. *Treatise on surgery, its principles and practice.* Philadelphia, PA: Henry C. Lea, 1876.

90. Duret H. *Expérimentales et clinique sur les traumatismes cérébreaux: Thèse pour le doctorat en médecine.* Paris: De la Haye, 1878.

91. Obersteiner H. Ueber Erschütterung des Rückenmarks. *Wien Med Jahrb* 1879;3–4:531.

92. Kocher T. *Chirurgische Operationslehre.* Jena, Germany: Fischer Verlag, 1892.

93. Kocher. Die Verletzungen der Wirbelsäule, zugleich ein Beitrag zur Physiologie des menschlichen Rückenmarks. *Mitt Grenzgeb Med Chir* 1896;1:415.

94. Gama JP. *Traité des plaies de tête et de l'encéphalite, principalement de celle: Qui leur est consécutive; ouvrage dans lequel sont discutées plusieurs questions relatives aux fonctions du système nerveux en générale [Treatise of head injuries and of encephalitis in which many questions concerning the functions of the nervous system are discussed].* Paris: Sedillot, 1830.

95. Alquié A. Étude clinique et expérimentale de la commotion traumatique ou ébranlement de l'encéphale. *Gaz Med Paris* 1865;20:226–230; 254–256; 314–319; 382–385; 396–398; 463–466; 500–504.

96. Goodwin J. Brainstem trauma, *NANOS* 1989. Available at content.lib.utah.edu:81/cgi-bin/showfile.exe?CISOROOT=/ehsl…

97. Koch W, Filehne W. Beiträge zur experimentellen Chirurgie, 3: Ueber die Commotio cerebri. *Arch f Klin Chir* 1874;17:190–231.

98. Kramer SP. A contribution to the theory of cerebral concussion. *Ann Surg* 1896;23:163–173.

99. La Faye Gd. *Principes de chirurgie.* Paris: Cavlier, 1761.

100. Baudens ML. *Clinique plaies d'armes à feu.* Paris: Bailliere, 1836.

101. Kocher T. Die Therapie des Hirndrucks. In: Hoelder A, editor. *Hirnerschuetterung, Hirndruck und chirurgische Eingriffe bei Hirnkrankheiten.* Vienna: 1901.

102. Hooke, R. *Micrographia, or some physiological descriptions of minute bodies made by magnifying glasses. With observations and inquiries thereupon.* London: Jo. Martyn and Ja. Allestry, 1665.

103. Ehrenberg CG. Notwendigkeit einer feineren mechanischen Zerlegung des Gehirns und der Nerven vor der chemischen, dargestellt aus Beobachtungen. *Ann Physik Chem* 1833;28:449–473.

104. Baillarger J. Recherches sur la structure de la couche corticale des circonvolutions du cerveau. *Mem Acad R Med* 1840;8:149–183.

105. Kushchayev SV, Moskalenko VF, Wiener PC, Tsymbaliuk VI, Cherkasov VG, Dzyavulska IV, et al. The discovery of the pyramidal neurons: Vladimir Betz and a new era of neuroscience. *Brain* 2011;135:285–300.

106. Verplaetse J. Moritz Benedikt's (1835–1920) localization of morality in the occipital lobes: Origin and background of a controversial hypothesis. *Hist Psychiatry* 2004;15:305–328.

107. Meynert T. *Vom Gehirn der Saugetiere.* In: Stricker S, editor. *Handbuch der Lehre von den Geweben des Menschen und Tiere.* Leipzig, Germany: Engelmann, 1872.

108. Betz W. Die Untersuchungsmethode des Centrainervensystems beim Menschen. *M Schultez's Arch Micr Anat* 1872;9:101–117.

109. Betz W. Anatomischer Nachweis zweier Gehirncentra. *Centralbl med Wissensch* 1874;12:578–580, 595–599.

110. Betz W. Methods of investigating the central nervous system in man. *Q J Microsc Sci* 1873;s2–13:343–350.

111. Betz W. *Morphology of osteogenesis (in old Russian).* Kiev, Russia: Kulzhenko Publishing, 1887.

112. Golgi C. Sulla struttura della sostanza grigia del cervelo. *Gazz Med Ital* 1873:33: 244–246.

113. Golgi C. *Opera Omnia. VoI II Istologia normale.* Milano: Ulrico Hoepli; Editore Libraio Dell Real Casa 1883–1902.

114. Witkowski L. Ueber Gehirnerschutterung. *ArchPath Anat* 1877;69:498–516.

115. Strich SJ. Shearing of nerve fibers as a cause of brain damage due to head injury, a pathological study of 20 cases. *Lancet* 1961;2: 443–448.

116. Scagliosi G. Uber die Gehirnerschütterung und die daraus im Gehim und Rückenmark hervorgerufenen histologischen Veränderungen. *Virchows Arch Pathol Anat* 1898;152: 487–525.

117. Luzenberger Ad. Su d'una special alterazione delle cellule gangliari prodotta da trauma sperimentale. *Neurol Centralbl* 1898;17:363.

118. Tillman. Die Theorie der Gehirn- und Rückenmarkserschütterung. *Arch Klin Chir* 1899;59.

119. Rosenblath W. Uber einen bemerkenswerten Fall von Hirnerschutterung. *Dtsch Arch Klin Med* 1899;64:406–424.

120. Skae FMT. Facuolation of the nuclei of nerve cells in the cortex. *Br Med J* 1894;19:1075–1076.

121. Harrison B. First annual message to the Senate and House of Representatives. (December 3, 1889). Available at http://millercenter.org/president/bharrison/speeches/speech-3765.

122. Savory WS. *Hysteria,* 2nd edition. London: Longmans, Green, 1870.

123. Putnam JJ. Recent investigations into the pathology of so-called concussion of the spine, with cases illustrating the importance of seeking for evidences of typical hysteria in the chronic as well as in the acute stages of the disease. *Boston Med Surg J* 1883;109:217–220.

124. Walton GL. Possible cerebral origin of the symptoms usually classed under "railway spine." *Boston Med Surg J* 1883;109:337–305.

125. Friedmann M. Ueber eine besondere schwere Form von Folgezustanden nach Gehirnerschtitterung und über den vasomotorischen Symptomencomplex bei derselben im allgemeinen. *Arch Psychiatry* 1892;23:230–267.

126. Hodges RM. So-called concussion of the spinal cord. *Boston Med Surg J* 1881;104:361–365.

127. Page HW. *Injuries of the spine and spinal cord without apparent mechanical lesion, and nervous shock, in their surgical and medico-legal aspects.* London: J. & A. Churchill, 1883.

128. Charcot JM. *Clinical lectures on diseases of the nervous system,* vol. III. London: Sydenham Society, 1889.

129. Gray LC. *A treatise on nervous and mental diseases.* Philadelphia, PA: Lea Brothers, 1893, pp. 570–571.

130. Micale M. Charcot and les névroses traumatiques. *J Hist Neurosci* 1995;4:101–119.

131. Evans RW. The postconcussion syndrome and the sequelae of mild head injury. *Neurol Clin* 1992;10:815–847.

132. Evans RW. The post-concussion syndrome: 130 years of controversy. *Semin Neurol* 1994;14:32–39.

133. Evans RW. Persistent post-traumatic headache, postconcussion syndrome, and whiplash injuries: The evidence for a non-traumatic basis with an historical review. *Headache* 2010; 50(4):716–724.

134. Guyton GP. A brief history of workers' compensation. *Iowa Orthop J* 1999;19:106–110.

135. Brooks JG. *Compulsory insurance in Germany: Including an appendix relating to compulsory insurance in other countries in Europe.* Washington, DC: US Government Printing Office, 1893.

136. Bikeles G. Zur pathologischen Anatomie der Hirn- und Rückenmarkserschütterung. *Neurol Centralbl* 1895;14:463–464.

137. Luzenberger Ad. Anatomie pathologique du traumatisme nerveux. *Arch Neurol* 1897.

138. Kirchgasser G. Experimentelle Untersuchungen über Rückenmarkserschütterung. *Deutsch Ztschr f Nervenh* 1897;11:406; 1898;13:422.

139. Jakob A. Experimentelle Untersuchungen über die traumatischen Schädigungen des Zentralnervensystems. *Histol Histopathol Arb Grosshirnrinde* 1912;5:182.

140. Tscherbak AE. On the value of anatomy and pathology of nervous system for physiological psychology. *Rev Psychiatry Neurol Exp Psychol (Russian)* 1898;10:809–810.

141. Cornil L. *Commotion méduallaire directe.* Paris: Librairie le François, 1921.

142. Schmauss H. Commotio spinalis. *Ergeb allg Pathol Pathol Anat* 1897;1:594.

143. Schterbach H. Des alterations de la moelle épinière chez le lapin sous l'influence de la vibration intensive. *Encéphale.* 1907;2:521.

144. Mott FW. The microscopic examination of the brains of two men dead of commotio cerebri (shell shock) without visible external injury. *BMJ* 1917;2:612.

145. Tanzi E, Lugaro G. *Malattie mentali,* 2nd edition. Milan, Italy: Società Editrice Libraria, 1914.

146. Osnato M, Giliberti N. Postconcussion neurosis-traumatic encephalitis: A conception of postconcussion phenomena. *Arch Neurol Psychiatry* 1927;18:181–214.

147. Cannon WB. Cerebral pressure following trauma. *Am J Physiol* 1901;6:91–121.

148. Obersteiner H. Diseases of the spinal cord. In: Sajous CH, editor. *Annual of the universal medical sciences and analytical index: A yearly report of the progress of general sanitary sciences throughout the world. Vol. II.* Philadelphia: FA Davis, 1896 (p. B53).

149. Meyer A. The anatomical facts and clinical varieties of traumatic insanity. *Am J Insanity* 1904;60:373–441.

150. Wrightson P. The development of a concept of mild head injury. *J Clin Neurosci* 2000;7:384–388.

151. Strich SJ. Diffuse degeneration of cerebral white matter in severe dementia following head injury. *J Neurol Neurosurg Psychiatry* 1956;19:163–185.

152. Aldich M. *Death rode the rails: American railroad accidents and safety, 1828–1965.* Baltimore, MD: Johns Hopkins University Press, 2009.

153. Schaller WF. Diagnosis in traumatic neurosis. *JAMA* 1918; 71:338–344.

154. Silverman RA. *Law and urban growth: Civil litigation in the Boston trial courts.* Princeton, NJ: Princeton University Press, 1981.

155. Bergstrom RE. *Courting danger: Injury and law in New York City, 1870–1910.* Ithaca, NY: Cornell University Press, 1992.

156. Hale NG. *The rise and crisis of psychoanalysis in the United States: Freud and the Americans, 1917–1985.* London: Oxford University Press, 1995.

157. Dercum FX. *Hysteria and accident compensation.* Philadelphia, PA: G.T. Bisel, 1916.

158. Jefferson G. Gunshot wounds of the scalp, with special reference to the neurological signs presented. *Brain* 1919;42:93–112.

159. Ferraro A. Experimental medullary concussion of the spinal cord in rabbits: Histologic study of the early stages. *Arch Neurol Psychiatry* 1927;18:357–373.

160. Army. *Report of the war office committee of enquiry into "shell-shock."* London: His Majesty's Stationery Office, 1922.

161. Elliott TR. *Biographical memoirs of Fellows of the Royal Society* vol. 3, no. 9 (Jan., 1941), pp. 325–344.

162. Trotter W. Certain minor injuries of the brain. *Lancet* 1924;1:935–939.

163. Phelps C. A clinico-pathological study of injuries of the head, with special reference to lesions of the brain's substance (read before the New York State Medical Association 4 Nov 1892). *N Y Med J* 1893;57:1–98.

164. Russell WR. Cerebral involvement in head injury: A study based on the examination of two hundred cases. *Brain* 1932;55:549–603.

165. Trotter W. Shell wound of head, 1915; persistent headache four years; operation; free opening of skull and dura in region of injury; contusion of brain found; relief of headache. *Brain* 1920;42:353–355.

166. Mohr JC. *Doctors and the law: Medical jurisprudence in nineteenth century America.* New York: Oxford University Press, 1994.

167. Romanis WHC, Mitchener PH. *The science and practice of surgery.* London: J. & A. Churchill, 1930.

168. Symonds CP. Functional or organic? Some points of view. *Lancet* 1926;207(5341):64–67.

169. Armour D. Some considerations on head injuries. *Brain* 1928;51:427–439.

170. Strauss I, Savitsky N. Head injury, neurologic and psychiatric aspects. *Arch Neurol Psychiatry* 1934;31:893.

171. Hall GW, MacKay RP. The posttraumatic neuroses. *JAMA* 1934;102:510–513.

172. Russel CK. The nature of the war neuroses. *Can Med Assoc J* 1939;41:549–554.

173. Munro D. The late effects of crania-cerebral injuries. *Ann Surg* 1943;117:544.

174. Munro D. The diagnosis and therapy of so-called posttraumatic neurosis following craniocerebral injuries. *Surg Gynecol Obstet* 1939;68:587–592.

175. Rand CW, Courville CB. Histological changes in the brain in cases of fatal injury to the head, part iii: Reactions of microglia and oligodendroglia. *Arch Neurol Psychiatry* 1932;27:605–644.

176. Rand CW, Courville CB. Histological changes in the brain in cases of fatal injury to the head, part vi: Cytoarchitectonic alterations. *Arch Neurol Psychiatry* 1936;36:1277–1293.

177. Rand CW, Courville CB. Histological changes in the brain in cases of fatal injury to the head, part vi: Cytoarchitectonic alterations. *Arch Neurol Psychiatry* 1936;36:1277–1293.

178. Rand CW, Courville CB. Histologic changes in the brain in cases of fatal injury to the head; alterations in nerve cells. *Arch Neurol Psychiatry* 1946;55:79–110.

179. Symonds CP. Mental disorder following head injury. *Proc R Soc Med* 1937;30:1081.

180. Goldstein K. Brain concussion: Evaluation of the after effects by special tests. *Dis Nerv Syst* 1943;4:325–334.

181. Greenwald RM, Chu JJ, Beckwith JG, Crisco JJ. A proposed method to reduce underreporting of brain injury in sports. *Clin J Sport Med* 2012;22:83–85.

182. Denny-Brown DE, Russell WR. Experimental cerebral concussion. *Brain* 1941;64:93–164.

183. Denny-Brown DE. Cerebral concussion. *Physiol Rev* 1945;25:296–325.

184. Marinesco G. Lésions commotionelles expérimentales. *Rev Neurol* 1918;34:329.

185. Carver A, Dinsley A. Some biological effects of high explosives. *Brain* 1919;42:113.

186. Mairet A, Durante G. Contribution a l'étude expérimentale de lesions commotionnelles. *Revue Neurol* 1919;36:97.

187. Zuckerman S. Discussion on the problem of blast injury. *Proc R Soc Med* 1941;34:171.

188. Tedeschi CG. Cerebral injury by blunt mechanical trauma. *Arch Neurol Psychiatry* 1945;53:333.

189. Eden K, Turner JW. Loss of consciousness in different types of head injury. *Proc R Soc Med* 1941;34:685.

190. Walker AE, Kollros JJ, Case TJ. The physiological basis of cerebral concussion: Trauma of the nervous system. *Assoc Res Nerv Ment Dis* 1945;24:437–472.

191. Tönnis W, Loew F. Einteilung der gedeckten Hirnschädigungen. *Arztl Prax* 1953;36:13–14.

192. Groat RA, Windle WF, Magoun IW. Functional and structural changes in the monkey's brain during and after concussion. *J Neurosurg* 1945;2:26.

193. Frey E. Commotio cerebri: Beitrage zur Frage der traumatischen Schwellung und Ödembildung des Gehrins. *Confin Neurol* 1947–1948;8:53–72.

194. Groat RA, Simmons JQ. Loss of nerve cells in experimental cerebral concussion. *J Neuropathol Exp Neurol* 1950;9:150–163.

195. Symonds CP. Concussion and its sequelae. *Lancet* 1962;1:1–5.

196. Groat RA, Windle WF, Magoun IW. Functional and structural changes in the monkey's brain during and after concussion. *J Neurosurg* 1945;2:26.

197. Meerloo AM. Cerebral concussion: A psychosomatic survey. *J Nerv Ment Dis* 1949;110(4):347–53.

198. Windle WF, Groat RA, Fox CA. Structural changes in the brain in experimental concussion. *Arch Neurol Psychiatry* 1946;55:162–164.

199. Windle WF, Groat RA, Fox CA. Experimental structural alterations in the brain during and after concussion. *J Gynecol Surg* 1944;79:561–572.

200. Miller Fisher C. Concussion amnesia. *Neurol* 1966;16:826–830.

201. Trotter W. *Instincts of the herd in peace and war.* London: T.F. Unwin, 1916.

202. Goldstein K. Das psycho-physische Problem in seiner Bedeutung fuer aerztliches Handeln. *Ther Gegenw* 1931; special issue, no. 1:1–11.

203. Goldstein K. *Aftereffects of brain injuries in war.* New York: Grune & Stratton, 1942.

204. Saucier J. Concussion: A misnomer. *J Can Med Assoc* 1955;72:816–820.

205. Johnson B, Zhang K, Gaya M, Neuberger T, Horovitz S, Hallett M, et al. Metabolic alterations in corpus callosum may compromise brain functional connectivity in MTBI patients: An 1H-MRS study. *Neurosci Lett* 2012;509:5–8.

206. Giza CC, Hovda DA. The neurometabolic cascade of concussion. *J Athl Train* 2001;36:228–235.

207. Anonymous. Microscopic lesions in head injury. *Lancet* 1968;292:1069.

208. Chen Y, Sutton B, Conway C, Broglio SP, Ostoja-Starzewski A. Brain deformation under mild impact: Magnetic resonance imaging-based assessment and finite element study. *Int J Numer Anal Model, Series B Comput Info* 2012;3:20–35.

209. Holbourn AHS. Mechanics of head injuries. *Lancet* 1943;2:438–441.

210. Holbourn AHS. The mechanics of brain injuries. *Br Med Bull* 1945;3:147–149.

211. Pudenz RH, Shelden CH. The lucite calvarium – a method for direct observation of the brain, part ii: Cranial trauma and brain movement. *J Neurosurg* 1946;3:487–505.

212. Peerless SJ, Rewcastle NB. Shear injuries of the brain. *Can Med Assoc J* 1967;96:577–582.

213. Signoretti S, Vagnozzi R, Tavazzi B, Lazzarino G. Biochemical and neurochemical sequelae following mild traumatic brain

injury: Summary of experimental data and clinical implications. *Neurosurg Focus* 2010;29:E1.

214. Signoretti S, Lazzarino G, Tavazzi B, Vagnozzi R. The pathophysiology of concussion. *PM&R* 2011;3:S359–S368.

215. Hicks R, Soares H, Smith D, McIntosh T. Temporal and spatial characterization of neuronal injury following lateral fluid-percussion brain injury in the rat. *Acta Neuropathol* 1996;91:236–246.

216. Barkhoudarian G, Hovda DA, Giza CC. The molecular pathophysiology of concussive brain injury. *Clin Sports Med* 2011;30:33–48.

217. Giza CC, Prins ML, Hovda DA, Herschman HR, Feldman JD. Genes preferentially induced by depolarization after concussive brain injury: Effects of age and injury severity. *J Neurotrauma* 2002;19:387–402.

218. Tang-Schomer MD, Johnson VE, Baas PW, Stewart W, Smith DH. Partial interruption of axonal transport due to microtubule breakage accounts for the formation of periodic varicosities after traumatic axonal injury. *Exp Neurol* 2012;233:364–372.

219. Creed JA, DiLeonardi AM, Fox DP, Tessler AR, Raghupathi R. Concussive brain trauma in the mouse results in acute cognitive deficits and sustained impairment of axonal function. *J Neurotrauma* 2011;28:547–563.

220. Kasahara K, Hashimoto K, Abo M, Senoo A. Voxel- and atlas-based analysis of diffusion tensor imaging may reveal focal axonal injuries in mild traumatic brain injury: Comparison with diffuse axonal injury. *Magn Reson Imaging* 2012;30:496–505.

221. Inglese M, Makani S, Johnson G, Cohen BA, Silver JA, Gonen O, et al. Diffuse axonal injury in mild traumatic brain injury: A diffusion tensor imaging study. *J Neurosurg* 2005;103:298–303.

222. Niogi SN, Mukherjee P, Ghajar J, Johnson C, Kolster RA, Sarkar R, et al. Extent of microstructural white matter injury in postconcussive syndrome correlates with impaired cognitive reaction time: A 3T diffusion tensor imaging study of mild traumatic brain injury. *AJNR Am J Neuroradiol* 2008;29:967–973.

223. Rutgers DR, Toulgoat F, Cazejust J, Fillard P, Lasjaunias P, Ducreux D. White matter abnormalities in mild traumatic brain injury: A diffusion tensor imaging study. *AJNR* 2008;29:514–519.

224. Ling JM, Pena A, Yeo RA, Merideth FL, Klimaj S, Gasparovic C, et al. Biomarkers of increased diffusion anisotropy in semi-acute mild traumatic brain injury: A longitudinal perspective. *Brain* 2012;135(Pt 4):1281–1292.

225. Lipton ML, Kim N, Park YK, Hulkower MB, Gardin TM, Shifteh K, et al. Robust detection of traumatic axonal injury in individual mild traumatic brain injury patients: Intersubject variation, change over time and bidirectional changes in anisotropy. *Brain Imaging Behav* 2012;6: 329–342.

226. Mayer AR, Ling JM, Yang Z, Pena A, Yeo RA, Klimaj S. Diffusion abnormalities in pediatric mild traumatic brain injury. *J Neurosci* 2012;32:17961–17969.

227. Shenton ME, Hamoda HM, Schneiderman JS, Bouix S, Pasternak O, Rathi Y, et al. A review of magnetic resonance imaging and diffusion tensor imaging findings in mild traumatic brain injury. *Brain Imaging Behav* 2012;6:137–192.

228. Niogi SN, Mukherjee P. Diffusion tensor imaging of mild traumatic brain injury. *J Head Trauma Rehabil* 2010;25:241–255.

229. McAllister TW, Ford JC, Flashman LA, Maerlender A, Greenwald RM, Beckwith JG, et al. Effect of head impacts on diffusivity measures in a cohort of collegiate contact sport athletes. *Neurology* 2014;82:63–69.

230. Niogi SN, Mukherjee P, Ghajar J, Johnson CE, Kolster R, Lee H, et al. Structural dissociation of attentional control and memory in adults with and without mild traumatic brain injury. *Brain* 2008;131:3209–3221.

231. Lo C, Shifteh K, Gold T, Bello JA, Lipton ML. Diffusion tensor imaging abnormalities in patients with mild traumatic brain injury and neurocognitive impairment. *J Comput Assist Tomog* 2009;33:293–297.

232. Geary EK, Kraus MF, Rubin LH, Pliskin NH, Deborah M, Little DM. Verbal learning differences in chronic mild traumatic brain injury. *J Int Neuropsychol Soc* 2010;16:506–516.

233. Cubon VA, Putukian M. A diffusion tensor imaging study on the white matter skeleton in individuals with sports-related concussion. *J Neurotrauma* 2011;28:189–201.

234. Rutgers DR, Fillard P, Paradot G, Tadié M, Lasjaunias P, Ducreux D, Diffusion tensor imaging characteristics of the corpus callosum in mild, moderate, and severe traumatic brain injury. *AJNR* 2008;29:1730–1735.

235. Slobounov S, Gay M, Johnson B, Zhang K. Concussion in athletics: Ongoing clinical and brain imaging research controversies. *Brain Imaging Behav* 2012;6:224–243.

236. Giza CC, Hovda DA. The neurometabolic cascade of concussion. *J Athletic Train* 2001;36:228–235.

237. Tavazzi B, Signoretti S, Lazzarino G, Amorini AM, Delfini R, Cimatti M, et al. Cerebral oxidative stress and depression of energy metabolism correlate with severity of diffuse brain injury in rats. *Neurosurg* 2005;56:582–589.

238. Dashnaw ML, Petraglia AL, Bailes JE. An overview of the basic science of concussion and subconcussion: Where we are and where we are going. *Neurosurg Focus* 2012;33:E5:1–9.

239. Kan EM, Ling EA, Lu J. Microenvironment changes in mild traumatic brain injury. *Brain Res Bull* 2012;87:359–372.

240. Shrey DW, Griesbach GS, Giza CC. The pathophysiology of concussions in youth. *Phys Med Rehabil Clin N Am* 2011;22:577–602.

241. Giza CC, Hovda DA. The new neurometabolic cascade of concussion. *Neurosurgery* 2014;75:S24–S33.

242. Giza CC, Hovda DA. Ionic and metabolic consequences of concussion. In: Cantu RC, Cantu RI, editors. *Neurologic athletic and spine injuries*. St Louis, MO: WB Saunders, 2000, pp. 80–100.

243. Biegon A, Fry PA, Paden CM, Alexandrovich A, Tsenter J, Shohami E. Dynamic changes in *N*-methyl-D-aspartate receptors after closed head injury in mice: Implications for treatment of neurological and cognitive deficits. *PNAS* 2004;101:5117–5122.

244. Macleod GHB. *Notes on the surgery of the war in Crimea with remarks on the treatment of gunshot wounds*. Philadelphia: JB Lippincott, 1862.

245. Bass CR, Panzer MB, Rafaels KA, Wood G, Shridharani J, Capehart B. Brain injuries from blast. *Ann Biomed Engineer* 2012;40:185–202.

246. Blennow K, Hardy J, Zetterberg H. The neuropathology and neurobiology of traumatic brain injury. *Neuron* 2012;76:886–899.

247. Rowbotham GF. *Acute injuries of the head: Their diagnosis, treatment, complications, and sequels*. Edinburgh, UK: E. & S. Livingstone, 1942.

248. Oppenheimer DR. Microscopic lesions in the brain following head injury. *Neurol Neurosurg Psychiatry* 1968;31:299–306.

249. Anonymous. Microscopical sequelae of head injury. *Br Med J* 1969;7:169.

250. Clark JM. Distribution of microglial clusters in the brain after head injury. *J Neurol Neurosurg Psychiatry* 1974;37:463–474.

251. Engel S, Wehner HD, Meyermann R. Expression of microglial markers in the human CNS after closed head injury. *Acta Neurochirurg* 1996;66:87–95.

252. Schmidt OI, Heyde CE, Ertel W, Stahel PF. Closed head injury – an inflammatory disease? *Brain Res Rev* 2005;48:388–399.

253. Czigner A, Mihály A, Farkas O, Büki A, Krisztin-Péva B, Dobó E, et al. Kinetics of the cellular immune response following closed head injury. *Acta Neurochir* 2007;149:281–289.

254. Morganti-Kossmann MC, Satgunaseelan L, Bye N, Kossmann T. Modulation of immune response by head injury. *Injury Int J Care Injured* 2007;38:1392–1400.

255. Cederberg D, Siesjö P. What has inflammation to do with traumatic brain injury? *Childs Nerv Syst* 2010;26:221–226.

256. Helmy A, De Simoni MG, Guilfoyle MR, Carpenter KL, Hutchinson PJ. Cytokines and innate inflammation in the pathogenesis of human traumatic brain injury. *Prog Neurobiol* 2011;352–372.

257. Tsai Y-D, Liliang P-C, Cho C-L, Chen J-S, Lu K, Liang C-L, et al. Delayed neurovascular inflammation after mild traumatic brain injury in rats. *Brain Inj* 2013;27:361–365.

258. Yang SH, Gangidine M, Pritts TA, Goodman MD, Lentsch AB. Interleukin 6 mediates neuroinflammation and motor coordination deficits after mild traumatic brain injury and brief hypoxia in mice. *Shock* 2013;40:471–475.

259. Weil ZM, Gaier KR, Karelina K. Injury timing alters metabolic, inflammatory and functional outcomes following repeated mild traumatic brain injury. *Neurobiol Dis* 2104;70:108–116.

260. Khuman J, Meehan WP, Zhu X, Qiu J, Hoffmann U, Zhang J, et al. Tumor necrosis factor alpha and Fas receptor contribute to cognitive deficits independent of cell death after concussive traumatic brain injury in mice. *J Cereb Blood Flow Metab* 2011;31:778–789.

261. Das M, Subhra Mohapatra S, Mohapatra SS. New perspectives on central and peripheral immune responses to acute traumatic brain injury. *J Neuroinflamm* 2012;9:236.

262. Acosta, SA, Tajiri N, Shinozuka K, Ishikawa H, Grimmig B, Diamond D. et al. Long-term upregulation of inflammation and suppression of cell proliferation in the brain of adult rats exposed to traumatic brain injury using the controlled cortical impact model. *PLoS One* 2013;8:e53376.

263. Abdul-Muneer PM, Chandra N, Haorah J. Interactions of oxidative stress and neurovascular inflammation in the pathogenesis of traumatic brain injury. *Mol Neurobiol* 2014. Available at www.researchgate.net/…Abdul_Muneer/…Interactions…/5417a3770cf22…

264. Corps KN, Roth TL, McGavern DB. Inflammation and neuroprotection in traumatic brain injury. *JAMA Neurol* 2015;72:355–362.

265. Karve IP, Taylor JM, Crack PJ. The contribution of astrocytes and microglia to traumatic brain injury. *Br J Pharmacol* 2016;173:692–702.

266. Lozano D, Gonzales-Portillo GS, Acosta S, de la Pena I, Tajiri N, Kaneko Y, Borlongan CV. Neuroinflammatory responses to traumatic brain injury: Etiology, clinical consequences, and therapeutic opportunities. *Neuropsychiatr Dis Treat* 2015;11:97–106.

267. Shoamenesh A, Pries SR, Beiser AS, Vasan RS, Benjamin EJ, Kase CS, et al. Inflammatory biomarkers, cerebral microbleeds, and small vessel disease: Framingham Heart Study. *Neurology* 2015;84:825–832.

268. Woodcock T, Morganti-Kossmann MC. The role of markers of inflammation in traumatic brain injury. *Front Neurol* 2013;4:18.

269. Coughlin JM, Wang Y, Munro CA, Ma S, Yue C, Chen S, et al. Neuroinflammation and brain atrophy in former NFL players: An in vivo multimodal imaging pilot study. *Neurobiol Dis* 2015;74:58–65.

270. Kreisl WC, Jenko KJ, Hines CS, Lyoo CH, Corona W, Morse CL, et al. A genetic polymorphism for translocator protein 18 kDa affects both in vitro and in vivo radioligand binding in human brain to this putative biomarker of neuroinflammation. *J Cereb Blood Flow Metab* 2013;33:53–58.

271. Kumar A, Loane DJ. Neuroinflammation after traumatic brain injury: Opportunities for therapeutic intervention. *Brain Behav Immun* 2012;26:1191–1201.

272. Patterson ZR, Holahan MR. Understanding the neuroinflammatory response following concussion to develop treatment strategies. *Front Cell Neurosci* 2012;6:1–10.

273. Hawrylycz MJ, Lein ES, Guillozet-Bongaarts AL, Shen EH, Ng L, Jeremy A, et al. An anatomically comprehensive atlas of the adult human brain transcriptome. *Nature* 2012;489:391–399.

274. Barr TL, Alexander S, Conley Y. Gene expression profiling for discovery of novel targets in human traumatic brain injury. *Biol Res Nurs* 2011;13:140–153.

275. Poulsen CB, Penkowa M, Borup R, Nielsen FC, Caceres M, Quintana A, et al. Brain response to traumatic brain injury in wild-type and interleukin-6 knockout mice: A microarray analysis. *J Neurochem* 2005;92:417–432.

276. Colak T, Cine N, Bamac B, Kurtas O, Ozbek A, Bicer U, et al. Microarray-based gene expression analysis of an animal model for closed head injury. *Injury Int J Care Injured* 2012;43:1264–1270.

277. Michael DB, Byers DM, Irwin LN. Gene expression following traumatic brain injury in humans: Analysis by microarray. *J Clin Neurosci* 2005;12:284–290.

278. Di Pietro V, Amin D, Pernagallo S, Lazzarino G, Tavazzi B, Vagnozzi R, et al. Transcriptomics of traumatic brain injury: gene expression and molecular pathways of different grades of insult in a rat organotypic hippocampal culture model. *J Neurotrauma* 2010;27:349–359.

279. Di Pietro V, Amorini AM, Tavazzi B, Hovda DA, Signoretti S, Giza CC, et al. Potentially neuroprotective gene modulation in an in vitro model of mild traumatic brain injury. *Mol Cell Biochem* 2013;375:185–198.

280. Barnes DE, Kaup A, Kirby KA, Byers AL, Diaz-Arrastia R, Yaffe K. Traumatic brain injury and risk of dementia in older veterans. *Neurology* 2014;83:312–319.

281. Cushing H. A study of a series of wounds involving the brain and its enveloping structures. *Br J Surg* 1917;5:558–684.

282. Martland HS. Punch drunk. *JAMA* 1928;19:1103–1107.

283. Van Den Heuvel C, Thornton E, Vink R. Traumatic brain injury and Alzheimer's disease. In: Weber JT, Maas AIR, editors. *Progress in brain research*, vol. 161. Amsterdam: Elsevier, 2007 (pp. 303–316).

284. Parker HL. Traumatic encephalopathy ('punch drunk') of professional pugilists. *J Neurol Psychopathol* 1934;15:20–28.

285. Victoroff J. Traumatic encephalopathy: Review and provisional research diagnostic criteria. *NeuroRehab* 2013;32:211–224.

286. Stern RA, Daneshvar DH, Baugh CM, Seichepine DR, Montenigro PH, Riley DO, et al. Clinical presentation of chronic traumatic encephalopathy. *Neurology* 2013;81:1122–1129.

287. McKee AC, Stein TD, Nowinski CJ, Stern RA, Daneshvar DH, Victor E, et al. The spectrum of disease in chronic traumatic encephalopathy. *Brain* 2012;1–22.

288. Mondello S, Schmid K, Berger R, Kobeissy F, Italiano D, Jeromin A, et al. The challenge of mild traumatic brain injury: Role of biochemical markers in diagnosis of brain damage. *Med Res Rev* 2014;34:503–531.

289. Kang JH, Lin HC. Increased risk of multiple sclerosis after traumatic brain injury: A nationwide population-based study. *J Neurotrauma* 2012;29:90–95.

290. Ling H, Hardy J, Zetterberg H. Neurological consequences of traumatic brain injuries in sports. *Mol Cell Neurosci* 2015;S1044–S7431

291. Beauchamp MH, Ditchfield M, Maller JJ, Catroppa C, Godfrey C, Rosenfeld JV, et al. Hippocampus, amygdala and global brain changes 10 years after childhood traumatic brain injury. *Int J Dev Neurosci* 2011;29:137–143.

292. Bigler ED, Farrer TJ, Pertab JL, James K, Petrie JA, Hedges DW. Reaffirmed limitations of meta-analytic methods in the study of mild traumatic brain injury: A response to Rohling et al. *Clin Neuropsychol* 2013;27:176–214.

293. Dean PJA, Sato JR, Vieira G, McNamara A, Sterr A. Multimodal imaging of mild traumatic brain injury and persistent postconcussion syndrome. *Brain Behav* 2015;5:e00292.

294. Al-Samsam RH, Alessandri B, Ross Bullock R. Extracellular N-acetyl-aspartate as a biochemical marker of the severity of neuronal damage following experimental acute traumatic brain injury. *J Neurotrauma* 2000;17:31–39.

295. Garnett MR, Blamire AM, Rajagopalan B, Styles P, Cadoux-Hudson TA. Evidence for cellular damage in normal-appearing white matter correlates with injury severity in patients following traumatic brain injury: A magnetic resonance spectroscopy study. *Brain* 2000;123:1403–1409.

296. Johnson B, Zhang K, Gaya M, Neuberger T, Horovitz S, Hallett M, et al. Metabolic alterations in corpus callosum may compromise brain functional connectivity in MTBI patients: An 1H-MRS study. *Neurosci Lett* 2012;509:5–8.

297. George EO, Roys S, Sours C, Rosenberg J, Zhuo J, Shanmuganathan K, et al. Longitudinal and prognostic evaluation of mild traumatic brain injury: A 1H-magnetic resonance spectroscopy study. *J Neurotrauma* 2014;31:1018–1028.

298. Vagnozzi R, Signoretti S, Cristofori L, Alessandrini F, Floris R, Isgro E, et al. Assessment of metabolic brain damage and recovery following mild traumatic brain injury: A multicentre, proton magnetic resonance spectroscopic study in concussed patients. *Brain* 2010;133:3232–3242.

299. Cohen BA, Inglese M, Rusinek H, Babb JS, Grossman RI, Gonen O. Proton MR spectroscopy and MRI-volumetry in mild traumatic brain injury. *AJNR* 2007;28:907–913.

300. Dean PJA, Otaduy MCG, Harris LM, McNamara A, Seiss E, Sterr A. Monitoring long-term effects of mild traumatic brain injury with magnetic resonance spectroscopy: A pilot study. *NeuroRep* 2013;24:677–681.

301. Johnson B, Gay M, Zhang K, Neuberger T, Horovitz SG, Hallett M, et al. The use of magnetic resonance spectroscopy in the subacute evaluation of athletes recovering from single and multiple mild traumatic brain injury. *J Neurotrauma* 2012;29:2297–2304.

302. Chen JK, Johnston KM, Frey S, Petrides M, Worsley K, Ptito A. Functional abnormalities in symptomatic concussed athletes: An fMRI study. *NeuroImage* 2004;22:68–82.

303. Chen JK, Johnston KM, Collie A, McCrory P, Ptito A. A validation of the post concussion symptom scale in the assessment of complex concussion using cognitive testing and functional MRI. *J Neurol Neurosurg Psychiatry* 2007;78:1231–1238.

304. Keightley ML, Sinopoli KJ, Davis KD, Mikulis DJ. Is there evidence for neurodegenerative change following traumatic brain injury in children and youth? A scoping review. *Front Human Neurosci* 2014;8:1–6.

305. McAllister TW, Sparling MB, Flashman LA, Guerin SJ, Mamourian AC, Saykin AJ. Differential working memory load effects after mild traumatic brain injury. *NeuroImage* 2001;14:1004–1012.

306. Jantzen KJ, Anderson B, Steinberg FL, Kelso JAS. A prospective functional MR imaging study of mild traumatic brain injury in college football players. *Am J Neuroradiol* 2004;25:738–745.

307. Scheibel RS, Newsome MR, Troyanskaya M, Lin X, Steinberg JL, Radaideh M, et al. Altered brain activation in military personnel with one or more traumatic brain injuries following blast. *J Int Neuropsychol Soc* 2012;18:89–100.

308. Jantzen KJ. Functional magnetic resonance imaging of mild traumatic brain injury. *J Head Trauma Rehabil* 2010;25:256–266.

309. McAllister TW, Flashman LA, McDonald BC, Saykin AJ. Mechanisms of working memory dysfunction after mild and moderate TBI: Evidence from functional MRI and neurogenetics. *J Neurotrauma* 2006;23:1450–1467.

310. Witt ST, Lovejoy DW, Pearlson GD, Stevens MC. Decreased prefrontal cortex activity in mild traumatic brain injury during performance of an auditory oddball task. *Brain Imaging Behav* 2010;4:232–247.

311. Gosselin N, Bottari C, Chen JK, Petrides M, Tinawi S, de Guise E, et al. Electrophysiology and functional MRI in postacute mild traumatic brain injury. *J Neurotrauma* 2011;28:329–341.

312. Matthews S, Simmons A, Strigo I. The effects of loss versus alteration of consciousness on inhibition-related brain activity among individuals with a history of blast-related concussion. *Psychiatry Res* 2011;191:76–79.

313. Matthews SC, Strigo IA, Simmons AN, O'Connell RM, Reinhardt LE, Moseley SA. A multimodal imaging study in U.S. Veterans of Operations Iraqi and Enduring Freedom with and without major depression after blast-related concussion. *NeuroImage* 2011;54:69–75.

314. McDonald BC, Saykin AJ, McAllister TW. Functional MRI of mild traumatic brain injury (mTBI): Progress and perspectives from the first decade of studies. *Brain Imaging Behav* 2012;6:193–207.

315. Chen J-K, Johnston KM, Petrides M, Ptito A. Neural substrates of symptoms of depression following concussion in male athletes with persisting postconcussion symptoms. *Arch Gen Psychiatry* 2008;65:81–89.

316. Slobounov SM, Gay M, Zhang K, Johnson B, Pennell D, Sebastianelli W, et al. Alteration of brain functional network at rest and in response to YMCA physical stress test in concussed athletes: RsFMRI study. *NeuroImage* 2011;55:1716–1727.

317. Chen C-J, Wu C-H, Liao Y-P, Hsu H-L, Tseng Y-C, Liu H-L, et al. Working memory in patients with mild traumatic brain injury: Functional MR imaging analysis. *Radiology* 2012;264:844–851.

318. Dettwiler A, Murugavel M, Putukian M, Cubon V, Furtado J, Osherson D. Persistent differences in patterns of brain activation after sports-related concussion: A longitudinal functional magnetic resonance imaging study. *J Neurottrauma* 2014;31:180–188.

319. Hillary FG. Neuroimaging of working memory dysfunction and the dilemma with brain reorganization hypotheses. *J Int Neuropsychol Soc* 2008;14:526–534.

320. Hillary FG, Genova HM, Medaglia JD, Fitzpatrick NM,Chiou KS, Wardecker BM et al. The nature of processing speed deficits in traumatic brain injury: Is less brain more? *Brain Imaging Behav* 2010;4:141–154.

321. Fazio VC, Lovell MR, Pardini JE, Collins MW. The relation between post concussion symptoms and neurocognitive performance in concussed athletes. *NeuroRehab* 2007;22:207–216.

322. Mayer AR, Yang Z, Yeo RA, Pena A, Ling JM, Mannell MV, et al. A functional MRI study of multimodal selective attention following mild traumatic brain injury. *Brain Imaging Behav* 2012;6:343–354.

323. Slobounov S, Sebastianelli W, Hallett M. Residual brain dysfunction observed one year post-mild traumatic brain injury: Combined EEG and balance study. *Clin Neurophysiol* 2012;123:1755–1761.

324. Abbas K, Shenk TE, Poole VN, Robinson ME, Leverenz LJ, Nauman EA, et al. Alteration of default mode network in high school football athletes due to repetitive subconcussive mild traumatic brain injury: A resting-state functional magnetic resonance imaging study. *Brain Connect* 2015;5:91–101.

325. Bigler ED, Maxwell WL. Neuropathology of mild traumatic brain injury: Relationship to neuroimaging findings. *Brain Imaging Behav* 2012;6:108–136.

326. Jennett B, Bond M. Assessment of outcome after severe brain damage. A practical scale. *Lancet* 1975;1:480–484.

327. Alexander MP. Mild traumatic brain injury: Pathophysiology, natural history, and clinical management. *Neurol* 1995;45: 1253–1260.

328. Pertab JL, James KM, Bigler ED. Limitations of mild traumatic brain injury meta-analyses. *Brain Inj* 2009;23:498–508.

329. Ruff RM, Crouch JA, Tröster AI, Marshall LF, Buchsbaum MS, Lottenberg S, et al. Selected cases of poor outcome following a minor brain trauma: Comparing neuropsychological and positron emission tomography assessment. *Brain Inj* 1994;8:297–308.

330. Ruff RM, Camenzuli L, Mueller J. Miserable minority: Emotional risk factors that influence the outcome of a mild traumatic brain injury. *Brain Inj* 1996;10:551–565.

331. Binder LM, Rohling ML, Larrabee GJ. A review of mild head trauma, part i: Meta-analytic review of neuropsychological studies. *J Clin Exp Neuropsychol* 1997;19:421–431.

332. Frencham KA, Fox AM, Maybery MT. Neuropsychological studies of mild traumatic brain injury: A meta-analytic review of research since 1995. *J Clin Exp Neuropsychol* 2005;27:334–351.

333. Rohling ML, Binder LM, Demakis GJ, Larrabee GJ, Ploetz DM, Langhinrichsen-Rohling J. A meta-analysis of neuropsychological outcome after mild traumatic brain injury: Reanalyses and reconsiderations of Binder et al. *Clin Neuropsychol* 2011;25:608–623.

334. Committee on Head Injury Nomenclature of the Congress of Neurological Surgeons. Glossary of head injury, including some definitions of injury to the cervical spine. *Clin Neurosurg* 1966;12:386–394.

335. American Academy of Neurology. Practice parameter: The management of concussion in sports (summary statement). Report of the Quality Standards Subcommittee. *Neurology* 1997;48:581–585.

336. Miller Fisher C. Concussion amnesia. *Neurology* 1966;16;826–830.

337. Aubry M, Cantu RC, Dvorak J, Graf-Baumann T, Johnston K, Kelly J, et al. Summary and agreement statement of the First International Conference on Concussion in Sport, Vienna 2001: Recommendations for the improvement of safety and health of athletes who may suffer concussive injuries. *Br J Sports Med* 2002;36:6–10.

338. McAllister TW. Evaluation and treatment of neurobehavioral complications of traumatic brain injury – have we made any progress? *Neurorehabil* 2002;17:263–264.

339. Alves WM, Coloban ART, O'Leary TJ, Rimel RW, Jane JA. Understanding posttraumatic symptoms after minor head injury. *J Head Trauma Rehabil* 1986;1:1–12.

340. Guskiewicz KM, Bruce SL, Cantu RC, Ferrara MS, Kelly JP, McCrea M, et al. National Athletic Trainers' Association position statement: Management of sport-related concussion. *J Athl Train* 2004;39:280–297.

341. Herring SA, Bergfeld JA, Boland A, Boyajian-O'Neill LA, Cantu RC, Hershman E. Concussion (mild traumatic brain injury) and the team physician: A consensus statement. *Med Sci Sports Exerc* 2006;38:395–399.

342. McCrory P, Johnston KM, Meeuwisse W, Aubry M, Cantu R, Dvorak J, et al. Summary and agreement statement of the 2nd International Conference on Concussion in Sport in Prague. *Br J Sports Med* 2005;39: 196–204.

343. McCrory P, Meeuwisse W, Johnston KM, Dvorak J, Aubry M, Molloy M, et al. Consensus statement on concussion in sport: The 3rd international conference on concussion in sport held in Zurich. *J Sci Med Sport* 2009;12:340–351.

344. McCrory P, Meeuwisse W, Aubry M, Cantu RC, Dvorak J, Echemendia RJ, et al. Consensus statement on concussion in sport: the 4th International Conference on Concussion in Sport held in Zurich, November 2012. *Br J Sports Med* 2013;47:250–258.

345. McCrory P, Meeuwisse W, Dvorak J, Aubry M, Bailes J, Broglio S, et al. Consensus statement on concussion in sport – the 5th International Conference on Concussion in Sport held in Berlin, October 2016. *Br J Sports Med* 2017;51:838–847.

346. Cantu RC. An overview of concussion consensus statements since 2000. *Neurosurg Focus* 2006;21:1–5.

347. Makdissi M. Is the simple versus complex classification of concussion a valid and useful differentiation? *Br J Sports Med* 2009;43:i23–i127.

348. Centers for Disease Control and Prevention. *Injury prevention and control: Traumatic brain injury*. 2013. Available at www.cdc.gov/concussion/sports/.

349. Brain Injury Association of America. *Sports concussions fact sheet*. 2010. Available at www.biausa.org/Default.aspx?SiteSearchID=1192&ID=/search-results.htm.

350. Bodin D, Yeates KO, Klamar K. Definition and classification of concussion. In Apps JN, Walter KD, editors. *Pediatric and adolescent concussion: Diagnosis, management, and outcomes*. New York: Springer, 2012.

351. Peloso PM, Carroll LJ, Cassidy D. Borg J. von Holst H, Holm L, Yates D. Critical evaluation of the existing guidelines on mild traumatic brain injury. *J Rehabil Med* 2004;Suppl. 43: 106–112.

352. Carroll LJ, Cassidy JD, Holm L, Kraus J, Coronado VG. Methodological issues and research recommendations for mild traumatic brain injury: The WHO Collaborating Centre Task Force on mild traumatic brain injury. *J Rehabil Med* 2004;Suppl. 43:113–125.

Chapter

2

Epidemiology of Concussive Brain Injury

Jeff Victoroff

Without accurate data, how can we begin to address the problem?

Anonymous CBI survivor testifying before
the U.S. Congress in 2001 [1]

Antelogium
What Counts?

Imagine omniscience. Three innocent 17-year-old girls play a brutal game of the dangerous "non-contact" sport, high school ice hockey. Steeling yourself, you monitor their brains. As Cindy, Mindy, and Malak slide, whirl, and crash into the boards, the ice, and each other, you assay everything important: regional cerebral blood flow, blood–brain barrier integrity, ionotropic glutamate receptor excitatory post-synaptic potentials, microglia activation, mitochondrial complex II electron transfer, microtubule buckling, axolemmal porosity, glymphatic clearance, Toll-like receptor binding, up-regulation in dentate gyrus mossy cell gene expression – you know, all the stuff we ought to measure. (Instead, we tap legs with rubber objects and call it a "neurological examination.")

Cindy tries to bodycheck Mindy but slips and bounces her helmet off Mindy's shoulder pad. Mindy careens off balance and slams her helmet into the glass. She trips Malak, who falls backwards, denting the ice with her helmet. Their coach, deeply concerned, rushes on to the ice and shouts at them to keep playing. The girls shake it off and get back to their unpaid university advertising jobs, while you check their telemetered head impact measures.

- Cindy's readout: the expression of 261 genes in her basolateral amygdala projection cells was up-regulated by 6.3–16.4% from pre-impact baseline. N-methyl-D-aspartate (NMDA) binding increased enough in the hippocampus that 13% of the magnesium ion control over calcium channels was impaired in 12% of CA3 neurons, leading to an average 9.5% increase in phosphorylation of three cytosolic protein kinase transcription factors. Some 7.2% buckling of the average microtubule in 7.3% of the axons bundled in the splenium of her corpus callosum led to a mean 11% decrement in the pace of vesicular transport along those tracts.
- Mindy's readout: the same as Cindy's, but 5% worse.
- Malak's readout: the same as Mindy's, but 5% worse.

All three girls later report they are not sure, but they *might* have been dazed at the moment of head impact. Which one had a brain injury?

This futuristic scenario exposes the root conceptual fallacy of brain injury science. Throughout Chapter 1, we discussed *injury* as if that term was anchored in objectivity. "This child was injured. That one wasn't." At the extremes, of course, clinicians are able to state that one person has been badly hurt and another has not. Death with decomposition, for example, can usually be distinguished from vibrant, happy life. This comports with the ancient Galenean/Oslerian approach to medical diagnosis – a strict and inviolable dichotomy between well and ill.

But that's not how biology works. Throughout many physiological systems and much of the body, structure and function are in constant flux. Nobody and no body is the same from one second to the next. Compromise defines many evolutionary solutions. So we are always undergoing changes that, left uncountered, would cause deterioration, but we counter them and do fine.

Not to perturb older clinicians, but the black-and-white dichotomy between health and disease taught in medical school is a fast-thinking heuristic most valuable for focusing energies on prevention or management of obvious threats. It is not a scientifically nuanced worldview. The real-life style of many biological systems is stress, repair, repeat. DNA damage is normal. Cell damage is normal. Brain damage is normal. Trouble comes when either repetitive workaday wear and tear or arrival of one extraordinary stress overwhelms our built-in repair systems.

Consider the little mitochondrion. Cells need it to generate energy. Yet, like a Volkswagen diesel, it also generates noxious byproducts – in this case, reactive oxygen species (ROSs). ROSs are prone to trigger peroxidation of the lipids in membranes, a step or two away from apoptosis and autophagy, the undesirable moment when the cell eats itself. Thankfully, white-knight antioxidants such as superoxide dismutases have evolved to launch rescue missions, saving cells from the natural stress of energy production. When confronted with everyday energy demands and assaulted by ROSs, does the cell recoil in fright and pray for deliverance from its cursed fate? No. The evidence suggests a cool aplomb.

Now consider the 17-year-girl playing ice hockey. As she races and stops and trips and collides, her rattling brain is somewhat stressed. The vast majority of those rattlings are borne with no cerebral grief. A few of the rattlings trigger atypical gene expression in metabolic, growth regulatory, and immunological pathways. A few stretch axons enough to change axolemmal permeability and jigger bundles of microtubules. A few provoke excitatory neurotoxicity with excess calcium influx. Very few may cause neuronal energy crisis and set apoptotic and anti-apoptotic enzymes at each other's throats. Is this traumatic brain damage? If the girl looks fine, feels fine, and tests fine but underwent a few million brain changes that would not have otherwise occurred, was this a concussion?

What is a brain injury? In a previous generation, the physiology of traumatic brain injury (TBI) was described in terms of a "neurometabolic cascade" – a hypothesized phenomenon in which abrupt impact above an injurious threshold triggers cationic influx and a chain reaction of further molecular embarrassments, sometimes resulting in apoptosis [2, 3]. Christopher Giza and David Hovda of UCLA promulgated that theory. They deservedly reign at the apogee of Western concussion science. They have vastly more laboratory experience than the present author, who cannot overstate his personal admiration and respect for these academic giants. The author, however, has so far failed to persuade the pair that, conceivably, hitting the rodent's actual head might better model hitting a human head than hitting the rodent's surgically exposed dura.[1]

The "neurometabolic cascade" hypothesis, at one time considered the standard model of concussion, is bedeviled by two major limitations. First, it implies a dichotomy that does not exist, separating concussion from non-concussion and injury from non-injury when the truth is a biological continuum, and the boundary properly named "injurious" has yet to be divined. Second, as we will show in forthcoming chapters, post-concussive brain change is not a one-way street. Rather than a "cascade" of molecular happenings splashing downstream toward a cataract of neuronal doom, an impact to the head is followed immediately by a complex melee of neurobiological skirmishing, a tug of war between damaging and reparative processes, many of which probably remain to be discovered.

Epidemiologists count. One thing they often count is the incidence of an injury. With guillotine wounds and lightning strikes, presence or absence of injury is not such a classification problem. With TBI, however, where should one draw the line between presence and absence? We know that injury can occur without loss of consciousness. For that reason, all three girls may have been injured. We know that illness can occur (for instance, rhinovirus) with no lasting harm and even some paradoxical benefit. For that reason, even if all the girls return to baseline after 72 h, they may all have been injured. The physiological changes listed for Cindy, Mindy, and Malak (an infinitesimal accounting of the real list we would get if we monitored each organelle in their heads) create biological stresses, just as normal healthful mitochondrial function creates biological stresses. At what point along this continuum of awesome biological variety should the omniscient athletic trainer check off "brain injury"? And, since the source of almost all of the epidemiologist's counts of sport-related brain injuries come from athletic trainers, how many brain injuries should the epidemiologist count?

The point is merely that the first and most irresolvable problem an epidemiologist faces, even if he or she were omniscient, is one of classification. There exists no biological threshold between brain-injured and not. We are forced, therefore, to pick an utterly, comically arbitrary classification rule, such as "only Malak had forgetfulness 31.43 h later. Thus, just one girl was injured." This chapter will show that it is impossible to know how many people suffer symptomatic concussions. But it is even less possible to know how many people suffer asymptomatic brain injuries. The author apologizes for mentioning this unmentionable conundrum. The author fully appreciates that clinical medicine demands practical decision making that ignores such philosophical nuance. But one cannot, in good conscience, embark on writing or reading a chapter on the epidemiology of CBI without noting that every published number is based on the assumption that we know when the brain is hurt, when in fact we do not.

Readers may wonder whether this is an abstraction worthy of our attention. It will become a practical, concrete question very shortly. Consider repetitive concussions and the average linebacker. He will suffer more than 500 brain impacts each season. None may cause symptoms, but he is nonetheless prone to develop early-onset dementia. His much-rattled brain, therefore, was probably injured. Should the epidemiologist pay attention? Even given perfect knowledge of every immediate biological change in our three brutalized high school girls, can we count the number of injuries? No. Epidemiologists enumerate the occasionally visible tip among an archipelago of icebergs.

Introduction and Apologia[2]

Nobody knows.

How many people will suffer a concussion each year? How many people will suffer a concussion in their lifetime?

---

[1] As every reader and many children know, concussive forces usually impact hair or fur. Whatever force is not absorbed by this multipurpose keratin helmet (manufactured from the same tough material as rhinoceros horn) is then transmitted through scalp to skull, whence it is dispersed in dazzlingly complex mechanical ways that have been idealized by finite element modeling to eventually affect the brain. In contrast, the UCLA team, and many other laboratories employing the fluid percussion model, first pops off a window of skull, then hits rodents directly on the dura of the brain and bravely assumes the results are similar to those of CBI.

[2] This introduction is intended to provide context for the available epidemiological data. Readers who are pressed for time and eager to get to the numbers should probably skip it! Note, however: the numbers are not what matters.

How many people are currently suffering disabling effects of a concussion? What is the magnitude of this human problem? Nobody knows.

That is the first and most important declaration to be made in any forthright chapter on the epidemiology of concussive brain injury (CBI). Due to impracticable diagnostic criteria, insensitive detection, and the impossibility of calculating point prevalence, nobody knows what proportion of this world's human population is likely to experience a concussion this year (incidence), how many will suffer a concussion in their lives (cumulative life incidence), what proportion of society currently suffers from either short- or long-term effects of a concussion (prevalence), or how to quantify the net damage to human well-being (global impact).

Our ignorance has profound implications. Evidence exists that CBI survivors live shorter lives [e.g., 4]. But to what degree is the average global cerebral capacity diminished by CBI? To what extent does CBI explain the grim global siege of dementia we are about to experience? Does the delay in scientific discovery – for instance, for precision cures to cancers or practical fusion energy – derive in part from the population effect of CBI on support for science education and collective intellectual potency? Can the common and socially disabling occurrence of depression, domestic violence, political partisanship, religious enmity, market catastrophes, hunger, international conflict, and nuclear jeopardy be attributed, to some extent, to CBI? Analyzing the psychopathy of leaders such as Vladimir Putin or Vlad the Impaler, what measure of their immorality, agonism, paranoia, and tyranny is justly attributed to CBI? (We'd need to ask their Moms.) What are the odds that your beautiful daughter or your handsome son will never fulfill his or her true potential and will die early and confused because of CBI?

Without any concrete scientifically based measure of this collective impact, it is hard to know whether the average citizen should regard brain trauma as a rare threat with mostly innocuous impact on the functioning of society (merely permanently disabling most of our high school football players and some of our cheerleaders), or a common threat with considerable deleterious impact on the human residents of Earth. *Untold damage* is the correct descriptor of the impact. And, as much as the various authors of this brief book may wish to be the tellers of the damage, we will fail. We are part of the nobody who knows.

Here is the problem: as explained in Chapter 1, concussion is a general term for a rattling impact. It was applied to medicine only lately, to describe, for example, spinal or pulmonary traumas due to visitation by abrupt external force. Heads experience the visitation of external forces daily. But the landing of a swallowtail butterfly or the caress of a lover is not the external force one needs fear. All available evidence suggests that it requires a certain minimum amount of abrupt external force before the shaking of the brain hurts that little organ. (By "hurts," one means, in the most non-quantifiable sense, harms, damages, and produces deleterious effects on.) Concussive external force is the main element of virtually all TBIs. The proportion of the damage due to external force is the concussive element of a brain injury. For instance, concussive force is a major part of the negative impact of a punch, but concussive force is a minor part of the negative impact of a penetrating small-caliber bullet, since it does less punching and brain rattling and more non-concussive skewering. Put simply – whether or not there is also a skull fracture, a brain penetration, or an intracerebral hemorrhage – transmission of damaging external force deflected and dispersed by the skull is CBI.

In epidemiological publications, the typical academic work-around to compensate for the toughness of identifying CBI (not usually acknowledged in candor) is to take some slice of the big pie of CBI and assign that slice a neat categorical title lacking in biological meaning (for instance, "mild traumatic brain injury" (mTBI)), then invent or come to consensus on arbitrary operational criteria for bounding that slice of the pie, and then study the epidemiology of that slice. This would be entirely defensible if the operational distinguishing criteria had any merit. Some do. For instance, if every victim undergoes a computed tomography (CT) scan, one can scientifically distinguish the subset with criteria A:

1. patient-reported subjective alteration in consciousness
2. no known skull penetration
3. no intracerebral bleed reported by the local radiologist
4. survival for at least a year.

Criteria such as A may not identify a biologically distinct group (that is, they lack validity in regard to specifying a neurobiologically homogeneous group) but would at least be reliable. Emergency room (ER) doctors in Brazil or Burkina Faso could apply criteria A with high interrater agreement. Instead, the Western literature is dominated by less practical criteria. The archons of the World Health Organization (WHO) [5] and the U.S. Centers for Disease Control and Prevention (CDC) [6], have nominated rules for diagnosing concussions, and some investigators employ ICD codes, but one of the most commonly applied algorithms was that proposed by several individuals and published in 1993 as the American College of Rehabilitation Medicine (ACRM) criteria [7]. Let us call it criteria B.

A patient with mild TBI is a person who has had a traumatically induced physiological disruption of brain function, as manifested by at least one of the following:

1. any period of loss of consciousness
2. any loss of memory for events immediately before or after the accident
3. any alteration in mental state at the time of the accident (e.g., feeling dazed, disoriented, or confused)
4. focal neurological deficit(s) that may or may not be transient, but where the severity of the injury does not exceed the following:

   - loss of consciousness of approximately 30 minutes or less
   - after 30 minutes, an initial Glasgow Coma Scale (GCS) of 13–15
   - post-traumatic amnesia not greater than 24 h.

The problems with operational (non-biological) criteria B are instantly apparent. First, rather than simply requiring that there be a subjectively reported change in consciousness, something that is readily ascertained, the ACRM dictates that there must have been actual loss of consciousness. Loss of consciousness is a somewhat specific, somewhat detectable neurological phenomenon. It cannot be reported accurately by the patient or by any observer who did not have a handy electroencephalograph at the moment of the accident. Second, once the doctor has listed the memories the patient should have, he or she can determine whether any are lost. But the doctor can never do this. What is the virtue of asking, "Please tell me all that occurred that you do not recall." It is impossible for anyone to know all that the victim's brain should recorded in a retrievable format. The best one can do is to determine whether an obvious gap occurs on retrieval – and retrieval of a memory is completely dissociable from formation and storage of a memory. Third, without meaning to be harsh, it is absurd to require that there be focal neurological deficits. These rarely (indeed, practically never) occur in the population with CBI. Moreover, the neurological examination is extremely challenging and unreliably performed, even by board-certified neurologists. Fourth, the criteria require a stopwatch for monitoring the duration of loss of consciousness and an expert for rating the GCS – which is unreliably documented by most ER personnel. Fifth: if you are a doctor, can you name a single case in the last 50 years of your practice when you have monitored PTA with a normed and validated instrument such as the Galveston Orientation and Amnesia Test [8] at the time of injury and again at exactly 24:00 h after the injury?

PTA is almost never measured, monitored, or recorded. When it is, the medical record is rarely accurate, since testing PTA is highly unreliable without a formal and expert examination. As Powell [9] opined, "it is all too easy to examine retrospectively the events surrounding an accident and find gaps in memory that can lead to the erroneous diagnosis of post-traumatic amnesia or to its overestimation" (p. 237). Thus, the final line of criteria B would by itself eliminate such criteria from serious consideration as practical specifiers of any medical condition.

All of these errors aside, the ACRM and its sibling criteria proffered by the WHO share a fatal flaw: they base severity on the examination at the time of injury. In 2009 the actress Natasha Richardson slipped on some snow. She bumped her head, got up, felt fine, and joked about her fall. Had a baker's dozen world-renowned brain surgeons instantly come to her aid, they would have begged for clinging selfies. But her neurological condition in the first hour was reported to be without complaint beyond mild chagrin. Thus, the neurosurgeons would probably have diagnosed Natasha with nothing. She did not even qualify for the "mild TBI" label as defined by the ACRM. She died of TBI a few hours later. The point is hopefully clear: it is outcome that matters. Initial presentation is no time for assigning a severity label. TBI severity criteria yoked to the early minutes have no merit.

The author does not mean to criticize! In 1993, when the ACRM criteria were proposed, little research had been published regarding the reliability of TBI assessment. It was only with the recent contribution of many earnest scholars that the fallacies of criteria B have become apparent. However, our apologia for the data in this chapter is largely due to the fact that one is obliged to summarize the results of studies of concussion that cannot be trusted. Since the old phrase "mild traumatic brain injury" has been popular for several decades, since practical operational criteria such as criteria A have never been employed to distinguish a subset of CBI cases for study, the literature reviewed is noxiously tainted by the untenable clinical judgments imposed by criteria B. As Barker-Collo and Feigin put it [10], "The data currently available in the literature does not reflect true incidence … [because] no standard methodological criteria exist for carrying out a population-based TBI incidence study." The author deeply regrets that the following review is, therefore, like a concatenation of corked wine.

Worse yet, the published investigations of CBI frequency, prevalence, and incidence fail to report the unreported cases. Unreported means two things: reported to the doctor, but not by the doctor; and not reported to the doctor. With regard to the first issue, one might hope that if you go to the hospital and declare that you have been knocked silly, someone would take note. That is not always the case. In a study by Powell et al. [11], "Fifty-six percent of mild TBI cases identified by study personnel did not have a documented mild TBI-related diagnosis in the ED [emergency department] record" (p. 1550). If this is typical, then a minority of those who get medical attention get counted. With regard to the second issue: if you are a physician who attended to 100 teenaged boys with complaints of being hit on the head this month, what proportion does this represent of the population of local teenaged boys who were hit on the head this month? 2%? 7½%? With sufficient video cameras in every square meter of the community, including auto interiors, closets, and bathrooms, one might respond to that question scientifically.

If self-report of past concussion in population-based surveys were reliable, one could respond quasi-scientifically by calculating the ratio of clinical visits to self-reports. In fact, one does not expect an accurate estimate until the counter-terrorism surveillance culture is complete. For this reason, we further apologize that our data are an amalgam of claims about an unknown sized cohort who have come to medical attention only to be categorized "mTBIs" in an unreliable and biologically meaningless way.

Apart from these minor caveats, we stand by our conclusions. To preview the denouement: this chapter will meticulously review data regarding:

- annual incidence
- prevalence
- lifetime cumulative incidence of concussion.

We will discuss both the insurmountable barriers to accurate estimates for any of these constructs, and the vast difference in the importance of each. Annual incidence has been studied a lot. The author pledges to work hard to distill a reasonable estimate of the proportion of adults in first-world nations who suffer a CBI each year. The chapter will reveal why this number by itself, even if accurate to the nth degree, has no conceivable clinical value. Prevalence, in contrast, has rarely been studied. Almost nothing can be said about it, except that it matters a lot. Lifetime cumulative incidence, when combined with knowledge about the prevalence of untoward effects, is what matters the most, but can, at best, be the subject of earnest guesswork. By the end of the chapter, readers will be among the best guessers on Earth.

Epidemiology of TBI in the United States: Deconstructing the CDC Pyramid

some patients may not have the above factors medically documented in the acute stage … Some patients may not become aware of, or admit, the extent of their symptoms until they attempt to return to normal functioning … Mild traumatic brain injury may also be overlooked in the face of more dramatic physical injury.

(Kay et al.1993 [7], p. 87)

Since Toynbee announced the arrival of post-modernism in 1939, the term "deconstruct" has been used with reckless abandon. It is, nonetheless, a worthwhile concept: investigating how the ambiguities of language debunk the conventional idea that words have a single meaning. Figure 2.1 is the CDC pyramid, an attempt to summarize the best available data about the epidemiology of TBI in the United States. It is the result of a sincere and laudable effort. Its authors, however, were at the mercy of circumstances beyond their control: only some CBI survivors see a doctor. Only some doctors recognize that their patient is a CBI survivor. On rigorous analysis, the meaning of the CDC's much-quoted sentence, "An estimated 1.7 million TBIs occur in the United States annually" begins to unravel. Our mission is to examine the origins of the numbers in the CDC pyramid and test their robustness in the face of impartial critique.

Typical CBIs are relatively mild. That is, although CBI encompasses a broad range of severity, humans most often experience the type that do not involve gross intracerebral hemorrhage visible on CT, prolonged coma, or immediate death, and that therefore roughly match the medically indefinable cohort commonly labeled with the phrase "mild TBI." To enumerate such typical CBIs, one merely has to know how

many total TBIs occur and what proportion of those are reasonably classified as occurring without prompt death, lengthy coma, or major bleed. (Later we will re-emphasize the point that any classification of severity based on initial presentation is misleading. For the time being, we will adopt this operational compromise. Readers will readily appreciate that the overwhelming majority of injuries diagnosed as TBIs are in fact typical CBIs.)

Therefore, to determine the annual incidence, lifetime cumulative incidence, and prevalence of typical CBIs, one might first look to the more general literature on TBIs. Several investigations have attempted to estimate the total annual incidence of TBIs in the United States. Figure 2.1 (or a variant) is the most popular depiction of annual national incidence. This pyramid comes from the CDC Blue Book [12], reporting U.S. data from 2002 to 2006. It asserts that about 1.7 million TBIs are diagnosed annually. Among these were allegedly 1.365 million ED visits and 275,000 hospitalizations.

Wherever did the CDC get these numbers? In 1989, the CDC's Division of Acute Care, Rehabilitation Research, and Disability Prevention launched the first U.S. population-based injury surveillance system for TBI [13]. The hope was that representative state data might permit extrapolation to the entire nation. Six years later, fortunately, the CDC realized that little is gained by counting cases without an agreed-upon definition of TBI. This realization led to the publication of *Guidelines for Surveillance of Central Nervous System Injury* [14], which essentially defined TBI as an injury to the head with associated signs or symptoms, such as skull fracture, decreased level of consciousness, or intracranial injury. In 1999, a decade after the surveillance initiative was launched, Thurman et al. presented their first *Report to Congress* [13]. That report was based on data from seven of the 50 states. It justifiably received attention because it offered, for the first time, an estimate both of annual incidence of TBIs and prevalence of TBI-related disability:

- "During 1990–1995, the mean annual incidence rate for persons hospitalized with TBI and survived was 99 per 100,000 population."
- "each year, approximately 35 percent (80,500) of the 230,000 hospitalized survivors of TBI experience the onset of long-term disability" ([15], p. 16).

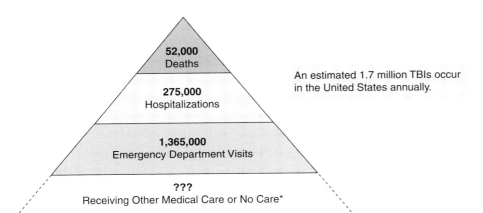

An estimated 1.7 million TBIs occur in the United States annually.

Fig. 2.1 Traumatic brain injury (TBI) in the United States: emergency department visits, hospitalizations, and deaths 2002–2006. *An estimated 439,000 TBIs treated by physicians during office visits and 89,000 treated in outpatient settings were not included in this report. In addition, TBIs with no medical advice sought, an estimated 25% of all mild and moderate TBIs, were not included ([12], p. 61).

Source: Faul et al., 2010 [12]. CDC, 2016. www.cdc.gov/traumaticbraininjury/tbi_ed.html

This CDC program has evolved into the main source of data regarding the U.S. national incidence of TBIs. Better yet, the CDC expanded the program from those early days when only hospitalized patients were counted in the National Hospital Discharge Survey (NHDS). Affiliate programs now count TBIs that present to ERs via the National Hospital Ambulatory Medical Care Survey (NHAMCS) [1] and to outpatient settings via the National Ambulatory Medical Care Survey (NAMCS) (www.cdc.gov/nchs/ahcd/about_ahcd.htm). These are the sources of the three numbers stacked in the pyramid of Figure 2.1. Most TBIs are CBIs. If one accepts the CDC's own estimate, 75% of survivors represented mild cases. (The WHO 2004 meta-analysis [16] put that figure at 70–90%.) Hence, about 1.023 million annual ED visits and 206,000 annual hospitalizations are attributable to injuries that are probably typical concussions.[3]

But before estimating the number of CBIs from this much-cited enumeration of TBIs, one wishes to assess the actual meaning of the numbers. Backtracking the reference trail reveals how the most recent data were gathered and subjected to mathematical manipulations [17–19]. The figure "275,000 hospitalizations" comes from NHDS. The credibility of this number is entirely dependent on factors of doubtful reliability: the recognition that an inpatient had a TBI and the formal documentation of that discovery in the discharge summary. That is, NHDS data depend on complete and accurate case ascertainment and case recording but other evidence shows that this is uncommon. The 1.365 million ED visits were based on the NHAMCS. A total of 364–398 hospitals were "sampled" during 1995 to 2001, yielding a total of a total of 2227 TBI-related ED visits. In this case, *sampling* means, "Hospital staff were asked to complete patient record forms for a systematic random sample of patient visits occurring during a randomly assigned 4-week reporting period" [1; see www.cdc.gov/nchs/ahcd/about_ahcd.htm]. One might be wary of accepting the numbers at face value.

Any serious attempt to study the epidemiology of concussion faces a raft of measurement barriers. The least ponderable is the number of concussive injuries never attended by a medical professional. We will address the conundrum of the patient who seeks no care momentarily. Yet even when concussed people visit medical facilities, five notorious barriers prevent a complete accounting of CBIs:

1. misuse of the GCS
2. infancy
3. sports
4. multi-trauma
5. misplaced faith in CT scans.

The misuse of the GCS will be discussed in more detail later in this essay. Suffice it to say that the GCS: (1) was never intended for use as a measure of TBI severity; (2) has little predictive validity for outcome from TBI; and (3) is not accurately measured by doctors or nurses [20–25]. The author of this chapter understands the GCS's stranglehold on emergency medicine tradition. We appreciate that few ED doctors have read the warning by the creators of the GCS that it must not be used as a measure of severity. We merely ask the reader to be open to the possibility that, even when the hospital staff troubles to fill in the blanks on the GCS form (skipped more often than one expects), those numbers are neither valid nor reliable. As a result, studies that employ review of GCS for the purposes of finding cases of "mTBI" are hamstrung. They cannot count missing scores, and they cannot trust scores that are present, so the detection of cases and the proportion of mild cases will never be altogether accurate.

The next difficult issue is accurate diagnosis of concussion in infants. As the graphs later in this chapter will show, people in the group aged 0–4 years are the most likely of all U.S. humans to arrive at an ED with a chief concern of head trauma – largely from accidental falls, sometimes from inflicted abuse. In most circumstances, the ED doctor can depend on historical reports from the patient. But infants cannot report. And while good parents sometimes witness and can report accidental falls, in a surprisingly large number of cases, parents have no idea that a concussion occurred and bring their infant to the ED because they note him or her to be listless or fussy. Inflicted TBI is the main cause of TBI-related death among infants, yet, in the absence of a head wound, not-so-good parents tend to deny and detection is often difficult. How, then, shall the busy ED physician enumerate brain injuries (let alone mild ones) in one-year-olds for whom there is no available history?

The answer, ideally, would be biomarkers – our highest research priority. For example, Berger et al. [26] conducted a prospective case–control study of 98 well-appearing infants who presented with no history of trauma. Serum or cerebro-spinal fluid (CSF) was collected in the ED for three putative markers of acute brain trauma: neuron-specific enolase (NSE), S100B, and myelin-basic protein (MBP). In all, 14–19 of the 98 cases were judged to be instances of inflicted TBI; five more were thought to have accidental brain injury. NSE levels were 77% sensitive and 66% specific for this problem. Of course, neither the consensus diagnosis of the child protection team nor the biomarkers represent gold standards, so we will never know the true proportion of those infants with abusive brain damage. This article is only cited because it illustrates a problem: a significant number of infants arrive at the ED with absolutely no history of head trauma but are in fact cases of CBI (in the Berger et al. [26] study, up to 24%). The national average proportion of infants with undetected head injury is unknown. Since diagnosis is especially difficult in this highest-risk human group, one suspects that many infant CBI cases go uncounted in epidemiological studies.

Sports-related concussion presents a different problem. Athletes are justifiably disinclined to report their concussions. Due to personal temperament and sociological pressures, they tend to deny that they have been hurt [27–29]. As a result, the accounting of sports-related concussions is inaccurate. Only

---

[3] The authors recognize that there are surely different proportions of mild cases among those who were treated and released from the ED versus those admitted.

some unknown (and probably small) proportion of concussed athletes visit the ED. There, the same sociological pressures apply. Many athletes correctly surmise that, if they tell the doctor, "I vomited twice, I'm still seeing double, and I can't remember my girlfriend's name," a notch will be cut from their image of invincibility and they will perhaps be restricted or banished from an identity-defining activity. Denial of injury presumably impacts the enumeration of injuries.

The fourth cause of missed cases is multi-trauma. It is well documented that persons evaluated in EDs for major trauma, especially spinal cord injury, are often misdiagnosed if they also have brain injuries. For instance, Macciocchi et al. [30] reviewed the literature on co-morbid brain and spinal injuries. These authors commented: "Not surprisingly, investigators also found that in many studies traumatic SCI [spinal cord injury] persons' rehabilitation records failed to document any TBI-related information" [30]. In their own study, they prospectively followed 198 patient with spinal cord injuries. Sixty percent were also found to have brain injuries – 57% of which were mild. Yet in 42% of cases, no GCS was ever recorded. They concluded, "In many cases, emergency medical service and/or acute care medical records did not contain basic information necessary to diagnose the presence and severity of TBI" ([30], p. 1355). Sharma et al. [31] reported that, among 92 patients with spinal cord injuries, missed diagnosis of TBI occurred in 58.5% of cases. In another study, Tolonen et al. [32] reported that only nine of 31 SCI patients were diagnosed with TBI at the acute hospital. However, 23 of 31 (745) actually met criteria for the diagnosis of TBI, so the acute trauma teams misdiagnosed 61% of TBI cases. Such findings suggest a troubling failure to detect TBIs during acute hospitalization.

Fifth, there is the problem of the CT scan. Later in this essay we will show why universal scanning might be life saving and cost-efficient. However (apart from misdiagnosis due to failure to scan), two frailties diminish one's faith in the reported results of CT scanning. One: CT is blind to almost all the neurobiological changes of TBI. Neither the neurometabolic/inflammatory cascades, nor the initiation of apoptosis, nor the disruption of axonal function appears on these scans. CT is an excellent ER measure, since it identifies patients likely to benefit from immediate neurosurgical intervention to evacuate threatening masses of blood. Otherwise, CT results are misleading. In fact, a normal CT is the expected finding after most concussions, with or without loss of consciousness. As most neuroradiologists would say, false negatives are the most common results from CT assessment of TBI. Moreover, whatever the findings, CT results are not predictive of outcome [33–37]. Jacobs et al. [34] summarized these observations: "We conclude that, although valuable for the identification of the individual mTBI patient at risk for deterioration and eventual neurosurgical intervention, CT characteristics are imperfect predictors of outcome after mTBI" (p. 655).

Two: those who read CT scans do not do so reliably. For all the faith and trust patients and other physicians put in radiologists, it is a widely known secret that interrater reliability for reading CT scans is less than ideal – even among specialists. Huff and Jahar [38] found that three experienced neuroradiologists only agreed on the diagnosis of intracerebral hematomas 55% of the time. As Laalo et al. [39] summarized the findings for CT diagnosis of acute TBI: "Experience increased accuracy, yet even between the reports of the most experienced readers, there were marked differences" (p. 2169). The combination of these two problems suggests that failure to perform a CT might lead to misdiagnoses, yet performing a CT will also lead to misdiagnoses.

The reader, by this point, may be gaining the impression that counting TBIs in the medical setting is hard. Due to their less obvious signs and symptoms, counting milder TBIs (such as typical concussions) is even harder. Pape et al. [40] summed up that problem:

> Findings indicate that no well-defined definition or clinical diagnostic criteria exist for mTBI and that diagnostic accuracy is currently insufficient for discriminating between mTBI and co-occurring mental health conditions for acute and historic mTBI. Findings highlight the need for research examining the diagnostic accuracy for acute and historic mTBI.
>
> ([40], p. 856)

In the light of these five barriers to complete accounting, when combined with the innate challenge of detecting mTBI, how many people *actually* visit hospitals due to CBI each year? The CDC estimate of 1.023 million seems very conservative. It is quite challenging to estimate how many cases are missed in the national surveillance program due to the collective degradation of the census by the circumstances listed above. However, one report provides a hint. Powell [41] conducted an interesting study: interviewers were trained and placed at two urban ERs for 10–16 h a day. Using data from ambulance records, emergency medical technicians, and the medical record, the interviewers identified subjects who, by virtue of the cause of injury and the GCS score, might meet the CDC's "conceptual" criteria for mTBI [6]. In all, 197 subjects underwent a structured clinical interview. Note that the interview actually included a brief mental status examination to determine whether the case met CDC criteria for memory loss.[4] Witnesses were also interviewed when available. Interviews were compared with the detection of mTBIs by the hospital staff, coded using ICD criteria. The result: "Fifty-six percent of mild TBI cases identified by study personnel did not have a documented mild TBI-related diagnosis in the ED record." That is, the hospital *only diagnosed 44% of mTBIs*. The authors speculated about one cause of the low detection rate by the ED staff: "Lack of diagnosis may also reflect reduced recognition by medical providers and the lay public of the potential for prolonged effects of a brain injury when the presenting symptoms appear to be minor." That is, in fact, one passionate theme of this essay.

---

[4] The fact that the interviewers performed a mental status exam, however brief, may help explain their much better success at TBI case detection. In a national survey, Schootman and Fuortes [42] found that mental status examinations were only performed in 33% of emergency room TBI cases. This suggests a striking, if not altogether surprising, lapse in typical American health care.

Candidly, there is no telling whether this worrisome finding is representative of case ascertainment rate across U.S. hospitals, or would necessarily apply to the cohort screened by the NHAMCS. In addition, the ICD coding process is known to be inaccurate for concussions [43]. However, if Powell's finding [41] is representative, then the number of persons seen in hospital ERs with CBI each year is not 1.023 million. It would perhaps be closer to 2.325 million.

The Three Question Marks

We still face the toughest job: estimating the number of persons who sustain a concussion and do not go to a medical facility. Looking again to the CDC pyramid (Figure 2.1), what number should replace the trio of question marks at the bottom? In its Report to Congress of 2003, the CDC acknowledged, "Both national surveillance systems and the SC DOH [South Carolina Department of Health] data underestimate the occurrence of TBI because they do not include injured people who received medical care in other facilities … or those who received no medical care for their injuries" [6]. But to estimate total U.S. annual TBIs, one needs to know how many additional concussed persons were seen away from the hospital or never seen.

At least four estimates have been published employing various methods to guess at that answer. In 1987, Fife reported results from 200,000 households surveyed during 1977–1981 for the National Health Interview Survey [44]. Respondents were asked about injuries in the preceding two weeks. The questions about TBI were arguably flawed: head injury was only recorded if there was a known non-fatal skull fracture or there was known "damage to the cranial contents." One suspects that few persons with recent concussion would answer "yes" to either question. (In fact, it is unlikely that most doctors could accurately comment on intracranial damage.) That concern aside, Fife found that 89% of those with recent skull fractures or known damaged cranial contents sought medical attention, implying that 11% did not.

Sosin et al. [45] employed similar methodology, using data collected in the Injury Supplement of the National Health Interview Survey for 1991. A total of 46,761 households participated in this door-to-door survey. This time, however, the brain injury questions seem to have been phrased more colloquially: the respondents were simply asked if someone in the household had suffered a head injury with loss of consciousness in the last 12 months. The results included an annual incidence of 618/100,000. Among those, 25% sought no medical help. The Sosin et al. study is probably the most-cited source of an estimate for the proportion of concussed persons who are missed by hospital-based surveys.

Boswell et al. [46] conducted a smaller prevalence survey: a trained interviewer administered a questionnaire about past head injuries to 601 consecutive ED patients at a level 1 trauma center. Forty-one percent of respondents acknowledged past head injuries. Half of these reported that their head injury involved loss of consciousness. Only 61% of those with histories of head injury had sought medical help, meaning that 39% did not. Of interest: if the head injury was sustained in

a motor vehicle accident 89% saw a doctor, "whereas those injured during a sports activity were least likely (47%)" ([46], p. 179).

Finally, in a non-peer-reviewed report, Abbott partnered with KRC Research in 2014 to conduct the Abbott Concussion IQ Survey [47]. Among more than 1000 adult respondents, 64% reported that they did not seek medical attention the last time they hit their head very hard, and only 11% said they would go to the ED if they thought they had a concussion (!).

The data in the above section concretize our initial statement. Nobody knows how many persons in the United States suffer concussions each year. Deconstructing the CDC pyramid, it appears that the totals reported for hospitalized and ED patients (275,000 and 1.365 million respectively) are likely underestimates compromised by multiple sources of error. Assuming that 75% of cases are mild (although WHO would say up to 90%), then the numbers for typical CBIs would be 206,250 hospitalized and 1.023 million ED visits. But if Powell's [41] discovery about missed diagnoses were valid, then a better estimate would be 468,750 CBIs hospitalized and 2.325 million ED cases. Then one must adjust somehow for all the people who decline to seek medical attention. If we take Sosin et al.'s frequently cited 1996 estimate [18], then the actual annual incidence of concussions leaps up to 625,000 hospitalized and 3.1 million in the ED. But what if the Abbott Concussion IQ Survey is the first candid report of medical help seeking after CBI? What if only 11% of concussed persons show up at the doctor's door? The annual incidence of hospitalized CBI hypothetically becomes 4,261,363. The annual ED visits balloon to 21.136 million!

The authors, and perhaps the readers, at this point take a deep breath. So many opportunities for large-scale error crowd the epidemiological dance floor that we simply cannot claim knowledge of the truth. Guessing – which is about all one can do, even with access to the very best published evidence and the most impartial of approaches – one must say that the CDC numbers are an underestimate – yet not so far off as Powell's data would predict [41]. Guessing, one might say that the proportion of concussed persons who do not go to the doctor is somewhat higher than Sosin et al.'s estimate of 25% [45]. Despite our best efforts to wring truth from the published data, our final conclusions must be festooned with caveats, bracketing the truth as best we can:

- **Rather conservative estimate:** assume that 75% of the CDCs cases were mild, that three-quarters of people with CBIs who came to the ER were correctly diagnosed, and that two-thirds of people with concussions went to the ER. Then 2.047 million U.S. persons are concussed each year.
- **Less conservative estimate** (closer to the author's observations): assume 85% of CDC's ER cases were mild, 66.7% were correctly diagnosed, and that 25% of concussed persons go to the ER. Then 6.96 million Americans are concussed each year.
- **More liberal estimate:** assume that 90% of TBIs in U.S. EDs are mild (WHO's upper estimate). Assume that Langlois et al.'s [48] (2006) estimate is correct: that more

than 3.8 million Americans may suffer sport-related concussions each year. Assume that Hanson et al.'s [49] (2013) report was accurate, and that sports-related TBIs only account for 15.4% of TBI cases seen in the ED.[5] In that case, 8.19 million Americans are concussed each year.

In simple terms, the best available published data are indisputably an underestimate of actual U.S. concussions. One can employ ancillary data to try to improve the CDC estimates, but the inconsistency of that ancillary data defies certainty. And even our best efforts to correct the U.S. data leaves out the Second and Third worlds, where unbelted motor vehicle accidents and poor construction safety standards are expected to magnify the risk. Let us retire the CDC's count of TBIs. By any reasonable recalculation, the real numbers are more daunting by far.

And lifetime cumulative incidence? If only the National Health Interview Surveys had asked one more question ("Have you ever had a head injury?"), we would have lifetime numbers. The most-cited estimates regarding lifetime incidence come from Anneger's et al.'s study of Olmsted County, Minnesota [50]: by age 75, 20% of U.S. males and 8% of U.S. females have suffered one or more TBIs. If everything else about the derivation of these estimates were trustworthy, they would be overestimates because the authors failed to adjust for cases of repeat concussions in one person. However, case ascertainment was incomplete in this study since it relied entirely on record review. Systematic consecutive ED interviews, such as those conducted by Boswell et al. [46] surely yield a more accurate estimate of lifetime incidence. In that study, 207 patients (41% of subjects) reported 321 past head injuries.

Is 41% a fair estimate of a U.S. person's lifetime risk of TBI? There is no easy way to tell. One expects the true lifetime risk to be higher than Boswell et al.'s number, since the mean age of that sample was 36.5 years, and people remain at risk of head injury for many more years. A rough estimate might be that one-third of TBIs occur in the second half of life, leading to the guess that about 61% of people experience a head injury at some point. On the other hand, people who were interviewed at an ED may be especially accident-prone. Given these added uncertainties, one has no mathematically robust way to derive the national or international lifetime cumulative risk of concussion. Perhaps it hovers in the neighborhood of 40–50%.

Risk Factors for TBI

By deconstructing the actual meaning of the CDC's pronouncements we have shown why their reported annual incidence of TBI must be an underestimate. Fortunately, we need not conduct such a recondite analysis of every concussion fact! Henceforth we are dealing mostly with *proportions* of that total. Demographic proportions might hold true no matter how far off the total counts.

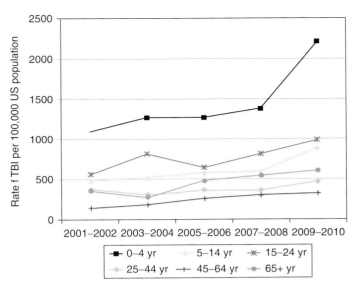

Fig. 2.2 Rates of traumatic brain injury (TBI)-related emergency department visits by age group: United States, 2001–2010.
Source: Centers for Disease Control and Prevention [51]. CDC, 2016. www.cdc.gov/traumaticbraininjury/data/rates_ed_byage.html

Age

Figure 2.2 illustrates the annual incidence of ED diagnoses of TBI for six age groups from 2001 to 2010. One might as easily have selected the graph for hospitalizations, but far more concussed persons visit the ED and go home.

Figure 2.2 illustrates the first major point about population distribution: as previously mentioned, persons aged 0–4 years are far and away the most likely to be brought to the ED with head injury. Two admonitions about this graph: first, the progressively rising incidence between 2001 and 2010 does not necessarily mean there were more injuries over time. It might reflect increased nervousness about brain troubles, inspired by a host of new reports about concussed football players. Second, the high rate observed among infants and toddlers does not necessarily mean that young children suffer that many more brain injuries. It may mean, at least in part, that 30-year-old parents with a fallen two-year-old are perhaps more likely to know about the fall and more likely to be worried than middle-aged parents with a fallen 15-year-old.

Sex

Figure 2.3 illustrates a second major point about the epidemiology of CBI: boys and men are more likely to suffer brain trauma than girls and women. Note that the sex difference depends on age. Among young children and the elderly, males and females have about the same rate of injury. For instance, at age 0–4 years, the incidence per 100,000 is about 1357 among boys and 1150 among girls – a sex ratio of 1.18. In contrast, at age 10–24 years, the mean incidence is about

---

[5] Some down-adjustment would be required, since Hanson et al.'s data [49] are weighted toward younger victims. But an up-adjustment would be required if Langlois et al. [54] are correct that 3.8 million is an underestimate.

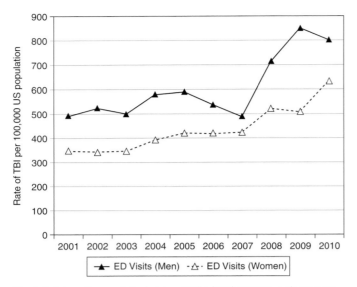

Fig. 2.3 Rates of traumatic brain injury (TBI)-related emergency deprtment (ED) visits by sex: United States, 2001–2010.

Source: Centers for Disease Control and Prevention [51]. CDC, 2016. www.cdc.gov/traumaticbraininjury/data/rates_ed_bysex.html

860 among males and 445 among females – a sex ratio of 1.93. This large increase in sex-related relative risk is thought to be because boys' hormone-driven risk-taking behavior is most exaggerated in adolescence. Boys calm down in their dotage: over age 65, males' mean TBI incidence is 389; females' is 393 – a virtually identical risk [12].

Race/Ethnicity

In its 2015 *Report to Congress*, the CDC acknowledged, "Another gap involves a lack of uniform race and ethnicity data in TBI data-systems, which makes examining trends in TBI incidence by race/ethnicity difficult" ([52], p. 23). The issue of race and ethnicity raises three questions. One, regardless of geographical location and socioeconomic status, might there be a biological difference such that persons of one race or ethnic or genetic group are more prone to concussion or more resilient in recovery? Two: in nations or geographic regions with multiracial or multiethnic populations, does the incidence of CBI vary according to those factors? Three: do persons of one racial or ethnic group receive different acute treatment, rehabilitation, or social reintegration after head injuries?

The first question has barely been considered. In part this reflects the sensible post World War II reconceptualization of race as a social construct rather than a biological trait. The rising tide of precision medicine, however, opens the door to finding systematic genetic differences in vulnerability to the effects of CBI (for example, the apparent elevated risk of post-traumatic dementia associated with bearing the APOE-ε4 allele) or conceivably differences in response to interventions. It remains to be seen if "racial" variation occurs in the neurobiology of CBI.

The second question has barely been studied. In the 1999 National Institutes of Health Consensus Development Conference on Rehabilitation of Persons with Traumatic Brain Injury, there appeared a brief appendix that mentioned both a rapid increase

in the rate of TBI among African Americans from 1980 to 1994, and a disproportionately higher rate of TBI-associated mortality in this group [53]. No explanation was offered apart from noting a race-related elevated risk of pedestrian-related fatalities.

The first peer-reviewed summary of race and TBI incidence may have been that of Langlois et al. [54]. The authors used data from the previously described NHDS and NHAMCS. They examined race-related TBI incidence from 1995 to 2001 for children aged 0–14 years. Blacks had a significantly higher rate of TBI-related death (6.0 vs. 4.3/100,000). Black children aged 0–4 years also had a higher rate of TBI-related hospitalizations (95.7 vs. 56.7). Rates of motor vehicle-related hospitalizations were higher among blacks aged 0–9 years. The authors concluded, "The TBI death and hospitalization rates for black children aged 0–4 years were nearly twice those for whites" [54]. Although no definite cause was identified, the authors speculated that the difference might be due to the significantly lower use of child safety restraints among blacks.

The third question has been studied more often. Several concerning findings:

- Blacks and Hispanics are less likely than whites to be referred to rehabilitation after TBI [55, 56]. This cannot be altogether explained by economic constraints: insured whites were more likely to be discharged to rehabilitation than insured blacks, Hispanics, or Asians [57].
- Blacks and Native Americans of all ages are significantly more likely than whites to experience violent TBI [58].
- Blacks have more depression and lower quality of life than whites two years after moderate to severe TBI [59].
- Blacks are less likely than whites to be gainfully employed 1–5 years after TBI [60, 61].
- Blacks have lower scores on community reintegration than whites six months after TBI, even after accounting for income [62].
- In South Carolina, black females are less likely to be admitted after TBI [63].
- Combat exposure is associated with higher rates of mTBI among blacks and Hispanics than among whites [64].

These findings suggest inequality in risk and inequity in the distribution of medical resources. The impact would seem clear in regard to risk of and treatment for severe injuries, where biased provision of care may lead to unnecessary deaths or inadequate rehabilitation. The impact of these inequities on the likelihood of persistent post-concussive problems is less clear. For instance: do blacks suffer more post-CBI depression due to pre-morbid stressors, biological differences in brain response, sufficiency of personal and community resources to enable resilience, or substandard care?

Cause

Figure 2.4 illustrates the proportion of brain injuries attributable to different causes among different age groups. The standout observation is that falls account for most injuries during the life eras of highest risk – childhood and old age. In contrast, accidentally being struck by or against an object is the most common cause in middle childhood, and motor vehicle

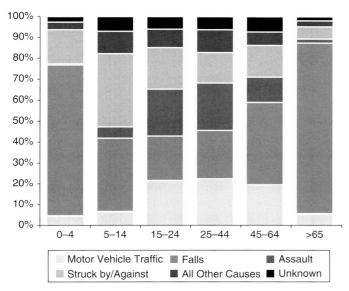

Fig. 2.4 Emergency department visits by age group and injury mechanism: United States, 2006–2010. [A black and white version of this figure will appear in some formats. For the color version, please refer to the plate section.]

Source: Centers for Disease Control and Prevention [65]. CDC, 2016. www.cdc.gov/traumaticbraininjury/data/dist_ed.html

Table 2.1 Centers for Disease Control and Prevention report regarding non-fatal traumatic brain injury (TBI)-related injuries for 2006–2010

- Men had higher rates of TBI hospitalizations and ED visits than women
- Hospitalization rates were highest among persons aged 65 years and older
- Rates of ED visits were highest for children aged 0–4 years
- Falls were the leading cause of TBI-related ED visits for all but one age group
  - Assaults were the leading cause of TBI-related ED visits for persons 15–24 years of age
- The leading cause of TBI-related hospitalizations varied by age:
  - Falls were the leading cause among children ages 0–14 and adults 45 years and older
  - Motor vehicle crashes were the leading cause of hospitalizations for adolescents and persons ages 15–44 years

ED: emergency department.

accidents account for most TBIs during the peak driving years, roughly ages 16–64 years. The authors strongly suspect that the age distribution of assaults, shown in dark blue on the figure, may not be accurate. As noted above, a completely unknown proportion of very young children brought to medical attention with head trauma are victims of abuse.

In brief and incomplete summary, and for the sake of citing a popular source, Table 2.1 lists the CDC's observations regarding risk of non-fatal TBI-related injuries. The overwhelming majority of these were CBIs.

Risk of Recurrence

Since no accurate count of CBIs is available, any estimate of the risk of suffering a second, third, or seventh CBI is empirically insecure. Still, as so much evidence exists that repetitive

concussions pose a threat that is greater than merely additive, one very much wishes to know how many concussed persons experience multiple concussions and why. Annegers et al. [50] attempted one of the most comprehensive population-based surveys – the review of Olmsted County/Mayo Clinic medical records from 1935 to 1974. Much of the data they reported pertained to the last decade of that time period. That paper reported the observed and expected rate of subsequent head injuries among survivors. Table 2.2 was derived from their data.

If the Mayo data are representative, then both males and females are at greatly increased risk of another CBI after their first. The age-related relative risks are intriguing. Note that a childhood head injury merely doubles the risk of another, but a teen or adult injury triples or quadruples the risk. It is also striking that persons with histories of two head injuries are almost an order of magnitude more likely to suffer another head injury compared with the general population. Annegers et al. neatly summarized the problem: "Among the groups at high risk of head trauma are those who have had head trauma previously"([50], p. 912).

Why do concussed people tend to be re-concussed? One can intuit many of the causal factors: child abuse, impulsivity, teen risk taking, dangerous neighborhoods, substance abuse, dangerous sports, military duty, risky occupations, sensory impairment (e.g., visual deficits), motor impairments (e.g., parkinsonism), and disequilibrium (e.g., vestibulopathies). Yet the authors again confess that too little empirical evidence exists to fully explain this phenomenon.

Data from the study reported by Boswell et al. [46] add nuance. Recall that this was a survey of ED cases in which 41% of subjects reported a past TBI. The questionnaire also investigated "repeat injury by the same mechanism." In their urban cohort of almost 200 TBI survivors, the highest incidence of repeat head injury occurred among victims of assaults: 35%. Repeated falls occurred in 16%. Repeated sports-related TBI was reported as 19%, but that number, like all reports of sports-related head traumas, is probably an understatement. Of interest: low household income was a risk factor for repeat injury. A further sign of inequality: subjects with repeat head injuries due to assault reported an income of less than $15,000. Subjects with repeat injuries due to sports reported household incomes of > $35,000.

In regard to sports-related CBIs, the risk of repeat injury exceeds that expected even for those risk-taking people who tend to engage in contact sports. That excess perhaps means that the dizziness, imbalance, incoordination, double vision, mental slowing, and compromised executive functions that so often persist make contact athletes highly vulnerable to further CBIs. However, the consequences of repetitive sports-related TBIs may be different depending on their timing.

As several studies have reported, a unique risk, referred to as the *second impact syndrome,* attends the first week or so after injury: not only is the athlete less physically and cognitively able to protect him- or herself, but also the brain is exquisitely vulnerable to more-than-additive harm because it has failed to re-establish metabolic homeostasis. For

Table 2.2 Relative risk of subsequent head injuries after one or two head injuries

	Patients	Expected	Observed	Relative risk
Risk of second head injury after first				
Males, overall	1842	45.3	130	2.8
Age at first injury				
< 15 years	742	24.4	53	2.1
15–24 years	523	11.5	34	2.9
25+ years	577	9.4	43	4.6
Females overall	935	9.4	28	3.0
Age at first injury				
< 15 years	394	5.8	11	2.0
15–24 years	257	1.9	8	4.2
25+ years	284	1.9	9	4.7
Risk of third or more head injury after second head injury				
Males	171	3.21	25	7.8
Females	32	0.22	2	9.3

instance, excessive intracellular calcium persists for about three to five days and abnormal cerebral blood flow persists for about ten days (see Chapter 3). As a result, those athletes whose subsequent concussions follow closely upon their first seem especially likely to suffer permanent brain damage [66–71]. Even without close temporal clustering, one suspects a vicious circle such that persons who become brain-damaged by sports have neurological impairments that increase their risk for more brain damage, which in turn increases the risk for even more CBIs and more brain damage – a *repeat-until-demented* cycle often encountered in professional boxers and football players.

Military Concussion

Collective intergroup aggression, such as war, reliably generates abrupt external forces that rattle the brain as well as stress. These effects of two can be hard to distinguish from one another. Penetrating injuries are easier to diagnose: commanders note that persons with sword or bullet holes in their heads or grossly depressed skull fractures have been hurt. Non-penetrating brain injuries, on the other hand, have been a source of contention for more than 100 years. A great deal of literature regarding both TBI and stress has been generated as a result of the Western invasions and occupations of Afghanistan and Iraq. Reviewing the recently reported epidemiology of military-related concussion requires recognizing that the exact tally of CBIs will never be known. Moreover, the overlap between the impacts of concussions and stress makes it very hard to pin the cause of persistent problems on one or the other. We humbly propose a moratorium on the publication of opinions about the relative contributions of each to post-deployment misery pending the availability of valid and reliable biomarkers.

As mentioned in Chapter 1 of this essay, World War I triggered a wave of scholarly debate about so-called "shell shock." In the early days of the war, Captain Charles Myers concluded that some British soldiers on the front lines in France were neurologically damaged by proximity to explosions [72]. In 1915 Captain Myers published a report in *The Lancet* of three cases under the title "A contribution to the study of shellshock. Being an account of the cases of loss of memory, vision, smell and taste admitted to the Duchess of Westminster's War Hospital, Le Touquet" [73]. The leading British neuropathologist of the time, Frederick Mott, was asked to investigate the cause. He concluded that head commotion disrupted "the delicate colloidal structures" of the brain and spinal cord [74]. The initial treatment was evacuation from the front.

Soon, however, the loss of manpower by evacuating shell-shock victims became a threat to battlefield success [72, 75]. Moreover, it became apparent that many British soldiers presenting with the same psychic and somatic symptoms had not been near explosions. An enduring description of those symptoms was penned by Turner [76]:

> a form of temporary "nervous breakdown" scarcely justifying the name of neurasthenia … ascribed to a sudden or alarming psychical cause such as witnessing a ghastly sight … the patient becomes "nervy", unduly emotional and shaky, and most typical of all his sleep is disturbed by bad dreams … of experiences through which he has passed. Even the waking hours may be distressful from acute recollections of these events.

By late 1916, the avalanche of complaining officers and soldiers, only some of whom had verifiable blast exposure, provoked a backlash. The term shell shock was banned. Captain Myers was forbidden to publish his follow-up article. The authorities' conclusion was published as the 1922 *Report of the War Office Committee of Enquiry into "Shellshock"* [77]. That inquiry concluded, for instance:

> No soldier should be allowed to think that loss of nervous or mental control provides an honourable avenue of escape from the battlefield, and every endeavour should be made to prevent slight cases leaving the battalion or divisional area, where treatment should be confined to provision of rest and comfort for those who need it and to heartening them for return to the front line.
>
> [77]

The commanders' dilemma is understandable. Brain injuries are an inconvenience to the military. An army's purpose is readiness for and execution of commands from civilian politicians. The disagreement most often cited since World War I can be crystallized: "His brain was rattled and he is hurt," versus "His spirit is weak and he prefers to avoid risk." Yet the striking clinical overlap between the effects of concussion and stress set off a debate that remains with us today: to what degree is non-fatal combat-associated neurobehavioral dysfunction attributable to brain rattling versus stress?

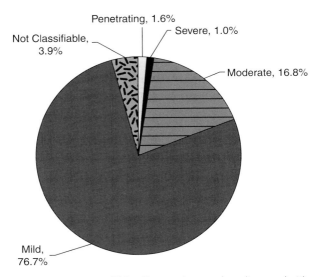

Fig. 2.5 Percentage of U.S. military service members diagnosed with a traumatic brain injury (TBI), by severity, 2000–2011 (n = 235,046).

Source: Centers for Disease Control and Prevention (CDC), National Institutes of Health (NIH), Department of Defense (DoD), Department of Veterans Affairs (VA) [83], p. 55. CDC, 2016. www.cdc.gov/traumaticbraininjury/pubs/congress_military.html

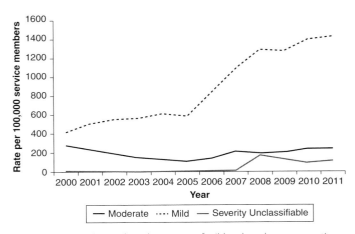

Fig. 2.6 Estimated annual incidence rates of mild and moderate traumatic brain injuries (TBIs) and TBIs with unclassifiable severity among active-duty U.S. military service members, 2000–2011.

Source: Centers for Disease Control and Prevention (CDC), National Institutes of Health (NIH), Department of Defense (DoD), Department of Veterans Affairs (VA) [83], p. 58. CDC, 2016. www.cdc.gov/traumaticbraininjury/pubs/congress_military.html

We will provide some mTBI/post-traumatic stress disorder (PTSD) numbers momentarily. But first, an overview of recent military TBI.

Figure 2.5 illustrates the classification of TBIs diagnosed in the U.S. military setting from 2000 to 2011. This corresponds roughly with the U.S.-led invasions and occupations of Afghanistan (Operation Enduring Freedom) and Iraq (Operation Iraqi Freedom). For several reasons, including improved personal protection equipment and rapid transfer to definitive care, conflict-related wounds have become more survivable [78]. With the introduction of Kevlar vests, the injury patterns have dramatically shifted from previous conflicts, with a much lower proportion of torso wounds and more head wounds [79, 80]. As Tanielian and Jaycox put it [81, p. 6]: "The current conflicts have witnessed the highest ratio of wounded to killed in action in U.S history … Wounded soldiers who would have likely died in previous conflicts are instead saved, but with significant physical, emotional, and cognitive injuries." One result has been an increase in survivors of TBIs. Bagalman [82] joined many observers who have commented that "Traumatic brain injury (TBI) has become known as a 'signature wound' of Operations Enduring Freedom and Iraqi Freedom (OEF/OIF)." However, it is not the broad diagnosis of TBI but instead typical CBIs (formerly mTBIs) that dominate the epidemiological findings. As shown in Figure 2.5, 76.7% of service members diagnosed with TBI had mild injuries.

The reported frequency of concussions among OEF/OIF veterans treated in the Veterans Administration system from October 2001 through December 2011 supports the conclusion that CBI has become the most common form of head injury in the U.S. military population. For instance, among

59,218 veterans with medical records coded for head injury, just 113 (0.2%) had skull fractures, while 36,412 – fully 61.5% – had concussions and 12,367 (20.9%) had "postconcussion syndrome"[6] [83]. Not obvious in the pie chart (Figure 2.5): in a post-deployment study of 1502 soldiers, 59% of those who reported mTBI reported more than one [84].

Figure 2.6 adds the temporal dimension. The overall rate of TBI more than doubled from 2000, when it stood at 720.3/100,000, to 2011, when it had leapt to 1811.4/100,000. Although none of the TBI epidemiology numbers are trustworthy due to the insurmountable counting problems already enumerated, note that total exceeds the highest CDC-reported civilian incidence rate, with the exception of recent ED visits by those aged 0–4 years. Readers will observe the big bump in mild cases. Moderate-severity TBIs remained stable. In contrast, the graph depicts a near quadrupling of the incidence of mild brain injuries over the same time period. What accounts for that dramatic increase in concussion counts? Proposed explanations include: (1) increased deployment; (2) improved pre-deployment screening; (3) increased awareness of the need to ask for help; (4) improved post-traumatic recording; and (5) education of providers with regard to injury coding.

While those incidence-related factors have probably increased the case detection of military TBIs, they have not served the much harder goal of analyzing prevalence. How many service members are affected by sequelae of brain traumas? The authors of the CDC's 2013 report [83] give an example of why the answer is unknown: if a soldier is treated for persistent headaches after his concussion, the diagnostic code is "headache." Even if the clinician takes the extra step of coding "history of TBI," there is literally no way for a chart reviewer to know that the clinician regards the headaches as a long-term consequence of head injury. As the CDC authors put it, "with

---

[6] Later chapters in this volume will explain why no "post-concussive syndrome" exists.

the exception of post-traumatic epilepsy, no process is in place for determining and recording long-term consequences" ([83], p. 60). Fortunately, an effort is currently under way to revise the codes and overcome this barrier to documenting the effects of concussions on military personnel. Until then, estimates of concussion-related long-term disability among soldiers and veterans remain unknown.

Understanding the Concussion–PTSD Relationship

At the outset of this section we noted that both concussion and stress are common in war. We have already demonstrated that "mTBI" has been common among U.S. forces in recent conflicts. Stress has also been common – and is equally hard to quantify. For instance, Hoge et al. [85] surveyed a representative sample of 3671 Army soldiers or marines after deployments to Iraq (OIF) or Afghanistan (OEF). The intensity of combat exposure was higher, on average, in Iraq (for instance, 71–86% of service members deployed to Iraq had been in a fire fight, compared with 31% of those deployed in Afghanistan). Subjects completed questionnaires that asked about 18 types of potentially stressful experiences. Ninety-five percent of those deployed to Iraq reported having been shot at; 92% reported being attacked or ambushed. In this cohort, PTSD was strongly associated with being shot at, having been wounded or injured, handling dead bodies, knowing someone who was killed, or killing enemy combatants.

A similar post-deployment questionnaire listing 36 potentially stressful experiences was administered to a different group of 768 OIF fighters [86]. The stability of recall was tested by comparing the subjects' responses at three and six months. In all, 85.2% reported "yes" at both surveys with regard to being attacked or ambushed and 86.9% reported yes to receiving small-arms fire. We submit that stressful experiences have been common among U.S. service members deployed in the previous decade.

Diagnostic confusion is inevitable because the symptoms of CBI and PTSD are virtually identical. "Overlap" is the term usually employed in the literature, but there is far more unity than difference. In multiple studies, fatigue, memory problems, concentration problems, anxiety, depression, irritability, and poor sleep comprise the most frequently reported symptoms in both conditions and in the combination of the two [84, 87–92]. Such symptoms are often labeled "post-concussive"; however, no evidence supports the claim that a particular symptom cluster identifies the consequences of concussion. As Lew et al. [93] noted, "In the postacute and chronic phases of recovery no symptom exists that is unique to or pathognomonic of mild TBI" (p. xii). Sayer [94] put it this way: "symptoms such as difficulty concentrating, irritability, anxiety, and sleep disturbance may be attributable to PTSD or depression, TBI sequelae, or both psychiatric disturbance and TBI" (p. 413).

The relationship between mTBI, PTSD, and so-called "post-concussive symptoms" (PC symptoms)in the military population has been studied. Schneiderman et al. [95] conducted a postal survey of 2235 OEF/OIF veterans. Based on self-report,

12.3% reported mTBIs and 11.2% screened positive for PTSD. The authors found that mTBI and PTSD were independently associated with three or more PC symptoms. However, "The strongest factor associated with postconcussive symptoms was PTSD, even after overlapping symptoms were removed from the PTSD score." Similarly, Brenner et al. [96] also found that mTBI or PTSD was independently associated with report of PC symptoms and that "PTSD and mTBI together were more strongly associated with having PC symptoms" than either diagnosis alone (p. 307).

This is not to conclude that the symptom profiles are identical. Potentially useful clinical differentiators: victims of concussion are more likely to report headache and victims of blast concussion are more likely to report hearing loss [97]. Otherwise, without a witness to loss of consciousness, the doctor cannot tell the cause since the residual distress from either problem is more or less the same. Moreover, among those with co-morbid concussion and PTSD, how might the doctor sensibly attribute some proportion of the symptoms to one, and another proportion to the other? Brenner et al. [87, pp. 242–243] commented on the doctor's dilemma:

> In the OEF/OIF cohort with delayed clinical presentation and multiple events that may have resulted in a mild TBI or posttraumatic stress, it is difficult to tease apart historical details and symptom onset and course to determine whether a TBI actually occurred … because of potential comorbidities and/or the late onset of symptoms, clinical presentations may be atypical. Moreover, parsing out the percent of current symptoms due to various comorbid conditions is not possible.

The author strongly agrees with Brenner et al.'s admonition. It would be illogical to try parsing out which of 16 symptoms (the usual number assessed in post-concussion research) is due to the head injury and which to the PC emotional state. The two are inextricable.

The Myth of Missing Traumatic Memory

How, then, might one understand the relationship between CBIs, PC symptoms, and PTSD? First (although this might seem unnecessary), it is necessary to dismantle a myth: some writers have opined that a +patient cannot develop PTSD as the result of a TBI [98–100]. This radical position is predicated on the hypothesis that "individuals who had been rendered unconscious or suffered amnesia due to a TBI are unable to develop PTSD because they would be unable to consciously experience the symptoms of fear, helplessness, and horror associated with the development of PTSD" [99, p. 63]. Setting aside the irrational basis of that claim, several early studies indeed reported that rates of PTSD were relative among cohorts with TBI [101–103], or that persons with comparable traumas might be *less* emotionally distressed if they also suffered an mTBI [104]. Indeed, one study reported that the less able the patient was to recall details of the accident, the lower the rate of PTSD [105] and another study reported that longer PTA was associated with lower rates of PTSD [106]. The claimants of the missing memory myth further propose that the reason so many other investigators find high rates of PTSD after concussion is a methodological error: both Sumpter and McMillan [100] and Sbordone and Ruff [99] declare that studies that use questionnaires find high rates of PC PTSD but studies based on diagnostic interviews find no such problem.

An abundance of more recent data rebuts the "TBI cannot trigger PTSD" bromide.

First: very low and very high rates of PC PTSD are reported, regardless of the method of data gathering. Self-report questionnaires have yielded rates of co-morbid mTBI and PTSD of 5–68%. Interview reports have yielded rates of 3–70% [107]. Betthauser et al. [108] justifiably urged that a concerted effort is needed to optimize the psychometric properties of instruments used to assess these two conditions. However, the currently available data do not support a claim of systematic differences in results due to self-report versus interview case ascertainment.

Second: PTSD indisputably occurs even when there is unconsciousness or PTA due to head injury [109–112, 113 (p. 1027), 114, 115]. In fact, unconsciousness perhaps predisposes to PTSD. As Mayou et al. [114] reported, "Post-traumatic stress disorder (PTSD) and depression and anxiety were more common at 3 months among those who had definitely been unconscious than in those who had not" (p. 540).

Third: among those exposed to trauma, the rate of PTSD is higher among the subset with mTBI. For instance, in the civilian setting, Bryant et al. [106] reported: "MTBI patients were more likely to develop PTSD than no-TBI patients, after controlling for injury severity (adjusted odds ratio: 1.86)." The evidence is even more striking in the military domain. Hoge et al. [116] reported the frequencies of concussion and PTSD among 2525 soldiers three to four months after returning from deployment to Iraq. Among those with injuries involving loss of consciousness, 43.9% met criteria for PTSD. By comparison, among those who only reported altered mental status, just 27.3% met PTSD criteria, and among those with no mTBI, only 9.1–16.2% had PTSD. This study has been justifiably criticized for failure to control for pre-morbid psychiatric status. Yet the results are similar to those of the RAND study of returning veterans: 19.5% had a probable mTBI; of those, 37.4% had co-morbid PTSD or depression [81].

In another large-scale study [96], a Brigade Combat Team of 3973 was assessed after a one-year deployment. A total of 1247 soldiers reported injuries. In all, 878 had "at least 1 clinician-confirmed TBI"; 399 did not. Thus, 71% of the injured soldiers (or 22.1% of the entire team) had confirmed mild TBIs. Among the 399 soldiers with non-TBI injuries, the rate of PTSD was 7%; among the 878 with mTBIs, the rate of PTSD was 26%. It seems reasonable to conclude that, among deployed U.S. service members, concussion increases the risk of PTSD.

The author of the present essay fully agrees with the statement that people do not consolidate detailed memories of events when they are comatose. But King [117] spelled out at least five ways the brain is influenced as a result of a traumatic concussion:

1. Many people have only a brief loss of consciousness and thus have conscious memories for virtually the entire traumatic event.
2. Islands of memory are known to form during the period of alleged PTA. (These also become apparent as retrograde amnesia shrinks over time.)
3. One need not lay down a fully formed, conscious, detailed memory of a trauma. The brain may implicitly store a stress response.
4. Imagined, reconstructed, or learned information about the accident can be terrifying and become woven into the PTSD phenomenology.
5. Events contingent upon or coincident to the concussion such as "painful medical procedures or frightening and confused perceptions while emerging from PTA" ([117], p. 2) could also provoke a stress response.

The radicals' position qualifies as a uniquely specious sophistry in contemporary writing about concussion. Sbordone and Ruff justified their hypothesis as follows:

> PTSD can develop if an individual with TBI is exposed to contiguous traumatic events while they are not experiencing retrograde or anterograde amnesia … Thus, two or more distinct and separate traumatic events or etiologies must occur for the diagnoses of MTBI and PTSD to coexist.
>
> [99, p. 70]

The error is self-evident: these authors have conflated the complex, multi-faceted, and sometime enduring life experience of a traumatic head injury with the few seconds of unconsciousness – never mind that ten seconds after the impact you are lying on the ground, retching violently, dizzy, with double vision, a terrible headache, confusion, and fear. That, opine the radicals, is a different life event than your brain injury. Let's say you have brought your extended family on a visit to Victoria Falls. You turn your back for 30 seconds to buy a Mazoe. The merchant screams. You look back at the edge of the cliff. No one is there. According to Sbordone and Ruff's logic, since you have no memory of your family's fall to their deaths, you had no conscious experience of trauma, and you will be blissfully spared any stress. Let us return to science.

How Common is PTSD After CBI?

Epidemiological data regarding the frequency of PTSD after concussion cannot be readily summarized with a single number. Military and civilian studies have both yielded diverse conclusions. In 2009, a Veterans Administration Consensus Conference collated the available data. Their systematic search unearthed 34 studies on co-morbid mTBI and PTSD. As the authors warn in their abstract: "None evaluated diagnostic accuracy or treatment effectiveness" (a finding that is unhappily common in concussion literature). Twenty of those articles reported incidence estimates. Figure 2.7 depicts the scattergram of results from these studies. Frequencies of mTBI/PTSD varied from 0 to 89% – testimony to the challenge of arriving at a single valid figure. However, the authors point out that three large military studies [81, 95, 116] arrived at similar

Frequency of post-traumatic stress disorder (PTSD) among study participants with mild traumatic brain injury (mTBI) history

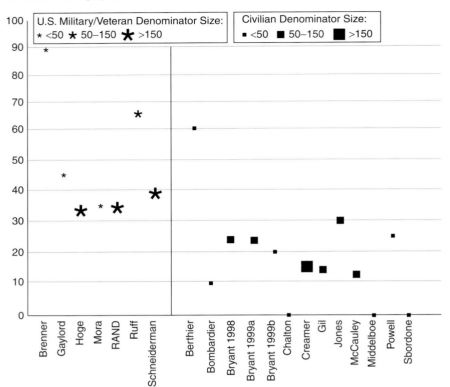

Fig. 2.7

Denominator size indicates the number of study participants with mTBI history used in the frequency estimates. Studies reporting more than one mTBI/PTSD frequency level over time are presented at the first time point. One study (RAND) did not explicitly report TBI severity but is assumed to have identified primarily mTBI history.

Source: Carlson et al., 2011 [107] with permission from Lippincott Williams & Wilkins, Inc./Wolters Kluwer

conclusions: the rate of PTSD among soldiers with mTBI is between 33 and 39%.

Why is Concussion so Strongly Associated with PTSD?

The data regarding the rate of PTSD after concussion, for all its variability, support the straightforward conclusion that these conditions are linked. King [117] called them "mutually exacerbating," which sounds reasonable. Yet one hopes for a more neurobiologically robust explanation for the very high rate of co-morbidity. Several have been proposed. Bryant [118] offered one plausible hypothesis:

The finding that mild traumatic brain injury is associated with an increased incidence of PTSD raises interesting possibilities about how mild traumatic brain injury may compound PTSD. Biologic models posit that a fundamental mechanism underpinning PTSD involves an exaggerated response of the amygdala, resulting in impaired regulation by the medial prefrontal cortex. Biologic models posit that a fundamental mechanism underpinning PTSD involves an exaggerated response of the amygdala, resulting in impaired regulation by the medial prefrontal cortex … It is possible that a person's capacity to regulate the fear reaction may be impaired after mild traumatic brain injury because the neural networks involved in the regulation of anxiety may be damaged as a result of the mild traumatic brain injury.

([118], p. 525)

Other contributors have posited other explanations. Kennedy et al. [112] reviewed the overlapping pathophysiologies of TBI and

PTSD from histological and imaging studies, neuroendocrine and neurochemical research, concluding, "A biological interface appears to be between TBI and PTSD. Many of the genetic, structural, endocrine, and neurochemical changes of TBI appear to have similar changes noted in the pathophysiology of PTSD" (p. 906). Chen et al. [119] suggested that a "volumetric blood surge" accompanied both physical and emotional trauma and produced secondary neuronal injury responsible for the matching symptoms of TBI and PTSD. Chapters 3 and 4 of this essay will summarize the neurobiology of concussion. As the reader will see, a great deal remains to be learned about the physiological, cellular, and molecular nature of CBI. A previous generation of neurologists discussed the "neurometabolic cascade" of concussion. Now it is apparent that concussion involves a conflict between innumerable harmful and helpful elements involving sudden and profound changes in gene expression, microvascular changes, and neuroimmunomodulatory functions that have barely been surveyed. The authors of the present essay suspect that the next generation will develop a better understanding of the concussion–PTSD link, using technologies we have yet to discover.

The Epidemiology of Sports-Related Concussion

American football players are similar to kittens. Genetically and behaviorally, they are almost indistinguishable. Both are more or less bilaterally symmetric vertebrates who seek food, reproduction, and defense against mortal threats. Why do they do what they do? When the football player moves the football or the kitten moves the yarn ball, neither behavior leads directly to calories. But play has indirect benefits, such as practice and maintenance of fitness for hunting and fighting, as well as demonstration to observers of reproductive fitness. So we should begin this brief overview of the epidemiology of sports-related concussion with the acknowledgment: play is an innate and adaptive animal behavior. And it cannot be put strongly enough that adult exercise (as opposed to "sports") is tremendously important for health and mental well-being, and may in fact be the single most important modifiable risk factor for dementia, heart disease, diabetes, depression, and death from "natural causes."

The problem: survival beyond age 35 was rare in the ancestral environment. For that reason, no selective pressure existed for the evolution of mechanisms to preserve brain function into late adulthood after cumulative play-, hunting-, or fighting-related brain injuries. Later chapters in this essay will address the implications for late life of those with concussions. For the time being, we simply note that play is natural, desirable, but somewhat risky. This section cannot possibly do justice to the wealth of new information on sports-related concussion discovered by the last decade of scholarship. For reviews, the reader might consider looking at Toth (2008) [120], Daneshvar et al. (2011) [121], Pfister et al. (2016) [122], or Zuckerman et al. (2015) [123]. If there is a take-home message, it is this: a vast unspoken conspiracy exists in which many players, fans, parents, coaches, university presidents, and corporations agree to ignore the problem of brain injury in sports. As in the case of tobacco, one expects a 50-year lag between alarmed scientists' public exposure of this conspiracy and significant behavioral change.

Barriers to Knowledge Regarding Sports-Related Concussions

Assuming an unlimited research budget, how might the world's best scientist count sports-related concussions? Despite the best intentions and the most rigorous efforts of scholars, certain barriers prevent an accurate count.

First and foremost: athletes underreport their head injuries [28, 124–129]. From high school through college and professional sports, members of teams tend to deny that their brains have been damaged. Can this problem be quantified? Following the lead of Rowson and Duma [130]: ask athletic trainers and you learn that 5% of high school football players are concussed. Ask the players using the word concussion and the rate jumps by a factor of 3–15%. But ask the players about concussion symptoms, leaving out the word, and the rate becomes 47%. Rowson and Duma consequently propose a correction factor: the actual number of sports-related concussions is about ten times the reported rate.

Athletes underreport for at least four reasons. In part, this is due to ignorance or obliviousness. A surprisingly large proportion of athletes do not know the symptoms of a concussion, do not realize they have been concussed, and do not appreciate the risk of lasting brain damage. As Daneshvar et al. [121] expressed it, "Because these impairments in neurologic

function often present with a rapid onset and resolve spontaneously, many concussions are neither recognized by athletes nor observed by coaches or athletic trainers. As a result, a large proportion of concussions are simply unreported" (p. 2).

The problem, in some cases, is simply language. As Buzzini and Guskiewicz [131] stated,

Coaches and the popular press use phrases such as "he had his bell rung" or "suffered a ding" to describe a blow to the head. Such descriptions can lead athletes and their families to assume that a concussion is part of the game.

This has practical consequences for CBI counting. Valovich-McLeod et al. [132] reported that the incidence of concussions varied by a factor of more than six depending on the phraseology of the interview question. Only 3.8% of high school athletes reported having been "knocked out," but 8.5% were "concussed," and 25% had their "bell rung." Similarly, one report documented an astonishing mismatch between concussion symptoms versus concussion diagnosis [133]. In all, 62.7% of college soccer players reported concussion symptoms in the previous year, and 81.7% of these had apparently suffered multiple concussions. But only 19.8% of these concussed players realized they'd been concussed (!). In the same study, 70.4% of college football players reported symptoms consistent with having been concussed in the last year and 84.6% reported more than one concussion, but only 23.4% of those players realized they had been concussed. Perhaps one should not be surprised at these findings. Given the fact that Western medicine has struggled to agree on a definition of concussion for more than 2000 years, it is unfair to expect young athletes to have a firm grasp of the meaning of the word. Still, reports such as this help to explain the scientific challenge of accurate and complete concussion counting. They also help to explain the high rate of recurrent concussion in sports. For example, in one study of high school football players, 81% of those who had sustained a concussion without loss of consciousness and 69% of those who had been knocked out returned to play on the same day [126].

The second reason for underreporting is unconscious denial. That is, in some cases, impacted athletes are driven to suppress conscious awareness that their brain has been rendered dysfunctional. Athletes are understandably disinclined to admit their brain injuries, even to themselves. For them to acknowledge somatic frailty is for them to undermine their own identity as invincible.

The third reason athletes underreport is so-called "subconcussive blows." One does not want to become embroiled in a semantic dust-up, but readers may wonder what that phrase could possibly mean. A concussion, in English, is a rattling blow. The authors of this essay urged fidelity to this original and actual meaning in Chapter 1 in the hopes of inspiring a logical approach to this medical problem. Rattling blows vary. It is not reasonable to limit them to "mildness" or restrict them to "rattling – but only a little bit." Better to simply note that concussive blows vary in force and effect. If one accepts this simple 400-year-old English use of concussion, then what would a "subconcussive blow" be? A blow with no force? We realize that some authors use subconcussive to mean "asymptomatic."

But such blows obviously involve concussive force. Rather than the problematic new adjective "subconcussive," we recommend a straightforward alternative: let's call asymptomatic blows asymptomatic. That having been said, *athletes almost never report asymptomatic head impacts.*

Fourth: in many cases, however, athletes who are well aware of episodes of brain injury deliberately decline to report them. The motivations for this dishonesty vary. In one study, 797 former collegiate athletes completed a questionnaire regarding their past concussions [134]. A total of 26.9% reported one or more CBIs, and 33.2% reported non-disclosure of at least one of their concussions. Men were significantly more likely than women to report non-disclosure (42.9% vs. 14.9%). Male football players were the most likely to report non-disclosure (68.3%), yet 42.9% of male track and field athletes, 35.7% of male wrestlers, and 35.7% of male lacrosse players also failed to disclose concussions. In order of frequency, the most common motivations were: (1) did not want to leave the game or practice (78.9%); (2) did not want to let the team down (71.8%); (3) did not know it was a concussion (70.4%); and (4) did not think it was serious enough to report (70.4%). For professional athletes, candor also threatens gainful employment. Millions of dollars may be at stake.

Coaches, athletic trainers, and other stakeholders in team success are also known to minimize the problem. Yet even the most willing coaches and supervisors may lack the resources to count injuries. As Buckley et al. [135] reported, National Collegiate Athletic Association (NCAA) Division II and III teams have inferior funding. This prevents hiring and training athletic trainers to employ the standardized concussion assessments advised by modern guidelines. Even the machinations the present author employed above in the hope of reporting an accurate range of estimates for total national concussion incidence are not equal to the task of counting health problems among people who deny them.

How on earth might one overcome these barriers? Until all cheerleaders, rodeo riders, and synchronized swimmers are outfitted with helmets bristling with accelerometers, there will never be an accurate accounting of the frequency of sports-related head impacts. And even then, it has yet to be determined at what lower limit of force, in people with what genome, head impacts yield brain-rattling injuries.

For the sake of argument, let's assume that linear and rotational head accelerations were monitored with great precision on every dusty *fútbol* field on every continent. That would fail to provide much useful data about CBI. Instrumented helmets, as they are called, only measure simple movements of head relative to hat. Innumerable mechanical factors (e.g., bulk modulus, shear strain, compressibility) complicate the effects on a brain exposed to a given combination of skull accelerations. Clinical research on football players wearing accelerometers reveals how weakly predictive such electronic measures are of acute symptoms and lasting disability. And, to date, no evidence permits one to translate accelerometry into measures of deleterious molecular cascades – let alone to predict risk of dementia 50 years hence. So, even after the Fédération Internationale de Football Association (FIFA) persuades all its players to wear five-kilo helmets with satellite up-links, this will only tell us something about external forces. It will reveal very little about brain rattling, and nothing whatsoever about cell damage or neurodegeneration.

As further discussion will reveal, we can vaguely enumerate impacts but will not, for the foreseeable future, accurately enumerate sports-related concussions. For these reasons, any document titled "epidemiology of sports-related concussion" needs to bow on to the stage with apologies. The numbers we have painstakingly compiled are wrong. The author's duty, therefore, is to report the best available data and qualify this report with caveats that will defend the reader from premature closure regarding that which is uncountable.

How Many People Play Sports?

The first question one must answer with reasonable confidence is: "How many people engage in sports?" Sport-related brain injury is a global issue. One wishes to present global data. Unfortunately, the hierarchy of sports participation recently compiled on the basis of figures submitted by each international sports federation [136] seems fudged: "#1: Volleyball; #2: Basketball; #3: Table Tennis; #4: Soccer; #5: Badminton; #6: Tennis; #7: Baseball; #8: Dragon Boat Racing …"

Dragon boat racing? The author of the present essay admits having failed to note the explosive gains in the popularity of dragon boat racing, which, according to this list, attracts more worldwide participation than going for a brisk walk. A more credible answer, for individuals, would seem to be running or dancing or bicycling, and for teams, "soccer." However, he shares the opinion that, "As yet there does not seem to be an accurate list of the most played sports around the world" [136]. Accepting a common academic problem – that peer-reviewed literature is disproportionately attentive to U.S. behaviors – the best one can do may be to summarize local trends. As ever, consistency is unavailable.

According to a 2008 estimate by the National Council of Youth Sports, 44 million children and adolescents participate in organized sports in the United States each year [137]. By comparison, the National Operating Committee of Standards for Athletic Equipment states, "Forty-five million kids and teens participate in organized youth sports each year" [138]. Counting adults is even harder, given the lack of any registry. Over a decade ago, the CDC estimated that about 170 million adults participate in physical activity, including sports [139]. Another source superficially seems to support that estimate for "physical activity" (not to say sports): in the summer of 2015, 55.5% (178 million) of Americans reported exercising 30+ minutes a day on three or more days per week [140]. Based on both the National Health Interview Survey for 2008–2010 and the 2015 Gallup poll, those who exercised most frequently were Hispanic or white, upper-income, aged 18–29 years. (Of possible interest, 63.6% of adults with graduate-level degrees met the 2008 guidelines for aerobic activity compared with 28.9% of those with high school educations. Readers of this essay will please refrain from *Schadenfreude.*) Yet the 2015 U.S. Physical Activity Council reported that, among 292 million Americans

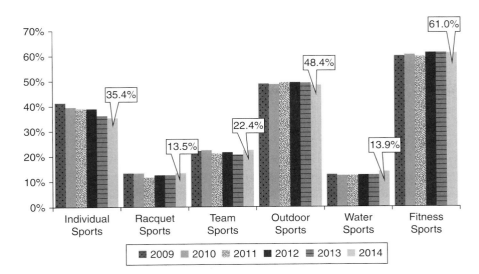

Fig. 2.8 Participation rates in sports: percentage of individuals aged 6+ years.

Source: Physical Activity Council [141]

age 6 years or older, just 83 million were "active" [141]. Figure 2.8, from that publication, illustrates the alleged distribution in participation by sport in the United States. Since the methods of counting were different in these various surveys, one cannot determine whether 83 million or 183 million is closer to the true nationwide rate of adult sports participation.

How Many Sport-Related Concussions Occur?

More important than total sports participation, how many people sustain CBIs playing sports each year? The correct answer is that nobody knows. That does not restrain guessing: readers may have encountered the echo chamber of scholarship citing the CDC's work:

- "the Centers for Disease Control estimates that 1.6 to 3.8 million concussions occur in sports and recreational activities annually" [121].
- "The CDC estimates approximately 1.6 to 3.8 million sports- and recreation-related concussions occur each year in the United States" [138].

These remarks are rather casual about attribution. The CDC has never proposed any such estimate! The actual source is Langlois et al. [48]: "Although a previous Centers for Disease Control and Prevention study estimated that approximately 300,000 such injuries occur each year, it included only TBIs for which the person reported a loss of consciousness" (pp. 375–376). However, as those writers noted, loss of consciousness reportedly occurs in roughly 8–19.2% of sports-related concussions [142, 143]. Based on those figures, Langlois et al. extrapolated: "a more accurate approximation may be that 1.6 million to 3.8 million sports-related TBIs occur each year, including those for which no medical care is sought. This estimate might still be low because many of these injuries go unrecognized and thus uncounted" [48]. Therefore, the most-cited estimate of total sports-related concussions in the United States each calendar year is a guess that the originators admitted may still be an underestimate.

One more objective estimate is derived from unambiguous documentation: about 11,000 people receive ED treatment each day for sports-related injuries. Forty-five percent of those visits involve children aged 15 or younger [144]. But, as noted in the first part of this chapter, one can only guess whether the number of ED visits is 10% or 50% of actual injuries. Perhaps the most forthright conclusion was that offered by the General Accounting Office in Congressional testimony in 2010 regarding the net number of high school sports-related concussions: "The overall estimate of occurrence is not available" [145].

Risk Factors for Sports-Related Concussions: Age, Sex, Recurrence, and Activity

Age-Related Differences in Vulnerability to Sports-Related Concussions

Evidence has been published suggesting that concussed middle school students or high school athletes suffer more severe and more persistent post-CBI dysfunction than do concussed college athletes [131, 146–150]. Field et al. [151] compared cohorts from each age group and reported significantly worse memory at seven days post-CBI among the high school students. Other evidence suggests that children take longer to recover from CBI [152]. In one study [153] boy and girl high school athletes who had suffered sports-related concussions continued to show memory deficits seven days post-injury, a significant difference from college athletes. Yet in one prospective study that compared baseline with post-injury scores, Lee et al. [154] found no age-related difference. As Gessel et al. [155] summarized the available data: "In all sports, collegiate athletes had higher rates of concussion than high school athletes, but concussions represented a greater proportion of all injuries among high school athletes" (Figure 2.9). Based on a systematic review (the closest thing we have to an authoritative source), Foley et al. [156] judged that younger players indeed suffer more persistent symptoms and cognitive impairments. However, it was not clear that they suffered significantly higher rates of very long-term neurobehavioral problems.

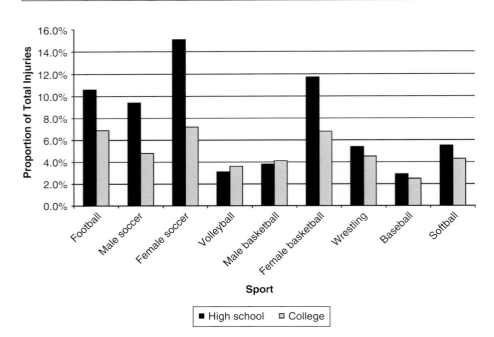

Fig. 2.9 Concussions as a percentage of total injuries sustained by high school and collegiate athletes, High School Sports-Related Injury Surveillance Study and National Collegiate Athletic Association Injury Surveillance System, United States, 2005–2006 school year.

Source: Gessel et al., 2007 [155]. Reproduced with permission from Gessel LM, Fields SK, Collins CL, Dick RW, Comstock RD.

Why might younger players be at higher risk? Thinner crania? Greater ratio of head to body weight? Weaker neck muscles? Less myelination? [131]. These and other factors have been proposed as explanations. None have been empirically tested. Animal models perhaps offer clues. For instance, McDonald and Johnston [157] reported that developing rodents were more prone to damage from post-traumatic release of excitatory neurotransmitters. Fan et al. [158] reported that immature mice fail to mount the antioxidant response observed after TBI among adults.

In the author's opinion, the issue is unresolved and potentially critical. Uncontrolled retrospective observations or short-term (less than 20-year) prospective observations are inadequate to provide useful information. The question is not whether objective cerebral dysfunction is different during the first year or two post-CBI, but whether suffering a single (or multiple) sport-related concussion in elementary school is more likely than similar brain damage in college to produce 70 years of adult neurological disadvantage.

Sex-Related Differences in Vulnerability to Sports-Related Concussions

Girls and women are more likely to suffer concussions in organized sports than boys and men. This is especially obvious in soccer and ice hockey [128, 159–161]. Moreover, multiple sources report that females exhibit more persistent subjective symptoms and more persistent objective cognitive impairments [153, 160, 162–165]. As part of the NCAA Injury Surveillance System, certified athletic trainers recorded concussion data during the 1997–2000 academic years. Across five sports, 9.5% of females were concussed during games compared with 6.4% of males. In a very short-term study [153], PC symptoms and cognitive changes were monitored for 14 days after concussion among 296 college athletes.

The women athletes had significantly more symptoms than the men (14.4 vs. 10.1) and the women had significantly worse scores on memory tests. The most striking and perhaps globally important statistic to emerge from this area of research: college women playing soccer were 13 times as likely to be concussed as college men [159].

The explanation for these sex differences remains unknown. Male doctors going back to Charcot and Babinsky have claimed that female hysteria explains more severe effects of minor injury [166–168]. Dick [160] suggested that the higher rate of symptom reporting may reflect females' higher levels of honesty. Neither theory explains females' objectively worse cognitive outcomes. One suspects a neurobiological explanation, but non-human animal experiments and clinical observations have yet to identify a single important factor. One possible factor: if a girl or woman experiences her concussion during the luteal phase when progesterone is high, there is a profound drop in this hormone. That drop (which does not occur in boys or men) is associated with more severe symptoms [169]. Some evidence suggests that female brains are more metabolically active, hence more prone to suffer when the mitochondrial energy crisis of concussion occurs (see Chapters 3–5). In a study comparing functional magnetic resonance imaging (MRI) findings six weeks after CBI (including cases of sports-related CBI), Hsu et al. [170] reported that brain regions associated with working memory were persistently hypoactive among concussed women but not men. Still, neither the neurobiological cause nor the long-term impact of this sex difference has been discovered.

In the author's opinion, Western society deserves great credit for advancing the cause of athletic participation among girls and women. Now it is time to count the cost. Although the lifetime cumulative incidence of concussion among women is probably less than half that among men, it is possible that the female's increased vulnerability to persistent cerebral damage

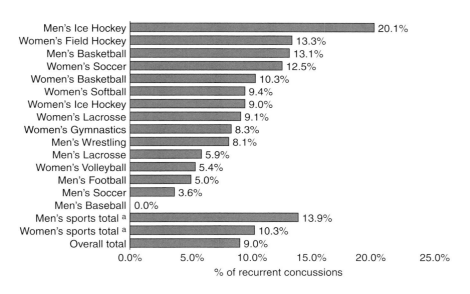

Fig. 2.10 Proportion of recurrent concussions among student athletes in 15 sports, National Collegiate Athletic Association Injury Surveillance Program, 2009–2010 to 2013–2014 academic years. [a]NCAA ISP: National Collegiate Athletic Association Injury Surveillance Program.

Source: Zuckerman et al., 2015 [123]. Reproduced with permission from SAGE

may lead to a disproportionate rate of sports-related post-traumatic dementia.

Recurrence

Recurrence of sports-related concussions, or repetitive concussions, are phrases that are used to refer ambiguously to three related problems. One is recurrence of unambiguous brain injury, subjectively apparent, within a short time frame – perhaps a matter of days. A player who gets hit and feels dazed (a subjective concussion) is more likely to get hit and feel dazed again soon, in which case he or she seems to face a risk of markedly worse outcome. The risk of the second impact is probably due to impairment of alertness, awareness, and balance, slowing of reaction time, and perhaps subtle diplopia due to the first hit. If those two hits are within a week or so of one another, there may be not only additive but dangerously synergistic harm, sometimes called the second impact syndrome [69, 70]. A second use of those phrases refers to the athlete with a remote history of concussion. He or she is also more prone to suffer subsequent concussions. Yet if they are separated by months or years, the second impact syndrome does not apply. Instead, unknown and probably highly individual factors determine how those two injuries interact, the net effect on current function, and the risk of later dementia. The third way these phrases are used is to discuss a different problem: repetitive "subconcussive" concussion, meaning trains of hundreds of brain-rattling impacts routinely survived by many young athletes playing football, soccer, ice hockey, or wrestling, that may cause little or no acute subjective symptoms but may progressively degrade brain health.

As mentioned in the introductory section, this third phenomenon is extremely difficult to analyze, because even if one equipped our trio of high school hockey players, Cindy, Mindy, and Malak, with perfect telemetry-monitored accelerometers, one does not know where to draw the line between injury and non-injury. Recurrence or repetition of all three varieties seems likely to be a major cause of persistent brain dysfunction. However, these three clinical scenarios are often conflated in the sports medicine literature, which often fails to distinguish between subjective and objective diagnosis and rarely reports individual time lapses between all injuries. Still, Zuckerman et al.'s [123] graphic (Figure 2.10) illustrates one data set from the NCAA Injury Surveillance Program. If these data are to be believed, then men's college ice hockey is associated with quadruple the recurrence rate compared with men's college football, and more women volleyball players suffer recurrent concussion than do men playing football. The author gladly provides the image, but cannot guarantee its worth.

Activity-Related Differences in Vulnerability to Sports-Related Concussions

It is commonly said that "contact" sports are especially likely to cause concussions. This is not the only factor of importance. As Hootman et al. [171] noted, "Sports that limit or restrict player contact, such as soccer, basketball, and women's ice hockey, still have a majority of their game injuries associated with player contact" (p. 314). Bicycling is not generally considered a contact sport but may be the most common cause of CBIs leading to ED visits in the United States. Globally speaking, American football is a trivial contributor to human activity. Far more concussions probably occur in the non-contact sport, soccer, because the rate of participation is hugely higher than that of football.

Readers will surely want to know what sports are most dangerous to the brain. Understanding the many factors that interfere with accuracy, Table 2.3 offers three perspectives. The first list ranks the ten sports or recreational activities responsible for the most ED visits in the United States. The second list ranks high school sports in order of concussion incidence per 1000 athlete exposures (AEs: one practice or game played by one athlete). The third list ranks a wider variety of sports in order of concussion incidence per 1000 AEs. The difference in rankings in each column helps to show why alternate approaches to counting yield different findings.

Many metrics are employed for determining concussion incidence. These include CBIs per 1000 athletic exposures,

Table 2.3 Three perspectives on the relative incidence of concussive brain injury in various sports and recreations

Rank	The ten sporting/recreational activities responsible for the largest number of ED visits for non-fatal TBIs among persons aged ≤ 19[a]	The ten high school or college sports responsible for the highest incidence of concussions[b]	The ten sporting/recreational activities with the highest incidence of concussions[c]
1	Bicycling	Girls' college soccer	Boxing/martial arts
2	Football	Boys' college football	Football
3	Playground	Boys' college soccer	Ice hockey
4	Basketball	Boys' high school football	Snowboarding/skiing
5	Soccer	Girls' college basketball	Wrestling
6	Baseball	Boys' college wrestling	Soccer
7	All-terrain vehicle riding	Girls' high school soccer	Basketball
8	Skateboarding	Boys' college basketball	Cheerleading
9	Swimming	Boys' high school soccer	Lacrosse
10	Hockey	Girls' high school basketball	Gymnastics

[a] Source: Gilchrist, 2011 [172].
[b] Source: Gessel et al., 2007 [155].
[c] Source: The present author's review.

ED: emergency department; TBI: traumatic brain injury.

per 100 or 1000 player hours or game hours, per hour of play, per 100 games, per 100 player season exposures, or per team per season. Table 2.4 was compiled by the author in the hope of enabling the reader to review comparable statistics across sports. The table lists popular sports and recreational activities alphabetically and according to the age and sex of participation, along with published estimates of the incidence of concussions per 1000 AEs. Also noted, when available, are the proportion of injuries in a given sport that are concussions, and the rate of recurrence.

Brief Observations Regarding Several Popular Sports

All-Terrain Vehicle (ATV) Riding

Some evidence suggests that brain injuries are common in ATV riding, especially among children [197]. For example, the CDC estimates more than 6300 ATV riding-related ED visits for non-fatal TBIs from 2001 to 2009 for ages ≤ 19 years [172]. Helmets probably reduce that risk among both ATV drivers and riders – up to 50% of whom report concussion symptoms [198]. Unfortunately, compliance with helmet use is spotty and the limited available surveillance prohibits estimates of incidence per exposure.

Baseball

The CDC estimates more than 9600 baseball-related ED visits for non-fatal TBIs from 2001 to 2009 for ages ≤ 19 years [172]. Concussions, however, are relatively uncommon in both men's baseball and women's softball. The concussion rate per 1000 AEs is often the lowest of all high school and college sports and is also low among professional players, among whom mTBI accounts for just 1% of injuries leading to time off [171,

175]. Note that these statistics were derived from athletic trainers or team physicians, not from self-report or objective observations, so the actual incidence is probably higher. Among professionals, catchers are especially vulnerable. One interesting study assayed performance in the two weeks after returning from concussion [199]. The players were not symptomatic. Nonetheless, batting average, on-base percentage, and slugging percentage were significantly depressed during that period.

Basketball

Basketball is one of the three most popular organized sports in the United States. The CDC estimates almost 14,000 basketball-related ED visits for non-fatal TBIs from 2001 to 2009 for ages ≤ 19 years [172]. It is therefore more likely to produce concussion than baseball but remains a relatively low-risk sport. Guards are the players most at risk during games. Girls and women are at higher risk of concussions than boys and men [120, 155]. Among girls, playing injuries are most common during ball handling and defending. Among boys, injuries are most common when chasing a loose ball and rebounding [155].

Bicycling

Bicycling is the most common cause of ED visits for non-fatal TBIs among children age 5–9 years and the second most common cause among other minors [172]. The CDC estimates more than 26,000 bicycling-related ED visits for non-fatal TBIs from 2001 to 2009 for ages ≤ 19 years [172]. Girls and women are more prone to serious injuries in off-road bicycling than are men [120]. Helmet use profoundly reduces the risk of bicycling-related CBIs. For instance, as Sosin et al. reported [45]:

An average of 247 traumatic brain injury deaths and 140,000 head injuries among children and adolescents

Table 2.4 Rate of concussive brain injuries in several popular sports

(At the time of writing, few data are available regarding concussive brain injuries (CBIs) among girls and women who box, wrestle, and play American-style tackle football)

Sport or recreation	CBIs per 1000 exposures	% of injuries that were CBIs	Recurrence rate[a]
Baseball, high school boys	0.08 games; 0.03 practice [155] 0.05 [161] 0.06 [173] 0.11 games; 0.01 practice [174]		
Baseball, college men	0.23 games; 0.03 practice [155] 0.2 [120] 0.07 [171] 0.12 games; 0.07 practice [123]	2.5% [171] 5% [120]	0%
Baseball, professional men	0.42 [175]		
Basketball, high school boys	0.11 game/0.06 practice [155] 0.11 [161] 0.10 [173] 0.39 games; 0.06 practice [174]		
Basketball, college men	0.45 games; 0.22 practice [155] 0.16 [171] 0.3 [120] 0.56 games; 0.34 practice [123]	3.2% [171]	13.1%
Basketball, high school girls	0.16 [161] 0.60 games; 0.06 practice [155] 0.16 [173] 0.55 games; 0.06 practice [174]		
Basketball, college women	0.85 (14.2 × practice) 0.22 [171] 1.09 games; 0.44 practice [123]	4.7% [171]	10.3%
Basketball, adult women	0.5 [120]		
Boxing, amateur men	11–77 [120]		
Boxing, professional men	186–251 [120] 171 [176]		
Cheerleading, youth	< 0.1 [120]		
Cheerleading, girls' high school	0.14 [177] < 0.1 [120] 0.06 [173] 0.12 games; 0.14 practice [174]		
Cheerleading, college sex not specified	0.29 [177]		
Field hockey, high school boys	1.1 [120]		
Field hockey, high school girls	0.09 [161] 0.5–0.7 [120] 0.10 [173] 0.41 games; 0.14 practice = [174]		
Field hockey, college women	0.18 [171] 1.11 games; 0.178 practice [123]	3.9% [171]	13.3%
Football, youth 8–12 years	6.16 games; 0.24 practice [178]		
Football, high school boys	0.59 [161] 1.55 games/0.21 practice [155] 2.58 games/ 0.25 practice [179] 1.3 [120] 0.60 [173] 2.29 games; 0.31 practice [174]		
Football, high school girls	N/A		
Football college men	3.35 games/0.46 practice [179] 3.02 games/0.39 practice [155] 0.37 [171] 2.3–6.1 [120] 3.0 games; 0.42 practice [123]	6.0% [171]	5.0%

(continued)

Table 2.4 (*Cont.*)

Sport or recreation	CBIs per 1000 exposures	% of injuries that were CBIs	Recurrence rate[a]
Spring football, college men	0.54 [171]	5.6% [171]	
Football, college women	N/A		
Football, professional men	16.2 (quarterbacks) 12.3 (wide receivers) [180]		
Gymnastics, high school girls	0.24 competition; 0.03 practice [174]		
Gymnastics, college women	0.16 [171] 0.4 [181] 0.48 competition; 0.24 practice [123]	2.3% [171]	8.3%
Ice hockey, girls 11–17 years	0.28 [182]	15.1% [183]	
Ice hockey, high school boys	3.6–3.9 [179] 3.6 [184] 1.46 games; 0.11 practice [174] 3.7 [120]		
Ice hockey "junior" males 16–21 years	21.5 [185]		
Ice hockey, college men	1.5 [179] 0.41 [171] 1.5–4.2 [120] 2.49 games; 0.25 practice [123]	7.9% [171]	20.1%
Ice hockey, college women	0.91 [171] 2.72 games; 0.33 practice [186] 2.7 [120] 14.93 (games) [187] 2.01 games; 0.30 practice [123]	18.3% [171]	9.4%
Ice hockey, men 20–36 years	6.6 [120]		
Ice hockey, adult women	0.49 [188]		
Ice hockey, professional men	6.5 [184]		
Karate, adult males	1.62 [179]		
Lacrosse, high school boys	0.30 [173] 0.29 [189] 1.04 games; 0.11 practice [174] 0.97 games; 0.28 practice [190]		
Lacrosse, college men	0.26 [171] 0.93 games; 0.19 practice [174]	5.6% [171]	5.9%
Lacrosse, high school girls	0.20 [173] 0.10 [189] 0.83 games; 0.13 practice [174] 0.55 games; 0.26 practice [190]		
Lacrosse, college women	0.25 [171] 0.82–1.37 games [159] 0.70 games; 0.15 practice [191]	6.3% [171]	9.1%
Rodeo, men	2.77 [192] 3.4 [193]		
Rugby, high school	3.8 [194]		
Rugby, professional men	9.05 [184]		
Skiing, sex and age not specified	2.1 [120]		
Snowboarding, sex and age not specific	6.1 [120]		
Soccer, high school boys	0.59 games; 0.04 practice [155] 0.18 [161] 0.18 [179] 0.17 [173] 0.53 games; 0.04 practice [174]		

Table 2.4 *(Cont.)*

Sport or recreation	CBIs per 1000 exposures	% of injuries that were CBIs	Recurrence rate[a]
Soccer, high school girls	0.97 games; 0.09 practice [155] 0.23 [161] 0.23 [179] 0.35 [173] 0.92 games; 0.08 practice [174]		
Soccer, college men	1.38 games; 0.24 practice [155] 0.28 [171] 1.1 [120] 0.97 games; 0.17 practice [123]	3.9% [171]	3.6%
Soccer, college women	1.80 games; 0.25 practice [155] 0.41 [171] 1.4 [120] 1.94 games; 0.21 practice [123]	5.3% [171]	12.5%
Softball, high school girls	0.10 [161] 0.11 [173] 0.29 games; 0.09 practice [174]		
Softball, high school no specified sex	0.04 games; 0.09 practice [155]		
Softball, college women	0.14 [171] 0.3 [120] 0.25 [195] 0.56 games; 0.17 practice = [123]	4.3% [171]	9.4%
Swimming, high school boys	0.01 practice [174]		
Swimming, high school girls	0.04 competition; 0.01 practice [174]		
Swimming, college men	0.01 competition; 0.04 practice [123]		
Swimming, college women	0.09 competition; 0.03 practice [123]		
Taekwondo, junior boys	5.1 [179] 5.11 [196]		
Taekwondo, junior girls	1.2 [179] 4.55 [196]		
Taekwondo, adult men	7.04–15.5 [179]		
Taekwondo, adult women	2.42–8.77 [179] 8.77 [184]		
Track and field, high school boys	0.03 competition; 0.02 practice [174]		
Track and field, high school girls	0.04 competition; 0.01 practice [174]		
Volleyball high school, sex unspecified	0.05 games; 0.05 practice		
Volleyball, high school girls	0.02 [161] 0.10 games; 0.05 practice [174]		
Volleyball, college women	0.09 [171] 0.57 games; 0.27 practice [123]	2.0% [171]	5.4%
Volleyball college sex not specified	0.13 games; 0.21 practice [155]		
Volleyball, age and sex not specified	0.1–0.2 [120]		
Wrestling, high school boys	0.25 [161] 0.32 matches; 0.13 practice [155] 0.17 [173] 0.48 matches; 0.13 practice [174]		
Wrestling, high school girls	N/A		
Wrestling, college men	1.00 matches; 0.35 practice [155] 0.25 [171] 1.3 [120] 5.55 matches; 0.57 practice [123]	3.3% [171]	8.1%

[a] Recurrence rates, source: Zuckerman et al., 2015 [123].

younger than 20 years were related to bicycle crashes each year in the United States. As many as 184 deaths and 116,000 head injuries might have been prevented annually if these riders had worn helmets.

Boxing

As reported in Chapter 1, the association between boxing and CBI has been studied for more than a century, and the link to dementia was established about 90 years ago. This popular recreational activity is unique in its unapologetic pursuit of a human's brain injury as the participant's most-desired goal (Figure 2.11). The very high risk of brain injury in boxing has been a provocation for research in the field of CBI, repetitive concussion, and the very common outcome of persistent or permanent traumatic encephalopathy. We will not belabor the point.

It is perhaps worth noting how very much more frequent CBI is in boxing than in virtually any other sport. For instance, Toth [120] reported a range of 11–77 CBIs per 1000 AEs among amateurs and 186–251 among professionals. Bledsoe et al.'s [176] review of professional boxing in Nevada yielded a comparable estimate of 171 concussions per 1000 AEs. (By way of comparison, college football, in the Toth review, was reported to generate just 2.3–6.1 CBIs/1000 AEs.) Strikes to the chin are the main mechanism of knockouts, because they rapidly twist the brainstem and disrupt the pontine ascending reticular activating system, often causing prompt loss of consciousness.

Substantial evidence suggests that boxers who carry one or more ε4 alleles of the gene for apolipoprotein E are more likely to develop post-CBI dementia [201, 202]. This confronts us with the obvious benefit of genetic screening and the potentially life-saving measure of discouragement of genetically at-risk persons from participation. The American Academy of Neurology, however, disapproves of testing. Hence, no momentum exists in the communities of medicine or boxing to capitalize on this knowledge.

Women also box. Given the evidence that females suffer more severe and lasting cerebral dysfunction after sports-related CBIs, one predicts a high rate of PC signs and symptoms in this cohort. Research, however, is sparse. Two Italian studies concluded that female boxing is "a safe sport" [203, 204]. That reassurance is not very persuasive, since neither study involved any assessment whatsoever of concussion symptoms, cognitive status, or brain integrity.

Cheerleading

About 3.3 million people, mostly girls and young women, participate in cheerleading in the United States each year [205]. Most popular in the southeastern states, cheerleading has recently gained in popularity with a doubling of participation since early 1990. That change has been attributed to the adoption of more gymnastic (that is, dangerous) maneuvers and the rise of cheerleading competitions dissociated from other sports – e.g., "All-Star" cheerleading [177]. These changes have been accompanied by a marked increase in injuries, including CBIs (Figure 2.12) [145].

About 6–6.3% of cheerleading injuries are concussions [207, 208]. Cheerleading is unique in that the majority of

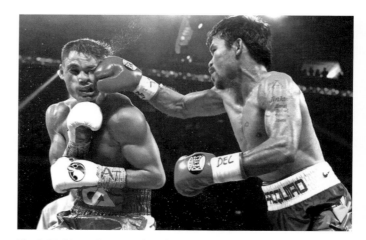

Fig. 2.11 Manny Pacquiao abruptly rotating the head of Chris Algieri en route to retaining his World Boxing Organization welterweight belt.
Source: Kin Cheung/AP images, 2014 [200]. Reproduced with permission from Associated Press/Kin Cheung

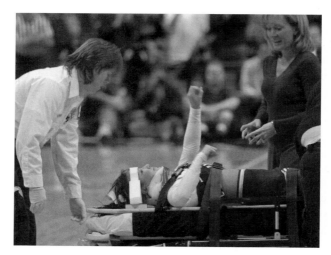

Fig. 2.12 Cheerleader Kristi Yamaoka after her 15 ft fall causing a concussion and cervical fracture.
Source: Associated Press, 2006 [206]

concussions occur in practice. In one study [174], for instance, the concussion rate was 0.12 per 100 AEs in games and 0.14 in practice. Concussion sometimes occurs during falls; however, 96% of cheerleading-related concussions occur during gymnastic stunts [208, p. 578; 209, p. 586]. In one report, two-level pyramids were responsible for almost two-thirds of concussions [207]. Although the *flyer* – the girl who is lifted or flung into the air – is more prone to catastrophic spinal injuries, the *basers* and *spotters* (girls who support, throw, or catch the flyers) are more prone to concussions. Higher body mass index, harder surfaces, and poorly trained coaches are known risk factors for cheerleading-related injuries [210].

Equestrian Sports

Head injuries are common among horseback riders, whether the horse is used for work or recreation [120]. The CDC estimates more than 3600 horseback riding-related ED visits for non-fatal TBIs from 2001 to 2009 for ages ≤ 19 years [172]. The popularity of riding varies considerably, both by region and socioeconomic group. For example, in Oklahoma in 1992–1993 horseback riding was that state's number one cause of sports-related TBIs. Ninety-five percent of those injuries were associated with falls from the horse [211]. A single study reported neuropsychological deficits after concussions among jockeys. Those with repetitive concussions exhibited persistent deficits in response inhibition and divided attention [212].

Football and the Sophistry of the "Concussion Threshold"

I shouldn't have to prove to anybody that there's something wrong with me. I'm not being vindictive. I'm not trying to reach up from the grave and get the N.F.L.[National Football League]. But any doctor who doesn't connect concussions with long-term effects should be ashamed of themselves.

Ted Johnson, 2009

American-style football is a team sport involving violent contention to move a prolate spheroid on a field marked with a grid.[7] Since about 1985, football has surpassed baseball to become the most popular sport in the United States. According to the National Federation of State High School Associations [213], in the 2014–2015 school year 1,083,617 boys and 1,565 girls participated. Add to that the 70,000 annual U.S. college players, 1700 U.S. professionals, plus about 20,000 participants in other countries, and the global total is probably somewhere short of 1.2 million. Evidence has rapidly accumulated during the past two decades that American-style football is an extremely dangerous sport that often causes permanent brain damage, early-onset dementia, and suicide. The overwhelming majority of football players are the recipients of hundreds of head impacts each season. Yet, perhaps to a greater degree than for any other organized sport in the world, the incidence of concussion in football is misrepresented in the literature. So, for instance, Table 2.4 dutifully cites several published estimates of the incidence of concussion in football, from youth to professional play. But one cannot put faith in any of these reports. Ignorance and dissimulation by players and trainers and coaches and team doctors and team executives trump scholarship in this matter.

To get a sense of the mismatch between reports authored by doctors employed by the football industry versus actual incidence of brain injuries, consider the report by Pellman et al. [180].[8] This publication purportedly summarized data from the NFL Injury Surveillance System for the seasons 1996–2001. Quarterbacks reportedly experienced mTBIs at a rate of 16.2 per 1000 game positions. Wide receivers reportedly experienced 12.3 mTBIs per 1000 game positions.

Are these numbers meaningful? The authors declared, "The system requires that each team record data on all concussions that occur"; "there were 787 reported cases of mTBI." These statements expose both faulty methodology and sophistic rhetoric: no system existed then or now that permitted athletic trainers, coaches, or team physicians to know when any concussions occurred, apart from inferences they might make from the small subset of obvious major head bangs that were both objectively observed and also documented by staff, or those subjective abrupt brain dysfunctions players elected to report and staff elected to document. In a professional boxing match, as many as ten experts monitor every instance of contact between a single pair of athletes at every moment. Concussion marks the win and often ends the match. In a football game, no such monitoring occurs. Detection of potentially neurologically significant application of force to each head is difficult, especially when multiple players collide in human piles during which each participant may receive multiple head impacts within several seconds. This difficulty of objective monitoring increases reliance on self-report, and self-report is known to be extremely unreliable. As previously noted, most concussed football players do not know when they have been concussed, and those who know often decline to report it, and disincentives exist that probably inhibit forthright reporting by athletic

---

[7] For readers who may not know the game: professional American-style football is an engaging gladiatorial circus. Evidence suggests it is likely to numb observers to violence and persuade them to purchase pick-up trucks [214–217]. The NFL, which profits from American-style football, "markets and manufactures controlled violence and mayhem better than any other league in the history of organized sports" [216]. The NFL, its medical staff, and executives have reportedly engaged in a conspiracy to deny the permanent brain damage that their business is certain to produce [218]. On January 7, 2017 the U. S. District Court for the Eastern District of Pennsylvania facilitated a settlement that obliges the NFL to compensate about one-quarter of brain-damaged players for football-related dementia. However, that settlement was written to preclude compensation for retired players living with chronic traumatic encephalopathy, or mood disorders, or depression consequent to football-related brain injuries [219]. Moreover, despite reported evidence of a massive, multi-year cover-up by the NFL and some of its apparently co-conspiratorial doctors, by settling without a trial, the NFL avoids confessing its mendacity or paying punitive damages [220]. Readers know from Chapter 1 that the causal link between repetitive concussions and early-onset neurodegenerative disease was established by 1927, for instance, with the publications of Giliberti and Osnato [221] and Martland [222]. It is not clear whether the court's reserving medical compensation for only a subset of players and its sidestepping the issue of liability ideally serve the goal of justice. On December 31, 2014, the author offered to provide an *amicus curiae* brief to the court impartially summarizing the relevant neuroscientific data. Judge Anita B. Brody declined to accept that brief. It remains to be seen whether the NFL will ever collect its just reward for (in the author's opinion) replicating the dynamic of the Tuskegee syphilis experiment [223], in which some men advanced their own agendas by willfully putting others at risk for a terrible health outcome about which they could not possibly know.

[8] The first author, Pellman, is reportedly a foreign-trained rheumatologist (and personal physician of a former commissioner of the league) who was paid by the NFL for his *neurological* expertise.

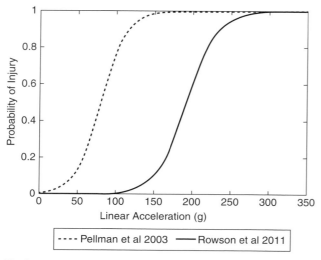
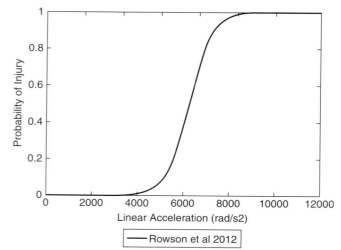

Fig. 2.13 Injury risk as a function of linear and rotational acceleration.
Source: Urban et al., 2013 [231]. Reprinted by permission from Springer

trainers. Considering these factors, how might one determine whether the 787 cases of football-related head injuries reported in the Pellman et al. paper represented 5%, 11%, or some other percent of the actual concussions? How might science circumvent the player–team conspiracy to hide concussions?

The standard reply is "telemetry." In fact, remote monitoring of helmet-mounted accelerometers is a legitimate way to count and measure those helmet–head interactions that are detectable with this equipment. Multiple investigators have published concussion risk curves ostensibly predicting the force required to harm a football player. However, this literature is not quite what it seems.

In one early study, 31 NFL head injuries were reconstructed based on game films and the estimated forces were inflicted upon Hybrid III crash test dummy heads [224, 225]. A threshold for the occurrence of "mTBI" was derived – but not based on athlete reports of having been dazed. The only impacts regarded as concussive were those documented on forms by team staff members. Peak linear accelerations causing "concussion" averaged 98 **g** (49–138 **g**); acceleration causing "no injury" averaged 60 **g** (19–85 **g**). As the reader might guess, there is no "threshold." Some 60-**g** hits caused concussion and some 80-**g** hits did not. According to the so-called NFL risk curve there is a 50% chance of concussion with an 85-**g** hit [226].

Funk et al. [227] adopted a different approach, outfitting college players with helmets instrumented with the Head Impact Telemetry (HIT) system – a device that situates six spring accelerometers between the helmet and the head. The system has been validated in the sense that, with corrections for errors, its recordings of linear accelerations approximate those recorded at the center of gravity of the Hybrid III head [228]. The advantage of this strategy was collection of data regarding 27,319 impacts, permitting determination of exposures per unit time. The authors set their device to ignore impacts less than 10 **g**. Almost 4000 recorded impacts exceeded 40 **g**; one reached 200 **g**. The authors state that just four concussions occurred in those > 27,000 head impacts – again, not based

on any systematic player interviews. Apparently using several sources other than the player to determine the occurrence of concussions, the authors concluded that the NFL curve was deeply flawed and that, instead, a hit of 165 **g** or more was required to create a 50% risk of concussion.

Rowson and Duma [229] published a curve that is similar to that of Funk et al. Figure 2.13 compares two of these concussion risk curves. A fourth study [230] determined that concussions, on average, were associated with a peak linear acceleration of 112.1 ± 35.5 **g**. Their curve predicts that a 95th percentile impact of 84.9 **g** generates 10.3 times greater risk of concussion compared with a 50th percentile hit of 38.9 **g**.

Hence, having not asked any players whether they were concussed or tested whether players were functional, these scholars determined that college football players' brains tolerate very high linear forces. Other studies have also generated risk curves or estimated threshold forces that produce brain injury [232–235]. Until recently, none of them have made an effort to determine whether these numbers correlate with brain injury or developed methods to address the problem of underreporting.

Matters are improving. Broglio et al. [238] deserve credit for their small 2011 study: 19 high school football players underwent baseline cognitive testing and were followed for four seasons. Twenty concussions were judged to have occurred. But no relationship was found between impact mechanics, cognitive scores, and post-CBI symptoms. This study raises a red flag: one can monitor relative movements between helmet and head. One can count impacts. It is not clear how this helps with our epidemiological goal: to assess the incidence of CBIs in football and the effect on public health.

Rowson and Duma [130] earnestly attempted to overcome the underreporting problem with their reasonable estimate that ten times as many concussions occur as players report. Combining linear and rotational acceleration data, analyzing more than 63,000 impacts and adjusting for expected underreporting, they produced a novel risk curve according to

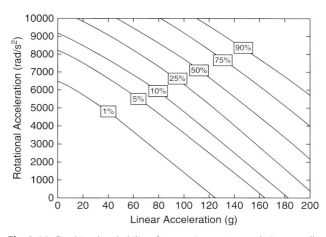

Fig. 2.14 Combined probability of concussion contours relating overall concussion risk to linear and rotational head acceleration.

Source: Rowson and Duma, 2013 [130]. Reproduced under the terms of the Creative Commons Attribution licence, CC-BY.

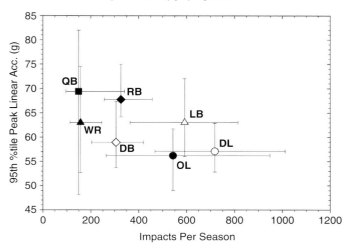

Fig. 2.15 Median (25–75%) of the 95th percentile of peak linear acceleration (**g**) as a function of the median (25–75%) number of head impacts per season greater than 10 **g** and categorized by player position. QB: quarterback; WR: wide receiver; RB: running back; DB: defensive back; LB: linebacker; DL: defensive lineman; OL: offensive lineman.

Source: Crisco et al., 2011 [232] with permission from Elsevier

which a 0-**g** linear acceleration yields about a 1% risk of CBI, an 89-**g** force yields a 10% risk, and a 115-**g** force yields a 50% risk. Figure 2.14 displays that curve.

With that curve in mind, please consider Figure 2.15. In 2011, Crisco et al. analyzed 286,636 head impacts among 314 college players over three seasons [232]. The graph shows the number and linear force of impacts per season per player. It is immediately striking to see how many hundreds of head impacts are regarded as par for the course.

A similar study was conducted by Broglio et al. [236]. They recorded 101,994 head impacts among 95 high school players across four seasons, finding that 652 impacts per season was average for this popular form of child's play. Even younger players are recipients of a worrisome number of head impacts: Daniel et al. [237] outfitted 17 middle school players aged 12–14 with instrumented helmets. These pre-teens and early teens averaged 275 ± 190 impacts apiece.

Another factor not well described in most of the existing literature is the disproportionate clustering of concussions among an unlucky subset: those who have been concussed. Zemper [238] tracked high school and college football players for two years. Those with no history of concussion had a 2.9% risk. Those with a history of concussion had a 16.5% risk. That is, brain-injured football players had 5.8 times the likelihood of brain injury.

At this point, one can set aside the debate regarding the risk curve, since we know that no publication is altogether accurate regarding the relationship between force and brain damage. For instance, at the time of this writing it is unknown how many football players with head impacts measured at 50 **g** would feel dazed, or exhibit cognitive change, or ultrastructural damage, or enhanced risk of early dementia. But at least we know that most middle school, high school, and college football players receive hundreds of head impacts each season, and quarterbacks tend to receive the fewest but some of the most

forceful impacts, while defensive linemen tend to receive less severe impacts, but an enormous number.[9]

Concussive Brain Injuries Classified as Non-Concussions

This brief section is merely intended to address the epidemiology of concussions in football, hoping to get a very rough sense of the incidence of injuries and public health implications of this violent game. For a quick numerical conclusion, one might simply take the incidences reported in Table 2.4 and apply the Rowson and Duma correction [130]: whenever someone cites a number of football-related concussions, the reader may safely assume that the correct total is about ten times as high. But two admonitions are in order: one, there is no concussion threshold. Two: even if there were a concussion threshold, so-called *clinical concussions* are merely a subset of clinically important sports-related brain injuries.

Regarding the first admonition, concussion risk curves – neatly drawn graphs such as Figure 2.14 – create the impression that scientific study has unveiled the amount of external brain-shaking force required to produce a clinical concussion. That impression is false. The relationship is not correlative; it is probabilistic. Since no two heads or brains exhibit the same geometry or biology, since no two bodies and cardiovascular-respiratory systems are identically yoked to those brains, no two CBIs are alike and no mechanical threshold for human concussions exists. There is no switch in the head that signals, "feel dazed" at a given level of force, and no known marker heralding a given level of long-term damage. Instead, every

---

[9] The NFL has generally forbidden telemetric monitoring of head impacts. The NFL's Medical Director (now terminated) justified this to the author stating that accurate counts and measures of concussive impacts "would confuse the trainers."

individual at every moment – depending on virtually infinite factors such as the way the individual's skull–brain interaction disperses forces, genetic variants, momentary levels of gene expression, life history of brain traumas, blood level of non-steroidal anti-inflammatories, current intravascular volume, momentary intrathoracic pressure, coagulation parameters, and sub-nanometer-scale differences in the relative position of each brain cell and organelle – should expect different brain changes in response to identical external forces. The subjective feeling of dazedness depends on whether or not the combined linear and rotational forces in a blow just so happen to perturb a couple of critical zones such as the pontine ascending reticular activating system. Surely there are blows that happen not to bother those particular cells, but devastate others, leaving the victim fully conscious yet significantly hurt.

In an insightful essay, Duhaime et al. [239] attempt to correct the common misperception that a concussion is a reliably diagnosable life event and that a given force produces a given result. Among collegiate athletes wearing instrumented helmets, no impact was recorded in 17 out of 48 cases of diagnosed concussion. "Half of all players diagnosed with concussions had delayed or unclear timing of onset of symptoms" ([239], p. 1092). The range of linear accelerations associated with clinical concussions varied from 16.5 to 177.9 **g**. The fallacy of a "concussion threshold" is altogether consistent with a major theme of this essay. People vary. Different players have different clinical outcomes from identical forces.

But that is not the most important correction to the tale implied by much of the older literature. That tale amounts to, "Impacts do not matter unless consciousness is subjectively altered." No *a priori* logic or empirical evidence supports that holding; it is a major conceptual error to assume that reportable concussions are what matter. To the contrary, increasing evidence proves that brain-rattling forces may fall far short of producing frank loss of consciousness yet produce cumulative damage that is just as bad as, or worse than, a couple of knockouts. For an epidemiologist to determine the damage done to the U.S. population by our collective uncritical enthusiasm for football, it might be tempting to limits one's investigation to all of the brain injuries athletes notice. Yet the dings we notice are just part of the problem. Repetitive "subconcussive" concussions – those that are virtually asymptomatic – possibly give rise to as much or more net cerebral dysfunction in the global population. Later chapters will provide better accounts. For now, the tip of the iceberg is all one needs to mention.

Consider three reports. The first was published by McAllister et al. [240]. The authors were not satisfied to count impacts reported by little springs. They investigated the impact of those impacts. Again, no biomarker measures brain injury, but MRI scanning with diffusion tensor imaging (DTI) is emerging as a useful guide to some forms of post-concussional white-matter change. Eighty college football players had zero known concussions. Both DTI and neuropsychological measures were obtained before and after the season. Not to mince words: non-concussion head impact correlated with persisting brain and behavioral abnormalities. In athletes exposed to impacts, white-matter diffusivity was altered in the hippocampus, amygdala, thalamus, hemispheric white matter, and corpus callosum. Changes in the corpus callosum correlated with inferior cognitive scores.

A second study by Davenport et al. [241] took the same tack but with youngsters. Twenty-four high school players were monitored for impacts over one season. None had "concussions." Fractional anisotropy was significantly associated with risk-weighted exposures to linear and rotational accelerations. In fact, all measures of head impact correlated with DTI abnormalities. What's more, post-season declines in memory correlated with DTI scores. The authors summarized: "We demonstrate that a single season of football can produce brain MRI changes in the absence of clinical concussion. Similar brain MRI changes have been previously associated with mild traumatic brain injury" (p. 1617).

In a third study, renowned Boston University neuropathologist Ann McKee announced on September 18, 2015 that 95.6% of former NFL players referred for autopsy suffered from dementia associated with a form of neurodegeneration recently labeled "chronic traumatic encephalopathy" [242].

Candidly, it is challenging to interpret such a finding. Since 1973, a succession of pathologists (e.g., Corsellis, Hof, and Geddes) [243–245] have reported oddly distributed neurofibrillary tangles in the brains of some persons believed to have been exposed to repetitive CBIs (rCBIs). A productive research group at Boston University deserves credit for replicating and greatly expanding upon the research programs of Corsellis, Hof, and Geddes. They collected a convenience sample of more than 100 brains from persons believed to have been exposed to rCBIs (although limited clinical information is available, apart from typically undocumented reports of the patient having experienced multiple blows to the head – devoid of virtually any account of acute signs or symptoms – at some time in the past), and found multiple brain changes that often, but not always, include some oddly distributed tangles. As discussed in Chapter 11, (1) it is unknown how often that pathological change occurs after exposure to rCBIs; (2) essentially none of these cases includes basic clinical information regarding each injury, or regarding the course between injuries, based on sequential medical examinations and controlling for plausible confounding factors; (3) almost all of these cases exhibit polypathology, not a tauopathy; (4) tau deposits, in themselves, may be harmless; (5) no uniform clinical presentation or symptom cluster characterizes persons with this brain change; and (6) evidence suggests that other exposures, such as temporal lobe epilepsy, are associated with the same or a similar neuropathological picture. Hence, it does not seem appropriate to opine that "Repetitive concussion causes a distinct neurodegenerative disease." Still, this scholarship may unveil important clues about how brain rattling interacts with genes and with other environmental variables to alter the course of time-passing-related brain change. And it seems legitimate to hope that, some day, these observations may inform effective interventions.

The likely cerebral dysfunction of many (possibly most) former NFL players is tragic. Due to their small numbers, it is not in itself a public health concern. The real problem is that, due to their risky behavior, these few men strongly encourage a million children to damage their brains each year. One wishes

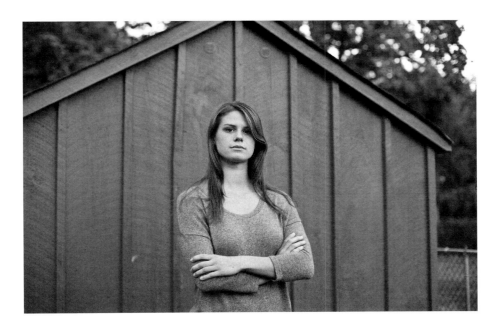

Fig. 2.16 Former US Olympic hockey star Josephine Pucci.

Source: Berkman, 2015 [250]. Reproduced with permission from New York Times/eyevine

to ask those who continue to deny the danger of football (especially the professional concussion deniers apparently employed by the NFL) which part of the mountain of smoking guns is hardest to smell. Like the death by a thousand cuts, football steadily chips away at the brain. This may not be ideal for development – and is certainly a strange focus of pride for an educational institution.

Ice Hockey

Ice hockey, like American football, is a dangerous sport associated with a high incidence of CBIs. Each season more than 1 million U.S. and Canadian children participate [246]. The CDC estimates more than 4400 ice hockey-related ED visits for non-fatal TBIs from 2001 to 2009 for ages ≤ 19 years [172]. Incidence estimates for concussions per 1000 AEs are listed in Table 2.4. As in football, underreporting is routine, making all of these published figures questionable [182, 183]. One notable report: when independent physicians actually observed games of junior hockey, the incidence of concussions was 21.5 per 1000 AEs [185]. Similarly, when athletic trainers were hired to continuously monitor players during tournaments, the concussion rate was 18.5 per 1000 player hours among high school boys, 10.7 per 1000 player hours among boys 14–15 years, and a rather concerning 23.1 concussions per 1000 player hours among boys aged 12–13 years [247]. Such figures are approximately ten times the rate reported by observers in other studies, and more consistent with Rowson and Duma's [130] proposed ten-times estimate for the ratio of actual versus reported sports-related concussions.

Unlike football, in which female participation rates remain low, many girls and women play ice hockey. Indeed, the popularity of girls' and women's ice hockey over the last two decades has increased by a factor of ten [183, 248]. As Abbott [183] observed, "Women's ice hockey has a high burden of concussion injuries, with a higher proportion of injuries due to

concussion than all other NCAA collegiate sports"(p. 378). The consequences of this dramatic change are beginning to become apparent. First, the physician-observed incidence of concussion was 14.93/1000 AEs in women's college ice hockey [187]. This is twice the rate among men and more than 16 times the rate reported by less rigorous observers [171]. Second, evidence is mounting that, despite far fewer impacts, girls are more prone to ice hockey-related concussion than boys [183, 249]. Third, as previously noted, girls and women tend to have more serious and lasting outcomes from sport-related concussions. As a result of these three factors, this sociological advance will probably provide a fresh wellspring of female cerebral dysfunction in North America. Cases include Amanda Kessel and Josephine Pucci (Figure 2.16). Both played on the U.S. Women's Olympic hockey team at Sochi. Ms. Pucci retired at age 24. Ms. Kessel retired at age 23. Concussion was the cause in both cases [250].

As in most organized sports, ice hockey games are much more dangerous to the brain than practices for both boys and girls [183]. Contact between players or with the boards is the usual cause of concussion. Fighting accounts for a low proportion of CBIs. Body checking is ostensibly forbidden in girls' and women's ice hockey. This rule probably reduces the rate of concussion, but not necessarily as much as expected. For instance, Emery et al. [251] reported that:

> Among 11- to 12-year-old ice hockey players, playing in a league in which body checking is permitted compared with playing in a league in which body checking is not permitted was associated with a 3-fold increased risk of all … categories of concussion, severe injury, and severe concussion.
>
> (p. 2265)

On the other hand, players with experience in body checking learn to anticipate and brace themselves for contact. As Abbott [183] speculated: "One theory for the higher rate of concussion in women's ice hockey is that the players' nonchecking leagues may not anticipate collisions due to legal body contact

123

and therefore may result in greater forces translated to the athlete" (p. 380). Within Canadian Pee-Wee hockey (age 11–12 years) the overall rate of injuries per 1000 player hours was 1.1 among girls who had yet to menstruate but 4.4 among those who were post-menarche. It seems worth considering that hormonal changes may trigger aggression and injury in this newly popular sport for young girls.

Helmet telemetry has enabled impact monitoring in ice hockey (although evidence exists that measurements with this system are even less accurate than those installed in football helmets) [252]. Consistent with the fact that no threshold exists, concussions and non-concussions are observed across an order of magnitude of linear and rotational forces. These biomechanical studies show that head impacts are most common in player-to-player contact, but the head accelerations are greatest with head-to-ice contact [249]. In one study [253], female collegiate players were concussed at an average linear acceleration of 43.0 **g** – a figure significantly lower than that typically measured for men's concussions – again suggesting sex-related vulnerability.

Persistent brain change associated with playing collegiate ice hockey has been documented in several studies. Koerte et al. [254] found altered diffusivity in the white matter of male players after one season. Changes were most prominent in the corpus callosum, corticospinal tracts, and superior longitudinal fasciculus. Helmer et al. [255] employed susceptibility-weighted MRI to scan men and women players before and after the collegiate season. A "hypointensity burden index" was derived to capture microbleeds. Men (but not women) exhibited significantly greater lesion burden two weeks after concussions. Figure 2.17 illustrates another study: Sasaki et al. [256] recruited 34 college-level ice hockey players – 18 men and 16 women. Among them, 16 had been concussed. Although cognitive scores did not distinguish the concussed group, DTI measures in multiple white-matter regions were significantly different.

These findings exemplify three points the reader will encounter throughout this essay on human CBI:

1. The boundary between brain injury and not brain injury is undefined.
2. Neuropsychological testing is insensitive to a significant proportion of the cerebral dysfunction caused by concussion.
3. Long-lasting brain changes are common after concussion.

In fairness, neuropsychology – like dream interpretation, clinical neurology, and phrenology – played an important historical role in the slow-growing understanding of the relationship between brain and behavior. Since neuropsychological findings fail to reveal the location, chemistry, electrophysiology, metabolism, or genetics of neural function, and since there is little correlation between neuropsychological findings and diagnosis of disease, the limits of neuropsychological inquiry have become clear. Yet this historically interesting enterprise remains useful because paper and pencil or machine-administered psychological to-and-fro better quantifies deficits in artificial constructs such as "visuo-spatial learning" or "speed of information processing" than does psychiatric interview. In the absence of a capable interviewer – for instance, in

settings with inadequate behavioral health care – testing is a cost-efficient way to screen for psychological distress. Testing enhances the objectivity of some behavioral assays thought to correlate with cerebral activity. This, when integrated with observation of biomarkers of such activity, holds promise for clinical–pathological correlation. Moreover, until biomarkers for response bias are found, neuropsychological examination remains a superior approach to detection of ambivalence or complex motives that invalidate tests.

As cognitive neuroscience informs neuropsychology, and as scientists seek better evidence of correlations between psychological pronouncements and biological function, the old paradigm of paper-and-pencil psychological testing is exposed as poorly reflective of neural activity. The prefix "neuro-" for these behavioral tests has become hard to justify. This discovery, however, should not be considered a criticism of this popular stop-gap approach to assessment, pending the development of scientific alternatives.

Karate/Taekwondo/Mixed Martial Arts (MMA)

Being kicked in the head seems an especially uncomfortable form of exercise. Data support this judgment. For instance, Fife et al. [257] instrumented Hybrid II or III crash test dummy heads to detect acceleration in three planes. Resultant linear head accelerations from boxing punches were 71 **g** for a hook punch and 24 **g** for an uppercut. By comparison, acceleration associated with a roundhouse kick was 130 **g** and for a clench axe kick was 162 **g** (Figure 2.18). As shown in Table 2.4, the incidence of concussion in taekwondo is among the highest in all sports. Therefore, although the rates of participation in the United States are modest, the risks are high.

MMA has enjoyed an explosion in popularity over the last 20 years. Hutchinson et al. [259] studied data and video from 844 MMA matches. The knockout incidence was 64 per 1000 AEs, but the technical knockout incidence due to repetitive strikes was even higher, at 95 per 1000 AEs. MMA is too recent an innovation to have generated much empirical data. However, efforts such as the Cleveland Clinic's longitudinal Professional Fighters Brain Health study, which employs 7-T MRI and aims to study more than 600 professional boxers and MMA fighters, are beginning to report findings that should clarify the neurological risks of this new form of recreation [260].

Lacrosse

Lacrosse, like cheerleading and female ice hockey, is a fast-growing sport in the United States. More than 170,000 high school boys and girls were participants in the 2011 season [190, 213]. Lacrosse is a full-contact sport and concussion incidence is relatively high, as reported in Table 2.4. Again, however, these figures are not based on either systematic self-report or objective observation. In the largest study published to date [190], the incidence of CBI among girls playing games was five times the rate during practice; CBI incidence among boys playing games was more than seven times the rate during practice. Rates are about 50% higher among boys than girls – making lacrosse an exception to the rule that girls are more

Diffusion tensor imaging reveals persistent white-matter microstructural abnormalities among concussed hockey players

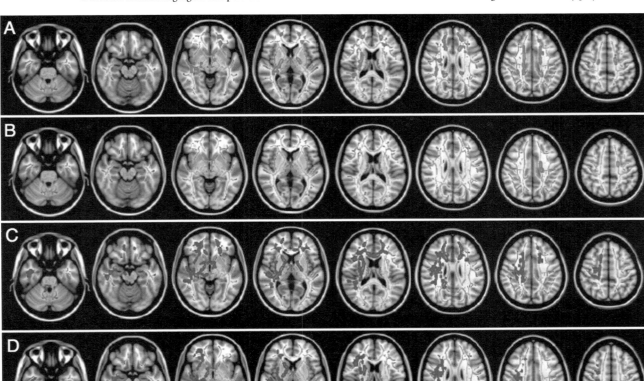

Fig. 2.17 Results of the tract-based spatial statistics analysis showing the clusters of significantly increased fractional anisotropy (A) and axial diffusivity (B) (red to yellow), and decreased radial diffusivity (C) and trace (D) (blue to light blue) for concussed players compared with non-concussed players ($p < 0.05$). Voxels are thickened into local tracts on the fractional anisotropy skeleton (green) and a T1-weighted template image. The left side in each image corresponds to the right hemisphere. [A black and white version of this figure will appear in some formats. For the color version, please refer to the plate section.]

Source: Sasaki et al., 2014 [256] with permission from the American Association of Neurological Surgeons

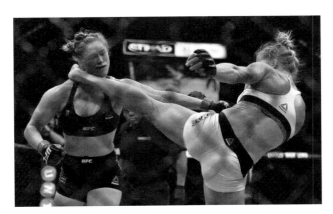

Fig. 2.18 Roundhouse kick causes rapid head rotation and loss of consciousness.

Source: Frankland, 2015 [258] with permission from Paul Crock/AFP/Getty Images

vulnerable in parallel settings. As with other sports that purport to protect girls by outlawing intentional contact, contact nonetheless occurs and is responsible for most concussions. Among both boys and girls, concussions are usually caused by contact with the stick (e.g., in one study 63.8% of concussions among high school girls playing lacrosse were due to contact with "playing apparatus" [190]). The high frequency of concussion and head and facial injuries has precipitated a small movement to equip female lacrosse players with helmets.

Rodeo

Rodeo performance is another very risky sport. "Rough stock" events (bull riding, bareback horse riding, and saddle bronc riding – attempting to remain on a saddled but uncooperative horse) account for most injuries. The event called wild horse racing is also associated with a very high injury density[10]

---

10   For non-cowboys: wild horse racing involves teams of three men, each team attempting to control one horse and move it across a finish line. "Amongst all the chaos, the shankman holds the horse in a position so that the mugger can move up the shank and grab the horse by the halter. The next moment, the rider sets the saddle on the horse and secures it by the quick cinch" [262].

[192, 261]. Estimates of concussion incidence are reported in Table 2.4. However, these numbers are controversial. Meyers and Laurent [193] summarized the concern:

> Reported injuries have included not only a high incidence of concussions, but a substantial incidence of orofacial trauma, similar to other high-collision sports. Isolated and non-isolated skull fractures with intracranial lesions, dentoalveolar trauma, oral and maxillofacial and fractures primarily involving orbital/zygomatic and mandibular regions, avulsed ears, retinal detachment, eye loss and soft tissue damage have been reported.
>
> ([193], p. 823)

It is possible that the proportion of concussions that go unreported among rodeo riders is especially high, since no athletic trainers are observing and no mechanism exists for injury documentation. So, for example, Meyers and Laurent [193] reported a concussion incidence of 3.4/1000 AEs but also reported that head and facial injuries occur 15 times per 1000 rides. Since most head or facial injuries rattle the brain, one suspects underreporting of CBIs. Contact with the ground or "unknown" are the most common mechanisms of rodeo-associated concussions [192].

Rugby

Rugby (aka rugby union) is another full-contact sport involving team efforts to move a ball. It is far more popular elsewhere (such as Australia, New Zealand, the United Kingdom, or South Africa) than in the United States. Girls' and women's rugby began to gain popularity about 15 years ago, but the rate of female participation is not so high (compared, for instance, to women's soccer or ice hockey) as to represent a significant burden on public health as yet. Like other contact sports, the incidence of concussions is unknown but probably high. Rates listed in Table 2.4 suggest that high school boys' rugby is among the most dangerous team sports for the developing brain and professional rugby perhaps exceeds American football in the routine brutality that causes CBIs [194]. Those playing forward are especially prone to concussions. One study compared cognitive function among 124 rugby payers across the age spectrum from high school to adult clubs with 102 non-contact sportsmen. More rugby players than controls had histories of two or more concussions. Visuomotor processing speed (which may be more sensitive to concussion than most conventional neuropsychological tests due to its dependence on white-matter integrity) was inferior among the rugby players.

Skateboarding

The CDC estimates more than 6000 skateboarding-related ED visits for non-fatal TBIs from 2001 to 2009 for ages ≤ 19 years [172]. According to data from the National Trauma Databank [263], TBIs represent a large proportion of skateboard-related injuries: 24.1% among riders less than age 10, 32.6% among riders 10–16 years, and 45.5% among older riders. Across age groups, 11.9% of injuries are due to concussions. Loss of balance and failed attempts at tricks are the most common mechanisms of injuries. Helmets are critical. The odds ratio

for TBIs among helmeted riders was 0.38 compared with those who did not wear a helmet. Unfortunately for their own health, for public health, and for the equanimity of their parents, many adolescent riders decline to wear helmets [264].

Skiing and Snowboarding

Concussions are frequent in skiing and even more frequent in snowboarding, especially among children and adolescents [265–267]. One review estimates that 11% of child skiers under age 14 years and 20% of skiers aged 15–19 years will suffer a head or neck injury each season [266]. Helmets help a lot. In a meta-analysis of 12 studies, the odds ratio for head injury among skiers and snowboarders wearing helmets compared with those without was 0.61–0.65 [268]. As with skateboarding adolescents, the question is compliance.

Soccer

Soccer is the world's most played team sport. Like American football, it involves violent competition over movement of an air bag. According to the FIFA Big Count, 265 million people played soccer and another five million refereed or officiated games during 2006 [269]. Soccer (aka association football) is the dominant sport in Germany, France, the United Kingdom, Italy, Brazil, Russia, Mexico, Spain, Turkey, the Netherlands, Nigeria, and Saudi Arabia. Although rates of participation vary by region and nation, about 4% of the world population plays this game, about 90% of whom are male and 10% female. Twenty-two million of the total are youth players. Thus, in round numbers, about 220 humans play soccer for each one who plays football. For this reason, even if the incidence of concussions and "subconcussive" brain injuries is higher in American football, soccer probably constitutes a massively greater threat to global cerebral health.

Table 2.4 lists several estimates of the incidence of soccer-related CBIs. As with other sports that have recently gained popularity among females, soccer is associated with a higher rate of concussions among high school girls and college women than among opposite-sex coeducational peers. Most concussions are associated with head-to-head contact as two players contend for control of the ball. Ball-to-head (not deliberate heading), elbow-to-head, and ground-to-head contact are also common CBI scenarios.

A question that has preoccupied TBI scholars for several decades is whether deliberate heading of the ball causes brain damage (Figure 2.19). Players head the ball about 6–12 times per game [270]. Forces in heading tend to fall in the range of 10–20 **g**, which is lower than the average force involved in concussions but not so low as to be dismissable. Until recently, investigations were based primarily on pre- and post-season neuropsychological testing – a dated approach that is known to be insensitive to the effects of concussion. (That is, as forthcoming chapters will discuss, few of the paper-and-pencil cognitive tests developed in the 1950s–1970s effectively detect the subtle but persistent brain dysfunction often produced by concussions.) As one would expect, the findings from that early work were inconsistent, with some reports detecting cognitive

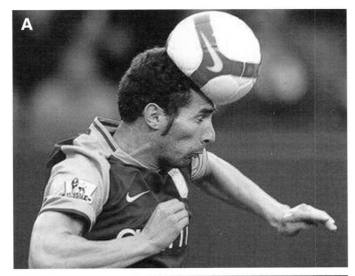

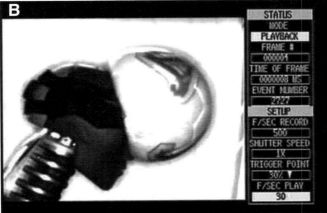

Fig. 2.19 (A) The force of impact between the ball and the player's cranium is directly related to the mass of the ball and the duration of impact (acceleration). A regulation-size and weight ball weighs approximately 0.45 kg, whereas the velocity of the ball can vary considerably. The force of impact causes considerable deformation of the ball as it strikes the head. (B) In biomechanical studies, the force of impact absorbed by the head can be measured directly with a force transducer, and the ball deflection can be measured with high-speed video.

Source: Spiotta et al., 2012 [270] by permission of Oxford University Press

decrements apparently associated with heading [150, 271, 272] and others not [273–275].

Two more objective approaches have recently been applied to the question. First, some fluid measures are regarded as possible biomarkers for brain injury. These include the glial calcium-binding protein, S-100B, and the cytoplasmic enzyme NSE. Stalnacke et al. [276] found that heading exposure in elite male soccer players was associated with elevations of both markers. The same research team reported that headers, falls, and collisions were associated with increases in those two putative biomarkers among elite female soccer players [277]. Yet Zetterberg et al. [278] found that a training session for male amateur players involving repetitive heading did not lead to increased serum S-100B.

The second modern research approach is imaging. Lipton et al. [279], for example, recruited 37 adult amateur soccer

players. By self-report, individuals had headed balls 32–5400 times in the prior 12 months. DTI revealed that players with heading histories above 1800 impacts had inferior memory and reduced fractional anisotropy in three regions of tempero-occipital white matter. Importantly, the results remained significant after controlling for concussion history (Figure 2.20). Forthcoming chapters in this essay will address the open question of what such DTI changes mean. Replication is required prior to conviction. In the meantime, these data support the view that repeatedly heading the soccer ball tends to cause persistent brain change.

Wrestling

According to the National High School Federation of Associations [280], a total of 258,208 boys participated in wrestling in the United States in 2015. That count puts wrestling at the rank of sixth among high school sports. Although the actual incidence of CBIs is not known, Table 2.4 lists some recent estimates. Those may not fully convey the concern. As Myers et al. reported [281]:

> Despite having only the sixth highest average annual participation of boys in high school sports, wrestling is second only to tackle football for frequency of injury in high school athletes. The risk of serious injury is significant in young athletes and includes permanent debilitation from fracture, traumatic brain injury and rarely, death.
> ([281], p. 442)

That study also reported a dramatically higher frequency of injuries among adolescent wrestlers compared with young boys, with 2352 ED visits for head or neck injuries from 2000 to 2006 among those aged 7–11 and 22,169 among those aged 12–17. The increased strength and violence of middle and high school boys may account for this difference. As shown in Table 2.4, college wrestling is probably associated with an even higher frequency of CBIs [123].

Professional wrestling is a different sport. Scripted and at least minimally rehearsed, the sequences of events and outcomes are pre-determined. Incidence figures of concussions are not published, although one might research the evocative term "chair shot" to better understand the cerebral destiny assigned to those redoubtable thespians.

Legal Implication of Sports-Related Concussion

The author cheers and revels in the freedoms of the West. The United States and other democratic countries, despite the intractable problem of inequality, represent gratifying advances over genocidal dictatorships with chattel slavery. It is nonetheless disheartening that sports-related brain injury is denied and covered up. The optimum balance between freedom of action and public health is not immediately obvious. The best way to liberate people to spend their time as they wish and yet support the social good of reciprocal altruism is not self-evident. As a starting point for discussion, the author supports freedom of

Exposure to heading over 12 months is associated with scattered foci of altered fractional anisotropy on diffusion tensor imaging

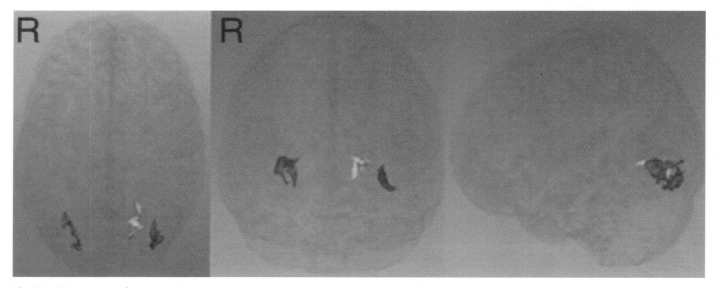

Fig. 2.20 Three regions of interest in the temporo-occipital white matter detected by the initial voxelwise linear regression of estimated prior 12 months of heading on fractional anisotropy, shown as color regions rendered in three-dimensional images and superimposed on T1-weighted axial (left), coronal (middle), and sagittal (right) images from the Montreal Neurological Institute template. [A black and white version of this figure will appear in some formats. For the color version, please refer to the plate section.]

Source: Lipton et al., 2013 [279] with permission by the Radiological Society of North America

religion, speech, and suicide. Therefore, fully informed adults who wish to box, play football, play ice hockey, or jump off cliffs should be free to do so. That having been said, two questions that scream for legal attention are:

1. What does fully informed mean? For instance, if executives of a for-profit corporation willfully lie to their employees about the brain damage they are knowingly producing for the sake of their own personal wealth, is that behavior better understood as socially desirable economic productivity or criminality?

2. How should social services deal with parents who knowingly multiply the risk of lasting brain damage in their children?

There will always be some who insist that childhood participation in violent sports is the sole effective parenting strategy to build character. However, the author has yet to encounter research showing that exposure to likely brain damage is the best route to character, or that mastery of violence is the best route to a peaceful, responsible adulthood. At some point in the coming decades, some U.S. parents may begin to consider these issues.

Prevalence of Concussion-Related Disability

How many persons in the world are currently disabled in some manner and to some degree by post-CBI cerebral problems, whether somatic, cognitive, or psychiatric? This section needs to be short, shy, and candid. For reasons about to be explained in the section on Cost, no useful estimate of prevalence will be published in the foreseeable future.

Cost

It is common to conclude a chapter on the epidemiology of a disease with a comment about cost. The comment is sometimes lyrically composed to alarm, e.g., "This illness costs Western society the equivalent of the gross national product of Denmark each month." Then the author offers a lifeline: "If only 'they' fund the research I recommend, society will save $X billion each year." But the author of the present essay must end the chapter as he began it. Nobody knows.

As an intellectual exercise, try to count up the dollars lost when a 14-year-old boy skateboards without his helmet, suffers a "mild traumatic brain injury," and exhibits a persistent impairment in several aspects of cognitive capacity such as speed of information processing, concentration under stress, and multitasking, and diminished libido due to pituitary dysfunction, as well as various degrees of post-CBI irritability, anxiety, depression, sleep disorder, and intermittent aggression. Clinicians who care for CBI survivors see it again and again. A promising child begins to fail at what used to be easy. A cycle of disadvantage replaces a cycle of advantage. Secure attachments become loose. Friendships dissolve. And each disappointment, frustration, or wound to self-esteem whittles away further at the boy's resilience and identity, increases his vulnerability to stress, and paves the way for an altered life – an inescapable rat-wheel of isolated dysthymia and painful effort with little perceptible progress. Even if he recovers his memory in time, even if his somatic problems of headache, dizziness, and blurred vision are long gone, this hiccup in his life trajectory may have permanent deleterious effects on his familial relationships, school success, work success, romantic success, and parenting. In simple terms: his well-being may be irreversibly degraded. And perhaps (although this remains to be sorted out) he will die early and confused due to accelerated neurodegeneration.

How often does that happen? The next three chapters will answer that question, in so far as the pitiful state of the science permits. How much does that cost? The author dares not even guess. What price a secure sense of self?

Turning to a more conventional analysis of the cost issue, several scholars have attempted to do the math. Olesen et al. [282], for instance, compiled data regarding costs of brain disorders in Europe. They estimated that 3.7 million persons were affected by TBI in 2010, that direct health care costs were €10.106, direct non-medical costs were €3.348, and indirect costs were €19.560 billion. This totaled €33.013 billion. The data, however, do not stratify by severity. The authors specify, "Our approach was prevalence based (in terms of 12-month diagnoses) as most brain disorders are long lasting or chronic and usually incur cost over many years" ([282], p. 156).

This focuses our attention on an irresolvable problem: accurately calculating the cost of disease depends on knowing its *prevalence*. That is, one must know how many people are afflicted by that disease today. Then one can multiply the costs (including acute, subacute, and chronic medical care, lost income, increased utilization of social services, missed life opportunities, depression treatment, broken families, early demise) by that prevalence. Concussion, however, is special. If the concussion minimizers are correct and almost everyone is restored to their exact pre-morbid condition within three months – with no subclinical deleterious impact on quality of life or longevity – then the prevalence is low. But if (as we will show to be the case in Chapter 5) about 30–50% of concussed persons are still struggling fruitlessly toward their pre-morbid baseline at one year or ten years post-CBI, then prevalence is very much higher.

This should not be controversial! Prevalence is hard to know but not impossible to estimate. Three barriers hunker like junk yard rhinoceri on the path to that knowledge:

One: had we simply started prospective longitudinal studies of concussion 50 years ago (when they were first suggested) we would know the spectrum of (extremely individually variable) outcomes according to *type* of PC trouble, *severity* of that type of trouble, and its *duration*, which would enable us to estimate prevalence with authority. For example, had we continued funding the National Children's Study or the historic Framingham Study and followed a large cohort of concussed persons for decades, we would be in a position to say, "Post-concussive depression of a sufficient magnitude to cause clinical dysfunction is expected in about 38% of CBI survivors at six months, 22% of survivors at three years, and 12% of survivors at 20 years post-CBI. Therefore, considering the incidence of concussions, the slope of the recovery curve, and the direct and indirect cost to self, family, and society of suffering from depression, CBI-related depression costs Americans *X* billion dollars each year." We have collectively failed to do any such prospective research.

Two: had we ever conducted a population-based study – for instance, strolling door to door through greater Brussels with a neurologist, neuropsychologist, physiatrist, and psychiatrist to examine everyone and take their concussion histories – we would be in a stronger position to opine regarding the prevalence of CBI-based troubles and likely costs. That modest proposal has yet to be funded.

Three: even if that population-based study had been submitted for publication, reviewers would be justifiably critical. There exists no biomarker permitting us to assay brain injury. One can ask a subject, "are you struggling with irritability and short-term memory and sleep disruption and have you had a concussion?" That does not prove a causal link. This fact should rivet our attention on the immediate highest priority for research: *we need a biomarker*.

Obviously, some approaches to seeking the necessary knowledge are more practical than others. The author understands that "mild traumatic brain injury" has been wrestling through the tiers of diseases to get attention and funding. It has not helped that completely resolvable disputes have riven the brain injury community. It would probably have helped if we had not waited until the 21st century to muster the conceptual maturity to say "TBI severity ratings are not scientific. 'Mild' has no biological meaning. The issue is the public health impact of brain-damaging trauma, the vast majority of which does not kill the victim but often leaves him or her disadvantaged in ways that are inscrutable to the survivor's compatriots." It would probably have helped if we had conducted even one large, controlled, prospective, longitudinal, population-based study that took the trouble to really determine who had been concussed and how it had affected him or her (not another uninformative exercise in paper-and-pencil testing or sophisticated neuropathological analysis with vanishingly little clinical information). If vision is ever harnessed to authority, we would be far closer to a robust and dignified consensus regarding the net health impact of CBIs, instead of wallowing aimlessly, as we do, in the tar pit of scholarly contention.

Conclusion

This completes our comprehensive summary of quantitative epidemiological ignorance. Many numbers have been typed. The author strived mightily to provide the reader with the highest-quality untrustworthy data. The reader is now incomparably qualified to speak with authority about that which is not known. At least, perhaps, a generation of young scholars will be well versed in the deeply entrenched sources of error and the barriers to definitive knowledge in this field. Only when a concerted and impartial effort breaks the logjam of misrepresentation – an event that may require new technology – will the epidemiology of concussion become a legitimate science.

Our next job is to do our best to reconcile the mismatch between the objective empiricism of the laboratory and the subjective empiricism of the clinic. Animal studies using multiple neurobehavioral assays show that concussions are harmful. Clinical studies using paper-and-pencil brain assays imply that concussions are benign. Yet finally, for perhaps the first time in history, sufficient data have been generated to dismiss the distractions of conventional neuropsychology and make progress in the direction of the globally important truth.

References

1. Langlois J, Rutland-Brown W, Thomas K. *Traumatic brain injury in the United States: Emergency department vists, hospitalizations and deaths*. Atlanta, GA: Centers for Disease Control and Prevention, National Center for Injury Prevention and Control, Division of Acute Care, Rehabilitation Research and Disability Prevention, National Center for Injury Prevention and Control, 2004.

2. Giza CC, Hovda DA. The neurometabolic cascade of concussion. *J Athl Train* 2001;36:228–235.

3. Giza CC, Hovda DA. The new neurometabolic cascade of concussion. *Neurosurgery* 2014;75(Suppl 4): S24–S33.

4. Brown AW, Leibson CL, Malec JF, Perkins PK, Diehl NN, Larson DR. Long-term survival after traumatic brain injury: A population-based analysis. *NeuroRehabilitation* 2004;19:37–43.

5. Carroll LJ, Cassidy JD, Holm L, Kraus J, Coronado VG, WHO Collaborating Centre Task Force on Mild Traumatic Brain Injury. Methodological issues and research recommendations for mild traumatic brain injury: The WHO Collaborating Centre Task Force on Mild Traumatic Brain Injury. *J Rehabil Med.* 2004: 113–25.

6. National Center for Injury Prevention and Control. *Report to Congress on mild traumatic brain injury in the United States: Steps to prevent a serious public health problem*. Atlanta, GA: Centers for Disease Control and Prevention, 2003.

7. Kay T, Harrington DE, Adams R, Anderson TJ, Berrol S, Cicerone KD, et al. Definition of mild traumatic brain injury. *J Head Trauma Rehabil* 1993;8:86–87.

8. Levin HS, O'Donnell VM, Grossman RG. The Galveston Orientation and Amnesia Test. A practical scale to assess cognition after head injury. *J Nerv Ment Dis* 1979;167:675–684.

9. Powell GE. Mild traumatic brain injury and postconcussion syndrome: The importance of base rates in diagnosis and clinical formulation. *J Neurol Neurosurg Psychiatry* 2008;79:237.

10. Barker-Collo SL, Feigin VL. Capturing. the spectrum: Suggested standards for conducting population-based traumatic brain injury incidence studies. *Neuroepidemiology* 2009;32:1–3.

11. Powell JM, Ferraro JV, Dikmen SS, Temkin NR, Bell KR. Accuracy of mild traumatic brain injury diagnosis. *Arch Phys Med Rehabil* 2008;89:1550–1557.

12. Faul M, Xu L, Wald MM, Coronado V. *Traumatic brain injury in the United States: Emergency department vists, hospitalizations and deaths 2002–2006*. Atlanta, GA: Centers for Disease Control and Prevention, 2010.

13. Thurman D, Alverson C, Browne D, Dunn K, Guerrero J, Johnson VE, et al. Division of acute care, rehabilitation research, and disability prevention. National Center for Injury Prevention and Control, Centers for Disease Control and Prevention, 1999.

14. Thurman DJ, Sniezek JE, Johnson D, Greenspane A, Smith SM. *Guidelines for surveillance of central nervous system injury*. Atlanta, GA: Centers for Disease Control and Prevention, 1995.

15. Centers for Disease Control and Prevention, National Center for Injury Prevention and Control. *Traumatic brain injury in the United States. A report to Congress*. Atlanta: Centers for Disease Control and Prevention, 1999.

16. Cassidy JD, Carroll LJ, Peloso PM, Borg J, Von Holst H, Holm L, et al. Incidence, risk factors and prevention of mild traumatic brain injury: Results of the WHO Collaborating Centre Task Force on Mild Traumatic Brain Injury. *J Rehabil Med* 2004;28–60.

17. Langlois JA, Kegler SR, Butler JA, Gotsch KE, Johnson RL, Reichard AA, et al. Traumatic brain injury-related hospital discharges. Results from a 14-state surveillance system, 1997. *MMWR Surveill Summ* 2003;52:1–20.

18. Pickelsimer EE, Selassie AW, Gu JK, Langlois JA. A population-based outcomes study of persons hospitalized with traumatic brain injury: Operations of the South Carolina Traumatic Brain Injury Follow-up Registry. *J Head Trauma Rehabil* 2006;21:491–504.

19. Sosin DM, Sniezek JE, Thurman DJ. Incidence of mild and moderate brain injury in the United States, 1991. *Brain Inj* 1996;10:47–54.

20. Crossman J, Bankes M, Bhan A, Crockard HA. The Glasgow Coma Score: Reliable evidence? *Injury* 1998;29:435–437.

21. Gill MR, Reiley DG, Green SM. Interrater reliability of Glasgow Coma Scale scores in the emergency department. *Ann Emerg Med* 2004;43:215–223.

22. Namiki J, Yamazaki M, Funabiki T, Hori S. Inaccuracy and misjudged factors of Glasgow Coma Scale scores when assessed by inexperienced physicians. *Clin Neurol Neurosurg* 2011;113:393–398.

23. Riechers RG, 2nd, Ramage A, Brown W, Kalehua A, Rhee P, Ecklund JM, et al. Physician knowledge of the Glasgow Coma Scale. *J Neurotrauma* 2005;22:1327–1334.

24. Rowley G, Fielding K. Reliability and accuracy of the Glasgow Coma Scale with experienced and inexperienced users. *Lancet* 1991;337:535–538.

25. Teasdale G, Jennett B. Assessment of coma and impaired consciousness. A practical scale. *Lancet* 1974;2:81–84.

26. Berger RP, Dulani T, Adelson PD, Leventhal JM, Richichi R, Kochanek PM. Identification of inflicted traumatic brain injury in well-appearing infants using serum and cerebrospinal markers: A possible screening tool. *Pediatrics* 2006;117: 325–332.

27. Kerr ZY, Register-Mihalik JK, Marshall SW, Evenson KR, Mihalik JP, Guskiewicz KM. Disclosure and non-disclosure of concussion and concussion symptoms in athletes: Review and application of the socio-ecological framework. *Brain Inj* 2014;28:1009–1021.

28. Mccrea M, Hammeke T, Olsen G, Leo P, Guskiewicz K. Unreported concussion in high school football players: Implications for prevention. *Clin J Sport Med* 2004;14:13–17.

29. Register-Mihalik JK, Guskiewicz KM, Mcleod TC, Linnan LA, Mueller FO, Marshall SW. Knowledge, attitude, and concussion-reporting behaviors among high school athletes: A preliminary study. *J Athl Train* 2013;48:645–653.

30. Macciocchi S, Seel RT, Thompson N, Byams R, Bowman B. Spinal cord injury and co-occurring traumatic brain injury: Assessment and incidence. *Arch Phys Med Rehabil* 2008;89:1350–1357.

31. Sharma B, Bradbury C, Mikulis D, Green R. Missed diagnosis of traumatic brain injury in patients with traumatic spinal cord injury. *J Rehabil Med* 2014;46:370–373.

32. Tolonen A, Turkka J, Salonen O, Ahoniemi E, Alaranta H. Traumatic brain injury is under-diagnosed in patients with spinal cord injury. *J Rehabil Med* 2007;39:622–626.

33. Deepika A, Munivenkatappa A, Devi BI, Shukla D. Does isolated traumatic subarachnoid hemorrhage affect outcome in patients with mild traumatic brain injury? *J Head Trauma Rehabil* 2013;28:442–445.

34. Jacobs B, Beems T, Stulemeijer M, Van Vugt AB, Van Der Vliet TM, Borm GF, et al. Outcome prediction in mild traumatic brain

injury: Age and clinical variables are stronger predictors than CT abnormalities. *J Neurotrauma* 2010;27:655–668.

35. Lannsjo M, Backheden M, Johansson U, Af Geijerstam JL, Borg J. Does head CT scan pathology predict outcome after mild traumatic brain injury? *Eur J Neurol* 2013;20:124–129.

36. Lee H, Wintermark M, Gean AD, Ghajar J, Manley GT, Mukherjee P. Focal lesions in acute mild traumatic brain injury and neurocognitive outcome: CT versus 3T MRI. *J Neurotrauma* 2008;25:1049–1056.

37. Yuh EL, Cooper SR, Mukherjee P, Yue JK, Lingsma HF, Gordon WA, et al. Diffusion tensor imaging for outcome prediction in mild traumatic brain injury: A TRACK-TBI study. *J Neurotrauma* 2014;31:1457–1477.

38. Huff JS, Jahar S. Differences in interpretation of cranial computed tomography in ED traumatic brain injury patients by expert neuroradiologists. *Am J Emerg Med* 2014;32:606–608.

39. Laalo JP, Kurki TJ, Sonninen PH, Tenovuo OS. Reliability of diagnosis of traumatic brain injury by computed tomography in the acute phase. *J Neurotrauma* 2009;26:2169–2178.

40. Pape TL, High WM, Jr., St Andre J, Evans C, Smith B, Shandera-Ochsner AL, et al. Diagnostic accuracy studies in mild traumatic brain injury: A systematic review and descriptive analysis of published evidence. *PM R* 2013;5:856–881.

41. Powell GE. Mild traumatic brain injury and postconcussion syndrome: The importance of base rates in diagnosis and clinical formulation. *J Neurol Neurosurg Psychiatry* 2008;79:237.

42. Schootman M, Fuortes LJ. Ambulatory care for traumatic brain injuries in the US, 1995–1997. *Brain Inj* 2000;14:373–381.

43. Bazarian JJ, Veazie P, Mookerjee S, Lerner EB. Accuracy of mild traumatic brain injury case ascertainment using ICD-9 codes. *Acad Emerg Med* 2006;13:31–38.

44. Fife D. Head injury with and without hospital admission: comparisons of incidence and short-term disability. *Am J Public Health* 1987;77:810–812.

45. Sosin DM, Sacks JJ, Webb KW. Pediatric head injuries and deaths from bicycling in the United States. *Pediatrics* 1996;98: 868–870.

46. Boswell JE, Mcerlean M, Verdile VP. Prevalence of traumatic brain injury in an ED population. *Am J Emerg Med* 2002;20:177–180.

47. Anonymous. New concussion survey reveals majority of adults are unable to recognize common concussion symptoms. Available at http://abbott.mediaroom.com/2015-08-24-New-Concussion-Survey-Reveals-Majority-of-Adults-are-Unable-to-Recognize-Common-Concussion-Symptoms.

48. Langlois JA, Rutland-Brown W, Wald MM. The epidemiology and impact of traumatic brain injury: A brief overview. *J Head Trauma Rehabil* 2006;21:375–378.

49. Hanson HR, Pomerantz WJ, Gittelman M. ED utilization trends in sports-related traumatic brain injury. *Pediatrics* 2013;132:e859–e864.

50. Annegers JF, Grabow JD, Kurland LT, Laws ER, Jr. The incidence, causes, and secular trends of head trauma in Olmsted County, Minnesota, 1935–1974. *Neurology* 1980;30:912–919.

51. Centers for Disease Control and Prevention. Rates of TBI-relates emergency department visits by age-group – United States, 2001–2010. www.cdc.gov/traumaticbraininjury/data/rates_ed_byage.html.

52. Centers for Disease Control and Prevention. *Report to Congress on traumatic brain injury in the United States: Epidemiology and rehabilitation.* Atlanta, GA: National Center for Injury Prevention and Control; Division of Unintentional Injury Prevention; 2015. Available at www.cdc.gov/traumaticbraininjury/pdf/tbi_report_to_congress_epi_and_rehab-a.pdf.

53. Dunn K, Thurman D, Alverson C. Appendix B: The epidemiology of traumatic brain injury among children and adolescents. NIH Consensus Development Conference on Rehabilitation of Persons with Traumatic Brain Injury, 1999.

54. Langlois JA, Rutland-Brown W, Thomas KE. The incidence of traumatic brain injury among children in the United States: Differences by race. *J Head Trauma Rehabil* 2005; 20: 229–38.

55. Heffernan DS, Vera RM, Monaghan SF, Thakkar RK, Kozloff MS, Connolly MD, et al. Impact of socioethnic factors on outcomes following traumatic brain injury. *J Trauma* 2011;70:527–534.

56. Meagher AD, Beadles CA, Doorey J, Charles AG. Racial and ethnic disparities in discharge to rehabilitation following traumatic brain injury. *J Neurosurg* 2015;122:595–601.

57. Asemota AO, George BP, Cumpsty-Fowler CJ, Haider AH, Schneider EB. Race and insurance disparities in discharge to rehabilitation for patients with traumatic brain injury. *J Neurotrauma* 2013;30:2057–2065.

58. Linton KF, Kim BJ. Traumatic brain injury as a result of violence in Native American and Black communities spanning from childhood to older adulthood. *Brain Inj* 2014;28:1076–1081.

59. Perrin PB, Krch D, Sutter M, Snipes DJ, Arango-Lasprilla JC, Kolakowsky-Hayner SA, et al. Racial/ethnic disparities in mental health over the first 2 years after traumatic brain injury: A model systems study. *Arch Phys Med Rehabil* 2014;95:2288–2295.

60. Arango-Lasprilla JC, Ketchum JM, Williams K, Kreutzer JS, Marquez De La Plata CD, O'Neil-Pirozzi TM, et al. Racial differences in employment outcomes after traumatic brain injury. *Arch Phys Med Rehabil* 2008;89:988–995.

61. Gary KW, Arango-Lasprilla JC, Ketchum JM, Kreutzer JS, Copolillo A, Novack TA, et al. Racial differences in employment outcome after traumatic brain injury at 1, 2, and 5 years postinjury. *Arch Phys Med Rehabil* 2009;90:1699–1707.

62. Sander AM, Pappadis MR, Davis LC, Clark AN, Evans G, Struchen MA, et al. Relationship of race/ethnicity and income to community integration following traumatic brain injury: Investigation in a non-rehabilitation trauma sample. *NeuroRehabilitation* 2009;24:15–27.

63. Selassie AW, Pickelsimer EE, Frazier L, Jr., Ferguson PL. The effect of insurance status, race, and gender on ED disposition of persons with traumatic brain injury. *Am J Emerg Med* 2004;22:465–473.

64. Dismuke CE, Gebregziabher M, Yeager D, Egede LE. Racial/ethnic differences in combat- and non-combat-associated traumatic brain injury severity in the Veterans Health Administration: 2004–2010. *Am J Public Health* 2015;105:1696–1702.

65. Centers for Disease Control and Prevention. Percent distributions of TBI-related emergency department visits by age group and injury mechanism – United States, 2006–2010. www.cdc.gov/traumaticbraininjury/data/dist_ed.html.

66. Cobb S, Battin B. Second-impact syndrome. *J Sch Nurs* 2004;20:262–267.

67. Gronwall D, Wrightson P. Cumulative effect of concussion. *Lancet* 1975;2:995–997.

68. Tavazzi B, Vagnozzi R, Signoretti S, Amorini AM, Belli A, Cimatti M, et al. Temporal window of metabolic brain vulnerability to concussions: Oxidative and nitrosative stresses – Part II. *Neurosurgery* 2007;61:390–395; discussion 395–396.

69. Vagnozzi R, Signoretti S, Tavazzi B, Cimatti M, Amorini AM, Donzelli S, et al. Hypothesis of the postconcussive vulnerable brain: Experimental evidence of its metabolic occurrence. *Neurosurgery* 2005;57:164–171; discussion 164–171.

70. Vagnozzi R, Tavazzi B, Signoretti S, Amorini AM, Belli A, Cimatti M, et al. Temporal window of metabolic brain vulnerability

to concussions: Mitochondrial-related impairment – Part I. *Neurosurgery* 2007;61:379–388; discussion 388–389.

71. Weinstein E, Turner M, Kuzma BB, Feuer H. Second impact syndrome in football: New imaging and insights into a rare and devastating condition. *J Neurosurg Pediatr* 2013;11:331–334.

72. Jones E, Fear NT, Wessely S. Shell shock and mild traumatic brain injury: A historical review. *Am J Psychiatry* 2007;164:1641–1645.

73. Myers C. A contribution to the study of shellshock. Being an account of the cases of loss of memory, vision, smell and taste admitted to the Duchess of Westminster's War Hospital, Le Touquet. *Lancet* 1915;185:316–320.

74. Mott FW. The microscopic examination of the brains of two men dead of commotio cerebri (shell shock) without visible external injury. *Br Med J* 1917;2:612–615.

75. Macleod AD. Shell shock, Gordon Holmes and the Great War. *J R Soc Med* 2004;97:86–89.

76. Turner W. Remarks on cases of nervous and mental shock. *BMJ* 1915;833–835.

77. *Report of the War Office Committee of Enquiry into "Shellshock".* London: HMSO, 1922.

78. Lew HL, Poole JH, Alvarez S, Moore W. Soldiers with occult traumatic brain injury. *Am J Phys Med Rehabil* 2005;84:393–398.

79. Okie S. Traumatic brain injury in the war zone. *N Engl J Med* 2005;352:2043–2047.

80. Owens BD, Kragh JF, Jr., Wenke JC, Macaitis J, Wade CE, Holcomb JB. Combat wounds in operation Iraqi Freedom and operation Enduring Freedom. *J Trauma* 2008;64:295–299.

81. Tanielian TL, Jaycox L. *Invisible wounds of war: Psychological and cognitive injuries, their consequences, and services to assist recovery.* Santa Monica, CA: Rand, 2008.

82. Bagalman E. *Health care for veterans: Traumatic brain injury.* Washington, DC: Congressional Research Service, 2015.

83. Centers for Disease Control and Prevention (CDC), National Institutes of Health (NIH), Department of Defense (DoD), Department of Veterans Affairs (VA). Report to Congress on traumatic brain injury in the United States: Understanding the public health problem among current and former military personnel. Centers for Disease Control and Prevention (CDC), National Institutes of Health (NIH), Department of Defense (DoD), Department of Veterans Affairs (VA), 2013.

84. Wilk JE, Herrell RK, Wynn GH, Riviere LA, Hoge CW. Mild traumatic brain injury (concussion), posttraumatic stress disorder, and depression in U.S. soldiers involved in combat deployments: Association with postdeployment symptoms. *Psychosom Med* 2012;74:249–257.

85. Hoge CW, Castro CA, Messer SC, Mcgurk D, Cotting DI, Koffman RL. Combat duty in Iraq and Afghanistan, mental health problems, and barriers to care. *N Engl J Med* 2004;351:13–22.

86. Garvey Wilson AL, Hoge CW, Mcgurk D, Thomas JL, Castro CA. Stability of combat exposure recall in Operation Iraqi Freedom veterans. *Ann Epidemiol* 2010;20:939–947.

87. Brenner LA, Ladley-O'Brien SE, Harwood JE, Filley CM, Kelly JP, Homaifar BY, et al. An exploratory study of neuroimaging, neurologic, and neuropsychological findings in veterans with traumatic brain injury and/or posttraumatic stress disorder. *Mil Med* 2009;174:347–352.

88. Bryant RA. Posttraumatic stress disorder and traumatic brain injury: Can they co-exist? *Clin Psychol Rev* 2001;21:931–948.

89. Sayer NA, Rettmann NA, Carlson KF, Bernardy N, Sigford BJ, Hamblen JL, et al. Veterans with history of mild traumatic brain injury and posttraumatic stress disorder: Challenges from provider perspective. *J Rehabil Res Dev* 2009;46:703–716.

90. Stein MB, McAllister TW. Exploring the convergence of posttraumatic stress disorder and mild traumatic brain injury. *Am J Psychiatry* 2009;166:768–776.

91. Tanev KS, Pentel KZ, Kredlow MA, Charney ME. PTSD and TBI co-morbidity: Scope, clinical presentation and treatment options. *Brain Inj* 2014;28:261–270.

92. Vanderploeg RD, Belanger HG, Curtiss G. Mild traumatic brain injury and posttraumatic stress disorder and their associations with health symptoms. *Arch Phys Med Rehabil* 2009;90:1084–1093.

93. Lew HL, Vanderploeg RD, Moore DF, Schwab K, Friedman L, Yesavage J, et al. Overlap of mild TBI and mental health conditions in returning OIF/OEF service members and veterans. *J Rehabil Res Dev* 2008;45:xi–xvi.

94. Sayer NA. Traumatic brain injury and its neuropsychiatric sequelae in war veterans. *Annu Rev Med* 2012;63:405–419.

95. Schneiderman AI, Braver ER, Kang HK. Understanding sequelae of injury mechanisms and mild traumatic brain injury incurred during the conflicts in Iraq and Afghanistan: Persistent postconcussive symptoms and posttraumatic stress disorder. *Am J Epidemiol* 2008;167:1446–1452.

96. Brenner LA, Vanderploe RD, Terrio H. Assessment and diagnosis of mild traumatic brain injury, posttraumatic stress disorder, and other polytrauma conditions: Burden of adversity hypothesis. *Rehab Psychol* 2009;54:239–246.

97. Belanger HG, Proctor-Weber Z, Kretzmer T, Kim M, French LM, Vanderploeg RD. Symptom complaints following reports of blast versus non-blast mild TBI: Does mechanism of injury matter? *Clin Neuropsychol* 2011;25:702–715.

98. Sbordone RJ, Liter JC. Mild traumatic brain injury does not produce post-traumatic stress disorder. *Brain Inj* 1995;9: 405–412.

99. Sbordone RJ, Ruff RM. Re-examination of the controversial coexistence of traumatic brain injury and posttraumatic stress disorder: Misdiagnosis and self-report measures. *Psychol Inj Law* 2010;3:63–76.

100. Sumpter RE, McMillan TM. Misdiagnosis of post-traumatic stress disorder following severe traumatic brain injury. *Br J Psychiatry* 2005;186:423–426.

101. Mayou R, Bryant B, Duthie R. Psychiatric consequences of road traffic accidents. *BMJ* 1993;307:647–651.

102. Middleboe T, Andersen HS, Birket-Smith M, Friis ML. Minor head injury: Impact on general health after 1 year. A prospective follow-up study. *Acta Neurol Scand* 1992;85:5–9.

103. Warden DL, Labbate LA, Salazar AM, Nelson R, Sheley E, Staudenmeier J, et al. Posttraumatic stress disorder in patients with traumatic brain injury and amnesia for the event? *J Neuropsychiatry Clin Neurosci* 1997;9:18–22.

104. Bryant RA, Harvey AG. The influence of traumatic brain injury on acute stress disorder and post-traumatic stress disorder following motor vehicle accidents. *Brain Inj* 1999;13:15–22.

105. Gil S, Caspi Y, Ben-Ari IZ, Koren D, Klein E. Does memory of a traumatic event increase the risk for posttraumatic stress disorder in patients with traumatic brain injury? A prospective study. *Am J Psychiatry* 2005;162:963–969.

106. Bryant RA, Creamer M, O'Donnell M, Silove D, Clark CR, Mcfarlane AC. Post-traumatic amnesia and the nature of posttraumatic stress disorder after mild traumatic brain injury. *J Int Neuropsychol Soc* 2009;15:862–867.

107. Carlson KF, Kehle SM, Meis LA, Greer N, Macdonald R, Rutks I, et al. Prevalence, assessment, and treatment of mild traumatic brain injury and posttraumatic stress disorder: A systematic review of the evidence. *J Head Trauma Rehabil* 2011;26:103–115.

108. Betthauser LM, Bahraini N, Krengel MH, Brenner LA. Self-report measures to identify post traumatic stress disorder and/or mild traumatic brain injury and associated symptoms in military veterans of Operation Enduring Freedom (OEF)/Operation Iraqi Freedom (OIF). *Neuropsychol Rev* 2012;22:35–53.

109. Feinstein A, Hershkop S, Ouchterlony D, Jardine A, Mccullagh S. Posttraumatic amnesia and recall of a traumatic event following traumatic brain injury. *J Neuropsychiatry Clin Neurosci* 2002;14:25–30.

110. Harvey AG, Brewin CR, Jones C, Kopelman MD. Coexistence of posttraumatic stress disorder and traumatic brain injury: Towards a resolution of the paradox. *J Int Neuropsychol Soc* 2003;9:663–676.

111. Hickling EJ, Gillen R, Blanchard EB, Buckley T, Taylor A. Traumatic brain injury and posttraumatic stress disorder: A preliminary investigation of neuropsychological test results in PTSD secondary to motor vehicle accidents. *Brain Inj* 1998;12:265–274.

112. Kennedy JE, Jaffee MS, Leskin GA, Stokes JW, Leal FO, Fitzpatrick PJ. Posttraumatic stress disorder and posttraumatic stress disorder-like symptoms and mild traumatic brain injury. *J Rehabil Res Dev* 2007;44:895–920.

113. Lew HL, Poole JH, Vanderploeg RD, Goodrich GL, Dekelboum S, Guillory SB, et al. Program development and defining characteristics of returning military in a VA polytrauma network site. *J Rehabil Res Dev* 2007;44:1027–1034.

114. Mayou RA, Black J, Bryant B. Unconsciousness, amnesia and psychiatric symptoms following road traffic accident injury. *Br J Psychiatry* 2000;177:540–545.

115. Ohry A, Rattok J, Solomon Z. Post-traumatic stress disorder in brain injury patients. *Brain Inj* 1996;10:687–695.

116. Hoge CW, Mcgurk D, Thomas JL, Cox AL, Engel CC, Castro CA. Mild traumatic brain injury in U.S. soldiers returning from Iraq. *N Engl J Med* 2008;358:453–463.

117. King NS. PTSD and traumatic brain injury: Folklore and fact? *Brain Inj* 2008;22:1–5.

118. Bryant RA. Disentangling mild traumatic brain injury and stress reactions. *N Engl J Med* 2008;358:525–527.

119. Chen Y, Huang W, Constantini S. Concepts and strategies for clinical management of blast-induced traumatic brain injury and posttraumatic stress disorder. *J Neuropsychiatry Clin Neurosci* 2013;25:103–110.

120. Toth C. The epidemiology of injuries to the nervous system resulting from sport and recreation. *Neurol Clin* 2008;26:1–31, vii.

121. Daneshvar DH, Nowinski CJ, Mckee AC, Cantu RC. The epidemiology of sport-related concussion. *Clin Sports Med* 2011;30:1–17, vii.

122. Pfister T, Pfister K, Hagel B, Ghali WA, Ronksley PE. The incidence of concussion in youth sports: A systematic review and meta-analysis. *Br J Sports Med* 2016;50:292–297.

123. Zuckerman SL, Kerr ZY, Yengo-Kahn A, Wasserman E, Covassin T, Solomon GS. Epidemiology of sports-related concussion in NCAA athletes from 2009–2010 to 2013–2014: Incidence, recurrence, and mechanisms. *Am J Sports Med* 2015;43:2654–2662.

124. Delaney JS, Al-Kashmiri A, Drummond R, Correa JA. The effect of protective headgear on head injuries and concussions in adolescent football (soccer) players. *Br J Sports Med* 2008;42:110–115; discussion 115.

125. Delaney JS, Lacroix VJ, Leclerc S, Johnston KM. Concussions during the 1997 Canadian Football League season. *Clin J Sport Med* 2000;10:9–14.

126. Gerberich SG, Priest JD, Boen JR, Straub CP, Maxwell RE. Concussion incidences and severity in secondary school varsity football players. *Am J Public Health* 1983;73:1370–1375.

127. Kaut KP, Depompei R, Kerr J, Congeni J. Reports of head injury and symptom knowledge among college athletes: Implications for assessment and educational intervention. *Clin J Sport Med* 2003;13:213–221.

128. Meehan WP, 3rd, Bachur RG. Sport-related concussion. *Pediatrics* 2009;123:114–123.

129. Williamson IJ, Goodman D. Converging evidence for the under-reporting of concussions in youth ice hockey. *Br J Sports Med* 2006;40:128–132; discussion 128–132.

130. Rowson S, Duma SM. Brain injury prediction: Assessing the combined probability of concussion using linear and rotational head acceleration. *Ann Biomed Eng* 2013;41:873–882.

131. Buzzini SR, Guskiewicz KM. Sport-related concussion in the young athlete. *Curr Opin Pediatr* 2006;18:376–382.

132. Valovich McLeod TC, Bay RC, Heil J, Mcveigh SD. Identification of sport and recreational activity concussion history through the preparticipation screening and a symptom survey in young athletes. *Clin J Sport Med* 2008;18:235–240.

133. Delaney JS, Lacroix VJ, Leclerc S, Johnston KM. Concussions among university football and soccer players. *Clin J Sport Med* 2002;12:331–338.

134. Kerr ZY, Hayden R, Dompier TP, Cohen R. Association of equipment worn and concussion injury rates in National Collegiate Athletic Association football practices: 2004–2005 to 2008–2009 academic years. *Am J Sports Med* 2015;43:1134–1141.

135. Buckley TA, Burdette G, Kelly K. Concussion-management practice patterns of National Collegiate Athletic Association division II and III athletic trainers: How the other half lives. *J Athl Train* 2015;50:879–888.

136. TopEnd Sports. Ultimate list of the world's most popular sports. Available at: www.topendsports.com/world/lists/popular-sport/final.htm.

137. National Council of Youth Sports. *Report on trends and participation. NCYS membership survey – 2008 edition.* Stuart, FL: National Council of Youth Sports, 2008.

138. Centers for Disease Control and Prevention. Behavioral Risk Factor Surveillance System (BRFSS) historical questions. Nutrition, physical activity, and obesity data portal. Available at: https://chronicdata.cdc.gov/browse?category=Nutrition%2C+Physical+Activity%2C+and+Obesity

139. Prevention CFDCA. *Behavioral risk factor surveillance system: Exercise.* 2006.

140. Riffkin R. So far in 2015, more Americans exercising frequently. 2015. www.gallup.com/poll/184403/far-2015-americans-exercising-frequently.aspx.

141. Physical Activity Council. *Participation report.* 2017. Available at www.physicalactivitycouncil.com/PDFs/current.pdf.

142. Collins MW, Iverson GL, Lovell MR, Mckeag DB, Norwig J, Maroon J. On-field predictors of neuropsychological and symptom deficit following sports-related concussion. *Clin J Sport Med* 2003;13:222–229.

143. Schulz MR, Marshall SW, Mueller FO, Yang J, Weaver NL, Kalsbeek WD, et al. Incidence and risk factors for concussion in high school athletes, North Carolina, 1996–1999. *Am J Epidemiol* 2004;160:937–944.

144. National Center for Injury Prevention and Control. CDC injury research agenda, 2009–2018. 2009. Atlanta, GA: U.S. Department of Health and Human Services. Centers for Disease Control and Prevention. Available at: https://stacks.cdc.gov/view/cdc/21769.

145. Jinguji TM, Krabak BJ, Satchell EK. Epidemiology of youth sports concussion. *Phys Med Rehabil Clin N Am* 2011;22:565–575, vii.

146. Grady MF. Concussion in the adolescent athlete. *Curr Probl Pediatr Adolesc Health Care* 2010;40:154–169.

147. Lovell MR, Collins MW, Iverson GL, Johnston KM, Bradley JP. Grade 1 or "ding" concussions in high school athletes. *Am J Sports Med* 2004;32:47–54.

148. Mcclincy MP, Lovell MR, Pardini J, Collins MW, Spore MK. Recovery from sports concussion in high school and collegiate athletes. *Brain Inj* 2006;20:33–39.

149. Sim A, Terryberry-Spohr L, Wilson KR. Prolonged recovery of memory functioning after mild traumatic brain injury in adolescent athletes. *J Neurosurg* 2008;108:511–516.

150. Webbe FM, Ochs SR. Recency and frequency of soccer heading interact to decrease neurocognitive performance. *Appl Neuropsychol* 2003;10:31–41.

151. Field M, Collins MW, Lovell MR, Maroon J. Does age play a role in recovery from sports-related concussion? A comparison of high school and collegiate athletes. *J Pediatr* 2003;142:546–553.

152. Makdissi M, Davis G, Jordan B, Patricios J, Purcell L, Putukian M. Revisiting the modifiers: How should the evaluation and management of acute concussions differ in specific groups? *Br J Sports Med* 2013;47:314–320.

153. Covassin T, Elbin RJ, Harris W, Parker T, Kontos A. The role of age and sex in symptoms, neurocognitive performance, and postural stability in athletes after concussion. *Am J Sports Med.* 2012;40:1303–1312.

154. Lee YM, Odom MJ, Zuckerman SL, Solomon GS, Sills AK. Does age affect symptom recovery after sports-related concussion? A study of high school and college athletes. *J Neurosurg Pediatr* 2013;12:537–544.

155. Gessel LM, Fields SK, Collins CL, Dick RW, Comstock RD. Concussions among United States high school and collegiate athletes. *J Athl Train* 2007;42:495–503.

156. Foley C, Gregory A, Solomon G. Young age as a modifying factor in sports concussion management: What is the evidence? *Curr Sports Med Rep* 2014;13:390–394.

157. McDonald JW, Johnston MV. Physiological and pathophysiological roles of excitatory amino acids during central nervous system development. *Brain Res Brain Res Rev* 1990;15:41–70.

158. Fan P, Yamauchi T, Noble LJ, Ferriero DM. Age-dependent differences in glutathione peroxidase activity after traumatic brain injury. *J Neurotrauma* 2003;20:437–445.

159. Covassin T, Swanik CB, Sachs ML. Sex differences and the incidence of concussions among collegiate athletes. *J Athl Train* 2003;38:238–244.

160. Dick RW. Is there a gender difference in concussion incidence and outcomes? *Br J Sports Med* 2009;43(Suppl 1):146–150.

161. Powell JW, Barber-Foss KD. Traumatic brain injury in high school athletes. *JAMA* 1999;282:958–963.

162. Broshek DK, Kaushik T, Freeman JR, Erlanger D, Webbe F, Barth JT. Sex differences in outcome following sports-related concussion. *J Neurosurg* 2005;102:856–863.

163. Covassin T, Schatz P, Swanik CB. Sex differences in neuropsychological function and post-concussion symptoms of concussed collegiate athletes. *Neurosurgery* 2007;61:345–350; discussion 350–351.

164. Covassin T, Swanik CB, Sachs M, Kendrick Z, Schatz P, Zillmer E, et al. Sex differences in baseline neuropsychological function and concussion symptoms of collegiate athletes. *Br J Sports Med* 2006;40:923–927; discussion 927.

165. Zuckerman SL, Apple RP, Odom MJ, Lee YM, Solomon GS, Sills AK. Effect of sex on symptoms and return to baseline in sport-related concussion. *J Neurosurg Pediatr* 2014;13:72–81.

166. Didi-Huberman G. *Invention of hysteria: Charcot and the photographic iconography of the Salpêtrière.* Cambridge, MA: MIT Press, 2003.

167. Gomes Mda M, Engelhardt E. Hysteria to conversion disorders: Babinski's contributions. *Arq Neuropsiquiatr* 2014;72: 318–321.

168. Micale MS. Charcot and *Les névroses traumatiques*: scientific and historical reflections. *J Hist Neurosci* 1995;4:101–119.

169. Wunderle K, Hoeger KM, Wasserman E, Bazarian JJ. Menstrual phase as predictor of outcome after mild traumatic brain injury in women. *J Head Trauma Rehabil* 2014;29:E1–E8.

170. Hsu HL, Chen DY, Tseng YC, Kuo YS, Huang YL, Chiu WT, et al. Sex differences in working memory after mild traumatic brain injury: A functional MR imaging study. *Radiology* 2015;276:828–835.

171. Hootman JM, Dick R, Agel J. Epidemiology of collegiate injuries for 15 sports: Summary and recommendations for injury prevention initiatives. *J Athl Train* 2007;42:311–319.

172. Gilchrist J. Nonfatal traumatic brain injuries related to sports and recreation activities among persons aged≤ 19 years – United States, 2001–2009. *MMWR Morb Mortal Wkly Rep* 2011;60:1337–1342.

173. Lincoln AE, Caswell SV, Almquist JL, Dunn RE, Norris JB, Hinton RY. Trends in concussion incidence in high school sports: A prospective 11-year study. *Am J Sports Med* 2011;39:958–963.

174. Marar M, Mcilvain NM, Fields SK, Comstock RD. Epidemiology of concussions among United States high school athletes in 20 sports. *Am J Sports Med* 2012;40:747–755.

175. Green GA, Pollack KM, D'Angelo J, Schickendantz MS, Caplinger R, Weber K, et al. Mild traumatic brain injury in major and minor league baseball players. *Am J Sports Med* 2015;43: 1118–1126.

176. Bledsoe GH, Li G, Levy F. Injury risk in professional boxing. *South Med J* 2005;98:994–998.

177. Shields BJ, Smith GA. Cheerleading-related injuries in the United States: A prospective surveillance study. *J Athl Train* 2009;44:567–577.

178. Kontos AP, Elbin RJ, Fazio-Sumrock VC, Burkhart S, Swindell H, Maroon J, et al. Incidence of sports-related concussion among youth football players aged 8–12 years. *J Pediatr* 2013;163:717–720.

179. Koh JO, Cassidy JD, Watkinson EJ. Incidence of concussion in contact sports: A systematic review of the evidence. *Brain Inj* 2003;17:901–917.

180. Pellman EJ, Powell JW, Viano DC, Casson IR, Tucker AM, Feuer H, et al. Concussion in professional football: Epidemiological features of game injuries and review of the literature – Part 3. *Neurosurgery* 2004;54:81–94; discussion 94–96.

181. Marshall SW, Covassin T, Dick R, Nassar LG, Agel J. Descriptive epidemiology of collegiate women's gymnastics injuries: National Collegiate Athletic Association Injury Surveillance System, 1988–1989 through 2003–2004. *J Athl Train* 2007;42:234–240.

182. Decloe MD, Meeuwisse WH, Hagel BE, Emery CA. Injury rates, types, mechanisms and risk factors in female youth ice hockey. *Br J Sports Med* 2014;48:51–56.

183. Abbott K. Injuries in women's ice hockey: Special considerations. *Curr Sports Med Rep* 2014;13:377–382.

184. Tommasone BA, Valovich McLeod TC. Contact sport concussion incidence. *J Athl Train* 2006;41:470–472.

185. Echlin PS, Tator CH, Cusimano MD, Cantu RC, Taunton JE, Upshur RE, et al. A prospective study of physician-observed concussions during junior ice hockey: Implications for incidence rates. *Neurosurg Focus* 2010;29:E4.

186. Agel J, Dick R, Nelson B, Marshall SW, Dompier TP. Descriptive epidemiology of collegiate women's ice hockey injuries: National Collegiate Athletic Association Injury Surveillance System, 2000–2001 through 2003–2004. *J Athl Train* 2007;42:249–254.

187. Echlin PS, Skopelja EN, Worsley R, Dadachanji SB, Lloyd-Smith DR, Taunton JA, et al. A prospective study of physician-observed concussion during a varsity university ice hockey season: Incidence and neuropsychological changes. Part 2 of 4. *Neurosurg Focus* 2012;33(E2): 1–11.

188. Dryden DM, Francescutti LH, Rowe BH, Spence JC, Voaklander DC. Epidemiology of women's recreational ice hockey injuries. *Med Sci Sports Exerc* 2000;32:1378–1383.

189. Hinton RY, Lincoln AE, Almquist JL, Douoguih WA, Sharma KM. Epidemiology of lacrosse injuries in high school-aged

girls and boys: A 3-year prospective study. *Am J Sports Med* 2005;33:1305–1314.

190. Xiang J, Collins CL, Liu D, McKenzie LB, Comstock RD. Lacrosse injuries among high school boys and girls in the United States: Academic years 2008–2009 through 2011–2012. *Am J Sports Med* 2014;42:2082–2088.

191. Dick R, Lincoln AE, Agel J, Carter EA, Marshall SW, Hinton RY. Descriptive epidemiology of collegiate women's lacrosse injuries: National Collegiate Athletic Association Injury Surveillance System, 1988–1989 through 2003–2004. *J Athl Train* 2007;42:262–269.

192. Butterwick DJ, Hagel B, Nelson DS, Lefave MR, Meeuwisse WH. Epidemiologic analysis of injury in five years of Canadian professional rodeo. *Am J Sports Med* 2002;30:193–198.

193. Meyers MC, Laurent CM, Jr. The rodeo athlete: Injuries – Part II. *Sports Med* 2010;40:817–839.

194. Marshall SW, Spencer RJ. Concussion in rugby: The hidden epidemic. *J Athl Train* 2001;36:334–338.

195. Marshall SW, Hamstra-Wright KL, Dick R, Grove KA, Agel J. Descriptive epidemiology of collegiate women's softball injuries: National Collegiate Athletic Association Injury Surveillance System, 1988–1989 through 2003–2004. *J Athl Train* 2007;42:286–294.

196. Pieter W, Zemper ED. Head and neck injuries in young taekwondo athletes. *J Sports Med Phys Fitness* 1999;39:147–153.

197. Larson AN, Mcintosh AL. The epidemiology of injury in ATV and motocross sports. *Med Sport Sci* 2012;58:158–172.

198. Luo TD, Clarke MJ, Zimmerman AK, Quinn M, Daniels DJ, Mcintosh AL. Concussion symptoms in youth motocross riders: A prospective, observational study. *J Neurosurg Pediatr* 2015;15:255–260.

199. Wasserman EB, Abar B, Shah MN, Wasserman D, Bazarian JJ. Concussions are associated with decreased batting performance among major league baseball players. *Am J Sports Med* 2015;43:1127–1133.

200. Keeney T. Pacquiao vs. Algieri results: Winner, recap and prize money split. 2014. Available at http://bleacherreport.com/articles/2277216-pacquiao-vs-algieri-results-winner-recap-and-prize-money-split.

201. Forstl H, Haass C, Hemmer B, Meyer B, Halle M. Boxing-acute complications and late sequelae: From concussion to dementia. *Dtsch Arztebl Int* 2010;107:835–839.

202. Jordan BD, Relkin NR, Ravdin LD, Jacobs AR, Bennett A, Gandy S. Apolipoprotein E epsilon4 associated with chronic traumatic brain injury in boxing. *JAMA* 1997;278:136–140.

203. Bianco M, Pannozzo A, Fabbricatore C, Sanna N, Moscetti M, Palmieri V, et al. Medical survey of female boxing in Italy in 2002–2003. *Br J Sports Med* 2005;39:532–536.

204. Bianco M, Sanna N, Bucari S, Fabiano C, Palmieri V, Zeppilli P. Female boxing in Italy: 2002–2007 report. *Br J Sports Med* 2011;45:563–570.

205. Statista. Number of participants in cheerleading in the United States from 2006 to 2013 (in millions). www.statista.com/statistics/191651/participants-in-cheerleading-in-the-us-since-2006/.

206. Anonymous. Cheerleader continues cheering after breaking neck. ESPN/Associated Press photo, March 6, 2006. Available at www.espn.com/mens-college-basketball/news/story?id=2356442.

207. Schulz MR, Marshall SW, Yang J, Mueller FO, Weaver NL, Bowling JM. A prospective cohort study of injury incidence and risk factors in North Carolina high school competitive cheerleaders. *Am J Sports Med* 2004;32:396–405.

208. Shields BJ, Smith GA. Epidemiology of cheerleading fall-related injuries in the United States. *J Athl Train* 2009;44:578–585.

209. Shields BJ, Fernandez SA, Smith GA. Epidemiology of cheerleading stunt-related injuries in the United States. *J Athl Train* 2009;44:586–594.

210. Labella CR, Mjaanes J, Fitness COSMA. Cheerleading injuries: Epidemiology and recommendations for prevention. *Pediatrics* 2012;130:966–971.

211. Archer P, Mallonee S, Lantis S. Horseback-riding-associated traumatic brain injuries – Oklahoma, 1992–1994. From the Centers for Disease Control and Prevention. *JAMA* 1996;275:1072.

212. Wall SE, Williams WH, Cartwright-Hatton S, Kelly TP, Murray J, Murray M, et al. Neuropsychological dysfunction following repeat concussions in jockeys. *J Neurol Neurosurg Psychiatry* 2006;77:518–520.

213. National Federation of State High School Associations. High school athletics participation survey. 2011–2012. www.nfhs.org/content.aspx?id=3282.

214. Bushman BJ, Anderson CA. Comfortably numb: Desensitizing effects of violent media on helping others. *Psychol Sci* 2009;20:273–277.

215. Carnagey NL, Anderson CA, Bushman BJ. The effect of video game violence on physiological desensitization to real-life violence. *J Exp Soc Psychol* 2007;43:489–496.

216. Rhoden W. Numb to violence? Fans, maybe, but not players. *N Y Times* 2014; January 21.

217. Thomas MH, Horton RW, Lippincott EC, Drabman RS. Desensitization to portrayals of real-life aggression as a function of exposure to television violence. *J Pers Soc Psychol* 1977;35:450–458.

218. Kain DJ. It's just a concussion: The National Football League's denial of a casual link between multiple concussions and later-life cognitive decline. *Rutgers LJ* 2008;40:697.

219. Stern, Declaration of Robert A, Civil action no. 2:14-cv-00029-AB.

220. Almond S. The NFL gets off easy in concussion settlement. *Boston Globe* 2014; June 27.

221. Giliberti V, Osnato M. Postconcussion neurosis-traumatic encephalitis: A conception of postconcussion phenomena. *Arch Neurol Psychiatry* 1927;18:181.

222. Martland HS. Punch drunk. *JAMA* 1928;91:1103–1107.

223. Centers for Disease Control and Prevention. U.S. Public Health Service syphilis study at Tuskegee. 2017. Available at www.cdc.gov/tuskegee/timeline.htm.

224. Pellman EJ, Viano DC, Tucker AM, Casson IR, Committee on Mild Traumatic Brain Injury NFL. Concussion in professional football: Location and direction of helmet impacts – Part 2. *Neurosurgery* 2003;53:1328–1340; discussion 1340–1341.

225. Pellman EJ, Viano DC, Tucker AM, Casson IR, Waeckerle JF. Concussion in professional football: Reconstruction of game impacts and injuries. *Neurosurgery* 2003;53:799–812; discussion 812–814.

226. Zhang L, Yang KH, King AI. A proposed injury threshold for mild traumatic brain injury. *J Biomech Eng* 2004;126:226–236.

227. Funk JR, Duma SM, Manoogian SJ, Rowson S. Biomechanical risk estimates for mild traumatic brain injury. *Annu Proc Assoc Adv Automot Med* 2007;51:343–361.

228. Beckwith JG, Greenwald RM, Chu JJ. Measuring head kinematics in football: Correlation between the head impact telemetry system and Hybrid III headform. *Ann Biomed Eng* 2012;40:237–248.

229. Rowson S, Duma SM. Development of the STAR evaluation system for football helmets: Integrating player head impact exposure and risk of concussion. *Ann Biomed Eng* 2011;39:2130–2140.

230. Beckwith JG, Greenwald RM, Chu JJ, Crisco JJ, Rowson S, Duma SM, et al. Head impact exposure sustained by football players on days of diagnosed concussion. *Med Sci Sports Exerc* 2013;45:737–746.

231. Urban JE, Davenport EM, Golman AJ, Maldjian JA, Whitlow CT, Powers AK, et al. Head impact exposure in youth football: high school ages 14 to 18 years and cumulative impact analysis. *Ann Biomed Eng* 2013;41:2474–2487.

232. Crisco JJ, Wilcox BJ, Beckwith JG, Chu JJ, Duhaime AC, Rowson S, et al. Head impact exposure in collegiate football players. *J Biomech* 2011;44:2673–2678.

233. Crisco JJ, Wilcox BJ, Machan JT, McAllister TW, Duhaime AC, Duma SM, et al. Magnitude of head impact exposures in individual collegiate football players. *J Appl Biomech* 2012;28:174–183.

234. Funk JR, Rowson S, Daniel RW, Duma SM. Validation of concussion risk curves for collegiate football players derived from HITS data. *Ann Biomed Eng* 2012;40:79–89.

235. Mihalik JP, Bell DR, Marshall SW, Guskiewicz KM. Measurement of head impacts in collegiate football players: An investigation of positional and event-type differences. *Neurosurgery* 2007;61:1229–1235; discussion 1235.

236. Broglio SP, Eckner JT, Surma T, Kutcher JS. Post-concussion cognitive declines and symptomatology are not related to concussion biomechanics in high school football players. *J Neurotrauma* 2011;28:2061–2068.

237. Daniel RW, Rowson S, Duma SM. Head impact exposure in youth football: middle school ages 12–14 years. *J Biomech Eng* 2014;136:094501.

238. Zemper ED. Two-year prospective study of relative risk of a second cerebral concussion. *Am J Phys Med Rehabil* 2003;82:653–659.

239. Duhaime AC, Beckwith JG, Maerlender AC, McAllister TW, Crisco JJ, Duma SM, et al. Spectrum of acute clinical characteristics of diagnosed concussions in college athletes wearing instrumented helmets: Clinical article. *J Neurosurg* 2012;117:1092–1099.

240. McAllister TW, Ford JC, Flashman LA, Maerlender A, Greenwald RM, Beckwith JG, et al. Effect of head impacts on diffusivity measures in a cohort of collegiate contact sport athletes. *Neurology* 2014;82:63–69.

241. Davenport EM, Whitlow CT, Urban JE, Espeland MA, Jung Y, Rosenbaum DA, et al. Abnormal white matter integrity related to head impact exposure in a season of high school varsity football. *J Neurotrauma* 2014;31:1617–1624.

242. McKee A. Interview by Tom Goldman T. National Public Radio; All things considered, July 25th 2017. Available at www.npr.org/2017/07/25/539198429/study-cte-found-in-nearly-all-donated-nfl-player-brains.

243. Corsellis J, Bruton C, Freeman-Browne D. The aftermath of boxing. *Psychol Med* 1973;3:270–303.

244. Hof PR, Knabe R, Bovier P, Bouras C. Neuropathological observations in a case of autism presenting with self-injury behaviour. *Acta Neuropathol* 1991;82:321–326.

245. Geddes JF, Vowles GH, Robinson SFD, Sutcliffe JC. Neurofibrillary tangles, but not Alzheimer-type pathology, in a young boxer. *Neuropathol Appl Neurobiol* 1996;22:12–16.

246. Bonfield CM, Wecht DA, Lunsford LD. Concussion in ice hockey. *Prog Neurol Surg* 2014;28:161–170.

247. Roberts WO, Brust JD, Leonard B. Youth ice hockey tournament injuries: Rates and patterns compared to season play. *Med Sci Sports Exerc* 1999; 31:46–51.

248. Forward KE, Seabrook JA, Lynch T, Lim R, Poonai N, Sangha GS. A comparison of the epidemiology of ice hockey injuries between male and female youth in Canada. *Paediatr Child Health* 2014;19:418–422.

249. Wilcox BJ, Machan JT, Beckwith JG, Greenwald RM, Burmeister E, Crisco JJ. Head-impact mechanisms in men's and women's collegiate ice hockey. *J Athl Train* 2014;49:514–520.

250. Berkman B. Women's hockey grows bigger, faster and dire. *N Y Times* 2015; December 18.

251. Emery CA, Kang J, Shrier I, Goulet C, Hagel BE, Benson BW, et al. Risk of injury associated with body checking among youth ice hockey players. *JAMA* 2010;303:2265–2272.

252. Allison MA, Kang YS, Maltese MR, Bolte JHT, Arbogast KB. Measurement of Hybrid III head impact kinematics using an accelerometer and gyroscope system in ice hockey helmets. *Ann Biomed Eng* 2015;43:1896–1906.

253. Wilcox BJ, Beckwith JG, Greenwald RM, Raukar NP, Chu JJ, McAllister TW, et al. Biomechanics of head impacts associated with diagnosed concussion in female collegiate ice hockey players. *J Biomech* 2015;48:2201–2204.

254. Koerte IK, Kaufmann D, Hartl E, Bouix S, Pasternak O, Kubicki M, et al. A prospective study of physician-observed concussion during a varsity university hockey season: White matter integrity in ice hockey players. Part 3 of 4. *Neurosurg Focus* 2012;33 (E3):1–7.

255. Helmer KG, Pasternak O, Fredman E, Preciado RI, Koerte IK, Sasaki T, et al. Hockey Concussion Education Project, part 1. Susceptibility-weighted imaging study in male and female ice hockey players over a single season. *J Neurosurg* 2014;120: 864–872.

256. Sasaki T, Pasternak O, Mayinger M, Muehlmann M, Savadjiev P, Bouix S, et al. Hockey Concussion Education Project, part 3. White matter microstructure in ice hockey players with a history of concussion: A diffusion tensor imaging study. *J Neurosurg* 2014;120:882–890.

257. Fife GP, O'Sullivan D, Pieter W. Biomechanics of head injury in Olympic taekwondo and boxing. *Biol Sport* 2013;30:263–268.

258. Frankland N. Holly Holm stuns Ronda Rousey with shocking KO. *Boston Globe* 2015; November 16, www.bostonglobe.com/sports/2015/11/15/holly-holm-stuns-ronda-rousey-with-round-knockout/Ahf4xzPEwTrx29NM2jxQPL/story.html.

259. Hutchison MG, Lawrence DW, Cusimano MD, Schweizer TA. Head trauma in mixed martial arts. *Am J Sports Med* 2014;42: 1352–1358.

260. Cleveland Clinic Lou Ruvo Center for Brain Health. Preliminary findings: Professional fighters brain health study. 2016. http://my.clevelandclinic.org/services/neurological_institute/lou-ruvo-brain-health/clinical-trials-research/research?utm_campaign=fighterstudy-url&utm_medium=offline&utm_source=redirect.

261. Brandenburg MA, Butterwick DJ, Hiemstra LA, Nebergall R, Laird J. A comparison of injury rates in organised sports, with special emphasis on American bull riding. *Int Sport Med J* 2007;8.

262. Mountain High Broncs and Bulls. Wild horse racing history. www.mountainhighrodeo.com/home/wild-horse-race-history/.

263. Lustenberger T, Talving P, Barmparas G, Schnuriger B, Lam L, Inaba K, et al. Skateboard-related injuries: Not to be taken lightly. A National Trauma Databank Analysis. *J Trauma* 2010;69:924–927.

264. Schieber RA, Olson SJ. Developing a culture of safety in a reluctant audience. *West J Med* 2002;176:E1–E2.

265. Diamond PT, Gale SD, Denkhaus HK. Head injuries in skiers: An analysis of injury severity and outcome. *Brain Inj* 2001;15:429–434.

266. Meyers MC, Laurent CM, Jr., Higgins RW, Skelly WA. Downhill ski injuries in children and adolescents. *Sports Med* 2007;37:485–499.

267. Sulheim S, Holme I, Ekeland A, Bahr R. Helmet use and risk of head injuries in alpine skiers and snowboarders. *JAMA* 2006;295:919–924.

268. Russell K, Christie J, Hagel BE. The effect of helmets on the risk of head and neck injuries among skiers and snowboarders: A meta-analysis. *CMAJ* 2010;182:333–340.

269. FIFA. FIFA big count. 2007. www.fifa.com/worldfootball/bigcount/allplayers.html.

270. Spiotta AM, Bartsch AJ, Benzel EC. Heading in soccer: Dangerous play? *Neurosurgery* 2012;70:1–11.

271. Matser JT, Kessels AG, Lezak MD, Troost J. A dose–response relation of headers and concussions with cognitive impairment in professional soccer players. *J Clin Exp Neuropsychol* 2001;23:770–774.

272. Rutherford A, Stephens R, Potter D, Fernie G. Neuropsychological impairment as a consequence of football (soccer) play and football heading: Preliminary analyses and report on university footballers. *J Clin Exp Neuropsychol* 2005;27:299–319.

273. Rieder C, Jansen P. No neuropsychological consequence in male and female soccer players after a short heading training. *Arch Clin Neuropsychol* 2011;26:583–591.

274. Rutherford A, Stephens R, Fernie G, Potter D. Do UK university football club players suffer neuropsychological impairment as a consequence of their football (soccer) play? *J Clin Exp Neuropsychol* 2009;31:664–681.

275. Straume-Naesheim TM, Andersen TE, Dvorak J, Bahr R. Effects of heading exposure and previous concussions on neuropsychological performance among Norwegian elite footballers. *Br J Sports Med* 2005;39(Suppl 1):i70–i77.

276. Stalnacke BM, Tegner Y, Sojka P. Playing soccer increases serum concentrations of the biochemical markers of brain damage S-100B and neuron-specific enolase in elite players: A pilot study. *Brain Inj* 2004;18:899–909.

277. Stalnacke BM, Ohlsson A, Tegner Y, Sojka P. Serum concentrations of two biochemical markers of brain tissue damage S-100B and neurone specific enolase are increased in elite female soccer players after a competitive game. *Br J Sports Med* 2006;40:313–316.

278. Zetterberg H, Jonsson M, Rasulzada A, Popa C, Styrud E, Hietala MA, et al. No neurochemical evidence for brain injury caused by heading in soccer. *Br J Sports Med* 2007;41:574–577.

279. Lipton ML, Kim N, Zimmerman ME, Kim M, Stewart WF, Branch CA, et al. Soccer heading is associated with white matter microstructural and cognitive abnormalities. *Radiology* 2013;268:850–857.

280. National Federation of State High School Associations. High school athletics participation survey. 2014–2015. www. nfhs.org/ParticipationStatics/ParticipationStatics.aspx/.

281. Myers RJ, Linakis SW, Mello MJ, Linakis JG. Competitive wrestling-related injuries in school aged athletes in U.S. emergency departments. *West J Emerg Med* 2010;11:442–449.

282. Olesen J, Gustavsson A, Svensson M, Wittchen HU, Jonsson B, Group CS, et al. The economic cost of brain disorders in Europe. *Eur J Neurol* 2012;19:155–162.

The Pathophysiology of Concussive Brain Injury

Stefano Signoretti, Barbara Tavazzi, Giuseppe Lazzarino, and Roberto Vagnozzi

Introduction

Concussion, is indeed the most common form of Traumatic Brain Injury (TBI) worldwide [1, 2], and has become a significant public health issue – as witnessed by the recent exponential increase of scientific reports focusing on this topic. According to a PubMed research (simply obtained by typing "concussion" as the keyword), more than 2500 papers have been published through the last 5 years, about 700 of which during 2015, providing competing definitions and clinical characterizations of this distinctive type of TBI.

Nevertheless, two notoriously misleading issues complicate the modern understanding of concussion: first, although the overwhelming majority of CBIs involve either no loss of consciousness or a brief (less than five minutes) loss of consciousness, CBI is not a synonym for so-called "mild traumatic brain injury" (mTBI). That unfortunate phrase arose partly due to a misinterpretation of the significance of the Glasgow Coma Scale (GCS). According to that scale, a TBI with a high GCS of 13–15 is labeled "mild." But a high GCS is *not* a measure of injury severity. It is merely a report indicating a "mildly affected level of consciousness at this particular moment." Yet that rhetorical usage of "mild" does not take into account either the condition of the brain or the consequences of the injury: mildly confused during the four minutes the emergency room doctor swings by the gurney does not mean mildly brain-damaged! Since *mildness* lacks biological specificity or predictive validity, "mTBI" is best avoided as a medical term. Second – contrary to the conventions adopted by clinical neurology in the previous century – new experimental, clinical, and imaging evidence suggests that a large proportion (at least one-third) of survivors of concussive injuries who come to medical attention experience persistent neurological and/or psychiatric problems. Terms such as "transient" or "self-limited" or "short-lived" fail to acknowledge this natural variation in neurobehavioral outcomes and must not be used to define human CBI.

The implications of these observations become more apparent in the light of the available epidemiological data [5–7]. This reveals some truly alarming statistics: for example, in European countries, approximately 235 people per 100,000 are admitted annually to hospital after TBI, 80% of whom are classified as belonging to the mTBI category or "concussed."

U.S. figures are very similar, with approximately 1.7 million people experiencing a TBI each year, with 75–90% of them being "mildly" injured patients [8]. Moreover, as discussed in Chapter 2, there is reason to suspect that these much-cited statistics seriously underestimate the true incidence. The combined significance of these observations is apparent and concerning: The social impact of this phenomenon appears evident when we consider that the proportion of severe and mild TBI is about 1:22 [2]; consequently the majority of the patients are labeled as "mildly-injured" and improperly grouped into a supposedly homogeneous but actually highly heterogeneous population, difficult to typify and further characterize only on the basis of the G.C.S. And if CBI is both more common and more persistent than claimed in traditional texts, the prevalence of post-concussive neurobehavioral problems and the magnitude of the public health impact of CBI may be much greater than previously assumed.

To date, due to the formidable challenge of studying this type of cerebral damage in the laboratory, basic science data collected from many bench studies have clarified only some aspects of this particular clinical entity. It appears that concussion symptoms and possible complications are mainly due to biochemical, molecular. and ultra-structural processes triggered by a truly peculiar traumatic insult that may not cause any discernible cell death, but that can obligate a person to spend prolonged periods off work or dependent on others and in some cases to suffer catastrophic consequences.

This chapter represents the authors' effort to piece together the crucial concepts and the most recent findings from previously published experimental works about the complex basic pathophysiology triggered and sustained by this traumatic injury (CBI).

External Force and the Metabolic Cascade: From Biomechanical to Biochemical

A considerable body of modern evidence keeps on showing that the traumatic insult, albeit "mild," is directly responsible for sudden alterations of the brain cellular networks, mainly caused by acute modification in biochemical signaling and subsequent depression of brain energy metabolism. To some degree, those immediate effects are stereotypical and similar from one brain to another (although, even in that hyperacute stage, genetically mediated biological differences may moderate and individualize the response).

Two fundamental questions require reasonable answers: by what series of events and physical laws does the mechanical energy generated from the external force on the head transfer to the cells, and how is the brain affected in response to this insult?

Briefly, two main categories of forces – contact and inertial – are included in the causal forces associated with CBIs. During the impact loading, both contact and inertial forces occur, while in the absence of the head striking an object, only inertial (acceleration) forces come to pass, generated by head motions. It is well established that the primary cause of concussive injuries is the inertial (or acceleration) loading experienced by the brain at the moment of impact. Additionally, with the head/neck motions that occur during a typical impact, two distinct components of this acceleration are taking place: linear and rotational acceleration. Linear acceleration-based brain injury is thought to result from a transient intracranial pressure gradient, while rotational acceleration-based injury is thought to result from a strain response [8]. Due to the intrinsic physical properties of the brain, it is clear enough that the strains induced by pressure gradients are of much less significance than the strains caused by rotational accelerations, primarily because the brain "material" deforms little in response to pressure. So, it happens that rapid head rotations that generate rotational accelerations have a high potential to cause shear-induced tissue damage. The importance of shear forces was confirmed in series of studies across different laboratories, leading to the conventional wisdom that shear deformation caused by rotational acceleration is the predominant mechanism of injury in concussion [9]. More recently, however, it has become apparent that stretch or strain, without frank shearing of axons, may explain much of the subsequent dysfunction [10–15].

Then, what happens when the mechanical energy from the external input (acceleration) is transferred to the brain? Several reviews refer to a "neurometabolic cascade" [16], and more recent evidence implicates both complex vascular and neuroimmunomodulatory/inflammatory changes that interact with cellular metabolism to produce the net effects of the inopportune external force [17–20]. Moreover, virtually simultaneous injurious and reparative effects initiate a competition for the welfare of brain cells. However, for the sake of coherence, we will first focus on the best-studied components of this newly appreciated biological competition.

The sudden stretching of the neuronal and axonal membranes sets off an indiscriminate flux of ions through previously regulated ion channels and transient physical membrane defects [21, 22]. While the precise process of the mechano-activation of receptors and channels remains to be fully described, the final result is an immediate, non-specific increase in plasma membrane permeability. This process is followed by a widespread release of a multitude of neurotransmitters, particularly excitatory amino acids (EAAs) [23], resulting in further changes of neuronal ionic homeostasis. Among the EAAs, glutamate plays the pivotal role by binding to the kainite, N-methyl-D-aspartate (NMDA) and D-amino-3-hydroxy-5-methyl-4-isoxazolepropionic acid (AMPA) ionic channels. NMDA receptor activation is responsible for a further depolarization, ultimately causing an influx of calcium ions into the cells. As clearly demonstrated in bench studies, these biochemical adverse events unfold immediately after injury and some of their effects are already detectable at one minute [24]. More recent studies showed that the voltage-gated sodium channels are truly mechano-activated from the stretch event and undergo rapid proteolysis that can lead to a sustained elevation of axoplasmic calcium [25]. Interestingly, this proteolysis is activated at stretch levels below the structural failure threshold and, the subsequent mitochondrial calcium overloading represents one of the essential points of the aforementioned post-traumatic ionic cellular derangement.

Three essential evidences are triggered as a consequence of mitochondrial calcium overfilling. The first is alteration of organelle membrane permeability and relative malfunctioning with uncoupling of oxidative phosphorylation. This initial mitochondrial impairment becomes the leading cause of the second event: generation of reactive oxygen species (ROS) [26], a phenomenon known as oxidative stress or ROS-mediated damage, mainly characterized by the onset of lipid peroxidation, a chain reaction that spontaneously propagates and causes significant irreversible modification to biological membranes and which has been demonstrated to occur at very early stages post-injury [27], even in TBI patients [28]. One target of ROS is the nicotinic coenzyme pool which is significantly depleted [29], further contributing to jeopardize all the oxido-reductive reactions, including those related to the cell energy supply.

In conjunction with oxidative stress, a contemporary phenomenon known as nitrosative stress takes place and it is defined as an overproduction of reactive nitrogen species (RNS) through the Ca^{2+}-dependent activation of neuronal nitric oxide (NO) synthase and of the expression of the inducible form of NO synthase [26, 30]. NO generation can either induce an increase of nitrosylation reaction of various fundamental biomolecules, particularly but not exclusively, of peptides (reduced glutathione) and proteins having the –SH group of cysteine residues available to react with NO, or react with ROS, giving rise to secondary, extremely reactive, radicals such as peroxynitrite and nitroxyl [31]. Both these RNSs have damaging effects on biomolecules and contribute to deplete tissue antioxidant defenses. Recent data indicate that neuroglobin, the newly discovered neuron-specific hexacoordinated hemoprotein capable of binding various ligands, including O_2, NO, and CO [32–35], with still unclear biological functions, is implicated in oxidative/nitrosative stress, acting as a neuropotector toward ROS and RNS-mediated damages [36–39]. However, experimental results in graded TBI, in which the gene and protein expression of neuroglobin was measured together with various parameters representative of ROS and RNS cell damage, did not support the role of neuroglobin as an endogenous neuroprotective antioxidant agent [40].

At this point, following the impact, to re-establish the pre-trauma ionic balance, the neuronal Na^+/K^+ adenosine triphosphate (ATP)-dependent pumps must work at maximal capacity, and a high level of glucose oxidation is urgently required to satisfy this sudden increased energy demand. Under normal aerobic conditions and correct mitochondrial functioning, most glucose consumption would be coupled to oxygen consumption, thus optimizing ATP generation. However, damaged by the calcium overloading and under multiple attacks from ROS and RNS, most of these oxido-reductive reactions are impaired, and the mitochondria cannot maintain their correct phosphorylating capacity. The imbalance between ATP consumption and production is the reason for the third fundamental observable fact: neurons are obligated to work overtime via the more rapid, but less efficient, oxygen-independent glycolysis, causing an almost paradoxical temporary increase in neuronal glucose consumption, notwithstanding a period of general metabolic depression. In many previous reports, local cerebral metabolic rates for glucose have indeed been documented to increase by 46% above control levels within the first 30 minutes after injury [41–43], and the marked post-traumatic increase in lactate/glucose ratio, along with reduced oxygen consumption and well-preserved cerebral blood flow [44], allows us to rule out any ischemic etiology, suggesting that the increase in anaerobic glycolysis is truly due to dysfunctional mitochondria and to the need to buffer ATP decrement.

The early post-concussion biochemical scenario can then be summarized in a rapid net decrease of the metabolites representative of the cell energy state (ATP and guanosine triphosphate (GTP)), mirrored by a proportional increase of their dephosphorylated products (i.e., adenosine diphosphate (ADP), adenosine monophosphate (AMP), guanosine diphosphate, guanosine monophosphate, nucleosides, and oxypurines). The rise in some of these intracellular compounds (AMP, ADP, inorganic phosphorus) acts as an efficient, positive signaling on some of the key regulatory enzymes of glycolysis such as phosphofructokinase, hexokinase, and pyruvate kinase, leading to an overall net temporary increase in the glycolytic rate.

CBI can then be considered as the most common mechanism by which trauma harms brains. The vast majority of the time, the degree of brain rattling is sublethal. No appreciable neuronal death is present and the immediate metabolic changes seem to be largely or completely reversible [24, 45]. It is then possible that this metabolic derangement and the post-mTBI "energy crisis" are chiefly responsible for the compromised synaptic plasticity and subsequent cognitive deficits [46]. The increasing awareness that concussions are often followed by long-term changes in brain and behavior raises the question: might other neurobiological changes (e.g., inflammation, neurodegeneration, microvascular change, microRNA expression, epigenetic change) perpetuate the problematic effects of concussion [47–52]? It is of course premature to claim that all the answers are available.

Measuring and Monitoring the Post-Concussive Metabolic Imbalance: Energy Metabolism and the Role of *N*-Acetyl Aspartate

Despite the fact that *N*-acetylaspartate (NAA) has been known since the late 1950s, and despite knowledge of its relevant cerebral concentration and complex mechanisms regulating its homeostasis, there is no unanimity regarding the exact biochemical functions of this "enigmatic" molecule. NAA is, by all means, a brain-specific metabolite and one of the most abundant low molecular weight compounds of the human brain, having concentrations (up to 15 mM) similar to those of the neurotransmitter glutamate [53, 54]. The the most accredited hypothesis indicates that the acetate source for oligodendrocyte lipid metabolism is the sole role of NAA [55]. To this purpose, it should however be underlined that: (1) free acetate for myelin biosynthesis must be converted into acetyl-coenzyme A (CoA); (2) NAA may generate only 2.5–4% of the total cerebral acetyl-CoA generated from glucose metabolism; and (3) the daily amount of acetate produced by NAA turnover greatly exceeds (by more than ten times) the daily amount of acetate consumed to satisfy daily myelin turnover. Altogether, these considerations render extremely doubtful the conclusions about NAA and reinforce the concept that this compound is still awaiting a precise role within brain metabolism. It is highly probable that NAA has more than one role and that its real function is a balanced combination of those mentioned previously.

NAA is synthesized in neurons from acetyl-CoA and aspartate by aspartate *N*-acetyl transferase, a membrane-bound enzyme identified as NAT8L (*N*-acetyltransferase 8-like) [56], which has been associated with endoplasmic reticulum [57] rather than mitochondria [58, 59], even if the mitochondrial localization of NAA biosynthesis appears strongly corroborated [58–61]. A significant amount of experimental evidence has been collected in the last two decades to assert that NAA biosynthesis is in strict correlation with mitochondrial function and cell energy state [62–64], while several clinical studies have clearly demonstrated that NAA is negatively affected by various acute and chronic states of neurodegeneration all having in common the malfunction of mitochondria [65].

Interestingly, research from these laboratories previously indicated that changes of NAA concentrations in the brain of TBI rats clearly mirror the time course variations of cerebral ATP and mitochondrial phosphorylating capacity (measured by the ATP/ADP ratio), with these three parameters being influenced either by the severity of TBI or, in the case of repeat head injuries, by the time between the two impacts [62, 63, 66, 67]. In these studies, it was also indicated, at least from a metabolic point of view, that 48 h post-injury was the minimal time point at which experimental mTBIs were clearly distinguishable from more severe traumatic insults; in fact, with respect to severe TBI and severe TBI with secondary insult, only mTBI rats clearly showed recovery of metabolites at this time point, thereby demonstrating the spontaneous reversibility of at least some biochemical alterations in this type of head injury. All these findings together suggest that NAA is indeed a valid surrogate marker for an indirect evaluation of the cerebral energy state, its synthesis being, beyond question, strictly dependent on the correct mitochondrial functioning.

To better understand this crucial point we must consider that NAA synthesis necessarily requires the availability and energy of hydrolysis of acetyl-CoA ($\Delta G = -31.2$ kJ/mol), working as the acetyl group and energy donor in the acetylation reaction of aspartate catalyzed by the aforementioned NAT8L. It is of primary importance to remember that when acetyl-CoA is used for NAA synthesis there is an indirect high energy cost to the cell, since in this case acetyl-CoA will not enter the citric acid cycle (Krebs cycle) and there will be a decrease in the production of reducing equivalents (3 NADH and 1 $FADH_2$) as the fuel for the electron transport chain (ETC), as well as a decrease in energy in terms of 1 GTP molecule/cycle. Since oxidative phosphorylation is stoichiometrically coupled to the amount of electron transferred to molecular oxygen by the ETC, the final result will be a net loss of 12 ATP molecules for each newly synthesized NAA molecule. NAA, then, is undeniably an "expensive" metabolite and to be maintained within physiological levels, the energetic metabolism of neurons must be very efficient.

Under physiological conditions, the high NAA cerebral concentration is kept within a strict oscillation range, even though it is regenerated 1.8 times/24 h with a calculated turnover rate of approximately 0.75 mmol/L water/hour [51]. Physiologically, to complete its metabolic cycle NAA must leave the neuron and change cellular compartment, reaching oligodendrocytes, where it is degraded into acetate and aspartate by aspartoacylase (ASPA) [66]. Therefore, NAA has a complex homeostasis, regulated by the rate of biosynthesis through NAT8L, outflow from neurons, uptake by oligodendrocytes and ultimately by degradation passing through ASPA (to date, no indications have been produced about the mechanisms regulating outflow from neurons and uptake by oligodendrocytes).

Recently, data from these laboratories indicated that in mild TBI changes in NAA levels were due to a combination of transient mitochondrial malfunctioning with energy crisis (limiting acetyl-CoA availability for NAA biosynthesis and causing temporary decrease in ATP and in the ATP/ADP ratio) and time post-injury-dependent modulation in the gene and protein levels of NAT8L (initial decrease and late increase with respect to pre-injury) and of ASPA levels (initial increase and rapid decrease with respect to pre-injury) [69]. The irreversible decrease in NAA following severe TBI was instead caused by profound mitochondrial malfunctioning with energy depletion (constant 65% decrease of ATP/ADP indicating permanent impairment of the mitochondrial phosphorylating capacity), dramatic steady down-regulation of the NAT8L gene (with remarkable decrease in the NAT8L protein levels), and concomitant remarkable overexpression in the ASPA gene and protein levels. This last phenomenon might be the consequence of the increased rate of NAA efflux from neurons [70] that per time

unit reaches the oligodendrocyte, where its degradation into aspartate and acetate is performed, exceeding the physiological ASPA-degrading capacity and representing the signal for the 2.3-times ASPA overexpression that has been described [69].

Then, the transient NAA decrement following concussion is probably caused by the combination of at least two factors: (1) a significant mitochondrial malfunctioning causing neuronal energy deficit and transient jam of NAA synthesis; and (2) an increased rate of NAA degradation in the oligodendrocyte compartment caused by an accelerated efflux from neurons and by an augmentation in the ASPA protein levels, now capable of efficiently providing NAA hydrolysis. Vice versa, recovery of mitochondrial functions (evidenced by normalization of ATP and ATP/ADP ratio), increase in gene expressions and protein levels of NAT8L, and decrease in those of ASPA simultaneously acted to produce the return of NAA cerebral concentrations to pre-impact values. These concomitant changes in parameters affecting NAA homeostasis at early and late stages post CBI are summarized in Figures 3.1 and 3.2, respectively.

Figure 3.1 illustrates the early phase of the post-concussive competition between harmful and protective mechanisms. Abrupt brain rattling triggers mitochondrial dysfunction and threatens an energetic crisis. The concomitant decrease in acetyl-CoA required for NAA biosynthesis causes a decrease in the rate of NAA production in this early post-injury period. To counteract that crisis, neurons modify their gene expressions – down-regulating genes of the ETC to avoid induction of oxidative/nitrosative stress, and modulating the expression of genes coding for proteins responsible for ATP-consuming processes, including the NAA-synthesizing enzyme NAT8L. In the oligodendrocyte compartment, the increased outflow of NAA from neurons provokes a higher rate of NAA inflow, exceeding the NAA-hydrolyzing capacity of physiologic ASPA. This leads to a transient NAA accumulation within the oligodendrocyte cytoplasm that possibly represents the signal causing the ASPA gene to up-regulate and to increase ASPA protein levels, a feedback mechanism adjusting the rate of NAA hydrolysis to the altered conditions.

The combination of this sequence of events causes the dysregulation of the mechanisms controlling NAA homeostasis during a period, or temporal window, of increased brain vulnerability to subsequent stressors (e.g., second impact), characterized by energy depression and decreased cerebral concentration of NAA. Experimentally (in concussed rats), this period lasts about 72 h.

Figure 3.2 illustrates a successive stage in the competition. Ultimately, recovery of NAA homeostasis is mediated by different mechanisms and is coincident to the normalization of energy metabolism and mitochondrial functions occurring with the closure of the window of metabolic brain vulnerability. In the concussed rat, this complex mechanism is completed about 5 days after injury.

All these findings evince a complex mechanism involving metabolic, genetic, and enzymatic changes that lead to homeostatic dysregulation of NAA following TBI. As in previous studies [62, 63, 66, 67], normalization of NAA homeostasis coincided with normalization of mitochondrial-dependent energy metabolism and was observed after "mTBI" only [69]. Therefore,

Figurative representation of most of the intracellular mechanisms influencing the *N*-acetyl aspartate (NAA) homeostasis during the first phase of brain vulnerability due to a concussive brain injury (CBI)

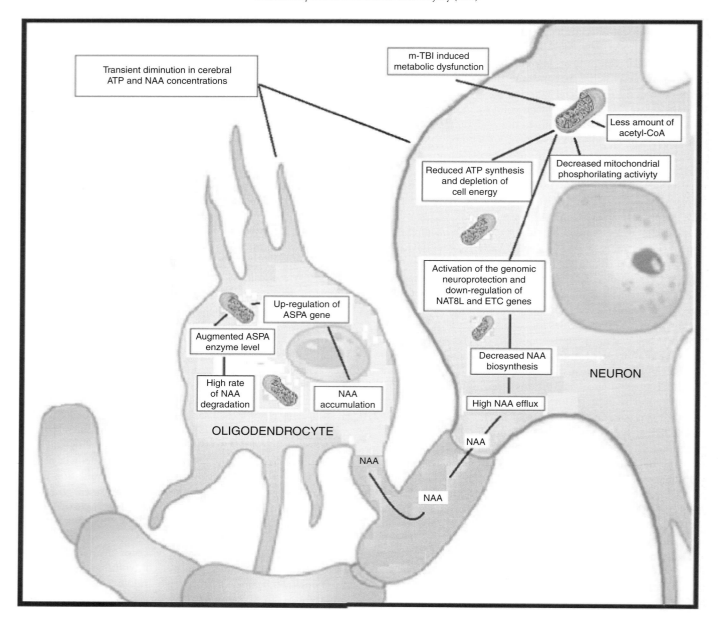

Fig. 3.1 In the neuron: sudden mitochondrial malfunctioning due to an ionic imbalance subsequent to CBI , coupled with a derangement ATP production/ consumption and consequent energetic cellular crisis. In the oligodendrocyte: NAA inflow exceeds the physiological enzymatic activity of aspartoacylase (ASPA) in hydrolyzing NAA Both contribute to an early, typically temporary, decrease in the availability of metabolic energy.

Abbreviations used: ATP: adenosine triphosphate; CoA: coenzyme A; ETC, electron transport chain; mTBI, mild traumatic brain injury; NAT8L, N-acetyltransferase 8-like.

Source: Signoretti, Tavazzi, Lazzarino, and Vagnozzi

measuring the decrease and recovery of NAA after a CBI potentially has the biochemical meaning not only of indirectly evaluating gene and protein expressions of NAT8L and ASPA, but, most importantly, of indirectly determining cerebral energy state (ATP) and mitochondrial functions (ATP/ADP ratio).

The aforementioned complex mechanism might be of relevance in the case of repeat concussions occurring during the delicate period of the NAA recovery process, coincident with the so-called window of brain vulnerability and characterized by transient dysfunctional mitochondria [62, 63, 66, 67].

The aforesaid bench data strongly supported the indication for a potential role of NAA in quantifying the post-traumatic metabolic neuronal damage and eventually were revealed to be of high clinical relevance since the use of proton magnetic resonance spectroscopy (^{1}H MRS) allows NAA to be measured noninvasively *in vivo*. Furthermore, beyond showing the profound TBI-induced modification in NAA homeostasis, this finding clearly demonstrated that different levels of "physical" injury correlated with different levels and kinetics of "biochemical" damage, which may be reversible in mTBI but irreversible in

Figurative representation of the intracellular mechanisms leading to the normalization the *N*-acetyl aspartate (NAA) homeostasis and to the closure of the brain vulnerability period

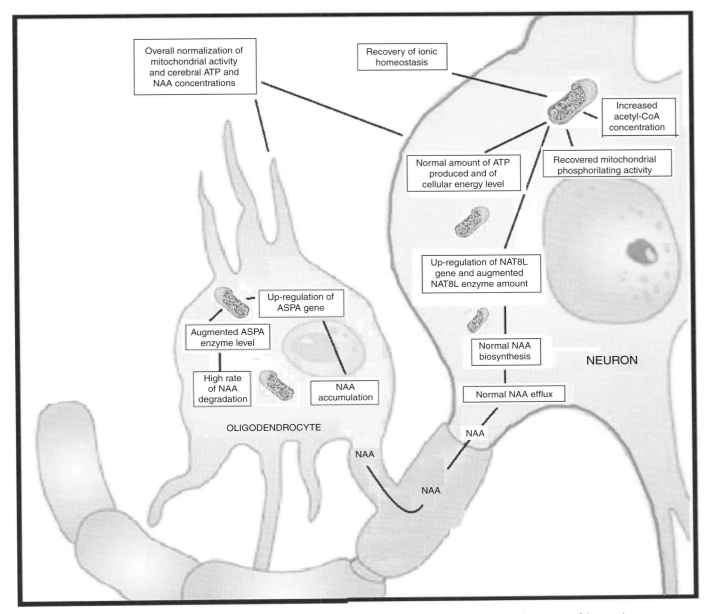

Fig. 3.2 In the neuron, recovery of mitochondrial activity is followed by the restoration of the cellularl energy state and the increase of the acetyl- coenzyme A utilization for NAA biosynthesis. This is favored by over-expression of N-acetyltransferase 8-like with consequent increase in NAT8L protein levels. In the oligodendrocyte, the restart of NAA inflow to pre-impact rate induces the ASPA gene expression reduction and recover ASPA protein levels to physiological values. Abbreviations used: ATP: adenosine triphosphate; CoA: coenzyme A; ETC, electron transport chain; mTBI, mild traumatic brain injury; NAT8L, N-acetyltransferase 8-like.

Source: Signoretti, Tavazzi, Lazzarino, and Vagnozzi

severe TBI [62, 63, 66, 67]. To complete the picture, even acetyl-CoA homeostasis has been proved to be affected by graded head injury, following a pattern very similar to those observed for both ATP and NAA [63]. For these reasons, in metabolic conditions of low ATP availability, when all of the pathways and cycles devoted to energy supply are operating at their maximal activity with the aim of replenishing ATP levels, acetyl-CoA will not be accessible for NAA synthesis. Only when the ATP deficiency is fully restored will acetyl CoA become available again to be shifted into the NAA "production" pathway.

A decrease in NAA concentration can then be seen as an indirect marker of post-traumatic metabolic energy impairment and it appears evident that if NAA is still below the physiological values after an mTBI, the concussive biochemical derangement, involving more complex pathways than the mere NAA homeostasis [16, 17, 23, 47, 71], cannot be considered to be resolved. Thus NAA represents a biochemical surrogate marker to monitor the overall neuronal metabolic status and it appears that, under conditions of decreased NAA, although the cells are functional, they are still experiencing energetic imbalance.

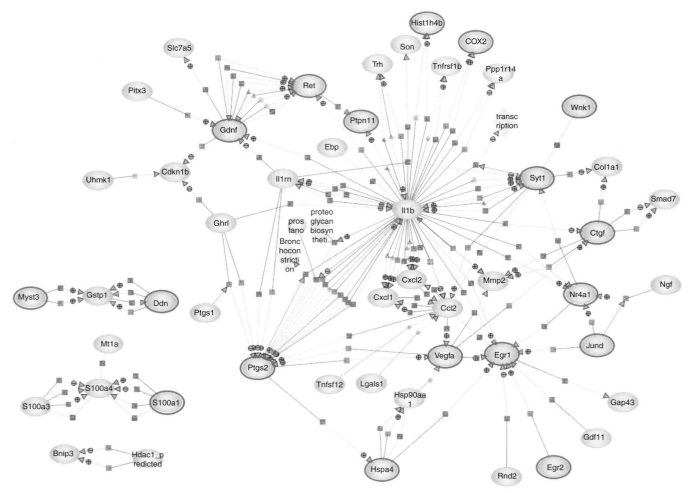

Fig. 3.3 Pathway analysis diagram showing interactions between various genes with differential expression for a "mild" traumatic brain injury (10% stretch). Source: Di Pietro et al., 2010 [72]. Reproduced with permission from Mary Ann Liebert, Inc.

Gene Modulation After Concussion: Visualizing the Post-Concussive Melee

The neurobiology of concussed mammal brains encompasses not only a "cascade" – a term that implies a unidirectional harmful chain reaction – but also a *competition* between pathways in which potentially damaging elements of the molecular/metabolic/inflammatory/vascular response to CBI and potentially neuroprotective elements vie for control of the outcome. One facet of this competition is mediated by, and reflected in, the rather astonishing number of genes that experience promptly altered transcription.

One approach to assessing that phenomenon involves employing complementary DNA microarray technology to monitor immediate post-concussive transcriptomics. Di Pietro et al. [72], for example, reported the consequences following abrupt stretch injury to hippocampal slice cultures (a tissue model intended to facilitate measurement of neurobiological response to graded TBI). As predicted, the expression of genes was altered in "mTBI" compared with controls. The altered genes clustered in the "biological process" group, which had been shown to be involved in the structural damage of cellular architecture. Figure 3.3 illustrates some of the genes affected and their biological relationships.

The findings depicted in Figure 3.3 help characterize the classes of molecular change that may be most relevant to the post-concussive melee (or tug of war) between degenerative and regenerative forces. For instance, proinflammatory cytokines appear to have a central role in molecular interactions following CBI. It can be clearly seen that interleukin-1β plays an important role and has numerous interactions with other genes. Prostaglandin endoperoxide synthase 2, also known as cyclooxygenase-2, also appears to be vital in 10% stretch, with many regulation, expression, and metabolism interactions with interleukin-1β. Yet most of the genes with altered transcription are involved in signal transducer activities, regulations of transcription, and cell communication. This indicates that, even after a "mild" injury, intense activity involving transcription and signaling exchange is initiated.

It has also been found that certain genes involved in the apoptotic process, such as Vdac1 (voltage-dependent anion-selective channel protein 1), Sh3glb1 (SH3-domain GRB2-like endophilin B1), Phlda1 (leckstrin homology-like domain, family A, member 1), Rock1 (Rho-associated coiled-coil containing protein kinase1), and Eif4g2-predicted (eukaryotic translation initiation factor 4 gamma2) were down-regulated. On the contrary, an up-regulation was seen in genes involved in the anti-apoptotic process, such as Ccl2 (chemokine [C-C motif] ligand 2), Vegfa (vascular endothelial growth factor A), BIRC3 (baculoviral IAP repeat-containing 3), Tsc22d3 (TSC22 domain family, member 3), Bnip3 (BCL2/adenovirus E1B 19-kD interacting protein 3), and Nr4a1 (nuclear receptor subfamily 4, group A, member 1). Interestingly, the majority of these expression changes were only found following "mild" injuries, suggesting that these cell cultures have activated protective and repair mechanisms.

As stated before, in line with mitochondrial dysfunction and increased energy demand, a clear condition of hypometabolism (decreased ATP, ATP/ADP, and nicotinic coenzymes) occurs following the early post-concussion period. However, lowering the rate of ATP biosynthesis, when cells are engaged in re-establishing homeostasis (e.g., ionic balance, oxidant/antioxidant balance) and in reparative processes (e.g., membrane restoration, refolding of unfolded proteins) would be extremely deleterious for the entire organ unless accompanied by a concomitant energy-conserving program.

Using the same model of *in vitro* stretch injury for rat hippocampal slice cultures, it has been demonstrated that, along with the hypometabolic state, a very peculiar pattern of gene modulation is also activated – a sort of "gene program" of neuroprotection, directly triggered by the traumatic insult [73]. Briefly, the gene expression of proteins involved in some relevant ATP-consuming processes (transcription, translation, and protein phosphorylation) is drastically down-regulated, indicating a complex adaptive strategy aimed at optimizing ATP consumption when ATP production is limited. The further observation of the down-regulation of genes encoding for several subunits of the ETC suggests that neurons also tend to reduce mitochondrial activity in a period of mitochondrial malfunctioning, most likely to avoid an overproduction of ROS and RNS, occurring during incorrect electron transfer through the ETC [74]. The transient malfunctioning of mitochondria is in fact also characterized by a decreased capacity to correctly handle the tetravalent reduction of molecular oxygen, generating oxygen and nitrogen radicals [74].

To avoid transitory damaged mitochondria working at a high rate in a period of increased cell energy demand, injured neurons trigger such a gene program of neuroprotection finalized to decrease the activities of complexes I, III, IV, and ATP synthase (complex V) and to minimize the risks of insurgence of oxidative/nitrosative stress [71, 74]. Concomitantly, a gene response aimed at optimizing ATP utilization during this time interval of decreased mitochondrial ATP supply

takes place [73]. For instance, restoring calcium homeostasis via ATP-independent mechanisms has been evidenced by the simultaneous up-regulation of Calm3 and Gap43. Both genes are involved in encoding for calmodulin-binding proteins to regulate intracellular calcium and to induce cell resistance to calcium-mediated toxicity, when overexpressed. Additionally, the up-regulation of the ionotropic GABA receptors and AMPA2 (GluR2) subunit of the AMPA receptor was observed; such an increase should reduce calcium entry into the cell and guard against excitotoxicity, as demonstrated by several previously published data. Similarly, the down-regulation of Grin2d encoding for the ionotropic NMDA2D glutamate receptor should counteract glutamate excitotoxicity, avoiding further calcium entry in post-injured cells. In all these cases, cell counteracted ionic imbalance via ATP-independent mechanisms.

To further contribute to saving ATP, neurons strategically down-regulate transcription and translation genes, thus ensuring significant decrease of energy-consuming processes, evidently of low priority when cells are engaged to recover after a traumatic insult. Recalling the indirect high energy expenditure for NAA biosynthesis, even the change in NAA homeostasis, caused by a combined metabolic, gene, and enzymatic mechanism, and leading to transient decrease in cerebral NAA [69], might be inserted into the "save energy program" occurring after mTBI.

All these findings support additional evidence that major molecular changes are triggered by a so-called "mild trauma," so profound as to be able to temporarily depress the basal metabolic rate and enter neurons into a hypometabolic or dormant state (similar to those observed in hibernators), through a targeted modulation of gene expression.

All these adaptive mechanisms, characterize the molecular bases of the period of time known as "window of brain vulnerability," originally suggested by Hovda et al. [75] (see below).

Post-Concussion Brain Vulnerability and the Second Impact Syndrome

Although scientifically attractive, all these biochemical modifications might appear, at first glance, of negligible clinical utility because they are spontaneously and generally fully reversible. However, despite the strong evidence favoring reversibility, a reasonable body of evidence clearly demonstrates that the "concussed" brain cells undergo a peculiar state of vulnerability for a yet-to-be-defined period of time, during which, if they sustain a second, typically non-lethal insult, they will suffer further, more severe damage, sometimes irreversible [59, 60]. This fascinating hypothesis, originally proposed by Hovda et al. [75], was tested in various bench studies [76, 77] and this period of time has now experimentally been well defined in mechanisms and duration.

Thanks to the high reproducibility of an experimental model of "mild" closed head injury [78, 79], it was possible to analyze the metabolic effects produced by two consecutive

CBIs, the second occurring at various intervals after the first, and to investigate how the temporal gap between traumatic events could influence the overall severity of injury.[1]

Measuring levels of NAA and ATP, and the ATP/ADP ratio after the second concussion, it was clearly demonstrated that maximal metabolic abnormalities were seen when the two mild injuries were separated by a three-day interval; in fact, the metabolic abnormalities in these animals were similar to those occurring after a single severe TBI [63, 67]. To explain the differences between the underlying metabolic dysfunction taking place after a concussion and those occurring after a severe TBI, it is again necessary to use bench data and consider the degrees of the NAA and energy metabolites decrements (ATP, creatine phosphate), which are approximately 20% following a single mTBI and 50% following a single severe TBI [24, 66, 80].

More importantly, the ADP concentration is only slightly increased after mTBI but it is substantially increased by 35% after severe TBI. Despite the significant ATP decrease by one-fifth, if the insult is "mild," the mitochondria are not irreversibly damaged, possessing a sufficient phosphorylating capacity (i.e., a modest decrease of the ATP/ADP ratio, which is a very good index for evaluating the mitochondrial phosphorylating activity) to allow later but spontaneous complete ATP restoration. This was fulfilled after approximately five days in the aforementioned experiments, when it was demonstrated that two mTBIs spaced by a five-day interval have the same effects on brain metabolism as those induced by a single mTBI [63, 67]. On the contrary, the 35% increase in ADP, found after more severe levels of injury, indicates a profoundly different situation with an altered capacity of mitochondria to support the cell energy requirements in terms of ATP synthesis (i.e., profound decrease in the ATP/ADP ratio).

Data reported in a histopathology study by Laurer et al. [77] showed the important cumulative effects of two episodes of mTBI (24 h apart) in mice, which led to pronounced cellular damage compared with animals that sustained a single trauma only. The authors concluded that, although the brain was not morphologically damaged after a single concussive insult, its vulnerability to a second impact was dangerously increased.

All these data provide the experimental demonstration of the exquisitely metabolic nature of "brain vulnerability" following a concussion and offer a unique contribution to the complex biochemical damage underlying the clinical scenario of a repeated concussive trauma, sometimes leading to catastrophic brain injury. In fact, the possibility of having a second concussive injury within an as-yet undefined period of time from the first (i.e., days or weeks) has been reported to

be even fatal in some instances, a phenomenon that Saunders and Harbaugh [81] called "the second-impact syndrome of catastrophic head injury," actually first described by Schneider [82]. A handful of published cases have reported on patients (mostly involved in sports-related activities) who, while still having symptoms from a previous head injury, experienced a second injury that unexpectedly and unpredictably led to sustained intracranial hypertension and catastrophic outcomes. The second blow may be remarkably minor, perhaps involving only a blow to the chest that indirectly injures the athlete's head by imparting accelerative forces to the brain [83–85].

So, what can be clinically considered the occurrence of malignant cerebral edema after a "mild" injury? From a patho-physiological point of view, it must be taken into account that we are most likely facing the result of a new concussion that unfortunately overlapped with an as-yet unresolved previous one [86, 87].

Several authors have asserted skepticism about the second impact syndrome [88, 89]. The major concern is that it seems to be an uncommon clinical condition when compared with the overall incidence of concussion, even though an elevated risk for subsequent head trauma exists among persons who are still recovering from a previous one [90–92]. If a second impact occurs at this stage it might have the most profound effects because of the minimal "metabolic buffering capacity" to counteract the known early changes reinitiated by the new CBI. With their biochemical homeostasis not yet re-established, the cells' ionic imbalance would prevail and massive cerebral swelling can take place [93, 94].

The key to avoiding such a complication seems rather simple: one must limit exposure to another concussion while still symptomatic from the first. Yet the topic is further complicated by the fact that the resolution of clinical symptoms does not necessarily coincide with the "closure" of the temporal window of brain metabolic imbalance "opened" by the first trauma [63, 67, 75, 77].

According to the experimental results previously summarized, mitochondrial-related changes progressively worsened with the time between concussions up to three days apart, when the metabolic abnormalities were similar to those occurring after a single severe TBI [63, 67]. With this experimental timeline in the rat, the third day after trauma was the point when the cell's energy-dependent recovery processes were at their maximal intensity. However, a direct translation to human beings is rendered difficult both because it is hard to compare the rat time and the human time and because many uncontrolled variables render each impact occurring to

---

[1] The forces that can produce a CBI vary greatly. No biological definition of mildness indeed exists. Yet, for the sake of discussing this experimental literature, we will refer to the biomechanics and pathophysiology originally described by Marmarou et al. [78, 79]. In the impact acceleration model, the distinction between a "mild" and a "severe" TBI was obtained by varying the height from which a 450-g weight fell. For severe TBI (450 g from 2 m), the acceleration developed was rather brief, lasting approximately 0.20 ms and approaching a peak magnitude of 900 **g**. For the 450-g–1-m injury the acceleration peak was lower, namely 630 **g**, with an identical profile, since in this model the acceleration patterns remain the same and increase only with increased height. At the 0.20 ms time point (one-half of the contact duration), compression of the skull (and thus of the brain) approached the maximum of 0.3 mm in 450 g–2 m and of 0.2 mm in 450 g–1 m. As the acceleration, the compression curves were identical for varying mass but varied directly with increases in height.

humans different from every other. This concept was clearly developed by Giza and Hovda [16], who showed that each physiologic parameter modified by a concussion has its own time frame, and each head injury can be very different from the next. Therefore, it is difficult to definitively state the true duration of vulnerability to a second injury and the question of whether the brain had fully recovered from the first concussive injury while experiencing the second one remains pivotal, but still unanswered. It was however clearly shown that concussed athletes with no history of previous concussions, undergoing serial (3, 15, 22, 30 days) ^{1}H MRS analyses, showed an initial remarkable decrease in cerebral NAA, as measured bilaterally in the frontal lobe white matter using the single-voxel mode [95, 96]. In both these cohorts, including the one in which subjects were enrolled at three neuroradiological centers and analyzed using different instrumental apparatuses and mode of spectrum acquisition [96], all athletes normalized their mitochondrial-related metabolism within 30 days post injury, as evaluated by measuring the surrogate marker of brain energy metabolism NAA [95, 96]. It is worth noting that these results also indicated that NAA recovery was not linearly related to time. Furthermore, data obtained in singly and doubly concussed athletes demonstrated that athletes who experienced a second concussion between the ninth and the 21st day after the first insult did not have second impact syndrome, nor did they demonstrate signs of severe TBI; however, they all had a significant delay in both symptom resolution and NAA normalization [97].

In other words, the effects of the second concussion were not fatal, but they were somehow not proportionate to the concussive insult. Most likely, the second concussion occurred when the brain cells were struggling toward recovery of impaired metabolic functions, and thus it only produced limited cumulative effects, however characterized by a significant delay of the clinical pictures and by a prolonged period of brain metabolic imbalance.

Hence, second impact syndrome should not be solely considered as an "all-or-none" phenomenon and should not be limited to those instances that result in death from malignant swelling. The concept of second impact syndrome should probably be extended to include all other occurrences in which a disproportion between the severity of the second injury and the concussive clinical features (i.e., intensity and/or time of resolution) or cerebral metabolic changes (i.e., extent of NAA decrease and/or delay in its normalization) is clearly observed. The degree of the "severity" of SIS will depend on which phase of the metabolic recovery the brain is in at the time of the second concussion. To verify this hypothesis, very recently, the effect of the time interval between repeat concussions has been demonstrated to affect the severity of the cognitive impairment in a group of 105 concussed athletes, thus confirming the results of previous animal and pilot human being studies [98].

Further Clinical Implications

At present, in the majority of Emergency Departments (EDs), the fundamental decision of whether to observe, discharge, or obtain imaging studies in mild-injured/concussed patients is logically focused essentially on identifying those individuals at risk for hemorrhagic complications that would threaten their lives – an eventuality that may occur in less than 0.1% of cases [99]. However, it is time that another danger from CBI, perhaps more common and certainly more modifiable than eventual post-traumatic intracranial hemorrhage, must be considered and this entails a completely different attention. The foremost clinical implications of all the reported experimental and clinical data are that, within days after injury, the metabolic effects of two concussions can be dangerously additive, and that it is very difficult to establish how long the aforementioned period of "brain vulnerability" will last, and when the occurrence of a second trauma would be uneventful. So the most important issue after a CBI would be that of avoiding a second concussion. Rest then can be brain saving and even life saving.

Risk of the second impact syndrome apart, however, the management of concussed patients is nowadays rather inconsistent and best practices remain unknown. So it happens that long beyond the classically reported recovery interval of less than months, at least 15% of persons with a history of concussion will continue to see their primary care physician because of persistent problems [99–101]. Many authors agree that this phenomenon of a "miserable minority" among concussion victims, characterized by long-lasting or even permanent distress, indeed exists, and can be observed even in rodent experiments.

Basic science data collected from the reported bench studies demonstrated that in a concussive type of injury the complex neurometabolic events are fully reversible and that different levels of trauma correspond to different kinetics of "biochemical" damage: reversible in mTBI and irreversible in severe TBI. However, the occurrence of persistent symptoms apparently raises other questions beyond the "neurometabolic" hypothesis. If concussion is a transient and reversible metabolic event with no permanent functional correlates, how are we to account for the "miserable minority" from a biochemical point of view? The only possible way to answer this question is to obtain objective measurements reliable enough to describe the actual metabolic status of the brain in these subjects suffering from persistent post-concussive syndrome.

Measuring NAA after an initial concussion and monitoring it until normalization might definitively represent a significant step in quantifying the amount of post-concussive metabolic disturbances. NAA levels are easily demonstrated by ^{1}H MRS, a technique based on the ability to localize the MR signal into a specific volume of tissue, thus providing a real-time "image" of the brain neurochemistry.

To date, our group has measured NAA by ^{1}H MRS in more than 150 singly concussed patients at three different neuroradiologic centers. Each patient was repeatedly analyzed up to normalization of mitochondrial-related metabolism, with very long longitudinal studies (up to one year). All cases we had the opportunity to evaluate experienced a single concussion for the first time and all demonstrated a significant decrease in NAA at the first ^{1}H MRS (3–15 days from impact), i.e., at present we never had a false negative. All subjects had full clinical recovery and normalization of mitochondrial-related metabolism, with significant delay between disappearance of symptoms (3–10 days) and metabolism normalization (25–45 days). In one case only, of a young athlete whose initial computed tomography scan was positive for signs of diffuse axonal injury, symptoms persisted for more than six months and metabolic pattern (NAA) never showed full recovery.

Excluding this last 16-year-old patient, our series apparently indicates that the percentage of this "miserable minority" is much lower than previously reported, possibly because some published studies have not selected patients strictly controlled for being at their first concussive episode. That is, the clinical history must be thoroughly ascertained before knowing where to include a patient: in the group of those with one, two, three, or more concussions. In addition, the time interval between those concussions may be critical in determining the likelihood of the lasting brain change: two 35-year-old men both having a history of two CBIs might exhibit rather different effects if one of those CBI subjects suffered two concussions in the same week, while the other suffered two concussions separated by 20 years. Such rigorously stratified data would advance our understanding of the circumstances that are more or less likely to provoke persistent dysfunction.

Furthermore, not all concussive injuries show the same biochemical derangement. This observation speaks directly to our concern about attention to individuality: given the very large number of genes that are up- or down-regulated after CBI, and given the indisputable observation of major variations in outcome after similar injuries, one must expect that a victim's genome moderates his or her brain's response. Indeed, a great deal of evidence suggests genetic (and even epigenetic) variation in response to TBI [102–109]; yet it remains to be seen at what point genome assessment will begin to usefully enhance predictions of outcome or guide clinical management.

Possibly relevant to that expectation of individual variation in response is a paper describing 11 cases of concussed athletes. It was pointed out that, in this sub-cohort of patients, alteration of brain metabolism involved not only NAA but also creatine [110]. This subgroup of athletes exhibited the classic early symptoms of concussion, but they seem to have suffered from a more problematic concussive event with a more pronounced imbalance of metabolism (change in both NAA and creatine concentrations) associated with a longer time in both metabolic and clinical recovery.

It is important to underline that if the determination of NAA levels (indirectly allowing energy metabolism evaluation) is of great relevance at a relatively short post-injury time to monitor the window of metabolic brain vulnerability and to reduce the risks of second impact syndrome, it may or may not be the best measure of cerebral status after CBI to monitor patients with long-lasting symptoms.

To date no studies have demonstrated continued abnormalities of NAA or creatine at ≥ one year after injury in such subjects. Although it is too early to judge whether patients with long-lasting somatic, cognitive, and non-cognitive behavioral dysfunction may have "energetically normal" brains, once the clinical history of these patients has been established with absolute certainty (one concussive episode only, eventual repeat concussions spaced by ≥ three months), it is entirely possible that NAA might normalize even as other neurobiological problems persist. Indeed, evidence suggests that clinically significant alterations of neural and glial function (although very difficult to detect) may begin later and last longer than the so-called "neurometabolic cascade." Multiple inflammatory, immunological, neurovascular, molecular genetic, and/or ultrastructural changes may continue long after energy metabolism has recovered. These factors perhaps correlate better with neurobehavioral outcome than measures of metabolism, even though they are of null utility to assess mitochondrial recovery and closure of the window of brain vulnerability.

Therefore, finding normal metabolism in a CBI patient with persistent problems would indeed suggest that he or she is out of the window of vulnerability to a second impact; but other factors must be found to explain his/her chronic disability, first of all his/her previous clinical history.

The subset of CBI subjects with persistent dysfunctions after their first episode of a single concussion remains hard either to be classified or to be quantified. It is however clear that, once the real existence of this subset of CBI patients with long-lasting symptoms after a first single concussive episode has been established, we have currently no biomarkers to analyze. Further translation research is needed to identify, first in animals, then in humans, the biological alterations most likely to account for persistent neurobehavioral impairments.

One study possibly hints at an avenue worthy of further investigation: a small cohort of concussed female athletes was scanned at a mean time of 18.9 months post injury. Significantly lower levels of myo-inositol, but not of NAA, were detected in the hippocampus and the primary motor cortices bilaterally [111]. This was accompanied by diffusion tensor imaging analysis using tract-based spatial statistics, with no difference in fractional anisotropy. However, a higher level of mean diffusivity in athletes with concussion was detected in large white-matter tracts (forceps minors, inferior/superior longitudinal fasciculi, inferior fronto-occipital fasciculus, cingulum, uncinate fasciculus, anterior thalamic radiations, and corticospinal tract), as well as a significantly lower level of fractional anisotropy in the segment containing fibers projecting to the primary motor cortices using a region-of-interest approach for the corpus callosum. The results of this study suggest that different patterns of metabolite change over specific time periods may be associated with persistence of post-concussive symptoms.

Additionally, one strongly suspects that individual genetic variability influences the probability and degree of post-injury recovery. Pilot evidences suggest that this includes not only APOE polymorphisms but also potentially hundreds of gene variants – from mitochondrial haplogroups [112] to clock genes [108]. Therefore, wide-ranging studies should genetically characterize the so-called "miserable minority" in the hopes of spotlighting differences that distinguish this subpopulation.

Key Issues for Future Studies

It is common experience that concussion-related impairments can persist well beyond six months. This is revealed when patients are assessed: (1) by more complex cognitive tasks [113]; (2) under circumstances of stress such as depression, pain, sleep deprivation, or high altitude [114–121]; (3) by functional neuroimaging; and (4) by electrophysiological measures [122, 123]. With regard to the last: a small number of studies have also provided support for long-term changes in functional brain activity after concussion by recording electroencephalograms and measuring the classic P300 event-related potential component. The P300 is thought to reflect a basic cognitive process by which incoming information is categorized and has also been linked to processes involved in updating the context of working memory [124]. This study showed that, long after a concussion, more sensitive electrophysiological measures can reveal subtle changes in brain activity during cognitive processing, including inefficient information-processing capacity during a working-memory task, and it would be of great interest to couple these data with metabolic measurements.

One of the biggest challenges of the next ten years will be to improve the applicability of advanced neuroimaging to concussion by determining its validity for reliably identifying biological changes that have clinical significance. Ultimately, the changes of greatest importance may occur at an ultrastructural level beyond the resolution of current non-invasive technologies. Yet the pace of progress in imaging is such that we may soon have a much finer-grained picture of post-CBI neurobiology. Advances in this domain will tremendously improve our comprehension of what happens to the neuronal architecture after a concussion. Coupling such data with those related to brain metabolism and neuro-behavior would enable a far more accurate and sophisticated analysis of the short- and long-term consequences of CBI.

As far as experimental analysis is concerned, the feeling is that new animal models are needed that more accurately and sophisticatedly replicate "typical" human concussion. This step is essential to accelerating our progress in understanding, defining, and developing effective interventions for CBI and CTE.

References

1. Bruns J Jr., Hauser WA. The epidemiology of traumatic brain injury: A review. *Epilepsia* 2003;44(Suppl 10):2–10.
2. Tagliaferri F, Compagnone C, Korsic M, Servadei F, Kraus J. A systematic review of brain injury epidemiology in Europe. *Acta Neurochir (Wien)* 2006;148:255–268.
3. McCrory P, Johnston K, Meeuwisse W, Aubry M, Cantu R, Dvorak J, et al. Summary and agreement statement of the 2nd International Conference on Concussion in Sport, Prague 2004. *Br J Sports Med* 2005;39: 196–204.
4. McCrory P, Meeuwisse W, Johnston K, Dvorak J, Aubry M, Molloy M, et al. Consensus statement on Concussion in Sport – the 3rd International Conference on Concussion in Sport held in Zurich, November 2008. *Clin J Sport Med* 2009;19:185–200.
5. Kristman VL, Borg J, Godbolt AK, Salmi LR, Cancelliere C, Carroll LJ, et al. Methodological issues and research recommendations for prognosis after mild traumatic brain injury: results of the International Collaboration on Mild Traumatic Brain Injury Prognosis. *Arch Phys Med Rehabil.* 2014;95(3 Suppl):S265–S277.
6. Roozenbeek B, Maas AI, Menon DK. Changing patterns in the epidemiology of traumatic brain injury. *Nat Rev Neurol* 2013;9:231–236.
7. Coronado VG, Xu L, Basavaraju SV, McGuire LC, Wald MM, Faul MD, et al. Surveillance for traumatic brain injury-related deaths – United States, 1997–2007. Centers for Disease Control and Prevention (CDC). *MMWR Surveill Summ* 2011;60:1–32.
8. Rowson S, Duma SM. Brain injury prediction: Assessing the combined probability of concussion using linear and rotational head acceleration. *Ann Biomed Eng.* 2013;41:873–882.
9. Meaney DF, Smith DH. Biomechanics of concussion. *Clin Sports Med* 2011;30:19–31.
10. Salvador E, Burek M, Forster CY. Stretch and/or oxygen glucose deprivation (OGD) in an in vitro traumatic brain injury (TBI) model induces calcium alteration and inflammatory cascade. *Front Cell Neurosci* 2015;9:323.
11. Magou GC, Pfister BJ, Berlin JR. Effect of acute stretch injury on action potential and network activity of rat neocortical neurons in culture. *Brain Res* 2015;1624:525–535.
12. Sullivan S, Eucker SA, Gabrieli D, Bradfield C, Coats B, Maltese MR, et al. White matter tract-oriented deformation predicts traumatic axonal brain injury and reveals rotational direction-specific vulnerabilities. *Biomech Model Mechanobiol* 2015;14:877–896.
13. Yap YC, Dickson TC, King AE, Breadmore MC, Guijt RM. Microfluidic culture platform for studying neuronal response to mild to very mild axonal stretch injury. *Biomicrofluidics* 2014;8:044110.
14. Ahmadzadeh H, Smith DH, Shenoy VB. Viscoelasticity of tau proteins leads to strain rate-dependent breaking of microtubules during axonal stretch injury: Predictions from a mathematical model. *Biophys J* 2014;106:1123–1133.
15. Pan Y, Sullivan D, Shreiber DI, Pelegri AA. Finite element modeling of CNS white matter kinematics: Use of a 3D RVE to determine material properties. *Front Bioeng Biotechnol* 2013;1:19.
16. Giza CC, Hovda DA. The neurometabolic cascade of concussion. *J Athl Train* 2001;36:228–235.
17. Johnson VE, Stewart JE, Begbie FD, Trojanowski JQ, Smith DH, Stewart W. Inflammation and white matter degeneration persist for years after a single traumatic brain injury. *Brain* 2013;136 (Pt 1):28–42.
18. Corps KN, Roth TL, McGavern DB. Inflammation and neuroprotection in traumatic brain injury. *JAMA Neurol* 2015;72(3): 355–362.
19. Balu R. Inflammation and immune system activation after traumatic brain injury. *Curr Neurol Neurosci Rep* 2014; 14(10):484.
20. Abdul-Muneer PM, Chandra N, Haorah J. Interactions of oxidative stress and neurovascular inflammation in the pathogenesis of traumatic brain injury. *Mol Neurobiol* 2015;51:966–979.
21. Kilinc, D, Gallo, G, Barbee, KA. Mechanically-induced membrane poration causes axonal beading and localized cytoskeletal damage. *Exp Neurol* 2008;212(2):422–430.
22. Barkhoudarian G, Hovda DA, Giza CC. The molecular pathophysiology of concussive brain injury. *Clin Sports Med* 2011;30:33–48.
23. Gilley JA, Kernie SG. Excitatory amino acid transporter 2 and excitatory amino acid transporter 1 negatively regulate calcium-dependent proliferation of hippocampal neural progenitor cells

and are persistently upregulated after injury. *Eur J Neurosci* 2011;34:1712–1723.

24. Vagnozzi R, Marmarou A, Tavazzi B, Signoretti S, Di Pierro D, del Bolgia F, et al. Changes of cerebral energy metabolism and lipid peroxidation in rats leading to mitochondrial dysfunction after diffuse brain injury. *J Neurotrauma* 1999;16:903–913.

25. von Reyn CR, Mott RE, Siman R, Smith DH, Meaney DF. Mechanisms of calpain mediated proteolysis of voltage gated sodium channel α-subunits following in vitro dynamic stretch injury. *J Neurochem* 2012;121:793–805.

26. Hall ED, Wang JA, Miller DM. Relationship of nitric oxide synthase induction to peroxynitrite-mediated oxidative damage during the first week after experimental traumatic brain injury. *Exp Neurol* 2012;238:176–182.

27. Nishio S, Yunoki M, Noguchi Y, Kawauchi M, Asari S, Ohmoto T. Detection of lipid peroxidation and hydroxyl radicals in brain contusion of rats. *Acta Neurochir Suppl* 1997;70:84–86.

28. Cristofori L, Tavazzi B, Gambin R, Vagnozzi R, Vivenza C, Amorini AM, et al. Early onset of lipid peroxidation after human traumatic brain injury: A fatal limitation for the free radical scavenger pharmacological therapy? *J Investig Med* 2001;49:450–458.

29. Morgan WA. Pyridine nucleotide hydrolysis and interconversion in rat hepatocytes during oxidative stress. *Biochem Pharmacol* 1995;49:1179–1184.

30. Cherian L, Hlatky R, Robertson CS. Nitric oxide in traumatic brain injury. *Brain Pathol* 2004;14:195–201.

31. Hall ED, Wang JA, Miller DM. Relationship of nitric oxide synthase induction to peroxynitrite-mediated oxidative damage during the first week after experimental traumatic brain injury. *Exp Neurol* 2012;238:176–182.

32. Kakar S, Hoffman FG, Storz JF, Fabian M, Hargrove MS. Structure and reactivity of hexacoordinate hemoglobins. *Biophys Chem* 2010;152:1–14.

33. Dewilde S, Kiger L, Burmester T, Hankeln T, Baudin-Creuza V, Aerts T, et al. Biochemical characterization and ligand binding properties of neuroglobin, a novel member of the globin family. *J Biol Chem* 2001;276:38949–38955.

34. Trent JT 3rd, Watts RA, Hargrove MS. Human neuroglobin, a hexacoordinate hemoglobin that reversibly binds oxygen. *J Biol Chem* 2001;276:30106–30110.

35. Hundahl CA, Kelsen J, Dewilde S, Hay-Schmidt A. Neuroglobin in the rat brain (II): Co-localisation with neurotransmitters. *Neuroendocrinology* 2008;88:183–198.

36. Shang A, Liu K, Wang H, Wang J, Hang X, Yang Y, et al. Neuroprotective effects of neuroglobin after mechanical injury. *Neurol Sci* 2012;33: 551–558.

37. Shang A, Feng X, Wang H, Wang J, Hang X, Yang Y, et al. Neuroglobin upregulation offers neuroprotection in traumatic brain injury. *Neurol Res* 2012;34:588–594.

38. Chuang PY, Conley YP, Poloyac SM, et al. Neuroglobin genetic polymorphisms and their relationship to functional outcomes after traumatic brain injury. *J Neurotrauma* 2010;27: 999–1006.

39. Lin X, Li M, Shang A, et al. Neuroglobin expression in rats after traumatic brain injury. *Neural Regen Res* 2012;5(25):1960–1966.

40. Di Pietro V, Lazzarino G, Amorini AM, et al. Neuroglobin expression and oxidant/antioxidant balance after graded traumatic brain injury in the rat. *Free Radic Biol Med* 2014;69:258–264.

41. Yoshino A, Hovda DA, Kawamata T, et al. Dynamic changes in local cerebral glucose utilization following cerebral conclusion in rats: Evidence of a hyper and subsequent hypometabolic state. *Brain Res* 1991;561:106–119.

42. Kawamata T, Katayama Y, Hovda DA, et al. Administration of excitatory amino acid antagonists via microdialysis attenuates the increase in glucose utilization seen following concussive brain injury. *J Cereb Blood Flow Metab* 1992;12:12–24.

43. Andersen BJ, Marmarou A. Post-traumatic selective stimulation of glycolysis. *Brain Res* 1992;585:184–189.

44. Levasseur JE, Alessandri B, Reinert M, et al. Fluid percussion injury transiently increases then decreases brain oxygen consumption in the rat. *J Neurotrauma* 2000;17:101–112.

45. Maruichi K, Kuroda S, Chiba Y, et al. Graded model of diffuse axonal injury for studying head injury-induced cognitive dysfunction in rats. *Neuropathology* 2009;29:132–139.

46. Wu A, Ying Z, Gomez-Pinilla F. Vitamin E protects against oxidative damage and learning disability after mild traumatic brain injury in rats. *Neurorehabil Neural Repair* 2010;24:290–298.

47. Meissner L, Gallozzi M, Balbi M, et al. Temporal profile of microRNA expression in contused cortex following traumatic brain injury in mice. *J Neurotrauma* 2016;33(8):713–720.

48. Wang WX, Visavadiya NP, Pandya JD, et al. Mitochondria-associated microRNAs in rat hippocampus following traumatic brain injury. *Exp Neurol* 2015;265:84–93.

49. Truettner JS, Motti D, Dietrich WD. MicroRNA overexpression increases cortical neuronal vulnerability to injury. *Brain Res* 2013;1533:122–130.

50. Sharma A, Chandran R, Barry ES, et al. Identification of serum microRNA signatures for diagnosis of mild traumatic brain injury in a closed head injury model. *PLoS One* 2014;7(9):e112019.

51. Liu L, Sun T, Liu Z, et al. Traumatic brain injury dysregulates microRNAs to modulate cell signaling in rat hippocampus. *PLoS One* 2014;4(9):e103948.

52. Jadhav SP, Kamath SP, Choolani M, et al. microRNA-200b modulates microglia-mediated neuroinflammation via the cJun/MAPK pathway. *J Neurochem* 2014;130:388–401.

53. Baslow MH, Guilfoyle DN. (2006) Functions of *N*- acetylaspartate and *N*-acetylaspartylglutamate in brain: evidence of a role in maintenance of higher brain integrative activities of information processing and cognition. *Adv Exp Med Biol* 2006;576:95–112.

54. Pan JW, Takahashi K. Interdependence of *N*-acetyl aspartate and high-energy phosphates in healthy human brain. *Ann Neurol* 2005;57:92–97.

55. Moffett JR, Ross B, Arun P, et al. *N*-acetylaspartate in the CNS: From neurodiagnostics to neurobiology. *Prog Neurobiol* 2007;81:89–131.

56. Wiame E, Tyteca D, Pierrot N, et al. Molecular identification of aspartate *N*-acetyltransferase and its mutation in hypoacetylaspartia. *Biochem J* 2010;425:127–136.

57. Tahay G, Wiame E, Tyteca D, et al. Determinants of the enzymatic activity and the subcellular localization of aspartate *N*-acetyltransferase. *Biochem J* 2012;441:105–112.

58. Ariyannur PS, Madhavarao CN, Namboodiri AM. *N*-acetylaspartate synthesis in the brain: Mitochondria vs. microsomes. *Brain Res* 2008;1227:34–41.

59. Arun P, Moffett JR, Namboodiri AM. Evidence for mitochondrial and cytoplasmic *N*-acetylaspartate synthesis in SH-SY5Y neuroblastoma cells. *Neurochem Int* 2009;55:219–225.

60. Jalil MA, Begum L, Contreras L, et al. Reduced *N*-acetylaspartate levels in mice lacking aralar, a brain- and muscle-type mitochondrial aspartate-glutamate carrier. *J Biol Chem* 2005;280: 31333–31339.

61. Satrústegui J, Contreras L, Ramos M, et al. Role of aralar, the mitochondrial transporter of aspartate-glutamate, in brain *N*-acetylaspartate formation and Ca(2+) signaling in neuronal mitochondria. *J Neurosci Res* 2007;85:3359–3366.

62. Signoretti S, Marmarou A, Tavazzi B, et al. *N*-Acetylaspartate reduction as a measure of injury severity and mitochondrial dysfunction following diffuse traumatic brain injury. *J Neurotrauma* 2001;18:977–991.

63. Vagnozzi R, Tavazzi B, Signoretti S, et al. Temporal window of metabolic brain vulnerability to concussions: Mitochondrial-related impairment – part I. *Neurosurgery* 2007;61:379–388.

64. Boumezbeur F, Mason GF, de Graaf RA, et al. Altered brain mitochondrial metabolism in healthy aging as assessed by in vivo magnetic resonance spectroscopy. *J Cereb Blood Flow Metab* 2010;30:211–221.

65. Lin MT, Beal MF. Mitochondrial dysfunction and oxidative stress in neurodegenerative diseases. *Nature* 2006;443:787–795.

66. Tavazzi B, Signoretti S, Lazzarino G, et al. Cerebral oxidative stress and depression of energy metabolism correlate with severity of diffuse brain injury in rats. *Neurosurgery* 2005;56:582–589.

67. Vagnozzi R, Signoretti S, Tavazzi B, et al. Hypothesis of the postconcussive vulnerable brain: Experimental evidence of its metabolic occurrence. *Neurosurgery* 2005;57:164–171.

68. Wijayasinghe YS, Pavlovsky AG, Viola RE. Aspartoacylase catalytic deficiency as the cause of Canavan disease: a structural perspective. *Biochemistry*. 2014;53(30):4970–4978.

69. Di Pietro V, Lazzarino G, Amorini AM, et al. The molecular mechanisms affecting N-acetylaspartate homeostasis following experimental graded traumatic brain injury. *Mol Med* 2014;20: 147–157.

70. Belli A, Sen J, Petzold A, et al. Extracellular N-acetylaspartate depletion in traumatic brain injury. *J Neurochem* 2006;96: 861–869.

71. Tavazzi B, Vagnozzi R, Signoretti S, et al. Temporal window of metabolic brain vulnerability to concussions: Oxidative and nitrosative stresses – part II. *Neurosurgery* 2007;61: 390–395.

72. Di Pietro V, Amin D, Pernagallo S, et al. Transcriptomics of traumatic brain injury: Gene expression and molecular pathways of different grades of insult in a rat organotypic hippocampal culture model. *J Neurotrauma* 2010;27:349–359.

73. Di Pietro V, Amorini AM, Tavazzi B, et al. Potentially neuroprotective gene modulation in an in vitro model of mild traumatic brain injury. *Mol Cell Biochem* 2013;375:185–198.

74. Musatov A, Robinson NC. Susceptibility of mitochondrial electron-transport complexes to oxidative damage. Focus on cytochrome c oxidase. *Free Radic Res* 2012;46(11): 1313–1326.

75. Hovda DA, Badie H, Karimi S, et al. Concussive brain injury produces a state of vulnerability for intracranial pressure perturbation in the absence of morphological damage. In: Avezaat CJ, van Eijndhoven JH, Maas AI, et al., editors. *Intracranial Pressure VIII.* New York: Springer-Verlag, 1983, pp. 469–472.

76. Longhi L, Saatman KE, Fujimoto S, et al. Temporal window of vulnerability to repetitive experimental concussive brain injury. *Neurosurgery* 2005;56:364–374.

77. Laurer HL, Bareyre FM, Lee VM, et al. Mild head injury increasing the brain's vulnerability to a second concussive impact. *J Neurosurg* 2001;95:859–870.

78. Marmarou A, Foda MA, van den Brink W, et al. A new model of diffuse brain injury in rats. Part I: Pathophysiology and biomechanics. *J Neurosurg* 1994;80:291–300.

79. Foda MA, Marmarou A. A new model of diffuse brain injury in rats. Part II: Morphological characterization. *J Neurosurg* 1994;80:301–313.

80. Signoretti S, Di Pietro V, Vagnozzi R, et al. Transient alterations of creatine, creatine phosphate, N-acetylaspartate and high-energy phosphates after mild traumatic brain injury in the rat. *Mol Cell Biochem* 2010;333:269–277.

81. Saunders RL, Harbaugh, RE. Second impact in catastrophic contact-sports head trauma. *JAMA* 1984;252:538–539.

82. Schneider RC. *Head and neck injuries in football: Mechanisms, treatment and prevention.* Baltimore, MD: Williams & Wilkins, 1973.

83. Cobb S, Battin B. Second-impact syndrome. *J School Nurs* 2004;20:262–267.

84. Logan SM, Bell GW, Leonard JC. Acute subdural hematoma in a high school football player after 2 unreported episodes of head trauma: A case report. *J Athl Training* 2001;36:433–436.

85. Mori T, Katayama Y, Kawamata T. Acute hemispheric swelling associated with thin subdural hematomas: Pathophysiology of repetitive head injury in sports. *Acta Neurochir Suppl* 2006;96:40–43.

86. Cantu RC. Malignant brain edema and second impact syndrome. In: Cantu RC, editor. *Neurologic athletic head and spine injuries.* Philadelphia, PA: WB Saunders, 2000, pp. 132–137.

87. Cantu RC, Gean AD. Second-impact syndrome and a small subdural hematoma: An uncommon catastrophic result of repetitive head injury with a characteristic imaging appearance. *J Neurotrauma* 2010;27:1557–1564.

88. McLendon LA, Kralik SF, Grayson PA, Golomb MR. The controversial second impact syndrome: A review of the literature. *Pediatr Neurol* 2016;62:9–17.

89. McCrory P, Davis G, Makdissi M. Second impact syndrome or cerebral swelling after sporting head injury. *Curr Sports Med Rep* 2012;11:21–23.

90. United States Centers for Disease Control and Prevention. Sports related recurrent brain injuries. *MMWR Morb Mortal Wkly Rep* 1997;46:224–227.

91. Guskiewicz KM, Weaver NL, Padua DA, et al. Epidemiology of concussion in collegiate and high school football players. *Am J Sports Med* 2000;28:643–650.

92. Lincoln AE, Caswell SV, Almquist JL, et al. Trends in concussion incidence in high school sports: A prospective "11-year study". *Am J Sports Med.* 2011;39(5):958–963.

93. Marmarou A, Signoretti S, Fatouros PP, et al. Predominance of cellular edema in traumatic brain swelling in patients with severe head injuries. *J Neurosurg* 2006;104:720–730.

94. Signoretti S, Marmarou A, Aygok GA, et al. Assessment of mitochondrial impairment in traumatic brain injury using high-resolution proton magnetic resonance spectroscopy. *J Neurosurg* 2008;108:42–52.

95. Vagnozzi R, Signoretti S, Tavazzi B, et al. Temporal window of metabolic brain vulnerability to concussion: A pilot 1H-magnetic resonance spectroscopic study in concussed athletes – Part III. *Neurosurgery* 2008;62:1286–1295.

96. Vagnozzi R, Signoretti S, Cristofori L, et al. Assessment of metabolic brain damage and recovery following mild traumatic brain injury: A multicentre, proton magnetic resonance spectroscopic study in concussed patients. *Brain* 2010; 133:3232–3242.

97. Vagnozzi R, Manara M, Tavazzi B, et al. The importance of restriction from physical activity in the metabolic recovery of concussed brain. In Agrawal A, editor.*Brain injury: Pathogenesis, monitoring, recovery and management.* Rijeka, Croatia: InTech, 2012, pp. 501–522.

98. Silverberg ND, Lange RT, Millis SR, et al. Post-concussion symptom reporting after multiple mild traumatic brain injuries. *J Neurotrauma* 2013;30:1398–1404.

99. Fabbri A, Servadei F, Marchesini G, et al. The changing face of mild head injury: Temporal trends and patterns in adolescents and adults from 1997 to 2008. *Injury* 2010;41:968–972.

100. Wood RL. Understanding the 'miserable minority': A diathesis-stress paradigm for post-concussional syndrome. *Brain Inj* 2004;18:1135–1153.

101. Shenton ME, Hamoda HM, Schneiderman JS, et al. A review of magnetic resonance imaging and diffusion tensor imaging findings in mild traumatic brain injury. *Brain Imaging Behav* 2012;6:137–192.

102. Lipsky RH, Lin M. Genetic predictors of outcome following traumatic brain injury. *Handb Clin Neurol* 2015;127:23–41.

151

103. McAllister TW. Genetic factors in traumatic brain injury. *Handb Clin Neurol* 2015;128:723–739.

104. Yuan F, Xu ZM, Lu LY, et al. SIRT2 inhibition exacerbates neuroinflammation and blood–brain barrier disruption in experimental traumatic brain injury by enhancing NF-κB p65 acetylation and activation. *J Neurochem* 2016;136: 581–593.

105. Merritt VC, Arnett PA. Apolipoprotein E (APOE) e4 allele is associated with increased symptom reporting following sports concussion. *J Int Neuropsychol Soc* 2015;22:89–94.

106. Davidson J, Cusimano MD, Bendena WG. Post-traumatic brain injury: Genetic susceptibility to outcome. *Neuroscientist* 2015;21:424–441.

107. Failla MD, Myrga JM, Ricker JH, et al. Posttraumatic brain injury cognitive performance is moderated by variation within ANKK1 and DRD2 genes. *J Head Trauma Rehabil* 2015; 30:E54–E66.

108. Hong CT, Wong CS, Ma HP, et al. PERIOD3 polymorphism is associated with sleep quality recovery after a mild traumatic brain injury. *J Neurol Sci* 2015;358:385–389.

109. Haghighi F, Ge Y, Chen S, et al. Neuronal DNA methylation profiling of blast-related traumatic brain injury. *J Neurotrauma* 2015;32:1200–1209.

110. Vagnozzi R, Signoretti S, Floris R. Decrease in *N*-acetylaspartate following concussion may be coupled to decrease in creatine. *J Head Trauma Rehabil* 2013;28:284–292.

111. Chamard E, Lassonde M, Henry L, et al. Neurometabolic and microstructural alterations following a sports-related concussion in female athletes. *Brain Inj* 2013;27:1038–1046.

112. Bulstrode H, Nicoll JA, Hudson G, et al. Mitochondrial DNA and traumatic brain injury. *Ann Neurol* 2014;75: 186–195.

113. Ozen LJ, Fernandes MA. Slowing down after a mild traumatic brain injury: A strategy to improve cognitive task performance? *Arch Clin Neuropsychol* 2012;27:85–100.

114. Temme L, Bleiberg J, Reeves D, et al. Uncovering latent deficits due to mild traumatic brain injury by using normobaric hypoxia stress. *Front Neurol* 2013;30(4):41.

115. Kamaraj DC, Dicianno BE, Cooper RA, et al. Acute mountain sickness in athletes with neurological impairments. *J Rehabil Res Dev* 2013;50:253–262.

116. Duclos C, Beauregard MP, Bottari C, et al. The impact of poor sleep on cognition and activities of daily living after traumatic brain injury: A review. *Aust Occup Ther J* 2015;62:2–12.

117. Lucke-Wold BP, Smith KE, Nguyen L, et al. Sleep disruption and the sequelae associated with traumatic brain injury. *Neurosci Biobehav Rev* 2015;55:68–77.

118. Chamelian L, Feinstein A. The effect of major depression on subjective and objective cognitive deficits in mild to moderate traumatic brain injury. *J Neuropsychiatry Clin Neurosci* 2006;18:33–38.

119. Mauri MC, Paletta S, Colasanti A, et al. Clinical and neuropsychological correlates of major depression following posttraumatic brain injury, a prospective study. *Asian J Psychiatr* 2014;12:118–124.

120. Hart T, Hoffman JM, Pretz C, et al. A longitudinal study of major and minor depression following traumatic brain injury. *Arch Phys Med Rehabil* 2012;93:1343–1349.

121. Vasterling JJ, Brailey K, Proctor SP, et al. Neuropsychological outcomes of mild traumatic brain injury, post-traumatic stress disorder and depression in Iraq-deployed US Army soldiers. *Br J Psychiatry* 2012;201:186–192.

122. Vavilala MS, Dorsch A, Rivara FP. Association between posttraumatic stress, depression, and functional impairments in adolescents 24 months after traumatic brain injury. *J Trauma Stress* 2012;25:264–271.

123. Broglio SP, Pontifex MB, O'Connor P, et al. The persistent effects of concussion on neuroelectric indices of attention. *J Neurotrauma* 2009;26:1463–1470.

124. Ozen LJ, Itier RJ, Preston FF, et al. Long-term working memory deficits after concussion: electrophysiological evidence *Brain Inj* 2013;27:1244–1255.

Chapter

4

What Happens to Concussed Animals?

Jeff Victoroff

The previous chapter of this brief, introductory text on concussion focused on neurobiological changes in the immediate aftermath of concussive brain injury (CBI). The next several chapters summarize what we know today about post-concussive changes in brain and behavior. We begin by discussing non-human animals because, having hit them, scholars are sure that they have been hit and, in so far as is currently known, animals do not feign neurological impairments for love or money.[1]

A conventional chapter might summarize the published results, assume that the methodology is trustworthy, and draw inferences. This chapter will first demonstrate that the methodology is not trustworthy, then – having insulated the reader from credulity – summarize findings from animal studies that do not legitimately model human CBI. In a nutshell: the standard experimental models do not accurately replicate typical human concussion. Rodents – the usual victims of the laboratory – never exhibit neurobehavioral problems that meaningfully model many of the problems routinely caused by CBI. Rodent brains do not age the way human brains age. Shockingly little controlled longitudinal research has been done.

That said, based on the remarkably skimpy portfolio of relevant reports, experimental concussion imposed upon healthy animals often leads to persistent brain change and long-term post-concussive neurobehavioral problems. We turn to humans in the following chapter. There the data will show – consistent with the fragmentary results from non-human animal experiments and exactly as the reader will predict having been armed with the arsenal of animal data: persistent post-concussive brain change and neurobehavioral problems are common.

Introduction

If the late syndrome of concussion were to occur in animals, it certainly could not be recognized by the same signs that characterize it in the human, which are largely subjective.

Apparatus used for the induction of mild traumatic brain injury in a sedated rat

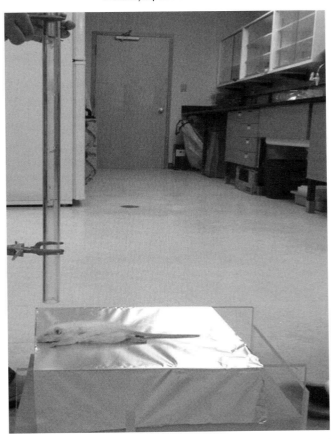

Fig. 4.1 The juvenile rat is placed chest down on the scored tin foil; the head is positioned directly below the falling weight.

Source: Mychasiuk et al., 2014 [1]. Reproduced with permission from Mary Ann Liebert, Inc.

---

[1] The author feels a duty to disclaim. Humans have used non-humans to help figure out human disease for a long time. The author cannot. He has tried. But youthful summers in laboratories at the National Institutes of Health, at Stanford, and at Harvard taught him that he lacks the capacity to ignore the fact that the animal he is carrying to the guillotine did not evolve for, did not elect, and does not (in any way one could perceive) savor this style of life and death. It would not be appropriate to discuss that issue in this essay at length. The author fully acknowledges the debt humanity owes to investigators who do this work, and to their unwitting subjects. He offers only that perhaps one should not take lightly the question of animal consciousness and the slippery slope of speciesism.

However, it is quite possible that the same underlying basis for the syndrome does exist in animals. This proposition is given considerable support by the following findings.

Groat and Simmons, 1950, pp. 152–153 [2]

In order to conclude with any confidence that a "mild" CBI (a typical clinically attended CBI) meaningfully, and perhaps lastingly, damages human brains, one might first ask, "Is there evidence that a relatively minor abrupt external force damages the brain of *any* living organism?" Chapter 1 offered several historically key animal studies demonstrating such post-concussive brain effects. There is somewhat more to be said. This chapter will assume that weighty duty. Hopefully, the drama of the story will outweigh its occasional lapses into technicalities and provide refreshing insights.

Second, one might demand evidence that the parts of the brain – the particular networks, cells, and molecules that are typically damaged in experimental CBI – are comparable to the brain parts that seem to mediate human post-concussive dysfunction and emotional distress. The answer is a qualified *yes*. An abrupt external force that shakes the brain of a non-human mammal tends to hurt many of the same brain parts implicated in human post-concussive neurobehavioral problems.

A third and more awkward question is whether lightly concussed animals suffer persistent or even permanent brain change. If a good answer had ever been seriously sought, it might have largely obviated the need for this textbook. The author confesses his personal abhorrence of cost–benefit ethical justifications for medical experiments on sentient beings. However, imagine that, in 1920, Air Vice Marshal and pioneering neurologist Sir Charles Putnam Symonds, KBE, CB [3], had established a large colony of free-living squirrel monkeys. If 1000 had been exposed to experimental concussion, and 1000 not, by 1935 he would have had the answer. Far better than rodents, old world monkeys exhibit recognizable irritability, anxiety, and depression – perhaps the most important disabling sequelae after traumatic brain injury (TBI). Monkeys do not develop "Alzheimer's Disease" (AD) (no non-human animal does), but they exhibit memory loss and neurodegeneration and could have been monitored for a lifetime of brain and behavior changes in 15 years. What's more, monkeys have personalities. Lasting change might have been detected. Dr. Symonds would not have been able to perform immunocytochemistry or *in vivo* tractography, or measure network efficiency or voxel-specific *N*-acetyl aspartate levels, but many neuropathological techniques were well in hand at that time, and he could have accomplished reasonably sophisticated clinico pathological correlations 85 years ago.

Rodents are harder to read. A similar rodent experiment might have been completed in two years, but the behavior and brain changes would have been less easily interpreted. Still, students reviewing the literature are routinely amazed to find that this simple, important project has yet to be done. In so far

as suggested by the disappointing scraps of available data, the tentative answer is *yes*, concussed animals develop persistent post-CBI brain changes.[2] This chapter will summarize relevant reports from laboratories around the world.

A fourth question might be, "Yes, one must acknowledge evidence of persistent post-CBI brain change in animals. Yet what of behavioral change?" The relevant data – which again happen to be remarkably thin on the ground – have been painstakingly harvested for presentation later in this chapter. Even winnowed and warmed, it makes a thin gruel. Readers can decide for themselves whether that evidence satisfies the natural hunger for adequate hypothesis testing.

Experiments with Abrupt External Force

In an earnest and well-intentioned effort to understand human concussion, investigators have beaten animals about the head for at least 150 years. That work exploded over the previous decade (not a pun), as investigators conducted many more experiments with blast injuries, less forceful blows, and repetitive blows, sometimes employing more ecologically valid models of both injury and post-concussive status. This chapter will describe the findings.[3] As previously mentioned, the time course of the effects of a concussive blow is not linear. The beaten brain does not reach a nadir of function immediately and then gradually recover. It hosts a battle, with colliding forces of competing damaging and reparative molecular processes and highly variable neurobehavioral consequences over different time periods. (Adumbrating one denouement: the good news from animal studies is recent confirmation of post-traumatic neurogenesis.)

Let us say that a 12-year-old boy, Henry, is beaned in a Little League baseball game and unresponsive for two minutes. Contrary to the common lore, one does not expect a linear trajectory of recovery. As addressed more fully in Chapter 5, different problems tend to come and go during different time periods. Whether or not his coach has the prudence to get him to a doctor, what is Henry likely to experience in the first day or two? Disorientation, headache, double vision, dizziness, and nausea, sometimes with vomiting. The first month or two? Thankfully, there is often a significant decrease in all of those symptoms except headache, but disinhibition, irritability, and new learning deficits often become overt. Three to nine months? Henry, whose parents and teachers have perhaps been wringing their hands from the first week, aware that Henry is falling behind, may himself finally become disconcerted as he gains insight into his own impairments. Such a patient will commonly report slowed and effortful mental processing, sometimes accompanied by depression, emotional dysregulation, and personality change. These last are the troubles that sometimes persist for a year, or for five years, or for life. Yet evidence also suggests late healing. Whether mediated by adaptation, or cellular repurposing, or resolution of inflammation, or

---

2 The present author hopes that, by the time this slender text wends its way through production in England, someone will have filled in this embarrassing scientific blank.

3 From this point forward, the colloquial term *animals* will be substituted for the scientific phrase *non-human animals*.

neurogenesis, or some other mechanism, thankfully, some CBI survivors continue to improve for as long as a decade.

That may or may not be the end of the story. Perhaps the greatest unresolved question about a single, typical, clinically attended concussion is whether such an injury alters the myriad processes that might collectively be called time-passing-related brain change. The traditional phrase for such changes is "late effects" [4]. One way to characterize the last 15 years of CBI research: it has become very clear and widely accepted that repetitive CBIs sometimes lead to late effects – meaning potentially disabling cognitive, psychiatric, or motor disorders perhaps 1–75 years post-exposure. In sharp contrast, it remains unknown whether, and how often, and by what pathophysiological mechanism a single CBI might alter brain and behavior many years after the fact. One piece of evidence supporting the guess that single CBIs trigger late effects: unless a first concussion changed the brain in ways that persisted for months or years, two or 20 concussions separated by months or years would not have any more effects than one. Yet they often seem to. This, added to the evidence from functional neuroimaging, debunks the theory promoted by some 20th-century neuropsychologists that single concussions have no lasting effects. But the pressing question, unanswered at the time of this writing due to a lack of funded longitudinal research in both animals and humans, is whether a single concussion increases the risk for late-life dementia.

If, indeed, single CBIs sometimes cause late effects, it is easy to see why they might be almost impossible to detect. Regarding Henry: assume that, absent his concussion, he would have begun to forget his shopping list and his grandchildren's names at age 82. Assume that, as a result of his concussion, his forgetfulness instead begins at age 76. How would one ever know? We cannot – certainly not in Henry's individual case, even if we had somehow daily tracked the well-being of each of his neurons. One might say "many cross-sectional studies have reported that people who survive a concussion are more likely to develop AD." However, as discussed in the chapter titled *Late Effects* (Chapter 11), the quality of peer-reviewed retrospective studies comparing mentation in persons with and without a history of concussion is so poor that no credible inference regarding whether a single CBI is a risk factor for dementia is possible.

Animal models have been devised primarily to approximate the short-term brain changes attributable to TBI/CBI. Properly done, they could provide vital clues regarding late effects. Yet experimental study of long-term effects has lagged. Success, to date, is fragmentary. (Readers, if they wish, may leap ahead to Table 4.2 and review the data themselves.) But the few available findings are intriguing, suggestive, and, to the author, affecting.

What this Chapter will Defer

This chapter focuses on changes in brain and cognition after experimental concussion. It will only mention non-cognitive changes such as depression, anxiety, and aggression in passing. That vital subject earned its own chapter: *Persistent Post-Concussive Psychiatric Problems* (Chapter 10). Nor will this chapter address neuroimaging in either humans or animals – an exciting domain of study experiencing exponential growth and inching us ever closer to measuring concussion with biomarkers. Again, coming chapters better summarize and synthesize that literature. In addition, this chapter will momentarily sidestep the compelling evidence that repetitive concussions may trigger devastating dementias. Other chapters better address the sad tale of human brain gauntlets, often self-selected. The goal of this chapter is ambitious enough: to distill and present in a digestible way the vital lessons learned from observing the effects of experimental concussions.

Five Serious Problems With Animal Models (and the Other Four)

As fascinating as the story is, as much as one would hope that animal experiments would unveil the mysteries of concussion, they don't. At least five caveats restrain our confidence that the animal findings apply to humans:

1. We do not know what force best approximates typical human concussion.
2. In the majority of laboratories, investigators seem to hit the wrong thing in the wrong way.
3. Animals cannot tell us how they feel.
4. The behaviors assessed are neither ecologically valid nor comparable to human behaviors.
5. Nobody wants to care for a brain-damaged mouse.

A *sixth* problem is that *individuality* is obvious among humans but not obvious among rodents. That is, in many societies, each of the ten children on a school bus T-boned by a big rig already has a written record of their medical and psychological uniqueness. Parents and doctors are able to detect change from those ten unique baselines. No medical person would claim that CBI does the same thing to any two people, and we fully expect to observe those individual differences. As Mychasiuk et al. put it, crystallizing a vital, often overlooked, conceptual insight, "an important hallmark characteristic of human TBI is symptom heterogeneity; individual responses to similar injuries vary substantially as a result of genetic, epigenetic, and environmental influences" [1].

In contrast, individual mice are rarely befriended and studied with care prior to injury, so it is hard to say whether mouse Alfredo is more aggressive than he was before his concussion, while mouse Benedict is less aggressive. This encourages the convenient fiction that mice are interchangeable and the marked differences in their reactions to identical injuries are due to happenstance or natural variation rather than the result of individual strengths and weaknesses that deserve study. For example, Creed et al. [5] exposed six mice to virtually identical forces. The outcomes were hardly identical; only two of those six mice developed focal brain hemorrhage beneath the impact site. Similarly, although some scholars report that amyloid deposition is expected in transgenic mice after repetitive concussions [6, 7], other scholars [8] report that this varies from mouse to mouse.

That raises a *seventh* problem: mice don't get AD. How then will hitting mice reveal the biological link between acute concussive brain change and later neurodegeneration? Admittedly, it is not yet known how single CBIs affect aging-related neurodegenerative processes – which are typically (if rather dubiously) thought of as specific "diseases" involving the deposition of one or more "toxic" proteins. (The new doubts about the discrete nature of classically labeled diseases such as "Alzheimer's" will be addressed in the *Late Effects* chapter, Chapter 11). It is also a matter of debate whether concussions provoke a special tauopathy some pathologists elect to call "chronic traumatic encephalopathy," or instead simply represent one of many environmental risk factors that accelerate brain aging – lowering the threshold for the many forms of time-passing-related brain change.

What's more, at the time of this writing, a long-overdue revolution in nosology is taking place. Neurologists are reconsidering the 20th-century assumption that aggregates of atypically folded proteins such as tau and amyloid β are neurotoxic. Evidence suggests that they are not – although they may hint at a threat from toxic oligomers. That discovery has clarified the fact that only by application of biologically arbitrary operational criteria might one claim a distinction between expected time-passing-related brain change and alleged "disease" [9, 10]. As a result, the old habit of labeling heterogeneous lumps of clinico pathological phenomena as specific diseases such as "Alzheimer's," "frontotemporal dementia," and "vascular dementia" is being reconceptualized as simplistic pigeon holing. Instead, it appears that there is an infinite spectrum of polypathological mixtures of time-passing-related brain alterations, the contribution of any particular protein to which is relative, not absolute. These paradigm-shifting conceptual concerns aside, it is a matter of importance (perhaps more honored in the breach than the observance) to employ transgenic mice with brains that can mimic some human changes (such as Aβ deposition), but not others.

An *eighth* problem: among the slings and arrows in the melee between injurious and reparative processes after concussion, something wonderful happens: neurogenesis. It has been exciting and heartening to detect post-CBI neurogenesis in rodents. It explains and it offers hope. But, since neurogenesis is very hard to see in living humans, we are left with our fingers crossed regarding whether that rodent boon applies to human recovery from CBI.

A *ninth* problem is that some scientists still make judgments of brain health based on the 1590's technology of the light microscope. We will return to this. But let's focus on the top five problems.

Problem 1: We Do Not Know What Force Best Approximates Typical Human Concussion

In animal models of TBI, the mechanism of MTBI [mild TBI] is the same for severe TBI; there is simply more damage in the severely injured cases.

Ucar et al., 2006 [11]

Although the term "mild" TBI is used often in the pre-clinical literature, clearly defined criteria for mild, moderate, and severe TBI in animal models have not been agreed upon.

Shultz et al., 2017 [12]

Imagine that one positioned the members of a large family of mice in such a way that their heads will be impacted at the same anatomical target with a reasonable degree of accuracy. The student might drop weights from a height of 40 cm on to all of those heads. He or she might start with one-tenth of a gram (0.1 g) for mouse #1. Then half a gram (0.5 g) for mouse #2. Keep escalating the weight. One gram, two grams, then perhaps 5, 10, 25 … say, up to 2 kg. One can reasonably intuit that 0.1 g will do no harm and 2 kg will kill. But at what point in this sequence of experiments did the student begin subjecting a mouse to a concussive force? And, if one has become habituated to the notion that concussion means something "mild," at what point in this sequence of events did the student *stop* exposing mice to a concussive force?

The physics of this thought experiment are trivial. One can readily calculate the linear accelerative force applied to each mouse. It is different at each weight. But one can only *guess* the force transmitted to the brain, because every brain/skull combination is different, so structural and functional damage will occur at different thresholds of force for different little mice. Even if the force hitting the brain was absolutely uniform and measured to three decimal places (the goal of the earnest scientists who employ fluid percussion and controlled cortical impact) the threshold of damage will still vary, since every mouse has its own brain microanatomy, ultrastructure, gene expression, and epigenetic fiddlings with those genes.

Of course, one can wager that very light force is benign and a very heavy force is fatal. Yet, apart from these extremes, it is not self-evident at what point one might expect what changes, to what degree, in the virtually innumerable biological parameters one might monitor, or in the hundreds of measures of short- or long-term behavioral change one might observe in a single mouse named Alfredo. If 100 mice of the same age, sex, and weight were exposed to the same brain-shaking force somewhere in the damaging-but-not-deadly range, it is critical to understand what the laboratory has revealed: the changes might be somewhat different in every cell in every mouse.

This thought experiment exposes a problem in the coherence of scholarly banter regarding concussion. The straightforward view of concussion, as the concept was employed for millennia, is a rattling or shaking blow. In neurology, that phenomenon might be described as *an abrupt external force that rattles the brain*. Prior to about 1924 any English-speaking doctor would as happily use the word *concussion* to describe both a lance impaling the royal brain and causing immediate death and an uppercut by a two-year-old. Both are rattling blows. The more recent use of *concussion* dramatically narrowed the concept, tossing out both extremes, very light and heavy – like Goldilocks, that insouciant trespasser – to focus on the middling.

This narrow point of view, so at odds with the original meaning of the word *concussion*, signaled a scientifically dubious mutation in definition urged by a few early-20th-century writers. As described in Chapter 1, Trotter and his acolytes said that concussion is a certain *amount* of *injury*: not too little; not too much; just enough to rattle the brain and impair consciousness without killing. According to their notion, a falling leaf, a toddler's boxing practice, or any similar trivial impact that shakes the brain without altering consciousness is not a concussion. At the same time, those early-20th-century writers also excluded fatal impacts. Many excluded impacts that fracture the skull. According to that thesis, concussion only refers to some narrow slice of the midrange along the infinite spectrum of possible forces, defined in a non-biological way such as "sufficient to trigger a subjective report that sounds like altered consciousness but not to produce a skull fracture."

In Chapter 1 we expressed concern that this Goldilocks thesis was dogmatic and divorced from science. In English, a concussion is simply a rattling or shaking blow. Respecting the logic of semantics, CBI is not "all those blows, but really only the little ones, but maybe not too little." The phrase *CBI* is simple – mechanically specific and theoretically agnostic. It denotes brain rattling across the spectrum of deleterious effects. As Russell put it in 1971:

> We are therefore faced with the problem of classification and, as far as closed accidental concussion of the acceleration type is concerned, it is simpler basically to look at all cases as being different grades of the one type of trauma caused by violent accelerations.
>
> [13, p. 2]

Unless biomarkers are some day discovered that meaningfully distinguish "grades," injurious brain rattling is injurious brain rattling. In animal research, it is tough enough to define the threshold between injury and non-injury let alone mumbling over criteria for ordinal rankings within the injury group. Indeed, only post-mortem examination can confirm "injury," and mouse pathologists may not even agree about the definitional cut-off for that phenomenon.

As much as it is human nature to assign qualifying adjectives to problems (e.g., "ghastly accident," "brutal assault"), no red lines appear in the data sets. Where is the boundary at which a "mild" mouse brain change becomes "moderate"? An injury involving ≥ 17.5 g when dropped from 80 cm? An injury involving ≥ 2.15 atmospheres of pressure with a brain deflection of 1.5 mm? An injury involving resolution of apnea in ≤ 6.5 seconds? An injury in which $\leq 14\%$ of the animals developed subdural hematomas? An injury that causes a 17–31% increase in foot faults on the rotarod test at 24 h? None of these hypothetical severity thresholds predicts good or bad outcome six months down the road.

From the viewpoint of evolutionary biology, one might propose a different approach: rate severity based on the impact on the animal's inclusive fitness (survival and reproduction measured over the two subsequent generations).

That might be a more scientifically compelling yardstick. Yet where should one draw the mild vs. moderate line along that stick?

On the one hand, certain laboratory observations have come to be employed as markers of severity [14–22]. In "mild to moderate" injury there is typically no apnea. The normal pedal withdrawal reflex returns about 17 s after ending anesthesia in sham-injured control rats, while in "mildly" injured rats that reflex recovers at about 24 s, and in "moderate" injury this occurs at about 32 s. The righting reflex usually comes back after sham injury at about 60 s; but after "mild" injury it requires about 100 s and after "moderate" injury about 180 s. Sham injury does not produce forepaw contraflexion (flexion posturing of the forepaw contralateral to the hemisphere that was impacted). "Mild" injury may produce it for one to three days; more severe injury, for a week or longer. Do any of these thresholds sound like legitimate signifiers of a categorical biological difference?

Investigators have also used survival to judge severity. Ucar et al. [11], for instance, exposed rats to weights of 300 g, 350g, or 450 g, all dropped from 1 m. It seems reasonable to regard the impact of the 450-g weight as "severe" given that 11 of 14 subjects died. It also seems reasonable to regard the 300-g impact as "milder," given that only one of 14 rats died, only three experienced apnea, and fewer exhibited subarachnoid hemorrhage.

The typical way investigators judge a hit's severity is by reference to *average* whole-animal behavioral responses, such as seconds of apnea, or duration of loss of righting reflexes, or proportion killed outright. On the other hand, since results of identical blows are quite variable, and since one can only predict what will happen to any individual within a wide range, again, *no red line divides mild from not mild*. For this reason, readers are admonished to be wary: if the writer says "Trust me, I hit my rodents mildly," it does not mean that any other lab would necessarily agree.

Now let us consider the actual results of graded exposure to concussive force. The goal of these protocols is to replicably mimic the spectrum of human TBI. Investigators label the injuries they produce as "mild," moderate," or "severe," but these labels really do not refer to a biologically identifiable injury threshold. Instead, as mentioned above and demonstrated below:

1. The same force produces different degrees of injury in different mice.
2. Different forces may produce the same degree of injury.
3. Some purportedly "mild" impacts cause death.

As in the thought experiment above, investigators in fact routinely expose animals to graded concussive forces. For example, Schwarzbold et al. [23] dropped weights of 10, 12.5, or 15 g on to the left parietal region of mice from 120 cm. The neurobiological severity scores (Figure 4.2) imply a roughly proportionate relationship between force of impact and harm. Yet a closer look at the data reveals that such linear relationships are merely statistical means that mask natural variations. That is, a given amount of force *does not mean*

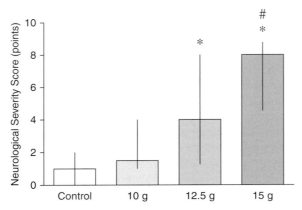

Effects of traumatic brain injury on neurological state of mice as measured by the Neurological Severity Scale

Fig. 4.2 A higher score indicates greater neurological impairment. Mice in the 12.5-g group had higher scores than controls. Mice in the 15-g group had higher scores than both 10-g groups and controls.

Source: Schwarzbold et al., 2010 [23]. Reproduced with permission from Mary Ann Liebert, Inc.

a given amount of brain damage. It only puts the little guy in a little more peril. It's a probabilistic threat to health and well-being.[4]

For instance, in Schwarzbold et al.'s experiment, mice exposed to 10-g weights had a 16.7% skull fracture rate and a 9% death rate. Those exposed to 12.5 g had a 53.5% skull fracture rate and a 51.2% death rate. Those exposed to 15 g had an 80% skull fracture rate and a 72.2% death rate. Thus, the effects of "mild" impact varied from none to death. What, then, is mild? Anyone can nominate a level on this scale and call it "mild" –but only if he or she ignores outcome: minor impact is a risk factor that sometimes leads to major harm, and vice versa.[5]

This is a crucial idea. Within the natural range of resilience, "exposure" to a head knock does not equate to brain injury, any more than exposure to a sneezing baby means a head cold. Exposure to a head knock is to brain cell death as driving fast is to a motor vehicle accident.

It's probabilistic.

It's unpredictable.

It's a matter of odds.

Similarly, in an effort to approximate the brain forces suffered by American football players, Viano et al. [24] devised a rat concussion model involving higher impact velocities and helmet-protected but freely moving rats. (As we will touch upon below, free movement is important. It is the natural circumstance when almost every concussion happens to almost

every animal.) A 50-g impactor was accelerated to 7.4, 9.3, or 11.2 m/s on the left side of a head protected by an aluminum helmet. These velocities were carefully selected in hopes of matching the mean velocity, plus or minus one standard deviation, of National Football League collisions causing concussion. Rats were exposed either to single or repetitive impacts, using impactors of either 50 or 100 g.

The results?

- No level of force guaranteed gross pathology.
- A bigger force did not mean a bigger degree of pathology.
- Instead, just as the reader expects from a probabilistic threat, a bigger force means a higher mathematical *risk* of pathology

– in this case, rising from 11% to 28% to 33%. Viano et al.'s finds are exactly consistent with shaking-head-blow-as-risk concept. Some animals receiving the lightest blows came away with nasty brain damage; some receiving the heaviest blows did not. These findings and those from similar studies of graded force [13, 18, 25–30] confirm that a given concussive force does not determine a given outcome. That hardly makes it safe.

Of course the reader (and this author) cannot contain our curiosity: among 16 mice exposed to identical forces and energy transfers, why did just two mice suffer gross brain damage? We are bound to think of our patients – or perhaps ourselves. Why do some individuals suffer more than others? As the upcoming chapters will discuss in more depth, the quick answer is that we do not know. Until we get a better handle on genetic factors affecting injury response, we are obliged to humbly admit the limits of our insight. However, abundant empirical evidence suggests that several patient-related, injury-related, and post-injury-related variables moderate the impact of a shaking blow on long-term well being. This observation is central to solving the ancient and mysterious observation: the effects of CBI vary greatly.

In partial conclusion: we witness and accept the simple fact that the same concussive force may have very different consequences. A force that one little head tolerates might produce disabling problems in another. This finding in animals has direct bearing on clinical practice. In human concussion, as we know, when big complaints follow modest hits, certain authorities rush to blame the patient. "You're not that bad off. You're just confusing matters due to your expectations, misattributions, imagination, exaggeration, faking, and 'litigation overlay.'" Indeed, some people are more fragile. But the wide variation in outcome after similar hits in genetically identical rodents cannot reasonably be attributed to frail egos or lust for dollars.

---

[4] The concept of probabilistic injury is easily mastered. What happens when one drops a China cup? It might break; it might not. Through diligent attention to his grandmother's material legacy, at about age seven the author determined that, from table height on to hardwood floor, the chances of shattering were about 33%. As he recalls, the odds of fragmentation increased to more than 50% when the flight was initiated by the cat, Midnight, from atop the refrigerator. That is a probabilistic injury. Due to individual conditions and chance, breakage might or might not follow exposure to a given force. The brain is the same.

[5] Perhaps contrary to intuition, Schwarzbold et al. also found that 10-g-impacted animals exhibited more anxiety at ten days post-CBI than those exposed to weightier injuries. This phenomenon of disproportionate psychiatric distress after "mild" injury will be explained in the chapter on *Persistent Post-Concussive Psychiatric Problems* (Chapter 10).

Problem 2: We Usually Hit the Wrong Thing in the Wrong Way

Although FP [fluid percussion] and CCI [controlled cortical impact] models employ highly reproducible mechanical inputs and can mimic many pathological features of human TBI, their predominantly focal tissue destruction and lack of head movement decreases their resemblance to the majority of human impact acceleration injuries, which most often occur without skull fracture and are chiefly characterized by diffuse axonal injury (DAI).

Namjoshi et al., 2017, p. 81 [31]

A 39-year-old woman named Rosabel is motoring to her office. A texting teenaged driver interrupts her progress. Rosabel's mobile head collides with her auto's steering wheel and door pillar. It is her hair that makes impact. Force is subsequently transmitted through that material and a bony vault. Finally, her brain is shaken against her skull – every cell affected in a different way. As with the Hybrid III crash test dummy, the distribution of forces to the internal detectors is significantly dependent on the complex mechanical properties of the shell.

A one-year-old mouse named Hermione is handled gently, apart from the intraperitoneal needle that induces stupor, and what follows. First, an accomplished technician cuts and peels away her scalp. Then, faithfully applying Incan research methodology, he trepans a hole in her skull. Hermione is chained such that her head sits on a block of something – wood, steel, foam. The technician attaches a tube to the big hole he made in her skull and, when all is well, shoots a high-pressure blast of fluid through the tube. Although her head hardly moves, although her skull is untouched, her brain is rattled (Figures 4.3 and 4.4).

Are these comparable life events?

A major problem with interpreting the findings from experimental brain injury is that hardly any investigators strive to reproduce a typical CBI. Among the deviations from that commonplace mammalian phenomenon:

1. The animal's head is fixed – rather than mobile, as occurs in nature.
2. The animal is sedated, hence, not exposed to the usual psychic trauma of CBI.
3. No abrupt external force impacts the head. Instead, in a manner that is grossly inconsistent with typical CBI, a force is administered that strikes the dura, bypassing the hair, scalp, and skull – which, in the natural world, is the mechanical transmitter and disperser of almost every harmful brain acceleration.

Popular (But Flawed) Experimental Models of Concussive Brain Injury

Neuroscientists are in a bind. They wish to do experiments that mimic concussion. But they are under the gun to do experiments that are uniform – for instance, hitting identical subjects in identical ways. These are competing agendas. As we have hopefully established, no two concussions are the same. Yet one can try to reduce the number of variables in an experiment.

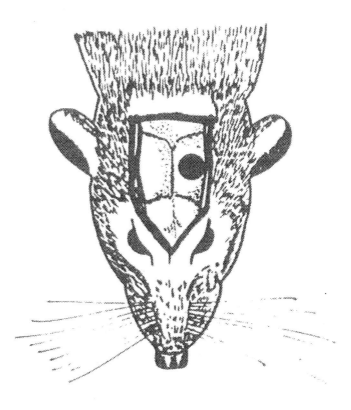

Fig. 4.3 Craniotomy exposing the dura of a rat in preparation for fluid percussion injury. The black dot represents the parasagittal target of the fluid pulse.
Source: McIntosh et al., 1989 [32] with permission from Elsevier

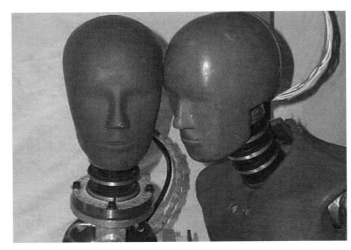

Fig. 4.4 Hybrid III 50th-percentile male instrumented dummy heads.
Source: Withnall et al., 2005 [33] with permission from BMJ Publishing Group Ltd

For instance, one can greatly reduce the affect of individual differences if all the subjects are from the same species, with the same size, weight, and age. One can further reduce variability by delivering the same punch to ten inbred mice. That is possible because lab mice of one strain are (almost) genetically identical to one another. Such steps permit one to say, "This is the spectrum of change observed when force X is applied to site Y on 27-g, 6-month-old, male C5BL/6 mice."

But one cannot draw conclusions about what happens to mice as a species, since the laboratory never tested any of the other > 400 inbred strains of mice such as BALB/Cs, CD-1s, SCIDs, A/Js. … In fact, one cannot even declare that the findings apply to the strain C5BL/6: purportedly "identical" strains from one mouse merchandiser (such as Charles River Laboratories) may be biologically different from those from another (such as Taconic Farms). Besides which: to understand human concussion one needs to study the range of effects it has on people with different genomes. Confine studies to a single genome? One will fail to discover the natural range of effects.

Similarly, one can greatly reduce anatomical variability of the injury by removing the skull before hitting the animal and aiming carefully. Yet that procedure rather cavalierly ignores a major mechanical element of concussion: the vast majority of concussions affect closed heads. Most CBIs involve force *transmitted through* and *dispersed by* bony skulls – within which the brain then rattles around. How can one replicate the effects of a pea shaken in a can without the can? Moreover, the investigator who studies the results of impacting one site – comprising, for instance, 3% of the dural surface – with one force in ten mice would have about 330 more experiments to run in order to claim having tested the effects of that one force, since he or she would wish to investigate the effects on each 3% of the dura.

One can also greatly increase the chances of hitting a chosen target by strapping the poor animal down. But it was noted more than 500 years ago that the neurological outcome is different when a fixed head gets crushed versus when a mobile head gets knocked. Moreover, one can certainly decrease variability if the strapped-down victim sustains a simple linear acceleration. Yet a human football player, for example, typically suffers concussions from hits producing not only a linear acceleration but also a rotational acceleration in all three planes of motion [34] – not to mention the mind-boggling distribution of strains.

The problem is that the more one's experimental model contorts itself to avoid natural variation in the interest of idealized research design, the less likely the findings will reflect nature. "Identical injuries" in nearly identical rodents are important for reducing the number of confounding variables. Yet they perhaps deter neuroscientists from understanding what neurologists see in the clinic: a remarkable variation of outcomes.

Six Models

no TBI model is currently able to reproduce pathological changes identical to those seen in human patients.
Romine et al., 2014, p. 1 [35]

Knowing all this, neuroscientists have earnestly attempted to devise a rodent model that accurately replicates human concussion [3, 15, 20–22, 32, 36–44]. Candidly, no animal model accurately reproduces the biomechanical effects, let alone the molecular effects, of concussion. Yet readers may wish to know the source of published claims.

The six most commonly employed models are: (1) the weight drop acceleration injury model [14, 45, 46]; (2) the impact acceleration injury model [16, 19]; (3) the fluid percussion injury (FPI) model [15, 32, 47]; (4) the controlled cortical impact (CCI) model [40, 48]; (5) the closed head impact model of engineered rotational acceleration (CHIMERA); and (6) some version of a blast injury. Figure 4.5 illustrates the first four.

The weight drop acceleration injury model is simple. The subject is positioned beneath a tube. A weight with a flat or hemispheric tip is dropped through the tube from a known distance, generating a known force, usually impacting the top or side of the head of a restrained animal. Although this is the easiest, least expensive method – and has largely been abandoned in favor of higher technology – it is one of the few methods that comes close to replicating a human concussion, since the target of the weight is the head, not the exposed dura or the brain.

Skull fractures sometimes occur with focal weight drop. For this reason, Marmarou et al. [19] devised a variation called the impact acceleration injury, in which a rigid plate is glued to the head. The weight strikes the plate. This disperses the force and reduces the complication of skull fracture. In this sense (like the animal experiments that actually employ helmets), it sacrifices fidelity compared with typical blunt force trauma, but is more likely to reproduce DAI and better replicates a typical football or military non-blast concussion in a helmeted victim.

The FPI protocol is perhaps the most commonly employed laboratory model of CBI, despite the dubious validity of its results. First, the anesthetized animal undergoes craniectomy with trephine, exposing an area of unprotected dura. Then a hub is installed that will receive and focus the coming fluid pulse. Then a calibrated pulse of fluid under pressure is forced through the tube, impacting a circular area of dura (Figure 4.6) (Also see Alder et al., 2011, for a video demonstration [49].) Although there is no universal standard, a pulse of 0.5–1.5 atm is often called a mild injury; > 2 atm is usually considered moderate or severe. The FPI can be administered either centrally or, more commonly, laterally (LFPI). The advantage is precision. The obvious drawback is that this injury is really very different from a natural CBI in which an external force impacts a somewhat hairy scalp covering a bony skull. FPI delivers a pulse of pressure directly to the unnaturally naked dura. There is no absorption or diffusion of force by the skull.

The FPI model provides a reasonable degree of reproducibility and perhaps mimics some aspects of CBI. Yet fluid percussion utterly fails to replicate the most basic dynamics of the event: what happens to the brain only does so after whatever complex tricks of energy absorption, transmission, and dispersion that the hair, scalp, galea, and bony skull play on the noxious quantum of external kinetic energy. A CBI is, by definition,

Four experimental models of traumatic brain injury

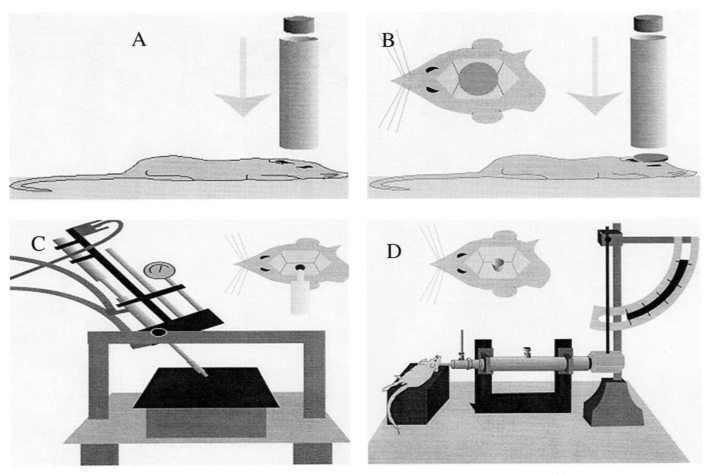

Fig. 4.5 A: weight drop model; B: impact acceleration model; C: controlled cortical impact model; D: fluid percussion injury model.
Source: Morales et al., 2005, p. 972 [20]. Reprinted by permission from Springer

the consequence of an abrupt visitation by an external force usually transmitted through the skull. Brain/skull biomechanics are extremely complex. The skull partially deforms, absorbing some force. It sometimes breaks, absorbing more force. It distributes the force, just as a helmet is intended to do, resulting in less focal damage and more widespread damage. Yet that damage is not "diffuse" in any mathematically rigorous way. It is distributed chaotically – the virtually impossible-to-predict consequence of not a single acceleration of a single object but the different accelerations over different nanoseconds in the brain rattling that surely impact each of 86 billion neurons and their neighboring glia and blood vessels somewhat differently, and then rebound a few times, not like the perfect shiny balls in a Newton's cradle but bouncing around against each other and the skull more like three boys rolling down a hill in a barrel. FPI does not represent CBI. As will be further explained in the commentary about finite element modeling (Chapter 7), it is impossible to reproduce the strains and stresses of a typical external force by directly hitting the brain's slip of dural lingerie.

As depicted in Figure 4.5C, in CCI a mechanically or pneumatically driven impactor strikes the head or brain of a restrained animal. Unilateral CCI was formerly thought

to produce a mostly focal injury, yet more recent evidence suggests that, when certain impact parameters are selected, CCI yields a diffuse white-matter injury similar to DAI [50, 51]. This hints at the advantage of CCI: investigators can control the brain-shaking blow far better than with weight drop or FPI by adjusting the velocity, depth of tissue deformation, and dwell time. With respect to velocity: speed itself is not a measure of force. Two injuries at the same velocity may be very different in severity. Moreover, a modest difference in velocity can produce a large difference in effect, since the kinetic energy is proportional to the square of the velocity ($KE = \frac{1}{2}\ mass \times (velocity)^2$), but kinetic energy can also be dissipated. The real question is what *change* of velocity is experienced by what masses in the head. Be that as it may, a piston velocity 2–6 m/s is often used in modeling mild injury and 6–7 m/s is often used in modeling moderate injury – understanding that a 6 m/s injury can be mild, moderate, or severe depending on the depth of the divot of dural deformation. Dural deformation can be varied precisely. About 1 mm is typical in a "mild" injury experiment, yet different laboratories use 0.2–1.5 mm for mild and 1–2.5 mm for "moderate" injuries. Dwell time refers to the time

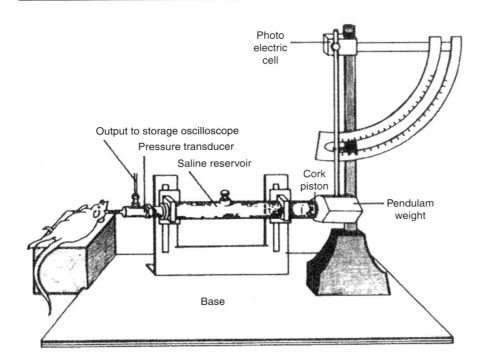

Fig. 4.6 Fluid percussion device adapted for rat concussive brain injury.

Source: McIntosh et al., 1989 [32] with permission from Elsevier

the piston or impactor remains at its depth in the deformed head. A typical CCI dwell time is about 50–500 ms, regardless of intended severity. However (as will be discussed in Chapter 7's brief commentary on finite element modeling), duration of contact at depth may be more important to replicating a typical concussion than previously thought. For all the precision of CCI, the findings can be just as hard to interpret as those from FPI: although some laboratories replicate natural CBI by striking a closed head, *most labs remove an area of skull and expose the dura.* Another problem is a lack of standardization; every laboratory chooses unique impact parameters they believe will replicate a "mild TBI."

CHIMERA is a recent addition. This model was introduced because open-skull focal injury models such as FPI and CCI do not replicate the basic mechanism of CBI, yet, in previous closed head injury models,

> the input parameters used to induce injury (e.g., mechanical loading, method of mechanical input, and response of the animal's head to mechanical loading) are often poorly controlled, which can contribute to the considerable experimental variation across cognitive, histological, and biochemical outcome measures.
>
> [52, p. 2]

The semi-automatic CHIMERA apparatus, which employs a solenoid-operated piston, overcomes several drawbacks of other designs by: (1) requiring no surgery and minimal isoflurane anesthesia; (2) permitting unconstrained head movement; and (3) allowing for unlimited adjustment of multiple biomechanical input parameters such as impact energy, velocity, and direction (Figure 4.7). Early results are impressive. The model faithfully generates many familiar features of CBI, including DAI with persistent axonal degeneration, microgliosis and inflammation, and increased tau phosphorylation [31, 52].

Another recent advance in experimental modeling of CBI has been dispensing altogether with sedation and administering injury to awake animals. That approach raises ethical questions but potentially eliminates a host of confounding factors. For example, isoflurane and other commonly employed anesthetic agents reportedly alter cerebral blood flow, glutamatergic and GABAergic neurotransmission, mitochondrial function, and apoptosis – all factors directly relevant to the pathophysiology of CBI [12]. Moreover, sedation obviates monitoring whatever component of the post-concussive stress response is related to the memory of the injury. Injuries to unanesthetized animals are thus more naturalistic in some respects (although memory of restraint-induced stress adds a complication).

Less commonly employed models are meant to mimic projectile or blast exposure, such as a projectile concussive impact device, a controlled blast protocol such as the Johns Hopkins University Applied Physics Laboratory shock tube system [37], or an open-field blast exposure model [51]. Figure 4.8 schematically illustrates a blast tube. Figure 4.9 illustrates mice restrained for an open-field blast. Sometimes, in order to better reproduce combat conditions, subject mice are even outfitted with a Kevlar vest (Figure 4.10). One advantage: like the weight drop model, blast experiments mimic the imposition of an abrupt external force on a brain encased, as it usually is, in a skull. A "mild" blast is determined by trial and error, seeking a neurologically impactful intervention that is less than lethal.

Briefly, then, FPI and CCI are by far the most commonly employed laboratory models of TBI. But what kind of injury do they replicate? In both cases, before impact, the investigator removes the inconvenient skull. His apparatus bangs a part of the body that virtually never gets banged: the 270-micron-thick dura mater encasing the brain. CCI replicates reasonably well what happens when a clumsy neurosurgeon, after performing a

CHIMERA device and mouse head positioning

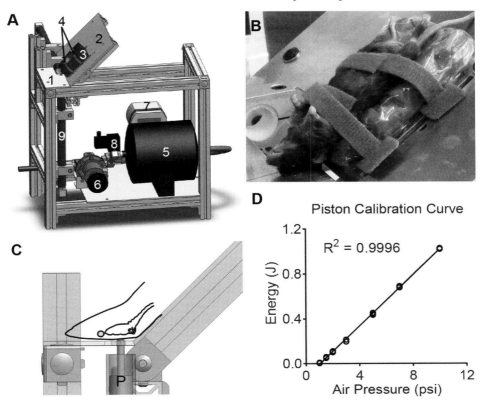

Fig. 4.7 (A) The CHIMERA device. 1: head plate; 2: body plate; 3: animal bed; 4: Velcro straps; 5: air tank; 6: air pressure regulator; 7: digital pressure gauge; 8: two-way solenoid valve; 9: vertical piston barrel. (B) Close-up view of animal strapped on the holding platform. (C) Location of impact relative to the mouse head and brain. P: impact piston. (D) Air pressure–energy calibration curve was obtained by driving a 50-**g** piston at increasing air pressure values and calculating the resultant impact energy. The graph depicts three measurements for each air pressure value.

Source: Namjoshi et al., 2014 [52]. Reproduced under the terms of the Creative Commons Attribution licence, CC-BY 4.0

A pressurized gas-driven shock tube apparatus

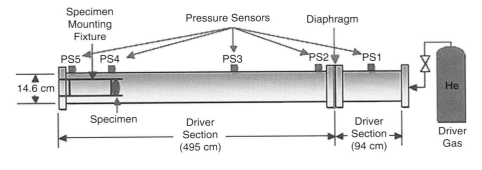

Fig. 4.8 Johns Hopkins University Applied Physics Laboratory shock tube system.

Source: Cernak et al., 2011 [37] with permission from Elsevier

Apparatus for experimental open-field blast injury

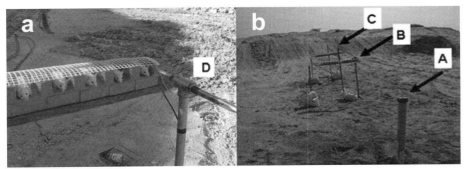

Fig. 4.9 (a) The anesthetized mice were placed in a loose restraint device on a platform, which was covered with white plastic mesh. Each platform had space for 12 anesthetized mice. (b) Photograph of the explosive charge (A) and mice immediately prior to detonation. A cast of 500 g TNT (A) was placed on a pedestal 1 meter above the ground. The 1-meter-high platforms constraining the anesthetized mice were situated 4 meters (B) and 7 meters (C) from the TNT charge. Two pressure gauges were mounted at the ends of each platform (D). [A black and white version of this figure will appear in some formats. For the color version, please refer to the plate section.]

Source: Rubovitch et al., 2011 [53] with permission from Elsevier

Experimental method recreating exposed head/protected torso in open-field blast

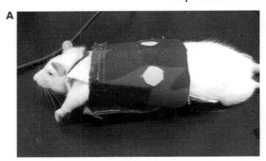
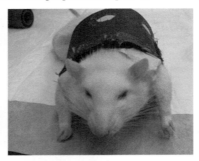

Fig. 4.10 (A) A Kevlar protective vest was secured with Velcro and completely encased the thorax and part of the abdomen. The head was left fully exposed. (B) For airblast exposures, the rats were anesthetized with isoflurane and placed in a transverse prone position in a wire mesh holder secured with stainless steel rods.

Source: Long et al., 2009 [54]. Reproduced with permission from Mary Ann Liebert, Inc.

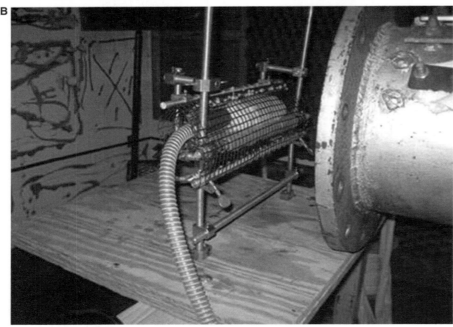

craniotomy, drops a steel tool into the opening. This, I rush to say, is blessedly infrequent.[6]

Thus, contrary to the insistent claim in scores of scientific publications, the work described is not accurately modeling concussion. The published findings – the post-traumatic brain changes painstakingly assayed with sophisticated and pricey methods at the expense of the animal's life – cannot be used to infer what CBI does to brains. Moreover, there has yet to be a well-designed comparison of the effects of forces applied to skulls and to dura. Therefore, one is unable to extrapolate in any rational way from the peer-reviewed results of FPI or CCI experiments to the damage that might have occurred if the investigators had concussed the head.

One quick-and-dirty strategy for culling the literature, in the hope of identifying the most valid and translatable findings, is to focus on experiments that, like human CBI, actually hit the head. However, even the infrequent experiments that hit an intact rodent skull lack ecological validity. Few humans are hit in the head while lying prone on the sidewalk or bed. The overwhelming majority of human CBIs involve a blow to a mobile head – whether in a motor vehicle injury, a fall, a sports-related injury, or an assault. Simple physics dictates that the effects of dynamic loading are quite different when imposed on a fixed versus mobile target. Although foam head beds used in some laboratories allow more natural motion than, for instance, wood or metal platforms, the strains on the typically mobile human head are best imitated by a model allowing free movement of the animal. The new CHIMERA system, described above, is one of few to accommodate free head movement – but still restrains the mouse. (The present author speculates that latter apparatus conceivably risks unintended cervical spine injuries, which could confound the interpretation of subsequent behaviors.)

One laboratory has devised a system that seems to circumvent this potentially important confounding factor: Figure 4.1 depicts the apparatus employed by Mychasiuk et al. [1]. The rodent is positioned on a previously scored (weakened) sheet of aluminum foil. This breaks at the moment of impact, permitting both body and head to move freely. Another clever workaround: give the animal freedom of movement, but partially constrain it in the drop zone with magnetic force [55].

---

6   Fluid percussion injury is even less faithful to the mechanism of typical CBIs. It more or less mimics the experiment of a demented surgeon who, after carefully sawing a hole in the patient's skull, hooks up a firehose.

Neuroscientists are (sometimes) candid in acknowledging that experimental rodent concussion is unlike human concussion. Liu et al. began their 2014 report: "Animal models of traumatic brain injury (TBI) are essential for testing novel hypotheses and therapeutic interventions. Unfortunately, due to the broad heterogeneity of TBI in humans, no single model has been able to reproduce the entire spectrum of these injuries." But this admission barely heeds the tip of the iceberg. The problem is not just that experimental brain injury fails to accurately replicate "the spectrum" of human injury; it fails to accurately replicate *any* human injury. Whether the investigator hits a closed head or an exposed brain, one must question the generalizability of findings with restrained animals. And even those very few laboratories that hit the right thing (the closed head) in the right way (permitting free movement) fail to replicate many aspects of a human concussion because, as finite element modeling demonstrates, the strains and stresses, rattling, shaking, and multiple rebounds of force galloping through a human brain when hit from the outside are incredibly complex and simply not possible to match in a 27-g mammal. A mere glance comparing the rodent with the human skull is enough to raise doubt that the tricks of energy dispersion expected with the geometry and the material properties of the tissue (e.g., fracture toughness, plasticity, tensile strength, shear strength, hydrodynamics) in one species would be comparable to those in the other. Therefore, it seems prudent to restrain enthusiasm regarding the fidelity of rodent models to human concussion.

Problem 3: Animals Cannot Tell us How They Feel

The author requests that this be accepted, pending enhanced interspecies dialogue, as axiomatic.

Problem 4: The Behaviors Assessed are Neither Ecologically Valid nor Comparable to Human Behaviors

It is impossible to observe in animals a direct counterpart of the altered consciousness in man.

Groat and Simmons, 1950, p. 151 [2]

Since we cannot verbally ask other mammals how they feel, and since our theory of mind and mirror neuron system seems most effective in giving us insight into and empathy for the subjectivity of members of our own species, we must be humble in guessing what an injury was like for a mouse. Evidence suggests that it is the non-cognitive psychiatric or behavioral sequelae of concussion that have the greatest impact on human well-being. Detecting post-concussive depression or anxiety in a rodent, one admits, involves our own subjectivity. Although laboratory methods have been developed in an effort to overcome this limitation (to be described in more detail in Chapter 10, *Persistent Post-Concussive Psychiatric Problems*), psychiatric distress in non-humans remains rather cryptic.

Post-concussive elementary sensory/motor changes are easier to measure. Two commonplace methods are beam walking and the rotarod test. In the beam-walking test, the rodent strives to escape a bright light and loud noise by walking along a slender elevated wooden beam toward a darkened goal box. Sometimes pegs on the beam add a challenge. Rodents are highly motivated to escape the stimulus, so their motor skills can be estimated from their time to reach the goal box. Figure 4.11B shows a concussed animal losing his or her footing on a beam – a typical sign of injury. Figure 4.11C displays the

Effect of mild and moderate controlled cortical impact (CCI) on fine motor coordination in the mouse: the beam-walking test

(A)
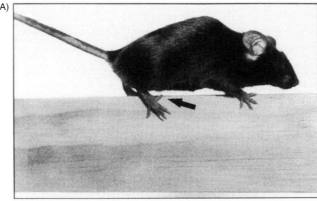

(B)
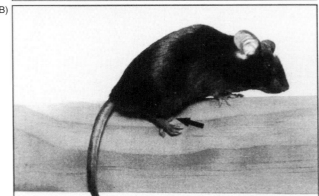

(C)
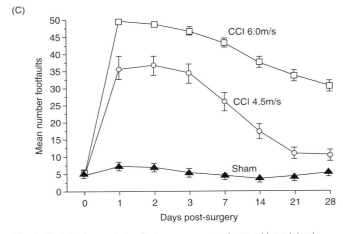

Fig. 4.11 Animals were trained to traverse a narrow beam with a minimal number of hindlimb footfaults, with each subject required to grip the edge of the beam with the innermost digit (arrow in A). Moderate injury resulted in a significant deficit in this task, with the contralateral hindlimb frequently slipping down the side of the beam (arrow in B). This deficit persisted for at least 28 days (C), although mildly injured mice performed significantly better 7–28 days post-CCI.

Source: Fox et al., 1998 [56]. Reproduced with permission from Mary Ann Liebert, Inc.

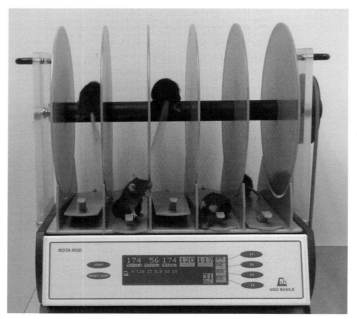

Fig. 4.12 Rotarod test of sensorimotor function, balance, and coordination after concussive brain injury.
Reproduced with permission of B.C. Mouzon

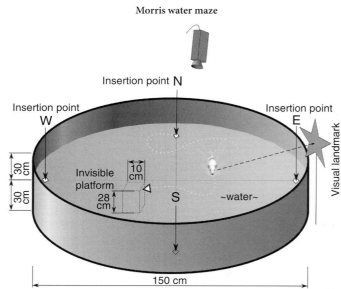

Fig. 4.13 The subject animal swims in opaque fluid, seeking the hidden platform, and learns to use visual cues to find it more quickly on subsequent trials.
Source: Wikimedia Commons. S. John, 2010. Reproduced under the terms of the Creative Commons Attribution licence, CC-BY-SA 3.0

experimental results. As expected, a more forceful injury was associated with longer recovery.

The rotarod is a device with a rotating bundle of rods arranged in a cylinder (the walking surface) between discs that inhibit lateral movement. The animal's ability to maintain balance is tested at progressively higher rotational speeds (Figure 4.12).

Regarding cognition, perhaps the most common persistent complaint after human concussion is memory difficulty. A large number of techniques for testing rodent memory have been standardized, normed, and validated by clinico pathological and clinical imaging studies. So one may be unable to listen sympathetically as a mouse complains of difficulty finding his or her car in a parking lot, or missing appointments, or leaving the kettle to melt, but we can obtain replicable measures of classical conditioning, working memory, associative memory, and procedural memory. A few examples will suffice to acquaint the reader with the most popular approaches.

In place avoidance tasks, animals must learn that a foot shock or other noxious stimulus is associated with a certain part of an arena, e.g., the northwest corner. Passive avoidance refers to learning to stay out. Active avoidance refers to learning to escape if some apparatus is moving into the noxious zone. The Morris water maze (Figure 4.13) may be the most frequently employed technique for testing rodent cognition – especially spatial learning. The animal is placed in a circular tank of milky

water.[7] Somewhere, just beneath the surface, is an escape platform. The subject swims about, learns the location of the platform, and forms an associative memory, using visual cues to find the platform again. Cognition is assessed by escape latency (time to reach the platform), path length, and cumulative distance swum before escaping. The T-maze is another swimming test. One arm leads to an escape platform; the other does not.[8] Drier tests include the radial arm maze, in which the animal must learn and remember which of eight routes leads to a food reward, or the Barnes maze, in which the animal must learn and remember which of multiple holes in a large round platform permits escape from bright lights (Figure 4.14).

This short list of popular rodent exercises is offered for two purposes. First, the reader may wish to be acquainted with the actual generators of the limited available data regarding the long-term effects of concussion in animals: experimental injuries that do not seem likely to imitate those in humans, in non-humans, the outcomes of which are assessed with methods lacking any ecological validity and quite different from those used to assess motor, cognitive, and psychiatric outcomes in humans. Second, the list demonstrates that, even if bioengineers hugely improved the biofidelity of animal experimental brain injuries with human CBI, we would *still* be at a loss to determine whether animals deteriorate or suffer as we do. We cannot ask them how they feel, or test whether the subtle changes in executive function, speed of information

---

[7] For rats, a typical tank is 180 cm in diameter and the water is 30 cm deep.
[8] Rodents can either be tested on the simple condition – remembering that it was safe if they turn left – or on a delayed non-matching condition – remembering that the safe direction switches sides every time [57].

The Barnes maze

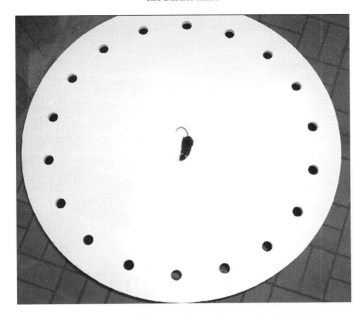

Fig. 4.14 The subject animal is exposed to a rather aversive brightly lit platform with 18 holes, one of which is an escape tunnel.

Source: Wikimedia Commons. Bd008, 2007. Reproduced under the terms of the Creative Commons Attribution licence, CC-BY-SA 3.0

processing, multitasking, irritability, or moodiness found in CBI survivors have a parallel in rodents. Moreover, the commonly administered tests owe a debt to the 20th-century model of neuropsychological testing: defining purportedly dissociable cognitive constructs and devising desktop exercises alleged to measure them. What matters to the mouse and the human is whether they can function in their usual circumstances – not whether they can mimic a log-rolling lumberjack on a rotarod or copy designs using plastic blocks.

In a laudable departure from conventional approaches, Nichols et al. [58] employed two tests of species-typical behavior pre and post CBI: marble burying and nestlet building. In the first, mice were monitored as they encountered objects of interest (in this case marbles) and instinctively dug holes to bury the objects. In the second test, mice were introduced to a new cage, permitted time to acclimatize, and observed as they undertook the first priority of a nomad (after finding water): constructing a dwelling place. Sleep was also observed. The present author opines that such naturalistic assessments may better reflect the fitness consequences of CBI than do the popular but artificial protocols.

These problems are massively exacerbated by problem 5.

Problem 5: Nobody Wants to Care for a Brain-Injured Mouse

This problem takes two forms, the first perhaps trivial, the second probably critical.

First, some human studies suggest that CBI survivors do better with a network of social support. It is not clear whether the benefit derives from emotional support actively enhancing brain healing, or caring giving the CBI survivor a time with

reduced duties during which he can rest and recover, or simply that supportive family and friends are accommodating, which permits lifestyle adaptation even without healing. Yet it seems worth asking whether some aspects of human post-concussion behavior may have evolved exactly as they did *because* the survivor's recovery depends, in part, on human pro-sociality and reciprocal altruism.

Consider a finding: brains often exhibit a week or more of post-CBI increase in GABAergic inhibition. Of course, this might merely be a feature of pathophysiological misfortune. However, inhibitory activity (depending very much on the circuit) sometimes has the behavioral effect of slowing us down. Post-concussive fatigue is almost universal. Let's guess, for a moment, that the current fragmentary evidence that post-CBI rest helps recovery turns out to be true. If so, that might be because depressing human activity for a while – a GABAergic trick the brain plays to fix itself by encouraging rest, in part to mitigate excitotoxic/oxidative damage – may possibly be an evolved, adaptive, reparative response to concussion.

In a Hobbesian state of nature, that's a bad thing. If humans did not care for one another, the CBI survivor – slowed, fatigued, forgetful, and inattentive – would be at considerable greater fitness risk due to his diminished capacity for hunting, gathering, socializing, lovemaking, and self-defense. But Hobbes neglected to read Darwin. Humans care. Parents of concussed children and many spouses of concussed spouses report that their CBI survivor exhibits, for a while, increased dependence on the aid and tolerance of others. They get it. As a result, in a highly social caregiving species like our own, a period of brain-enforced rest may have little or no impact on survival. Perhaps post-CBI slowing neatly dovetails with hominid cooperation to optimize recovery. (In fact, when skeptics dismiss subjective complaints of fatigue, one may wish to suggest the possibility of an evolved silver lining.)

Mice are different. Even in the most commensal of house mice, there is nothing akin to human empathy for the ill. Nobody in their mouse group wants to care for a brain-damaged mouse. One does not see solicitous grooming (let alone hear encouraging words). Therefore, to whatever degree the match between human recovery needs and human sociality affects CBI outcome, animal experiments fail to model it.

The second problem with non-caring for brain-damaged mice is a much bigger issue in translational concussion research and testimony to the near-sightedness of neuroscience.

No biological marker identifies a threshold between "mild" and "not mild" TBI. The same is true for humans and mice. At the same time, the most common CBIs in humans are those that do not cause prolonged coma. It is legitimate to focus on that short-coma subgroup – the typical concussed human – in the hope of better understanding the chain of causality that leads, in some cases, to persistent post-concussive problems. However, one cannot study persistent problems if one sacrifices one's subject before those problems have time to emerge. The persistent problems are the ones we desperately need to understand, prevent, and treat. Why do animal experimenters almost always kill their brain-damaged animals long before those animals would otherwise die? Why do they forego, or ignore, or dismiss the precious opportunity to study the long-term consequences of CBI? Why are there so very, very few prospective longitudinal studies of TBI?

It is costly to house and feed animals. It is costlier if one is making an effort to be humane. Once an animal has been deliberately subjected to a brain-damaging laboratory intervention, care becomes somewhat more challenging, time consuming, and expensive. In addition, during the preceding 75 years or so, there has been tremendous resistance to acknowledging that concussive injury causes long-term problems. How often does that happen? Who knows? A collection of good studies has never been attempted in any species.

Nobody wants to care for a mouse for a year or two after having hit it in the head. Laboratory work is disheartening enough. If you are an assistant professor, why on earth would you subject yourself to witnessing the ghastly aftermath of the brain injuries you have inflicted for month after month – especially if you can get neither decent funding nor serious attention from peer reviewers? For all of their limitations, for all of their dubious representation of typical human CBI, animal studies might have been much, much more helpful than they have been. All those mice. All dead, and so little learned. Maybe it's better that way?

Problem 6 (individuality) was mentioned in passing. Sparing the reader, that will do. But problem 7 – the fact that mice do not naturally develop so-called AD – deserves comment because it exposes the unnatural lengths we go to in hopes of investigating the relationship between concussion and dementia, and problem 8 deserves comment since it prefigures the impending doom of an entire profession: the eagle-eyed neuropathologist.

Problem 7: Rodents Don't Get "Alzheimer's Disease"

There are currently no effective treatments for improved recovery and long-term rehabilitation of survivors of TBI, in part owing to lack of clinically relevant experimental models of TBI (particularly those that model TBI-induced increased risk for AD).

Abrahamson et al., 2013 [59]

As this essay will discuss later, evidence is very strong that TBI increases the risk of neurodegenerative disease in humans.[9] But how can today's community of clinicians and scientists make progress in understanding the relationship between concussion and dementia without conducting long-term animal experiments looking for signs of post-concussive neurodegeneration? This looks to be low-hanging fruit! It

would be the labor of only about 20 months to expose adult rodents to CBI and follow them prospectively into their senium – checking to see whether some animals exhibit persistent, or delayed-onset, or progressive brain dysfunction. Why is this so rarely done?

There are multiple practical and scientific answers. An important one is simple: rodents don't get AD.[10]

The conventional model of neurodegeneration argues that proliferation and dissemination of putatively toxic proteins, some prone to folding into β-pleated sheet conformation and fibrillization (e.g., Aβ, tau, TDP-43. ubiquitin, synuclein, prion protein (PrP^{Sc})) is the *sine qua non* of human aging-related "neurodegenerative disease." Moreover, immunohistochemistry in humans demonstrates that amyloid deposition begins within hours after TBI in about one-third of cases [60–64]. As in virtually every aspect of TBI, first, the likelihood of this occurring varies, and second, genotype makes a difference: both APOE and neprilysin polymorphisms alter the odds [65–67]. Later chapters will address the frequently overlooked challenge of scientifically defining *aging, degeneration*, and *disease*. The point is that a useful animal model of TBI needs to mimic this occurrence.

Early work with wild-type (natural genome) rats produced authentically thrilling findings: Iwata et al. [68] exposed rats to moderate FPI. Within two days, there was increased expression of the gene for the amyloid precursor protein (APP). By one month after injury, there was widespread accumulation of Aβ in damaged axons. And – in a potentially critical finding that remains mysterious – one year later the brain was still peppered with dense accumulations of Aβ. Yet by that time, the expression of the APP gene had subsided to baseline. This experiment was interpreted as evidence that TBI triggers a burst of production of Aβ, then Aβ becomes a long-lived feature of the brain. Although most post-traumatic Aβ seems to be the shorter, more soluble, better-tolerated Aβ40, traumatized mice also express the longer, less soluble, and more damaging Aβ42. TBI even generates spherical senile amyloid plaques, although these are usually the "diffuse" type, lacking the paired helical filaments found in the "neuritic" type [56, 69–71]. Question answered. TBI causes "AD" – or at least some of the brain changes that some 20th-century neuropathologists opined were markers of "neurodegenerative disease."

Maybe. The story turns out to be both more convoluted and less probative.

Other rodent studies, especially with wild-type mice, failed to replicate the finding of long-lived Aβ. In fact, wild-type mice exposed to CCI more often exhibit a prompt burst of Aβ

---

[9] Post-modernism alert: if you are a neurologist trained in the 1970s and grew up puzzled by the illogic of claims that Aβ and tau depositions define neurodegenerative diseases, you may be relieved to learn that Aβ and tau deposition, neurodegeneration, and mental incapacity are now widely acknowledged to be three dissociable phenomena. It is commonplace to find examples in which any one occurs without the others. At this point in the infant history of neuroscience, we are obliged to guess how deposition of various atypically folded proteins relates to the vastly more complex and diverse phenomena of time-passing-related brain change, and the threshold between normal and diseased change, and the threshold at which brain or behavior change meaningfully impacts inclusive fitness. We have about as persuasive evidence that plaques and tangles explain dementia as we do to that endocannabinoids explain love.

[10] As discussed in the chapter *Late Effects* (Chapter 11), pending the discovery of some credible principle of biological classification distinguishing "Alzheimer's disease" from "non-Alzheimer's disease," it seems most prudent to regard that entity as hypothetical – or perhaps indefinable.

production, but an almost-as-prompt *vanishing* of that excess Aβ, with levels returning to baseline in about a week [72, 73]. Vanishing Aβ hardly seems a set-up for neurodegeneration.

At the same time, one cannot assume that findings in wild-type mice apply to humans; in the state of nature, mice just do not make enough APP (not to mention tau), or slice that precursor protein up into Aβ fragments in the same way that humans do. Thus, it frustrated neuroscientists for decades that the level of Aβ in wild-type rodent brains is so low that accumulation into plaques is infrequent [74].

Single, Double, Triple

The standard work-around, since we could do it, has been the creation of transgenic animals – rodents with added human genes that permit the expression of Aβ, tau, or both. Initial experiments were done with single-transgenics – mutant mice bearing the whole human APP domain that chronically overexpress human APP and spontaneously deposit Aβ. (This occurred in an era when the amyloid hypothesis of AD was still given credence.) Some early results of single-mutation APP-transgenic mouse models were rather baffling. Sometimes hitting these mice led to a burst of Aβ production and accumulation, sometimes not [56]. In fact, in one report, mice exhibited a decrease in such deposits after trauma [75].

However, an impressive recent APP-transgenic study by Kokiko-Cochran et al. [76] was especially informative because the investigators permitted the subject to live 120 days after a mild (1 atm) FPI. These mice would have been expected to develop aging-related Aβ plaques without TBI; the question was whether TBI made a difference. Three findings were notable. First, in both the short and long term, these mice exhibited not only APP accumulation but also persistent activation of microglia, cytokine generation associated with macrophages, proliferation of circulating monocytes, and other signs of inflammation. This confirms the suspicion that (1) APP is an immunomodulator and (2) neuroimmunomodulation is important in concussive brain damage. Second, the investigators tested for behavior. In these mice expressing human APP, concussion caused an apparent acceleration in age-related impairment of working memory at 90 days and inferior carry-over of spatial learning at 120 days. Third, "immunohistochemistry suggested that TBI did not advance the appearance of Aβ plaques as no aggregates of APP could be detected." In other words, transgenic mice indeed accumulated more APP but *did not exhibit more Aβ plaques.* Without putting faith in a single study, these very interesting results suggest that concussion does accelerate dementia – a behavioral issue – but not necessarily by boosting Aβ deposition. Increasingly, it seems, one must be open to the possibility that Aβ, neurodegeneration, and dementia are three dissociable phenomena.

A variation on the single-transgenic APP theme was make mice with *knocked-in* human APP. These are not technically transgenic since they lack the human promoter and do not spontaneously generate Aβ plaques. Nonetheless, controlled cortical injury doubled production of Aβ40 and Aβ42 [69]. What's more, some single transgenic APP mice have been kitted

out with the addition of human APOE genes. As in humans, presence of the APOEε4 allele exacerbates these post-traumatic degenerative changes, *even in mild injuries* [70, 77–79].

In an effort to enhance the model, some investigators have built *double*-transgenic APP + PS1 mice (that is, mice expressing both the human β-APP and the human presenilin-1 mutation). The results have tracked closer to the human sequence, but are mixed. In 2013, Tajiri et al. [80] published the first experimental evidence that TBI causes double-transgenic presymptomatic AD mice to develop both neurodegenerative and cognitive changes. Webster et al. [81], like Kokiko et al., showed that closed head injury produced inflammation and cognitive loss in such double-transgenic mice. Yet not every double-transgenic study has been as compelling [82].

The amyloid hypothesis of AD in its pioneer iteration ("amyloid deposition kills neurons and explains AD") has been abandoned. Still, amyloid seems to play some role. A recent reconceptualization of the data suggests that neither amyloid nor tau is altogether up to the job of neurodegeneration, but that tau and amyloid interact, conspire, or "crosstalk" to harm brains [83–86]. Therefore, if one's animal model fails to include human tau, it is really not mimicking sporadic human AD. Innovators have responded. Since 2003 [87, 88] triple-transgenic mice have been available. These are the triple-transgenic 3XTg-AD mice bearing genes for human APP, PS1, and microtubule-associated protein. 3XTg-AD mice enable virtually complete expression of the pathological changes expected in sporadic AD: senile plaques and neurofibrillary tangles. Using such animals, studies have confirmed that head trauma initiates intra-neuronal Aβ and phospho-tau immunoreactivity within hours, suggesting that trauma tremendously accelerates AD-like pathologies [89, 90]. Moreover, damaged axons seem to be the major site of Aβ accumulation [91].

One might justifiably be tempted to celebrate this innovation and these findings. TBI indisputably triggers accumulation of Aβ40 and 42 and generation of extracellular spherical amyloid plaques. Damaged axons are the main site. Scientists can mimic some features of "AD" by hitting mice.

For Better or for Worse?

Again, however, applause is premature. As promising as this laboratory legerdemain seems, even after the invention of triple transgenics, confusion reigns over the mouse-hitting literature. Five sub-caveats bear consideration. First: most experiments seeking to understand the relationship between head trauma and neurodegeneration have been too short and too severe to translate into useful explanations of the persistent effects of concussion. Moderate, severe, and repetitive mild TBI often triggers Aβ and sometimes triggers tau accumulation [8, 9]. Sometimes those deposits persist for months [68]. But (perhaps the major caveat of this textbook) the long-term outcome from a single "mild" trauma has not been tested rigorously.

Second, some results are inconsistent with the simple narrative "TBI causes neurodegenerative Aβ deposits." For example, Schwetye et al. [73] reported a *decrease* in extracellular soluble Aβ after TBI. "These results support the alternative hypothesis that post-injury extracellular soluble Aβ levels are acutely decreased" (p. 555). In another head scratcher, Nakagawa et al. [92] exposed single-transgenic APP mice to TBI. These were old mice, so they had *already* developed abundant Aβ plaques. The astonishing effect of TBI, in the authors' own words: "there was also a remarkable regression in the Aβ amyloid plaque burden in the hippocampus ipsilateral to TBI" (p. 244). That is, contrary to expectations, old mice with AD-like brains were serendipitously deprived of their neurodegenerative lesions by being hit in the head! Moreover, only some animals with damaged axons exhibit Aβ, and axonal APP-related pathologies are quite phenomenologically variable [93].

Third, the emergence of AD lesions in transgenic animals may not follow the same pathway as in humans: "While end-stage amyloid and tau pathologies in 3xTG-AD mice are similar to those observed in sporadic AD, the pathophysiological mechanisms leading to these lesions are quite different." [87, p. 361]. A question that has yet to be answered: how well do such genetically manipulated little neo-pseudo-rodents serve as models for investigating the long-term brain change after concussion? If the change permits the rodent to respond to TBI more like a human, it is likely to help us understand concussion. Yet if the change creates a hippogriff that responds neither like a rodent nor like a human, we remain in the dark.

Fourth, it is completely unknown what, if anything, these early protein deposits have to do with later neurodegeneration. Multiple investigators have observed that acute Aβ clears by about seven days post-injury [e.g., 91]. As one scholar lamented, "Whether and how these acute accumulations contribute to subsequent AD development is not known" [89, p. 9513]. To rephrase this concern in the most unvarnished terms: *we remain uncertain what Aβ and tau have to do with human health.*

The near-universal occurrence of these proteins inspires the question: why do we make them? Would one not expect there to be some adaptive advantage that explains their persistence in the genome? The large APP, so widely expressed in mammalian brains, presumably has *some* fitness benefit. Perhaps the net cost or benefit depends on what other genes you carry, and how you slice it. Supporting that hypothesis, one APP fragment called soluble APP-alpha apparently has multiple neuroprotective, neurotrophic, and cell adhesion functions [94–96]. If one administers exogenous soluble APP-alpha to a concussed mouse, it improves both pathological and functional outcome [95, 96]. Indeed – in something of a proof of principle – mice deprived of their APP gene fare considerably worse after head trauma [97]. As Thornton et al. [96] opined, "APP can be both beneficial or detrimental depending on the way in which it is posttranslationally processed within cells" (p. 39). Perhaps contrary to instinct, the fact that head trauma promptly up-regulates expression of the APP gene should not be presumed to be either a component of brain injury or a herald of neurodegeneration. APP generation, and even Aβ accumulation, may represent an adaptive trick that helps concussed brains.

Fifth – and closely related to our ignorance of the role of these proteins in health and disease – we do not understand how a little Aβ or a little tau in a couple of places turns into a lot in many places.

In 2000, Kane et al. [98] found a clue. He did not hit mice. He merely injected a bit of "Alzheimeric" brain extract into brains of single-transgenic APP mice. Five months later, the ipsilateral hemisphere exhibited "profuse Aβ-immunoreactive senile plaques and vascular deposits." What is this? Alzheimer's infection? Kane called it "seeding." In 2002, Walker et al. [99] took this line of inquiry a step further. They commented, with innocent prescience, "Except for the prionoses, the initiation and propagation of these proteinopathies *in vivo* remains poorly understood." Walker et al.'s mice helped advance that understanding. Like Kane et al., they merely injected a bit of "Alzheimeric" extract. Five months later, there was widespread Aβ – but the deposits were *bilateral*. The spread after seeding seemed to follow neuronal pathways, suggesting, "the possible spread of seeded pathology from the injection site via neuronal transport mechanisms." In other words, like the prionoses, the initial Aβ exposure perhaps acts as a template for the generation and dissemination of more and more, ultimately causing neurodegeneration.

Soon thereafter, a host of studies confirmed this paradigm-shifting idea – that prion-like neuron-to-neuron spread of neurodegenerative proteins is common and may in fact be an important part of brain aging [100–107]. In a related study, a rather shocking finding has arisen from Creutzfeldt–Jakob disease research: Aβ, like prion infection, was apparently transmitted via surgical instruments [108]. The dizzying possibility of infectious transmission of brain aging aside, it remains to be seen whether seeding and prion-like spreading of problematic proteins occur after human concussion. To the best of this author's knowledge, this exact occurrence has yet to be demonstrated in mice – again limiting the value of the current models.

Mice do, however, exhibit significantly increased cellular prion protein (PrP^c) near the site of TBI [108]. Marciano et al. speculated, "the increase in PrP^c-immunopositive cells we observed in the dentate gyrus of the hippocampus … may have important consequences for posttraumatic cellular vulnerability" [108, p. 2874]. A very different line of research also links this molecule to TBI: Pham et al. [109] exposed adult rats to simulated blast injury and reported that plasma-soluble PrP^c significantly increased, making this assay another potential TBI biomarker. The same research group demonstrated that plasma PrP^c also increased among concussed university athletes [110]. Yet the role of PrP^c in short- or long-term brain change after CBI is unclear.

PrP^c is a detergent-soluble glycosyl phosphatidylinositol-anchored cell surface protein that occurs widely in mammalian cells, especially in the brain. This normal molecule must be distinguished from its protease-resistant toxic isoform, PrP^{Sc}. The former has the α-sheet conformation; the latter has the β-pleated-sheet conformation. Only cells bearing PrP^c can become "infected" by PrP^{Sc}, since the benign protein provides the template for manufacture of its malignant cousin. Yet the physiological role of PrP^c remains unknown. Several vertebrate species seem to live untroubled by the loss of this protein.

However, based on observations in knockout models, in 2015 Chiesa [111] summarized:

> mammalian PrP^c has been assigned roles in many biological processes, including neurotransmission, olfaction, proliferation and differentiation of neural precursor cells, myelin maintenance, copper and zinc ion transport, and calcium homeostasis, as well as neuroprotective activities against several toxic insults, such as oxidative and excitotoxic damage.
>
> (p. 1)

Several recent findings possibly suggest ways in which PrP^c might be involved in either the offensive or the defensive sides of the post-concussive melee. First, as already mentioned, this molecule seems to block excitotoxicity. PrP^c reportedly moderates both N-methyl-D-aspartate (NMDA) excitotoxicity (perhaps in concert with copper) and inflammation [112]. Second, PrP^c binds to Aβ oligomers, a phenomenon that may have multiple consequences. For instance, PrP^c accumulates within neuritic plaques with Aβ cores [113]. The effect of this binding is not clear – whether, for example, it represents a defensive response to cellular threat, an enhancement of Aβ's potential toxicity, or even a facilitation of fibrillization. However, AD transgenic mice lacking PrP^c have normal survival and normal memory, suggesting that such binding may be central to Aβ toxicity [114]. In addition, Pflanzner et al. [115] reported that PrP^c binding to Aβ enhances the movement of Aβ across the blood–brain barrier. Again, it is unknown whether the net result of altered transcytosis is increased movement of Aβ into the brain or clearance. However, after "severe" closed head injury in mice, both T-tau and P-tau levels are reportedly associated with PrP^c levels, and tau phosphorylation seems to be associated with PrP^c [114]. Collectively, these findings implicate PrP^c in the pathophysiological events after CBI – and conceivably a new avenue for therapeutic investigations.

Another recently discovered facet of basic cell biology, also prion-related, may also be worth considering in explorations of CBI pathophysiology: ribonucleoprotein (RNP) granules. (The author mentions this in an altogether speculative vein. He is unaware of empirical evidence linking RNP granules to post-concussive neurodegeneration.) The fine points of transcription and translation are slowly yielding to study. Epigenetic regulation of transcription by histone proteins is widely known and rather revolutionary, opening the door to inheritance of acquired traits. In a somewhat analogous way, regulation of translation appears to be under the control of RNPs, which bind to mRNAs upon transcription, and which potently dictate whether translation occurs or does not.

When RNPs are free in the cytosol, they are reportedly prone to liquid–liquid phase transition, forming condensed but membrane-less organelles – like drops of oil in water. Within such organelles, RNPs participate in the formation of several types of intracytoplasmic granules, which "often contain both RNA binding domains as well as sequences that have been variously termed prion-related, low complexity or intrinsically disordered" [116]. The "low complexity" regions of RNPs appear to prompt potentially pathological fibrillization [116–118]. RNP-associated granules include Cajal bodies, processing bodies and stress granules (SGs) [119]. Like that of PrP^c, the physiological role of RNP granules remains obscure. One presumes they have adaptive value. Some evidence suggests that SGs are formed when RNPs are interrupted or "stalled" in the course of initiating translation, which occurs under stressful conditions.

Several observations suggest possible links between RNPs, SGs, and the sometimes long-lived brain pathology seen after CBI. First, mechanical shear injury can trigger the generation of SGs [117]. Second, as Molliex et al. [118] concluded, "Liquid–liquid phase separation by RNA binding proteins harboring low complexity sequence domains is the molecular basis for stress granule assembly, and persistent stress granules promote pathological protein fibrillization" (Figure 4.15). Third, inherited forms of neurodegenerative conditions, including amyotrophic lateral sclerosis and frontotemporal dementia are associated with mutations in RNPs, with altered dynamics of SGs, and with pathological fibrillization, which suggests that SGs facilitate fibrillization-related neurodegeneration [118]. Fourth, Gunawardana et al. [120] reported a surprising and strong association between tau and RNP complexes. Those authors also found that tau co-isolated with 27 RNA-recognition motif (RMM) domain-containing proteins. "The RRM family is notorious for its high proportion of members predicted to be able to acquire prion-like properties" (p. 3011). There is not, as yet, a smoking gun. Still, the discovery that neuronal stress (in particular, shear) is associated with abnormalities in translational machinery that are, in turn, associated with tau, prion-like activity, and fibrillization, is surely worthy of attention in animal studies of CBI.

It is perhaps an assignment for the next generation to unravel the interactions between Aβ, tau, PrP^c, their many proteinaceous cousins, inflammation, vascular change, and human well-being. In the meantime, this author must humbly acknowledge: one does not know exactly what to make of the animal concussion literature as it pertains to aging-related neurodegeneration of the "Alzheimer" type. It nonetheless seems plausible that exploring this avenue might lead to an intervention we very much need: interrupting a putative sequence from CBI through atypically folded proteins to early dementia.[11]

Problem 8: Rodents Fix Themselves, in Part, by Making New Neurons

there was tremendous skepticism and frank disbelief in these data, and I was finding it increasingly difficult to move forward. I was beginning to realize that it might become

---

[11] One preliminary study encourages such hope: Sawmiller et al. [122] exposed transgenic Aβ-expressing mice to a moderate TBI. Untreated mice developed the expected storm of APP, Aβ, and inflammatory cytokines. Mice treated with the flavanoid luteolin (found in celery and green peppers) were spared this dangerous squall.

Membrane-less organelles formed by ribonucleoproteins host assembly of stress granules that promote fibrillization

Model for Normal and Pathological RNP Granule Assembly by Phase Separation

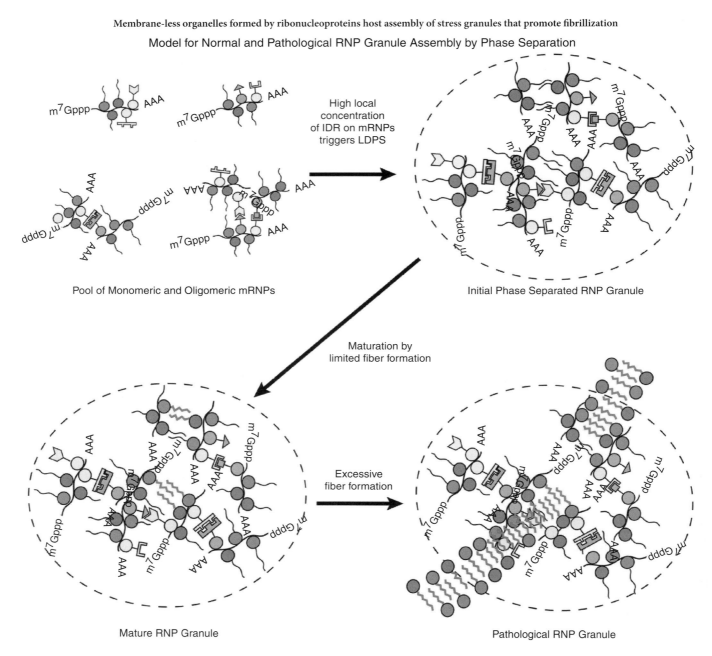

Fig. 4.15 Liquid–liquid phase separation by RNA-binding proteins (RNPs) harboring low-complexity sequence domains is the molecular basis for stress granule assembly, and persistent stress granules promote pathological protein fibrillization. IDR: innate defense regulator; LDPS: phospholipids and associated proteins; mRNPs: messenger ribonucleoprotein complexes. [A black and white version of this figure will appear in some formats. For the color version, please refer to the plate section.]

Source: Molliex et al., 2015 [118] with permission from Elsevier

impossible for me to continue in this particular career direction.

Kaplan, 2001 [121]

Most of the nine problems with experimental concussion listed in this chapter cause scholarly headaches because one doubts the mouse hitters have faithfully mimicked human CBI. Post-traumatic neurogenesis is a problem of a different sort. In this special case, we may be perfectly confident that

the brain rattling was similar in the mouse and the man. But these post-CBI brain changes so hearteningly detected in rodents – new neurons – are devilishly hard to detect in living concussed people. That plaint will be addressed shortly.

The "no new neurons" dogma was a cornerstone of 20th-century neuroscience, carved into granite and tattooed on to the foreheads (well, perhaps the forebrains) of every graduating resident neurologist. The claim that neurogenesis only happens in development was stoutly defended and stubbornly clung to

Adult neurogenesis in the hippocampus

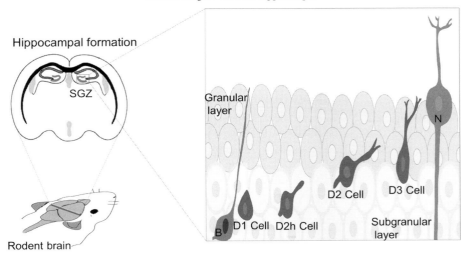

Fig. 4.16 Schematic drawing that represents the cytoarchitecture of the subgranular zone SGZ of the adult hippocampus. The neural progenitor cells (in blue), also known as type-1 cells or type-B cells, give rise to type-2 cells (in red), also known as type-D cells. Intermediate progenitors migrate locally and undergo different maturation stages (D2h, D2, D3 cells) to finally differentiate into functional granular neurons (N). [A black and white version of this figure will appear in some formats. For the color version, please refer to the plate section.]

Source: Gonzalez et al., 2012 [132] with permission from Elsevier

in the face of its counterfactuality. Like other wars between conservatism and science, the no-new-neurons war provoked passionate partisanship.[12]

In 1988, birdbrain expert Fernando Nottebohm reported the discovery of new neurons in adult canary heads. Alvarez-Buylla's and Nottebohm's famous paper [123] was not, however, the first to announce this astonishing discovery. That honor arguably belongs to Joseph Altman and his colleagues. These scholars published a string of elegant experiments beginning with Altman's 1962 *Science* paper titled, "Are new neurons formed in the brains of adult mammals?" [124–128]. Altman's earth-shaking studies were ignored. Another early contributor, Michael Kaplan, was essentially hounded out of academia in 1982. Dogmatists, martialed by Pasko Rakic of Yale, simply denied that Kaplan was looking at neurons [121]. In the early 1980s Shirley Bayer published impressive data confirming Altman's and Kaplan's findings [129]. She too was largely ignored. It was perhaps 1998, and a paper by Eriksson et al. showing new neurons in adult cancer survivors, when the new paradigm finally began gaining ground against the closed-minded conservative blockade [130].

Adult neurogenesis in humans was finally, though grudgingly, accepted circa 1999. It was indeed breath-taking news that many animals retain a reservoir of neural stem cells in convenient storage sites in the brain well into middle age, and routinely nurture these infant cells into new working neurons. However, a legitimate question arose that still requires an answer: in humans and other adult mammals, the two most prominent reservoirs of neural stem cells appear to be the subgranular zone of the hippocampus and the subventricular zone of the lateral ventricles (Figure 4.16). How, then, can repair and rebuilding occur at some distance from these precious reserves? Two answers apply. First, it is clear that

newborn neurons can migrate from these labor and delivery zones to damaged cortex elsewhere in the head. Second, some evidence suggests that the rest of the brain is not altogether lacking in neuron-birthing competence: in 1999, Gould et al. [131] became the first to publish evidence that adult neurogenesis in primates seemingly occurred widely in the neocortex.

A rich vein of empirical effort confirmed these early observations in humans and other species. True, as late as 2006, a few scholars failed to see what they judged to be strong enough data, and continued resisting the new-neurons paradigm [133]. In fairness, outcomes vary with methods. Yet the preponderance of the evidence made the discovery of adult neurogenesis one of the principal neurobiological advances of the late 20th century [134–136].

Suffice it to say that the once-controversial discovery of human adult neurogenesis is now regarded as established fact. The author only digresses to mention this drama because it so perfectly parallels the recent course of the concussion debate. And Dr. Kaplan's experience as an eager young scholar sadly illustrates the human cost of truth seeking during science wars.

Neurogenesis Helps Overcome the Deleterious Effects of TBI

Just at the very cusp of acceptance of the new-neurons paradigm (~ 1999), neuroscientists were already trying to figure out whether neurogenesis helped to explain recovery after concussion. The analogy of the melee remains heuristically helpful: just as a blow to the head triggers a battle between pro- versus anti-apoptotic gene expression, and pro- and anti-inflammatory activity, there seems to be a battle pitting apoptosis against neurogenesis. That battle may determine whether the outcome will be a net gain or a net loss in brain cells [137].

---

[12] The author perhaps unwittingly risked his place in the Harvard neurology residency when, the day of his interview, he alerted a renowned Crimson professor to the paper by Nottebohm reporting the discovery of new neurons in adult canary heads. "Adult neurogenesis?" recoiled the august interlocutor. "So you're saying all my education was wrong?"

This is one leg of today's new paradigm: whatever a CBI survivor has left in his head after a year or two may depend on the relative vigor of these competing forces.

In 1997, Scott and Hansen [138] became among the first to show this in the laboratory. Within several years, multiple colleagues confirmed that moderate or severe TBI triggers neurogenesis, and that this neurogenesis appears to be reparative. Many of these studies reported local proliferation of new neurons and focal incorporation of those neurons into functional circuits of the hippocampus. Others reported that new neurons can migrate from their birthplaces in the dentate gyrus or subventricular zones to needful regions in the cortex [139–152]. Cui et al. [153] reported that the transcription factor FoxJ1 is up-regulated after TBI in rats. That may be pertinent, since FoxJ1 triggers the differentiation of stem cells in the subventricular zone to be differentiated into astrocytes, oligodendrocytes, and neurons.

Critically, it has been shown that new neurons are associated with both incorporation into circuits and functional improvement [149, 154]. Villasana et al. [154], for example, showed in 2015 that post-traumatic adult-born neurons are integrated into the hippocampus (Figure 4.17). Not to put too fine a point on a study that requires replication, neurogenesis seems to help fix concussed brains.

Post-TBI neurogenesis appears to peak about three days after injury. Its longest duration is not yet clear, but Chen et al. [155] reported persistent neurogenesis and gliogenesis for at least *a year* after brain trauma in rats. As Yu et al. [152] opined in 2008, "This work suggests that injury-induced hippocampal remodeling following brain injury likely requires sustained activation of quiescent early progenitors." A slew of related studies demonstrated that neurogenesis not only births new cells but also enhances cognitive recovery after injury [144, 155–160]. In fact, in a reasonably strong proof of principle, it has been shown not only that post-TBI neurogenesis improves cognition but also that blocking such neurogenesis does the opposite [148, 156].

All of these studies inflicted CBIs in the strict sense of an external brain-shaking blow. However, few laboratories employed "mild" blows, as typically quantified. That inspires the obvious question: does post-TBI neurogenesis also occur after "mTBI?" Attempting to answer that astute question exemplifies how very recently humans have come around to studying mild injuries: the only quality data come from work published from 2015 onwards. Wang et al. [150] did not find enhanced neurogenesis in mice after mild TBI. Zhang [161], in an idiosyncratic report, actually found that mild TBI *decreased* hippocampal neurogenesis. Yet Chohan et al. [157] reported that a mild CCI (5 m/s; 1.5 mm) produced the same phenomenon that moderate injury does: a burst of dentate gyral neurogenesis.

This handful of findings is so inconsistent that one begs leave to defer an answer for a few months. That is how close we seem to be to a major advance.

Multiple studies have sought the endogenous and exogenous factors that enhance this encouraging post-TBI cell proliferation. Table 4.1 offers a preliminary list in rough chronological order of discovery. The reader need not grant this Table 4.1 more than a passing glance. It was compiled with a view toward the future, for the benefit of clinical researchers looking for a project and perhaps even for pharmaceutical entrepreneurs. At some point soon, the ghastly social impact of concussions will

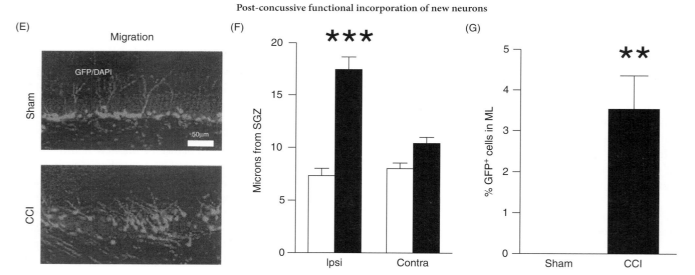

Fig. 4.17 E: Representative images of GFP+ cell dispersion in the granule cell layer of the ipsilateral dentate gyrus. F: Traumatic brain injury mice had increased cell migration away from the subgranular zone on the injured hemisphere compared with sham mice. G: A greater percentage of GFP+ cells from traumatized mice migrated into the molecular layer (ML) of the ipsilateral dentate gyrus. CCI: controlled cortical impact; DAPI: 4'6-diamidino-2-phenylindole; GFP: green fluorescent protein. [A black and white version of this figure will appear in some formats. For the color version, please refer to the plate section.]

Table 4.1 Endogenous and exogenous agents reported to enhance post-traumatic brain injury neurogenesis

Primarily endogenous agents	Source
• Nitric oxide[a]	Scott and Hansen [138]
• Erythropoietin[a]	Lu et al. [144], Xiong et al. [164]
• Fibroblast growth factor 2	Yoshimura et al. [151], Thau-Zuchman et al. [165]
• Neurotrophin 4/5	Royo et al. [166]
• Brain-derived neurotrophic factor (BDNF)	Kazanis et al. [167]
• Glial cell-derived neurotrophic factor (GDNF)	Conte et al. [168]
• Nerve growth factor	Conte et al. [168]
• SB-100[a]	Kleindienst et al. [143]
• Basic fibroblast growth factor	Sun et al. [160]
• Vascular endothelial growth factor	Thau-Zuchman et al. [165]; Lee and Agoston et al. [169]
• Insulin-like growth factor-1[a]	Carlson et al. [170]; Madathil and Saatman [171]

Primarily exogenous agents	
• DEtA/NONOate, a nitric oxide donor	Lu et al. [144]
• Brain cooling	Kuo et al. [172]
• Fluoxetine	Wang et al. [173]
• Statins	Lu et al. [174]; Wu et al. [175], Xie et al. [176]
• Agmatine	Kuo et al. [177]
• Imipramine	Han et al. [178]
• Exercise	Itoh et al. [179], Piao et al. [180]
• Hyperbaric oxygen	Lin et al. [181]
• Etanercept	Cheong et al. [182]
• Survivin	Zhang et al. [183]
• LM11A-31, a p75 neurotrophin receptor ligand	Shi et al. [184]
• P7C3-A20, an aminopropyl carbazole agent	Blaya et al. [185]
• Tissue plasminogen activator	Meng et al. [158]
• MLC901, a traditional Chinese medicine	Quintard et al. [186]
• Cerebrolysin	Zhang et al. [161]
• Tissue plasminogen activator*	Meng et al. [158]
• Peptide 6, a peptide based on a biologically active region of human ciliary neurotrophic factor	Chohan et al. [157]

[a] Agents that are naturally occurring but may also be administered exogenously.

become so obvious that funding for clinical trials of TBI therapies will blossom (or, hopefully, explode). At that point – since boosting our in-built reparative systems is one of our most tantalizing therapeutic options and the human benefits will be tremendous – one speculates a good deal of effort to be expended winnowing agents such as those listed in Table 4.1 (or, for the profit-minded, trying to jury-rig patentable analogues).

Since our goal is, at least, to do no harm, it is also important to know what factors depress or inhibit post-traumatic neurogenesis. These include stress, ganciclovir, and propofol [162, 163]. Concussed persons are unlikely to encounter ganciclovir. However, propofol use is widespread in the inpatient setting. If that finding is replicated, it might oblige hospitals to rethink sedation after TBI. And if stress (perhaps associated with excess corticotropin-releasing hormone) interferes with post-TBI neuron production and brain repair, this discovery – which is completely consistent with the observed benefits of rest – has direct, practical, low-cost, high-benefit applicability.

In addition to the wealth of new data regarding neurogenesis, two other potentially brain-fixing factors have attracted much attention: post-TBI gliagenesis (aka gliogenesis) and angiogenesis. Readers will be familiar with the pejorative implications of the phrase "reactive astrocytosis." The appearance of new astrocytes has long been considered a bane to damaged brains. What if, instead, it was a boon? Recent research has inspired reconsideration of the conventional wisdom. Scholars now ask whether newborn astrocytes are beneficial or detrimental [187, 188]. The answer is not clear and may depend very much on the genomic milieu into which these cells are thrust. Early reports, however, suggest that many neural stem cells become glia after brain injury, and that this is a salubrious event [186]. The same is perhaps true of post-TBI angiogenesis [164, 177, 181]. Time will tell.

This section was introduced with the plaint that post-TBI neurogenesis is hard to confirm in humans. It has been done *in vitro*: in 2013, Zheng et al. [189] reported convincing evidence that neurogenesis indeed occurs during recovery from human TBI (Figure 4.18).

It remains to be determined at what threshold of severity, or in persons with what biological traits, post-CBI neurogenesis might be expected. However, indirect neuroimaging tactics are already available that should soon enable investigators to visualize human neurogenesis *in vivo*. First, evidence suggests that the density of neural precursor cells in rodent hippocampus is detectable as a spectroscopic metabolite peak resonating at 1.28 ppm. (In fairness, the peak is also associated with apoptosis [190].) Using proton magnetic resonance spectroscopy (^{1}H MRS), Manganas et al. [191] scanned human subjects and detected the same resonant peak. "Our findings thus open the possibility of investigating the role of NPCs [neural precursor cells] and neurogenesis in a wide variety of human brain disorders"(p. 1). Second, high-resolution magnetic resonance imaging (MRI) can detect changes in dentate gyrus cerebral blood flow, apparently reflecting post-exercise neurogenesis [192]. If these techniques are validated and optimized, they may soon unleash a vital new research enterprise. Investigators will finally be able to monitor the natural history of spontaneous human post-concussive neurogenesis. More clinically important, they will be able to conduct randomized controlled trials of the many agents already shown to enhance

Post-concussive neurogenesis

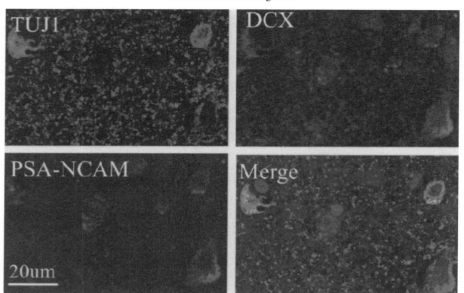

Fig. 4.18 Triple immunostaining shows that TUJ1 (green) is expressed in the DCX (red)- and PSA-NCAM (purple)-positive cells in the cortical regions of adult human brain after traumatic brain injury. [A black and white version of this figure will appear in some formats. For the color version, please refer to the plate section.]

Source: Zheng et al., 2013 [189]. Reproduced with permission from Mary Ann Liebert, Inc.

neurogenesis, testing safety and efficacy for genuinely disease-modifying subacute management of CBI.[13] At the risk of injudicious sanguinity, the prospect of discovering the first effective biological concussion treatment is stirring.

Based on the available data, one can summarize the yes-new-neurons paradigm shift as follows:

- Mammals that suffer a TBI – mild, moderate, or severe – quickly start birthing new brain cells.
- In rodents, these new cells are strongly associated with better recovery.
- This phenomenon probably helps explain what we have seen in the clinic for 2000 years: a gratifying trend toward recovery that is individually variable in timing and degree.
- Clinical neuroscientists, employing new techniques to measure neurogenesis *in vivo*, may soon provide even better news: safe and effective post-acute treatments for victims of concussion.

Problem 9: The Limits of the Accessorized Human Eye

The major component of neuropathological technique – using a microscope to make judgments about organic tissue – is a 1590's technology. Several minor improvements have been made in the last 400 years. For example, stains have been

found to enhance visualization of biologically interesting features. As a result of such advances, judgments about the health or sickness of brain cells, neurons, and glia, have changed, changed, and changed again. In other words, every time someone cooks up a new batch of stain, we must rethink last year's conclusions. Given this iterative progress, when can we say the microscope has showed us the truth? We are forced to admit that optical microscopic assessment can never be definitive, since:

1. It attends to dead things in the hope of understanding live things.
2. Its resolution is limited by the reasonably firm laws of optics.
3. We are at the mercy of today's stains.[14]

Any present-day study that examines the same brain tissue with different stains makes it vividly apparent that we are at the mercy of this year's available arsenal of coloring agents. Gao and Chen [194], for example, subjected mice to a very mild CCI (2.8 m/s; deformation 0.2 mm). They sacrificed the animals after three days and examined the brains with several dyes. If they had stopped with crystal violet, one would sigh with relief and infer that concussion does not kill neurons: "Staining with crystal violet showed that cortical tissue was generally intact without dramatic lesions … These data indicate that the cortex does not show major tissue lesions after mTBI" (p. 185).

---

[13] This need not involve risky, exotic, or costly agents. Several neurogenesis-promoting agents are already in widespread clinical use, e.g., serotonin reuptake-inhibiting antidepressants [173] and statins such as simvastatin and atorvastatin [174–176] are generally safe, generally well tolerated in long-term use, relatively inexpensive, and might be prescribed off-label at low risk.

[14] Hence, whatever the microscope gazer announces in 1720 or 2020 must be taken with a grain of salt. In 2050, when we will have *in vivo* neuroimaging technology capable of video monitoring real-time neuronal function at the sub-molecular level, gorgeous still-deaths such as those published since *Micrographia* [193] may be relegated to history.

"Mild" traumatic brain injury may cause extensive neurodegeneration

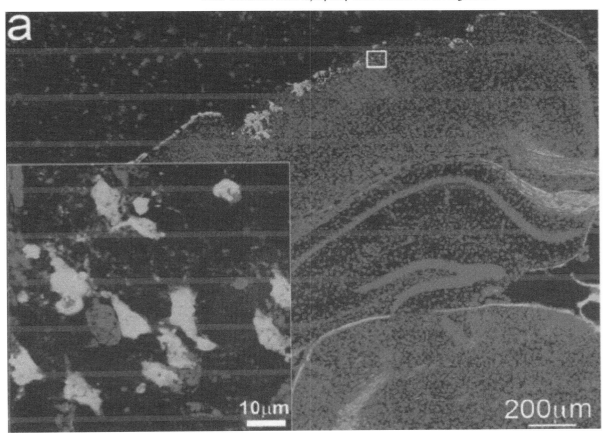

Fig. 4.19 Cell death in the neocortex of mice with mild traumatic brain injury (mTBI). (a) Fluoro-Jade B (FJB)-positive cells are green in the epicenter on the ipsilateral side of the neocortex. [A black and white version of this figure will appear in some formats. For the color version, please refer to the plate section.]

Source: Gao and Chen, 2011 [194], by permission of Oxford University Press

However, when those authors applied different dyes to the same tissue, the denouement changed. As illustrated in Figure 4.19, the authors found that mTBI in fact triggers cell death: "Fluoro-Jade B staining is a widely used method to detect dying cells in the cortex … Animals with a mild level of CCI injury exhibited FJB-positive neurons (green) in the epicenter on the lesioned side of the neocortex."

Moreover, even when these authors applied the conventional Golgi stain (Figure 4.20), they found that mTBI caused extensive degenerative change:

> The density of the Golgi-stained neurons in the outlined area of the injury brain was significantly decreased compared with the corresponding position of the control brains, consistent with the finding that mTBI induced cell death … and decreased cell density in the injury area.

In fact, the authors discovered that the region in which these degenerative-but-not-fatal changes occurred was 10.3 times the volume of the lesion – the zone of dead neurons (Figure 4.21). This is perhaps the most telling finding from this study. mTBI

"Mild" traumatic brain injury may cause extensive degeneration in neural processes

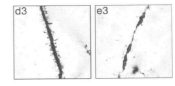

Fig. 4.20 Golgi staining revealed that surviving neurons exhibited dendritic beading and loss of spines. d3: control; e3: mild injury.

Source: Gao and Chen, 2011 [194] by permission of Oxford University Press

causes some dead cells, but a lot of nearly dead cells (also please see the section below regarding cell death after CBI).

Which of these changes matters for the well-being of the animal?

That is – leaping somewhat ahead in our story – two observations confront us. One: concussions sometimes kill neurons. Two: many people develop persistent post-concussive behavioral changes. Does the one cause the other? If a medical student (or a mouse) named Hermione were to be concussed and, a year later, suffers from slowed thinking and depression, is that because some neurons died in Hermione's brain? In order to devise preventive treatments – in order to save

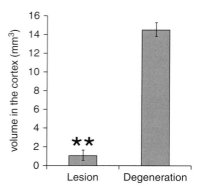

Fig. 4.21 Comparison between volume of mild traumatic brain injury lesion and volume of neurodegenerative change. **$p < 0.005$.

Source: Gao and Chen, 2011 [194] by permission of Oxford University Press

Hermione from slowed thinking and depression – we ought to know whether long-term behavioral changes are due to cell death. Gao and Chen's study, finding both sick and dead brain cells, does not provide the answer. Still, it might provide a clue: mTBI may cause a lot more sick cells than dead cells. If you only have a dead cell stain, you may be seeing the tip of the iceberg of concussion-induced brain change.

Given that different stains yield different answers about cell loss, the most earnest neuropathologist working with the wrong box of paints might be excused for failing to see and acknowledge the dire effects of "mild" concussions. In essence, the scores of peer-reviewed scientific articles reporting "intact" brains after concussion may simply be telling the same misleading story as the old reports based on conventional neuropsychological tests:

"Using insensitive methods, we found nothing. Therefore concussion is benign."

Perhaps the fundamental inference from the available data is a caveat that, at this point in history, should not require discussion: light microscopic examination is limited. When a laboratory reports, "we did not see any changes," some might be tempted to interpret that as, "there was no brain damage." Such a conclusion would be equivalent to opining that, since plain X-rays do not show human disc herniations, disc herniations do not occur in humans. Indisputable evidence of persistent post-CBI brain dysfunction, not possibly due to expectation, feigning, hypochondriasis, or litigation, is apparent to any reader of the animal literature. Just don't expect it to show up under your table-top Zeiss.[15]

Science marches on. As this essay will show, when authentically sensitive assays are employed it becomes apparent that *even very mild CBI causes lasting brain damage and initiates neurodegeneration that may or may not be reversible.* That discovery helps explain the subject of our worries: long-term, disabling post-concussive neurobehavioral change. One simply has to be alert to the perceptive limits of one's technology.

What Experimental Studies With Non-Human Animals Reveal

Readers, rejoice! We have completed the introduction to the animal chapter. We can now commence the animal chapter. Having squeezed the last drop out of the rock of caveats, having explained why the animal data fail to answer many questions, it seems about time to impartially review that data.

We begin with evidence supporting three simple conclusions:

1. Animal CBI immediately triggers competing waves of harmful and helpful brain change.
2. Animal CBI tends to disproportionately hurt the very brain cells known to mediate human post-concussive problems.
3. Animal CBI kills neurons.

1. Animal CBI Immediately Triggers Competing Waves of Harmful and Helpful Brain Change

The immediate post-concussive melee of brain damage and brain repair was discussed in Chapters 1 and 2. A brief review will suffice.

When an abrupt external force is visited upon a head, if that force shakes the brain, and if that shaking is sufficient to trigger clinically meaningful change, certain events seem to occur with awful reliability. As Giza and Hovda described in 2001 [195], a molecular "cascade" commences as excitatory neurotransmitters bind to post-synaptic receptors, permitting excessive calcium to deluge the interior of brain cells. This causes potassium to exit, which requires energy from the ionic pumps, which get their energy from burning glucose, which requires effective operation of many cell parts, including glucose transporters and mitochondria, which hanker for more energy at a time when it is not available, which stresses the brain cell at the same time that the excess calcium is switching on production of pro-apoptotic enzymes and threatening axons with axolemmal (the axon's skinny scabbard), neurofilament, and microtubule disorder – all of this under the gun from changes in cytoskeletal proteins, inflammatory mediators, and neurotrophic factors – these events all being linked to measurable micro- and macro-vascular changes. Simultaneously, brain-defense-or-repair mechanisms we have just begun to appreciate go to work.

The popular phrase *neurometabolic cascade of concussion*, therefore, is a partial descriptor. The actual suite of events might more accurately (if less pithily) be called *abrupt external force-related neuronal/glial change altering the molecular genetics and metabolic operations of cells, and brain metabolism, and axoplasmic integrity, and inflammatory and immune processes, and vascular function, and activation of protein aggregation akin to neurodegeneration.* Or, to abbreviate, let's call it *the*

---

[15] Optical microscopists, with regrets: your time might be nie. (Lurian-oriented behavioral neurologists like the author will convivially join you in idle obsolescence.) But there's a bright side: the moment we have motion-compensated *in vivo* neuroimaging machines with a resolution of about 0.01 micron (good enough to watch mitochondria breath), we can all retire to fly-fish for cutthroats in Montana. The author speculates that our professions will continue to offer gainful employment for several years.

neurometabolic/inflammatory-immunomodulatory/vascular/ neurodegerative cascade of concussion.

Yet, like an Iliad without Trojans, this only depicts one side of the battle. As Giza and Hovda [195] put it, "Each wave of gene expression and subsequent protein synthesis may, in turn, trigger secondary and tertiary waves of molecular change in the brain, both as a direct response to damage and to effect repair of injured neural systems" (p. 388). That is, the brain's ecology is subjected to a dust-up of competing harmful and reparative events, down to the ultrastructural, molecular, and possibly atomic level.

For example, as previously mentioned, among the roughly 1000 genes known to be up- or down-regulated in the minutes after concussion, some tend to increase cell death, other to decrease it. Pro- and anti-apoptotic enzymes face off. Pro- and anti-inflammatory cytokines go nose to nose. The volcanic eructations of the excitatory transmitter glutamate are corked, to some degree, by the inhibitory redoubts of gamma-aminobutyric acid (GABA). On a longer time scale: release of dangerous reactive oxygen species by the limping mitochondria is countered by native antioxidants. Some aspects of astrocytosis may be cleaned up by activated microglia. Rapid deposition of Aβ-42 protein is apparently followed by some clearance. Moreover, evidence exists that when one struggling little neuron is unidirectionally connected to another, deafferentation spreads dysfunction from the first cell to its target cells. Yet, gratifyingly, that deafferentation may be balanced by post-deafferentation denervation-induced axonal sprouting [196].

Yet it is probably erroneous to imagine this battle as shock and awe eventually followed by rally and counterattack. A more accurate view credits the remarkably quick reflexes of defensive biology: brain self-defense perhaps swings into action within a second after impact. For many dangerous changes that develop over the succeeding days and weeks, the brain has an answer. As mentioned in Chapters 1 and 2, animal experiments are the main source of this realization. Might we nominate a more accurate name than "neurometabolic cascade"? It's hardly a cascade. More a maelstrom. In the light of progress since Giza and Hovda's seminal 2001 paper, one flounders for as nifty a headline. The author confesses to preferring: "*the neurobiological melee of concussion.*"

2. Animal CBI Tends to Disproportionately Hurt the Very Brain Cells Known to Mediate Human Post-Concussive Problems

Few head-injured patients complain of apoptosis. They're more likely to complain of disabilities such as memory loss or distress such as sadness. In order to gain confidence that animal experiments mimic human concussion, one would want to see evidence that first, the same parts of the brain tend to be damaged in animals and humans and second, those are the very parts of the brain that help mediate post-concussive troubles such as memory and sadness. Both predictions seem to be true.

For background purposes (and asking the reader's forbearance for this telegraphic abridgement of 150 years of discovery): the dorsolateral prefrontal cortex (DLPFC) helps mediate working memory. The anterior cingulate gyrus and DLPFC together mediate planning. The ventromedial prefrontal cortex helps mediate self-control and social comportment. The hippocampus helps mediate acquisition and retrieval of memories for facts and events. The amygdala helps mediate memories for anxiety and fear. The hippocampus, amygdala, and thalamus collectively help mediate depression. We even know a little about the mechanics. For instance, hippocampal cells that are critical for laying down a new associative memory are the large pyramidal cells in the two regions called CA3 and CA1. Communication between these two relies on the excitatory neurotransmitter glutamate. (That turns out to be a slightly risky business, since excessive depolarization due to glutamatergic transmission causes excitotoxicity and neuronal death.)

Remember too: since the skull disseminates injurious force and every brain cell is shaken when the brain is shaken, the focal site of a blunt injury is a relatively minor factor. No matter where one hits the little volunteer, certain brain parts take the brunt of the blow.

First: in moderate to severe TBI, are the same brain parts damaged in mice and humans? Yes. These are the ipsilateral cortex, the medial temporal lobe (especially the hippocampus and amygdala), the thalamus, the cingulate gyrus, and the long axons [197–204]. Within the hippocampus, it seems that the dentate hilus is especially sensitive to force [205, 206]. Groat and Simmons crystalized this concept in 1950: "the concussive action is spatially discontinuous on a microscopic scale" [2, p. 160].

Second: are these brain parts also prone to damage in milder injury, such as the work-a-day concussion without prolonged coma? Yes. Consider the hippocampus. Lowenstein et al. [205] and Nawashiro et al. [207], for example, both demonstrated that hippocampal neurons in the CA3 region are extraordinarily vulnerable to death-by-TBI. In contrast, CA1 neurons exhibit exquisite vulnerability to ischemia. Yet the primarily unidirectional flow of information from CA3 to CA1 means that traumatic damage to CA3 will likely cause deafferentation damage to CA1. Giza et al. [208] reported that TBI-associated depolarization induces immediate early genes associated with cell death specifically in the hippocampus. Tweedie et al. [209] also reported that "mTBI" alters the expression of the hippocampal transcriptome in mice – but interestingly, that mild physical impact and mild blast had somewhat different effects.

Third: are these fragile brain parts in fact the very parts associated with the post-concussive neurobehavioral symptoms? Yes. The reader may simply compare the list of fragile regions to the list of behaviorally critical regions. And there are nuances worthy of mention. As noted above, the dentate hilus of the hippocampus is highly vulnerable to traumatic brain strain. It also plays a unique role in regulating the flow of information from the entorhinal cortex via the perforant pathway into the hippocampus. Excessive activation (and, for instance, seizures) seems to be restrained by multiple GABAergic systems [210]. Therefore – to oversimplify in good faith – the hippocampus is a big part of the braking and acceleration system for memory and emotion:

- Dentate hilus = brakes.
- Pyramidal cells = accelerator.

In consequence, depending on the relative degree of damage in these different zones of the hippocampus, one expects memory loss and/or emotional disinhibition.

Fourth: can these injuries persist? Yes. These deleterious regional effects are not only persistent but sometimes progressive: Smith et al. [204] exposed rats to FPI. The authors called the force "high severity" (although their 2.5-atm injury is often regarded as moderate). Periodic examination of the brain revealed pathological changes of *progressive* neurodegeneration and brain atrophy up to one year after the injuries. Dixon et al. [211] exposed rats to CCI. (The velocity of 4 m/s would usually be regarded as mild to moderate; the deformation of 2.5 mm as moderate to severe.) Histological examination revealed an average hemispheric volume loss of 30.4 mm^3 at three weeks, but nearly double that, 50.5 mm^3, at one year. Similarly, ventricular expansion increased dramatically between three weeks and one year. Both findings again suggest *progressive* post-concussive brain change. Hence, we know that concussing a rodent head tends to deleteriously, lastingly, and perhaps *progressively* impact neurobehaviorally sensitive areas. Indeed, the majority of experimental studies of mTBI damage focus on assessments of the post-concussional health of the medial temporal lobe. Exactly as the reader might guess, these memory- and emotion-impacting brain changes persist – even after lesser forces of impact.

Fifth: when we say "brain damage," do we mean dead neurons? No, not necessarily. In less-severe concussions, the almost inescapable hippocampal injuries may be more functional than structural, but that hardly lets the brain off the hook. Recall Gao and Chen's 2011 results [194]: mTBI indeed kills neurons, but it renders ten times as many dysfunctional as dead. Cell loss, surprisingly, may be the least of one's worries. The main problem may be years of ongoing abnormal activity of the remaining circuitry. As Cohen et al. [212, p. 143] put it:

> While neuronal death has been considered to be a major factor, the pervasive memory, cognitive and motor function deficits suffered by many mild TBI patients do not always correlate with cell loss. Therefore, we assert that functional impairment may result from alterations in surviving neurons.

The term *functional* might be confused with *benign*. However, if functional change persists, so does disability. For instance, the electrophysiological correlate of associative memory in the hippocampus is long-term potentiation (LTP). We know that moderate injury disrupts LTP, rendering memory ineffectual [196]. In 1992, Miyazaki et al. [213] reported the same problem after mTBI. That is, even though mTBI more often produces sub-lethal than lethal damage to hippocampal pyramidal cells, it nonetheless suppresses LTP. Wu et al. [57] not only confirmed that mTBI suppresses LTP but also showed that concussion decreases brain-derived neurotrophic factor, which is necessary for survival of some neurons and memory, as well as synaptophysin 1, which is a marker for pre-synaptic integrity in the hippocampus. Thus, a CBI may toss wrenches into several parts of the electrochemical engine of memory and emotion. And Darwish et al. [214] provided evidence that such changes are not limited to the hyper-acute period. His rats still showed spatial learning impairments and abnormal hippocampal synaptophysin density 25 days after mTBI.

One way to conceptualize the electrophysiological effects of a blow to the head is to say that TBI throws off the healthy balance between excitement and inhibition. At the same time TBI down-regulates excitatory LTP in the CA1, it up-regulates inhibitory synaptic efficacy in the dentate hilus [215]. For example, using whole-cell patch clamp recording, Toth et al. [216] determined that a moderate concussion not only kills dentate hilar granular cells but also specifically disarms GABAergic inhibitory control, causing months of hyperexcitability. Santhakumar et al. [217] confirmed that TBI causes both longer-lasting depolarizations in dentate granular cells and also excessive responses of mossy cells to perforant pathway stimulation.

More recent technical advances enable direct visualization of these functional changes. In something of a *tour de force*, Smith et al. [218] exposed mice to LFPI, tracked what happened to behavior, assessed changes in synaptic networks of single hippocampal cells, and then used voltage-sensitive dye imaging to study the spatiotemporal dynamics of these changes. Moreover, in a potentially important announcement, Cole et al. [219] also exposed mice to LFPI. The subjects exhibited the expected disruption of hippocampal synaptic efficiency as well as cognitive impairment. The authors claim, however, that dietary treatment with branched-chain amino acids (direct precursors of temporal lobe glutamate synthesis) *restored* cognition. Such clinically startling reports, in this author's opinion, cry out for strict scrutiny and replication.

Why is the Hippocampus so Fragile?

For orientation: Figure 4.22 is a photomicrograph and overlaid schematic depicting the hippocampus. The hilus is the region embraced medial to the crook of the dentate gyrus.

Why the hippocampus? Readers may be less than satisfied by the declaration, "Trust me; these neurons are fragile." Given the central duties of this little apparatus, one cannot help wonder how nature could leave it so exposed to mechanical injury. The author does not know the answer, but McCarthy [220] offered several reasons why these memory- and emotion-critical neurons are so vulnerable to concussion:

1. CA1 neurons are unusually sensitive to glutamatergic excitotoxicity and to hypoxic/ischemic compromise.
2. CA3 and dentate hilus neurons are unusually sensitive to mechanical forces.
3. Tumor necrosis factor-alpha, an inflammatory cytokine, is locally up-regulated.
4. Gap junctions contribute to the spread of cell death.

A horizontal section through the hippocampus

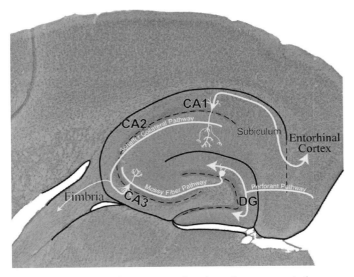

Fig. 4.22 The major pathways are in yellow. Axons from neurons in the entorhinal cortex project via the perforant pathway to synapse on dentate granular cells. The dentate hilus is the area embraced within the crook of the dentate gyrus (DG). These project via mossy fibers to synapse with CA3 pyramidal neurons, which, in turn, project via Schaffer collaterals to CA1 pyramidal neurons. [A black and white version of this figure will appear in some formats. For the color version, please refer to the plate section.]
Source: Smith et al., 2012 [218]. Reproduced with permission from A. Cohen

5. Increased inositol phosphate may exacerbate the dangers of calcium influx.

6. Hippocampal pyramidal cells exhibit slower rebound in energy stores as compared with neocortical neurons.

7. A high local density of NMDA and AMPA receptors as well as L-type voltage-gated calcium channels all favor excessive calcium influx.

8. The unidirectional connections between CA3 and CA1 make it more likely that damage in the first zone will cause deafferentation damage in the second.

9. Glucocorticoid receptors make hippocampal neurons uniquely vulnerable to stress-induced saturation.

The amygdala is a close neighbor to the hippocampus. Its cells are perhaps a little more resilient in the face of traumatic or ischemic threats. Yet the two tend to share the stress of concussion. For instance, Abrous et al. [221] reported that mild FPI directed at the right lateral parietal lobe of rats selectively and consistently provokes the expression of inducible transcription factors, c-Fos, c-Jun, JunB, and Krox-24, thus altering immunoreactivity in the amygdala and hippocampus while sparing multiple other brain regions. Reger et al. [222] reported that mTBI in rats upregulated NMDA receptors, especially in the basolateral amygdala. Meyer et al. [223] reported that mTBI in rats was associated with changes in neuron counts related to apoptosis specifically in the CA1 region of the dorsal hippocampus and in the basolateral amygdala, but not in many other parts of the cortex/isocortex. As the authors put it: "The most sensitive zones for trauma were anterior cingulate cortex and CA3 area of hippocampus" (p. 197).

Of course, our ignorance outweighs our knowledge: are all the changes found after concussion in the hippocampus necessarily bad? Dash et al. [224] showed that TBI increased phosphorylation of the memory-linked transcription factor cyclic AMP response element-binding protein (CREB) in the hippocampus. While the immediate effect of hyperphosphorylation of CREB might be suboptimal associative learning, the net effect might actually be reparative: phosphorylation of CREB has been linked to up-regulation of the neuroprotective factors BCl-2 and brain-derived neurotrophic factor [220]. A concussion with a duration of less than one second can be thought of as provoking an hours- to months-long fight for the survival of hippocampal pyramidal cells. In this corner are the physical and chemical peculiarities of these neurons that give them something of a glass jaw. In that corner are a host of trainers and cut men – neuroprotective humors and mechanisms. Whatever goes wrong, nature has tried to evolve a defense.

Evidence also exists that there is a direct relationship between this regionally selective brain damage and cognitive impairment. For example, Lyeth et al. [225] exposed rats to FPI in the mild to moderate range. Prior to sacrifice at 25 days, the rats were tested for memory in a radial arm maze. "[M]ildly injured rats exhibited significant working memory deficits within the first five days after injury"(p. 254). Tang et al. [46] exposed mice to a "concussive-like" brain injury short of skull fracture. Learning and memory were "profoundly impaired" at one week and still impaired at two weeks, although these deficits typically vanished after three weeks. Henninger et al., exposed rats to a mild concussive force and reported spatial learning deficits on the Morris water maze, even though no change was visible on MRI. In a similar model, Spain et al. [226] reported persistence of spatial learning deficits three weeks after mild concussion. Creed et al. [5] exposed mice to a closed head injury judged as mild based on the brevity of the apnea and prompt recovery of the righting reflex. Concussed mice exhibited deficits in working memory and spatial learning on the Morris water maze on days 1–3, although they typically recovered by days 7–9. Such studies confirm that learning and memory deficits, almost universally described by human survivors of concussion, are objectively verifiable in animal models. However, the reviewed experiments suggest recovery in less than one month – a common maximum duration for housing beaten rodents prior to sacrifice. (The duration of clinically significant damage will only become clear when more investigators wait a couple years before decapitating their subjects.)

Detecting non-cognitive emotional disturbance is more challenging, yet it is critical to understanding human postconcussive change, since persistence of symptoms is strongly associated with emotional distress. (This issue will receive more attention in the upcoming chapter titled *Persistent Post-Concussive Psychiatric Problems*, Chapter 10). One animal model of depression is forced swimming, also known as the Porsolt test [227]: a rodent is confined to a narrow tube filled with water 6 cm deep. Healthy mice will keep swimming for several minutes, perhaps hoping to find an exit. When mice with no motor deficits give up trying to swim prematurely, it is interpreted as a "loss of hope," or learned helplessness, analogous to human depression. Just as we see in the neurology clinic, sadness may be the main post-concussive problem. Tweedie et al. [228], for instance, exposed mice to mild concussion. Injured mice could not be distinguished from healthy mice on the basis of any neurological deficit. Yet they were significantly more likely to exhibit "depression" on this test.

A broader range of animal protocols investigates post-concussive anxiety, driven by the need to better understand the co-morbidity of concussion and post-traumatic stress disorder in humans. Reger et al. [222], for example, reported that "mTBI" in rats was associated with not only an increase in fear conditioning but also an *overgeneralization* of fear to stimuli that would not ordinarily provoke this response. That is strikingly akin to the reaction of many wounded warriors. Meyer et al. [223] also reported that weight drop "mTBI" in rats increased conditioned fear and anxiety-like behaviors. Getting closer to a biopsychological mechanism, other evidence suggests that animals exhibit increased vulnerability to stress in the aftermath of experimental CBI. For instance, Griesbach et al. [229] reported that injured adult male rats exhibit heightened hypothalamic–pituitary stress responses for at least two weeks after mild FPI.

In partial conclusion, concussive force has a predilection for harming the very cells and circuits that support working memory, consolidation of declarative, episodic, and semantic memory, and emotional regulation. In other words, so-called "mild TBI" often harms the exact brain regions crucial for typical post-concussive behavioral decay.

The clinical implications are huge. Countless times, patients have told me "Doc, I don't have a 'short fuse.' I have *no* fuse! How could such a little bump on the head do that?"

I doodle a cartoon. "Here's your Ford F-150 truck. Here's a rock. Your truck bounces over the rock. You hear a little bang and maybe feel a moment of concern. But you soon decide, 'Hell, it can't be that bad.' Here is your brake line. What if the only thing that rock did was cut your brake line?"

Much has been made of the "trivial" cell loss after CBI. But what if those cells regulated the brakes for emotions and memory? What if (as just happens to be the case) the crucial dentate hilus – the braking system of the hippocampus – is the most brittle straw in the cerebral haystack – the first to break when exposed to a rattling blow?

Flashbulb memory is generational. A member of the author's generation can recite, within inches, where he or she stood upon learning that President Kennedy had been shot. Millennials seem to be able to do the same for New York's tragic 9/11. That awful event offers a salient analogy to the grim mechanics of human concussion: a very small but critically placed structural injury can trigger functional catastrophe.

3. Concussion (aka, "mTBI") Sometimes Kills Neurons

it is evident that some cell loss will occur in all concussions, even in extremely light ones, and in some subconcussions.

Groat and Simmons, 1950, p. 162 [2]

This section fleshes out an idea we introduced above: CBI damages brains; cell death is part of that story. However, death may not be this horror story's denouement. If human CBI often has long-term effects (as it seems to), and if some exceptional young investigator ever meaningfully mimics human concussion with her rodent experiments and waits a while to see what occurs, one expects the brains of those animals to show *something* more than just temporary harm. What does that something look like? What long-lived brain change accounts for our *bête noire* – persistent human neurobehavioral dysfunction? Three possibilities:

1. lasting brain dysfunction without cell death
2. lasting brain dysfunction with cell death, but without irreversible neurodegeneration
3. irreversible neurodegeneration.

The reader might legitimately hope that we know which of these three occurs with what frequency after what severity of injury. The author currently speculates that the neurometabolic/inflammatory-immunomodulatory/vascular melee triggers a complex tissue reaction such that acute changes (with or without cell death) plus subacute changes (such as APP production and transient circuit disruption and inflammation) set up a perilous state, and multiple individual factors determine not only the degree of peril but also the success of rescue. But we really do not know.

Acknowledging today's ignorance, one of these three is more amenable to study than the other two: we have lots of data on brain cell death after experimental brain injury. Let us begin there. If you or your rat survive a concussion, will your brain cells all survive, or will some die?

Moderate and Severe

Before we tackle the mysteries of "mild," let us settle the question: does a moderate-to-severe TBI typically kill neurons? Yes. Abundant evidence supports the conclusion that moderate or severe TBI can cause lasting deleterious changes in brain and behavior. Multiple techniques confirm the sorry fate of neurons in concussed heads. However, a subtlety warrants attention: there is a difference between dying and dead.

Early in every biological career, one is taught to look through his or her microscope, detect classic cell changes, and declare that cell a goner. However, some cells that appear to be on death's door may recover. Ooigawa et al. [230], for example, looked at different signs of cell "death" after TBI in the hippocampus versus the neocortex. In both brain regions, many neurons were regarded as lost because they stained dark with Nissl. Another, perhaps more specific, measure of life or death was also used: immunohistochemistry with phosphorylated extracellular signal-regulated protein kinase (pERK) antibody. In the hippocampus the Nissl-stained dark neurons were confirmed dead with pERK. Yet in the cortex, many Nissl dark cells did *not* exhibit pERK reactivity – suggesting that *Nissl staining need not mean doom*. These findings force us to remember that what we call "dead" is a function of technique. It may be more accurate to say: some techniques reveal critical injury. Others reveal downright death.

Critical injury is visible using the antique optical microscope. Within hours of a blow to the head one detects:

1. *pyknosis* (irreversible condensation of chromatin, which makes the nucleus look like a spotted fruit and more or less guarantees that neuron will die soon)
2. *chromatolysis* (a sometimes-reversible state in which the Nissl substance of the cell is lost or dispersed)
3. *loss of synaptophysin density* (a sign that axonal transport is probably impaired to the point of collapse)
4. *apoptosis.*

Our state-of-the-art neurometabolic/inflammatory-immunomodulatory/vascular/neurodegenerative melee concept predicts that, with sufficient membrane damage, excessive calcium entry, and mitochondrial energy crisis, neurons will undergo apoptosis. Note, however, that apoptosis is a process, not an endpoint. It is, to be sure, a ghastly threat to neuronal survival due to the triggering of gene-mediated suicide pathways. But apoptosis does not always kill.

Degenerating neurons and their processes are sensitive to silver staining (one variety of which remains the old Golgi method). Fluoro-Jade B staining is probably even more sensitive, with a higher signal-to-noise ratio. Apoptosis (so-called cellular "suicide") can be detected in several ways. One is the presence of activated caspase 3, a key enzymatic marker of neuronal suicidal. Another is to look for neurons that stain positive with TUNEL (terminal deoxynucleotidyl-transferase-mediated biotin-dUTP nick end labeling). Note that these methods detect apoptosis in progress – fearsome but not always fatal. When we see it, we can assume that *some* afflicted cells are doomed (subsequent cell death has been confirmed using various measurement methods), but the prudent conclusion and realistic hope are that, a week later, some TUNEL-stained neurons may recover.

Downright death is also optically visible. There is a distinctly ghost-like microscopic appearance to dead neurons that have yet to be dissolved completely. As Groat and Simmons [2, p. 160] put it:

> Since the severity of the concussive action is mirrored by the extent and intensity of chromatolysis as well as by the number of cells that later disappear, the latter phenomenon is proportional to the former. These cells which appear as ghosts early in concussion certainly drop out.

Another approach is to estimate neuron numbers with immunocytochemistry, such as the activity of mitogen-activating protein kinase 2 (MAP2). More to the point for quantifying neuronal death, one can count every neuron in a carefully selected region, then compare the average number of cells found in control (non-injured) animals to those found in concussed animals. All of these methods confirm that moderate-to-severe experimental TBI kills neurons [e.g., 186]. While apoptosis may abate within several days, some of its effects are lasting. Momentarily setting aside the rugged individual cells that perhaps defeat the apoptotic hordes, many cells that experience apoptosis in progress will be lost forever.

For instance, Pierce et al. [231] subjected rats to severe TBI. Structural changes were apparent in the hippocampus, and axonal degeneration was observed in the striatum, corpus callosum, and cortex, even a year later. Moreover (as briefly noted before), these deleterious effects may be not only *persistent* but also *progressive*. After Smith et al. [190] exposed rats to moderate TBI, periodic sacrifice revealed histopathological changes of *progressive* neurodegeneration and brain atrophy up to one year after injury. A plurality of studies suggests that hippocampal CA3 pyramidal neurons are the most immediately vulnerable to concussive force. However, their sister cells – CA1 neurons connected to the CA3s – are also at risk because of *deafferentation*. This refers to the fact that sometimes a neuron in the CA3 region connects to and supports the survival of a neuron in the CA1 region. Under those circumstances, the death of neuron #1 risks the death of neuron #2.

How About "Mild" Injuries? Answering the Sometimes Question

Multiple investigators have exposed rodents to concussion or "mTBI." Several laboratories report no evidence of cell death in the cortex or hippocampus on short-term follow-up [38, 56, 213, 232]. Yet the opposite result has also been found – for instance, as reported by Corrigan et al. [97] in a study showing that wild-type (normal) mice exposed to mTBI exhibit cortical cell loss under the impact site. This leads to our *sometimes* question. The point is not to demand that every experiment demonstrate dead cells. The point is to ask: when one peeks at brain slices showing fatally wounded neurons, ghost neurons, or missing neurons – when one looks for signs of death after sacrificing the subject at one hour or one year post-injury, based on 80 years of experimental concussion research – is there strong evidence that concussion/"mTBI" *sometimes* kills neurons?

Yes.

Since this point was once hotly contested, it is again worth noting that different outcomes in different laboratories may simply and innocently be a matter of different techniques. Rather than doubting the moral compass of investigators who have come to opposite conclusions, one must fairly acknowledge that: (1) species vary; (2) strains vary; (3) individuals vary; (4) head-hitting methods vary; (5) assays searching for dead cells vary in sensitivity and specificity; and (6) (a giant technical hurdle), although we could count every person before and after plague, *we never count every neuron before and after concussion.* Each laboratory adopts its favorite method of figuring out whether cells died or not. Several positive reports suffice to answer our *sometimes* question.

In a remarkably eloquent – indeed, prescient – paper, Groat and Simmons [2] described a very small, very carefully conducted experiment. Five guinea pigs were the subjects. Two were anesthetized but not struck. Three were both anesthetized and struck a single blow on the head with what the authors called "a moderate, a moderately severe, and a severe concussion" (p. 154). (Severity was based on how long it took the animals to recover corneal reflexes and breathing, and was in all cases less severe than in a previous paper by this research team [233].) In a rare feat of patience, the investigators waited

13 months before sacrificing the animals. The results: a 19.4–38.8% loss of neurons in the reticular formation, a 13.2–15.9% loss in the lateral vestibular nucleus, and a 4.7–33.2% loss in the red nucleus.

This early experiment, by itself, does not answer our question. The number of animals was so small and the description of severity so ambiguous that the "neuronal loss" seen after concussion might have been due to sampling errors. Yet the paper gains seminal authority from two traits. First, the period of follow-up was much longer than usual for rodent TBI experiments. Second, the findings were part of a series of studies using the same technique, so the results can be compared across a large subject pool. Across experiments, this research group made several key observations. One was that, even in quite mild blows, there is both multifocal and diffuse damage in which some cells and regions are more vulnerable than others. The authors stated:

> The regional distribution of concussive action and this determines the regional pattern of functional alteration and cell damage and loss. But there are factors that operate on a microscopically local scale to involve neighboring groups of cells, and neighboring cells within a group, differentially … A logical explanation appears to incorporate two aspects … Firstly, cells are both differentially susceptible to the concussive action, and differentially capable of recovery. … Secondly, the concussive action is spatially discontinuous on a microscopic scale.

([2], p. 160)

Another observation across their experiments was that, in the mildest concussion, the number of early ghost cells is the same as the number of neurons that ultimately died. This implies that, after a minimal TBI, what you see is what you get. The hope of self-repair notwithstanding, some cells are gone. No "progressive" process was detected in that historic study, but the scholars neither used transgenic animals capable of displaying human-like neurodegeneration, nor waited for aging. In contrast, after a more severe concussion, the number of ghosts is not nearly as high as the number that die on long-term follow-up. This worrisome finding implies, again, that what you see early may be just the tip of the iceberg. When more investigators explore the whole story with delayed sacrifices, we will know better how light a concussion it takes to trigger degeneration.

Newer techniques confirm that concussed cells degenerate after mild injury. For example, Tashlykov et al. [29] exposed mice to mild graded impacts caused by dropping weights of 5, 10, 20, 25, and 30 g on to the right side of the animals' heads from a height of 80 cm. The investigators examined the brains at 72 h employing silver stains to detect degenerating neurons and TUNEL staining to detect apoptosis. Silver-impregnated neurons (argyrophilic) regarded as makers of neurodegenerative change were observed in the cortex and hippocampus. There was a 2.7–15 times increase in argyrophilic cells in different regions and sub-regions. As shown in Figure 4.23, there was a roughly linear relationship between force and damage; the greater the weight – the higher the force – the greater the number of hippocampal neurons thought to be degenerating on the basis of silver impregnation. Within

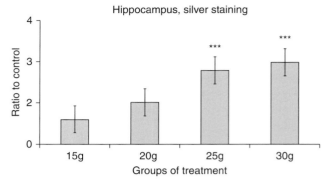

Fig. 4.23 The number of silver-impregnated neurons was elevated gradually in cerebral cortex and hippocampus after traumatic impact due to increase of plummet weight. The impact of 20–25 g plummet weights was the threshold for neurodegeneration in the hippocampus.

Source: Tashlykov et al., 2007 [29] with permission from Elsevier

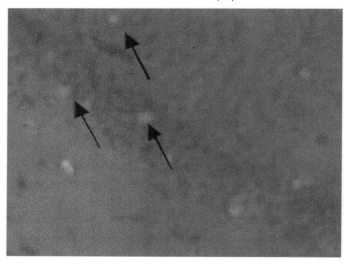

Fig. 4.24 Arrows identify TUNEL-staining neurons in the CA3 hippocampus after mild TBI. [A black and white version of this figure will appear in some formats. For the color version, please refer to the plate section.]

Source: Tashlykov et al., 2007 [29] with permission from Elsevier

the hippocampus, CA3 neurons were most affected. TUNEL staining revealed apoptotic change in that region (Figure 4.24). Within the cortex, the anterior cingulate gyrus was most seriously affected. As shown in Figure 4.25, the greater the force, the greater the number of apoptotic cortical neurons.

This relatively straightforward experiment provides multiple clues to the neuropathology of post-concussive brain change. It confirms that:

1. Architectonically different regions exhibit differential vulnerability to force.
2. Different regions displaying similar architectonics exhibit different vulnerabilities.

Increasing numbers of apoptotic neurons in the anterior cingulate cortex with increasing dropped weight in "minimal" traumatic brain injury

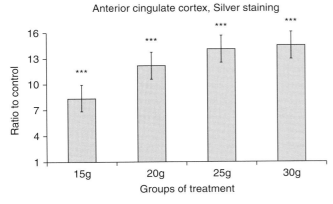

Fig. 4.25 The largest number of stained cells was observed in anterior cingulate cortex. The impact of 10–15 g weights was the threshold to activation of neurodegeneration in cortex. In some regions, the damage did not increase in the high end of the weight trauma. ***$p < 0.001$.
Source: Tashlykov et al., 2007 [29] with permission from Elsevier

3. Within the same architectonic region, different subregions exhibit different vulnerability.

These findings support the speculation that, even within the minimal part of the spectrum of mild TBI, greater force is associated with greater brain injury. The CBI-related brain changes are not just "functional" but structural, and of the type associated with permanent brain damage.

How little injury is enough to flip the degeneration switch? The force at the lower threshold for cell death has yet to be established – and perhaps represents a false summit: even if rigorous investigation determined the average lower limit of rotational acceleration to kill exactly one little cornu ammonis cell among six-month-old male C5BL/6 mice, it would not apply to all of them, or to any other mouse strain, or to any other species. Still, one can seek to answer that question by inflicting the most minimal of hits and then looking for absent, dead, or critically injured neurons. Fujiki et al. [234], for instance, exposed rats to a closed mTBI (the most faithful model) using the weight drop method. After nine days, concussed rats exhibited an 18.5% loss of CA1 hippocampal neurons compared to controls. But this lab employed the hematoxylin and eosin stains – not the best for neuron hunting. Darwish et al. [214] used a better method: immunofluorescence. They exposed rats to "mild TBI." After 25 days, using MAP2 as a specific marker of neurons (mostly found in dendrites), these authors observed loss of neurons in the CA3 region and dentate gyri of the hippocampus bilaterally. Moreover, "mild" CBI was associated with a drop in synaptophysin density in the dentate gyrus bilaterally – potentially indicating disruption of axonal transport.

Other investigators have turned to the "sick-neuron" methods, silver staining, fluoro-Jade B staining, and TUNEL staining, to look for dying/degenerating cells. As briefly mentioned, Lowenstein et al. [205] exposed rats to a really minimal FPI of 0.5–1.2 atm. A week later, silver staining found a marked decrease in the number of healthy hippocampal neurons, especially in the ipsilateral dentate hilus. Raghupathi et al. [235] also subjected rats to a mild injury. Not only was cell death noted in the CA3 region of the hippocampus, but also TUNEL-positive cells indicated apoptosis in the thalamus and ipsilateral parietal cortex and white matter. We have already summarized the study by Gao and Chen [194]. Using high-resolution silver staining, "The cortex volume showing dendritic degeneration was surprisingly large … The volume of neuronal degeneration was 10.3 times larger than the tissue lesion volume" (p. 187). Similarly, as noted above, Tashlykov et al. [29] subjected mice to graded severity of injury. A threshold was identified. Based on silver stain, 10–15 g was sufficient to provoke degenerative change in the cortex; ≥20 g produced this effect in the CA3 hippocampus. A 20-g weight drop also seemed to be the lower threshold at which cortical and bilateral hippocampal cells exhibited TUNEL staining.

The results of these studies regarding death or dying after "mild" CBI present a challenge. Why do some labs see dead neurons, and others not? We have already credited the probability that differences in technology are often to blame. In addition, one expects differences in the resilience of particular mouse strains, differences in the resilience between each animal sitting in the same box, and differences in the resilience of different regions or even individual neurons in the same animal's head. The most logical conclusion is again the teacup analogy: occurrence of sequelae such as subdural hematoma, skull fracture, fatality, memory loss, and emotional upset is probabilistic, not determinative. Knock ten mice on the head in what you think is an "identical" way; expect ten outcomes. In the same way, one expects variation in the neuron loss after "mild" injury. This mandates a red-flag warning: peer-reviewed articles often throw the data in a grinder and crank out an average. It might be better if investigators emphasized stochasticism: hitting 50 mice is an opportunity to gauge the diversity of effects, which better reflects the reality of human concussion than a mathematical average.

As remarked at the outset of this chapter, no agreed definition of *mild*, *moderate*, or *severe* has been accepted across animal TBI laboratories. In the absence of such an agreement, one must qualify any conclusion regarding the occurrence of neuronal loss in "mild" TBI as dependent upon investigators' rhetoric. That caveat in mind, it is accurate to state that:

1. Experimental TBIs arbitrarily designated as "mild" indeed kill neurons.
2. Both the *presence* of cell death and the *degree* of cell death vary – probably depending on factors such as location, mass, velocity, acceleration, mechanical properties of the myriad affected tissues (including perhaps 17 types of cortical neurons), genetic variants conditioning the innumerable degenerative and protective responses of that individual, rearing, hydration status, nutritional status, and perhaps even the emotional/stress status of the mouse.

So What?

The late phase is a residual state, characterized by loss of neural elements which underwent irreparable change in the basic phase, and often, also, by an altered functional capacity.

Groat and Simmons, 1950, p. 151 [2]

Given the multiplicity of replications, it seems reasonably well established that concussion or "mTBI" is sometimes followed by neuronal death. If cell death is observed in the minutes, hours, or days after concussion, one presumes those cells do not return to life over the next year. Therefore, immediate post-TBI observations of irreversibly fatal changes in a neuron or other evidence of necrosis or apoptosis (two pathways to death) is reasonably sound proof of structural brain damage. In fact, some evidence exists that the neuronal loss suffered in the early phase is not the end of cellular fatality. And again, this death of neurons tends to occur in the regions known to mediate the human memory and emotional regulation – the very domains of function about which people most often express post-concussive complaints.

Having rifled a library of discoveries to determine that mild injury sometimes kills neurons, the author must confess a concern: does it matter? The concern has two faces. First, given the embarrassing lack of scientific meaning of the term "mild," one can hardly countenance a triumphalism phrased, "See? Mild injury does kill cells!" Second, even if we rephrase this conclusion in a more rational way, where does it get us? "See? CBI toward the lower end of the multidimensional spectrum of outcomes kills neurons!" Apart from the trivial job of overthrowing 100 years of dogma – the claim that concussion is a "functional" not a "structural" disease – is this clinically important news?

Consider the first concern: the time may come when the neuroscience community arrives at a consensus definition of "mild" TBI based on biology. That may not be an advance. Medical nosology is often the brainchild of splitters. Typically, these are professors temperamentally desperate for cognitive closure and cavalier about the tyranny of arbitrary choices. Hence, for example, neurology still suffers from committees that have foisted definitions of AD upon us that rest on arbitrary dividing lines and do not, by any logical analysis, distinguish between that condition and aging. So what might a biological red line for mild TBI look like? Given thousands of potentially measurable parameters, one would have to be selected. Let's pick "neuronal loss" because it rings of quantifiable finality. Next, a cleaver would have to be dangled over the diversity of change in both biology and time, and dropped at will. Imagine the press release:

We, the Lord High arbiters of neuro-nosography, hereby declare and command that "mild traumatic brain injury" shall henceforth and forever refer to CBI followed by 4.7–13.3% neuron loss in the dentate hilus observed within the first 26.9 days.

In fact, advances in neuroimaging render this kind of quantitative standard entirely feasible (if miraculously silly, since any such standard will fail to predict anything that matters, such as degree of disability, return to work, quality of life, time to dementia. or survival of the victim's marriage). In the meantime, the author predicts that journal editors will continue to publish reports from investigators who claim that they have administered "mild" TBIs – even though the forces called "mild" are different from lab to lab, and the effects observed are different from mouse to mouse.

As an aside: the author fully appreciates the abiding desire, in some quarters, for a scientifically meaningful and technically detectable definition of mild TBI. As mentioned before, we suspect this is primarily an interest of attorneys, insurance executives, and those in need of cognitive closure. Yet, based on years of teaching, it may be impossible to comfort all of those who need "mild" by pointing to the amazing, extremely intriguing diversity and continuum of the biological melee. Therefore, one is tempted (being pushed daily by stakeholders) to satisfy that "mild" urge. Symptoms are a blind alley. Deficits do not lend themselves to red lines. Cell loss requires arbitrary borderlines (not to mention the challenge of having counted every cell pre-injury by anticipatory autopsy). So how about the following as one of many conceivable operational definitions that might, some day, be non-invasively determinable?

A Mild Concussive Brain Injury is One in Which no Biological Signaling Attempts to Trigger Reactive Neurogenesis

One cannot nominate this candidate definition in full faith, since some brains are surely better than others in lighting the signal fires, pleading with the subgranular zone of the dentate and the subventricular zone to mount up fresh cellular recruits. And the exact signal to look for is up in the air. As we noted above, more than a dozen agents are thought to play a role in priming the pump for post-traumatic neurogenesis [171, 236]. In addition, aging tends to impair brain neurogenesis [237, 238], so older people's CBIs might be misclassified as "mild" simply because they cannot react. The above definition is merely offered in the spirit of demonstrating how hard it is, based on the present state of the art, to scientifically classify severity.

As a bottom line, applying our "sometimes" guideline: yes. Indisputably, neuronal death *sometimes* occurs after a typical CBI (meaning, for lack of a better qualifier, one not causing long-term coma).

Which leaves the second concern: so what?

Just because a mouse named Frank loses 42 or 420 or 4200 neurons after his concussion does not necessarily mean that Frank's behavioral changes are either due to or proportional to that cell death. And just because we have shown that mild injury kills brain cells does not mean we have explained persistent post-concussive problems among human survivors of CBI. Brains are dynamic. If we have gained anything from the last century of behavioral neuroscience, it is astonishment at the brain's capacity for plasticity. Neuronal recovery, remodeling, transfer of function, and neurogenesis occur. Maybe the brain can shrug off a 5–15% loss of hippocampal neurons (after a recovery period) without the slightest impairment in function, without obliging the brain to use more energy to do the same work, and without increased risk of neurodegenerative disease. Or maybe such a loss is irrelevant to daily function but highly relevant to function under stress. Until we know what happens to the concussed animal in the year or two after the event, under different conditions and challenges, we are forced to guess whether the effects of "mild" injury – the hundreds of alterations in gene expression, the metabolic, neurochemical, vascular, and inflammatory changes, the straining of axons, the apoptosis and death of neurons in behaviorally vital places – are problematic or not.

Ultimately, one wants to see a clear, statistically robust association between an objective marker of concussive damage and long-lasting behavior change. But is "dead cells" that marker? When Groat and Simmons gravely warn of "irreparable" loss of neural elements, one must ask, "Is loss of brain cells really the main reason for loss of function?" Is that why a woman is forgetful and sad, or a man is sluggish and irritable, a year after their respective concussions?

Although "neuron loss" sounds undesirable, it may not be the best measure of lasting brain dysfunction.

First, is the total number of neurons a useful metric for brain health? Consider this: for decades it was clear that human adolescence was a time of synaptic pruning [239]. In 2007, Stevens et al., soon joined by others, advanced the surprising premise that microglia and complement help orchestrate plasticity and specifically this adolescent-era elimination of less robust synapses – a topiary view of development [240–244] (This, by the way, raises the question: "what are all those microglia and immunomodulatory factors doing in the weeks after TBI? Dismantling weak synapses?"). One consequence of synaptic defenestration seems to be a significant loss of prefrontal cortical gray matter: human prefrontal lobes reach their apex of cellularity at about age 12; it's downhill from there, although the lost volume is replaced in the head by the teen's still-myelinating white matter [245, 246]. It now seems that mammals lose more than just connections: about a decade ago, new evidence from rodent research supported the speculation that normal development involves *neuronal loss* [247–250]. The same may be true for humans: for example, in 2007 Abitz et al. [251] reported that medial dorsal thalamic neuron numbers are cut roughly in half from birth to adulthood, while glial numbers triple. This is hardly to trumpet the benefits of neuron loss. It is merely to inquire whether post-CBI pruning of synapses and even cell bodies might have an adaptive aspect.

Second, the "dead cells equal permanent brain damage" perspective fails to consider the brain's resilience. What if concussed brains often restore themselves to full function after "mild" TBI, with or without their pre-morbid complement of neurons? That is – just as the post-adolescent brain finds a way to function reasonably well with fewer neurons – might the evolved concussion repair system be so good that post-concussive cell loss is irrelevant to behavioral outcome? Neurodegeneration sounds serious, but it can be reversible or irreversible. Many organelles, membrane elements, ultrastructural elements, even synapses and dendrites can regenerate. Delays in that process may disrupt established circuit-dependent functions such as memories or skills, but one might intuit that those effects would be non-catastrophic and the end result, after reparations, should be an effective brain.

Third, perhaps cell death, or recovery from cell death, is not the main cause of post-concussive behavioral changes. Might physiological changes occur that do not involve cell death, but nonetheless play a major role in lasting behavioral impairment?

Consider three alternative foci of research attention: sickly cells, missed connections, and wayward genes.

Sickly Cells

Remember Gao and Chen [194]? The *dead* neuron zone may be less than one-tenth the size of the *degenerate* neuron zone. Reconsider the sorry-looking little fellow in Figure 4.19. We have no idea how long degenerative changes persist after typical "mild" CBI. We have no idea how often the presence of such wizened, decrepit little cells heralds cell mortality, cell recovery, or circuit breakdown. Still, if a CBI survivor's brain is hosting a bunch of sickly cells like those, one would not be surprised if his behavior is suboptimal. At this very early stage in brain injury research, the best we can say is, "Traumatically killing off neurons possibly explains the problems of CBI survivors. Traumatically *not* killing off neurons possibly explains the problems of CBI survivors."

Missed Connections

Take a giant squid. Borrow an axon (gently). Stretch it. At about 10%, one begins to see the threshold between recoverable and unrecoverable damage. As previously noted, axonal stretch (or strain) seems to be the best predictor of brain harm in finite element models. Diffusion tensor imaging, which assesses the health of axons, is arguably the most sensitive current MR technique for detecting concussive injury. And connectivity plays a role in cell survival. Especially in the hippocampus, given its unique unidirectional projections, changes in connectivity can cause death of the downstream cell, either by virtue of excitotoxicity or the opposite, loss of activity-dependent trophism [220].

Wayward Genes

Some animal studies of post-concussive gene expression examine only a few genes. For instance, Chen et al. [38] found up-regulation of glial acidic fibrillary protein production in the hippocampus and up-regulation of ubiquitin carboxyl-terminal hydrolase L1 in the cortex. A more global strategy is to employ multi-gene probing with a cDNA microarray, either applied to hippocampal tissue dissected from an animal after mTBI or to a hippocampal slice culture after exposure to mild injury – in other words, to try to figure out what happens to every gene you can.

Tweedie et al. [252], for example, exposed closed-headed mice to either a mild physical impact or mild blast. The physical mTBI provoked the up-regulation of 122 genes and down-regulation of 156. The blast provoked up-regulation of 215 and down-regulation of 127 genes. As di Pietro et al. reported [253], mild (10%) stretch in hippocampal slice cultures provoked the up-regulation of 210 and down-regulation of 789 hippocampal genes. On the whole, the authors interpreted the altered expression of these 999 genes as healthful. Many down-regulated genes were pro-apoptotic; many up-regulated genes were anti-apoptotic. One of many things that remain to be determined: to what extent do these changes in gene expression trigger behavioral effects? To what extent does genetic variation interact with post-CBI gene expression to generate a spectrum of outcomes?

Any or all of these factors plausibly influence outcome. These factors occur in virtually infinite permutations and combinations. So what really matters? At the risk of sounding like a skipping LP (for younger readers, this was a slender platter of black plastic that, historically, coded sounds): we need a biomarker, or an algorithm combining markers, that explains, predicts, and measures clinically meaningful post-concussive brain change.

The crying shame of modern TBI research is the fact that *so few long-term animal studies have been done testing the hypothesis that "mild" injury may produce lasting harm.* Although that is changing, and more may be discovered by the time the ink is dry in this page, as of late 2017 one can search high and low and not find a handful of high-quality studies that report the brain and behavioral conditions of rodents a year after mTBI.

This embarrassing knowledge gap has serious consequences for our goal, to figure out whether or not, and how often, concussion/"mTBI" harms a person for years or for life. Not only does this knowledge gap represent a barrier to interpreting the persistent behavioral changes reported in animals and humans, it represents a virtually insurmountable barrier for answering questions that have gained burning status in recent years: multiple investigators, from Martland [254] to McKee et al. [255], have reported dementia in humans after repetitive concussions. Victoroff [256, reproduced in this volume] offered evidence that (1) the typical clinical course of chronic traumatic encephalopathy after repetitive sports-related concussion involves neither immediate onset nor relentless deterioration, but instead may begin any time between the years of exposure to decades later (with an average 15-year delay in onset of symptoms after CBI exposure in the classic literature), and (2) the majority of cases exhibit *progressive* rather than mere static encephalopathy. Other investigators have noted evidence that TBI – even a single hit, and even a "mild" one – presents the most important modifiable environmental risk factor for AD [257–259]. Yet that evidence of a definitive association between a single typical CBI and later dementia is not consistent [260], owing to a variety of conceptual and methodological confounds, to be discussed in the chapter titled *Late Effects* (Chapter 11).

We need to know whether this happens, how often, and why in order to learn how to intervene effectively. A great deal

is at stake in delaying the onset of dementia. Misgivings about animal research aside, better experimental models of CBI would probably accelerate progress toward finding what works. Toward that end, it might be a precious service to humanity if more investigators were to humanely care for their transgenic mice after experimental concussion and up until those reluctant little subjects die of "aging"-related causes. Then we can better see what we are up against.

Medium- to Long-Term Change: The Data

Having explained why animal studies have doubtful value, having bemoaned the paucity of long-term studies, the chapter now turns to reviewing the longest available studies. Bucking tradition, several meritorious investigators of experimental concussion have followed their injured animals for weeks or months after injury. Some have focused on brain changes, some on behavioral change (cognitive or psychiatric). A brief review offers a tantalizing glimpse of what we could have been learning, had more laboratories housed and fed their injured subjects for a while after hitting them.[16]

With Regard to Brain Change

Dixon et al. [211] were among the first to care for their subjects long after they hit them. The authors imposed CCI (4 m/s., 2.5-mm deformation) on ten rats.[17] The rats were examined histologically at three weeks and 12 months. As noted above, there was progressive hemispheric volume loss and ventricular enlargement over the year after concussion.

Santhkumar et al. [263] was another one of the first teams to keep their concussed rats alive for extended testing. Rather than cell death, these investigators assayed risk for seizures (which, in fact, are rare after a CBI without prolonged coma). They employed FPI @ 2.0–2.2 atm. (nominally a lower-moderate severity).

> These results demonstrate that a single episode of experimental closed head trauma induces long-lasting alterations in the hippocampus. These persistent structural and functional alterations in inhibitory and excitatory circuits are likely to influence the development of hyperexcitable foci in posttraumatic limbic circuits.
>
> ([263], p. 708)[18]

The authors raised the same question we raise about cognitive impairment: is the defect only obvious under stressful conditions? "Is it possible that this recovery is incomplete, and that when the neuronal network is challenged with stronger

---

16 The forthcoming review excludes repetitive injuries. With the explosion of interest in sport-related CBI, multiple laboratories have recently sought to replicate that exposure in rodent models. For instance, in 2017, Chen et al. [261] reported that adult male mice exposed to CHIMERA-induced concussions for three consecutive days exhibited persistent cognitive impairments as well as astrogliosis and microgliosis at six months. Also see Petraglia et al., 2014 [262]. But permanent brain damage after repetitive injuries is not controversial. The present review focuses on single typical CBIs.

17 As previously mentioned, this combination of relatively low velocity but relatively deep deformation is not a typical "mild" experimental force. It might be called moderate (or maybe moderate to severe, depending on dwell time.)

18 One recognizes the possibility that this neurophysiological change might lower the seizure threshold. However, might it also contribute to emotional irritability?

stimuli, the system reveals a persistently decreased seizure threshold?" (p. 711). Unfortunately, behavior was not assessed. Any neuropsychiatrist would want to know whether this long-lasting physiological hyperexcitability translates into irritability, acquired deficits of attention, or cognitive trouble that is only apparent under stress.

Kasturi and Stein [264] permitted their rats to live for two months after a CCI at a velocity of 2.5 m/s, deforming the dura by 2.5 mm, dwelling for 500 ms (very mild in terms of velocity but at least moderate in terms of deformation). Their interest was neuroendocrinology. Since the hypothalamic–pituitary–adrenal apparatus is both key to behavior and routinely harmed by CBI, and since growth hormone may be the endocrine change most commonly seen after concussion, they assayed growth hormone. Injured rats exhibited a significant decrease in serum growth hormone compared with sham-injured controls ($p = 0.0167$).

Spain et al. [226] exposed their mice to a mild LFPI of 0.9 atm, then let them live for four to six weeks. At four weeks the CBI mice had significantly higher numbers of axonal bulbs (highly consistent with axonal damage) in the external capsule ($p = 0.041$), and at six weeks they had significantly higher numbers of axonal bulbs in both the external capsule ($p = 0.041$) and thalamus ($p < 0.001$). One despairs that the investigators did not wait a year before decapitating their little subjects. Although the axonal changes perhaps predicted unrecoverable stretching, we really need to know whether an injury this mild produces permanent brain change.

Goldstein et al. [265] administered blasts to their mice.[19] The subjects were permitted to survive for a month. At that point, persistent changes were detected in both electrophysiology and pathology. The authors reported: "marked impairments of stimulus-evoked LTP in mouse slices prepared … 1 month after blast exposure." LTP is the electrical signature of hippocampal memory consolidation. Although behavior was not tested, the implications for cognition are evident: "These results indicate that exposure to single blast impaired long-term activity-dependent synaptic plasticity for at least 1 month after blast exposure." The authors seemed even more impressed by the microscopic findings:

Blast-exposed mice demonstrated phosphorylated tauopathy, myelinated axonopathy, microvasculopathy, chronic neuroinflammation, and neurodegeneration in the absence of macroscopic tissue damage or hemorrhage.

[265]

These findings may be compared with those of Shetty et al. [266], who reported that low-intensity blast also has significant vascular effects. It swells astrocyte end-feet, eliminates pericytes, damages the basement membrane, and disrupts tight junctions in brain microvessels (Figure 4.26).

Although some have interpreted such results as evidence that mild blast can trigger chronic traumatic encephalopathy,

the present author is more conservative. Protein deposition promptly after concussion – which some authorities refer to as "neurodegenerative" – might be temporary. If so, despite the striking resemblance of these mouse changes to the permanent brain damage sometimes seen in athletes after repetitive concussions, it is premature to conclude that "mild" blast provokes progressive and inescapable neurodegeneration.

In recent years – perhaps because of residual sensitivities about the failure of the old ischemic theory of concussion – relatively less experimental research has focused on vascular and blood–brain barrier changes after CBI. Findings such as Shetty et al.'s may revive that interest. Some evidence supports the hypothesis that cerebrovascular change plays a critical role in the pathophysiology of AD [267–271]. We truly do not understand whether, or how, or under what circumstances a single concussive injury triggers this or any other element of neurodegeneration. Yet it is interesting to note that both concussion and "AD" involve microvascular change. One hypothesis is that traumatic vascular disruption, along with traumatic production of protein aggregates, is a causal factor linking head blows to later dementia [272]. At the same time, recovery from CBI might be related, at least in part, to restoration of microvascular integrity. (Without concluding that there is direct relevance: as previously mentioned, CBI is associated with increased PrP^c. One rodent study reported that PrP^c may be necessary for brain microvascular endothelial cells to migrate into sites of cerebral injury [273]. That finding conceivably identifies PrP^c as a defensive fighter in the post-CBI melee.)

The author demurs. It remains opaque whether there are any long-term consequences either of CBI microvascular damage or of CBI-related generation of amyloid. For instance, intra-axonal APP accumulation is thought to be a marker of lasting axonal injury and some investigators [e.g., 226] suggest that this marks or parallels observed deficits in spatial learning. However, other studies show that this neuropathological change is dissociable from behavioral change. For instance, Tweedie et al. [228] found APP accumulations but no learning deficit, and Longhi et al. [274] observed the onset of depression-like behavior but no APP accumulation in wild-type mice.

One more medium-term animal study also raises the possibility that very mild brain injury causes permanent damage with persistent clinical effects. Washington et al. [275] exposed their mice to CCI with a velocity of 5.25 m/s, deformation of 1.5 mm, and dwell of 0.1 s. Mild injury was associated with significant loss of brain volume ($p < 0.001$) and with a 22% loss of hippocampal volume ($p > 0.05$) 26 days after injury. That seems worrisome.

What, then, of rodent *behavior*? Table 4.2 summarizes many of the available findings from the very small number of published medium- to long-term studies of "mild" injury in which the animals have been permitted to live for two weeks to 11 months after CBI prior to sacrifice.[20] In very brief summary

---

[19] Severity of the injury in this case was somewhat difficult to assess: the Mach was 1.26, the wind velocity 50m/s, and the peak average radial head acceleration was 954 krad/s². Since this is lower than similar measures in other blast studies, the term "mild" perhaps applies.

[20] This review was conducted using PubMed, reviewing papers in which the title or abstract contained the terms "mild traumatic brain injury" or "concussion" and "animal," "mouse," "mice," "rat," or "rodent." To call the search *systematic* would be too generous. *Focused* might be more accurate.

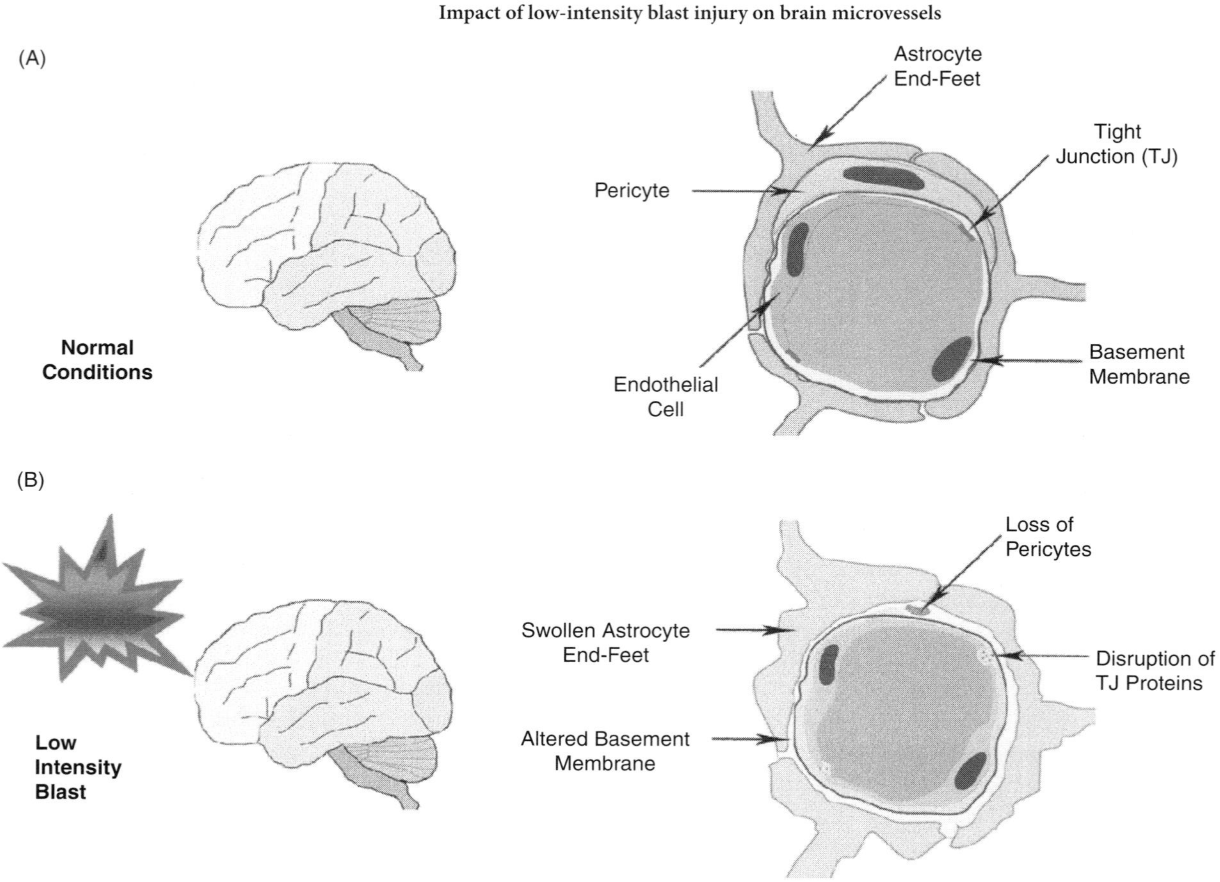

Impact of low-intensity blast injury on brain microvessels

Fig. 4.26 In brain microvessels, low-intensity blast swells astrocyte end-feet, eliminates pericytes, damages the basement membrane, and disrupts tight junctions (TJ). (A) Normal conditions; (B) low-intensity blast. [A black and white version of this figure will appear in some formats. For the color version, please refer to the plate section.]

Source: Shetty et al., 2014 [266]. Reproduced under the terms of the Creative Commons Attribution licence, CC-BY.

of this literature: in order to establish some criterion for inclusion of studies worthy of attention, one is obliged to make a guess at the upper limits of mildness. The reasons that such a limit is biologically meaningless have already been stated. Moreover, one cannot equate or compare FPI's atmospheres of pressure (expressed, for instance, as kg/m²) with the weight drop acceleration injury force of a fall (expressed in newtons, or kg-m/s²), or with CCI's velocity (m/s). The author therefore candidly acknowledges that the inclusion criteria employed in this review were arbitrary:

1. The injury should be mild. In the case of a mouse, perhaps that means a falling weight producing ≤ 200 N, a pressure hose generating ≤ 1.5 atm, or a piston deforming tissue by ≤ 1.5 mm.

2. The follow-up should be ≥ 14 days (since this exceeds the estimated time for the resolution of calcium influx and cerebral blood flow change).

3. Ideally, the target should be a closed head.

4. Ideally, the closed head should be mobile.

5. Blasts are excluded because the entire body is shaken and it is especially difficult to guess at the limits of mildness.

Table 4.2 is offered with misgivings. It represents a sincere effort to compile the highest-quality available data, emphasizing the recent past. Yet the introductory narrative of this chapter has hopefully disabused the reader of taking these reports at face value. Too many compromises degrade the resemblance between these experiments and real-world concussion. Little is known about the relevance of these studies to human CBI. The most meticulous study and most sophisticated statistical manipulations of this data cannot overcome the doubts about its validity. In a different textbook, the author might attempt an eloquent narrative, hoping to distill core lessons from this substantive body of peer-reviewed research. Instead, mindful of the serious barriers to meaningful inference about humans from this bricolage of claims, perhaps one should confine oneself to generalities:

First: no clear and convincing threshold of force leaps out as the lower limit at which impact becomes injurious.

Second: despite widespread use of several popular injury methods (e.g., weight drop) and popular behavior tests (e.g., the elevated plus maze), and despite a great deal of overlapping work, few (if any) experiments have been replicated across laboratories.

Table 4.2 Persistent neurobehavioral or neurobiological change in rodents exposed to experimental "mild traumatic brain injury"

Author, year	Species	Injury model (open vs. closed = O vs. C)	Impact parameters	Behavioral tests	Follow-up period	Findings
Abdel Baki et al., 2009 [276]	R	CCI/O	V: 3 m/s Def: 1 mm	Active place avoidance	3 weeks	Mildly-injured rats failed to learn to avoid shock, while controls learned ($p < 0.001$)
Baskin et al., 2003 [277]	M	CCI/O Anterior, middle, and posterior subjects	V: 6.87 m/s Def: 1 mm	Spontaneous forelimb use task	5 months	"anterior and posterior insult animals favored the use of their ipsilateral limb for at least 5 months following TBI relative to baseline" (p. 90)
Bree and Levy, 2016 [278]	M	WDAI/C	Weight 250 g Height 80 cm	Open-field Novel object recognition Tactile pain hypersensitivity	2 weeks	1. Open-field: no deficits @ 7 days except reduced exploratory vertical rearing 2. Novel object recognition: no deficit @ 7 days 3. Cephalic tactile pain hypersensitivity: increased @ 7 days; not @ 14 days
Chen et al., 1996 [14]	M	WDAI/C	Weight: 333 g Height: 2–3 cm (2 cm: ~ 52 N; 3 cm: ~ 78 N)	Beam walk	30 days	"Some residual deficit, mainly of motor function, persists 30 days postinjury" (p. 562)
Darwish et al., 2012 [214]	R	CCI/O	V: 4 m/s Def: 1.5 mm	MWM	25 days	1. Escape latency signicantly longer for mild vs. controls ($p = 0.04$) consistent with delayed spatial learning abilities not apparent at days 1–5 2. "On day 25 post-injury the animals with mild injury did not recover their spatial learning abilities"(p. 161).
Dixon et al., 1999 [211]	R	CCI/O	V: 4 m/s Def: 2.5 mm Dw: 50 ms	MWM	12 months	1. Escape latency significantly longer than controls @ 1 year ($p < 0.021$) 2. Progressive hippocampal atrophy 3. Neurotransmitter changes
Emmerich et al., 2017 [279]	M	Electromagnetic CCI/C	V: 5 m/s Def: 1 mm Dw: 200 ms	Measures of plasma phospholipid profle	Up to 24 months	Multiple phospholipids from several major classes were persistently decreased after mTBI
Fox et al., 1998 [280]	M	CCI/O	"Mild" V: 4.5 m/sec Def: 1mm Dw: 400 ms "Moderate" V: 6 m/s	Beam walk Rotarod MWM	2–4 weeks	"Mild" injury associated with 1. Beam walk deficit @ 2 weeks, not 4 weeks 2. No rotarod deficit @ 2 weeks 3. No MWM deficit @ 21 days 4. Injury to deep somatosensory cortex; necrosis of subcortical white matter "Moderate" injury associated with: 1. Beam walk deficit @ 2 and 4 weeks 2. No rotarod deficit @ 2 weeks 3. MWM deficit @ 21 days 4. Extensive cortical and subcortical damage; many TUNEL + apoptotic cells
Fox et al., 1998 [56]	M	CCI/O	"Moderate" V: 6 m/s Def: 1mm Dw: 400 ms	Beam walk Barnes maze	28 days	"Moderate" injury associated with: 1. Significant deficit on beam walking @ 28 days ($p < 0.0001$) 2. Deficit on maze for 10 days (no later test)

(continued)

Table 4.2 (Cont.)

Author, year	Species	Injury model (open vs. closed = O vs. C)	Impact parameters	Behavioral tests	Follow-up period	Findings
Goldstein et al., 2012[a] [265]	M	Blast/C	Mach = 1.26; wind V = 50 m/s; peak average radial head acceleation = 954 krad/s^2	Barnes maze	30 days	"blast-exposed mice exhibited significantly longer escape latencies … (P < 0.05) … and poorer memory retrieval"
Guley et al., 2016 [281]	M	High-pressure air blast/C	20–60 psi	Rotarod Open-field Optokinetic response	2–3 weeks	25–40 psi mice @ 2 weeks: no significant deficits in rotarod or most open-field measures except total distance 50–60 psi mice @ 2 weeks: no significant deficits in rotarod. But significantly impaired on most open-field measures
Hamm et al., 1992 [282]	R	CCI/O	"Moderate"V: 6 m/s Def: 1.5–2 mm	MWM	30–34 days	"brain-injured rats exhibited significant deficits (p < 0.05) in maze performance at both testing intervals" (p. 11)
Heim et al., 2017 [283]	M	WDAI/C	Weight: 10, 30, 50, or 70 g Height: 80 cm	Staircase test Rotarod FST EPM Novel Object Recognition Y-Maze	30 days	No deficits at any weight on staircase motor test No deficits at any weight on rotarod Increased immobility at 50 or 70 g on FST No change at any weight on EPM Significantly impaired performance for 30, 50, and 70 g on Novel Object Recognition Significantly impaired performance for 30, 50, and 70 g on Y-maze
Heldt et al., 2014 [284]	M	High-pressure air blast/C	20–60 psi	Open-field Acoustic startle Prepulse inhibition Tail suspension Fear conditioning	Up to 8 weeks	25–40 psi mice: @ 7 days, significantly avoided the midfield; @ 14 days, this effect was no longer significant 50–60 psi mice: @ 7 days, did **not** significantly avoid midfield; @ 14 days, trended toward avoiding midfield; @ 6–8 weeks showed increased acoustic startle, and reduced prepulse inhibition (seen in schizophrenia), and increased immobility on tail suspension (compared with depression)
Kokiko-Cochran et al., 2015 [76]	M (wild-type and Aβ-expressing Tg)	CCI/O	V: 4 m/sec. Def: 1.5 mm	Rotarod @ 90 days Y-maze @ 90 days MWM @ 120 days	6 months	1. Wild-type and Tg mice expressing Aβ both had persistent deficits in rotarod performance 2. Tg mice had persistent spatial working-memory deficits on Y-maze 3. Tg mice had significantly inferior overnight recall of MWM
Levy et al., 2016 [285]	M	1. WDAI/C 2. Blast	Weight: 30 g Height: 80 cm Blast wave pressure ~ 5.5 psi	N/A	30 days	Dural mast cell degranulation increased at 30 days after both WDAI and blast
Lindner et al., 1998 [286]	R	CCI/O	V: frontal 2.25 m/s Lateral 3.22 m/s Def: 2 mm	RAM: 6–7 months MWM: 7.5–11 months Rot = 11 months	6–11 months	1. Lateral injury, but not frontal association with significantly worse performance on RAM @ 6–9 months 2. Frontal injury, but not lateral association with significantly worse performance on reinforcement test @ 10–12 months 3. Lateral injury associated with significantly worse performance on MWM @ 10–12 months

Table 4.2 (Cont.)

Author, year	Species	Injury model (open vs. closed = O vs. C)	Impact parameters	Behavioral tests	Follow-up period	Findings
Lyeth et al., 1990 [225]	R	Sagittal FPI/O	"Mild + moderate" (no measures)	Beam walk; RAM	25 days	"Mild" injury associated with: 1. Beam walk deficit only 5 days 2. No RAM deficit beyond 5 days "Moderate" injury associated with: 1. Beam walk deficit only 5 days 2. RAM deficit @ 15 days
Milman et al., 2005 [287]	M	WDAI/C	Weight = 30 g Height = 80 cm (~188 N)	Swim T-maze (spatial learning); Passive avoidance (non-spatial learning	7–90 days	1. At 30 days, mTBI mice significantly impaired on passive avoid learning ($p < 0.001$). No significant difference from sham at 60 or 90 days 2. At 30 days, mTBI mice significantly impaired on spatial learning ($p < 0.05$). No significant difference from sham at 60 or 90 days
Milman et al., 2008 [288]	M	WDAI/C	Weight = 30 g Height = 80 cm (~188 N)	Passive avoidance (non-spatial learning	7–90 days	1. At 30 ($p < 0.05$) and 60 days ($p = 0.01$), mTBI mice significantly impaired in non-spatial learning. No significant difference @ 90 days
Namjoshi et al., 2017 [289]	M	CHIMERA/C	0.1, 0.3, 0.4, 0.5, 0.6, or 0.7 J of energy via steel piston	Rotarod Open-field	14 days	Rotarod latency @ 14 days: reduced Open-field thigmotaxis (anxiety-related tendency to remain close to walls) @ 7 days: increased
Nichols et al., 2016 [58]	M	WDAI on to steel disc/C	Weight = 100 g Height 70 cm (~ 686 N)	MWM EPM FST Marble burying Nestlet shredding	3 weeks	mTBI associated with: 1. Greater distance traveled to find MWM platform (3 weeks) 2. Reduced marble burying (10 days) 3. Poorer nest building (11 days) No significant association with: 1. EPM 2. FST
Ojo et al., 2014[b] [290]	M	Electromagnetic-controlled impact device/C	V: 5 m/s Def: 1 mm Dw: 200 ms	Rotarod RAM (water) EPM Open-field	22 days	mTBI associated with: 1. Anxiety per open-field test ($p = 0.002$) 2. Increased GFAP (marker of astroglial activation) in corpus callosum ($p = 0.038$), hippocampus and cortex ($p = 0.022$) 3. Increased Th17 cytokine (interleukin-17A) levels No significant association with: 1. Spatial learning and memory 2. Anxiety per elevated plus maze 3. Motor activity or coordination 4. NFL (marker of axonal injury) or ICAM-1(marker of inflammation) 5. Brain weight
Petraglia et al., 2014 [262]	M	CCI/C + helm. No anesthesia	V: 5 m/s Dw: 100 ms	MWM EPM FST	1 month 6 months	mTBI associated with: 1. MWM deficits at 1 month 2. EPM at 14 days No significant association with: 1. MWM at 6 months 2. EPM at 1 month, or 6 months 3. FST at 1 month

(continued)

Table 4.2 (Cont.)

Author, year	Species	Injury model (open vs. closed = O vs. C)	Impact parameters	Behavioral tests	Follow-up period	Findings
Rubovitch et al., 2011 [53]	M	Blast/O	2.5 psi (milder) or 5.5 psi overpressure	Staircase test (motor + anxiety); Object recognition Test; Y-maze (spatial memory)	30 days	1. 2.5 psi-exposed mice significantly more rearing events ($p < 0.01$) and on staircase test 2. 2.5 psi-exposed mice significantly reduced preference for novel objects ($p < 0.05$) 3. 2.5 psi-exposed mice: no significant difference in Y-maze spatial memory
Scheff et al., 1997 [291]	R	CCI/O	V: 3.5 m/s Def: 1 mm	MWM	14 days	"Mildly injured animals manifest a significant behavioral deficit in the MWM" (p. 621)
Schneider et al., 2016 [292]	M	Electromagnetically driven impactor/C	V: 5 m/s Def: 1 mm Dw: 100 ms	Conditioned fear acquisition/extinction	25 days	mTBI associated with: 1. Increased acquisition of conditioned fear 2. Decreased extinction 3. Decreased GABA/Glu in hippocampus [c]
Shultz et al., 2011 [293]	R	FPI/O	Mean = 1.20 atm	MWM	4 weeks	1. No significant difference in acquisition training 2. Injured mice significantly less decrease in search times vs. controls ($p < 0.01$)
Shultz et al., 2012 [294]	R	Lateral FPI/O	0.5–0.99 "subconcussive"	MWM Beam walk	4 weeks	1. No significant difference in acquisition or reversal training on MWM 2. No significant difference on beam walk
Spain et al., 2010 [226]	M	FPI/O	0.9 atm	MWM	2–3 weeks	1. No significant difference in learning cued task 2. Injured mice failed to improve learning over 5 days: significantly worse than controls @ day 4 ($p = 0.046$) and day 5 ($p = 0.028$)
Tweedie et al., 2016 [295] [d]	M	WDAI/C	Weight: 30 g Height: 80 cm	N/A	14 days	Molecular function of gene ontologies @ 14 days: 413 gene probes observed 143 genes were significantly up-regulated and 223 genes were significantly down-regulated
Washington et al., 2012 [275]	M	CCI/O	V: 5.25 m/s Def: 1.5 mm (mild); 2.0 mm (moderate); 2.5 mm (severe) Dw: 0.1 s	MWM	22–26 days	1. Day 25: mild injury associated with longer escape latency, although this did not reach significance (control mean = 9.9 s; injured mean = 26.1 s) 2. Day 26: mild injury associated with significantly less time in correct quadrant on probe trial ($p < 0.05$)
Zohar et al., 2003 [30]	M	WDAI/C	Weight: 20, 25, 30 g Height: 80 cm (very mild)	MWM	Up to 90 days	Learning rate – the rate of improving escape latency performance on consecutive trials on a given day – was significantly worse for all degrees of very mild injury; control mice improved 77%; injured mice improved 45–50% ($p < 0.001$)

Table 4.2 (Cont.)

Author, year	Species	Injury model (open vs. closed = O vs. C)	Impact parameters	Behavioral tests	Follow-up period	Findings
Zohar et al., 2011 [296]	M	WDAI/C	Weight: 20, 25, 30 g Height: 80 cm	MWM Passive avoidance T-maze	90 days	1. On the MWM (spatial learning), 20 g and 25 g injury associated with significant decrease in learning ($p < 0.001$). 2. On the MWM probe trial (free swim, missing platform) all injured mice significantly worse than controls at locating platform ($p < 0.05$). 3. On passive avoidance (non-spatial learning): injured mice (all degrees) learning was decreased vs. control (non-significant) 4. On T-maze (working memory), injured mice (all degrees) had significant learning deficit ($p < 0.001$)

[a] Re. Goldstein et al., 2012 [265]: the abstract reports memory deficits at one month, but the text fails to report the timing of Barnes Maze testing.
[b] Re. Ojo et al., 2014 [290]: "we also consider that the highly rigorous training schedule giving to the animals prior to the stress and concussive head injury paradigm might have been counterproductive and precluded detection of some of the subtle effects in response to trauma and head injury." (p. 13).
[c] Re. Schneider et al., 2016 [292]: The authors opined, "These neurochemical changes are consistent with early TBI-induced PFC [prefrontal cortex] hypoactivation facilitating the fear learning circuit and exacerbating behavioral fear responses" (p. 1614).
[d] RE. Tweedie et al., 2016 [295]: Altered gene regulation was concentrated in molecular pathways associated with inflammation, neurodegeneration, and neurogenesis.

atm: atmospheres; Barnes: Barnes maze; CCI: controlled cortical impact; CHIMERA: closed head impact model of engineered rotational acceleration; Def: deformation; Dw: dwell time; EPM: elevated plus maze; FPI: fluid percussion injury; FST: forced swim test; GABA, gamma-aminobutyric acid; GFAP, glial fibrillary acid protein; Glu, glutamate; Helm: helmeted subjects; Height: height for weight drop; M: mouse; mTBI, mild traumatic brain injury; MWM: Morris water maze; R: rat; RAM: radial arm maze; TBI: traumatic brain injury; V: velocity; WDAI: weight drop acceleration injury; Weight: weight for weight drop

Third: in so far as studies can be compared, the outcomes from similar experiments (e.g., type and duration of deficits) do not seem to be consistent.

Fourth: behavioral tests believed to reflect a common psychological construct (e.g., the open-field test or elevated plus maze to assess "anxiety") often have inconsistent results.

Fifth: dose–response effects have been observed within laboratories for one outcome, but not for other outcomes. And outcomes that do or do not exhibit dose–response effects vary from lab to lab.

At the risk of oversimplifying – and missing pearls hidden in this chest of treasures – the present author might narrow his conclusions to two. One: experimental concussion has promise. That promise has yet to be realized. The widespread employment of dated injury methods – those that simply do not represent naturalistic concussion – and the rank poverty of longitudinal observations both seem wasteful and disrespectful to the spirit of minimizing animal sacrifice and maximizing human benefit. One wonders whether pursuit of academic advantage and defense of intellectual property have been disincentives to coordination across laboratories, encouraging unnecessarily duplicative efforts. Moore's law (1965) and the movement toward open publishing have perhaps made it possible to orchestrate global coordination of experimental work in the interest of minimizing the number of animals used and developing synergistic initiatives. Fewer mice, concussed

more scientifically and observed more extensively, might tell us more.

Two: admitting that it is impossible to guess the full human implications of the data summarized in this chapter, sufficient experimental findings have been published to justify the conclusion that "mild" TBIs have measurable, deleterious effects on cognition, emotion, and multiple aspects of brain function for as long as one lets the animal live. Put another way: no matter how long one waits after administering a "mild" blow, there is evidence of lasting harm.

Table 4.2 is, to the best of this author's knowledge, the first compilation of results from 34 studies that investigated the effect of concussion on rodent behavior in the two to 52 weeks after injury. It fairly shouts its main lesson: we could have done better.

First, it would have been extremely helpful if more laboratories had employed Aβ + tau transgenics and cared for their animals into old age prior to sacrifice. Second, almost no laboratories retain world-class experts in behavioral, neurophysiological, neuroimaging, and neuropathological assessment. One often encounters reports in which the quality of attention to these diverse aspects of scientific investigation is uneven. As a result, it is often nearly impossible to interpret negative reports. For instance, Scheff et al. [291] stated, "mildly injured subjects demonstrated no obvious tissue destruction, but did manifest significant behavioral change" (p. 615). Was that because there was no tissue destruction, or because the laboratory did not

Table 4.3 Results of experiments employing "mild" injuries, assessed at ≥ 30 days post concussive brain injury

Positive findings

- Cognition: Dixon (12 months); Goldstein (30 days); Heim (30 days); Kokino (6 months); Lindner (6–12 months); Milman, 2005 (30 days); Milman, 2008 (30–60 days); Rubovitch (30 days); Schultz (4 weeks); Zohar, 2003 (up to 90 days); Zohar, 2011 (90 days)
- Behavior: Heldt (6–8 weeks); Heim (30 days); Rubovitch (30 days)
- Motor: Baskin (5 months); Chen (30 days); Kokino (6 months)
- Biomarkers: Dixon (12 months); Emmerich et al. (24 months); Levy (30 days); Schneider (30 days)

Negative findings

- Cognition: Petraglia (6 months)
- Behavior: N/A
- Motor: N/A
- Biomarkers: N/A

support a graduate student versed in TUNEL labeling? Third, too few studies involved administration of a blow to a closed head; those that produced focal insults to the dura cannot be regarded as representative of CBI. Fourth, the reader can see why the possibility of gaining deeper insight from meta-analysis is obviated: no two laboratories used the same method.

Methodological limitations aside, one might condense the findings into a digestible format, as shown in Table 4.3. In brief, 21 of 34 studies reported findings after "mild" injuries in which the subjects were assessed at ≥ 30 days post-CBI. Twelve studies assessed cognition. Persistent cognitive deficits were reported in 11 of the 12. Three studies assessed behaviors (e.g., anxiety or depression); all three reported persistent impairments. Three studies assessed motor function; all reported persistent impairments. Four studies assessed biomarkers; all reported persistent impairments. Only ten studies of "mild" injury were identified that followed up subjects at ≥ 90 days post-CBI [30, 76, 211, 262, 277, 279, 286–288, 296]. All except Petraglia reported persistent neurobehavioral or biological problems.

This analysis, however, cannot be regarded as probative evidence that "mild" experimental TBI necessarily causes persistent abnormalities (indeed, up to 24 months, the natural lifespan of many mice) in multiple aspects of health and behavior. It is biased both by restriction to longer-term studies (which excludes studies that perhaps stopped examining their subjects because no deficits were found early on), and by likely publication bias. Again, one is rather hamstrung by the quality of the data. Perhaps two non-scientific interpretations are equally appropriate: where there is smoke, there is fire (that is, multiple reports of persistent problems perhaps reflect an authentic association between "mTBI" and persistent deleterious change), and where there is smoke and mirrors (that is, where dubious methods compromise quality), the truth is beclouded.

Conclusion

Scholars have hit thousands upon thousands of animals on the head to see what happens. Most subjects were hit hard enough to alter their level of consciousness but not to render them comatose all day. Admitting our nine caveats regarding the conceptual and methodological limitations that have bedeviled this work, admitting the uncertainty of conclusions from small numbers of observations, admitting our astonishing collective failure to rigorously test the hypothesis that late effects follow single concussions, within the bounds of reasonable inference, one must conclude that CBI of the sort that is sometimes somewhat similar to typical human CBI is often followed by persistent brain damage and neurobehavioral deficits in rodents.

Afterword: In Praise of Fact Finders

Readers have accomplished a great deal if they have made it to this sentence. One should be rewarded for such conscientious effort. The reward is confidence. Close readers are in an enviable position: they now know as much as, or more than, many a self-professed expert in experimental concussion. What is to be gained? These hard-won findings are – in a rough-hewn way – probably pertinent to typical human concussion. This overview, ideally, will fire up young scientists to fill in the giant factual gaps.

The author must now and forever confess his limited contribution and parasitic role. Like many plodding thinkers, he rarely generates data; he consumes it. He has always depended upon the generosity of fact finders – like the Blanche DuBois of the neuroscience agora.

Graduate students are the main finders of facts. These are the unheralded knights of humanity's forever war between science and conservatism. Subsisting on left-over pizza, microwaved coffee, and gossamer dreams of discovery, forgoing the hedonic allure of material comforts, social life, matrimonial security, and economic stability, laboring late into many nights in cramped and dismal labs bedizened with broken equipment, at the mercy of distracted mentors and stingy funders, facing a promotion system that is Dickensian in design and Kafkaesque in execution, they accept self-abnegation to seek truth. Let's remember them.

The mice should be remembered too.

Now, what about humans?

References

1. Mychasiuk R, Farran A, Esser MJ. Assessment of an experimental rodent model of pediatric mild traumatic brain injury. *J Neurotrauma* 2014;31:749–757.
2. Groat RA, Simmons JQ. Loss of nerve cells in experimental cerebral concussion. *J Neuropathol Exp Neurol* 1950;9:150–163.
3. Symonds CP. Prognosis in cerebral concussion and contusion. *Lancet* 1936;1:854–856.
4. Walker AE, Caveness WF, Critchley M. *The late effects of head injury.* Springfield, IL: CC Thomas, 1969.
5. Creed JA, Dileonardi AM, Fox DP, Tessler AR, Raghupathi R. Concussive brain trauma in the mouse results in acute cognitive deficits and sustained impairment of axonal function. *J Neurotrauma* 2011;28:547–563.
6. Conte V, Uryu K, Fujimoto S, Yao Y, Rokach J, Longhi L, et al. Vitamin E reduces amyloidosis and improves cognitive function in Tg2576 mice following repetitive concussive brain injury. *J Neurochem* 2004;90:758–764.

7. Uryu K, Laurer H, Mcintosh T, Pratico D, Martinez D, Leight S, et al. Repetitive mild brain trauma accelerates Abeta deposition, lipid peroxidation, and cognitive impairment in a transgenic mouse model of Alzheimer amyloidosis. *J Neurosci* 2002;22:446–454.

8. Yoshiyama Y, Uryu K, Higuchi M, Longhi L, Hoover R, Fujimoto S, et al. Enhanced neurofibrillary tangle formation, cerebral atrophy, and cognitive deficits induced by repetitive mild brain injury in a transgenic tauopathy mouse model. *J Neurotrauma* 2005;22:1134–1141.

9. Chen M, Maleski JJ, Sawmiller DR. Scientific truth or false hope? Understanding Alzheimer's disease from an aging perspective. *J Alzheimers Dis* 2011;24:3–10.

10. Whitehouse PJ, George DR, D'Alton S. Describing the dying days of "Alzheimer's disease." *J Alzheimers Dis* 2011;24:11–13.

11. Ucar T, Tanriover G, Gurer I, Onal MZ, Kazan S. Modified experimental mild traumatic brain injury model. *J Trauma* 2006;60:558–565.

12. Shultz SR, McDonald SJ, Vonder Haar C, Meconi A, Vink R, van Donkelaar P, et al. The potential for animal models to provide insight into mild traumatic brain injury: Translational challenges and strategies. *Neurosci Biobehav Rev* 2017;76:396–414

13. Russell WR. *The traumatic amnesias*. Oxford: Oxford University Press, 1971.

14. Chen Y, Constantini S, Trembovler V, Weinstock M, Shohami E. An experimental model of closed head injury in mice: Pathophysiology, histopathology, and cognitive deficits. *J Neurotrauma* 1996;13:557–568.

15. Dixon CE, Lyeth BG, Povlishock JT, Findling RL, Hamm RJ, Marmarou A, et al. A fluid percussion model of experimental brain injury in the rat. *J Neurosurg* 1987;67:110–119.

16. Foda MA, Marmarou A. A new model of diffuse brain injury in rats. Part II: Morphological characterization. *J Neurosurg* 1994;80:301–313.

17. Lighthall JW. Controlled cortical impact: A new experimental brain injury model. *J Neurotrauma* 1988;5:1–15.

18. Lighthall JW, Goshgarian HG, Pinderski CR. Characterization of axonal injury produced by controlled cortical impact. *J Neurotrauma* 1990;7:65–76.

19. Marmarou A, Foda MA, Van Den Brink W, Campbell J, Kita H, Demetriadou K. A new model of diffuse brain injury in rats. Part I: Pathophysiology and biomechanics. *J Neurosurg* 1994;80:291–300.

20. Morales DM, Marklund N, Lebold D, Thompson HJ, Pitkanen A, Maxwell WL, et al. Experimental models of traumatic brain injury: Do we really need to build a better mousetrap? *Neuroscience* 2005;136:971–989.

21. O'Connor WT, Smyth A, Gilchrist MD. Animal models of traumatic brain injury: A critical evaluation. *Pharmacol Ther* 2011;130:106–113.

22. Xiong Y, Mahmood A, Chopp M. Animal models of traumatic brain injury. *Nat Rev Neurosci* 2013;14:128–142.

23. Schwarzbold ML, Rial D, De Bem T, Machado DG, Cunha MP, Dos Santos AA, et al. Effects of traumatic brain injury of different severities on emotional, cognitive, and oxidative stress-related parameters in mice. *J Neurotrauma* 2010;27:1883–1893.

24. Viano DC, Hamberger A, Bolouri H, Saljo A. Concussion in professional football: Animal model of brain injury – Part 15. *Neurosurgery* 2009;64:1162–1173; discussion 1173.

25. Kallakuri S, Cavanaugh JM, Ozaktay AC, Takebayashi T. The effect of varying impact energy on diffuse axonal injury in the rat brain: A preliminary study. *Exp Brain Res* 2003;148:419–424.

26. Liu P, Li YS, Quartermain D, Boutajangout A, Ji Y. Inhaled nitric oxide improves short term memory and reduces the inflammatory reaction in a mouse model of mild traumatic brain injury. *Brain Res* 2013;1522:67–75.

27. Nilsson B, Ponten U. Exerimental head injury in the rat. Part 2: Regional brain energy metabolism in concussive trauma. *J Neurosurg* 1977;47:252–261.

28. Signoretti S, Marmarou A, Tavazzi B, Lazzarino G, Beaumont A, Vagnozzi R. *N*-Acetylaspartate reduction as a measure of injury severity and mitochondrial dysfunction following diffuse traumatic brain injury. *J Neurotrauma* 2001;18:977–991.

29. Tashlykov V, Katz Y, Gazit V, Zohar O, Schreiber S, Pick CG. Apoptotic changes in the cortex and hippocampus following minimal brain trauma in mice. *Brain Res* 2007;1130:197–205.

30. Zohar O, Schreiber S, Getslev V, Schwartz JP, Mullins PG, Pick CG. Closed-head minimal traumatic brain injury produces long-term cognitive deficits in mice. *Neuroscience* 2003;118:949–955.

31. Namjoshi DH, Cheng WH, Bashir A, Wilkinson A, Stukas S, Martens KM, et al. Defining the biomechanical and biological threshold of murine mild traumatic brain injury using CHIMERA (Closed Head Impact Model of Engineered Rotational Acceleration). *Exp Neurol* 2017;292:80–91.

32. McIntosh TK, Vink R, Noble L, Yamakami I, Fernyak S, Soares H, et al. Traumatic brain injury in the rat: Characterization of a lateral fluid-percussion model. *Neuroscience* 1989;28:233–244.

33. Withnall C, Shewchenko N, Gittens R, Dvorak J. Biomechanical investigation of head impacts in football. *Br J Sports Med* 2005;39(Suppl I):i49–i57.

34. Rowson S, Duma SM, Beckwith JG, Chu JJ, Greenwald RM, Crisco JJ, et al. Rotational head kinematics in football impacts: An injury risk function for concussion. *Ann Biomed Eng* 2012;40:1–13.

35. Romine J, Gao X, Chen J. Controlled cortical impact model for traumatic brain injury. *J Vis Exp* 2014;90:e51781.

36. Brody DL, Mac Donald C, Kessens CC, Yuede C, Parsadanian M, Spinner M, et al. Electromagnetic controlled cortical impact device for precise, graded experimental traumatic brain injury. *J Neurotrauma* 2007;24:657–673.

37. Cernak I, Merkle AC, Koliatsos VE, Bilik JM, Luong QT, Mahota TM, et al. The pathobiology of blast injuries and blast-induced neurotrauma as identified using a new experimental model of injury in mice. *Neurobiol Dis* 2011;41:538–551.

38. Chen Z, Leung LY, Mountney A, Liao Z, Yang W, Lu XC, et al. A novel animal model of closed-head concussive-induced mild traumatic brain injury: Development, implementation, and characterization. *J Neurotrauma* 2012;29:268–280.

39. Dewitt DS, Perez-Polo R, Hulsebosch CE, Dash PK, Robertson CS. Challenges in the development of rodent models of mild traumatic brain injury. *J Neurotrauma* 2013;30:688–701.

40. Dixon CE, Clifton GL, Lighthall JW, Yaghmai AA, Hayes RL. A controlled cortical impact model of traumatic brain injury in the rat. *J Neurosci Methods* 1991;39:253–262.

41. Morganti-Kossmann MC, Yan E, Bye N. Animal models of traumatic brain injury: Is there an optimal model to reproduce human brain injury in the laboratory? *Injury* 2010;41:10–13.

42. Petraglia AL, Dashnaw ML, Turner RC, Bailes JE. Models of mild traumatic brain injury: Translation of physiological and anatomic injury. *Neurosurgery* 2014;75(Suppl 4):S34–S49.

43. Rostami E, Davidsson J, Ng KC, Lu J, Gyorgy A, Walker J, et al. A model for mild traumatic brain injury that induces limited transient memory impairment and increased levels of axon related serum biomarkers. *Front Neurol* 2012;3:115.

44. Zhang YP, Cai J, Shields LB, Liu N, Xu XM, Shields CB. Traumatic brain injury using mouse models. *Transl Stroke Res* 2014;5:454–471.

45. Feeney DM, Boyeson MG, Linn RT, Murray HM, Dail WG. Responses to cortical injury: I. Methodology and local effects of contusions in the rat. *Brain Res* 1981;211:67–77.

46. Tang YP, Noda Y, Hasegawa T, Nabeshima T. A concussive-like brain injury model in mice (II): Selective neuronal loss in the cortex and hippocampus. *J Neurotrauma* 1997;14:863–873.

47. Mcintosh TK, Noble L, Andrews B, Faden AI. Traumatic brain injury in the rat: Characterization of a midline fluid-percussion model. *Cent Nerv Syst Trauma* 1987;4:119–134.

48. Smith DH, Soares HD, Pierce JS, Perlman KG, Saatman KE, Meaney DF, et al. A model of parasagittal controlled cortical impact in the mouse: Cognitive and histopathologic effects. *J Neurotrauma* 1995;12:169–178.

49. Alder J, Fujioka W, Lifshitz J, Crockett DP, Thakker-Varia S. Lateral fluid percussion: Model of traumatic brain injury in mice. *J Vis Exp* 2011;22(54):pii:3063.

50. Hall ED, Bryant YD, Cho W, Sullivan PG. Evolution of post-traumatic neurodegeneration after controlled cortical impact traumatic brain injury in mice and rats as assessed by the de Olmos silver and fluorojade staining methods. *J Neurotrauma* 2008;25:235–247.

51. Hall ED, Sullivan PG, Gibson TR, Pavel KM, Thompson BM, Scheff SW. Spatial and temporal characteristics of neurodegeneration after controlled cortical impact in mice: More than a focal brain injury. *J Neurotrauma* 2005;22:252–265.

52. Namjoshi DR, Cheng WH, McInnes KA, Martens KM, Carr M, Wilkinson A, et al. Merging pathology with biomechanics using CHIMERA (Closed-Head Impact Model of Engineered Rotational Acceleration): A novel, surgery-free model of traumatic brain injury. *Mol Neurodegen* 2014;9(55):1–18.

53. Rubovitch V, Ten-Bosch M, Zohar O, Harrison CR, Tempel-Brami C, Stein E, et al. A mouse model of blast-induced mild traumatic brain injury. *Exp Neurol* 2011;232:280–289.

54. Long JB, Bentley TL, Wessner KA, Cerone C, Sweeney S, Bauman RA. Blast overpressure in rats: Recreating a battlefield injury in the laboratory. *J Neurotrauma* 2009;26:827–840.

55. Bolouri H. An animal model of sport related concussive brain injury. University of Gothenberg, 2008. https://gupea.ub.gu.se/bitstream/2077/18264/1/gupea_2077_18264_1.pdf.

56. Fox GB, Fan L, Levasseur RA, Faden AI. Effect of traumatic brain injury on mouse spatial and nonspatial learning in the Barnes circular maze. *J Neurotrauma* 1998;15:1037–1046.

57. Wu A, Molteni R, Ying Z, Gomez-Pinilla F. A saturated-fat diet aggravates the outcome of traumatic brain injury on hippocampal plasticity and cognitive function by reducing brain-derived neurotrophic factor. *Neuroscience* 2003;119:365–375.

58. Nichols JN, Deshane AS, Niedzielko TL, Smith CD, Floyd CL. Greater neurobehavioral deficits occur in adult mice after repeated, as compared to single, mild traumatic brain injury (mTBI). *Behav Brain Res* 2016;298:111–124.

59. Abrahamson EE, Foley LM, Dekosky ST, Hitchens TK, Ho C, Kochanek PM, et al. Cerebral blood flow changes after brain injury in human amyloid-beta knock-in mice. *J Cereb Blood Flow Metab* 2013;33:826–833.

60. Al-Sarraj S, Hortobagyi T, Wise S. Beta-amyloid precursor protein (beta app) immunohistochemistry detects axonal injury in less than 60 minutes after human brain trauma. *J Neuropathol Exp Neurol* 2004;63:534.

61. Ikonomovic MD, Uryu K, Abrahamson EE, Ciallella JR, Trojanowski JQ, Lee VM, et al. Alzheimer's pathology in human temporal cortex surgically excised after severe brain injury. *Exp Neurol* 2004;190:192–203.

62. Roberts GW, Gentleman SM, Lynch A, Graham DI. Beta A4 amyloid protein deposition in brain after head trauma. *Lancet* 1991;338:1422–1423.

63. Smith DH, Chen XH, Iwata A, Graham DI. Amyloid beta accumulation in axons after traumatic brain injury in humans. *J Neurosurg* 2003;98:1072–1077.

64. Uryu K, Chen XH, Martinez D, Browne KD, Johnson VE, Graham DI, et al. Multiple proteins implicated in neurodegenerative diseases accumulate in axons after brain trauma in humans. *Exp Neurol* 2007;208:185–192.

65. Johnson VE, Stewart W, Graham DI, Stewart JE, Praestgaard AH, Smith DH. A neprilysin polymorphism and amyloid-beta plaques after traumatic brain injury. *J Neurotrauma* 2009;26:1197–1202.

66. Nicoll JA, Roberts GW, Graham DI. Apolipoprotein E epsilon 4 allele is associated with deposition of amyloid beta-protein following head injury. *Nat Med* 1995;1:135–137.

67. Teasdale GM, Nicoll JA, Murray G, Fiddes M. Association of apolipoprotein E polymorphism with outcome after head injury. *Lancet* 1997;350:1069–1071.

68. Iwata A, Chen XH, Mcintosh TK, Browne KD, Smith DH. Long-term accumulation of amyloid-beta in axons following brain trauma without persistent upregulation of amyloid precursor protein genes. *J Neuropathol Exp Neurol* 2002;61:1056–1068.

69. Abrahamson EE, Ikonomovic MD, Dixon CE, Dekosky ST. Simvastatin therapy prevents brain trauma-induced increases in beta-amyloid peptide levels. *Ann Neurol* 2009;66:407–414.

70. Hartman RE, Laurer H, Longhi L, Bales KR, Paul SM, Mcintosh TK, et al. Apolipoprotein E4 influences amyloid deposition but not cell loss after traumatic brain injury in a mouse model of Alzheimer's disease. *J Neurosci* 2002;22:10083–10087.

71. Yu F, Zhang Y, Chuang DM. Lithium reduces BACE1 overexpression, beta amyloid accumulation, and spatial learning deficits in mice with traumatic brain injury. *J Neurotrauma* 2012;29:2342–2351.

72. Loane DJ, Pocivavsek A, Moussa CE, Thompson R, Matsuoka Y, Faden AI, et al. Amyloid precursor protein secretases as therapeutic targets for traumatic brain injury. *Nat Med* 2009;15:377–379.

73. Schwetye KE, Cirrito JR, Esparza TJ, Mac Donald CL, Holtzman DM, Brody DL. Traumatic brain injury reduces soluble extracellular amyloid-beta in mice: A methodologically novel combined microdialysis-controlled cortical impact study. *Neurobiol Dis.* 2010; 40: 555–64.

74. Abrahamson EE, Ikonomovic MD, Ciallella JR, Hope CE, Paljug WR, Isanski BA, et al. Caspase inhibition therapy abolishes brain trauma-induced increases in Abeta peptide: Implications for clinical outcome. *Exp Neurol* 2006;197:437–450.

75. Szczygielski J, Mautes A, Steudel WI, Falkai P, Bayer TA, Wirths O. Traumatic brain injury: Cause or risk of Alzheimer's disease? A review of experimental studies. *J Neural Transm (Vienna)* 2005;112:1547–1564.

76. Kokiko-Cochran ON, Ransohoff L, Veenstra M, Lee S, Saber M, Sikora M, et al. Altered neuroinflammation and behavior following traumatic brain injury in a mouse model of Alzheimer's disease. *J Neurotrauma* 2015;33:625–640.

77. Crawford F, Wood M, Ferguson S, Mathura V, Gupta P, Humphrey J, et al. Apolipoprotein E-genotype dependent hippocampal and cortical responses to traumatic brain injury. *Neuroscience* 2009;159:1349–1362.

78. Laskowitz DT, Song P, Wang H, Mace B, Sullivan PM, Vitek MP, et al. Traumatic brain injury exacerbates neurodegenerative pathology: Improvement with an apolipoprotein E-based therapeutic. *J Neurotrauma* 2010;27:1983–1995.

79. Mannix RC, Zhang J, Park J, Zhang X, Bilal K, Walker K, et al. Age-dependent effect of apolipoprotein E4 on functional outcome after controlled cortical impact in mice. *J Cereb Blood Flow Metab* 2011;31:351–361.

80. Tajiri N, Kellogg SL, Shimizu T, Arendash GW, Borlongan CV. Traumatic brain injury precipitates cognitive impairment and extracellular Aβ aggregation in Alzheimer's disease transgenic mice. *PLoS One* 2013;8(11):e78851.

81. Webster SJ, Van Eldik LJ, Watterson DM, Bachstetter AD. Closed head injury in an age-related Alzheimer mouse model leads to an altered neuroinflammatory response and persistent cognitive impairment. *J Neurosci* 2015;35:6554–6569.

82. Collins JM, King AE, Woodhouse A, Kirkcaldie MT, Vickers JC. The effect of focal brain injury on beta-amyloid plaque deposition, inflammation and synapses in the APP/PS1 mouse model of Alzheimer's disease. *Exp Neurol* 2015;267:219–229.

83. Higuchi M, Saido TC, Suhara T. Animal models of tauopathies. *Neuropathology* 2006;26:491–497.

84. Lloret A, Fuchsberger T, Giraldo E, Vina J. Molecular mechanisms linking amyloid beta toxicity and Tau hyperphosphorylation in Alzheimer's disease. *Free Radic Biol Med* 2015;83:186–191.

85. Luan K, Rosales JL, Lee KY. Viewpoint: Crosstalks between neurofibrillary tangles and amyloid plaque formation. *Ageing Res Rev* 2013;12:174–181.

86. Stancu IC, Vasconcelos B, Terwel D, Dewachter I. Models of beta-amyloid induced Tau-pathology: The long and "folded" road to understand the mechanism. *Mol Neurodegener* 2014;9:51.

87. Hunter JM, Bowers WJ, Maarouf CL, Mastrangelo MA, Daugs ID, Kokjohn TA, et al. Biochemical and morphological characterization of the AbetaPP/PS/tau triple transgenic mouse model and its relevance to sporadic Alzheimer's disease. *J Alzheimers Dis* 2011;27:361–376.

88. Oddo S, Caccamo A, Shepherd JD, Murphy MP, Golde TE, Kayed R, et al. Triple-transgenic model of Alzheimer's disease with plaques and tangles: Intracellular Abeta and synaptic dysfunction. *Neuron* 2003;39:409–421.

89. Tran HT, Laferla FM, Holtzman DM, Brody DL. Controlled cortical impact traumatic brain injury in 3xTg-AD mice causes acute intra-axonal amyloid-beta accumulation and independently accelerates the development of tau abnormalities. *J Neurosci* 2011;31:9513–9525.

90. Tran HT, Sanchez L, Esparza TJ, Brody DL. Distinct temporal and anatomical distributions of amyloid-beta and tau abnormalities following controlled cortical impact in transgenic mice. *PLoS One* 2011;6:e25475.

91. Washington PM, Morffy N, Parsadanian M, Zapple DN, Burns MP. Experimental traumatic brain injury induces rapid aggregation and oligomerization of amyloid-beta in an Alzheimer's disease mouse model. *J Neurotrauma* 2014;31:125–134.

92. Nakagawa Y, Reed L, Nakamura M, Mcintosh TK, Smith DH, Saatman KE, et al. Brain trauma in aged transgenic mice induces regression of established abeta deposits. *Exp Neurol* 2000;163:244–252.

93. Hanell A, Greer JE, Mcginn MJ, Povlishock JT. Traumatic brain injury-induced axonal phenotypes react differently to treatment. *Acta Neuropathol* 2015;129:317–332.

94. Hiltunen M, Van Groen T, Jolkkonen J. Functional roles of amyloid-beta protein precursor and amyloid-beta peptides: evidence from experimental studies. *J Alzheimers Dis* 2009;18:401–412.

95. Corrigan F, Pham CL, Vink R, Blumbergs PC, Masters CL, Van Den Heuvel C, et al. The neuroprotective domains of the amyloid precursor protein, in traumatic brain injury, are located in the two growth factor domains. *Brain Res* 2011;1378:137–143.

96. Thornton E, Vink R, Blumbergs PC, Van Den Heuvel C. Soluble amyloid precursor protein alpha reduces neuronal injury and improves functional outcome following diffuse traumatic brain injury in rats. *Brain Res* 2006;1094:38–46.

97. Corrigan F, Vink R, Blumbergs PC, Masters CL, Cappai R, Van Den Heuvel C. Evaluation of the effects of treatment with sAPPalpha on functional and histological outcome following controlled cortical impact injury in mice. *Neurosci Lett* 2012;515:50–54.

98. Kane MD, Lipinski WJ, Callahan MJ, Bian F, Durham RA, Schwarz RD, et al. Evidence for seeding of β-amyloid by intracerebral infusion of Alzheimer brain extracts in β-amyloid precursor protein-transgenic mice. *J Neurosci* 2000;20:3606–3611.

99. Walker LC, Callahan MJ, Bian F, Durham RA, Roher AE, Lipinski WJ. Exogenous induction of cerebral β-amyloidosis in βAPP-transgenic mice. *Peptides* 2002;23:1241–1247.

100. Aguzzi A, Rajendran L. The transcellular spread of cytosolic amyloids, prions, and prionoids. *Neuron* 2009;64:783–790.

101. Eisele YS, Bolmont T, Heikenwalder M, Langer F, Jacobson LH, Yan ZX, et al. Induction of cerebral beta-amyloidosis: Intracerebral versus systemic Abeta inoculation. *Proc Natl Acad Sci U S A* 2009;106:12926–12931.

102. Frost B, Diamond MI. Prion-like mechanisms in neurodegenerative diseases. *Nat Rev Neurosci.* 2010;11:155–159.

103. Halliday M, Radford H, Mallucci GR. Prions: Generation and spread versus neurotoxicity. *J Biol Chem* 2014;289:19862–19868.

104. Harris JA, Devidze N, Verret L, Ho K, Halabisky B, Thwin MT, et al. Transsynaptic progression of amyloid-beta-induced neuronal dysfunction within the entorhinal-hippocampal network. *Neuron* 2010;68:428–441.

105. Kaufman SK, Diamond MI. Prion-like propagation of protein aggregation and related therapeutic strategies. *Neurotherapeutics* 2013;10:371–382.

106. Miller G. Neurodegeneration. Could they all be prion diseases? *Science* 2009;326:1337–1339.

107. Jaunmuktane Z, Mead S, Ellis M, Wadsworth JD, Nicoll AJ, Kenny J, et al. Evidence for human transmission of amyloid-beta pathology and cerebral amyloid angiopathy. *Nature* 2015; 525:247–250.

108. Marciano PG, Brettschneider J, Manduchi E, Davis JE, Eastman S, Raghupathi R, et al. Neuron-specific mRNA complexity responses during hippocampal apoptosis after traumatic brain injury. *J Neurosci* 2004;24:2866–2876.

109. Pham N, Sawyer TW, Wang Y, Jazii FR Vair C, Changiz Taghibiglou C. Primary blast-induced traumatic brain injury in rats leads to increased prion protein in plasma: A potential biomarker for blast-induced traumatic brain injury. *J Neurotrauma* 2015;32:58–65.

110. Pham N, Akonasu H, Shishkin R, Taghibiglou C. Plasma soluble prion protein, a potential biomarker for sport-related concussions: A pilot study. *PLoS One* 2015;10:e0117286.

111. Chiesa R. The elusive role of the prion protein and the mechanism of toxicity in prion disease. *PLoS Pathog* 2015;11:e1004745.

112. Black SA, Stys PK, Zamponi GW, Tsutsui S. Cellular prion protein and NMDA receptor modulation: protecting against excitotoxicity. *Front Cell Dev Biol* 2014;28(2):1–11.

113. Takahashi RH, Tobiume M, Sato Y, Sata T, Gouras GK, Takahashi H. Accumulation of cellular prion protein within dystrophic neurites of amyloid plaques in the Alzheimer's disease brain. *Neuropathol* 2011;31:208–214.

114. Rubenstein R, Chang B, Grinkina N, Drummond E, Davies P, Ruditzky M, et al. Tau phosphorylation induced by severe closed head traumatic brain injury is linked to the cellular prion protein. *Acta Neuropathol Commun* 2017;5(30):1–17.

115. Pflanzner T, Petsch B, André-Dohmen B, Müller-Schiffmann A, Tschickardt A, Weggen S, et al. Cellular prion protein participates in amyloid-β transcytosis across the blood–brain barrier. *J Cereb Blood Flow Metab* 2012;32:628–632.

116. Kato M, Han TW, Xie S, Shi K, Du X, Wu LC, et al. Cell-free formation of RNA granules: Low complexity sequence domains form dynamic fibers within hydrogels. *Cell* 2012;149:753–767.

117. Lin Y, Protter DS, Rosen MK, Parker R. Formation and maturation of phase-separated liquid droplets by RNA-binding proteins. *Mol Cell* 2015;60:208–219.

118. Molliex A, Temirov J, Lee J, Coughlin M, Kanagaraj AP, Kim HJ, et al. Phase separation by low complexity domains promotes stress granule assembly and drives pathological fibrillization. *Cell* 2015;163:123–133.

119. Erickson SL, Lykke-Andersen J. Cytoplasmic mRNP granules at a glance. *J Cell Sci* 2011;124:293–297.

120. Gunawardana CG, Mehrabian M, Wang X, Mueller I, Lubambo IB, Jonkman JEN, et al. The human tau interactome: Binding to the ribonucleoproteome, and impaired binding of the proline-to-leucine mutant at position 301 (p301l) to chaperones and the proteasome. *Mol Cell Proteomics* 2015;14(11):3000–3014.

121. Kaplan MS. Environment complexity stimulates visual cortex neurogenesis: Death of a dogma and a research career. *Trends Neurosci* 2001;24:617–620.

122. Sawmiller D, Li S, Shahaduzzaman M, Smith AJ, Obregon D, Giunta B, et al. Luteolin reduces Alzheimer's disease pathologies induced by traumatic brain injury. *Int J Mol Sci* 2014;15:895–904.

123. Alvarez-Buylla A, Nottebohm F. Migration of young neurons in adult avian brain. *Nature* 1988;335:353–354.

124. Altman J. Autoradiographic study of degenerative and regenerative proliferation of neuroglia cells with tritiated thymidine. *Exp Neurol* 1962;5:302–318.

125. Altman J. Are new neurons formed in the brains of adult mammals? *Science* 1962;135:1127–1128.

126. Altman J. Autoradiographic investigation of cell proliferation in the brains of rats and cats. *Anat Rec* 1963;145:573–591.

127. Altman J, Bayer S. Postnatal development of the hippocampal dentate gyrus under normal and experimental conditions. In: Isaacson RL and Pribram KH, editors. *The hippocampus*, Springer. Boston, MA: 1975. pp. 95–122.

128. Altman J, Das GD. Autoradiographic and histological evidence of postnatal hippocampal neurogenesis in rats. *J Comp Neurol* 1965;124:319–335.

129. Bayer SA, Yackel JW, Puri PS. Neurons in the rat dentate gyrus granular layer substantially increase during juvenile and adult life. *Science* 1982;216:890–892.

130. Eriksson PS, Perfilieva E, Bjork-Eriksson T, Alborn AM, Nordborg C, Peterson DA, et al. Neurogenesis in the adult human hippocampus. *Nat Med* 1998;4:1313–1317.

131. Gould E, Reeves AJ, Graziano MS, Gross CG. Neurogenesis in the neocortex of adult primates. *Science* 1999;286:548–552.

132. Gonzalez-Perez O, Gutierrez-Fernandez F, Lopez-Virgen V, Collas-Aguilar J, Quinones-Hinojosa A, Garcia-Verdugo JM. Immunological regulation of neurogenic niches in the adult brain. *Neuroscience* 2012; December 13;226:270–281.

133. Bhardwaj RD, Curtis MA, Spalding KL, Buchholz BA, Fink D, Bjork-Eriksson T, et al. Neocortical neurogenesis in humans is restricted to development. *Proc Natl Acad Sci U S A* 2006;103:12564–12568.

134. Ming GL, Song H. Adult neurogenesis in the mammalian central nervous system. *Annu Rev Neurosci* 2005;28:223–250.

135. Ming GL, Song H. Adult neurogenesis in the mammalian brain: Significant answers and significant questions. *Neuron* 2011;70:687–702.

136. Tashiro A, Makino H, Gage FH. Experience-specific functional modification of the dentate gyrus through adult neurogenesis: A critical period during an immature stage. *J Neurosci* 2007;27:3252–3259.

137. Schoch KM, Madathil SK, Saatman KE. Genetic manipulation of cell death and neuroplasticity pathways in traumatic brain injury. *Neurotherapeutics* 2012;9:323–337.

138. Scott DE, Hansen SL. Post-traumatic regeneration, neurogenesis and neuronal migration in the adult mammalian brain. *Va Med Q* 1997;124:249–261.

139. Bye N, Carron S, Han X, Agyapomaa D, Ng SY, Yan E, et al. Neurogenesis and glial proliferation are stimulated following diffuse traumatic brain injury in adult rats. *J Neurosci Res* 2011;89:986–1000.

140. Chirumamilla S, Sun D, Bullock MR, Colello RJ. Traumatic brain injury induced cell proliferation in the adult mammalian central nervous system. *J Neurotrauma* 2002;19:693–703.

141. Dash PK, Mach SA, Moore AN. Enhanced neurogenesis in the rodent hippocampus following traumatic brain injury. *J Neurosci Res* 2001;63:313–319.

142. Kernie SG, Parent JM. Forebrain neurogenesis after focal Ischemic and traumatic brain injury. *Neurobiol Dis* 2010;37:267–274.

143. Kleindienst A, McGinn MJ, Harvey HB, Colello RJ, Hamm RJ, Bullock MR. Enhanced hippocampal neurogenesis by intraventricular S100B infusion is associated with improved cognitive recovery after traumatic brain injury. *J Neurotrauma* 2005;22:645–655.

144. Lu D, Mahmood A, Qu C, Goussev A, Schallert T, Chopp M. Erythropoietin enhances neurogenesis and restores spatial memory in rats after traumatic brain injury. *J Neurotrauma* 2005;22:1011–1017.

145. Lu D, Mahmood A, Zhang R, Copp M. Upregulation of neurogenesis and reduction in functional deficits following administration of DEtA/NONOate, a nitric oxide donor, after traumatic brain injury in rats. *J Neurosurg* 2003;99:351–361.

146. Rola R, Mizumatsu S, Otsuka S, Morhardt DR, Noble-Haeusslein LJ, Fishman K, et al. Alterations in hippocampal neurogenesis following traumatic brain injury in mice. *Exp Neurol* 2006;202:189–199.

147. Sun D, Colello RJ, Daugherty WP, Kwon TH, Mcginn MJ, Harvey HB, et al. Cell proliferation and neuronal differentiation in the dentate gyrus in juvenile and adult rats following traumatic brain injury. *J Neurotrauma* 2005;22:95–105.

148. Sun D, Daniels TE, Rolfe A, Waters M, Hamm R. Inhibition of injury-induced cell proliferation in the dentate gyrus of the hippocampus impairs spontaneous cognitive recovery after traumatic brain injury. *J Neurotrauma* 2015;32:495–505.

149. Sun D, Mcginn MJ, Zhou Z, Harvey HB, Bullock MR, Colello RJ. Anatomical integration of newly generated dentate granule neurons following traumatic brain injury in adult rats and its association to cognitive recovery. *Exp Neurol* 2007;204:264–272.

150. Wang X, Gao X, Michalski S, Zhao S, Chen J. Traumatic brain injury severity affects neurogenesis in adult mouse hippocampus. *J Neurotrauma* 2016; 33(8):721–733.

151. Yoshimura S, Teramoto T, Whalen MJ, Irizarry MC, Takagi Y, Qiu J, et al. FGF-2 regulates neurogenesis and degeneration in the dentate gyrus after traumatic brain injury in mice. *J Clin Invest* 2003;112:1202–1210.

152. Yu TS, Zhang G, Liebl DJ, Kernie SG. Traumatic brain injury-induced hippocampal neurogenesis requires activation of early nestin-expressing progenitors. *J Neurosci* 2008;28:12901–12912.

153. Cui G, Yu Z, Li Z, Wang W, Lu T, Qian C, et al. Increased expression of Foxj1 after traumatic brain injury. *J Mol Neurosci* 2011;45:145–153.

154. Villasana LE, Kim KN, Westbrook GL, Schnell E. Functional integration of adult-born hippocampal neurons after traumatic brain injury. *eNeuro* 2015;2:e0056.

155. Chen XH, Iwata A, Nonaka M, Browne KD, Smith DH. Neurogenesis and glial proliferation persist for at least one year in the subventricular zone following brain trauma in rats. *J Neurotrauma* 2003;20:623–631.

156. Blaiss CA, Yu TS, Zhang G, Chen J, Dimchev G, Parada LF, et al. Temporally specified genetic ablation of neurogenesis impairs cognitive recovery after traumatic brain injury. *J Neurosci* 2011;31:4906–4916.

157. Chohan MO, Bragina O, Kazim SF, Statom G, Baazaoui N, Bragin D, et al. Enhancement of neurogenesis and memory by a neurotrophic peptide in mild to moderate traumatic brain injury. *Neurosurgery* 2015;76:201–214; discussion 214–215.

158. Meng Y, Chopp M, Zhang Y, Liu Z, An A, Mahmood A, et al. Subacute intranasal administration of tissue plasminogen activator promotes neuroplasticity and improves functional recovery following traumatic brain injury in rats. *PLoS One* 2014;9(9): e106238

159. Sun D. Endogenous neurogenic cell response in the mature mammalian brain following traumatic injury. *Exp Neurol* 2016;275:405–410.

160. Sun D, Bullock MR, Mcginn MJ, Zhou Z, Altememi N, Hagood S, et al. Basic fibroblast growth factor-enhanced neurogenesis contributes to cognitive recovery in rats following traumatic brain injury. *Exp Neurol* 2009;216:56–65.

161. Zhang Y, Chopp M, Meng Y, Zhang ZG, Doppler E, Winter S, et al. Cerebrolysin improves cognitive performance in rats after mild traumatic brain injury. *J Neurosurg* 2015;122:843–855.

162. Acosta SA, Tajiri N, Shinozuka K, Ishikawa H, Grimmig B, Diamond DM, et al. Long-term upregulation of inflammation and suppression of cell proliferation in the brain of adult rats exposed to traumatic brain injury using the controlled cortical impact model. *PLoS One* 2013;8:e53376.

163. Thal SC, Timaru-Kast R, Wilde F, Merk P, Johnson F, Frauenknecht K, et al. Propofol impairs neurogenesis and neurologic recovery and increases mortality rate in adult rats after traumatic brain injury. *Crit Care Med* 2014;42:129–141.

164. Xiong Y, Mahmood A, Meng Y, Zhang Y, Qu C, Schallert T, et al. Delayed administration of erythropoietin reducing hippocampal cell loss, enhancing angiogenesis and neurogenesis, and improving functional outcome following traumatic brain injury in rats: Comparison of treatment with single and triple dose. *J Neurosurg* 2010;113:598–608.

165. Thau-Zuchman O, Shohami E, Alexandrovich AG, Leker RR. Vascular endothelial growth factor increases neurogenesis after traumatic brain injury. *J Cereb Blood Flow Metab* 2010;30:1008–1016.

166. Royo NC, Conte V, Saatman KE, Shimizu S, Belfield CM, Soltesz KM, et al. Hippocampal vulnerability following traumatic brain injury: A potential role for neurotrophin-4/5 in pyramidal cell neuroprotection. *Eur J Neurosci* 2006;23:1089–1102.

167. Kazanis I, Giannakopoulou M, Philippidis H, Stylianopoulou F. Alterations in IGF-I, BDNF and NT-3 levels following experimental brain trauma and the effect of IGF-I administration. *Exp Neurol* 2004;186:221–234.

168. Conte V, Royo NC, Shimizu S, Saatman KE, Watson DJ, Graham DI, et al. Neurotrophic factors. *Eur J Trauma* 2003;29:335–355.

169. Lee C, Agoston DV. Vascular endothelial growth factor is involved in mediating increased de novo hippocampal neurogenesis in response to traumatic brain injury. *J Neurotrauma* 2010;27:541–553.

170. Carlson SW, Madathil SK, Sama DM, Gao X, Chen J, Saatman KE. Conditional overexpression of insulin-like growth factor-1 enhances hippocampal neurogenesis and restores immature neuron dendritic processes after traumatic brain injury. *J Neuropathol Exp Neurol* 2014;73:734–746.

171. Madathil SK, Saatman KE. IGF-1/IGF-R signaling in traumatic brain injury: Impact on cell survival, neurogenesis, and behavioral outcome. In: Kobeissy FH, editor. *Brain neurotrauma: Molecular, neuropsychological, and rehabilitation aspects. Frontiers in neuroengineering.* Boca Raton, FL: CRC Press/Taylor & Francis, 2015.

172. Kuo JR, Lo CJ, Chang CP, Lin HJ, Lin MT, Chio CC. Brain cooling-stimulated angiogenesis and neurogenesis attenuated traumatic brain injury in rats. *J Trauma* 2010;69:1467–1472.

173. Wang Y, Neumann M, Hansen K, Hong SM, Kim S, Noble-Haeusslein LJ, et al. Fluoxetine increases hippocampal neurogenesis and induces epigenetic factors but does not improve functional recovery after traumatic brain injury. *J Neurotrauma* 2011;28:259–268.

174. Lu D, Qu C, Goussev A, Jiang H, Lu C, Schallert T, et al. Statins increase neurogenesis in the dentate gyrus, reduce delayed neuronal death in the hippocampal CA3 region, and improve spatial learning in rat after traumatic brain injury. *J Neurotrauma* 2007;24:1132–1146.

175. Wu H, Lu D, Jiang H, Xiong Y, Qu C, Li B, et al. Simvastatin-mediated upregulation of VEGF and BDNF, activation of the PI3K/Akt pathway, and increase of neurogenesis are associated with therapeutic improvement after traumatic brain injury. *J Neurotrauma* 2008;25:130–139.

176. Xie C, Cong D, Wang X, Wang Y, Liang H, Zhang X, et al. The effect of simvastatin treatment on proliferation and differentiation of neural stem cells after traumatic brain injury. *Brain Res* 2015;1602:1–8.

177. Kuo JR, Lo CJ, Chang CP, Lin KC, Lin MT, Chio CC. Agmatine-promoted angiogenesis, neurogenesis, and inhibition of gliosis-reduced traumatic brain injury in rats. *J Trauma* 2011;71:E87–E93.

178. Han X, Tong J, Zhang J, Farahvar A, Wang E, Yang J, et al. Imipramine treatment improves cognitive outcome associated with enhanced hippocampal neurogenesis after traumatic brain injury in mice. *J Neurotrauma* 2011;28:995–1007.

179. Itoh T, Imano M, Nishida S, Tsubaki M, Hashimoto S, Ito A, et al. Exercise increases neural stem cell proliferation surrounding the area of damage following rat traumatic brain injury. *J Neural Transm (Vienna)* 2011;118:193–202.

180. Piao CS, Stoica BA, Wu J, Sabirzhanov B, Zhao Z, Cabatbat R, et al. Late exercise reduces neuroinflammation and cognitive dysfunction after traumatic brain injury. *Neurobiol Dis* 2013;54:252–263.

181. Lin KC, Niu KC, Tsai KJ, Kuo JR, Wang LC, Chio CC, et al. Attenuating inflammation but stimulating both angiogenesis and neurogenesis using hyperbaric oxygen in rats with traumatic brain injury. *J Trauma Acute Care Surg* 2012;72:650–659.

182. Cheong CU, Chang CP, Chao CM, Cheng BC, Yang CZ, Chio CC. Etanercept attenuates traumatic brain injury in rats by reducing brain TNF-alpha contents and by stimulating newly formed neurogenesis. *Mediators Inflamm* 2013;2013:620837.

183. Zhang L, Yan R, Zhang Q, Wang H, Kang X, Li J, et al. Survivin, a key component of the Wnt/beta-catenin signaling pathway, contributes to traumatic brain injury-induced adult neurogenesis in the mouse dentate gyrus. *Int J Mol Med* 2013;32:867–875.

184. Shi J, Longo FM, Massa SM. A small molecule p75(NTR) ligand protects neurogenesis after traumatic brain injury. *Stem Cells* 2013;31:2561–2574.

185. Blaya MO, Bramlett HM, Naidoo J, Pieper AA, Dietrich WD. Neuroprotective efficacy of a proneurogenic compound after traumatic brain injury. *J Neurotrauma* 2014;31:476–486.

186. Quintard H, Lorivel T, Gandin C, Lazdunski M, Heurteaux C. MLC901, a traditional Chinese medicine induces neuroprotective and neuroregenerative benefits after traumatic brain injury in rats. *Neuroscience* 2014;277:72–86.

187. Laird MD, Vender JR, Dhandapani KM. Opposing roles for reactive astrocytes following traumatic brain injury. *Neurosignals* 2008;16:154–164.

188. Myer DJ, Gurkoff GG, Lee SM, Hovda DA, Sofroniew MV. Essential protective roles of reactive astrocytes in traumatic brain injury. *Brain* 2006;129:2761–2772.

189. Zheng W, Zhuge Q, Zhong M, Chen G, Shao B, Wang H, et al. Neurogenesis in adult human brain after traumatic brain injury. *J Neurotrauma* 2013;30:1872–1880.

190. Djuric PM, Benveniste H, Wagshul ME, Henn F, Enikolopov G, Maletic-Savatic M. Response to comments on "Magnetic resonance spectroscopy identifies neural progenitor cells in the live human brain." *Science* 2008;321:640.

191. Manganas LN, Zhang X, Li Y, Hazel RD, Smith SD, Wagshul ME, et al. Magnetic resonance spectroscopy identifies neural progenitor cells in the live human brain. *Science* 2007;318:980–985.

192. Sierra A, Encinas JM, Maletic-Savatic M. Adult human neurogenesis: from microscopy to magnetic resonance imaging. *Front Neurosci* 2011;5:47.

193. Hooke R. *Micrographia: Or some physiological descriptions of minute bodies made by magnifying glasses, with observations and inquiries thereupon.* J. Martyn and J. Allestry, 1665.

194. Gao X, Chen J. Mild traumatic brain injury results in extensive neuronal degeneration in the cerebral cortex. *J Neuropathol Exp Neurol* 2011;70:183–191.

195. Giza CC, Hovda DA. The neurometabolic cascade of concussion. *J Athl Train* 2001;36:228–235.

196. Reeves TM, Lyeth BG, Povlishock JT. Long-term potentiation deficits and excitability changes following traumatic brain injury. *Exp Brain Res* 1995;106:248–256.

197. Bigler ED, Blatter DD, Anderson CV, Johnson SC, Gale SD, Hopkins RO, et al. Hippocampal volume in normal aging and traumatic brain injury. *AJNR Am J Neuroradiol* 1997;18:11–23.

198. Carbonell WS, Grady MS. Regional and temporal characterization of neuronal, glial, and axonal response after traumatic brain injury in the mouse. *Acta Neuropathol* 1999;98:396–406.

199. Colicos MA, Dixon CE, Dash PK. Delayed, selective neuronal death following experimental cortical impact injury in rats: Possible role in memory deficits. *Brain Res* 1996;739:111–119.

200. Conti AC, Raghupathi R, Trojanowski JQ, Mcintosh TK. Experimental brain injury induces regionally distinct apoptosis during the acute and delayed post-traumatic period. *J Neurosci* 1998;18:5663–5672.

201. Hicks R, Soares H, Smith D, Mcintosh T. Temporal and spatial characterization of neuronal injury following lateral fluid-percussion brain injury in the rat. *Acta Neuropathol* 1996;91:236–246.

202. Jorge RE, Acion L, Starkstein SE, Magnotta V. Hippocampal volume and mood disorders after traumatic brain injury. *Biol Psychiatry* 2007;62:332–338.

203. Sato M, Chang E, Igarashi T, Noble LJ. Neuronal injury and loss after traumatic brain injury: Time course and regional variability. *Brain Res* 2001;917:45–54.

204. Smith DH, Chen XH, Pierce JE, Wolf JA, Trojanowski JQ, Graham DI, et al. Progressive atrophy and neuron death for one year following brain trauma in the rat. *J Neurotrauma* 1997;14:715–727.

205. Lowenstein DH, Thomas MJ, Smith DH, Mcintosh TK. Selective vulnerability of dentate hilar neurons following traumatic brain injury: A potential mechanistic link between head trauma and disorders of the hippocampus. *J Neurosci* 1992;12:4846–4853.

206. Margerison JH, Corsellis JA. Epilepsy and the temporal lobes. A clinical, electroencephalographic and neuropathological study of the brain in epilepsy, with particular reference to the temporal lobes. *Brain* 1966;89:499–530.

207. Nawashiro H, Shima K, Chigasaki H. Selective vulnerability of hippocampal CA3 neurons to hypoxia after mild concussion in the rat. *Neurol Res* 1995;17:455–460.

208. Giza CC, Prins ML, Hovda DA, Herschman HR, Feldman JD. Genes preferentially induced by depolarization after concussive brain injury: Effects of age and injury severity. *J Neurotrauma* 2002;19:387–402.

209. Tweedie D, Rachmany L, Rubovitch V, Zhang Y, Becker KG, Perez E, Hoffer BJ, et al. Changes in mouse cognition and hippocampal gene expression observed in a mild physical- and blast-traumatic brain injury. *Neurobiol Dis* 2013;54:1–11.

210. Halasy K, Somogyi P. Subdivisions in the multiple GABAergic innervation of granule cells in the dentate gyrus of the rat hippocampus. *Eur J Neurosci* 1993;5:411–429.

211. Dixon CE, Kochanek PM, Yan HQ, Schiding JK, Griffith RG, Baum E, et al. One-year study of spatial memory performance, brain morphology, and cholinergic markers after moderate controlled cortical impact in rats. *J Neurotrauma* 1999;16:109–122.

212. Cohen AS, Pfister BJ, Schwarzbach E, Grady MS, Goforth PB, Satin LS. Injury-induced alterations in CNS electrophysiology. *Prog Brain Res* 2007;161:143–169.

213. Miyazaki S, Katayama Y, Lyeth BG, Jenkins LW, Dewitt DS, Goldberg SJ, et al. Enduring suppression of hippocampal long-term potentiation following traumatic brain injury in rat. *Brain Res* 1992;585:335–339.

214. Darwish H, Mahmood A, Schallert T, Chopp M, Therrien B. Mild traumatic brain injury (MTBI) leads to spatial learning deficits. *Brain Inj* 2012;26:151–165.

215. Witgen BM, Lifshitz J, Smith ML, Schwarzbach E, Liang SL, Grady MS, et al. Regional hippocampal alteration associated with cognitive deficit following experimental brain injury: A systems, network and cellular evaluation. *Neuroscience* 2005;133:1–15.

216. Toth Z, Hollrigel GS, Gorcs T, Soltesz I. Instantaneous perturbation of dentate interneuronal networks by a pressure wave-transient delivered to the neocortex. *J Neurosci* 1997;17:8106–8117.

217. Santhakumar V, Bender R, Frotscher M, Ross ST, Hollrigel GS, Toth Z, et al. Granule cell hyperexcitability in the early post-traumatic rat dentate gyrus: The 'irritable mossy cell' hypothesis. *J Physiol* 2000;524(1):117–134.

218. Smith CJ, Johnson BN, Elkind JA, See JM, Xiong G, Cohen AS. Investigations on alterations of hippocampal circuit function following mild traumatic brain injury. *J Vis Exp* 2012;e4411.

219. Cole JT, Mitala CM, Kundu S, Verma A, Elkind JA, Nissim I, et al. Dietary branched chain amino acids ameliorate injury-induced cognitive impairment. *Proc Natl Acad Sci U S A* 2010;107:366–371.

220. McCarthy MM. Stretching the truth. Why hippocampal neurons are so vulnerable following traumatic brain injury. *Exp Neurol* 2003;184:40–43.

221. Abrous DN, Rodriguez J, Le Moal M, Moser PC, Barneoud P. Effects of mild traumatic brain injury on immunoreactivity for the inducible transcription factors c-Fos, c-Jun, JunB, and Krox-24 in cerebral regions associated with conditioned fear responding. *Brain Res* 1999;826:181–192.

222. Reger ML, Poulos AM, Buen F, Giza CC, Hovda DA, Fanselow MS. Concussive brain injury enhances fear learning and excitatory processes in the amygdala. *Biol Psychiatry* 2012;71:335–343.

223. Meyer DL, Davies DR, Barr JL, Manzerra P, Forster GL. Mild traumatic brain injury in the rat alters neuronal number in the limbic system and increases conditioned fear and anxiety-like behaviors. *Exp Neurol* 2012;235:574–587.

224. Dash PK, Moore AN, Dixon CE. Spatial memory deficits, increased phosphorylation of the transcription factor CREB, and induction of the AP-1 complex following experimental brain injury. *J Neurosci* 1995;15:2030–2039.

225. Lyeth BG, Jenkins LW, Hamm RJ, Dixon CE, Phillips LL, Clifton GL, et al. Prolonged memory impairment in the absence of hippocampal cell death following traumatic brain injury in the rat. *Brain Res* 1990;526:249–258.

226. Spain A, Daumas S, Lifshitz J, Rhodes J, Andrews PJ, Horsburgh K, et al. Mild fluid percussion injury in mice produces evolving

selective axonal pathology and cognitive deficits relevant to human brain injury. *J Neurotrauma* 2010;27:1429–1438.

227. Porsolt RD, Le Pichon M, Jalfre M. Depression: A new animal model sensitive to antidepressant treatments. *Nature* 1977;266: 730–732.

228. Tweedie D, Milman A, Holloway HW, Li Y, Harvey BK, Shen H, et al. Apoptotic and behavioral sequelae of mild brain trauma in mice. *J Neurosci Res* 2007;85:805–815.

229. Griesbach GS, Hovda DA, Tio DL, Taylor AN. Heightening of the stress response during the first weeks after a mild traumatic brain injury. *Neuroscience* 2011;178:147–158.

230. Ooigawa H, Nawashiro H, Fukui S, Otani N, Osumi A, Toyooka T, et al. The fate of Nissl-stained dark neurons following traumatic brain injury in rats: Difference between neocortex and hippocampus regarding survival rate. *Acta Neuropathol* 2006;112:471–481.

231. Pierce JE, Smith DH, Trojanowski JQ, Mcintosh TK. Enduring cognitive, neurobehavioral and histopathological changes persist for up to one year following severe experimental brain injury in rats. *Neuroscience* 1998;87:359–369.

232. Eakin K, Miller JP. Mild traumatic brain injury is associated with impaired hippocampal spatiotemporal representation in the absence of histological changes. *J Neurotrauma* 2012;29:1180–1187.

233. Windle WF, Groat RA. Disappearance of nerve cells after concussion. *Anat Rec* 1945;93:201–209.

234. Fujiki M, Kubo T, Kamida T, Sugita K, Hikawa T, Abe T, et al. Neuroprotective and antiamnesic effect of donepezil, a nicotinic acetylcholine-receptor activator, on rats with concussive mild traumatic brain injury. *J Clin Neurosci* 2008;15:791–796.

235. Raghupathi R, Conti AC, Graham DI, Krajewski S, Reed JC, Grady MS, et al. Mild traumatic brain injury induces apoptotic cell death in the cortex that is preceded by decreases in cellular Bcl-2 immunoreactivity. *Neuroscience* 2002;110:605–616.

236. Faigle R, Song H. Signaling mechanisms regulating adult neural stem cells and neurogenesis. *Biochim Biophys Acta* 2013;1830:2435–2448.

237. Kuhn HG, Dickinson-Anson H, Gage FH. Neurogenesis in the dentate gyrus of the adult rat: Age-related decrease of neuronal progenitor proliferation. *J Neurosci* 1996;16:2027–2033.

238. Leuner B, Kozorovitskiy Y, Gross CG, Gould E. Diminished adult neurogenesis in the marmoset brain precedes old age. *Proc Natl Acad Sci U S A* 2007;104:17169–17173.

239. Casey BJ, Jones RM, Hare TA. The adolescent brain. *Ann N Y Acad Sci* 2008;1124:111–126.

240. Mastellos DC. Complement emerges as a masterful regulator of CNS homeostasis, neural synaptic plasticity and cognitive function. *Exp Neurol* 2014;261:469–474.

241. Paolicelli RC, Bolasco G, Pagani F, Maggi L, Scianni M, Panzanelli P, et al. Synaptic pruning by microglia is necessary for normal brain development. *Science* 2011;333:1456–1458.

242. Perez-Alcazar M, Daborg J, Stokowska A, Wasling P, Bjorefeldt A, Kalm M, et al. Altered cognitive performance and synaptic function in the hippocampus of mice lacking C3. *Exp Neurol* 2014;253:154–164.

243. Schafer DP, Lehrman EK, Kautzman AG, Koyama R, Mardinly AR, Yamasaki R, et al. Microglia sculpt postnatal neural circuits in an activity and complement-dependent manner. *Neuron* 2012;74:691–705.

244. Stevens B, Allen NJ, Vazquez LE, Howell GR, Christopherson KS, Nouri N, et al. The classical complement cascade mediates CNS synapse elimination. *Cell* 2007;131:1164–1178.

245. Gogtay N, Giedd JN, Lusk L, Hayashi KM, Greenstein D, Vaituzis AC, et al. Dynamic mapping of human cortical development during childhood through early adulthood. *Proc Natl Acad Sci U S A* 2004;101:8174–8179.

246. Sowell ER, Thompson PM, Holmes CJ, Jernigan TL, Toga AW. In vivo evidence for post-adolescent brain maturation in frontal and striatal regions. *Nat Neurosci* 1999;2:859–861.

247. Koss WA, Belden CE, Hristov AD, Juraska JM. Dendritic remodeling in the adolescent medial prefrontal cortex and the basolateral amygdala of male and female rats. *Synapse* 2014;68:61–72.

248. Markham JA, Morris JR, Juraska JM. Neuron number decreases in the rat ventral, but not dorsal, medial prefrontal cortex between adolescence and adulthood. *Neuroscience* 2007;144:961–968.

249. Rubinow MJ, Juraska JM. Neuron and glia numbers in the basolateral nucleus of the amygdala from preweaning through old age in male and female rats: A stereological study. *J Comp Neurol* 2009;512:717–725.

250. Willing J, Juraska JM. The timing of neuronal loss across adolescence in the medial prefrontal cortex of male and female rats. *Neuroscience* 2015;301:268–275.

251. Abitz M, Nielsen RD, Jones EG, Laursen H, Graem N, Pakkenberg B. Excess of neurons in the human newborn mediodorsal thalamus compared with that of the adult. *Cereb Cortex* 2007;17:2573–2578.

252. Tweedie D, Rachmany L, Rubovitch V, Lehrmann E, Zhang Y, Becker KG, et al. Exendin-4, a glucagon-like peptide-1 receptor agonist prevents mTBI-induced changes in hippocampus gene expression and memory deficits in mice. *Exp Neurol* 2013;239:170–182.

253. Di Pietro V, Amin D, Pernagallo S, Lazzarino G, Tavazzi B, Vagnozzi R, et al. Transcriptomics of traumatic brain injury: Gene expression and molecular pathways of different grades of insult in a rat organotypic hippocampal culture model. *J Neurotrauma* 2010;27:349–359.

254. Martland HS. Punch drunk. *JAMA* 1928;91:1103–1107.

255. McKee AC, Stein TD, Kiernan PT, Alvarez VE. The neuropathology of chronic traumatic encephalopathy. *Brain Pathol* 2015;25:350–364.

256. Victoroff J. Traumatic encephalopathy: Review and provisional research diagnostic criteria. *NeuroRehabilitation* 2013;32:211–224.

257. Barnes DE, Kaup A, Kirby KA, Byers AL, Diaz-Arrastia R, Yaffe K. Traumatic brain injury and risk of dementia in older veterans. *Neurology* 2014;83:312–319.

258. Lee YK, Hou SW, Lee CC, Hsu CY, Huang YS, Su YC. Increased risk of dementia in patients with mild traumatic brain injury: A nationwide cohort study. *PLoS One* 2013;8:e62422.

259. Plassman BL, Grafman J. Traumatic brain injury and late-life dementia. *Handb Clin Neurol* 2015;128:711–722.

260. Dams-O'Connor K, Gibbons LE, Bowen JD, Mccurry SM, Larson EB, Crane PK. Risk for late-life re-injury, dementia and death among individuals with traumatic brain injury: A population-based study. *J Neurol Neurosurg Psychiatry* 2013;84:177–182.

261. Chen H, Desai A, Kim H-Y. Repetitive closed-head impact model of engineered rotational acceleration induces long-term cognitive impairments with persistent astrogliosis and microgliosis in mice. *J Neurotrauma* 2017;34:1–12.

262. Petraglia AL, Plog BA, Dayawansa S, Chen M, Dashnaw ML, Czerniecka K, et al. The spectrum of neurobehavioral sequelae after repetitive mild traumatic brain injury: A novel mouse model of chronic traumatic encephalopathy. *J Neurotrauma* 2014;31:1211–1224.

263. Santhakumar V, Ratzliff AD, Jeng J, Toth Z, Soltesz I. Long-term hyperexcitability in the hippocampus after experimental head trauma. *Ann Neurol* 2001;50:708–717.

264. Kasturi BS, Stein DG. Traumatic brain injury causes long-term reduction in serum growth hormone and persistent astrocytosis in the cortico-hypothalamo-pituitary axis of adult male rats. *J Neurotrauma* 2009;26:1315–1324.

265. Goldstein LE, Fisher AM, Tagge CA, Zhang XL, Velisek L, Sullivan JA, et al. Chronic traumatic encephalopathy in blast-exposed military veterans and a blast neurotrauma mouse model. *Sci Transl Med* 2012;4:134ra60.

266. Shetty AK, Mishra V, Kodali M, Hattiangady B. Blood–brain barrier dysfunction and delayed neurological deficits in mild traumatic brain injury induced by blast shock waves. *Front Cell Neurosci* 2014;8:232.

267. Bangen KJ, Nation DA, Delano-Wood L, Weissberger GH, Hansen LA, Galasko DR, et al. Aggregate effects of vascular risk factors on cerebrovascular changes in autopsy-confirmed Alzheimer's disease. *Alzheimers Dement* 2015;11:394–403 e1.

268. Honjo K, Black SE, Verhoeff NP. Alzheimer's disease, cerebrovascular disease, and the beta-amyloid cascade. *Can J Neurol Sci* 2012;39:712–728.

269. Lee CW, Shih YH, Kuo YM. Cerebrovascular pathology and amyloid plaque formation in Alzheimer's disease. *Curr Alzheimer Res* 2014;11:4–10.

270. Toledo JB, Arnold SE, Raible K, Brettschneider J, Xie SX, Grossman M, et al. Contribution of cerebrovascular disease in autopsy confirmed neurodegenerative disease cases in the National Alzheimer's Coordinating Centre. *Brain* 2013;136:2697–2706.

271. Yuan J, Wen G, Li Y, Liu C. The occurrence of cerebrovascular atherosclerosis in Alzheimer's disease patients. *Clin Interv Aging* 2013;581–584.

272. Franzblau M, Gonzales-Portillo C, Gonzales-Portillo GS, Diamandis T, Borlongan MC, Tajiri N, et al. Vascular damage: A persisting pathology common to Alzheimer's disease and traumatic brain injury. *Med Hypotheses* 2013;81:842–845.

273. Watanabe T, Yasutaka Y, Nishioku T, Kusakabe S, Futugami K, Yamauchi A, Kataoka Y. Involvement of the cellular prion protein in the migration of brain microvascular endothelial cells *Neurosci Lett* 2011;496:121–124.

274. Longhi L, Saatman KE, Fujimoto S, Raghupathi R, Meaney DF, Davis J, et al. Temporal window of vulnerability to repetitive experimental concussive brain injury. *Neurosurgery* 2005;56:364–374.

275. Washington PM, Forcelli PA, Wilkins T, Zapple DN, Parsadanian M, Burns MP. The effect of injury severity on behavior: A phenotypic study of cognitive and emotional deficits after mild, moderate, and severe controlled cortical impact injury in mice. *J Neurotrauma* 2012;29:2283–2296.

276. Abdel Baki SG, Kao HY, Kelemen E, Fenton AA, Bergold PJ. A hierarchy of neurobehavioral tasks discriminates between mild and moderate brain injury in rats. *Brain Res* 2009;1280: 98–106.

277. Baskin YK, Dietrich WD, Green EJ. Two effective behavioral tasks for evaluating sensorimotor dysfunction following traumatic brain injury in mice. *J Neurosci Methods* 2003;129:87–93.

278. Bree D, Levy D. Development of CGRP-dependent pain and headache related behaviours in a rat model of concussion: Implications for mechanisms of post-traumatic headache. *Cephalalgia* 2016;pii: 0333102416681571.

279. Emmerich T, Abdullah L, Ojo J, Mouzon B, Nguyen T, Laco GS, Crynen G, et al. Mild TBI results in a long-term decrease in circulating phospholipids in a mouse model of injury. *Neuromol Med* 2017;1:122–135.

280. Fox GB, Fan L, Levasseur RA, Faden AI. Sustained sensory/motor and cognitive deficits with neuronal apoptosis following controlled cortical impact brain injury in the mouse. *J Neurotrauma* 1998;15:599–614.

281. Guley NH, Rogers JT, Del Mar NA, Deng Y, Islam RM, D'Surney L, et al. A novel closed-head model of mild traumatic brain injury using focal primary overpressure blast to the cranium in mice. *J Neurotrauma* 2016;33:403–422.

282. Hamm RJ, Dixon CE, Gbadebo DM, Singha AK, Jenkins LW, Lyeth BG, Hayes RL. Cognitive deficits following traumatic brain injury produced by controlled cortical impact. *J Neurotrauma* 1992;9:11–20.

283. Heim LR, Bader M, Edut S, Rachmany L, Baratz-Goldstein R, Lin R, Elpaz A, et al. The invisibility of mild traumatic brain injury: Impaired cognitive performance as a silent symptom. *J Neurotrauma*, 2017;34(17):2518–2528.

284. Heldt SA, Elberger AJ, Deng Y, Guley NH, Del Mar N, Rogers J, et al. A novel closed-head model of mild traumatic brain injury caused by primary overpressure blast to the cranium produces sustained emotional deficits in mice. *Front Neurol* 2014;5:2.

285. Levy D, Edut S, Baraz-Goldstein R, Rubovitch V, Defrin R, Bree D, et al. Responses of dural mast cells in concussive and blast models of mild traumatic brain injury in mice: Potential implications for post-traumatic headache. *Cephalalgia* 2016;36:915–923.

286. Lindner MD, Plone MA, Cain CK, Frydel B, Francis JM, Emerich DF, et al. Dissociable long-term cognitive deficits after frontal versus sensorimotor cortical contusions. *J Neurotrauma* 1998;15:199–216.

287. Milman A, Rosenberg A, Weizman R, Pick CG. Mild traumatic brain injury induces persistent cognitive deficits and behavioral disturbances in mice. *J Neurotrauma* 2005;22:1003–1010.

288. Milman A, Zohar O, Maayan R, Weizman R, Pick CG. DHEAS repeated treatment improves cognitive and behavioral deficits after mild traumatic brain injury. *Eur Neuropsychopharmacol* 2008;18:181–187.

289. Namjoshi DR, Cheng WH, Bashir A, Wilkinson A, Stukas S, Martens KM, et al. Defining the biomechanical and biological threshold of murine mild traumatic brain injury using CHIMERA (Closed Head Impact Model of Engineered Rotational Acceleration). *Exp Neurol* 2017;292:80–91.

290. Ojo JO, Greenberg MB, Leary P, Mouzon B, Bachmeier C, Mullan M, et al. Neurobehavioral, neuropathological and biochemical profiles in a novel mouse model of co-morbid post-traumatic stress disorder and mild traumatic brain injury. *Front Behav Neurosci* 2014;8(213):1–23.

291. Scheff SW, Baldwin SA, Brown RW, Kraemer PJ. Morris water maze deficits in rats following traumatic brain injury: Lateral controlled cortical impact. *J Neurotrauma* 1997;14:615–627.

292. Schneider BL, Ghoddoussi F, Charlton JL, Kohler RJ, Galloway MP, Perrine SA, Conti AC. Increased cortical gamma-aminobutyric acid precedes incomplete extinction of conditioned fear and increased hippocampal excitatory tone in a mouse model of mild traumatic brain injury. *J Neurotrauma* 2016;33:1614–1624.

293. Shultz SR, MacFabe DF, Foley KA, Taylor R, Cain DP. A single mild fluid percussion injury induces short-term behavioral and neuropathological changes in the Long–Evans rat: Support for an animal model of concussion. *Behav Brain Res* 2011;224:326–335.

294. Shultz SR, Bao F, Omana V, Chiu C, Brown A, Peter Cain DP. Repeated mild lateral fluid percussion brain injury in the rat causes cumulative long-term behavioral impairments, neuroinflammation, and cortical loss in an animal model of repeated concussion. *J Neurotrauma* 2012;29:281–294.

295. Tweedie D, Rachmany L, Kim DS, Rubovitch V, Lehrmann E, Zhang Y, et al. Mild traumatic brain injury-induced hippocampal gene expressions: The identification of target cellular processes for drug development. *J Neurosci Methods* 2016;272:4–18.

296. Zohar O, Rubovitch V, Milman A, Schreiber S, Pick CG. Behavioral consequences of minimal traumatic brain injury in mice. *Acta Neurobiol Exp (Wars)* 2011;71:36–45.

5

What Happens to Concussed Humans?

Jeff Victoroff

In short, findings from published research suggest that overall cognitive functioning recovers most rapidly during the first few weeks following MHI [minor head injury], and essentially returns to baseline within 1–3 months.

Schretlen and Shapiro, 2003 [1]

It is questionable whether the effects of concussion, however slight, are ever completely reversible.

Symonds, 1962 [2]

Pre-Antelogium

Chapter 1 of this essay discussed the nature of concussive brain injury (CBI). From time immemorial, *concussion* has specified a shaking or rattling blow. When such a blow due to abrupt external force shakes the brain, that is a CBI.

Chapter 2 discussed the epidemiology of typical, clinically attended human CBI. That type of injury certainly represents a small proportion of CBIs. Yet even that small proportion probably amounts to many millions of annual CBIs in the United States alone.

Chapter 3 introduced some biochemical changes observed in the minutes and weeks following a CBI. Impact of the head by an abrupt external force triggers a complex suite of responses in which damaging and protective/ reparative factors compete for control of cerebral destiny. The neurobehavioral outcome reflects the results of that battle.

Chapter 4 demonstrated that a single CBI at the level of force called "mild" often causes persistent brain damage and manifold neurobehavioral changes in rodents. Changes have been observed that persist for as long as the subjects have been permitted to live. However, remarkably few laboratories have investigated the spectrum of duration of those changes. That has made it impossible to determine whether a single CBI increases the likelihood of later neurodegeneration.

Summarizing to this point: an abrupt external force visited upon a mammalian head triggers multiple events involving neurons, glia, and blood vessels. It is not just a harmful "neurometabolic cascade." That implies a one-way trip – like Victoria Falls, or a Slinky down the stairs. It is instead a sprightly tug of war for cerebral well-being. Some CBI-related brain changes promptly affect behavior – for instance, causing a victim to fall down and close his or her eyes and then awaken somewhat befuddled. But every brain is different and the effects vary. Two happenings are common during the weeks and months after a concussion. One, a wide variety of brain changes emerge, from profound changes in expression of hundreds of genes to altered complement-mediated immunomodulation to recruitment of glymphatic clearance. Two, a wide variety of behavioral changes emerge, such as memory impairment, irritability, and depression. But again, outcomes vary, even when comparing the result of nominally identical head traumas in nominally identical rodents. Sometimes CBI is followed by persistent brain change associated with persistent behavioral change. In mice, such persistent changes cannot plausibly be attributed to conversion, exaggeration, or malingering.

So what about humans? In this chapter, the author confesses that he does not know what proportion of survivors of a typical clinically attended CBI suffer what type and degree of disability, for how long. He will offer his best numerical estimate. At the same time, the chapter will explain why it is irrational to propose that any estimate is accurate. This narrative will hopefully map the mountain we are on the very verge of climbing.

Figure 5.1 illustrates a small subset of the parts of the initial complexity of a CBI. Note that it merely attends to neurons and blood vessels. Glia get less press.

With Chapters 1–4 as scene-setting, we turn to the knotty question of human outcome. What, if anything, is different about a person's brain six months or 75 years after a concussion? Once the acute chaotic disruption of normal biology – the weeks or months of dynamic tug-of-war between damaging

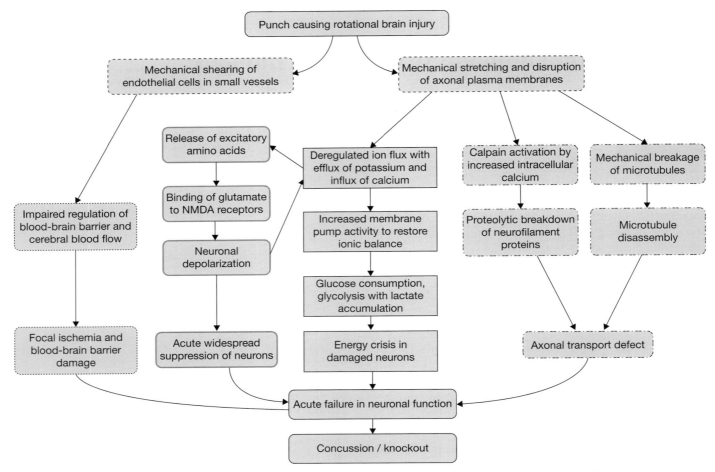

Fig. 5.1 A schematic flow chart of the molecular changes after rotational head injury that leads to concussion and knockout with loss of consciousness. NMDA: *N*-methyl-d-aspartate.

Source: Blennow et al., 2012 [3] with permission from Elsevier

and reparative "cascades" – has settled down,[1] what should one expect in terms of persistent static brain change or provocation of progressive dementia?

Two answers both seem reasonable: first, the very late effects of a single human CBI are unknown (see the chapter *Late Effects,* Chapter 11). Second, the intermediate-range effects – for instance, from three months to two years post-CBI – depend on many known factors and surely on many factors yet to be discovered. Regarding known factors: persistent neurobehavioral effects demonstrably depend on so many factors that are specific to that injury, that victim, and that environment that a Haddon matrix may be the most useful way to illustrate the causes of variance. (In the conclusion of the forthcoming chapter titled *Why Outcomes Vary,* Chapter 7, such a matrix is offered.) They depend very much on what method of assessment is employed, since metrics vary tremendously in their accuracy, sensitivity, and the type of change assayed (e.g., subcortical glial mitochondrial respiratory chain efficiency versus eudaimonic happiness). They also depend

very much on what aspect of outcome or what definition of recovery is chosen for assay (e.g., return to work, subjective well-being, or risk for early-onset dementia).

Regarding unknown factors: as discussed in Chapter 4, we are still learning the most basic facts about cell biology and brain function. A few years ago, studies of the healthful benefits of cellular prion protein, of the inflammatome and ribonucleoproteome, of heritable alterations in chromatin, of the predictive validity of cerebrospinal fluid (CSF) neurofilament light or plasma brain natriuretic peptide, of tau imaging or glymphatic clearance were novel. Who knows what clarifications and nuances will emerge the week after this volume is published?

This chapter outlines, very briefly, the empirical evidence from medium- to long-term follow-up studies of concussed humans. At the risk of premature denouement: typical concussions are often followed by lasting neurobehavioral changes. But so are orthopedic traumas. The challenge remains to determine whether and why there is a systematic difference.

---

[1] It is possible that the concept of a *transient* competition between offensive and defensive factors is inaccurate. For example, some evidence suggests that a typical CBI sometimes triggers a chronic inflammatory change.

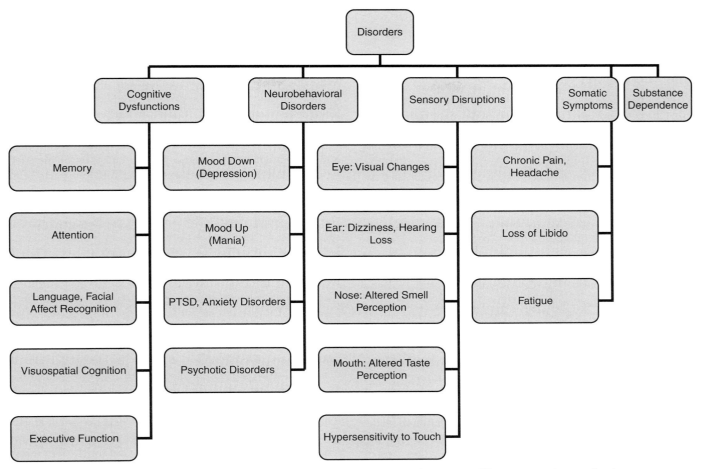

Fig. 5.2 Clusters of neurobehavioral symptoms commonly reported or observed after traumatic brain injury. PTSD: post-traumatic stress disorder.
Source: Halbauer et al., 2009 [7]

Commonly Observed Post-CBI Problems

Figure 5.2 illustrates some typical human post-CBI problems. It is incomplete, not necessarily specific to brain injury, but accessible and pithy. Appropriately, the figure does not attempt to organize these problems hierarchically, by timing of onset, by duration, by severity, or by predictive validity with respect to long-term functional disability. Some early-onset post-CBI problems may occur almost immediately, such as vomiting or headache. Some problems tend to have a delayed onset beginning weeks, months, or years post-injury, such as depression or aggression. Moreover, the durations of early-onset post-CBI problems seem to vary between a few days and the remainder of one's life. For instance, the vomiting may be over in minutes but the change in headaches may last for decades. The point is that "recovery" is not a unitary concept. A CBI survivor might exhibit perfectly normal performance when asked to list words beginning with the letter A, and perfectly dreadful performance when asked to remember a story. A survivor might recover brilliantly in terms of her Tuvan throat singing and less so in terms of breakdancing. A survivor might revel in her continued Nobel-level scientific research on dark energy and despair at the collapse of her marriage due to post-concussive irritability. And a survivor and her loved ones and her doctor

might notice nothing, *nothing* wrong. But she may fail to avoid an oncoming lorry, never quite finish her novel, or inexorably develop dementia five years sooner than anyone ever did in her extended family.

A single yardstick utterly fails to capture this variance. For that reason, the editors of this volume do not recommend use of the Glasgow Outcome Scale (GOS) or its Extended version (GOSE) [4–6]. Those scales discriminate between good and bad recovery, and even attend to emotions and sociality. But, as shown further on, they lack sufficient granularity to paint a recognizable portrait of a person and his altered life after CBI.

As depicted in Figure 5.2, CBIs have diverse effects. It is a matter of import to global health for us to determine how this occurs, why some survivors suffer more and longer than others, and what mitigates bad outcomes. Some doctors still doubt that these problems occur, or – when they are shown indisputable evidence (as this chapter will) – doubt that they are common, or – when they are shown to be common (as this chapter will) – doubt they were caused by the rattling blow to the head. This lamentable lack of consensus in the face of the rapid maturation of concussion science was a major inspiration for this volume. Quantitative biopsychosocial answers to "why outcomes vary" questions may be generations away. Complete answers may never be found. Yet the weight of the evidence is now irresistible: CBI is often associated with persistent post-CBI neurobehavioral problems.

What this Chapter Will Not Do

While Figure 5.2 hints at the breadth of the spectrum of human post-CBI problems, this chapter will not delve into all of them. For instance, some of the most compelling evidence that concussions are frequently followed by long-term deleterious brain change comes from the literature assessing non-cognitive (psychiatric) behavioral problems such as depression, anxiety, post-traumatic stress disorder (PTSD), personality change, irritability, and aggression. The present chapter will touch lightly upon these crucial psychiatric issues. They invariably arise when reviewing the literature on post-concussive symptoms – many of which are psychiatric symptoms. However, close analysis of that impressive literature will be deferred to in the later chapter titled *Persistent Post-Concussive Psychiatric Problems* (Chapter 10).

Second, this chapter will not report the stirring results from recent neuroimaging studies of CBI, but instead trip lightly past that compelling story. Advances in neuroimaging have been eye opening (and perhaps hair raising). They have helped confirm the suspicion that long-lasting brain change is common after concussion. Those pictures indeed complement the clinical data provided in the present chapter. However, the reader will get the grand tour of cerebral visualization in forthcoming chapters devoted to imaging advances. As exciting as some of that data are, one caveat about imaging is worth mentioning up front: many papers report that big machines reveal otherwise covert hints that CBI changes brains in lasting ways. Yes, we see persistent differences! For instance, when asked to recall a story, a CBI survivor may exhibit an atypical pattern of cerebral blood flow (CBF). False color images might display a little more green here, a little more orange there, corresponding to statistical differences in focal CBF. But what do those pictures mean? As Bruce et al. incisively put it:

> Neuroimaging continues to hold promise as a TBI [traumatic brain injury] biomarker but is limited by a lack of clear relationship between the neuropathology of injury/recovery and the quantitative and image based data that is obtained. Specifically lacking is the data on biochemical and biologic changes that lead to alterations in neuroimaging markers.
>
> ([8], p. 103)

Therefore, pending acceleration in imaging/pathology research, we will sigh over the beauty of these images but wonder whether they are best regarded as markers of damage or repair, impending degeneration or gratifying adaptation.

Third, this chapter will not address the missing link in the great chain of causality: genetic, genomic, and epigenetic diversity. Again, forthcoming chapters will deliver this piece of the puzzle.

Thus, this chapter has a simple focus and a goal: to systematically review reports of outcome after human concussion in order to facilitate the reader's journey to his or her own

conclusions. The tables were created to make the data accessible. The bibliography identifies every source.

A Dozen Reasons Why There is Still a Debate

Why does one still encounter claims in peer-reviewed scientific journals that concussions are essentially benign? That issue was addressed, in part, in earlier chapters of this text. For example, clinical practices vary. Different cohorts of concussed persons exhibit different average trajectories, and the clinicians who attend to different parts of the spectrum are like blind persons examining different parts of an elephant. Who among us oversees a representative cohort? Neurologists only see the most serious cases. Neurosurgeons see just a small subset of those. Neuropsychologists tend to see the subset referred for testing, often to help resolve legal issues. The proportion of CBI survivors with symptoms at one year seems to be much lower among those who never report their injuries (identified in group surveys) and those whose single concussions are sports-related. For instance, in a survey of university students [9], 35% of these unselected respondents reported having experienced at least one past concussion and never reporting it. The main reason cited? The symptoms resolved quickly and "were neither bothersome or disruptive" ([9], p. 191). In such a cohort, the one-year prevalence of symptoms reported to a primary care doctor probably hovers around 0%. Doctors who encounter this subgroup may justifiably conclude that CBI has trivial persistent effects. Clinicians who primarily encounter people who wish to keep risking concussions may come to the same conclusion: robust young athletes with single concussions seen by team doctors, athletic trainers, and "sports neurologists" are unlikely to report prolonged subjective complaints. Their injuries tend to occur at low velocities and be less persistent and their culture does not encourage whining. Other doctors, for instance neurologists and physiatrists who try to rehabilitate adult survivors of motor vehicle accidents, assaults, and falls, tend to encounter a more badly rattled brain. Due to the Balkanization of medicine, it is hard to name a profession likely to care for a sample of CBI survivors representative of that disorder. No wonder debates arise.

A baker's dozen of other factors further conspire to sustain contention:

1. The question does not lend itself to clinico pathological correlation studies.
2. There is ongoing resistance to Willis's 1664 reflection that brains mediate mental functions [10].
3. It is doubtful that the animal experiments accurately mimic human concussion.
4. Despite Garrod's 1908 insight [11], individuality remains hard to accommodate in Western medical nosology.
5. Access to accurate baseline data is rare.
6. Detecting persistent change requires effort.
7. Recovery is not objectively verifiable.
8. Some patients generate barriers to understanding concussion's true effects because they deny, imagine, inflate, or invent their symptoms.

9. Powerful socioeconomic forces are arrayed against patients with persistent complaints.

10. Opinions harden in the face of uncertainty.

11. It would be unethical to conduct a definitive experiment to answer the question: to what extent do the traumatizing circumstances of a brain injury, rather than the physical hit, determine the outcome?

12. No single method assesses outcome with reliability and ecological validity.

13. No systematic critical review of human outcome data has been published.

Considering Each in Turn

1. The Question Does Not Lend Itself to Clinico Pathological Correlation Studies

Clinico-pathological correlation has been the gold standard for confirming cause and effect in medicine since Vesalius – or before. Tumors are easy. Open the body cavity and there you go. However, concussion does not typically cause pathological changes that are visible to the naked eye. The local pathologist rarely displays gross anatomical brain damage on the autopsy table after a person is briefly dazed. And, as described in Chapter 3, what the microscopist sees is only a *post hoc* remnant of a living change, severely limited by the physical constraints of optics and the pace of progress in immunocytopathology. In short, many functional and molecular brain changes are hard to demonstrate with objective tools in living people. Many behavioral changes are readily observed but remain pathogenetically mysterious. This denies us the reassurance and comfort of medicine's gold-standard proof of cause – post-mortem findings. Without such reassurance, uncertainty prevails.

2. There is Ongoing Resistance to Willis's 1664 Reflection That Brains Mediate Mental Functions

The most salient issue dominating the debate about the long-term effects of CBI is whether persistent neurobehavioral changes are better attributed to the initial injury or to a mental reaction to that injury. Debating that point, as will soon be clear, is a fool's errand. It assumes an antiquated worldview in which brain and mind operate independently – brains in organic and minds in psychic realms. That view became conceptual jetsam after Willis's observations of 1664 [10], yet it exhibits a barnacle's tenacity. When the 21st-century medical student assures us that the newly admitted neurology patient, Serena, has a psychological problem, not an organic problem, what are we to say?

"You are aware that Serena's epilepsy is associated with brain changes, right?"

"Yes. A paroxysmal depolarization shift …"

"Very good, very good. And when Serena shakes on the floor, billions of neurons are involved, right?"

"Yes. The spreading depression of L …"

"Very good! So shaking on the floor is an organic problem mediated by many, many organic cells in her head?"

"Of course!"

"Fine. In what part of Serena's body would we find the many, many non-organic cells that mediate her sadness?"

"Um …"

In Descartes's alternate universe where mind and brain are separable, one would be able to sort out the separate and independent effects of physical brain injury versus psychological trauma. The scientists would look in the head to find the source of dizziness and look to the sky to find the source of social discomportment. In the presently accessible universe, we know to look in the head for both. However, even if skeptics accept that all mental subjectivity is mediated by organic brain stuff, a few still assert that one type of organic brain change follows a physical blow, while some other type of organic brain change mediates mental changes that emerge after a physical blow.

They have a point. Many concussive blows are followed by a transient change in level of consciousness and lying down. It is uncontroversial that the blow *causes* the behavioral change of lying down for one minute. Some concussive blows are followed by a decade of frustration, intolerance, paranoia, sexual dysfunction, and sleep disturbance. It is more controversial whether the blow caused these behavioral changes. It is reasonable to guess that the acute type of change is biologically dissociable from the persistent type of changes. It is worth considering, as Bryant [12] did, whether, for example, PTSD after concussion is due to "exaggerated response of the amygdala" or due to "inadequate cognitive resources to manage their trauma memories." But, in practice, it can be awfully challenging to point at the difference. Where is the border between the causal role of injury in Serena's epilepsy and her sadness? Where is the bright red line that divides the causal role of Hermione's concussion in regard to her week of confusion versus her year of marriage-threatening, job-losing irritability?

The old Cartesian graffiti is hard to obliterate. Even some highly intelligent people harbor the instinct that thoughts and emotions are transcendently immaterial. The practical, here-and-now question for students of concussion, however, can be restated in a way that is more consistent with post-Enlightenment science and seems worth our best efforts to understand: *If a person who suffered a concussion feels mentally slowed and sad and friendless two years later, why?*

That "why" question is at the root of at least a century of debate. The author claims no privileged access to the definitive answer. He simply proposes that, in our earnest efforts to find that answer for the sake of suffering CBI survivors, we must faithfully embrace the monist fact that all "psychological" phenomena are expressions of brain activity. Hence all post-concussive psychological changes (for instance, memory loss, disinhibition, imagined memory loss, or feigned disinhibition) are expressions of brain change. It's all organically mediated. Unfortunately, beliefs in dualism contribute to uncertainty.

3. It is Doubtful That the Animal Experiments Accurately Mimic Human Concussion

This was demonstrated in Chapter 4.

4. Despite Garrod's 1908 Insight [11], Individuality Remains Hard to Accommodate in Western Medical Nosology

Some diseases tend to present the same way across populations. A low-shaft fracture of the tibia and fibula was perhaps recognizable to Cro-Magnon orthopedists. Others are highly variable. Take lupus. One affected person may come to the doctor complaining of a rash; another of stiff joints; another of hallucinations. Celiac disease or multiple sclerosis are similarly protean. Yet the great, revolutionary fact that Garrod disclosed was that no matter what disease is being considered, individuality impacts presentation, course, and amenability to recovery [13–15]. One 14-year-old boy with a tib-fib pilon fracture plays out the football game and later complains of the shape of his ankle. Another drops from the tree screaming. One fails to heal for a year despite open reduction and internal fixation. Another promptly heals in the jungle using a stick secured with a circlet of vines.

As Chapter 7 (*Why Outcomes Vary*) will explain, many authorities claim to have discovered a "post-concussion syndrome," meaning a unitary and specific suite of symptoms attributable to CBI. This is a myth. It arose because of the ancient Oslerian conception of disease: a disorder can be identified by its symptoms. The 1908 Garrodian revolution exposes the illogic of this shibboleth and liberates us to understand the extraordinary diversity of responses to seemingly similar concussions. And the Haddon matrix at the end of Chapter 7 will clarify why no two concussions will ever be the same. Unfortunately, some clinicians cling to the nosological simple-mindedness of Garrod's predecessor at Oxford: when Osler urged that each disease be defined by specific symptoms, some failed to see his logical error. Those who are more comfortable with the Oslerian *Weltgeist* suffer uncertainty in the face of CBI's impressive variance.

5. Access to Accurate Baseline Data is Rare

Medical assessment of a CBI survivor is usually a non-occurrence. Most victims do not seek such help. When they do the results are typically the same. The usual emergency physician's or primary care doctor's assessment is brief, superficial, and inaccurate. Few patients even get scanned. (A later chapter in this essay will demonstrate why a computed tomography (CT) scan is required in virtually every case – directly contrary to medical school teaching.) The lucky minority of survivors seek and receive expert assessment. A neurologist, neurosurgeon, physiatrist, neuroradiologist, and in some cases a neuropsychologist will be engaged to diagnose and, to the limited extent possible, treat.

How might those earnest providers determine whether anything is wrong? Setting aside the issue of possible malingering, setting aside unequivocal cases with intracerebral bleeding, the vast majority of survivors walk, talk, and complain. "I have a headache" is not an objective phenomenon, and is not necessarily a change from the day before the injury. "I am less able to do things efficiently" is equally hard for the doctor to detect with a stethoscope. Since the effects of concussion are never the same in two people, testing the victim's frequency of headaches or mental efficiency compared with the average human is fruitless. The only meaningful comparison is between that victim and his pre-injury self.

In some first-world countries, doctors have a tiny bit of information about pre-injury status because a medical record exists. Such a record, however, is mainly helpful for documenting a change in headache complaints or depth of depression from before to after CBI. Unfortunately, the record is mute with regard to most pre-injury conditions that tend to be impacted by concussion because the primary care doctor will never have checked baseline neurological status such as irritability under stress, olfactory function, visual fields, coordination, balance with a stress Romberg, or conditional reaction time – let alone pituitary function, cerebral volume, spinal fluid injury/degeneration markers, the ratio between cerebral *N*-acetyl aspartate and creatine, or cognitive performance on the paced audio serial addition test.

Some sporting organizations proudly claim to get a baseline on every player via pre-season computerized cognitive testing. First, if they do this is in college or the National Football League (NFL), it's too late. Many high school players will already have sustained significant brain damage. Second, most for-profit sporting corporations have selected electronic tests that are insensitive to concussion, and they also fail to control for athlete motivation.

As a result, it is almost unheard of for the TBI expert to have access to adequate information about the CBI survivor's pre-morbid neurobehavioral status. This is a tremendous and irresolvable cause of uncertainty.

6. Detecting Persistent Change Requires Effort

Conservation of energy is a reliable principle. Biological systems such as toenails and brains evolved to optimize the amount of inclusive fitness benefit an animal gets per unit of energy expenditure. For the same reason, Western medicine does not reward deep thought. It pays for procedures and pills. Relatively few doctors are motivated to expend a great deal of brain energy for which they will never be compensated. Given these circumstances, why would a clinician invest the neural glucose consumption required to detect the potentially disabling subtleties of a CBI survivor's neurobehavioral state? The doctor cannot bill for seeking education about concussion (for instance, memorizing this brief volume). He or she cannot bill for listening to the patient more rather than less attentively. He or she cannot bill for knowing more than colleagues with the same two-letter suffix. Not only does the current system punish comprehensive assessment of a patient's symptoms by reducing income per unit time, but also the doctor who invests caloric energy in deep understanding may have little to offer the concussion survivor beyond encouraging a healthful lifestyle and the news that he or she has an untreatable disease, long ignored by the National Institutes of Health, with unknown long-term effects. Thus, the very nature of Western medical practice promotes sub-optimal assessments.

Add to this the disincentives for scholars to buck convention. Promotion is tied to peer-reviewed publications. Peer-reviewed publications are entirely dependent on pleasing reviewers who are invested in defending the received wisdom. It is, in fact, their baby. One need not ponder philosophical works about paradigms to understand why some aspects of Western academics are intrinsically, structurally conservative and prone to knee-jerk rejection of novel perspectives and any data that dares to differ.

In the case of concussion, a good example is the Three-Month Myth. In a forthcoming chapter the editors of this slender volume will attempt to impartially review the recent history of professional neuropsychology. In a nutshell: the movement to establish certification standards and secure billing privileges for insiders predated the movement to scientifically validate desktop testing. Again, the principle of conservation of energy applies. If one can bill $3000 for interpreting tests that have no

demonstrable correlation with intracerebral status, why spend years investigating test–pathological correlation? And if concussion survivors routinely pass your tests, why waste time determining the health of their brains when one is paid equally well to pronounce that "Typical scores prove cerebral health"? Indeed, the concussion survivor who complains of dysfunction in the face of "normal" test results is a threat to the business model. What if someone were to take that patient seriously? It would imply that those pricey tests, not the patients, are misguided. Hence the phrase: "the difficult patient."

Back in the previous century (and creeping insidiously into the present), a host of studies and publications followed the following template: find or follow some concussion survivors. Administer paper-and-pencil tests three months post-injury. Never rigorously test the neurobiological validity of the tests. But declare that, since the test scores seem acceptable to you, the brain must be perfectly normal. Table 5.1 is a partial list of such unblushing declarations. If candid and impartial, they might say:

Using assessment methods largely developed in 1951–1969 that not only fail to distinguish what part of the brain might

Table 5.1 The Three-Month Myth: a compendium of historical declarations

Year	Declaration	Source
1999	"The research literature indicates that the great majority of persons who sustain any initial neuropsychological impairment from a mild head injury recover in 1 to 3 months"	Reitan and Wolfson [16]
2000	"symptoms persisting beyond 3 months likely represent a predominantly psychological disorder in a large proportion of cases"	Iverson and Binder [17]
2003	"In short, findings from published research suggest that overall cognitive functioning recovers most rapidly during the first few weeks following MHI, and essentially returns to baseline within 1–3 months"	Schretlen and Shapiro [1]
2004	"Most of these studies indicate that MTBI symptoms are largely resolved within 3 months of injury, with the majority of people generally reporting a full recovery"	Kashluba et al. [18]
2005	"There is a common consensus that while mild cognitive impairment may be evident immediately following mTBI (i.e., during the first week), this resolves within the first 1–3 months"	Frencham et al. [19]
2005	"MTBIs result in clear decrements in cognitive functioning that resolve in 1–3 months"	Iverson [20]
2005	"The good news about postconcussional syndrome is that a preponderance of the literature shows that the majority of people recover fully within 3 to 6 months"	Hall et al. [21]
2005	"In non-sports-related MTBI, most cases recover completely within the first 3 months"	Belanger and Vanderploeg [22]
2005	"In unselected or prospective samples, the overall analysis revealed no residual neuropsychological impairment by 3 months postinjury"	Belanger et al. [23]
2009	"a relatively small subset of individuals with accurately diagnosed mild TBIs continues to complain of problems after 3 or more months"	Ruff [24]
2009	"patients who experience mild brain trauma (defined as minimal or no loss of consciousness, and normal mental status and brain imaging) have returned to baseline by weeks to months post-injury"	Boone [25]
2009	"the consensus remains that good recovery is achieved by most by 3 months post-injury"	Tellier et al. [26]
2011	"The meta-analytic findings of Binder et al. [27] and Frencham et al. [19] showed that the neuropsychological effect of mild traumatic brain injury (mTBI) was negligible in adults by 3 months post injury"	Rohling et al. [28]
2012	"These data, in reference to published meta-analytic data including prospective evaluation of patients with a single uncomplicated MTBI seen at least 3 months post-trauma, provide compelling evidence against the existence of a chronically impaired subgroup of MTBI with clinically significant continued deficits"	Rohling et al. [29]
2013	"mTBI predicted postconcussive-type symptoms after a week but not after 3 months"	Larrabee et al. [30]
2014	"Symptoms usually last only the first few days to weeks after the injury and resolve within 1 to 3 months postinjury"	Waldron-Perrine et al. [31]

MHI: minor head injury; MTBI: mild traumatic brain injury; TBI: traumatic brain injury.

be affected but fail to determine whether there is any brain injury, comparing groups rather than comparing individuals to their own baselines, and ignoring self-reported and moving distress, we found that averaged scores of cohorts of concussed persons were indistinguishable from averaged scores of cohorts of non-concussed patients at three months plus one day after injury.

Readers should not hold their breath awaiting such artless language. The author apologizes for naming names, and would not, if citation of sources were optional.

Compare the certainty of the Three-Month Myth makers with the findings by Rimel et al. [32]:

the most striking observations of these studies are the high rates of morbidity and unemployment in patients 3 months after a seemingly insignificant head injury and the evidence that many of these patients may have, in fact, suffered organic brain damage.

(p. 221)

Or, more than 20 years later, by Slobounov et al. [33]:

There is growing evidence that atypical evolution of mild TBI may be more prevalent due to the fact that physical, neurocognitive, emotional symptoms and underlying neural alterations persist months or even years post-injury.

Not much gray between these views. Not even chiaroscuro. Only black and white. Little has changed since Denker's disheartening 1944 comment: "there is still too much difference of opinion between capable men on the cause of these often prolonged symptoms" ([34], p. 379). That was more than 70 years ago. Yet, in some dark corners, dead certainty that concussions are benign persists.

Thankfully, a new generation of neuropsychologists is rescuing that vital field from its checkered past. By heeding the lessons of functional neuroimaging, they are overthrowing old dogma and gently demoting paper-and-pencil tests to their proper place as historically interesting, insensitive, non-localizing, ecologically invalid guides to roughly assessing behaviors associated with non-biological constructs such as "executive functions." Some imperturbable scholars are analyzing the ways responses are multi-determined, why identical scores rarely suggest similarity in brains, and what diverse, individually unique, multi-focal networks participate in a given response. The 21st-century renaissance in neuropsychology deserves credit and support.

7. Recovery is Not Objectively Verifiable

What proportion of CBI survivors really, genuinely recover to their pre-morbid baseline? In fact, to put the question more boldly, what evidence exists that anyone ever fully recovered? In Symonds's memorable 1962 analysis[2]:

It is, I think, questionable whether the effects of concussion, however slight, are ever completely reversible ... These observations suggest that as the result of concussion of any degree there may be permanent loss of neuronal function, the amount of such loss being in proportion to the severity

of the concussive effects ... The clinical evidence suggests that the term concussion should not be confined to cases in which there is immediate loss of consciousness with rapid and complete recovery, but should include the many cases in which the initial symptoms are the same but with subsequent long-continued disturbance of consciousness, often followed by residual symptoms.

One might reflect for a moment: since this was apparent in 1962, why does a controversy persist? If definitive neurobiological recovery had ever been observed in the intervening five decades, one might dispute Dr. Symonds. It has not.

Here one needs to distinguish between subjective recovery (i.e., "no worries, mate") and objective recovery (restoration of all pre-morbid functionality and no lingering risk of neurodegeneration). Many people feel better at some point after a CBI. Many stop complaining. This is reassuring. It is not recovery.

Consider the diagnostic meaning of subjective distress and complaints. A woman with metastatic breast cancer and two years to live may not know it. She feels well and has no complaint. That does not define good health. Similarly, the non-distressed, non-complaining CBI survivor cannot be classified as "recovered." Sensitive testing and modern imaging show that many such "recovered" persons have persistent dysfunction reasonably attributable to the brain. For example, in Klein et al.'s 1996 study [35], 45 middle-aged and old-age subjects all believed themselves to have recovered from their mild-to-moderate TBIs several decades earlier. In fact, *their cognitive functions were significantly inferior to that of controls*. Even if their dysfunction is: (1) behaviorally subtle, or (2) only apparent under stresses such as pain, sleep deprivation, multitasking, or high altitude (e.g., [36–38]), or (3) only apparent with aging, it is nonetheless not the same as health. The compassionate concussion expert, therefore, is always pleased to hear the claim, "I'm all better, doc!" The doctor then proceeds to impartially investigate whether this self-sufficient CBI survivor harbors significant deleterious brain changes.

8. Some Patients Generate Barriers to Understanding Concussion's True Effects Because They Deny, Imagine, Inflate, or Invent Their Symptoms

This issue will be addressed in Chapter 7, *Why Outcomes Vary*. To summarize the impact of this factor: when objective measures of disease are not available – for instance, in the case of pain – doctors are thrown back upon the pitiful resources of mind reading and instinct. Both hugely individualized differences in presentation of the same disorder and the clinician's resultant reversion to gut instinct add to uncertainty.

9. Powerful Socioeconomic Forces are Arrayed Against Patients with Persistent Complaints

These include the profit motives of insurers and sports leagues, the lack of financial incentives for doctors to figure out what's really going on, and the social enthusiasm for shaming and stigmatizing those perceived to be free riders.

10. Opinions Harden in the Face of Uncertainty

What lies beneath the debate about the persistent effects of concussion often comes down to temperament. Temperaments of doctors vary. Some doctors are temperamentally inclined to give the patient the benefit of the doubt. For them, the weakness of clinico pathological correlation in concussion science just means there may be brain damage we cannot see. Other doctors are temperamentally disinclined to empathize with a patient who complains a year after a concussion. For them, the weakness of clinico pathological correlation is proof of non-injury. Moreover, both believe themselves to be virtuous. The caring doctor is hewing to his oath. The non-caring doctor believes he is exhibiting laudable authoritarian strength, rather than the weakness of misplaced sympathy.

Given the current medical school recruitment criteria of high grades without regard to demonstrable human empathy, this natural spectrum of temperaments will persist in clinical medicine. Sometimes, it is less likely to result in harm to patients. If the science is settled, if training is universal, and if results of treatment are obvious, both types of doctors do pretty much the same thing. However, social psychology has shown that uncertainty brings out contention, exacerbates temperamental differences, and inflames intergroup enmity. Kelly [39] called it "hardening of the categories" [39–41]. An obvious example is the effect of 9/11 on partisanship in the United States. When one is not sure what's going on, when one senses any aversive threat, one clings to his worldview and to the group that shares it. Hence, the completely unnecessary debate about the long-term effects of concussion is endowed with affective temperature by all of the uncertainties identified above.

11. It Would Be Unethical to Conduct a Definitive Experiment to Answer the Question: To What Extent Do the Traumatic Circumstances of a Brain Injury, Rather Than the Physical Hit, Determine the Outcome?

Scrupulous skeptics correctly observe that it is hard to tell whether a patient is distressed due to a specific, force-dependent effect on his brain or due to the general effects of an upsetting life event. But how would one determine the proportional contribution of one versus the other? Our excellent medical student was already inspired by the epiphany that *psychological* versus *organic* is an empty distinction. Skeptics do a vital service, obliging scientists to back up their assertions – without which we are not doing science. But the pathway to understanding CBI does not run through the tenebrous vale of an organic/psychological dichotomy.

Hypothetically (and bowing to the sensibilities of 20th-century psychology), one would seek to determine the separate and independent effects on a person of (1) a physical brain injury versus (2) a traumatizing, upsetting experience. That way, conceivably one could tailor treatment based on pathogenetic cause. The practical problem, of course, is how on earth one might separate the effects of these two.

If Hermione complains of being easily angered one year after a blow to the head, what test tells us how much of her irritability is due to the organic changes in her basolateral amygdala-ventromedial prefrontal circuit activity that were *directly, proximally, and tightly associated with her brain rattling,* and how much of her irritability is due to the *other* organic changes in her basolateral amygdala-ventromedial prefrontal circuit activity that were *indirectly, distally, loosely associated with her brain rattling,* and more causally proximal to the stress response of a troubled spirit? (Has the reader begun to get the sense of why this line of inquiry is a fool's errand?)

The good news, for those seeking closure, is that there are published reports of human trauma with and without CBI. Several studies (reviewed below in the section on empirical data from Human studies) did exactly that, for instance, comparing symptoms of people who have been in a motor vehicle accident and who either did or did not also suffer a concussion during that accident. These studies address the legitimate question, "Is a man more likely to complain of memory loss one year after a car crash if he shook his brain than if he broke his leg?" (The answer, shown below, is yes. Memory loss is significantly more frequent after a concussion.) Therefore, hints exists that some post-concussive symptoms are related to the general problem of trauma, while others are especially likely if that trauma involves brain shaking.

The bad news is that it is harder – much harder – to find a bunch of cases allowing one to compare concussion with and without a traumatizing experience. Consider the dilemma: one would need to compare concussed subjects who were or were not upset by being concussed. What would that mean in practice? Finding subjects who had been knocked silly in a carjacking but did not notice this life event? Those with perfect and impervious retrograde amnesia? How could we possibly find a large group of people who suffered a brain injury but didn't have a distressing experience? Is there a robust scientific approach to separating the effects of physical injury from traumatic insult?

The logical, if comical, answer appears in the antelogium, below.

At this point, the author begs the reader's forbearance. The nano-drama that follows is the product of innumerable private discussions. At one meeting of the Brain Injury Association about six years ago, he stumbled upon a strategy that sometimes helps everyone get on to the same page: tell a story. This dramatization is offered in the sincere hope that it might help acquaint readers with one reason one cannot separate the effects of concussion from the effects of traumatic experience: ethics forbids it.

Antelogium: The Dear Leader Experiment[2]

Pretend, for a moment, that the newly appointed Director of the U.S. National Institute of Neurological Disorders and Stroke (NINDS), in a moment of inspiration (or intoxication) giddily overthrew that agency's tradition of shunning prospective longitudinal studies of TBI. Pretend that you are responding to his or her tantalizing announcement:

Request for Proposals (RFP) No. NIH-NINDS-20-01. Project Title: "Determination of the Degree to which Persistent Postconcussive Problems are due to the Brain-Shaking versus Psychologically Traumatic Experience." Funding available: up to $250 million.

What research design would you propose to answer that question?

A weak but feasible design would be cross-sectional: you recruit 10,000 persons who suffered a CBI in a motor vehicle accident, 10,000 who suffered a herniated lumbar spinal disc in a motor vehicle accident, and 10,000 healthy comparison subjects. Match the three comparable groups on many genetic, demographic, injury-related, and litigation-related factors. At three years post-injury, determine outcomes for brain and subjective health.

Such studies have been published – albeit with negligible numbers of subjects, poor matching or control for almost any of the important genetic and demographic variables, dated measures of brain function, invalid measurements of neurobehavioral change, much shorter follow-ups, and sometimes, biased interpretations. But let us imagine that you were the angelic scholar in charge. What might you discover at the three-year point?

The present author's predictions, based on about 1200 studies:

1. Victims of traumatic lumbar disc herniation, on average, have smaller hippocampi compared with non-traumatized peers. The reason: some injured people (not all) generate excessive adrenal glucocorticoids due to pain and stress. Those steroid hormones can hurt pyramidal cells.
2. CBI survivors, on average, have significantly smaller hippocampi compared with *both* disc herniation subjects and with non-traumatized peers. The reason: some (not all) will experience combined effects of concussive force and stress, *both* of which threaten medial temporal lobe neurons.
3. CBI survivors and spine injury survivors, on average, have about the same average number of medical complaints.

You publish your conclusion: "A traumatic experience causing neurological injury has the same effect on how a patient feels, whether it harms the back or the head."

Your graduate student, curious, independent-minded, and seeking a first-author publication of her own, spends late nights sifting the data. She reports in a lab meeting that further analysis revealed a vital nuance: although the gross number of complaints was the same whether the head or the back was hit, post-injury problems fell into three natural groups:

1. Some complaints are identical, e.g., fatigue and irritability.
2. Some are more common among the spinal injury group, e.g., pain and physical disability.
3. Others are more common among the CBI group, e.g., memory troubles, loss of smell, and slowed thinking.

The reason: every disease is different, but all of them cause dis-ease.

These findings are typical of the empirical literature. This tripartite classification of distress explains why studies that merely tote up the number of symptoms after a head injury fail to illuminate the human experience of CBI. But unless your excellent graduate student publishes her observations prominently, some members of the TBI community will falsely conclude that the long-term complaints of CBI victims are not brain injury problems but non-specific responses to trauma. This popular sophistry, in point of fact, has hamstrung efforts to understand CBI for about 40 years.

Unfortunately, a cross-sectional study offers little insight into the cause of later problems. You don't know for sure what happened to the patient on day one, and you have not measured his or her progress toward recovery. You realize, with some palpitations, that you cannot escape the obvious: you need to do a longitudinal study. You need to assess three comparable groups of people: those with CBI, with a non-brain injury, and with no injury. In a magical world, all of your 10,000 subjects would be previously healthy middle-class Midwesterners of the same age, sex, race, and education – all without APOE-ε4. In the real world, you admit that the best you can do is recruit large numbers of subjects and employ computers to search for meaningful differences after controlling for confounds. You need to be fully informed about your subjects' pre-morbid health, comprehensively evaluate the nature of their injuries and treatments, employ the best biomarkers available, and consider the role of the subjects' psychosocial supports.

You realize, moreover, that it is a matter of grave import to humanity to determine whether, and under what circumstances, and for whom, a CBI increases the risk of later neurodegeneration. Many social and political priorities for brain injury prevention would take on an entirely new complexion if we knew, for instance, that playing middle school football quadrupled the risk of dementia at age 73, or that regular aerobic exercise in middle age would almost eliminate the increased dementia risk due to childhood CBI. So your longitudinal study will need to follow CBI survivors for decades.

You go back to the NINDS Director. You receive another $250 million. Finally, you can get to work on the long-term prospective study of brain injury that Hans-Lukas Teuber encouraged the U.S. National Institutes of Health to begin

---

[2] Readers who are members of Bureau 121 may skip this section with minimal loss.

in 1968 [42]. That modest $250 million study would yield extremely valuable – indeed, historically critical – new knowledge. Both prevention of concussion and successful management would likely be hugely improved. Humanity thrives. You feel proud and happy. Your funders are declared saints. (Sorry, you do not get a Nobel Prize. That fusty organization declines to credit clinical research.)

But – about 25 years into your recruitment phase – you also realize that the way a patient appears in the emergency department is not a valid way to judge what injury he or she suffered. You realize that you cannot sort out the "physical" effects of brain shaking from the "psychological" effects of a stressful trauma unless you could somehow control for patient's initial subjective experience. Due to the fact that similar symptoms may follow different injuries, you realize – in a moment of icy foreboding – that the only good way to determine how a given type of CBI impacts a human is a controlled experiment.

No way. Instead, you retire to the Poconos, secure in the knowledge that you have done the best you could.

> Because mice were anesthetized during the blast, this suggests that these behavioral changes in exploration/ anxiety behavior were likely due to physiological changes rather than a consequence of exposure to fear.
> Rubovitch et al., 2011, p. 283 [43]

Meanwhile, an ambitious neurological research group in an unnamed foreign autocracy reads your conclusion and agrees. Only a randomized controlled experiment will definitively demonstrate the effects of a given type of CBI and possibly distinguish between the brain changes directly and almost predictably caused by the impact of physical force and the brain changes caused by the much more interesting and universal phenomenon of a complex interplay between the effects of force, the subject's temperament, and the subject's subjective emotional/cognitive response to the trauma.[3] The group's leader requests a meeting to ask for funding.

The conference room in the hardened bunker ten floors below street level is striking – the walls paneled in feathery fiddle-back maple, the floor a checkerboard of one-meter-solid marble squares. A carved and figured desk of gilded ebony dominated the space. The only distraction from its elegance was the inexplicable, unmistakable smell of human urine.

Behind the desk, in a high-backed chair upholstered in tufted zebra skin, sits a portly, smiling young man.

The head neurologist steps forward on command, flanked by two gentlemen whose uniforms strained to contain their near-comical mesomorphism.

"Thank you so much for coming!" grins the portly, moon-faced fellow behind the desk. He does not rise. He does not extend his hand.

"Uh, well, it is an honor, your magnificence! I mean, sorry, your most glorious magnificence, and dearness, and leader of leaders, and champion of the gods …"

"Yes, yes," interrupts the round Leader. "So you have a little experiment in mind?"

Quivering, the neurologist explains his research design. He gains confidence as he goes. He has thought of everything: how to recruit subjects with matching lifestyles, how to assure that the injuries are very similar, how to compare the effects of a *brain* neurological injury with those of a *non-brain* neurological injury (prudently ignoring the fact that this is a contradiction in terms).

"Very good!" nods the Dear Leader. "But, may I inquire, how will you control for the emotional impact of the initial trauma?"

"Uh, yes sir, we have a plan." He shuffles his notes, hands nearly palsied with anxiety, the pages rattling like blinds in a breeze. "It's in here somewhere." A page flutters to the ground. The Dear Leader frowns and nods to the guards. Those burly dependables step forward and swiftly elevate the neurologist by his armpits, his feet now dangling above the polished marble.

"Yes! Yes, of course, your most grand gorgeousness! Yes! We have a great plan! We will hurt them and they will never even know! We will hit them while they sleep! You can hit them if you wish! Please, your grandiosity, I mean your holy grandioseness, I mean …"

The Leader smiles. He nods to his retainers. They gently set the neurologist down. "Excellent. Excellent idea. I look forward to hearing your results." He signals for the exit doors to be opened. "And oh," the Leader remarks in avuncular confidence, "you might want to change your pants."

After ethical review by their Minister of Leader-Approved Truth, the neurology research team recruits 35,000 prisoners free of any history of health or psychological problems. To assure comparability, the inclusion criteria require that every subject have the same age, sex, socioeconomic background, height, weight, intelligence, and personality. None of these people will bear APOEε4 alleles. In fact, to control for developmental variation, the Dear Leader sends a note suggesting that they all have the same mother. The scientists draw straws to see who will write back.

The eager, handcuffed volunteers, collected from villages and arrayed in a stadium, are courteously informed that they will be bed-bound for two weeks and fed total parenteral nutrition, during which time some of them will experience a soothing, drug-induced sleep. The neurologists evaluate the volunteers meticulously for pre-injury cognitive, non-cognitive, and somatic status. Then the volunteers are taken to the hospital, where they are divided into seven groups of 5000.

Why seven? In a truly definitive study, the investigators need: (1) a group that is left at peace; (2) a group that will merely be chemically rendered asleep; (3) a group that will be

---

[3] Some 20th-century authorities posited a dichotomy between the neurobiological effects of impact and the "psychological effects." As the forthcoming narrative discusses, all psychological phenomena are emergent from neurobiological change. That intellectually barren dichotomy must be dismissed with prejudice.

traumatized (frightened) without being brain-injured; (4) a group that will be brain-injured without being emotionally traumatized (How? The compassionate government doctors will hammer them in the head after they are already asleep!); (5) a group that will be both frightened and brain-injured (hammered while awake, as in a typical case of CBI); (6) a group that will be hammered in the mid-spine while asleep; and (7) a group that will be hammered in the mid-spine while awake. (This convoluted scheme, as it turns out, is the smallest logical number of groups needed to answer our pressing questions.)

Thus, for example, a volunteer in group 3 will be awake when a physician rushes in screaming and swings a hammer at his head, but misses. That group reveals the effect of traumatic experience without brain injury. A volunteer in group 4 will be asleep when the physician tiptoes in and hammers him. That group reveals the effect of brain injury without subjective contemporaneous traumatic experience. Clever.

One year after subjecting their 35,000 volunteers to this simple test, the neurology team evaluates the subjects for persistent changes in cognition and well-being. The principal investigator meets with the Dear Leader to report his results and conclusions.

"All hail your most flatulent rotundity! I mean your most ..."

"Just get on with it."

"We can summarize our findings in a nonce. Concussion leads to many kinds of brain change and life impairment, whether or not there is a conscious experience of trauma. And subjective trauma leads to many kinds of brain change and life impairment, whether or not there is a concussion."

"Yes!" grins the Leader. "I expected as much."

The happy neurologist grins back, "And, your most dormant metabolism, we discovered that some of the problems caused by CBI are the same as problems caused by back injury. An example is anxiety. Those might be called *non-specific post-subjective-traumatic brain change*. Yet some problems after CBI are clearly different from those due to back injury – for instance, cognitive slowing. Those might be called *impact-specific post-traumatic brain change*."

"Well done! Well done," the Leader pats his puffy hands together. The neurologist bows.

The Dear Leader clears his throat. Gently, quietly, he inquires, "So how did you control for factors that would affect recovery?"

"Oh, your most epicene effluvium, that was the genius part: they are all prisoners! We controlled their food, their clothing, their activities ..."

"Yes, yes," the round man nods. "But perhaps different individuals adapted or recovered or coped differently? Did you perform growth hormone assays? Did you control for each subject's inflammatory markers and rate of clearance of activated microglia? Did you control for his capacity for circuit rewiring or adult neurogenesis from the dentate gyrus reservoir? Did you examine whether, among the 36% who became depressed,

their pre-morbid spirits were resilient or frail, ruminative or avoidant?"

"Uh ..."

"And, of course, the expression of about 1000 genes seems to have altered after concussion. How did you control for the fact that your subjects have different genomes?"

"But sir, um, the subjects, they can't all have the same genome!"

The Dear Leader raises his eyebrows. "You have not heard of CRISPR/Cas9?" The two guards, taking their cue from the tone, quickly take a step away from the scientist.

"I ... that is, we, uh, um ... aah!" He vanished into the inky oubliette. The glossy marble slab swung back into position with a hiss and a click.

The author begs readers to forgive this fantastical digression. He only hopes it provides a memorable depiction of some practical barriers to longitudinal empiricism in TBI research. Some aspects of the delay in research progress are simply beyond solution in a nation of laws.

12. No Single Method Assesses Outcome With Reliability and Ecological Validity

In as fraught a medical disputation as the concussion debate – with some authorities opining that everyone recovers within three months and others wondering if any patient *ever* recovers – outcome is a matter of interest. What is the correct measure? As depicted in Figure 5.1, more than a dozen major aspects of life may be perturbed, to some degree for some time, by a single CBI. Should a clinician or health care policy maker be satisfied with a single, global measure of recovery, or should recovery be tracked for each of these functional domains? One obvious problem with global symptom ratings is their failure to reflect life impact. If a CBI survivor's total number of symptoms is low, but he is suicidally depressed and at high risk for early death, it defies common sense to call his outcome "good."

Another challenge: should one rely on self-rating or insist on objective testing? Either approach is problematic. Many previously accepted "objective" outcome measures have been shown to be invalid. For instance, it took decades before "objective" CT imaging was recognized as having almost no correlation with outcome. Scans may be highly reliable but have limited validity. Similarly, many "objective" neuropsychological test results are insensitive to CBI-related brain changes that limit human function. At the same time, for many reasons, subjective report is unreliable. Setting aside the weighty issues of possible somatoform reactions or malingering, insight is one of the brain duties vulnerable to physical damage. As Sasse et al. [44] opined, "a key issue is the extent to which estimates of HRQOL [health-related quality of life] are affected by the clinical phenomenon of anosognosia, that is, impaired self-awareness" (p. 464). Since some patients are unaware of their impairments and others deny them, how much weight should self-report be granted?[4]

---

[4] Insight into one's emotional status is individually variable, even without injury, because of alexithymic traits in mood disorder. Insight into one's cognitive status is perhaps more injury-dependent: some evidence suggests that full awareness of memory loss improves roughly three to six months post-injury.

Table 5.2 Outcome measures frequently employed in peer-reviewed studies of "mild traumatic brain injury"

General health symptom surveys

- Short Form-36 Health Survey [59, 60]
- Health and Behavior Inventory [61, 62]
- Sickness Impact Profile Questionnaire [63–65]
- Patient Health Questionnaire-15 [66]
- General Health Questionnaire [67]
- Illness Representation Questionnaire-Revised (IPQ-R) [68]
- Brief Illness Perception Questionnaire (BIPQ) [69]

Global judgments of outcome

- Glasgow Outcome Scale (GOS) [4, 70]
- Glasgow Outcome Scale-Extended (GOSE) [6]

Pre-injury condition surveys

- Stressful Life Events Questionnaire (SLESQ) [71]
- CES-D [72]

Presence versus absence of "postconcussive syndrome"

- DSM-III, IV, or IV-TR criteria for "postconcussional disorder" [73–75]
- ICD-9 or ICD-10 criteria for post-concussive disorder [76, 77]
- Cut-off scores on post-concussive symptom surveys such as the RPQ

Post-concussive symptom surveys

- Problem Checklist from the New York Head Injury Family Interview [78]
- Post Concussion Syndrome Checklist (PCSC) [79]
- Rivermead Post-concussion Symptoms Questionnaire (RPQ) [80–82]
- Postconcussion Syndrome Questionnaire [83]
- ImPACT Postconcussion Symptoms Inventory (ImPACT) [84]
- Graded Symptoms Checklist (GCS) [85]

Neuropsychiatric or psychological symptoms surveys

- Center for Epidemiological Studies Depression scale (CES-D) [72]
- Brief Symptom Inventory (BSI) [86, 87]
- Minnesota Multiphasic Personality Inventory-2 (MMPI-2) [88, 89]
- Post-traumatic Stress Disorder Checklist (PCL) [90, 91]
- Neurobehavioral Symptom Inventory (NSI) [92–94]
- Neurobehavioral Functioning Inventory [95, 96]
- Neurobehavioral Rating Scale-Revised (NRS) [97, 98]
- Hospital Anxiety and Depression Scale (HADS) [99, 100]
- Behavior Response to Illness Questionnaire (BRIQ) [101]

Disability rating instruments

- Disability Rating Scale (DRS) [53]
- Functional Independence Measures (FIMs) [54–56]
- Craig Handicap Assessment and Reporting Technique (CHART) or
- Craig Handicap Assessment and Reporting Technique, Short Form (CHART-SF) [102]
- Rivermead Head Injury Follow-up Questionnaire (RHFUQ) [103]

Community and work integration surveys

- Katz Adjustment Scale (KAS) [104, 105]
- Revised Social Readjustment Rating Scale [106, 107]
- Reintegration into Normal Living Scale [108]
- Community Integration Questionnaire (CIQ) [109]
- Functional Status Examination [110]

Quality-of-life measures

- Satisfaction with Life Scale [111, 112]
- Perceived Quality of Life (PQOL) [113]
- Quality of Life After Brain Injury (QOLIBRI) [114, 115][a]
- Perceived Self-efficacy and Life Satisfaction after Traumatic Brain Injury [116]
- LiSat11 = Life satisfaction[117]

Self-awareness measures

- Patient Competency Rating Scale for Neurorehabilitation (PCRS-NR) [118][b]

Cognitive test results

- Wechsler Adult Intelligence Scale [119, 120]
- Wechsler Intelligence Scale for Children [121]
- Halstead Impairment Index [122, 123]
- Neuropsychological tests or batteries too numerous to tabulate

Motor test results

- Gait
- Finger tapping
- Grooved pegboard

[a] The Quality of Life After Brain Injury (QOLIBRI) is not represented in the papers meeting inclusion criteria.
[b] The Patient Competency Rating Scale for Neurorehabilitation (PCRS-NR) is not represented in the papers meeting inclusion criteria.

And *when* should one assess outcome? Concussion may accelerate time-passing-related neurodegeneration. That unfortunate outcome may only be detectable after a long dormant period, during which this sequela is invisible to doctor and patient. At what time point can one confidently exclude lasting effects?

It is beyond the scope of this chapter to review the strengths and weaknesses of each popular outcome measure. Reviews are widely available [44–51]. But to interpret the universe of data (and again to explain the inapplicability of meta-analysis), one needs a sense of the striking diversity of these measures. Table 5.2 lists the most commonly employed concussion/mild TBI ("mTBI") outcome measures. Some instruments are excluded – such as the Barthel Index [52], the Disability Rating Scale [53], the Functional Independence Measures [54–55], the Mayo-Portland Adaptability Inventory [57], and the JFK Coma Recovery Scale-Revised [58] – because these are better applied to the assessment of severe cases.

Students of concussion reasonably ask: "What is the gold standard?" A later chapter in this volume summarizes the Common Data Elements project – a major NINDS initiative to establish standard approaches to assessing outcome after "concussion/mildTBI" [124]. That project recommends the GOSE [6, 125]. The GOSE is an acceptable way to formulate a rough-and-ready summary judgment of recovery, good or bad. That judgment, however, lacks the resolution to offer more than a black, gray, and white picture of a rainbow.

The Rivermead Post-concussion Symptoms Questionnaire (RPSQ) [81] is the most-cited outcome instrument. Its 16 items comprise a helpful checklist to gather data about commonly reported problems. Unfortunately, (1) many of the 16 problems are reported by healthy people and most of them occur in multiple medical or psychiatric disease states; (2) only four of those 16 problems (double vision, light sensitivity, noise sensitivity, taking longer to think) may be marginally specific to brain injury; and (3) the RPSQ fails to assess aggression. It might better be called the *Rivermead Several Types of Human Distress Questionnaire*. Moreover, two identical total scores may describe very different outcomes: one survivor may be severely depressed, irritable, and frustrated, but have excellent vision. Another may have persistent problems with forgetfulness, taking longer to think, and dizziness, but not feel sad.

This exposes the essential conundrum with devising a measure of outcome: brain injury tends to impact many aspects of life. It seems imprudent to confine outcome assessment to a handful of problems that may or may not be especially common after CBI. That approach invariably de-emphasizes other problems that are slightly less common but equally important to quality of life. In fact, in the author's opinion, seeking a "post-concussion" measure is not a valid pursuit any more than devising an *American College of Chest Physicians Post-Pneumonia Scale* or *National Institutes of Allergy and Infectious Diseases Post-Lyme Disease Rating Scale*. Every illness potentially affects many cells, and changes life in many ways.

Two ideas deserve dissociation: one idea is "what effect did the abrupt external force have on the brain?" A completely different idea is, "What effect did that abrupt external force have on the person's life?" To date, no biomarker has emerged of much utility in measuring brain outcome. Little has changed since Lidvall et al.'s 1974 lament: "No diagnostic method can disclose with complete accuracy all transitory or persistent cerebral dysfunction" ([126], p. 7). Resting functional connectivity on functional magnetic resonance imaging is one possibility. Recent evidence suggests that serum neurofilament light assays are somewhat reflective of brain injury [127]. The author's personal guess is that one could only properly weight effects on brain and life with measures that attend to both intermediate and long-term outcomes. A valid quantitative measure of intermediate outcome? Perhaps some assay of the extent to which, compared with pre-injury scanning, the survivor's brain is capable of making agile, energy-efficient adaptive adjustments in connectivity in response to experience. Long-term? Perhaps a measure of acceleration in time-passing-related neurodegeneration. A valid global measure? The best outcome measure for CBI would simply be an outcome measure for a human life in all its imponderable dimensions.

Acknowledging that no one scale is perfect, and that subjectivity colors the most honest tailor's tape measures, the author values the Achenbach Behavior Checklists [128]. This suite of instruments enables self-rating and caregiver rating, with separate versions for children and adults, and opens its eyes to much of the human condition. As a principle, the Hippocratic clinician has a straightforward duty. It is not to count how many symptoms, or how many animals, the patient can name. It is to determine how the patient is doing.

13. No Systematic Critical Review of Human Outcome Data has Been Published

At last, a soluble problem! Among the 13 listed barriers to consensus regarding the long-term effects of CBI, we have finally come to one that is tractable. What at first may seem a Herculean labor becomes humanly manageable on application of the lever of scholarship.

Empirical Data From Human Studies

Introduction to, and for, Humans

The above brief introduction leaves us with the question: how common is it for concussion survivors to experience persistent neurobehavioral problems? Drake et al., for example, asserted, "The rate of these symptoms varies widely across studies, with estimate ranging between 7% and 84% of MTBI patients reporting continued problems" ([129], p. 1104). This is hardly a useful conclusion. One wishes to know, based on the most impartial and meticulous attention to the best available data, whether a substantial proportion of survivors of CBI suffers from lasting problems due to abrupt brain shaking, or not.

The reader has arrived at the white-hot nuclear core of this textbook. Co-editor Erin D. Bigler and the present author confess our hope: that this narrative sufficiently harnesses the power of data that it improves neurological knowledge, and perhaps even neurological practice. If so, a little of that power might derive from our devoted multi-year writing effort. Yet most of that power must derive from verifiable facts. This next section offers a compilation of facts.

As with the review of animal experiments summarized in Chapter 4, the following review cannot be regarded as comprehensive in the sense of a Cochrane Database project. But it was, in its way, systematic. The author searched three decades of PubMed (January 1986–December 2016) for peer-reviewed publications with the title/abstract terms "concussion," or "mild traumatic brain injury," that appeared after applying the specifier "human" (4721), and "journal article" (4474). Review of all accessible abstracts led to a selective download of full-texts. Review of the bibliographies of those texts prompted further search. A second and third round of search and review added more relevant studies. In the end, 1898 abstracts and 566 full-text articles were reviewed, yielding the papers listed in Table 5.3–5.5.

Fully eluci those tables would be like asking the reader to plow through Deuteronomy, in Latin, in small print, in a cave. The number of studies, methods, subject pools, claims, and caveats about each is eye glazing. Who has time to read the whole story? An effort has been made to identify every important contribution to this field, and to present those findings in an accessible format. The author confesses mortality; he surely missed or misunderstood some data. But the months of study that the present author invested in assembling this compilation will have been well worth it if the tables of empirical findings help neurologists and neuropsychologists to overthrow the dangerous 20th-century error that concussions are invariably benign.

The Basis for Selection of the Tabulated Peer-Reviewed Articles

At What Moment Post-Injury Should One Assess Outcome?

Henry, a square-jawed, jokey 14-year-old boy, Captain of the Junior Varsity track team and founder of the Robotics Club, forgot to wear his helmet on the day he rode his skateboard into a car. He was knocked out and awoke at the hospital. Two neurologists, a neurosurgeon, and an emergency physician gathered around his gurney to stroke their chins.

One might approach such a troupe and ask three questions about Henry: "How will he do today?" "How will he do next month?" "How will he do next year?"

The experts would largely agree, and be largely correct, when predicting Henry's symptoms that day: confusion, nausea, vomiting, headache, dizziness, a slightly tippy gait, and diplopia (he also had anosmia, but, as usual, no one checked). The most common symptoms in the day or week after a CBI are reasonably predictable and have been described in innumerable publications. Although there is no uniform "syndrome," patients tend to exhibit one or more of these highly predictable symptoms. The three experts would also be likely to agree if asked to predict Henry's medical course over the next two to three months: probable rapid recovery from confusion and steady improvement in most other functional domains, with the possible exception of insidiously increasing moodiness and growing awareness of his own cognitive deficits.

Yet those self-same experts are much less likely to agree if one dared to ask them to predict Henry's life course any time after the three-month point. (Try this at your hospital. Have an exit plan ready in case the debate becomes physical.) Chapters 1 and 2 primarily discussed the first minutes or days after CBI. But that is not the nidus of neurology's embarrassing dispute. It is the Three-Month Myth. From the acre-feet of publications, how should one select the few papers most likely to help bring insight and peace to neurology's concussion war? The search did not dwell on that which is widely agreed: CBI survivors typically exhibit their most prominent symptoms during – and tend to improve steadily over – the first three months. The goal is to resolve the mystery that has bedeviled neurology for the last 150 years: what happens next? For that reason, the first selection mandate of this project was to find every English-language empirical report offering data from a documented follow-up interval of ≥ three months post-injury.

What Was the Medical Problem Called?

Second, as explained in Chapter 1, concussion simply means a *shaking hit* or *rattling blow*. Brain injuries with fractured skulls, extensive intracranial bleeding, cerebral penetration, lobectomy or hemi-resection, permanent coma, or immediate death almost always involve concussion. Impalement of the swimmer's head on a snorkeling narwhal's tooth involves concussion. Still, the most typical, clinically attended concussions – those that numerically dominate the attention of patients, doctors, public health agencies, and social leaders – do *not* exhibit those features. For more than two decades it has been popular to designate a small subgroup of concussion victims as concussion victims. The stereotypical designator has been "mild TBI." The most commonly employed operational criteria for mildness are those of the American Congress of Rehabilitation Medicine, 1993 [130]. Other identified mildness standards included: (1) the European Federation of Neurological Societies definition [131]; (2) the World Health Organization criteria [132]; (3) the U.S. Department of Defense criteria [133]; and (4) the Mayo Clinic criteria [134–135]. In fact, however, at least *37 different inclusion criteria were employed by investigators leading these various studies* – all of whom labeled their subjects "mTBI."

The articles in Tables 5.3–5.5 were selected because they either focus on or include that subgroup. Therefore, hoping to focus attention on that most common and typical variety of CBI, which is also the largest threat to public health, papers were selected that identified their subjects with terms such as "mTBI" or "minor head injury."

Age Range

Third, this textbook is primarily devoted to understanding adult CBI. Most of the selected papers report studies of subjects ≥16 years old. However, like the extraordinary paper by Klonoff et al. [136], several reports of long-term studies of pediatric CBI survivors are included for reference and comparison.

Number

Fourth, although there is urgency to understanding the outcomes of repetitive CBIs – since some societies may wish to reassess the virtue of pressing girls and boys to participate in that which will likely damage their brains – the initial focus is on the outcome after a single concussion. For this reason, many reports of sports-related CBIs, varying in rigor, were excluded because a large proportion of subjects had survived multiple concussions, in some cases more than ten [102, 137–140]. Exceptions occurred if the results were stratified, permitting one to extract data describing the subset of athletes thought to have suffered a single brain injury. Yet (admittedly violating our own criteria), a few especially interesting studies were included, even though some subjects had a history of two concussions. For instance, Broglio et al. [141] reported on a cohort with an average of 1.7 concussions. Also see Hugenholtz et al., 1988 [142] and Mickeviciene et al., 2002 [143].

Rejecting Tunnel Visions

A number of very intriguing papers have been excluded because their methodology made their claims uninterpretable. For example, some researchers (e.g., [144–150]) pre-selected CBI survivors with disappointing outcomes – either on the basis of a larger number of post-concussive symptoms or because they were referred for neuropsychological testing due to poor recovery. As Russell [151] described them: "Chronic cases which have been previously treated in other hospitals;

many of these have been transferred because their progress, judged by expectation, has been unsatisfactory, and they therefore form a highly selected group" (p. 13). A highly selected group with atypically bad outcome, by definition, is not representative of the concussed population. Those studies were excluded. Conversely, some studies recruited an atypically good-outcome group. The most glaring example is research confined to college students (e.g., [77], [152]). How can one generalize from findings among the subgroup of CBI survivors who are active, healthy, intellectually engaged, and recently selected for superior academic promise? This is analogous to testing the hypothesis that cancer is harmful by studying the subgroup that was cured. Those studies were excluded.

Some studies (e.g., [153]) are less useful because, rather than comparing CBI survivors with a healthy or injured group, they bifurcate the CBI subjects into those with and without multiple post-concussive complaints, and then look for group differences. This approach completely defeats any effort to determine the long-term effects across a representative group. It typically produces conclusions that amount to: "The subjects with more problems were more likely to have problems."

Some studies were excluded because they only compared one cohort of "mTBI" subjects with another (e.g., [32]) and therefore offer no comparison between CBI survival and good health. Other studies (e.g., [154]) bifurcated the CBI subjects according to whether or not they met criteria for some other diagnosis, such as PTSD, but then failed to calculate the frequency of outcome variables by diagnosis. This means no information is reported about how CBI itself impacts people. (In a few such cases, published data tables enabled *post hoc* reconstruction and analysis.) Several studies were excluded because of other recruitment biases (e.g., [155]).

Another problem was that some studies compared athletes with and without acknowledged concussions (e.g., [156, 157]). Since college and professional athletes tend not to acknowledge their own concussions [158–160] one must take results reported in such studies with a large grain of salt. Given the average of 300–400 impacts per season, one must question whether a "non-concussed football player" cohort exists. (As of September 18, 2015, 87 of 91 (95%) deceased brain-donating NFL football players have tested positive for the neurodegenerative condition popularly called "chronic traumatic encephalopathy" [161].)

The author fears the reader will share the author's impatience if he or she is asked to plows through all the qualifiers, exceptions, and special circumstances that were considered in building this compilation. However, it may be worthwhile mentioning a few more source selection problems to explain why meta-analysis of this data, as enticing as that might seem, would be like counting clouds during a tempest.

Avoiding a Seductive Mistake

No two studies from different research groups studied subjects with the same demographic profile. No two studies report on cohorts with the same distribution of severities. Recruitment methods varied from the rigorous (systematic prospective longitudinal capture of consecutive patients in a tertiary emergency

department) to the cavalier (any respondents to a newspaper advertisement). Many papers declared, "All subjects met criteria for 'mTBI,'" but some groups studied patients with an initial Glasgow Coma Scale (GCS) of 13–15, others studied patients with GCS 14 or 15, and many failed to report those scores. Some groups selected subjects on the basis of duration of post-traumatic amnesia, most not. Mechanism of injury (i.e., proportion of falls, motor vehicle accidents, sports-related injury, assaults, or blasts) varied greatly between studies. Some groups excluded subjects with "positive CT" results. Most did not, and "positive" was never defined the same way twice. Some groups claim to have excluded subjects with a pre-morbid neuropsychiatric diagnoses or prior TBI. But few reported how they did this, and other groups, arguing it is vital to be "representative," specifically *included* such subjects. Some studies excluded litigants; others did not. No two studies that used injury controls recruited them with the same methods, and no two studies matched their comparison group with their CBI group in the same way. Research designs varied from prospective longitudinal studies of reasonably representative CBI patients and reasonably selected comparison patients to uncontrolled retrospective studies with egregiously biased samples. Readers can be confident: articles on this challenging subject with "meta-analysis" in their titles are mainly good for kindling.

Sven's Admonitions

Finally – before unleashing the reader to leap on to this mountain of gems – the author advises consideration of one single study and its deep implications.

Sven's Admonition Number 1: Please Do Not Judge the Effect of a Disease by Comparing Groups With and Without That Disease

In 1954, Sven J. Dencker and his team in southern Sweden began to examine concussion survivors [162]. They worked from a list of 14,647 consecutive cases of concussion contusion, skull fracture, scalp wounds, or post-concussional state among persons born between 1880 and 1946 who suffered concussions between 1920 and 1953. The authors judged that CBI occurred in every case. Thirty-seven pairs of monozygotic twins were identified in which one twin, the proband, had been concussed, the other not. Regarding severity: 33/37 (89.2%) of concussed twins exhibited post-traumatic amnesia of ≤ 24 h and 28/37 (75.7%) had disability lasting less than two months. After limiting the cohort to those aged 10–60 years, excluding those who declined to be tested, and excluding twin pairs in which both had been brain-injured, there were 28 pairs in the study. All underwent electroencephalograms; none exhibited abnormalities. It is reasonable, in the author's opinion, to regard this as a typical cohort of almost exclusively "mild" concussion survivors.

The investigators examined both members of each twin pair at between three and 34 years after the concussions; this follow-up period averaged ten years. The investigators administered cognitive testing (this paper predated the post-1960 enthusiasm for the term *neuropsychology*). The authors selected 15 tests presumed to be sensitive to organic brain injury. The special and historic virtue of this study should be instantly apparent: "as monozygotic twins are generally assumed to be genetically identical, any difference in the test results between probands and partners were probably due to the head injury" ([162], p. 6). It's not the Dear Leader experiment; but, as the only concussion study to control for genetics, it's an extraordinary contribution.

Results:

1. *When the concussed twin was compared with his healthy twin*, on four of these tests, the concussed twin was significantly inferior: (1) a mirror drawing test intended to assess ability to shift mode of performance; (2) a sorting test regarded as a measure of ability to abstract; (3) a visual perceptual testing requiring making rapid figure/ground distinctions on tachistoscopic presentation; and (4) a continuous performance test intended to assess mental fatigability.
2. *When the whole group of concussed twins was compared with the whole group of non-concussed twins*, there was no difference.

It would be hard to overstate the vital importance of Sven's study. First, by controlling for the billions of genetic differences that might influence response to an abrupt external force, the authors vanquished the toughest confounding factor in this research area. Second, as this chapter has already hinted and will further show, only some tests are sensitive to the effects of concussion; using insensitive tests is a waste of time. Third – and here is *Sven's first admonition* – if scholars compare a bunch of brain-injured people to a bunch of non-brain-injured people, they are doing the wrong research project. The question is not "Does the average score of these 28 people with head injury differ from the average score of those 28 people without?" The question is, "Did Henry get worse?"

Hence, *none of the studies we are about to review studied what matters: objectively verifiable individual change.*

An analogous inspiration for clinical caution: the present author once cared for an engineering professor who came to the clinic having diagnosed himself with Alzheimer's disease. The nurse saw him first. She came out unconvinced: "His Mini Mental State Exam score is perfect, 30 out of 30." As soon as the author entered the exam room, the engineer theatrically unfurled a scroll of computer printouts. "See!" he said. "Right there!" He pointed at one term in a grand equation. He stated it was an error. He stated he did not make errors. He concluded that, therefore, he must have Alzheimer's disease. Two years later, the rest of us finally appreciated that he was right.

Neurobehavioral disorders are not reliably identifiable using an absolute scale, because nervous systems differ. A ten-hour battery of cognitive tests tell us absolutely nothing about whether that guy's brain is doing better or worse than the day before. Sometimes a concussed person scores well, and the tester will mistakenly opine, "All the results are within normal limits. Thus, there is no evidence of traumatic brain injury." A perfect score never means "no evidence of brain injury."

Sven's Admonition Number 2: Please Stop Predicting Long-Term Outcome

Medical students get it instantly: it is one thing to say that an event is associated with a 30% decline in function; it is entirely different to say that event is associated with a 30% chance of decline in function. For the sake of discussion, let us say we care for 100 cardiac patients. One cardiologist may declare, "A patient whose circumflex coronary artery is completely clogged has an average 19% decline in ejection fraction." That comment predicts a clinical problem of a certain magnitude in each and every one of our patients – 100 out of 100 who have that blockade. It is an entirely different concept for the cardiologist to state, "A patient whose circumflex coronary artery is completely clogged has a 19% chance of a heart attack in the next three years." That comment predicts a clinical problem in just 30 of our patients.

Sven Dencker and his team observed that, if you have a group of 28 people who have suffered a concussion and compare them with 28 people who have not suffered a concussion, *one should not expect any difference in the two groups' performance.* That is because, rather than a concussion leading to an average 30% decline in function in everybody – a deterministic result – it is far more accurately conceptualized as causing a 30% *chance* of cognitive decline – a probabilistic result that pertains to only eight people in the group of 28. The change in function that matters is not relative to all the folks in your village, *it is relative to your pre-injury self* (or, if you happen to have one, your monozygotic twin).

In the long run, concussion does not reliably do anything. The long-term effects of a concussion vary so much, and depend so much on human individuality, that it is grossly inappropriate to predict (or even describe) outcome as a percent of lost function. Until we can predict every molecular event in one another, it is unwise and unkind to tell a concussed person: "You will have a mild memory loss for six months." That would be every bit as honest and useful as the meteorologist announcing that the rain will stop at 3:27 p.m. A scientifically defensible statement would be more along the lines of "You have about a 22–44% chance of some degree of memory problem three years from now."

What Each Table Offers

Three tables summarize the results of the selected reports. The first is Table 5.3, which compiles the results of uncontrolled long-term follow-up studies after so-called "mild traumatic brain injury" (or "minor TBI," or "minor head injury"). The tempting conclusion from these studies: yes, many CBI survivors report or are judged to have persistent post-concussive problems at one year or longer post-injury.[5] Scrupulous skeptics will correctly

---

[5] Note that "symptoms" or "complaints" are suboptimal words, since many injured people inflate, deny, or lack awareness of their CBI-related problems. *Problems* include, for instance, mental slowing that reorients avocational engagement, or irritability that erodes sociality, or subclinical imbalance that leads to more downhill-skiing tumbles, or – the looming unknown – accelerated neurodegeneration.

Table 5.3 Uncontrolled studies of human adults with concussion or mild traumatic brain injury ("mTBI"): the proportion reporting persistence of one or more post-concussive symptoms at different time points

Source	n Diagnosis	Syptoms @ 3 months	Symptoms @ 6 months	Symptoms @ 1 year	Symptoms @ 1–2 years	Symptoms @ ≥ 3 years
Adler, 1945 [a] [183]	200 "closed head injury"		31.5% @ 6 months			
Alves et al., 1986 [184]	847 "mild traumatic brain injury"	66% @ 3 months	50% @ 6 months	46% @ 1 year		
Alves et al., 1993 [185]	587 "Uncomplicated" mTBI	63% @ 3 months	44% @ 6 months	40% @ 1 year		
Anderson and Catroppa, 2005 [186]	27 "mTBI" pediatric subjects				14% arithmetic below grade level @ 24 months	
Barlow et al., 2015 [187]	461	11.8% @ 3 months				
Barth et al., 1983 [b] [188]	71 "mild head injury"	62% @ 3 months				
Bryant et al., 2010 [189]	817 "mTBI"			31% psychiatric disorder; (22% new disorder) @ 1 year		
Cartlidge, 1978 [190]	372 "acute head injury"				18–24% @ 2 years	
Chan and Feinstein, 2015 [192]	374 "mTBI"			53.7% sleep-disordered @ 1 year		
De Kruijk et al., 2002 [193]	79 "mTBI"		28% @ 6 months			
Demakis et al., 2010 [9]	191 "treated" mTBI	20.4% @ ≥ 3 months				
Denker, 1944 [34]	100 (excluded litigants)			33% @ 1 year		
Eisenberg et al., 2014 [194]	207 "concussion" (pediatric subjects)	15%				
Erez et al., 2009 [195]	13 "mTBI"	23.1–84.6% activity restrictions (mean = 4.7 months)				
Faux et al., 2011 [196]	107 "mTBI"	35.1% post-concussive syndrome @ 3 months				
Fenton et al., 1993 [197]	43 "mild head injury"	3	48.8% symptoms @ 6 months			
Guthkelch, 1980 [c] [198]	398 "head injury" (mixed severity)		33.7% absent from work > 6 months			
Haagsma et al., 2015 [199]	282 "mTBI"			12.8% depression or post-traumatic stress disorder @ 12 months		
Hanlon et al., 1999 [200]	100 "mTBI"			67% poor or modified vocation @ 12 months		
Hartvigsen et al., 2014 [201]	1158 "mTBI"			"More than half" @ 1 year		

Table 5.3 (*Cont.*)

Source	n Diagnosis	Syptoms @ 3 months	Symptoms @ 6 months	Symptoms @ 1 year	Symptoms @ 1–2 years	Symptoms @ ≥ 3 years
Hessen et al., 2007 [202]	119 mTBI (45 children; 74 adults)					@ 23 years, the cohort had an average of 4/24 impaired cognitive test scores
Hou et al., 2012 [203]	107 "mTBI"		21% post-concussive syndrome @ 6 months			
Ingebrigsten et al., 1998 [204]	100 "minor head injury"	62% symptoms at 3 months 40% post-concussive syndrome				
Jakobsen et al., 1987 [205]	55 "concussion"	22% "PC syndrome" @ 3 months				
King et al., 1995 [81]	46 "head injured"	3	"Fewer than half" @ 6 months			
Klonoff et al., 1993 [206]	159 mTBI (as children)					31% @ 23 years
Kumar et al., 2005 [207]	30 "mild head injury"		86.7% post-concussive symptoms @ mean = 5 months			
Lange et al., 2014 [d] [208]	1600 "mild-to-moderate TBI"		65.75% @ mean = 5 months			
Lannsjo et al., 2009 [209]	2523 "mTBI"	44% at 3 months				
Levin et al., 1987 [210]	32 "minor head injury"	47% headache, 22% decreased energy, 22% dizziness				
Lidvall et al., 1974 [126]	83 "concussion"	24% @ 3 months				
Lingsma et al., 2015 [e] [211]	386 "mTBI"		48.7% @ 6 months			
Lundin et al., 2006 [212]	112 "mTBI"	49% @ 3 months				
Maestas et al., 2014 [213]	187 "mTBI"	@ 3 months: 27% depressed; 24.6% anxiety				
Mahon and Elger, 1989 [214]	67 "multiple trauma with mild head injury"	60% @ 3 months	21% @ 6 months			
Max et al., 2013 [215]	79 "mTBI"			28% novel psychiatric disorder @ 12 months		
Mazzucchi et al., 1992 [216]	27 "mTBI"			32.8% "evidence of deterioration" @ mean = 10.4 months		
McMahon et al., 2014 [217]	199 "mTBI"			82% @ 12 months		
Middleboe et al., 1992 [218]	28 "mTBI"			50% "PC syndrome" @ 1 year		

(continued)

Table 5.3 (*Cont.*)

Source	n Diagnosis	Syptoms @ 3 months	Symptoms @ 6 months	Symptoms @ 1 year	Symptoms @ 1–2 years	Symptoms @ ≥ 3 years
Mittenberg and Strauman, 2000 [219]	58 "mild head injury"		67% post-concussive syndrome @ 6 months			
Montgomery et al., 1991 [220]	25 "minor head injury"		48% @ 6 months			
Nolin and Heroux, 2006 [221]	85 "mTBI"					57.6% @ 1–3 years
Petersen et al., 2008 [222]	10 "mTBI"	30% @ 5 months				
Relander et al., 1972 [223]	59 "concussion"			39% @ 1 year		
Ricard et al., 2013 [191]	795 "m TBI"		11.7% @ 6 months			
Rickels et al., 2010 f [165]	4202 "mTBI"			50% "required Tx" 21.3% not doing well at jobs		
Rimel et al., 1981 [32]	424 "minor head trauma"	84% @ 3 months				
Røe et al., 2009 [224]	52 "mTBI"			42% post-concussive syndrome @ 12 months		
Ruffolo et al., 1999 [225]	50 "mTBI"		58% not returned to work @ 7 months			
Rutherford et al., 1979 g [226]	41 "mild concussion"			16.1% @ 1 year		
Sawyer et al., 2015 [227]	212 "mTBI"			77% headache @ 12 months		
Scholten et al., 2012 [228]	364 "mTBI"			34.8% GOSE ≤ 7 @ 12 months		
Scott et al., 2016 [229]	50 "mTBI"	54% other than good outcome @ 3 months				
Sigurdardottir et al., 2009 [230]	40 "mTBI"	40% @ 3 months		27.3% @ 1 year		
Schneiderman et al, 2008 [231]	275 mTBI	35% "PC syndrome" @ ~ 4–5 months				
Snell et al., 2015 [232]	125 "mTBI"		25% @ 6 months			
Stålnacke, 2007 [233]	163 "mTBI"					68% @ 3 years
Steadman and Graham, 1970 h [234]	415 "head injury"					18% "unwell" @ 5 years
Stulemeijer et al., 2008 [235]	201 mTBI		33% @ 6 months			
Theadom et al., 2015 [236]	341 "mTBI"			47.9% had ≥ 4 symptoms @ 1 year		
Wilkinson et al., 2012 [237]	26 mTBI			42% with HPA hormone abnormalities @ 1 year		

Table 5.3 (*Cont.*)

Source	*n* Diagnosis	Syptoms @ 3 months	Symptoms @ 6 months	Symptoms @ 1 year	Symptoms @ 1–2 years	Symptoms @ ≥ 3 years
Wrightson and Gronwall, 1981 [238]	66 "minor head injury" 44 @ 90 days; 8 @ 2 years	20% @ 3 months				50% of those with symptoms @ 3 months still had symptoms @ 2 year
Zemek et al., 2013 [239]	59 "concussion"	46% @ 3 months				
Zumstein et al., 2011 [240]	86 "mTBI"					37.2% decreased life quality @ 10 years

a Re Adler, 1945 [183]: severity varied. A total of 173/200 (86.5%) were disoriented for < 12 h. Follow-up varied from one month to > 12 months; 155/200 (77.5%) were followed up at four to nine months.

b Re Barth et al., 1983 [188]: 44/71 (62%) subjects exhibited mild to severe impairment on the Halstead Impairment Index; 22/71 exhibited "minimal" impairment.

c Re Guthkelch, 1980 [198]: mixed-severity cohort.

d Re Lange et al., 2014 [208]: 80.7% mild; this study failed to stratify results by severity.

e Re Lingsma et al., 2015 [211]: preselected for available 6-month outcome data. GOSE of 8 regarded as "complete recovery" (102/386 subjects) "some remaining symptoms (GOS-E, 7)." A total of 188/386 survived, had data, and had less than full recovery.

f Re. Rickels et al., 2010 [165]: 90.2% of subjects with "mTBI"; failed to stratify findings by severity.

g Re Rutherford et al., 1979 [226]: the author claimed a cohort of 131. They contacted 118 @ 12 months. Nineteen of 118 (16.1%) of those contacted by mail @ 12 months had persistent symptoms. Nineteen of 41 (46.3%) of those directly assessed at 12 months had persistent symptoms.

h Re Steadman and Graham, 1969 [234]: 85% were mild in the sense that loss of consciousness < 1 hour.

GOSE, Glasgow Outcome Scale-Extended; HPA: hypothalamic–pituitary–adrenal; PC, post-concussive; Tx, treatment.

admonish, "Wait. Just because almost half of CBI survivors complain of symptoms or are diagnosed with persistent post-concussive problems one full year after their head injuries, that's not evidence that brain injuries are harmful. Perhaps all you have done is find the base rate of daily symptoms among humans – with or *without* injury."

The author agrees. So Table 5.4 summarizes the studies comparing CBI survivors with matched healthy controls. The conclusion from these controlled studies: yes. Persistent post-concussive problems are more commonly reported by, or diagnosed in, CBI survivors than in healthy persons. Scrupulous skeptics will again correctly point out, "Just because significantly more CBI survivors are distressed or impaired at one year after injury, that is not evidence that an abrupt force transmitted to the brain is harmful. Perhaps all the long-term impairment and distress we see are non-specific effects of a traumatic experience."

Again, the author takes the point. As depicted in the Dear Leader experiment, without controlling for trauma one cannot pin symptoms on a particular organ.

So Table 5.5 lists the studies that compared victims of brain trauma with victims of non-brain trauma – those who have suffered an injury (perhaps associated with a psychic trauma) but no apparent brain damage. The conclusion from these other-injury-controlled studies: indeed, both brain and non-brain trauma are strongly associated with persistent post-concussive problems that persist for one or more years. However, (1) multiple controlled studies show that CBI survivors have more persistent or serious problems (both emotional and cognitive) than survivors of other injuries; and (2) the most frequent problems in the two groups are somewhat different. For instance, sleep disturbance, irritability, and even headache may be equally common among brain injury and orthopedic patients, but visual disturbance, disequilibrium, slowed thought, and degraded high-level executive functions seem to be more common among CBI survivors.

A popular explanation has emerged. A simple dichotomy is alleged:

- Some problems are non-specific effects of the traumatic stress response that Cannon described in his famous 1915 text [163].
- Other problems are biologically specific to brain trauma.

But, as discussed momentarily, that commonplace may over-simplify a more compelling story.

After Tables 5.3–5.5 are widely reviewed, one hopes there will be fewer skeptics. The remaining resistance to the conclusion that concussive brain rattling is often associated with lasting troubles begins to sound defensive and dogmatic. This text may be a generation shy of meaty physiological evidence, but multiple empirical clues tend to swing the compass in the same direction, favoring a more nuanced view:

- Some problems are reported with roughly the same frequency after either CBI or non-brain injury. But it is premature and implausible to state that this is entirely explained by a non-specific, universal stress response. Instead, one suspects that, despite their superficial similarity, symptoms in different patients may be mediated by different biological phenomena. For example: sleep disturbance is extremely common in the months after trauma. Yet post-concussive sleep disorder linked to anterior hypothalamic damage is likely a different problem than post-fracture pain-related insomnia.

Table 5.4 Medium- to long-term studies of post-concussive problems employing healthy controls

Author year	Study type	n CBI survivors	n healthy subjects	Follow-up	Results
Alexander et al., 2015 [a] [247]	Prosp. long.	45 rugby-playing teens w concussion 21 w/o concussion	30 non-rugby-playing teens	Mean = 4.8 years	1. Rugby subjects (with or without CBI) had significantly worse scores on: WISC-III coding incidental immediate recall ($p = 0.04$) WISC-III similarities ($p = 0.03$) 2. Non-rugby subjects had significantly superior academic scores at study completion ($p = 0.001$). (Inclusion controlled for pre-injury neurological/psychiatric conditions)
Baldassarre et al., 2015 [b] [242]	Observ.	188 veterans "mTBI"	210 healthy	Mean = 4.8 years	1. CBI survivors had more total sxs (mean = 16.7 vs. mean = 9.4) 2. CBI survivors (based on incident rate ratios) had 30% more sxs ($p < 0.001$) - 34% more somatic sxs ($p < 0.001$) - 22% more cognitive sxs ($p < 0.05$) - 15% more affective sxs ($p < 0.05$) - 59% more vestibular sxs (p. < 0.001) 3. Anxiety and insomnia predicted # of sxs
Bernstein, 2002 [c] [248]	X-sect.	13 "mild head injury"	10 healthy	Mean = 8 years (1–16.5 years)	1. CBI survivors reported significantly more sleep problems ($p < 0.05$) 2. CBI survivors had significantly worse scores on digit symbol ($p < 0.05$) 3. No significant difference on most conventional NΨ tests
Broglio et al., 2009 [141]	X-sect.	46 h of concussion	44 healthy	Mean = 3.4 years	1. No significant difference on ImPACT test 2. No significant difference in number of symptoms (Inclusion controlled for prior neurological disorders)
Catale et al., 2009 [169]	Prosp. long.	15 "mTBI" children	15 healthy	1 year	1. CBI survivors had significantly fewer correct responses on selective attention task ($p = 0.02$) but no difference in incorrect responses 2. CBI survivors had significantly lower accuracy on auditory selective attention ($p = 0.04$) but no difference on false responses 3. CBI survivors had significantly lower accuracy on divided attention ($p = 0.03$) but no difference for incorrect responses 4. CBI survivors had significantly fewer correct responses on working memory ($p = 0.04$) but no difference in reaction time for correct responses 5. No significant difference on WISC-III subtests 6. No significant difference on simple reaction time (Inclusion controlled for pre-injury learning disability or neurological disorder)
Cicerone, 1996 [d] [36]	X-sect.	15 "mTBI"	9 healthy	Mean = 18.6 months (6–30 months)	1. CBI survivors had significantly slower processing ($p = 0.000$) 2. CBI survivors were significantly more impaired by adding a task that competed for their attention ($p < 0.01$) 3. No significant difference on the standard condition of the Extended 2 and 7 Selective Attention Test

Table 5.4 (*Cont.*)

Author year	Study type	n CBI survivors	n healthy subjects	Follow-up	Results
Clarke et al., 2012 e[177]	X-sect.	21 "mTBI"	19 healthy	3–12 months	1. CBI survivors significantly worse cognitive complaints ($p = 0.004$) 2. CBI survivors significantly higher average neuroticism ($p = < 0.001$) 3. CBI survivors with poorer NΨ results had significantly more cognitive complaints ($p < 0.01$), affective distress ($p < 0.05$), and PCS ($p < 0.01$) 4. Both CBI and healthy subjects showed significant association between affective distress and cognitive complaints 5. Both CBI and healthy subjects showed significant association between cognitive complaints and PCS 6. Both CBI and healthy subjects showed significant association between affective distress and PCS 7. No significant difference on conventional NΨ tests (Excluded CBI subjects with any other neurological condition)
Cossette et al., 2014 [249]	Retrosp.	7 "mTBI"	7 Healthy	Mean = 158 days	1. CBI survivors had significantly slower gait ($p = 0.004$) 2. CBI survivors had a significantly larger relative change in gait speed when a cognitive task was combined (executive function) ($p = 0.001$) (Inclusion controlled for neurological, cognitive, or substance abuse problems)
Dean et al., 2012 [250]	Retrosp. X-sect.	119 "mTBI" (with and w/o diagnosis of PCS)	246 Healthy (with and w/o diagnosis of PCS)	Mean = 7.8–8.5 years	1. CBI survivors had significantly more cognitive complaints ($p = 0.001$) 2. CBI survivors more likely to c/o headache, dizziness, nausea, light sensitivity, double vision 2. No significant difference in "PC syndrome" diagnosis (ICD-10 criteria) (CBI = 31%; control = 34%) ($p = 0.6$) 4. Only c/o headache distinguished CBI + PCS from healthy + PCS (Inclusion controlled for pre-injury TBI)
Dikmen et al., 1986 [164]	X-sect.	19 "minor head injury"	19 uninjured friends	12 months	1. CBI survivors significantly more likely to be limited in recreational/leisure activities (31.6% vs. 0%) 2. No significant difference on conventional NΨ tests (Inclusion controlled for pre-injury neurological or psychiatric problems)
Donnell et al., 2012 [178]	X-sect.	154 "mTBI"	3001 healthy	~8 years	CBI survivors more likely to have "PC syndrome" (DSM-IV criteria: 32% vs. 13%; ICD-10 criteria: 27% vs. 10%)
Ellemberg et al., 2007 f [251]	X-sect.	10 female soccer w concussion	12 female soccer w/o concussion	6–8 months	1. CBI survivors had significantly slower speed of information processing (1.3–2.0 times slower for concussed on four of eight tests. Effect size 1.67–3.29) 2. No significant difference on verbal learning, letter fluency, digits

(continued)

Table 5.4 (*Cont.*)

Author year	Study type	*n* CBI survivors	*n* healthy subjects	Follow-up	Results
Emanuelson et al., 2003 [252]	Pop.; case–control	101 adult "mTBI"	2424 age, gender-matched healthy	1 year	CBI survivors had significantly more impaired scores on all dimensions of the SF36
Ettenhofer and Barry, 2012 [179]	X-sect.	256 "mTBI"	2280 healthy	Mean = 3.59 years	1. CBI survivors significantly more likely to have somatic symptoms ($p = 0.022$), dizziness ($p < 0.001$), and cognitive symptoms ($p = 0.03$) 2. CBI survivors reported slightly higher PC total symptom scores (NS; $p = 0.16$) (Inclusion controlled for past TBI, pre-injury psychotic or neurological illness)
Ewing et al., 1980 [37]	Case–control	10 concussed	10 healthy	M – 2.2 years (1–3 years)	1. CBI survivors had significantly lower scores on a vigilance task ($p < 0.05$), and a memory task ($p < 0.05$) at simulated altitude 2. No significant difference on the PASAT
Fay et al., 1993 [253]	Case–control	53 peds. "mTBI"	53 classroom controls	1 year	1. CBI survivors had significantly lower scores on coding (WISC-R) 2. No significant difference on other NΨ tests 3. No significant difference on Achenbach CBCL
Fay et al., 1994 [9] [254]	Case–control	40 peds. "mTBI"	40 classroom controls	3 years	"children with mild injuries demonstrated negligible differences from their matched controls" (p. 735) on NΨ. But no significance data were provided
Geary et al., 2010 [170]	X-sect.	40 "mTBI"	35 healthy	Mean = 5.29 years	1. CBI survivors significantly more likely to have cognitive complaints (82.5% vs. 0%) 2. CBI survivors had significantly worse scores on CVLT-II list A, trial 1 ($p = 0.02$) 3. CBI survivors had significantly lower learning rates ($p = 0.014$) 4. The differences were not attributable to depression, anxiety, or apathy 5. No difference on other CVLT-II scores (Inclusion controlled for litigation, pre-injury neurological or psychiatric conditions, and response bias)
Hanten et al, 2013 [180]	Prosp. long.	59 "mTBI" young adults	27 healthy	3 months	CBI survivors significantly worse on KeepTrack task, categories correct ($p = 0.0009$–0.0349) "suggesting no recovery in mTBI up to 90 days" (p. 618) (Inclusion controlled for pre-injury neurological or major psychiatric problems)
Heitger et al., 2007 [148]	Prosp. long.	31 "mTBI"	31 healthy matched for age, sex, education	12 months	1. CBI survivors had significantly higher RPSQ scores 2. No difference on conventional NΨ tests 3. Marginal differences on selected eye and limb movement tasks (Inclusion controlled for pre-injury neurological or major psychiatric problems and litigation)

Table 5.4 (*Cont.*)

Author year	Study type	*n* CBI survivors	*n* healthy subjects	Follow-up	Results
Hoge et al., 2008 [h][181]	X-sect.	384 "mTBI"	1706 healthy	> 4 months	CBI survivors were divided into those with and without LOC 1. CBI survivors with LOC were significantly more likely to report poor overall health ($p = 0.04$) and elevated health problem scores ($p < 0.001$) 2. CBI survivors with LOC reported significantly more missed work days ($p = 0.02$), medical visits ($p = 0.005$), headaches ($p < 0.001$), chest pain ($p < 0.001$), dizziness ($p = 0.01$), heart pounding ($p < 0.001$), shortness of breath ($p = 0.02$), bowel problems ($p = 0.006$), fatigue ($p < 0.001$), and sleep disturbance ($p = 0.001$) 3. CBI survivors with LOC reported significantly more memory problems ($p = 0.005$), balance problems ($p = 0.02$), ringing in the ears ($p = 0.01$), concentration problems ($p = 0.002$), and irritability ($p < 0.001$) 4. After control for depression and PTSD, the only remaining significant differences were in regard to headache and heart pounding
Hugenholtz et al., 1988 [142]	Prosp. case–control	22 mild concussion	22 matched healthy	3 months	No significant difference in simple or choice reaction time
Jakola et al., 2007 [i][255]	Retrosp. case–control	28 "mild head injury"	28 matched random	5–7 years	1. CBI survivors had significantly more PC sxs ($p = 0.017$) 2. CBI survivors had significantly lower quality-of-life scores ($p = 0.008$)
Kashluba et al., 2004 [18]	X-sect.	110 "mTBI"	118 healthy	Mean = 98 days (73–164 days)	1. CBI survivors significantly more likely to report poor balance, doing things slowly, fatiguing quickly (Bonferroni-adjusted significance 0.0116) 2. CBI survivors c/o significantly greater severity for poor balance, doing things slowly, problems with coordination, fatiguing quickly, headaches, difficulty thinking clearly and efficiently, difficulty planning, irritability, sleep disturbance, changed personality (Bonferroni-adjusted significance 0.0116) 3. 39% of CBI survivors (vs. 15% of controls) endorsed ≥ 1 severe symptom
Kashluba et al., 2008 [256]	X-sect.	110 mTBI	118 healthy	Mean = 98 days (73–164 days)	20% of CBI survivors had average symptom severity score > 2 across 43 sxs vs. 8% of controls
Keller et al., 2000 [257]	X-sect.	12 mTBI	11 healthy	Mean = 38 months (10–70 months)	1. CBI survivors had significantly worse on-time responses on the first of two conditional reaction time tasks 2. CBI survivors also had significantly worse on-time responses on the second of two conditional reaction time tasks 3. CBI survivors remained significantly worse on the second task after a motivation ($p = 0.03$). However, CBI scores were within published norms and as good as controls prior to motivation (Inclusion controlled for history of psychiatric illness; no litigants)

(*continued*)

Table 5.4 (*Cont.*)

Author year	Study type	n CBI survivors	n healthy subjects	Follow-up	Results
Killam et al., 2005 [j] [156]	X-sect.	11 concussed athletes	8 healthy non-concussed 9 athletes "non-concussed"	5 recently concussed (mean = 2.4 months); 6 non-recent (mean = 5.2 years)	1. Athletes ("non-concussed" or recently concussed) had significantly worse scores on immediate and delayed memory (p = < 0.05). 2. Athletes ("non-concussed," recently or non-recently concussed) had significantly worse RBANS total scores (p < 0.01 to < 0.05)
Klein et al., 1996 [k] [35]	X-sect. case–control	Group A: 25 middle-aged "uncomplicated mild to mod." Group B: 20 "old"	45 matched healthy	Group A: mean = 26.4 years (1–52 years) Group B: mean = 35.7 years (2–63 years)	1. CBI survivors performed significantly worse on word recall (p < 0.001), learning (p < 0.001), delayed recall (p < 0.001), and retrieval ((p < 0.05). 2. CBI survivors performed significantly worse on the Stroop Color Word Test (p < 0.01) 2. Age was associated with significantly lower scores for memory (p < 0.05), learning (p < 0.05), the Stroop test (p < 0.001) (Inclusion controlled for previous brain damage and major psychiatric disease)
Konrad et al., 2011 [258]	X-sect.	33 "mTBI"	33 healthy	Mean = 6 years (4.75–7.25 years)	CBI survivors had significantly worse results on tests of acquisition of episodic memory (p < 0.01–0.05), retention of episodic memory (p < 0.001–0.05), working memory (p < 0.001), attention (p < 0.001–0.01), word fluency (p < 0.001–0.01) (Inclusion controlled for depression, litigation, and response bias)
Lee et al., 2008 [259]	X-sect.	28 "mTBI"	18 healthy	12 months	CBI survivors had significantly worse scores on CVLT total recall (p = 0.007), and long delay cued recall (p = 0.031) (Inclusion controlled for pre-injury neurological or psychiatric problems)
Levin et al., 1987 [210]	Prosp. long. Case–control	32 "minor head injury"	56 healthy	3 months	No significant difference on conventional NΨ tests (Inclusion controlled for past neurological diagnosis or psychiatric hospitalization)
Levine et al., 1998 [260]	Prosp. long.	11 "mTBI"	10 healthy	~1.5 years	1. CBI survivors significantly worse on phonemic fluency (p < 0.05) 2. No significant difference on most conventional NΨ tests
Lundin et al., 2006 [212]	Prosp. long.	102 "mTBI"	35 healthy	3 months	1. 25% of CBI survivors reported dysfunction in ≥ 1 domain of life (no data reported for controls) 2. No difference in proportion of each group reporting ≥ 1 symptom; however 3. CBI survivors reported higher mean symptom intensity (6.5 vs. 3.9)
Mangels et al., 2002 [261]	Prosp. long.	11 "mTBI"	10 healthy	3.6 years	1. CBI survivors significantly worse on free recall divided attention (p < 0.05). 2. CBI survivors significantly *better* performance on digit monitoring (p < 0.02) 3. No significant difference on recall (Inclusion controlled for "serious medical or psychiatric illness")
Massagli et al., 2004 [262]	Prosp. cohort case–control	490 "mTBI"	1470 healthy	3 years	1. CBI survivors with no psychiatric history were significantly more likely to develop psychiatric disorders (26% vs. 16%; p < 0.001) 2. Among those with pre-morbid psychiatric history, no significant difference in later psychiatric disorder

Table 5.4 (*Cont.*)

Author year	Study type	*n* CBI survivors	*n* healthy subjects	Follow-up	Results
Mayer et al., 2015 [263]	X-sect.	11 "mTBI" (adolescent)	12 healthy	4 months	CBI survivors had a "significant trend" for worse processing speed (p = 0.09; classified here as NS) (Inclusion controlled for pre-injury neurological or psychiatric problems)
McHugh et al., 2006 [264]	X-sect.	26 "mTBI"	20 healthy	4 months	CBI survivors had significantly worse verbal fluency (p = 0.02), physical symptoms (p = 0.02), and pain (p = 0.01) (Inclusion controlled for response bias)
Moore et al., 2014 [265]	X-sect.	19 asymptomatic concussion	21 healthy	Mean = 7.1 years	1. CBI survivors had lower response accuracy on flanker task and electrophysiological changes c/w "deficits in allocation of attentional resources" 2. No significant difference in mood, fatigue, satisfaction with life
O'Jile et al., 2006 [266]	X-sect.	67 "mild head injury"	60 healthy	Mean = 5 years	1. CBI survivors exhibited a significantly inferior practice benefit (p > 0.05) 2. No difference in most measures of processing speed per PASAT
Oldenburg et al., 2016 [267]	Prosp.	82 "mTBI"	31 healthy	3 months	1. CBI survivors significantly worse than controls on all measures of Selective Reminding Task except multiple choice (p = 0.001–0.025) 2. No significant difference on other NΨ tests
Papoutsis et al., 2014 [268]	X-sect.	52 "mTBI" (peds.) (34 complicated; 18 uncomplicated)	33 healthy	Mean = 96 months	1. "Complicated mTBI" significantly worse on divided attention 2. No significant group differences on WISC-IV coding, block design, digit span
Pieper and Garvan, 2014 [167]	Prosp.	25 "mTBI" (peds).	38 healthy (28 non-brain injury_	12 months	1. CBI surviving children self-reported significantly more cognitive fatigue than either control group (p = 0.047) 2. No significant difference in reported physical or psychosocial health
Pontifex et al., 2012 [269]	X-sect.	38 college athletes with "mTBI"	42 without "mTBI"	Mean = 3.6 years	On Flanker task: 1. CBI survivors had significantly worse response accuracy (p = 0.006) 2. CBI survivors had significantly more omission errors (p = 0.01) 3. No significant group difference in reaction time (Inclusion controlled for neurological and cardiovascular disorders)
Potter et al., 2001 [270]	X-sect.	24 "mTBI"	24 healthy	M= 12 months (≤ 5 years)	1. CBI survivors had significantly lower scores on paired associates, hard (p = 0.014) and digit symbol (p = 0.036) 2. No significant difference on paired associates, easy; Trails A and B; digit span
Potter et al., 2002 [271]	X-sect.	24 "mTBI"	24 healthy	< 3 years Median = 6 months	1. CBI survivors significantly worse on AVLT (p = 0.004–0.019) 2. CBI survivors had significantly slower reaction times (p = 0.044) 3. CBI survivors had significantly more incongruent errors (p = 0.01) 4. CBI survivors significantly higher on Eysenck lie scale (p = 0.018) 5. No significant difference on Trails; digit span 6. No significant difference on measures of depression or anxiety

(*continued*)

Table 5.4 *(Cont.)*

Author year	Study type	*n* CBI survivors	*n* healthy subjects	Follow-up	Results
Rabinowitz et al., 2015 [182]	X-sect.	66 "mTBI"	38 healthy; 63 orthopedic injury	3 months	1. CBI survivors significantly more likely to have poor cognitive outcome (36.4% vs. 15.8%; $p = 0.0064$) 2. CBI survivors significantly more likely to have poor symptomatic outcome (52% vs. 13%; $p = 9.991e\text{-}05$)
Schoenhuber and Gentilini, 1988 [272]	X-sect.	35 "MHI"	35 matched healthy	Mean = 9 months (5–17 months)	1. CBI survivors significantly more likely to be depressed ($p = 0.001\text{--}0.002$) 2. No significant difference on anxiety scores
Segalowitz et al., 2001 [273]	X-sect.	10 "mTBI"	12 healthy	Mean = 6.4 years (1–13 years)	1. CBI survivors had lower scores on a difficult oddball task 2. CBI survivors had significantly reduced P300 amplitudes 3. No significant difference on conventional NΨ tests
Singh et al., 2014 [140]	X-sect.	25 concussed college football players	25 "non-concussed" players	Mean = 270 days (1–1672 days)	1. No significant difference on conventional NΨ tests
Sinopoli et al., 2014 [274]	X-sect.	13 male "mTBI" (adolescent)	14 "without known history of mTBI"	3–6 months	1. CBI survivors had significantly worse dual-task reaction times ($p = 0.03$) 2. No significant difference on dual-task accuracy or cost 3. No significant difference on more conventional NΨ tests (Inclusion controlled for pre-injury neurological or psychiatric conditions)
Sterr et al., 2006 [275]	X-sect.	38 "mTBI"	38 matched healthy	Mean = 6.55–7 years (≥ 12 months)	CBI survivors significantly more likely to meet criteria for diagnosis of "PC syndrome" (29% vs. 0%) (Inclusion controlled for pre-injury neurological or psychiatric conditions)
Styrke et al., 2013 [276]	X-sect	163 "mTBI"	461 healthy for PC symptoms 2533 healthy for life satisfaction	3 years	1. CBI survivors had significantly higher median RPSQ scores ($p < 0.001$) 2. CBI survivors were significantly more likely to report "almost all" PC symptoms 3. CBI survivors were significantly less likely to report life satisfaction (56% vs. 70%, $p < 0.001$) 4. Within CBI survivors, females were significantly more likely to report headache ($p = 0.001$), dizziness ($p = 0.029$), nausea/vomiting ($p = 0.042$), noise sensitivity ($p = 0.035$), fatigue ($p = 0.022$), depression ($p = 0.009$), taking longer to think ($p = 0.042$), and spinal pain ($p = 0.002$)
Tay et al., 2010 [277]	X-sect.	31 "mTBI"	31 healthy	3 months	CBI survivors had significantly worse prospective memory ($p < 0.01$)
Vanderploeg et al., 2005 [174]	X-sect.	254 "minor or mild uncomplicated head injuries" in motor vehicle accidents	3214 healthy	Mean = 8 years (≤ 16 years)	1. CBI survivors had significantly worse continuation trial 3 on PASAT ("a difficult measure of concentration and working memory") (OR = 1.32) 3. CBI survivors had significantly worse effect of proactive interference on working memory ($p < 0.01$) 3. No significant difference on more conventional NΨ tests

Table 5.4 (*Cont.*)

Author year	Study type	*n* CBI survivors	*n* healthy subjects	Follow-up	Results
Vanderploeg et al., 2007 [175]	X-sect.	254 "minor or mild uncomplicated head injuries" in motor vehicle accidents	3214 healthy	Mean = 8 years (≤ 16 years)	1. CBI survivors had significantly higher frequency of "PC syndrome" (adjusted OR 1.80–1.99) 2. CBI survivors had significantly more balance or dizziness problems (adjusted OR = 2.43), light sensitivity (adjusted OR = 1.92), headaches (adjusted OR = 1.94), trouble sleeping (adjusted OR = 1.85), double vision (adjusted OR = 1.81, and fatigue (adjusted OR = 1.42) 3. CBI survivors had significantly more periods of confusion or memory loss (adjusted OR = 2.80), memory problems (adjusted OR = 1.75), and irritability (OR = 1.36) 4. CBI survivors had significantly more peripheral visual imperceptions (adjusted OR = 1.98) and impaired tandem gait (adjusted OR = 2.93) 5. No significant difference in olfaction 6. CBI survivors significantly more likely to be unmarried (adjusted OR = 2.01), employed less than full time (adjusted OR = 1.89), have incomes < $10,000/year (adjusted OR = 1.88), and have self-reported disability (adjusted OR = 2.90) (Analyses controlled for demographics and pre-injury medical, neurological, and psychiatric conditions)
Vanderploeg et al., 2009 [176]	X-sect.	254 "minor or mild uncomplicated head injuries" in motor vehicle accidents	3214 healthy	Mean = 8 years (≤ 16 years)	1. CBI survivors more likely to have memory problems (adjusted OR = 1.31), headaches (adjusted OR = 1.30), and sleep problems (adjusted OR = 1.37) 2. CBI survivors more likely to have somatic sxs (adjusted OR = 1.34) 3. CBI survivors more likely to meet criteria for "PC syndrome" (Analyses controlled for demographics and pre-injury medical, neurological, and psychiatric conditions)
Waljas et al., 2015 [278]	X-sect.	103 "mTBI"	36 matched healthy controls	12 months	1. No difference in diagnosis of "mild or greater" "PC syndrome" (ICD-10 criteria; CBI survivors = 37.9%; controls = 30.6%) 2. CBI survivors significantly more likely to have "moderate or greater" "PC syndrome" (ICD-10 criteria; CBI survivors = 12%; controls = 0%; p = 0.036) 3. CBI survivors had significantly higher total RPSQ scores than controls (p = 0.015) 3. CBI survivors were more likely to complain of 1–10 post-concussive symptoms (50.5% vs. 24.1%) (Inclusion controlled for litigation; analyses controlled for prior TBI)

(continued)

Table 5.4 (*Cont.*)

Author year	Study type	*n* CBI survivors	*n* healthy subjects	Follow-up	Results
Wright and Telford, 1996 [279]		42 "predom. minor head injury"	42 healthy	6 months	1. CBI survivors had significantly higher General Health Questionnaire scores (6.2 vs. 1.1; *p* < 0.01) 2. CBI survivors were more likely to report high levels of distress (48% vs. 0% controls)

[a] Re Alexander et al., 2015 [247]: (1) 1 Students who elected non-contact sports had higher baseline intellect than those who elected rugby. (2) Seven rugby subjects and three non-rugby subjects had prior concussions. (3) None of the rugby playing teens without *known* concussions can be assumed to have healthy brains. Contact sport players routinely underreport concussions and are prone to suffer sub-clinical cognitive impairments in the absence of a diagnosable concussion. See [156].

[b] Re Baldassarre et al., 2015 [242]: (1) The flow sheet for the parent study states there were 196 "TCR screen positive" and 242 "TCR screen negative." *TCR screen* is not translated. (2) The text (p. 850) states that "188 veterans endorsed a history of mTBI and 201 did not." (3) Table 3 (p. 851) states that 210 had mTBI and 188 had no mTBI. Therefore, it is impossible to determine how many cases and controls were recruited for this study.

[c] Re Bernstein, 2002 [248]: seven of 13 subjects reported more than one concussion.

[d] Re Cicerone, 1996 [36]: this study did not assess a representative sample of CBI patients. The subjects had been referred because of persistent problems. It is nonetheless included because it illustrates the importance of using sensitive tests.

[e] Re Clarke et al., 2012 [177]: results on cognitive and non-cognitive measures did not differ by time interval since injury, from 3 to 12 months. The Clarke study is too small to have probative value, but the authors deserve credit for the creativity of their analyses.

[f] Re Ellemberg et al., 2007 [251]: none of the female soccer teen players without *known* concussions can be assumed to have healthy brains.

[g] Re Fay et al., 1994 [254]: the authors reported the significance of differences across levels of severity. The significance of the differences between mild cases and controls was not reported.

[h] Re Hoge et al., 2008 [181]: the authors did not report the time from injury to assessment.

[i] Re Jakola et al., 2007 [255]: the control group was randomly selected; those subjects cannot be assumed to be healthy.

[j] Re Killam et al., 2005 [156]: the group identified as "athletes/non-concussed" cannot be presumed to be a healthy normal group because: (1) contact post players tend to underreport concussions; and (2) as Killam et al., state: "More provocatively, the data also suggest that participation in contact sports may produce sub-clinical cognitive impairments in the absence of a diagnosable concussion presumably resulting from the cumulative consequences produced by multiple mild head trauma" (p. 599).

[k] Re Klein et al., 1996 [35]: this study was accepted because, although the authors included several cases of "moderate severity," their "method" implies that those cases perhaps fall into a border-zone between mild and moderate. First, moderate cases were included if they were "uncomplicated" and excluded if there was a skull fracture. Second, the severity of the injuries is hard to infer because the authors employed an idiosyncratic grading system: patients were asked to report their duration of coma, degree of memory loss, and duration of post-concussive complaints, each on a four-point scale. "The subsequent summation of the scores on the three scales yielded a crude measure of the severity of TBI" (p. 461).

[l] Re Segalowitz et al., 2001 [273]: seven mTBI subjects reported more than one head injury.

[m] Re Singh et al., 2014 [140]: no credible reason exists to assume that "non-concussed players" had not been concussed.

AVLT: Auditory Verbal Learning Test; CBCL: Child Behavior Checklist; CBI: concussive brain injury; c/o: complain of; CVLT: California Verbal Learning Test [243, 244]; c/w: compared with; ImPACT: ImPACT Postconcussion Symptoms Inventory; LOC: loss of consciousness; MHI: minor head injury; NΨ: neuropsychological; NS: not significant; Observ.: observational study; OR: odds ratio; PASAT: Paced Auditory Serial Addition Task [245, 246]; PCS: post-concussion syndrome; Pop.: population-based study; Prosp. long.: prospective longitudinal study; RBANS: Repeatable Battery for the Assessment of Neuropsychological Status; Retrosp.: retrospective study; RPSQ: Rivermead Postconcussion Symptom Questionnaire; SF36: Short Form 36; sxs: symptoms; TBI: traumatic brain injury; w: with; WISC: Wechsler Intelligence Scale of Children; w/o: without; X-sect.: cross-sectional study.

- Other problems seem to occur more frequently after CBI than after non-brain damage. A reasonable explanation is that these are, in fact, specific to brain injury (e.g., diplopia).

Unfortunately, it is almost unheard of for scholars to make these distinctions. The plurality of published studies is content to compare total RPSQ scores without fussing with questions of global life impact or pathophysiology.

One more explanation for the elevated prevalence of persistent symptoms among CBI survivors deserves consideration: *brain injury* is affectively loaded. The phrase seems more likely to trigger fears and spark litigious quiverings. That might indeed account for some of the difference in self-reported symptoms. But that would hardly account for the published differences in objectively measured impairments.

At this point, the present author is left with gently requesting that the remaining skeptics look at the inclusion and exclusion criteria and analytic controls employed in these studies. Although very few good studies have controlled for all of the commonly suspected confounding variables, multiple studies have controlled for the two most important confounds: prior TBI and pre-morbid psychiatric history. As the author will propose further on in this chapter: the commonsense conclusion from the available body of controlled long-term research is that, no matter how scholars have tested the hypothesis, no matter how many confounding factors they have excluded, a strong body of peer-reviewed reports suggests that CBI survivors often exhibit disproportionate, measurable, persistent problems – problems that are most parsimoniously explained as the consequence of brain shaking.

Pre-Emptively Curbing Enthusiasm

As remarked at the outset of this chapter, it would be medically precious to credibly determine what proportion of CBI survivors suffer what type and duration of post-concussive sequelae. However, no single analytic method commends itself for extracting lessons from the wealth of hard-won data in Tables 5.3–5.5. Ask your neighborhood biostatistician. He or she may laugh. For example, what helpful procedure exists to quantitatively compare or synthesize a study of 249 motor vehicle

Table 5.5 Medium- to long-term studies of post-concussive problems employing injured or ill controls

Author, year	Type of study	n CBI survivors	n non-TBI injury subjects	Follow-up	Results
Bazarian et al., 1999 [291]	Prosp. long.	65 minor head injury	59 orthopedic	6 months	1. 25% of CBI survivors met criteria for "PC syndrome" vs. 34% of controls
Boake et al., 2005 [292]	Prosp. long.	160 TBI M GCS = 14.6	97 general trauma	6 months.	1. CBI survivors "tended to report greater difficulty" at work 2. No significant difference in employment rate (CBI survivors = 61%, trauma = 62%) 3. No significant difference in jobs performed pre- and post-injury (CBI = 79%; trauma = 80%) (Inclusion controlled for past TBI hospitalization, substance dependence, mental retardation, psychosis)
Bohnen et al., 1994 [293]	Case–control	152 mild head injury	152 general practice patients	1–5 years	1. CBI survivors had significantly higher scores on cognitive performance complaints ($p < 0.001$) and somatic complaints ($p < 0.001$) 2. Results accounted for, in part, by pre-existing emotional status and injury-related neurological complications
Bohnen et al., 1995 [294]	Case–control	231 MHI	231 general practice patients	1–5 years (mean = 2.1 years)	CBI survivors reported significantly more sxs than controls on 21/41 items
Brooks et al., 2016 [295]	Prosp.	77 youth "mTBI"	28 orthopedic	3 months	CBI survivors were significantly more likely to be "not recovered" (13.7% vs. 7.1%) "significantly higher PCSI total scores and very large effect sizes for the "mTBI not recovered" group compared to … OIC groups at each time point" (p. 382)
Bryant and Harvey, 1999 [154]	Prosp. long.	46 "mTBI" motor vehicle	56 motor vehicle	6 months	1. CBI survivors were more likely to be irritable (68% vs. 30.5%) 2. CBI survivors were more likely to have headaches (37% vs. 27%) 3. CBI survivors were more likely to have dizziness (15% vs. 7%) 2. Non-CBI patients were more likely to be diagnosed with PTSD (28% vs. 20%)
Clarke et al., 2012 [177]		21 "mTBI"	19 spinal injury	3–12 months	1. No significant difference on conventional NΨ tests 2. No difference re cognitive complaints 3. No difference re neuroticism 4. Both CBI and spinal subjects showed significant association between affective distress and PC symptoms 5. Both CBI and spinal subjects showed significant association between cognitive complaints and PC symptoms 6. CBI subjects with poorer NΨ results had more cognitive complaints ($p < 0.01$), affective distress (p< 0.05), and PC symptoms ($p < 0.01$)
De Leon et al., 2009 [296]	Prosp. X-sect.	58 "mild head injury"	128 "mild nonhead injury"	12 months	Injury type did not predict fatigue
Dikmen et al., 2001 [110]	Prosp. long.	157 "mTBI"	109 trauma	12 months	1. CBI survivors had lower Selective Reminding Test sum of recall scores when controlled for pre-injury traits 2. No significant difference on other NΨ tests
Dikmen et al., 2010 [a] [286]	Prosp. long.	365 "mTBI" 68 mild 1 297 mild 2	111 general trauma	12 months	CBI "Mild 2" subjects had significantly worse complaints re memory ($p = 0.000$), temper ($p = 0.002$), dizziness ($p = 0.003$), and total sxs ($p = 0.000$) (Inclusion partly controlled for pre-injury medical conditions)
Donnell et al., 2012 [178]	X-sect.	154 "mTBI"	MDD = 58; GAD = 141; somatiz. D = 21; alcohol abuse = 391; PTSD = 130	~ 8 years	1. CBI survivors (with 32%) had a lower frequency of DSM-IV "PC syndrome" than subjects with MDD (55%), GAD (50%), somatiz D. (91%), PTSD (40%) 2. CBI survivors (32%) had a higher frequency of DSM-IV "PC syndrome" than subjects with alcohol abuse (26%)

(continued)

Table 5.5 (*Cont.*)

Author, year	Type of study	n CBI survivors	n non-TBI injury subjects	Follow-up	Results
Edna, 1987 [297]	Prosp. long.	361 MHI	110 acute appendicitis	3–5 years Mean = 4 years	CBI survivors had significantly more complaints ($p = 0.03$)
Edna and Cappelen, 1987 [b] [298]	X-sect.	485 (430 with "mTBI")	93 acute appendicitis	3–5 years Mean = 4 years	1. 51% of CBI survivors had new (post-injury onset) symptoms 3–5 years post injury 2. Within CBI survivors: females more likely to complain of headache (38% vs. 18%; $p < 0.01$), dizziness (31% vs. 14%, $p < 0.01$), irritability to noise, light (24% vs. 16%, $p < 0.05$), insomnia (20% vs. 11%; $p < 0.01$), depression (13% vs. 85; $p < 0.05$), and anxiety (12% vs. 6%; $p < 0.05$) (Controlled for pre-injury complaints)
Ettenhofer and Abeles, 2009 [280]	X-sect.	63 "mTBI"	63 orthopedic	Mean = 34.3 months	1. CBI survivors had significantly lower scores on trails letter sequencing ($p < 0.05$), but not on other NΨ tests 2. No significant group difference on self-reported PC sxs or psychiatric sxs
Ettenhofer and Barry, 2012 [c] [179]	X-sect.	256 "mTBI"	491 orthopedic	CBI: mean = 3.59 years Orthopedic: mean = 2.81 years	1. CBI survivors had significantly higher PC symptom scores ($p = 0.016$) 2. CBI survivors significantly more likely to have somatic symptoms ($p = 0.022$), dizziness ($p < 0.001$), cognitive symptoms ($p = 0.03$) (Inclusion controlled for past TBI, pre-injury psychotic, or neurological illness)
Friedland and Dawson, 2001 [299]	Prosp. long.	64 "mTBI" in MVA	35 MVA	9 months	1. No difference in perception of disability, satisfaction with return to normal living, or rate of return to work 2. CBI survivors had significantly higher scores on stress ($p < 0.05$) and more dysfunction on psychosocial scores ($p = 0.01$)
Hajek et al., 2010 [300]	Prosp. long.	167 "mTBI" children	84 orthopedic	12 months	1. 19% of both CBI survivors and controls were diagnosed with "PC syndrome" 2. CBI survivors had greater cognitive symptoms than controls 3. Controlling for PTSD, CBI survivors had significantly higher PC symptom scores ($p = 0.000$) and higher cognitive impairment scores ($p = 0.005$) (Analysis controlled for PTSD)
Hanten et al, 2013 [180]	Prosp. long.	59 "mTBI" young adults	58 orthopedic	3 months	No significant difference on a working-memory task
Heltemes et al., 2012 [301]	X-sect.	473 "mTBI"	656 minor non-TBI injury	6 months	CBI survivors were significantly more likely to report a "major negative change" in self-rated health: - CBI: 41.3% - Other injury 16.5% ($p = 0.001$)
Hoge et al., 2008 [d] [181]	X-sect.	124 "mTBI" w LOC 260 "mTBI" w altered mental status	435 other injury	> 4 months	1. CBI survivors were divided into those with and without LOC 2. CBI survivors with LOC were significantly more likely to report poor overall health ($p = 0.04$) and elevated health problem scores ($p < 0.001$) 3. CBI survivors with LOC were more likely to report significantly more missed work days ($p = 0.02$), medical visits ($p = 0.005$), headaches ($p < 0.001$), chest pain ($p < 0.001$), dizziness ($p = 0.01$), heart pounding ($p < 0.001$), shortness of breath ($p = 0.02$), bowel problems ($p = 0.006$), fatigue, ($p < 0.001$), and sleep disturbance ($p = 0.001$). 4. CBI survivors with LOC reported significantly more memory problems ($p = 0.005$), balance problems ($p = 0.02$), ringing in the ears ($p = 0.01$), concentration problems ($p = 0.002$), and irritability ($p < 0.001$) CBI survivors with altered mental status reported more heart pounding ($p = 0.01$) and irritability ($p = 0.006$) 6. After controlling for depression and PTSD, the only remaining significant differences pertained to headache and heart pounding

Table 5.5 (*Cont.*)

Author, year	Type of study	*n* CBI survivors	*n* non-TBI injury subjects	Follow-up	Results
Kraus et al., 2005 [302]	Prosp. long.	235 "mTBI"	235 non-head injuries	6 months	1. CBI survivors reported more headaches (ARR = 1.31), dizziness (ARR = 1.50), blurred vision (ARR = 1.50), double vision (ARR = 1.81), noise bothersome (ARR = 1.35), memory problems (ARR = 1.52), learning problems (ARR = 1.52), and lower alcohol tolerance (ARR = 1.88) (all 90% confidence intervals and after adjustment for history of concussion, alcohol use, and mechanism of injury) 2. Other medical subjects more likely to be troubled by sleep disturbance (relative risk = 0.84)
Kraus et al., 2009 [e][303]	Prosp. long.	454 "mTBI" (?)	795 non-head-injured ED patients	3 months	1. CBI survivors were significantly more likely to have "PC syndrome" (32% vs. 19%; $p < 0.0001$) 2. CBI survivors had significantly higher total RPSQ scores (mean = 7.17 vs. 4.04; $p < 0.01$) 3. CBI survivors significantly more likely to complain re sleep quality (mean = 6.35 vs. 5.82; $p < 0.05$)
Kraus et al., 2014 [f] [304]	Prosp. long.	368 "mTBI" (?)	596 non-head-injured ED patients	6 months	1. CBI survivors reported more PC symptoms in each of 16 categories 2. CBI survivors had higher RPQ mean scores (5.97 vs. 3.61) 3. CBI surivors had higher rates per 100 adults reporting ≥ 3 sxs (28.12 vs. 17.15)
Levin et al., 2013 [305]	Prosp.	102 "mTBI"	85 orthopedic	3 months	1. CBI survivors had significantly higher symptom composite scores ($p = 0.0001$) 2. CBI survivors had lower cognitive processing speed, which was also significantly age-related ($p = 0.0014$) 3. No difference in verbal or visual memory (Excluded subjects with prior neurological disorder, bipolar disorder, schizophrenia, or substance abuse)
Losoi et al., 2015 [g] [306]	Prosp.	60 "mTBI"	29 orthopedic	12 months	CBI survivors had significantly more PCS, fatigue, and stress sxs @ 12 months ($p < 0.01$) (Excluded subjects with pre-injury medical, psychiatric, or neurological problems)
Losoi et al., 2016 [g] [168]	Prosp.	60 "mTBI"	20 orthopedic	12 months	1. CBI survivors had slightly higher mean PCS sxs (6.9 vs. 4.4, NS) 2. Somewhat more CBI survivors met criteria for persistent "PC syndrome" (31.7% vs. 20.6%, NS) 3. No significant difference on quality of life 4. No significant difference on life satisfaction (Excluded subjects with pre-injury medical, psychiatric, or neurological problems)
Masson et al., 1996 [307]	X-sect.	114 minor head injury	64 lower-limb injury	5 years	1. CBI survivors had significantly more somatic sxs: headache ($p < 0.001$), memory problems ($p < 0.05$), dizziness ($p < 0.01$), and sleep disturbance ($p < 0.05$) 2. CBI survivors had significantly more psychiatric sxs: depression ($p < 0.01$), anxiety ($p < 0.01$), and irritability ($p < 0.01$) 3. Lower-limb injury subjects had more pain ($p < 0.001$)
McLean et al., 2009 [h] [166]	Prosp. X-sect.	251 "CDC mTBI"	168 other injury	12 months	CBI survivors had "a significantly higher incidence of PC syndrome and reported cognitive symptoms" ($p < 0.001$) (p. 185)
Meares et al., 2011 [308]	Prosp. long.	62 "mTBI"	58 non-brain-injured trauma	3 months	1. CBI survivors significantly more likely to be aggravated by noise ($p = 0.004$) 2. No difference in frequency of "PC syndrome" (CBI survivors = 46.8%; trauma = 46.3%) (Inclusion controlled for psychosis, pre-injury cognitive impairment, response bias)

(*continued*)

Table 5.5 (*Cont.*)

Author, year	Type of study	*n* CBI survivors	*n* non-TBI injury subjects	Follow-up	Results
Mickeviciene et al., 2002 [143]	X-sect. Case–control	131 "mTBI"	146 minor non-head injury	22–35 months (mean= 28 months)	1. CBI survivors significantly more likely to report depression ($p = 0.002$) and intolerance of alcohol ($p = 0.04$) 2. CBI survivors marginally more likely to report sporadic memory problems ($p = 0.052$) 3. No significant difference in reported headaches, dizziness, concentration, and nine other PC symptoms
Mickeviciene et al., 2004 [309]	Prosp. long. Case–control	192 "mTBI"	215 minor injury	12 months	1. CBI survivors significantly more likely to have memory problems ($p = 0.01$), concentration problems ($p = 0.01$), tiredness ($p = 0.01$), and depression ($p = 0.05$) 2. No significant difference in reported headaches, dizziness, and eight other PC symptoms (Inclusion controlled for "significant" pre-injury neurological and psychiatric conditions)
Nash et al., 2014 [310]	Prosp. long.	89 "mTBI"	70 "seriously injured non-TBI"	12 months	1. CBI survivors had significantly worse memory disorders ($p < 0.001$), attention ($p < 0.05$), initiative $p < 0.05$), and anxiety ($p < 0.05$) 2. No significant difference on trail-making test
Pieper and Garvan, 2014 [167]	Prosp.	24 "mTBI" children	27 matched "mild non-brain injuries"	12 months	No significant difference on physical health, psychosocial health, or cognitive fatigue
Ponsford et al., 2000 [311]	X-sect.	84 "mTBI"	53 other minor injury	3 months	1. CBI survivors had significantly worse headaches ($p = 0.013$) and more concentration difficulties ($p = 0.024$) 2. 24% of "mTBI" subjects had "ongoing problems" vs. 0% of injured controls 3. No significant difference on conventional NΨ tests
Ponsford et al., 2011 [312]	Prosp. long.	90 "mTBI"	80 matched minor injury	3 months	1. CBI survivors had: - significantly worse visual memory composite scores ($p = 0.015$) - significantly more post-concussive symptoms ($p < 0.0001$) - significantly more reports of cognitive impairment ($p = 0.003–0.016$) 2. CBI survivors had non-significant trend for more sadness and fatigue 4. No significant difference on composite scores for verbal, memory, motor speed, or reaction time (Inclusion controlled for pre-injury neurological or psychiatric conditions)
Ponsford et al., 2012 [313]	Prosp. long.	90 "mTBI"	80 matched minor injury	3 months	1. No significant difference in frequency of "PS syndrome" 2. No significant. difference in level of anxiety and depression (HADS) (Inclusion controlled for pre-injury neurological or psychiatric conditions)
Rabinowitz et al., 2015 [182]	Prosp.	66 "mTBI"	68 orthopedic	3 months	1. CBI survivors were significantly more likely to have prolonged elevated symptomatology (52% vs. 17%; $p = 3.905e-05$) 2. No significant difference in cognitive scores
Sheedy et al., 2009 [314]	Prosp. long.	76 "mTBI"	89 minor non-head injury	3 months	1. CBI survivors had significantly more PC symptoms ($p < 0.001$) 2. CBI survivors significantly more likely to have "PC syndrome" (25.6% vs. 2.2%; $p < 0.001$) (Excluded subjects with pre-injury history of psychosis)
Smith-Seemiller et al., 2003 [315]	X-sect.	32 "mTBI"	63 chronic pain	Mean = 12.3 months	1. CBI survivors significantly more likely to have memory problems ($p = 0.004$), concentration problems ($p = 0.05$), taking longer to think ($p = 0.01$), light sensitivity ($p = 0.001$), noise sensitivity ($p = 0.01$), and double vision ($p = 0.04$) 2. No significant difference in total PC symptom scores 3. Pain subjects significantly more likely to report sleep problems ($p = 0.0003$), depression ($p = 0.02$), and restlessness ($p = 0.005$)

Table 5.5 (*Cont.*)

Author, year	Type of study	*n* CBI survivors	*n* non-TBI injury subjects	Follow-up	Results
Studer et al., 2014 [316]		37 pediatric "mTBI"	34 orthopedic	4 months	1. No significant difference on conventional NΨ tests 2. No significant difference in sociobehavioral problems (Excluded subjects with pre-existing psychiatric or neurological disorders except ADHD)
Stulemeijer et al., 2008 [i] [235]	Prosp. long.	201 "mTBI"	287 wrist/ankle injury	6 months	More CBI survivors had elevated PC symptoms (24.4% vs. 6%)
Taylor et al., 2010 [62]	X-sect.	169 "mTBI" children	84 orthopedic	12 months	1. CBI survivors had significantly higher parent ratings of cognitive symptoms 2. CBI survivors had significantly higher self-rated symptoms
Vanderploeg et al., 2005 [174]	X-sect.	254 "minor or mild uncomplicated head injuries" in MVAs	539 MVAs without TBI	Mean = 8 years (≤ 16 years)	1. CBI survivors significantly worse on continuation trial 3 of PASAT (OR 1.53) 2. No significant difference on more conventional NΨ tests
Vanderploeg et al., 2007 [175]	X-sect.	254 "minor or mild uncomplicated head injuries" in MVAs	539 MVAs without TBI	Mean = 8 years (≤ 16 years)	1. CBI survivors had higher frequency of DSM-IV "PC syndrome" vs. MVA (40.9% vs. 25.2%; adjusted OR 1.80–1.99) 2. CBI survivors had more headaches (adjusted OR = 1.94), and trouble sleeping (adjusted OR = 1.85) 3. CBI survivors had more periods of confusion or memory loss (adjusted OR = 2.80), and memory problems (adjusted OR 1.75) 4. CBI survivors had more peripheral visual imperceptions (adjusted OR = 1.98) and impaired tandem gait (adjusted OR = 2.93) 5. No significant difference in olfaction CBI survivors more likely to be unmarried (adjusted OR = 2.01), employed less than full time (adjusted OR 1.89), and have incomes < $10,000/year (adjusted OR = 1.88) (Analyses controlled for demographics and pre-injury medical, neurological, and psychiatric conditions)
Vanderploeg et al., 2009 [176]	X-sect.	254 "minor or mild uncomplicated head injuries" in MVAs	539 MVAs without TBI	Mean = 8 years (≤ 16 years)	1. CBI survivors had more memory problems (adjusted OR = 1.31), headaches (adjusted OR = 1.30), and sleep problems (adjusted OR = 1.21) 2. CBI survivors more likely to fulfill DSM diagnosis criteria for PCS (41.4% vs. 25.2%; adjusted OR = 1.37) 3. CBI survivors more likely to faint (adjusted OR = 1.80) 4. CBI survivors more likely to have persistent PTSD after 16 years (11.5% vs. 5.8%; adjusted OR = 1.41) (Analyses controlled for demographics, medical conditions, and any current psychiatric conditions, i.e., depression, PTSD, alcohol abuse)
Webb et al., 2015 [317]	X-sect.	5065 "mTBI"	44,733 other-injured	≥ 180 days	CBI survivors more likely to have memory loss (HR 4.00; *p* = 0.05), cognitive disorders NOS (HR 10.75; *p* = 0.05), sleep disorders (HR 1.30; *p* = 0.05), epilepsy (HR 3.28; *p* = 0.05) and pain disorders (HR 1.44; *p* = 0.05) (Analyses controlled for depression and PTSD)

[a] Re Dikmen et al., 2010 [286]: the "mTBI" group was divided into "mild 1" (normal CT; PTA < 24 h) and "mild 2" (abnormal CT or PTA > 24 h). Unfortunately, no analyses were reported or could be reconstructed regarding the entire "mTBI" group.

[b] Re Edna, 1987 [297] vs. Edna and Cappelen, 1987 [298]: (a) The first study excluded subjects with intracranial hematomas. A total of 361/504 subjects responded to recruitment. Comparisons were reported between post-traumatic symptoms of CBI and control subjects. The second study included subjects with intracranial hematomas. In all, 430 of 569 subjects responded. The prevalence of symptoms among control subjects was not reported. Although the text states, "The frequencies of … complaints … in the control group compared largely with the frequencies of preinjury complaints in the head injury group," that frequency was *also* not reported. (2) The second study was included despite the possible inclusion of some "moderately" brain-injured subjects. A total of 88% of 351 males and 90% of 134 females were "mild" cases, so the study is credited with 430 mild subjects. Oddly, no comparisons are reported regarding post-traumatic symptoms of the two subject groups. Moreover, the time between acute illness and symptom report is unclear for the comparison subjects.

[c] Re Ettenhofer and Barry, 2012 [179]: like many studies comparing groups with different injuries, this one failed to assess the two groups at the same time post

(continued)

Table 5.5 (*Cont.*)

accident survivors aged 35–70 followed for an average 4.8 years of whom 54% had reduced life satisfaction with a study of 126 teenaged survivors of sport-related CBI followed for an average of 2.1 years of whom 32% had three or more persistent post-concussive symptoms? Arithmetic creates the illusion of facts. The present author defers to those with superior numeracy who might devise a magical analytic method that avoids bias and accommodates the fact that no two studies by different research groups were methodologically comparable.

One major conundrum is the difficulty of authentically assessing the life-changing impact of these injuries. If one counts so-called "post-concussive symptoms," the study is likely to overestimate the impact of the injury, since many of those symptoms are common among healthy people and those with other illnesses. If one assays cognition with desktop neuropsychological tests, the study is likely to underestimate the life impact, since such testing is ecologically invalid and often insensitive to the functionally limiting effects of CBI. Even if two studies employed the same outcome measure – for example, the GOSE as recommended by NINDS – such instruments are blunt tools that simply do not communicate the impact of the injury. For instance, two CBI survivors may both be accurately scored as "lower moderate disability" on the GOSE. One maintains his pre-morbid IQ of 143 and works at his nuclear fusion research job, although his wife left him and he's been arrested for brawling in a tavern. The other is an amiable companion, sweet as a kitten, but forgot how to put his garbage truck in reverse. The point: even within the same study, matching outcome scores hardly mean matching outcomes.[6]

How then might the most well-meaning and impartial team of scholars extract significance from Tables 5.3–5.5? Many analytic approaches conceivably add knowledge, but caveats abound.

For instance, one can enumerate studies that came to certain conclusions (e.g., "48 cross-sectional studies were positive and 12 were negative"). That provides a technically accurate overview of the literature. Yet such numbers have limited value, since not only do the cohort sizes vary greatly, but so do the demographic profiles, mechanisms of injuries, diagnostic methods, inclusion criteria, and assessment methods. For example, among the 24 studies that reported the proportion of CBI survivors with persistent problems at 12 months, the concussed cohorts varied from 19 [164] to 4202 [165]. These two reports cannot be granted equal weight. Yes, one can overcome the cohort size issue when studies report the frequency of an outcome by summing the absolute numbers of subjects affected in all studies. But that strategy fails to accommodate differences in outcome constructs and is prone to bias if one large study skews the results. Moreover, even if that mathematical trick would reduce the size-related bias, it presumes the two studies are equally right and true. (And all this leaves out the massive influence of the file drawer problem and positive publication bias.) This analytic project is perhaps akin to surveying the fauna in a vast rain forest: no single expedition is likely to have captured a full and accurate picture. One might precisely average the reports of geckos per square furlong, but which data set has what degree of reptilian validity with respect to the whole forest?

Another research approach would be to count controlled long-term studies of a given kind and determine whether a majority of studies found that CBI survivors were more affected than controls. As the reader will see, 53 controlled studies followed injured subjects for one year or more (range 12 months to 35.7 years) and reported whether one or more post-concussive problems was measurably greater among CBI survivors. Thirty-three of those long-term studies

---

6 This data chaos would be only slightly reduced if there is some day global compliance with the NINDS Common Data Elements initiative, since the only core outcome measure they support is the GOSE.

compared CBI with healthy subjects. Twenty compared CBI with non-brain-injured subjects. One of the 33 studies with healthy controls [141] and three of the 20 studies with injured controls [166–168] failed to report at least one significantly greater problem among CBI subjects on long-term follow-up. Thus, 99.2% of published studies report that concussed people have more problems than controls, persisting for one to almost 36 years. One might be tempted to conclude, "The evidence for persistent post-concussive problems is overwhelming!" The author demurs. So much pressure exists in academia favoring positive publications that this extraordinary result must be viewed with caution. Moreover, so many comparisons are represented that some differences surely arise from chance.

The Effect of Controlling for Suspected (Rarely Verified) Pre-Morbid Neurobehavioral Conditions

The present author strongly agrees with the widely expressed concern that pre-morbid status is an important conditioner of outcome. In fact, he speculates that the two largest confounding factors for long-term outcome may be prior TBI and pre-morbid psychiatric problems. (Prior TBI, in particular, is a well-established risk factor for poor outcome – which even skeptics acknowledge is itself compelling evidence that prior injury, however remote in time, *must* generate lasting deleterious effects.) He does not, however, subscribe to the transparent fallacy that pre-morbid neurobehavioral problems are grounds to dismiss the disabilities of CBI survivors, any more than one should dismiss a broken hip in a patient with osteoporosis. Since the magnitude of the influence of pre-morbid problems has yet to be determined (and is surely individual), another analytic approach might be to compare the prevalence of persistent problems in studies that did or did not exclude subjects with pre-morbid troubles. Of course, that exercise is easier contemplated than performed, because some studies are much more exclusive than others. For instance, Broglio et al. [141] excluded subjects with prior neurological disorders, Catale et al. [169] excluded subjects with pre-injury learning disability or neurological disorders, and Geary et al. [170] excluded all subjects involved in litigation, those with pre-injury neurological or psychiatric conditions, and those suspected of response bias. In addition, the disorders included by a stated category of exclusion are rarely specified. (Does Catale et al.'s phrase "neurological disorders" include childhood unreported concussions [169]?)

All that aside, excluding subjects with pre-morbid ills is a seductive error.

What happens when one confines his or her attention to the subset of subjects perfectly free of pre-morbid neurobehavioral conditions? That exclusion is popular among skeptics who suspect (with good reason) that long-term post-concussive complaints are influenced by pre-existing traits, and editors accept that selection maneuver with placid complacence. Yet the conceptual costs and benefits of this research maneuver deserve comment. If one's life goal is to determine the impact of concussion on the ideal specimen of human vigor and mental

equipoise, the exclusion is required. But what if, instead, one's goal is to determine the effects of concussion in a representative human population?

Consider the implications of one recent rodent experiment. In 2017 Peña et al. [171] reported on C57BL/6J mice that were exposed to early-life stress and later tested for vulnerability to adult stress. Those authors found that early stress alters the function of ventral tegmental "reward" area in a way that renders the brain permanently susceptible to later stress. That change was due to altered transcriptional programming of the ventral tegmental area, a change that seems to be mediated by an early-life decrease in the developmental transcription factor, orthodenticle homeobox 2 (*Otx2*). In an apparent proof of principle, they also found that overexpression of *Otx2* reverses the adult vulnerability caused by early-life stress – thus describing for the first time a specific physiological mechanism that explains individual variation in stress responsiveness. That is, in addition to our awareness that genetic variants predispose some individuals to stress, one can now point to a pathophysiological sequence by which environment does the same. As the present author will urge in a forthcoming chapter, the traditional Western paradigm of disease fails to accommodate the central role of individual differences in response to a biological challenge. A new paradigm was introduced by Garrod in 1908 [172] and has finally gained traction with the innovation of precision medicine. A disease is not an identifiable insult that impacts a patient. It is an interaction between a challenge and individual biology, yielding a broad spectrum of results, only some of which cause undesirable life perturbation (dis-ease).

Therefore, the tactic of confining attention to the previously optimum brain is bound to mislead in two ways. First, to exclude those with pre-morbid troubles means to study the effects of concussion on a special subset of humans. One might as well study the effects of otitis media among toddlers, but exclude all toddlers who had ever had otitis media. In other words, the enthusiasm for excluding subjects with pre-morbid TBI or neuropsychiatric troubles in favor of focusing on ideal specimens obviates any possibility of understanding how concussion affects the human species, since about half of humans will be erased from the record [173]. Second, such exclusion also obviates investigating the possibility that pre-morbid status itself somehow affects the risk of concussion (as shown in Chapter 2). Confining research attention to a special subgroup of robust, resilient, ever-healthy people may mean drawing conclusions from a population that has a systematically different physiological response to abrupt external force. Put simply, excluding people with a history of any of a large number of common human conditions is hard-to-defend medical discrimination.

Acknowledging these admonitions, studies that excluded persons with prior TBIs and/or pre-morbid psychiatric problems were identified. The results of that subset of studies were analyzed separately for Tables 5.4 and 5.5. Readers, forearmed with this discussion, can judge for themselves how that curious data might be interpreted.

The Tables

A total of 166 publications met the stated inclusion and exclusion criteria. Three of those apparently reported different data from the same cohort and are therefore regarded as a single study [174–176]. Eight studies provided data suitable for listing in more than one table [167, 174–182]. This review therefore systematically identified and tabulated results from 152 unique studies.

Table 5.3 is offered in the spirit of a systematic, if not necessarily comprehensive, review of the available data from uncontrolled research on medium- to longer-term outcomes after CBI. It will hopefully comprise a reference that will spare other scholars months of labor. But, in the present author's opinion, there is no scientific way to derive confident conclusions about the typical course of typical, clinically attended CBI from this data. Far too many methodological frailties and uncontrolled confounds are present to put much faith in even one of these reports. Since almost none of the studies shared methodology, meta-analysis would not be appropriate. Since so-called "post-concussive" symptoms are not unique to CBI, it is literally impossible to know what proportion of reported subjective complaints or objective impairments are attributable to brain rattling. And this is setting aside the freighted question of how to distinguish between direct effects of cerebral rattling versus the inevitable interactions between rattling, pre-morbid traits, and post-traumatic reactions. Therefore, as much as one might be impressed by the magnitude of this collective effort and proliferation of findings, one must take every reported numerical result with a large grain of salt.

Analytic Comments Regarding Table 5.3: Uncontrolled Studies of Concussion Survivors

Sixty-four peer-reviewed empirical papers reported outcomes among cohorts of concussion survivors consisting of 10–4202 subjects assessed at three months to 23 years post-injury. One duty of this volume is to impartially examine the Three-Month Myth – the notion popularized by some 20th-century writers that the overwhelming majority of CBI victims "recover" within three months. The uncontrolled data in Table 5.3 are not definitive in any way. However, limiting one's attention to the 20 studies that assayed neurobehavioral outcomes at one year post-injury, excluding the single endocrine report, and ignoring the substantive differences in the definitions of caseness, 12.8–82% of subjects remained symptomatic. Simple summation (not worthy of the label *meta-analysis*) reveals that 4624 of 9855 survivors remained symptomatic at one year, yielding a weighted average of 46.9% with persistent complaints, problems, or impairments.[7] If one performed the same analysis of the eight longer-term studies that reported the proportion persistently affected, then 405/1373 or 29.5% remained affected at a median of 2.5 years.

These figures are the result of a systematic and replicable review. They are not, however, offered as a milestone

discovery, or even an accurate estimate. To sum the findings and weight them according to cohort size assumes each study was equally accurate and representative. That could not possibly be the case. Therefore, although this chapter's figures may be far more credible than the boilerplate textbook guess of "10% remain affected beyond three months," they do not deserve a shrine.

Reading these papers, realizing the human effort involved, including the discommodious treatment of hundreds of subjects, one is disheartened at the waste. The scrupulous skeptics are entirely correct to doubt the value of this literature. Despite the compassion of the clinicians, the acuity of their observations, and the eloquence of their prose, one cannot conclude from this uncontrolled literature whether concussions cause the problems with which they are associated. Perhaps the principal virtue in studying this work is recognizing how exacting and familiar are the many early descriptions of post-concussive distress. Little has changed since Denker's comment, "The symptoms complained of were remarkably similar: headaches, dizziness and a heterogeneous group of 'Nervous' changes, such as irritability, weakness, difficulty in concentration, insomnia, antisociablity, hyperaccussis etc." ([241], p. 379).

Approaching Table 5.4

Better science has been done. Table 5.4 compiles the findings from all medium- to long-term studies of post-concussive problems identified by the search that employed healthy/normal controls and met inclusion criteria for review. Figure 5.3 illustrates a representative result from this kind of controlled, long-term study. Baldassarre et al. [242] compared persistent post-concussive symptoms among 188 military veterans with a history of "mTBI" at an average of 4.8 years post-injury versus 210 healthy controls. The CBI survivors expressed an average of 16.7 such symptoms; the healthy group expressed an average of 9.4.

The results in Figure 5.3 are not to be regarded as either definitive or representative. The picture is provided only to illustrate the important fact that medical complaints are a human commonplace. Knowing that, one knows better than to attribute every post-injury complaint to the injury. Table 5.4, nonetheless, is revealing.

Analytic Comments Regarding Table 5.4: Comparing Concussion Survivors With Healthy Persons

Unless the investigators massaged their findings (which perhaps occurs more often than is generally advertised), the data reported in Table 5.4 are facts. For the purposes of our analysis, we are obliged to take them at face value – always awaiting verification and replication. If these are the facts, then readers can judge for themselves whether persistent neurobehavior problems are more

---

[7]   Hartvigsen et al. [201] reported that "more than half" of 1128 subjects had three or more symptoms at 12 months. A conservative estimate might be 51% or 591. The final proportion 46.9% is based on that estimate. If the correct figure for Hartvigsen et al. were 60%, one would estimate 695 with symptoms. In that case, the in that study, the total final figure would have been 4728/9855 = 49%.

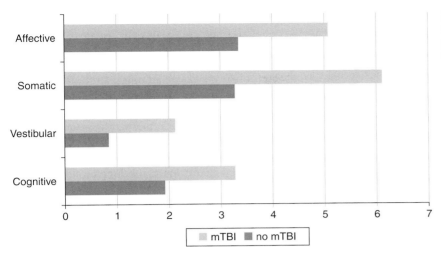

Fig. 5.3 Mean number of symptoms: mild traumatic brain injury (mTBI) versus no mTBI.
Source: Baldassarre et al., 2015 [242] with permission from Elsevier

common after CBI than in everyday life.[8] Of course, one must beware the *post hoc ergo propter hoc* fallacy; we have yet to scratch the surface of the many reasons a symptom might temporally follow a CBI. Yet the elevated prevalence compared with similarly assessed healthy subjects at least requires one to acknowledge an association between concussion and long-term distress.

Fifty-eight studies were identified that met the search criteria. However, Vanderploeg et al. composed three of them [174–176], seemingly based on the same cohort. Thus, 56 unique studies are included. Analysis of the collective findings might be divided into results pertaining to cognitive deficits and results pertaining to non-cognitive symptoms or impairments.

Cognitive Outcomes

The mTBI individuals had significant impairments in all cognitive domains compared to the healthy control subjects. Effect sizes of cognitive deficits were medium to large, and could not be accounted for by self-perceived deficits, depression, compensation claims or negative response bias.

(Konrad et al., 2011, [258], p. 1197)

Thirty-seven of these 56 studies reported results of cognitive testing. Among those, 29 (78.4%) reported that one or more test results were significantly inferior among CBI survivors. (Those 29 included 11 studies in which all results were inferior among CBI survivors and 18 in which only some test results were inferior in the injured group.) Nine of 37 studies (23.4%) reported no significant group difference in cognitive test results. Superficially these findings might be taken to imply that concussion is more likely than not to result in long-lasting cognitive impairments above and beyond those detected in a healthy group. However, several factors make one wary. First, no easy way exists to control for multiple comparisons. It is possible that, when a long battery of tests is administered to two groups,

one group will be significantly more impaired on one or more comparisons by chance. Second, summing papers is not scientific. Unless the studies have equal quality and matched cohorts, it is irrelevant if more papers find CBI victims to exhibit significant mental impairments. Third, although it is tempting to put faith in conclusions from comparing large groups, such findings may obfuscate the measurement of systematically different subgroups. Fourth, and most important, cognitive tests have no clear meaning. Although the results of a few individual desktop tests perhaps correlate weakly with activity in functional networks currently being investigated as contributors to given cognitive operations (replacing the 19th-century localizationist theories), no evidence has been produced elucidating the cerebral correlates of any collection of findings on any neuropsychological battery. The evidence from Table 5.4 is smoke, hinting that concussions cause lasting cognitive deficits, but not proving it.

In addition, seven studies compared the frequencies of subjective cognitive complaints [18, 170, 176, 177, 179, 280, 281]. Collectively, these studies included 1184 CBI subjects and 7618 healthy subjects. All seven studies reported significantly more complaints among CBI survivors than among healthy persons. At the extreme: Geary et al. [170] compared 40 "mTBI" subjects with 35 healthy persons at a mean of 5.29 years post-injury. A total of 82.5% of the CBI survivors had cognitive complaints; 0% of the healthy subjects did. It is widely understood in medicine that a complaint is not a disease.

One cannot conclude with confidence that lasting cerebral damage explains this dramatic difference in the prevalence of complaints. Surely, complainers include some exaggerators, imaginers, and inventors of symptoms. On the other hand, multiple studies show that subjective cognitive complaints antedate measurable deficits and brain degeneration in "mild cognitive impairment" and impending "Alzheimer's disease" [282–285]. One cannot shrug off the strong implications of these data: concussion often causes the persistent feeling of being impaired, which is plausibly due to being impaired.

---

8   Several tabulated studies enrolled both healthy controls and injured controls. In those cases, the results of comparisons with healthy controls appear in Table 5.4 and the results of comparisons with injured controls appear in Table 5.5.

Symptomatic Outcomes

Symptomatic outcomes (excluding cognition) include somatic, emotional, motor, functional, quality-of-health, and quality-of-life measures. (The author would add the closely related construct of subjective well-being, aka happiness, but that was not studied.) Since many studies reported total RPSQ scores but failed to enumerate which of those 16 symptoms differ to what extent, one cannot sum the subjects for whom each of these aspects of subjectivity was assessed. Eighteen studies reported symptoms, not otherwise specified (for instance, significant difference on RPSQ total scores). Fourteen of those (77.7%) reported that CBI survivors had significantly more or more severe symptoms. Two reported no significant difference between concussed and healthy subjects, and two reported mixed results. Nine studies explicitly compared somatic symptoms; all nine found those significantly greater among CBI survivors. Twelve studies reported emotional symptoms. Ten of those (83.3%) found significantly more symptoms among CBI survivors. Four studies reported motor symptoms; three of those found more symptoms in the concussed patients. Four studies reported subjective quality of health (for instance, Short Form 36 total scores); three of those found more global health concerns among the concussed. Three studies each reported functional and quality-of-life symptoms. In both cases, two of three studies found more symptoms among the concussed subjects.

Again, the neurobiological significance of these findings is unknown. One is obliged to absorb the information and speculate. The overwhelmingly greater symptom burden reported by CBI survivors is hard to ignore. As discussed elsewhere in this volume, the false dichotomy between psychological and neurological mediation of symptoms must be dismissed with prejudice. These findings probably indicate that typical concussion is likely to lead to long-term subjective distress due to changes in the brain.

Twenty independent studies reported in 22 publications were controlled in this way (although the exclusions varied between studies and the methods of exclusion were almost never revealed) [116, 148, 169, 170, 174–176, 180, 246, 248, 257–259, 261, 269, 274, 275, 278, 280, 286–288]. Within this subgroup, 16 studies employed neuropsychological testing. Five of those reported that CBI survivors performed worse than controls in all or most domains tested [35, 180, 247, 257, 259] and six reported CBI survivors performed worse on some tests but not others [169, 170, 174, 261, 269, 274]. Only two of 16 studies (12.5%) explicitly reported no significant group differences [177, 288]. These findings suggest that concussion causes lasting cognitive loss, even among the healthiest, but are not conclusive.

Among the same 20 narrowly focused studies, ten assessed persistent symptoms. In three of three studies that measured symptoms not otherwise specified (usually with the RPSQ total score) CBI was associated with significantly more symptoms compared with healthy controls [175, 275, 278]. In four of four studies that assessed cognitive complaints, CBI was associated with more [170, 175–177, 280]. In five of five studies that assessed persistent emotional symptoms, CBI was associated

with more [148, 170, 175–177, 280]. And in five of five studies that assessed somatic or physical symptoms, CBI was associated with more symptoms than controls [148, 175, 177, 249, 280].

Together, the findings from narrowly focused studies are interesting and possibly even meaningful. Without crediting the quality of the work, one can at least conclude that, when controlled for pre-existing conditions, many long-term cognitive changes – and *all* long-term non-cognitive changes – are significantly worse among the concussed. Three conceivable interpretations come to mind. One: cognitive tests are less valid measures of outcome than symptom assessment after CBI. As a result, studies employing desktop tests are less likely to detect the lasting effects of concussion. Two: cognitive tests are *more* valid than symptom assessment, so the mixed results among the cognitive papers are more representative of the truth. Three: the assessments are equally valid, but perhaps measurable cognitive problems are more likely to resolve in a year, while non-cognitive symptoms are more likely to persist. The author does not pretend to know which of these three is the most accurate.

In partial conclusion: our attempted rigorous review and analysis of the data comparing CBI survivors with healthy persons lead to a puzzle box of hints. When biomarkers are readily available, scholars will look back on convoluted exercises such as ours and feel pity. Innumerable mysteries will be promptly resolved. In the meantime, Table 5.4 confronts us with a great deal of inconclusive evidence supporting the hypothesis that concussion often leads to multiple long-term clinically significant neurobehavioral problems mediated by brain change.

Approaching Table 5.5

The incidence of symptoms at three months varies between 24% and 84%.

> (Rutherford, 1989 [289], p. 220)

sadly as many as 64% will experienced prolonged symptoms.
> (Bay and Liberzon, 2009 [290], p. 42)

If we consider all concussions/MTBIs, the percentage of people with poor outcome is likely very small (i.e. clearly less than 5%).

> (Iverson, 2005 [20], p. 306)

The data in Table 5.4, taken as a whole, are superficially compelling. In all, 51/56 (91%) studies reported that concussed persons either reported or exhibited one or more significantly worse long-term outcomes compared with healthy persons. Yet any scientist would require better data before arriving at a conclusion about the effects of CBI. It is easy to conjure up a list of potentially confounding factors that raise realistic doubts about the meaning of these data. Simply having been identified as a patient – regardless of the presence or absence of disease or severity of biological disruption – increases the likelihood of complaints.

Still, more than 75% of the 37 studies that administered neuropsychological tests reported some inferiority among CBI patients at a mean follow-up interval of 35.7 months. More than 80% of the 26 studies that assessed symptoms reported more symptoms among CBI patients at a mean of

30.3 months post-injury. Boiled down and admittedly over-simplified, Table 5.4 demonstrates that most peer-reviewed publications reporting empirical research found that cohorts of CBI survivors are significantly more likely than healthy persons to report or exhibit neurobehavioral problems more than two years after concussion.

That finding is not proof of long-term force-related brain damage. But it is also not compatible with the much-cited claim that "recovery" is complete at three months. Unlike the uncontrolled reports tabulated in Table 5.3, these controlled studies provide an abundance of data supporting the conclusion that concussions are often associated with long-term neurobehavioral distress above and beyond that experienced in the normal course of life. True, the papers report only statistical associations. Some third factor may be cryptically operative. However, without tormenting ourselves with an exegesis of Aristotle's theory of causality, to a reasonable degree of certainty one may conclude that a brain-rattling injury represents a risk factor – or biological trigger, or provocateur – but for which CBI survivors would not have exhibited such an excess of long-lasting troubles compared with healthy controls.

Is brain injury unique? Are commonly listed "post-concussive symptoms" specific to concussion? Or instead, might any traumatizing experience trigger more or less the same effects in a non-specific way? As previously mentioned (cf. the Dear Leader experiment), an even better way to evaluate the long-term impact of a concussion might be to compare CBI survivors with survivors of non-brain traumas, injuries, or other potentially distressing medical emergencies. This research strategy receives strong support in the recent literature. The author agrees that injury-controlled studies may be very helpful in determining whether there exist any unique or disproportionately common long-lasting problems after concussion – especially if those problems are more plausibly explained by brain damage than by ankle damage (e.g., diplopia). This helps (less than some writers have proposed) in drawing a distinction between symptoms that are almost universal after human trauma versus those that are especially common after CBI. Yet the rhetoric in the conclusion sections of some of these papers inspires two caveats.

First caveat: what value is there in comparing the *number of symptoms* in two diseases? The conceptual rationale for doing these studies is essentially flawed. In order to understand the effects of stroke on humans, shall we count how many symptoms stroke survivors have at one year and compare them with the number of symptoms reported by heart attack survivors? The inspiration implicit in many injury-controlled studies is, "Well, somebody claimed that brain concussion is associated with an average of 16 symptoms, some of which seem to be very logically explained by CBI. I will prove that wrong, showing that back injury may also cause 16 symptoms." The investigators would have more justification for publishing if, instead, they had asked, first, is long-term distress common or uncommon after head injury and back injury? It is unimportant how the prevalence of distress compares in the two illnesses. Second, does evidence exist that some problems are more common after head injury, others more common after back injury, and

others roughly equally common? That question makes common sense – but every reader already knows the answer without plowing through this prickly pack of papers. The principal drive behind this literature seems to have come from psychologists who wished to demonstrate that long-term survivors of CBI and survivors of non-brain injuries exhibit comparable performance on dated, conventional, desktop neuropsychological tests. Granted. That finding has been helpful in exposing the invalidity of those tests as measures of concussive effects. But it is not relevant to the question of whether CBI survivors have long-term brain damage – an issue that must be studied by test–pathophysiological correlation.

Second caveat: similar symptoms do not mean similar biological changes. Let's say a symptom is equally common one year after brain injury, leg injury, or low-back injury. Irritability seems to be one example. Multiple writers, making this observation, have leapt to the conclusion that irritability (which represents a brain change in every case) arises from the same chain of causality regardless of the anatomical locus of injury. They presume "stress is irritating." That conclusion is not necessarily true. Overtly expressed irritability is a complex behavior, a final common pathway that looks the same to the observer, and perhaps even feels the same to the subject, whether it occurs in a nun who is thwarted in opening a cloister door or a child with attention deficit-hyperactivity disorder trying to understand *Sesame Street*. A chronic pain patient may be irritable because peripheral inflammatory cytokines are tormenting a nerve root in a foramen. A brain-injured person may be irritable because his amygdalofugal pathway is physically disrupted. Symptoms are not causes. Thus, it is illogical to claim that equal prevalence of symptoms, or even identical symptoms, proves the effect is a "non-specific" process.

No single study carries much weight. However, Figure 5.4 illustrates results from one of multiple controlled studies that found more persistent symptoms after CBI than after other injuries. McLean et al. [166] followed 251 CBI survivors and 168 victims of other injuries. At one, three, and 12 months, the proportion of subjects with post-concussive symptoms was higher in the CBI group.

The point is not in any way to imply that the typical laundry list of so-called "post-concussive symptoms" is collectively specific to concussion. It is not. As explained in Chapter 7, no good evidence supports the existence of a "post-concussive syndrome." Findings such as these are only to say, "There is something about concussion. It often leaves victims more lastingly distressed than does a comparably 'mild' non-brain injury. Moreover, some of those symptoms are far better explained by brain rattling than by non-brain events."

The question is ultimately best addressed after reviewing Table 5.5 – summarizing the findings from another systematic review employing the same three-step search methodology as for Tables 5.3 and 5.4. One note of possible relevance to analyzing this data: most investigators compared two types of abrupt mechanical trauma (e.g., brain vs. orthopedic injury). A few compared brain trauma with a non-traumatic illness such as appendicitis – a different kettle of fish. The implications are discussed below.

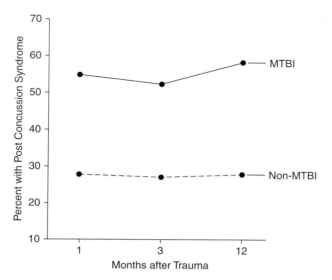

Fig. 5.4 Percentage of individuals with post-concussive syndrome one, three, and 12 months after injury, according to mild traumatic brain injury (MTBI) status.

Source: McLean et al., 2009 [166] with permission from Elsevier

Narrative Comments Regarding Table 5.5: Comparisons of Concussion Survivors With Survivors of Other Injuries

Forty-six articles meeting inclusion criteria reported 44 unique studies comparing concussed persons with otherwise medically traumatized controls. (Again, the three papers by Vanderploeg et al., 2005, 2007, 2009 [174–176] were regarded as a single study.) Four of the papers exclusively reported data on children (Hajek et al. [300], Pieper and Garvan [167], Studer et al. [316], and Taylor et al. [62]). Those are tabulated for the edification of readers but their findings were not included in the summary statistics. Hence, 40 unique studies compared the medium- to long-term outcomes of adult CBI survivors with those of survivors of other adult traumas.

Unlike Table 5.4, which includes several studies that extended for decades, the average follow-up interval for the 40 adult papers in Table 5.5 was somewhat shorter. No exact calculation is possible because specificity varied. For instance, Hoge et al. [181] only suggested that their interval exceeded four months. The largest study, Webb et al. [317], involved 49,789 subjects and only reported a follow-up of "≥ 180 days." If one guesses that Hoge's cohort was assessed at a mean of six months (and avoids the massive bias that would be introduced by guessing the size of Webb et al.'s cohort), the average time elapsed from CBI to assessment was 15.86 months.

Cognitive Outcomes

Among the 40 injury-controlled studies, 12 employed neuropsychological testing. Eight of those 12 (66.7%) found that CBI survivors had inferior scores on one or more tests compared with other-injury subjects (two reporting all tests inferior among the concussed; six reporting mixed results). A minority

of four studies found no significant group-wise difference. Sixteen studies reported subjective cognitive impairment. Fourteen of those (87.5%) reported that concussed persons were significantly more likely to report ongoing cognitive problems at an average of more than one year post-injury compared with survivors of non-brain traumas.

This evidence, again, is not probative. Perhaps the fairest conclusion is that, among peer-reviewed publications of this type, the majority employing desktop tests report some evidence of excess "objective" cognitive dysfunction after CBI. However, the multiplicity of comparisons reduces one's confidence in this finding. More persuasively, the overwhelming majority of such research reports that CBI survivors are more likely to *perceive* themselves to be impaired at more than one year post-injury. The question, of course, is whether their perceptions are usually correct, like those of older persons with memory complaints, or not.

Symptomatic Outcomes

Among the 40 adult studies, 27 assessed symptoms not otherwise specified, in most cases administering the RPSQ. Seventeen of 27 (63%) reported that CBI survivors had significantly more long-term symptoms. In six studies, the results for total symptom scores were mixed or equivocal. In four studies, other-injury subjects complained of as many or more total persistent symptoms as did CBI subjects [281, 291, 313, 315]. Seventeen of 40 studies reported somatic complaints. Thirteen of 17 (76.5%) found significantly more long-term somatic complaints among CBI subjects. Fifteen studies reported on emotional symptoms. Ten of 15 (66.7%) of those studies reported more persistent emotional symptoms among CBI subjects. Five studies reported quality-of-life outcomes. Three of five reported more symptoms among CBI subjects.

Readers are surely aware that a count of symptoms is not a good measure of outcome. (Victims of the common cold check off more symptoms on a written list than do victims of coma, even though the latter condition is usually more disabling.) Readers will also divine that – exactly as in the case of cognitive findings – some non-cognitive symptoms are equally common in the compared groups, while other symptoms are more common in one group. These observations hint at the rickety logical scaffold of many reports – which unaccountably embraced the number of items selected from the RPSQ smorgasbord as a measure of distress.

A few studies, however, reported results regarding specific symptoms. Friedland and Dawson [299] found that, while concussed and non-concussed survivors of motor vehicle accidents had about the same perceptions regarding disability and the same rate of return to work, the CBI patients were more stressed and socially dysfunctional. This echoes Boake et al. [292], who reported that job holding was equally impacted by brain and non-brain trauma, but that CBI survivors reported greater "difficulty" at work. Even after controlling for PTSD, in several studies concussed people were more likely to report persistent cognitive and non-cognitive impairment. Masson et al. [307] found that lower-limb injury survivors had more pain, while CBI survivors had more headache, dizziness, sleep disturbance, anxiety, irritability, and "depressive temper." Meares et al. [308] found that CBI survivors were significantly more likely to be bothered by noise. Mickeviciene et al.'s two reports [143, 309] stand out. In these large, reasonably long, reasonably well-designed case–control studies, no difference was found regarding the prevalence of 11 symptoms (interestingly, including headache and dizziness). Yet CBI survivors exhibited significantly more memory problems, concentration problems, fatigue, and depression. These findings do not yield any obvious pattern. They are mentioned only to emphasize that earnest investigators, often employing the same outcome questionnaire, virtually never arrive at the same conclusion about a cluster of symptoms unique to concussion.

Acknowledging these limitations, a tentative conclusion is that a clear majority of injury-controlled studies find that total symptoms, somatic symptoms, and emotional symptoms are all more prevalent at more than one year post-injury among concussed persons than among persons who have suffered non-brain injuries. For rehabilitation doctors who follow both types of patients, this is not likely to come as a surprise.[9]

Although these injury-controlled studies may be a good way to search for a signal specific to brain change (as opposed to a non-specific reaction to trauma), the strategy is imperfect for reasons previously explained. For instance, just because both an orthopedic victim and a depressed and brain-injured person both have trouble sleeping does not mean that brain injury has no biological effect on the brain's sophisticated sleep and arousal apparatus. Different diseases may produce matching symptoms in different ways.

Excluding Subjects With Histories of Neurological and Psychiatric Conditions

Among the 40 adult studies, 12 excluded subjects with certain pre-morbid neurobehavioral problems [168, 175, 179, 286, 293, 298, 306, 308, 309, 313, 314, 319]. Some writers have opined that this type of study (controlling for both pre-existing conditions and for trauma) might be the least confounded and best for objectively answering questions about concussion. However, as in the case of Table 5.4, the exclusion criteria were not uniform and the methods used in each study to confirm neuropsychiatric diagnoses (that may or may not have been made years before) are rarely reported. These studies might have contributed to understanding the effects of concussion among a biased sample of especially healthy people had they selected representative, validly diagnosed subjects, been authentically prospective (following cohorts with matched comparison subjects assessed *before* and after injury), been somewhat longer-term (involving periodic follow-up assessments for at least two years), and if outcome

had been assessed with biologically quantitative or, at least, ecologically valid methods (yet to be discovered). None were. Put simply: our very best studies are not very good.

Still, in the interest of completion: among studies that systematically dismissed the effects on about half of the human population (those with a life history of neurobehavioral problems), only one administered limited cognitive tests [144, 313]. The results were mixed; concussed persons exhibited measurably excessive deficits in visual but not verbal memory. Six studies assessed subjective cognitive integrity [175, 179, 286, 293, 309, 312]. All six found more reports of impairment among the concussed. Eleven studies assessed total symptoms. In seven of those 11 studies (63.6%), CBI survivors were more symptomatic [175, 179, 286, 298, 306, 312, 314]. In three studies [168, 308, 309] the results were mixed, and in one study [313] there was no significant difference in diagnosis of a persistent "post-concussive syndrome." (As a forthcoming chapter will show, the preponderance of the evidence does not support the existence of such a syndrome.)

Hoping not to dishearten the undaunted reader who has courageously followed the logical thread through this Minotaur's cavern of data: the author's systematic review fails to unearth conclusive evidence of any scientific discovery. In fact, its main value may be to disabuse us all of the simplistic certainties that dominate textbooks and peer-reviewed publications. No reasonable analyst could step back from these data and conclude that concussion and other injury lead to comparable outcomes. Yet no one could conclude that we fully understand the frequently observed group-related differences. Probably, the affective weight of *brain injury*, the effect of litigation, and the interaction between neuro-atypicality (e.g., premorbid depression) and injury account for both some of the discrepancies between group outcomes and some of the inconsistencies between studies. That explanation comports with a major theme of this book: it's not just the hit. It's the head. Individual differences in response to CBI are tremendously diverse.

Imagine, for a moment, what Table 5.5 would look like if every concussion were as similar to every other as two mildly displaced midshaft fractures of the humerus. Would one expect this superfluity of incomparable outcome measures? This divergence of results and interpretations? The reported variance of symptom duration from days to nearly a decade? As a young research volunteer asked as we rappelled into a cavernous archive to find the first volume of a patient's chart, "Why is it so hard to arrive at clear answers in this field?" It is so hard because brain science is infant, longitudinal research is underfunded, and outcomes vary. Why do outcomes vary? The answer, in so far as the present author can divine at this scientifically primitive time in the evolution of concussion research, is summarized in Chapter 7.

---

[9]   Not meaning to rely on an argument *ad hominem*, the present author treated a variety of patients in a renowned neurorehabilitation hospital for more than 20 years. He wonders whether the choice of orthopedic patients as a comparison group is optimal, since there seems to be a large difference in the variance of recovery trajectories. Orthopedic patients tend to return to subjective well-being in roughly four to 16 weeks. Concussed persons? Hours to years.

A Number

The reader has now reviewed data from 152 systematically selected studies. He or she should have gained confidence that the preponderance of the evidence supports two conclusions: CBI is often associated with persistent neurobehavioral problems, whether reported or observed. CBI is more likely to be associated with such lasting problems than non-brain injuries of ostensibly similar severity.

Still, counting studies with a given result is not a good way to decide a scientific question. And meta-analysis is inapplicable due to the diversity of methodologies. Retreating to middle school arithmetic, one quantitative approach is to sum the absolute numbers of CBI cases and controls that were assessed in studies that reported the frequency of persistent post-concussive problems (symptoms or cognitive deficits) matched for the same follow-up period – a tactic that permits isolation of a reasonably comparable subset of studies – and compare those proportions.

Twenty-four studies assessed CBI survivors at 12 months and reported the proportion of those with persistent symptoms or impairments (20 uncontrolled studies, two studies comparing CBI survivors with healthy controls, and two comparing CBI victims with victims of other injuries). These studies collectively reported on the 12-month outcome of 10,762 CBI survivors. A total of 5017 of those (46.6%) reported or exhibited persistent neurobehavioral problems – including somatic, cognitive, and psychiatric problems. As described above, this mathematical analysis could be biased if one or more very large studies had outlying results. Indeed, the data in our analysis are dominated by two large studies: Rickels et al. [165] with 4202 "mTBI" subjects and Hartvigsen et al. [201], with 1716 "mTBI" subjects. Excluding those two, 2101 out of 4844 CBI survivors remained symptomatic at 12 months. That yields a lower number: 43.4% CBI of typical, clinically attended survivors have neurobehavioral sequelae persisting for at least a year post-injury (and sometimes much longer). It seems reasonable, and perhaps even conservative, to conclude that more than *40% of CBI survivors report or exhibit neurobehavioral problems at one year post-injury.*[10]

Readers might pause for a moment to contemplate that number. In 20th-century textbooks one might read that "only about 10%" of CBI survivors remain symptomatic at three months. That much-cited number is grossly inconsistent with the available data.

It is important to qualify any numerical conclusion to the hilt. Having symptoms or cognitive deficits does not mean having brain damage caused by concussion. The remainder of this textbook will strive to address *why* so many people report or exhibit persistent problems. Multiple scientific and conceptual barriers block the route to an answer. Absent a biomarker for CBI, one cannot state, "33.4% of Jeremiah's slowed thinking is due to axon damage, 29.6% is due to psychomotor retarded depression." Absent a scientifically falsifiable analytic

approach to mental causation, one cannot state, "7.3% of Jeremiah's depression is due to harsh parenting, 16.8% due to his divorce, 22.5% due to persistent post-concussive inflammation, 5.1% due to post-traumatically misfolded proteins, 9.0% due to the stress of CBI-related cognitive disability, 3.3% due to perturbed insulin signaling." It seems high time for neuropsychiatry to confess its utter bafflement with the inevitable multi-determination of symptoms, the certainty that symptoms are associated with imponderably complex feedback and feed-forward interactions (e.g., subjective responses to circumstances change the brain which in turn changes subjective responses), and the certainty that absolute uniqueness of genes and environments guarantees that no two humans will ever respond to similar concussions in the same way. In addition, given the abundant evidence that subjective cognitive complaints correlate with objective biomarkers of preclinical "Alzheimer's disease," it seems a bit mean-spirited for skeptics to reflexively reject similar complaints by concussion survivors. Please: let us suspend judgment during this awkward sophomore era pending biomarkers of TBI.

Recovery or Adaptation?

At one year post-injury, a little more than half of CBI survivors will neither report nor exhibit (in any grossly apparent way) persistent neurobehavioral dysfunction. Without awakening a sleeping dragon of contention, it is legitimate to ask how best to characterize that slight majority. Have they (or some of them) truly recovered? Have they partially recovered, but sufficiently so that neither the patient nor the doctor is aware of the residual deficits that might only become evident under stress or using sensitive imaging? Or have they adapted?

Adaptation is an amorphous concept. In this case – the brain's management of interactions with the world – adaptation might refer to either cerebral work-arounds that make up for degraded cells or networks (e.g., via neurogenesis or recruitment of spare resources or migration of functions), or to a less mechanically understood psychological phenomenon. A fragment of evidence often cited in favor of the adaptation hypothesis is a striking finding readers will have noticed in their review of Tables 5.3–5.5: reported distress is very common at one year, yet reported functional disability is less common. The present review is by no means the first to document that finding. In fact, the hypothesis that brains do not *recover* from concussion so much as *adapt* can be readily traced back through the layers of academic sediment. In 2016 Losoi et al. [168] wrote:

> According to Heitger and coworkers, this discrepancy between post-concussion symptoms and relatively normal functionality and quality of life could suggest that the "good recovery" from MTBI may involve a behavioral adaptation rather than a complete return to a previous health status.
>
> (p. 774)

---

[10] The present author has no stake in this or any number. It has been his impression, based on decades in neurorehabilitation, that many survivors of typical, clinically attended concussions have persistent problems. But he gladly yields to whatever the data reveal. He welcomes, indeed urges, that accomplished armies of impartial biostatisticians have at the universe of available data and undertake more sophisticated analyses.

They are referring to Heitger et al.'s 2007 remark [148]:

> variations in the literature on the occurrence and degree of persistent problems with post-concussional symptoms and problems on everyday tasks may … reflect … Bernstein's suggestion that "good recovery" after mCHI may actually present a behavioural adaptation rather than a return to pre-injury levels of functioning.
>
> ([148], p. 619)

That refers to Bernstein's 1999 statement: "'good recovery' may actually represent a behavioural adaptation rather than a return to pre-injury levels of functioning … Indeed, Seymonds [sic] … questioned the reversibility of any concussion, regardless of severity [320]."[11] This returns us to Symonds's bold 1962 paper [2], previously cited in this volume. One might be inspired to reflect for a moment. If definitive neurobiological recovery had once been observed in the intervening five decades, one might relieve Symonds's doubts that recovery ever occurs. It has not. By a small margin, the majority of CBI patients are asymptomatic at one year post-injury. However, it is not demonstrable that these patients have "recovered."

Very Brief Conclusions

> It appears that an apparently "innocent" MHI can produce a neurobehavioral residue in terms of suboptimal physical and mental health conditions. … It can be concluded that 1–5 years after trauma MHI may produce symptoms often indistinguishable from ordinary everyday stresses or discomforts, but to a much higher degree than in a non-concussed control population.
>
> Bohnen et al., 1994 [293], p. 707

What should a fair-minded, scientifically trained person conclude from this, or any, systematic documentation of the research effort and wealth expended to date – ostensibly in an impartial effort to figure out whether a single concussion has lasting effects? In the author's considered opinion, respectful of the expertise and best intentions of the cited investigators, a great deal of time, money, and effort has been wasted. Patients have been needlessly inconvenienced. Most studies have been poorly designed, poorly controlled, failed to employ sensitive, reliable, ecologically valid or biologically confirmed outcome assessments, and were too short. Most readers of this book could write the outline of a superior and feasible study in ten minutes. Moreover, as readers will instantly detect,[12] most reviews of these studies have been incomplete and either too selective (cherry picking) or insufficiently selective (encouraging bad research to breed on). Many reviewers have either tiptoed around academic sensibilities by declining to enumerate gross methodological deficiencies, or advocated unjustifiably for an extreme position. In the bitter end, it much comes down to the word "common." Are persistent neurobehavioral problems *common* after typical CBI? What is the universally agreed medical definition of common?

The animal and human data summarized in Chapters 4 and 5 of this volume are consistent. The combination of the two provides some of the strongest evidence regarding the long-term course of a brain disorder available in the annals of neurology. And this chapter does not even include the overwhelming neuroimaging evidence! To a first approximation, critical readers will conclude that typical human concussions often have lasting effects.

Yet what level of confidence do we have that the very broad spectrum of natural courses after concussion is known, or that our survey has been representative? One has reason to doubt. First, the cited papers perhaps document the best available studies; that does not mean any are good. The combination of unsettled diagnostic criteria and disappointing methodological quality does not inspire great confidence in the published findings. Second, aside from research teams that replicated themselves, no two studies are comparable, obviating any statistical magic to extract an overarching effect size. Third, subject selection was not only poorly specified in most reports but probably biased to load the cohort with more seriously concussed subjects: in addition to the fact that clinically attended concussion tends to be more severe than unreported injury, many studies focused on hospitalized patients, and compliance with follow-up is probably more common among those who remain symptomatic. Fourth, once again: the virtual non-existence of population-based authentically prospective longitudinal research leaves us hanging, twisting in the wind without a granite empirical platform. If these were not reason enough to question the perfection of our "> 40% at one year" figure, consider publication bias and file drawer archives invisible to database searches.

The author does not intend that "> 40% at one year" become a rallying cry. He has been persuaded by the animal studies that there is no known end to post-concussive biological disruption and behavioral dysfunction. He has been persuaded by the disheartening weight of the human evidence that controlled, intermediate- to long-term follow-up reliably reveals multiple forms of persistent distress, reported or observed. He strongly agrees that subjective complaints are an unsatisfactory metric. Yet he strongly disagrees that self-report should be dismissed. In fact, when a neurologist is prone to minimize the CBI survivor's persistent complaints, that professional displays all the wisdom and compassion he or she would when dismissing the pleas of all patients with chronic pain. Whatever the pathophysiological mechanism, whatever the best estimate of prevalence, neurobehavioral distress persists for many months in a substantial proportion of those who present for medical attention after surviving a concussion.

---

[11] Bernstein also anticipated the present review in 1999: "The evidence for long-lasting (i.e. more than 1 year), subtle neurobehavioural impairment after MHI indicates that additional research is required on MHI 1 year or more after injury" [317].

[12] This is the subject of a separate systematic review, not printed here because it adds no medically helpful empirical data.

Let us hope that every clinician would agree:

1. External forces sometimes visit human heads. The abruptness and the mechanical forces involved vary greatly.
2. Some instances of abrupt external force present virtually no risk of lasting harm. Example: the alighting of a swallowtail butterfly.
3. In other instances, the force is certain to cause lasting harm. Example: a five-pound brick falling 50 feet.
4. But in many instances, lasting brain change is both plausible and impossible to confirm.

The seductive question about which debate has roiled: if a person survives the visiting force – and especially if the survivor gets up and walks away – what is the mathematical likelihood that he or she will suffer long-term deleterious brain change? Few would tussle over the likely fates of those impacted by flying butterflies and bricks. The shamefully vituperous dispute concerns forces between such extremes. The obvious answer is – it depends! A millennium of increasingly precise observations testifies that apparently identical forces yield different outcomes in both human and non-human animals. It is high time to set aside the obstreperous contest between concussion believers and concussion deniers. Both have a point, because *outcomes vary*. It is exciting to realize that we have finally leapt the hurdle on the route to discovering why. Chapter 7, *Why Outcomes Vary*, will narrate our progress on that journey.

One must also confess a compelling interest in the very long-term or "late effects" of CBI. The data presented so far give us confidence that some survivors suffer for years. The data do not, however, number those years. Can a concussion produce permanent brain damage? Or (and this is beginning to seem more likely) might a concussion sometimes cause a bimodal illness with an initial phase of injury and imperfect recovery followed later in life by the insidious acceleration of late-life time-passing-related brain change? The forthcoming chapter titled *Late Effects* (Chapter 11) will present the best available evidence regarding whether a single CBI is a risk factor for early-onset dementia.

We are also rambling closer to shining a light into the living heads of CBI survivors. How can one objectively assess brain function in a victim of concussion with persistent symptoms? Symptoms are subjective. Some sick people don't feel sick. Others don't want the doctor to know they feel well. Primary neurological signs are infrequent in CBI. Autopsy is usually premature. But non-invasive imaging would help, if it were proven to have sufficient sensitivity, specificity, validity, and reliability. Readers can judge for themselves after reading the next chapter, Chapter 6.

References

1. Schretlen DJ, Shapiro AM. A quantitative review of the effects of traumatic brain injury on cognitive functioning. *Int Rev Psychiatry* 2003; 15: 341–9.
2. Symonds C. Concussion and its sequelae. *Lancet* 1962; 279: 1–5.
3. Blennow K, Hardy J, Zetterberg H. The neuropathology and neurobiology of traumatic brain injury. *Neuron* 2012; 76: 886–99.
4. Jennett B, Snoek J, Bond MR, Brooks N. Disability after severe head injury: observations on the use of the Glasgow Outcome Scale. *J Neurol Neurosurg Psychiatry* 1981; 44: 285–93.
5. Pettigrew LE, Wilson JT, Teasdale GM. Assessing disability after head injury: improved use of the Glasgow Outcome Scale. *J Neurosurg* 1998; 89: 939–43.
6. Wilson JT, Pettigrew LE, Teasdale GM. Structured interviews for the Glasgow Outcome Scale and the extended Glasgow Outcome Scale: guidelines for their use. *J Neurotrauma* 1998; 15: 573–85.
7. Halbauer JD, Ashford JW, Zeitzer JM, Adamson MM, Lew HL, Yesavage JA. Neuropsychiatric diagnosis and management of chronic sequelae of war-related mild to moderate traumatic brain injury. *J Rehabil Res Dev* 2009; 46: 757–96.
8. Bruce ED, Konda S, Dean DD, Wang EW, Huang JH, Little DM. Neuroimaging and traumatic brain injury: state of the field and voids in translational knowledge. *Mol Cell Neurosci* 2015; 66: 103–113.
9. Demakis GJ, Hammond FM, Knotts A. Prediction of depression and anxiety 1 year after moderate-severe traumatic brain injury. *Appl Neuropsychol* 2010; 17: 183–9.
10. Willis T. *Cerebri anatome cui accessit nervorum descriptio et usus.* London: James Flesher, Joseph Martyn, and James Allestry, 1664.
11. Garrod AE. The Croonian lectures on inborn errors of metabolism. Delivered before the Royal College of Physicians on June 18th, 23rd, 25th, and 30th. *Lancet* 1908; 172(4427): 1–7; 172(4428): 73–79; 172(4429): 142–148; 172(4430): 214–230.
12. Bryant RA. Disentangling mild traumatic brain injury and stress reactions. *N Engl J Med* 2008; 358: 525–7.
13. Weaver IC. Integrating early life experience, gene expression, brain development, and emergent phenotypes: unraveling the thread of nature via nurture. *Adv Genet* 2014; 86: 277–307.
14. Weaver IC. Epigenetics: integrating genetic programs, brain development and emergent phenotypes. *Cell Dev Biol* 2014; 3: 1–11.
15. Weaver SM, Chau A, Portelli JN, Grafman J. Genetic polymorphisms influence recovery from traumatic brain injury. *Neuroscientist* 2012; 18: 631–44.
16. Reitan RM, Wolfson D. The two faces of mild head injury. *Arch Clin Neuropsychol* 1999; 14: 191–202.
17. Iverson GL, Binder LM. Detecting exaggeration and malingering in neuropsychological assessment. *J Head Trauma Rehabil* 2000; 15: 829–58.
18. Kashluba S, Paniak C, Blake T, Reynolds S, Toller-Lobe G, Nagy J. A longitudinal, controlled study of patient complaints following treated mild traumatic brain injury. *Arch Clin Neuropsychol* 2004; 19: 805–16.
19. Frencham KA, Fox AM, Maybery MT. Neuropsychological studies of mild traumatic brain injury: a meta-analytic review of research since 1995. *J Clin Exp Neuropsychol* 2005; 27: 334–51.
20. Iverson GL. Outcome from mild traumatic brain injury. *Curr Opin Psychiatry* 2005; 18: 301–17.
21. Hall RC, Hall RC, Chapman MJ. Definition, diagnosis, and forensic implications of postconcussional syndrome. *Psychosomatics* 2005; 46: 195–202.
22. Belanger HG, Vanderploeg RD. The neuropsychological impact of sports-related concussion: a meta-analysis. *J Int Neuropsychol Soc* 2005; 11: 345–57.
23. Belanger HG, Curtiss G, Demery JA, Lebowitz BK, Vanderploeg RD. Factors moderating neuropsychological outcomes following mild traumatic brain injury: a meta-analysis. *J Int Neuropsychol Soc* 2005; 11: 215–27.
24. Ruff R. Best practice guidelines for forensic neuropsychological examinations of patients with traumatic brain injury. *J Head Trauma Rehabil* 2009; 24: 131–40.

25. Boone KB. The need for continuous and comprehensive sampling of effort/response bias during neuropsychological examinations. *Clin Neuropsychol* 2009; 23: 729–41.

26. Tellier A, Marshall SC, Wilson KG, Smith A, Perugini M, Stiell IG. The heterogeneity of mild traumatic brain injury: where do we stand? *Brain Inj* 2009; 23: 879–87.

27. Binder LM, Rohling ML, Larrabee GJ. A review of mild head trauma. Part I: Meta-analytic review of neuropsychological studies. *J Clin Exp Neuropsychol* 1997; 19: 421–31.

28. Rohling ML, Binder LM, Demakis GJ, Larrabee GJ, Ploetz DM, Langhinrichsen-Rohling J. A meta-analysis of neuropsychological outcome after mild traumatic brain injury: re-analyses and reconsiderations of Binder et al. (1997), Frencham et al. (2005), and Pertab et al. (2009). *Clin Neuropsychol* 2011; 25: 608–23.

29. Rohling ML, Larrabee GJ, Millis SR. The "Miserable Minority" following mild traumatic brain injury: who are they and do meta-analyses hide them? *Clin Neuropsychol* 2012; 26: 197–213.

30. Larrabee GJ, Binder LM, Rohling ML, Ploetz DM. Meta-analytic methods and the importance of non-TBI factors related to outcome in mild traumatic brain injury: response to Bigler et al. (2013). *Clin Neuropsychol* 2013; 27: 215–37.

31. Waldron-Perrine B, Hennrick H, Spencer RJ, Pangilinan PH, Bieliauskas LA. Postconcussive symptom report in polytrauma: influence of mild traumatic brain injury and psychiatric distress. *Milit Med* 2014; 179: 856–64.

32. Rimel RW, Giordani B, Barth JT, Boll TJ, Jane JA. Disability caused by minor head injury. *Neurosurgery* 1981; 9: 221–8.

33. Slobounov S, Gay M, Johnson B, Zhang K. Concussion in athletics: ongoing clinical and brain imaging research controversies. *Brain Imaging Behav* 2012; 6: 224–43.

34. Denker P. The postconcussion syndrome: prognosis and evaluation of the organic factors. *NY State J Med* 1944; 44: 379–84.

35. Klein M, Houx PJ, Jolles J. Long-term persisting cognitive sequelae of traumatic brain injury and the effect of age. *J Nerv Ment Dis* 1996; 184: 459–67.

36. Cicerone KD. Attention deficits and dual task demands after mild traumatic brain injury. *Brain Inj* 1996; 10: 79–89.

37. Ewing R, Mccarthy D, Gronwall D, Wrightson P. Persisting effects of minor head injury observable during hypoxic stress. *J Clin Exp Neuropsychol* 1980; 2: 147–55.

38. Temme L, Bleiberg J, Reeves D, Still DL, Levinson D, Browning R. Uncovering latent deficits due to mild traumatic brain injury by using normobaric hypoxia stress. *Front Neurol* 2013; 4: 41.

39. Kelly G. *Personal construct psychology*. New York: Norton, 1955.

40. Holbrook C, Sousa P, Hahn-Holbrook J. Unconscious vigilance: worldview defense without adaptations for terror, coalition, or uncertainty management. *J Pers Soc Psychol* 2011; 101: 451–66.

41. Mcgregor I, Zanna MP, Holmes JG, Spencer SJ. Compensatory conviction in the face of personal uncertainty: going to extremes and being oneself. *J Pers Soc Psychol* 2001; 80: 472–88.

42. Teuber H-L. Neglected aspects of the posttraumatic syndrome. In Walker AE, Caveness WF, Critchley M, editors. *Late effects of head injury*. Springfield, IL: Charles C. Thomas, 1969, pp. 13–34.

43. Rubovitch V, Ten-Bosch M, Zohar O, Harrison CR, Tempel-Brami C, Stein E, et al. A mouse model of blast-induced mild traumatic brain injury. *Exp Neurol* 2011; 232: 280–9.

44. Sasse N, Gibbons H, Wilson L, Martinez-Olivera R, Schmidt H, Hasselhorn M, et al. Self-awareness and health-related quality of life after traumatic brain injury. *J Head Trauma Rehabil* 2013; 28: 464–72.

45. Hall KM, Bushnik T, Lakisic-Kazazic B, Wright J, Cantagallo A. Assessing traumatic brain injury outcome measures for long-term follow-up of community-based individuals. *Arch Phys Med Rehabil* 2001; 82: 367–74.

46. Hudak AM, Caesar RR, Frol AB, Krueger K, Harper CR, Temkin NR, et al. Functional outcome scales in traumatic brain injury: a comparison of the Glasgow Outcome Scale (Extended) and the Functional Status Examination. *J Neurotrauma* 2005; 22: 1319–26.

47. Nichol AD, Higgins AM, Gabbe BJ, Murray LJ, Cooper DJ, Cameron PA. Measuring functional and quality of life outcomes following major head injury: common scales and checklists. *Injury* 2011; 42: 281–7.

48. Paniak C, Phillips K, Toller-Lobe G, Durand A, Nagy J. Sensitivity of three recent questionnaires to mild traumatic brain injury-related effects. *J Head Trauma Rehabil* 1999; 14: 211–19.

49. Shukla D, Devi BI, Agrawal A. Outcome measures for traumatic brain injury. *Clin Neurol Neurosurg* 2011; 113: 435–41.

50. Van Baalen B, Odding E, Van Woensel MP, Roebroeck ME. Reliability and sensitivity to change of measurement instruments used in a traumatic brain injury population. *Clin Rehabil* 2006; 20: 686–700.

51. Wilde EA, Whiteneck GG, Bogner J, Bushnik T, Cifu DX, Dikmen S, et al. Recommendations for the use of common outcome measures in traumatic brain injury research. *Arch Phys Med Rehabil* 2010; 91: 1650–60 e17.

52. Mahoney FI, Barthel DW. Functional evaluation: the Barthel Index. *Md State Med J* 1965; 14: 61–5.

53. Rappaport M, Hall KM, Hopkins K, Belleza T, Cope DN. Disability rating scale for severe head trauma: coma to community. *Arch Phys Med Rehabil* 1982; 63: 118–23.

54. Dodds TA, Martin DP, Stolov WC, Deyo RA. A validation of the Functional Independence Measurement and its performance among rehabilitation inpatients. *Arch Phys Med Rehabil* 1993; 74: 531–6.

55. Hamilton B, Granger C, Sherwin F, Zielezny M, Tashman J. Uniform national data system for medical rehabilitation. In: Fuhrer M, editor. *Rehabilitation outcomes: analysis and measurement*. Baltimore, MD: Brookes, 1987, pp. 137–47.

56. Linacre JM, Heinemann AW, Wright BD, Granger CV, Hamilton BB. The structure and stability of the Functional Independence Measure. *Arch Phys Med Rehabil* 1994; 75: 127–32.

57. Malec J, Lezak M. Manual for the Mayo-Portland adaptability inventory (MPAI-4) for adults, children and adolescents. 2003 4/15/14. Available from: www.tbims.org/combi/mpai/.

58. Giacino J, Kalmar K. *Coma Recovery Scale-revised. Administration and scoring guidelines*. Edison, NJ: Center for Head Injuries, 2004.

59. Jenkinson C, Coulter A, Wright L. Short Form 36 (SF36) health survey questionnaire: normative data for adults of working age. *BMJ* 1993; 306: 1437–40.

60. Ware JE, Jr., Sherbourne CD. The MOS 36-item short-form health survey (SF-36). I. Conceptual framework and item selection. *Med Care* 1992; 30: 473–83.

61. Ayr LK, Yeates KO, Taylor HG, Browne M. Dimensions of postconcussive symptoms in children with mild traumatic brain injuries. *J Int Neuropsychol Soc* 2009; 15: 19–30.

62. Taylor HG, Dietrich A, Nuss K, Wright M, Rusin J, Bangert B, et al. Post-concussive symptoms in children with mild traumatic brain injury. *Neuropsychology* 2010; 24: 148–59.

63. Bergner M, Bobbitt RA, Carter WB, Gilson BS. The Sickness Impact Profile: development and final revision of a health status measure. *Med Care* 1981; 19: 787–805.

64. De Bruin AF, Buys M, De Witte LP, Diederiks JP. The sickness impact profile: SIP68, a short generic version. First evaluation of the reliability and reproducibility. *J Clin Epidemiol* 1994; 47: 863–71.

65. Post MW, De Bruin A, De Witte L, Schrijvers A. The SIP68: a measure of health-related functional status in rehabilitation medicine. *Arch Phys Med Rehabil* 1996; 77: 440–5.

66. Kroenke K, Spitzer RL, Williams JB. The PHQ-15: validity of a new measure for evaluating the severity of somatic symptoms. *Psychosom Med* 2002; 64: 258–66.

67. Golderberg D, Williams P. *A user's guide to the General Health Questionnaire.* Windsor, UK: NFER-Nelson, 1988.

68. Moss-Morris R, Weinman J, Petrie K, Horne R, Cameron L, Buick D. The revised illness perception questionnaire (IPQ-R). *Psychol Hlth* 2002; 17: 1–16.

69. Broadbent E, Petrie KJ, Main J, Weinman J. The brief illness perception questionnaire. *J Psychosom Res* 2006; 60: 631–7.

70. Jennett B, Bond M. Assessment of outcome after severe brain damage. *Lancet* 1975; 1: 480–4.

71. Goodman LA, Corcoran C, Turner K, Yuan N, Green BL. Assessing traumatic event exposure: general issues and preliminary findings for the Stressful Life Events Screening Questionnaire. *J Trauma Stress* 1998; 11: 521–42.

72. Radloff LS. The CES-D scale: a self-report depression scale for research in the general population. *Appl Psychol Meas* 1977; 1: 385–401.

73. American Psychiatric Association. *Diagnostic and statistical manual of mental disorders*, 4th edition, text revision. Arlington, VA: American Psychiatric Association, 2000.

74. American Psychiatric Association. *Diagnostic and statistical manual of mental disorders (DSM-5)*, 5th edition. Washington, D.C.: American Psychiatric Publishing, 2013.

75. Mccauley SR, Boake C, Pedroza C, Brown SA, Levin HS, Goodman HS, et al. Postconcussional disorder: are the DSM-IV criteria an improvement over the ICD-10? *J Nerv Ment Dis* 2005; 193: 540–50.

76. The Centers for Medicare and Medicaid Services (CMS) and the National Center for Health Statistics (NCHS). ICD-9-CM official guidelines for coding and reporting. 2011. Available at www.cdc.gov/nchs/data/icd/icd9cm_guidelines_2011.pdf.

77. *ICD-10. Classification of mental and behavioural disorders. Diagnostic criteria for research.* Geneva: World Health Organization, 2015.

78. Kay T, Cavallo MM, Ezrachi O, Vavagiakis P. The Head Injury Family Interview: a clinical and research tool. *J Head Trauma Rehabil* 1995; 10: 12–31.

79. Gouvier WD, Cubic B, Jones G, Brantley P, Cutlip Q. Postconcussion symptoms and daily stress in normal and head-injured college populations. *Arch Clin Neuropsychol* 1992; 7: 193–211.

80. Herrmann N, Rapoport MJ, Rajaram RD, Chan F, Kiss A, Ma AK, et al. Factor analysis of the Rivermead Post-Concussion Symptoms Questionnaire in mild-to-moderate traumatic brain injury patients. *J Neuropsychiatry Clin Neurosci* 2009; 21: 181–8.

81. King N, Crawford S, Wenden F, Moss N, Wade D. The Rivermead Post Concussion Symptoms Questionnaire: a measure of symptoms commonly experienced after head injury and its reliability. *J Neurol* 1995; 242: 587–92.

82. Potter S, Leigh E, Wade D, Fleminger S. The Rivermead Post Concussion Symptoms Questionnaire: a confirmatory factor analysis. *J Neurol* 2006; 253: 1603–14.

83. Axelrod BN, Fox DD, Lees-Haley PR, Earnest K, Dolezal-Wood S, Goldman RS. Latent structure of the Postconcussion Syndrome Questionnaire. *Psychol Assess* 1996; 8: 422–7.

84. Lovell MR, Collins MW. Neuropsychological assessment of the college football player. *J Head Trauma Rehabil* 1998; 13: 9–26.

85. Piland SG, Motl RW, Guskiewicz KM, McCrea M, Ferrara MS. Structural validity of a self-report concussion-related symptom scale. *Med Sci Sports Exerc* 2006; 38: 27–32.

86. Derogatis LR. *Symptom checklist SCL-90-R.* Towson, MD: Clinical Psychometric Research, 1975.

87. Derogatis LR, Melisaratos N. The Brief Symptom Inventory: an introductory report. *Psychol Med* 1983; 13: 595–605.

88. Butcher J, Atlis M, Hahn J. The Minnesota Multiphasic Personality Inventory-2 (MMPI-2). In: Hilsenroth M, Segal D, Hersen M, editors. *Comprehensive handbook of psychological assessment*, volume 2: *Personality assessment*. New York: John Wiley, 2004, pp. 30–38.

89. Butcher J, Dahlstrom W, Graham J, Tellegen A, Kaemmer B. *Minnesota Multiphasic Personality Inventory-2 (MMPI-2): manual for administration and scoring*. Minneapolis, MN: University of Minnesota Press, 1989.

90. Blanchard EB, Jones-Alexander J, Buckley TC, Forneris CA. Psychometric properties of the PTSD Checklist (PCL). *Behav Res Ther* 1996; 34: 669–73.

91. Weathers F, Litz B, Herman D, Huska J, Keane T. The PTSD Checklist (PCL): reliability, validity, diagnostic utility. Paper Presented at the 9th Annual Conference for the International Society for Traumatic Stress Studies, San Antonio, TX, 1993.

92. Caplan LJ, Ivins B, Poole JH, Vanderploeg RD, Jaffee MS, Schwab K. The structure of postconcussive symptoms in 3 US military samples. *J Head Trauma Rehabil* 2010; 25: 447–58.

93. Cicerone KD, Kalmar K. Persistent postconcussion syndrome: the structure of subjective complaints after mild traumatic brain injury. *J Head Trauma Rehabil* 1995; 10: 1–17.

94. King PR, Donnelly KT, Donnelly JP, Dunnam M, Warner G, Kittleson CJ, et al. Psychometric study of the Neurobehavioral Symptom Inventory. *J Rehabil Res Dev* 2012; 49: 879–88.

95. Kreutzer JS, Marwitz JH, Seel R, Serio CD. Validation of a neurobehavioral functioning inventory for adults with traumatic brain injury. *Arch Phys Med Rehabil* 1996; 77: 116–24.

96. Seel RT, Kreutzer JS, Sander AM. Concordance of patients' and family members' ratings of neurobehavioral functioning after traumatic brain injury. *Arch Phys Med Rehabil* 1997; 78: 1254–9.

97. Vanier M, Mazaux JM, Lambert J, Dassa C, Levin HS. Assessment of neuropsychologic impairments after head injury: interrater reliability and factorial and criterion validity of the Neurobehavioral Rating Scale-Revised. *Arch Phys Med Rehabil* 2000; 81: 796–806.

98. Mccauley SR, Boake C, Levin HS, Contant CF, Song JX. Postconcussional disorder following mild to moderate traumatic brain injury: anxiety, depression, and social support as risk factors and comorbidities. *J Clin Exp Neuropsychol* 2001; 23: 792–808.

99. Bjelland I, Dahl AA, Haug TT, Neckelmann D. The validity of the Hospital Anxiety and Depression Scale. An updated literature review. *J Psychosom Res* 2002; 52: 69–77.

100. Zigmond AS, Snaith RP. The Hospital Anxiety and Depression Scale. *Acta Psychiatr Scand* 1983; 67: 361–70.

101. Spence M, Moss-Morris R, Chalder T. The Behavioural Responses to Illness Questionnaire (BRIQ): a new predictive measure of medically unexplained symptoms following acute infection. *Psychol Med* 2005; 35: 583–93.

102. Chen JK, Johnston KM, Collie A, Mccrory P, Ptito A. A validation of the post concussion symptom scale in the assessment of complex concussion using cognitive testing and functional MRI. *J Neurol Neurosurg Psychiatry* 2007; 78: 1231–8.

103. Crawford S, Wenden FJ, Wade DT. The Rivermead head injury follow up questionnaire: a study of a new rating scale and other measures to evaluate outcome after head injury. *J Neurol Neurosurg Psychiatry* 1996; 60: 510–14.

104. Goran DA, Fabiano RJ. The scaling of the Katz Adjustment Scale in a traumatic brain injury rehabilitation sample. *Brain Inj* 1993; 7: 219–29.

105. Katz MM, Lyerly SB. Methods for measuring adjustment and social behavior in the community: I. Rationale, description, discriminative validity and scale. *Dev Psychol Rep* 1963; 13: 503–35.

106. Holmes TH, Rahe RH. The Social Readjustment Rating Scale. *J Psychosom Res* 1967; 11: 213–18.

107. Horowitz M, Schaefer C, Hiroto D, Wilner N, Levin B. Life event questionnaires for measuring presumptive stress. *Psychosom Med* 1977; 39: 413–31.

108. Wood-Dauphinee SL, Opzoomer MA, Williams JI, Marchand B, Spitzer WO. Assessment of global function: the Reintegration to Normal Living Index. *Arch Phys Med Rehabil* 1988; 69: 583–90.

109. Dijkers M. Measuring the long-term outcomes of traumatic brain injury: a review of the Community Integration Questionnaire. *J Head Trauma Rehabil* 1997; 12: 74–91.

110. Dikmen S, Machamer J, Miller B, Doctor J, Temkin N. Functional status examination: a new instrument for assessing outcome in traumatic brain injury. *J Neurotrauma* 2001; 18: 127–40.

111. Diener E, Emmons RA, Larsen RJ, Griffin S. The Satisfaction With Life Scale. *J Pers Assess* 1985; 49: 71–5.

112. Pavot W, Diener E. The affective and cognitive context of self-reported measures of subjective well-being. *Soc Indicators Res* 1993; 28: 1–20.

113. Patrick DL, Danis M, Southerland LI, Hong G. Quality of life following intensive care. *J Gen Intern Med* 1988; 3: 218–23.

114. Von Steinbuechel N, Petersen C, Bullinger M, QOLIBRI Group. Assessment of health-related quality of life in persons after traumatic brain injury – development of the Qolibri, a specific measure. *Acta Neurochir Suppl.* 2005; 93: 43–9.

115. Von Steinbuchel N, Wilson L, Gibbons H, Hawthorne G, Hofer S, Schmidt S, et al. Quality of Life after Brain Injury (QOLIBRI): scale validity and correlates of quality of life. *J Neurotrauma* 2010; 27: 1157–65.

116. Cicerone KD, Azulay J. Perceived self-efficacy and life satisfaction after traumatic brain injury. *J Head Trauma Rehabil* 2007; 22: 257–66.

117. Fugl-Meyer AR, Melin R, Fugl-Meyer KS. Life satisfaction in 18- to 64-year-old Swedes: in relation to gender, age, partner and immigrant status. *J Rehabil Med* 2002; 34: 239–46.

118. Borgaro SR, Prigatano GP. Modification of the Patient Competency Rating Scale for use on an acute neurorehabilitation unit: the PCRS-NR. *Brain Inj* 2003; 17: 847–53.

119. Wechsler D. *The measurement of adult intelligence.* Baltimore, MD: Williams & Wilkins, 1939.

120. Wechsler D. *Wechsler Adult Intelligence Scale – fourth edition (WAIS-IV).* San Antonio, TX: Pearson Assessments, 2008.

121. Wechsler D. *Wechsler Intelligence Scale for Children – fifth edition.* San Antonio, TX: Pearson Assessments, 2014.

122. Halstead WC. *Brain and intelligence; a quantitative study of the frontal lobes.* Chicago, IL: University of Chicago Press, 1947.

123. Matarazzo JD, Wiens AN, Matarazzo RG, Goldstein SG. Psychometric and clinical test–retest reliability of the Halstead impairment index in a sample of healthy, young, normal men. *J Nerv Ment Dis* 1974; 158: 37–49.

124. NINDS. NINDS Common Data Elements. 2016. https://commondataelements.ninds.nih.gov/projreview.aspx#tab=Introduction.

125. Teasdale GM, Pettigrew LE, Wilson JT, Murray G, Jennett B. Analyzing outcome of treatment of severe head injury: a review and update on advancing the use of the Glasgow Outcome Scale. *J Neurotrauma* 1998; 15: 587–97.

126. Lidvall HF, Linderoth B, Norlin B. Causes of the post-concussional syndrome. *Acta Neurol Scand Suppl* 1974; 56: 3–144.

127. Shahim P, Zetterberg H, Tegner Y, Blennow K. Serum neurofilament light as a biomarker for mild traumatic brain injury in contact sports. *Neurology* 2017; 88: 1788–94.

128. Achenbach T. Achenbach System of Empirically Based Assessment (ASEBA). 2016. April 12, 2014. Available from: www.aseba.org/adults.html.

129. Drake AI, Gray N, Yoder S, Pramuka M, Llewellyn M. Factors predicting return to work following mild traumatic brain injury: a discriminant analysis. *J Head Trauma Rehabil* 2000; 15: 1103–12.

130. American Congress of Rehabilitation Medicine. Definition of mild traumatic brain injury. *J Head Trauma Rehabil* 1993; 8: 86–87.

131. Vos PE, Battistin L, Birbamer G, Gerstenbrand F, Potapov A, Prevec T, et al. EFNS guideline on mild traumatic brain injury: report of an EFNS task force. *Eur J Neurol* 2002; 9: 207–19.

132. Borg J, Holm L, Cassidy JD, Peloso PM, Carroll LJ, Von Holst H, et al. Diagnostic procedures in mild traumatic brain injury: results of the WHO Collaborating Centre Task Force on Mild Traumatic Brain Injury. *J Rehabil Med* 2004: 61–75.

133. The Management of Concussion–Mild Traumatic Brain Injury Working Group. VA/DOD clinical practice guideline for the management of concussion-mild traumatic brain injury. Version 2.0. 2016. Available at www.healthquality.va.gov/guidelines/Rehab/mtbi/mTBICPGFullCPG50821816.pdf.

134. Malec JF, Brown AW, Leibson CL, Flaada JT, Mandrekar JN, Diehl NN, et al. The Mayo classification system for traumatic brain injury severity. *J Neurotrauma* 2007; 24: 1417–24.

135. National Center for Injury Prevention and Control. *Report to Congress on mild traumatic brain injury in the United States: steps to prevent a serious public health problem.* Atlanta, GA: Centers for Disease Control and Prevention, 2003.

136. Klonoff H, Low MD, Clark C. Head injuries in children: a prospective five year follow-up. *J Neurol Neurosurg Psychiatry* 1977; 40: 1211–19.

137. Chen JK, Johnston KM, Frey S, Petrides M, Worsley K, Ptito A. Functional abnormalities in symptomatic concussed athletes: an fMRI study. *NeuroImage* 2004; 22: 68–82.

138. King NS, Kirwilliam S. Permanent post-concussion symptoms after mild head injury. *Brain Inj* 2011; 25: 462–70.

139. Lippa SM, Pastorek NJ, Benge JF, Thornton GM. Postconcussive symptoms after blast and nonblast-related mild traumatic brain injuries in Afghanistan and Iraq war veterans. *J Int Neuropsychol Soc* 2010; 16: 856–66.

140. Singh R, Meier TB, Kuplicki R, Savitz J, Mukai I, Cavanagh L, et al. Relationship of collegiate football experience and concussion with hippocampal volume and cognitive outcomes. *JAMA* 2014; 311: 1883–8.

141. Broglio SP, Pontifex MB, O'Connor P, Hillman CH. The persistent effects of concussion on neuroelectric indices of attention. *J Neurotrauma* 2009; 26: 1463–70.

142. Hugenholtz H, Stuss DT, Stethem LL, Richard MT. How long does it take to recover from a mild concussion? *Neurosurgery* 1988; 22: 853–8.

143. Mickeviciene D, Schrader H, Nestvold K, Surkiene D, Kunickas R, Stovner LJ, et al. A controlled historical cohort study on the post-concussion syndrome. *Eur J Neurol* 2002; 9: 581–7.

144. Hartlage LC, Durant-Wilson D, Patch PC. Persistent neurobehavioral problems following mild traumatic brain injury. *Arch Clin Neuropsychol* 2001; 16: 561–70.

145. Chan RC. Attentional deficits in patients with persisting postconcussive complaints: a general deficit or specific component deficit? *J Clin Exp Neuropsychol* 2002; 24: 1081–93.

146. Chan RC. How severe should symptoms be before someone is said to be suffering from post-concussion syndrome? An exploratory study with self-reported checklist using Rasch analysis. *Brain Inj* 2005; 19: 1117–24.

147. Solbakk AK, Reinvang I, Svebak S, Nielsen CS, Sundet K. Attention to affective pictures in closed head injury: event-related brain potentials and cardiac responses. *J Clin Exp Neuropsychol* 2005; 27: 205–23.

148. Heitger MH, Jones RD, Frampton CM, Ardagh MW, Anderson TJ. Recovery in the first year after mild head injury: divergence of symptom status and self-perceived quality of life. *J Rehabil Med* 2007; 39: 612–21.

149. Johansson B, Berglund P, Ronnback L. Mental fatigue and impaired information processing after mild and moderate traumatic brain injury. *Brain Inj* 2009; 23: 1027–40.

150. Robb Swan A, Nichols S, Drake A, Angeles A, Diwakar M, Song T, et al. Magnetoencephalography slow-wave detection in patients with mild traumatic brain injury and ongoing symptoms correlated with long-term neuropsychological outcome. *J Neurotrauma* 2015; 32: 1510–21.

151. Russell WR. *The traumatic amnesias*. Oxford, England: Oxford University Press, 1971.

152. Sawchyn JM, Brulot MM, Strauss E. Note on the use of the Postconcussion Syndrome Checklist. *Arch Clin Neuropsychol* 2000; 15: 1–8.

153. Dean PJ, Sterr A. Long-term effects of mild traumatic brain injury on cognitive performance. *Front Hum Neurosci* 2013; 7: 30.

154. Bryant RA, Harvey AG. Postconcussive symptoms and posttraumatic stress disorder after mild traumatic brain injury. *J Nerv Ment Dis* 1999; 187: 302–5.

155. Mccullagh S, Feinstein A. Outcome after mild traumatic brain injury: an examination of recruitment bias. *J Neurol Neurosurg Psychiatry* 2003; 74: 39–43.

156. Killam C, Cautin RL, Santucci AC. Assessing the enduring residual neuropsychological effects of head trauma in college athletes who participate in contact sports. *Arch Clin Neuropsychol* 2005; 20: 599–611.

157. Moser RS, Schatz P. Enduring effects of concussion in youth athletes. *Arch Clin Neuropsychol* 2002; 17: 91–100.

158. Mccrea M, Hammeke T, Olsen G, Leo P, Guskiewicz K. Unreported concussion in high school football players: implications for prevention. *Clin J Sport Med* 2004; 14: 13–17.

159. Sefton J, Pirog K, Capitao A, Harackiewicz D, Cordova M. An examination of factors that influence knowledge and reporting of mild brain injuries in collegiate football. *J Athl Train* 2004; 39: S52–S53.

160. Shuttleworth-Edwards AB, Noakes TD, Radloff SE, Whitefield VJ, Clark SB, Roberts CO, et al. The comparative incidence of reported concussions presenting for follow-up management in South African rugby union. *Clin J Sport Med* 2008; 18: 403–9.

161. Breslow J. New: 87 Deceased NFL players test positive for brain disease. 2015 09/18/2015. Available from: www.pbs.org/wgbh/frontline/article/new-87-deceased-nfl-players-test-positive-for-brain-disease/.

162. Dencker SJ, Lofving B. A psychometric study of identical twins discordant for closed head injury. *Acta Psychiatr Neurol Scand Suppl* 1958; 122: 1–50.

163. Cannon WB. *Bodily changes in pain, hunger, fear and rage*. New York, NY: D. Appleton, 1915.

164. Dikmen S, McLean A, Temkin N. Neuropsychological and psychosocial consequences of minor head injury. *J Neurol Neurosurg Psychiatry* 1986; 49: 1227–32.

165. Rickels E, Von Wild K, Wenzlaff P. Head injury in Germany: a population-based prospective study on epidemiology, causes, treatment and outcome of all degrees of head-injury severity in two distinct areas. *Brain Inj* 2010; 24: 1491–504.

166. McLean SA, Kirsch NL, Tan-Schriner CU, Sen A, Frederiksen S, Harris RE, et al. Health status, not head injury, predicts concussion symptoms after minor injury. *Am J Emerg Med* 2009; 27: 182–90.

167. Pieper P, Garvan C. Health-related quality-of-life in the first year following a childhood concussion. *Brain Inj* 2014; 28: 105–13.

168. Losoi H, Silverberg ND, Wäljas M, Turunen S, Rosti-Otajärvi E, Helminen M, et al. Recovery from mild traumatic brain injury in previously healthy adults. *J Neurotrauma* 2016; 33: 766–76.

169. Catale C, Marique P, Closset A, Meulemans T. Attentional and executive functioning following mild traumatic brain injury in children using the Test for Attentional Performance (TAP) battery. *J Clin Exp Neuropsychol* 2009; 31: 331–8.

170. Geary EK, Kraus MF, Pliskin NH, Little DM. Verbal learning differences in chronic mild traumatic brain injury. *J Int Neuropsychol Soc* 2010; 16: 506–16.

171. Peña CJ, Kronman HG, Walker DM, Cates HM, Bagot RC, Purushothaman I, et al. Early life stress confers lifelong stress susceptibility in mice via ventral tegmental area OTX2. *Science* 2017; 356: 1185–8.

172. Garrod A. The Croonian lectures on inborn errors of metabolism. *Lancet* 1908; 172: 1–7.

173. Kessler RC, Berglund P, Demler O, Jin R, Merikangas KR, Walters EE. Lifetime prevalence and age-of-onset distributions of DSM-IV disorders in the National Comorbidity Survey Replication. *Arch Gen Psychiatry* 2005; 62: 593–602.

174. Vanderploeg RD, Curtiss G, Belanger HG. Long-term neuropsychological outcomes following mild traumatic brain injury. *J Int Neuropsychol Soc* 2005; 11: 228–36.

175. Vanderploeg RD, Curtiss G, Luis CA, Salazar AM. Long-term morbidities following self-reported mild traumatic brain injury. *J Clin Exp Neuropsychol* 2007; 29: 585–98.

176. Vanderploeg RD, Belanger HG, Curtiss G. Mild traumatic brain injury and posttraumatic stress disorder and their associations with health symptoms. *Arch Phys Med Rehabil* 2009; 90: 1084–93.

177. Clarke LA, Genat RC, Anderson JF. Long-term cognitive complaint and post-concussive symptoms following mild traumatic brain injury: the role of cognitive and affective factors. *Brain Inj* 2012; 26: 298–307.

178. Donnell AJ, Kim MS, Silva MA, Vanderploeg RD. Incidence of postconcussion symptoms in psychiatric diagnostic groups, mild traumatic brain injury, and comorbid conditions. *Clin Neuropsychol* 2012; 26: 1092–101.

179. Ettenhofer ML, Barry DM. A comparison of long-term postconcussive symptoms between university students with and without a history of mild traumatic brain injury or orthopedic injury. *J Int Neuropsychol Soc* 2012; 18: 451–60.

180. Hanten G, Li X, Ibarra A, Wilde EA, Barnes A, Mccauley SR, et al. Updating memory after mild traumatic brain injury and orthopedic injuries. *J Neurotrauma* 2013; 30: 618–24.

181. Hoge CW, McGurk D, Thomas JL, Cox AL, Engel CC, Castro CA. Mild traumatic brain injury in U.S. soldiers returning from Iraq. *N Engl J Med* 2008; 358: 453–63.

182. Rabinowitz AR, Li X, McCauley SR, Wilde EA, Barnes A, Hanten G, et al. Prevalence and predictors of poor recovery from mild traumatic brain injury. *J Neurotrauma* 2015; 32: 1488–96.

183. Adler A. Mental symptoms following head injury: a statistical analysis of two hundred cases. *Arch Neurol Psychiatry* 1945; 53: 34–43.

184. Alves WM, Colohan AR, O'Leary TJ, Rimel RW, Jane JA. Understanding posttraumatic symptoms after minor head injury. *J Head Trauma Rehabil* 1986; 1: 1–12.

185. Alves W, Macciocchi SN, Barth JT. Postconcussive symptoms after uncomplicated mild head injury. *J Head Trauma Rehabil* 1993; 8: 48–59.

186. Anderson V, Catroppa C. Recovery of executive skills following paediatric traumatic brain injury (TBI): a 2 year follow-up. *Brain Inj* 2005; 19: 459–70.

187. Barlow KM, Crawford S, Brooks BL, Turley B, Mikrogianakis A. The incidence of postconcussion syndrome remains stable following mild traumatic brain injury in children. *Pediatr Neurol* 2015; 53: 491–7.

188. Barth JT, Macciocchi SN, Giordani B, Rimel R, Jane JA, Boll TJ. Neuropsychological sequelae of minor head injury. *Neurosurgery* 1983; 13: 529–33.

189. Bryant RA, O'Donnell ML, Creamer M, McFarlane AC, Clark CR, Silove D. The psychiatric sequelae of traumatic injury. *Am J Psychiatry* 2010; 167: 312–20.

190. Cartlidge NE. Post-concussional syndrome. *Scott Med J* 1978; 23: 103.

191. Ricard C, Casez P, Gstalder H, Mawazini S, Gauthier V, Fontanel A, et al. Six-month outcome of 795 patients admitted to Annecy hospital emergency department for mild traumatic brain injury. *Santé Publique (Vandoeuvre-les-Nancy, France)* 2013; 25: 711–18.

192. Chan LG, Feinstein A. Persistent sleep disturbances independently predict poorer functional and social outcomes 1 year after mild traumatic brain injury. *J Head Trauma Rehabil* 2015; 30: E67–E75.

193. De Kruijk JR, Leffers P, Menheere PP, Meerhoff S, Rutten J, Twijnstra A. Prediction of post-traumatic complaints after mild traumatic brain injury: early symptoms and biochemical markers. *J Neurol Neurosurg Psychiatry* 2002; 73: 727–32.

194. Eisenberg MA, Meehan WP, 3rd, Mannix R. Duration and course of post-concussive symptoms. *Pediatrics* 2014; 133: 999–1006.

195. Erez AB, Rothschild E, Katz N, Tuchner M, Hartman-Maeir A. Executive functioning, awareness, and participation in daily life after mild traumatic brain injury: a preliminary study. *Am J Occup Ther* 2009; 63: 634–40.

196. Faux S, Sheedy J, Delaney R, Riopelle R. Emergency department prediction of post-concussive syndrome following mild traumatic brain injury – an international cross-validation study. *Brain Inj* 2011; 25: 14–22.

197. Fenton G, McClelland R, Montgomery A, Macflynn G, Rutherford W. The postconcussional syndrome: social antecedents and psychological sequelae. *Br J Psychiatry* 1993; 162: 493–7.

198. Guthkelch AN. Posttraumatic amnesia, post-concussional symptoms and accident neurosis. *Eur Neurol* 1980; 19: 91–102.

199. Haagsma JA, Scholten AC, Andriessen TM, Vos PE, Van Beeck EF, Polinder S. Impact of depression and post-traumatic stress disorder on functional outcome and health-related quality of life of patients with mild traumatic brain injury. *J Neurotrauma* 2015; 32: 853–62.

200. Hanlon RE, Demery JA, Martinovich Z, Kelly JP. Effects of acute injury characteristics on neuropsychological status and vocational outcome following mild traumatic brain injury. *Brain Inj* 1999; 13: 873–87.

201. Hartvigsen J, Boyle E, Cassidy JD, Carroll LJ. Mild traumatic brain injury after motor vehicle collisions: what are the symptoms and who treats them? A population-based 1-year inception cohort study. *Arch Phys Med Rehabil* 2014; 95: S286–94.

202. Hessen E, Nestvold K, Anderson V. Neuropsychological function 23 years after mild traumatic brain injury: a comparison of outcome after paediatric and adult head injuries. *Brain Inj* 2007; 21: 963–79.

203. Hou R, Moss-Morris R, Peveler R, Mogg K, Bradley BP, Belli A. When a minor head injury results in enduring symptoms: a prospective investigation of risk factors for postconcussional syndrome after mild traumatic brain injury. *J Neurol Neurosurg Psychiatry* 2012; 83: 217–23.

204. Ingebrigtsen T, Waterloo K, Marup-Jensen S, Attner E, Romner B. Quantification of post-concussion symptoms 3 months after minor head injury in 100 consecutive patients. *J Neurol* 1998; 245: 609–12.

205. Jakobsen J, Baadsgaard SE, Thomsen S, Henriksen PB. Prediction of post-concussional sequelae by reaction time test. *Acta Neurol Scand* 1987; 75: 341–5.

206. Klonoff H, Clark C, Klonoff PS. Long-term outcome of head injuries: a 23 year follow up study of children with head injuries. *J Neurol Neurosurg Psychiatry* 1993; 56: 410–15.

207. Kumar S, Rao SL, Nair RG, Pillai S, Chandramouli BA, Subbakrishna DK. Sensory gating impairment in development of post-concussive symptoms in mild head injury. *Psychiatry Clin Neurosci* 2005; 59: 466–72.

208. Lange RT, Brickell TA, Kennedy JE, Bailie JM, Sills C, Asmussen S, et al. Factors influencing postconcussion and posttraumatic stress symptom reporting following military-related concurrent polytrauma and traumatic brain injury. *Arch Clin Neuropsychol* 2014; 29: 329–47.

209. Lannsjo M, Af Geijerstam JL, Johansson U, Bring J, Borg J. Prevalence and structure of symptoms at 3 months after mild traumatic brain injury in a national cohort. *Brain Inj* 2009; 23: 213–19.

210. Levin HS, Mattis S, Ruff RM, Eisenberg HM, Marshall LF, Tabaddor K, et al. Neurobehavioral outcome following minor head injury: a three-center study. *J Neurosurg* 1987; 66: 234–43.

211. Lingsma HF, Yue JK, Maas AI, Steyerberg EW, Manley GT, Including T-TI, et al. Outcome prediction after mild and complicated mild traumatic brain injury: external validation of existing models and identification of new predictors using the TRACK-TBI pilot study. *J Neurotrauma* 2015; 32: 83–94.

212. Lundin A, De Boussard C, Edman G, Borg J. Symptoms and disability until 3 months after mild TBI. *Brain Inj* 2006; 20: 799–806.

213. Maestas KL, Sander AM, Clark AN, Van Veldhoven LM, Struchen MA, Sherer M, et al. Preinjury coping, emotional functioning, and quality of life following uncomplicated and complicated mild traumatic brain injury. *J Head Trauma Rehabil* 2014; 29: 407–17.

214. Mahon D, Elger C. Analysis of posttraumatic syndrome following a mild head injury. *J Neurosci Nurs* 1989; 21: 382–4.

215. Max JE, Pardo D, Hanten G, Schachar RJ, Saunders AE, Ewing-Cobbs L, et al. Psychiatric disorders in children and adolescents six-to-twelve months after mild traumatic brain injury. *J Neuropsychiatry Clin Neurosci* 2013; 25: 272–82.

216. Mazzucchi A, Cattelani R, Missale G, Gugliotta M, Brianti R, Parma M. Head-injured subjects aged over 50 years: correlations between variables of trauma and neuropsychological follow-up. *J Neurol* 1992; 239: 256–60.

217. McMahon P, Hricik A, Yue JK, Puccio AM, Inoue T, Lingsma HF, et al. Symptomatology and functional outcome in mild traumatic brain injury: results from the prospective TRACK-TBI study. *J Neurotrauma* 2014; 31: 26–33.

218. Middleboe T, Andersen HS, Birket-Smith M, Friis ML. Minor head injury: impact on general health after 1 year. A prospective follow-up study. *Acta Neurol Scand* 1992; 85: 5–9.

219. Mittenberg W, Strauman S. Diagnosis of mild head injury and the postconcussion syndrome. *J Head Trauma Rehabil* 2000; 15: 783–91.

220. Montgomery EA, Fenton GW, McClelland RJ, Macflynn G, Rutherford WH. The psychobiology of minor head injury. *Psychol Med* 1991; 21: 375–84.

221. Nolin P, Heroux L. Relations among sociodemographic, neurologic, clinical, and neuropsychologic variables, and vocational status following mild traumatic brain injury: a follow-up study. *J Head Trauma Rehabil* 2006; 21: 514–26.

222. Petersen C, Scherwath A, Fink J, Koch U. Health-related quality of life and psychosocial consequences after mild traumatic brain injury in children and adolescents. *Brain Inj* 2008; 22: 215–21.

223. Relander M, Troupp H, Af Bjorkesten G. Controlled trial of treatment for cerebral concussion. *Br Med J* 1972; 4: 777–9.

224. Røe C, Sveen U, Alvsåker K, Bautz-Holter E. Post-concussion symptoms after mild traumatic brain injury: influence of demographic factors and injury severity in a 1-year cohort study. *Disabil Rehabil* 2009; 31: 1235–43.

225. Ruffolo CF, Friedland JF, Dawson DR, Colantonio A, Lindsay PH. Mild traumatic brain injury from motor vehicle accidents: factors associated with return to work. *Arch Phys Med Rehabil* 1999; 80: 392–8.

226. Rutherford WH, Merrett JD, Mcdonald JR. Symptoms at one year following concussion from minor head injuries. *Injury* 1979; 10: 225–30.

227. Sawyer K, Bell KR, Ehde DM, Temkin N, Dikmen S, Williams RM, et al. Longitudinal study of headache trajectories in the year after mild traumatic brain injury: relation to posttraumatic stress disorder symptoms. *Arch Phys Med Rehabil* 2015; 96: 2000–6.

228. Scholten JD, Sayer NA, Vanderploeg RD, Bidelspach DE, Cifu DX. Analysis of US Veterans Health Administration comprehensive evaluations for traumatic brain injury in Operation Enduring Freedom and Operation Iraqi Freedom veterans. *Brain Inj* 2012; 26: 1177–84.

229. Scott KL, Strong CA, Gorter B, Donders J. Predictors of postconcussion rehabilitation outcomes at three-month follow-up. *Clin Neuropsychol* 2016; 30: 66–81.

230. Sigurdardottir S, Andelic N, Roe C, Jerstad T, Schanke AK. Post-concussion symptoms after traumatic brain injury at 3 and 12 months post-injury: a prospective study. *Brain Inj* 2009; 23: 489–97.

231. Schneiderman AI, Braver ER, Kang HK. Understanding sequelae of injury mechanisms and mild traumatic brain injury incurred during the conflicts in Iraq and Afghanistan: persistent postconcussive symptoms and posttraumatic stress disorder. *Am J Epidemiol* 2008; 167: 1446–52.

232. Snell DL, Surgenor LJ, Hay-Smith EJC, Williman J, Siegert RJ. The contribution of psychological factors to recovery after mild traumatic brain injury: is cluster analysis a useful approach? *Brain Inj* 2015; 29: 291–9.

233. Stålnacke B-M. Community integration, social support and life satisfaction in relation to symptoms 3 years after mild traumatic brain injury. *Brain Inj* 2007; 21: 933–42.

234. Steadman JH, Graham JG. Head injuries: an analysis and follow-up study. *Proc R Soc Med* 1970; 63: 23–8.

235. Stulemeijer M, Van Der Werf S, Borm GF, Vos PE. Early prediction of favourable recovery 6 months after mild traumatic brain injury. *J Neurol Neurosurg Psychiatry* 2008; 79: 936–42.

236. Theadom A, Parmar P, Jones K, Barker-Collo S, Starkey NJ, McPherson KM, et al. Frequency and impact of recurrent traumatic brain injury in a population-based sample. *J Neurotrauma* 2015; 32: 674–81.

237. Wilkinson CW, Pagulayan KF, Petrie EC, Mayer CL, Colasurdo EA, Shofer JB, et al. High prevalence of chronic pituitary and target-organ hormone abnormalities after blast-related mild traumatic brain injury. *Front Neurol* 2012; 3: 11.

238. Wrightson P, Gronwall D. Time off work and symptoms after minor head injury. *Injury* 1981; 12: 445–54.

239. Zemek R, Clarkin C, Farion KJ, Vassilyadi M, Anderson P, Irish B, et al. Parental anxiety at initial acute presentation is not associated with prolonged symptoms following pediatric concussion. *Acad Emerg Med* 2013; 20: 1041–9.

240. Zumstein MA, Moser M, Mottini M, Ott SR, Sadowski-Cron C, Radanov BP, et al. Long-term outcome in patients with mild traumatic brain injury: a prospective observational study. *J Trauma Acute Care Surg* 2011; 71: 120–7.

241. Denker PG. The post-concussion syndrome. Prognosis and evaluation of the organic factors. *NY State Med J* 1944;44:379–84.

242. Baldassarre M, Smith B, Harp J, Herrold A, High WM, Jr., Babcock-Parziale J, et al. Exploring the relationship between mild traumatic brain injury exposure and the presence and severity of postconcussive symptoms among veterans deployed to Iraq and Afghanistan. *PM R* 2015; 7: 845–58.

243. Delis DC, Freeland J, Kramer JH, Kaplan E. Integrating clinical assessment with cognitive neuroscience: construct validation of the California Verbal Learning Test. *J Consult Clin Psychol* 1988; 56: 123–30.

244. Delis DC, Kramer JH, Kaplan E, Ober BA. *The California Verbal Learning Test*. San Antonio, TX: Psychological Corporation, 1987.

245. Gronwall DMA, Sampson H. *The psychological effects of concussion*. Auckland: Oxford University Press, 1974.

246. Tombaugh TN. A comprehensive review of the Paced Auditory Serial Addition Test (PASAT). *Arch Clin Neuropsychol* 2006; 21: 53–76.

247. Alexander DG, Shuttleworth-Edwards AB, Kidd M, Malcolm CM. Mild traumatic brain injuries in early adolescent rugby players: long-term neurocognitive and academic outcomes. *Brain Inj* 2015; 29: 1113–25.

248. Bernstein DM. Information processing difficulty long after self-reported concussion. *J Int Neuropsychol Soc* 2002; 8: 673–82.

249. Cossette I, Ouellet MC, McFadyen BJ. A preliminary study to identify locomotor-cognitive dual tasks that reveal persistent executive dysfunction after mild traumatic brain injury. *Arch Phys Med Rehabil* 2014; 95: 1594–7.

250. Dean PJ, O'Neill D, Sterr A. Post-concussion syndrome: prevalence after mild traumatic brain injury in comparison with a sample without head injury. *Brain Inj* 2012; 26: 14–26.

251. Ellemberg D, Leclerc S, Couture S, Daigle C. Prolonged neuropsychological impairments following a first concussion in female university soccer athletes. *Clin J Sport Med* 2007; 17: 369–74.

252. Emanuelson I, Andersson Holmkvist E, Björklund R, Stålhammar D. Quality of life and post-concussion symptoms in adults after mild traumatic brain injury: a population-based study in western Sweden. *Acta Neurol Scand* 2003; 108: 332–8.

253. Fay GC, Jaffe KM, Polissar NL, Liao S, Martin KM, Shurtleff HA, et al. Mild pediatric traumatic brain injury: a cohort study. *Arch Phys Med Rehabil* 1993; 74: 895–901.

254. Fay GC, Jaffe KM, Polissar NL, Liao S, J'may BR, Martin KM. Outcome of pediatric traumatic brain injury at three years: a cohort study. *Arch Phys Med Rehabil* 1994; 75: 733–41.

255. Jakola AS, Muller K, Larsen M, Waterloo K, Romner B, Ingebrigtsen T. Five-year outcome after mild head injury: a prospective controlled study. *Acta Neurol Scand* 2007; 115: 398–402.

256. Kashluba S, Hanks RA, Casey JE, Millis SR. Neuropsychologic and functional outcome after complicated mild traumatic brain injury. *Arch Phys Med Rehabil* 2008; 89: 904–11.

257. Keller M, Hiltbrunner B, Dill C, Kesselring J. Reversible neuropsychological deficits after mild traumatic brain injury. *J Neurol Neurosurg Psychiatry* 2000; 68: 761–4.

258. Konrad C, Geburek AJ, Rist F, Blumenroth H, Fischer B, Husstedt I, et al. Long-term cognitive and emotional consequences of mild traumatic brain injury. *Psychol Med* 2011; 41: 1197–211.

259. Lee H, Wintermark M, Gean AD, Ghajar J, Manley GT, Mukherjee P. Focal lesions in acute mild traumatic brain injury and neurocognitive outcome: CT versus 3T MRI. *J Neurotrauma* 2008; 25: 1049–56.

260. Levine B, Stuss DT, Milberg WP, Alexander MP, Schwartz M, Macdonald R. The effects of focal and diffuse brain damage on strategy application: evidence from focal lesions, traumatic brain injury and normal aging. *J Int Neuropsychol Soc* 1998; 4: 247–64.

261. Mangels JA, Craik FI, Levine B, Schwartz ML, Stuss DT. Effects of divided attention on episodic memory in chronic traumatic brain injury: a function of severity and strategy. *Neuropsychologia* 2002; 40: 2369–85.

262. Massagli TL, Fann JR, Burington BE, Jaffe KM, Katon WJ, Thompson RS. Psychiatric illness after mild traumatic brain injury in children. *Arch Phys Med Rehabil* 2004; 85: 1428–34.

263. Mayer AR, Hanlon FM, Ling JM. Gray matter abnormalities in pediatric mild traumatic brain injury. *J Neurotrauma* 2015; 32: 723–30.

264. McHugh T, Laforce R, Jr., Gallagher P, Quinn S, Diggle P, Buchanan L. Natural history of the long-term cognitive, affective, and physical sequelae of mild traumatic brain injury. *Brain Cogn* 2006; 60: 209–11.

265. Moore RD, Hillman CH, Broglio SP. The persistent influence of concussive injuries on cognitive control and neuroelectric function. *J Athl Train* 2014; 49: 24–35.

266. O'Jile JR, Ryan LM, Betz B, Parks-Levy J, Hilsabeck RC, Rhudy JL, et al. Information processing following mild head injury. *Arch Clin Neuropsychol* 2006; 21: 293–6.

267. Oldenburg C, Lundin A, Edman G, Nygren-De Boussard C, Bartfai A. Cognitive reserve and persistent post-concussion symptoms – a prospective mild traumatic brain injury (mTBI) cohort study. *Brain Inj* 2016; 30: 146–55.

268. Papoutsis J, Stargatt R, Catroppa C. Long-term executive functioning outcomes for complicated and uncomplicated mild traumatic brain injury sustained in early childhood. *Dev Neuropsychol* 2014; 39: 638–45.

269. Pontifex MB, Broglio SP, Drollette ES, Scudder MR, Johnson CR, O'Connor PM, et al. The relation of mild traumatic brain injury to chronic lapses of attention. *Res Q Exerc Sport* 2012; 83: 553–9.

270. Potter DD, Bassett MR, Jory SH, Barrett K. Changes in event-related potentials in a three-stimulus auditory oddball task after mild head injury. *Neuropsychologia* 2001; 39: 1464–72.

271. Potter DD, Jory SH, Bassett MR, Barrett K, Mychalkiw W. Effect of mild head injury on event-related potential correlates of Stroop task performance. *J Int Neuropsychol Soc* 2002; 8: 828–37.

272. Schoenhuber R, Gentilini M. Anxiety and depression after mild head injury: a case control study. *J Neurol Neurosurg Psychiatry* 1988; 51: 722–4.

273. Segalowitz SJ, Bernstein DM, Lawson S. P300 event-related potential decrements in well-functioning university students with mild head injury. *Brain Cogn* 2001; 45: 342–56.

274. Sinopoli KJ, Chen JK, Wells G, Fait P, Ptito A, Taha T, et al. Imaging "brain strain" in youth athletes with mild traumatic brain injury during dual-task performance. *J Neurotrauma* 2014; 31: 1843–59.

275. Sterr A, Herron KA, Hayward C, Montaldi D. Are mild head injuries as mild as we think? Neurobehavioral concomitants of chronic post-concussion syndrome. *BMC Neurol* 2006; 6: 7.

276. Styrke J, Sojka P, Bjornstig U, Bylund PO, Stalnacke BM. Sex-differences in symptoms, disability, and life satisfaction three years after mild traumatic brain injury: a population-based cohort study. *J Rehabil Med* 2013; 45: 749–57.

277. Tay SY, Ang BT, Lau XY, Meyyappan A, Collinson SL. Chronic impairment of prospective memory after mild traumatic brain injury. *J Neurotrauma* 2010; 27: 77–83.

278. Waljas M, Iverson GL, Lange RT, Hakulinen U, Dastidar P, Huhtala H, et al. A prospective biopsychosocial study of the persistent post-concussion symptoms following mild traumatic brain injury. *J Neurotrauma* 2015; 32: 534–47.

279. Wright JC, Telford R. Postconcussive symptoms and psychological distress. *Clin Rehabil* 1996; 10: 334–6.

280. Ettenhofer ML, Abeles N. The significance of mild traumatic brain injury to cognition and self-reported symptoms in long-term recovery from injury. *J Clin Exp Neuropsychol* 2009; 31: 363–72.

281. Hoge CW, Castro CA, Messer SC, McGurk D, Cotting DI, Koffman RL. Combat duty in Iraq and Afghanistan, mental health problems, and barriers to care. *N Engl J Med* 2004; 351: 13–22.

282. Cantero JL, Iglesias JE, Van Leemput K, Atienza M. Regional hippocampal atrophy and higher levels of plasma amyloid-beta are associated with subjective memory complaints in nondemented elderly subjects. *J Gerontol Ser A: Biomed Sci Med Sci* 2016; 71: 1210–15.

283. Lee SD, Ong B, Pike KE, Kinsella GJ. Prospective memory and subjective memory decline: a neuropsychological indicator of memory difficulties in community-dwelling older people. *J Clin Exp Neuropsychol* 2017; 1–15.

284. Seo EH, Kim H, Choi KY, Lee KH, Choo IH. Association of subjective memory complaint and depressive symptoms with objective cognitive functions in prodromal Alzheimer's disease including pre-mild cognitive impairment. *J Affect Disord* 2017; 217: 24–8.

285. Teipel SJ, Cavedo E, Weschke S, Grothe MJ, Rojkova K, Fontaine G, et al. Cortical amyloid accumulation is associated with alterations of structural integrity in older people with subjective memory complaints. *Neurobiol Aging* 2017; 57:143–52.

286. Dikmen S, Machamer J, Fann JR, Temkin NR. Rates of symptom reporting following traumatic brain injury. *J Int Neuropsychol Soc* 2010; 16: 401–11.

287. Levin HS, High WM, Goethe KE, Sisson RA, Overall JE, Rhoades HM, et al. The neurobehavioural rating scale: assessment of the behavioural sequelae of head injury by the clinician. *J Neurol Neurosurg Psychiatry* 1987; 50: 183–93.

288. Mayer AR, Ling JM, Yang Z, Pena A, Yeo RA, Klimaj S. Diffusion abnormalities in pediatric mild traumatic brain injury. *J Neurosci* 2012; 32: 17961–9.

289. Rutherford W. Postconcussion symptoms: relationship to acute neurological indices, individual differences, and circumstances of injury. In: Levin H, Eisenberg H, Benton A, editors. *Mild head injury*. New York: Oxford University Press, 1989, pp. 217–28.

290. Bay EH, Liberzon I. Early stress response: a vulnerability framework for functional impairment following mild traumatic brain injury. *Res Theory Nurs Pract* 2009; 23: 42–61.

291. Bazarian JJ, Wong T, Harris M, Leahey N, Mookerjee S, Dombovy M. Epidemiology and predictors of post-concussive syndrome after minor head injury in an emergency population. *Brain Inj* 1999; 13: 173–89.

292. Boake C, McCauley SR, Levin HS, Pedroza C, Contant CF, Song JX, et al. Diagnostic criteria for postconcussional syndrome after mild to moderate traumatic brain injury. *J Neuropsychiatry Clin Neurosci* 2005; 17: 350–6.

293. Bohnen N, Van Zutphen W, Twijnstra A, Wijnen G, Bongers J, Jolles J. Late outcome of mild head injury: results from a controlled postal survey. *Brain Inj* 1994; 8: 701–8.

294. Bohnen NJ, Wijnen G, Twijnstra A, Van Zutphen W, Jolles J. The constellation of late post-traumatic symptoms of mild head injury patients. *Neurorehabil Neural Repair* 1995; 9: 33–9.

295. Brooks BL, Daya H, Khan S, Carlson HL, Mikrogianakis A, Barlow KM. Cognition in the emergency department as a predictor of recovery after pediatric mild traumatic brain injury. *J Int Neuropsychol Soc* 2016; 22: 379–87.

296. De Leon MB, Kirsch NL, Maio RF, Tan-Schriner CU, Millis SR, Frederiksen S, et al. Baseline predictors of fatigue 1 year after mild head injury. *Arch Phys Med Rehabil* 2009; 90: 956–65.

297. Edna TH. Disability 3–5 years after minor head injury. *J Oslo City Hosp* 1987; 37: 41–8.

298. Edna TH, Cappelen J. Late post-concussional symptoms in traumatic head injury. An analysis of frequency and risk factors. *Acta Neurochir (Wien)* 1987; 86: 12–17.

299. Friedland JF, Dawson DR. Function after motor vehicle accidents: a prospective study of mild head injury and post-traumatic stress. *J Nerv Ment Dis* 2001; 189: 426–34.

300. Hajek CA, Yeates KO, Gerry Taylor H, Bangert B, Dietrich A, Nuss KE, et al. Relationships among post-concussive symptoms and symptoms of PTSD in children following mild traumatic brain injury. *Brain Inj* 2010; 24: 100–9.

301. Heltemes KJ, Holbrook TL, Macgregor AJ, Galarneau MR. Blast-related mild traumatic brain injury is associated with a decline in self-rated health amongst US military personnel. *Injury* 2012; 43: 1990–5.

302. Kraus J, Schaffer K, Ayers K, Stenehjem J, Shen H, Afifi AA. Physical complaints, medical service use, and social and employment changes following mild traumatic brain injury: a 6-month longitudinal study. *J Head Trauma Rehabil* 2005; 20: 239–56.

303. Kraus J, Hsu P, Schaffer K, Vaca F, Ayers K, Kennedy F, et al. Preinjury factors and 3-month outcomes following emergency department diagnosis of mild traumatic brain injury. *J Head Trauma Rehabil* 2009; 24: 344–54.

304. Kraus JF, Hsu P, Schafer K, Afifi AA. Sustained outcomes following mild traumatic brain injury: results of a five-emergency department longitudinal study. *Brain Inj* 2014; 28: 1248–56.

305. Levin H, Li X, Mccauley SR, Hanten G, Wilde EA, Swank PR. Neuropsychological outcome of mTBI: a principal component analysis approach. *J Neurotrauma*. 2013; 30: 625–632.

306. Losoi H, Wäljas M, Turunen S, Brander A, Helminen M, Luoto TM, et al. Resilience is associated with fatigue after mild traumatic brain injury. *J Head Trauma Rehabil* 2015; 30: E24–32.

307. Masson F, Maurette P, Salmi LR, Dartigues JF, Vecsey J, Destaillats JM, et al. Prevalence of impairments 5 years after a head injury, and their relationship with disabilities and outcome. *Brain Inj* 1996; 10: 487–97.

308. Meares S, Shores EA, Taylor AJ, Batchelor J, Bryant RA, Baguley IJ, et al. The prospective course of postconcussion syndrome: the role of mild traumatic brain injury. *Neuropsychology* 2011; 25: 454–65.

309. Mickeviciene D, Schrader H, Obelieniene D, Surkiene D, Kunickas R, Stovner LJ, et al. A controlled prospective inception cohort study on the post-concussion syndrome outside the medicolegal context. *Eur J Neurol* 2004; 11: 411–19.

310. Nash S, Luaute J, Bar JY, Sancho PO, Hours M, Chossegros L, et al. Cognitive and behavioural post-traumatic impairments: what is the specificity of a brain injury? A study within the ESPARR cohort. *Ann Phys Rehabil Med* 2014; 57: 600–17.

311. Ponsford J, Willmott C, Rothwell A, Cameron P, Kelly AM, Nelms R, et al. Factors influencing outcome following mild traumatic brain injury in adults. *J Int Neuropsychol Soc* 2000; 6: 568–79.

312. Ponsford J, Cameron P, Fitzgerald M, Grant M, Mikocka-Walus A. Long-term outcomes after uncomplicated mild traumatic brain injury: a comparison with trauma controls. *J Neurotrauma* 2011; 28: 937–46.

313. Ponsford J, Cameron P, Fitzgerald M, Grant M, Mikocka-Walus A, Schonberger M. Predictors of postconcussive symptoms 3 months after mild traumatic brain injury. *Neuropsychology* 2012; 26: 304–13.

314. Sheedy J, Harvey E, Faux S, Geffen G, Shores EA. Emergency department assessment of mild traumatic brain injury and the prediction of postconcussive symptoms: a 3-month prospective study. *J Head Trauma Rehabil* 2009; 24: 333–43.

315. Smith-Seemiller L, Fow NR, Kant R, Franzen MD. Presence of post-concussion syndrome symptoms in patients with chronic pain vs mild traumatic brain injury. *Brain Inj* 2003; 17: 199–206.

316. Studer M, Simonetti BG, Joeris A, Margelisch K, Steinlin M, Roebers CM, et al. Post-concussive symptoms and neuropsychological performance in the post-acute period following pediatric mild traumatic brain injury. *J Int Neuropsychol Soc* 2014; 20: 982–93.

317. Webb TS, Whitehead CR, Wells TS, Gore RK, Otte CN. Neurologically-related sequelae associated with mild traumatic brain injury. *Brain Inj* 2015; 29: 430–7.

318. Stulemeijer M, Werf SPVD, Jacobs B, Biert J, Vugt ABV, Brauer JM, et al. Impact of additional extracranial injuries on outcome after mild traumatic brain injury. *J Neurotrauma* 2006; 23: 1561–9.

319. Ponsford J, McLaren A, Schonberger M, Burke R, Rudzki D, Olver J, et al. The association between apolipoprotein E and traumatic brain injury severity and functional outcome in a rehabilitation sample. *J Neurotrauma* 2011; 28: 1683–92.

320. Bernstein DM. Recovery from mild head injury. *Brain Inj* 1999; 13: 151–72.

Chapter

6

Neuroimaging Biomarkers for the Neuropsychological Investigation of Concussive Brain Injury (CBI) Outcome

Erin D. Bigler and Jeff Victoroff

Introduction

This essay, so far, has hopefully accomplished three goals. First: we have clarified that *concussion* means an abrupt impact or rattling blow. It is a general term, as applicable to medicine and mining as to nuclear ballistics. A concussive brain injury (CBI) is a brain injury attributable to such a rattling blow.

Second: the majority of CBIs receive no clinical attention and seem to run a benign course with an apparent spontaneous return to baseline level of function without any systematic treatment. In the absence of an enduring neurological deficit of the sort detectable on physical examination, a guess promoted by some 20th-century neuropsychologists was that no post-concussion cognitive change, behavioral change, or functional change reflects permanent neuropathology. A common reason cited for that guess was that many of those who experience a CBI seem to return to pre-injury baseline and resume typical function – at least based on conventional paper-and-pencil neuropsychological measures. Indeed, prior to about 1940, transient perturbation of neuronal physiology seemed a plausible explanation that fit well with both the available neurobiological investigations (using neurochemically, metabolically, and molecularly insensitive assays to look for changes in non-human animals concussed in mechanically non-comparable ways) and the high rate of apparently good outcomes documented in "mild traumatic brain injury" (mTBI) research.[1] However, we have provided abundant evidence from experimental and clinical/pathological literature (Chapters 3–5) that when mammals suffer a CBI, whether or not the force has been labeled "mild," many of those mammals exhibit lasting changes in brain and in neurobehavioral function. Those impairments effect three popularly distinguished domains: somatic integrity, cognitive behavior, and non-cognitive behavior. A substantial proportion of humans who receive some kind of clinical attention after a CBI either experience or exhibit impairments for a year – and sometimes much longer.

Third, diverse and hard-to-predict changes in brain and behavior may become apparent at different time intervals after the rattling blow. However, neuroscience has not progressed so far as to reveal the chain of causality explaining each post-concussive problem. If Antoine, a 43-year-old man, walks into a beam at work and briefly loses consciousness, one possible outcome one year later is a combination of persistent headaches, job-threatening disequilibrium, difficulty multitasking, and relationship-threatening irritability – none of which are apparent to his primary care doctor or on conventional desktop neuropsychological testing. Some neuropsychologists have resorted to a dualist sophistry: "Antoine's long-lasting distress is not the result of his concussion. It is the result of his personality." To be fair, it is a seductive question: "To what degree are each of Antoine's problems directly attributable to the neurobiological changes that would have happened even if he had no psychological reaction to his head injury?" That is, according to a popular 16th–19th-century position, one can separate the universal and invariable brain effects of the rattling blow from the way that blow resonates for that individual, considering his particular genes, development, environmental exposures, psychological predispositions, and current life circumstances. One cannot. The organic/psychological dichotomy must be dismissed as an antiquated misconception. As Garrod's principle explains (1908) [2], the moment the beam hits Antoine's forehead, the impact on his life is a unique phenomenon resulting from the on-going interactions between that force and all that is Antoine.

At the outset of this discussion, it is important to acknowledge that many (perhaps most) victims of CBI decline to pursue medical evaluation. It is possible that a large proportion of those struck on the head experience symptoms that are brief and tend to run a benign course – perhaps similar to the experience of one of the authors.[2] (That cannot be asserted with confidence, however, since few prospective longitudinal studies have

---

[1] In this chapter, TBI simply denotes *traumatic brain injury*. Based on the International and Interagency Initiative toward Common Data Elements for Research on Traumatic Brain Injury and Psychological Health, "TBI is defined as an alteration in brain function, or other evidence of brain pathology, caused by an external force" ([1], p. 1637). CBI is used to specify the most common type of TBI: that caused by external force transmitted through and diffused by the skull. CBIs therefore vary in severity from innocuous to fatal. CBIs that do not cause gross intracranial bleeding roughly correspond to the spectrum of injuries previously called "mild" without a specified biological metric. "mTBI" is used to credit the work of other authors who have employed that historically popular but biologically undefined phrase.

[2] Dr. Bigler sustained a sports-related concussion playing high school football in 1966. He must have displayed significant post-traumatic amnesia and confusion on the sideline because he was taken to the emergency room for evaluation and subsequently hospitalized overnight for

studied such subjects.) This review is primarily concerned with the subset of CBI victims who have sought medical attention, because this is manifestly the group for which substantive data exist. Many suffer for years or for life.

Despite the potency of the evidence reviewed so far, some skeptics dismiss the implications of the best experimental and clinical/pathological research. They cling with unseemly rigidity to the opinion that concussions are benign – based on superficial appearances. Furthermore, the position espoused by those who claim that CBI cannot result in any permanent pathology fails to consider what evolutionarily adaptive neural strategies have been at play when the brain is acutely injured [3]. It is possible, for example, that a trade-off was selected, favoring biological processes likely to rescue short-term function at the risk of long-term dementia. A critical distinction must here be drawn between the *appearance* of return to baseline and the actuality. A great deal is at stake. It must become universal medical knowledge that CBI often produces lasting brain damage.

This chapter will report one small step forward on that path, summarizing how modern neuroimaging is rapidly converting the last of the skeptics, providing impressive objective evidence of long-term post-concussive neurobiological change.

The Dark Ages

This essay has already discussed the drama of the debate between skeptics and scholars about the long-term dangers of concussion. Frankly, the clinical data were available for many years dismissing the skeptical argument that few, if any, CBI survivors suffered long-term problems. In the previous chapter, we provided abundant evidence for the reader demonstrating the fallacy of that position. However – at the risk of a moment of repetition – one might begin the story of neuroimaging's promising historical contribution by briefly revisiting the dark ages of pre-imaging concussion science.

From the 1960s through about 2005, the understanding of concussion was dominated by mythology. "She seems fine to me" was the essence of the neuropsychological position. Ignoring the conflicting evidence, a small but noisy cadre of writers recited the Three-Month Myth – that almost all victims recover completely within 90 days of their brain injuries (e.g., [4–6]). But that early literature was based on several untenable assumptions. One: that dated test techniques are sensitive to CBI-related cognitive changes; two: that group averages suffice to describe the spectrum of individual responses; three: that the concussive injury itself (as opposed to the interaction between the rattling blow and myriad biological responses) is a sufficient independent variable that characterizes the injury; and four: that cognitive changes are what matter – ignoring the fact that non-cognitive behavioral changes are clearly more important in terms of well-being and community reintegration.

To this day, a few holdouts keep the faith. Their radical camp views CBI as a transient physiological event with no lasting sequelae. Their position is captured by Greiffenstein's statement that mTBI "is a self-contained condition that resolves quickly without special treatment, a generally accepted conclusion by fair-minded neuropsychologists" [7]. As another example of this perspective, Boone [8] states, "The field [referring to neuropsychology] as a whole is taking the position that there is no long-term cognitive consequence from mTBI" (p. 275). Note that these positions rely on neuropsychological tests that were never developed to specifically assess CBI, use paper-and-pencil techniques, and measure processing speed in seconds to minutes rather than neural processing speed that is measured in milliseconds. Furthermore, the neuropsychological examination is mostly focused on cognitive assessment whereas complex human behavior and emotional functioning are more than just conscious mentation. Mood changes, drive, motivation, sensitivity to pain, disruption in sleep all occur with CBI, that would be overlooked if one just examined cognition with a battery of neuropsychological tests. Additionally, from an anatomical perspective, if upper brainstem and thalamic as well as cerebellar areas including their white-matter tracts have been stretched or structurally altered, subtle symptoms of coordination, postural instability, dizziness, pupillary response, and ocular accommodation could all be present and completely overlooked by the psychologist who only assesses cognition.

The scholars' camp acknowledges that many people who experience CBI *appear* to return to pre-injury baseline – at least, in so far as the patient is self-aware and in so far as that can be measured by conventional neuropsychological methods. However, even using those dated assessment methods, some careful investigators have reported contrary findings. As Ponsford et al. [9] observed in a longitudinal study involving adults who sustained CBI, some did exhibit ongoing impairment in memory function after three months and "at least a proportion of these mTBI participants did have subtle residual cognitive sequelae 3 months post-injury" (p. 945). In children, Barlow et al. [10] found in a prospective longitudinal cohort of 670 children who presented to the emergency room and were assessed to have sustained mTBI, 13.7% had persisting symptoms at three months or longer post-injury when compared to a consecutive case-controlled cohort of children who sustained an extracranial injury but were not diagnosed with mTBI. Similarly, in a prospective cohort study of concussion (all types) and resolution of symptoms that enrolled 280 patients over 12 months, Eisenberg et al. [11] showed that 15% remained symptomatic at three months.

In an adult sample, followed up to 14 years post-TBI that contained a substantial number of patients with "mTBI," McMillan et al. [12] found persistence of disability based on the Glasgow Outcome Scale-Extended. In another study, Levin et al. [13] identified 102 CBI patients at baseline within four

---

observation. He is amnestic to those events, but it was recorded on an 8-mm tape. However, he recovered rapidly, as the injury was on a Friday and he practiced Monday and played in the next game on the following Friday. This, of course, was long before return-to-play guidelines but for him, subjective post-concussion symptoms were minimal and short-lived.

days of injury and tracked them for three months compared to similarly tracked *orthopedically injured* (OI) controls. At three months, using a conservative cut-point for symptom endorsement of post-concussive symptoms (PCS), about 10% of the CBI sample had PCS compared to under 2% of the OI subjects. Importantly, at three months the CBI patients in Levin et al.'s study [13] did differ from OI controls on a computer-based measure of processing speed but not on traditional neuropsychological measures.

The studies above, and others [14–17], demonstrate that some with CBI endorse persisting cognitive and neurobehavioral problems beyond three months. (See Chapter 5 for a review.) However, are the complaints and impairments specific to brain injury or related to some other factor? Abundant literature discusses a host of pre-morbid personality and emotional factors that purportedly predispose the individual who sustains a CBI to misattribute residual symptoms to the injury rather than a pre-existing condition [18], but the problem with *all* such research is that without some independent objective biomarker of possible persistent neural damage/dysfunction associated with CBI, how would the clinician and/or research ever be able to distinguish true attribution versus misattribution?

Some criticize the CBI neuropsychological literature because of not controlling for depression, litigation, and effort. However, Heitger et al. [19] controlled for all of these factors and observed subtle cognitive deficits associated with CBI after six months. Hanten et al. [20], in a well-designed, within-subjects longitudinal study of mTBI compared to OI and non-injured controls that tracked 59 mTBI patients (cognitive testing at < one week, one and three months post-injury), found persisting memory problems to three months in some of those with mTBI. Konrad et al. [21] examined 33 mTBI patients on average six years post-injury, all of whom passed symptom validity testing but nonetheless demonstrated persisting, chronic cognitive and emotional dysfunction. Dean and Sterr [14] have also controlled for these factors, finding residual subtle cognitive impairments associated with CBI beyond three months post injury. So, as shown in Chapter 5, the best, most rigorous cognitive research has been exposing the fallacy of the Three-Month Myth for many years. Yet the skeptics still raise a legitimate query: how is it possible that CBI should result in such a diversity of effects? If concussion is a unique, discrete, knowable entity, why is it that only a subgroup exhibits long-lasting problems? Why do outcomes vary so much? Chapter 7 will answer that question. In the meantime, we return to the historic story of the neuroimaging revolution.

A Light Begins to Glimmer at the Far End of the Tunnel

As the limitations of paper-and-pencil tests of neuronal activity became more and more obvious, the need for a biomarker became more and more clear. Cipolotti and Warrington [22] summarized this point over two decades ago: if neuropsychological assessment is to provide unique information about a condition and its relationship to underlying neurological impairment, there must be a method to independently define the pathophysiology and/or "brain damage" of that condition or objectively rule it out. In other words to use neuropsychological measures as dependent variables to characterize a disorder, the independent variable reflecting neurological impairment must be specific to the condition being examined. Once established, hypotheses about how brain impairment or damage which may selectively disrupt some components of a cognitive or behavioral system can then be examined. This is how neuropsychology has demonstrated neurocognitive and neurobehavioral correlates with many of the major neurological and neuropsychiatric disorders. To date this has *never* happened for CBI or "mild TBI" because there has been no independent marker of brain pathology, other than the event of having sustained a "mild head injury." Multiple studies report a failure to find neuropsychological impairments after CBI, but almost all of those studies have utilized the injury itself as the only independent factor to classify the condition. If the mere fact of sustaining a CBI is insufficient to identify a specific neural condition with potential lasting sequelae, then the event by itself becomes an inadequate criterion related to outcome. Obviously, what is needed is a biomarker that validly identifies those with persistent brain change among those who have suffered closed head injuries.

Unfortunately, the data reviewed so far neither convince all the skeptics nor satisfy our burning desire to fully understand the chains of causality linking the external force to the long-lasting brain change. The most compassionate clinician, the best-trained cognitive tester, or the most insightful patient cannot measure brain function. Diagnosis, prognosis, and perhaps efficacious treatment depend on access to data we cannot get by asking questions or tapping knees. This is where biomarkers become indispensable. In brief, we propose:

1. Clinical criteria on initial or subacute examination are not valid or reliable for classifying TBI severity; outcome is what counts.
2. Neuropsychological testing is woefully inappropriate, inadequate, and misleading as a measure of outcome.
3. Since neither the patient nor any doctor can accurately diagnose typical CBI-related brain change, objective biomarkers such as neuroimaging are desperately needed to advance clinical research and care.

Although fluid biomarkers in serum or CSF and neurophysiological markers show promise, neuroimaging biomarkers seem more likely to provide the next level of progress for identifying pathophysiological factors at play following CBI. Indeed, without identifying the presence or absence of underlying brain change after CBI, how could neuropsychological findings be interpreted?

To this end, the review that follows examines the potential role that neuroimaging biomarkers of brain change will play in the next decade of CBI outcomes research. The history of neuroimaging in CBI and contemporary methods, including underlying magnetic resonance (MR) physics, have been reviewed elsewhere (e.g., [23]). This chapter will forgo a detailed recapitulation of that history. Nonetheless, the drama of the story of how imaging is revolutionizing concussion science would be less vivid without a passing reference to the trial and error that has led to a new and realistic hope: we will soon have definitive non-invasive testing for CBI.

Computed Tomography

Computed tomography (CT) scanning was developed by Hounsfield beginning in 1967 and the first brain CT scan was performed in October of 1971. Commercial machines became widely available in U.S. hospitals by 1980 [24, 25]. As with pneumoencephalography (1919) and electroencephalography (EEG) (1924), the arrival of CT was hailed as both the end of the mystery of the brain and the end of neurology. Who needs a reflex tapper when you can look at the living brain? Scholars of concussion became hopeful. At last! A biomarker!

Yet, as we quickly discovered, CT failed to exhibit the slightest change after many CBIs. Throughout the 1980s and early 1990s, apparent confirmation of no identifiable gross neuropathology was the conclusion of the majority of "mTBI" cases who underwent CT imaging [26]. This discovery seemed to support the skeptical view that such injuries were noninjurious. Even when cognitive studies were published demonstrating long-lasting cognitive impairments, the negative CTs of those impaired patients were sometimes taken as evidence that no real harm had been done. For example, Hanten et al.'s 2012 study [20] (described above) found persistent memory problems in their subjects but no CT abnormalities. The skeptics could reasonably argue that persistent memory loss must have some other cause – e.g., imagination or pretense. Since the CTs were normal, clearly the brain damage was irrelevant.

Since CT scanning utterly failed to advance the debate toward resolution, it was merely a dim glint of light at a great remove in a dark tunnel. The *idea* of a definitive way to visualize damage in the living brain was thrilling. The chance that it would settle the issue of whether CBI caused lasting brain damage was entirely plausible. Why, then, did the advent of CT fail to settle this ancient debate? Because CT shows some pathologies and is utterly blind to others. We might have known as much, had clinical doctors heeded the dramatic progress in the basic science of CBI. Going back to the mid-1960s, neuroscientists could have told clinicians to curb their enthusiasm and not expect their big new machines to be much good for assessing head trauma. CT simply cannot visualize the things that were discovered to be wrong with the concussed mammalian brain. It can't see what matters.

For perspective, it bears recalling a three-step revolution that occurred in the mid 20th century.

The White-Matter Three-Step

Step One

During the last 200–300 years, many neurologists opined that the widespread damage found after traumatic head injury indicated hypoxia or ischemia. If that theory were true, then of

course CTs would be useful detectors; they are reasonably good at detecting strokes, which are hypoxic/ischemic injuries. So if the pre-1965 understanding of concussion were true, then the skeptics would be persuasive in declaring that a negative CT means a lack of brain injury.

There were, however, dissidents from the hypoxic/ischemic theory of concussion. As early as 1830, Gama speculated that damage to axons might better explain mental changes: "fibres as delicate as those of which the organ of the mind is composed are liable to break as a result of violence to the head" [27, 28]. Increasingly, the dissidents noted that the hypoxic/ischemic theory did not jibe with typical autopsy findings. Pathologists saw that white matter was often damaged more than gray matter – and very unequally across the brain – in patterns that made no sense for hypoxic/ischemic harm. In 1943, the physicist AHS Holbourn supported Gama's guess, observing that post-mortem findings could be far better explained by *mechanical damage* to the brain's various long fibers, including axons and blood vessels, due to *stretching, rotation,* and *shear strain* [29].

Step Two

In 1956, neuropathologist Sabrina Strich studied five brains and concluded that Holbourn was probably right [30]. Yet she hesitated to publish that claim based on so few cases. She gained confidence after examining 20 brains and, in 1961, she wrote, "The results of the microscopic examination were startling ... active mylein and nerve-fibre degeneration was seen ... large numbers of ... retraction balls – evidence that the fibres had been severed" [31]. As Strich pointed out, death of neuronal cell bodies was completely inadequate to account for this superabundance of white-matter changes. In her historic words: "The nerve-fibre degeneration in the white matter ... accounted for the neurological signs and mental state of the patients" (p. 445).

Step Three

Yet Strich's bold inference was only that. Retraction balls *imply* axon damage; they do not show it. Finally, in 1967, Peerless and Rewcastle published dramatic photomicrographs actually showing the stages of stretching/shearing leading to the final break of a traumatized axon [32]. As those authors speculated:

concussion depends upon varying degrees of damage to the axon as well as the neuron. The current definition of concussion – immediate loss of consciousness with rapid and complete recovery of cerebral function – should not exclude the fact that a small number of neurons may have been permanently disconnected or have perished.

([32], p. 577)

A good 132 years were required to prove Gama right.

Since then, the concept of shear lesions became central to the understanding of rattled brains. That discovery, in turn, became the foundation for a dramatically novel notion of why TBI is disabling: You can't function if your white matter suffers widespread dilapidation. *Diffuse axonal injury* thus explains many sequelae of TBI – from dizziness to death [33]. Moreover, the discovery of the importance of axonal damage turned out to be a giant leap toward settling the burning question, "For how long does concussion hurt the brain?" But how might one measure the health of white matter in a living person?

We will return to white matter in a page or two. But let us briefly review the neuroscience of Chapters 1–3. By the early 1980s, the neurometabolic cascade was discovered. In essence, this observation crystallizes a great deal of bench evidence that concussed mammals experience a waterfall of bad events, starting with the mechanical blow, leading to calcium invasion of neurons, leading to mitochondrial energy crisis and activation of apoptotic threat, and rapidly triggering multi-faceted axonal dysfunction – from stretching-related ultrastructural wreckage of the axolemma and axoskeleton to frank, complete shearing. (It is only more recently that we have realized that inflammatory, immunological, and microvascular disturbances are probably at least as important.)

Thus, at the very moment CT scanning became clinically available, neuroscientists could have taught neurologists, neuropsychologists, neurosurgeons, and radiologists that all they need do is image subtle changes in white matter and the impact of molecular energy crisis on circuits. Hence, CT was doomed to be virtually useless for visualizing the critical damage done by CBI. High hopes were dashed. The great debate was not settled, because that hulking, spinning X-ray beast is totally incapable of seeing catastrophic changes in the molecular biology of neurons and microscopic jeopardy to axons.

Slouching Toward Authentic Knowledge

Fortunately, engineers kept working. Better imaging methods were invented. True, we remain in the dark. The deep molecular pathology of concussions remains invisible in the clinic. But some light is beginning to shine. Neuroimaging improvements have resulted in a number of techniques that appear to be sensitive in detecting subtle pathology associated with CBI [34–38]. Because of the objectivity that accompanies neuroimaging and image analysis techniques, neuroimaging findings may serve a biomarker role for the investigation of cognitive and neurobehavioral outcome from CBI [39].

Indeed, advances in neuroimaging technology have inspired important questions about the utility of histopathological examination for determining brain change. On the one hand, a neuropathologist can visualize a small piece of brain under high-power light microscopy and even higher-power electron microscopy. On the other, at least in human cases, the pathologist is not examining the brain, but a dramatically altered formerly human tissue that has died, been removed from its cranial nest, been steeped in chemicals, and then sliced fine. In regard to the relative accuracy of imaging versus histopathology, a distinction should be made between structural and functional imaging. Structural neuroimaging of a living person, already possible at the sub-millimeter level of resolution, cannot (yet) match the optical resolution of pathological

examination. No currently available structural imaging technology can reveal the health of individual neurons or glia. Even at 0.1 mm with 0.1-s temporal resolution – the standard expected soon – a magnetic resonance imaging (MRI) scanner is visualizing about 1000 neurons, whereas microscopes can unveil the well-being of sub-cellular organelles. This becomes even more daunting when the standard resolution of 1 mm^3 is considered; this is the typical imaging thickness in conventional imaging as this chapter is being written. If a conventional MRI is done with no gap to generate a $1 \times 1 \times 1$-mm voxel there will be an estimated 80,000 neuron count and 4.5 million synapses within a single voxel [40]. Thus, we acknowledge from the outset that there is a trade-off – our best scanner see things invisible to pathologists, and our best pathologists see things invisible to scanners, but an *in vivo* biomarker is more likely to have clinical utility.

To highlight the various points made in this review, individual cases with CBI with several types of neuroimaging abnormalities will be presented. From a clinical neuropsychological perspective, clinical decision making must occur on an individual basis – all the while understanding what group data analyses may show. Where individual cases are used in this review, they were carefully selected to reflect findings based on larger studies and not just case studies.

Candidate Neuroimaging Biomarkers

Forthcoming chapters will address functional neuroimaging technologies that also have potential to serve as biomarkers in CBI, especially functional MRI and magnetic resonance spectroscopy (MRS) (also see reviews: [41–43]). This chapter will focus on structural imaging techniques. Although one hopes and expects that imaging will eventually enhance clinical management, this chapter will not attempt to anticipate exactly how improved neuroimaging biomarker identification of CBI will improve treatment outcomes, except to predict in general terms: once we are sure we can measure what is wrong, it should significantly enhance our ability to determine which interventions make things right.

Structural MRI

MRI (originally called nuclear magnetic resonance (NMR) imaging until that phrase was exorcised by manufacturers due to the scary word "nuclear") was introduced in 1976 and became widely used by 1985 [44, 45]. Its potential is far from fully realized. Advance after advance has turned it from a superior detector of structural change to a remarkable detector of moment-by-moment focal brain activity. As neuroimaging studies move more and more toward revealing white-matter integrity, microstructure, and regional function, more and more neuroimaging-based investigations with a wide spectrum of modalities show changes in the brains of CBI survivors. The advantage of MR over CT is why the previously mentioned Hanten et al. [20] and Hellyer et al. [46] studies are classic, if not archetypical. The Hanten et al. investigation was longitudinal, obtaining baseline imaging within 96 h, and followed up at one and three months post injury. The study also included

Table 6.1 Potential MRI biomarkers of mTBI

Imaging modality	Measures
DTI	Quantitative water diffusion metrics like FA, voxel and tract-based comparisons
SWI	Hypointensities reflective of blood by-products (i.e., hemosiderin)
FLAIR	WMHs indicating WM signal abnormality and/or increased perivascular space
Quantitative MRI	Volume, thickness, shape, and/or contour quantitative measurements

DTI: diffusion tensor imaging; FA: fractional anisotropy; FLAIR: fluid-attenuated inversion recovery; MRI: magnetic resonance imaging; mTBI: mild traumatic brain injury; SWI: susceptibility-weighted imaging; WM: white matter; WMHs: white-matter hyperintensities.

OI subjects as well as non-injured controls who were all imaged with high-field 3-T MRI. Nineteen of the 59 (32%) CBI subjects had identifiable trauma-related pathology on follow-up MRI, even though none had identifiable day-of-injury CT abnormalities. And despite the fact that MRI findings were based only on qualitative ratings by a neuroradiologist, clinically identifiable pathology involving the frontal lobes was associated with persisting deficit in an executive function (EF) working-memory task in the CBI patients (also see the study by Raz et al. (2011) [47] that shows MRI correlates with impaired EF performance in CBI). In the Hellyer et al. [46] investigation the MRI "classifier" not only distinguished CBI subjects, as well as those with more severe injury, from controls but also related performance to EF measures in TBI patients on average almost three years post injury.

Acknowledging that the very long-term predictive validity of such observed brain changes has yet to be determined, all of these studies support the conclusion that persistent brain injury occurs in some victims of CBI.

Numerous MR techniques currently identify trauma-related neuropathology [48, 49], with potential candidate biomarkers of CBI listed in Table 6.1. The MRI method known as diffusion tensor imaging (DTI) [50] has become the most frequently employed MRI metric in CBI research [34–36, 51]. DTI is an established neuroimaging procedure used diagnostically and in research across a variety of neurological diseases and disorders, especially those that predominantly influence white-matter integrity [52–58]. As will be discussed in this review, CBI may be viewed, to a significant extent, as a disruption in white-matter neural networks [59–64], where damage or disruption of myelin integrity and oligodendrocytes may characterize a significant amount of of the pathology that comes from TBI when chronic problems persist [65]. The key element in networks is pathways [66], and fundamental to all pathways is *axon integrity*. In regard to contemporary neuroimaging,

DTI provides the best visualization and MR metrics of water diffusion that directly assess axon integrity [67]. Indeed, the research and clinical applications of DTI are well established, including its use in providing *in vivo* visualization and analysis of white-matter integrity in CBI [68]. As such, DTI findings will be among the major technologies discussed as potential biomarkers of underlying neural pathology in concussion.

Figure 6.1 shows CT and MR images from two cases of pediatric CBI, as well as a model of connectivity taken from Qiu et al. [69], derived from structural and functional neuroimaging techniques that permit a parcellation and regionalization of the brain – highlighting reconstructed white-matter paths, nodes, and integration of brain networks, as shown in Figure 6.2. This technology is the basis for the Human Connectome Project [70], which is investigating more basic and general questions than those addressed in this text, but nonetheless helps to understand why two children with CBIs that are apparently similar may have quite different outcomes. Derived from advanced neuroimaging techniques, connectomic methods provide unique insights and ways to visualize how neural networks are damaged in TBI [71]. In these two cases, we start with visible traumatic lesions so there is no debate about whether the brain was injured.

Figure 6.1 depicts the CT and MRI findings in these two children to illustrate how different white-matter lesions (WMLs) may differentially damage brain networks. Both children had only "mild" injuries as traditionally defined. Child A's injury was from a fall from a bicycle and he had an emergency department-assessed Glasgow Coma Scale (GCS) of 14. Child B's injury was from a motor vehicle accident and he had an emergency department GCS of 15. Both had identifiable traumatically induced hemorrhagic pathology on day-of-injury CT (which, according to one system of classification, meets criteria for "complicated" mTBI).[3] The hemorrhagic lesions in child B were not associated with indicators of white-matter damage on follow-up MRI, whereas the injury in child A had positive findings for white-matter damage. Furthermore, the white-matter hyperintense (WMH) signal abnormality in child A occurred within the distribution of presumed contrecoup forces from the skull fracture and surface contusions that occurred in the opposite hemisphere. The strategic location of the WMH (Figure 6.1, upper right image) in the left frontal lobe is in a position to disrupt inter-hemispheric transmission across the corpus callosum (CC) as well as long-coursing anterior–posterior pathways of the superior longitudinal fasciculus.

Reviewing the network map in the lower right of Figures 6.1 and 6.2, a WML in deep white matter of the frontal lobe would have the potential to disrupt major networks and pathways.[4] No WMHs were observed in child B. While WMHs are not

---

[3]   In the past, some writers urged a distinction between *simple* and *complicated* concussion. Williams et al. [73] proposed, for example, that a concussion without neurological signs, skull fracture, or CT abnormalities be regarded as "simple." Little evidence suggests that this distinction has clinical utility or predictive validity (e.g., [74, 75]).

[4]   In Figure 6.1, the white-matter hyperintensity in child A had dimensions that approximated 3 mm³. Based on previously discussed estimates, such a lesion could affect 200,000+ axons. Yet because of its strategic hub location, this lesion could adversely influence billions of neural cells.

Computed tomography (CT) and magnetic resonance imaging (MRI) images of two child survivors of "mild TBI" (traumatic brain injury)

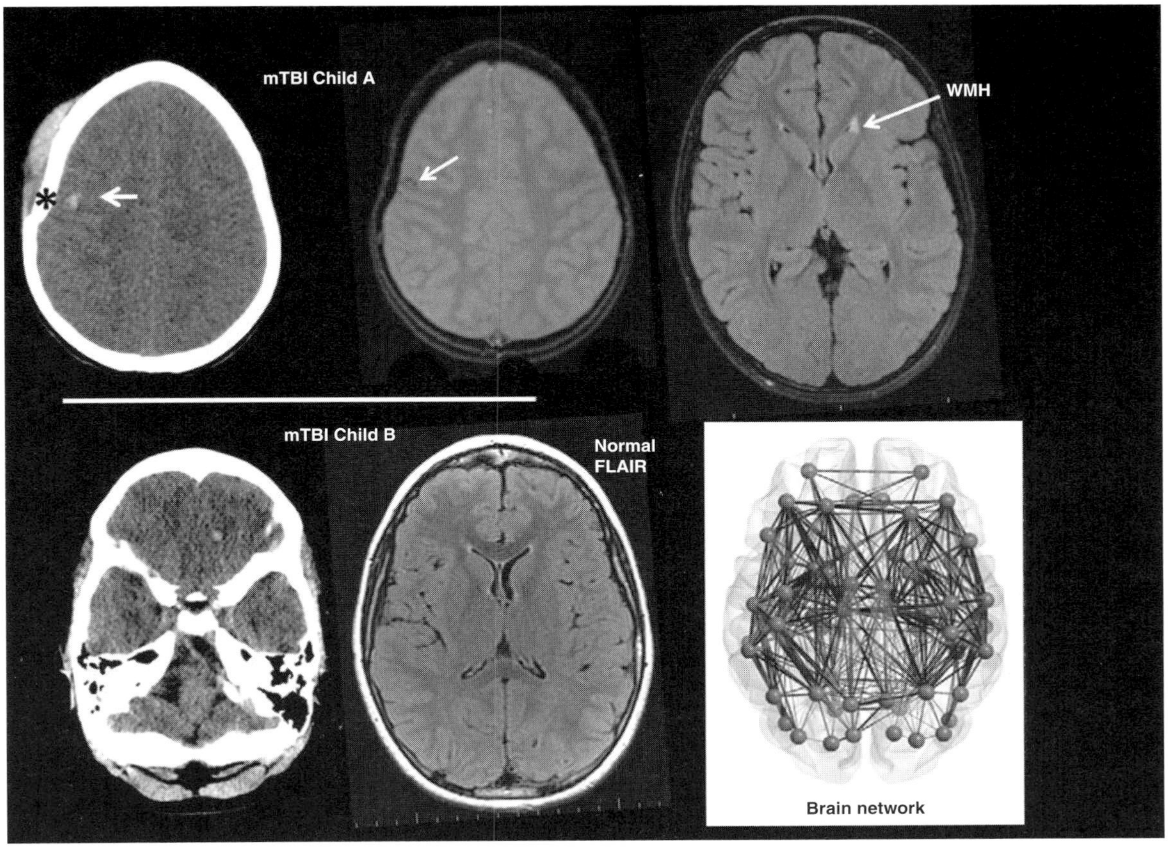

Fig. 6.1 Top: Child A had a Glasgow Coma Scale of 14, but sustained a skull fracture on the day-of-injury CT (black asterisk). The top middle scan is gradient-recalled echo that shows residual blood by-product in the same region on MRI done two years post injury. Just as importantly, the fluid-attenuated inversion recovery (FLAIR: top right) shows prominent white-matter hyperintensities (WMH) in the contralateral frontal white matter adjacent to the anterior horn of the lateral ventricle, plausibly part of a contrecoup injury. Child B's case is illustrated by the images on the bottom left. The leftmost image is the day-of-injury CT scan (Glasgow Coma Scale =15). It shows multiple petechial hemorrhages in the inferior frontal region. However, on the MRI 2.5 years post injury there was no detectable hemosiderin on the gradient-recalled echo sequence, and no discernible WMHs, although the overall volume of FLAIR frontal white matter was reduced. The diagram on the lower right depicts a network of tracts and nodes derived from streamline tractography. Note that actual tracts cannot be visualized. The presumed space path of a tract can be estimated as a curve derived from regressing information from multiple adjacent voxels. Technically, the black lines represent mathematically derived "edges" of linkage, where the weight of an edge stands for the number of "streamlines" (lines created by connecting pixels sharing a preferred direction of diffusivity) linking nodes. In informal terms, black lines depict connectivity and red circles depict nodes and hubs. [A black and white version of this figure will appear in some formats. For the color version, please refer to the plate section.]

Sources: CTs and MRIs are original images from E.D. Bigler's research program. The brain connectivity diagram is from Qiu et al., 2015 [69]

necessarily specific to TBI, they do occur with higher frequency in those with a history of TBI and may reflect a focal WML from traumatic injury [76]. (Note that the contemporary view of lesion analysis in neuroimaging puts less emphasis on where the lesion resides and more emphasis on how it affects the functional networks in which it plays a part [37].)

Returning to Figure 6.1: while both children have sustained an mTBI, the patterns of "damage" are different: the damage in child A probably involves major hub areas of deep white-matter pathways that are damaged but were not in child B. Small lesions in the periphery of a network may damage the network but network rearrangement and adaption may create a "work-around," at least in theory. And in fact, in the case of child B, although there is not fluid-attenuated inversion recovery (FLAIR) evidence of residual injury, the MRI gradient-recalled echo (GRE) sequence did show a few residual microbleeds.

Shear-strain sufficient to result in microbleeds within brain parenchyma is certainly sufficient to produce axonal injury.

Figure 6.3 [77] captures the complexity of what is being attempted with advanced neuroimaging and how it provides our best glimpse at the living brain, in terms of structure and function [78].

Fortunately, because of major improvements, present-day imaging methods provide an array of techniques not available a decade ago (see [34], and discussed in part in Chapter 16 on structural neuroimaging). Advanced neuroimaging methods can assess the brain *in situ* and *in vivo* – circumstances far more useful for detecting changes in function than post-mortem brain cutting. Improvements in DTI already transcend mere assays of regional white matter and permit tractography that would be horrendously laborious for a pathologist. DTI methods linked with improvements in the standardization of

How diffusion-weighted imaging data can be used to map the connectome

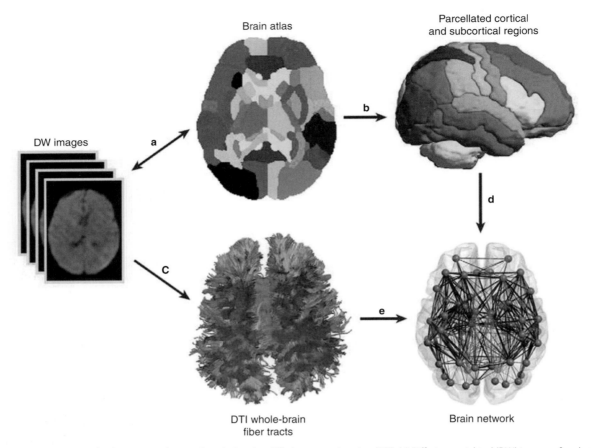

Fig. 6.2 The major processes involved in structural network analysis using diffusion tensor imaging (DTI). (a) Diffusion-weighted (DW) images of each subject are aligned to those of the brain atlas. (b) The parcellation of cortical and subcortical regions using the brain atlas. (c) The whole-brain tractography using DTI deterministic tractography. (d) Nodes (red spheres) representing cortical and subcortical regions. (e) Weighted edges (black lines) obtained using the tract information. (Figure adapted with permission from Ratnarajah et al. (2013) [72].) [A black and white version of this figure will appear in some formats. For the color version, please refer to the plate section.]

functional MRI protocols will soon enable comparative measurement of an individual CBI patient versus a matched non-CBI subject's connectivity and responses to stimuli in ways that are impossible with histopathology. Similarly, improvements in NMR, now referred to as MRS, already facilitate regional chemical assays impossible to perform in the post-mortem exam. And improvements in ligands for use with nuclear medicine devices steadily enhance the capacity to visualize the distribution and burden of neurobiological factors such as pathological proteins in real time. As a result, for the purpose of accurately monitoring many aspects of cerebral biology, imaging already trumps information derived from the patient's complaints, the neurologist's physical examination, the psychologist's queries, and the pathologist's cutlery.

Moreover, precise biomechanical finite element studies, like those of Chatelin et al. [81], empirically show where the greatest strains occur in the brain when subjected to head impact and/or acceleration/deceleration movement, as depicted in Figure 6.4 (see also [82–84]). Most importantly, as shown in Figure 6.4, note that these regions of greatest axonal elongation, stress, and

strain occur in the very regions where acute DTI changes are well documented in mTBI [85, 86] as well as during the chronic phase [87–89]. To date much of the biomechanical studies in mTBI have been with acceleration/deceleration and blunt-force traumas, but blast injury also produces similar mechanical deformation of the axon, although the distribution of pathology appears to be different [90]. Regardless of whether blast or more conventional methods of inducing CBI are involved, neuroimaging studies that are sensitive to white-matter integrity may be of particular importance in understanding mild brain injuries [91].

Current neuroimaging methods now indisputably show that a subgroup of "mTBI"/CBI patients have more than a transient physiological disruption in neural function, but instead an identifiable underlying and persistent cerebral change [36, 38, 51, 59, 92–99].

In fairness, it is legitimate to ask, "What are we looking at?" "What is the long-term functional significance of these newly visible changes?" That is, one must restrain the impulse to call all visible changes neuropathological. One requires more

The brain at seven orders of magnitude

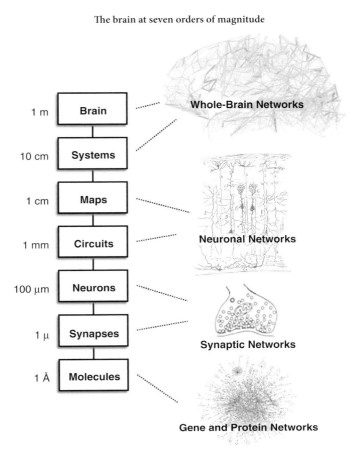

Fig. 6.3 Schematic representation of levels of structure within the nervous system. The large-scale analyses discussed in the paper focus on the levels of areas/maps and systems, but network ideas clearly extend down to the level of neuronal circuits and populations, individual neurons and synapses, as well as genetic regulatory and protein interaction networks. (Adapted from a similar illustration in Churchland and Sejnowski, 1992 [79]; Sejnowski and Churchland, 1989 [80].)

Source: Petersen and Sporns, 2015 [77] with permission from Elsevier

and better imaging-pathological correlation studies to be able to opine with confidence that a difference is a disorder. For example, DTI provides voxel-level data regarding fractional anisotropy (FA, a measure of the degree to which diffusion is restricted to just one direction versus less restricted) and apparent diffusion coefficient (ADC, a measure of average magnitude of water movement in a voxel). These concepts will be more fully explain below. But what is the normal range of FA and mean diffusivity for a given brain voxel, and what exact biological problems are being revealed when FA or mean diffusivity deviates from that range? Are we seeing pictures of increased axolemmal permeability, microtubule derangement with disrupted axoplasmic flow, demyelination-related increase in radial diffusivity, stretch, shear, losses of connectivity that are reparable either via regeneration or substitution, irrevocable losses of connectivity that adaptive remodeling can never fully mitigate, changes that predict later encephalomalacia and/or acceleration of neurodegeneration – or are we seeing changes that will cause diverse outcomes depending on other biological (e.g., genetic) characteristics of the individual?

That caveat in mind, the trend in animal research seems to be filling in this knowledge gap. We are approaching the ability to accurately identify the neurobiological meaning of newly visible imaging changes. And if a particular neuroimaging change is proven to correlate with persistent, biologically problematic abnormalities associated with CBI then, for the CBI patient with that documented neuroimaging abnormality, the view of CBI being nothing more than a transient event is incorrect.

DTI and CBI

DTI is based on the properties of water diffusion nicely demonstrated by the anisotropy coefficient referred to as FA. Figure 6.5 diagrammatically shows that, as water is unconstrained, FA approaches zero with water molecules equally diffusing in all directions. In contrast, if an axon membrane (axolemma) constrains the direction that water molecules may flow inside the membrane, their direction of flow would be parallel to the constraint applied by the axolemma. Note in Figure 6.5 the long and slender appearance of water diffusion with the highest FA. From this kind of restriction in water diffusion, the inference can be made about axonal orientation as shown for the CC assessed with DTI in the mid-sagittal plane in Figure 6.6. The aggregate tracts of axons, thousands of them that bundle together and identified through a process referred to as tractography, are shown in Figure 6.6. As an example of how tractography and measuring FA can detect abnormalities, in Figure 6.6 from an mTBI patient (injury sustained from a fall) using the FA metric, FA values along the entire axonal projections across the forceps minor can be tracked and show a region of abnormally low FA at the end of the projection stream in the left frontal lobe where this child had sustained a small contusion. As can be visualized, FA values should generally be symmetric across the two hemispheres, but as the tracts get closer to where cortical deformation occurred from the head injury, FA drops into the gray zone within the left frontal lobe, being lower than where it should normally be.

Hulkower et al. [102] conducted an impressive review based on the first 100 published DTI studies that examined the ability of DTI to detect differences between controls and TBI, and included over 30 studies that specifically assessed "mTBI." The authors concluded, "DTI effectively differentiates patients with TBI and controls, regardless of the severity and timeframe following injury" (p. 2064). As an index of white-matter integrity, DTI metrics may serve as biomarkers of the health of white-matter connections in CBI [36, 103–106]. As noted above, for neuroimaging findings to serve as biomarkers in TBI, and particularly its most common manifestation, CBI, there must be neuropathological confirmation of the relationship between what is observed from neuroimaging with that viewed histologically [107]. Animal studies of TBI with *in vivo* DTI metrics, compared to histological confirmation, provide the necessary neuropathological foundation to infer in the living human what a particular DTI finding may mean at the histological level [108–110]. Likewise, in cases of epilepsy and cerebral neoplasm, there is pre-surgical and post-surgical confirmation of how DTI changes relate to damaged neural

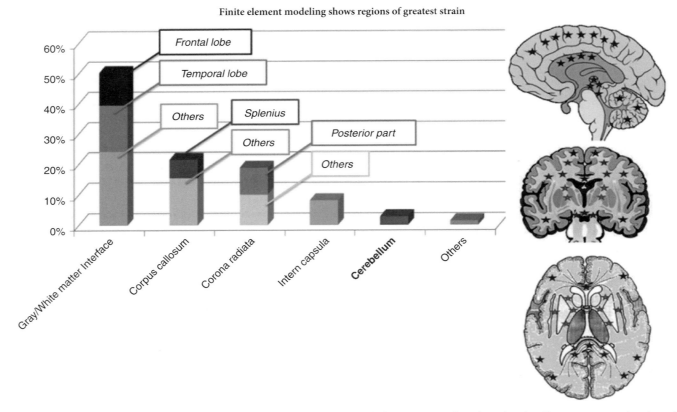

Fig. 6.4 Main diffuse axonal injury (DAI) locations in human brain. Data summarize results from various epidemiological studies. The most common locations of DAI are represented by stars. [A black and white version of this figure will appear in some formats. For the color version, please refer to the plate section.]
Source: Chatelin et al., 2011 [81] with permission from Elsevier

tissue [111, 112]. Given the status of DTI research and clinical findings, DTI is one of several neuroimaging methods that meet criteria for use as a biomarker of white-matter integrity.

Specific to CBI, in a study that examined only CC DTI findings, Aoki et al. [113] demonstrated in a meta-analysis of 15 "mTBI" studies that DTI consistently demonstrated differences between mTBI groups and controls. The consistency of these findings across studies allowed Aoki et al. to conclude that DTI metrics were sufficient "to detect white matter damage in the CC of mTBI patients" (p. 870). Aoki et al. focused on the CC because of its vulnerability in CBI to stretch and strain [84, 114], but many other studies have also shown the vulnerability of other long-coursing tracts in the brain, such as the superior longitudinal fasciculus and tracts within frontal and temporal lobe regions [23]. Differences in the biomechanics of CBIs probably help explain differences in short- and long-term outcomes [115], yet other factors may be equally influential. For instance, typical complaints after a single sports-related concussion differ from – and are often subdued when compared with – complaints after motor vehicle or auto–pedestrian CBIs. This may be because of differences in typical linear and angular accelerations, but it is also because (1) athletes fail to recognize that they've suffered a concussion and (2) athletes are strongly incentivized to underreport their concussions [116–120]. Nonetheless, even in sports concussion, which may produce the mildest of injuries (or at least, the

fewest voiced complaints), DTI seems capable of distinguishing those with significant parenchymal injury and those without, at least in the acute and early sub-acute stages [42, 121–127].

A meta-analysis of DTI studies involving what Eierud et al. [35] define as mTBI from any type of etiology graphically shows a consistent distribution of abnormal findings, as shown in Figure 6.7. Combining these meta-analytic findings with the above-mentioned finite element modeling provides confirmation that the neuroimaging methods are sensitive to detecting white-matter changes associated with CBI that more likely occur in the anterior CC and cingulate gyrus.

DTI shows increasing promise as a complement to neuropsychological outcome research in CBI. For instance, Sorg et al. [128] examined 30 war veterans with a history of mTBI (on average more than two years post injury) with a subgroup of 13 showing impaired neuropsychological performance – defined as performance at least one standard deviation below the mean – on at least one EF measure. Figure 6.8 plots out DTI-detected white-matter differences that related to reduced EF performance in the mTBI group, importantly showing that these regions of reduced EF performance corresponded with reduced white-matter integrity in the ventral prefrontal white matter, posterior cingulum bundle, genu, and splenium of the CC. These regions are all well known to participate in EF networks and likewise, to be vulnerable to mechanical deformation during head injury [81]. Most importantly, the

Visualization of the fractional anisotropy (FA) of diffusion tensors

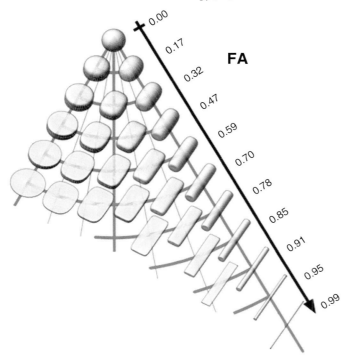

Fig. 6.5 This figure represents different hypothetical tensor shapes that may be associated with different FA values. Note that the lowest FA would be rendered as a perfect sphere, where water molecules are free to move equally in any direction. In contrast, the highest FA values would be reflected by tensor shapes that are cylindrical, where the motion of water molecules preferentially follow one direction. Also note that tensors of different shapes can have the same FA. (Adapted from Ennis and Kindlmann, 2006 [100].)

Source: Wilde et al., 2015 [91]. Reprinted by permission from Springer

Sorg et al. study [128] replicates findings of other studies that investigated the impact of CBI on these brain regions and EF [129, 130]. Hence, the DTI findings provide novel information about brain–behavior relations that could never be gleaned from neuropsychological data, both because group averaging of cognitive findings may obscure those with impairment and because cognitive testing is blind to pathophysiology.

Hellyer et al. [46] took a different approach. The authors studied TBI subjects, the majority of whom had "mild" TBI and showed no visible abnormality on conventional MRI. They used machine learning to identify DTI and other MR metrics that could segregate TBI patients. The MRI-based machine learning classifier extracted from the CC achieved 86% correct classification of those with TBI. Moreover, these classifiers positively correlated with impairments in EF and speed of processing. This is a very different approach from the way Sorg et al. [128] used MR metrics of TBI, yet the studies have convergence, both demonstrating that neuroimaging provides added information regarding the neural basis of concussive effects.

The presence of DTI findings in cases of CBI has also been used to predict outcome. For example, Rao et al. [131] obtained DTI at one month post injury and subsequently discovered that certain frontotemporal DTI findings were associated with clinically significant depression at one year post injury. Messe et al. [87, 132] used DTI findings in the subacute (8–21 days)

timeframe compared to chronic phase (~6 months), reporting that persistence of abnormal DTI findings was associated with persistence of "post-concussion syndrome." Yet DTI metrics after brain trauma are dynamic; they seem to change over time post injury. For this reason, one cannot assume that a given MR biomarker for CBI will appear the same in the acute, sub-acute, and chronic/recovery stages. Moreover, simultaneous changes may impact different tissues in different ways, literally leading to opposite changes in the same biomarker. For example, a great deal of confusion has attended the measurement of post-concussive FA on DTI. At the sub-acute stage of injury, some investigators report increases and others report decreases in this parameter.

Figure 6.9 perhaps helps to explain these inconsistencies. This diagram depicts a hypothetical, idealized estimate of change with time in multiple aspects of post-CBI neurobiology, showing how those changes perhaps affect FA. At post-injury day four, edema, membrane permeability dysfunction, and restricted blood flow all might increase FA, while disruption of axonal integrity might decrease FA – a mix of changes that would depend on the relative degree of change in each aspect of biology – the proportions varying on an individual basis and rendering net visualized FA changes baffling to interpret. Three months later one might still observe a hard-to-interpret mix of increased and decreased FA, but at that point the contributing biology might include inflammation and reparative processes not shown in the schematic [36]. Put simply, hopes for a simple DTI biomarker of "injury" may not be realistic.

A number of obstacles remain for research to overcome before DTI methods are fully implemented in the clinical assessment of TBI [133]. Still, as a research tool to advance our understanding of CBI, DTI methods have already provided important insights into the nature of traumatic injury. One anticipates that this method will also facilitate tracking of recovery and, potentially, help to select and monitor the efficacy of interventions.

Detection of Hemosiderin

Several other candidate measures as neuroimaging biomarkers of CBI, as listed in Table 6.1, include detection of hemosiderin as an indication of shear force injury, currently best detected using *susceptibility-weighted imaging* (SWI; [134]). Presence of shear injury may be associated with WMH and focal atrophy, and when the three are together in the CBI patient they are most likely the best, and most accepted, indicators of TBI. However, hemosiderin deposition, WMH, and either regional or whole-brain atrophy may occur independently of one another. When one or two of these findings are observed, but not the triad, it is less clear that TBI was the cause.

For example, the case in Figure 6.10 shows both the WMH and hemosiderin deposition in a patient injured in a high-speed motor vehicle collision with an initial GCS of 14, but 15 when assessed in the emergency department. Day-of-injury CT demonstrated a small hemorrhage in the region of the left globus pallidus. Because of persisting symptoms this patient was scanned using MRI approximately a year post injury, where SWI

Diffusion tensor imaging (DTI) tractography shows decreased fractional anisotropy (FA) in the forceps minor of the corpus callosum after frontal traumatic brain injury

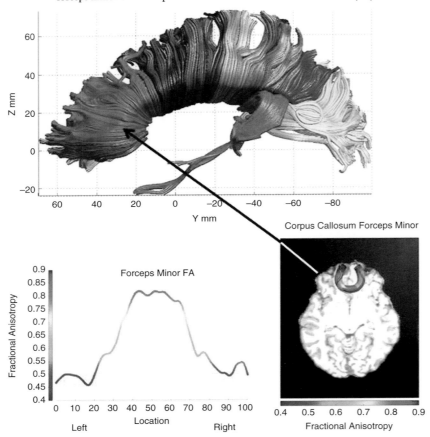

Fig. 6.6 The upper colorized tractography image depicts the projection territory of aggregated corpus callosum fiber tracts (anterior projection in red and green, with posterior projections in yellow, temporal projections in violet, with posterior frontal in purple to orange and parietal projections in orange to aquamarine blue). This child sustained a concussive brain injury which involved a documented frontal contusion. Plotting the tractography results across the forceps minor shows that FA significantly drops in the region where the contusion appeared, whereas normal values were observed in other regions of the tract. The combination of tractography and advanced methods in DTI analysis may revolutionize how microstructural abnormalities are defined in concussive brain injury. [A black and white version of this figure will appear in some formats. For the color version, please refer to the plate section.]

Source: original image adapted from Bigler et al., 2016 [101]

shows multiple hemorrhagic findings, beyond the small initial hemorrhage noted on CT. This case is another demonstration of how improved image resolution detects smaller and smaller abnormalities associated with CBI.

As will be discussed further below, cerebral microvasculature is just as small and delicate as neural tissue and therefore susceptible to deformation injury [135]. Vascular damage is intrinsic to TBI and post-concussive petechial hemorrhages have been described for more than a century. These are visible by light microscopy and sometimes even on gross inspection. Such intraparenchymal microbleeds are almost always seen when there is subdural or subarachnoid bleeding, but frequently occur in the absence of any gross hemorrhage [136]. As early as 1985, Hekmatpanah and Hekmatpanah observed that these tiny bleeds are not only a sign of mechanical damage but are also suspected of heralding secondary injury: "The torn vascular walls caused petechial hemorrhages which dissected through the neural tissues causing further nerve damage remote from the site of the vascular tear" ([137], p. 892).[5]

Although microbleeds may continue for three months post injury, after that point they are typically surrounded by glial scars and hemosiderin deposits [138].

This phenomenon makes another form of neuroimaging fruitful: MRI detection of hemosiderin. In individuals with no risk factors for cerebrovascular disease and under 50 years of age, MRI signs of hemosiderin are unlikely unless there is injury or disease [49, 139, 140]. Yet Bigler et al. [141] found MRI evidence of cerebral hemosiderin in 12 of 41 children with "mTBI" versus none of 52 children with OI. Like hemosiderin, white-matter signal abnormalities (often referred to as WMHs because of their appearance on T2-weighted MRI) are relatively uncommon among individuals under age 50 [147, 148], but have been noted to occur with increased frequency after TBI [36, 149].

Another technique that involves white matter is *diffusion kurtosis imaging* [150], which provides another metric shown to be affected in CBI [151–153]: because of biological constraints in normal tissue, water diffusion metrics like those visualized

---

5   Petechial hemorrhages only hint at the microvascular harm caused by CBI. Experimental TBI in multiple species reveals that, short of frank hemorrhage, abrupt traumatic force causes mechanical damage to the vessel walls, with folding, cratering, and flattening of the lumen, vacuolation, degeneration, endothelial cell apoptosis, swelling of perivascular astrocytes, transcription of inflammatory factors, microglial activation, and blood–brain barrier disruption [142–145]. Moreover, evidence suggests reciprocal dysfunction, such that microvascular damage disrupts neural function and abnormal neural function causes microvascular damage [146].

White-matter regions colored to indicate the number of publications reporting abnormalities

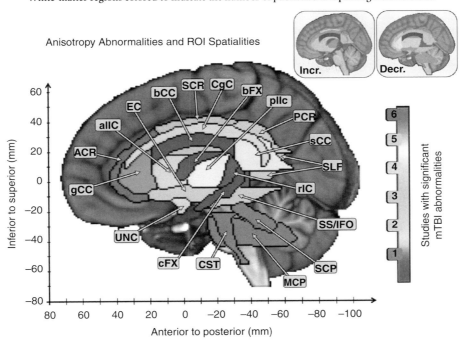

Fig. 6.7 Shown are the International Consortium of Brain Mapping (ICBM-81) white-matter regions, colored to indicate the number of publications reporting white-matter abnormalities (regions with no abnormal findings in the literature are not shown). The Montreal Neurological Institute (MNI-152) template is added for anatomical reference. Using the center of mass for each ICBM-81 structure, we determined that a significant anterior-to-posterior relationship exists between frequency in the literature and anatomical location. Note that since more lateral structures are only partially visible, the anatomical labels point to a convenient, visible location and do not necessarily reflect a structure's center of mass. For example, SLF is mostly covered by more medial structures and is only visible at its most posterior-inferior part. Coordinates are displayed in MNI-152 space. ACR: anterior corona radiata; aIIC: anterior limb of internal capsule; bCC: body of corpus callosum; bFX: body of fornix; cFX: fornix crus; CgC: cingulate cortex; CST: corticospinal tract; EC: entorhinal cortex; gCC: genu of corpus callosum; MCP: middle cerebellar peduncle; PCR: posterior corona radiata; pIIC: posterior limb of internal capsule; rIC: retrolenticular part of internal capsule; ROI: region of interest; SCC: splenium of corpus callosum; SCP: superior cerebellar peduncle; SCR: superior corona radiata; SLF: superior longitudinal fasciculus; SS/IFO: superior stratum/inferior fronto-occipital fasciculus; UNC: uncinate fasciculi. [A black and white version of this figure will appear in some formats. For the color version, please refer to the plate section.]

Source: Eierud et al., 2014 [35] with permission from Elsevier

with kurtosis imaging should have a rather uniform distribution, but would be expected to deviate in the shape of the distribution when damage occurs. Small focal contusions occur in CBI and may result in focal areas of atrophy [141]. Regions of focal atrophy may be quantified, as may whole-brain volumetric changes. Indeed, longitudinal volumetric studies that provide quantitative metrics show whole-brain volume loss over time in CBI subjects [154–156].

In a recent study of 251 pediatric mTBI cases [101], only a few children with CBI exhibited focal encephalomalacia. However, when it occurred in this cohort it was either in the frontal or temporal polar regions, as shown in Figure 6.11. Figure 6.11 also shows the distribution of focal areas of hemosiderin deposition as well as the location of WMHs. Note the frontotemporal distribution of these CBI-related abnormalities.

Magnetic Resonance Spectroscopy

MRS derives chemical signals, or metabolites, from a brain region of interest (ROI) where a spectrum of peaks reflects a particular chemical concentration within brain parenchyma that can be used as biomarkers of CBI [157, 158]. The beauty of the MRS plot is that (1) it is a non-invasive method using conventional MR sequences capable of assaying multiple

neurometabolic factors pertinent to brain integrity, and (2) it is sensitive to the effects of TBI [157, 159]. Figure 6.12 depicts the six spectroscopic peaks most commonly examined:

1. *N*-acetyl aspartate (NAA): NAA is an amino acid derivative synthesized in neurons and transported down axons. A decrease in the NAA signal (often summing NAA with *N*-acetyl aspartyl glutamate) is regarded as an indicator of either neuronal loss, dysmetabolism, or myelin repair [160].

2. Glutamate and glutamine (combined abbreviation: Glx): glutamate is the primary excitatory neurotransmitter in the brain and is tightly coupled to glutamine, which is found in the astrocytes. Post-concussive release of excessive glutamate is neurotoxic, and evidence suggests that the Glx signal is sensitive to "mTBI" [161, 162].

3. Choline (Cho): Cho is a marker of membrane lipid metabolites. Decreased Cho is thought to reflect axonal damage [163].

4. Myo-inositol (mI): this is an astrocyte marker and osmolyte that is also involved in the metabolism of phosphatidyl inositol, a membrane phospholipid. Increased mI levels are thought to reflect membrane

Atlas-based region-of-interest placement and group comparisons of fractional anisotropy values

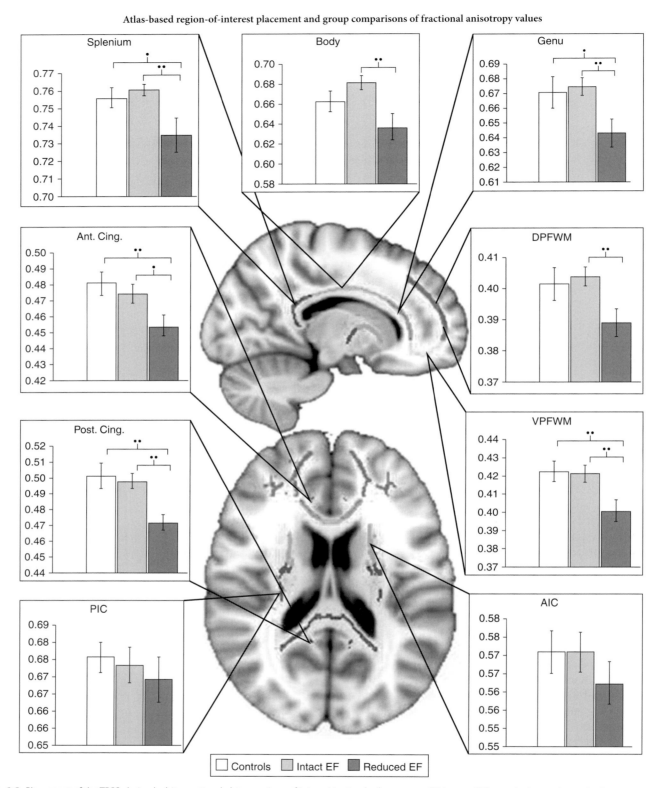

Fig. 6.8 Placement of the TBSS-derived white-matter skeleton regions of interest in standard space on a T1 image. AIC: anterior internal capsule; Ant. Cing.: anterior cingulum bundle; DPFWM: dorsal prefrontal white matter; EF: executive functions; PIC: posterior internal capsule; Post. Cing.: posterior cingulum bundle; TBSS, tract-based spatial statistics; VPFWM: ventral prefrontal white matter. Error bars represent s e m. a: corrected $p < 0.10$; b: corrected $p < 0.05$. [A black and white version of this figure will appear in some formats. For the color version, please refer to the plate section.]

Source: Sorg et al., 2014 [128] with permission from Lippincott Williams & Wilkins, Inc./Wolters Kluwer

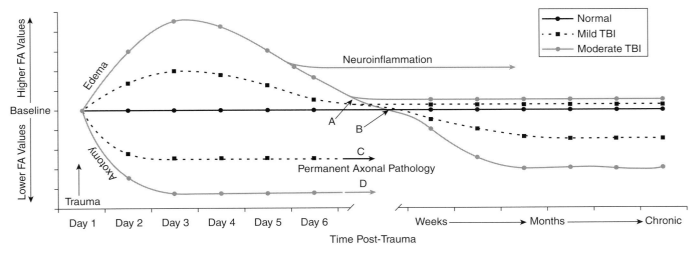

Fig. 6.9 Graph depicts the relationship between fractional anisotropy (FA) observed on functional magnetic resonance imaging and longitudinal changes in brain physiology after traumatic brain injury (TBI). In mild injury (typical concussive brain injury): (1) elevated FA values may identify regions that exhibit edema in the first week. (2) Depressed FA may identify regions at risk for axotomy. (3) Persistently elevated FA values (after the first week) may identify regions exhibiting chronic inflammation. (4) Persistently depressed FA may indicate permanent axonal pathology and atrophy. All of these changes may occur in the same individual; the differences are dependent on the time post-injury and local pathophysiological changes influencing neuronal health and axonal integrity. A reflects a theoretical return to baseline where "normal" functionality occurs. B reflects theoretical axonal pathology that evolves after inflammation where cellular function would be impaired. C reflects initial pathological changes indicating axon degradation after injury which ultimately progresses to axon damage. D reflects immediate shear axotomy from point of initial injury with immediate loss of axon integrity and function.

Source: original, Dr. Bigler

damage or to represent a glial marker, and are found after concussive injury [162].

5. Glutathione (GSH): reduced GSH is the major antioxidant in astrocytes. GSH measures may therefore provide insights into the antioxidant status of white matter [164].

6. Creatine (Cr): Cr is often used as an internal reference for the measurement of other peaks. Most MRS studies report ratios such as NAA/Cr, Cho/Cr, and mI/Cr. However, some evidence suggests that neither the Cr signal nor the ratio between Cr and phosphocreatine are constants, "rendering interpretation of ratio scores problematic" ([165], p. 2).

The remarkable heterogeneity of CBI is emphasized throughout this volume. Although recognizing the diversity of concussive injuries helps to explain otherwise mysterious inconsistencies in the literature, it also represents a limitation for current MRS studies. For example, one cannot reasonably expect the same biological change in one particular brain region across all concussions. Yet past CBI MRS studies have typically been limited in the number of regions of interest examined. This risks both false-positive and false-negative findings. A case in point is the multicenter CBI study by Vagnozzi et al. [167]. Young athletes with sports-related CBI underwent MRS within three days of injury and were followed systematically. At one of three sites, data were exclusively obtained from a single prefrontal lobe white-matter voxel. (Figure 6.13 depicts the single frontal voxel examined in this investigation.) The location of the region of interest was chosen to maximize the chance of detecting a change, given that this white-matter region is often impacted by

CBI. Initially depressed after the injury, the NAA/Cr ratio in that one voxel gradually returned to normal. And indeed, the report seems to suggest that sports-related concussion causes parenchymal damage that, to some degree, is reparable: the return of the NAA/Cr ratio to control baseline correlated roughly with improved clinical status. MRS was therefore proposed as a possible indicator of safe return to play. A potential problem with this approach: assaying the biochemistry of a single voxel fails to consider that individuals might vary in the locus or distribution of traumatic chemical disturbance [168–170].

Also using MRS, George et al. [171] reported a different outcome. The authors examined a more diverse CBI clinical population that encompassed multiple mechanisms of injury – including motor vehicle accidents and participants with "complicated mild TBI" (meaning with abnormal CT results on the day of injury). While all subjects met criteria for "mTBI" with no GCS below 13 and the mean GSC scores hovering around 14.5, the multi-voxel approach by George et al. showed that, in some regions, MRS values following CBI do *not* return to baseline, perhaps reflecting permanent pathology.

This is consistent with the findings of Yeo et al. [165]: 30 "mTBI" survivors were studied at the subacute stage. Conventional neuropsychological measures failed to detect any difference between the concussed group and matched controls, but, at a mean of 13 days post injury, CBI survivors exhibited significantly elevated white-matter Cre and Glx and depressed gray-matter Glx. Moreover, at a mean of 120 days post injury, CBI survivors showed recovery in gray-matter Glx, but continued abnormalities in white-matter Glx and Cre.[6] Such

---

6   Intriguingly, Yeo et al. [165] also found that estimated pre-morbid intelligence predicted metabolic normalization. That, is, cognitively superior subjects recovered better. Replication and further research will be required to determine why.

Magnetic resonancec findings in a patient with persistent symptoms one year post-concussion

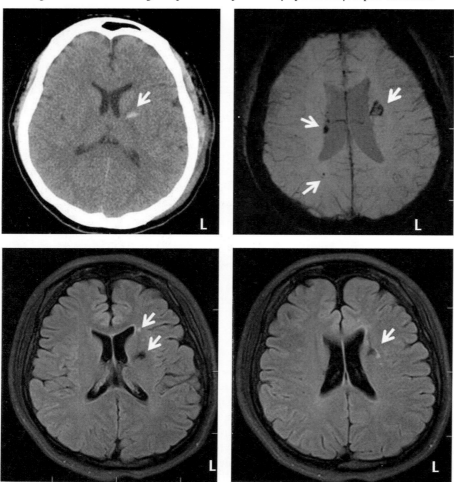

Fig. 6.10 On the day-of-injury computed tomography scan the patient had only a solitary small hemorrhage (top left: arrow). Subsequent magnetic resonance imaging revealed classic multifocal hemorrhagic and white-matter lesions (arrows).

Source: original, Dr. Bigler

reports suggest that MRS measures are substantially more sensitive than conventional cognitive testing, and have potential as biomarkers for both acute and chronic CBI [172].

Network Analyses That Integrate Structural and Functional Neuroimaging

As introduced in Figures 6.1 and 6.2, neuroimaging-based methods that assess the integrity of brain networks by *combining* structural and functional neuroimaging methods are being developed specifically to assess CBI [173]. Network analyses hold great promise, with the potential to better address the diversity of lesion presentation in CBI and individual differences in injury [91, 174].

Individualized Neuroimaging Biomarker Detection

Research benefits aside, the practical goal for most neuroimaging techniques is to develop them for clinical use, permitting health care providers to identify the type and location of pathology in individual CBI patients. Ideally, one hopes to find imaging markers that (1) have predictive validity and (2) identify modifiable risk factors for persistent post-concussive problems.

Figure 6.14 illustrates a general schematic of how this could be achieved. Neuroimaging metrics will differ by the type of scan obtained but the basic principle of image analysis will be the same where a normative range of values is determined by broadly sampling a typically developed, healthy, non-injured control sample. That control sample will permit normative values to be established for each measurable metric. (In the case of Figure 6.14, it is DTI.) When the CBI patient's values differ significantly, those values will be plotted on a representative scan image. In this way the clinician or researcher will be able to visualize where in the brain, and to what degree, differences from the norm can be observed. Progress toward that goal will still require a daunting research effort, combining imaging–pathological correlation studies with clinical inference to make sense out of the observed differences. But that multi-disciplinary, multi-institutional project will facilitate another step forward in understanding CBI-related brain change.

Magnetoencephalography

Magnetoencephalography (MEG) also has potential as a biomarker [175–177], although the limited availability and expense

Magnetic resonance imaging changes at 3 T in three survivors of pediatric traumatic brain injury

Fig. 6.11 Three cases from the Pediatric mTBI study highlight the independently identified magnetic resonance imaging abnormalities (blinded to group) observed in the first 251 patients screened for participant inclusion. Research magnetic resonance imaging studies were obtained all from the same GE 3-T scanner and included a sagittal-plane volume acquisition T1 IR-SPGR sequence (TR: 7.15 ms, TE: 2.90 ms, 1.2 mm slice thickness), T2-fluid-attenuated inversion recovery sequence (TR: 8000 ms, TE: 140.58 ms, 3.0 mm slice thickness) and a three-dimensional susceptibility-weighted imaging sequence (TR: 30 ms, TE: 23 ms, 1.0 mm slice thickness). Each abnormality was neuroradiologically defined as a region of interest generated by hand tracing the lesion boundaries on to a template image using Mango (http://ric.uthscsa.edu/mango/). Then, a surface model was generated to represent each lesion area in three-dimensional space. The regions of interest represent the relative location where lesions were located. Small white-matter hyperintensities and regions of hemosiderin deposition were slightly enlarged to improve visualization. [A black and white version of this figure will appear in some formats. For the color version, please refer to the plate section.]

Source: Bigler et al., 2016 [101] with permission from Lippincott Williams & Wilkins, Inc./Wolters Kluwer

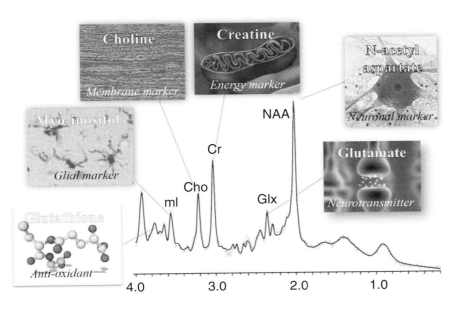

Fig. 6.12 The six MRS spectroscopic peaks most commonly measured. Cho: choline; Cr: creatine; Glx: glutamate; ml: myoinositol; NAA: *N*-acetyl aspartate. [A black and white version of this figure will appear in some formats. For the color version, please refer to the plate section.]

Source: Koerte et al., 2015 [166] © Georg Thieme Verlag KG. Reproduced with permission

Top: axial magnetic resonance imaging (MRI) showing one frontal voxel and its magnetic resonance spectroscopy (MRS) spectrum

Bottom: recovery of *N*-acetyl aspartate (NAA) measures in 40 athletes and 30 controls

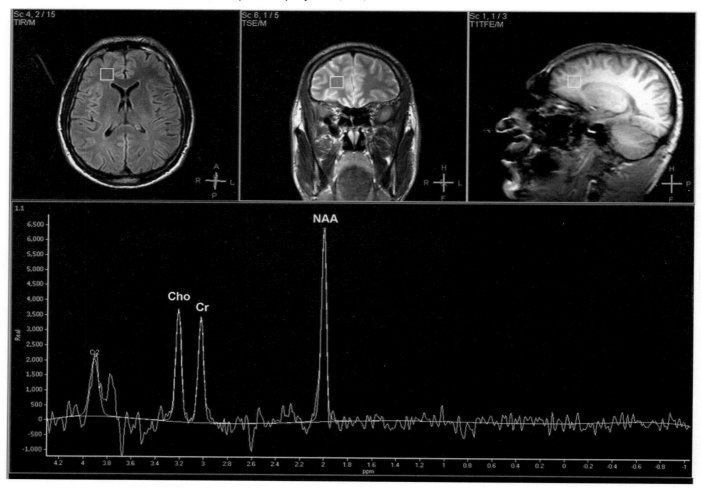

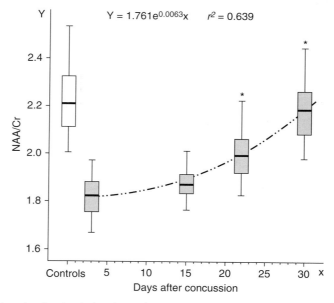

Fig. 6.13 Top: axial MRI of a normal volunteer showing the single volume of interest (single voxel) located in the right frontal lobe, along with the corresponding proton spectrum. The tallest peak on the right represents NAA, the middle peak creatine-containing compounds (Cr), and leftmost choline-containing compounds (Cho).

Bottom: box plot showing the recovery of the NAA/Cr-containing compound ratio occurring in 40 athletes following concussion and reporting the equation and the best-fit curve to the data (indicated by a dash-dotted line). Each box is the mean value determined in 30 healthy controls and 40 concussed athletes. Confidence intervals (95%) are represented by vertical bars. *$p < 0.01$ with respect to three days.

Source: Vagnozzi et al., 2010 [167] by permission of Oxford University Press

A schematic showing how individuals can be compared with norms

Individual Subject Testing

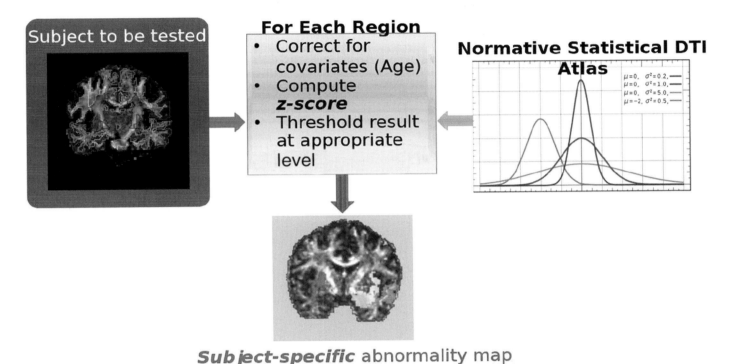

Subject-specific abnormality map

Fig. 6.14 A coronal diffusion tensor imaging (DTI) color map depicting the raw fractional anisotropy data for an individual subject is depicted in the upper left. A voxel-by-voxel comparison is made with a normative statistical DTI atlas where various demographic variables are taken into consideration, as shown in the middle box. The subject-specific output is displayed as a "heat map," showing where the most significant statistical deviations occur in the individual patient with concussive brain injury compared to the healthy, typically developing normative sample. [A black and white version of this figure will appear in some formats. For the color version, please refer to the plate section.]

Source: illustration courtesy of Sylvain Bouix, Ph.D. and Martha E. Shenton, Ph.D., Psychiatry Neuroimaging Lab, Brigham and Women's Hospital and Harvard Medical School

of MEG are currently rate-limiting factors for the widespread use of this technique. Nonetheless, it appears to be an exceptionally sensitive detector of abnormalities associated with TBI [98]. Although positron emission tomography and single-photon emission tomography imaging techniques provide biomarker identifiers for mTBI [178], expense and exposure to radiation are limiting factors for the biomarker research, especially for sequential imaging to track findings over time.

Near-Infrared Spectroscopy

Lastly, near-infrared spectroscopy technology has been quickly improving, and this technique may have a biomarker role in assessing CBI [179]. The procedure is portable and inexpensive. Unfortunately, current technology is only capable of assessing a limited number of cortical regions and does not directly assess white matter.

General Commentary

These examples hopefully illustrate important ways in which neuroimages may serve as biomarkers of CBI. It is a matter

of some urgency that valid and reliable biomarkers be identified, since the clinical impact on the human population may be massive and growing, and since the dated clinical criteria of so-called "mTBI" do not correlate with or predict somatic, cognitive, or behavioral sequelae [36, 180]. We by no means propose that currently available imaging is sensitive and specific enough to decipher the protean pathophysiology of an individual CBI, to predict persistent post-concussive problems, to identify those at greatest risk for late-onset post-concussive neurodegeneration, or to guide therapy. That would be hyperventilation – as short-sighted as some early claims about the boundless promise of pneumoencephalography and EEG. The sensitivity of imaging technology is sure to improve, so a textbook (like a consensus guideline) must not yoke diagnosis to findings from some momentarily state-of-the-art device. The principle is what matters: there are good reasons to believe that imaging has already surpassed the sensitivity of cognitive testing for the detection of clinically problematic persistent post-traumatic brain change. It remains to be seen: (1) what the predictive validity of currently visualized changes is for future patient function; (2) what future imaging might permit one to conclude about future patient function; and (3) what proportion of those with CBIs genuinely recover to their pre-morbid baseline, without exhibiting non-obvious yet deleterious long-term changes, such as:

1. preserved performance on conventional, if antiquated, testing as well as on more sophisticated and concussion-sensitive testing, and absence of any subjective sense of cognitive or non-cognitive impairment, due to recovery of salvageable neurons, adaptive remodeling circumventing neuronal losses, and neurogenesis that permits *true* return to baseline performance – albeit at a higher cost in energy efficiency, which might lead to untoward consequences such as increased mitochondrial stress, production of reactive oxygen species, and premature brain aging, even if the patient looks and feels as good as new for the first 50–70 years after his concussion

2. preserved performance on conventional testing and absence of any subjective sense of cognitive or non-cognitive impairment, together creating the false impression of return to "baseline," contradicted by the presence of detectable declines from baseline when exposed to: (1) sophisticated and concussion-sensitive neuropsychological tests; or (2) performing at or near the limits of capacity; or (3) under circumstances such as divided attention

3. preserved performance on conventional testing creating the false impression of return to baseline, but imperfect salvage of damaged neural and glial elements, imperfect adaptive remodeling and insufficient neurogenesis adaptation, causing subjective feelings that cognitive work that formerly was straightforward has become more effortful. (This is perhaps the most common scenario in which the clinician is at risk of failing to understand his or her patient)

4. preserved performance on conventional testing *and* on more sophisticated neuropsychological testing, as well as absence of any subjective sense of cognitive difficulty whatsoever, in the presence of some degree of emotional dysregulation that impairs quality of life, subjective well-being, social relations, and resilience in the face of stress – whether or not that emotional dysregulation is subjectively or clinically detectable

5. preserved performance on conventional testing *and* on more sophisticated neuropsychological testing, as well as absence of any subjective sense of cognitive difficulty or emotional dysregulation whatsoever … for the first 50–70 years after the concussion, in the presence of acceleration of one or more of the very large number of known (or suspected) aging-associated neurobiological changes, perhaps beginning within minutes after the concussion

6. preserved performance on conventional testing *and* on more sophisticated neuropsychological testing, as well as absence of any subjective sense of cognitive difficulty or emotional dysregulation whatsoever … for the first 50–70 years after the concussion.

In other words, we are on the very cusp of a new clinical paradigm of CBI in which, rather than declaring with supercilious brass that hard-to-see damage does not exist, we are open-minded about the possibility that hard-to-detect damage not only exists but is clinically important. Neuroimaging – as early and primitive as it is – opens the door to awareness of such previously imperceptible damage. Yes, it is a little too soon to interpret visible changes on scans (e.g., mysterious changes in echo intensity or anisotropy or chemical spectra or magnetic fields or ligand binding) as *biomarkers* that validly and reliably localize and measure the most worrisome sorts of brain damage. But we are getting closer every day.

Over the Horizon

One is eager to see what the future holds for non-invasive brain imaging, but hard-pressed to guess which technology will deliver the CBI biomarker breakthroughs we urgently need. What, after all, do we wish to know? Is the brain healthy? Answering that question might include analysis of functionality and potentiality over many orders of magnitude – from "Do electrons get transported efficiently by the mitochondria?" to "Does the connectome respond to experience as it should?" That which best reflects the occurrence of and response to typical CBI might be some molecular anomaly of neuronal organelles, spines, axons, synapses, glia, clearance, neurogenesis, transneuronal spread of atypical protein folding, immunoregulation – or perhaps an emergent property such as plasticity or connectivity. We may already have the big machine that offers the answer and just need to up our analytic game. Or the most pertinent metric might require detection at unheard-of levels of precision.

For example, one of many innovations likely to come online is enhanced spatial and spectral resolution of NMR spectroscopy. The resolution and sensitivity of conventional MRI have been limited by its reliance on perturbing nuclear spins – considered collectively across multicellular swathes of tissue – with an external magnet, and measuring their rotation frequency with nearby inductive coils. Novel methods are pushing the envelope toward detecting a single nuclear spin. That would theoretically enhance precision by 12–13 orders of magnitude [181]). New nano-NMR technology capitalizes on the capacity of sensors to optically read spin qubits formed by negatively charged nitrogen vacancy defects in diamonds. Employing that technology, Bucher et al. [182] may have been the first to report successful detection of chemical shifts at the level of a single protein in ~ 1-pL liquid samples. The precision of such sensors depends on accumulating coherent signals over time. Hence, better spectroscopy requires longer qubit coherence time. Schmitt et al. [183] reported a protocol permitting them to leapfrog that limitation, sensing nanoscale magnetic fields (such as those that accompany chemical shifts in single proteins) with a frequency resolution eight orders of magnitude narrower than the qubit coherence time. Boss et al. [184] employed stroboscopic periodic sampling to extract signals "reaching a frequency resolution of 70 mHz and a precision of 260 nHz with SNR [signal-to-noise ratio] > 104" (p. 837). And

Aslam et al. [185] recently reported an NMR linewidth of about 1 ppm in a 20-zL sample. This technology perhaps opens the door to videos of individual proteins folding within a neuron.

Of course, translating this benchtop method to the clinical setting poses fearsome engineering challenges. For instance, how would one sufficiently decrease the distance between the sensor and the sample without invading the brain? And one may soon face the cable-TV question: "Honey, which of the 6353 proteins expressed in each of the 16 billion neocortical neurons shall we watch tonight?"[7] Long before we exhaust the potential findings regarding the brain's proteome, even with current technology, we will exhaust the Earth's entire computational power. Such conundra notwithstanding, the astonishing pace of progress in metrology hopefully presages an entirely new generation of *in vivo* brain assays.

References

1. Menon DK, Schwab K, Wright DW, Maas AI, on behalf of The Demographics and Clinical Assessment Working Group of the International and Interagency Initiative toward Common Data Elements for Research on Traumatic Brain Injury and Psychological Health. Position statement: definition of traumatic brain injury. *Arch Phys Med Rehabil* 2010; 91: 1637–40.

2. Garrod AE. The Croonian lectures on inborn errors of metabolism. Delivered before the Royal College of Physicians on June 18th, 23rd, 25th, and 30th, (1908). *Lancet* 1908; 172(4427): 1–7; 172(4428): 73–79; 172(4429): 142–148; 172(4430): 214–230.

3. Bigler ED. Mild traumatic brain injury: the elusive timing of "recovery." *Neurosci Lett* 2012; 509: 1–4.

4. Carroll LJ, Cassidy JD, Holm L, Kraus J, Coronado VG, WHO Collaborating Centre Task Force on Mild Traumatic Brain Injury. Methodological issues and research recommendations for mild traumatic brain injury: The WHO Collaborating Centre Task Force on Mild Traumatic Brain Injury. *J Rehabil Med* 2004; 113–25.

5. Larrabee GJ, Binder LM, Rohling ML, Ploetz DM. Meta-analytic methods and the importance of non-TBI factors related to outcome in mild traumatic brain injury: response to Bigler et al. (2013). *Clin Neuropsychol* 2013; 27: 215–37.

6. Rohling ML, Binder LM, Demakis GJ, Larrabee GJ, Ploetz DM, Langhinrichsen-Rohling J. A meta-analysis of neuropsychological outcome after mild traumatic brain injury: re-analyses and reconsiderations of Binder et al. (1997), Frencham et al. (2005), and Pertab et al. (2009). *Clin Neuropsychol* 2011; 25: 608–23.

7. Greiffenstein MF. Foreword. In: Carone DA, Bush SS (eds.) *Traumatic brain injury: symptom validity assessment and malingering*. New York: Springer, 2013, p. xiii.

8. Boone KB. *Clinical practice of forensic neuropsychology*. New York: Guilford, 2013.

9. Ponsford J, Cameron P, Fitzgerald M, Grant M, Mikocka-Walus A. Long-term outcomes after uncomplicated mild traumatic brain injury: a comparison with trauma controls. *J Neurotrauma* 2011; 28: 937–46.

10. Barlow KM, Crawford S, Stevenson A, Sandhu SS, Belanger F, Dewey D. Epidemiology of postconcussion syndrome in pediatric mild traumatic brain injury. *Pediatrics* 2010; 126: e374–81.

11. Eisenberg MA, Andrea J, Meehan W, Mannix R. Time interval between concussions and symptom duration. *Pediatrics* 2013; 132: 8–17.

12. McMillan TM, Teasdale GM, Stewart E. Disability in young people and adults after head injury: 12–14 year follow-up of a prospective cohort. *J Neurol Neurosurg Psychiatry* 2012; 83: 1086–91.

13. Levin H, Li X, McCauley SR, Hanten G, Wilde EA, Swank PR. Neuropsychological outcome of MTBI: a principal component analysis approach. *J Neurotrauma* 2013; 30(8): 625–32.

14. Dean PJ, Sterr A. Long-term effects of mild traumatic brain injury on cognitive performance. *Front Hum Neurosci* 2013; 7: 30.

15. Kumar S, Rao SL, Chandramouli BA, Pillai S. Reduced contribution of executive functions in impaired working memory performance in mild traumatic brain injury patients. *Clin Neurol Neurosurg* 2013; 115: 1326–32.

16. Pontifex MB, Broglio SP, Drollette ES, Scudder MR, Johnson CR, O'Connor PM, et al. The relation of mild traumatic brain injury to chronic lapses of attention. *Res Q Exerc Sport* 2012; 83: 553–9.

17. Tallus J, Lioumis P, Hamalainen H, Kahkonen S, Tenovuo O. TMS-EEG responses in recovered and symptomatic mild traumatic brain injury. *J Neurotrauma* 2013; 30(14): 1270–7.

18. Silver JM. Effort, exaggeration and malingering after concussion. *J Neurol Neurosurg Psychiatry* 2012; 83: 836–41.

19. Heitger MH, Jones RD, Macleod AD, Snell DL, Frampton CM, Anderson TJ. Impaired eye movements in post-concussion syndrome indicate suboptimal brain function beyond the influence of depression, malingering or intellectual ability. *Brain* 2009; 132: 2850–70.

20. Hanten G, Li X, Ibarra A, Wilde EA, Barnes AF, Mccauley SR, et al. Updating memory after mild TBI and orthopedic injuries. *J Neurotrauma* 2012; 30 (8): 618–24.

21. Konrad C, Geburek AJ, Rist F, Blumenroth H, Fischer B, Husstedt I, et al. Long-term cognitive and emotional consequences of mild traumatic brain injury. *Psychol Med* 2010; 1–15.

22. Cipolotti L, Warrington EK. Neuropsychological assessment. *J Neurol Neurosurg Psychiatry* 1995; 58: 655–64.

23. Shenton ME, Hamoda HM, Schneiderman JS, Bouix S, Pasternak O, Rathi Y, et al. A review of magnetic resonance imaging and diffusion tensor imaging findings in mild traumatic brain injury. *Brain Imaging Behav* 2012; 6: 137–92.

24. Beckmann EC. CT scanning: the early days. *Br J Radiol* 2006; 79: 5–8.

25. Robb WL. Perspective on the first 10 years of the CT scanner industry. *Acad Radiol* 2003; 10: 756–60.

26. Bigler ED, Snyder JL. Neuropsychological outcome and quantitative neuroimaging in mild head injury. *Arch Clin Neuropsychol* 1995; 10: 159–74.

27. Gama JP. *Traité des plaies de tête et de l'encéphalite, principalement de celle: qui leur est consécutive; ouvrage dans lequel sont discutées plusieurs questions relatives aux fonctions du système nerveux en général [Treatise of head injuries and of encephalitis in which many questions concerning the functions of the nervous system are discussed].* Paris: Sedillot; 1830.

28. Feinsod MA. Flask full of jelly: the first in vitro model of concussive head injury – 1830. *Neurosurg* 2002; 50: 386–391.

29. Holbourn AHS. Mechanics of head injuries. *Lancet* 1943; 2: 438–41.

30. Strich SJ. Diffuse degeneration of cerebral white matter in severe dementia following head injury. *J Neurol Neurosurg Psychiatry* 1956; 19: 163–85.

---

[7] According to one estimate, if that scientist couple were to check for gene expression of each gene in each neuron at the rate of one gene–cell pair per second, their project would require more than 100 million years [186].

31. Strich SJ. Shearing-of nerve fibers as a cause of brain damage due to head injury, a pathological study of 20 cases. *Lancet* 1961; 2: 443–8.

32. Peerless SJ, Rewcastle NB. Shear injuries of the brain. *Can Med Assoc J* 1967; 96: 577–82.

33. Adams JH. Diffuse axonal injury in non-missile head injury. *Injury* 1982; 13: 444–5.

34. Amyot F, Arciniegas DB, Brazaitis MP, Curley KC, Diaz-Arrastia R, Gandjbakhche A, et al. A review of the effectiveness of neuroimaging modalities for the detection of traumatic brain injury. *J Neurotrauma* 2015; 32: 1693–721.

35. Eierud C, Craddock RC, Fletcher S, Aulakh M, King-Casas B, Kuehl D, et al. Neuroimaging after mild traumatic brain injury: review and meta-analysis. *NeuroImage Clin* 2014; 4: 283–94.

36. Bigler ED. Neuroimaging biomarkers in mild traumatic brain injury (mTBI). *Neuropsychol Rev* 2013; 23: 169–209.

37. Bigler ED. Structural image analysis of the brain in neuropsychology using magnetic resonance imaging (MRI) techniques. *Neuropsychol Rev* 2015; 25: 224–49.

38. Mutch WA, Ellis MJ, Ryner LN, Ruth Graham M, Dufault B, Gregson B, et al. Brain magnetic resonance imaging CO stress testing in adolescent postconcussion syndrome. *J Neurosurg* 2015; 1–13.

39. Kou Z, Wu Z, Tong KA, Holshouser B, Benson RR, Hu J, et al. The role of advanced MR imaging findings as biomarkers of traumatic brain injury. *J Head Trauma Rehabil* 2010; 25: 267–82.

40. Insel TR, Landis SC. Twenty-five years of progress: the view from NIMH and NINDS. *Neuron* 2013; 80: 561–7.

41. Bryer EJ, Medaglia JD, Rostami S, Hillary FG. Neural recruitment after mild traumatic brain injury is task dependent: a meta-analysis. *J Int Neuropsychol Soc: JINS* 2013; 1–12.

42. Slobounov S, Gay M, Johnson B, Zhang K. Concussion in athletics: ongoing clinical and brain imaging research controversies. *Brain Imaging Behav* 2012; 6: 224–43.

43. Zhou Y, Lui YW. Changes in brain organization after TBI: evidence from functional MRI findings. *Neurology* 2013; 80: 1822–3.

44. Damadian R, Minkoff L, Goldsmith M, Stanford M, Koutcher J. Field focusing nuclear magnetic resonance (FONAR): visualization of a tumor in a live animal. *Science* 1976; 194: 1430–2.

45. Geva T. Magnetic resonance imaging: historical perspective. *J Cardiovasc Magn Reson* 2006; 8: 573–80.

46. Hellyer PJ, Leech R, Ham TE, Bonnelle V, Sharp DJ. Individual prediction of white matter injury following traumatic brain injury. *Ann Neurol* 2013; 73: 489–99.

47. Raz E, Jensen JH, Ge Y, Babb JS, Miles L, Reaume J, et al. Brain iron quantification in mild traumatic brain injury: a magnetic field correlation study. *Am J Neuroradiol* 2011; 32: 1–14.

48. Duhaime AC, Holshouser B, Hunter JV, Tong K. Common data elements for neuroimaging of traumatic brain injury: pediatric considerations. *J Neurotrauma* 2012; 29: 629–33.

49. Hunter JV, Wilde EA, Tong KA, Holshouser BA. Emerging imaging tools for use with traumatic brain injury research. *J Neurotrauma* 2012; 29: 654–71.

50. Fox WC, Park MS, Belverud S, Klugh A, Rivet D, Tomlin JM. Contemporary imaging of mild TBI: the journey toward diffusion tensor imaging to assess neuronal damage. *Neurol Res* 2013; 35: 223–32.

51. Strauss S, Hulkower M, Gulko E, Zampolin RL, Gutman D, Chitkara M, et al. Current clinical applications and future potential of diffusion tensor imaging in traumatic brain injury. *Top Magn Reson Imaging* 2015; 24: 353–62.

52. Alexander AL, Lee JE, Lazar M, Field AS. Diffusion tensor imaging of the brain. *Neurotherapeut: J Am Soc Exper NeuroTherapeut* 2007; 4: 316–29.

53. Chanraud S, Zahr N, Sullivan EV, Pfefferbaum A. MR diffusion tensor imaging: a window into white matter integrity of the working brain. *Neuropsychol Rev* 2010; 20: 209–25.

54. Chapman CH, Nagesh V, Sundgren PC, Buchtel H, Chenevert TL, Junck L, et al. Diffusion tensor imaging of normal-appearing white matter as biomarker for radiation-induced late delayed cognitive decline. *Int J Radiat Oncol Biol Phys* 2012; 82: 2033–40.

55. Sundgren PC, Dong Q, Gomez-Hassan D, Mukherji SK, Maly P, Welsh R. Diffusion tensor imaging of the brain: review of clinical applications. *Neuroradiol* 2004; 46: 339–50.

56. Travers BG, Adluru N, Ennis C, Tromp Do PM, Destiche D, Doran S, et al. Diffusion tensor imaging in autism spectrum disorder: a review. *Autism Res* 2012; 5: 289–313.

57. Wycoco V, Shroff M, Sudhakar S, Lee W. White matter anatomy: what the radiologist needs to know. *Neuroimaging Clin N Am* 2013; 23: 197–216.

58. Zappala G, Thiebaut De Schotten M, Eslinger PJ. Traumatic brain injury and the frontal lobes: what can we gain with diffusion tensor imaging? *Cortex* 2012; 48: 156–65.

59. Mayer AR, Ling JM, Yang Z, Pena A, Yeo RA, Klimaj S. Diffusion abnormalities in pediatric mild traumatic brain injury. *J Neurosci* 2012; 32: 17961–9.

60. Pandit AS, Expert P, Lambiotte R, Bonnelle V, Leech R, Turkheimer FE, et al. Traumatic brain injury impairs small-world topology. *Neurology* 2013; 80: 1826–33.

61. Shumskaya E, Andriessen TM, Norris DG, Vos PE. Abnormal whole-brain functional networks in homogeneous acute mild traumatic brain injury. *Neurology* 2012; 79: 175–82.

62. Stevens MC, Lovejoy D, Kim J, Oakes H, Kureshi I, Witt ST. Multiple resting state network functional connectivity abnormalities in mild traumatic brain injury. *Brain Imaging Behav* 2012; 6: 293–318.

63. Tang L, Ge Y, Sodickson DK, Miles L, Zhou Y, Reaume J, et al. Thalamic resting-state functional networks: disruption in patients with mild traumatic brain injury. *Radiology* 2011; 260: 831–40.

64. Voelbel GT, Genova HM, Chiaravalloti ND, Hoptman MJ. Diffusion tensor imaging of traumatic brain injury review: implications for neurorehabilitation. *NeuroRehabilitation* 2012; 31: 281–93.

65. Maxwell WL. Damage to myelin and oligodendrocytes: a role in chronic outcomes following traumatic brain injury? *Brain Sci* 2013; 3: 1374–94.

66. Catani M, Thiebaut De Schotten M. *Atlas of human brain connections.* Oxford: Oxford University Press, 2012.

67. Mori SVZ, Peter CM, Oishi K, Faria AV. *MRI atlas of human white matter,* 2nd edition. New York: Elsevier, 2012.

68. Huston JM, Field AS. Clinical applications of diffusion tensor imaging. *Magn Reson Imaging Clin N Am* 2013; 21: 279–98.

69. Qiu A, Mori S, Miller MI. Diffusion tensor imaging for understanding brain development in early life. *Annu Rev Psychol* 2015; 66: 853–76.

70. Van Essen DC, Barch DM. The human connectome in health and psychopathology. *World Psychiatry* 2015; 14: 154–7.

71. Irimia A, Goh SY, Torgerson CM, Vespa P, Van Horn JD. Structural and connectomic neuroimaging for the personalized study of longitudinal alterations in cortical shape, thickness and connectivity after traumatic brain injury. *J Neurosurg Sci* 2014; 58: 129–44.

72. Ratnarajah N, Rifkin-Graboi A, Fortier MV, Chong YS, Kwek K, et al. Structural connectivity asymmetry in the neonatal brain. *NeuroImage* 2013; 75: 187–94.

73. Williams DH, Levin HS, Eisenberg HM. Mild head injury classification. *Neurosurgery* 1990; 27(3): 422–8.

74. Korinthenberg R, Schreck J, Wesera J, Lehmkuhlb G. Posttraumatic syndrome after minor head injury cannot be predicted by neurological investigations. *Brain Devel* 2004; 26: 113–17.

75. McCrory P, Meeuwisse W, Johnston K, Dvorak J, Aubry M, Molloy M, et al. Consensus statement on concussion in sport – the 3rd International Conference on Concussion in Sport, held in Zurich, November 2008. *J Clin Neurosci* 2009; 16: 755–63.

76. Riedy G, Senseney JS, Liu W, Ollinger J, Sham E, Krapiva P, et al. Findings from structural MR imaging in military traumatic brain injury. *Radiology* 2015: 150438.

77. Petersen SE, Sporns O. Brain networks and cognitive architectures. *Neuron* 2015; 88: 207–19.

78. Sporns O, Betzel RF. Modular brain networks. *Annu Rev Psychol* 2016; 67: 613–40.

79. Churchland PS, Sejnowski TJ. *The computational brain.* Cambridge, MA: MIT Press, 1992.

80. Sejnowski TJ, Churchland PS. Brain and cognition. In: Posner M (ed.) *Foundations of cognitive science.* Cambridge, MA: MIT Press, 1989, p. 888.

81. Chatelin S, Deck C, Renard F, Kremer S, Heinrich C, Armspach JP, et al. Computation of axonal elongation in head trauma finite element simulation. *J Mech Behav Biomed Mater* 2011; 4: 1905–19.

82. Post A, Hoshizaki TB, Gilchrist MD, Brien S, Cusimano M, Marshall S. Traumatic brain injuries: the influence of the direction of impact. *Neurosurgery* 2015; 76: 81–91.

83. Sullivan S, Eucker SA, Gabrieli D, Bradfield C, Coats B, Maltese MR, et al. White matter tract-oriented deformation predicts traumatic axonal brain injury and reveals rotational direction-specific vulnerabilities. *Biomech Model Mechanobiol* 2015; 14: 877–96.

84. Bayly PV, Clayton EH, Genin GM. Quantitative imaging methods for the development and validation of brain biomechanics models. *Annu Rev Biomed Eng* 2012; 14: 369–96.

85. Wilde EA, McCauley SR, Hunter JV, Bigler ED, Chu Z, Wang ZJ, et al. Diffusion tensor imaging of acute mild traumatic brain injury in adolescents. *Neurology* 2008; 70: 948–55.

86. Chu Z, Wilde EA, Hunter JV, McCauley SR, Bigler ED, Troyanskaya M, et al. Voxel-based analysis of diffusion tensor imaging in mild traumatic brain injury in adolescents. *AJNR Am J Neuroradiol* 2010; 31: 340–6.

87. Messe A, Caplain S, Pelegrini-Issac M, Blancho S, Montreuil M, Levy R, et al. Structural integrity and postconcussion syndrome in mild traumatic brain injury patients. *Brain Imaging Behav* 2012; 6: 283–92.

88. Koerte IK, Hufschmidt J, Muehlmann M, Lin AP, Shenton ME. Advanced neuroimaging of mild traumatic brain injury. In: Laskowitz D, Grant G (eds.) *Translational research in traumatic brain injury.* Boca Raton (FL): Frontiers in Neuroscience, 2016.

89. Metting Z, Cerliani L, Rodiger LA, Van Der Naalt J. Pathophysiological concepts in mild traumatic brain injury: diffusion tensor imaging related to acute perfusion CT imaging. *PLoS One* 2013; 8: e64461.

90. Bandak FA, Ling G, Bandak A, De Lanerolle NC. Injury biomechanics, neuropathology, and simplified physics of explosive blast and impact mild traumatic brain injury. *Handb Clin Neurol* 2015; 127: 89–104.

91. Wilde EA, Bouix S, Tate DF, Lin AP, Newsome MR, Taylor BA, et al. Advanced neuroimaging applied to veterans and service personnel with traumatic brain injury: state of the art and potential benefits. *Brain Imaging Behav* 2015; 9: 367–402.

92. Jang SH, Seo JP. Damage to the optic radiation in patients with mild traumatic brain injury. *J Neuroophthalmol* 2015; 35: 270–3.

93. Davenport ND, Lim KO, Sponheim SR. White matter abnormalities associated with military PTSD in the context of blast TBI. *Hum Brain Mapp* 2015; 36: 1053–64.

94. Shin SS, Pathak S, Presson N, Bird W, Wagener L, Schneider W, et al. Detection of white matter injury in concussion using high-definition fiber tractography. *Prog Neurol Surg* 2014; 28: 86–93.

95. Yuh EL, Cooper SR, Mukherjee P, Yue JK, Lingsma HF, Gordon WA, et al. Diffusion tensor imaging for outcome prediction in mild traumatic brain injury: a TRACK-TBI study. *J Neurotrauma* 2014; 31: 1457–77.

96. Wang X, Wei XE, Li MH, Li WB, Zhou YJ, Zhang B, et al. Microbleeds on susceptibility-weighted MRI in depressive and non-depressive patients after mild traumatic brain injury. *Neurol Sci* 2014; 35: 1533–9.

97. Xiong KL, Zhu YS, Zhang WG. Diffusion tensor imaging and magnetic resonance spectroscopy in traumatic brain injury: a review of recent literature. *Brain Imaging Behav* 2014; 8: 487–96.

98. Lewine JD, Davis JT, Bigler ED, Thoma R, Hill D, Funke M, et al. Objective documentation of traumatic brain injury subsequent to mild head trauma: multimodal brain imaging with MEG, SPECT, and MRI. *J Head Trauma Rehabil* 2007; 22: 141–55.

99. Niogi SN, Mukherjee P, Ghajar J, Johnson C, Kolster RA, Sarkar R, et al. Extent of microstructural white matter injury in postconcussive syndrome correlates with impaired cognitive reaction time: a 3T diffusion tensor imaging study of mild traumatic brain injury. *AJNR Am J Neuroradiol* 2008; 29: 967–73.

100. Ennis DB, Kindlmann G. Orthogonal tensor invariants and the analysis of diffusion tensor magnetic resonance images. *Magn Reson Med* 2006; 55(1): 136–46.

101. Bigler ED, Abildskov TJ, Goodrich-Hunsaker NJ, Black G, Christensen ZP, Huff T, et al. Structural neuroimaging findings in mild traumatic brain injury. *Sports Med Arthrosc* 2016; 24(3): e42–52.

102. Hulkower MB, Poliak DB, Rosenbaum SB, Zimmerman ME, Lipton ML. A decade of DTI in traumatic brain injury: 10 years and 100 articles later. *AJNR Am J Neuroradiol* 2013; 34 (11): 2064–74.

103. Bigler ED, Bazarian JJ. Diffusion tensor imaging: a biomarker for mild traumatic brain injury? *Neurology* 2010; 74: 626–7.

104. Kuo JR, Lo CJ, Chang CP, Lin HJ, Lin MT, Chio CC. Brain cooling-stimulated angiogenesis and neurogenesis attenuated traumatic brain injury in rats. *J Trauma* 2010; 69: 1467–72.

105. Ling JM, Pena A, Yeo RA, Merideth FL, Klimaj S, Gasparovic C, et al. Biomarkers of increased diffusion anisotropy in semi-acute mild traumatic brain injury: a longitudinal perspective. *Brain* 2012; 135: 1281–92.

106. Niogi SN, Mukherjee P. Diffusion tensor imaging of mild traumatic brain injury. *J Head Trauma Rehabil* 2010; 25: 241–55.

107. Bigler ED, Maxwell WL. Neuroimaging and neuropathology of TBI. *NeuroRehabil* 2011; 28: 63–74.

108. Bennett RE, Mac Donald CL, Brody DL. Diffusion tensor imaging detects axonal injury in a mouse model of repetitive closed-skull traumatic brain injury. *Neurosci Lett* 2012; 513: 160–5.

109. Budde MD, Janes L, Gold E, Turtzo LC, Frank JA. The contribution of gliosis to diffusion tensor anisotropy and tractography following traumatic brain injury: validation in the rat using Fourier analysis of stained tissue sections. *Brain* 2011; 134: 2248–60.

110. Hylin MJ, Orsi SA, Zhao J, Bockhorst K, Perez A, Moore AN, et al. Behavioral and histopathological alterations resulting from mild fluid percussion injury. *J Neurotrauma* 2013; 30: 702–15.

111. Abdullah KG, Lubelski D, Nucifora PG, Brem S. Use of diffusion tensor imaging in glioma resection. *Neurosurg Focus* 2013; 34: E1.

112. Liu P, Li YS, Quartermain D, Boutajangout A, Ji Y. Inhaled nitric oxide improves short term memory and reduces the inflammatory reaction in a mouse model of mild traumatic brain injury. *Brain Res* 2013; 1522: 67–75.

113. Aoki Y, Inokuchi R, Gunshin M, Yahagi N, Suwa H. Diffusion tensor imaging studies of mild traumatic brain injury: a meta-analysis. *J Neurol Neurosurg Psychiatry* 2012; 83: 870–6.

114. McAllister TW, Ford JC, Ji S, Beckwith JG, Flashman LA, Paulsen K, et al. Maximum principal strain and strain rate associated with concussion diagnosis correlates with changes in corpus callosum white matter indices. *Ann Biomed Eng* 2012; 40: 127–40.

115. Breedlove EL, Robinson M, Talavage TM, Morigaki KE, Yoruk U, O'Keefe K, et al. Biomechanical correlates of symptomatic and asymptomatic neurophysiological impairment in high school football. *J Biomech* 2012; 45: 1265–72.

116. McCrea M, Hammeke T, Olsen G, Leo P, Guskiewicz K. Unreported concussion in high school football players: implications for prevention. *Clin J Sport Med* 2004; 14: 13–17.

117. Miyashita TL, Diakogeorgiou E, Hellstrom B, Kuchwara N, Tafoya E, Young L. High school athletes' perceptions of concussion. *Orthop J Sports Med* 2014; 2: 2325967114554549.

118. Register-Mihalik JK, Guskiewicz KM, McLeod TC, Linnan LA, Mueller FO, Marshall SW. Knowledge, attitude, and concussion-reporting behaviors among high school athletes: a preliminary study. *J Athl Train* 2013; 48: 645–53.

119. Taylor ME, Sanner JE. The relationship between concussion knowledge and the high school athlete's intention to report traumatic brain injury symptoms: a systematic review of the literature. *J Sch Nurs* 2017; 33(1): 73–81.

120. Valovich McLeod TC, Bay RC, Heil J, Mcveigh SD. Identification of sport and recreational activity concussion history through the preparticipation screening and a symptom survey in young athletes. *Clin J Sport Med* 2008; 18: 235–40.

121. Bazarian JJ, Zhu T, Blyth B, Borrino A, Zhong J. Subject-specific changes in brain white matter on diffusion tensor imaging after sports-related concussion. *Magn Reson Imaging* 2012; 30: 171–80.

122. Cubon VA, Putukian M, Boyer C, Dettwiler A. A diffusion tensor imaging study on the white matter skeleton in individuals with sports-related concussion. *J Neurotrauma* 2011; 28: 189–201.

123. Gardner A, Kay-Lambkin F, Stanwell P, Donnelly J, Williams WH, Hiles A, et al. A systematic review of diffusion tensor imaging findings in sports-related concussion. *J Neurotrauma* 2012; 29: 2521–38.

124. Koerte IK, Ertl-Wagner B, Reiser M, Zafonte R, Shenton ME. White matter integrity in the brains of professional soccer players without a symptomatic concussion. *JAMA* 2012; 308: 1859–61.

125. Koerte IK, Kaufmann D, Hartl E, Bouix S, Pasternak O, Kubicki M, et al. A prospective study of physician-observed concussion during a varsity university hockey season: white matter integrity in ice hockey players. Part 3 of 4. *Neurosurg Focus* 2012; 33 (E3): 1–7.

126. Maugans TA, Farley C, Altaye M, Leach J, Cecil KM. Pediatric sports-related concussion produces cerebral blood flow alterations. *Pediatrics* 2012; 129: 28–37.

127. Virji-Babul N, Borich MR, Makan N, Moore T, Frew K, Emery CA, et al. Diffusion tensor imaging of sports-related concussion in adolescents. *Pediatr Neurol* 2013; 48: 24–9.

128. Sorg SF, Delano-Wood L, Luc N, Schiehser DM, Hanson KL, Nation DA, et al. White matter integrity in veterans with mild traumatic brain injury: associations with executive function and loss of consciousness. *J Head Trauma Rehabil* 2014; 29(1): 21–32.

129. Jorge RE, Acion L, White T, Tordesillas-Gutierrez D, Pierson R, Crespo-Facorro B, et al. White matter abnormalities in veterans with mild traumatic brain injury. *Am J Psychiatry* 2012; 169: 1284–91.

130. Wada T, Asano Y, Shinoda J. Decreased fractional anisotropy evaluated using tract-based spatial statistics and correlated with cognitive dysfunction in patients with mild traumatic brain injury in the chronic stage. *AJNR Am J Neuroradiol* 2012; 33: 2117–22.

131. Rao V, Mielke M, Xu X, Smith GS, McCann UD, Bergey A, et al. Diffusion tensor imaging atlas-based analyses in major depression after mild traumatic brain injury. *J Neuropsychiatr Clin Neurosci* 2012; 24: 309–15.

132. Messe A, Caplain S, Paradot G, Garrigue D, Mineo JF, Soto Ares G, et al. Diffusion tensor imaging and white matter lesions at the subacute stage in mild traumatic brain injury with persistent neurobehavioral impairment. *Hum Brain Mapp* 2011; 32: 999–1011.

133. Douglas DB, Iv M, Douglas PK, Anderson A, Vos SB, Bammer R, et al. Diffusion tensor imaging of TBI: potentials and challenges. *Top Magn Reson Imaging* 2015; 24: 241–51.

134. Benson RR, Gattu R, Sewick B, Kou Z, Zakariah N, Cavanaugh JM, et al. Detection of hemorrhagic and axonal pathology in mild traumatic brain injury using advanced MRI: implications for neurorehabilitation. *NeuroRehabilitation* 2012; 31: 261–79.

135. Bigler ED. Neuropsychological results and neuropathological findings at autopsy in a case of mild traumatic brain injury. *J Int Neuropsychol Soc: JINS* 2004; 10: 794–806.

136. Oppenheimer DR. Microscopic lesions in the brain following head injury. *J Neurol Neurosurg Psychiatry* 1968; 31: 299–306.

137. Hekmatpanah J, Hekmatpanah CR. Microvascular alterations following cerebral contusion in rats. Light, scanning, and electron microscope study. *J Neurosurg* 1985;62:888–897.

138. Glushakova OY, Johnson D, Hayes RL. Delayed increases in microvascular pathology after experimental traumatic brain injury are associated with prolonged inflammation, blood–brain barrier disruption, and progressive white matter damage. *J Neurotrauma* 2014; 31: 1180–93.

139. Kubal WS. Updated imaging of traumatic brain injury. *Radiol Clin North Am* 2012; 50: 15–41.

140. Sharp DJ, Ham TE. Investigating white matter injury after mild traumatic brain injury. *Curr Opin Neurol* 2011; 24: 558–63.

141. Bigler ED, Abildskov TJ, Petrie J, Farrer TJ, Dennis M, Simic N, et al. Heterogeneity of brain lesions in pediatric traumatic brain injury. *Neuropsychology* 2013; 27: 438–51.

142. Dietrich WD, Alonso O, Halley M. Early microvascular and neuronal consequences of traumatic brain injury: a light and electron microscopic study in rats. *J Neurotrauma* 1994; 11(3): 289–301.

143. Golding EM. Sequelae following traumatic brain injury. The cerebrovascular perspective. *Brain Res Rev* 2002; 38(3): 377–88.

144. Sangiorgi S, De Benedictis A, Protasoni M, Manelli A, Reguzzoni M, Cividini A, et al. Early-stage microvascular alterations of a new model of controlled cortical traumatic brain injury: 3D morphological analysis using scanning electron microscopy and corrosion casting. *J Neurosurg* 2013; 118(4): 763–74.

145. Glushakova OY, Johnson D, Hayes RL. Delayed increases in microvascular pathology after experimental traumatic brain injury are associated with prolonged inflammation, blood–brain barrier disruption, and progressive white matter damage. *J Neurotrauma* 2014; 31(13): 1180–93.

146. Ueda Y, Walker SA, Povlishock JT. Perivascular nerve damage in the cerebral circulation following traumatic brain injury. *Acta Neuropathol* 2006; 112(1): 85–94.

147. Hopkins RO, Beck CJ, Burnett DL, Weaver LK, Victoroff J, Bigler ED. Prevalence of white matter hyperintensities in a young healthy population. *J Neuroimag* 2006; 16: 243–51.

148. Ylikoski A, Erkinjuntti T, Raininko R, Sarna S, Sulkava R, Tilvis R. White matter hyperintensities on MRI in the neurologically nondiseased elderly. Analysis of cohorts of consecutive subjects aged 55 to 85 years living at home. *Stroke* 1995; 26: 1171–7.

149. Marquez De La Plata C, Ardelean A, Koovakkattu D, Srinivasan P, Miller A, Phuong V, et al. Magnetic resonance imaging of diffuse axonal injury: quantitative assessment of white matter lesion volume. *J Neurotrauma* 2007; 24: 591–8.

150. Zhou Y, Milham MP, Lui YW, Miles L, Reaume J, Sodickson DK, et al. Default-mode network disruption in mild traumatic brain injury. *Radiology* 2012; 265: 882–92.

151. Grossman EJ, Ge Y, Jensen JH, Babb JS, Miles L, Reaume J, et al. Thalamus and cognitive impairment in mild traumatic brain injury: a diffusional kurtosis imaging study. *J Neurotrauma* 2012; 29: 2318–27.

152. Grossman EJ, Jensen JH, Babb JS, Chen Q, Tabesh A, Fieremans E, et al. Cognitive impairment in mild traumatic brain injury: a longitudinal diffusional kurtosis and perfusion imaging study. *AJNR Am J Neuroradiol* 2013; 34: 951–7, S1–3.

153. Stokum JA, Sours C, Zhuo J, Kane R, Shanmuganathan K, Gullapalli RP. A longitudinal evaluation of diffusion kurtosis imaging in patients with mild traumatic brain injury. *Brain Inj* 2015; 29: 47–57.

154. Mackenzie JD, Siddiqi F, Babb JS, Bagley LJ, Mannon LJ, Sinson GP, et al. Brain atrophy in mild or moderate traumatic brain injury: a longitudinal quantitative analysis. *AJNR Am J Neuroradiol* 2002; 23: 1509–15.

155. Ross DE, Ochs AL, Seabaugh JM, Demark MF, Shrader CR, Marwitz JH, et al. Progressive brain atrophy in patients with chronic neuropsychiatric symptoms after mild traumatic brain injury: a preliminary study. *Brain Inj* 2012; 26: 1500–9.

156. Zhou Y, Kierans A, Kenul D, Ge Y, Rath J, Reaume J, et al. Mild traumatic brain injury: longitudinal regional brain volume changes. *Radiology* 2013; 267:880–90.

157. Lin KC, Niu KC, Tsai KJ, Kuo JR, Wang LC, Chio CC, et al. Attenuating inflammation but stimulating both angiogenesis and neurogenesis using hyperbaric oxygen in rats with traumatic brain injury. *J Trauma Acute Care Surg* 2012; 72: 650–9.

158. Papa L, Ramia MM, Edwards D, Johnson BD, Slobounov S. Systematic review of clinical studies examining biomarkers of brain injury in athletes following sports-related concussion. *J Neurotrauma* 2014; 32: 661–73.

159. Babikian T, Freier MC, Ashwal S, Riggs ML, Burley T, Holshouser BA. MR spectroscopy: predicting long-term neuropsychological outcome following pediatric TBI. *J Magn Reson Imaging: JMRI.* 2006; 24: 801–11.

160. Moffett JR, Ross B, Arun P, Madhavarao CN, Namboodiri AM. *N*-acetylaspartate in the CNS: from neurodiagnostics to neurobiology. *Prog Neurobiol* 2007; 81: 89–131.

161. Gasparovic C, Yeo R, Mannell M, Ling J, Elgie R, Phillips J, et al. Neurometabolite concentrations in gray and white matter in mild traumatic brain injury: an 1H-magnetic resonance spectroscopy study. *J Neurotrauma* 2009; 26: 1635–43.

162. Kierans AS, Kirov II, Gonen O, Haemer G, Nisenbaum E, Babb JS, et al. Myoinositol and glutamate complex neurometabolite abnormality after mild traumatic brain injury. *Neurology* 2014; 82: 521–8.

163. Brooks WM, Stidley CA, Petropoulos H, Jung RE, Weers DC, Friedman SD, et al. Metabolic and cognitive response to human traumatic brain injury: a quantitative proton magnetic resonance study. *J Neurotrauma* 2000; 17: 629–40.

164. Harris JL, Choi IY, Brooks WM. Probing astrocyte metabolism in vivo: proton magnetic resonance spectroscopy in the injured and aging brain. *Front Aging Neurosci* 2015; 7: 202.

165. Yeo RA, Gasparovic C, Merideth F, Ruhl D, Doezema D, Mayer AR. A longitudinal proton magnetic resonance spectroscopy study of mild traumatic brain injury. *J Neurotrauma* 2011; 28: 1–11.

166. Koerte IK, Lin AP, Willems A, Muehlmann M, Hufschmidt J, Coleman MJ, et al. A review of neuroimaging findings in repetitive brain trauma. *Brain Pathol* 2015; 25(3): 318–49.

167. Vagnozzi R, Signoretti S, Cristofori L, Alessandrini F, Floris R, Isgro E, et al. Assessment of metabolic brain damage and recovery following mild traumatic brain injury: a multicentre, proton magnetic resonance spectroscopic study in concussed patients. *Brain* 2010; 133: 3232–42.

168. Dimou S, Lagopoulos J. Toward objective markers of concussion in sport: a review of white matter and neurometabolic changes in the brain after sports-related concussion. *J Neurotrauma* 2014; 31: 413–24.

169. Gardner A, Iverson GL, Stanwell P. A systematic review of proton magnetic resonance spectroscopy findings in sport-related concussion. *J Neurotrauma* 2014; 31: 1–18.

170. Kubas B, Lebkowski W, Lebkowska U, Kulak W, Tarasow E, Walecki J. Proton MR spectroscopy in mild traumatic brain injury. *Pol J Radiol* 2010; 75: 7–10.

171. George EO, Roys S, Sours C, Rosenberg J, Zhuo J, Shanmuganathan K, et al. Longitudinal and prognostic evaluation of mild traumatic brain injury: a 1H-magnetic resonance spectroscopy study. *J Neurotrauma* 2014; 31: 1018–28.

172. Tremblay S, Beaule V, Proulx S, Marjanska M, Doyon J, Lassonde M, et al. Multimodal assessment of primary motor cortex integrity following sport concussion in asymptomatic athletes. *Clin Neurophysiol* 2014; 125: 1371–9.

173. Messe A, Caplain S, Pelegrini-Issac M, Blancho S, Levy R, Aghakhani N, et al. Specific and evolving resting-state network alterations in post-concussion syndrome following mild traumatic brain injury. *PLoS One* 2013; 8: e65470.

174. Wintermark M, Coombs L, Druzgal TJ, Field AS, Filippi CG, Hicks R, et al. Traumatic brain injury imaging research roadmap. *AJNR Am J Neuroradiol* 2015; 36: E12–23.

175. Da Costa L, Robertson A, Bethune A, Macdonald MJ, Shek PN, Taylor MJ, et al. Delayed and disorganised brain activation detected with magnetoencephalography after mild traumatic brain injury. *J Neurol Neurosurg Psychiatry* 2015; 86(9): 1008–15.

176. Huang MX, Nichols S, Baker DG, Robb A, Angeles A, Yurgil KA, et al. Single-subject-based whole-brain MEG slow-wave imaging approach for detecting abnormality in patients with mild traumatic brain injury. *NeuroImage Clin* 2014; 5: 109–19.

177. Lee RR, Huang M. Magnetoencephalography in the diagnosis of concussion.*Prog Neurol Surg* 2014; 28: 94–111.

178. Yuh EL, Hawryluk GW, Manley GT. Imaging concussion: a review. *Neurosurgery* 2014; 75 (Suppl 4): S50–63.

179. Kontos AP, Huppert TJ, Beluk NH, Elbin RJ, Henry LC, French J, et al. Brain activation during neurocognitive testing using functional near-infrared spectroscopy in patients following concussion compared to healthy controls. *Brain Imaging Behav* 2014; DOI 10.1007/s11682-014-9289-9.

180. Bigler ED. Neuroinflammation and the dynamic lesion in traumatic brain injury. *Brain* 2013; 136: 9–11.

181. Bar-Gill N, Retzker A. Observing chemical shifts from nanosamples. *Science* 2017; 357(6346): 38.

182. Bucher DB, Glenn DR, Lee J, Lukin MD, Park H, Walsworth RL. High resolution magnetic resonance spectroscopy using solid-state spins. *Quant Physics* 2017; arXiv: 1705.08887.

183. Schmitt S, Gefen T, Stürner FM, Unden T, Wolff G, Müller C, et al. Submillihertz magnetic spectroscopy performed with a nanoscale quantum sensor. *Science* 2017; 356: 832–7.

184. Boss JM, Cujia KS, Zopes J, Degen CL. Quantum sensing with arbitrary frequency resolution. *Science* 2017; 356 (6340): 837–40.

185. Aslam N, Pfender M, Neumann P, Reuter R, Zappe A, Fávaro De Oliveira F, et al. Nanoscale nuclear magnetic resonance with chemical resolution. *Science* 2017; 357 (6346): 67–71.

186. Goldin R. Genetic expression in the human brain: the challenge of large numbers. Genetic Literacy Project April 15, 2013. Available at https://geneticliteracyproject.org/2013/04/15/genetic-expression-in-the-human-brain-the-challenge-of-large-numbers/.

7

Why Outcomes Vary

Jeff Victoroff

How many survivors of single, typical, clinically attended concussive brain injuries (CBIs) suffer lasting deleterious effects? Chapter 5 summarized the available empirical evidence. The conclusion came highly qualified, scintillating with an aura of reasonable doubt. Only some CBIs can be included in any analysis. Almost nothing is known about the large cohort of concussed people that does not seek, or fails to receive, documented clinical attention. Confining our estimate, therefore, to the subset of survivors who seek clinical attention and provoke documentation – and hopefully providing a replicable factual advance upon opinions sometimes expressed in the pre-scientific era of concussion studies – more than 40% of CBI survivors continue to express or exhibit clinical problems for a year or longer. Somewhat fewer will report or experience those problems for as long as they live.[1] Since the numbers are neither 100% nor 0%, and since they vary mind-bogglingly from one person and one study to the next, it is safe to conclude that outcomes vary.

Why? There is nothing novel about the observation that outcomes from CBI vary. One suspects it was apparent to the average adult *Homo erectus*, if not to the common ancestor of humans and chimpanzees. But why this astonishing heterogeneity of outcomes? That is the question to be addressed by this chapter of our collaborative essay.

Consider Figure 7.1. This is a typical illustration, a commonplace of every textbook on traumatic brain injury, an unashamed depiction of the conventional wisdom. It purportedly depicts a recovery curve – a picture of the natural history of traumatic encephalopathy after human CBI, implying that "mild" injuries never have lasting effects and that, no matter what the severity (including immediate death?), everyone recovers nearly to his or her baseline. Show this cartoon to a medical student. He or she will infer, and memorize for the test, that concussions get better.

Idealized and minimized course of traumatic encephalopathy

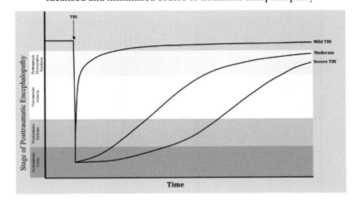

Fig. 7.1 Typical courses of progression through the stages of post-traumatic encephalopathy following mild, moderate, and severe traumatic brain injury (TBI). The lines illustrating these courses for each level of injury severity are idealized; there is substantial variability in outcome at all levels of initial injury severity which, for the purpose of diagrammatic simplicity, is not illustrated here.
Source: Arciniegas, 2011 [2]. Reproduced with permission from Healio

Yet fantastic schematics such as Figure 7.1 are idealized. Like Chinese *shuimohua* mountain water paintings, graphs of this species are simple, lovely, pleasing, monochromatic, and blithely divorced from nature's reality. This graph does not depict recovery after any actual concussion, but theoretical outcome after a theoretical concussion.[2] It is like a band of gray across the sky submitted by a fine arts student. The professor asks, "What is this?" The student replies, "A rainbow." The professor looks quizzical. The student explains: "I averaged."

Figure 7.2, on the other hand, depicts data. At first glance, it may appear more complex. It is certainly messier. On reflection it is far more consistent with our everyday experience of

---

[1]   The author invites readers who have not yet done so to read the source articles for the quantitative estimates in Chapter 5. Within six months of starting, one would surely begin to get a sense for the problems with the reported data. Multiple methodological limitations in the original sources mandate caution in considering the estimates derived by Chapter 5's analysis, but our conclusions are at least based on a systematic review, and seem to dovetail with the most recent credible evidence [1].

[2]   In the author's opinion, one of the grievous errors in the education of medical students is inordinate exposure to deeply misleading graphs such as Figure 7.1. That practice is tantamount to a confession that textbook writers and professors do not trust our most capable young people to understand human heterogeneity. Doctors-in-training would probably be less shocked when they encounter actual suffering humans by early and frequent exposure to graphs like Figure 7.2.

Actual trajectories of recovery after traumatic brain injury

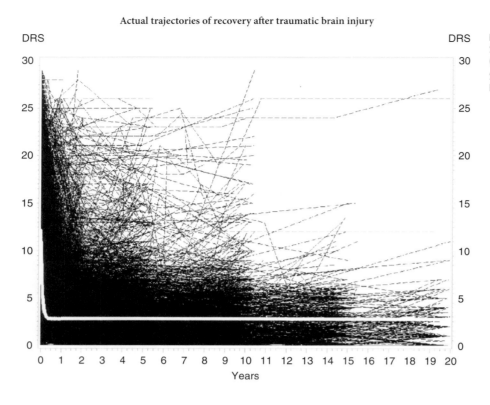

Fig. 7.2 Average trajectory for the Disability Rating Scale (solid white line) with individual trajectories (black dashed lines).

Source: Pretz et al., 2013 [3] with permission from Elsevier

human phenomena. This is a straightforward, accurate, immediately accessible visualization of the post-concussion course. It varies.

The Scientific Problem, in Perspective

So far, this brief essay has hopefully provided robust evidence to support three strong conclusions.

Conclusion Number One

Abrupt external force impacting the head sometimes changes brain function. It is not necessarily true that a given amount or direction of force yields a particular brain change (think *perching butterfly*), or that the brain change attendant upon forceful impact is necessarily deleterious (think *awareness of perching butterfly*). Complex intracerebral processes swing into action at the moment of impact that counter one another at the molecular level, some tending to be deleterious or produce stress on neurons and glia, others tending to relieve that stress. However, at a point that remains to be scientifically defined, the net result is "injury." Appreciating that "injury" lacks either a universally accepted conceptual definition or a biological measure, for the sake of medical discussion one might simply say that "brain injury" is change that is not conducive to survival or reproduction.

By far the most common scenario for that maladaptive change is visitation by an abrupt external force on the head, subsequently transmitted and dispersed by the six intervening tissues (hair, scalp skin, galea, skull, dura, cerebrospinal fluid) to rattle the brain. Although a very wide range of forces may technically "concuss" the brain, from the wafting of a leaf to

the inconvenient descent of a large asteroid, the medically important part of that range is the injurious part. *That* is a CBI. It is self-evident that the degree of injury varies continuously across an infinitely divisible spectrum. For that reason (except to please attorneys and comfort those who need dichotomies), no rational basis exists to divide severity of CBI into mild versus not mild. However, in so far as emergency room or clinic visits reflect actual incidence, the overwhelming majority of CBIs involve: (1) either no loss of consciousness or brief loss of consciousness (no upper boundary in minutes is biologically meaningful, hence "brief" awaits a useful definition); (2) no brain penetration (although that can certainly occur since CBI is sometimes accompanied by parenchymal intrusion, e.g., with a sharp needle or a dull axe); and (3) no intracerebral hemorrhage (ICH) of the sort that is visible with a computed tomography (CT) scan and likely to benefit from immediate neurosurgical intervention (although that too occurs in a subset of brain-rattling injuries).

Conclusion Number Two

The epidemiology of CBI is unfathomable. For reasons outlined in Chapter 2, it is not currently possible, nor will it be possible in the foreseeable future, to count the number of persons who have survived CBI. An unknown proportion of the total number of concussed persons never comes to medical attention. Among those who do seek medical care, roughly a third are improperly diagnosed. We can try, and Chapter 2 comprehensively summarized the findings from such trials, to infer preliminary conclusions about the subset of CBI survivors who come to medical attention. Yet even the most scrupulous prospective longitudinal study with 100% reporting from birth to death would fail to determine the incidence or prevalence of medically unreported concussions or the magnitude of their effect on public health, since case ascertainment requires a biomarker and none exists. That is one reason the discovery of a valid and reliable biomarker tops the global research agenda.

Conclusion Number Three

Outcomes vary. That observation is surely apparent to every reader who is a clinician. Some CBI survivors are literally unaware of any deleterious effect a few minutes after the event (although, in some of these asymptomatic survivors, imaging or long-term follow-up reveals lasting brain change). Others – an unknown but substantial proportion of those who seek medical attention, and far more than the 20th-century literature acknowledged – both feel and display persistent or permanent impairments in somatic, cognitive, or non-cognitive behavioral function.

Explaining why outcomes vary compares well with cleaning the Augean stables. The literature is piled high, and redolent with academic excretions. That hefty pile lists risk factors that have been statistically associated with poor outcome and/or later post-concussive dementia in one or more empirical studies of widely varying worth [4–26]. That information is a necessary step toward insight, but insufficient for our purposes. It is, respectfully, mere epidemiology. If one's goal is to help concussed persons and help prevent concussion, one must march on beyond associations and find causes. Millions of already-concussed brains are presently at risk. It is a matter of some urgency to discover modifiable aspects of the pathophysiological mechanisms that *cause* poor outcome, vulnerability to worse outcome on subsequent exposure, and progression to dementia.

That effort must not be mired in the muck of 20th-century mistakes. For example, many early concussion writings erroneously attended to clinical "recovery" as if the patient's saying "I'm fine" and the neuropsychologist's saying "He's fine" meant that the patient was fine. Multiple lines of 21st-century evidence reveal that clinical recovery is a mirage. For example, as Johnson et al. [27] put it, "These findings demonstrate a distinct dissociation between clinical findings of restoration of function and advanced imaging abnormalities" (p. 516). To be frank, clinical recovery is reassuring to the patient but irrelevant to the brain. The subjective feeling of "I'm fine" means that the damaged brain – sometimes permanently and dangerously disordered, exquisitely vulnerable to excessive further damage, and highly prone to progressive dementing degeneration – is temporarily functional enough to pass for normal in the insensitive appraisal of its owner and the local quizmaster. Only by setting aside the mythology of recovery can we push for sophisticated assessments with markers that will reveal the covert biology of persistent injury, without which clinical researchers are impotent to search for effective interventions.

Another 20th-century mistake (with somewhat earlier roots) is contaminated inference. When social tradition is substituted for science, data may be accurately collected and abysmally misinterpreted. Example: unequivocal data show that females tend to have more severe and prolonged post-concussive problems. That difference was attributed to hysteria 150 years ago. Nineteenth-century French experts knew that such hysterical symptoms were due to disordered reproductive tracts starved for orgasm [28]. As recently as 2010, one group of authors [6] explained women's excess post-concussive complaints by reference to their relatively greater use of analgesics, which revealed the true nature of the sex difference: "Compared to males with mTBI, females were … more likely to be on analgesics before injury (*surrogate for poor coping style*) [emphasis added]" (p. 530). Although the author of the present essay is open to the possibility that "poor coping style" is the key neurobiological explanation for women's elevated rate of persistent post-concussive problems, he suggests investigating other possible factors – for instance, known differences in brain anatomy and physiology – before resorting to the Victorian enthusiasm for blaming the victim.

A Brief Outline of What is to Come

Such muddy thinking is sadly common. The author lacks the wherewithal to divert the Alpheus and Peneus through such scholastic stables. But his job is to somehow provide a robust conceptual framework that makes sense out of the variety of outcomes.

To that end he will rely on one defensible scientific axiom with potent implications: differences in concussion outcome are due to biological variation that is innate, biological variation that is acquired, or the interaction between these two. (Readers may safely assume that this is the author's sole contribution and feel free to skip to other chapters after reading the last five words of the conclusion. Those who wish to know *why* the author has arrived at this conclusion, please grant me a few pages for exegesis. I promise to do my best.) That fundamental axiom undergirds five organizing concepts:

1. No two human brains are alike.
2. Force, time since injury, genes, and at least seven other factors seem to influence outcome after CBI. All factors that influence outcome do so because they impact the unique brain's unique organic response to concussion.
3. As previously established, several empirical observations support the conclusion that persistent or lifelong brain disorder is common among CBI survivors: (a) persistent symptoms; (b) persistent signs (e.g., on imaging or autopsy); (c) vulnerability to excess dysfunction after subsequent trauma; and (d) evidence of accelerated neurodegenerative dementia. In most cases, present technology cannot detect or quantify that persistent or lifelong brain disorder. Yet these four observations strongly suggest the existence of a threshold, *a point of no return* in the course of the neurometabolic-vascular-inflammatory melee at which brains fail to contain the effects of the initial concussion. In other words, in the course of the competition between degenerative and regenerative forces, excess degeneration can do lasting harm the brain can neither repair nor accommodate.

When we find a modifiable biological factor that causes a CBI to pass that point of no return, we will hugely mitigate the global problem of concussion.

4. CBI survivors with neurons and glial harmed beyond the point of no return complain of or display lasting symptoms. For the foreseeable future, scholars will attempt to list "risk factors" for that unfortunate end result. Many such risk factors have been championed by experts to account for the vast difference in perceived health of people who have suffered similar head impacts, from skull thickness, to pre-morbid personality, to "litigation overlay." Some of these proposed risk factors have stood up to empirical scrutiny better than others. This chapter will impartially review the evidence for and against each proposed risk factor. But more importantly, the chapter will explain why risk factor is a misleading phrase. It implies "this factor increases the risk by this much." As Garrod [29, 30] explained more than 100 years ago, no illness is ever attributable to a risk factor. Illness only results when there occurs the unfortunate combination of a risk factor with an individual and unique biological vulnerability to that factor.

Warning: Some scholars have been unable to resist calling some risk factors "psychological." For instance, persistent complaints are occasionally attributed to "pre-existing psychiatric problems." Psychological terminology such as *psychiatric problems* facilitates casual chat about familiar subjective percepts. However, no organic/psychological dichotomy exists in nature. Every "psychological" construct and label is some scholar's shorthand for yet-to-be-determined biological states and happenings.

This has practical implications for transcending the *drama of attribution* – the divisive and unnecessary debate about why a CBI survivor is distressed or impaired. All post-concussive change is organic change. Of course pre-injury neurobiology (such as the biology of depression or resilience) influences post-concussive neurobiology (such as the biology of apparent prompt recovery or permanent problems). But it is a fool's errand to assign proportional attribution of post-CBI variation to the influence of one organic element versus another. Rhetoric such as "She has persistent memory loss and headaches because she was sad before the accident" inflames the drama of attribution and reflects a profound conceptual error. She has persistent memory loss and headaches because of a collusion of biological factors so complex as to befuddle the best thinking and technology known to humankind.

5. Since outcomes vary, there is no "post-concussion syndrome." Readers who are clinicians probably discovered this long ago. The wild diversity of presentations after concussion escapes any neat package. Yet the phrase *post-concussion syndrome* has been hard to retire, since certain symptoms are indeed seen repeatedly,

alone or in combination. The author proposes that, rather than a syndrome, the similarities and differences between patients are better accommodated by a Haddon matrix. A Haddon matrix is simply a pragmatic conceptual model – not a finished biological account but a heuristic device readers can use to figure out why a patient exhibits his or her unique response to concussion. It may seem daunting that such responses are infinitely variable and multi-determined. A modified Haddon matrix is a handy, visualizable chessboard to organize the pieces that play white and black roles in the post-concussive melee.

"Outcomes" is Plural

Outcome is often misunderstood. One reads literally hundreds of 20th-century articles on concussion that use *outcome* as if it were a fixed address along the alley of destiny between good and bad. As the reader probably intuits, there is no single outcome from a concussion. There are outcomes. This chapter is the author's best effort to unearth a useful idea or two from the academic literature that uses the word *outcome* as if it were a unitary and scalable phenomenon. It is not. A more patient-oriented framework will conceivably help free us from the conceptual straightjacket of the old conventional view, liberating the doctor from the strictures of documenting a simplistic outcome score (good or bad) to listen to the CBI survivor and take note of the many different ways and degrees to which a brain injury may impact a human life.

Consider just two symptoms in realistic clinical depth.

Georgia is a 29-year-old Hispanic college graduate, inner-city high school teacher, and equestrienne.[3] In the ten years before her concussion in a fall from Sandy – a blood bay 16 hands at the withers – Georgia was nauseated on average once every eight months, or, to simplify for the purposes of discussion, one-210th time per day. On post-CBI day 2 she was nauseated every six minutes, or 240 times per day. Hence, her *day 2 concussion-related nausea outcome* was 57,840% of baseline. Georgia was nauseated four times during the ninth month after CBI. Therefore, Georgia's *month 9 post-concussion nausea outcome* was 3200% of baseline – a gratifying improvement, but not a full recovery. Every day over the next year her concussion nausea outcome varied but remained somewhat above 100% of baseline. Finally, after 2.5 years, her frequency of nausea matched her baseline. Recovery status at three to five years post-CBI is pretty close to lifetime outcome. Hence, to a reasonable degree of certainty, Georgia's *long-term post-concussion nausea outcome* was full recovery.

Consider Georgia's mood. In the ten years prior to her CBI she was dysthymic (sad) for 29 months (24.2% of the time) and depressed to the point of disability for 11 months (9.2% of the time). During her second month after CBI she was dysthymic for 13 days and disabled by depression for two days. Georgia's *month 2 post-concussion mood outcome* was therefore dysthymia at 179% of baseline and depression at 73% of baseline. Depression often peaks about 6–12 months post-CBI. During

---

[3] This is a case reported from the author's clinic. The identifying data were revised to preserve confidentiality.

post-CBI month 9 Georgia was dysthymic for all 30 days and disabled by depression for 18 days – a *month 9 post-concussion mood outcome* of dysthymia at 413% of baseline and depression at 652% of baseline. Now at the four-year anniversary of her injury, Georgia is dysthymic half the time and depressed about four days per month. That means Georgia's *long-term post-concussion mood outcome* is a 65% increase from baseline in dysthymia and a 45% increase in depression.

We have considered just two of Georgia's post-CBI problems. In a recent study, Tator et al. [31] reported that the average number of persistent post-concussive symptoms was 8.1, most commonly headache, memory deficits, concentration difficulties, imbalance, and dizziness. But in order to assess the impact of a concussion on a survivor, at a minimum one expects the TBI doctor to perform this type of time-and-severity assessment for the 16 symptoms addressed by the Rivermead Post-Concussion Symptoms Questionnaire [32].[4] Such a patient-sensitive review of common problems is required not only to discover dismay beyond the chief complaint but also to take into account health variables that are often overlooked but critical to patient well-being: (1) the multiplicity of symptoms; (2) the degree of disability; (3) the time since injury; and (4) the change from baseline for each symptom.

If you know a doctor who routinely assesses his or her concussion survivors in this depth, raise your hand. I know three in the United States.

In the author's opinion, a lack of conceptual sophistication and, not to put too fine a point on it, physician sloth may be barriers to clinical assessments of the depth and rigor required to accelerate discovery. In-depth assessment as exemplified above would make outcomes research vastly more scientific. Rather than a fruitless quest for the single answer to a multi-determined problem, one would be in a far better position to tease out what causes what and what helps what. This chapter, unfortunately, can only summarize the superficial glimpse of CBI survivors provided by the state of the art of recent scholarship. That said, the author will attempt to summarize the latest findings and crystalize his best guesses.

With that perspective in mind, the present chapter will reject mere epidemiological reportage, raise questions about undisciplined assumptions, and attempt to organize the knowledge we have, little though it may be, about the biological underpinnings of risk factors for bad outcome that have, in some cases, been reported but not explained for more than a century. Along our way we will overcome two ancillary errors that have delayed resolution of the great concussion debate. First, medical nosology is largely beholden to an antiquated perspective, exemplified by Galen and still in common use. The essence: "A disease is a particular problem." Fortunately, the solution to that fallacious perspective has been available since 1908. Second, psychology is half-born. That is, this vital, even thrilling, discipline devoted to abstracting human nature and classifying aspects of mind was conceived and gestated before neurobiology was available to endow it with any tether to material fact. Fortunately, the solution to that problem has been available since 1664.

Measures of Outcome

Outcome is used three different ways in the medical literature. *The first approach*: outcome might be conceptualized as an absolute assessment of function rated on a universal metric. Examples include the Glasgow Outcome Scale (GOS) [33] or total Functional Independence Measures (FIM) score [34–37]. This use of *outcome* is problematic for two reasons. First, it tends to have a low ceiling. A person who is doing perfectly in terms of functional independence can walk and talk and eat and bathe but may remain impaired in domains not evaluated by the FIM. More importantly, universal metrics ignore individuality. The GOS underspecifies the diversity of outcomes. If a neurosurgeon and a short-order cook are both concussed, a year later they might both exhibit IQs of 100. But the neurosurgeon's pre-morbid IQ was 145 while the cook began at 100. The cook returned to work. The neurosurgeon lost her job and plunged into despair. How shall we rank their GOS? Two of the five levels of recovery described by the GOS: "disabled but independent" means "independent as far as daily life. Disabilities include varying degrees of dysphasia, hemiparesis, or ataxia as well as intellectual and memory deficits and personality changes." *Good recovery* means "resumption of normal activities even though there may be minor neurological or psychological deficits." The jobless, hopeless neurosurgeon has no dysphasia, hemiparesis, ataxia, intellectual or memory deficits. The neuropsychologist who tested her for the insurance company reported "completely normal IQ." Yet she will never resume her normal activities. Something precious about human health is betrayed by this presumptuous oversimplification. A GOS score ignores: (1) the multiplicity of symptoms; (2) the degree of disability from each symptom; (3) the time elapsed since injury with respect to each symptom; and (4) change from baseline function for each symptom. We are better doctors than that.

The *second approach*: given the problems with absolute metrics, a superior understanding of outcome requires a *relative* measure in which the patient's pre-morbid capacity is considered as the baseline. This approach is far more sensitive to the impact of the injury, enabling the clinician to explore whether there has been a loss or not. For that reason (leaping ahead somewhat) the author recommends that doctors do their best to estimate pre-morbid and post-concussion disability using an instrument such as the World Health Organization's Disability Assessment Schedule 2.0 (WHODAS 2.0) [38, 39].

Again, there are drawbacks. A single measure of change in human capacity, such as "a 25% decline on the WHODAS 2.0" hardly captures the innumerable ways in which a CBI may affect a survivor. The cook may have no drop in IQ and remain employed, but become divorced due to irritability and arrested

---

4 Headaches, dizziness, nausea/vomiting, noise sensitivity, sleep disturbance, fatigue, irritability/anger proneness, depression, frustration, memory problems, concentration problems, taking longer to think, blurred vision, light sensitivity, double vision, and restlessness.

for exposure due to disinhibition. The neurosurgeon may have no drop in IQ but suffer slowed multi-tasking and diminished dexterity – having suffered a massive drop from being in the top 0.1% of human nimbleness to the top 2%. She is 20 times less dexterous, but some psychologists might say, "recovery complete; extremely high-level functioning."

The *third approach*, therefore, is to assess change from baseline in multiple aspects of function. For this purpose, the 16-item Rivermead Post-Concussion Symptoms Questionnaire [32, 40] has become the go-to instrument in English speaking countries. In practical terms, it would represent a terrific advance if this instrument were familiar to and utilized by every general practitioner. The author must express a concern and personal preference: insight varies. CBI survivors are not always the ones most aware of how they have changed, so self-report is incomplete and sometimes dangerously inaccurate. A superior assessment requires parallel instruments that also gather the observations of a family member or caregiver. In addition, aggression is a major psychosocial problem after CBI. The Rivermead only asks about subjective irritability, failing to assess threatening or aggressive behavior. For these reasons (and due to its open-ended questions), the author uses and recommends the Achenbach System of Empirically Based Assessment [41, 42]. Normed and validated instruments are available for every age bracket, are cross-culturally applicable, and predict long-term outcomes [43–52].[5] The problem is that these proprietary instruments cost money. For serious scholars, it's a trivial investment. For clinicians, the Achenbach system will never achieve the popularity it deserves because it is too effortful to administer and score by a family doctor. A later chapter in this book introduces an alternative: the National Institutes of Health Toolbox [53] is a very carefully selected suite of instruments for assessing the impact of traumatic brain injury (TBI). All are free (in the common domain) and iPad-ready.

Contrary to Instinct and Conventional Wisdom, Similar Forces are Followed by Different Effects

Visualize a remote scrub desert, tawny, dusty, and sun-blasted. Imagine you were the emergency department doctor at the Greater Mootwingee International Urgent Care Center in western New South Wales. It might so happen that two vacationing pharmacists from Burkina Faso named Maxime and Guillaume are brought to your clinic after having both been punched in the head by the same red kangaroo (named Lucinda). Witnesses attest that the force and direction of the blows seemed much the same. The dusty paw prints near their temples look very much the same. To a first approximation, let us assume exactly identical forces impacting identical

sites. Maxime, after a chagrined recovery to his feet, felt a headache for several minutes and then, fine. Guillaume is still disoriented. You monitor them carefully for a year (they elect, as some pharmacists do, to retire early to Mootwingee). Twelve months after their receipt of identical concussive forces, now it is Maxime who is more distressed! He complains of subtle slowing in his thinking, occasional embarrassing irritability, and somewhat more frequent headaches than he had before the incident. Guillaume is asymptomatic. Any textbook on concussion must make an earnest effort to explain this story, because it is a distillation of facts that every neurologist and almost everyone else knows: outcomes vary from similar accidents.

"Vary" hardly does justice to the medical phenomenon under discussion. "Vary" is such a frail descriptor, e.g., "The temperature varies in Bora Bora as much as 4 degrees." Or "Patterns on the Glory of the Seas seashell vary between small brown triangles and smaller brown triangles." CBIs are followed by a tremendous diversity of alternate clinical pathways. If concussion produced only a single symptom – for instance, headache – then the neurologist would be obliged to consider at least ten types of variation, including: (1) the number of weeks before emergence of a new headache pattern; (2) severity; (3) frequency; (4) location; (5) duration; (6) quality (e.g., throbbing or non-throbbing); (7) associated symptoms (e.g., photophobia, sonophobia); (8) triggers (e.g., stress or sleep deprivation); (9) relievers of headaches within that pattern; and (10) variation in the time course (months, years) over which that new bothersome headache pattern might, in the best of circumstances, subside. The permutations and combinations of these ten standard headache characteristics mean that even the seemingly simple problem of post-concussion *headache* exhibits extraordinary clinical variability. We then recall that the Rivermead Post-Concussion Symptoms Questionnaire [32] lists 16 frequent post-concussion symptoms. Like headache, each of these varies along the continuous dimension of severity and each also varies along its own symptom-specific dimensions (for instance, the multiple classifications of sleep disorder). The net result is that the number of alternative clinical pathways after a concussion is infinite. Literally and indisputably infinite. What is the best a brain injury expert might assert with conviction? "Please look at Figure 7.2, above. Should you suffer a concussion, your clinical course will fall somewhat along one of these curves, or not."

A Blow to the Head is Not a Disease

To avoid the risk of going back to old controversies of sending back patients complaints to their personalities, one cannot do else but subscribe to a multifactorial vision of the constitution of PCS [post-concussional syndrome], in terms of vulnerability factors. The first of these factors remains the brain trauma.

Fayol et al. 2009 [54], p. 500

---

[5] For patients aged 18–59 years, the author recommends pairing the *Achenbach Adult Self-report* (ASR) with the *Adult Behavior Checklist* (ABCL, for observers). Children can be comprehensively assessed using the *Child Behavior Checklist* self-report, parent report, and teacher report. Older adults can be assessed with the *Older Adult Assessments*.

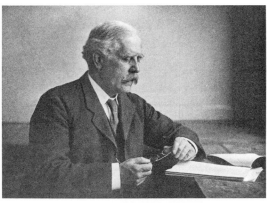

Fig. 7.3 Sir Archibald Edward Garrod, KCMG, FRS.
Source: Wellcome Collection. Reproduced under the terms of the Creative Commons Attribution license, CC-BY 4.0

A blow to the head is not a disease. A "brain injury," mentioned without qualification, is not a disease. Since the outcome of a non-fatal blow is probabilistic, since the lasting consequences could be happy good health or rapid death, a blow to the head sufficient to affect the brain is best conceptualized as a risk factor for deleterious brain change. That brain change, in all its infinite individuality, is often but not always associated with human distress, dysfunction, or dis-ease.

What, then, is a disease? As ever, the author begs the reader's toleration of a brief detour into the entrancing domain of ideas.

One of the great barriers to resolution of the concussion debate is simply that there is an old and a new understanding of disease. According to the old idea (pre-1908), a disease is an external insult to the body and CBI is a single problem – not a universe of different problems held together by the gravitational pull of common physical provocation, like the billion stars in a galaxy, but one single disorder. That dated idea of disease, by itself, explains where many early concussion writers understandably went awry: people naturally find it hard to accept that there is an infinitude of possible outcomes if they think a CBI is one single problem. Seeing beyond the one-disease error, which springs from an ancient and biologically impossible view of disease, explains why the consequences of a blow to the head are so profoundly variable.

In his 1908 Croonian lectures [29], Archibald E. Garrod delivered the concept of inborn errors of metabolism (Figure 7.3). He published his insight in a book one year later [30]. His conceptual contribution is grander than is usually acknowledged. It represents a profound, yet to be fully appreciated paradigm shift in the concept, "disease."

Garrod's predecessor in the Regius Professorship of Medicine at Oxford was one William Osler. Dr. Osler conceived of a disease just as Galen did – something assaulting the body from without, diagnosed by recognizing a reliable cluster of symptoms, i.e., a syndrome. Garrod overthrew Galenic/Oslerian dogma, making the disruptive observation that people are individuals. Thus, even though a single provocateur (for example, a bacterium) might infect ten people, no two of them should be expected to exhibit the exact same symptoms because *human dis-ease always involves the interplay between the triggering factor (e.g., infection or trauma) and the patient's unique biological identity.*

Garrod's insight left Osler in the dust. Osler's approach, inferring a diagnosis from an observed syndrome, is clearly untenable. A doctor seeking to identify a distinctive cluster of symptoms by pattern recognition and attribute that pattern to a specific disease will often mislead him- or herself, since the same etiology generates a somewhat different response in every case and different etiologies are clinical mimics [55]. Galen's and Osler's concept of "disease" is equally untenable. The Oslerian, for example, might observe that a noxious external factor (smoking tobacco) is often associated with a syndrome (coughing and wasting) and a pathological change (pulmonary neoplasm). That Oslerian then opines, "Smoking tobacco causes lung cancer."

"Nonsense," responds the Garrodian. "Smoking tobacco, in and of itself, never 'caused' a case of lung cancer. Smoking tobacco is a risk factor. It provokes. It triggers. It interacts with a person's individual human vulnerabilities and defenses. It does not affect any two humans in the very same way. *However*, on average across the billions of available human genomes, it appears to increase the likelihood of lung cancer by a factor of about 20." Pointing out this difference between cause and risk factor, pointing out the uniqueness of every disease–patient interaction, Garrod anticipated precision medicine by a century.

Embracing Garrod's modern [29] concept of illness as the interplay between an unwelcome guest and an unhappy host, accepting that there must be an infinite number of possible interactions between the brain-rattling force and the victim, and accepting that the concussive event is merely a risk factor for brain change, are there risk factors that predictably moderate this risk factor? If so, one guesses that some of those risk factors pertain to the traits of the injury, some to the traits of the patient, and some to the traits of the environment. We will return to this conceptual triad when we assemble our modified Haddon matrix. In the meantime, let us investigate what has been empirically discovered about the reasons outcomes vary.

Risk (or Predictive) Factors for Worse Outcome After CBI

In the 20th century it was sometimes claimed that initial severity predicted outcome after concussion. Many peer-reviewed papers on from the 1970s through the 1990s perpetuated that claim, sometimes accompanied by empirical data, rarely accompanied by valid and reliable measures of clinical observations or outcome. In fact, the misunderstanding that the Glasgow Coma Scale (GCS) [56] – a measure of awakeness – had something to do with the long-term impact of the injury was used to justify the mistake of misapplying that awakeness scale as if it were a severity scale. In a linked deviation from defensible science, for about four decades, medical students were taught that there is a "mild" variety of TBI, identified by the numbers 13, 14, and 15 on that Glasgow awakeness scale. In the Introduction and Chapters 1–5 of this essay it was demonstrated that no measures of initial severity, especially not the GCS, bear any trustworthy relationship to the effects of a concussion on a person's life. Duration of post-traumatic amnesia (PTA) was briefly nominated as a better predictor, until sufficient evidence accumulated showing that accurate and reliable measurement of PTA is a clinical anomaly. So, before discussing factors that do help explain variation in outcomes, one must begin by disabusing readers of the old mythology. Presence vs. absence of loss of consciousness, duration of loss of consciousness, GCS at the scene, GCS after a fixed time interval, occurrence or duration of retrograde amnesia, occurrence or duration of PTA, skull fracture, CT scan results, "complicated" mildness, or any other initial clinical observation does not predict outcome. It has also been claimed, sometimes supported by empirical data, that early symptoms are predictive. Again, weak and inconsistent evidence suggests that early headache, dizziness, light or noise sensitivity, or neuropsychological test results are risk factors for delayed recovery. Without repeating data previously presented, suffice it to say that none of these factors reliably predict outcome.

What does? The author of the present essay has no privileged access to the answer. This chapter is merely one more attempt to distill something true from the cloudy beaker of claims. At least, however, the forthcoming analysis is meant to be systematic, comprehensive, and transparent. In the end, the reader will know a great deal about the difference between factors likely to affect outcome versus factors previously claimed to affect outcome. Two simple conclusions will stand out.

First, every victim is a unique individual. Every concussion is a unique, a one-off-in-all-of-history event. Simply put, the differences between outcomes from similar blows to the head are due to the interaction of genetic, epigenetic, and environmental variables currently beyond human reckoning.

Second, since there are differences in outcome – major, complex, sometimes baffling differences that add up to dazzling clinical heterogeneity – it is profoundly misleading to postulate a post-concussion syndrome.

All caveats aside, what explains the variations in outcome? *Brain variation, force, time after impact, genes, and six other factors.*

On Human Brain Variation

What Does "The Human Brain" Mean?

To ask, "What does 'the human brain' mean"? may seem rhetorically precious. No art is intended. The question is just a simple way to draw attention to a definitional issue that is rarely considered, and that conceivably helps us to organize our thoughts about the fact that outcomes vary after typical CBI.

Of course, to a first approximation, the human brain is the semi-solid organ that occupies most of the intracranial space – the *skull offal* in Egyptian terms. Yet one finds a large number of peer-reviewed studies reporting variations in individual brain anatomy and fewer such papers regarding variation in

human liver anatomy. That, one guesses, may be less because the variations in brain shape are more common and more odd than those of liver shape, and more because of the importance that has been attributed to the brain as the seat of identity, consciousness, and will. The advent of phrenology, and then the localizationist hypothesis of the 19th century – the partially correct claim that different brain parts have different functions – probably added affective weight to the interest in individual anatomical variation because, unlike minor liver shape variations, minor brain shape variations have been suspected of perhaps having profound behavioral significance. (There are, to be fair, a handful of simple sensorimotor functions that depend on obligate participation from somewhat localizable brain parts. But no conscious thought has ever sprung from a place.)

This question requires a momentary revisit to our discussion of same and different. The more all instances of a class or category are self-evidently alike – such as "black Labrador retrievers," the steadier one feels in discussing the typical traits of that entity: intelligent, biddable, loyal, good with children, keen hearing, 21.5–24.5 inches in height, black. The more heterogeneous a category, such as "landscapes," the more challenging it is to list universal traits. To state, "there is a human brain" implies universal traits. And indeed, there are many. In the brainstem one finds a relatively uniform design. However, the brain's phylogenetically and ontogenetically later pieces vary more.

The History of Localizationism

Until the year 1870, it was generally believed that the cerebral cortex was inexcitable to electrical stimuli, that all parts of it were in fact of equal value, and that no definite part could be pointed to as the seat of any special function. In the year named Fritsch and Hitzig demonstrated electrically the motor area of the dog's brain and inaugurated a new era of cerebral research.

Jefferson, 1916 [57], p. 30

Medical students are routinely exposed to the simplistic and fallacious Swiss Watch Theory of Behavioral Neurology: the notion that there exist architectonically differentiable subunits of human neocortex devoted to given higher cortical functions. Some introductory textbooks lead off with Gall's creative phrenological map, an 18th-century invention based on the correct guess that brain parts have different functions, and the incorrect guess those functions can be quantified by examining the skull [58]. Figure 7.4 exemplifies the fanciful "science" of that time.

The next image in many basic neurology textbooks is often Brodmann's 1909 map (Figure 7.5) [60]. Brodmann reported having examined human brains stained with Nissl's method. He reported having painstakingly determined the location of 52 areas distinguished by cytoarchitectonic features. Figure 7.5 is from Brodmann's 1909 text. (His data were never published, leading to doubts. More credibility is attached to the 1925 map by von Economo and Koskinas [61].)

Soon after the Brodmann map circulated, neurologists commenced coloring it in, assigning specific functions to specific brain pieces. Figure 7.6 depicts a typical schematic of this kind.

Such maps are valuable heuristics. They bring a sense of mechanical order to the brain, an appropriate metaphor for the industrial age.[6] They are, however, similar to Gall's phrenology maps in idealistically demarcating places with purported functions – an inevitable consequence of the Swiss Watch Fallacy. They are a natural product of their times.

One hundred and fifty years ago, three scholarly approaches were applied to determined the function of brain parts: (1) ablation studies in animals; (2) stimulation studies in animals and humans; and (3) clinicopathological correlations. Thus, for example, Flourens removed pieces of rabbit and pigeon brains and reported his findings in 1825. Fritsch and Hitzig inserted electrified probes into the brains of dogs, successfully mapping some functions. Ferrier expanded on that technique, confirming 15 functional cortical areas in dogs and monkeys by first stimulating, then surgically removing, the parts.

In 1861, Auburtin [62] boldly demonstrated that speech production seemed dependent on the anterior frontal lobes. A gentleman shot himself in the head and then visited the good doctor. Dr. Auburtin commenced doing experiments as the patient lay dying. Pressing a "large spatula" against the exposed brain could cut off speech mid-word – early evidence of a special relationship between verbal productivity and prefrontal function. Broca, Wernicke, and others subsequently published cases of relatively circumscribed behavioral change associated with relatively circumscribed ablative brain damage. And German neurosurgeon Feodor Krause was among the first to map human cortex via intraoperative electrostimulation [58, 63, 64]. The limitations of these early efforts notwithstanding (for instance, extrapolating from one brain to all of humanity), a lore developed.

Two lines of research have dispelled the old claim that there exists a uniform human brain in which functions are assigned to locations. First, there is the discovery, confirmed with the help of twins, that no two human brains are alike. Second, there has been the steady march of increasingly sophisticated tests of the hypothesis that a given brain place has a function. Localizationism is, generally speaking, wrong.

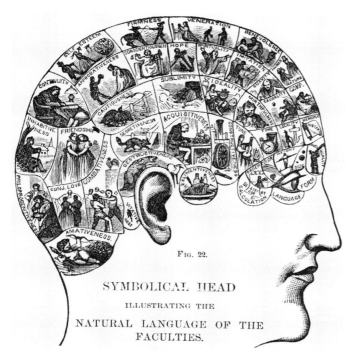

Fig. 7.4 Nineteenth-century example of phrenological localization. Source: Wells [59]

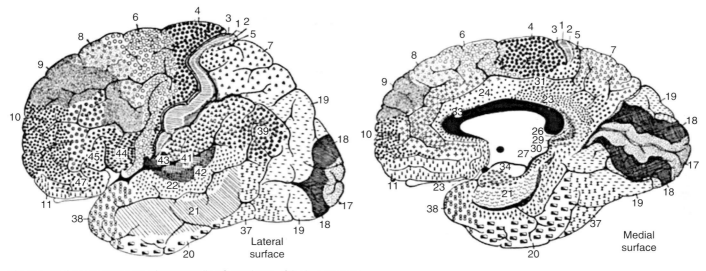

Fig. 7.5 Brodmann's 1909 cytoarchitectonically informed map of the human cortex. Source: Brodmann, 1909 [60]

---

6   About the same year, Freud began his own campaign to account for human behavior with metaphors suiting the *Weltgeist* of the industrial age, characterizing mind in terms of Helmholtzian mechanics.

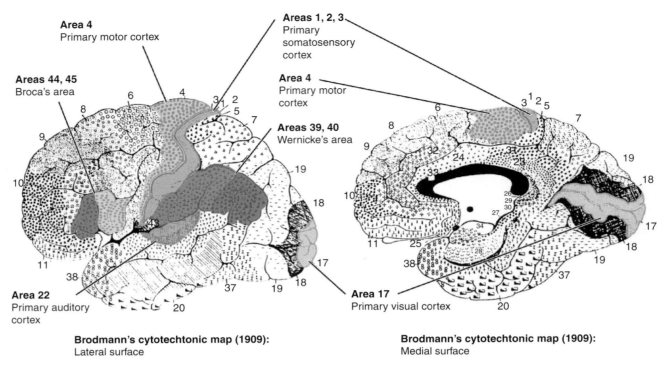

Area 4
Primary motor cortex

Areas 44, 45
Broca's area

Areas 1, 2, 3
Primary somatosensory cortex

Area 4
Primary motor cortex

Areas 39, 40
Wernicke's area

Area 22
Primary auditory cortex

Area 17
Primary visual cortex

Brodmann's cytotechtonic map (1909):
Lateral surface

Brodmann's cytotechtonic map (1909):
Medial surface

Fig. 7.6 Brodmann's map, colored to highlight purported functional areas. [A black and white version of this figure will appear in some formats. For the color version, please refer to the plate section.]

First: No Two Human Brains are Alike

Twins are never identical. Monozygotic (MZ) twins reared together have different genomes. Therefore, even if there were no effect of twin-to-twin transfusion syndrome in monochorionic pairs or birth order, and even if shared postnatal environment were identical in every way, one would not expect MZ twins to have brains with the same structures or localizations of functions. And if MZ twins do not have the same brains, then even the most perfectly replicated external concussive force could never be expected to produce the same brain changes or symptoms in any two humans.

Phenotypic discordance between MZ twins has perhaps been observed for centuries. Medical documentation that "identical" twins sometimes exhibit striking differences in brain and behavior became apparent about 50 years ago when multiple MZ twins pairs were reported to be discordant for schizophrenia [65–67]. More recently, it has become apparent that multiple environmental and genetic factors account for MZ neurobehavioral discordance [68–70].

"Environmental" differences were suspected long ago. Even in twins reared together, there occurs a literal infinitude of different environmental exposures. But the discovery of epigenetic chromatin modification blurs the distinction between genetic and environmental etiologies. Hence, some "environmental" causes of discordance affect gene expression via impact on transcription, while others affect gene expression via epigenetic changes [71–73]. There are also post-fertilization effects with an uncertain relationship to the environment, such as chromosomal mosaicism and post-zygotic mutagenesis [70, 74].

As one result, identical twin brains are never identical. It has been apparent since the early days of magnetic resonance imaging (MRI) that gyral and sulcal patterns are indisputably different in every MZ twin pair [75–77]. Subcortical structures, such as the massive white-matter bundles of the corpus callosum that are especially vulnerable to CBI, are also different between twins [78].

This is not to deny heritability of some aspects of brain anatomy. As a general rule, in studies comparing MZ and dizygotic (DZ) twin cohorts to estimate heritability, two conclusions seem to be justified: (1) studies that compare very large brain regions show higher heritability than those comparing smaller regions; (2) there is evidence of more heritable comparability of prefrontal anatomy, less of hippocampal anatomy, and even less of medial brain areas [79–82]. Some evidence suggests that heritability increases from childhood to adulthood, but that the aging-associated deterioration is less heritable [83, 84]. That is, despite a relatively high heritability of late-life brain structure, there is a lower heritability of cognitive impairment – suggesting that mid-life environmental factors may be more important for dementia [85].[7] More recent twin research has suggested that the asymmetry of homologous cerebral regions

---

[7] Chapter 11 of this volume is titled Late Effects. In that chapter, the author will hesitantly propose a speculative reconceptualization of aging. One phenomenon predicted by his hypothesis is that heritability of deleterious brain change with the passing of time will diminish after the usual age range of reproduction.

(except in the globus pallidus and nucleus accumbens) is independent of genetic control [86], although one report found that genetics has a much stronger influence on left- than right-hemisphere development [87]. Interestingly, in a Dutch sample gross anatomical measures were more heritable than white-matter measures made with diffusion tensor imaging (DTI) and magnetization transfer imaging [88]. Yet, even within the domain of white matter, there seem to be differences. As Shen et al. [89] reported: "Inter-hemispheric connections tended to be more heritable than intra-hemispheric and cortico-spinal connections" (p. 628). Another issue is the inter-individual variability of brain structure heritability. For example, although Vuoksimaa et al. [90] declare that white-matter structures in middle age are highly heritable, the heritability of fractional anisotropy (FA) of individual tracts varied from 0 to 82%.

Functional imaging also supports the expectation of MZ twin discordance for cerebral processing [84]. Results from functional MRI (fMRI) activation studies (as always) have reportedly varied by region and task and cohort. For instance, Polk et al. [91] reported significant heritability (MZ > DZ correlation) of ventral visual pathway activity in response to faces but not to pseudo-words. Matthews et al. [92] found evidence of heritability of response to an interference task in the dorsal anterior cingulate cortex (ACC) but not in the ventral ACC. Similar regionally dependent degrees of heritability were reported by Silverman et al. [93]: among 46 pairs of adolescent MZ twins, there was significant similarity in anticipation of reward-related activity, but in only three of 18 regions. The heritability of resting fMRI has also been investigated. For instance, Glahn et al. [94] estimated the heritability of the default mode network at a modest 42%.

Although the author felt obliged to offer the above summary of the state of the art (and to gently hint at its resistance to simple interpretation), readers will justifiably ask: "What is the bottom line regarding MZ twins and brains?" The main conclusion should stand the test of time: One reason that outcomes from concussion vary is that, even under the closest-to-ideal theoretical experimental circumstances – identical forces arriving at identical skull locations in identical twins – it would be illogical to expect the same outcome since no two human brains have the same structure or function.

Second: Localizationism is, Generally Speaking, Wrong

Whoever calmly considers the question cannot long resist the conviction that different parts of the brain must, *in some way or other* [emphasis in the original], subserve different kinds of mental action. Localization of function is the law of all organization whatever; and it would be marvellous were there here an exception.

Spencer, 1855 [95], p. 204

Back in the 19th, and even the early 20th, century, some neurologists honestly believed that certain parts of the neo-cortex had dedicated functions. There was, for example, the concept of the "motor strip" or primary cortical motor area. It was, at that time in history, claimed that the pre-central gyrus was devoted to transmitting motor signals from giant layer V Betz cells down the corticospinal tract. Recent research has perhaps only scratched the surface of the many functionalities of the pre-central gyrus – from perceiving the amplitudes of movements [96], to maintaining working memories [97], to facets of emotional intelligence such as sensitivity to others' movements in the context of anger [98]. Textbooks tend to be late to the party. Many still pronounce that: (1) ensembles of neurons and glia occupying a certain part of a certain gyrus do a particular job; (2) the cells in that place do no other jobs; and (3) the cells in other places never do that job.

That concept is untrue. Long before the advent of functional neuroimaging, Wilder Penfield and others reported that the location of brain pieces that, when stimulated, elicited a given motor response differed between individuals. Resistance to localizationism on empirical grounds in fact goes back to the mid 19th century. As early as 1914, von Monakow [99] urged attention to hodological effects such as diaschisis – the fact that injury in one place often disrupts function at distant sites sharing network connections – a discovery that raised doubts about the special job of any three-dimensional brain piece.[8] But progress toward resolution of this debate was extremely slow prior to high-resolution *in vivo* neuroimaging.

Progress has recently been faster. Yet the explosion of 21st-century data has not, in every case, been informative. As the editors of this brief essay have repeatedly cautioned, most MRI-based functional neuroimaging reports cannot be taken at face value. The lack of standardization of every facet of most protocols (hardware, software, stimulus, and elected threshold of significance) has been a frustrating barrier to credible replication. In structural imaging, DTI has become controversial because the FA measured in a given tract is routinely reported to be exactly opposite that found in another study. (Perhaps diffusion kurtosis imaging will earn a better track record than DTI.) In functional imaging, it is not just reproducibility that is doubted, but validity. (Perhaps earnest adjustment for multiple comparisons will enhance the field's reputation.) For now, we must acknowledge that reports of thinking in a dead salmon suggest imperfect technology [100].

Still, for the foreseeable future, functional imaging remains more promising than clinico pathological correction for assaying patterns of cerebral activity such as blood flow or metabolism in response to a given stimulus. Mapping of activity with this technology almost instantly antiquated the concept of localization that hails back to well before the 1855 manifesto ([95], cited above) by amateur sociologist, philosopher, and psychologist, Herbert Spencer. Had Spencer's prediction come true, there would have been a host of publications on the heels of Auburtin, Broca, and Wernicke, each reporting unique behavioral changes associated with focal strokes. That did not occur. Nor did intraoperative electrostimulation move the field

---

8   Every CBI has focal, multi-focal, and diffuse effects. However, it would be difficult to determine whether a given neuron is dysfunctional because of (a) primary or secondary traumatic injury; (b) disrupted connectivity due to axonal damage; or (c) authentic diaschisis.

much beyond reports of twitches. Moreover, reviewing the early results of functional neuroimaging in behavioral neurology may not be helpful. Papers from the 1980s and 1990s reporting positron emission tomography (PET) cerebral blood flow (CBF) activations in response to tasks simply hinted at what would soon become indisputable at higher resolutions: no task ever activates just one piece of brain. Instead, no matter how carefully the investigators tried to isolate a mental operation by subtracting control task from experiment task-related CBF, mentation usually provokes the activation of multiple gyri.

Seeking to advance the understanding of localization of mental functions, some psychologists turned to fMRI. This was not a mistake. Minding their limitations, the data are informative. It is, however, a serious error to assume that any fMRI scan represents either the way a given subject processes a given stimulus, or the way any other subject processes that stimulus [101–104]. One problem: seeing especially tall trees in the normal, healthy neural forest requires two types of mathematical manipulation: (1) restricting attention to a few small areas with greater-than-arbitrarily-defined threshold change in activity (e.g., via statistical parametric mapping), and (2) lumping together results from multiple subjects and reporting the *average* location as the *real* location, a misleading homogenization of the truth called "group-level analysis." This last deserves clarification. Investigators typically recruit multiple volunteers to perform tasks while monitored. But that individual data are almost never reported. To optimize the chances of publishing a persuasive paper, professors routinely agglomerate findings from many subjects and call that mash-up the "locus of activity."

Manuel, for instance, volunteers for an activated fMRI experiment. He performs a mental task (for instance, calculations) alternating with a control task meant to subtract lower-level processing (such as seeing the question on a screen) with the hope of localizing calculation-specific processing. His scan is successful: based on statistical parametric mapping, it reveals 18 areas of significantly increased activation. The next day, Manuel returns. He does the same task. The new scan now reveals 15 areas of activation. Eight of them are in places similar to yesterday's scan. The other seven are not.

That is the expected result. It would be a perpetuation of an old fallacy to imagine that Manuel's brain, or anyone's, uses the same pieces in the same way to do the same job twice. As Song et al. [105] put it:

Note that fMRI data exhibit a nonstationary nature due to long-term neuro-physiological effects, such as sensory/learning-induced neuronal plasticity and functional reorganization …, and short-term factors, such as subjects' task strategy, attention, fatigue, mood, movement, physiological fluctuation, and machine instability.

(p. 3)

This phenomenon is called *intra-subject variability*. It disabuses scholars of the Swiss Watch Fallacy by demonstrating that much mental processing is not only distributed rather than localized, but also variably distributed.

Now invite Igor. His scan shows 11 "significant" sites of activation. Of course, his cortical topography is not the same

as Manuel's so one can only guess which of Igor's gyri derive from the same developmental source as which of Manuel gyri. Still, if one squints, five of the activated sites in Igor's scan are arguably homologous to sites activated in one or another of Manuel's scans. The differences are called *inter-subject variability* – another lesson in the updated catechism of behavioral neurology. See Song et al. [105] : "considerable variation in amplitude and spatial extent of fMRI activations exist across subjects and sessions even using a consistent task paradigm and identical imaging conditions" (p. 3).

A picture may be helpful. Figure 7.7 depicts fMRI measures of brain activation from two healthy subjects scanned while performing the same mental tasks. As previously noted, a few simple sensorimotor operations are somewhat localizable. Thinking is not.

Figure 7.7 is typical – for those rare instances when investigators publish individual results. The cortical activity mediating thinking appears as scattered as the spots on a Dalmatian. And every Dalmatian has different spots. Splitting the difference between Manuel and Igor does not reveal how the human brain works. It reveals a hippogriff.

The main conceptual advance in localizationism in recent years has probably been an idea advanced by Mesulam in his seminal 1990 paper, "Large-scale neurocognitive networks and distributed processing for attention, language, and memory" [107]. Mesulam and his younger colleagues deserve credit for a paradigm shift (which, by the way, is compatible with von Monakow's 1914 observations about distant effects of local damage [99]): rather than each piece of cortex having a function, *networks* have functions [108–111]. One only wishes Dr. Mesulam had added an asterisk: "These are impressionist schematics. They do not accurately reflect behavioral neuroanatomy of any human." Figure 7.8 depicts this connectionist hypothesis.

The concept of functional networks is an extremely important advance. The present author has the utmost respect for Dr. Mesulam and his team. Yet readers may be mildly bemused. Yet again, neurology shies from the truth of individuality. Like the coloring used to vivify Brodmann's old maps, purporting to delineate functionally dedicated brain pieces, one now finds idealized coloring overlying idealized neuroimages. This updates and modernizes the Swiss Watch Fallacy of Behavioral Neurology. These cartoons – based in almost all cases on group-level analysis of functional imaging data – replace the oversimplification that brain parts have given jobs with the oversimplification that brain circuits, readily localized down to the millimeter, have given jobs. Again, such schematics are valuable for introducing medical students to the brain. But for understanding why outcomes from concussions vary, they perpetuate the mythology of localizationism.

This eagerness for clear pictures, in the author's opinion, remains a stiff barrier to progress in clinical neurobehavior. One cannot expect to understand human nature or human disease by ignoring variation. The author humbly asks that professors tell medical students the truth. Dr. Wernicke's report was quite interesting, but there is no "understanding language" area. There is far too much individual variation in the neuronal/

Functional magnetic resonance imaging activation maps of two subjects performing the same tasks

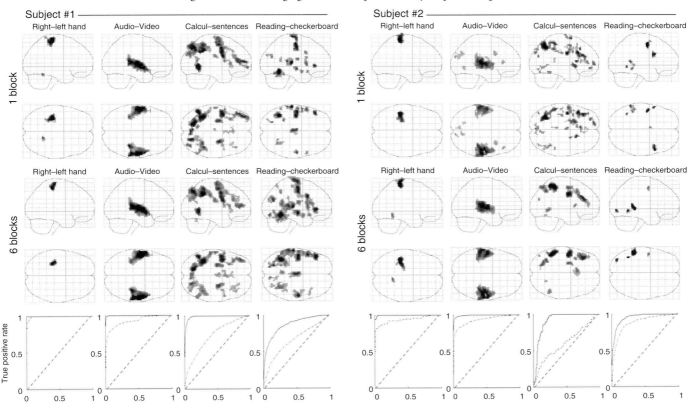

Fig. 7.7 Individual functional information captured in 5 min. Illustration of functional information captured in one 5-min session (one block) compared with a 30-min-long session (six blocks), for two subjects. Individual correlates of four tasks are plotted (sagittal and axial view) at $p < 10-3$ uncorrected (cluster extent 10 voxels) for the one-block analysis. Similar correlates are plotted at $p < 10-3$ corrected (cluster extent 10 voxels) for the six-block analysis. Below are plotted receiver operating characteristic (ROC) curves of each subject's contrast images. Solid line represents curve obtained using the t-value map of the corresponding subject, while dotted line represents curve obtained using the t-value map of the same contrast but of the other subject. Diagonal lines represent the ROC curves that would be obtained in the case of a non-informative random map.

Source: Pinel et al., 2007 [106]. Reproduced under the terms of the Creative Commons Attribution license, CC-BY 2.0

glial ensembles that contribute to various aspects of mentation to sustain the mythology of gyral purpose.

Why does every brain differ from every other in both structure and function? The previous subsection of this essay provided a hint: genomes vary.[9] That variation explains some of the diversity. For example, variants in the genes for brain-derived neurotrophic factor (BDNF) [112], the oxytocin receptor [113], the calcium voltage-gated channel subunit alpha1 C (CACNA1C) [114], and an unnamed linkage peak at 12q24 [115] have all been reported to explain variation in brain architecture. It was previously noted in this text that genetic variation surely helps explain variation in concussion outcome; that variation surely includes gene-mediated variation in the size and shape of brain parts.

In partial summary of this section of the chapter, one reason outcomes do and will always vary after a typical, clinically attended CBI is that – contrary to industrial metaphor – there

is no fixed, uniform, predictably functioning human brain. There are billions. Two recent reports make this point with eloquent grace. They respectively overthrow the dogma that the cortex and the subcortex have a species-specific structure and function.

As part of the Human Connectome Project, Tavor et al. [116] scanned subjects with fMRI at rest in response to several tasks. As they described their project: "We investigated the possibility that individual differences in brain activation are inherent features of individuals and, to a large degree, independent of volatile factors" (p. 216). In other words, the investigators surmised that if each individual exhibits his or her own unique baseline brain activity, the additional activity required for a given task will be somewhat predictable on the basis of known relationships between network activity and task activity. Figure 7.9 illustrates some results. Impressively, resting activity did enable the investigators to roughly predict

---

9 The author must restrain himself from proposing a deeper answer. Why brains vary is a burning issue in evolutionary science. Mutations presumably arise because they facilitate natural selection. Yet some scholars have asked whether diversity in cerebral function adds resilience to social groups. This touches upon the third rail of group-level selection, and will not be discussed here.

Proposed large-scale networks for cognition and behavior

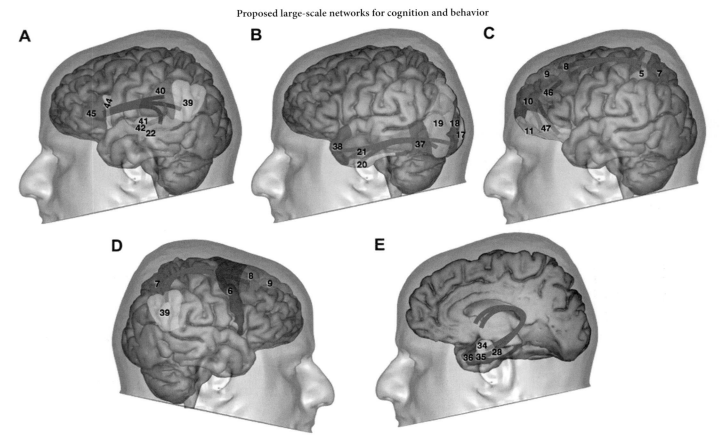

Fig. 7.8 (A) A left-hemisphere-dominant language network with epicenters in Wernicke's and Broca's areas. (B) A face object identification network with epicenters in occipitotemporal and temporopolar cortex. (C) An executive function comportment network with epicenters in lateral prefrontal cortex, orbitofrontal cortex, and posterior parietal cortex. (D) A right-hemisphere-dominant spatial attention network with epicenters in dorsal posterior parietal cortex, the frontal eye fields, and the cingulate gyrus. (E) A memory emotion network with epicenters in the hippocampal-entorhinal regions and the amygdaloid complex. [A black and white version of this figure will appear in some formats. For the color version, please refer to the plate section.]

Source: Catani et al., 2012 [111] with permission from Elsevier

stimulated activity. For the purposes of this essay, however, that study's take-home finding is simpler: no two subjects, either at rest or in response to any task, employ the same brain parts.

Hibar et al. [117] published a complementary study. As part of the Enhancing Neuro Imaging Genetics through Meta-Analysis (ENIGMA) consortium, those investigators explored the hypothesis that genetic individuality impacts development and structure of seven subcortical structures: the nucleus accumbens, caudate, putamen, pallidum, amygdala, hippocampus, and thalamus. It does. In a sophisticated series of experiments, those authors compared genotypes with MRI-determined structures in a sample of 30,717 individuals aged 9–97 years. Among the most dramatic results was the finding that four loci influence the volume and shape of the putamen. The single-nucleotide polymorphisms (SNPs) impacting putamen structure were largely in genes affecting apoptosis, axon guidance, and vesicle transport – which the authors interpreted as evidence of genetic control over neuronal size and dendritic complexity. Figure 7.10 illustrates the individual variability in putamen structure generated by these genetic variants in a subset of 1541 young and healthy subjects.

Reports such as these will hopefully grant perspective to maps such as Brodmann's, and to the neurobehavioral coloring books that followed. Idealized brains, depicted in textbooks as if they corresponded to any living human, will continue to assist beginners in visualizing the skull offal. But they probably contribute to the psychological rigidity that has perhaps delayed understanding why outcomes vary after CBIs. The combination of genetic variation, epigenetic variation, and environment-dependent plasticity secures the wonder of human uniqueness. It is liberating to discard the dogma of brain uniformity. It opens the door to unfettered thought about the medical implications of human diversity. These reports may thus help 21st-century doctors to finally embrace Garrod's 1908 wisdom: Human dis-ease is *never* a uniform, externally imposed problem. It is *always* the result of an interplay between risk factors and individual nature.

Informed by these basic tenets of neuroscience, even lay persons will immediately realize the impossibility of any two concussions producing the same results. One might theoretically administer forces, identical to the nearest nano-newton, to the same place on two skulls, identical to the nearest

Predicting individual variations in task maps

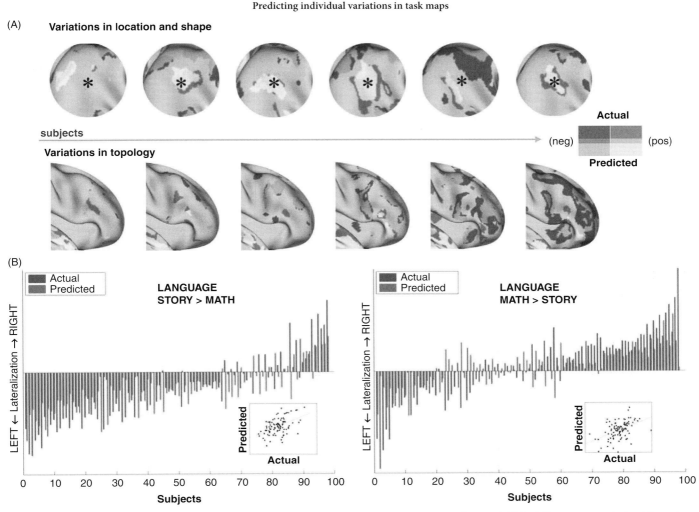

Fig. 7.9 (A) Variations in location, shape, and topology are predicted by the model (contrast: language math > story). (B) Peak Z scores were calculated for each hemisphere to examine how well the model can predict the amount of activation for each subject. A lateralization index (difference between right and left peak activation levels) is then calculated for each subject for both predicted and actual data and is shown as red and blue bars, respectively (language task). The model is able to predict individual subjects' lateralization index for both contrasts, including the case where the majority of the subjects are left-lateralized. Statistical tests: math > story (correlation coefficient (r) = 0.47, $p < 10−5$), story > math ($r = 0.48$, $p < 10−6$). [A black and white version of this figure will appear in some formats. For the color version, please refer to the plate section.]

Source: Tavor et al., 2016 [116]. Reprinted with permission from AAAS.

nanometer. Brain individuality in both structure and function predicts different outcomes.

On Force

In animal research, two factors consistently correlate with the likelihood or severity of post-CBI problems. One is the force of the impact. The other is the time after impact. Neither is determinative. That is, as shown in Chapter 4, ten mice exposed to 2.0 atm impacts will have ten different degrees of impairment on a dozen different measures. However, the proportion killed or the *average* outcome of survivors will indeed vary according to force. Similarly, animals (including humans) that survive concussions tend to get better over time. Ten mice who survive the first several days after a 2.0 atm impact will exhibit better performance at week two and even better performance

at week eight. Again these are *average* outcomes, since some individuals will lag much more than others in recovery. Both of these factors, force and time, are also predictive of the average human outcome after CBI. However, in both cases, the relationship between the risk factors and the outcome is complex and interesting.

Consider force. As discussed in Chapter 6, when two college football players experience a helmet-moving brain-rattling blow, the forces measured by accelerometers poised between their helmets and their hair are weak predictors of both subjective concussion (feeling dazed) and outcome. In part, this is the result of innumerable individual differences in molecular neurobiology. But in part, it is a matter of mechanics. Force is not a single number but shorthand for the incredibly complex intracerebral mechanics of a bump on the hair (in those with hair).

Genetically influenced individual variation in the human putamen

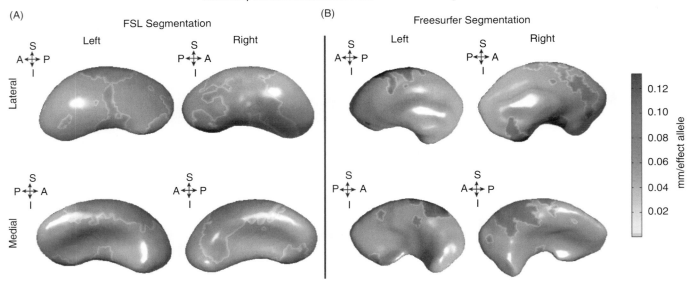

Fig. 7.10 Shape analysis in 1541 young healthy subjects shows consistent deformations of the putamen regardless of segmentation protocol. (a, b) The distance from a medial core to surfaces derived from FSL FIRST (a) or FreeSurfer (b) segmentations was derived in the same 1541 subjects. Each copy of the rs945270-C allele was significantly associated with an increased width in colored areas (false discovery rate corrected at q50.05) and the degree of deformation is labeled by color. The orientation is indicated by arrows. A: anterior; I: inferior; P: posterior; S: superior. Shape analysis in both software suites gives statistically significant associations in the same direction. Although the effects are more widespread in the FSL segmentations, FreeSurfer segmentations also show overlapping regions of effect, which appears strongest in anterior and superior sections. [A black and white version of this figure will appear in some formats. For the color version, please refer to the plate section.]

Source: Hibar et al. [117]. Reprinted by permission from Macmillan

The most popular commercially available instrumented helmet is the Head Impact Telemetry System (HITS) [118–120]. In one study [121], Division I college football players wore HITS-outfitted helmets capable of recording linear and rotational acceleration. Concussions occurred at anywhere from 60.51–168.71 **g** of linear acceleration, and symptoms *were not related to force*. For example, a player who sustained a hit of 60.51 **g** had a neurological symptoms change score of 27 (a scaled change in neurological status over the 48 h after concussion compared with pre-season baseline). Another player took a hit of about the same force, 63.84 **g**, but exhibited a neurological change of only 8. Similarly, one player suffered a hit of 99.74 **g** with a neurological change of 30; another suffered a hit of 100.36 **g** with a change score of 0. As explained in Chapter 5, the authors appropriately concluded that it is doubtful one can establish a threshold for the force that produces a human concussion; *the same force yields dramatically different results in different people*. In another study [122] of 486,594 impacts to the head of 450 college athletes, 44 concussions were reported. Concussions occurred with linear accelerations as low as 16.5 **g** and as high as 177.9 **g**, and with rotation accelerations as low as 183 and as high as 7589 rad/s². Again, force did not predict outcome. Why not?

It is simplistic to discuss concussion as a high school physics experiment, considering the heft of a ball bearing or how far it fell before contacting a furry head. The head is not spherical. Its contents include all sorts of different deformable materials. As the force is diffused and dispersed by fur, scalp skin, galea, skull, spinal fluid, and dura on its way to the brain, predicting

the number of newtons that will arrive at a particular piece of the brain such as the medial hippocampus or pontine tegmentum (both critical to symptomatic results) becomes almost impossible.

However, one can obtain a somewhat closer approximation than the high school physic class if we employ finite element modeling (FEM). This technique involves mathematical approximation. As a weak analogy: let's say you wished to determine the circumference of an oak tree, but all you had was a yardstick. The stick will not bend. But you might walk around the tree measuring successive six-inch nearly flat segments, adding them to approximate the curved circumference. FEM allows one to take multiple straight measurements and approximate, to a fair degree of fidelity, the measure of any curve. FEM assumes that two human brains are structurally alike, though of course they are not. Still, the exercise is useful since the impact of an external force on a brain cannot be realistically described as "this amount of linear acceleration" or "that amount of rotational acceleration." A CBI is not like a hammer hitting a bowling ball. The head is not a perfect astronomical sphere. It is an odd, irregular, bulky, complex container of solid, liquid, and gas. As a result, knowing that one hit a head in one place with a given force gives us very little information about the way that force was really transmitted, dispersed, and rebounded throughout the many rattling tissues of the battered brain. In point of fact, a concussion shakes every brain cell in a unique way. Although FEM does not get us to that microscopic level, it provides a more realistic estimate of the effects of a blow than a model conceiving

Finite-element modeling of traumatic brain injury

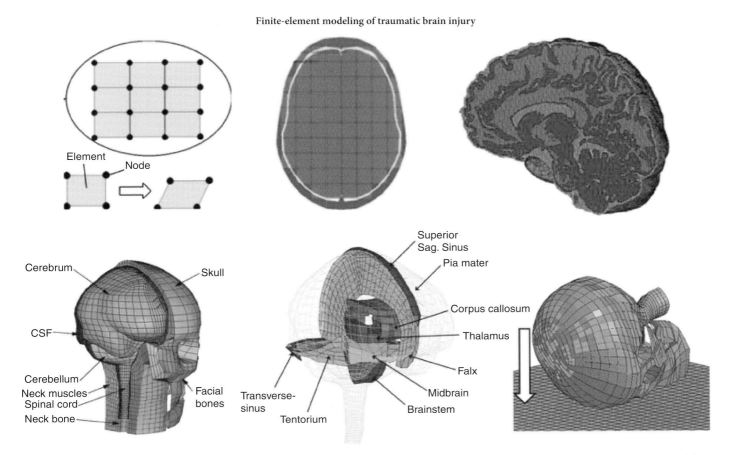

Fig. 7.11 The continuum of a tissue mass is approximated by many finite elements connected at nodes. The two pictures on the lower left illustrate the model's division into tissue types. The image on the right depicts a simulated right frontal head injury. CSF: cerebrospinal fluid. [A black and white version of this figure will appear in some formats. For the color version, please refer to the plate section.]

concussion as a Newtonian baseball hitting a Platonic orb. Figure 7.11 illustrates one FE model.

Beyond mere acceleration, FEM allows estimation of multiple aspects of intracerebral stress and strain. Oeur et al. [124] recently reconstructed human concussions, comparing the brain strains among CBI survivors whose symptoms resolved within nine days versus those who remained symptomatic at 18 months (persistent post-concussive symptoms). The measures overlapped. "No significant differences were found between groups for either brain tissue measures of maximum principal strain [elastic limit] or von Mies stress [strain accounting for volume and shape]." One conclusion: the same concussive force may possibly produce mild, moderate, or severe, short-, medium-, or long-term changes to brains and behaviors. To be clear, force on the hair, skull, or even the dura is a weak predictor of outcome.

Another caveat deserves attention: animal experiments almost always compare a known amount of linear and/or rotational force with clinically observed outcomes. What if neither linear nor rotational force is predictive of brain harm or behavioral change? That must be true, given the variance in outcomes with identical forces. However, biomechanical modeling also hints that we are perhaps making insufficiently sophisticated approximations of real brain strain. For example, von Holst

and Li [123] mathematically reconstructed a human brain injury due to a fall. They attempted to determine what mechanical parameters might best predict cerebral metabolic compromise – linear or rotational acceleration? Neither.

> rather than suggesting another predictor, we propose that the external kinetic energy transferred to the head during an accident may result in at least three sequential impacts to the brain tissue defined as the immediate dynamic triple peak impact factor.
>
> (von Holst and Li [123], p. 7)

Three different impacts? This exemplifies how FEM suggests nuances of brain harm that are hard to capture with a typical laboratory apparatus. In another study, Post et al. [125] mathematically and experimentally reconstructed 20 human falls for which clinical data were available. They too found that neither peak linear nor peak rotational acceleration accounted for brain lesions. Instead, "the majority of the variance was accounted for by *duration* of the resultant and component linear and rotational acceleration [emphasis added]." Thus, while very few rodent studies dwell on dwell time (the time the impactor lounges deep in the head), that neglected parameter of experimental brain injury may be important for judging

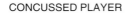

Contours of principal strain during simulation of a concussion

UNHARMED PLAYER   CONCUSSED PLAYER

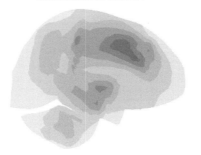 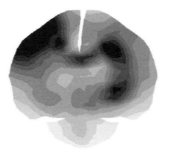 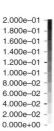

```
2.000e−01
1.800e−01
1.600e−01
1.400e−01
1.200e−01
1.000e−01
8.000e−02
6.000e−02
4.000e−02
2.000e−02
0.000e+00
```

Fig. 7.12 Large strain can be seen in the corpus callosum, left temporal and parietal lobes, and right dorsal cortex.

Source: Giordano and Kleiven, 2014 [128] by permission from The Stapp Association

whether the laboratory is replicating a mild or severe human injury.

Together the offerings of these engineers give us fair warning: concussions are not a simple matter of a linear pulse punching an exposed patch of dura. A CBI is less like kicking a soccer ball or punching a sand bag and more like shaking a peach in a can. Brain/skull interplay and multiple components of force and rebound contribute to outcome. The many labs that pop open an animal's head so they can directly pound on the brain are not modeling concussion. By circumventing the skull and taking away head movement, experiments that hit the dura of a strapped-down mouse have perhaps been misleading us for 40 years.

Note, however, that even these elegant FE models oversimplify. The reader will please forgive a brief dip into the sometimes-frosty pool of engineering.

Most FE models treat the brain as if it were both homogeneous and isotropic – that is, equal stuff in all directions, like gelatin in a mold. It is most certainly not! Tissue densities, elasticities, bulk moduli, and so forth are highly inhomogeneous across the many varieties of tissue. And axons render the whole thing *anisotropic*. (That simply means *direction matters* [126].) It turns out that strains running *along* the axons may have completely different effects on our brains than strains running *perpendicular* to the axons. This is strikingly important, since *stretching of axons may be the most important single mechanical predictor of behavioral outcome.* Can a computer model that ignores axon stretch truly predict the impact of a CBI on a patient's life, health, and happiness? Not likely. We need a better model.

And we have it.

Giordano and Kleiven [127, 128] cleverly devised a somewhat more naturalistic brain injury model that accounts for both inhomogeneity and anisotropy: they began with old National Football League data. Fifty-eight accidents were videotaped. Twenty-five of these involved concussions. Viewers did their best to estimate the velocity and direction of impact when the players were struck. Those data were used to reconstruct the sporting accident using a Hybrid III crash test dummy head. Data collected from the dummy's accelerometers were applied to a model brain. Figure 7.12 illustrates the distribution of principal strain in one case. The real muscularity of this report

is its bold effort to estimate the strain on the axons – that is, taking into account axon directionality in the brain. Indeed, the authors compared the predictive power of maximum axonal strain (MAS) with five other strain measures: maximum principal strain, anisotropic equivalent strain, cumulative strain damage, brain injury criteria, and head injury criterion. Just as they had suspected, "On average, MAS has the highest predictive power" ([128], p. 50).

Figure 7.13 summarizes the comparison between MAS experienced among football players who were concussed versus those who were not. The error bars between concussion and non-concussion overlap for every region, more evidence that force does not predict individual outcome.

In addition, the strains apparently required to induce clinical concussion are *different in each part of the brain*. This confirms the commonsense predictions that axonal strain predicts outcome and that more force is more likely than less force to produce concussion. But it hardly lends credence to the notion of a specific human "concussion threshold." The tiniest change in the angle of attack or the careening of intracranial strains subverts the engineer's most rigorous math.

FEM is introduced not with the expectation that it will ever predict clinical outcome with accuracy, but merely to acquaint the reader with state-of-the-art efforts to estimate what happens in rattled brains. With these experiments in mind, one reason that outcomes vary is immediately apparent. Even if all else were equal in two CBIs that involved absolutely identical forces arriving from the same direction at the same location on human head hair, hair-measured force is only an extremely rough predictor of outcome. On the other hand, as soon as we can monitor force as the ultrastructural level – for example, in microtubules of hippocampal Schaeffer collaterals – force might become a useful predictor.

On Time

The second reliable predictor of difference in outcome is simply when outcome is measured – the time gap after impact. Earlier in the essay we demonstrated that a substantial proportion of concussed people will exhibit persistent symptoms for months or years after their injuries. Indeed, Figure 7.2 implies that there is an infinite variation in post-concussive clinical

Maximal axonal strain by tissue type

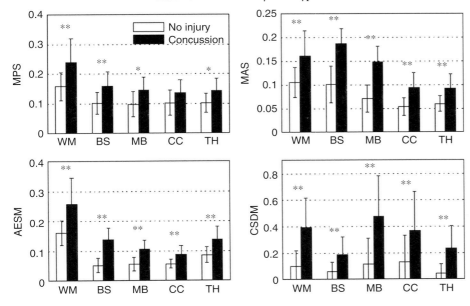

Fig. 7.13 A summary of the mean values and standard deviations observed in the simulations for strain-based predictors. The values are shown in black for concussed ($n = 25$) and white for non-injured ($n = 33$) National Football League players for various anatomical regions of the brain model. Top left: maximum principal Green–Lagrange strain. MPS: maximum principal strain. Top right: maximum axonal strain (MAS), Bottom left: maximum anisotropic equivalent strain measure (AESM). Bottom right: maximum values of the cumulative strain damage measure (CSDM) for a principal strain of 0.1. Statistical differences in t-tests are reported ($*p < 0.01$; $**p < 0.001$). Maximal axonal strain appears in the white matter (WM), brainstem (BS), midbrain (MB), corpus callosum (CC), and thalamus (TH).

Source: Giordano and Kleiven, 2014 [128] by permission from The Stapp Association

courses. But it is nonetheless true, and good for patients and doctors to know, that things tend to improve, especially over the first 6–18 months. Hence – in answer to the question "why do outcomes vary? – *time* after CBI accounts for a substantial amount of that variance.

We know even more. Different symptoms are common at different time points after CBI.

It is immediately apparent on reviewing the universe of available research that some symptoms are especially common after CBI. However, as multiple scholars have observed [129–132], it is equally apparent to clinicians that the symptoms that are common at one point after CBI – for instance, the first hour – are not necessarily those that are common at another time point – say the five-year follow-up visit. This, by the way, is one of many empirical observations undermining popular claims of a unitary, diagnosable post-concussion syndrome. (The syndrome notion will be debunked later in this chapter.) It would be very helpful to summarize which symptoms are common when. The author would very much like to provide readers with that intriguing and clinically valuable information. But that's easier said than done.

One approach would be a rigorous quantitative analysis of the prevalence of symptoms in published reports. Unfortunately, just as we showed (Chapter 5) in the case of the proportion of survivors with persistent symptoms, the diversity of cohorts and methods in the literature regarding post-CBI symptoms renders meta-analysis infeasible. Another approach would be pedestrian and replicable: one might scrutinize the papers cited in Tables 5.4–5.6 in Chapter 5, and count the number of manuscripts that report a given symptom at a given time point. Unfortunately, that would also yield scientifically dubious conclusions, because: (1) almost all of the cited studies were hamstrung by the investigators'

narrow, pre-conceived notions of what symptoms deserved assessment; and (2) not one of those studies was based on comprehensive, open-ended clinical evaluations by an experienced neurobehaviorist.

The author, therefore, has applied a hybrid approach to deriving this data. With apologies for seeking to extract truth from inadequate data, Table 7.1 lists the most common symptoms in each post-CBI era, based on a systematic review of the literature as previously described, but adjusted by: (1) attention to scholars who attended to these issues [21, 129–138]; (2) experience; and, hopefully, (3) common sense.

Another observation pertains to the *number* of symptoms reported at different post-CBI eras. Overwhelming evidence supports the conclusion that, on average, the intensity of distress peaks early – probably in the first 500 msec to ten days. Equally strong evidence suggests that substantial improvement is both subjectively felt and objectively observed (on average across large unselected cohorts) during the first three months. However, some evidence exists [139] that CBI survivors exhibit an increase in the *number* of post-concussive symptoms between about two months and six months after injury, followed by a decrease between six months and one year. Why the roller-coaster? With respect to depression, the author speculates that evolving insight is a factor in the increase after several months, and natural resolution, adaptation, or (rarely) treatment in the decrease over a year. With respect to post-traumatic stress disorder (PTSD), the literature is less consistent. Reports exist of the emergence of PTSD as a continuation of a day-one acute stress reaction, or with onset delayed up to several years post accident. Note that this curve hardly corresponds with the typical trajectory of litigation [140]. Nor does this curve ever approach a baseline. As McMahon et al. observed:

Table 7.1 The most common post concussive brain injury symptoms at different follow-up times

Assessment era	Cognitive behavioral symptoms	Non-cognitive behavioral symptoms	Somatic symptoms and signs
First few hours or days	• Unconsciousness • Somnolence • Lethargy • Disorientation • Confusion • Retrograde amnesia • Anterograde amnesia • Confabulation	• Agitation • Subjective stress • Anxiety and fearfulness • Combativeness/non-directed	• Headache • Nausea/vomiting • Double or blurred vision • Abnormal extra-ocular movements • Subjective dizziness • Objective disequilibrium/imbalance • Dysosmia • Sensitivity to light and noise • Sleep disturbance
First few weeks	• ↓ Attention • ↓ Concentration • Distractibility • Slowed thinking • Some awareness of memory impairment	• Subjective stress • Anxiety and fearfulness • Irritability • Emotional dysregulation • Lability • Disinhibition	• Headache • Double or blurred vision • Subjective dizziness • ↑ Fatigue • Sleep disturbance • Slowed simple reflexes • Dysosmia
First few months	• ↓ Attention • ↓ Concentration • Distractibility • Slowed thinking • ↑ Explicit learning and memory problems (working, episodic, semantic) • Impaired multitasking/divided attention • Impaired cognition under stress • Slowed conditional reflexes	• Increasing insight • Anxiety and fearfulness • Increasing depression • Irritability or easily angered • Increasing aggression/directed • Emotional dysregulation • Lability • Frustration • Disinhibition • Social awkwardness and withdrawal	• ↓ Headache • ↓ Dizziness • ↓ Visual disturbance • ↓ Sensitivity to light and noise • Fatigue • Sleep disturbance • Dysosmia
Persistent or permanent	• Slowed thinking • Stable but impaired learning and memory • Impaired multitasking/divided attention • Impaired cognition under stress	• Increasing insight • Anxiety • Dysphoria or depression • Irritability, easily angered • ↓ Disinhibition • Frustration • Overt aggression • Emotional dysregulation • Social awkwardness and withdrawal	• ↓ Sleep disturbance • ↓ Dysosmia • Fatigue

The results of this study indicate that recovery from mTBI is a nonlinear process and the time course to full recovery for some may be protracted. This supports the possibility that, in a subpopulation of patients, full recovery may not ever be achieved.

([139], p. 32)

That prediction is supported not only by the large number of studies reporting no resolution at one year, but also by the neurophysiological and neuroimaging evidence. Just one example: Slobounov et al.'s [138] authentically prospective study – in which an at-risk population of 380 student athletes was tested before concussion. None of the 49 subsequently concussed youngsters had a single post-concussive complaint. Yet a single concussive blow led to significantly altered alpha suppression on electroencephalogram, and "MTBI [mild TBI] subjects, who experienced 20% and higher alpha suppression … (on day 7 post-MTBI) did not return to pre-injury status … during the year of observation" ([138], p. 5).

Much has been made of the fact that, in some surveys, survivors of "mild" brain injuries report a higher average number of complaints than do survivors of "severe" brain injuries. One interpretation has been (without putting too fine a point on the covert meaning of the published rhetoric): "You see, complaining concussion survivors are all either pre-morbidly psychiatrically impaired or malingering crooks." Long and Novack [141] questioned the integrity of this assault on the integrity of patients:

If premorbid psychiatric weaknesses are a causal factor in the development of postconcussion symptoms, the prevalence of such difficulties among mildly injured patients would suggest that this group is selectively predisposed. There is no evidence, however, to support the presumption that psychiatrically unstable individuals are more likely to have a mild, as opposed to severe, head injury.

([141], p. 729)

This comment facilitates transition to the next section of the chapter: a discussion of the factors other than force and time that explain variation in outcomes after CBI.

On Genes

Alfred Russell Wallace [142] reviews an 1869 book by Sir Charles Lyell, using that as a springboard to comment on Mr. Darwin's 1859 opus: a thirty-second reflection:

> Mr. Darwin's theory is based on a very few groups of observed facts, and on one demonstrable principle. The first group of facts is the *variability* of all organisms descended from the same parents; a variability not confined to external form or colour, but extending to every part of the structure, and even to constitutional and mental characteristics. Every one knows from his own experience that *no two individuals of a family, whether human or animal, are absolutely alike* [emphasis added].
>
> ([142], p. 382)

> the moral and higher intellectual nature of man is as unique a phenomenon as was conscious life on its first appearance in the world, and the one is almost as *difficult to conceive as originating by any law of evolution as the other.* We may even go further, and maintain that *there are certain purely physical characteristics of the human race which are not explicable on the theory of variation and survival of the fittest.* The brain, the organs of speech, the hand, and the external form of man, offer some special difficulties in this respect [emphasis added].
>
> ([142], p. 391)

Mr. Wallace was completely right about individuality. *No two individuals are alike in body or mind.* Wallace was completely wrong when he declared that the human brain could never be explained by natural selection. In his 1869 book report regarding Sir Charles Lyell's 1869 book *On Geological Climates and the Origin of Species*, Wallace's religion obliged him to "find the true reconciliation of Science with Theology." His solution was to state that every living thing on earth and sea evolved except us. That opinion is perhaps the only excuse one might use for denying the fact that the outcomes of concussion depend on genetic variation. The author of the present essay mentions this history for a reason: there still exist writers who claim that the major reason that some people complain of memory problems or depression three years after a concussion is imagination (hysteria) or immorality (malingering). It is entirely reasonable to posit that those factors sometimes play a role. It is not reasonable to emphasize those factors, having failed to first examine the influence of natural variation. As early as it is in our progress toward understanding the molecular biology of CBI, it is not premature to summarize the very strong evidence that virtually every aspect of outcome from concussion varies depending on the survivor's genome.

By a strict count of peer-reviewed TBI publications over the last 40 years (judged subjectively by this author and impossible to verify) the central issue of genetics has not received the attention it deserves. That seems to be less a matter of an oversight than of a late-maturing technology. Breathtaking advances in computational biology and massively parallel processing have rapidly replaced Sanger sequencing with whole-genome shotgun pairwise end sequencing, and then with ultra-high-throughput next-generation sequencing. Let us skip over the algorithms. The message is merely that neurogeneticists long ago recognized the likelihood that variation in concussion outcome was probably due to genetic variation, but the tools for proving that hypothesis are new to market.

Transcriptomics

Over more than a decade, multiple laboratories have reported changes in expression of hundreds of genes shortly after TBI [143–154]. Even "mild" TBI provokes almost immediate up- or down-regulation of up to 999 genes [144–146, 153–155]. It seems reasonable to infer that the response to head injury evolved, that the genes involved and the cell's transcriptome response to injury was subject to selection, and that variations in the genes and their response are relevant to variations in the efficacy of that response – hence, likely to influence outcome.

Abundant evidence has also been generated demonstrating that genetic variation indeed influences outcome after TBI. Excellent reviews are available discussing the influence of genetic variation on outcome [156–162]. One conceptual model for this remarkable set of nearly simultaneous changes in transcription was advanced by Di Pietro et al. [145]. "In this study, we investigated the hypothesis that mild traumatic brain injury (mTBI) triggers a controlled gene program as an adaptive response finalized to neuroprotection, similar to that found in hibernators and in ischemic preconditioning" (p. 185). Setting aside the intriguing hibernation hypothesis, this concept is consistent with the present essay's encouragement that post-traumatic brain change is better understood not as a cascade of damaging events but as an evolved, adaptive *competition* between injurious and defensive factors (the latter hopefully dominating) selected over hundreds of millions of years to optimize outcome and perhaps, with luck, prevent lasting harm.

The goal of concussion transcriptomics and finding gene variants associated with better outcome is to help CBI survivors. Insights from this work might slightly widen the crack in the door to finding effective therapies by implicating approachable targets for medical mitigation [163, 164]. Approachability, of course, is a relative thing. Knowing that nerve growth factor (NGF) is neuroprotective, one way to rescue a traumatized brain is to engraft cells capable of expressing NGF [165, 166]. That may not be practical in the primary care clinic. Similarly, knowing that expression of calpains is important in the competition between oxidative stressors and defenses and influential in TBI outcome, Yamada et al. [167] showed that altering calpain 1 expression (in this case, by devising calpain 1 null mice) led to significant protection from traumatic neural degeneration and apoptosis. In a similar experiment Kabadi et al. [168] showed that Cyclin D1–null mice exhibited much less post-traumatic inflammation and neurodegeneration. Although these experiments have been educational, such genetic intervention techniques do not lend themselves to direct clinical application.

A more accessible approach: by 2005 evidence had been published that progesterone alters post-traumatic expression of apoptotic genes [169]. In 2011, Anderson et al. [170] reported that low-dose progesterone changes expression of 551 genes involved in apoptosis and inflammation. The net effect seems to be beneficial. Replication might inspire an effective medicinal treatment for concussion. As interventions to modulate gene expression improve, the long list of genes that undergo traumatic expression changes will be winnowed and some transcription is likely to be amenable to clinical optimization without germ line management.

Another practical application: just as an environmental factor (abrupt external force) can threaten the brain and provoke massive changes in gene expression, so can other environmental factors alter post-traumatic gene expression in ways that enhance neuroprotection and recovery: Shin et al. [171], for instance, reported that environmental enrichment (analogous to rehabilitation) mitigates the expression of dozens of genes in the substantia nigra and ventral tegmental area, leading to better outcome. This finding would appear to have therapeutic implications, if only we can translate mouse to human "environmental enrichment" (shared cages? corporate gyms?).

Consistent with the now-familiar observations of research in neurobehavioral genetics, one does not expect any single genetic variant such as an SNP or one variable number tandem repeat (VNTR) to account for much of the variance in clinical outcome. (As discussed below, the striking exception is the gene for apolipoprotein E.) Instead, it appears that a great many genes acting in a large number of pathways produce differences on the order of 1–3% in any measurable phenotype. Moreover, four complications restrain the hope of telling a simple story about gene variation and concussion variation:

1. epistasis (gene–gene interaction)
2. gene–environment (GxE) interaction
3. epigenetics
4. three-dimensional spatial patterns of gene expression.

Regarding Gene–Gene Interactions

As a general rule in neurobehavioral genetics, the effect of SNPs and VNTRs identified in early studies as risk factors influencing clinical outcome will increasing be shown to be either mediated or moderated by other genes. For example, p11 (S100A10) gene variation by itself is associated with proneness to depression [172–174]. BNDF gene variation also impacts proneness to depression [175]. New evidence suggests that the effect of variation in the BDNF gene on affective disorder depends on variation in the p11 gene [176, 177]. Hitting upon such discoveries was initially a matter of serendipity or brute force, exhaustive trial and error. More recently laboratories employ data mining and machine learning facilitated by increasing sophisticated software packages [178, 179]. The point is merely that papers announcing the influence of a single allele on outcome after a blow to the head may soon be considered naive.

Regarding Gene–Environment Interaction

To understand how genetic variation helps explain variation in concussion outcome, one must also consider the gene–environment interactions – including those predating the injury that molded the victim's predispositions and vulnerabilities, and those after the injury. For instance, evidence exists that a genetic variant one might fully expect to reduce the impact of concussion may or may not do so depending on prior life events: the G-allele of a common variant (rs53576) in the oxytocin receptor gene (OXTR) has been associated with a more adaptive response to stress [180]. One might therefore expect carriers to be more resilient in the face of concussion. Paradoxically however, maltreated children carrying this polymorphism show the opposite behavioral effects; they are apparently *more* vulnerable to stress and depression [181, 182]. Dannlowski et al. [113] recently reported that the effect of early maltreatment on a child's brain anatomy is also moderated by variation in this SNP. People with the G-allele and histories of childhood adversity have altered limbic structure and function. One suspects that this kind of structural-plus-functional limbic disadvantage would be especially problematic for people exposed to concussion, since the affected phenotypes belong to neuroanatomical and behavioral domains often implicated in persistent post-CBI dysfunction. But nobody knows. And a strong caution is in order: recent critical reviews expose the fact that the *candidate gene approach* (testing correlations between a behavior and a gene that, nominated by informed guesswork, seems likely to be related) and *gene–environment studies* both have rotten records of replicability [183–187]. The principle is unassailable – that gene variants and *gene–environment* interactions influence clinical outcomes. The conclusions are not ready to take to the bank.

Nonetheless, the trajectory of discovery is clear. Given such data at the cutting edge of neurobehavioral science, one looks back on the 20th-century comments that firmly reject an organic basis and instead blame CBI survivors with prolonged symptoms for their "psychological" weakness, and shudders. As the author began, so he will maintain: genes make some brains more fragile. Bad parenting damages brains. Stress damages brains. It may even so happen that a physical blow damages parts of the brain, that the stress reaction to that trauma further damages the brain, that that additional physical damage exacerbates stress … and so forth in a *reciprocating trauma* of mind and brain (see the conclusion of this chapter). Simply put, all differences in concussion outcome are due to biological variation that is innate, biological variation that is acquired, or the interaction between these factors.

Regarding Epigenetics

Beware! The ghost of Lamarck seeks revenge! Contrary to Mr. Darwin's opus (and replacing the present author's first 50 years of education), inheritance of acquired characteristics is now proved, a veritable Phoenix from the ashes of premature scholarly closure. Since histone proteins envelope strands of DNA, they can modify gene expression, and since they are vulnerable to the impact of environment, it is possible to acquire heritable change in the expression of nuclear DNA. As a result, neuropsychiatry is evolving (acquiring?) a new perspective on mental disorders. In particular, stress vulnerability, affective regulation, mood disorders, and response to treatment appear to be associated with epigenetic change [188–192]. That discovery is probably relevant, to some unknown extent, to the project of determining innate differences that explain variation in outcome after concussion. That is, the heritable factors that influence whether a CBI survivor feels well after six months or poorly after six years are probably not confined to genes but may also be explained by epigenes. While this has no immediate practical application, it is conceivable that public health policy will eventually take into account the effects of given stressors on population-wide vulnerability to lasting impairment after commonplace head impact.[10]

Regarding Three-Dimensional Patterns of Gene Expression

There have been many reports of associations between gene variants and concussion outcome. They sometimes mention that a particular gene is active in a particular brain locale – such as dopamine (DA) receptor gene expression in the basal ganglia – but they rarely include molecular-resolution photographs of brain-wide expression of that gene. In the same way, many reports on post-traumatic transcriptomics provide schematic maps intended to help visualize the functional relationships among clusters of genes expressed after concussion. They do not, however, provide real-time videos of gene expression occurring across the brain. This is common in neurobehavioral studies: the artificial separation of investigations between what Benson [193] called soups versus wires – studies of neurochemistry versus studies of anatomical and network structure. The problem with this dichotomy: brain measures of gene expression may have little biological meaning without knowing exactly which cells where are rich or poor in those agents; and detailed anatomical tractography may contribute little unless one knows that the tracts are biochemically/electrophysiologically active.

For instance, when one discusses the discovery that "The X allele of the gene for protein A is associated with delayed recovery after concussion," one is discussing a functionally significant biological difference between two individuals. The unfortunate patient who carries the X allele is predicted to suffer from memory problems longer than the patient who does not carry that allele. Yet such reports isolate the chemical assay from the wires – the places in the brain and connections between them where the changes occur. As a result, a gross chemical assay fails to illuminate what is really happening: after a blow to the head, in certain specific brain sites connected in astonishingly complex three-dimensional patterns, the gene for protein A will be expressed. If it happens to be the X version of the A gene, and it happens to be expressed in particular places and times, there will be less successful competition between injurious and beneficial gene change. Those brain places (cells and networks) will not work as well. Memory may still be a problem after a year.

How might one visualize this crucial, much-neglected space- and time-dependent aspect of genetic individuality?

The author has occasionally tried to help medical students and residents imagine the molecular movie of a simple blow to the head. He confesses: it's a tough job. The ideas under consideration are not readily illustrated with a white-board cartoon. One needs a video of a transparent rattled brain showing the ebb and flow of gene transcription in three dimensions. Until videos are embedded in textbooks, and admitting the author's limited knowledge and capacity for communication, he will do his best to describe the action.

Recall our peripatetic pharmacists, Maxime and Guillaume, visiting the kangaroo-petting zoo in western New South Wales. Before their unfortunate accidents, each had an intact brain. Maxime, for example, had billions of neurons forming a three-dimensional network of networks. Gene expression was ongoing but different during every moment in each of his billions of neurons. In an effort to facilitate visualizing this dynamic brain state, Hawrylycz et al. [194] combined histological analysis with microarray profiling of 911 neuroanatomical regions. Figure 7.14 is an explanatory figure from that study. This montage is bursting with information, but presented here only for its heuristic value: in the ghostly image at lower right, one readily sees that different cortical regions display different transcriptomes. As the authors explained, "Transcriptional regulation varies enormously by anatomical location."

To make this concept concrete, consider two brain loci – let's say Maxime's motor cortex versus his striatum. His motor cortex transcriptome will be enriched in the neurofilament proteins needed for long-range projection neurons, such as NEFL and NEFM. In contrast, his ventral tegmental area transcriptome will be enriched in the tyrosine hydroxylase needed for DA metabolism. Thus, as advertised, enormous variation by location. Figure 7.14, of course, is an oversimplification. Rather than a few hundred loci in a few hundred neurons, try to imagine an anatomically accurate, slow-motion, color-coded video depicting all the transcription events in every neuron in the brain. When one considers that: (1) hundreds of genes will be transcribed simultaneously in each of those billions of neurons; and (2) the amount and time course of that transcriptional activity spread over three dimensions will be different in every cell, it becomes hard to doodle the picture for medical students.

Now consider what is the same and what is different about gene expression in two different people. Hawrylycz et al. [194] discovered that "different regions and their constituent cell types displaying robust molecular signatures that are highly conserved between individuals" (p. 1). In other words, an image of gene expression across Guillaume's brain will also exhibit variation by location, but his variations will be comparable to those of his friend. The genes he expresses in his motor cortex and his ventral tegmental area will be similar to genes being expressed in those places in Maxime. That, however, oversimplifies human

---

10 The following speculation is offered as a conceptual example, not a prediction of medical fact: let us assume that common behavioral/environment-linked problems such as obesity, metabolic syndrome, or excessive weight gain during pregnancy will be found to influence the expression of inflammatory genes, and that these are among the hundreds of genes that respond to brain injury. Due to epigenetic transmission, hypothetically at least, one might witness more resilience and improved concussion outcomes in children by improving their parents' diets.

The geography of the transcriptome: regional gene expression in three dimensions

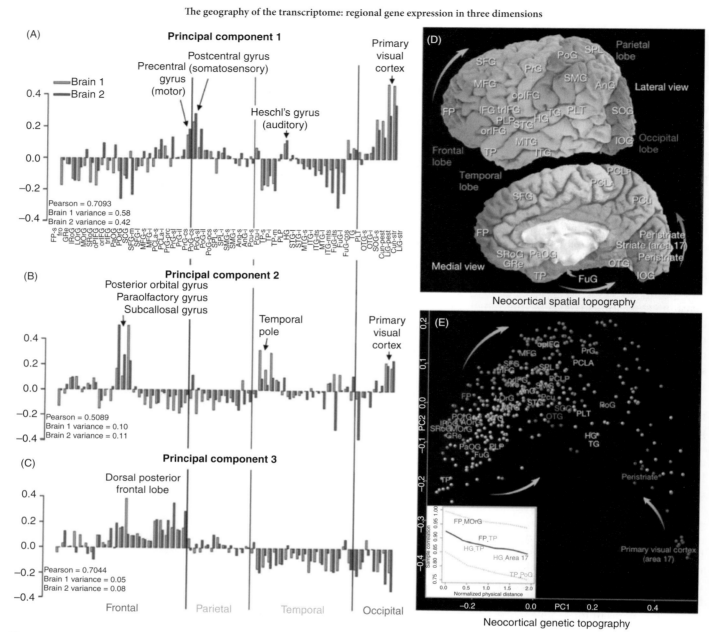

Fig. 7.14 The neocortical transcriptome reflects primary sensorimotor specialization and *in vivo* spatial topography. (a–c) First three neocortical principal components, plotted across 57 cortical divisions ordered roughly from rostral to caudal (frontal to occipital pole), are highly reproducible between brains. PC1 (Pearson r = 0.71) is selective for primary sensory and motor areas (a). PC2 (Pearson r = 0.51) is differential for specific subdivisions of the frontal, temporal, and occipital poles (b), whereas PC3 (Pearson r = 0.70) is selective for the caudal portion of the frontal lobe (c). (d, e) Relationship between the (x, y, z) location of sampled cortical gyri and their transcriptional similarities. Native brain 1 magnetic resonance imaging is shown in (d) with major gyri labeled. (e) Multidimensional scaling (MDS) applied to the same cortical samples, where distance between points reflects similarity in gene expression profiles. Median samples for major gyri are labeled. Samples cluster by lobe, and both lobe positions and gyral positions generally mirror the native spatial topography, emphasized by arrows in (d) and (e). Inset panel in (e) plots the relationship (mean ± 1 sd) between three-dimensional (3D) MDS-based similarity and 3D *in vivo* sample distance, demonstrating correlations that are stronger between proximal samples and multi-dimensional scaling applied to cortical samples, where distance between points reflects similarity in gene expression profiles. Median samples for major gyri are labeled. Samples cluster by lobe, and both lobe positions and gyral positions generally mirror the native spatial topography, emphasized by arrows in d and e. Inset panel in e plots the relationship (mean ± 1 sd) between 3D MDS-based similarity and 3D in vivo sample distance, demonstrating correlations that are stronger between proximal samples and decrease with distance. Selected gyral pairs are labeled. [A black and white version of this figure will appear in some formats. For the color version, please refer to the plate section.]

Source: Hawrylycz et al., 2012 [194]. Reprinted by permission from Macmillan

individuality. In an impressive feat, the authors also compared two brains. Figure 7.15 helps to visualize the differences in three-dimensional transcriptomes between two individuals.

Again, the details of this illustration are fascinating (and worth the interested reader's attention) but the figure is offered merely to assist in illustrating three simple ideas:

Structural variation in gene expression, comparing two human brains

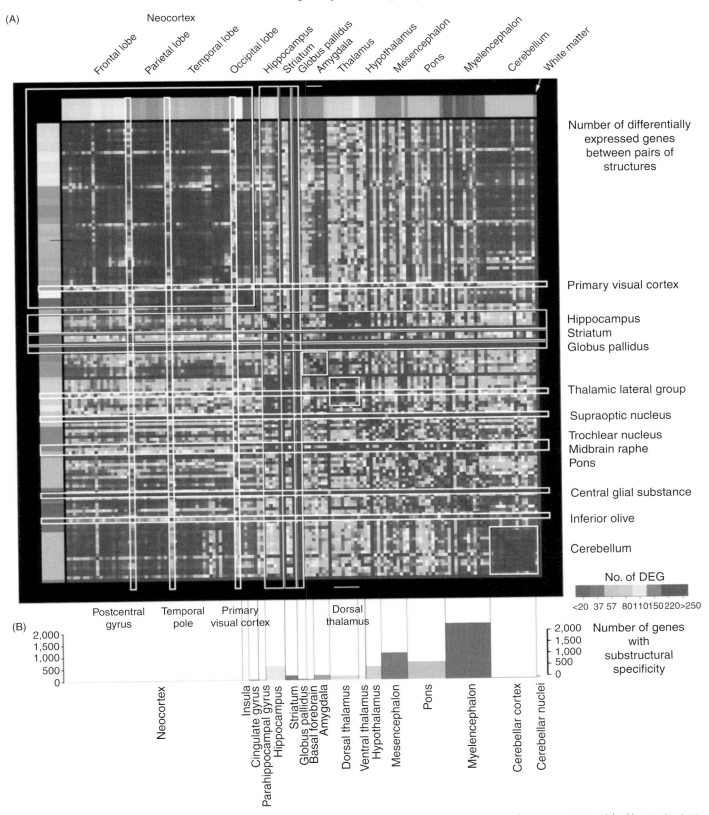

Fig. 7.15 (a) Matrix of differential expression between 146 regions in both brains. Each point represents the number of common genes enriched in one structure over another in both brains (Benjamini–Hochberg-corrected *p* < 0.01, log2(fold change) > 1.5). DEG: differentially expressed genes. Several major regions exhibit relatively low internal variation (blue), including the neocortex, cerebellum, dorsal thalamus, and amygdala. Subcortical regions show highly complex differential patterns between specific nuclei. (b) Frequency of marker genes with selective expression in specific subdivisions of major brain regions (greater than twofold enrichment in a particular subdivision compared to the remaining subdivisions). [A black and white version of this figure will appear in some formats. For the color version, please refer to the plate section.]

Source: Hawrylycz et al., 2012 [194]. Reprinted by permission from Macmillan

1. Within a single brain: transcriptomes vary enormously from one place to the next.
2. Across two brains: transcriptomes are similar in homologous areas.
3. However, vast and complex differences, numbering almost beyond comprehension, characterize the difference between one person's four-dimensional transcriptome and another's.

Therefore, despite considerable overlap, the maps of healthy day-to-day gene expression from Maxime and Guillaume will display an almost incomprehensibly gigantic number of differences.

Now recall Chapter 2's omniscient athletic trainer – the remarkable sideliner who monitors every athlete's brain changes in real time. Imagine he or she happened to be scanning tourists at the kangaroo-petting zoo. Maxime and Guillaume, jovial and sanguine, stride purposefully across the dust to confront the biggest marsupial. The monitor is pointed at Maxime. Although the device can show everything from mitochondrial electron transport to arteriolar vasospasm, it is tuned to show only gene expression in three dimensions. When Maxime is punched in the head, what would the read-out on the concussion-monitoring screen look like? The picture would be dizzyingly complex because, as explained in Chapter 3, *a typical concussion seems to provoke up- or down-regulation of about 999 genes.*

A Pause to Smell the Roses

The foregoing is a lot to absorb. A simple summary may be handy. For millions of years, keen-eyed hominids have surely observed that two different great apes who suffer similar blows to the head sometimes experience quite different symptoms and longer or shorter periods of distress. We all want to understand why. *Force* and *time* since the injury are two good explanations. *Heritable difference* is a third good explanation.

In the 21st century, the phrase "heritable differences" has become rich to overflowing with new and fascinating connotations. The author is about to offer a table listing gene variants that plausibly, and only to a small extent, explain differences in the outcome after concussion. Yet he wants to communicate both the infancy of the effort and the remarkable, dazzling integrated inner workings of the gene/epigene/environment watch, which neuroscience inspects in ever more amazing detail, only to confirm how far we are from understanding.

The problem, in a nutshell, is that we are not *Pisum sativum* – Mendel's peas. The classical laws of inheritance that underlie genetics were relatively accessible to Friar Mendel because several readily visible pea traits are largely controlled by single genes. Human behavior, in contrast, seems to be influenced to a very small degree by a very large number of genes. The typical effects found to date are on the order of 1–3%. Can one effectively study the genetics of a 1.5% difference in post-concussive irritability? Our enthusiasm must be tempered by this challenge.

Several approaches to finding behavior-modifying genes have dominated the literature for decades. One is the *candidate gene* approach. A common example: knowing that serotonin is involved in emotional regulation, it makes sense to test whether variations in genes affecting serotonin metabolism or transmission correlate with variations in mood. Another approach is the *gene × environment* approach. This type of research acknowledges that a gene by itself may have unpredictable effects; the *interaction* between a susceptibility gene and an environmental trigger may better explain a behavioral trait. Much of the data in the forthcoming table derives from one or another of these two research strategies. Warning: please do not expect to read in next week's *Green* journal: "CBI survivors with allele *X* are likely to suffer memory loss and anxiety for twice as long as those with allele *Y*." Any such report would merely be a thread on a loom – and a fragile one at that. The tapestry of the genetic explanation for the difference in concussion outcome includes interweavings of gene–gene, gene–environment, epigenetic, and intracerebral architectural variation. And the threads in Table 7.2 cannot be altogether trusted because – as has recently become glaringly apparent to our widespread chagrin – *few candidate gene and gene–environment studies in behavioral genetics are replicated.* It is, at best, a first step.

Table 7.2 is one more result of a systematic search. The *left-hand column* lists phenotypes, meaning either biological or behavioral differences that are probably relevant to inter-individual differences in concussion outcome. The *right-hand column* lists genes with variants reported to influence concussion outcome. For example, it seems plausible that a person who is more vulnerable to depression might suffer more or longer after a blow to the head. And, as it happens, a variation in a gene associated with vulnerability to depression (*FAAH*) is reportedly also associated with worse mTBI outcome [195]. Along the same lines, inflammation seems to play a very important role in concussion outcome. Two gene variations pertinent to the brain's inflammatory response (APOE and Visfatin) have been reported to influence concussion outcome [196–199]. Note, however: inflammation per se is probably not deleterious. Evidence is mounting that there are productive, tissue-rescuing inflammatory responses and counterproductive tissue-damaging inflammatory responses [200]. Hence, as one visualizes the competition between degenerative and regenerative forces immediately after an abrupt force affects the head, it would be simplistic to characterize this as pro- vs. anti-inflammatory battle. Instead the competition is between inflammatory/immunomodulatory factors with net beneficial versus net harmful effects (reserving the suspicion that brain response to CBI may involve short-term benefits and long-term side-effects).

Table 7.2 is not intended as a reference or final answer. Even if the reader has memorized the first six chapters of this little essay, please resist the urge to memorize Table 7.2. It is merely today's state of the art; one absolutely expects the list to change; as research advances, many of the listed associations may fail replication and many new associations will be added. All of the effort to compile Table 7.2 was really to make a simple but vital point: genes that vary between individual people have already been reported to influence more than a dozen aspects of concussion outcome. This list, however, is far from settled. It has

Table 7.2 Some genes with variants that appear to influence outcome after traumatic brain injury (TBI)

Phenotype	Genes or loci
Vulnerability to depression	• FAAH [195]
Proneness to exhibiting irritability or aggression	• MAO-A [201]
TBI outcome (e.g., Glasgow Outcome Score)	• APOE-ε4 [202–208] • APOE-ε4 [202–208] • APOE-G-219T [209, 210] • Aromatase [211] • ABCB1 [212] • Gsta4 [213] • NGB [214] • TNFA [215]
Proneness to worse cognitive outcome after TBI	• ACE [216] • ANKK1 [217, 218] • APOE-ε4 [219–228] • BDNF [229, 230] • COMT [218, 231, 232] • DD2R [217, 218, 233] • KIBRA [234] • VMAT [218]
Female proneness to worse outcome	• APOE-ε4 [235]
Post-traumatic edema	• Aquaporin 4 [236] • ISG15 [237]
Proneness to metabolic stress	• APOE-ε4 [238] • PARP-1 [239]
Proneness to excitatory neurotoxicity	• APOE-ε4 [240]
Proneness to apoptosis	• p53 [241] • BCL2 [242–244] • PARP-1 [239]
Proneness to amyloid and/or tau deposition	• APOE-ε4 [245–247] • Neprilysin [248]
Proneness to "Alzheimer's disease"	• APOE-ε4 [249, 250]
Proneness to pituitary dysfunction	• APOE-ε4 [251]
Proneness to hippocampal injury	• APOE-ε4 [202, 252, 253]
Proneness to axonal injury	• APOE-ε4 [254]
Proneness to inflammation	• APOE-ε4 [196–198] • Visfatin [199]
Blood–brain barrier integrity	• ISG15 [237]
Proneness to vascular disorders or complications (e.g., hemorrhage)	• APOE-ε4 [161, 255–258] • NOS3 [259] • IL-1RN and IL-1B [260]
Proneness to lipid peroxidation	• Gsta4 [213]

ACE: angiotensin-converting enzyme; ANKK1: ankyrin repeat and kinase domain containing 1; APOE-ε4: the epsilon 4 polymorphic variant in the apolipoprotein E gene-coding region; APOE-G-219T: the G-219T polymorphic variant in the apolipoprotein E promoter region (of interest: some evidence also suggests that this polymorphism is associated with an increased risk of sports-related concussion [210, 261]; ABCB1: ATP-binding cassette B1; BCL2: (oncogene); BDNF: brain-derived neurotrophic factor; COMT: catechol-*O*-methyltransferase; DD2R: dopamine D2 receptor T allele; FAAH: fatty-acid amide hydrolase; Gsta4: glutathione-S-transferase alpha 4; IL-1RN and IL-1B: interleukins 1RN and 1B; ISG15: interferon-stimulated gene 15; KIBRA: kidney brain protein; MAO-A: monoamine oxidase-A; NGB: neuroglobin; NOS3: endothelial nitric oxide gene; p53: (tumor suppressor gene); PARP-1: poly(ADP-ribose) polymerase-1; TNFA: tumor necrosis factor-α; Visfatin: (aka pre-B-cell colony-enhancing factor); VMAT: vesicular monoamine transporter.

a manifest destiny. It will grow rapidly, and it will gain clinical meaning as laboratories transcend the conceptual bounds of candidate gene studies and probe gene/epigene/environment complexes.

Missing Links

The gene variants in Table 7.2 have already been linked to aspects of TBI. Yet many other promising variants have yet to be studied. Consider: depression, anxiety, intellect, and other behaviors often impacted by concussion have been studied for decades in populations *without* TBI; now it remains to be tested whether gene variants that influence these behaviors in *non-concussed* persons also help explain persistent problems after concussion.

In addition, the replication crisis in behavioral genetics has inspired new thinking about the best way to find genes that matter. Scholars have learned not to expect big effects from single-gene variants. Instead, we will have to do a job that might have driven Mendel to nervous fits: we must figure out the way that many different genes with tiny effects combine to moderate complex human behaviors. We no longer say, "She's nervous. Nervousness involves serotonin. Let's study serotonin genes" (the candidate gene approach). Instead, we bow to the human genome in humility, admitting that we need to interrogate the whole thing in our quest for genes relevant to clinical phenomena that almost certainly have multifactorial etiologies. Toward that end, genome-wide association studies (GWAS) are increasingly employed [262]. In GWAS, one abandons the presumption that we know which genes to study and we just ask the question, "What is the difference in genomes of people who do or do not have this trait?"

The bad news: what trait shall we study? What is our independent variable – the result caused by the genetic variant? The job is easier for scientists studying relatively homogeneous traits like yellow peas or major depression. The job is much tougher for scientists who want to discover why some people have long-term problems after concussion – because *long-term problems after concussion* is not one thing. One CBI survivor will suffer frequent headaches, irritability, and forgetfulness for a year and a half. Another will be fearful and mentally slow for a decade. A third will seem to recover but later become demented. What is our specific and measurable outcome? The best-funded lab on Earth with access to 10,000 CBI survivors cannot do a GWAS study unless they can identify a homogeneous trait. In addition, *long-term problems after concussion* are likely to be caused by multiple gene–environment interactions, in which an environmental force visiting a human head causes different problems in folks with different genomes. The bottom line and inescapable barrier to discovery: there is no post-concussion syndrome. Therefore, there is no post-concussion syndrome gene.

What then can we do? How might one figure out the role of genetic variation in concussion outcome? The answer may be to study intermediate variables – the missing biological links between the neurometabolic–vascular–inflammatory melee and prolonged symptoms. To clarify: a dozen troubled

CBI survivors will have a dozen different symptom profiles, but all of them might exhibit hippocampal atrophy, or excessive stress responsiveness, or abnormal microglial reactivity, or demyelination-related slowing of information processing. These are relatively homogeneous and potentially measurable traits. The author, not a geneticist and gladly deferring to those who know better, merely speculates that research may be more productive if GWAS search for correlations between gene variants and clearly identifiable neurobiological traits such as these. To narrow the search: genetic susceptibility has already been reported in regard to several brain problems that are directly relevant to concussion outcome. It would seem reasonable and feasible to test the hypothesis that one or more of these already-identified gene variants predicts who is most likely to suffer persistent post-concussive distress. Possible targets follow.

Brain Structure

For example, consider the first factor that explains differences in concussion outcome: *force*. FEM assumes that two human brains are structurally alike, though of course they are not [263].[11] Genetic variations are known to explain some of the variation in human brain structure. For example, variants in the genes for BDNF [112], the oxytocin receptor [113], the calcium voltage-gated channel subunit alpha1 C (CACNA1C) [114], and an unnamed linkage peak at 12q24 [115] have all been reported to explain variation in brain architecture. It does not seem a stretch to posit that genetic variation in brain structure is a factor influencing concussion outcome.

Emotion

Similarly, abundant research suggests that "psychosocial stress" is a risk factor for worse concussion outcome. But – contrary to the early-20th-century model – *psychosocial stress is not an environmental variable*. There is no fixed and measured amount of stress associated with lost dog, divorce, or war. Stress is a biological phenomenon dependent on the degree to which a given brain, with all its genetic, epigenetic, and developmental backgrounds, exhibits a baseline trait that might or might not be impacted by new life circumstances. Variation in vulnerability to stress under identical life circumstances (for instance, a concussion and emergency department visit and months of impaired cognition and worry) is associated with gene variation.

According to reports derived from studies using varying methods (therefore, plausible but imperfectly credible), stress vulnerability is linked to variation in the genes for: (1) the promoter of the serotonin transporter gene (5-HTTLPR) [264, 265]; (2) corticotropin-releasing hormone receptor 1 (CRHR1) [266–268]; (3) BDNF [269, 270]; (4) adenyate cyclase 7 (ADCY7) [271]; (5) FK506-binding protein 51 (FKBP51) [272]; (6) the phosphoribosyl transferase domain containing 1 gene (PRTFDC1) [273]; and (7) the neutral amino acid transporter,

SLC6A15 [274]. Proneness to depression is associated with variants in genes for: (1) 5-HTTLPR [275–277]; (2) neuropeptide Y [278]; and (3) ADCY7 [271]. However, some evidence suggests that a genetic association might be strongest with respect to narrow aspects of the depression phenotype. For instance, among depressed persons, links are reported between somatic anxiety and variation in the trytophan hydroxylase (TPH) gene [279], and between suicidality and variants of the TPH gene [280, 281] or the genes for MAPK1 and CREB1 [282]. The latter two gene variants conceivably warrant special attention in concussion, since they influence not only behavior but also inflammation and neuroplasticity.

Proneness to anxiety is associated with variation in 5-HTTLPR [283–287]. There is even evidence that 5-HTTLPR gene variants explain proneness to *neuroticism* [279, 288, 289] and proneness to *somatization* [276, 290].

Beyond these findings, many discovered via candidate gene research, GWAS have recently unearthed evidence of a host of variants impacting depression proneness, stress responsiveness, neuroticism, well-being, and academic achievement [291–297].

The author offers the very tentative suggestion that it may be worth determining whether survivors of concussion who carry these genetic variants are more prone to persistent problems. At the same time, he must confess uncertainty about the efficacy of this work. In the case of the link between APOE-ε4 alleles and TBI outcome, the effect size is concerning and it may be critical to modify clinical practice according to genome (see upcoming subsection). In the case of dozens or maybe hundreds of smaller genetic influences on outcome, it is not clear whether the benefits to patients will ever justify the outlay of effort.

In the light of these data and the great enterprise of modern neuroscience, calling psychological explanations for concussion outcome "non-organic" is exposed as anti-scientific. Human behavioral traits are profoundly products of the natural, material world. We may or may not ever paint the high-resolution molecular portrait of our patient's persistent post-concussive sadness. But empirical evidence tells us to expect it, and biological evidence tells us that DNA is involved. To attribute that sadness to a psychological construct like "expectation" or "conversion" is missing the point. Mentation and emotion, like vision and hearing, are abstract constructs we use to talk about how brains do their job of negotiating the slings and arrows of life in the interests of gene replication. Each three-pound lump of cells in the head does the best it can, its wings tangled in the kraal of its genes.

In brief summary: concussion science is late to the party. Twenty-first-century genetic observations, the baby steps toward so-called "precision medicine," have long since alerted doctors that when they see a clinical difference in health or well-being, it is simplistic to search for "psychological" explanations. Yes, abstract psychological constructs such as "depression" are useful for lay discussions. Yes, psychotherapeutic interventions

---

[11] Even identical twins have altogether different brain structures; side by side on the table, you would never guess [262].

blind to biology often have tremendous practical benefits. But the pathophysiological processes that explain persistent post-concussive problems only occur in brains.

Polymorphisms of the APOE Gene: Readers Are Urgently Recruited to Answer a Weighty Practical Question

Evidence has been available for more than 20 years that persons who carry either one or two APOE-ε4 alleles are likely to have worse outcome after a single or multiple concussions [202, 203, 205, 206, 208, 226, 298–302].[12] The impact of ε4 on outcome appears to have two effects: a near-term increase in post-traumatic symptoms and a long-term increase in the incidence of post-traumatic dementia [202, 224, 300, 303–307].[13] The empirical findings with regard to ε4 are not in perfect harmony [312]. Two meta-analyses and one systematic review somewhat clarify the issue. Based on 14 cohort studies, Zhou et al. [208] concluded that APOE-ε4 indeed predicts lower GOS scores six months after CBI. Based on 13 cohort studies, Zeng et al. [313] agreed that the APOE-ε4 carriers do worse after CBI. The 2015 review by Lawrence et al. [301] provides a slightly different perspective. The authors reviewed 65 studies. They divided the investigations into those claiming to address "mild" TBI versus those claiming to address other-than-mild TBI.[14] Among 24 studies of "mTBI," ε4 was associated with worse outcome in nine, no difference in 14, and a benefit in one. Among 33 studies of "severe" TBI, ε4 was associated with worse outcome in 21, no difference in nine, and a benefit in three. Four out of seven studies confirmed a link to dementia. Perhaps the ε4/concussion data can be summarized by acknowledging that inconsistency currently forestalls certainty, but that a great deal of evidence supports the conclusion that it is riskier to have a head injury (or many head injuries) with ε4 than without. That makes this APOE gene variant the most important genetic susceptibility finding known to concussion science, and perhaps to all of neuropsychiatry.

APOE genotype is also linked to vascular disease. Although the data are weaker than the dementia findings [314], multiple studies have found that ε4 carriers are more prone to elevated lipid levels, cardiovascular disease, vascular dementia, mixed Alzheimer's disease (AD)/vascular dementia, and the impact of vascular risk factor on cognitive loss [212, 315–320]. In fact, evidence has emerged that at least part of the mechanism by which ε4 raises the risk of post-concussive dementia is via the variant gene's effect on cerebrovascular integrity [301] (apparently not via increasing the risk of acute traumatic hemorrhage or later amyloid angiopathy) [255, 321]. APOE-ε4 occurs in 14% of Caucasians, 12% of Hispanics, 19% of Africans, and 0.09% of Asians [322]. Hundreds of millions of people are at risk. Should they know?

Who, if Anyone, Should be Tested?

There are three reasons to test a person's genotype. One: to assist in the diagnosis of a disorder. Two: to predict a person's future health. Three: to empower a person to delay his or her fate. The author has no quarrel with the argument that pre-emptive APOE testing does little to advance goals one and two. Goal three is an entirely different kettle of fish. Knowledge of APOE genotype is power. We must firmly reject the paternalistic policy of concealing crucial, even life-saving health information from patients and from the parents of at-risk children. If you know you have epilepsy, you might wisely hesitate to take up ocean swimming. If you know you have diabetes, you might hesitate to make fudge brownies your primary diet. If you know your cholesterol is 350 mg/dL, you may select the tuna sub instead of the liver-and-bacon special. If you know you are ε4-positive, you may think twice about a career in football or a hobby of mixed martial arts. If you know your teenaged daughter is ε4-positive, you might recommend almost any sport other than ice hockey. Yet, slavishly compliant with outdated reasoning, many TBI writers, even some neurologists, advise secrecy. Would you go to a doctor who refused to tell you your cholesterol?

In 1997, Jordan et al. published their seminal paper, "Apolipoprotein E epsilon 4 associated with chronic traumatic brain injury in boxing" [203]. Those authors may be forgiven for having thought that they had done something beneficial. As Jordan and Relkin put it in a letter [323]: "We hope that identification of APOE e4 as a genetic susceptibility factor for chronic traumatic brain injury will provide novel inroads for predicting, diagnosing, treating, and ultimately preventing the long-term neurologic sequelae of head trauma" (p. 2143). Absolutely nothing has come of this sentiment. No movement exits within U.S. neurology likely to overcome the dogged resistance of our conservative leadership, which persists in their refusal to promote genetic testing prior to participation in violent sports. Boxing commissions, football leagues, and high schools did not rush to test their athletes. Instead,

---

[12] Evidence also exists that carriers of the g-219t polymorphism in the promoter region of the APOE gene are more likely to experience worse outcome [208, 209].

[13] At the time of this writing, a new debate has roiled the neuroscientific community. The exceptional team of scholars at Boston University [307] strongly opine that concussions are associated with two entirely different and neatly distinguishable types of dementia: so-called "*Alzheimer's disease*" – which is itself an insupportable, unscientific abstract construct that (according to a rapidly diminishing cadre of older authorities) is allegedly distinguishable with a microscope from normal aging and from every other type of brain change [308], versus so-called "*chronic traumatic encephalopathy*" – a putative neurodegenerative "disease," its title borrowed without attribution from a 1934 paper by Parker [309], which (according to one panel of experts) is allegedly distinguishable from "Alzheimer's disease" (which does not exist) and from every other brain change [310]. Later chapters will help the reader test the logic of that proposed dichotomy.

[14] For reasons previously stated, perhaps to the point of perseveration, this is a scientifically indefensible distinction. Classification according to this false dichotomy may confound the conclusions reported in the Lawrence et al. review [300].

the association between APOE-ε4, head trauma, and "AD" provoked a flurry of breathless warnings best summarized as, "Pay no attention to that man behind the curtain." Sports authorities urged willful ignorance. Physicians and even researchers were forcefully dissuaded from testing their patients. In 1995 the American College of Medical Genetics/American Society of Human Genetics Working Group on ApoE and Alzheimer's Disease [324] published the following recommendation regarding genotyping: "at the present time it is not recommended for use in routine clinical diagnosis nor should it be used for predictive testing" (p. 1627). The American Academy of Neurology published a practice parameter [325]: "Routine use of APOE genotyping in patients with suspected AD is not recommended at this time."

Ethicists weighed in. Fleck [326], for example, asked this question about APOE testing: "Does it offer enough in the way of benefit or probability of benefit relative to cost that a just and caring society would be morally obligated to assure that all who had the relevant medical need would have access to this technology …?" (p. 128). He answered his own question: "We concluded that predictive APOE genotyping for AD cannot be defended as a health care need; and, therefore, no one has a just claim to social resources for securing access to that test." The preponderance of published recommendations during the intervening 20 years have perpetuated that view. Examples of the logic:

- "APOE status is a very poor predictor of AD risk and should not be used as a predictive test … There is no medical justification for such predictive testing. No grave threats could be averted by encouraging patients to receive that information" [327].
- "Some authorities in the field, including the influential Nuffield Council on Bioethics [328], have taken the stance that the decision to offer or to recommend genetic testing should turn on two factors: the availability of effective interventions for the tested disorder and the predictive accuracy of the test … This approach has led major professional organizations to take the position that apolipoprotein E gene (APOE) testing for susceptibility to late-onset Alzheimer's disease (AD) is not clinically indicated … of course, *prophylactic interventions are not available*" (emphasis added) ([329], p. 6).
- "testing is best deferred until adulthood unless preventive interventions exist" [329].

Adding insult to injury, the 2011 joint practice guidelines of the American College of Medical Genetics and the National Society of Genetic Counselors [330] state, "Patients should be informed that currently there are no proven pharmacologic or lifestyle choices that reduce the risk of developing AD or stop its progression" (p. 7).

Oh? To adopt the language of the U.S. Supreme Court: the author respectfully dissents. As the reader surely noticed, all of these recommendations are rooted in a completely false premise. The committees that birthed and published them sincerely thought "no lifestyle choices reduce the risk." That is not true. To be charitable, that was the state of the art of knowledge back in the 20th century. Three discoveries have made the do-not-test recommendation obsolete.

1. *TBI* is the most robustly researched and confirmed modifiable environmental risk factor for AD [331–334].
2. *Vascular disease* (including cardiovascular disease, cerebrovascular disease, and other threats to vascular health such as diabetes, obesity, and inactivity) is the second most robustly researched and confirmed modifiable risk factor for AD [335–339].
3. *Exercise* is the most robustly researched and confirmed activity that, if adopted, will significantly reduce the risk of so-called AD [340–343].

The fact that exercise helps prevent AD is the most recent and (in the author's opinion) the most exciting of the three discoveries. It offers a practical path to prevention and it clearly interdigitates with the relatively recent acknowledgment that so-called "AD" is largely due to vascular changes, and that lifestyle modification to reduce vascular risk (such as exercise) also reduces the risk of AD.

The earliest study contributing to this conclusion began in 1939 [344]. A cohort of Harvard undergraduate men agreed to have their health monitored indefinitely. At age 90, 40 survivors were cognitively intact and 44 had dementia. If the man had a warm childhood relationship with his mother or exercised at age 60, or both, he was significantly more likely to be cognitively intact. For those of us in middle age, it is perhaps a little late to modify our childhood relationships with our mothers. But we can exercise. The efficacy of exercise to prevent AD and other dementias has been demonstrated by multiple cross-sectional cohort/population-based studies [345–347] and by multiple prospective longitudinal studies [344, 348–351].

Even rodents benefit [352] – and that benefit is not only because exercise mitigates vascular risk factors that underlie neurodegeneration. Animal research shows that exercise promotes adult hippocampal neurogenesis [353, 354]. This finding possibly explains the observation that people who exercise have larger hippocampal gray-matter volumes [355]. In effect, it appears that exercise not only slows degeneration but also enhances neuronal reserve.

To summarize the new knowledge in our toolbox:

1. Concussion increases the risk of AD.
2. That risk is much higher among persons who are ε4+.
3. Avoiding concussion helps prevent AD.
4. That is especially true among persons who are e4+.
5. Vascular risk factors increase the risk of AD.
6. The risk of vascular disease is higher among persons who are ε4+.
7. Exercise reduces the risk of both AD and of vascular disease.

In the revelatory light of this suite of 21st-century discoveries, *why not warn people who are ε4+?* Contrary to the assumptions of the 20th century, people who carry ε4 are neither doomed nor helpless. Again, we read antique bluster published as recently as 2012 ("of course, prophylactic interventions are not available") [329] and try to remain calm. It is safe to consign such reasoning to the ashcan of history. But … is it safe to test?

Is There Any Harm in Disclosing APOE Genotype?

As noted above, in the heady days when APOE genotype testing first became available, many writers and organizations discouraged testing, warning that disclosure to asymptomatic patients would cause serious harm such as depressive reactions, anxiety, social stigmatization, job loss, insurance denial, and even suicide. The "keep it secret" cabal was extrapolating from the research on disclosing risk of Huntington's disease. First, no lifestyle choices can reduce the risk of Huntington's; lifestyle choices clearly reduce the risk of AD. Second, the original grim forecasts have been proven inaccurate.

For instance, in the REVEAL study [356] 162 adult children of AD patients were tested and then randomized to receive or not receive their genotypes. Learning that one was ε4+ produced no more anxiety than non-disclosure, either immediately or at one year. As Arribas-Ayllon [357] interpreted these results: "The new evidence … on the effects of … APOE testing of AD suggests that professionals' ethical concerns about presumed psychosocial harms are not entirely justified" (p. 17). Still, the design of the REVEAL study has been criticized. One problem is that the control group was tested but not informed. Gordon and Landa [358] argued: "From a policy perspective, one would wish to compare persons who were tested and provided results with those who were not tested at all; no one advocates testing and withholding results" (p. 181). Another problem with the REVEAL study: the intervention was not just disclosure but also *counseling*. This may have confounded the experiment – although it seems to have inadvertently revealed that counseling mitigates the stress of testing [357]. In a more recent trial [359], disclosure by genetic counselors was compared with disclosure by physicians. Neither approach generated a problematic emotional reaction, suggesting both the relative benignity of testing and the acceptability of disclosure by one's personal physician.

In a more sophisticated study [360], subjects who received APOE disclosure were counseled regarding 12 potential advantages or "pros" of obtaining this genetic information and 11 potential disadvantages or "cons." At 12 months, subjects judged that the pros strongly outweighed the cons – more evidence that the early predictions of harm from disclosure were inflated and misleading.

Given the superfluity of evidence that exercise helps prevent AD, one might surmise that learning one is ε4+ would be a motivator. Data support that prediction. Chao et al. [361] conducted an extension of the REVEAL study. Subjects were randomized to received their genotype or not. Although they were "informed that no proven preventive measures for AD existed," they were given a sheet with information about promising preventive therapies. The results: subjects who learned they were ε4+ were 2.73 times more likely than ε4– subjects to adopt health-promoting behaviors in the following year.[15]

The author understands the conditional recommendation laid out by many ethicists 20 years ago: if prevention of a genetically influenced disease is impossible, disclosure may be pointless. But if prevention is possible, disclosure is desirable. *At the time of this writing (2016) the ethical conditions for disclosure have been amply fulfilled.* We know that people can take simple actions and reduce their risk of dementia. We know that, when people learn their genotype, they take those actions. One by one, rational objections to APOE testing have blown away like willow tufts in the breeze of discovery. What's the hold-up? Probably intellectual Ludditism [362].

Humpty Goes to Camp: A Nanodrama

SEVEN-YEAR-OLD HUMPTY: "Mom! Dad! I just got a flyer inviting me to go to Pop Warner Football Camp!"
DAD: "Good job!"
MOM: "That's nice, dear."
HUMPTY: "So, can I go?"
DAD AND MOM: "Well …"
HUMPTY: "Hey, I'm a big boy now. I even checked it out on the web! Here are the facts:

1. I will probably suffer 200–700 concussive impacts to my head each year.
2. The proportion of those impacts that will exceed the threshold to produce lasting damage (as a single event) or that will, in combination with a second impact within the same month combine to produce lasting brain damage, is finite but currently unfathomable. [Many seven-year-olds talk like this in California.]
3. My helmet will not protect my brain.
4. The statistical likelihood of my suffering permanent brain damage is currently unknown because no American agency, especially not the National Institutes for Neurological Disease, has ever funded a high-quality prospective research project.
5. However, strong evidence suggests that: (a) any boy who played football before entering college is likely to have hippocampal atrophy whether or not he had a reportable concussion [363]; and (b) the chances of permanent brain damage are hugely increased if I happen to carry one or more APOE-ε4 alleles. Thus, it seems reasonable to predict that, genotype aside, playing football during my youth will significantly increase the probability of my suffering both permanent brain damage and my exhibiting inferior brain functioning for the rest of my life, compared with that which I would have otherwise exhibited; and if you fail to check my genotype in advance, and I'm ε4+, you may be assuring that grisly end to my short life. So, how about it?" [Big, cute, endearing grin.]

[15] A different APOE disclosure study [361] was negative. But in that project subjects were not told about the risk of Alzheimer's disease and did not get counseling.

DAD: "Gosh, I mean …"

MOM: "Honey, let's see …"

HUMPTY: "Oh, and by the way: despite our family trip summiting K-2 last summer and my after-school job wrestling alligators, ever since I got that B+ in English, 216 million kids on social media have been calling me a four-eyed nerd-wimp."

DAD AND MOM [IN UNISON AND HARMONY]: "Go for it!"

Without in any way dramatizing what is at stake, the reader is recruited to help in a thinking project: how should wealthy societies with access to genetic testing address the fact that children who carry APOE-ε4 alleles are significantly more likely to become drooling, incontinent, demented wrecks earlier in life if they play football, ice hockey, or any of about ten other sports? Based on an unemotional, impartial analysis of the currently available evidence, no honest scientist can dispute that fact. In the author's observation, however, many people invested in sports deliberately ignore such facts and even lie under oath to deny such facts because they derive personal gains by denying such facts. This is not a criticism, just a neutral comment about psychopathology.

Human nature compels many parents, coaches, and business persons to hide from or battle against medical truth. It seems invariable that certain men (and some women), having become parents, strive to compensate for their insecurities and perceived failures of social standing by pushing their children to participate in activities likely to cause permanent brain damage. Such parasitic pride is a low-risk behavior for the parents. The fathers will probably die before they have to start changing the diapers of their children again should those children, having been exhorted to suffer brain damage, again need someone to change their diapers. Facing that little chore, therefore – not to mention dooming their family to multi-generational neurobehavioral disadvantage – is no disincentive and will never tarnish the imagined glow of a bookshelf of trophies, short-sighted bragging opportunities, and (rarely) a small savings on college costs when a scholarship is dangled as an inducement to Saturday self-destruction for the amusement of intoxicated alumni.

Society must answer two questions. One: how much freedom should parents (and coaches and school principals) have to encourage and facilitate children's participation in very dangerous sports? Two: does a duty exist to better determine a child's risk by a pre-season medical evaluation? Regarding question one: genes aside, the news has been out for about a decade: the violent sports that routinely cause many concussions also routinely cause permanent brain damage. Adults, of course, are free to ignore the facts. What about children? In the 21st century, parents and educators who encourage and facilitate a child's participation in a neurologically dangerous sport deliberately and self-consciously put the child at elevated risk for diminished cerebral function and early death. Is that a good thing? Society, a social contract, necessarily balances free will against communal welfare. Long tradition and democratic consensus favor the least interference in family affairs compatible with minimal protections of child welfare. For that reason, laws only restrain parental behavior when the risk to the child is, by

consensus, perceived as grave. The problem with this principle of decision making: risk is literally impossible to measure and hard to understand. In addition, family dynamics vary but laws cannot be personalized for different levels of parental intellect, parental caring, and child maturity. As a result, the legal system sets down arbitrary but enforceable red lines, usually inflexibly yoked to age. For instance (in so far as the author understands law) statutes in many U.S. states currently forbid serving Jack Daniels at toddlers' birthday parties although that is legal if the children are age 21 or over. It is discouraged for a mother to strap her eight-year-old daughter into a 600-horsepower top-fuel funny car at a drag race and command her to stamp on the accelerator, although that might be OK if the girl were a little older. It would be frowned upon for parents to hand a ten-year-old boy a live hand grenade and mention to him that he should probably throw it after he pulls the pin, but the government legally and daily imposes this scenario on 18-year-olds. Thus, despite our love of freedom and preference not to interfere, we restrict some adult actions with respect to children. The reason that it is illegal to encourage children to do deadly dangerous things is not because we know the risks with mathematical certainty, but because society has judged some fun recreations too risky by common sense.

High school football is similar – although, in fact, we can provide a more accurate mathematical risk assessment in this case. The parents of a 15-year-old linebacker named George are rarely concussion authorities. They may or may not know that they are encouraging George to suffer 200–700 blows to his head each season. They may or may not know that George has a substantial risk of developing brain atrophy even *before* college. In fact, McKee et al. [364] reported neuropathological changes of traumatic encephalopathy in the brain of 17-year-old Nathan Stiles – a high school player in the last game of his senior year who walked off the field, screamed that his head hurt, and died. But, today, the parents probably know: (1) George is likely to suffer multiple concussions; and (2) the risk of early dementia is higher for football players who survive multiple concussions.

Back in the 20th century, the legally responsible parties such as fathers and university presidents could have credibly claimed ignorance. No longer. Increasingly, knowledge of the medical facts is widespread enough that parents, coaches, and school administrators cannot plausibly deny awareness of the consequences of their actions. This inspires moral and even legal rumination: does enthusiastically encouraging a sport widely known to doom some children to permanent brain damage and early dementia represent good parenting, suboptimal but acceptable parenting, or child abuse?

And what, the anthropologist from Mars might ask, motivates this behavior? Given the stakes, why do tens of thousands of North American parents encourage and facilitate hugely elevating the risk that their own flesh and blood will suffer permanent brain damage? Based on an informal survey of 18 fathers at a California high school football game, the most common rationalization was, "It builds character."

Character? Evidence indeed exists from social psychology (and from studies of programs such as Outward Bound) that participation in group activities that push young people to perform beyond the limits they previously perceived may enhance self-esteem, strengthen in-group affiliation, and reduce anxiety in the face of future challenges [139, 365, 366]. The question is whether, for optimum efficacy, those activities need to frequently cause brain damage. In his 2012 [367] essay in the *Chronicle of Higher Education* praising football and himself, Mark Edmundson opined, "Plato would probably approve the way athletics function in our culture – they let the most thymotic of us express their hunger for conquest, rather harmlessly, and they allow the rest of us to get their hit of glory through identification." Indeed, violent sports channel the activity of, and reward, violent boys. But the claim of harmlessness is counter-factual. And the harm is not limited to the boys. It harms society.

Consider, for instance, the culture of American-style football versus the well-being of American women. U.S. college boys who participated in violent high school sports are more likely to engage in sexual aggression [368]. College boy athletes are consistently overrepresented as alleged assailants in cases of acquaintance rape [369]. At 20 universities, boy athletes were named as the perpetrators of sexual assaults at a significantly higher frequency then boy non-athletes [370]. What's more, college football is especially associated with extreme deviant behavior [371]. College football players commit more sexual aggression than non-athletes or athletes in non-violent sports such as track and field or crew [372]. These behaviors are both well known and expected within university communities. National Collegiate Athletic Association (NCAA) Division 1 football games are associated with a 28% increase in daily reports of rape among 17–24-year-old girls by 17–24-year-old boys [373]. As Gage [372] explained,

> Sports have been highlighted as a site where a unidimensional, hegemonic understanding of masculinity is nurtured, if not mandated … Because of the money they produce as well as their historical prominence within university culture, center sports [i.e., football and ice hockey] are often immune to, or protected against, external sanctions that would otherwise discourage deviant behavior by their athletes.
>
> (p. 1016)

The facts are indisputable – yet rarely discussed with candor. Western boys trained in violent sports are at high risk for brain damage and at elevated risk for becoming rapists.[16] What is not clear is the extent to which the routine immunity of elite professional athletes from prosecution for rapes and beatings of women impacts the mental development of Western boys and, as a result, degrades the average quality of life of Western girls. Suffice it to say that the benefits to character are open to question.

The foregoing digression may help us contemplate what is at stake in the decisions adults make regarding children's activities they encourage versus activities they discourage. Some literature suggests, and the author strongly agrees, that some children benefit from participation in challenging, supervised activities, including team sports. However, parents who wish to enhance their offspring's self-esteem obviously have many alternatives to violent sports that, apart from other grisly social consequences from which society tends to avert its gaze, routinely damage brains.

A Modest Proposal

Returning to our conundrum of medical ethics: who should be tested for APOE genotype?

The 20th-century objections to revealing the truth to patients do not stand up to scrutiny. The cost is trivial. The risk of harm is trivial. The evidence shows that informed people take health-promoting action based on this simple piece of information about their bodies. Apart from Luddite devotion to irrational tradition and resistance from those who wish to make money from violent sports, who favors hiding this medical information? Certainly not the medical ethicists. Their consensus clearly favors disclosure if it can help people. Blacker [374] predicted this eventuality in a 2000 essay, opining, "APOE testing might become important in the future if it helps to define the need for intervention." It has become important.

The author, therefore, offers an opinion and a modest proposal for the reader's consideration. Testing is advantageous. It should be widely available and covered by health insurance. For clarity, it seems reasonable to make a distinction between disclosure policies for adults and for children.

Regarding Adults

Knowledge of one's blood pressure and cholesterol level (or, for that matter, blood counts, thyroid hormone levels, or liver functions) exposes patients to the stress of knowing they are at risk of early death and gives them a powerful incentive to avoid that fate. Preventive interventions are readily available. APOE genotype does the same. The overwhelming weight of the evidence suggests that failing to test for, or hiding, APOE genotype violates patient autonomy. Testing and counseling are safe and effective, cheap and easy. This should become a routine part of primary health care.

Regarding Children

As noted above, in 2012 Hoge and Appelbaum [329] opined, "testing is best deferred until adulthood unless preventive interventions exist" (p. 1547). Agreed. Fine. Preventive interventions exist. But that will not be enough to change the culture. Given the illusion of character building, the pressure from fans whose enthusiasm for seeing injuries outweighs their empathy for players, the U.S. devaluation of

---

[16] The author is not aware of any methodologically sound estimate of the proportion of high school and college football players who are sex offenders. The point is not that football makes boys rapists. The point is that football is a subculture – like, for example, Silicon Valley, Hollywood, or Islamic State – that devalues women, attracting and nurturing those who share its particular worldview.

education, and the billions of dollars up for grabs, the author predicts that violent sports will remain popular and lucrative in the United States for approximately four to five more decades. Like smoking and racism, mesolimbic comforts are resistant to the influence of knowledge. As a result, knowing that many thousands of children are doomed to irreversible brain damage via the ongoing collusion of unwitting parents, ignorant schools, and psychopathic sports organizations, the medical community must reconsider its position with regard to APOE testing.

Parents have a legal duty, in many countries, to act on behalf of their children's good health. Religious exceptions occur, but football and ice hockey have yet to qualify. Generally speaking, Western parents are expected to heed common sense and/or the pediatrician's advice regarding matters such as providing food, defending from high falls, and deferring access to semi-automatic weapons until at least age six. If parents have been informed that their child has a special health problem they are expected to make accommodations. So imagine that, in some remarkable future breakthrough, neuroscientists discovered that certain people are genetically prone to suffer disabling brain damage if they pursue a certain behavior. What if a simple test could find those people, so that the parents could be warned of the risk? Should doctors do the test? More than half the readers of this book have already had such a test.

Pheneylketonuria (PKU) is a genetic condition. Like people carrying the APOE ε4 variant, those carrying the PKU gene variant have a high risk of developing serious brain damage. But their brains may be fine for many years so long as they avoid certain behaviors. In the case of PKU, one should avoid foods that contain large amounts of phenylalanine, meaning high-protein foods such as milk, meat, fish, and poultry, eggs and nuts. Yes, avoiding serious brain damage means a restraint on freedom of behavior. "The diet allows extremely limited choices ... and interferes with the social and cultural aspects of eating" ([375], p. 988). In spite of this downside, Western societies do this test on every infant and have done so since the mid-1960s [376]. Brain saving was considered important at that time. Doctors do not refuse to do the PKU test. Doctors do not deny their patients vital knowledge that could save their brains. In fact, in many countries law *requires* doctors to do the test and disclose the results. It saves brains from damage. Knowledge of APOE genotype can do the same.

What if parents would rather not know? Then schools have a duty. Schools routinely obtain medical evaluations before permitting children to participate in violent sports. The examination is typically perfunctory and involves the heart, lungs, and scrotum. Children revealed to have a high risk of harm are excluded from

participation. Will it require a multi-million-dollar tort to inspire Western schools to also check APOE genotype before "clearing" a child to bang his or her head repeatedly? In brief, and with deep sadness, the author predicts the answer is "yes."

Universities face different responsibilities. It is becoming increasingly difficult for those who profit from college football to maintain their awkward head-in-the-sand posture. Mez et al. [377], for example, recently published colorful images of a 25-year-old former college football player, his brain riddled with widespread traumatic encephalopathy pathology.

Although they act *in loco parentis* for minors, most scholarship-paid college players of violent sports are technically "adults." The author has little legal knowledge. It is outside his purview to answer such topical questions such as: "Are U.S. college players of violent sports *employees* whose health and welfare come under the jurisdiction of the National Labor Relations Board (NLRB) and the Occupational Safety and Health Administration (OSHA)?" If these young athletes are employees and OSHA investigates, one can only guess the federal reaction given that OSHA's published list of employer's responsibilities begins with the words, "Provide a workplace free from serious recognized hazards" [378]. In fact, in 2014 the College Athletes Players Association (CAPA) asked the NLRB to permit Northwestern University football players to unionize. In 2015, the NLRB declined to exercise its jurisdiction, stating that the question of whether athletes are employees "does not have an obvious answer" [379]. CAPA understandably expressed concern at this dodge: "Northwestern and its [allies] have enormous self-interest in maintaining the system whereby the universities, coaches and athletic directors, the NCAA, and others – who do not risk concussion and other injury – share multi-millions in revenue generated by the players' labor" [379].[17]

In the reader's most considered opinion, what should society do?

The Other Seven Factors

Force, time, and genes have been addressed. At this early era of CBI research it is not possible to estimate what proportion of the variance in concussion outcome is explained by those three factors. Moreover, it is impossible to calculate (or perhaps even to contemplate) the number of permutations and combinations of clinical outcomes potentially due to variant *mélanges* of the three factors, since each occurs along an infinitely divisible spectrum.

These three are *not*, however, the factors that have received the most attention. Seven other risk factors are actually more commonly cited in peer-reviewed publications to explain

---

[17] At the time of writing, Max Nikias was the president of my university, the University of Southern California (USC). He was also, in a perfect irony, both chair of the USC Health System Board and chair of the College Football Playoff Board of Managers [379]. He reportedly earned $ 4 million dollars per year. It is not clear whether Max fully appreciated that his gainful employment involved helping to guarantee permanent brain injuries among USC undergraduate students – not his most effective pursuit of the good.

Table 7.3 The seven risk factors for bad outcome after concussive brain injury most commonly cited in peer-reviewed literature

1. History of prior TBI

2. History of pre-morbid neurological or psychiatric symptoms, diagnosis, or treatment other than prior TBI

3. Co-morbid non-TBI physical injury, especially neck injury

4. Female sex

5. Age (especially younger than 12 or older than 65 years)

6. Response bias associated with, for example, imagination, poor motivation, misattribution, low expectations, or litigation

7. Social disadvantage or adversity, including low socioeconomic status, low education, low occupational status, low social standing, low freedom of self-determination, minority membership, and other social stressors or adversities that may be pre-morbid or ongoing

TBI: traumatic brain injury.

variation in outcome, assuming a given force of impact, time after impact, and identical genes.[18] These are listed in Table 7.3. We have yet to fully sort out the biological processes and mechanisms that explain links between these seven factors and risk of post-CBI problems, but we can, at least, list them and assess them in the clinic. The list is roughly ordered in terms of the frequency of 20th-century publications claiming that they matter [380]. Note: just as no antemortem biomarker exists confirming occurrence of concussion, no biomarker of badness of outcome (number, frequency, duration, or severity of post-CBI problems considered collectively) exists. Moreover, one cannot reliably distinguish between the survivors who *complain* of many impairments and those who *have* many impairments. Therefore, "bad outcome" will forever be subjective.

Whence comes this list? It represents the author's best effort to compile those factors most often discussed in the literature in rough order of occurrence, based on a systematic review.[19] More than 50 empirical studies have made finding factors that predict outcome their explicit goal. Unfortunately, as noted regarding the entire domain of concussion studies, almost none of the published research mathematically correlates well-designed, well-controlled, long-term assessments of functional or biological outcome (understanding that no valid measure for that is universally accepted) with: (1) *injury-related* risk factors (e.g., force); (2) *patient-related* risk factors (e.g., age); or (3) *environmental* risk factors (e.g., socioeconomic circumstances). As a result of this research gap, as Reuben et al. (2014) remarked,

There is little guidance available on which patients, if any, with mTBI should be followed-up routinely or indeed whether there are any reliable acute-phase predictors which would deem a head-injury patient to be at "high-risk" of developing PCS in the future.

([381], p. 74)

These caveats forever restraining "expert" certainty, students of concussion might nonetheless consider the better among the published reports. In the spirit of transparency, and entirely open to alternative analyses, the author has compiled a wealth of sources.[20]

Selection Criteria

Table 7.4 summarizes a systematic review that began with targeted searches in PubMed and Ovid MEDLINE, followed by review of all bibliographies of the identified papers, followed by review of all the bibliographies of those papers represented in all the bibliographies. Empirical studies were identified that reported risk factors or predictors of outcome upon follow-up of "mild" TBI or concussion ≥ three months. Studies were excluded that consisted of selected case reports [382] or that reported on cohorts of mixed severity and did not stratify analyses to reveal that which pertained to the mild cases (e.g., [383–385], or that reported correlations among post-concussion problems without seeking predictors [129, 130, 386–388], or that failed to report factors that distinguished between better and worse outcome [389], or that confined their observations to cohorts pre-selected for persistent symptoms or neuropsychological testing referral (typically for litigation) [390–398].

Several studies sought to determine whether pre-injury neuropsychiatric conditions predicted long-term outcome. Some did this in more credible ways than others. For instance, Luis et al. [18] and Kashluba et al. [399] were more selective, considering there to have been pre-injury emotional trouble only if there was an unambiguous history of pre-injury psychiatric treatment. Other published reports were included with misgivings. For example, readers should be wary of projects that assessed "pre-injury" psychiatric condition based on examinations *after* the injury (e.g., [400, 401]); it seems methodologically suboptimal to base a scientific conclusion on asking a brain-injured patient, "Please provide an accurate account of your mental health over the 20 years prior to today's brain injury." Fewer investigators took the trouble to gather

---

[18] To the best of the author's knowledge, none of the empirical publications that suggest the effect of another risk factor (e.g., litigation) explain that the effect of that putative factor could only be isolated definitively if force, time, and genes are matched between survivors with and without that factor.

[19] The review was systematic but not comprehensive. PubMed and Ovid MEDLINE were searched from 1980 to 2015. Search terms included combinations of *traumatic brain injury*, *concussion*, *mild*, *outcome*, and *risk factor*. Thirty-eight English-language studies were identified that were self-identified as attempts to find risk factors impacting outcome. An additional 14 studies were identified on reviewing the bibliographies.

[20] As in previous chapters, the author strives to present the best available data in an easily reviewed format. The goal is to eschew the too-common academic practice of cherry picking. Readers can judge whether the data have been reasonably selected and accurately transcribed.

that possibly useful information from a more reliable source such as the medical records or the caregiver [389].

Quality matters. So how should one weigh the relative credibility of these reports? For example, might one construct a hierarchy of trustworthiness based on the strategy of data collection or expertise of the collector? Many outcomes were determined by whether or not telephone calls reached a subset of the subjects. Those calls were made by people of widely varying training, using measures as sophisticated as structured interviews to, literally, "Any problems?" [402]. Other outcomes were determined on the basis of self-report forms, para-professional interviews, neuropsychological testing, or (in rare cases) comprehensive neuropsychiatric examinations. Each approach might be rated more or less likely to obtain accurate and useful data. Neuropsychological testing, for instance, can be informative, so long as a perfect score is never misinterpreted as evidence of good health or "recovery."

Most studies were prospective. Several retrospective studies are included if the independent variables were judged likely to have been assessed in a valid way [12, 403, 404]. As noted in Table 7.4, methods of assessment and measures of outcome varied significantly, again precluding meta-analysis (idiosyncrasies are described in the alphabetical footnotes). Please note: those factors determined *not* to predict outcome are every bit as important to know as those predicting outcome, and were also tabulated. This empowers the reader to judge the credibility of the risk factors nominated by competing authorities.

Table 7.4, of course, is necessarily daunting and virtually unreadable. It was not included for its narrative charm. It was compiled as a reference. In an essay of this type, there is a risk that writers will be consciously or unconsciously biased and that readers will find themselves exhorted by opinion. The author heartily encourages readers to independently analyze the universe of data, including the studies that failed the inclusion criteria due to methodological questions, and arrive freely at their own conclusions.

A Brief Reminder About the Non-Existence of an Organic/Psychological Dichotomy

Disagreement still prevails in regard to the etiology and pathogenesis of the post-concussional syndrome (PCS). Some investigators believe that this syndrome is essentially due to traumatic brain lesion, while others consider it a psychoneurosis.

(Lidvall et al., 1974 [131], p. 7)

The reader has already been introduced to (and perhaps long since acknowledged) the non-existence of an organic/psychological dichotomy. At the risk of overlap with previous chapters, this critical matter possibly warrants a brief reprise here, because the idea reappears in the writing about post-concussional symptoms with unseemly regularity, like fleas on a feral cat. There are quires and reams and bundles and bales

of 20th-century articles discussing risk factors for bad outcome after concussion. Unfortunately, a certain segment of that writing ignores the rather thrilling discovery that brain makes mind.

One commonplace that echoes from the barren canyons of the early literature:

It is presumed that functional factors are playing a significant role if post-concussion symptoms persist beyond a few months.

([141], p. 729)

That is, in the 20th century a vocal subset of TBI writers declared that the early symptoms after a brain injury were due to the brain injury, but any persistent symptoms were to be explained by "mental" or "psychological" factors, to be dismissed as imagination or malingering. Relatively few modern clinicians subscribe to this old saw in its unregenerate form. Still, even in the 21st century, there remain professors of neurology who publicly opine that post-concussive phenomena are either "organic-and-real" or "psychogenic-and-imagined." Modern students are still occasionally exposed to doctrinaire rhetoric along the lines of "Susan is not complaining because of her brain injury but because of her psychological state *before* the brain injury and her psychological reaction *after* her brain injury." What would that mean? That her doctor put her in a scanner that identified the ways in which each of her ~86 billion neurons was affected by the blow to the head during the subsequent neurometabolic–vascular–inflammatory–degenerative melee (inevitably the product of interplay between those changes and the totality of Susan's nature leading up to the moment of the impact), and then identified how each of those changes differed from the changes detected in each of those 86 billion cells that would have occurred if, instead, she had not recently been in a stressful romance – or if, instead of her brain, she broke her leg? Medical students and neurology residents will instantly appreciate the conceptual bankruptcy of such distinctions. Psychiatrists raised in the Freudian era may need a moment or two.

The author absolutely regards the phenomenology of emotional distress as central to human health. But time is past due to insist on a simple clarification: emotions emerge from tissue – what, given our lack of a satisfactory understanding of the roles of neurons and glia, one might call *brain stuff*. When life events provoke the brain change-mediating subjectivities we label "emotions," two things tend to happen:

1. Some aspects of brain function and structure change for a short time (e.g., post-traumatic depression is partly mediated by complex genetically conditioned changes in fronto-limbic activity).

2. Other aspects of brain function and structure may change for a long time (e.g., the initial fronto-limbic change may be part of a complex genetic/epigenetic/developmental/environmental response with innumerable determinants, mediators, and modifiers that sum to produce both

Table 7.4 Risk factors for, or predictors of, persistent post-concussive neurobehavioral problems

Source	n	Design	Follow-up	Predictive risk factors	Non-predictive factors	Outcome measure
Adler, 1945 [133]	200	Prosp. long.	77.5% 4–9 months	1. Older age 2. Female sex 3. If male, married 4. Latin or Slavic "national stock" 5. Industrial accident 6. Psychotic family history 7. Pre-injury mental problems 8. Litigation	Duration of LOC	Mental symptoms
Alves et al., 1993 [4]	189	Prosp. long.	12 months	Female sex + GCS (combined)	1. Older age 2. GCS 3. Pre-injury psychiatric 4. Pre-injury substance abuse	PC symptoms
Barth et al., 1983[a] [405]	71	Random selection	3 months	Re. Halstead–Reitan: Older age and less education (combined) Re. psychopathology on SCL-90: Older age	Re. Halstead–Reitan: 1. Duration of LOC 2. PTA	1. Halstead–Reitan Battery 2. SCL-90
Bazarian et al., 1999[b] [7]	71	Prosp. long.	6 months	None	1. Mechanism 2. Locus of impact 3. LOC 4. Amnesia 5. Neck pain 6. NΨ tests 7. Blaming 8. Sueing	PC syndrome
Bohnen et al., 1994 [406]	231	Retrosp.	1–5 years	For all three scales: 1. Female sex 2. Pre-existing emotional problems 3. Neurological complications For dysthymic and somatic: Co-morbid disorder For dysthymic only: Alcohol intoxication For somatic only: 1. Education 2. Orthopedic fracture 3. Hospitalization For cognitive only: Older age	For all three scales: 1. Compensation claim 2. Previous head injury 3. Neck trauma 4. Skull fracture 5. Smoking	1. Dysthymic scale 2. Somatic scale 3. Cognitive scale
Carlsson et al., 1987[c] [403]	1112	Retrosp.	NR	1. Duration of LOC 2. Alcohol abuse 3. Smoking	Skull fracture	Sequelae Score

(continued)

Table 7.4 (*Cont.*)

Source	*n*	Follow-up	Design	Predictive risk factors	Non-predictive factors	Outcome measure
Cassidy et al., 2014 [407]	1476	12 months	Prosp. long.	1. Age > 50 2. Education < high school 3. Poor expectation 4. Early depression 5. Early arm numbness 6. Early headaches 7. Early back pain 8. Early hearing problems	1. LOC 2. PTA	"Recovery"
de Kruijk et al., 2002[d] [408]	79	6 months	Prosp. long.	1. ≥ 3 symptoms in ED 2. Headache in ED 3. Dizziness in ED 4. Nausea in ED 5. ↑ Serum neuron-specific enolase 6. ↑ S-100B	Neck pain in ED	Post-traumatic complaints
Denker, 1944 [409]	100	Mean = 36 months	Prosp. long.	Age > 40	LOC	Prolonged symptoms (excluded litigants]
Dikmen et al., 1995[e] [410]	261	12 months	Prosp. long.		Litigation	NΨ test results
Dischinger et al., 2009 [11]	110	3 months	Prosp. long.	1. Female sex 2. Early "baseline" (≤3 days) anxiety 3. Initial depression 4. Initial noise sensitivity 5. Initial light sensitivity 6. Initial trouble thinking 7. Initial memory problems 8. Initial irritability	1. Older age 2. Education 3. Previous brain injury 4. Lifetime alcohol dependence 5. Mechanism; 6. "Baseline" (≤3 days) Headache 7. Dizziness 8. Fatigue 9. Extracranial injury	PC syndrome
Drag et al., 2012[f] [404]	167	Mean = 41.93 months	Retrosp.	PTA and or/LOC (vs. only disorientation)	PTA and or/LOC (vs. only disorientation)	Psychiatric outcome; subjective ↓ cognitive; not objective ↓ cognitive
Edna, 1987 [411]	361	3–5 years (mean = 4)	Prosp. long.	1. Prior head injury 2. Skull fracture 3. PTA	1. Duration of LOC 2. "Most of the pre-injury complaints"	PC symptoms
Edna and Cappelen, 1987[g] [12]	485	3–5 years (mean = 4 years)	Retrosp.	1. Female sex 2. Prior head injury 3. Skull fracture	Pre-injury PC symptoms	≥ 4 persistent PC symptoms
Faux et al., 2011[h] [412]	155	3 months	Prosp. long.	1. Previous neck injury 2. Immediate recall 3. More severe headache in ED	1. Female sex 2. Pre-injury psychiatric conditions 3. Chronic headaches	DSM-IVTR post-concussive disorder

(continued)

Study	N	Follow-up	Design	Predictors	Predictors	Outcome
Fenton et al., 1993 [413]	45	6 months	Prosp. long.	1. Older age; 2. Chronic social adversity	1. Pre-morbid social adjustment; 2. Social support; 3. Life events in the prior year	≥ 3 persistent PC symptoms
Hessen and Nestvold, 2009 [414]	97	23 years	Prosp. long.	1. PTA > 30 months; 2. PTA > 30 months + abnormal @ EEG ≤ 24 h (combined)	1. Pre-injury somatic/psychological Illness; 2. Early headache; 3. Skull fracture; 4. Abnormal neurological exam	Elevated MMPI-2 Hysteria scale
Hou et al., 2012[i] [415]	107	6 months	Prosp. long.	1. Negative mTBI perceptions; 2. Early subjective distress; 3. Early anxiety; 4. Early depression; 5. "All-or-nothing behavior"	1. Social support; 2. Litigation	Post-concussional syndrome
Ingebrigtsen et al., 1998 [416]	100	3 months	Prosp. long.	Sick leave	1. Older age; 2. Female sex; 3. Mechanism; 4. GCS; 5. PTA; 6. Alcohol	RPQ score
Jacobs et al., 2010[j] [14]	1069	6 months	Prosp. long.	1. Older age; 2. Extracranial injuries; 3. Alcohol intoxication; 4. CT facial fractures and # of hemorrhagic contusions	1. GCS; 2. PTA; 3. LOC	GOSE
Jakobsen et al., 1987 [417]	55	3 months	Prosp. long.	Early reaction time		PC symptoms
Kashluba et al., 2008[k] [399]	110	3–4 months		1. Compensation; 2. # of pre-injury life stressors; 3. Pre-injury psychological treatment; 4. Pre-injury analgesic, psychopharmologic, or neurologic medications	1. Female sex; 2. Married; 3. Student; 4. Prior head injury; 5. Extracranial injury; 6. Prior neurological hospitalization	Problem Checklist
King, 1996[l] [418]	45	3 months	Prosp. long.	1. Early RPQ score; 2. Early HADS anxiety score; 3. Early HADS depression score; 4. Early IES intrusions score; 5. Early IES avoidance score; 6. Early SOMC score	1. PTA; 2. Early PASAT score; 3. Early AMIPB score; 4. Early Stroop score	RPQ score
King et al., 1999[m] [419]	57	6 months	Prosp. long.	Early HADS anxiety score	1. PTA; 2. RPQ @ 7–10 d; 3. IES avoidance score @ 7–10 days; 5. SOMC score @ 7–10 days	RPQ score

Table 7.4 (Cont.)

Source	n	Follow-up	Design	Predictive risk factors	Non-predictive factors	Outcome measure
Larson and McIntosh, 2012 [420]	155	Mean = 24 years	Retrosp.	1. Pre-morbid concentration ability 2. Attributing symptoms to concussion		RPQ score
Lidvall et al., 1974[n] [131]	83	3 months	Prosp. long.	1. Early worry about extracranial injuries 2. Stress at work 3. Difficulties in the home [4. Having been told to rest]	1. PTA 2. Pre-injury anxiety 3. Pre-injury tendency to react with somatic or other symptoms 4. Pre-injury adjustment to work 5. Fear of further misfortunes 6. Apprehension of decreased work capacity	PC symptoms NΨ tests
Luis et al., 2003 [18]	532	~ 8 yr.	Retrosp.	1. LOC 2. Pre-injury internalizing psychiatric difficulties 3. Lower pre-injury intelligence 4. Low perceived social support 5. LOC + low intellect 6. No pre-morbid psychiatric difficulties + low perceived social support		PC syndrome
Lundin et al., 2006 [135]	102	3 months	Prosp. long.	RPQ symptoms at day 1		RPQ symptoms
Maestas et al., 2014 [421]	187	3 months	Prosp. long.	"Avoidant coping" (per WOCQ)		BSI 36-item SF-36
McMahon et al., 2014[o] [139]	199	1 year	Prosp. long.		1. Older age 2. Sex 3. GCS 4. CT positive	PC symptoms GOSE
Meares et al., 2011[p] [137]	62	~3 months	Prosp. long.		1. Sex 2. PTA	PC syndrome
Nolin and Heroux, 2006[q] [422]	85	12–35 months	Prosp. long.		1. Older age 2. Female sex 3. GCS 4. RA 5. PTA 6. # of initial symptoms	RTW
Ponsford et al., 2000[r] [21]	84	~3 months	Prosp. long.	Unmarried	1. Older age 2. Education 3. Socioeconomic status 4. PTA 5. Student 6. Pre-morbid neuropsychological problems 7. History of learning difficulties 8. History of prior head injury 9. Estimated pre-injury SCL-90-R	SCL-90-R PCSC

Study	N	Follow-up	Design			Outcome
Ponsford et al., 2012[s] [423]	90	3 months	Prosp. long.	Older age	1. Female sex 2. Education 3. Pre-injury physical health 4. Pre-injury mental health 5. GCS 6. PTA	ImPACT
Rao et al., 2010 [424]	43	12 months	Prosp. long.	1. Older age 2. Frontal subdural hemorrhage	1. Female sex 2. Education 3. Race 4. Married 5. Working 6. Mechanism 7. CT positive	Depression
Rimel et al., 1981[t] [425]	424	3 months	Prosp. long.	1. Older age [2. Education] [3. Prior employment] [4. Income] 5. Lower socioeconomic status 6. Greater pre-injury life stress	1. Insured 2. Prior head trauma 3. LOC 4. GCS	Employment/return to work
Russell, 1932[u] [426]	72	6 months	Prosp. long.	Older age (dizzy/memory) Younger age (headache, nervousness)		PC symptoms (excluded litigants)
Russell, 1971 [427]				Older age		
Rutherford et al., 1979[v] [402]	118/41			"All other positive neurological findings at 24h … considered as a single group"		
Schneiderman et al., 2008[w] [428]	275	≥ 5 months	X-sect.	1. Older age 2. ≥ 3 injury mechanisms 2. "Level 2"	1. Female sex 2. Iraq vs. Afghanistan 3. Blast exposure 4. High energy injury exposure	≥ 3 PC symptoms
Sheedy et al., 2009[x] [429]	78	3 months	Prosp. long.	1. Mechanism [2. Occupational satisfaction] [3. Occupation] [4. Immediate memory in ED] [5. Delayed memory in ED] 6. Headaches severity in ED [7. Balance error score in ED] [8. Demographic model: occupational + occupational satisfaction + education] 9. Cognitive model: immediate memory + delayed memory + headache		# of RPQ symptoms

(continued)

Table 7.4 (Cont.)

Source	n	Follow-up	Design	Predictive risk factors	Non-predictive factors	Outcome measure
Stalnacke et al., 2005y [397]	69	15 ± 4 months	Prosp. long.	For RHIFU: 1. S-100B 2. Dizziness at ED For LiSat-11: Nausea in ED	For RPQ: 1. Headache in ED 2. Nausea in ED 3. Dizziness in ED 4. S-100B levels	RPQ symptoms RHIFU LiSat-11
Stulemeijer et al., 2008z [400]	152	6 months	Prosp. long.	For both RPQ symptoms and RTW: [1. Education] 2. Early RPQ severe complaints For RPQ symptoms only: 1. Pre-morbid physical co-morbidities 2. Early stress (IES) For RTW only: [1. Education] 2. Extracranial injuries	For both RPQ symptoms and RTW: 1. Older age 2. Female sex 3. Prior head injury 4. Mechanism 5. LOC 6. PTA 7. Early headache 8. Nausea/vomit. For RPQ symptoms: Extracranial injury	Low RPQ symptoms Full RTW
Styrke et al., 2013 [430]	163	3 years	Pop. based	Re. RPQ: Female sex Re. Disability (RHFUQ): For women: 1. Injured in traffic 2. Back pain For men: Back pain Re. LiSat11: Both sexes: living alone		RPQ symptoms RHFUQ Li-Sat11
van Veldhoven et al., 2011aa [401]	186	3 months	Prosp. long.	1. Early depression (CES-D) predicted BSI depression and anxiety and SF-36 physical health 2. SLESQ predicted BSI depression and anxiety and SF-36 physical and mental health 3. Early stress (PCL) predicted SF-36 physical health	1. Older age 2. CT results	BSI SF-36
Whittaker et al., 2007bb [431]	73	3 months	Prosp. long.	[RPQ score + timeline + consequences] (combined) IPQ-R	1. LOC 2. GCS 3. PTA	PC syndrome
Wrightson and Gronwall, 1981cc [432]	63	3 months	Prosp. long.	Alcohol	1. Age 2. PTA 3. Occupation/salary 4. Mechanism 5. Counseling	RTW

a Re Barth et al., 1983: the subjects were randomly selected from among 1248 with closed head injuries. It is not clear whether they were followed prospectively.

b Re Bazarian et al., 1999: univariate statistics identified multiple factors with positive predictive values but no input variables fit the regression model at 6 months

c Re Carlsson et al, 1987: the follow-up interval was not reported in this population-based survey. Most subjects would be classified as mild. Among the 347 patients in the group called "head-trauma restricted," 240 (69%) had LOC < 30 min.

d Re de Kruijk et al, 2002: vomiting in the ED was associated with a seven times increase in later dizziness.

e Re Dikmen et al, 1995: the authors comment (p. 87) that litigation had no apparent effect on NΨ outcome. This comment pertains to the entire cohort of 436, only 261 of whom were "mild" cases. But the authors describe the compensation-seeking and non-seeking groups as "very similar in … severity distribution."

f Re Drag et al, 2012: report of PTA and or LOC at the time of injury (as opposed to mere disorientation) predicted psychiatric outcome and subjective cognitive outcome but not objective cognitive dysfunction.

g Re Edna and Cappelen, 1987: 89% of subjects had sustained "mild"TBIs.

h Re Faux et al, 2011: assault and being intoxicated at the time of injury were associated with risk of post-concussive disorder at 3 months.

i Re Hou et al, 2012: the tabulated results report to the univariate analysis. On regression, when cognitive and behavior factors were added to the model, emotional factors (anxiety, depression) were no longer predictive of outcome. Only all-or-nothing behavior (a pattern of over-activity then rest) on the Behavior Response to Illness Questionnaire (BRIQ) [433] and perception of illness on the Brief Illness Perception Questionnaire (BIPQ) [434] predicted six-month outcome.

j Re Jacobs et al, 2010: alcohol intoxication on the day of injury was a predictor of *favorable* outcome.

k Re Kashluba et al, 2008: Problem Checklist [435].

l Re King, 1996: the subjects had "mild and moderate" injuries; all except two had PTAs < 24 h; the comparisons are between assessments at 7–10 days and at 3 months. Tabulated findings are based on univariate analysis. Multiple regression led to a model in which eight early measures combined to account for 74% of the variance in RPQ score.

m Re King et al, 1999: the subjects had "mild and moderate" injuries; all had PTAs < 24 h; the comparisons are between assessments at 7–10 days and at 6 months. Univariate analysis showed only the HADS anxiety score to be predictive; multiple regression showed that [HADS anxiety + RPQ @ 7–10 days + PTA] together accounted for 23% of the variance.

n Re Lidvall et al, 1974: the association between likelihood PC symptoms and (1) stress at work or (2) difficulties at home cannot be interpreted as a risk factor because the questionnaire inquired about problems at the time of the injury "or later during the observation period" (p. 79). One factor was associated with a *lower* risk of PC symptoms: "The C-group [comparison group of concussed subjects who were judged free of PC symptoms at two weeks post injury] more often than the PCS-group had been told that one should keep quiet and rest in bed for some time after a head trauma." (p. 77).

o Re Maestas et al, 2014: the findings are suspect because assessment of "pre-injury" coping style was done within two weeks post injury.

p Re Meares et al, 2011: the authors reported that, if they mixed mild traumatic brain injury subjects with non-brain-injured controls, then pre-injury depressive or anxiety disorder or stress at five days post injury predicted PC syndrome at three months. Unfortunately, they failed to stratify results by group.

q Re Nolin and Heroux, 2006: of interest, there was no significant association between NΨ scores and return to work.

r Re Ponsford et al, 2000: for reasons that are not clear, having shown history of sex, prior head injury, history of neurological or psychiatric problems, and student status *not* to be significant predictors, the authors of this paper claimed these were predictors in their abstract.

s Re Ponsford et al, 2012: ImPACT Postconcussion Symptoms Inventory [444]

t Re Rimel et al, 1981: almost all reported associations pertained to the full sample of 424. The claim that pre-injury life stress was a risk factor pertained to a subgroup of 59.

u Re Russell, 1932: age was differently associated with different PC symptoms: age < 40 associated with headaches and nervousness; age > 40 associated with dizziness and memory loss.

v Re Rutherford et al, 1979: the significance of the reported predictive factors is suspect. The authors claimed a cohort of "131." They actually contacted 118. They assessed only 41 in the clinic. The remainder (77) reportedly replied "no problems" when called on the telephone.

w Re Schneiderman et al, 2008: "level 2" mild TBI = loss of consciousness, amnesia, self-reported head injury; "high energy" = blasts, shrapnel, motor vehicle accident, falls, air/water transport.

x Re Sheedy et al, 2009: factors 1–7: significant univariate correlation. Factors 8 + 9: regression analyses: A. Demographic model = [occupation + occupation satisfaction + education] = 45% sensitive and 82.8% specific. Cognitive model = [immediate memory + delayed memory + headache severity in ED] = 80% sensitive and 76% specific.

y Re Stalnacke et al, 2005: the authors separately report associations of risk factors with three outcome measures: RPQ, RHIFU, and LiSat-11.

z Re Stulemeijer et al, 2008: tabulated factors report univariate findings. In a final multivariate model, low 6-month PCS was predicted by: [no pre-morbid physical comorbidity + low early PCS + low scores on early IES (Impact Event Scale; measure of stress)]. Return to work was predicted by: [higher education + no early nausea/vomiting + no extracranial injuries + no early severe pain].

aa Re van Veldhoven et al, 2011: "baseline" data were gathered "within 2 weeks" of concussive brain injury. That is, the authors collected data about pre-injury depression post injury, yet stated that this was a valid assessment of pre-injury mental health.

bb Re Whittaker et al, 2007: univariate correlations were not reported. IPQ-R = Illness Perception Questionnaire-Revised. [449] Timeline = beliefs regarding the expected duration of the illness. Consequences = beliefs concerning the effects of illness on well-being.

cc Re Wrightson and Gronwall, 1981: older age was a risk factor among (1) those with longer PTA and (2) those with shorter PTA + alcohol.

Note: Tabulated predictive risk factors were significantly and positively associated with worse outcome. Some factors predict a *better* outcome. Those are enclosed in square brackets. Factors that were determined **not** to be significantly associated with outcome are tabulated in the non-predictive column. Tabulated **n** refers to those assessed at the time of follow-up. AMIPB: information processing subtest, adult memory and information processing battery [440]; BSI: depression and anxiety subscales of the Brief Symptom Inventory; CES-D: Center for Epidemiological Studies Depression scale [447]; CT: computed tomography; ED: emergency department; EEG: electroencephalogram; GCS: Glasgow Coma Scale; GOSE: Glasgow Outcome Scale-Extended; HADS: Hospital Anxiety and Depression Scale [436]; IES: Impact of Event Scale [437]; ImPACT: International Mission on Prognosis Analysis of Clinical Trials in Traumatic Brain Injury; LOC: loss of consciousness; LiSat-11: Life satisfaction [446]; M: mean; MMPI-2: Minnesota Multiphasic Personality Inventory-2; NΨ: neurological; mTBI: mild traumatic brain injury; PASAT: Paced Auditory Serial Addition Task [439]; PC: post-concussion; PCL: Post-traumatic Stress Disorder Checklist; PCSC: Post Concussion Syndrome Checklist [443]; Pop. based: population-based; Prosp. long.: prospective longitudinal; PTA: post-traumatic amnesia; RA: Retrosp.: retrospective; RHFUQ: Rivermead Head Injury Follow-up Questionnaire; RHIFU: Rivermead Head Injury Follow Up [445]; RPQ: Rivermead Post-concussion Symptoms Questionnaire; SF-36 = physical and mental component scores of the 36-item Short Form Health Survey (SFHS); SLESQ: Stressful Life Events Questionnaire [448]; SOMC: Short Orientation Memory and Concentration Test [438]; RTW: return to work; SCL-90: SCL-90-R = Symptom Checklist 90 Revised [442]; WOCQ: Ways of Coping Questionnaire [441]; X-sect: cross-sectional.

specific changes to cells and circuits (the way a forest fire incinerates specific trees) and changes to the trajectory of brain health (the way a fire alters the destiny of the forest). For example, one might experience both laminar hippocampal atrophy and accelerated multifaceted degeneration.

One should feel free to invoke abstract psychological concepts to "emotions" to describe these tissue changes. It's hard to see what those abstractions add to the quest for safe and effective treatment.

In addressing the seductive error of an organic/psychological dichotomy, two issues deserve differentiation: the *straw man* and the *earnest query*. I will address the straw man first.

By the straw man, I refer to the patently non-scientific claim that a CBI produces only brief "biological" effects and that whatever persists beyond a month or three is "psychological." When the opinion is stated in such a naked and cavalier format, it is a trivial matter to correct the speaker: "You wish to tar the distress of CBI survivors with the transparently derogatory label 'psychogenic.' But your organic/psychogenic dichotomy harks back to the ancient error that mind was independent from brain. Sorry; Cartesian dualism crashed and burned centuries ago."

That rebuttal is robustly supported not only by common sense (that is, acceptance of natural science and a material universe) but also by many lines of empirical evidence. There is nothing new about recognizing that all mental activity and behavior is mediated by brain. The author will not belabor the point that Willis [450] corrected Descartes's division of mind from brain before 1664. Imagination, indeed the very soul, Willis said, is a property of brain. By the mid 19th century, the issue was settled science. Ferrier [451], for example, wrote, "That the brain is the organ of mind, and that mental operations are possible only in and through the brain, is now so thoroughly well established and recognized that we may without further question start from this as an ultimate fact" (p. 255). As legendary behavioral neurologist D. Frank Benson pithily aphorized, "There may be some mindless brains, but there are no brainless minds" ([452], p. 5). All that is called *behavior*, *thought*, or *mental* is the product of bubbling brain stuff.

Concussion experts have long since dismissed efforts to rehabilitate Mr. Descartes. Strauss and Savitksy said in 1934 [453]: "It is necessary for once to abandon the specious dichotomy, organic and psychogenic, in an approach to head injury". They meticulously reviewed the then-available data and concluded:

The clinical features – headache, dizziness, irascibility, abnormal reaction to effort, vasomotor instability, fatigability, intolerance to intoxicants and to changes in the weather – as we have shown are evidence in almost all cases of alteration of the activity of the intracranial tissues.

([453], p. 948)

Dr. Symonds was equally firm in trouncing the perpetuators of non-material causality. He wrote in 1942 [454]:

As to the distinction between the physiogenic and the psychogenic factors in a given case, they appear in most cases so closely intertwined that to separate them is unnatural … It will be understood from what I have said that I regard the practice of dividing the post-contusional cases into two groups, labeling the one organic and the other functional, or neurotic, as unprofitable and misleading.

([454], p. 604)

Bohnen and Jolles added in 1992 [129]: "It may be clear that there is no place for dualistic thinking in the paradigm of MHI [minor head injury] today" (p. 690).

Thus, dismantling the straw man – the simplistic claim that vagaries of psyche explain post-CBI distress – is effortless.

Enough.

The Cartesian fantasy that mind occurs separate from brain has no place in serious human discourse. It is especially harmful when permitted to creep into medical dialogue. In the author's observation, there is a strong correlation between those who reject the oneness of mind and brain and those who blame the victims of brain disorders for their behaviors. The time has long since passed when scientists could conjure humors and souls to cover their bafflement. One must admit our profound ignorance of the exact mechanisms by which concussion/mTBI triggers short- and long-term behavioral change. But one cannot rationally attribute any of that change to disembodied spirits.

The Medical Student Saves the Baby From the Bath Water

Yet that rebuttal fails to respond to an earnest query. To simply point out the obvious – that all mentation is organic – threatens to throw out the baby with the bath water. One must not be distracted by the dated term "psychogenic." Lurking behind that shadow is an earnest and completely legitimate query about an incredibly challenging mystery: how does an abrupt external force interact with all that we are to change us?

The thoughtful 21st-century medical student rightly says:

Yes, yes, I know and agree! Of course all mental, emotional, and psychological matters are merely products of bubbling brain stuff. Of course a concussion involves an interaction between a force and an individual's unique biological self. I'm just wondering how it works. Doesn't brain stuff process different CBI symptoms in different ways?

For instance, when a baseball inexplicably detours from the strike zone to batter Joe's left temple, I propose that some brain changes are rapid. There is of course a unique force–individual biology interaction. But the most obvious brain change when he's staggering at home plate is not the soon-to-arrive interaction of the external force with the cells of Joe's brain that mediate his cognition, emotions, or personality. It's the immediate interaction of the force with biological factors such as: (1) how well Joe's neck muscles preserve consciousness by keeping his brainstem from twisting; (2) how well perfused his ascending reticular activating system is at that moment; (3) his hydration status; (4) how tight his middle fossa happens to be; (5) how agile his cerebrovascular autoregulation happens to be; and (6) how stretchy his pontine axons are that day. The physics and biology would stagger a supercomputer, but the overt human behavior is not terribly complex: over the course of about one second the interactions between the inopportune external force and Joe's personal biological nature knock the poor guy silly.

But lots more force–individual biology interactions are coming. For instance, when Joe awakens on the trainer's bench and grabs his head, it's because the brain stuff that was rattled six minutes ago is interacting with the brain stuff that mediates Joe's long-standing predisposition to migraines. Eight months after his concussion, when Joe is ripping up his half-completed tax return in frustration, it's because the initial force-related brain changes and the brain's attempt to repair them are interacting with the brain stuff that has mediated Joe's weakness in math and feisty temperament since birth, as moderated by his good experience with his eighth-grade math tutor and by an upsetting recent experience with his girlfriend.

I get that these are not "psychogenic" changes. *Of course* it's all due to changes in brain stuff.

She pauses to take a breath.

But shouldn't we acknowledge that some of Joe's impact-related brain-mediated behavioral changes are more temporary, universal, and force-dependent (like falling insensible into the dirt), while others may be more lasting and more dependent on the interaction between the force, the brain's early response to the force, and all the brain's functional apparatus underpinning Joe's selfhood?

I fully and happily acknowledge that the psychogenic/organic perspective is conceptually bankrupt. I agree that persistent post-concussive symptoms are due to physical brain change. I realize that these symptoms result from the inopportune arrival of an external force as it interacts with a host of brain traits, including:

1. the brain stuff that mediates the emergent mental phenomena we call Joe's pre-morbid psychology
2. the brain stuff that mediates Joe's emotional response to injury
3. the brain stuff associated with Joe's adaptive, if imperfect, reparative mechanisms
4. the brain stuff that mediates Joe's solicitation of empathy and response to social supports
5. the brain stuff that mediates the phenomena we call free riding – Joe's temptation to exploit his injury for gain, consciously or unconsciously.

Winded but valiant, the student concludes: "So just tell me: setting aside the mythology of 'psychogenic', isn't it the case that the causal pathway to different post-CBI symptoms is different?"

Wow. Well said. The only scientifically respectful answer to the medical student's earnest query the author could ever offer would be a hearty yes.

The force–individual biology interactions that lead to the astonishing spectrum of post-concussive brain and behavior changes documented in the above literature are remarkably complex. The mechanisms that explain them are far beyond our current scientific ken. Since we are really not able to describe the brain stuff changes, it is perfectly understandable that many revert to abstract psychological terms. Yet all the somewhat ephemeral constructs of psychology – such as "cognition" and "emotion" – have material bases. The student is right, but her heartfelt question is not currently answerable. History finds us poised halfway along a lofty tightrope: we have left behind the fiction of "psychogenic," but we are still far from arriving safely at knowledge of how the brain does its magic.

Thus we find Marcus, a year after his CBI, staring at the ring of wet mahogany left by his beer mug on the bar, only half aware of the lady in the red sweater down the counter, pondering why he cannot get along with people any more. Who amongst us dares to estimate the proportion of that feeling "caused" by the accident versus the proportion "caused" by his innate personality? To frame our clinical concerns in terms of such false dichotomies is a fallow exercise. We need a few hundred years to fill in the blanks. But the data no longer leave room for doubt: the brain changes that underlie persistent post-concussion problems are physical, organic, and common.

> It is not only the kind of injury that matters, but the kind of head.
>
> (Symonds, 1937 [455], p. 1092)

#1: On the Risk Factor Called *History of Prior TBI*

Some evidence suggests that prior TBI increases the risk of worse outcome after concussion in both adults [12, 411, 456, 457] and children. Yet more studies have not found that association [11, 21, 399, 400, 406, 425]. Before attempting to make sense of these inconsistent findings, a bit of conceptual housekeeping is needed to clarify the four patterns of injury to which the phrase "prior TBI" is applied.

Pattern #1. More-Than-One-But-Less-Than-Many Concussions with Cumulative Effects Seen Relatively Soon

As shown in Table 7.4, a few epidemiological studies have identified one (or more) prior TBIs/CBIs (earlier in life) as a risk factor for worse outcome after a subsequent concussion.

Typical Pattern

One or more CBIs at age two to 75. Then a subsequent CBI some time after the initial injury or injuries. The subsequent CBI is followed by a worse than usual or longer than usual post-concussive course. (Example: one concussion at age 11 in which the symptoms last a few months, then another CBI at age 26 in which the symptoms last two years.) Some evidence suggests that this scenario of several concussions increases the risk of dementia more than a single TBI.

Pattern #2. One TBI/CBI With Later-Life Effects

The phrase "prior TBI" has also been applied to circumstances in which a *single* prior TBI seems to increase the risk of neurodegeneration that may only become overt years later [12, 247, 411, 456–459].

Possible Exemplary Pattern

One lifetime TBI somewhere between age two and 75, followed by a time gap with apparent health, later followed by onset of a dementia purportedly similar to "AD."

Pattern #3: Multiple Recurrent Concussions

Evidence emerged in the 1920s that recurrent concussions can lead to permanent brain damage [460]. That sequence was originally called *dementia pugilistica* due to its association with boxers. That term was abandoned in the mid 20th century because the same disorder has been associated with a variety of other head injury exposures, including other sports (especially American football, ice hockey, wrestling, and karate) [461–467] as well as military exposures [468, 469].

Typical Pattern

In the sports-related CBI literature, the term "recurrent concussion" typically refers to five to 100 CBIs spread over five to 20 years [470]. This pattern of injury exposure may be followed promptly by neurobehavioral disability that ends the athletic career, or there is sometimes a period of apparent health lasting for up to 15–20 years before the onset of overt dementia. Late in the 20th century some neuropathologists began to label that dementia with the catchy slogan (perhaps borrowed from Parker [310]), *chronic traumatic encephalopathy*, CTE.

Pattern #4: Multiple Concussions in Quick Succession

Many animal experiments have attempted to replicate the human problem of recurrent concussion [471–477]. In the author's opinion, these investigators do not accurately replicate any of the human patterns #1–3. In fact (with the possible exception of persons with epilepsy [478], a second TBI after an interval of hours to days is infrequent among humans. When it does occur, there is so much disorder in the brain from the first injury that the second injury is sometimes fatal – a tragic phenomenon called the second impact syndrome [479, 480].

Typical Laboratory Pattern

Strike a rodent; wait minutes to days (rather than months or a year); strike him again; wait several minutes or hours

(rather than waiting for him to grow old); and then look at his brain. Pending trials of experimental sequences and methods that better mimic human cases, it is unknown whether such "second-impact" lab experiments generate useful conclusions about the more common human scenarios of repeated injury.

In a rush to judgment, recent literature tends to discuss patterns 2 and 3 as if they were neatly dichotomous disorders: there can either be one TBI followed by AD or many CBIs followed by CTE.[21] Indeed, the label CTE has achieved global memetic fixation, despite its inaccuracy. Traumatic encephalopathy is *not* usually chronic. As previously noted, survivors of multiple concussions often exhibit a period of apparent mental health lasting for years or decades before the onset of dementia, and the dementia is more often progressive than chronic [470]. A more accurate descriptor would therefore be "late-onset progressive post-traumatic encephalopathy." (But LOPPTE is, admittedly, less fetching.)

Whatever the name, in 2015 neuropathologists neared a consensus that the tau-predominant neurodegeneration that follows many concussions is different from the classic AD that can allegedly follow a single TBI [481]. Both conditions exhibit deposits of hyperphosphorylated tau (P-tau) and β–, yet in "CTE" the tau deposits reportedly tend to be perivascular and in the depths of the sulci – a pattern not usually seen in AD [482]. That observation about P-tau indeed suggests genuinely different entities.

Yet the AD vs. CTE theory of post-traumatic brain degeneration may not accurately reflect the data. For instance, CTE is invariably called a "tauopathy," but the majority of CTE brains are dappled with Aβ [308, 482, 483]. And post-TBI dementia is often called "AD" but the distribution of pathological changes is different [484]. In the light of the evolving knowledge base, Hay et al. [482] summarized misgivings about the purported dichotomy:

> Both historically and currently, TBI-associated dementia has been subdivided based on whether it follows a single, moderate or severe TBI (sTBI) or repetitive, mild TBI (rTBI), with the associated clinical syndromes considered distinct. In particular, despite compelling literature to the contrary, there is a general presumption that CTE is limited to patients exposed to rTBI, most often athletes. This misperception may be due in part to a complete absence of comparative research or clinicopathological studies looking at material from both sTBI and rTBI patients in parallel. As such, considering late neurodegenerative outcomes from an sTBI and rTBI as different syndromes is, at best, premature and, arguably, flawed.

([482], p. 23)

Another factor raising eyebrows about the "single TBI → AD while many concussions → CTE" theory: in most reports of

---

[21] Missing from this classification scheme, and rarely studied, is a third very common pattern of TBI: the person who survives two or three concussions in his or her lifetime.

post-traumatic AD neither the clinical picture nor the pathological data have been rigorously described and in most cases of post-repetitive concussion CTE the clinical data are poorly documented. In point of fact, the supposedly AD-like dementia following a single moderate to severe TBI does *not* mimic clinical AD; it tends to exhibit more motor and neuropsychiatric problems – making the clinical phenomenology more akin to that seen in traumatic encephalopathy after many concussions [482, 485, 486]. The author strongly agrees with Hay et al. [482] and with Furst and Bigler [484] that, given the overlaps between and deviations from classical pathological profiles, it is perhaps premature to immortalize a "single TBI → AD while many concussions → CTE" dichotomy. Further research is needed, particularly the long-delayed initiation of prospective longitudinal studies collecting more complete and credible clinical data.

Returning to the issue of prior TBI as risk factor: whether the pattern begins with one blow or many, whether it ends in one form of degeneration or another, the question is: why does it happen? Chapters 2–4 of this essay distilled the pathophysiological essence of concussion: external force triggers a battle between harmful degenerative and beneficial regenerative changes affecting neurotransmission, metabolism, axonal integrity and axoplasmic flow, microvascular function, myelination, hormonal function, and immunomodulatory/inflammatory functions – for short, the *neurometabolic-vascular–degenerative–inflammatory melee*. Back in the 20th century the focus was on the metabolic crisis and the first ten days. That framework must be gently dismissed. It utterly fails to explain the clinical changes we know last for years or decades after CBI. Twenty-first-century work, in contrast, attends to long-term brain change in gene expression, inflammatory markers, microvascular status, axon integrity, and protein deposition. For instance, fMRI and DTI detect abnormalities up to 39 years after "mild TBI"[487–492]; MRS detects abnormalities up to one year after "mTBI" [493]. Widespread deposition of Aβ and tau has been detected up to 47 years after TBI [494–496]; reactive microglia have been detected in 28% of TBI survivors up to 18 years post-concussion [495, 496]. But lasting changes do not seem to be either uniform or universal. Nor is it known which long-term post-CBI change explains worse outcome after the next concussion and/or accelerated neurodegeneration. Axon damage? Neuronal loss? Transcriptome deviance? Deposition or prion-like spread of toxic proteins? Chronic inflammation?

Let us consider a patient I saw, a boy named Raul who fell from a swing and was concussed at age seven. One year later, he had a minor memory problem. Bad luck: Raul was concussed again in a motor vehicle accident at age 17. One year after his second concussion, Raul exhibited a surprisingly problematic recovery with nearly-disabling slowing of thought and a tripling in the frequency of his occasional headaches. His neurologist might be correct to write: "Raul is not recovering well because of his prior TBI." But *why*? What has been lurking in his brain during the intervening decade? As noted in the introduction to this chapter, knowing that a statistical association exists between prior trauma and worse outcome is not practically helpful. But if we can discover the biological change that explains that epidemiological association, we might hone in on why brain injury can lead to dementia and what targets are most promising for intervention. That discovery would change the world.

In the hope of stumbling upon the key change that explains risk from prior TBI, one might study each element of the three-ring biological circus of events after concussion.

Axonal Stretch and Derailed Amyloid Precursor Protein

The first change, of course, is visitation by a *force*. Force, however, has already been shown to be a disappointing predictor of outcome. The next change one might consider is *axonal stretch*. This holds more promise as an explanation for brain degeneration since stretch disrupts the biology of both Aβ and tau.

That is, when Raul fell off that swing in childhood, he stretched his axons. Visualize an axon as a freeway, with microtubule lanes (tubulin dimers stabilized by tau, like rails stabilized by cross-ties) open to molecular traffic. Among the vehicles rolling down the tubulin road are the ingredients one needs to manufacture Aβ: amyloid precursor protein (APP) along with enzymes that include presenilin-1 and β-site–APP-cleaving enzyme [494, 497]. When Raul's axons were stretched, the tau cross-ties also broke loose from the tubulin rails. This may occur because hyperphosphorylated P-tau undergoes a conformation change that makes it breaks loose from the microtubule [498]. Raul's damaged microtubules impaired fast axonal transport such that APP and its companion enzymes literally became stuck on the broken rails. Forced into intimacy, these ingredients did what comes naturally, building excess Aβ within hours. The excess Aβ migrates toward the cell body and aggregates, forming plaques.

One might surmise, "Aha! So this starts the process of AD in Raul's brain, even at age seven!" Maybe. But some reports made that sequence seem doubtful. For one, in Roberts et al.'s renowned study of traumatized brains from the Corsellis Archive, post-concussive plaques were noted to be *diffuse* – hence, different from the neuritic plaques associated with AD [459, 499]. For another, evidence was published in 2009 that this acute post-CBI proliferation of Aβ may fail to form plaques and may vanish after weeks or months (presumably by effective clearance) [500]. If trauma makes the wrong kind of plaques and, in any case, these get cleared up pretty soon, how could this element of the post-concussive melee explain long-lasting brain vulnerability?

As touched upon above, one clue was perhaps embedded in a paper by Johnson et al. [247] titled, "Widespread tau and amyloid-β pathology many years after a single traumatic brain injury in humans." This case-controlled study of 39 people who survived a single moderate or severe TBI provided two surprises regarding amyloid: (1) contrary to the expectation that post-concussive Aβ vanishes, Aβ plaques were found in the brains of TBI survivors from 1 to 47 years post injury

331

(as well as in controls)[22]; and (2) contrary to the expectation that TBI only generates diffuse plaques, 64% of TBI survivors had neuritic plaques (or mixed plaques) versus none of the controls. These findings suggest that *long-lasting typical AD-like pathological change occurs in a substantial subset of survivors of single TBIs.*

Although this study focused on more severe cases, microtubule damage also occurs in typical concussions [501, 502]. That opens the door to the possibility that stretched axons → broken microtubules → derailed amyloid production material → inappropriate Aβ production → plaque deposition (and perhaps subsequent prion-like spread) is the chain of causality that puts the brain on track for multiple bad outcomes. And it would seem to support the "single TBI → AD" hypothesis.

Recent evidence inspires reserve. In a small but intriguing study, Scott et al. [503] examined nine CBI survivors using: (1) 11C-Pittsburgh compound B (11C-PiB) PET; (2) structural MRI; (3) DTI; and (4) cognitive testing.[23] TBI survivors exhibited more binding than normal persons in posterior cingulate cortex (PCC) and cerebellum and more binding than AD subjects in the cerebellum. The excess Aβ correlated with damage to the white matter (axons) on DTI. Consistent with our proposed pathway, these findings suggest that TBI → axon damage → excess Aβ burden. An additional finding: the longer the time elapsed since TBI, the greater the Aβ burden in the precuneus/pPCC. How did the Aβ get there? The authors speculated that prion-like transsynaptic spread enabled Aβ to migrate along the cingulum bundle, carrying the noxious, toxic Aβ from the original site of axonal rattling in the posterior cingulate forward to the PCC. "The implication for TBI is that the WM [white matter] may be both a source of Aβ and a conduit for Aβ diffusion" ([503], p. 826).

So far, the story hangs together and buttresses our theory of a road to ruin in which TBI → axon damage → excess Aβ burden → "AD." In a nutshell: axonal trauma apparently gives the human head a head start on the normal, natural, inescapable path to aging-related degeneration.

But inconsistencies need explaining. For one, Pittsburgh compound B binding (hence, Aβ burden) was high in the *cerebellum* of TBI survivors. Cerebellar change means the distribution of degeneration is not the same as seen in AD [484, 504]. If this is a representative finding, then single TBI does *not* lead to the condition popularly called "AD." It leads to something else, something perhaps unique and different from

both garden-variety aging-related neurodegeneration and from the tau-heavy encephalopathy reported after repetitive concussions.

Furst and Bigler [484] neatly phrased the mystery that has remained a head scratcher for decades: "Amyloid plaques in TBI: incidental finding or precursor for what is to come?" They agreed that Scott et al.'s findings are exciting, but they also pointed out reasons for caution. For instance, consider the anatomy: the bundle of axons called the cingulum follows a C-shaped path curving forward to the PCC and back to the entorhinal cortex/hippocampus. If the build-up of Aβ in the PCC is due to prion-like spread forward to the cingulate, surely it would also spread back to the entorhinal cortex/hippocampus. But there is no corresponding Aβ accumulation back there in the TBI subjects.

Why? At the time of this writing, the answer is unknown.

How About Tau?

Just as axon stretch discomfits microtubules and provokes Aβ production, so too it liberates P-tau. Until recently, tau proliferation and aggregation were *not* expected consequence in the days after concussion [505]. New findings from both animal and clinical research suggest that, in fact concussions are often followed by deposition and spread of P-tau or tau oligomers.[24]

Gerson et al. [506], for example, recently reported three relevant findings. First, contrary to previous claims, tau oligimers were found to form promptly after both fluid percussion injury and blast brain injuries. Second, injecting those tau nits into the hippocampi of Htau mice (mice that express human tau) accelerates cognitive deficits, a link to clinical dementia. Third, the nits injected into the hippocampi spread, like lice on a pre-school head, to the cerebellum, consistent with the observation that spatial dissemination occurs, perhaps due to prion-like mechanisms.

Another recent animal experiment demonstrated that even mild TBI provokes tau excess, and there is a link to neuroinflammation: Gyoneva et al. [507] also reported that lateral fluid percussion leads mice to generate P-tau promptly in the hippocampus. But these mice were special. The authors set out to explore the interaction between concussion, tau, and inflammation, so they disrupted the chemokine (C-C motif) receptor 2 (CCR2) (a regulator of monocyte infiltration). The result: although microglial reaction did not seem affected, P-tau was diverted to the cell body in both neocortex and hippocampus.

---

[22] Plaque distribution seemed wider and plaque density higher among TBI survivors. For example, 38% of controls versus 73% of TBI survivors exhibited high plaque density. But this trend did not reach statistical significance.

[23] The brain injuries were called "moderate-to-severe," so the relevance to typical concussions is unknown.

[24] As Ward et al. [497] reviewed the 20th-century model of AD, "For many years, it was assumed that NFTs [neurofibrillary tangles] were the cause of neuronal toxicity, since they correlate very well with cognitive decline and neuronal loss" (p. 667). It was also noted that caspases may cleave tau to produce a form that is highly prone to aggregate; hence cleaved tau became a new suspect. However, it has been observed that animals overexpressing tau can exhibit neurodegeneration without NFTs. This has drawn attention to an alternate suspect as the neuron-harming agent: tau oligomers – fragments of tau that have not formed fibrils. At the time of this writing it is not known how microtubule-associated tau harms brains.

Neurofibrillary tangles in the fusiform gyrus of a 27-year-old man 1.5 years after traumatic brain injury (TBI): comparison with similar lesions in other conditions

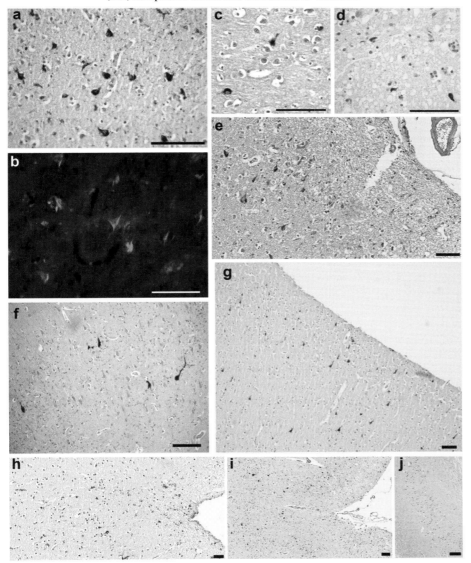

Fig. 7.16 Representative immunohistochemical and thioflavine-S staining for neurofibrillary tangles (NFTs). (A) NFTs in the parahippocampal gyrus of a 49-year-old male 1 year post-TBI. (B) Representative thioflavine-S positive staining in the same case as a. (C) NFTs in the fusiform gyrus of a 27-year-old male 1.5 years after TBI. (D) NFTs in the frontal lobe of a case of advanced Alzheimer's disease (positive control). (E, G) Representative images showing prevalent NFTs in the superficial layers of the cortex of the medial temporal lobe. (F) Extensive neuropil threads and occasional NFTS in a 53-year-old individual who died 8 years following TBI. (H-I) representative images showing Isolated clusters of NFTs within the depth of sulci. (J) Uninjured control case displaying no neurons positive for tau immunostaining in the hippocampal region CA1. All scale bars approx. 100 µm. [A black and white version of this figure will appear in some formats. For the color version, please refer to the plate section.]

Source: Johnson et al., 2012 [247] with permission from John Wiley & Sons

Those were single TBI experiments. Repetitive experimental concussion also triggers tau proliferation and aggregation: Xu et al. [508] exposed transgenic mice (with the tau P301S transgene associated with frontotemporal dementia) to repetitive mild trauma. "We found that the density of tau pS422 (+) retinal ganglion cells (RGCs) increased twenty fold with one mTBI hit, a little over fifty fold with four mTBI hits and sixty fold with 12 mTBI hits."

Finally, completing the story by showing that post-concussive tau causes cognitive problems, Cheng et al. [509] mildly hit mice twice. Mice that could make tau did so and developed deficits in spatial learning and memory. Mice lacking the capacity for tau production were spared those cognitive deficits. Another relevant finding: Aβ is suspected of triggering tau toxicity [510]. Hence, the generation of both Aβ and P-tau after microtubule damage may be synergistic. This combination of recent laboratory findings strongly bolsters the story that concussion → axon damage → excess Aβ and P-tau (or perhaps tau oligomers) → behavioral impairment.

Humans also exhibit post-concussive tau. As previously mentioned, Johnson et al. [247] found excessive tau after a single TBI – even in young people and even as early as one year later (Figure 7.16). Neurofibrillary tangles (NFTs, made from filaments of tau) were found in 34% of in the brains of TBI survivors under age 60, but in only 9% of young controls ($p = 0.015$). Moreover, NFT distribution after a single TBI was more extensive than that found in the controls (which more resembled normal aging than degeneration).

Johnson et al. opined,

The apparent delayed appearance of NFTs after trauma suggests that even a single TBI may, in the long-term, be associated with a neurodegenerative process. Moreover, this finding provides a potential pathological substrate for the epidemiological observation of an increased risk of developing syndromes of cognitive impairment, such as AD, following TBI.

([247], p. 5)

But, if P-tau (or tau oligomers) does not aggregate acutely after brain injury, how did the tau get there a year later? Autopsy and imaging evidence is sparse, but indirect evident suggests that, as in rodents, tau does in fact appear promptly after human concussions and in fact that serum or plasma tau is a potential biomarker for mTBI [511]. CSF tau is thought to roughly quantify axonal damage and has been found to predict one-year outcome after TBI [512, 513]. Olivera et al. [514] studied 70 soldiers who reported TBI on the Warrior Administered Retrospective Casualty Assessment Tool. Not only was plasma tau elevated in the 70 participants, but also the level correlated with post-concussive symptoms. As co-author Gill expressed the promise of this discovery: "Our findings suggest that tau elevations relate to chronic symptoms, and could facilitate the identification of individuals at risk and the provision of interventions to mitigate these risks" (quoted in Fyfe, 2015 [515]).

The foregoing data point in one direction. Contrary to previous assumptions, tau indeed commonly blossoms and spreads after concussion and probably contributes to worse outcome and later dementia.

It is tempting, in the face of such neatly dovetailing experimental and clinical reports, to champion a seductive story of a uniform post-concussive pathophysiology. "Now we know how it works! External force → microtubule damage → excess toxic proteins → persistent symptoms and risk for dementia." However, *none of the above reports found the same results in every mouse or every human*. None of them considered alternative explanations – factors such as microvascular or gene expression or demyelinating or counterproductive inflammatory change that may, alone or in combination with degenerative change, account for persistence of dysfunction. That is, the research findings regarding concussion and tau are frankly inconsistent. Rather than try to wish away the conflicting results by attributing inconsistency to methodological error or artifact, it seems more prudent to develop a theory that accommodates these inconsistencies, based on the guiding principle of this chapter: variation in findings is exactly what biological individuality predicts. That caveat in mind, it appears that both of the major pathological protein aggregates associated with AD pepper the brain in roughly a third of cases of CBI.

Is it possible that we have stumbled upon the key explanation for variation in clinical outcome? It is interesting to note how close the proportions are to a match: about 33% of CBIs exhibit degenerative change and more than 40% of typical, clinically attended concussions are followed by long-term problems. Might these two recent discoveries represent cause and effect? Let us restrain our enthusiasm. The neurobiological factors sustaining brain dysfunction during the first year might be completely dissociable from those explaining late effects. And without high-quality, large-scale, long-term prospective research, all of the research frailties previously discussed counsel hesitation before leaping in the direction of such a speculation. Still, it seems scientifically justifiable to consider that the observed difference in early production and spread of neurotoxic proteins might be a partial answer to this chapter's guiding question, why do outcomes vary?

But Why Does Post-Concussive Degeneration Vary?

Parents of a five-year-old know the drill. Answer one *but why* question and you will unleash a catena of *but why*s that only end in the Big Bang (or a nap). If post-CBI generation and spread of toxic proteins are inconsistent, if they vary from brain to brain, why? As always, one likely suspect is genetic variation. We have already discussed the association between APOE-ε4 and worse outcome from TBI. GWAS have identified other genetic polymorphisms that also increase the risk for AD [480, 516, 517]. In addition, more than 40 mutations have been identified that influence tau production, aggregation, and clearance [518].

A related possibility: Iliff et al. [489] examined tau clearance by the recently identified glymphatic pathway. Elimination of this potentially harmful protein indeed seems to depend on that pathway. The authors opined: "These findings suggest that chronic impairment of glymphatic pathway function after TBI may be a key factor that renders the post-traumatic brain vulnerable to tau aggregation and the onset of neurodegeneration." Without claiming to know the details, it seems conceivable that natural human variation in production and clearance of Aβ and tau may leave some CBI survivors, not others, with more toxic protein than their brain can clear.

All hope abandon ye who enter here.

Dante Alighieri, c. 1306, translated by
H. F. Cary, 1814 [519]

A Theory of the Point of No Return

The author does not claim to know exactly why some concussions are followed by prolonged neurobehavioral problems and neurodegenerative changes, other apparently not. But he can offer a heuristic model. It may even be true. Consider the gestalt of post-concussive biology: the brain is rattled. Every neural and glial and vascular and blood cell is rattled. Although one is accustomed to saying there is *brain damage*, that would be like saying, "having broken his ankle, the patient has *skeleton damage*." At the molecular and infrastructural level, every individual cell inside the skull exhibits its own unique response. Each suffers one of three fates: no molecular change with any functional consequences, molecular change with transient and reversible consequences, or molecular change with permanent consequences. In cell populations two and three, the battle commences between degenerative forces – led by axonal stretch, excitatory neurotransmission, energy crisis, pro-apoptotic, pro-counterproductive inflammatory, and pro-degenerative agents, perhaps disseminated by prion-like spread – versus forces counterposed to resist those harmful factors (e.g., antiapoptotic enzymes), or to regenerate cells (e.g., hippocampal dentate neurogenesis), or to permit functional accommodation for permanent loss of some tissue (e.g., circuit repurposing). Thus, the brain's self-rescue mechanisms act at the molecular, cellular, and connectome levels. No matter how grievous the magnitude of the abrupt external force, it is rare (if ever) that *all* of the cells in the brain are damaged. Certain tissue is especially prone to injury, such as long white-matter tracts and certain hippocampal cells. Yet no two parts of the brain are exactly equally harmed and (with the exception of extraordinarily severe cases) no part of the brain is totally ablated. Example: perhaps a CBI survivor suffers derangement of 16.7% of the microtubules in the rostrum of his corpus callosum. One would not expect that he suffered exactly 16.7% injury to the microtubules genu, truncus, isthmus, or splenium of his corpus callosum, let alone 16.7% injury to the axons of his superior longitudinal fasciculus or uncinate fasciculus.

Concussion, from this perspective, is not an all-or-none lesion to a particular anatomic place but *a threat to many billions of places*. In some cases and some places, the brain's resuscitative powers are equal to the task. With luck, even though microtubules are derailed, Aβ produced, tau released, myelin is stripped, and microglia activated, even though billions of brain changes occur during the neurometabolic-vascular–degenerative–inflammatory melee (which may, in the normal course of things, taper off in about a year), the regenerative forces successfully counter the degenerative forces, and damage never progresses so far as to be irreversible. The result for that single cell or circuit is absolutely perfect recovery. That cell or circuit – or the entire brain – did not change in any way that makes it more vulnerable to the three bad outcomes we have considered: prolonged symptoms, excessive dysfunction after a second concussion, or later neurodegeneration. In other cases, the damage overwhelms the rescue systems because excessive degenerative forces push the threatened part beyond the point of no return – a theoretical tipping point after which a cell or functional circuit is helpless to rescue itself or be effectively replaced.

If this is an accurate conceptualization, one suspects that the process involves several features. One: there is no single dark force or evil humor. It's not just a matter of measuring apoptosis or Aβ or activated microglia. Multiple dangerous mechanisms operate simultaneously. Two: genes, epigenetic modifications, development, and environmental factors all impact both the likelihood of and the course of post-concussive excess degeneration. Three: since the permutations and combinations of brain injury are, for all practical purposes, beyond number, no two individuals will ever suffer the same outcome. Four: no known clinical, psychological, or biological variable predicts which patients' brains will suffer such irreversible *excess degeneration*. The remarkable diversity described here helps explain why loss of consciousness, GCS, PTA, and other superficial clinical markers have such weak predictive validity. Five: a logical corollary (and deep theoretical problem)

that the reader has probably anticipated: the long-sought gold-standard biomarker for TBI may be a hunt for a snipe. Although we may be able to detect and quantify cell death, axon dysfunction, or neurodegenerative changes, given the barely conceivable degree of biological diversity due to cell-by-cell variation in post-concussive change, *where should one mark the threshold between brain injury versus brain non-injury?* That is a profound and disconcerting question. Candidly, it may take another generation of work and thought before we have a good answer.

> The patient with a minor head injury … is looked at often in a cursory fashion by a casualty officer in a hospital … When the patient returns complaining of headache, vertigo, and inability to think clearly and to concentrate, the doctor … insists that the symptoms are nervous and that the patient need not return to him again.
>
> (Kelly, 1975 [140], p. 21)

#2. On the Risk Factor Called *History of Pre-Morbid Neuropsychiatric Problems*

As displayed in Table 7.4, evidence supports the conclusion that persons with pre-injury neuropsychiatric problems such as attention deficit disorder, learning disability, anxiety, depression, or substance abuse are more likely to suffer more serious, more numerous, or more prolonged post-concussive problems. There can be no argument about the statistical findings. Indeed, most lay people would make the same prediction, since common sense suggests that a person with a behavioral problem at time *A* is more likely to have a problem at time *B*. The question of interest is not whether pre-injury psychiatric/behavioral problems are a risk factor for occurrence or persistence of post-injury problems, but what this means. To the confirmed skeptic, the data demonstrate that hitting the brain does not cause neurobehavioral distress lasting more than a month or two, because no biological harm could possibly last that long, so persistent complaints must be attributed to pre-morbid fragility, imagination, or feigning.

That position is problematic for several reasons.

First, the rhetoric used to make the argument that concussion does not cause lasting harm often rests on fidelity to two errors: (1) unfamiliarity with the data on persistent brain damage; and (2) the Cartesian dogma of the separateness of mind and brain. History helps explain the infiltration of the latter dogma into American medicine – a detour from the admirable trajectory toward impartial science we have yet to live down. With the evolution of theories of hysteria at the turn of the 20th century, it was common for psychologists to distinguish purportedly *psychological* versus *organic* causes of illness. Medicine, at the time, was less wedded to that dichotomy. In fact, "most physicians practiced neurology and psychiatry as a combined specialty in the 1930s" [520]. In 1934, the Section on Nervous and Mental Disease of the American Medical Association joined with other stakeholders to found the American Board of Psychiatry and Neurology. That board initially offered certification in neuropsychiatry – a single, unified specialty reflecting the scientifically robust position that this is a single domain of human illness. That unanimity began to unravel with the rise of the Nazis and World War II. Those sad events provoked the migration of many psychoanalytically oriented psychiatrists to the United States. As a result of pressure for a unique professional identity, the two disciplines split. As Grinker explained in 1959 [521]: "that decision was based on realistic recognition that neuropsychiatry has become separated into neurology and psychiatry as distinct clinical specialties." The result was an unfortunate Balkanization of a coherent medical domain such that one discipline assumed ownership of the psychological, and the other grabbed the organic. Thus, the indefensible Cartesian mind/brain dichotomy became concretized in separate medical guilds.

That divisive division helps explain the perspective of 20th-century opinions about post-concussive behavioral problems. Most of the early papers reporting the statistical association between pre-morbid behavior problems and post-concussive symptoms employ the terms "psychological" and "organic" in the semantic usage of 1900. The reader sees the conceptual error: since psychological constructs are labels for brain states and traits, there is no biological basis for this mind/brain differentiation. If a previously depressed person suffers a concussion and remains symptomatic for years, that is a brain problem.

Second, the majority of those publications suffer from an obvious methodological weakness: due to the paucity of prospective population-based research, it is uncommon for concussion investigators to know what was actually wrong with the CBI survivor in the decade prior to injury. There may be a doctor's note that the patient once fell and struck her head, or a nurse's note that the patient once seemed sad. There may be self-report questionnaires of varying validity. Yet a close review of the articles in Table 7.4 that reported statistical association between pre-injury and post-injury problems reveals that, in almost every publication, the conclusions are not supported by a definitive pre-morbid diagnosis, let alone stratification by diagnosis. Just one example: a recent study of three-month post-CBI outcome [503] included interviews to probe for "a history of mood problems, substance abuse, or personal trauma" (p. 71). That non-specific and unconfirmed reportage about pre-injury status was coded in the variable: "presence or absence of psychiatric history." Thus, suicidal depression and occasional marijuana use would be equated. This kind of variable lumping may prevent statistical detection of important associations. Without better efforts to diagnose specific pre-morbid disorders and stratify analysis of the correlations between those disorders and CBI outcome, the vast majority of reported findings have nominal significance.

A single recent paper deserves attention for breaking that mold. Nelson et al. [522] prospectively assessed 2055 high school and college athletes using measures of cognition, symptoms, balance, and well-being, including the Brief Symptom Inventory-18 somatization scale [523]. According to the observations of athletic trainers, 127 subjects were subsequently concussed. Follow-up was pursued for 45 days post injury. Duration of complaints was predicted by pre-injury somatization scores. As the first authentic prospective study of its kind, these findings possibly support the hypothesis that pre-morbid perceived physical distress is associated with post-concussion symptoms. However, confidence in the findings is limited by the fact that the authors only studied school-affiliated athletes – a group that notoriously misrepresents their own symptoms – and followed up very briefly, obviating any conclusion about persistent problems. Moreover, the authors did not assess brain change. The justifiable conclusion: boys who are willing to express feelings about their bodies before a concussion are willing to express feelings about their bodies after a concussion. A proper prospective longitudinal study awaits doing.

Third, a plurality of 20th-century papers on this subject discuss post-traumatic symptoms as if they were universal. That is, investigators have correctly noted that, three months after a concussion or a limb fracture, the number of complaints is about the same. This factual observation is then used to support a logical error: some investigators concluded that the psychological impact of trauma itself, not physical brain change, must therefore explain prolonged post-concussive problems. That argument would be worthy of consideration if all traumatic injuries were followed by the same symptoms. They are not. Indeed, there will be considerable overlap between the symptoms listed by the survivor of an accident with a broken leg or a shaken brain; the signs of traumatic stress (anguished or blank facial expressions, sweat, tremor, agitation, distraction) have surely been recognizable to adult hominids since bipedalism. But brain injury has unique effects not expected in other trauma, such as double vision, dizziness, impaired new learning with preserved declarative memory, slowed thinking, and imbalance. The main point is simple: the relationship between pre-morbid behavioral traits and brain injury is different from the relationship between pre-morbid behavioral traits and non-specific trauma in two obvious ways: (1) unlike in the circumstances of other traumas (e.g., scary accidents that injure limbs), the shaken brain was *already* atypical; CBI then paints on a pre-figured canvas; (2) unlike in other traumas, the tissue that is wrenched and disconcerted mediates feelings.

Let us briefly compare the two. Recall Georgia, the 29-year-old high school teacher and equestrienne discussed at the beginning of this chapter. She began with a disadvantage. In the 120 months prior to her concussion she was dysthymic for 29 months and depressed to the point of disability for 11 months. That is, before her fall from Sandy, she already had atypical brain function, perhaps affecting the ventromedial prefrontal–medial temporal lobar circuitry of emotional regulation as well as a large number of functionally connected parts from her lower brainstem to her frontal convexities. What would have happened if, in her fall, Georgia's primary tissue injury was a broken leg? That painful, stressful event would have impacted the function of her hypothalamic–pituitary–adrenal (HPA) axis and her already-abnormal limbic tissue. Arousal and stress would have provoked changes in neurotransmission involving amines and steroids, ions and receptors. It would have been no surprise if she expressed more pain and emotional upset than average after her fracture. One cannot argue with the view that pre-morbid emotional sensitivity tends to be associated with a higher likelihood of post-traumatic distress.

What in fact happened when Georgia suffered her equestrian-related CBI? Again – a universal mammalian stress response – this event impacted her HPA axis and limbic tissue. But in addition to the commonplace changes in transmitters and hormones, she probably up- or down-regulated expression of about a thousand neuronal and glial genes. Her neurons suffered Ca^{2+}-associated excitatory neurotoxicity, axonal stretch, microtubule disarray, liberated P-tau, excess Aβ production, microglial activation, apoptosis, demyelination, microvascular damage – too many CBI-associated changes to list. Just as in the case of a leg fracture, sensitive Georgia was at risk for a more prolonged recovery simply because acute stress is hard on a fragile brain.

However, *above and beyond* the circumscribed brain changes after a broken leg, CBI tends to physically damage the cerebral circuits of memory, balance, and eye movements, as well as the tissue that mediates subjective response – the limbic and peri-limbic circuits of emotional regulation. Abundant research supports this prediction, although it may require a decade or more to refine the technology to visualize these differences. In the meantime, it is a plausible hypothesis: when the brain of a neurobehaviorally atypical person is rattled by an abrupt external force in a traumatic event, the resulting brain changes represent a double hit (stress plus mechanical shaking) on already-atypical circuits.

Note: this analysis is not to imply that pre-morbid depression has a particular uniform biological basis and therefore, for instance, depression-plus-concussion yields a predictable result. Far from it. Neuroatypicality is infinitely variable and unique to every organism. To say, "Georgia has a history of depression" means, "Georgia has had periods of subjective distress reflecting molecular happenings unique to her in all the world and far beyond our capacity to analyze. For practical clinical purposes it seems reasonable to equate her unique condition with a familiar category of distress – an abstract ideal type we call 'depression' that seems to exhibit some degree of homogeneity, although it is better considered an overt (observable) phenotypic destination of multiple genetic and environmental pathways that differ from one sad person to the next." Georgia's depression, for example, might have been associated with a particular genetic polymorphism that affects amine transport, or an inflammatory response, or some other aspect of cerebral integrity in a way that interacted with the post-CBI

biological melee. A different person who also had a history of "pre-morbid depression" and survived a biologically identical CBI down to the last integrin might have an altogether different outcome.

The question often arises, "Is Georgia's long-term post-CBI depression caused by her pre-morbid depression or by her brain injury?" We will return to the illogic of such a question below when we revisit the drama of attribution. The author only asks that the reader consider his or her answer to that question. Can one meaningfully apportion causality to one of these factors or the other? If so, how?

In brief summary: it seems very reasonable that some pre-morbid neuropsychiatric traits are risk factors and help to explain some of the variance in outcome. Studies (of widely varying quality) support the conclusion that a history of learning disability or attention deficit-hyperactivity disorder [26, 524, 525], anxiety [11, 19, 23, 25], depression [19, 22, 25], or PTSD [24, 526] increases the likelihood of more or longer post-CBI problems.[25] One need not review the specific evidence for each, or critique the methodology of the weaker contributions. The fact that human distress tends to make a brain injury harder to bear would be predicted simply on the basis of the overlapping neurobiology, if it were not already obvious based on common sense. In the author's opinion, the last stains of controversy about these matters are rapidly fading. Our conclusions should not provoke debate:

1. Yes, pre-morbid neuropsychiatric problems are risk factors for worse outcome after CBI.
2. No, pre-morbid neuropsychiatric problems do not fully explain worse outcome after CBI.
3. Most important: post-concussive neuropsychiatric problems are somewhat treatable. Rather than blaming the victim for his or her delayed recovery, TBI experts should perhaps focus on alleviating his or her distress.

#3. On the Risk Factor Called *Female Sex*

Sex differences have been reported in outcomes after TBIs of all severities, but the findings are not altogether consistent. With regard to moderate and severe TBI, one meta-analysis reported that women fared worse than men on 85% of measures [527]. Another meta-analysis reported that women fared worse in two of eight high-quality studies but no sex difference was found in the other six studies [528]. At least one study reports that cognitive outcome was actually superior among women [529]. Research on "mild TBI" has also produced inconsistent findings. One 2016 opinion piece [530] concluded that the evidence of sex differences after "mTBI" was not persuasive, claiming, "Most studies did not find a sex difference for postconcussion symptoms in children and adults" (p. S5). Unfortunately, that commentary

---

[25] It also deserves mention that causality works in more than one way: attention deficit-hyperactivity disorder (ADHD) and substance abuse (and perhaps PTSD) are risk factors for TBI, and TBI is a risk factor for PTSD (and perhaps ADHD).

confined its attention to a small subset of the literature and misrepresented the few studies it reviewed.[26] In actuality, the majority of peer-reviewed follow-up studies report that females aged 15–55 are more likely to have worse outcome after concussion. Teen and adult women typically report a larger number of complaints for a longer average period of time [4–7, 10–12, 19, 21, 534–541].

It is also important to consider the nature of the problems diagnosed among CBI survivors of the two sexes. Teen girls and adult women are prone to post-concussive neuropsychiatric problems, especially depression. This is consistent with findings regarding the long-term impact of TBI regardless of severity. For instance, Scott et al. [542] reported that many adults of both sexes who had suffered TBI in childhood (mild, moderate, or severe) exhibited long-term neurobehavioral problems, but that females tended to develop internalizing disorders (e.g., depression) while males tended to develop externalizing disorders (e.g., aggression). For these reasons, rather than assessing outcome by the number of complaints, the present author urges attention to quality of life. Sex differences in concussion outcome are not absolute or consistent. Sex differences seem to be larger or smaller in different age groups and between alternate mechanisms of injury. Nonetheless, strong evidence suggests that, despite a lower incidence of CBI through most life stages as well as a lesser average injury severity, concussed teen girls and women suffer more than concussed teen boys and men.

The female sex risk factor deserves attention not only because it may inspire discoveries in the neurobiology of CBI but also because it has practical medical implications. At the time of this writing, no treatment is known to produce a benefit after acute TBI. Is that because a single fix should not be expected to work for a heterogeneous problem? Given the wealth of evidence of sex differences in response to concussion, it seems vital that clinical investigators consider that different treatments may be optimal for men and for women.

That is the principal take-home finding from a systematic review. However, that summary statement oversimplifies an increasingly intriguing biological story about sex and the brain. Our goal in this section is again to quest beyond the merely epidemiological association and explain *why* sex differences occur. In this case, a fine-grained analysis of epidemiology provides hints regarding the biological basis of the sex-related differences in outcome. To foreshadow our denouement: females indeed exhibit worse outcome – *but only during a particular stage of life*.

History

The historical progress in explanation for sex-related difference in outcome from head trauma, or from any trauma, has tracked closely with the progress in overthrowing both Cartesian dogma (mind/brain or psychological/organic separateness) and sexist prejudice. Impartial clinicians have observed for centuries that women (1) have a higher incidence of emotional illnesses than men, and (2) have a higher incidence of emotional complications of other illnesses. The frequency of Axis I mood and anxiety disorders is indisputably higher [543–550]. Again, the question is why? A century ago many medical men would have confidently attributed feminine predisposition to emotional problems to innate weakness or to "hysteria." Figure 7.17 depicts two giants of 19th-century neurology, Drs. Charcot and Babinsky, during an 1880s lecture and demonstration on that subject at the renowned Pitié-Salpêtrière Hospital in Paris.

The emphasis on hysteria as the explanation for sex differences in certain mental disorders persisted well into the tawdry mid-20th-century era during which American psychiatry was distracted by psychodynamic thought. Unfortunately, an important scientific fact – the sex difference in the incidence of disabling depression – was co-opted by some persons seeking evidence of supposed female fragility.

Sex is often listed in epidemiological reports about brain injury as a "demographic" trait. But sex should not be classified among traits such as zip code and household income; it is a biological trait unique to a subset of animals. Although most people realize without academic input that sex has profound implications for individual and group behavior among social species, it has recently become evident that sex and associated biological differences profoundly influence vulnerability to and resilience in the face of the same diseases [549, 553, 554]. Moreover, contrary to a 1960s political claim of perfect neurobiological equality, there are systematic sex differences in many aspects of brain structure and function. Before readers revolt, the author does not mean to resurrect the puerile biases of mid-20th-century North America. The goal is merely to credit the scientific observations of the 21st century. In the author's opinion, the persistence of references to female psychological fragility, even in late-20th-century TBI writing, reflects nostalgia for an unapologetically sexist era. Rather than reflexive resort to dogma, a better approach might be to carefully attend to the growing host of known neurobiological concomitants of gender – surely the first place one should search for mechanisms explaining difference in disease risk.

Sexual Dimorphism

Among potential scientific explanations for different outcomes after a blow to the head, the most obvious question is whether male and female heads (and head contents) differ. They do. To begin with, "the forehead of the skull is one of the human parts

---

[26] These writers reached their conclusion based on counting up studies that did and did not report sex differences from within a tiny and non-systematically selected subset of the existing literature. Even so, they misrepresented their own cherry-picked data. For instance, they included a study as proof of no sex difference in outcomes that never addressed that question [530]. They included a study that judged post-concussive symptoms less than one month after injury [531]. They included a study the outcome of which was unrelated to health or well-being [532]. Most concerningly, they included a study that clearly reported that females had worse outcome ("Female athletes performed worse than male athletes on visual memory (mean, 65.1% and 70.1%, respectively; $P = .049$) and reported more symptoms (mean, 14.4 and 10.1, respectively) after concussion ($P = .035$") [533] but claimed that that study *did not* report sex differences. The same authors wrote, "No sex difference was found for risk of dementia." This is another serious misstatement of the scientific evidence, as a later chapter of this essay will demonstrate.

Charcot explains women's health

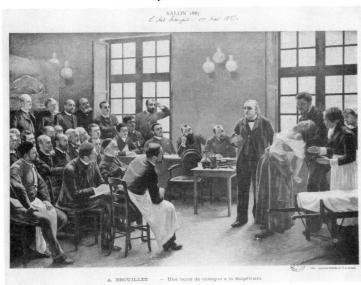

Fig. 7.17 Charcot demonstrating hypnosis on a "hysterical" Salpêtrière patient, Blanche Wittmann, who is supported by Dr. Joseph Babiński (rear). Each of the 30 individuals represented in this painting has been identified.

Source: *Une leçon clinique à la Salpêtrière*: Pierre Aristide, André Brouillet, 1887 [551, 552] with permission from BIU Santé (Paris) / CIPC0011

that show remarkable sex difference" [555]. Although skull thickness is not systematically different, a variety of geometric measures reliably distinguish male from female skulls [556]. An inescapable prediction is that if identical abrupt external forces visit identical skull loci in a man and a woman, their skulls will differently disperse that force to the brain.

Sexual dimorphism is also reported both for total brain volume (9–12% larger in males) and for regional anatomy. Note, however, that those sex differences are age-dependent [496, 557–561]. The differences reported below are those found in mature adult women, typically between age 18 and 59. Table 7.5 briefly summarizes the major gross anatomical findings, emphasizing those reported in Riugrok et al.'s 2014 meta-analysis of regional differences [561–564]. Figure 7.19 displays the regions of reported anatomical sex differences based on that analysis. Note that most brain regions do not exhibit obvious sexual dimorphism. As one might intuit, some evidence suggests a correlation between the density of sex hormone receptors and the regions exhibiting the greatest degree of sex-related difference [564, 565].

Frankly, most of this knowledge regarding regional sexual dimorphisms does not answer, in any obvious way, why CBI is more harmful to women – any more than knowing that the corresponding parts of two Swiss watches are different sizes explains different vulnerability to being dropped. Still, the consistent reports that men have larger hippocampi at least raise the question of brain reserve: the hippocampus is both uniquely vulnerable to CBI and uniquely important for emotional and memory processes. Might men's bigger hippocampi and amygdali confer an advantage when confronted with a rattling external force? At the very least, known differences in both skull and brain anatomy suggest that FEM should be sex-specific.

Remaining at the level of regional analysis (before considering chemical, microscopic, or molecular factors), some evidence suggests that emotional disorders differentially impact

Table 7.5 Regions of the brain reported to exhibit average sex differences in volume, controlled for total brain size

Regions of reported female superiority in gray-matter volume	Regions of reported male superiority in gray-matter volume
Bilateral inferior and middle frontal gyri	Right frontal pole
Bilateral pars triangularis	Bilateral amygdalae
Bilateral thalami	Bilateral putamen
Broca's area	Bilateral temporal poles
Bilateral anterior cingulate gyri	Bilateral posterior cingulate gyri
Bilateral planum temporale/parietal operculum	Bilateral angular gyri
Left parahippocampal gyrus	Bilateral anterior parahippocampal gyri
Bilateral insular cortex	Bilateral precuneus
Bilateral caudate nucleus	Bilateral cerebellum: VIIb, VIIIa, and crus I
Heschl's gyrus	Bilateral hippocampi
Superior division of the lateral occipital cortex	Left cerebellum: VI; right cerebellum: crus II

brain structure. For instance, depressed women reportedly exhibit emotional dysregulation as well as structural abnormalities in ACC, inferior orbital frontal cortex, and anterior insula [566, 567]; it is not clear whether such findings represent premorbid risk factors or pathological consequences of depression.

One might also consider the recently available data that strongly suggest sex differences in the connectome – the map of cerebral connectivity. For instance, Sun et al. [568] used DTI to visualize global and regional patterns of connectivity among adults aged 21–59. The authors reported that males had a higher total number of white-matter fibers and that, controlling for both brain size and fiber numbers, males exhibited superior processing efficiency. This methodology also permits localization of critical cerebral "addresses" that function as hubs or nodes for information processing. Among 15 hubs examined, most were found in both sexes. However, only scans of males detected functional nodes in four regions: the left superior frontal gyrus, left lingual gyrus, left fusiform gyrus, and right inferior temporal gyrus. In contrast, only scans of females detected nodes in the left post-central gyrus, left superior temporal gyrus, right middle cingulate gyri, and right cuneus (Figure 7.18).[27]

In a comparable study ten times the size, Ingalhalikar et al. [569] assayed the connectomes of 949 healthy young people, aged eight to 22. The data suggested greater connectivity *between* hemispheres among females but greater connectivity *within* hemispheres among males. The authors interpreted their data as follows: "The observations suggest that male brains are structured to facilitate connectivity between perception and coordinated action, whereas female brains are designed to facilitate communication between analytical and intuitive processing modes." In the present author's opinion, it seems imprudent to abstract lessons about sex differences by resorting to psychological constructs that imply valid and reliable localization of specific cognitive functions (not to mention the unfortunate reference to "design"). "Intuitive," for instance, is not known to be a tissue trait. Still, taking the rhetoric with a grain of salt, these connectome studies support the hypothesis that males and females successfully accomplish survival-relevant information processing using different brain structures and functions.

Theoretically speaking (and awaiting empirical testing), these sex differences observed in the connectome could help explain females' vulnerability to worse outcome after concussion in at least two ways. One: if a man begins with more white-matter fibers he may have more of a reserve in regard to axon damage. Two: if a woman's information processing is more reliant on long-distance white-matter connectivity, her brain may be more prone to axonal injury because long tracts are more vulnerable to mechanical forces.

Cytoarchitectonic dimorphism is also observed. Men tend to have more neurons, higher neuronal density, and more synapses, even controlling for body size. Ruigrok et al.'s [561] meta-analysis reported that men exhibit consistently higher gray-matter density in the left amygdala, hippocampus, insular cortex, pallidum, putamen, claustrum, and one sub-region in area VI of the right cerebellum. Women tend to have significantly higher gray-matter density in the left frontal pole [561], perhaps higher neuronal densities in the granular cortical layers [564], and possibly larger neurons than men, especially in the left hemisphere [570]. Again, the observation that men tend to have large hippocampi with denser complements of neurons conceivably makes male brains more resilient in the face of partial hippocampal cell loss.[28]

Evidence also suggests that depression and anxiety among adult females are associated with hormonal and genetic factors.

Nodes of functional connectivity exhibiting sex differences on diffusion tensor imaging

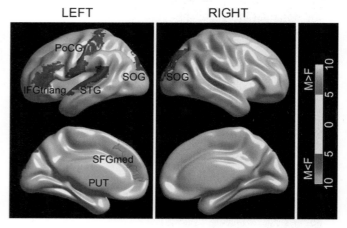

Fig. 7.18 The spatial distribution of cortical regions showing significant gender effect. The color bar represents F values of group comparison. Left and right represent left and right hemispheres, respectively. IFGtriang: inferior frontal gyrus (triangular); PoCG: post-central gyrus; PUT: putamen; SFGmed: superior frontal gyrus (medial); SOG: superior occipital gyrus; STG: superior temporal gyrus. [A black and white version of this figure will appear in some formats. For the color version, please refer to the plate section.]
Source: Sun et al., 2015 [568]. Reproduced under the terms of the Creative Commons Attribution licence, CC-BY.

Multiple studies attribute the excess vulnerability to emotional distress to steroid hormones, or to the fluctuation of hormone levels [571–573]. Other evidence suggests a link between female stress vulnerability and a combination of steroid hormone and amine transmitter differences [574]. Recently, several studies have reported associations between emotional distress among women and polymorphisms of the gene for catechol-O-methyltransferase [575–577].

It is premature to generate a unitary theory explaining girls' and women's increased emotional vulnerability, and the interaction between biological and environmental/social causes of stress has yet to be explored. It is conceivable that female excess of post-concussive problems merely reflects a difference in stress reactivity. However, this author guesses that matters may be more complex; perhaps – in addition to differential stress sensitivity – the specific neurometabolic–vascular–inflammatory changes of CBI synergize with sex-related biological differences to create an extraordinary risk to emotion-related systems. For many reasons, that risk may impact men and women differently. One study, for example, recruited men and women – all with prefrontal cortical brain damage. Given the location of the damage, one would suspect some alteration in their stress responsiveness. All were exposed to the same stressors in a laboratory. Despite their similar brain lesions, women systematically differed from men in their self-reported stress, their cortisol responses, and their heart rate reactivity [578]. We are only beginning to explore how sex differences in brain lead to sex differences in human distress.

---

[27] The authors also tested for within-subject aging-related change. They report that males and females exhibit different trajectories of evolving connectivity in the insula, superior temporal gyrus, cuneus, putamen, and parahippocampal gyrus.

[28] Note, however, that some investigators have reported women to have larger hippocampi than men after correction for brain size [561].

Voxel-based regional sex differences in grey matter volume based on a meta-analysis

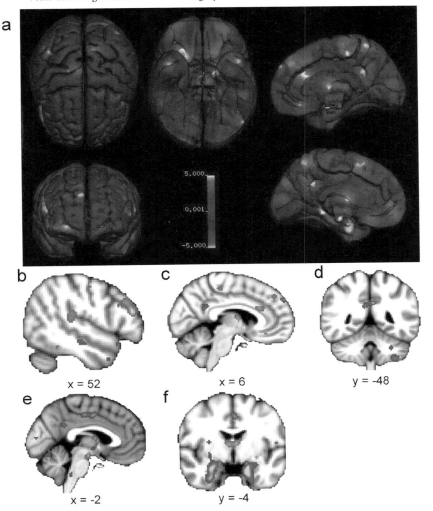

Fig. 7.19 Female > Male in red, and Male > Female is in blue. Panel a, rendered overview of uncorrected regional sex differences in grey matter volume. All other panels are thresholded at FDR q < 0.01. Panels b–f display areas of larger volume in females (red) including (b) the right inferior and middle frontal gyri, pars triangularis and planum temporale; (c) thalamus and right anterior cingulate gyrus; and (f) left and right thalamus; and areas of larger volume in males (blue), including (c) the anterior cingulate gyrus; (d) bilateral posterior cingulate gyrus and precuneus and left cerebellum; (e) anterior and posterior cingulate gyri; and (f) left and right amygdalae, hippocampi and parahippocampal gyri. [A black and white version of this figure will appear in some formats. For the color version, please refer to the plate section.]

Source: Ruigrok et al., Elsevier 2014 [561]. Reproduced under the terms of the Creative Commons Attribution licence, CC-BY.

Sex Differences Observed in Concussed Brains

Surprisingly few experimental (animal) studies report sex differences in the immediate aftermath of concussion. However, Acaz-Fonseca et al. [200] published a sophisticated investigation of a sex difference in the post-CBI inflammatory response. Recall previous comments in this chapter: markers of inflammation such as microglia do not, by themselves, comprise a threat. There seem to be both helpful and harmful aspects to the post-CBI inflammatory response. Acaz-Fonseca et al. [200] inflicted a penetrating TBI on adult mice and assayed three elements of that response.[29] Males exhibit both a more robust inflammatory reaction and less neuronal loss than females.

To make sense of this result, two details must be mentioned. One: microglia and macrophages are not all alike. As they invade through the damaged blood–brain barrier, these cells can adopt a pro-inflammatory "classic" M1 phenotype or a non-inflammatory M2 phenotype. Two: recruitment of these cells to the site of an injury depends on the chemokine CCL2. The authors of this experiment found that female mice were CCL2-deficient. Assembling these blocks into an understandable form: adult female mice failed to recruit the non-inflammatory microglia they needed to help contain and heal the wound and suffered more neuron loss as a result. It remains to be seen if this is a key explanation for worse outcome among adult human females [579].[30]

---

[29] Using antibodies against glial fibrillary acidic protein to mark total astrocytes, vimentin to mark activated astrocytes, and ionized calcium binding adaptor molecule 1 (IbA1) as a marker of macrophages and microglia.

[30] One DTI study reported sex differences in human post-CBI brain change: Fakhran et al. [578] found: (1) that females showed less of a decrease in FA in the uncinate fasciculus; and (2) that decrease correlated with time to recovery. However, recovery in this study was measured by conventional neuropsychological tests, not by sensitive markers of brain health.

On Beyond Dimorphism

Among females, mean adjusted PCS scores exceed those of males beginning around menarche, peak during the child-bearing years, and then return to the level of males after menopause … This observation suggests that post-mTBI outcome may be more physiological than sociological.

Bazarian et al., 2010 [6], p. 534

We have established that there exist sexual dimorphisms in the head (skull) and its contents (brain). Average sex differences in white matter and hippocampus are possible factors relevant to the observed differences in average CBI outcome. Yet gross anatomical dimorphisms and cell counts may be less important than molecular differences in determining whether a given brain degenerates beyond the point of no return. A more promising avenue of inquiry may be to focus on differences in the post-concussive melee, such as the sex difference in the traumatic inflammatory response reported above. One expects rapid advances in this domain, especially as neuroscientists graduate from the neurometabolic cascade paradigm to the paradigm of a competition between degeneration and regeneration.

However, the author offers a prediction: a full understanding of the clinical variation observed in outcome requires attention to another basic difference: men have brains that exhibit similar biological traits day after day. Women have brains that cycle. As implied by the above citation from Bazarian et al. [6], it is not all females who are prone to worse outcomes after concussion; *it is menstruating women who are at risk.*

Why?

One might begin to address that question by first noting the baffling inconsistencies between animal and human data. In experimental TBI, strong evidence suggests that adult female status, estrogen, and progesterone are all neuroprotective. Female rodents exhibit superior post-concussive cerebral blood flow and *less* edema [580]. Estrogen has anti-excitatory neurotoxic, anti-oxidant, anti-apoptotic, anti-Aβ and anti-inflammatory effects [581]. Recent data suggest that estradiol's anti-inflammatory effect is mediated by up-regulation of neuroglobin [200].[31] Progesterone therapy has demonstrated efficacy for preserving neurons and functions in multiple animal trials [582–587]. In contrast, and dishearteningly, progesterone therapy has *not* demonstrated efficacy in multiple trials for the management of human TBI [559, 588, 589]. Although those trials have been critiqued for failure to employ sensitive outcome assessments [587], it remains unproven that (1) women have better outcomes than men or (2) women derive any benefit from progesterone intervention. Thus, there are unexplained species differences.

Second, if female sex hormones have neuroprotective effects, it is logical to expect that cyclic differences in hormone levels would impact outcome. For example, given the strong evidence that progesterone is protective in animals, one would predict that concussion in the luteal phases (when progesterone is high) would be less injurious. Wagner et al. [581] tested this hypothesis in adult rats: "No significant differences were found

on any task between injured females regardless of estrous cycle stage" (p. 113). Yet females exhibited superior performance compared with males in post-injury motor function. The authors interpreted those results as suggesting that presence of circulating female hormones itself is sufficient for protection, but cyclic variation is not sufficient to produce detectable differences. In contrast, a human study [580] reported that women injured in the luteal phase had *lower* quality-of-life ratings at one month compared with women injured during the follicular phase. This is exactly the opposite of the result one would expect based on the animal literature.

Given these inconsistencies, it remains mysterious why cycling women seem to have worse post-concussive outcomes. No simple and consistent "progesterone is neuroprotective" conclusion is possible. One suspects that something about the cycling of women's brains – either a factor present throughout the cycle or at a particular phase – renders them more vulnerable to one or more of the harmful facets of the post-concussive melee. But which one?

It is conceivable that the focus on sex steroids and neurons has distracted us from other female- or cycle-related biology that might answer this question. For example, even without reference to diagnosable Axis I disorders, women on average experience more negative and anxious feelings than men, exhibit more fear and distress after trauma, have higher rates of depression, and are perhaps more prone to PTSD [590–593]. Some evidence links PTSD to aspects of HPA response to stress, including baseline variation in glucocorticoid metabolism and cortisol production at the time of acute stress [594, 595].

The story, however, is not "women generate larger cortisol bumps than men in response to stress and are therefore more likely to get sad or anxious." To the contrary, young men tend to have larger stress-related cortisol reaction than young women [592, 596]. Instead, *women's brains may respond differently to the same levels of cortisol*, perhaps due to differences in hormone receptor distribution or endocrine feedback loops, or perhaps because of sex-related differences in inflammatory cytokine production [597]. Recent research suggests another link between female sex and HPA reactivity: (1) estrogen triggers the production of corticotropin-releasing-hormone (CRH) in the paraventricular hypothalamic nucleus; (2) estrogen response elements have been reported in the promoter region of the gene for CRH; and (3) many of the CRH neurons active in the source of mood disorders co-express estrogen receptors [598]. More generally speaking, evidence shows that women's and men's brains process stress differently at the subcortical level and that, among women, that subcortical stress response is menstrual phase-dependent [599].

Both baseline and stress-related glucocorticoid production also seem to be phase-dependent. Like progesterone, this is highest during the mid luteal phase [600]. Thus, young women in the luteal phase match men in cortisol reactions to stress [596, 601]. Moreover, both the HPA response to stress and the influence of cortisol on memory consolidation are

---

[31] The reader is reminded, however, that anti-inflammation may not be desirable, since there are probably helpful aspects to inflammation.

also elevated during the luteal phase [601–603]. In addition, women exhibit negative emotional bias for information processing and enhanced emotionality of memories consolidated during the luteal phase – for instance, reporting more spontaneous intrusive memories – a finding also associated with progesterone levels [600, 604–607]. These findings join a host of others strongly supporting the conclusion that phase of menstrual cycle does, in fact, somewhat impact the mind [600, 603, 608]. One treads gently. The point is not that women are mental slaves to a carnival ride of neurobiological fluctuation but that subtle variation in some domains may marginally alter thresholds of vulnerability to disease.

In a report that seemingly weaves these observations together in a coherent and plausible way, Bryant et al. [600] evaluated the emotional reaction of 138 women to traumatic injuries, including TBI. After controlling for age, type of injury, and severity of injury, women who had been in the luteal phase at the time of the injury were almost five times as likely to suffer flashbacks. The authors concluded: "Increased glucocorticoid release associated with the luteal phase of the menstrual cycle may facilitate consolidation of trauma memories" (p. 398). Note that the finding of worse outcome after luteal-phase trauma matches that of Wunderle et al. [580]. It therefore seems worth considering that cycling-related factors *other than* the impact of sex hormones on neuronal survival explain women's increased vulnerability to concussion. Emotional processing – influenced by the phase-dependent combination of elevated glucocorticoids and progesterone – may trump mere brain cell survival as a factor in quality of life after concussion.

Another factor of possible relevance: Laskowski et al. [609] recently summarized the evidence that DA signaling is altered, DA receptor expression is increased, and DA-related changes may be implicated in working-memory deficits after concussion. Other evidence from fMRI studies implicates DA transmission rate in the efficacy of working memory [610]. Luteal phase-related change in DA transmission may therefore make the female brain more vulnerable to trauma during that phase – another potential disadvantage when cycling is combined with concussion. Yet another factor of possible interest: data suggest that post-traumatic cerebral edema is more common and more severe in women up to age 50 [611].

Taken together, these findings hint at several pathophysiological mechanisms by which adult women, but not necessarily female mice, could experience worse outcome after concussion. Neurobiological differences may tip the balance of forces in the direction of degeneration, especially during the luteal phase. Women possibly exhibit more post-concussive emotional and cognitive problems due to the interplay of external force with cerebral factors that may not occur (or may not be detectable) in rodents.

In brief summary, at the time of this writing – and admittedly based on inconsistent empirical data – female sex appears to be statistically associated with worse outcome after CBI among humans roughly aged 13–58 because menstruating girls and women are at higher risk for brain harm, especially if concussed during the luteal phase. Simply put, men and women from early teens through middle age may have slightly different responses to CBI because men and luteal-phase menstruating women have slightly different brains.

If this explanation is confirmed by high-quality prospective longitudinal studies, two implications come to mind. One is practical: these observations may enhance the theoretical sophistication of further treatment trials. It is possible that men and women in this age group would benefit from slightly different interventions and, conceivably, that women injured at the luteal phase might benefit from somewhat different treatment from those injured in the follicular phase. The other is a practical, immediately applicable conclusion that is highly unlikely to be heeded: although one does not expect many athletes to use the rhythm method to organize their sporting schedules, neurologists conceivably have a duty to warn girls and women of these observations.

#4. On the Risk Factor Called *Age*

Most aging-and-TBI research has focused on the moderate-to-severe cohort. One cannot assume that the published findings apply to so-called "mild" events that comprise the overwhelming majority of CBIs. Nonetheless, a brief review suggests a more sophisticated final answer than "old people do worse."

It is reasonably well established that, following a single moderate or severe TBI, persons in the youngest and oldest cohorts are prone to more post-concussive problems – whether this is measured on a functional scale such as the GOS or a symptom survey such as the Rivermead [31]. Children younger than age four[32] and adults over age 65 reportedly exhibit more disability and higher rates of mortalities than persons injured in between those extremes of age. One visualizes an inverted-U-shaped curve of vulnerability. However, there are nuances to this standard curve that inspire contemplation. For one: although elderly victims of TBI are more likely to die than younger victims, this claim may merely reflect the fact that elderly persons are more likely to die. It is a truism, not a discovery that reveals an interaction between the biologies of aging and brain injury. For another: although older victims of TBI exhibit worse overall outcomes, they may have better neuropsychiatric outcomes – an observation that has yet to be explained.

First, some studies have reported that older victims of moderate to severe TBI are more likely to die [613–617]. Other studies do not report this association [618–620]. That inconsistency may be explained by Nott et al. [621]: "Crude mortality rates, which do not account for the naturally increasing rate of death associated with ageing, artificially inflate estimates of age-related mortality risk following TBI" (p. E1). A more important finding may be that the relative increase in mortality is much greater among young TBI survivors than

---

[32] Experimental research suggests that increased vulnerability to oxidative stress may partially account for the unique sensitivity of children under age four [611]. However, human data are not available.

among older survivors [621]. In fact, as Harrison-Felix et al. reported, "Teenagers, young, and middle-aged adults are particularly at risk for early mortality" ([615], p. E53), and, "The age stratified SMR [standardized mortality ratio] was largest among those 15 to 19 years of age. This indicates that individuals with TBI between 15 to 19 years of age at the time of injury were almost 5 times more likely to die than individuals of similar age, gender, and race in the general population" ([615], p. E48). To date, however, no large-scale prospective study has meaningfully addressed the question, "does concussion (aka 'mild TBI') at any particular age of injury increase the subsequent mortality rate?" For the time being, no answer is available.

Second, it is widely and consistently reported that older victims of moderate to severe TBI are more likely to have poor functional outcomes [14, 622–630]. In a typical report: Hukkelhoven et al. [631] found, "the odds for a poor outcome increased by 40 to 50% per 10 years of age" (p. 666). This finding may reflect, in part, elderly victims exhibiting larger average lesion volumes [632]. Some of the cited studies included mild cases [622, 628, 629], but none stratified results by severity, making it impossible to determine whether the reported negative relationship between age and outcome applied to that subgroup. However, Jacobs et al. [14] found that older age also predicted worse outcome after "mild traumatic brain injury."

Various animal research findings are possibly pertinent to the observed excess vulnerability of the elderly. For instance, one study reported that elderly mice exhibit a hyper-inflammatory response to traumatic injury [633]. Another study reported that synaptic mitochondria are more susceptible to disrupted function after TBI [634]. A third study found that elderly animals exhibit a deficit in synaptic plasticity in response to mild TBI, apparently related to decreased cyclic adenosine monophosphate signaling [635]. One expects more such findings with further research. But these pathophysiological details may all contribute to a final common pathway.

Another finding of possible relevance: TBI aside, older persons are more vulnerable to primary ICH and more likely to suffer lasting consequences of ICH [636–639]. The reasons are not entirely clear, in part because few epidemiological studies control for subtype of ICH, use of platelet-modifying agents, family history, amyloid angiopathy, or other potential confounders. One possible explanation is a change in the inflammatory response to bleeding [640, 641]. Although it has yet to be settled how sex impacts this aging-related increase in bleeding risk, some evidence suggests that the vulnerability is greatest among post-menopausal women [642–645]. Conceivably (revisiting sex differences in brains) this reflects the fact that sexual dimorphisms in vascular function, inflammation, and other traits are somewhat aging-related [646]. One

suspects that a higher risk of hemorrhage in CBI contributes to the observed worse outcome among the elderly.

In the light of these findings, the author tentatively proposes a simple overarching explanation for worse outcome among the elderly: aging means a greater vulnerability to the degenerative, vascular, and inflammatory elements of concussion and a lower capacity for plasticity/neurogenesis. These are not co-morbid "diseases." One need not posit, for instance, that Aβ and tau deposition are *disorders*. These universal aging-related biological phenomena, like wrinkly skin, simply exemplify the inescapable nature of the passage of time after birth[33] [336, 338, 647–650, 652–655]. Both accelerated degeneration and impaired reactive plasticity mean progressive loss of functional reserve and resilience. Thus, up to a point, one can continue to learn and perform all of the life tasks essential to survival despite losses in neuron, synapses, brain size, and neurogenetic prowess. After that point – an observation surely obvious in the Neolithic and documented since the dawn of writing – there is loss of ability to learn and other forms of functional impairment. Elderly persons have less reserve, so additional CBI-caused loss of adaptability is more apparent.

Some data support this hypothesis. Chen et al. [656], for instance, recently reported that concussion harmed functional brain activation and working memory. However, younger survivors of CBI were significantly more likely to exhibit partial recovery of functional patterns and resolution of post-concussion symptoms. The authors opined, "These findings … supported that younger patients have better neural plasticity and clinical recovery than do older patients."

Third, if outcome is exploded into its diverse components and attention is paid to psychological health and well-being rather than, for instance, paper-and-pencil test scores, then age has a more complex effect. Deb and Burns [657], for example, found that "18–65 year old patients are likely to be at a greater risk of psychiatric morbidity following TBI than over 65 year olds" (p. 301). Similarly, Senathi-Raja et al. [629] found that younger adults displayed more anxiety and depression with longer time after brain injury, while older adults actually displayed *less* psychiatric distress with the passage of time. And Juengst et al. [658] reported, "We found that those over 60, when compared with those under 30, were most likely to have high satisfaction and were more likely to have improving satisfaction, even if it was initially low" (p. 359). Comparable results have been reported for typical concussions. For instance, Rapoport et al. [659] found that older adults were less likely than younger adults to exhibit major depression after CBI.

The reason for elderly patients' apparent psychiatric resilience in the face of TBI is not known. Juengst et al. [658] speculated (but did not find data supporting this speculation) that religious participation might be the explanation. The present author offers his own guess: up to half of the members of a study cohort under age 60 consists of menstruating women.

---

[33] To date, no evidence has emerged supporting the existence of a biologically discrete disorder corresponding to the popular phrase "Alzheimer's disease." Instead, state-of-the-art data, impartially interpreted, suggest that a large number of aging-related brain changes are universal, although they vary between individuals [335, 337, 646–654].

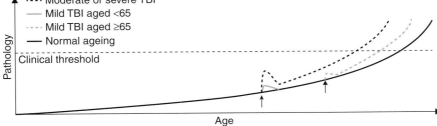

Fig. 7.20 Many of the neurodegenerative pathologies described in TBI survivors might also arise through "normal" ageing (black solid line). The data presented by Gardner et al. (2014) [674] support the hypothesis of an accelerated accumulation of neurodegenerative pathology following a single moderate or severe TBI regardless of age at time of injury (black dashed line), so crossing a threshold to clinical symptoms (dotted line) at an earlier age. By contrast, increased dementia risk after mild TBI was only present in patients aged ≥65 years (gray dashed line), implying no meaningful acceleration in neurodegenerative pathologies in patients aged <65 years (gray dashed line). Arrows indicate the occurrence of a TBI.

Source: Johnson and Stewart, 2015 [673]. Reprinted by permission from Macmillan

As previously shown, strong evidence supports the hypothesis that menstruating women are more prone to neurobehavioral sequelae after TBI. Hence, a plurality of subjects in every younger adult cohort are indeed at higher risk for psychiatric sequelae – a fact that would shift the relative risk for the entire cohort including both sexes. Again, the antique 20th-century interpretation of this finding – that women are emotionally weak – reflects a male bias favoring stoics. Yes, on average, the sexes differ. Women's brains have apparently evolved to be more sensitive. Multiple studies report female superiority in empathy (although some evidence suggests that this superiority is artifactual, reflecting a self-conscious effort to appear empathetic) [660–663]. Men are superior at upside-down map reading [664–668]. The author defers to a better sage to compare the values of these two capacities.

Fourth: although this section will not address the issue of TBI-related dementia in any depth, there appears to be an association between the age of injury and the likelihood that a typical concussion ("mild TBI") will provoke early-onset dementia. To begin with, multiple studies have reported that a single CBI increases the risk of dementia [669–672]. However, legitimate questions have been raised regarding the methodological soundness of those reports [673]. Gardner et al. [674] found that mTBI does significantly increase the risk of dementia but *only among persons injured after age 65*. As Johnson and Stewart [673] commented, the available data seem to support the conclusion that a single "mild TBI" will not accelerate neurodegeneration or provoke early-onset dementia unless it occurs after age 65. Figure 7.20 schematically illustrates the trajectories of TBI-associated increase in brain deterioration proposed by those authors.

The reader will immediately see the flaw: absent a scientifically valid and reliable marker of mildness, knowing that popular clinical definitions of "mild TBI" are untethered from the findings from modern imaging, from neuropathology, and from long-term outcomes, one cannot accept those authors' guess about the differential consequences of mild injury. Although Johnson and Stewart [673] raise sensible questions about the quality of data that rebuts their own speculation, it seems premature to reject all of that data and hang a black-and-white opinion on the shaky hook of some alleged but never proven absolute difference between the biology of mild and other-than-mild.

The present author offers a different proposal: regardless of emergency department GCS, regardless of which of the many criteria for "mild" an injury fulfills on the first day, some CBIs produce excess degeneration beyond that particular brain's point of no return; others do not. The author proposes that a biological discriminator such as this – if measurable – will predict whether an injury will increase the pace of aging-related brain degeneration far better than any clinical criteria for mildness. We are rapidly approaching the day when that hypothesis can be tested. All that is required is quantitative monitoring of the brain's molecular condition and functional integrity during the year or two after concussion.

#5. On the Risk Factor Response Bias Associated With, for Example, Imagination, Poor Motivation, Misattribution, Low Expectations, or Litigation

Consider, to begin, three declarations:

- "Persistent post-concussion syndrome (PCS) is considered as a somatoform presentation, influenced by the non-specificity of PCS symptoms which commonly occur in non-TBI samples and co-vary as a function of general life stress, and psychological factors including symptom expectation, depression and anxiety" (Larrabee and Rohling, 2013 [675], p. 686).
- "The weight of evidence suggests very strongly that there is an organic basis to the PCS. This evidence, from many different disciplines, has gathered volume and strength over the past 20 years. The more precise and accurate the tests become, from whatever specialty, the more likely it seems that organic dysfunction will be found" (Robertson, 1988 [676], p. 401).
- "As to the distinction between the physiogenic and the psychogenic factors in a given case, they appear in most cases so closely intertwined that to separate them is unnatural" (Lewis and Symonds, 1942 [677]).

This domain of CBI research, to say the least, is fraught with contention. A separate essay would be necessary to even introduce the conceptual matters at stake and to critically analyze the limited existing data available from the tenebrous closet of problematic research. This section will merely hint at factors worthy of consideration as the reader encounters distressed CBI survivors.

Multiple scholars have discussed, but few have investigated, why some CBI survivors complain of more problems, or longer-lasting problems, than other survivors. One thread of discussion claims that "psychological" factors confound the clinical presentation, leading patients to inflate or deflate their complaints. (Less attention is given to the equally important issue of symptom denial, especially by athletes and soldiers.) Those factors include theoretically (not actually) *unconscious* forces such as so-called "conversion disorder" and theoretically (not actually) *conscious* forces such as malingering or factitious disorder. The most commonly cited specific risk factors in this species of skeptical psychological commentary are "litigation overlay" (increase in complaints attributed to compensation seeking), diagnosis threat (worse test performance after reminders of the potential harm of CBI), cognitive biases (e.g., negative expectations regarding the impact of concussion, misattribution of symptoms to the head injury, and the good-old-days bias – a tendency to retrospectively inflate the quality of life prior to injury), somatoform disorders, and malingering [129, 675, 676, 678–696].

The author offers his personal perspective upfront: he enthusiastically supports all impartial, methodologically sound research to enhance our understanding of risk factors. He strongly agrees that people vary in their resilience when exposed to trauma. He notes, however, three barriers to discovery:

First Barrier

The current nosology of psychiatry is almost completely bereft of neuroscientific validity. The field has struggled for decades to replace psychoanalytic theory with scientific classification. Yet the relationship between the definition of disease and the classification of mental disorders remains unresolved [697–703]. In 1966 Abely [698] published an essay titled, "Has the time come to revise psychiatric nosology? If so, why and how? If not what must we wait for?" We are still waiting. Several themes dominate the debate: is the goal of classification epidemiology, clinical diagnosis, or research [704–706]? Should classification be based on purported categories (e.g., schizophrenia versus bipolar disorder) or instead on transdiagnostic dimensions of illness (e.g., psychosis) [707–710]? Does science in fact support the existence of the currently popular categories [711–714]? Is the Western classification system culture-bound [715–720]? Since all mentation is cerebral, should classification be based on a neural signature [721–727]? On genetic differentiation or imaging markers [728–736]? Has DSM-5 exposed the rejection of science intrinsic to the American Psychiatric Association's theory-less, symptom-based approach [737–740]? Despite progress in the last century, humans are far from understanding how mind emerges from brain, or what alters that emergence

among the mentally ill. As a result, the pathophysiology of atypical and seemingly maladaptive thought and mood has yet to be determined. Without this foundational information it is impossible to describe how CBI-related brain change acts differently on atypical brains.

A separate essay (in progress) is perhaps required to prove this point. For the sake of concision, a comparison with the rest of clinical science will have to do: one wishes to understand why a symptom is present. In many cases, the answer is already available. A million years ago, a doctor could have accurately explained the causal chain leading to the symptom, limping, by noting that the patient was missing a foot. More recently, a doctor could analyze the cause of a cough by detecting fluid in the lungs, and sometimes even the cause of that cause, e.g., inflammatory consequences of tubercular infection. But no doctor can satisfactorily specify the biological chain of causality explaining despair or poor reality testing. The 20th-century literature that lists abstract American Psychiatric Association-vetted constructs such as "major depression" or "generalized anxiety" as risk factors for worse outcome after concussion draws conclusions without having specified any neuroscientifically valid independent variable.

Second Barrier

Much of the literature on psychological risk factors requires that clinicians read minds. That is the inescapable presumption undergirding a classification of medically unexplained symptoms as conscious versus unconscious, since making that determination requires divining a patient's motives. Formerly, this conundrum applied to both conversion disorder and malingering, with the former requiring the doctor to determine the presence of an unconscious motive and the latter requiring determination of a conscious motive. To their credit, in 2013 the American Psychiatric Association reconceptualized conversion, both because motives are inaccessible to examiners and because "The reliability of determining that a somatic symptom is medically unexplained is limited, and grounding diagnosis on the absence of an explanation is problematic and reinforces mind–body dualism" ([741], p. 309). That professional guild failed, however, to overcome the same issues with regard to the diagnosis of malingering. "The essential feature of malingering is the intentional production of false or grossly exaggerated physical or psychological symptoms, motivated by external incentives" ([741], p. 726). It is not usually possible for a clinician to measure intentionality. Hence, although we certainly smell smoke when, for example, a patient cannot walk during an office examination but can jog when he thinks he is unobserved, no practical method exists to diagnose the fire of malingering with certainty.

Third Barrier

With deep regret, the author feels morally obliged to point out that some persons who represent themselves as TBI experts display a bias so extreme as to render their work unacceptable and even dangerous. For the lack of a better clinical descriptor, or a psychiatric diagnosis, or criminal label, one might call these *professional concussion deniers* (PCDs). A PCD is a individual for whom a major source of income is testifying under oath that post-concussive symptoms prolonged beyond three months represent either self-delusion (conversion) or fraud (malingering).[34] PCDs have authored several much-cited publications disseminating this falsehood. It is shocking that such anti-scientific writing satisfied peer review (although the term "peer" explains the phenomenon). As knowledge about the spectrum of natural histories of concussion grows, those publications will be dismissed as artifacts of an embarrassing lapse in Enlightenment progress (like Freudianism) and a cultural tolerance of victim blamers.

Fourth Barrier

Motivations are private. As this essay has previously discussed, humans are not mind readers. It is natural and useful to suspect that persons who complain of illness may not have illness or may be exaggerating their subjective symptoms. Society must defend itself from free-riders and con persons. Apparently deliberate, self-conscious feigning is observed, of course. Sometimes the putative goal is financial – a typical inspiration for malingering. Sometimes the goal is to limn the sick role in order to receive benefits such as sympathy or support or excusal from work or military duties – a typical inspiration for factitious disorder. However, the strict dichotomy of conscious and unconscious symptoms exaggeration is passé. Despite energetic attempts by researchers with large magnets, no laboratory method is yet available to detect lying or to divine another person's motives. Therefore, with rare exceptions (such as watching a man who complains of quadriplegia run a marathon) it is not possible for a clinician to state with utter certainty that medically unexplained symptoms are altogether and entirely feigned. Moreover, motivations are private from oneself. Brains elect behavioral strategies by calculating net benefits, but little of that cerebral activity is accessible to or controlled by conscious will. Therefore, the old distinction between *conversion disorder* (a discredited diagnosis that can only be made by a mind reader with magical access to the patient's unconscious invention of medically unexplained symptoms) and *malingering* (a justifiable construct pertaining to cheaters or free-riders on the social contract, although rarely diagnosable with certainty) is best abandoned.

Even the American Psychiatric Association, despite its historical resistance to scientific nosology, has reformed somewhat in regard to this matter. In 2013 the DSM-5 replaced the DSM-IV [741]. In addition to their discovery of Arabic numerals, the writers reconsidered listing criteria for medically unexplained symptoms that attributed these to internal unhealthy mental processes (separate from brain operations) to which psychiatrists purportedly had privileged professional access. In their rationale for a new somatic symptoms disorder (SSD), that organization stated:

> While DSM-IV was organized centrally around the concept of medically unexplained symptoms, DSM-5 criteria

instead emphasize the degree to which a patient's thoughts, feelings and behaviors about their somatic symptoms are disproportionate or excessive … In this sense, SSD is like depression; it can occur in the context of a serious medical illness … This change in emphasis removes the mind–body separation implied in DSM-IV and encourages clinicians to make a comprehensive assessment and use clinical judgment rather than a check list … .

[741]

In other words, every clinician will encounter CBI survivors whose symptoms seem excessive to that clinician (although TBI experts familiar with the data in Chapter 5 are less likely to encounter such patients, knowing that persistent symptoms are common, biologically based, and expected). But no rule or regulation endows any clinician with access to the patient's mind. It is far more honest to say, "I do not understand why this patient is so distressed," than to say:

> I know exactly where the line sits between normal and excessive distress in response to this post-concussive brain change; I also know which molecular and atomic changes were caused by the abrupt external force and which were not; thus I know exactly why this particular patient claims this distress.

"Psychological" explanations for worse outcomes after concussion are therefore difficult to discuss. The most impartial and rigorous effort will be hamstrung, perhaps for centuries, by our limited knowledge of the biology of complex behaviors. Pending advances in neuroscience, humans will cling to poorly defined but familiar concepts such as depression or emotional frailty. As a result of today's limits, one should perhaps not dismiss all the psychology of persistent symptoms claims out of hand. Setting aside the motives of those who report psychological explanations (a bias toward minimizing neurobiological change), and acknowledging that one is discussing abstractions, it may be heuristically helpful to report observed associations between measures of abstract mental states and post-CBI symptoms. Even without knowing why people are sad or nervous, there may be value in devising measures for those constructs and testing hypotheses to the effect that such people are more likely to experience persistent symptoms.

For instance, some writers have pointed to evidence that some concussed patients *expected* to feel badly after a brain injury, and do so [682, 687]. Some writers have pointed to evidence that some concussed patients with other reasons for symptoms focus on their concussion, misattributing current problems to that injury [696, 743–746]. Some writers declare that concussed patients harken back to the good old days, exaggerating the difference between their misperceived formerly perfect health and their current illness [692, 693]. All of these seem reasonable ideas, readily intuited by psychologically minded observers entirely without empirical data. None of

---

[34] PCDs hurt society. One hopes that this essay will assist courts in detecting PCDs' failure to comport with minimal standards of scientific responsibility, such as the Daubert standard – (Daubert *v.* Merrell Dow Pharmaceuticals, 1993 [741]) – not to mention their empty oaths to tell the truth.

them lends itself to objective verification, except by reference to non-validated measures of unknown cerebral operations.

What's the Use?

The author accepts that psychological labels such as "depression" or "psychosis" serve as useful stopgaps as we await better brain science. The author agrees with the likelihood that certain cognitive biases and behavioral traits increase the chances of prolonged symptoms after CBI. Yet the raft of recent publications regarding psychological "causes" of prolonged symptoms do not seem more profound than common sense, and do not seem more advanced than those of a century past. In 1918 Schaller [747] conducted one of the first systematic surveys of post-concussive complaints. He inspired a Stanford medical student, G.F. Helsley, to drive 6000 miles around California seeking 50 of Schaller's former patients and assessing outcomes about two years after concussion. Assuming young Mr. Helsley's examinations were accurate, Schaller came to conclusions similar to those in some modern commentaries, and equally immune to biologically falsifiability: "A case of traumatic neurosis existing over one year, with marked symptoms affecting earning capacity, is to be regarded as one in which there are serious psychic factors present unfavorable to recovery" (p. 344). How could Schaller opine that prolonged symptoms always indicate neurosis, and never indicate brain injury? The same way Miller did in 1961 [748] and some neuropsychologists do today: he defined persistent injury out of existence. As Miller declared: "Whatever the cause of accident neurosis, it is not the result of physical injury" ([748], p. 992).

Setting aside quibbles about the reification of abstract constructs, what is the use of claims regarding the psychological cause of persistent post-CBI symptoms? What if it were established, with all the certainty of gravity, that baseline emotional sensitivity, bad expectations, diagnosis threat, misattribution, and misremembering of the good old days all sometimes affect reporting of post-concussive symptoms?

Consider the patient who confirms every one, announcing, "Gosh, doc, I've always been oversensitive, I expected this head injury to cause serious problems, I know my injury will make me do poorly on tests, my lifetime migraines have nothing to do with my current headaches even though the symptoms are identical, and I wonder if I'm chocolate coating my life before the injury?" Given this testimony, does the doctor know whether the patient is still sad and forgetful a year after the accident because of her personal psychology, or because of her tumor necrosis factor-α gene polymorphism and slight endoglin deficiency? In what way have publications promoting the importance of these factors contributed to prevention, diagnosis, or treatment of this patient, or any patient? We can say "expectation might play a role in this case." We could have said that without reading a study. And the role of expectation remains impossible for us to determine. Hence, the main contribution of this pile of literature seems to be conducting research to

confirm that which is self-evident and inflaming the drama of attribution – the little theater in which stakeholders line up to emotively support or dismiss the victim's complaints.

Compensation, Litigation, and Post-Concussive Brain Dysfunction

A compensation neurosis is a state of mind, born out of fear, kept alive by avarice, stimulated by lawyers, and cured by a verdict.

Kennedy, 1946 [749]

The diagnosis of accident neurosis, malingering, or conversion neurosis should be made with a great deal of caution because some patients with seemingly hysterical signs and symptoms may actually have underlying organic disease

Evans, 1992 [680], p. 838

All hysterics die of organic disease.

D. Frank Benson, 1988, personal communication.

Compensation is a zero-sum game. When people take sides, as on any battlefield, one side's win is the other's loss. Stakeholders in litigation either win or lose. Justice either wins or loses. It need not be this way. It will, however, remain so until the distant day when outcome is measurable.

What is knowable about concussion outcome? This question may seem oblique to the issue of the relationship between compensation systems and post-concussive symptoms. In fact, it is the central quandary. Consider: if clinicians could state with certainty and indisputable accuracy the precise degree of distress and disability suffered by a CBI survivor, there would be no need for further discussion or for the unseemly intrusion of lawyers into medical matters. Compensation would be based on knowledge. The only reason that compensation is fraught with contention is the lack of a scientifically meaningful measure of outcome. As a result, it is impossible to determine whether the CBI survivor's complaints are less than, equal to, or greater than his or her distress and disability.[35]

There are just three observations one can report with confidence: verbatim quotes of complaints, test results (accurate or not), and behaviors (feigned or not), which run the gamut from walking to building a vaccine for Zika virus. None of these observations measures outcome. Yet the essential premise of compensation is that we measure loss and try to make up for it. Put in its starkest terms: fair compensation depends on knowing outcome. *Outcome is unknowable.* Contention arises.

A Priori, Compensation Incites Deviation From the Social Contract

As previously mentioned, Bismarck introduced historic reforms in 1884 that quickly crossed the Atlantic, establishing mechanisms to compensate persons injured in occupational

---

[35] Note that distress refers to a subjective loss while disability refers to a loss that has both subjective and objective elements. Outcome will forever be debated because some clinicians are more willing than others to acknowledge that subjective misery is an outcome.

accidents [750].[36] As also mentioned, human nature being what it is, that system creates perverse incentives. If one offers money and leisure to a person so long as he or she remains sick (or claims to be sick), many persons, not just draft dodgers and psychopaths, will be influenced at some level of consciousness to feel sick, to appear sick, or both. As Schaller put it [747]: "Of all the factors which enter into the course and duration of accident neuroses, the question of compensation is one of the most important, and its great psychic influence in a considerable proportion of cases cannot be denied" (p. 341).

Given the inevitability that some persons will be influenced by a compensation system to inaccurately report their symptoms, the literature has embraced a moral dichotomy: if one genuinely *feels* sick (and is not in the midst of a cavalry charge), it is socially acceptable to complain and *appear* sick. However, if one *feels* well, then adopting the appearance, behaviors, or identity of a sick person violates the social contract. Let there be no doubt: society must defend itself from free-riders who willfully prey upon the reciprocal altruism of others for personal gain. But again, it is simplistic to draw a phosphorescent line between conscious versus unconscious symptom production. Even the patient cannot be sure.

In the light of such incurable uncertainty, the impact of compensation on post-CBI symptom reporting can be considered in two ways: common sense and empirical investigation. The neuroscience community could be spared the second if it were comfortable with the first. Who could doubt that the prospect of money and leisure influences human behavior? And, since motives are not knowable, what can one realistically expect from a research program? The author suspects that the most comprehensive and insightful review of the available data leads to the same place as common sense: (1) some people will report symptoms inaccurately due to the influence of compensation systems; but (2) current science precludes any effort to determine who is doing so and the degree to which their report deviates from what it would otherwise be. Therefore, although this subsection is well intended and hopefully useful, it would be unnecessary if the community of TBI scholarship had matured beyond middle-school-level debates.

For the sake of simplicity (meaning, setting aside deep analysis), there are three explanations for persistent post-concussive complaints. One: as Oppenheimer proposed as early as 1892 [751], many survivors suffer a combination of molecular brain change and traumatic stress. The result is persistent impairment without gross structural damage. Two: the allure of compensation may influence behavior in the absence of mendacity. A person who feels shocked, broken, and/or victimized, in many cases with good reason, may understandably value an opportunity for recompense. It does not require evil intention for the brain to latch on to strategies for possible relief. That decision by the brain is not always accessible to consciousness. Three: some people will consciously seek more than fair compensation. The author fully agrees with

those who bemoan the disreputable histrionics of scoundrels and rapscallions. The author fully agrees that malingering occurs and is an intolerable violation of the social contract. The author agrees that compensation systems surely incite bias, massage ruminations of revenge, and trigger adoption of the sick role in vulnerable individuals. Beyond that, all bets are off. The debate about the role of compensation seeking in post-CBI symptoms is one more unnecessary drag on the serious work of TBI scholarship. It exposes prejudice on both sides, and unseemly personal attacks on patients about whose motivations one cannot possibly know. This section is intended to end the debate. It will fail. The very existence of compensation systems creates advocates and adversaries. With money on the table, stakeholders emerge and emotions run high. The best one can hope to do is to make the limitations of our knowledge crystal clear and plead for opinions to be leashed to that which can be known.

Does the Existence of Compensation Systems Demonstrably Cause Misreport of Symptoms?

A worker who is brain-damaged on the job will ideally receive medical and financial help precisely titrated to compensate for his or her losses. The brain-injured victim of a reckless driver or a malicious robber is justified in wanting to be restored, in so far as possible, to the life he or she led before. Does the existence of a system with that goal cause some CBI survivors to exaggerate or invent their symptoms? To save time and deflate the bombast, yes. As Schaller cautioned in 1918 [747]: "in the mental make-up of certain persons an accident neurosis may be unfavorably influenced, even perpetuated and aggravated by the pension system" (p. 341). It does not require psychological training or 7-T magnets to predict that a subset of humans will succumb to the allure of the compensated sick role. So, attending to the core issue, when blame can be laid for a CBI, one can classify survivors *a priori* into those who prefer to receive less than fair compensation (cases do occur), those who prefer to receive fair compensation, and those who prefer to receive more than fair compensation.

Common sense and *a priori* theses aside, the stakes are high and one wants evidence regarding whether, and to what extent, compensation systems cause inaccurate symptom report. The reader can immediately think of experimental designs that might help determine whether – on average across a demographically and medically homogeneous population of CBI survivors – financial incentives influence symptom reporting after concussion. Keep in mind that compensation seeking is often a routine, automatic element of employment, about which the employee makes no decision. Thus, only the subgroup willfully acting to get money belong in our study. In addition, most compensation systems involve a one-time decision by a board or a court, after which the die is cast. Our interest is not in the symptoms of those who have gained compensation; they have

---

[36]   Let us not blame Bismarck for the resulting 1.4 centuries of litigation. His intention seemed sincere. Yet this bold government innovation puts one in mind of Samuel Johnson's couplet: "How small, of all that human hearts endure, That part which laws or kings can cause or cure."

little incentive to complain. Our question is whether the carrot of compensation incentivizes excessive symptom reporting. We must focus on money seekers.

How would the reader conduct a high-quality study to address this question? What does one know, and what must one guess? One may know with certainty that a CBI survivor is party to a civil tort. Beyond that, the investigator is on thin ice. Can one say, "That patient deliberately elected to file a civil tort, utterly free from the influence of her brain damage on her decision-making capacity, utterly independent of the aggressive blandishments of an ambulance-chasing attorney, and completely independent of pressure from an angry niece and a greedy nephew"? That is not to say that being party to a suit commonly occurs against the patient's will. It is only to remark that brain injury may influence thinking, and that more than one brain may have influenced the decision.

Having determined that one knowable fact, that the CBI survivor is engaged in litigation, and assuming, not unreasonably, that his or her brain was one of the deliberators behind the decision to file litigation, what does the investigator know about the survivor's brain's motives? First, one must determine the time of the decision to engage in litigation with respect to the injury and symptoms. Is it scientifically acceptable to lump together subjects *seeking* compensation with subjects *receiving* compensation? Obviously not. Seekers, by nature, are driven to obtain something. Receivers are not seekers. Receivers, in fact, may never have been seekers: in many countries, workers' compensation, negotiated by unions, kicks in without litigation, without demands, without even willful action by the receiver. An investigation of the influence of financial seeking must not be contaminated by inclusion of non-seekers.

Second, might it matter what motivates the subjects in this investigation consider to be their own? That is, ignoring the human unconscious (an obvious research weakness), should the investigator stratify the study by self-reported motives? One subset of compensation seekers has been injured by persons cited for drunken and reckless driving, or by criminal assailants, or by others to whom any reasonable person would attribute blameworthiness. Another subset of compensation seekers might face daunting medical bills without inadequate insurance, hence, unarguably needing a large amount of money they do not have. Another subset might feel pain – ongoing, unrelenting physical pain. Any combination of such factors, and many more, is possible. Should the investigator wire all three into the same bale of presumed motivation? That is another issue condemning the researcher who elects to remain ignorant of subject heterogeneity.

Third, assume that the earnest and fair-minded investigator has properly identified a large cohort of CBI survivors, matched for demographic variables including socioeconomic status (SES), all of whom were injured in circumstances in which any reasonable victim would blame the perpetrator, none of whom face extraordinary financial hardship, and none of whom have pain. The ideal (albeit unrealistic) study: find two large groups of genetically identical patients with identical life histories (same neighborhood, school, job, spouse, and mother) all of whom have neurobiologically identical injuries.

Do the 50 who are willfully seeking compensation have more complaints than the 50 who are not? That study would be the beau ideal of rational science. Pending advances in cloning, it is impractical. Scholars are obliged to compromise, finding two cohorts that are somewhat similar in baseline traits and injuries, and accepting that the results are confounded by a great deal of heterogeneity.

Fourth, with that compromise cohort in hand, what research design seems likely to tease out the effect of compensation seeking on symptom persistence? One requires that this vaguely homogeneous group be divisible according to a behavior that is present or absent. For instance, the scholar might compare symptoms at one year post concussion between subjects all of whom remain symptomatic, who are actively seeking compensation via litigation (apparently by their own choice) and have yet to receive any compensation, versus subjects who are not and never were seeking compensation.

These, the reader will recognize, are relatively minimal basic requirements for a study intended to compare symptoms between seekers and non-seekers. A study conducted with these design elements has some hope of being interpretable. It will not reveal *why* the subject sought compensation, but at the least it will compare apples (seekers rationally justified in feeling harmed) with apples. These basic and commonsense requirements for a good study, the reader will discover, have almost never been met in the empirical realm.

An inferior but still scientific study: does evidence exist that, upon initiating litigation, CBI survivors display significantly more self-reported misery and, upon receiving compensation, do their complaints significantly decrease? Several studies adopted that design. Miller [752] stated:

> Up to the present time only two toilers in this field have followed up groups of such patients after settlement of their claims – Sir Farquhar Buzzard in 1928 and myself in 1961. Our results were similar. Nearly all these patients recover completely and without treatment after the case is settled.
>
> ([752], p. 258)

His opinion does not accurately predict empirical findings. First, in other studies [753, 754], disability persisted long after settlement. Mendelson [754], for instance, reported, "Up to 75% of those injured in compensable accidents may fail to return to gainful employment two years after legal settlement." The theory of cure by settlement is not supported by the data. Second, other research reports that recovery routinely occurs *before* settlement [755]. Both findings militate against Miller's hypothesis.

Another scientific design: as mentioned above, when a subject fails a cognitive test so breathtakingly that he scores worse than chance, he is "faking bad." People who score below chance, it may be fairly inferred, are exaggerating cognitive disability. This may be the chief utility of desktop testing. Although psychological tests are too insensitive to measure subtle brain injury, it is valuable to know that a patient is actively trying to persuade the examiner of his or her problems. That does not mean he does not have all the symptoms about which he complains. He very well may. Yes, flailing with theatrical intensity is one way hurting people ask for help. Nonetheless, deliberately feigning a cognitive impairment inspires suspicion. Binder [756] employed the Portland Digit Recognition Test (PDRT) in such a project. They found that 26% of those with compensable minor head injuries scored lower than the worst-performing non-compensable subject, indicating poor motivation. The present author agrees: that is strong evidence of response bias. It hardly proves good health. If Binder had only examined biomarkers and demonstrated a significant correlation between faking bad and no brain injury, the case would be settled! Absent that small additional step, our only conclusion is that some survivors of brain injuries fake bad on the PDRT. They may have permanent and disabling brain damage or not.

Indeed, a similar study [685] found that exaggeration of cognitive dysfunction on testing of attention and memory was "unrelated to symptom overreport." That means one is ill advised to generalize from evidence of exaggeration on one test. Although it is clearly imprudent to extrapolate beyond one's findings, some psychologists adopt the legal principle *falsus in uno, falsus in omnibus* – the presumption that if a witness misrepresents one fact, he or she is misrepresenting everything. Two facts counsel against such extrapolation. One: genuinely sick people often seek help by symptom exaggeration. Two: no reason exists to assume that pretense of a cognitive problem such as memory loss is scientific proof of pretense of non-cognitive symptoms such as headache, dizziness, and depression. By all means, let the index of suspicion be raised. But one must not draw conclusions beyond those the data support.

Another somewhat promising design: when a compensation system is universal, it is impossible to test whether variations in the incentives created by that system cause variations in symptom reporting. But what if the rules change in the middle of the game? Cassidy et al. [757] cleverly assessed the impact of a dramatic change in the Saskatchewan Government Insurance program on January 1, 1995. The province switched from tort to no fault and stopped paying money for pain and suffering after traffic-related mTBI. Claims for disability decreased by 25%. That finding indeed supports the contention that CBI survivors complain more when there is money on the line. It offers, however, less than meets the eye: why complain when no one listens? The results only show that *complaints* decrease, not that *symptoms* decrease.

Alternatives to Science

Instead of scientifically rational designs, a plurality of psychological literature on "litigation overlay" rests perilously on the illogical platform famously promulgated by one of neurological history's most notorious victim blamers: Henry Miller. In his 1961 Milroy lectures [748] he began with an intellectually respectable observation: a correlation is sometimes found between post-CBI symptoms and compensation claims. Miller then lectured that correlation proves causation. He repeatedly declared that a concussion survivor claims to suffer *because he or she seeks compensation*. Miller and those who followed in his pharisaic wake failed to consider that an alternative arrow of causality is equally plausible: might it be, instead, that some concussion survivors are more likely to seek compensation *because they are suffering*? Does one really expect an identical rate of compensation seeking among those who feel ill and well? Of course not. Between the alternative interpretations of the observed correlation, Miller's choice to blame the patient perhaps reveals more about his nature than about the nature of CBI.

Readers who are new to this literature may be surprised to learn the popularity of Miller's views. Instead of studying the broad spectrum of human responses to compensation, many peer-reviewed articles launch from the platform that seeking compensation is a problem or a sin. Such writings typically dichotomize compensation seekers into (1) ne'er-do-wells who consciously exaggerate symptoms and (2) the deluded who unconsciously do so. If one invests a few seconds of thought, it quickly becomes clear that such writings are simplistic. Humans are more interesting and complex. However, the strong thread of opinion that condemns complainers makes for interesting reading. Since workers' compensation originated in Northern Europe, that is the source of most late-19th-century writing about the problems with this system. Setting aside Ericksen and a few others, the American contribution was late. Making up for lost time, Miller published two Milroy lectures in 1961 [678, 748], thus winning notoriety as the spokesman for the cynic's worldview. Miller's seminal lectures mix data with opinions regarding 200 cases – all referred to him by insurance companies defending against claims. His rhetoric verges on the lyrical:

> The patient's attitude is one of martyred gloom, but he is also very much on the defensive, and exudes hostility, especially at any suggestions that his condition may be improving … The most consistent clinical feature is the subject's unshakeable conviction of unfitness for work.
>
> ([748], p. 922)

Dr. Miller apparently harbored negative feelings about compensation seekers. But his feelings are not at issue. The scientific question is whether he correctly identified a systematic problem such that compensation provoked widespread corruption. To answer that question brings us straight back to the original quandary: no valid method exists to determine whether a complaint is consistent with or inconsistent with outcome, so how did Dr. Miller classify patients as exaggerators? Miller himself admitted that bias might cause diagnostic error. "The subject is so fraught with prejudice that it demands a conscious effort to maintain a clear distinction between fact and interpretation" ([748], p. 919). What then shall we make of Miller's success in his conscious effort to diagnose neurotic exaggeration without prejudice? He diagnosed "accident neurosis" among CBI survivors whenever (1) they were absent from work for six months but (2) had no skull fracture. Skull fracture is almost entirely unrelated to brain injury; hence, Miller's diagnoses lacked validity. He further reveals his methods:

> Gross dramatization of symptoms … may be evident in … the patient's slumping forward with head in hands …

requesting a glass of water. I had long regarded this as a pathognomonic sign of accident neurosis, but I understand that it is often seen in women requesting termination of pregnancy on psychiatric grounds.

([748], p. 922)

The present author was unable to determine what form of statistical analysis Dr. Miller employed to show that malingering is best diagnosed on the basis of a request for water.

Ironically, Miller's study provided potent data supporting the conclusion that long-term brain problems are common after concussion. He claims to have analyzed 4000 medicolegal cases before his lectures (which would have required assessing a new legal case about once a day for 12 years, including Sundays and holidays). He claims to have performed a follow-up assessment on 175 closed head injury cases an average of 14 months post-concussion. Eighty-four of those (48% of the total) had persistent symptoms. Miller diagnosed "accident neurosis" in 11 of those 84. That means Miller judged 73 – that is, 42% of his closed head injury patients – to have *organically* based long-term post-concussion symptoms. This finding jibes well with the present text's best estimate of more than 40% (similar to the recent findings of de Koning et al. [1]). For some reason, Miller's advocates have neglected to mention that fact for more than 50 years.

Miller's lectures are intriguing since his language is so eloquent and the fallacies of his analysis are so apparent. Yet a review of this important subject need not harp on such extremists. Miller inspired a cavalcade of more academically savvy cynics. Binder and Rohling, for instance, carried the candle for Miller in their 1996 review [758] of litigation and symptoms they titled "Money matters." Although the duo called their paper a "meta-analysis," it was an opinion piece mathematically unworthy of that label since no methodological comparability was present between any two of their sources. Those writers claimed to have analyzed 18 studies that tested the hypothesis that compensation seeking inflates symptom reporting. They calculated an average "moderate" effect size of 0.47 favoring their hypothesis – and they reassured the reader that the two coauthors agreed with one another "100%" (!). In the interest of ethical correction, momentarily consider studies analyzed by Binder and Rohling.

Their first citation was Adler (1945) [759], who followed 200 patients after TBIs. Sixty-three developed mental symptoms. "Problems in relation to litigation and compensation" was called an "environmental" cause of those symptoms. Adler, somewhat remarkably, assumed that the mental symptoms in the presence of "litigation problems" were imaginary *regardless of their significance in the opinion of the psychiatrist*" (emphasis added). That is, his analysis dismissed professional judgment regarding whether any relationship existed between the brain injury and the complaints. Adler's summary observation was that about half of the patients with symptoms had "litigation problems." Contrary to Binder and Rohling's representation, nothing about the *causal* impact of litigation can be inferred from such data. It is merely correlative.

Binder and Rohling's second citation was to Steadman and Graham (1970) [760] who gathered information about 415

patients after head injury. Fifty (12%) had symptoms at five years. As a non-significant trend, survivors with more severe injuries (based on longer PTA) received more money. What upset those last authors was that, "One-quarter of patients without PTA claimed compensation; this figure seems remarkably high" ([760], p. 27). Those authors stated, "Against a background of previous studies of the influence of PTA this would suggest that these claims were tainted by malingering" ([760], p. 27). In other words, Steadman and Graham declared that receiving money without amnesia proves ignominy. That is absurd.

Binder and Rohling's third and fourth citations were to Russell's (1971) book [427]. Russell made the same illogical assumption as Steadman and Graham. He reports with shock, "There were 20 compensation cases in which the duration of loss of consciousness was less than one hour" (p. 11). That is, Russell assumed that if a patient was knocked out for 58 minutes and received money, he was malingering for money. This paragon of logical perversity was accorded an effect size of 0.82 by Binder and Rohling.

The fifth paper cited by Binder and Rohling was Cook (1972) [761]. He mailed questionnaires asking whether CBI survivors had *considered* claims for compensation. (Not, "Did you pursue compensation?" Not, "Did you request compensation?" Not even, "Do you want compensation?" Just, "Did you consider …?") Cook's predictable result: those who *considered* seeking compensation spent more time out of work. Is any reader surprised? Isn't it reasonable that people who are out of work *consider* their options for financial support? Remember: the study tracked no action, behavior, or symptom. It only reported a thought, "Hmm, I wonder if I should request compensation?" Binder and Rohling's interpretation of this as proof that financial incentives lead to symptom exaggeration lacks logical integrity.

They also cited Cartlidge and Shaw's otherwise very good book [762], which includes an analysis of two post-concussive symptoms: headache and dizziness. The authors made the following assumption: if a patient did not complain of headache or dizziness *at the time of the injury*, any later complaint indicates that the patient inflated his symptoms to seek compensation. That assumption is obviously invalid – a fact not addressed by Binder and Rohling. Collectively, those authors' systematic misrepresentation of the studies they cited begs for ethical assessment.

The present author will not trouble the reader with more of Binder and Rohling's artifice. Those who relish uncovering academic hijinks may effortlessly expose those writers' claims by reading their sources. Suffice it to say that, far beyond the shenanigans of Miller and Binder and Rohling, few writings that besmirch the virtue of patients who seek compensation are scientifically sound.

Yes, *of course, absolutely, money matters*. The glint of gold leads many astray. When parties take sides, it is best to be wary because, in the Solomonic aphorism of Harvard neurologist Steve Massaquoi, "Truth bends in proximity to money" (1988, personal communication). But no neurologist or psychologist has the supernatural power to divine the proportion of motivation that is conscious or unconscious, litigious, or venal, or simply desperate. No study can quantify the influence of money seeking and no machine can measure it in any given case. Moreover, counterexamples prevail in the literature:

> Dikmen et al. (1995) [410]: "Litigation did not appear to have systematic effects on neuropsychological outcome in this study."

> Konrad et al. (2011) [763]: "individuals who had sustained a minor trauma more than half a decade ago continue to have long-term cognitive and emotional sequelae … cognitive deficits were medium to large and could not be accounted for by … compensation claims or negative response bias."

Actual data such as this will hopefully vaccinate most medical and psychology students against exposure to Dr. Miller and his acolytes. Yet one suspects there will always be those who stigmatize distressed concussion survivors. This despite the repeated exposure of Miller's fallacies. Minderhoud et al.'s [764] epitaph for Dr. Miller's contribution to medical science:

> In contrast to the statement of Miller (1961 and 1966) that long lasting sequelae of minor head injuries (the post-concussional syndrome) result from the need of financial compensation, it is now more generally held that the aetiology of these sequelae is multifactorial. … For some reason Miller's statement has been used with respect to all kinds of patients who continue to have complaints after minor head injuries for a period of time longer than was expected, and 'it has been quoted by doctors as an excuse for inactivity and by lawyers in the courts as though it is the gospel according to Saint Henry'.

> ([764], p. 127)

The conclusions we can trust: (1) malingering is rare; (2) exaggeration is common in medicine, with or without a tort; (3) compensation probably influences some survivors; but (4) motivations are private. Crying piteously in the doctor's office is human nature in the face of change, fear, and uncertainty. As the author exhorts medical students: if you cannot empathize with patients who beg for help via theater, it is best to consider a different profession.

Seven Ways Compensation Systems Probably Influence Symptom Reporting

One hopes to start fresh. There seem to be at least seven ways that compensation systems influence symptom report after concussion:

One: The prospects of lucre and a life of Riley may inspire flagrant, self-conscious malingering. Malingering is sometimes neurologically certain. More often, there is an element of uncertainty and the diagnosis is prone to be influenced by observer bias.

Two: The opposite occurs: some CBI survivors consciously under-represent their symptoms. Athletes, soldiers, and stoics may do this.

Three: The possibility of compensation acts at a less than fully conscious level. Since the cerebral processes are inaccessible to study, the degree to which the minimization or exaggeration of a complaint is conscious versus unconscious is unknowable to the patient or to anyone else. And since (1) no relevant biomarker of damage exists and (2) subjective response to a given injury varies, the degree to which a complaint deviates from the "normal" response is also unknowable. This latter point deserves attention. At the risk of stating the obvious: different people experience different amounts of distress when exposed to similar stressful circumstances or illnesses [765–769]. Thresholds of perception of and tolerance of pain or dismay vary greatly – not only between individuals but within individuals based on diurnal or menstrual phase [770–772]. Two sisters hit on the head with identical external forces will not only have biological responses that differ in thousands of ways, but – even if their brain changes were magically identical down to the last excitatory post-synaptic potential – would not be expected to experience identical feelings. A clinician may pride himself on estimating how much distress is "normal" for a given medical problem, but that is knowledge beyond human ken. Since these matters are both infinitely variable and literally unknowable, how would one ever detect symptom report deviation?[37] Confronted by a trauma, the victim's brain's decision-making apparatus juggles multiple survival and well-being goals. These include everything from a reasonable expectation that compensation will help pay for rehabilitation, to the misguided belief that compensation will relieve distress, to the misguided belief that wealth is associated with happiness, to misattribution of pre-existing distress to the injury, to desire for revenge, rescue from poverty, sympathetic embraces, or morally driven pursuit of justice. The net influence of all of these incentives on exaggeration or minimization of symptoms seems to depend on many factors, such as:

1. pre-morbid traits and experiences
2. conviction that someone else was at fault in an accident
3. the will required to trigger a compensation-seeking process (in many cases, the question of incentivized symptom exaggeration is moot and prone to misunderstanding by researchers. Many injured persons *make no choice* because their employer, union, or insurance company automatically seeks redress)
4. social standing (e.g., whether one likes or dislikes working; whether one labors for a faceless corporation or one's family business; whether one's education permits alternative employment if injury eliminates one's first job)
5. financial security (and the elusive variation in human belief that money leads to eudaimonic happiness)
6. incitement by an aggressive attorney, and so forth …

---

[37] Readers will encounter statements to the effect that 40–60% of concussion survivors exaggerate. Those are guesses, since it is impossible to measure symptom exaggeration. At the same time, the author suspects that many people seeking relief from uncertainty, privation, or pain – from crying babies to hungry teenagers to terminal cancer victims – overstate their subjective distress as a low-cost way of enhancing their odds of being heard and helped.

Each of these factors, and probably many others, seems to contribute in various combinations and degrees that are probably unique to each individual, ultimately becoming overt in the difference between "It's been terrible" and *It's been terrible!*
Four: Direct effects of external force on emotional regulatory circuits.

Five: Complex effects on behavior, probably involving interactions between genetic predisposition, childhood influences, horror regarding the accident, direct effects of external force, reaction to stress, treatment, and available social supports – all playing a role in the possible development of depression or anxiety. Those emotional changes in turn lower the threshold for perceived incapacitation.

Six: Iatrogenic influences (for instance, due to cynical reception of authentic symptoms or a mismatch between a clinician's rosy prognosis and grim actuality).

Seven: Compensation system-induced stress [773]. This is similar to the "secondary neurosis" proposed by Rumpf and Horn in 1912 [774]: stress arising from the struggle for a pension.

In clinical or medicolegal practice, these seven compensation-related influences may affect symptom report in any magnitude or combination. Has any doctor or "expert" ever accurately determined the contribution of each? Better for us all to profess humble bafflement than proud certainty.

What Proportion of Compensation Seekers Exaggerates?

> Many of the claimants are not only consciously but even frankly and obsessively preoccupied with the question of financial compensation.
>
> Miller, 1966 [752]

> Although the question of simulation deals particularly with diagnosis, it may be here stated that we have found frank simulation a rare condition, although exaggeration not infrequent.
>
> Schaller, 1918 [747], p. 340

There are two ways to come by money: honestly and the other way. One may elect a career as a ditch digger, drug dealer, politician, or medical director of the National Football League. The first job can be performed honestly. The author would vastly prefer promotion from professor to ditch digger over demotion to the other three jobs. Accordingly, if you pay people to say they are suffering, some people will say they are suffering. That is the downside to Bismarck's great innovation, injury compensation [775, 776]: it smooths the road for victims, but also grooms a path for society's corrupt. One need not deal drugs or become Governor of Illinois. One can feign pain. For this reason, suspicion about complaints is altogether reasonable. The challenge is avoiding bias in either direction.

What proportion of concussed people prevaricate for profit? Perhaps about the same proportion as those who choose any other antisocial career: blessedly few. Schaller's (1918) study was among the first to attempt empirical rigor [747]. As noted above, he reported, "we have found frank simulation

a rare condition." Cartlidge and Shaw [777] replicated that observation more than 60 years later: "what of malingering? In our experience, true conscious malingering for financial or other personal gain is a rare phenomenon" (p. 153). Or Evans [680]: "Compensation neurosis or malingering in patients with litigation or claims pending is quite uncommon" (p. 838).

Malingering may be rare, but many survivors of concussions express more distress than the clinician intuits they should. The injury seemed trivial. Why the long face? Some studies even report that complaints seem inversely proportional to estimated head injury severity [678, 747]. The problem, again, is the lack of a scientific method to assess whether complaints are proportionate to the severity of the accident: we cannot measure severity and we cannot prejudge how distressing that amount of injury should be.

Even without conscious awareness that one is being influenced, it seems natural that distress may polish the hook of the compensation system. The possibility of unconscious symptom magnification is very important. But how shall we detect it? If a woman says, "My pain is seven out of ten," what machine should the neuropsychologist attach to her to determine that, in fact, she is imagining her pain to be two points higher than what she actually feels, which the machine knows to be five? In this respect, the author agrees with Dr. Miller [748]: "Differentiation between conscious and unconscious purpose is quite insusceptible to any form of scientific inquiry, and that it depends on nothing more infallible than one man's assessment of what is probably going on in another man's mind" (p. 993).

The question, indeed, often comes down to separating willful deceit from cognitive bias. In some cases, that is easy. Neurologists are trained to detect feigned symptoms and some are unequivocal to the point of *opera buffa*. In the case of the man who crawls about the office floor and jogs to his car, it is fair to infer duplicity. However, Gould et al. [778] showed the many standard neurological examination tricks purported to identify functional signs frequently detect "hysteria" in patients with proven neurological disease. Again, the wisdom of Cartlidge and Shaw [777]:

> In the context of medicolegal examination these performances are apt to be attributed to attempted deception for the basest of motives, yet how often are they encountered in everyday practice where "functional overlay" is readily accepted on the basis of anxiety or diminished expectation of performance in a genuinely impaired member.
>
> (p. 153)

This raises a subtle point: Miller [748] complained that lawyers make much of the conscious versus unconscious distinction. He asserted that it does not matter for purposes of compensation: "To compensate a man financially because he is stated to be deceiving himself as well as trying to deceive others is strange equity and stranger logic" (p. 993). This is carping cavil. The self-deceiver is absolutely *not* trying to deceive others. And self-deceit can be the natural product of awful depression or anxiety – no less a hardship due to injury than memory loss or pain.

The author hopes that this brief discussion of the compensation issue accurately reports the core considerations. Humans are diverse. Motivations are private. Research cannot determine the proportion of CBI survivors who exaggerate, any more than research can expose the proportion of TBI "experts" who are biased against science. Such studies would require mind reading. Academic debate aside, it is only good sense to assume that, if money or social advantage is dangled like a carrot, some people will bite. And dishonest money-seeking is not confined to malingerers and Ossetian oligarchs. Some of those who earn money testifying about the benignity of concussions seem to be hard-hearted, lacking in both medical and self-insight, wreathed in florid sanctimony, eager to prioritize public moralizing over acknowledgment of our limited access to ultimate truths. These too have chosen the dark side – seeking income by misrepresenting science. I trust our better angels: most readers, most clinicians, and most CBI survivors elect decency.

The compensation system cries out for reform. It needs a dramatic kick toward an ideal in which: (1) diagnosis is objective; (2) health is assessed independently of fault; (3) recovery is facilitated and incentivized; and (4) experts *never* serve plaintiffs or defense, only courts and truth. The moment society accomplishes those modest, overdue goals, cynical psychologists will repent and trial lawyers will hopefully abandon their practices to pursue world peace. In the meantime, clinicians must reject unscientific exhortations to assume that persistent misery after CBI is evidence of fraud, devil worship, Episcopalianism, or any other personal trait.

#7.   On the Risk Factor of Social Disadvantage or Adversity

We have come, at last, to the seventh major factor that has been reported to influence concussion outcome: social disadvantage or adversity. *Social disadvantage* is used in this section as shorthand. Multiple risk factors, individually or in combination, have been reported to cause bad outcome after concussion that (broadly speaking) pertain to sociality. These include minority status, low educational achievement, low SES, low occupational status, low social standing, low job independence, being unmarried, and "social adversity," not otherwise specified.

All of these are social stressors – potentially. "Potentially" is a necessary qualifier since people differ in the degree to which they regard themselves as disadvantaged. For some, being unmarried is a preference – or a cure. "Low occupational status" only seems to be a stressor when it reflects unrealized expectations: middle-class Amish farmers reportedly have high levels of subjective well-being equaling those of Fortune 500 CEOs. "Minority status" is a stressor in societies riven by prejudice (e.g., the United States), less so in more egalitarian communities (e.g., Sweden). Poverty may harm subjective well-being more in rich countries than in poor countries because the underlying stressor is inequality – an issue to which we must return [779–782]. Therefore, factors listed as socially disadvantaged are not universally problematic.

Nor are these factors neatly differentiable. One epidemiological study may report that *minority members* have worse outcome; another study may report that persons with *low education* have worse outcome; a third study might find the same regarding *low SES*. But which of these is a *cause*, which a mediator, and which a moderator? Before summarizing the social disadvantage data, it may be useful to consider why doctors should be suspicious when any one social factor is claimed to cause bad outcome. Consider "race." What causes what?

Being black or Hispanic in North America (or being a minority in other white-dominated societies) is associated with worse outcome after moderate to severe TBI. Investigators have variously attributed this observation to higher rates of head injuries due to violence [783, 784]; lower rates of insurance [785]; non-referral to rehabilitation [786, 787]; post-injury unemployment [788, 789]; lower likelihood of follow-up [790]; or post-injury depression [791]. This finding holds even after controlling for SES, education, marital status, pre-injury employment, and injury characteristics [783, 792]. In the light of this wealth of data on race/minority status and outcome after more severe injuries, it is striking how few data have been published about race and typical concussions. The Vanderploeg et al. [793] study is one of very few: they found that minority Army veterans with mTBI had inferior long-term employment outcomes.

Such epidemiological data are convincing, as well as completely blind to the real mechanism or mechanisms involved. That matters. If the true underlying cause is modifiable, the disparity is curable. But the scholar who wants to know *why* race is a risk factor is doomed, at present, to woe.

Closing his or her eyes, the reader can list a dozen plausible reasons that persons of a given race might suffer more, not one of which is readily measurable in the clinic. Do African Americans tend to experience worse post-injury distress or disability because of differences in the frequency of genes regulating traumatic microglial response? Or due to epigenetic variations in ribosomal gene silencing that became heritable due to five generations of suboptimal nutrition and high levels of stress? Or due to inadequate prenatal care with statistically greater chances of intrauterine exposure to alcohol, tobacco, fevers or viruses, low folate, gestational diabetes, or pre-eclampsia? Or due to higher rates of unnecessary cesarean section or birth hypoxia or uncontrolled infant fever or seizure? Or due to inferior toddler nutrition, weak pediatric oversight, lead exposure, or diesel fume exposure? Harsh parenting? Paternal absence? Lack of availability of affordable fresh fruits and vegetables? Higher incidence of childhood obesity, inflammation, and diabetes? Lower average fitness due to dangerous neighborhoods? Inferior educational opportunities? Repetitive exposure to violence? Less cognitively stimulating jobs? Lack of decision-making latitude at work? Inferior preventive health care, inferior trauma care, and a demonstrably lower chance of rehabilitation? Greater susceptibility to subconscious or conscious seduction by the sick role? Greater vulnerability to plaintiff's attorneys who coerce retreat to the sick role? Lower compensation success rates compromising access to health care? Greater skeptical rejection of symptoms by white upper-middle-class physicians? Shall we resort to a grab bag called "chronic stress due to social deprivation"? Or shall we admit that, in every case, perhaps 20 such factors act in some unique combination?

The author explains his concern about the superficiality of current scholarship to disseminate his sentiment: surely we can do better. Readers who plan to gain expertise in this field will regularly encounter statements such as "poverty is associated with worse outcome." As demonstrated by the previous paragraph, such words are empty of biological meaning and useless for devising effective interventions. One small assignment for the next generation is to probe beyond the present vacuity and figure out the actual risk factors. Some can hopefully be fixed.

With that as an introduction, in addition to minority status, several other traits that might reasonably be labeled "social disadvantage" have also been empirically implicated in a more problematic or prolonged post-concussive course. For instance, lower SES has been repeatedly associated with worse outcome [425, 680, 794]. Lower level of education is strongly associated with worse outcome. Of interest, just as in neurodegenerative dementia, the largest excess risk is associated with failure to complete high school[400, 406, 407, 425, 795]. Pre-morbid social adversity or stressful life events are also associated with worse outcome [401, 413]. Poor social support is also a risk factor [18, 796]. Conceivably, that factor underlies the relationship between worse outcome and unmarried status at the time of injury [797]. One theory raises the specter of a vicious circle: Schalen et al. [798] noted that some TBI survivors tend to withdraw from the very social supports they need due to irritability and/or difficulty following conversations [798]. Although that finding was made among persons with more severe injuries, it possibly occurs after typical concussions as well.

Low social standing is another proven risk factor [799]. Note that this is not equivalent to poverty and may be moderated by self-esteem. Bakey and Glasauer [799], for example, observed that "the urban poor react more strongly to their symptoms than the farmer rooted in the soil" (p. 387). Their comment introduces the fact that multiple features of occupational status predict worse outcome. These include pre-morbid unemployment [797], low occupational category [425, 797, 800, 801], low occupational satisfaction, limited independence, and limited decision making at work [131, 678, 800]. In this regard, the author overlooks Dr. Miller's cynicism and credits his insight: "The relation of accident neurosis to a lack of social responsibility is supported by its infrequency in workers who take pride in an important job, and its predilection for those human cogs in the industrial machine whose employments afford little opportunity for any kind of satisfaction or self-fulfillment" ([748], p. 993). Lidvall et al. [131], in 1974, were among the first to confirm this connection: "Patients in the PCS [post-concussive symptoms] group displayed ... a lower general satisfaction at work ... and a more negative attitude to

working tasks ... fellow workers ... and to their supervisors" (p. 77). Ruffolo et al. [801] specifically noted that mTBI survivors were less likely to return to work (RTW) if their jobs had less decision-making latitude (an observation echoed by Cancelliere et al. [795]). A related finding was reported by Rutherford, 1977 [800]: "Post-concussion symptoms were more frequent in ... those who blamed their employers or large impersonal organisations for their accidents" (p. 1), in essence a combination of negativity toward their jobs and fault finding.

Another issue pertaining to occupation deserves analysis. What are the cause and effect of failure to RTW? Failure to RTW is conventionally considered an outcome variable – supposedly a marker of incomplete recovery, failure to adapt, or shirking. It is not, however, a meaningful sign of brain health because not everyone likes working, and some people like their jobs more than others. Walker et al. [802], for example, found that "the best prospect of RTW was among people with professional/managerial jobs." Similarly, Forslund et al. [797] reported that persistent unemployment was more common among blue-collar workers up to five years after injury. In fact, failure to RTW is also a risk factor for poor outcome in itself. That is, of course some CBI survivors are too disabled to RTW, even with accommodations. Some have painful extracranial injuries and never receive accurate diagnosis or effective interventions for their ancillary disabilities.[38] Some have jobs that expose them to unbearable stresses likely to exacerbate post-concussive distress and slow recovery. Premature RTW, in particular, is self-defeating.

On the other hand, for many people work lends structure and meaning to life and self. Income aside, it offers diverse rewarding and mentally stabilizing merits, from opportunities to feel productive and display mastery, to preservation of a family role, to reliable socialization, and even to healthful circadian *Zeitgebers* (external clues that synchronize one's biorhythms with the Earth's 24-h cycle). Strong evidence exists that failure to RTW – whether from fear, anger, lack of self-awareness, sloth, misguided expectation of the joys of idleness, or misguided pressure from attorneys – can make life worse after CBI [803]. Although sparse empirical research is available to buttress that argument, the present author cannot restrain expressing his personal conviction: far too few concussed persons receive the education, rehabilitation, occupational therapy consultation, work-hardening, emotional support, and – frankly – passionate exhortation from clinicians, family, and friends required to get them back on the horse. This is sometimes the paradoxical consequence of litigation. Some CBI survivors suffer more as a result.

Why is Social Disadvantage Associated With Worse Outcome?

This question might seem rhetorical, or even circular, like, "why is a bad life associated with a bad life?" The author only

---

[38] Just as empirical evidence shows that co-morbid orthopedic injuries tend to distract emergency ward doctors from diagnosing concussions (see Chapter 2), the author's impression from two decades at an inpatient neurorehabilitation center is that patients admitted with the diagnosis of TBI sometimes languish for months before a proper orthopedic examination unveils a fracture.

means to explore the possibility that some common biological factor underlies the mountain of evidence that diverse aspects of disadvantage complicate recovery. "Stress" is frequently mentioned as that common theme; that may be as close as one can get to a medical explanation. Yet some of the factors listed above are more obviously stressful than others. For instance, an 11th-grade education is not intrinsically a stressor. Race or ethnicity may or may not be stressful; some minority communities flourish. Might there be another cause? A final common cerebral pathway linking social life, pre-morbid brain health, and concussion outcome? The present author confesses ignorance of good empirical data and offers only a tentative hypothesis: recovery after CBI depends on brain reserve – for instance, in terms of redundancy of circuits, plasticity, adult neurogenetic capacity, and emotional resilience. Social disadvantage potentially limits such reserve not only by all of the unequivocally damaging effects of stress but also perhaps by compromised capacity for adaptation in the face of cell loss or circuit disruption. Just as a better-educated middle-aged adult with a more cognitively challenging job tends to maintain his or her brain fitness longer in the face of neurodegeneration, so might socially advantaged people tend to have brains fitter to regenerate from the neurometabolic melee.

Plausible, as a concept. But what does "brain reserve" mean in terms of tissue – cells and organelles and molecules? Higher density of dendritic spines? More agile incorporation of dentate gyrus pluripotential stem cells into functional hippocampal circuits? Or perhaps a factor only coincidentally associated with social status, such as likely race-related difference in the frequency of genetic variants – such as the BDNF Val66Met polymorphism associated with mood and stress responsiveness, or new variants recently discovered to correlate with mood, neuroticism, well-being, or academic achievement on GWAS [291, 292, 294–296]? The author should not guess. He defers to the forthcoming generation of neuroscientists who will hopefully be dissatisfied with platitudes and push the envelope to find root physiological mediators.

That, however, will not solve the problem. It may be decades before we understand the neurobiology of social disadvantage. Even then, a unitary neurobiological process is both unlikely to explain the jeopardy of the underclass and unlikely to be amenable to post-injury treatment. But we already know the principal cause of social disadvantage: inequality. Pending easing of inequality, many health outcomes will forever be worse among our disadvantaged.

On the Drama of Attribution

The defense attorney assumes his gravest visage:

> She is depressed because she expected a bad outcome. She is depressed because she imagines herself to be more depressed than she was before the accident. She is depressed because her husband had an affair. She is depressed because she wants money. And her neuropsych testing was within normal limits so it's *impossible* that she has brain damage! Trust me. I can tell. The accident had no effect.

Any reader who already is or will soon become an expert in the domain of TBI will hear nonsense to this effect on a regular basis. In the literature, the clinic, and the forensic setting, one still encounters prickly clashes between those who are wedded to one explanation for a symptom versus those who are wedded to another. It is disheartening, but expected. So long as there is money or blame to be dispensed, there will be a drama of attribution.

The drama of attribution is the affect-laden effort to assign proportional causality. Back in the 20th century a writer could always find peers who would permit publication of a claim that only 10% of concussed persons exhibit long-term dysfunction. Some writers could even publish claims that prolonged symptoms could not possibly be due to damaged brain tissue, and therefore must be due to imagination or fakery. This essay, this book, is just one of many recent resources offering a step up from that slough of anti-science. Hopefully, editors and reviewers and judges and juries will henceforth reject such egregious misrepresentations of the empirical facts.

Still, pressures remain for clinicians to make attributions. The question "Why does this CBI survivor have her current symptoms?" is worthy of concerted investigation. It is entirely possible that a large number of factors other than immediate tissue change due to abrupt external force are operative. It is very much in the patient's interest to sort this out, in so far as one is able to, since individualized diagnosis, prognosis, and choice of the most effective treatments may hinge on identifying modifiable factors that may not be obvious in the emergency department. Although the research has yet to be done, some day we will know whether persons with pre-morbid anxiety and post-concussive PTSD or a given genetic polymorphism are significantly more likely to benefit from a given medication or therapy than those without those traits.

Attribution is not, however, amenable to black-and-white answers along the lines of "organic" versus "psychological," "neurological" versus "functional," or "conscious" versus "unconscious." And it is certainly not amenable to quantitative attribution of proportional causality. If the boastful pronouncement "It is because she was depressed before" were not silly enough, then "She is mostly depressed because she was depressed before but somewhat depressed because she is upset about her accident" is hysterical. What detracts from the humor is that clinicians sometimes say such things aloud as if medical knowledge was being invoked in good faith. Pending a remarkable advance in our ability to parse human distress, humility is the guiding byword.

By way of illustration, please again consider Georgia, our injured 29-year-old teacher and equestrian enthusiast. In both my clinic and in court, there were persons who opined "Georgia's difficult and prolonged post-CBI course is due to her pre-morbid psychiatric problems" versus those who opined "Her difficult and prolonged post-CBI course is due to the brain injury." This is obviously a false dichotomy. As previously noted: can one really apportion causality to one or the other factor when the two are inextricably intertwined?

A numerical example may help. Using the 36-item WHODAS 2.0 [38, 804], the author estimated that Georgia's average pre-morbid disability was roughly nine, which means that she was more disabled than all but 30% of the population. At one year post-CBI, Georgia was dysthymic 18 days in the month and depressed eight days. She missed days at work, stopped virtually all recreational and avocational activities, and put her marriage plans on hold. My best estimate was a WHODAS score of about 20, meaning she was more disabled than all but 17% of the population.

On interview it seemed that some of the environmental factors contributing to her on-again-off-again depression in the decade prior to trauma were ongoing – such as an emotionally withdrawn father and critical mother – and others were variable – such as the attentiveness of her current boyfriend and her performance evaluations by the new school principal. Her parents provided superficial support after the injury, showing the flag a couple of times at the hospital. Her boyfriend and boss were both more understanding. Discussing the impact of the concussion, she expressed what seemed to be somewhat excessive concerns that she would never ride again (bad expectations). At the same time, she seemed realistically aware, and hopeful, that her memory problems were improving. During her sadder clinical visits, she described her life before the injury and her life after the injury as night and day. This did not seem so much a good-old-days bias as a negative and pessimistic appraisal of her genuine progress toward recovery. Getting a lawyer at the behest of her parents did not seem to help or hurt; her self-reports followed the same uneven trajectory of slow improvement before and after she entered litigation – until her deposition when she was exposed to a cruelly accusatory insurance attorney, after which her depression deepened.

What possible virtue would there be in estimating the degree to which her change in baseline WHODAS was attributable to her various problems? How could the world's most insightful team of doctors divvy up her distress by its causes? What neurologist on earth would venture to say: "Georgia exhibits a 13 percentile increase from her pre-morbid dysfunctionality. I attribute four of those disability points to her pre-morbid depression, five to her brain injury, two to her emotional reaction to her brain injury, one half-point to her parents' lack of compassionate support, and one and a half disability points to litigation overlay"? Would any clinician dare to say, "If not for her pre-morbid depression, her disability score today would be only 12.3." If the neurologist learns that she failed a grade in elementary school or had a rough break-up with her ninth-grade boyfriend, should he or she recalculate the number of points on the disability scale attributable to those pre-morbid factors and correspondingly decrease attribution to her brain injury? If she happens to carry the short allele of the gene for 5HTTLPR, should her doctor attribute 2.7 points of her current disability to that risk factor?

No. Georgia's post-concussive condition is the product of her brain injury interacting with all that she is. This is the rational concept of the individuality of disease Garrod introduced in 1908. She is disabled because of all of the above. It is literally impossible to divvy up causality. Only a fool or a lawyer would seek to attribute a given amount of her troubles to each of the many contributing factors. The author earnestly implores that neurology set aside such empty dramas and fruitless debates.

The Haddon Matrix

A Haddon matrix [651, 805, 806] is a simple table, a format invented to permit epidemiologists to spell out the interplay among multiple factors causing an illness. The premise is that one cannot control an epidemic if one narrowly attends to just one or two of its many causes. For instance, who gets cholera depends on patient-related factors (such as personal hygiene and immune competence), illness-related factors (the virulence and transmissibility of the strain of cholera), and environmental factors (the communal use of a single water pump). A Haddon matrix further divides these causal factors according to the point in time when they act. For example, the communal pump was an environmental factor that acted *prior* to the infection. Environmental factors that might impact the course of the illness *after* the infection could include the availability of clean water, medical care, family support, soup, and soap. With some misgivings, the author proposes that the concepts in this chapter might be summarized usefully with such a matrix.

The Haddon matrix is conceptually imperfect. For instance, one is required to differentiate between *patient-related factors* and *environment-related factors*. This invariably creates a superfluity of words. If, for example, a fetus was exposed to a virus during the second trimester, the *viral exposure* was *environmental* but the *viral infection* was *patient-related*. This obliges one to list these related phenomena in both the "environment" and "patient" columns. Is poverty a patient- or environment-related factor? Similarly, *patient* and *environmental* factors both overlap with *injury-related* factors. For instance, a 90-**g** blow to the parietal head is imposed by the *environment* (e.g., standing in proximity to moving baseballs). The resulting *injury* arises from a complex interaction between that force and the Little League player.

Let us presume that a returned pitch caused a boy to suffer a 7.3% average stretch of fibers in his cingulum. It would require a semantic contortionist to separate aspects of the tissue change that are "injury-related" from those that are "patient-related." Naturally speaking, the 7.3% stretch is an "injury-related factor." Yet, due to the unique physics of every patient's head and brain, the same 90-**g** force might have caused a 4.2% or 11.6% stretch in a different patient – making the degree of stretch a "patient-related factor" and again requiring duplicative listing.

Moreover, almost all of the *patient-related* factors present *before* the injury remain influential both *during* and *after* the injury (e.g., genes, sex, race, education, prior health). Resilience to trauma, for instance, is a before-the-injury patient trait, yet its influence acts primarily after the injury. Need one list such traits three times in the rows for pre-injury, during injury, and post-injury influence? And some environmental factors present before an injury (e.g., poverty, inequality, and low education increase the risk of injury in advance by restricting the victim's residential and occupational options) are also influential in different ways after the injury (e.g., poverty, inequality, and low

Table 7.6 Factors known or reasonably suspected to influence outcome after a concussive brain injury (CBI): a modified Haddon matrix

Before the injury	Patient factors	Injury factors	Environmental factors
	Genetic variation Epigenetic variation Intrauterine environment and health Birth trauma Infant maternal bonding, health, and nutrition "Race" Sex Parenting Overall health from childhood to injury Stress exposure from fetal life to injury Brain injury (toxic, infectious, vascular, inflammatory, epileptogenic, traumatic) prior to index CBI Physical properties of the brain (see "during the injury") Psychological properties, including emotional regulation and resilience, subjective well-being, self-esteem, independence, "personality," thought and cognitive properties, and history of episodic atypicality of any of these History of exposures to atypical stressors and adversities Socioeconomic status Educational achievement Occupational history Social standing Level of alertness Helmet	Not applicable	**Built-environment factors** (e.g., heights, asphalt, traffic, potholes, lighting, tools/machines, unsecured or obstructive objects, area rugs, non-social distractors such as glare, unusual occurrences) **Weather-related factors** (e.g., rain, snow, ice, wind, heat) **Social environment factors** (e.g., child abuse, sports participation, poverty, assaults, military enlistment, social distractors such as cell phones; socio-sexual incentives to risk brain injury) **Factors involving both social and built environments** (e.g., altitude, exposure to personal or public vehicles) **Toxic factors** (e.g., alcohol, medications, illicit drugs) **Educational factors** (e.g., sufficient quality education to discourage participation in street crime and obtain a low-brain-risk job; brain safety training at home or elsewhere, including training of supervisors of sports and training of doctors; media depictions of TBI) **Cultural factors** (e.g., tolerance of fighting or domestic abuse; prejudice and bigotry; pressure for athletic participation and other rewards for risk taking; pervasiveness of gang influence; tolerance of speeding; tolerance of inequality; safety culture (helmet or seatbelt popularity) **Health care delivery factors** (e.g., proximity to hospitals or clinics; availability of TBI experts; availability of rehabilitation facilities)
During the injury	1. Position and fit of the helmet at the moment of impact 2. The momentary state of the brain, e.g., psychological status (including fear), hydration status, hormonal status, blood flow, energy status, ionic/electrochemical status, and transcriptional activity of each cell and synapse and larger unit of analysis at the moment of impact 3. The shape, size, and intensive and extensive physiochemical properties of each molecule and larger unit of analysis of the victim's head and its contents (e.g., hardness, density, malleability, friability, conductivity, volume, mass, specific weight and specific gravity, compressibility or bulk modulus, shear modulus, Young's modulus, Poisson's ratio, and intermolecular forces	The locus, number, and temporal sequence of the multiple waves of impact from a single blow The linear and rotational acceleration, force, and linear strain, shear strain, and volume strains of each impact on each molecule or unit of tissue comprising the head and neck	Temperature, barometric pressure, humidity, and wind speed at the moment of impact Physical properties of any surface encountered by the head Presence and capabilities of witnesses
After the injury	All of the above plus the post-injury changes in the brain – from structural perturbation, to altered gene transcription, to energy, ionic, vascular, hormonal, inflammatory, and other changes at the level of tissue, circuit, cellular and molecular responses Brain–mind *reciprocating trauma* emergent from the initial impact of tissue change (the post-concussive melee) on conscious and unconscious perceptions and all that comprises identity Functional sequelae		Emergency management in the field Emergency management at a medical facility Follow-up care or rehabilitation Responses of the social milieu (e.g., family, friends, co-workers, acquaintances) Responses of the occupational milieu Economic and legal sequelae including possible changes in socioeconomic status, residence, or occupation

education decrease the availability of care, rehabilitation, work accommodation, and alternative gainful employment.)

For reasons such as these, the author cannot commend the Haddon matrix as an elegant heuristic model. He merely hopes that this table summarizes the state of the art in a visually friendly format (Table 7.6).

The reader will encounter a novel phrase in the matrix describing what happens to the CBI survivor after the accident: brain–mind *reciprocating trauma*. The author has cast about for years, hoping to hit upon a pithier and more self-explanatory phrase that captures the phenomenon in question. He apologizes for the awkwardness of this one, and will gladly welcome almost any substitute.

As explained throughout this chapter, the available data do not lend themselves to a before-and-after analysis of brain injury. "Before" was not a fixed brain state but a dynamic, ever-changing physiochemical flow. "After" is the same. Prior to the moment of impact, the brain of the victim – and the mind that brain mediates – were both different every moment since their fetal fruition. Starting at the moment of injury, the brain and the mind continue to change, although the degree of change per unit time is admittedly more dramatic than the previous moment-by-moment change. Indeed, due to the neurometabolic-vascular–inflammatory melee the brain might change quite profoundly during the first several months, and possibly continue to change each moment – but along a new trajectory – until death.[39]

But brain and mind are as gracefully entwined as yin and yang. A change in one requires a change in the other. Consider a woman who strikes her head. Now she has a brain impacted by abrupt external force. That changed brain leads to changes in function and perception and mood and cognition. None of these are static. Changes in brain produce changes in mind and, somewhat like the swinging balls in Newton's cradle, changes in mind cause changes in brain. A commonplace example: the woman's medial temporal lobe was harmed by the forces of the accident. She has memory loss and irritability. Over the three months after injury, she may progressively realize that her memory loss and irritability are not improving as much as she had hoped. Insight of loss may provoke depression. Depression and stress will alter her aminergic transmission and HPA. Glucocorticoids and other biological aspects of stress may further injure her medial temporal lobe. This further injury may impact her memory and mood, which in turn might perpetuate the vicious cycle of stress and damage. "Brain–mind reciprocal stress," or something of that sort, is the best the present author can do at the moment.

Conclusion

The debate about the prognosis after TBI is literally ancient history. In the *Aphorisms* [807], Hippocrates opined that a wound involving the brain is fatal. Galen famously countered, "ἐγκέφαλον δε τρωθένντα εἴδομεν ἰνδέντα" ("but I have seen

a severely wounded brain healed") [808]. The present author hopes that some of the reasons for this 2000-year-old argument have become more clear: Hippocrates and Galen *both* made credible observations. But they saw different patients. To a degree that seems infrequently matched by other protean medical disorders, *CBIs vary*. Ill-conceived attempts to gloss over the awe-inspiring heterogeneity of TBI by such sophistries as dichotomizing the continuum of severity have been exposed. The present author offers his own aphorism: when in doubt, be in doubt. Only harm attends the pretense that we understand all the ways in which an external force that rattles the brain may change a life. Despite the last decade's squall of empirical fervor, despite the sacrifices of innumerable patients to our well-meant, half-baked science, despite the intellectual paradigm shifts reported so far in this book, we should regard ourselves as beginners – Darwins on the dock in Plymouth, about to set foot on the *Beagle*. Our heads may be largely empty, but they are prepared.

The goals of this brief chapter are modest. The author has tried to compile and systematically organize what is known and what seems likely regarding the uniqueness of every concussion. Abundant citations will hopefully make it easy for readers to explore further. New discoveries are sure to improve this part of the textbook. The essential message, however, is both so ferociously debated as to have seriously delayed the global enterprise of trying to help victims of concussion, and so simple it might be printed on a postage stamp with room to spare: people vary so outcomes vary.

References

1. de Koning ME, Scheenen ME, van der Horn HJ, Hageman G, Roks G, Spikman JM, et al. Non-hospitalized patients with mild traumatic brain injury: the forgotten minority. *J Neurotrauma* 2016; 34(1):257–261.

2. Arciniegas DB, Frey KL, Newman J, Wortzel HS. Evaluation and management of posttraumatic cognitive impairments. *Psychiatr Ann* 2010; 40:540–552.

3. Pretz CR, Malec JF, Hammond FM. Longitudinal description of the disability rating scale for individuals in the National Institute on Disability and Rehabilitation Research traumatic brain injury model systems national database. *Arch Phys Med Rehabil* 2013; 94(12):2478–2485.

4. Alves W, Macciocchi SN, Barth JT. Postconcussive symptoms after uncomplicated mild head injury. *J Head Trauma Rehabil* 1993; 8(3):48–59.

5. Bazarian JJ, Atabaki S. Predicting postconcussion syndrome after minor traumatic brain injury. *Acad Emerg Med* 2001; 8(8):788–795.

6. Bazarian JJ, Blyth B, Mookerjee S, He H, McDermott MP. Sex differences in outcome after mild traumatic brain injury. *J Neurotrauma* 2010; 27(3):527–539.

7. Bazarian JJ, Wong T, Harris M, Leahey N, Mookerjee S, Dombovy M. Epidemiology and predictors of post-concussive syndrome after minor head injury in an emergency population. *Brain Inj* 1999; 13(3):173–189.

8. Benson BW, Meeuwisse WH, Rizos J, Kang J, Burke CJ. A prospective study of concussions among National Hockey

---

[39] Please refer to the chapters discussing the likelihood that one or more concussions may cause lifelong brain changes that accelerate dementia.

League players during regular season games: the NHL-NHLPA Concussion Program. *Can Med Assoc J* 2011; 183(8):905–911.

9. Binder LM. Persisting symptoms after mild head injury: a review of the postconcussive syndrome. *J Clin Exp Neuropsychol* 1986; 8(4):323–346.

10. Carroll LJ, Cassidy JD, Holm L, Kraus J, Coronado VG, the WHO Collaborating Centre Task Force on Mild Traumatic Brain Injury. Methodological issues and research recommendations for mild traumatic brain injury: the WHO Collaborating Centre Task Force on Mild Traumatic Brain Injury. *J Rehabil Med* 2004; (43 Suppl):113–125.

11. Dischinger PC, Ryb GE, Kufera JA, Auman KM. Early predictors of postconcussive syndrome in a population of trauma patients with mild traumatic brain injury. *J Trauma* 2009; 66(2):289–296; discussion 296–297.

12. Edna TH, Cappelen J. Late post-concussional symptoms in traumatic head injury. An analysis of frequency and risk factors. *Acta Neurochir (Wien)* 1987; 86(1–2):12–17.

13. Field M, Collins MW, Lovell MR, Maroon J. Does age play a role in recovery from sports-related concussion? A comparison of high school and collegiate athletes. *J Pediatr* 2003; 142(5):546–553.

14. Jacobs B, Beems T, Stulemeijer M, van Vugt AB, van der Vliet TM, Borm GF, et al. Outcome prediction in mild traumatic brain injury: age and clinical variables are stronger predictors than CT abnormalities. *J Neurotrauma* 2010; 27(4):655–668.

15. Jotwani V, Harmon KG. Postconcussion syndrome in athletes. *Curr Sports Med Rep* 2010; 9(1):21–26.

16. King NS, Kirwilliam S. Permanent post-concussion symptoms after mild head injury. *Brain Inj* 2011; 25(5):462–470.

17. Leininger S, Strong CA, Donders J. Predictors of outcome after treatment of mild traumatic brain injury: a pilot study. *J Head Trauma Rehabil* 2014; 29(2):109–116.

18. Luis CA, Vanderploeg RD, Curtiss G. Predictors of postconcussion symptom complex in community dwelling male veterans. *J Int Neuropsychol Soc* 2003; 9(7):1001–1015.

19. McCauley SR, Boake C, Levin HS, Contant CF, Song JX. Postconcussional disorder following mild to moderate traumatic brain injury: anxiety, depression, and social support as risk factors and comorbidities. *J Clin Exp Neuropsychol* 2001; 23(6):792–808.

20. McCrory P, Meeuwisse WH, Aubry M, Cantu B, Dvorak J, Echemendia RJ, et al. Consensus statement on concussion in sport: the 4th International Conference on Concussion in Sport held in Zurich, November 2012. *Br J Sports Med* 2013; 47(5):250–258.

21. Ponsford J, Willmott C, Rothwell A, Cameron P, Kelly AM, Nelms R, et al. Factors influencing outcome following mild traumatic brain injury in adults. *J Int Neuropsychol Soc* 2000; 6(5):568–579.

22. Scott KL, Strong CA, Gorter B, Donders J. Predictors of postconcussion rehabilitation outcomes at three-month follow-up. *Clin Neuropsychol* 2016; 30(1):66–81.

23. Silverberg ND, Gardner AJ, Brubacher JR, Panenka WJ, Li JJ, Iverson GL. Systematic review of multivariable prognostic models for mild traumatic brain injury. *J Neurotrauma* 2015; 32(8):517–526.

24. Wall PL. Posttraumatic stress disorder and traumatic brain injury in current military populations: a critical analysis. *J Am Psychiatr Nurses Assoc* 2012; 18(5):278–298.

25. Wojcik SM. Predicting mild traumatic brain injury patients at risk of persistent symptoms in the Emergency Department. *Brain Inj* 2014; 28(4):422–430.

26. Zemek RL, Farion KJ, Sampson M, McGahern C. Prognosticators of persistent symptoms following pediatric concussion: a systematic review. *JAMA Pediatr* 2013; 167(3):259–265.

27. Johnson B, Zhang K, Gay M, Horovitz S, Hallett M, Sebastianelli W, et al. Alteration of brain default network in subacute phase of injury in concussed individuals: Resting-state fMRI study. *NeuroImage* 2012; 59: 511–518.

28. Maines RP. *The technology of orgasm: "hysteria," the vibrator, and women's sexual satisfaction*. Baltimore, MD: JHU Press, 1999.

29. Garrod A. The Croonian lectures on inborn errors of metabolism. Delivered before the Royal College of Physicians on June 18th, 23rd, 25th, and 30th (1908). *Lancet* 172(4427): 1–7; 172(4428): 73–79; 172(4429): 142–148; 172(4430): 214–230.

30. Garrod A. *Inborn errors of metabolism*. London, England: Frowde, Hodder & Stoughton, 1909.

31. Tator CH, Davis HS, Dufort PA, Tartaglia MC, Davis KD, Ebraheem A, et al. Postconcussion syndrome: demographics and predictors in 221 patients. *J Neurosurg* 2016; 1–11.

32. King NS, Crawford S, Wenden FJ, Moss NE, Wade DT. The Rivermead Post Concussion Symptoms Questionnaire: a measure of symptoms commonly experienced after head injury and its reliability. *J Neurol* 1995; 242(9):587–592.

33. Jennett B, Bond M. Assessment of outcome after severe brain damage. *Lancet* 1975; 1(7905):480–484.

34. Hamilton B, Granger C, Sherwin F, Zielezny M, Tashman J. Uniform national data system for medical rehabilitation. In: Fuhrer M, editor. *Rehabilitation outcomes: analysis and measurement*. Baltimore, MD: Brookes, 1987, pp. 137–147.

35. Keith RA, Granger CV, Hamilton BB, Sherwin FS. The Functional Independence Measure: a new tool for rehabilitation. *Adv Clin Rehabil* 1987; 1:6–18.

36. *Guide for the Uniform Data Set for Medical Rehabilitation (Adult FIM), version 4.0*. Buffalo, NY: State University of New York at Buffalo, 1993.

37. Corrigan JD, Smith-Knapp K, Granger CV. Validity of the functional independence measure for persons with traumatic brain injury. *Arch Phys Med Rehabil* 1997; 78(8):828–834.

38. World Health Organization (WHO). *WHODAS II – Disability Assessment Schedule training manual: a guide to administration*. Geneva: World Health Organization, 2004. Available from: www.who.int/icidh/whodas/training_man.pdf.

39. Üstün TB, Kostanjsek N, Chatterji S, Rehm J. *Measuring health and disability: manual for WHO Disability Assessment Schedule WHODAS 2.0*. Geneva: World Health Organization, 2010.

40. Eyres S, Carey A, Gilworth G, Neumann V, Tennant A. Construct validity and reliability of the Rivermead Post-Concussion Symptoms Questionnaire. *Clin Rehabil* 2005; 19(8):878–887.

41. Achenbach T. Achenbach system of empirically based assessment (ASEBA). April 12, 2014 [cited 2017 August 17]. Available from: www.aseba.org/adults.html.

42. Achenbach TM. *Achenbach System of Empirically Based Assessment (ASEBA): development, findings, theory, and applications*. Burlington, VT: University of Vermont, Research Center of Children, Youth & Families, 2009.

43. Achenbach T, Rescorla L. *Manual for the ASEBA adult forms and profiles*. Burlington, VT: University of Vermont, Research Center for Children, Youth, and Families, 2003.

44. Achenbach TM. *Manual for the Child Behavior Checklist/4–18 and 1991 profile*. Burlington, VT: University of Vermont, Department of Psychiatry, 1991.

45. Achenbach TM. *Integrative guide to the 1991 CBCL/4–18, YSR, and TRF profiles*. Burlington, VT: University of Vermont, Department of Psychiatry, 1991.

46. Achenbach TM, Becker A, Döpfner M, Heiervang E, Roessner V, Steinhausen HC, et al. Multicultural assessment of child and adolescent psychopathology with ASEBA and SDQ instruments: research findings, applications, and future directions. *J Child Psychol Psychiatry* 2008; 49(3):251–275.

47. Achenbach TM, Edelbrock CS. *Manual for the Teacher's Report Form and Teacher Version of Child Behavior Profile*. Burlington, VT: University of Vermont, Department of Psychiatry, 1986.

48. Achenbach TM, Ruffle TM. The Child Behavior Checklist and related forms for assessing behavioral/emotional problems and competencies. *Pediatr Rev* 2000; 21(8):265–271.

49. Brigidi BD, Achenbach TM, Dumenci L, Newhouse PA. Broad spectrum assessment of psychopathology and adaptive functioning with the Older Adult Behavior Checklist: a validation and diagnostic discrimination study. *Int J Geriatr Psychiatry* 2010; 25(11):1177–1185.

50. Reef J, Diamantopoulou S, van Meurs I, Verhulst F, van der Ende J. Predicting adult emotional and behavioral problems from externalizing problem trajectories in a 24-year longitudinal study. *J Eur Child Adolesc Psychiatry* 2010; 19(7):577–585.

51. Reef J, van Meurs I, Verhulst FC, van der Ende J. Children's problems predict adults' DSM-IV disorders across 24 years. *J Am Acad Child Adolesc Psychiatry* 2010; 49(11):1117–1124.

52. Rescorla L, Achenbach T, Ivanova MY, Dumenci L, Almqvist F, Bilenberg N, et al. Behavioral and emotional problems reported by parents of children ages 6 to 16 in 31 societies. *J Emot Behav Disord* 2007; 15(3):130–142.

53. National Institutes of Health. NIH Tool Box for the assessment of neurological and behavioral function. 2016. [cited 2017 August 17]. Available from: www.nihtoolbox.org/Pages/default.aspx.

54. Fayol P, Carriere H, Habonimana D, Dumond JJ. Preliminary questions before studying mild traumatic brain injury outcome. *Ann Phys Rehabil Med* 2009; 52(6):497–509.

55. Bearn AG. *Archibald Garrod and the individuality of man*. Oxford: Clarendon Press, 1993.

56. Teasdale G, Jennett B. Assessment of coma and impaired consciousness. A practical scale. *Lancet* 1974; 2(7872):81–84.

57. Jefferson G. Notes on cortical localization. *Can Med Assoc J* 1916; 6(1):30–38.

58. Sabbatini RM. Phrenology: the history of brain localization. [Internet]. *Brain Mind* 1997 [cited 2017 August 17]. Available from: www.cerebromente.org.br/n01/frenolog/frenologia.htm.

59. Wells SR. *How to read character: a new illustrated hand-book of phrenology and physiognomy, for students and examiners; with a descriptive chart*. New York: Samuel R. Wells, 1874.

60. Brodmann K. *Vergleichende Lokalisationslehre der Grosshirnrinde in ihren Prinzipien dargestellt auf Grund des Zellenbaues [Brodmann's localization in the cerebral cortex]*. Leipzig: Barth, 1909.

61. von Economo CF, Koskinas GN. *Die Cytoarchitektonik der Hirnrinde des erwachsenen Menschen [The cyto-architectonics of the cerebral cortex of adult man]*. Vienna: Julius Springer, 1925. Edited and translated by Garey LJ. New York: Springer, 2006.

62. Auburtin S. Reprise de la discussion sur la forme et le volume du cerveau [Resuming debate on the shape and volume of the brain]. *Bull Soc Anthropol* 1861; 2:209–220.

63. Jefferson G. The prodromes to cortical localization. *J Neurol Neurosurg Psychiatry* 1953; 16(2):59.

64. Gross CG. The discovery of motor cortex and its background. *J Hist Neurosci* 2007; 16(3):320–331.

65. Hoaken PC. Monozygotic twins discordant for schizophrenia. Similarities and differences in life patterns. *Psychiatr Q* 1969; 43(4):612–621.

66. Reveley AM, Reveley MA, Clifford CA, Murray RM. Cerebral ventricular size in twins discordant for schizophrenia. *Lancet* 1982; 1(8271):540–541.

67. Suddath RL, Christison GW, Torrey EF, Casanova MF, Weinberger DR. Anatomical abnormalities in the brains of monozygotic twins discordant for schizophrenia. *N Engl J Med* 1990; 322(12):789–794.

68. Kato T, Iwamoto K, Kakiuchi C, Kuratomi G, Okazaki Y. Genetic or epigenetic difference causing discordance between monozygotic twins as a clue to molecular basis of mental disorders. *Mol Psychiatry* 2005; 10(7):622–630.

69. Machin G. Non-identical monozygotic twins, intermediate twin types, zygosity testing, and the non-random nature of monozygotic twinning: a review. *Am J Med Genet C Semin Med Genet* 2009; 151C(2):110–127.

70. Silva S, Martins Y, Matias A, Blickstein I. Why are monozygotic twins different? *J Perinat Med* 2011; 39(2):195–202.

71. Singh SM, Murphy B, O'Reilly R. Epigenetic contributors to the discordance of monozygotic twins. *Clin Genet* 2002; 62(2):97–103.

72. Haque FN, Gottesman, II, Wong AH. Not really identical: epigenetic differences in monozygotic twins and implications for twin studies in psychiatry. *Am J Med Genet C Semin Med Genet* 2009; 151C(2):136–141.

73. Dempster EL, Pidsley R, Schalkwyk LC, Owens S, Georgiades A, Kane F, et al. Disease-associated epigenetic changes in monozygotic twins discordant for schizophrenia and bipolar disorder. *Hum Mol Genet* 2011; 20(24):4786–4796.

74. Zwijnenburg PJ, Meijers-Heijboer H, Boomsma DI. Identical but not the same: the value of discordant monozygotic twins in genetic research. *Am J Med Genet B Neuropsychiatr Genet* 2010; 153B(6):1134–1149.

75. Weinberger D, Bartley A, Jones D, Zigun J, editors. Regional cortical gyral variations in human monozygotic twins. *Soc Neurosci Abstr* 1992.

76. Steinmetz H, Herzog A, Huang Y, Hacklander T. Discordant brain-surface anatomy in monozygotic twins. *N Engl J Med* 1994; 331(14):952–953.

77. Biondi A, Nogueira H, Dormont D, Duyme M, Hasboun D, Zouaoui A, et al. Are the brains of monozygotic twins similar? A three-dimensional MR study. *Am J Neuroradiol* 1998; 19(7):1361–1367.

78. Oppenheim JS, Skerry JE, Tramo MJ, Gazzaniga MS. Magnetic resonance imaging morphology of the corpus callosum in monozygotic twins. *Ann Neurol* 1989; 26(1):100–104.

79. Peper JS, Brouwer RM, Boomsma DI, Kahn RS, Pol H, Hilleke E. Genetic influences on human brain structure: a review of brain imaging studies in twins. *Hum Brain Mapp* 2007; 28(6):464–473.

80. Schmitt JE, Eyler LT, Giedd JN, Kremen WS, Kendler KS, Neale MC. Review of twin and family studies on neuroanatomic phenotypes and typical neurodevelopment. *Twin Res Hum Genet* 2007; 10(5):683–694.

81. Eyler LT, Chen CH, Panizzon MS, Fennema-Notestine C, Neale MC, Jak A, et al. A comparison of heritability maps of cortical surface area and thickness and the influence of adjustment for whole brain measures: a magnetic resonance imaging twin study. *Twin Res Hum Genet* 2012; 15(3):304–314.

82. Batouli SA, Trollor JN, Wen W, Sachdev PS. The heritability of volumes of brain structures and its relationship to age: a review of twin and family studies. *Ageing Res Rev* 2014; 13:1–9.

83. Pedersen NL, Miller BL, Wetherell JL, Vallo J, Toga AW, Knutson N, et al. Neuroimaging findings in twins discordant for Alzheimer's disease. *Dement Geriatr Cogn Disord* 1999; 10(1):51–58.

84. Jansen AG, Mous SE, White T, Posthuma D, Polderman TJ. What twin studies tell us about the heritability of brain development, morphology, and function: a review. *Neuropsychol Rev* 2015; 25(1):27–46.

85. Lee T, Sachdev P. The contributions of twin studies to the understanding of brain ageing and neurocognitive disorders. *Curr Opin Psychiatry* 2014; 27(2):122–127.

86. Eyler LT, Vuoksimaa E, Panizzon MS, Fennema-Notestine C, Neale MC, Chen CH, et al. Conceptual and data-based investigation of genetic influences and brain asymmetry: a twin study of multiple structural phenotypes. *J Cogn Neurosci* 2014; 26(5):1100–1117.

87. Yoon U, Fahim C, Perusse D, Evans AC. Lateralized genetic and environmental influences on human brain morphology of 8-year-old twins. *NeuroImage* 2010; 53(3):1117–1125.

88. Brouwer RM, Mandl RC, Peper JS, van Baal GC, Kahn RS, Boomsma DI, et al. Heritability of DTI and MTR in nine-year-old children. *NeuroImage* 2010; 53(3):1085–1092.

89. Shen K-K, Rose S, Fripp J, McMahon KL, de Zubicaray GI, Martin NG, et al. Investigating brain connectivity heritability in a twin study using diffusion imaging data. *NeuroImage* 2014; 100:628–641.

90. Vuoksimaa E, Panizzon MS, Hagler Jr DJ, Hatton SN, Fennema-Notestine C, Rinker D, et al. Heritability of white matter microstructure in late middle age: a twin study of tract-based fractional anisotropy and absolute diffusivity indices. *Hum Brain Mapp* 2017; 38(4):2026–2036.

91. Polk TA, Park J, Smith MR, Park DC. Nature versus nurture in ventral visual cortex: a functional magnetic resonance imaging study of twins. *J Neurosci* 2007; 27(51):13921–13925.

92. Matthews SC, Simmons AN, Strigo I, Jang K, Stein MB, Paulus MP. Heritability of anterior cingulate response to conflict: an fMRI study in female twins. *NeuroImage* 2007; 38(1):223–227.

93. Silverman MH, Krueger RF, Iacono WG, Malone SM, Hunt RH, Thomas KM. Quantifying familial influences on brain activation during the monetary incentive delay task: an adolescent monozygotic twin study. *Biol Psychol* 2014; 103:7–14.

94. Glahn DC, Winkler AM, Kochunov P, Almasy L, Duggirala R, Carless MA, et al. Genetic control over the resting brain. *Proc Natl Acad Sci U S A* 2010; 107(3):1223–1228.

95. Spencer H. *The principles of psychology*. London: Longman, Brown, Green and Longmans, 1855.

96. Kenzie JM, Semrau JA, Findlater SE, Yu AY, Desai JA, Herter TM, et al. Localization of impaired kinesthetic processing post-stroke. *Front Hum Neurosci* 2016; 10:505.

97. Kambara T, Brown EC, Jeong JW, Ofen N, Nakai Y, Asano E. Spatio-temporal dynamics of working memory maintenance and scanning of verbal information. *Clin Neurophysiol* 2017; 128(6):882–891.

98. Ferri F, Ebisch SJ, Costantini M, Salone A, Arciero G, Mazzola V, et al. Binding action and emotion in social understanding. *PLoS One* 2013; 8(1):e54091.

99. von Monakow C. *Die Lokalisation im Grosshirn und der Abbau der Funktion durch kortikale Herde [The localization in the cerebrum and the reduction of the function by cortical head]*. Wiesbaden: JF Bergmann, 1914.

100. Bennett CM, Baird AA, Miller MB, Wolford GL. Neural correlates of interspecies perspective taking in the post-mortem Atlantic Salmon: an argument for multiple comparisons correction [Internet]. 2009. Presented at Organization for Human Brain Mapping Annual Conference, San Francisco [cited 2017 August 17]. Available from: www.wired.com/2009/09/fmrisalmon/.

101. McGonigle DJ, Howseman AM, Athwal BS, Friston KJ, Frackowiak RS, Holmes AP. Variability in fMRI: an examination of intersession differences. *Neuroimage* 2000; 11(6 Pt 1):708–734.

102. Wei X, Yoo SS, Dickey CC, Zou KH, Guttmann CR, Panych LP. Functional MRI of auditory verbal working memory: long-term reproducibility analysis. *NeuroImage* 2004; 21(3):1000–1008.

103. Yoo SS, Wei X, Dickey CC, Guttmann CR, Panych LP. Long-term reproducibility analysis of fMRI using hand motor task. *Int J Neurosci* 2005; 115(1):55–77.

104. Plichta MM, Schwarz AJ, Grimm O, Morgen K, Mier D, Haddad L, et al. Test–retest reliability of evoked BOLD signals from a cognitive-emotive fMRI test battery. *NeuroImage* 2012; 60(3):1746–1758.

105. Song X, Panych LP, Chou YH, Chen NK. A study of long-term fMRI reproducibility using data-driven analysis methods. *Int J Imaging Syst Technol* 2014; 24(4):339–349.

106. Pinel P, Thirion B, Meriaux S, Jobert A, Serres J, Le Bihan D, et al. Fast reproducible identification and large-scale databasing of individual functional cognitive networks. *BMC Neurosci* 2007; 8:91.

107. Mesulam MM. Large-scale neurocognitive networks and distributed processing for attention, language, and memory. *Ann Neurol* 1990; 28(5):597–613.

108. Mesulam M-M. *Principles of behavioral and cognitive neurology*. Oxford: Oxford University Press, 2000.

109. Mesulam M. Imaging connectivity in the human cerebral cortex: the next frontier? *Ann Neurol* 2005; 57(1):5–7.

110. Ross ED. Cerebral localization of functions and the neurology of language: fact versus fiction or is it something else? *Neuroscientist* 2010; 16(3):222–243.

111. Catani M, Dell'acqua F, Bizzi A, Forkel SJ, Williams SC, Simmons A, et al. Beyond cortical localization in clinico-anatomical correlation. *Cortex* 2012; 48(10):1262–1287.

112. Pezawas L, Verchinski BA, Mattay VS, Callicott JH, Kolachana BS, Straub RE, et al. The brain-derived neurotrophic factor Val66Met polymorphism and variation in human cortical morphology. *J Neurosci* 2004; 24(45):10099–10102.

113. Dannlowski U, Kugel H, Grotegerd D, Redlich R, Opel N, Dohm K, et al. Disadvantage of social sensitivity: interaction of oxytocin receptor genotype and child maltreatment on brain structure. *Biol Psychiatry* 2015; 80(5):398–405.

114. Perrier E, Pompei F, Ruberto G, Vassos E, Collier D, Frangou S. Initial evidence for the role of CACNA1C on subcortical brain morphology in patients with bipolar disorder. *Eur Psychiatry* 2011; 26(3):135–137.

115. Sprooten E, Gupta CN, Knowles EE, McKay DR, Mathias SR, Curran JE, et al. Genome-wide significant linkage of schizophrenia-related neuroanatomical trait to 12q24. *Am J Med Genet B Neuropsychiatr Genet* 2015; 168(8):678–686.

116. Tavor I, Parker Jones O, Mars RB, Smith SM, Behrens TE, Jbabdi S. Task-free MRI predicts individual differences in brain activity during task performance. *Science* 2016; 352(6282):216–220.

117. Hibar DP, Stein JL, Renteria ME, Arias-Vasquez A, Desrivieres S, Jahanshad N, et al. Common genetic variants influence human subcortical brain structures. *Nature* 2015; 520(7546):224–229.

118. Beckwith JG, Chu JJ, Greenwald RM. Validation of a non-invasive system for measuring head acceleration for use during boxing competition. *J Appl Biomech* 2007; 23(3):238–244.

119. Beckwith JG, Greenwald RM, Chu JJ. Measuring head kinematics in football: correlation between the head impact telemetry system and Hybrid III headform. *Ann Biomed Eng* 2012; 40(1):237–248.

120. Greenwald R, Chu JJ, Crisco JJ, Finkelstein JA. *Head impact telemetry system (HITS) for measurement of head acceleration in the field*. Lebanon, NH: Simbex, 2003.

121. Guskiewicz KM, Mihalik JP, Shankar V, Marshall SW, Crowell DH, Oliaro SM, et al. Measurement of head impacts in collegiate football players: relationship between head impact biomechanics and acute clinical outcome after concussion. *Neurosurgery* 2007; 61(6):1244–1252; discussion 1252–1253.

122. Duhaime AC, Beckwith JG, Maerlender AC, McAllister TW, Crisco JJ, Duma SM, et al. Spectrum of acute clinical characteristics of diagnosed concussions in college athletes

wearing instrumented helmets: clinical article. *J Neurosurg* 2012; 117(6):1092–1099.

123. von Holst H, Li X. Consequences of the dynamic triple peak impact factor in traumatic brain injury as measured with numerical simulation. *Front Neurol* 2013; 4:23.

124. Oeur RA, Karton C, Post A, Rousseau P, Hoshizaki TB, Marshall S, et al. A comparison of head dynamic response and brain tissue stress and strain using accident reconstructions for concussion, concussion with persistent postconcussive symptoms, and subdural hematoma. *J Neurosurg* 2015; 123(2):415–422.

125. Post A, Hoshizaki TB, Gilchrist MD, Brien S, Cusimano M, Marshall S. The dynamic response characteristics of traumatic brain injury. *Accid Anal Prev* 2015; 79:33–40.

126. Carlsen RW, Daphalapurkar NP. The importance of structural anisotropy in computational models of traumatic brain injury. *Front Neurol* 2015; 6:28.

127. Giordano C, Cloots RJ, van Dommelen JA, Kleiven S. The influence of anisotropy on brain injury prediction. *J Biomech* 2014; 47(5):1052–1059.

128. Giordano C, Kleiven S. Evaluation of axonal strain as a predictor for mild traumatic brain injuries using finite element modeling. *Stapp Car Crash J* 2014; 58:29–61.

129. Bohnen N, Jolles J. Neurobehavioral aspects of postconcussive symptoms after mild head injury. *J Nerv Ment Dis* 1992; 180(11):683–692.

130. Bohnen N, Twijnstra A, Jolles J. Post-traumatic and emotional symptoms in different subgroups of patients with mild head injury. *Brain Inj* 1992; 6(6):481–487.

131. Lidvall HF, Linderoth B, Norlin B. Causes of the post-concussional syndrome. *Acta Neurol Scand Suppl* 1974; 56:3–144.

132. Rutherford W. Postconcussion symptoms: relationship to acute neurological indices, individual differences, and circumstances of injury. In: Levin H, Eisenberg H, Benton A, editors. *Mild head injury.* New York: Oxford University Press, 1989, pp. 217–228.

133. Adler A. Mental symptoms following head injury: a statistical analysis of two hundred cases. *Arch Clin Neuropsychol* 1945; 53(1):34–43.

134. Dikmen S, Machamer J, Fann JR, Temkin NR. Rates of symptom reporting following traumatic brain injury. *J Int Neuropsychol Soc* 2010; 16(3):401–411.

135. Lundin A, de Boussard C, Edman G, Borg J. Symptoms and disability until 3 months after mild TBI. *Brain Inj* 2006; 20(8):799–806.

136. M M. *Postcommotionelle Klager.* Copenhagen: Munksgaard, 1967.

137. Meares S, Shores EA, Taylor AJ, Batchelor J, Bryant RA, Baguley IJ, et al. The prospective course of postconcussion syndrome: the role of mild traumatic brain injury. *Neuropsychology* 2011; 25(4):454–465.

138. Slobounov S, Sebastianelli W, Hallett M. Residual brain dysfunction observed one year post-mild traumatic brain injury: combined EEG and balance study. *Clin Neurophysiol* 2012; 123(9):1755–1761.

139. McMahon P, Hricik A, Yue JK, Puccio AM, Inoue T, Lingsma HF, et al. Symptomatology and functional outcome in mild traumatic brain injury: results from the prospective TRACK-TBI study. *J Neurotrauma* 2014; 31(1):26–33.

140. Kelly R. The post-traumatic syndrome: an iatrogenic disease. *Forensic Sci* 1975; 6(1–2):17–24.

141. Long CJ, Novack TA. Postconcussion symptoms after head trauma: interpretation and treatment. *South Med J* 1986; 79(6):728–732.

142. Wallace AR. Sir Charles Lyell on geological climates and the origin of species. *Q Rev* 1869; 126(252):359–394.

143. Colak T, Cine N, Bamac B, Kurtas O, Ozbek A, Bicer U, et al. Microarray-based gene expression analysis of an animal model for closed head injury. *Injury* 2012; 43(8):1264–1270.

144. Di Pietro V, Amin D, Pernagallo S, Lazzarino G, Tavazzi B, Vagnozzi R, et al. Transcriptomics of traumatic brain injury: gene expression and molecular pathways of different grades of insult in a rat organotypic hippocampal culture model. *J Neurotrauma* 2010; 27(2):349–359.

145. Di Pietro V, Amorini AM, Tavazzi B, Hovda DA, Signoretti S, Giza CC, et al. Potentially neuroprotective gene modulation in an in vitro model of mild traumatic brain injury. *Mol Cell Biochem* 2013; 375(1–2):185–198.

146. Giza CC, Prins ML, Hovda DA, Herschman HR, Feldman JD. Genes preferentially induced by depolarization after concussive brain injury: effects of age and injury severity. *J Neurotrauma* 2002; 19(4):387–402.

147. Lei P, Li Y, Chen X, Yang S, Zhang J. Microarray based analysis of microRNA expression in rat cerebral cortex after traumatic brain injury. *Brain Res* 2009; 1284:191–201.

148. Michael DB, Byers DM, Irwin LN. Gene expression following traumatic brain injury in humans: analysis by microarray. *J Clin Neurosci* 2005; 12(3):284–290.

149. Natale JE, Ahmed F, Cernak I, Stoica B, Faden AI. Gene expression profile changes are commonly modulated across models and species after traumatic brain injury. *J Neurotrauma* 2003; 20(10):907–927.

150. Raghavendra Rao VL, Dhodda VK, Song G, Bowen KK, Dempsey RJ. Traumatic brain injury-induced acute gene expression changes in rat cerebral cortex identified by GeneChip analysis. *J Neurosci Res* 2003; 71(2):208–219.

151. Rojo DR, Prough DS, Falduto MT, Boone DR, Micci MA, Kahrig KM, et al. Influence of stochastic gene expression on the cell survival rheostat after traumatic brain injury. *PLoS One* 2011; 6(8):e23111.

152. Shimamura M, Garcia JM, Prough DS, Dewitt DS, Uchida T, Shah SA, et al. Analysis of long-term gene expression in neurons of the hippocampal subfields following traumatic brain injury in rats. *Neuroscience* 2005; 131(1):87–97.

153. Tweedie D, Rachmany L, Rubovitch V, Lehrmann E, Zhang Y, Becker KG, et al. Exendin-4, a glucagon-like peptide-1 receptor agonist prevents mTBI-induced changes in hippocampus gene expression and memory deficits in mice. *Exp Neurol* 2013; 239:170–182.

154. Tweedie D, Rachmany L, Rubovitch V, Zhang Y, Becker KG, Perez E, et al. Changes in mouse cognition and hippocampal gene expression observed in a mild physical- and blast-traumatic brain injury. *Neurobiol Dis* 2013; 54:1–11.

155. Tweedie D, Rachmany L, Kim DS, Rubovitch V, Lehrmann E, Zhang Y, et al. Mild traumatic brain injury-induced hippocampal gene expressions: The identification of target cellular processes for drug development. *J Neurosci Methods* 2016; 272:4–18.

156. Dardiotis E, Fountas KN, Dardioti M, Xiromerisiou G, Kapsalaki E, Tasiou A, et al. Genetic association studies in patients with traumatic brain injury. *Neurosurg Focus* 2010; 28(1):E9.

157. Diaz-Arrastia R, Baxter VK. Genetic factors in outcome after traumatic brain injury: what the human genome project can teach us about brain trauma. *J Head Trauma Rehabil* 2006; 21(4):361–374.

158. Finnoff JT, Jelsing EJ, Smith J. Biomarkers, genetics, and risk factors for concussion. *PM R* 2011; 3(10 Suppl 2):S452–S459.

159. Kurowski B, Martin LJ, Wade SL. Genetics and outcomes after traumatic brain injury (TBI): what do we know about pediatric TBI? *J Pediatr Rehabil Med* 2012; 5(3):217–231.

160. McAllister TW. Genetic factors modulating outcome after neurotrauma. *PM R* 2010; 2(12 Suppl 2):S241–S252.

161. Waters RJ, Nicoll JA. Genetic influences on outcome following acute neurological insults. *Curr Opin Crit Care* 2005; 11(2):105–110.

162. Weaver SM, Chau A, Portelli JN, Grafman J. Genetic polymorphisms influence recovery from traumatic brain injury. *Neuroscientist* 2012; 18(6):631–644.

163. Barr TL, Alexander S, Conley Y. Gene expression profiling for discovery of novel targets in human traumatic brain injury. *Biol Res Nurs* 2011; 13(2):140–153.

164. Shen F, Wen L, Yang X, Liu W. The potential application of gene therapy in the treatment of traumatic brain injury. *Neurosurg Rev* 2007; 30(4):291–298.

165. Longhi L, Watson DJ, Saatman KE, Thompson HJ, Zhang C, Fujimoto S, et al. Ex vivo gene therapy using targeted engraftment of NGF-expressing human NT2N neurons attenuates cognitive deficits following traumatic brain injury in mice. *J Neurotrauma* 2004; 21(12):1723–1736.

166. Watson DJ, Longhi L, Lee EB, Fulp CT, Fujimoto S, Royo NC, et al. Genetically modified NT2N human neuronal cells mediate long-term gene expression as CNS grafts in vivo and improve functional cognitive outcome following experimental traumatic brain injury. *J Neuropathol Exp Neurol* 2003; 62(4):368–380.

167. Yamada KH, Kozlowski DA, Seidl SE, Lance S, Wieschhaus AJ, Sundivakkam P, et al. Targeted gene inactivation of calpain-1 suppresses cortical degeneration due to traumatic brain injury and neuronal apoptosis induced by oxidative stress. *J Biol Chem* 2012; 287(16):13182–13193.

168. Kabadi SV, Stoica BA, Loane DJ, Byrnes KR, Hanscom M, Cabatbat RM, et al. Cyclin D1 gene ablation confers neuroprotection in traumatic brain injury. *J Neurotrauma* 2012; 29(5):813–827.

169. Yao XL, Liu J, Lee E, Ling GS, McCabe JT. Progesterone differentially regulates pro- and anti-apoptotic gene expression in cerebral cortex following traumatic brain injury in rats. *J Neurotrauma* 2005; 22(6):656–668.

170. Anderson GD, Farin FM, Bammler TK, Beyer RP, Swan AA, Wilkerson HW, et al. The effect of progesterone dose on gene expression after traumatic brain injury. *J Neurotrauma* 2011; 28(9):1827–1843.

171. Shin SS, Bales JW, Yan HQ, Kline AE, Wagner AK, Lyons-Weiler J, et al. The effect of environmental enrichment on substantia nigra gene expression after traumatic brain injury in rats. *J Neurotrauma* 2013; 30(4):259–270.

172. Svenningsson P, Chergui K, Rachleff I, Flajolet M, Zhang X, El Yacoubi M, et al. Alterations in 5-HT1B receptor function by p11 in depression-like states. *Science* 2006; 311(5757):77–80.

173. Svenningsson P, Kim Y, Warner-Schmidt J, Oh YS, Greengard P. p11 and its role in depression and therapeutic responses to antidepressants. *Nat Rev Neurosci* 2013; 14(10):673–680.

174. Warner-Schmidt JL, Flajolet M, Maller A, Chen EY, Qi H, Svenningsson P, et al. Role of p11 in cellular and behavioral effects of 5-HT4 receptor stimulation. *J Neurosci* 2009; 29(6):1937–1946.

175. Verhagen M, van der Meij A, van Deurzen PA, Janzing JG, Arias-Vasquez A, Buitelaar JK, et al. Meta-analysis of the BDNF Val66Met polymorphism in major depressive disorder: effects of gender and ethnicity. *Mol Psychiatry* 2010; 15(3):260–271.

176. Park SW, Nhu le H, Cho HY, Seo MK, Lee CH, Ly NN, et al. p11 mediates the BDNF-protective effects in dendritic outgrowth and spine formation in B27-deprived primary hippocampal cells. *J Affect Disord* 2016; 196:1–10.

177. Warner-Schmidt JL, Chen EY, Zhang X, Marshall JJ, Morozov A, Svenningsson P, et al. A role for p11 in the antidepressant action of brain-derived neurotrophic factor. *Biol Psychiatry* 2010; 68(6):528–535.

178. Cordell HJ. Detecting gene–gene interactions that underlie human diseases. *Nat Rev Genet* 2009; 10(6):392–404.

179. Koo CL, Liew MJ, Mohamad MS, Salleh AH. A review for detecting gene-gene interactions using machine learning methods in genetic epidemiology. *Biomed Res Int* 2013; 2013:432375.

180. Rodrigues SM, Saslow LR, Garcia N, John OP, Keltner D. Oxytocin receptor genetic variation relates to empathy and stress reactivity in humans. *Proc Natl Acad Sci U S A* 2009; 106(50):21437–21441.

181. Hostinar CE, Cicchetti D, Rogosch FA. Oxytocin receptor gene polymorphism, perceived social support, and psychological symptoms in maltreated adolescents. *Dev Psychopathol* 2014; 26(2):465–477.

182. McQuaid RJ, McInnis OA, Stead JD, Matheson K, Anisman H. A paradoxical association of an oxytocin receptor gene polymorphism: early-life adversity and vulnerability to depression. *Front Neurosci* 2013; 7:128.

183. Colhoun HM, McKeigue PM, Davey Smith G. Problems of reporting genetic associations with complex outcomes. *Lancet* 2003; 361(9360):865–872.

184. Duncan LE, Keller MC. A critical review of the first 10 years of candidate gene-by-environment interaction research in psychiatry. *Am J Psychiatry* 2011; 168(10):1041–1049.

185. Keller MC. Gene × environment interaction studies have not properly controlled for potential confounders: the problem and the (simple) solution. *Biol Psychiatry* 2014; 75(1):18–24.

186. Lee JJ, McGue M. Why behavioral genetics matters: comment on Plomin et al. *Perspect Psychol Sci* 2016; 11(1):29–30.

187. Turkheimer E. Weak genetic explanation 20 years later: reply to Plomin et al. *Perspect Psychol Sci* 2016; 11(1):24–28.

188. Hodes GE, Pfau ML, Purushothaman I, Ahn HF, Golden SA, Christoffel DJ, et al. Sex differences in nucleus accumbens transcriptome profiles associated with susceptibility versus resilience to subchronic variable stress. *J Neurosci* 2015; 35(50):16362–16376.

189. Le Francois B, Soo J, Millar AM, Daigle M, Le Guisquet AM, Leman S, et al. Chronic mild stress and antidepressant treatment alter 5-HT1A receptor expression by modifying DNA methylation of a conserved Sp4 site. *Neurobiol Dis* 2015; 82:332–341.

190. McGowan PO, Kato T. Epigenetics in mood disorders. *Environ Health Prev Med* 2008; 13(1):16–24.

191. Vialou V, Feng J, Robison AJ, Nestler EJ. Epigenetic mechanisms of depression and antidepressant action. *Annu Rev Pharmacol Toxicol* 2013; 53:59–87.

192. Zannas AS, West AE. Epigenetics and the regulation of stress vulnerability and resilience. *Neuroscience* 2014; 264:157–170.

193. Benson DF. Neuropsychiatry and behavioral neurology: past, present, and future. *J Neuropsychiatry Clin Neurosci* 1996; 8(3):351–357.

194. Hawrylycz MJ, Lein ES, Guillozet-Bongaarts AL, Shen EH, Ng L, Miller JA, et al. An anatomically comprehensive atlas of the adult human brain transcriptome. *Nature* 2012; 489(7416):391–399.

195. Pardini M, Krueger F, Koenigs M, Raymont V, Hodgkinson C, Zoubak S, et al. Fatty-acid amide hydrolase polymorphisms and post-traumatic stress disorder after penetrating brain injury. *Transl Psychiatry* 2012; 2:e75.

196. Kokiko-Cochran ON, Ransohoff L, Veenstra M, Lee S, Saber M, Sikora M, et al. Altered neuroinflammation and behavior following traumatic brain injury in a mouse model of Alzheimer's disease. *J Neurotrauma* 2015; 33(7):625–640.

197. Lynch JR, Tang W, Wang H, Vitek MP, Bennett ER, Sullivan PM, et al. APOE genotype and an ApoE-mimetic peptide modify the systemic and central nervous system inflammatory response. *J Biol Chem* 2003; 278(49):48529–48533.

198. Lynch JR, Wang H, Mace B, Leinenweber S, Warner DS, Bennett ER, et al. A novel therapeutic derived from apolipoprotein E reduces brain inflammation and improves outcome after closed head injury. *Exp Neurol* 2005; 192(1):109–116.

199. Weng JF, Chen J, Hong WC, Luo LF, Yu W, Luo SD. Plasma visfatin, associated with a genetic polymorphism −1535C>T, is correlated with C-reactive protein in Chinese Han patients with traumatic brain injury. *Peptides* 2013; 40:8–12.

200. Acaz-Fonseca E, Duran JC, Carrero P, Garcia-Segura LM, Arevalo MA. Sex differences in glia reactivity after cortical brain injury. *Glia* 2015; doi: 10.1002/glia.22867.

201. Pardini M, Krueger F, Hodgkinson C, Raymont V, Ferrier C, Goldman D, et al. Prefrontal cortex lesions and MAO-A modulate aggression in penetrating traumatic brain injury. *Neurology* 2011; 76(12):1038–1045.

202. Isoniemi H, Tenovuo O, Portin R, Himanen L, Kairisto V. Outcome of traumatic brain injury after three decades – relationship to ApoE genotype. *J Neurotrauma* 2006; 23(11):1600–1608.

203. Jordan BD, Relkin NR, Ravdin LD, Jacobs AR, Bennett A, Gandy S. Apolipoprotein E epsilon4 associated with chronic traumatic brain injury in boxing. *JAMA* 1997; 278(2):136–140.

204. Moran LM, Taylor HG, Ganesalingam K, Gastier-Foster JM, Frick J, Bangert B, et al. Apolipoprotein E4 as a predictor of outcomes in pediatric mild traumatic brain injury. *J Neurotrauma* 2009; 26(9):1489–1495.

205. Ponsford J, McLaren A, Schonberger M, Burke R, Rudzki D, Olver J, et al. The association between apolipoprotein E and traumatic brain injury severity and functional outcome in a rehabilitation sample. *J Neurotrauma* 2011; 28(9):1683–1692.

206. Teasdale GM, Nicoll JA, Murray G, Fiddes M. Association of apolipoprotein E polymorphism with outcome after head injury. *Lancet* 1997; 350(9084):1069–1071.

207. Willemse-van Son AH, Ribbers GM, Hop WC, van Duijn CM, Stam HJ. Association between apolipoprotein-epsilon4 and long-term outcome after traumatic brain injury. *J Neurol Neurosurg Psychiatry* 2008; 79(4):426–430.

208. Zhou W, Xu D, Peng X, Zhang Q, Jia J, Crutcher KA. Meta-analysis of APOE4 allele and outcome after traumatic brain injury. *J Neurotrauma* 2008; 25(4):279–290.

209. Lendon CL, Harris JM, Pritchard AL, Nicoll JA, Teasdale GM, Murray G. Genetic variation of the APOE promoter and outcome after head injury. *Neurology* 2003; 61(5):683–685.

210. Terrell TR, Bostick RM, Abramson R, Xie D, Barfield W, Cantu R, et al. APOE, APOE promoter, and Tau genotypes and risk for concussion in college athletes. *Clin J Sport Med* 2008; 18(1):10–17.

211. Garringer JA, Niyonkuru C, McCullough EH, Loucks T, Dixon CE, Conley YP, et al. Impact of aromatase genetic variation on hormone levels and global outcome after severe TBI. *J Neurotrauma* 2013; 30(16):1415–1425.

212. Wang R, Fratiglioni L, Laukka EJ, Lovden M, Kalpouzos G, Keller L, et al. Effects of vascular risk factors and APOE epsilon4 on white matter integrity and cognitive decline. *Neurology* 2015; 84(11):1128–1135.

213. Al Nimer F, Strom M, Lindblom R, Aeinehband S, Bellander BM, Nyengaard JR, et al. Naturally occurring variation in the glutathione-S-transferase 4 gene determines neurodegeneration after traumatic brain injury. *Antioxid Redox Signal* 2013; 18(7):784–794.

214. Chuang PY, Conley YP, Poloyac SM, Okonkwo DO, Ren D, Sherwood PR, et al. Neuroglobin genetic polymorphisms and their relationship to functional outcomes after traumatic brain injury. *J Neurotrauma* 2010; 27(6):999–1006.

215. Waters RJ, Murray GD, Teasdale GM, Stewart J, Day I, Lee RJ, et al. Cytokine gene polymorphisms and outcome after traumatic brain injury. *J Neurotrauma* 2013; 30(20):1710–1716.

216. Ariza M, Matarin MD, Junque C, Mataro M, Clemente I, Moral P, et al. Influence of angiotensin-converting enzyme polymorphism on neuropsychological subacute performance in moderate and severe traumatic brain injury. *J Neuropsychiatry Clin Neurosci* 2006; 18(1):39–44.

217. McAllister TW, Flashman LA, Harker Rhodes C, Tyler AL, Moore JH, Saykin AJ, et al. Single nucleotide polymorphisms in ANKK1 and the dopamine D2 receptor gene affect cognitive outcome shortly after traumatic brain injury: a replication and extension study. *Brain Inj* 2008; 22(9):705–714.

218. Myrga JM, Failla MD, Ricker JH, Dixon CE, Conley YP, Arenth PM, et al. A dopamine pathway gene risk score for cognitive recovery following traumatic brain injury: methodological considerations, preliminary findings, and interactions with sex. *J Head Trauma Rehabil* 2015; 31(5):E15–E29.

219. Anderson GD, Temkin NR, Dikmen SS, Diaz-Arrastia R, Machamer JE, Farhrenbruch C, et al. Haptoglobin phenotype and apolipoprotein E polymorphism: relationship to post-traumatic seizures and neuropsychological functioning after traumatic brain injury. *Epilepsy Behav* 2009; 16(3):501–506.

220. Ariza M, Pueyo R, Matarin Mdel M, Junque C, Mataro M, Clemente I, et al. Influence of APOE polymorphism on cognitive and behavioural outcome in moderate and severe traumatic brain injury. *J Neurol Neurosurg Psychiatry* 2006; 77(10):1191–1193.

221. Chen Y, Lomnitski L, Michaelson DM, Shohami E. Motor and cognitive deficits in apolipoprotein E-deficient mice after closed head injury. *Neuroscience* 1997; 80(4):1255–1262.

222. Crawford FC, Vanderploeg RD, Freeman MJ, Singh S, Waisman M, Michaels L, et al. APOE genotype influences acquisition and recall following traumatic brain injury. *Neurology* 2002; 58(7):1115–1118.

223. Han SD, Drake AI, Cessante LM, Jak AJ, Houston WS, Delis DC, et al. Apolipoprotein E and traumatic brain injury in a military population: evidence of a neuropsychological compensatory mechanism? *J Neurol Neurosurg Psychiatry* 2007; 78(10):1103–1108.

224. Kutner KC, Erlanger DM, Tsai J, Jordan B, Relkin NR. Lower cognitive performance of older football players possessing apolipoprotein E epsilon4. *Neurosurgery* 2000; 47(3):651–657; discussion 657–658.

225. Muller K, Ingebrigtsen T, Wilsgaard T, Wikran G, Fagerheim T, Romner B, et al. Prediction of time trends in recovery of cognitive function after mild head injury. *Neurosurgery* 2009; 64(4):698–704; discussion 704.

226. Noe E, Ferri J, Colomer C, Moliner B, Chirivella J. APOE genotype and verbal memory recovery during and after emergence from post-traumatic amnesia. *Brain Inj* 2010; 24(6):886–892.

227. Ponsford J, Rudzki D, Bailey K, Ng KT. Impact of apolipoprotein gene on cognitive impairment and recovery after traumatic brain injury. *Neurology* 2007; 68(8):619–620.

228. Shadli RM, Pieter MS, Yaacob MJ, Rashid FA. APOE genotype and neuropsychological outcome in mild-to-moderate traumatic brain injury: a pilot study. *Brain Inj* 2011; 25(6):596–603.

229. Krueger F, Pardini M, Huey ED, Raymont V, Solomon J, Lipsky RH, et al. The role of the Met66 brain-derived neurotrophic factor allele in the recovery of executive functioning after combat-related traumatic brain injury. *J Neurosci* 2011; 31(2):598–606.

230. McAllister TW, Tyler AL, Flashman LA, Rhodes CH, McDonald BC, Saykin AJ, et al. Polymorphisms in the brain-derived

neurotrophic factor gene influence memory and processing speed one month after brain injury. *J Neurotrauma* 2012; 29(6):1111–1118.

231. Lipsky RH, Sparling MB, Ryan LM, Xu K, Salazar AM, Goldman D, et al. Association of COMT Val158Met genotype with executive functioning following traumatic brain injury. *J Neuropsychiatry Clin Neurosci* 2005; 17(4):465–471.

232. Winkler EA, Yue JK, McAllister TW, Temkin NR, Oh SS, Burchard EG, et al. COMT Val 158 Met polymorphism is associated with nonverbal cognition following mild traumatic brain injury. *Neurogenetics* 2016; 17(1):31–41.

233. McAllister TW, Rhodes CH, Flashman LA, McDonald BC, Belloni D, Saykin AJ. Effect of the dopamine D2 receptor T allele on response latency after mild traumatic brain injury. *Am J Psychiatry* 2005; 162(9):1749–1751.

234. Wagner AK, Hatz LE, Scanlon JM, Niyonkuru C, Miller MA, Ricker JH, et al. Association of KIBRA rs17070145 polymorphism and episodic memory in individuals with severe TBI. *Brain Inj* 2012; 26(13–14):1658–1669.

235. Ost M, Nylen K, Csajbok L, Blennow K, Rosengren L, Nellgard B. Apolipoprotein E polymorphism and gender difference in outcome after severe traumatic brain injury. *Acta Anaesthesiol Scand* 2008; 52(10):1364–1369.

236. Romeiro RR, Romano-Silva MA, De Marco L, Teixeira AL, Jr., Correa H. Can variation in aquaporin 4 gene be associated with different outcomes in traumatic brain edema? *Neurosci Lett* 2007; 426(2):133–134.

237. Rossi JL, Todd T, Daniels Z, Bazan NG, Belayev L. Interferon-stimulated gene 15 upregulation precedes the development of blood–brain barrier disruption and cerebral edema after traumatic brain injury in young mice. *J Neurotrauma* 2015; 32(14):1101–1108.

238. Ferguson S, Mouzon B, Kayihan G, Wood M, Poon F, Doore S, et al. Apolipoprotein E genotype and oxidative stress response to traumatic brain injury. *Neuroscience* 2010; 168(3):811–819.

239. Sarnaik AA, Conley YP, Okonkwo DO, Barr TL, Fink EL, Szabo C, et al. Influence of PARP-1 polymorphisms in patients after traumatic brain injury. *J Neurotrauma* 2010; 27(3):465–471.

240. Kerr ME, Ilyas Kamboh M, Yookyung K, Kraus MF, Puccio AM, DeKosky ST, et al. Relationship between apoE4 allele and excitatory amino acid levels after traumatic brain injury. *Crit Care Med* 2003; 31(9):2371–2379.

241. Martinez-Lucas P, Moreno-Cuesta J, Garcia-Olmo DC, Sanchez-Sanchez F, Escribano-Martinez J, del Pozo AC, et al. Relationship between the Arg72Pro polymorphism of p53 and outcome for patients with traumatic brain injury. *Intens Care Med* 2005; 31(9):1168–1173.

242. Clark RS, Kochanek PM, Chen M, Watkins SC, Marion DW, Chen J, et al. Increases in Bcl-2 and cleavage of caspase-1 and caspase-3 in human brain after head injury. *FASEB J* 1999; 13(8):813–821.

243. Graham SH, Chen J, Clark RS. Bcl-2 family gene products in cerebral ischemia and traumatic brain injury. *J Neurotrauma* 2000; 17(10):831–841.

244. Hoh NZ, Wagner AK, Alexander SA, Clark RB, Beers SR, Okonkwo DO, et al. BCL2 genotypes: functional and neurobehavioral outcomes after severe traumatic brain injury. *J Neurotrauma* 2010; 27(8):1413–1427.

245. Hartman RE, Laurer H, Longhi L, Bales KR, Paul SM, McIntosh TK, et al. Apolipoprotein E4 influences amyloid deposition but not cell loss after traumatic brain injury in a mouse model of Alzheimer's disease. *J Neurosci* 2002; 22(23):10083–10087.

246. Johnson VE, Stewart W, Smith DH. Traumatic brain injury and amyloid-beta pathology: a link to Alzheimer's disease? *Nat Rev Neurosci* 2010; 11(5):361–370.

247. Johnson VE, Stewart W, Smith DH. Widespread tau and amyloid-beta pathology many years after a single traumatic brain injury in humans. *Brain Pathol* 2012; 22(2):142–149.

248. Johnson VE, Stewart W, Graham DI, Stewart JE, Praestgaard AH, Smith DH. A neprilysin polymorphism and amyloid-beta plaques after traumatic brain injury. *J Neurotrauma* 2009; 26(8):1197–1202.

249. Jellinger KA, Paulus W, Wrocklage C, Litvan I. Effects of closed traumatic brain injury and genetic factors on the development of Alzheimer's disease. *Eur J Neurol* 2001; 8(6):707–710.

250. Mauri M, Sinforiani E, Bono G, Cittadella R, Quattrone A, Boller F, et al. Interaction between apolipoprotein epsilon 4 and traumatic brain injury in patients with Alzheimer's disease and mild cognitive impairment. *Funct Neurol* 2006; 21(4):223–228.

251. Tanriverdi F, Taheri S, Ulutabanca H, Caglayan AO, Ozkul Y, Dundar M, et al. Apolipoprotein E3/E3 genotype decreases the risk of pituitary dysfunction after traumatic brain injury due to various causes: preliminary data. *J Neurotrauma* 2008; 25(9):1071–1077.

252. Crawford F, Wood M, Ferguson S, Mathura V, Gupta P, Humphrey J, et al. Apolipoprotein E-genotype dependent hippocampal and cortical responses to traumatic brain injury. *Neuroscience* 2009; 159(4):1349–1362.

253. Han SH, Chung SY. Marked hippocampal neuronal damage without motor deficits after mild concussive-like brain injury in apolipoprotein E-deficient mice. *Ann N Y Acad Sci* 2000; 903:357–365.

254. Gentleman SM, Nash MJ, Sweeting CJ, Graham DI, Roberts GW. Beta-amyloid precursor protein (beta APP) as a marker for axonal injury after head injury. *Neurosci Lett* 1993; 160(2):139–144.

255. Leclercq PD, Murray LS, Smith C, Graham DI, Nicoll JA, Gentleman SM. Cerebral amyloid angiopathy in traumatic brain injury: association with apolipoprotein E genotype. *J Neurol Neurosurg Psychiatry* 2005; 76(2):229–233.

256. Mannix R, Meehan WP, Mandeville J, Grant PE, Gray T, Berglass J, et al. Clinical correlates in an experimental model of repetitive mild brain injury. *Ann Neurol* 2013; 74(1):65–75.

257. Mannix RC, Zhang J, Berglass J, Qui J, Whalen MJ. Beneficial effect of amyloid beta after controlled cortical impact. *Brain Inj* 2013; 27(6):743–748.

258. Smith C, Graham DI, Murray LS, Stewart J, Nicoll JA. Association of APOE e4 and cerebrovascular pathology in traumatic brain injury. *J Neurol Neurosurg Psychiatry* 2006; 77(3):363–366.

259. Robertson CS, Gopinath SP, Valadka AB, Van M, Swank PR, Goodman JC. Variants of the endothelial nitric oxide gene and cerebral blood flow after severe traumatic brain injury. *J Neurotrauma* 2011; 28(5):727–737.

260. Hadjigeorgiou GM, Paterakis K, Dardiotis E, Dardioti M, Aggelakis K, Tasiou A, et al. IL-1RN and IL-1B gene polymorphisms and cerebral hemorrhagic events after traumatic brain injury. *Neurology* 2005; 65(7):1077–1082.

261. Tierney RT, Mansell JL, Higgins M, McDevitt JK, Toone N, Gaughan JP, et al. Apolipoprotein E genotype and concussion in college athletes. *Clin J Sport Med* 2010; 20(6):464–468.

262. Bush WS, Moore JH. Genome-wide association studies. *PLoS Comput Biol* 2012; 8(12):e1002822.

263. Hulshoff Pol HE, Posthuma D, Baare WF, De Geus EJ, Schnack HG, van Haren NE, et al. Twin–singleton differences in brain structure using structural equation modelling. *Brain* 2002; 125(2):384–390.

264. Capello AE, Markus CR. Differential influence of the 5-HTTLPR genotype, neuroticism and real-life acute stress exposure on appetite and energy intake. *Appetite* 2014; 77:83–93.

265. Elmore AL, Nigg JT, Friderici KH, Jernigan K, Nikolas MA. Does 5HTTLPR genotype moderate the association of family environment with child attention-deficit hyperactivity disorder symptomatology? *J Clin Child Adolesc Psychol* 2016; 45(3):348–360.

266. Grimm S, Gartner M, Fuge P, Fan Y, Weigand A, Feeser M, et al. Variation in the corticotropin-releasing hormone receptor 1 (CRHR1) gene modulates age effects on working memory. *J Psychiatr Res* 2015; 61:57–63.

267. Hsu DT, Mickey BJ, Langenecker SA, Heitzeg MM, Love TM, Wang H, et al. Variation in the corticotropin-releasing hormone receptor 1 (CRHR1) gene influences fMRI signal responses during emotional stimulus processing. *J Neurosci* 2012; 32(9):3253–3260.

268. Labermaier C, Kohl C, Hartmann J, Devigny C, Altmann A, Weber P, et al. A polymorphism in the CRHR1 gene determines stress vulnerability in male mice. *Endocrinology* 2014; 155(7):2500–2510.

269. Razzoli M, Domenici E, Carboni L, Rantamaki T, Lindholm J, Castren E, et al. A role for BDNF/TrkB signaling in behavioral and physiological consequences of social defeat stress. *Genes Brain Behav* 2011; 10(4):424–433.

270. Yu H, Wang DD, Wang Y, Liu T, Lee FS, Chen ZY. Variant brain-derived neurotrophic factor Val66Met polymorphism alters vulnerability to stress and response to antidepressants. *J Neurosci* 2012; 32(12):4092–4101.

271. Joeyen-Waldorf J, Nikolova YS, Edgar N, Walsh C, Kota R, Lewis DA, et al. Adenylate cyclase 7 is implicated in the biology of depression and modulation of affective neural circuitry. *Biol Psychiatry* 2012; 71(7):627–632.

272. Wagner KV, Marinescu D, Hartmann J, Wang XD, Labermaier C, Scharf SH, et al. Differences in FKBP51 regulation following chronic social defeat stress correlate with individual stress sensitivity: influence of paroxetine treatment. *Neuropsychopharmacology* 2012; 37(13):2797–2808.

273. Nievergelt CM, Maihofer AX, Mustapic M, Yurgil KA, Schork NJ, Miller MW, et al. Genomic predictors of combat stress vulnerability and resilience in U.S. marines: a genome-wide association study across multiple ancestries implicates PRTFDC1 as a potential PTSD gene. *Psychoneuroendocrinology* 2015; 51:459–471.

274. Santarelli S, Wagner KV, Labermaier C, Uribe A, Dournes C, Balsevich G, et al. SLC6A15, a novel stress vulnerability candidate, modulates anxiety and depressive-like behavior: involvement of the glutamatergic system. *Stress* 2016; 19(1):83–90.

275. Hariri AR, Drabant EM, Munoz KE, Kolachana BS, Mattay VS, Egan MF, et al. A susceptibility gene for affective disorders and the response of the human amygdala. *Arch Gen Psychiatry* 2005; 62(2):146–152.

276. Lesch KP, Mossner R. Inactivation of 5HT transport in mice: modeling altered 5HT homeostasis implicated in emotional dysfunction, affective disorders, and somatic syndromes. *Handb Exp Pharmacol* 2006; (175):417–456.

277. Pezawas L, Meyer-Lindenberg A, Drabant EM, Verchinski BA, Munoz KE, Kolachana BS, et al. 5-HTTLPR polymorphism impacts human cingulate-amygdala interactions: a genetic susceptibility mechanism for depression. *Nat Neurosci* 2005; 8(6):828–834.

278. Mickey BJ, Zhou Z, Heitzeg MM, Heinz E, Hodgkinson CA, Hsu DT, et al. Emotion processing, major depression, and functional genetic variation of neuropeptide Y. *Arch Gen Psychiatry* 2011; 68(2):158–166.

279. Du L, Bakish D, Hrdina PD. Gender differences in association between serotonin transporter gene polymorphism and personality traits. *Psychiatr Genet* 2000; 10(4):159–164.

280. Rujescu D, Giegling I, Sato T, Hartmann AM, Moller HJ. Genetic variations in tryptophan hydroxylase in suicidal behavior: analysis and meta-analysis. *Biol Psychiatry* 2003; 54(4):465–473.

281. Souery D, Van Gestel S, Massat I, Blairy S, Adolfsson R, Blackwood D, et al. Tryptophan hydroxylase polymorphism and suicidality in unipolar and bipolar affective disorders: a multicenter association study. *Biol Psychiatry* 2001; 49(5):405–409.

282. Antypa N, Souery D, Tomasini M, Albani D, Fusco F, Mendlewicz J, et al. Clinical and genetic factors associated with suicide in mood disorder patients. *Eur Arch Psychiatry Clin Neurosci* 2016; 266(2):181–193.

283. Lesch K-P, Bengel D, Heils A, Sabol SZ, Greenberg BD, Petri S, et al. Association of anxiety-related traits with a polymorphism in the serotonin transporter gene regulatory region. *Science* 1996; 274(5292):1527–1531.

284. Mazzanti CM, Lappalainen J, Long JC, Bengel D, Naukkarinen H, Eggert M, et al. Role of the serotonin transporter promoter polymorphism in anxiety-related traits. *Arch Gen Psychiatry* 1998; 55(10):936–940.

285. Morey RA, Hariri AR, Gold AL, Hauser MA, Munger HJ, Dolcos F, et al. Serotonin transporter gene polymorphisms and brain function during emotional distraction from cognitive processing in posttraumatic stress disorder. *BMC Psychiatry* 2011; 11:76.

286. Munafo MR, Clark T, Flint J. Does measurement instrument moderate the association between the serotonin transporter gene and anxiety-related personality traits? A meta-analysis. *Mol Psychiatry* 2005; 10(4):415–419.

287. Sen S, Burmeister M, Ghosh D. Meta-analysis of the association between a serotonin transporter promoter polymorphism (5-HTTLPR) and anxiety-related personality traits. *Am J Med Genet B Neuropsychiatr Genet* 2004; 127(1):85–89.

288. Greenberg BD, Li Q, Lucas FR, Hu S, Sirota LA, Benjamin J, et al. Association between the serotonin transporter promoter polymorphism and personality traits in a primarily female population sample. *Am J Med Genet* 2000; 96(2):202–216.

289. Hu S, Brody CL, Fisher C, Gunzerath L, Nelson ML, Sabol SZ, et al. Interaction between the serotonin transporter gene and neuroticism in cigarette smoking behavior. *Mol Psychiatry* 2000; 5(2):181–188.

290. Hennings A, Zill P, Rief W. Serotonin transporter gene promoter polymorphism and somatoform symptoms. *J Clin Psychiatry* 2009; 70(11):1536–1539.

291. Genetics of Personality Consortium, de Moor MH, van den Berg SM, Verweij KJ, Krueger RF, Luciano M, et al. Meta-analysis of genome-wide association studies for neuroticism, and the polygenic association with major depressive disorder. *JAMA Psychiatry* 2015; 72(7):642–650.

292. Hosang GM, Shiles C, Tansey KE, McGuffin P, Uher R. Interaction between stress and the BDNF Val66Met polymorphism in depression: a systematic review and meta-analysis. *BMC Med* [Internet]. 16 January 2014; [cited 17 August 2017]. Available from: www.ncbi.nlm.nih.gov/pubmed/24433458.

293. Luciano M, Huffman JE, Arias-Vasquez A, Vinkhuyzen AA, Middeldorp CM, Giegling I, et al. Genome-wide association uncovers shared genetic effects among personality traits and mood states. *Am J Med Genet B Neuropsychiatr Genet* 2012; 159B(6):684–695.

294. Okbay A, Baselmans BM, De Neve JE, Turley P, Nivard MG, Fontana MA, et al. Genetic variants associated with subjective well-being, depressive symptoms, and neuroticism identified through genome-wide analyses. *Nat Genet* 2016; 48(12):1591.

295. Rietveld CA, Medland SE, Derringer J, Yang J, Esko T, Martin NW, et al. GWAS of 126,559 individuals identifies genetic variants associated with educational attainment. *Science* 2013; 340(6139):1467–1471.

296. Ware EB, Mukherjee B, Sun YV, Diez-Roux AV, Kardia SL, Smith JA. Comparative genome-wide association studies of a depressive symptom phenotype in a repeated measures setting by race/ethnicity in the Multi-Ethnic Study of Atherosclerosis. *BMC Genet* 2015; 16:118.

297. Ware EB, Smith JA, Mukherjee B, Lee S, Kardia SL, Diez-Roux AV. Applying novel methods for assessing individual- and neighborhood-level social and psychosocial environment interactions with genetic factors in the prediction of depressive symptoms in the Multi-Ethnic Study of Atherosclerosis. *Behav Genet* 2016; 46(1):89–99.

298. Alexander AL, Lee JE, Lazar M, Field AS. Diffusion tensor imaging of the brain. *Neurotherapeutics* 2007; 4(3):316–329.

299. Houlden H, Greenwood R. Apolipoprotein E4 and traumatic brain injury. *J Neurol Neurosurg Psychiatry* 2006; 77(10):1106–1107.

300. Isoniemi H, Kurki T, Tenovuo O, Kairisto V, Portin R. Hippocampal volume, brain atrophy, and APOE genotype after traumatic brain injury. *Neurology* 2006; 67(5):756–760.

301. Lawrence DW, Comper P, Hutchison MG, Sharma B. The role of apolipoprotein E episilon (epsilon)-4 allele on outcome following traumatic brain injury: a systematic review. *Brain Inj* 2015; 29(9):1018–1031.

302. Sundstrom A, Marklund P, Nilsson LG, Cruts M, Adolfsson R, Van Broeckhoven C, et al. APOE influences on neuropsychological function after mild head injury: within-person comparisons. *Neurology* 2004; 62(11):1963–1966.

303. Jordan BD. Chronic traumatic brain injury associated with boxing. *Semin Neurol* 2000; 20(2):179–185.

304. Koponen S, Taiminen T, Kairisto V, Portin R, Isoniemi H, Hinkka S, et al. APOE-epsilon4 predicts dementia but not other psychiatric disorders after traumatic brain injury. *Neurology* 2004; 63(4):749–750.

305. Luukinen H, Jokelainen J, Kervinen K, Kesaniemi YA, Winqvist S, Hillbom M. Risk of dementia associated with the ApoE epsilon4 allele and falls causing head injury without explicit traumatic brain injury. *Acta Neurol Scand* 2008; 118(3):153–158.

306. Maroon JC, Winkelman R, Bost J, Amos A, Mathyssek C, Miele V. Chronic traumatic encephalopathy in contact sports: a systematic review of all reported pathological cases. *PLoS One* 2015; 10(2):e0117338.

307. Plassman BL, Grafman J. Traumatic brain injury and late-life dementia. *Handb Clin Neurol* 2015; 128:711–722.

308. Stein TD, Montenigro PH, Alvarez VE, Xia W, Crary JF, Tripodis Y, et al. Beta-amyloid deposition in chronic traumatic encephalopathy. *Acta Neuropathol* 2015; 130(1):21–34.

309. Hyman BT, Phelps CH, Beach TG, Bigio EH, Cairns NJ, Carrillo MC, et al. National Institute on Aging-Alzheimer's Association guidelines for the neuropathologic assessment of Alzheimer's disease. *Alzheimers Dement* 2012; 8(1):1–13.

310. Parker HL. Traumatic encephalopathy ('punch drunk') of professional pugilists. *J Neurol Psychopathol* 1934; 15(57):20–28.

311. Shen H. Researchers seek definition of head-trauma disorder. *Nature* 2015; 518(7540):466–467.

312. Maiti TK, Konar S, Bir S, Kalakoti P, Bollam P, Nanda A. Role of apolipoprotein E polymorphism as a prognostic marker in traumatic brain injury and neurodegenerative disease: a critical review. *Neurosurg Focus* 2015; 39(5):E3.

313. Zeng S, Jiang JX, Xu MH, Xu LS, Shen GJ, Zhang AQ, et al. Prognostic value of apolipoprotein E epsilon4 allele in patients with traumatic brain injury: a meta-analysis and meta-regression. *Genet Test Mol Biomarkers* 2014; 18(3):202–210.

314. Heijmans BT, Slagboom PE, Gussekloo J, Droog S, Lagaay AM, Kluft C, et al. Association of APOE epsilon2/epsilon3/epsilon4 and promoter gene variants with dementia but not cardiovascular mortality in old age. *Am J Med Genet* 2002; 107(3):201–208.

315. Bennet AM, Di Angelantonio E, Ye Z, Wensley F, Dahlin A, Ahlbom A, et al. Association of apolipoprotein E genotypes with lipid levels and coronary risk. *JAMA* 2007; 298(11):1300–1311.

316. Irie F, Fitzpatrick AL, Lopez OL, Kuller LH, Peila R, Newman AB, et al. Enhanced risk for Alzheimer disease in persons with type 2 diabetes and APOE epsilon4: the Cardiovascular Health Study Cognition Study. *Arch Neurol* 2008; 65(1):89–93.

317. Irie F, Masaki KH, Petrovitch H, Abbott RD, Ross GW, Taaffe DR, et al. Apolipoprotein E epsilon4 allele genotype and the effect of depressive symptoms on the risk of dementia in men: the Honolulu-Asia Aging Study. *Arch Gen Psychiatry* 2008; 65(8):906–912.

318. Mou C, Han T, Wang M, Jiang M, Liu B, Hu J. Correlation of polymorphism of APOE and LRP genes to cognitive impairment and behavioral and psychological symptoms of dementia in Alzheimer's disease and vascular dementia. *Int J Clin Exp Med* 2015; 8(11):21679–21683.

319. Song Y, Stampfer MJ, Liu S. Meta-analysis: apolipoprotein E genotypes and risk for coronary heart disease. *Ann Intern Med* 2004; 141(2):137–147.

320. Zlokovic BV. Cerebrovascular effects of apolipoprotein E: implications for Alzheimer disease. *JAMA Neurol* 2013; 70(4):440–444.

321. Bell RD, Winkler EA, Singh I, Sagare AP, Deane R, Wu Z, et al. Apolipoprotein E controls cerebrovascular integrity via cyclophilin A. *Nature* 2012; 485(7399):512–516.

322. Alzforum. AlzGene – meta-analysis of all published ad association studies (case-control only) APOE_e2/3/4. [Internet] (updated 29 January 2010). [cited 2017 August 17]. Available from: www.alzgene.org/meta.asp?geneID=83.

323. Jordan BD, Relkin NR. Reply to letter. *JAMA* 1997; 276:2143.

324. American College of Medical Genetics, American Society of Human Genetics Working Group on ApoE and Alzheimer Disease. Statement on use of apolipoprotein E testing for Alzheimer disease. American College of Medical Genetics/American Society of Human Genetics Working Group on ApoE and Alzheimer disease. *JAMA* 1995; 274(20):1627–1629.

325. Knopman DS, DeKosky ST, Cummings JL, Chui H, Corey-Bloom J, Relkin N, et al. Practice parameter: diagnosis of dementia (an evidence-based review). Report of the Quality Standards Subcommittee of the American Academy of Neurology. *Neurology* 2001; 56(9):1143–1153.

326. Fleck LM. Just caring: the moral and economic costs of APOE genotyping for Alzheimer's disease. *Ann N Y Acad Sci* 1996; 802:128–138.

327. Greely HT. Special issues in genetic testing for Alzheimer disease. *Genet Test* 1999; 3(1):115–119.

328. Nuffield Council on Bioethics. *Mental disorders and genetics: The ethical context.* West Sussex, UK: RPM Reprographics, 1998.

329. Hoge SK, Appelbaum PS. Ethics and neuropsychiatric genetics: a review of major issues. *Int J Neuropsychopharmacol* 2012; 15(10):1547–1557.

330. Goldman JS, Hahn SE, Catania JW, LaRusse-Eckert S, Butson MB, Rumbaugh M, et al. Genetic counseling and testing for Alzheimer disease: joint practice guidelines of the American College of Medical Genetics and the National Society of Genetic Counselors. *Genet Med* 2011; 13(6):597–605.

331. Guo Z, Cupples LA, Kurz A, Auerbach SH, Volicer L, Chui H, et al. Head injury and the risk of AD in the MIRAGE study. *Neurology* 2000; 54(6):1316–1323.

332. Mortimer JA, French LR, Hutton JT, Schuman LM. Head injury as a risk factor for Alzheimer's disease. *Neurology* 1985; 35(2):264–267.

333. Mortimer JA, van Duijn CM, Chandra V, Fratiglioni L, Graves AB, Heyman A, et al. Head trauma as a risk factor for Alzheimer's disease: a collaborative re-analysis of case-control studies. EURODEM Risk Factors Research Group. *Int J Epidemiol* 1991; 20 (Suppl 2):S28–S35.

334. O'Meara ES, Kukull WA, Sheppard L, Bowen JD, McCormick WC, Teri L, et al. Head injury and risk of Alzheimer's disease by apolipoprotein E genotype. *Am J Epidemiol* 1997; 146(5):373–384.

335. Bangen KJ, Nation DA, Delano-Wood L, Weissberger GH, Hansen LA, Galasko DR, et al. Aggregate effects of vascular risk factors on cerebrovascular changes in autopsy-confirmed Alzheimer's disease. *Alzheimers Dement* 2015; 11(4):394–403. e391.

336. Honjo K, Black SE, Verhoeff NP. Alzheimer's disease, cerebrovascular disease, and the beta-amyloid cascade. *Can J Neurol Sci* 2012; 39(6):712–728.

337. Kornhuber HH. Prevention of dementia (including Alzheimer's disease). *Gesundheitswesen* 2004; 66(5):346–351.

338. Toledo JB, Arnold SE, Raible K, Brettschneider J, Xie SX, Grossman M, et al. Contribution of cerebrovascular disease in autopsy confirmed neurodegenerative disease cases in the National Alzheimer's Coordinating Centre. *Brain* 2013; 136(9):2697–2706.

339. Yuan J, Wen G, Li Y, Liu C. The occurrence of cerebrovascular atherosclerosis in Alzheimer's disease patients. *Clin Interv Aging* 2013; 8:581–584.

340. Davey DA. Alzheimer's disease and vascular dementia: one potentially preventable and modifiable disease? Part II: management, prevention and future perspective. *Neurodegener Dis Manag* 2014; 4(3):261–270.

341. Iwamoto T. Prevention of dementia on the basis of modification of lifestyle and management of lifestyle-related diseases. *Nihon Rinsho* 2014; 72(4):612–617.

342. Paillard T. Preventive effects of regular physical exercise against cognitive decline and the risk of dementia with age advancement. *Sports Med Open* 2015; 1(1):4.

343. Schlosser Covell GE, Hoffman-Snyder CR, Wellik KE, Woodruff BK, Geda YE, Caselli RJ, et al. Physical activity level and future risk of mild cognitive impairment or dementia: a critically appraised topic. *Neurologist* 2015; 19(3):89–91.

344. Vaillant GE, Okereke OI, Mukamal K, Waldinger RJ. Antecedents of intact cognition and dementia at age 90 years: a prospective study. *Int J Geriatr Psychiatry* 2014; 29(12):1278–1285.

345. Fan LY, Sun Y, Lee HJ, Yang SC, Chen TF, Lin KN, et al. Marital status, lifestyle and dementia: a nationwide survey in Taiwan. *PLoS One* 2015; 10(9):e0139154.

346. Kim SM, Seo HJ, Sung MR. Factors affecting dementia prevalence in people aged 60 or over: a community based cross-sectional study. *J Korean Acad Nurs* 2014; 44(4):391–397.

347. Wei CJ, Cheng Y, Zhang Y, Sun F, Zhang WS, Zhang MY. Risk factors for dementia in highly educated elderly people in Tianjin, China. *Clin Neurol Neurosurg* 2014; 122:4–8.

348. Buchman AS, Boyle PA, Yu L, Shah RC, Wilson RS, Bennett DA. Total daily physical activity and the risk of AD and cognitive decline in older adults. *Neurology* 2012; 78(17):1323–1329.

349. Kishimoto H, Ohara T, Hata J, Ninomiya T, Yoshida D, Mukai N, et al. The long-term association between physical activity and risk of dementia in the community: the Hisayama Study. *Eur J Epidemiol* 2016; 31(3):267–274.

350. Lee AT, Richards M, Chan WC, Chiu HF, Lee RS, Lam LC. Intensity and types of physical exercise in relation to dementia risk reduction in community-living older adults. *J Am Med Dir Assoc* 2015; 16(10):e891–899.

351. Llamas-Velasco S, Contador I, Villarejo-Galende A, Lora-Pablos D, Bermejo-Pareja F. Physical activity as protective factor against dementia: a prospective population-based study (NEDICES). *J Int Neuropsychol Soc* 2015; 21(10):861–867.

352. Parle M, Vasudevan M, Singh N. Swim every day to keep dementia away. *J Sports Sci Med* 2005; 4(1):37–46.

353. Inoue K, Okamoto M, Shibato J, Lee MC, Matsui T, Rakwal R, et al. Long-term mild, rather than intense, exercise enhances adult hippocampal neurogenesis and greatly changes the transcriptomic profile of the hippocampus. *PLoS One* 2015; 10(6):e0128720.

354. Nokia MS, Lensu S, Ahtiainen JP, Johansson PP, Koch LG, Britton SL, et al. Physical exercise increases adult hippocampal neurogenesis in male rats provided it is aerobic and sustained. *J Physiol* 2016; 594(7):1855–1873.

355. Killgore WD, Olson EA, Weber M. Physical exercise habits correlate with gray matter volume of the hippocampus in healthy adult humans. *Sci Rep* 2013; 3:3457.

356. Green RC, Roberts JS, Cupples LA, Relkin NR, Whitehouse PJ, Brown T, et al. Disclosure of APOE genotype for risk of Alzheimer's disease. *N Engl J Med* 2009; 361(3):245–254.

357. Arribas-Ayllon M. The ethics of disclosing genetic diagnosis for Alzheimer's disease: do we need a new paradigm? *Br Med Bull* 2011; 100:7–21.

358. Gordon SC, Landa D. Disclosure of the genetic risk of Alzheimer's disease. *N Engl J Med* 2010; 362(2):181–182; author reply 182.

359. Green RC, Christensen KD, Cupples LA, Relkin NR, Whitehouse PJ, Royal CD, et al. A randomized noninferiority trial of condensed protocols for genetic risk disclosure of Alzheimer's disease. *Alzheimers Dement* 2015; 11(10):1222–1230.

360. Christensen KD, Roberts JS, Uhlmann WR, Green RC. Changes to perceptions of the pros and cons of genetic susceptibility testing after APOE genotyping for Alzheimer disease risk. *Genet Med* 2011; 13(5):409–414.

361. Chao S, Roberts JS, Marteau TM, Silliman R, Cupples LA, Green RC. Health behavior changes after genetic risk assessment for Alzheimer disease: the REVEAL study. *Alzheimer Dis Assoc Disord* 2008; 22(1):94–97.

362. Hietaranta-Luoma H-L, Luomala H, Puolijoki H, Hopia A. Using ApoE genotyping to promote healthy lifestyles in Finland – psychological impacts: randomized controlled trial. *J Genet Couns* 2015; 24(6):908–921.

363. Singh R, Meier TB, Kuplicki R, Savitz J, Mukai I, Cavanagh L, et al. Relationship of collegiate football experience and concussion with hippocampal volume and cognitive outcomes. *JAMA* 2014; 311(18):1883–1888.

364. McKee AC, Stern RA, Nowinski CJ, Stein TD, Alvarez VE, Daneshvar DH, et al. The spectrum of disease in chronic traumatic encephalopathy. *Brain* 2013; 136(1):43–64.

365. Herskowitz RD. Outward bound, diabetes and motivation: experiential education in a wilderness setting. *Diabet Med* 1990; 7(7):633–638.

366. Kirkcaldy BD, Shephard RJ, Siefen RG. The relationship between physical activity and self-image and problem behaviour among adolescents. *Soc Psychiatry Psychiatr Epidemiol* 2002; 37(11):544–550.

367. Edmundson M. Do sports build character or damage it? *The Chronicle Rev* Washington DC. [Internet]. January 15 2012

[cited 16 July 2016]. Available at: www.chronicle.com/article/Do-Sports-Build-Character-or/130286.

368. Forbes GB, Adams-Curtis LE, Pakalka AH, White KB. Dating aggression, sexual coercion, and aggression-supporting attitudes among college men as a function of participation in aggressive high school sports. *Violence Against Women* 2006; 12(5):441–455.

369. Frintner MP, Rubinson L. Acquaintance rape: the influence of alcohol, fraternity membership, and sports team membership. *J Sex Educ Ther* 1993; 19(4):272–284.

370. Crosset TW, Benedict JR, McDonald MA. Male student-athletes reported for sexual assault: a survey of campus police departments and judicial affairs offices. *J Sport Soc Issues* 1995; 19(2):126–140.

371. Humphrey SE, Kahn AS. Fraternities, athletic teams, and rape. *J Interpers Violence* 2000; 15(12):1313–1322.

372. Gage EA. Gender attitudes and sexual behaviors: comparing center and marginal athletes and nonathletes in a collegiate setting. *Violence Against Women* 2008; 14(9):1014–1032.

373. Lindo JM, Siminski PM, Swensen ID. *College party culture and sexual assault. Am Econ J Appl Econ* 2018; 10:236–265.

374. Blacker D. New insights into genetic aspects of Alzheimer's disease. Does genetic information make a difference in clinical practice? *Postgrad Med* 2000; 108(5):119–122, 125–126, 129.

375. Brosco JP, Paul DB. The political history of PKU: reflections on 50 years of newborn screening. *Pediatrics* 2013; 132(6):987–989.

376. Dales D. Infant PKU tests made mandatory. *N Y Times* 1964.

377. Mez J, Solomon TM, Daneshvar DH, Stein TD, McKee AC. Pathologically confirmed chronic traumatic encephalopathy in a 25-year-old former college football player. *JAMA Neurol* 2016; 73(3):353–355.

378. United States Department of Labor. Employer responsibilities. Occupational Safety and Health Administration [cited 17 August 2017]. Available from: www.osha.gov/as/opa/worker/employer-responsibility.html.

379. Farrey T. Northwestern players denied request to form first union for athletes. ESPN, 2015 (updated August 17, 2015). [cited 17 August 2017]. Available from: espn.go.com/espn/print?id=13455477&type=HeadlineNews&imagesPrint=off.

380. University of Southern California. C. L. Max Nikias expanded biography. [Internet]. 2015. [cited 10 July 2017]. Available from: www.president.usc.edu/biography/expanded/.

381. Reuben A, Sampson P, Harris AR, Williams H, Yates P. Postconcussion syndrome (PCS) in the emergency department: predicting and pre-empting persistent symptoms following a mild traumatic brain injury. *Emerg Med J* 2014; 31(1):72–77.

382. Ruff RM, Levin HS, Marshall LF. Neurobehavioral methods of assessment and the study of outcome in minor head injury. *J Head Trauma Rehabil* 1986; 1(2):43–52.

383. Klonoff PS, Costa LD, Snow WG. Predictors and indicators of quality of life in patients with closed-head injury. *J Clin Exp Neuropsychol* 1986; 8(5):469–485.

384. Klonoff PS, Snow WG, Costa LD. Quality of life in patients 2 to 4 years after closed head injury. *Neurosurgery* 1986; 19(5):735–743.

385. Lange RT, Brickell T, French LM, Ivins B, Bhagwat A, Pancholi S, et al. Risk factors for postconcussion symptom reporting after traumatic brain injury in U.S. military service members. *J Neurotrauma* 2013; 30(4):237–246.

386. Bohnen N, Twijnstra A, Wijnen G, Jolles J. Tolerance for light and sound of patients with persistent post-concussional symptoms 6 months after mild head injury. *J Neurol* 1991; 238(8):443–446.

387. Bohnen NJ, Wijnen G, Twijnstra A, van Zutphen W, Jolles J. The constellation of late post-traumatic symptoms of mild head injury patients. *Neurorehabil Neural Repair* 1995; 9(1):33–39.

388. Lange RT, Iverson GL, Rose A. Depression strongly influences postconcussion symptom reporting following mild traumatic brain injury. *J Head Trauma Rehabil* 2011; 26(2):127–137.

389. Robertson Jr E, Rath B, Fournet G, Zelhart P, Estes R. Assessment of mild brain trauma: a preliminary study of the influence of premorbid factors. *Clin Neuropsychol* 1994; 8(1):69–74.

390. Merskey H, Woodforde JM. Psychiatric sequelae of minor head injury. *Brain* 1972; 95(3):521–528.

391. Leininger BE, Gramling SE, Farrell AD, Kreutzer JS, Peck EA, 3rd. Neuropsychological deficits in symptomatic minor head injury patients after concussion and mild concussion. *J Neurol Neurosurg Psychiatry* 1990; 53(4):293–296.

392. Nemeth AJ. Behavior-descriptive data on cognitive, personality, and somatic residua after relatively mild brain trauma: studying the syndrome as a whole. *Arch Clin Neuropsychol* 1996; 11(8):677–695.

393. Cicerone KD, Kalmar K. Does premorbid depression influence post-concussive symptoms and neuropsychological functioning? *Brain Inj* 1997; 11(9):643–648.

394. Evered L, Ruff R, Baldo J, Isomura A. Emotional risk factors and postconcussional disorder. *Assessment* 2003; 10(4):420–427.

395. Chan RC. How severe should symptoms be before someone is said to be suffering from post-concussion syndrome? An exploratory study with self-reported checklist using Rasch analysis. *Brain Inj* 2005; 19(13):1117–1124.

396. Mooney G, Speed J, Sheppard S. Factors related to recovery after mild traumatic brain injury. *Brain Inj* 2005; 19(12):975–987.

397. Stalnacke BM, Bjornstig U, Karlsson K, Sojka P. One-year follow-up of mild traumatic brain injury: post-concussion symptoms, disabilities and life satisfaction in relation to serum levels of S-100B and neurone-specific enolase in acute phase. *J Rehabil Med* 2005; 37(5):300–305.

398. Franke LM, Czarnota JN, Ketchum JM, Walker WC. Factor analysis of persistent postconcussive symptoms within a military sample with blast exposure. *J Head Trauma Rehabil* 2015; 30(1):E34–E46.

399. Kashluba S, Hanks RA, Casey JE, Millis SR. Neuropsychologic and functional outcome after complicated mild traumatic brain injury. *Arch Phys Med Rehabil* 2008; 89(5):904–911.

400. Stulemeijer M, van der Werf S, Borm GF, Vos PE. Early prediction of favourable recovery 6 months after mild traumatic brain injury. *J Neurol Neurosurg Psychiatry* 2008; 79(8):936–942.

401. van Veldhoven LM, Sander AM, Struchen MA, Sherer M, Clark AN, Hudnall GE, et al. Predictive ability of preinjury stressful life events and post-traumatic stress symptoms for outcomes following mild traumatic brain injury: analysis in a prospective emergency room sample. *J Neurol Neurosurg Psychiatry* 2011; 82(7):782–787.

402. Rutherford WH, Merrett JD, McDonald JR. Symptoms at one year following concussion from minor head injuries. *Injury* 1979; 10(3):225–230.

403. Carlsson GS, Svardsudd K, Welin L. Long-term effects of head injuries sustained during life in three male populations. *J Neurosurg* 1987; 67(2):197–205.

404. Drag LL, Spencer RJ, Walker SJ, Pangilinan PH, Bieliauskas LA. The contributions of self-reported injury characteristics and psychiatric symptoms to cognitive functioning in OEF/OIF veterans with mild traumatic brain injury. *J Int Neuropsychol Soc* 2012; 18(3):576–584.

405. Barth JT, Macciocchi SN, Giordani B, Rimel R, Jane JA, Boll TJ. Neuropsychological sequelae of minor head injury. *Neurosurgery* 1983; 13(5):529–533.

406. Bohnen N, Van Zutphen W, Twijnstra A, Wijnen G, Bongers J, Jolles J. Late outcome of mild head injury: results from a controlled postal survey. *Brain Inj* 1994; 8(8):701–708.

407. Cassidy JD, Boyle E, Carroll LJ. Population-based, inception cohort study of the incidence, course, and prognosis of mild traumatic brain injury after motor vehicle collisions. *Arch Phys Med Rehabil* 2014; 95(3 Suppl):S278–S285.

408. De Kruijk J, Leffers P, Menheere P, Meerhoff S, Rutten J, Twijnstra A. Prediction of post-traumatic complaints after mild traumatic brain injury: early symptoms and biochemical markers. *J Neurol Neurosurg Psychiatry* 2002; 73(6):727–732.

409. Denker P. The postconcussion syndrome: prognosis and evaluation of the organic factors. *NY State J Med* 1944; 44:379–384.

410. Dikmen SS, Machamer JE, Winn HR, Temkin NR. Neuropsychological outcome at 1-year post head injury. *Neuropsychology* 1995; 9(1):80–90.

411. Edna TH. Disability 3–5 years after minor head injury. *J Oslo City Hosp* 1987; 37(5):41–48.

412. Faux S, Sheedy J, Delaney R, Riopelle R. Emergency department prediction of post-concussive syndrome following mild traumatic brain injury – an international cross-validation study. *Brain Inj* 2011; 25(1):14–22.

413. Fenton G, McClelland R, Montgomery A, MacFlynn G, Rutherford W. The postconcussional syndrome: social antecedents and psychological sequelae. *Br J Psychiatry* 1993; 162:493–497.

414. Hessen E, Nestvold K. Indicators of complicated mild TBI predict MMPI-2 scores after 23 years. *Brain Inj* 2009; 23(3):234–242.

415. Hou R, Moss-Morris R, Peveler R, Mogg K, Bradley BP, Belli A. When a minor head injury results in enduring symptoms: a prospective investigation of risk factors for postconcussional syndrome after mild traumatic brain injury. *J Neurol Neurosurg Psychiatry* 2012; 83(2):217–223.

416. Ingebrigtsen T, Waterloo K, Marup-Jensen S, Attner E, Romner B. Quantification of post-concussion symptoms 3 months after minor head injury in 100 consecutive patients. *J Neurol* 1998; 245(9):609–612.

417. Jakobsen J, Baadsgaard SE, Thomsen S, Henriksen PB. Prediction of post-concussional sequelae by reaction time test. *Acta Neurol Scand* 1987; 75(5):341–345.

418. King NS. Emotional, neuropsychological, and organic factors: their use in the prediction of persisting postconcussion symptoms after moderate and mild head injuries. *J Neurol Neurosurg Psychiatry* 1996; 61(1):75–81.

419. King NS, Crawford S, Wenden FJ, Caldwell FE, Wade DT. Early prediction of persisting post-concussion symptoms following mild and moderate head injuries. *Br J Clin Psychol* 1999; 38 (1):15–25.

420. Larson AN, McIntosh AL. The epidemiology of injury in ATV and motocross sports. *Med Sport Sci* 2012; 58:158–172.

421. Maestas KL, Sander AM, Clark AN, van Veldhoven LM, Struchen MA, Sherer M, et al. Preinjury coping, emotional functioning, and quality of life following uncomplicated and complicated mild traumatic brain injury. *J Head Trauma Rehabil* 2014; 29(5):407–417.

422. Nolin P, Heroux L. Relations among sociodemographic, neurologic, clinical, and neuropsychologic variables, and vocational status following mild traumatic brain injury: a follow-up study. *J Head Trauma Rehabil* 2006; 21(6):514–526.

423. Ponsford J, Cameron P, Fitzgerald M, Grant M, Mikocka-Walus A, Schonberger M. Predictors of postconcussive symptoms 3 months after mild traumatic brain injury. *Neuropsychology* 2012; 26(3):304–313.

424. Rao V, Bertrand M, Rosenberg P, Makley M, Schretlen DJ, Brandt J, et al. Predictors of new-onset depression after mild traumatic brain injury. *J Neuropsychiatry Clin Neurosci* 2010; 22(1):100–104.

425. Rimel RW, Giordani B, Barth JT, Boll TJ, Jane JA. Disability caused by minor head injury. *Neurosurgery* 1981; 9(3):221–228.

426. Russell W. Cerebral involvement in head injury. A study based on the examination of two hundred cases. *Brain* 1932; (55):549–603.

427. Russell WR. *The traumatic amnesias*. Oxford, England: Oxford University Press, 1971, ix, 84.

428. Schneiderman AI, Braver ER, Kang HK. Understanding sequelae of injury mechanisms and mild traumatic brain injury incurred during the conflicts in Iraq and Afghanistan: persistent postconcussive symptoms and posttraumatic stress disorder. *Am J Epidemiol* 2008; 167(12):1446–1452.

429. Sheedy J, Harvey E, Faux S, Geffen G, Shores EA. Emergency department assessment of mild traumatic brain injury and the prediction of postconcussive symptoms: a 3-month prospective study. *J Head Trauma Rehabil* 2009; 24(5):333–343.

430. Styrke J, Sojka P, Bjornstig U, Bylund PO, Stalnacke BM. Sex-differences in symptoms, disability, and life satisfaction three years after mild traumatic brain injury: a population-based cohort study. *J Rehabil Med* 2013; 45(8):749–757.

431. Whittaker R, Kemp S, House A. Illness perceptions and outcome in mild head injury: a longitudinal study. *J Neurol Neurosurg Psychiatry* 2007; 78(6):644–646.

432. Wrightson P, Gronwall D. Time off work and symptoms after minor head injury. *Injury* 1981; 12(6):445–454.

433. Spence M, Moss-Morris R, Chalder T. The Behavioural Responses to Illness Questionnaire (BRIQ): a new predictive measure of medically unexplained symptoms following acute infection. *Psychol Med* 2005; 35(4):583–593.

434. Broadbent E, Petrie KJ, Main J, Weinman J. The Brief Illness Perception questionnaire. *J Psychosom Res* 2006; 60(6):631–637.

435. Kay T, Cavallo MM, Ezrachi O, Vavagiakis P. The Head Injury Family Interview: a clinical and research tool. *J Head Trauma Rehabil* 1995; 10(2):12–31.

436. Zigmond AS, Snaith RP. The Hospital Anxiety and Depression Scale. *Acta Psychiatr Scand* 1983; 67(6):361–370.

437. Horowitz M, Wilner N, Alvarez W. Impact of Event Scale: a measure of subjective stress. *Psychosom Med* 1979; 41(3):209–218.

438. Katzman R, Brown T, Fuld P, Peck A, Schechter R, Schimmel H. Validation of a short Orientation-Memory-Concentration test of cognitive impairment. *Am J Psychiatry* 1983; 140(6):734–739.

439. Gronwall DM. Paced auditory serial-addition task: a measure of recovery from concussion. *Percept Mot Skills* 1977; 44(2):367–373.

440. Coughlan A, Hollows S. *The Adult Memory and Information Processing Battery (AMIPB)*. Leeds, UK: Psychology Department, St. James University Hospital, 1985.

441. Folkman S, Lazarus RS. *Ways of Coping questionnaire*. Palo Alto, CA: Consulting Psychologists Press, 1988.

442. Derogatis LR. *Symptom checklist SCL-90-R*. Towson, MD: Clinical Psychometric Research, 1975.

443. Gouvier WD, Cubic B, Jones G, Brantley P, Cutlip Q. Postconcussion symptoms and daily stress in normal and head-injured college populations. *Arch Clin Neuropsychol* 1992; 7(3):193–211.

444. Lovell MR, Collins MW. Neuropsychological assessment of the college football player. *J Head Trauma Rehabil* 1998; 13(2):9–26.

445. Crawford S, Wenden FJ, Wade DT. The Rivermead Head Injury Follow Up questionnaire: a study of a new rating scale and other measures to evaluate outcome after head injury. *J Neurol Neurosurg Psychiatry* 1996; 60(5):510–514.

446. Fugl-Meyer AR, Melin R, Fugl-Meyer KS. Life satisfaction in 18- to 64-year-old Swedes: in relation to gender, age, partner and immigrant status. *J Rehabil Med* 2002; 34(5):239–246.

447. Radloff LS. The CES-D scale a self-report depression scale for research in the general population. *Appl Psychol Meas* 1977; 1(3):385–401.

448. Goodman LA, Corcoran C, Turner K, Yuan N, Green BL. Assessing traumatic event exposure: general issues and preliminary findings for the Stressful Life Events Screening Questionnaire. *J Trauma Stress* 1998; 11(3):521–542.

449. Moss-Morris R, Weinman J, Petrie K, Horne R, Cameron L, Buick D. The revised illness perception questionnaire (IPQ-R). *Psychol Health* 2002; 17(1):1–16.

450. Willis T. *Cerebri anatome cui accessit nervorum descripto et usus.* London: James Flesher, Joseph Martyn, and James Allestry, 1664.

451. Ferrier D. *The functions of the brain.* [Internet]. Waterloo Place, London: Smith, Elder, 1876 [cited 17 August 2017]. Available from: https://archive.org/details/functionsofbrain1876ferr.

452. Victoroff J. *Saving your brain: the revolutionary plan to boost brain power, improve memory, and protect yourself against aging and Alzheimer's.* New York: Bantam Books, 2002.

453. Strauss I, Savitsky N. Head injury: neurologic and psychiatric aspects. *AMA Arch NeurPsych* 1934; 31(5):893–955.

454. Symonds C. Discussion on differential diagnosis and treatment of post-contusional states. *Proc R Soc Med* 1942; 35(9):601–614.

455. Symonds CP. Mental disorder following head injury: section of psychiatry. *Proc R Soc Med* 1937; 30(9):1081–1094.

456. Gronwall D, Wrightson P. Cumulative effect of concussion. *Lancet* 1975; 2(7943):995–997.

457. Ponsford J, Willmott C, Rothwell A, Cameron P, Ayton G, Nelms R, et al. Cognitive and behavioral outcome following mild traumatic head injury in children. *J Head Trauma Rehabil* 1999; 14(4):360–372.

458. Roberts GW, Gentleman SM, Lynch A, Graham DI. Beta A4 amyloid protein deposition in brain after head trauma. *Lancet* 1991; 338(8780):1422–1423.

459. Roberts GW, Gentleman SM, Lynch A, Murray L, Landon M, Graham DI. Beta amyloid protein deposition in the brain after severe head injury: implications for the pathogenesis of Alzheimer's disease. *J Neurol Neurosurg Psychiatry* 1994; 57(4):419–425.

460. Martland HS. Punch drunk. *JAMA* 1928; 91(15):1103–1107.

461. Guskiewicz KM, Weaver NL, Padua DA, Garrett WE, Jr. Epidemiology of concussion in collegiate and high school football players. *Am J Sports Med* 2000; 28(5):643–650.

462. Guskiewicz KM, Marshall SW, Bailes J, McCrea M, Cantu RC, Randolph C, et al. Association between recurrent concussion and late-life cognitive impairment in retired professional football players. *Neurosurgery* 2005; 57(4):719–726; discussion 719–726.

463. Guskiewicz KM, Marshall SW, Bailes J, McCrea M, Harding HP, Jr., Matthews A, et al. Recurrent concussion and risk of depression in retired professional football players. *Med Sci Sports Exerc* 2007; 39(6):903–909.

464. Thornton AE, Cox DN, Whitfield K, Fouladi RT. Cumulative concussion exposure in rugby players: neurocognitive and symptomatic outcomes. *J Clin Exp Neuropsychol* 2008; 30(4):398–409.

465. Kerr ZY, Marshall SW, Harding HP, Jr., Guskiewicz KM. Nine-year risk of depression diagnosis increases with increasing self-reported concussions in retired professional football players. *Am J Sports Med* 2012; 40(10):2206–2212.

466. Ford JH, Giovanello KS, Guskiewicz KM. Episodic memory in former professional football players with a history of concussion: an event-related functional neuroimaging study. *J Neurotrauma* 2013; 30(20):1683–1701.

467. Hart J, Jr., Kraut MA, Womack KB, Strain J, Didehbani N, Bartz E, et al. Neuroimaging of cognitive dysfunction and depression in aging retired National Football League players: a cross-sectional study. *JAMA Neurol* 2013; 70(3):326–335.

468. Miller KJ, Ivins BJ, Schwab KA. Self-reported mild TBI and postconcussive symptoms in a peacetime active duty military population: effect of multiple TBI history versus single mild TBI. *J Head Trauma Rehabil* 2013; 28(1):31–38.

469. Spira JL, Lathan CE, Bleiberg J, Tsao JW. The impact of multiple concussions on emotional distress, post-concussive symptoms, and neurocognitive functioning in active duty United States Marines independent of combat exposure or emotional distress. *J Neurotrauma* 2014; 31(22):1823–1834.

470. Victoroff J. Traumatic encephalopathy: review and provisional research diagnostic criteria. *NeuroRehabilitation* 2013; 32(2):211–224.

471. Laurer HL, Bareyre FM, Lee VM, Trojanowski JQ, Longhi L, Hoover R, et al. Mild head injury increasing the brain's vulnerability to a second concussive impact. *J Neurosurg* 2001; 95(5):859–870.

472. Longhi L, Saatman KE, Fujimoto S, Raghupathi R, Meaney DF, Davis J, et al. Temporal window of vulnerability to repetitive experimental concussive brain injury. *Neurosurgery* 2005; 56(2):364–374.

473. Vagnozzi R, Signoretti S, Tavazzi B, Cimatti M, Amorini AM, Donzelli S, et al. Hypothesis of the postconcussive vulnerable brain: experimental evidence of its metabolic occurrence. *Neurosurgery* 2005; 57(1):164–171.

474. Vagnozzi R, Tavazzi B, Signoretti S, Amorini AM, Belli A, Cimatti M, et al. Temporal window of metabolic brain vulnerability to concussions: mitochondrial-related impairment – Part I. *Neurosurgery* 2007; 61(2):379–388; discussion 388–389.

475. Bennett RE, Mac Donald CL, Brody DL. Diffusion tensor imaging detects axonal injury in a mouse model of repetitive closed-skull traumatic brain injury. *Neurosci Lett* 2012; 513(2):160–165.

476. Kane MJ, Angoa-Perez M, Briggs DI, Viano DC, Kreipke CW, Kuhn DM. A mouse model of human repetitive mild traumatic brain injury. *J Neurosci Methods* 2012; 203(1):41–49.

477. Prins ML, Alexander D, Giza CC, Hovda DA. Repeated mild traumatic brain injury: mechanisms of cerebral vulnerability. *J Neurotrauma* 2013; 30(1):30–38.

478. Saunders LL, Selassie AW, Hill EG, Horner MD, Nicholas JS, Lackland DT, et al. Pre-existing health conditions and repeat traumatic brain injury. *Arch Phys Med Rehabil* 2009; 90(11):1853–1859.

479. Wetjen NM, Pichelmann MA, Atkinson JL. Second impact syndrome: concussion and second injury brain complications. *J Am Coll Surg* 2010; 211(4):553–557.

480. Weinstein E, Turner M, Kuzma BB, Feuer H. Second impact syndrome in football: new imaging and insights into a rare and devastating condition. *J Neurosurg Pediatr* 2013; 11(3):331–334.

481. McKee AC, Cairns NJ, Dickson DW, Folkerth RD, Keene CD, Litvan I, et al. The first NINDS/NIBIB consensus meeting to define neuropathological criteria for the diagnosis of chronic traumatic encephalopathy. *Acta Neuropathol* 2016; 131(1):75–86.

482. Hay J, Johnson VE, Smith DH, Stewart W. Chronic traumatic encephalopathy: the neuropathological legacy of traumatic brain injury. *Annu Rev Pathol* 2016; 11:21–45.

483. Stein TD, Montenigro PH, Alvarez VE, Xia W, Crary JF, Tripodis Y, et al. Beta-amyloid deposition in chronic traumatic encephalopathy. *Acta Neuropathol* 2015; 130(1):21–34.

484. Furst AJ, Bigler ED. Amyloid plaques in TBI: incidental finding or precursor for what is to come? *Neurology* 2016; 86(9):798–799.

485. Dams-O'Connor K, Spielman L, Hammond FM, Sayed N, Culver C, Diaz-Arrastia R. An exploration of clinical dementia phenotypes among individuals with and without traumatic brain injury. *NeuroRehabilitation* 2013; 32(2):199–209.

486. Sayed N, Culver C, Dams-O'Connor K, Hammond F, Diaz-Arrastia R. Clinical phenotype of dementia after traumatic brain injury. *J Neurotrauma* 2013; 30(13):1117–1122.

487. Bartnik-Olson BL, Harris NG, Shijo K, Sutton RL. Insights into the metabolic response to traumatic brain injury as revealed by (13)C NMR spectroscopy. *Front Neuroenergetics* 2013; 5:8.

488. Monti JM, Voss MW, Pence A, McAuley E, Kramer AF, Cohen NJ. History of mild traumatic brain injury is associated with deficits in relational memory, reduced hippocampal volume, and less neural activity later in life. *Front Aging Neurosci* 2013; 5:41.

489. Iliff JJ, Chen MJ, Plog BA, Zeppenfeld DM, Soltero M, Yang L, et al. Impairment of glymphatic pathway function promotes tau pathology after traumatic brain injury. *J Neurosci* 2014; 34(49):16180–16193.

490. Westfall DR, West JD, Bailey JN, Arnold TW, Kersey PA, Saykin AJ, et al. Increased brain activation during working memory processing after pediatric mild traumatic brain injury (mTBI). *J Pediatr Rehabil Med* 2015; 8(4):297–308.

491. Astafiev SV, Shulman GL, Metcalf NV, Rengachary J, MacDonald CL, Harrington DL, et al. Abnormal white matter blood-oxygen-level-dependent signals in chronic mild traumatic brain injury. *J Neurotrauma* 2015; 32(16):1254–1271.

492. Astafiev SV, Zinn KL, Shulman GL, Corbetta M. Exploring the physiological correlates of chronic mild traumatic brain injury symptoms. *NeuroImage Clin* 2016; 11:10–19.

493. Dean PJ, Otaduy MC, Harris LM, McNamara A, Seiss E, Sterr A. Monitoring long-term effects of mild traumatic brain injury with magnetic resonance spectroscopy: a pilot study. *Neuroreport* 2013; 24(12):677–681.

494. Chen XH, Siman R, Iwata A, Meaney DF, Trojanowski JQ, Smith DH. Long-term accumulation of amyloid-beta, beta-secretase, presenilin-1, and caspase-3 in damaged axons following brain trauma. *Am J Pathol* 2004; 165(2):357–371.

495. Johnson VE, Stewart JE, Begbie FD, Trojanowski JQ, Smith DH, Stewart W. Inflammation and white matter degeneration persist for years after a single traumatic brain injury. *Brain* 2013; 136(1):28–42.

496. Brain Development Cooperative Group. Total and regional brain volumes in a population-based normative sample from 4 to 18 years: the NIH MRI Study of Normal Brain Development. *Cereb Cortex* 2012; 22(1):1–12.

497. Smith DH, Chen XH, Iwata A, Graham DI. Amyloid beta accumulation in axons after traumatic brain injury in humans. *J Neurosurg* 2003; 98(5):1072–1077.

498. Ward SM, Himmelstein DS, Lancia JK, Binder LI. Tau oligomers and tau toxicity in neurodegenerative disease. *Biochem Soc Trans* 2012; 40(4):667–671.

499. Roberts G, Gentleman S, Lynch A, Graham D. βA4 amyloid protein deposition in brain after head trauma. *Lancet* 1991; 338(8780):1422–1423.

500. Chen XH, Johnson VE, Uryu K, Trojanowski JQ, Smith DH. A lack of amyloid beta plaques despite persistent accumulation of amyloid beta in axons of long-term survivors of traumatic brain injury. *Brain Pathol* 2009; 19(2):214–223.

501. Saatman KE, Graham DI, McIntosh TK. The neuronal cytoskeleton is at risk after mild and moderate brain injury. *J Neurotrauma* 1998; 15(12):1047–1058.

502. Li S, Kuroiwa T, Ishibashi S, Sun L, Endo S, Ohno K. Transient cognitive deficits are associated with the reversible accumulation of amyloid precursor protein after mild traumatic brain injury. *Neurosci Lett* 2006; 409(3):182–186.

503. Scott KL, Strong C-AH, Gorter B, Jacobus Donders J. Predictors of post-concussion rehabilitation outcomes at three-month follow-up. *Clin Neuropsychol* 2016; 30:66–81.

504. Spanos GK, Wilde EA, Bigler ED, Cleavinger HB, Fearing MA, Levin HS, et al. Cerebellar atrophy after moderate-to-severe pediatric traumatic brain injury. *AJNR Am J Neuroradiol* 2007; 28(3):537–542.

505. Smith C, Graham DI, Murray LS, Nicoll JA. Tau immunohistochemistry in acute brain injury. *Neuropathol Appl Neurobiol* 2003; 29(5):496–502.

506. Gerson J, Castillo-Carranza DL, Sengupta U, Bodani R, Prough DS, DeWitt DS, et al. Tau oligomers derived from traumatic brain injury cause cognitive impairment and accelerate onset of pathology in Htau mice. *J Neurotrauma* 2016; 33(22):2034–2043.

507. Gyoneva S, Kim D, Katsumoto A, Kokiko-Cochran ON, Lamb BT, Ransohoff RM. Ccr2 deletion dissociates cavity size and tau pathology after mild traumatic brain injury. *J Neuroinflamm* 2015; 12:228.

508. Xu L, Ryu J, Nguyen JV, Arena J, Rha E, Vranis P, et al. Evidence for accelerated tauopathy in the retina of transgenic P301S tau mice exposed to repetitive mild traumatic brain injury. *Exp Neurol* 2015; 273:168–176.

509. Cheng JS, Craft R, Yu GQ, Ho K, Wang X, Mohan G, et al. Tau reduction diminishes spatial learning and memory deficits after mild repetitive traumatic brain injury in mice. *PLoS One* 2014; 9(12):e115765.

510. Stancu IC, Vasconcelos B, Terwel D, Dewachter I. Models of beta-amyloid induced Tau-pathology: the long and "folded" road to understand the mechanism. *Mol Neurodegener* 2014; 9:51.

511. Bulut M, Koksal O, Dogan S, Bolca N, Ozguc H, Korfali E, et al. Tau protein as a serum marker of brain damage in mild traumatic brain injury: preliminary results. *Adv Ther* 2006; 23(1):12–22.

512. Zemlan FP, Rosenberg WS, Luebbe PA, Campbell TA, Dean GE, Weiner NE, et al. Quantification of axonal damage in traumatic brain injury: affinity purification and characterization of cerebrospinal fluid tau proteins. *J Neurochem* 1999; 72(2):741–750.

513. Ost M, Nylen K, Csajbok L, Ohrfelt AO, Tullberg M, Wikkelso C, et al. Initial CSF total tau correlates with 1-year outcome in patients with traumatic brain injury. *Neurology* 2006; 67(9):1600–1604.

514. Olivera A, Lejbman N, Jeromin A, French LM, Kim HS, Cashion A, et al. Peripheral total tau in military personnel who sustain traumatic brain injuries during deployment. *JAMA Neurol* 2015; 72(10):1109–1116.

515. Fyfe I. Traumatic brain injury: long-term tau elevation linked to chronic symptoms after brain injury. *Nat Rev Neurol* 2015; 11(9):485.

516. Kolsch H, Jessen F, Wiltfang J, Lewczuk P, Dichgans M, Teipel SJ, et al. Association of SORL1 gene variants with Alzheimer's disease. *Brain Res* 2009; 1264:1–6.

517. Morgan K, Carrasquillo MM, editors. *Genetic variants in Alzheimer's disease*. New York: Springer-Verlag, 2013, VIII.

518. Dujardin S, Colin M, Buee L. Invited review: animal models of tauopathies and their implications for research/translation into the clinic. *Neuropathol Appl Neurobiol* 2015; 41(1):59–80.

519. Dante Alighieri. *The vision; or hell, purgatory, and paradise*. HF Cary, translator. London: Taylor and Hessey, 1814.

520. Scheiber SC, Madaan V, Wilson DR. The American Board of Psychiatry and Neurology: historical overview and current perspectives. *Psychiatr Clin North Am* 2008; 31(1):123–135.

521. Grinker RR. Editorial. *AMA Arch Gen Psychiatry* 1959; 1(1):1–2.

522. Nelson LD, Tarima S, LaRoche AA, Hammeke TA, Barr WB, Guskiewicz K, et al. Preinjury somatization symptoms

contribute to clinical recovery after sport-related concussion. *Neurology* 2016; 86(20):1856–1863.

523. Derogatis LR. *BSI 18, Brief Symptom Inventory 18: administration, scoring and procedures manual.* Bloomington, MN: NCS Pearson, 2001.

524. Donders J, Strom D. The effect of traumatic brain injury on children with learning disability. *Pediatr Rehabil* 1997; 1(3):179–184.

525. Biederman J, Feinberg L, Chan J, Adeyemo BO, Woodworth KY, Panis W, et al. Mild traumatic brain injury and attention-deficit hyperactivity disorder in young student athletes. *J Nerv Ment Dis* 2015; 203(11):813–819.

526. Brown EA, Kenardy JA, Dow BL. PTSD perpetuates pain in children with traumatic brain injury. *J Pediatr Psychol* 2014; 39(5):512–520.

527. Farace E, Alves WM. Do women fare worse: a metaanalysis of gender differences in traumatic brain injury outcome. *J Neurosurg* 2000; 93(4):539–545.

528. Slewa-Younan S, van den Berg S, Baguley IJ, Nott M, Cameron ID. Towards an understanding of sex differences in functional outcome following moderate to severe traumatic brain injury: a systematic review. *J Neurol Neurosurg Psychiatry* 2008; 79(11):1197–1201.

529. Eramudugolla R, Bielak AA, Bunce D, Easteal S, Cherbuin N, Anstey KJ. Long-term cognitive correlates of traumatic brain injury across adulthood and interactions with APOE genotype, sex, and age cohorts. *J Int Neuropsychol Soc* 2014; 20(4):444–454.

530. Cancelliere C, Donovan J, Cassidy JD. Is sex an indicator of prognosis after mild traumatic brain injury? A systematic analysis of the findings of the World Health Organization Collaborating Centre Task Force on Mild Traumatic Brain Injury and the International Collaboration on Mild Traumatic Brain Injury Prognosis. *Arch Phys Med Rehabil* 2016; 97(2 Suppl):S5–S18.

531. Paniak C, Reynolds S, Toller-Lobe G, Melnyk A, Nagy J, Schmidt D. A longitudinal study of the relationship between financial compensation and symptoms after treated mild traumatic brain injury. *J Clin Exp Neuropsychol* 2002; 24(2):187–193.

532. Paniak C, Reynolds S, Phillips K, Toller-Lobe G, Melnyk A, Nagy J. Patient complaints within 1 month of mild traumatic brain injury: a controlled study. *Arch Clin Neuropsychol* 2002; 17(4):319–334.

533. Kristman VL, Cote P, Yang X, Hogg-Johnson S, Vidmar M, Rezai M. Health care utilization of workers' compensation claimants associated with mild traumatic brain injury: a historical population-based cohort study of workers injured in 1997–1998. *Arch Phys Med Rehabil* 2014; 95(3 Suppl):S295–302.

534. Covassin T, Schatz P, Swanik CB. Sex differences in neuropsychological function and post-concussion symptoms of concussed collegiate athletes. *Neurosurgery* 2007; 61(2):345–350; discussion 350–351.

535. Bazarian J, Hartman M, Delahunta E. Minor head injury: predicting follow-up after discharge from the emergency department. *Brain Inj* 2000; 14(3):285–294.

536. Kirkness CJ, Burr RL, Mitchell PH, Newell DW. Is there a sex difference in the course following traumatic brain injury? *Biol Res Nurs* 2004; 5(4):299–310.

537. Corrigan JD, Lineberry LA, Komaroff E, Langlois JA, Selassie AW, Wood KD. Employment after traumatic brain injury: differences between men and women. *Arch Phys Med Rehabil* 2007; 88(11):1400–1409.

538. Bay E, Sikorskii A, Saint-Arnault D. Sex differences in depressive symptoms and their correlates after mild-to-moderate traumatic brain injury. *J Neurosci Nurs* 2009; 41(6):298–309.

539. Dick RW. Is there a gender difference in concussion incidence and outcomes? *Br J Sports Med* 2009; 43 (Suppl 1):i46–i50.

540. Preiss-Farzanegan SJ, Chapman B, Wong TM, Wu J, Bazarian JJ. The relationship between gender and postconcussion symptoms after sport-related mild traumatic brain injury. *PM R* 2009; 1(3):245–253.

541. Ahman S, Saveman BI, Styrke J, Bjornstig U, Stalnacke BM. Long-term follow-up of patients with mild traumatic brain injury: a mixed-method study. *J Rehabil Med* 2013; 45(8):758–764.

542. Scott C, McKinlay A, McLellan T, Britt E, Grace R, MacFarlane M. A comparison of adult outcomes for males compared to females following pediatric traumatic brain injury. *Neuropsychology* 2015; 29(4):501–508.

543. Earls F. Sex differences in psychiatric disorders: origins and developmental influences. *Psychiatr Dev* 1987; 5(1):1–23.

544. Kessler RC, McGonagle KA, Swartz M, Blazer DG, Nelson CB. Sex and depression in the National Comorbidity Survey. I: Lifetime prevalence, chronicity and recurrence. *J Affect Disord* 1993; 29(2–3):85–96.

545. Kessler RC, Sonnega A, Bromet E, Hughes M, Nelson CB. Posttraumatic stress disorder in the National Comorbidity Survey. *Arch Gen Psychiatry* 1995; 52(12):1048–1060.

546. Leibenluft E. *Gender differences in mood and anxiety disorders: from bench to bedside.* Washington, D.C.: American Psychiatric Publishing, 1999.

547. Kessler RC. Epidemiology of women and depression. *J Affect Disord* 2003; 74(1):5–13.

548. Marcus SM, Young EA, Kerber KB, Kornstein S, Farabaugh AH, Mitchell J, et al. Gender differences in depression: findings from the STAR*D study. *J Affect Disord* 2005; 87(2–3):141–150.

549. Snow RC. *Sex, gender and vulnerability.* Contract no.: 07-628. University of Michigan Population Studies Center, 2007. Available at www.psc.isr.umich.edu/pubs/pdf/rr07-628.pdf.

550. Stranieri G, Carabetta C. Depression and suicidality in modern life. *Psychiatr Danub* 2012; 24 Suppl 1:S91–S94.

551. Brouillet A. Une leçon clinique à la Salpêtrière.jpg [a clinical lesson at the Salpêtrière] [Internet]. 1887 [painting]. [cited 17 August 2017]. Available from: http://commons.wikimedia.org/wiki/File:Une_le%C3%A7on_clinique_%C3%A0_la_Salp%C3%AAtri%C3%A8re.jpg.

552. Harris JC. A clinical lesson at the Salpêtrière. *Arch Gen Psychiatry* 2005; 62(5):470–472.

553. Anker M, World Health Organization (WHO). Addressing sex and gender in epidemic-prone infectious diseases. Departments of Gender, Women and Health; Epidemic and Pandemic Alert and Response. Geneva: World Health Organization, 2007 [cited 2016 July 16]. Available from: www.who.int/iris/handle/10665/43644.

554. Barth C, Villringer A, Sacher J. Sex hormones affect neurotransmitters and shape the adult female brain during hormonal transition periods. *Front Neurosci* 2015; 9:37.

555. Inoue M. Fourier analysis of the forehead shape of skull and sex determination by use of computer. *Forensic Sci Int* 1990; 47(2):101–112.

556. Inoue M, Inoue T, Fushimi Y, Okada K. Sex determination by discriminant function analysis of lateral cranial form. *Forensic Sci Int* 1992; 57(2):109–117.

557. Koolschijn PC, Crone EA. Sex differences and structural brain maturation from childhood to early adulthood. *Dev Cogn Neurosci* 2013; 5:106–118.

558. Lenroot RK, Gogtay N, Greenstein DK, Wells EM, Wallace GL, Clasen LS, et al. Sexual dimorphism of brain developmental trajectories during childhood and adolescence. *NeuroImage* 2007; 36(4):1065–1073.

559. Li LM, Menon DK, Janowitz T. Cross-sectional analysis of data from the U.S. Clinical Trials database reveals poor translational

clinical trial effort for traumatic brain injury, compared with stroke. *PLoS One* 2014; 9(1):e84336.

560. Pfefferbaum A, Rohlfing T, Rosenbloom MJ, Chu W, Colrain IM, Sullivan EV. Variation in longitudinal trajectories of regional brain volumes of healthy men and women (ages 10 to 85 years) measured with atlas-based parcellation of MRI. *NeuroImage* 2013; 65:176–193.

561. Ruigrok AN, Salimi-Khorshidi G, Lai MC, Baron-Cohen S, Lombardo MV, Tait RJ, et al. A meta-analysis of sex differences in human brain structure. *Neurosci Biobehav Rev* 2014; 39:34–50.

562. Goldstein JM, Seidman LJ, Horton NJ, Makris N, Kennedy DN, Caviness VS, Jr., et al. Normal sexual dimorphism of the adult human brain assessed by in vivo magnetic resonance imaging. *Cereb Cortex* 2001; 11(6):490–497.

563. Amunts K, Armstrong E, Malikovic A, Homke L, Mohlberg H, Schleicher A, et al. Gender-specific left–right asymmetries in human visual cortex. *J Neurosci* 2007; 27(6):1356–1364.

564. Lenroot RK, Giedd JN. Sex differences in the adolescent brain. *Brain Cogn* 2010; 72(1):46–55.

565. Neufang S, Specht K, Hausmann M, Gunturkun O, Herpertz-Dahlmann B, Fink GR, et al. Sex differences and the impact of steroid hormones on the developing human brain. *Cereb Cortex* 2009; 19(2):464–473.

566. Mak AK, Wong MM, Han S-h, Lee TM. Gray matter reduction associated with emotion regulation in female outpatients with major depressive disorder: a voxel-based morphometry study. *Prog Neuropsychopharmacol Biol Psych* 2009; 33(7):1184–1190.

567. Liu CH, Jing B, Ma X, Xu PF, Zhang Y, Li F, et al. Voxel-based morphometry study of the insular cortex in female patients with current and remitted depression. *Neuroscience* 2014; 262:190–199.

568. Sun Y, Lee R, Chen Y, Collinson S, Thakor N, Bezerianos A, et al. Progressive gender differences of structural brain networks in healthy adults: a longitudinal, diffusion tensor imaging study. *PLoS One* 2015; 10(3):e0118857.

569. Ingalhalikar M, Smith A, Parker D, Satterthwaite TD, Elliott MA, Ruparel K, et al. Sex differences in the structural connectome of the human brain. *Proc Natl Acad Sci USA* 2014; 111(2):823–828.

570. Rabinowicz T, Petetot JM, Gartside PS, Sheyn D, Sheyn T, de CM. Structure of the cerebral cortex in men and women. *J Neuropathol Exp Neurol* 2002; 61(1):46–57.

571. Young EA, Altemus M. Puberty, ovarian steroids, and stress. *Ann N Y Acad Sci* 2004; 1021:124–133.

572. Ter Horst GJ, Wichmann R, Gerrits M, Westenbroek C, Lin Y. Sex differences in stress responses: focus on ovarian hormones. *Physiol Behav* 2009; 97(2):239–249.

573. ter Horst JP, de Kloet ER, Schachinger H, Oitzl MS. Relevance of stress and female sex hormones for emotion and cognition. *Cell Mol Neurobiol* 2012; 32(5):725–735.

574. Lokuge S, Frey BN, Foster JA, Soares CN, Steiner M. Depression in women: windows of vulnerability and new insights into the link between estrogen and serotonin. *J Clin Psychiatry* 2011; 72(11):e1563–1569.

575. Stein MB, Fallin MD, Schork NJ, Gelernter J. COMT polymorphisms and anxiety-related personality traits. *Neuropsychopharmacology* 2005; 30(11):2092–2102.

576. Hettema JM, An SS, Bukszar J, van den Oord EJ, Neale MC, Kendler KS, et al. Catechol-O-methyltransferase contributes to genetic susceptibility shared among anxiety spectrum phenotypes. *Biol Psychiatry* 2008; 64(4):302–310.

577. Hatzimanolis A, Vitoratou S, Mandelli L, Vaiopoulos C, Nearchou FA, Stefanis CN, et al. Potential role of membrane-bound COMT gene polymorphisms in female depression vulnerability. *J Affect Disord* 2013; 148(2–3):316–322.

578. Buchanan TW, Driscoll D, Mowrer SM, Sollers JJ, 3rd, Thayer JF, Kirschbaum C, et al. Medial prefrontal cortex damage affects physiological and psychological stress responses differently in men and women. *Psychoneuroendocrinology* 2010; 35(1):56–66.

579. Fakhran S, Yaeger K, Collins M, Alhilali L. Sex differences in white matter abnormalities after mild traumatic brain injury: localization and correlation with outcome. *Radiology* 2014; 272(3):815–823.

580. Wunderle K, Hoeger KM, Wasserman E, Bazarian JJ. Menstrual phase as predictor of outcome after mild traumatic brain injury in women. *J Head Trauma Rehabil* 2014; 29(5):E1–E8.

581. Wagner AK, Willard LA, Kline AE, Wenger MK, Bolinger BD, Ren D, et al. Evaluation of estrous cycle stage and gender on behavioral outcome after experimental traumatic brain injury. *Brain Res* 2004; 998(1):113–121.

582. Singh M. Mechanisms of progesterone-induced neuroprotection. *Ann N Y Acad Sci* 2005; 1052:145–151.

583. Gibson CL, Gray LJ, Bath PM, Murphy SP. Progesterone for the treatment of experimental brain injury; a systematic review. *Brain* 2008; 131(2):318–328.

584. Stein DG, Wright DW. Progesterone in the clinical treatment of acute traumatic brain injury. *Expert Opin Investig Drugs* 2010; 19(7):847–857.

585. Stein DG. Is progesterone a worthy candidate as a novel therapy for traumatic brain injury? *Dialogues Clin Neurosci* 2011; 13(3):352–359.

586. Luoma JI, Stern CM, Mermelstein PG. Progesterone inhibition of neuronal calcium signaling underlies aspects of progesterone-mediated neuroprotection. *J Steroid Biochem Mol Biol* 2012; 131(1–2):30–36.

587. Geddes RI, Peterson BL, Stein DG, Sayeed I. Progesterone treatment shows benefit in female rats in a pediatric model of controlled cortical impact injury. *PLoS One* 2016; 11(1):e0146419.

588. Skolnick BE, Maas AI, Narayan RK, van der Hoop RG, MacAllister T, Ward JD, et al. A clinical trial of progesterone for severe traumatic brain injury. *N Engl J Med* 2014; 371(26):2467–2476.

589. Wright DW, Yeatts SD, Silbergleit R, Palesch YY, Hertzberg VS, Frankel M, et al. Very early administration of progesterone for acute traumatic brain injury. *N Engl J Med* 2014; 371(26):2457–2466.

590. Craske MG. *Origins of phobias and anxiety disorders: why more women than men?* Oxford: Elsevier, 2003.

591. Olff M, Langeland W, Draijer N, Gersons BP. Gender differences in posttraumatic stress disorder. *Psychol Bull* 2007; 133(2):183–204.

592. Kelly MM, Tyrka AR, Anderson GM, Price LH, Carpenter LL. Sex differences in emotional and physiological responses to the Trier Social Stress Test. *J Behav Ther Exp Psychiatry* 2008; 39(1):87–98.

593. Bao AM, Swaab DF. Sex differences in the brain, behavior, and neuropsychiatric disorders. *Neuroscientist* 2010; 16(5):550–565.

594. Hauger RL, Olivares-Reyes JA, Dautzenberg FM, Lohr JB, Braun S, Oakley RH. Molecular and cell signaling targets for PTSD pathophysiology and pharmacotherapy. *Neuropharmacology* 2012; 62(2):705–714.

595. van Zuiden M, Geuze E, Willemen HL, Vermetten E, Maas M, Amarouchi K, et al. Glucocorticoid receptor pathway components predict posttraumatic stress disorder symptom development: a prospective study. *Biol Psychiatry* 2012; 71(4):309–316.

596. Kudielka BM, Kirschbaum C. Sex differences in HPA axis responses to stress: a review. *Biol Psychol* 2005; 69(1):113–132.

597. Rohleder N, Schommer NC, Hellhammer DH, Engel R, Kirschbaum C. Sex differences in glucocorticoid sensitivity of proinflammatory cytokine production after psychosocial stress. *Psychosom Med* 2001; 63(6):966–972.

598. Bao AM, Meynen G, Swaab DF. The stress system in depression and neurodegeneration: focus on the human hypothalamus. *Brain Res Rev* 2008; 57(2):531–553.

599. Goldstein JM, Jerram M, Abbs B, Whitfield-Gabrieli S, Makris N. Sex differences in stress response circuitry activation dependent on female hormonal cycle. *J Neurosci* 2010; 30(2):431–438.

600. Bryant RA, Felmingham KL, Silove D, Creamer M, O'Donnell M, McFarlane AC. The association between menstrual cycle and traumatic memories. *J Affect Disord* 2011; 131(1–3):398–401.

601. Kajantie E, Phillips DI. The effects of sex and hormonal status on the physiological response to acute psychosocial stress. *Psychoneuroendocrinology* 2006; 31(2):151–178.

602. Andreano JM, Arjomandi H, Cahill L. Menstrual cycle modulation of the relationship between cortisol and long-term memory. *Psychoneuroendocrinology* 2008; 33(6):874–882.

603. Ossewaarde L, Hermans EJ, van Wingen GA, Kooijman SC, Johansson IM, Backstrom T, et al. Neural mechanisms underlying changes in stress-sensitivity across the menstrual cycle. *Psychoneuroendocrinology* 2010; 35(1):47–55.

604. Dreher JC, Schmidt PJ, Kohn P, Furman D, Rubinow D, Berman KF. Menstrual cycle phase modulates reward-related neural function in women. *Proc Natl Acad Sci U S A* 2007; 104(7):2465–2470.

605. Ferree NK, Kamat R, Cahill L. Influences of menstrual cycle position and sex hormone levels on spontaneous intrusive recollections following emotional stimuli. *Conscious Cogn* 2011; 20(4):1154–1162.

606. Mareckova K, Perrin JS, Nawaz Khan I, Lawrence C, Dickie E, McQuiggan DA, et al. Hormonal contraceptives, menstrual cycle and brain response to faces. *Soc Cogn Affect Neurosci* 2014; 9(2):191–200.

607. Sacher J, Okon-Singer H, Villringer A. Evidence from neuroimaging for the role of the menstrual cycle in the interplay of emotion and cognition. *Front Hum Neurosci* 2013; 7:374.

608. Andreano JM, Cahill L. Menstrual cycle modulation of medial temporal activity evoked by negative emotion. *NeuroImage* 2010; 53(4):1286–1293.

609. Laskowski R, Creed J, Raghupathi R. Pathophysiology of mild TBI: implications for altered signaling pathways. In: Kobeissy FH, editor. *Brain neurotrauma: molecular, neuropsychological, and rehabilitation aspects.* Boca Raton, FL: CRC Press/Taylor & Francis, 2015.

610. Jacobs E, D'Esposito M. Estrogen shapes dopamine-dependent cognitive processes: implications for women's health. *J Neurosci* 2011; 31(14):5286–5293.

611. Farin A, Deutsch R, Biegon A, Marshall LF. Sex-related differences in patients with severe head injury: greater susceptibility to brain swelling in female patients 50 years of age and younger. *J Neurosurg* 2003; 98(1):32–36.

612. Fan P, Yamauchi T, Noble LJ, Ferriero DM. Age-dependent differences in glutathione peroxidase activity after traumatic brain injury. *J Neurotrauma* 2003; 20(5):437–445.

613. Susman M, DiRusso SM, Sullivan T, Risucci D, Nealon P, Cuff S, et al. Traumatic brain injury in the elderly: increased mortality and worse functional outcome at discharge despite lower injury severity. *J Trauma* 2002; 53(2):219–223; discussion 223–224.

614. Harrison-Felix C, Whiteneck G, DeVivo M, Hammond FM, Jha A. Mortality following rehabilitation in the traumatic brain injury model systems of care. *J Head Trauma Rehabil* 2004; 19(1):45–54.

615. Harrison-Felix C, Kolakowsky-Hayner SA, Hammond FM, Wang R, Englander J, Dams-O'Connor K, et al. Mortality after surviving traumatic brain injury: risks based on age groups. *J Head Trauma Rehabil* 2012; 27(6):E45–E56.

616. Flaada JT, Leibson CL, Mandrekar JN, Diehl N, Perkins PK, Brown AW, et al. Relative risk of mortality after traumatic brain injury: a population-based study of the role of age and injury severity. *J Neurotrauma* 2007; 24(3):435–445.

617. El-Matbouly M, El-Menyar A, Al-Thani H, Tuma M, El-Hennawy H, AbdulRahman H, et al. Traumatic brain injury in Qatar: age matters – insights from a 4-year observational study. *Sci World J* 2013; 2013:354920.

618. Colantonio A, Escobar MD, Chipman M, McLellan B, Austin PC, Mirabella G, et al. Predictors of postacute mortality following traumatic brain injury in a seriously injured population. *J Trauma* 2008; 64(4):876–882.

619. Harrison-Felix CL, Whiteneck GG, Jha A, DeVivo MJ, Hammond FM, Hart DM. Mortality over four decades after traumatic brain injury rehabilitation: a retrospective cohort study. *Arch Phys Med Rehabil* 2009; 90(9):1506–1513.

620. Ventura T, Harrison-Felix C, Carlson N, Diguiseppi C, Gabella B, Brown A, et al. Mortality after discharge from acute care hospitalization with traumatic brain injury: a population-based study. *Arch Phys Med Rehabil* 2010; 91(1):20–29.

621. Nott MT, Gates TM, Baguley IJ. Age-related trends in late mortality following traumatic brain injury: a multicentre inception cohort study. *Australas J Ageing* 2015; 34(2):E1–E6.

622. Livingston DH, Lavery RF, Mosenthal AC, Knudson MM, Lee S, Morabito D, et al. Recovery at one year following isolated traumatic brain injury: a Western Trauma Association prospective multicenter trial. *J Trauma* 2005; 59(6):1298–1304; discussion 1304.

623. Testa JA, Malec JF, Moessner AM, Brown AW. Outcome after traumatic brain injury: effects of aging on recovery. *Arch Phys Med Rehabil* 2005; 86(9):1815–1823.

624. Willemse-van Son AH, Ribbers GM, Verhagen AP, Stam HJ. Prognostic factors of long-term functioning and productivity after traumatic brain injury: a systematic review of prospective cohort studies. *Clin Rehabil* 2007; 21(11):1024–1037.

625. Marquez de la Plata C, Hewlitt M, de Oliveira A, Hudak A, Harper C, Shafi S, et al. Ethnic differences in rehabilitation placement and outcome after TBI. *J Head Trauma Rehabil* 2007; 22(2):113–121.

626. Marquez de la Plata CD, Hart T, Hammond FM, Frol AB, Hudak A, Harper CR, et al. Impact of age on long-term recovery from traumatic brain injury. *Arch Phys Med Rehabil* 2008; 89(5):896–903.

627. Tokutomi T, Miyagi T, Ogawa T, Ono J, Kawamata T, Sakamoto T, et al. Age-associated increases in poor outcomes after traumatic brain injury: a report from the Japan Neurotrauma Data Bank. *J Neurotrauma* 2008; 25(12):1407–1414.

628. Wu X, Hu J, Zhuo L, Fu C, Hui G, Wang Y, et al. Epidemiology of traumatic brain injury in eastern China, 2004: a prospective large case study. *J Trauma* 2008; 64(5):1313–1319.

629. Senathi-Raja D, Ponsford J, Schonberger M. Impact of age on long-term cognitive function after traumatic brain injury. *Neuropsychology* 2010; 24(3):336–344.

630. Pedersen AR, Severinsen K, Nielsen JF. The effect of age on rehabilitation outcome after traumatic brain injury assessed by the Functional Independence Measure (FIM). *Neurorehabil Neural Repair* 2015; 29(4):299–307.

631. Hukkelhoven CW, Steyerberg EW, Rampen AJ, Farace E, Habbema JD, Marshall LF, et al. Patient age and outcome following severe traumatic brain injury: an analysis of 5600 patients. *J Neurosurg* 2003; 99(4):666–673.

632. Schonberger M, Ponsford J, Reutens D, Beare R, O'Sullivan R. The relationship between age, injury severity, and MRI findings after traumatic brain injury. *J Neurotrauma* 2009; 26(12):2157–2167.

633. Sandhir R, Berman NE. Age-dependent response of CCAAT/enhancer binding proteins following traumatic brain injury in mice. *Neurochem Int* 2010; 56(1):188–193.

634. Gilmer LK, Ansari MA, Roberts KN, Scheff SW. Age-related mitochondrial changes after traumatic brain injury. *J Neurotrauma* 2010; 27(5):939–950.

635. Titus DJ, Furones C, Kang Y, Atkins CM. Age-dependent alterations in cAMP signaling contribute to synaptic plasticity deficits following traumatic brain injury. *Neuroscience* 2013; 231:182–194.

636. Ariesen MJ, Claus SP, Rinkel GJ, Algra A. Risk factors for intracerebral hemorrhage in the general population: a systematic review. *Stroke* 2003; 34(8):2060–2065.

637. Thanvi B, Robinson T. Sporadic cerebral amyloid angiopathy – an important cause of cerebral haemorrhage in older people. *Age Ageing* 2006; 35(6):565–571.

638. Bejot Y, Osseby GV, Gremeaux V, Durier J, Rouaud O, Moreau T, et al. Changes in risk factors and preventive treatments by stroke subtypes over 20 years: a population-based study. *J Neurol Sci* 2009; 287(1–2):84–88.

639. van Asch CJ, Luitse MJ, Rinkel GJ, van der Tweel I, Algra A, Klijn CJ. Incidence, case fatality, and functional outcome of intracerebral haemorrhage over time, according to age, sex, and ethnic origin: a systematic review and meta-analysis. *Lancet Neurol* 2010; 9(2):167–176.

640. Wasserman JK, Yang H, Schlichter LC. Glial responses, neuron death and lesion resolution after intracerebral hemorrhage in young vs. aged rats. *Eur J Neurosci* 2008; 28(7):1316–1328.

641. Lively S, Schlichter LC. Age-related comparisons of evolution of the inflammatory response after intracerebral hemorrhage in rats. *Transl Stroke Res* 2012; 3(Suppl 1):132–146.

642. Feldmann E, Broderick JP, Kernan WN, Viscoli CM, Brass LM, Brott T, et al. Major risk factors for intracerebral hemorrhage in the young are modifiable. *Stroke* 2005; 36(9):1881–1885.

643. Umeano O, Phillips-Bute B, Hailey CE, Sun W, Gray MC, Roulhac-Wilson B, et al. Gender and age interact to affect early outcome after intracerebral hemorrhage. *PLoS One* 2013; 8(11):e81664.

644. Zhou J, Zhang Y, Arima H, Zhao Y, Zhao H, Zheng D, et al. Sex differences in clinical characteristics and outcomes after intracerebral haemorrhage: results from a 12-month prospective stroke registry in Nanjing, China. *BMC Neurol* 2014; 14:172.

645. Gokhale S, Caplan LR, James ML. Sex differences in incidence, pathophysiology, and outcome of primary intracerebral hemorrhage. *Stroke* 2015; 46(3):886–892.

646. Engman J, Ahs F, Furmark T, Linnman C, Pissiota A, Appel L, et al. Age, sex and NK1 receptors in the human brain – a positron emission tomography study with [(1)(1)C]GR205171. *Eur Neuropsychopharmacol* 2012; 22(8):562–568.

647. Chen M, Maleski JJ, Sawmiller DR. Scientific truth or false hope? Understanding Alzheimer's disease from an aging perspective. *J Alzheimers Dis* 2011; 24(1):3–10.

648. Drachman DA. The amyloid hypothesis, time to move on: amyloid is the downstream result, not cause, of Alzheimer's disease. *Alzheimers Dement* 2014; 10(3):372–380.

649. Ferreira ST, Clarke JR, Bomfim TR, De Felice FG. Inflammation, defective insulin signaling, and neuronal dysfunction in Alzheimer's disease. *Alzheimers Dement* 2014; 10(1 Suppl):S76–83.

650. Ferrer I. Defining Alzheimer as a common age-related neurodegenerative process not inevitably leading to dementia. *Prog Neurobiol* 2012; 97(1):38–51.

651. Haddon W, Jr. On the escape of tigers: an ecologic note. *Am J Public Health Nations Health* 1970; 60(12):2229–2234.

652. Morris GP, Clark IA, Vissel B. Inconsistencies and controversies surrounding the amyloid hypothesis of Alzheimer's disease. *Acta Neuropathol Commun* 2014; 2:135.

653. Mullane K, Williams M. Alzheimer's therapeutics: continued clinical failures question the validity of the amyloid hypothesis – but what lies beyond? *Biochem Pharmacol* 2013; 85(3):289–305.

654. Neill D. Should Alzheimer's disease be equated with human brain ageing? A maladaptive interaction between brain evolution and senescence. *Ageing Res Rev* 2012; 11(1):104–122.

655. Whitehouse PJ, George DR, D'Alton S. Describing the dying days of "Alzheimer's disease." *J Alzheimers Dis* 2011; 24(1):11–13.

656. Chen DY, Hsu HL, Kuo YS, Wu CW, Chiu WT, Yan FX, et al. Effect of age on working memory performance and cerebral activation after mild traumatic brain injury: a functional MRI study. *Radiology* 2016; 278(3):854–862.

657. Deb S, Burns J. Neuropsychiatric consequences of traumatic brain injury: a comparison between two age groups. *Brain Inj* 2007; 21(3):301–307.

658. Juengst SB, Adams LM, Bogner JA, Arenth PM, O'Neil-Pirozzi TM, Dreer LE, et al. Trajectories of life satisfaction after traumatic brain injury: influence of life roles, age, cognitive disability, and depressive symptoms. *Rehabil Psychol* 2015; 60(4):353–364.

659. Rapoport MJ, McCullagh S, Streiner D, Feinstein A. Age and major depression after mild traumatic brain injury. *Am J Geriatr Psychiatry* 2003; 11(3):365–369.

660. Eisenberg N, Lennon R. Sex differences in empathy and related capacities. *Psychol Bull* 1983; 94(1):100.

661. Graham T, Ickes W. When women's intuition isn't greater than men's. In: Ickes W, editor. *Empathetic accuracy*. New York, NY: Guilford Press, 1997, pp. 117–143.

662. Baron-Cohen S, Wheelwright S. The empathy quotient: an investigation of adults with Asperger syndrome or high functioning autism, and normal sex differences. *J Autism Dev Disord* 2004; 34(2):163–175.

663. Sucksmith E, Allison C, Baron-Cohen S, Chakrabarti B, Hoekstra RA. Empathy and emotion recognition in people with autism, first-degree relatives, and controls. *Neuropsychologia* 2013; 51(1):98–105.

664. Maccoby EE, Jacklin CN. *The psychology of sex differences*. Stanford, CA: Stanford University Press, 1974.

665. Voyer D, Voyer S, Bryden MP. Magnitude of sex differences in spatial abilities: a meta-analysis and consideration of critical variables. *Psychol Bull* 1995; 117(2):250–270.

666. Collins DW, Kimura D. A large sex difference on a two-dimensional mental rotation task. *Behav Neurosci* 1997; 111(4):845–849.

667. Kaufman SB. Sex differences in mental rotation and spatial visualization ability: can they be accounted for by differences in working memory capacity? *Intelligence* 2007; 35(3):211–223.

668. Quinn PC, Liben LS. A sex difference in mental rotation in young infants. *Psychol Sci* 2008; 19(11):1067–1070.

669. Graves AB, White E, Koepsell TD, Reifler BV, van Belle G, Larson EB, et al. The association between head trauma and Alzheimer's disease. *Am J Epidemiol* 1990; 131(3):491–501.

670. Schofield PW, Tang M, Marder K, Bell K, Dooneief G, Chun M, et al. Alzheimer's disease after remote head injury: an incidence study. *J Neurol Neurosurg Psychiatry* 1997; 62(2):119–124.

671. Lee YK, Hou SW, Lee CC, Hsu CY, Huang YS, Su YC. Increased risk of dementia in patients with mild traumatic brain injury: a nationwide cohort study. *PLoS One* 2013; 8(5):e62422.

672. Nordstrom P, Michaelsson K, Gustafson Y, Nordstrom A. Traumatic brain injury and young onset dementia: a nationwide cohort study. *Ann Neurol* 2014; 75(3):374–381.

673. Johnson VE, Stewart W. Traumatic brain injury: age at injury influences dementia risk after TBI. *Nat Rev Neurol* 2015; 11(3):128–130.

674. Gardner RC, Burke JF, Nettiksimmons J, Kaup A, Barnes DE, Yaffe K. Dementia risk after traumatic brain injury vs nonbrain trauma: the role of age and severity. *JAMA Neurol* 2014; 71(12):1490–1497.

675. Larrabee GJ, Rohling ML. Neuropsychological differential diagnosis of mild traumatic brain injury. *Behav Sci Law* 2013; 31(6):686–701.

676. Robertson A. The post-concussional syndrome then and now. *Aust N Z J Psychiatry* 1988; 22(4):396–402.

677. Lewis A, Symonds CP, editors. Discussion on differential diagnosis and treatment of post-contusional states. *Proc R Soc Med* 35; 1942:607.

678. Miller H. Accident neurosis. *Br Med J* 1961; 1(5230):919–925.

679. Lishman WA. Physiogenesis and psychogenesis in the 'post-concussional syndrome'. *Br J Psychiatry* 1988; 153:460–469.

680. Evans RW. The postconcussion syndrome and the sequelae of mild head injury. *Neurol Clin* 1992; 10(4):815–847.

681. Merskey H. Psychiatric aspects of the neurology of trauma. *Neurol Clin* 1992; 10(4):895–905.

682. Mittenberg W, DiGiulio DV, Perrin S, Bass AE. Symptoms following mild head injury: expectation as aetiology. *J Neurol Neurosurg Psychiatry* 1992; 55(3):200–204.

683. Jacobson RR. The post-concussional syndrome: physiogenesis, psychogenesis and malingering. An integrative model. *J Psychosom Res* 1995; 39(6):675–693.

684. Karzmark P, Hall K, Englander J. Late-onset post-concussion symptoms after mild brain injury: the role of premorbid, injury-related, environmental, and personality factors. *Brain Inj* 1995; 9(1):21–26.

685. Gasquoine PG. Postconcussion symptoms. *Neuropsychol Rev* 1997; 7(2):77–85.

686. Weight DG. Minor head trauma. *Psychiatr Clin North Am* 1998; 21(3):609–624.

687. Ferguson RJ, Mittenberg W, Barone DF, Schneider B. Postconcussion syndrome following sports-related head injury: expectation as etiology. *Neuropsychology* 1999; 13(4):582–589.

688. Mittenberg W, Strauman S. Diagnosis of mild head injury and the postconcussion syndrome. *J Head Trauma Rehabil* 2000; 15(2):783–791.

689. Suhr JA, Gunstad J. "Diagnosis threat": the effect of negative expectations on cognitive performance in head injury. *J Clin Exp Neuropsychol* 2002; 24(4):448–457.

690. Suhr JA, Gunstad J. Further exploration of the effect of "diagnosis threat" on cognitive performance in individuals with mild head injury. *J Int Neuropsychol Soc* 2005; 11(1):23–29.

691. Ettenhofer ML, Abeles N. The significance of mild traumatic brain injury to cognition and self-reported symptoms in long-term recovery from injury. *J Clin Exp Neuropsychol* 2009; 31(3):363–372.

692. Iverson GL, Lange RT, Brooks BL, Rennison VL. "Good old days" bias following mild traumatic brain injury. *Clin Neuropsychol* 2010; 24(1):17–37.

693. Lange RT, Iverson GL, Rose A. Post-concussion symptom reporting and the "good-old-days" bias following mild traumatic brain injury. *Arch Clin Neuropsychol* 2010; 25(5):442–450.

694. Ozen LJ, Fernandes MA. Effects of "diagnosis threat" on cognitive and affective functioning long after mild head injury. *J Int Neuropsychol Soc* 2011; 17(2):219–229.

695. Trontel HG. Diagnosis threat in a mild traumatic brain injury population. Paper 317. 2012. Theses, dissertations, professional papers. Missoula, MT: ScholarWorks at University of Montana. Available at https://scholarworks.umt.edu/cgi/viewcontent.cgi?article=1336&context=etd.

696. Broshek DK, De Marco AP, Freeman JR. A review of post-concussion syndrome and psychological factors associated with concussion. *Brain Inj* 2015; 29(2):228–237.

697. Haun P. A rational approach to psychiatric nosology. *Psychiatr Q* 1949; 23(2):308–316.

698. Abely P. Has the time come to revise psychiatric nosology? If so, why and how? If not what else must we wait for? *Ann Med Psychol (Paris)* 1966; 124(4):568–578.

699. Faraone SV, Tsuang MT. Measuring diagnostic accuracy in the absence of a "gold standard." *Am J Psychiatry* 1994; 151(5):650–657.

700. Mack AH, Forman L, Brown R, Frances A. A brief history of psychiatric classification. From the ancients to DSM-IV. *Psychiatr Clin North Am* 1994; 17(3):515–523.

701. Smolik P. Validity of nosological classification. *Dialogues Clin Neurosci* 1999; 1(3):185–190.

702. Berganza CE, Mezzich JE, Pouncey C. Concepts of disease: their relevance for psychiatric diagnosis and classification. *Psychopathology* 2005; 38(4):166–170.

703. Stein DJ. What is a mental disorder? A perspective from cognitive-affective science. *J Psychiatry* 2013; 58(12):656–662.

704. Veith I. Psychiatric nosology: from Hippocrates to Kraepelin. *Am J Psychiatry* 1957; 114(5):385–391.

705. Weissman MM, Klerman GL. Psychiatric nosology and Midtown Manhattan Study. *Arch Gen Psychiatry* 1980; 37(2):229–230.

706. Grob GN. Origins of DSM-I: a study in appearance and reality. *Am J Psychiatry* 1991; 148(4):421–431.

707. Blacker D, Tsuang MT. Contested boundaries of bipolar disorder and the limits of categorical diagnosis in psychiatry. *Am J Psychiatry* 1992; 149(11):1473–1483.

708. Kumbier E, Herpertz SC. Helmut Rennert's universal genesis of endogenous psychoses: the historical concept and its significance for today's discussion on unitary psychosis. *Psychopathology* 2010; 43(6):335–344.

709. London EB. Categorical diagnosis: a fatal flaw for autism research? *Trends Neurosci* 2014; 37(12):683–686.

710. Van Os J. The transdiagnostic dimension of psychosis: implications for psychiatric nosology and research. *Shanghai Arch Psychiatry* 2015; 27(2):82–86.

711. Hettema JM. The nosologic relationship between generalized anxiety disorder and major depression. *Depress Anxiety* 2008; 25(4):300–316.

712. Faravelli C, Castellini G, Landi M, Brugnera A. Are psychiatric diagnoses an obstacle for research and practice? Reliability, validity and the problem of psychiatric diagnoses. The case of GAD. *Clin Pract Epidemiol Ment Health* 2012; 8:12–15.

713. Faraone SV. Attention-deficit hyperactivity disorder and the shifting sands of psychiatric nosology. *Br J Psychiatry* 2013; 203(2):81–83.

714. Pearlson GD. Etiologic, phenomenologic, and endophenotypic overlap of schizophrenia and bipolar disorder. *Annu Rev Clin Psychol* 2015; 11:251–281.

715. Karp I. Deconstructing culture-bound syndromes. *Soc Sci Med* 1985; 21(2):221–228.

716. Aderibigbe YA, Pandurangi AK. Comment: the neglect of culture in psychiatric nosology: the case of culture bound syndromes. *Int J Soc Psychiatry* 1995; 41(4):235–241.

717. Parzen MD. Toward a culture-bound syndrome-based insanity defense? *Cult Med Psychiatry* 2003; 27(2):131–155.

718. Kirmayer LJ. Culture, context and experience in psychiatric diagnosis. *Psychopathology* 2005; 38(4):192–196.

719. Wurzman R, Giordano J. Differential susceptibility to plasticity: a 'missing link' between gene-culture co-evolution and neuropsychiatric spectrum disorders? *BMC Med* 2012; 10:37.

720. Lewis-Fernandez R, Aggarwal NK. Culture and psychiatric diagnosis. *Adv Psychosom Med* 2013; 33:15–30.

721. Panzetta AF. Toward a scientific psychiatric nosology. Conceptual and pragmatic issues. *Arch Gen Psychiatry* 1974; 30(2):154–161.

722. Murray RM, Murphy DL. Drug response and psychiatric nosology. *Psychol Med* 1978; 8(4):667–681.

723. de la Fuente JR. Towards a molecular psychiatry. *Acta Psiquiatr Psicol Am Lat* 1988; 34(2):101–108.

724. Kendler KS. Toward a scientific psychiatric nosology. Strengths and limitations. *Arch Gen Psychiatry* 1990; 47(10):969–973.

725. Robert JS. Gene maps, brain scans, and psychiatric nosology. *Camb Q Healthc Ethics* 2007; 16(2):209–218.

726. Gillihan SJ, Parens E. Should we expect "neural signatures" for DSM diagnoses? *J Clin Psychiatry* 2011; 72(10):1383–1389.

727. Goodkind M, Eickhoff SB, Oathes DJ, Jiang Y, Chang A, Jones-Hagata LB, et al. Identification of a common neurobiological substrate for mental illness. *JAMA Psychiatry* 2015; 72(4):305–315.

728. Torgersen S. Contribution of twin studies to psychiatric nosology. *Prog Clin Biol Res* 1978; 24A:125–130.

729. Zerbin-Rudin E. Psychiatric genetics and psychiatric nosology. *J Psychiatr Res* 1987; 21(4):377–383.

730. Ban TA. Neuropsychopharmacology and the genetics of schizophrenia: a history of the diagnosis of schizophrenia. *Prog Neuropsychopharmacol Biol Psychiatry* 2004; 28(5):753–762.

731. Robert JS, Plantikow T. Genetics, neuroscience and psychiatric classification. *Psychopathology* 2005; 38(4):215–218.

732. Kendler KS. Reflections on the relationship between psychiatric genetics and psychiatric nosology. *Am J Psychiatry* 2006; 163(7):1138–1146.

733. Craddock N, O'Donovan MC, Owen MJ. Genes for schizophrenia and bipolar disorder? Implications for psychiatric nosology. *Schizophr Bull* 2006; 32(1):9–16.

734. McGrath CL, Kelley ME, Holtzheimer PE, Dunlop BW, Craighead WE, Franco AR, et al. Toward a neuroimaging treatment selection biomarker for major depressive disorder. *JAMA Psychiatry* 2013; 70(8):821–829.

735. Smoller JW. Disorders and borders: psychiatric genetics and nosology. *Am J Med Genet B Neuropsychiatr Genet* 2013; 162B(7):559–578.

736. Jeste SS, Geschwind DH. Disentangling the heterogeneity of autism spectrum disorder through genetic findings. *Nat Rev Neurol* 2014; 10(2):74–81.

737. Insel TR. Disruptive insights in psychiatry: transforming a clinical discipline. *J Clin Invest* 2009; 119(4):700–705.

738. de Leon J. Is it time to awaken Sleeping Beauty? European psychiatry has been sleeping since 1980. *Rev Psiquiatr Salud Ment* 2014; 7(4):186–194.

739. Peterson BS. Editorial: Research Domain Criteria (RDoC): a new psychiatric nosology whose time has not yet come. *J Child Psychol Psychiatry* 2015; 56(7):719–722.

740. Cuthbert BN. Research Domain Criteria: toward future psychiatric nosologies. *Dialogues Clin Neurosci* 2015; 17(1):89–97.

741. American Psychiatric Association. *Diagnostic and statistical manual of mental disorders*, 5th edition. Arlington, VA: American Psychiatric Publishing, 2013.

742. Daubert *v.* Merrell Dow Pharmaceuticals, Inc. United States Supreme Court. Docket 92–102: 509 U.S. 579; 1993.

743. Barsky AJ, Klerman GL. Hypochondriasis, bodily complaints, and somatic styles. *Am J Psychiatry* 1983; 140(3):273–283.

744. Davis CH. Self-perception in mild traumatic brain injury. *Am J Phys Med Rehabil* 2002; 81(8):609–621.

745. Malec JF, Testa JA, Rush BK, Brown AW, Moessner AM. Self-assessment of impairment, impaired self-awareness, and depression after traumatic brain injury. *J Head Trauma Rehabil* 2007; 22(3):156–166.

746. Rohling ML, Larrabee GJ, Millis SR. The "Miserable Minority" following mild traumatic brain injury: who are they and do meta-analyses hide them? *Clin Neuropsychol* 2012; 26(2):197–213.

747. Schaller WF. Diagnosis in traumatic neurosis. *JAMA* 1918; 71(5):338–347.

748. Miller H. Accident neurosis (part II). *Br Med J* 1961; 1(5231):992–998.

749. Kennedy F. The mind of the injured worker: its effect on disability periods. *Compens Med* 1946; 1:19–21.

750. Guyton GP. A brief history of workers' compensation. *Iowa Orthop J* 1999; 19:106–110.

751. Oppenheimer H. Die traumatischen Neurosen nach den Verletzung [The traumatic neuroses after injury]. In: Hirschwald A, editor. *Der Nervenklinik der Charite in den 8 Jarhren 1883–1891*. Berlin: A. Hirschwald, 1892.

752. Miller H. Mental after-effects of head injury. *Proc R Soc Med* 1966; 59(3):257–261.

753. Fee CR, Rutherford WH. A study of the effect of legal settlement on post-concussion symptoms. *Arch Emerg Med* 1988; 5(1):12–17.

754. Mendelson G. Not "cured by a verdict" effect of legal settlement on compensation claimants. *Med J Aust* 1982; 2(3):132–134.

755. Kelly R, Smith BN. Post-traumatic syndrome: another myth discredited. *J R Soc Med* 1981; 74(4):275–277.

756. Binder LM. Assessment of malingering after mild head trauma with the Portland Digit Recognition Test. *J Clin Exp Neuropsychol* 1993; 15(2):170–182.

757. Cassidy JD, Carroll LJ, Peloso PM, Borg J, von Holst H, Holm L, et al. Incidence, risk factors and prevention of mild traumatic brain injury: results of the WHO Collaborating Centre Task Force on Mild Traumatic Brain Injury. *J Rehabil Med* 2004; (43 Suppl):28–60.

758. Binder LM, Rohling ML. Money matters: a meta-analytic review of the effects of financial incentives on recovery after closed-head injury. *Am J Psychiatry* 1996; 153(1):7–10.

759. Adler A. Mental symptoms following head injury: a statistical analysis of two hundred cases. *Arch Neurol Psychiatry* 1945; 53:34–43.

760. Steadman JH, Graham JG. Head injuries: an analysis and follow-up study. *Proc R Soc Med* 1970; 63:23–28.

761. Cook JB. The postconcussional syndrome and factors influencing recovery after minor head injury admitted to hospital. *Scand J Rehabil Med* 1972; 4:27–30.

762. Cartlidge NEF, Shaw DA. *Head injury*. London: W.B. Saunders, 1981.

763. Konrad C, Geburek AJ, Rist F, Blumenroth H, Fischer B, Husstedt I, et al. Long-term cognitive and emotional consequences of mild traumatic brain injury. *Psychol Med* 2011; 41(6):1197–1211.

764. Minderhoud JM, Boelens ME, Huizenga J, Saan RJ. Treatment of minor head injuries. *Clin Neurol Neurosurg* 1980; 82(2):127–140.

765. Frankel BG, Nuttall S. Illness behaviour: an exploration of determinants. *Soc Sci Med* 1984; 19(2):147–155.

766. Millar K, Purushotham AD, McLatchie E, George WD, Murray GD. A 1-year prospective study of individual variation in distress, and illness perceptions, after treatment for breast cancer. *J Psychosom Res* 2005; 58(4):335–342.

767. Fagg J, Curtis S, Stansfeld S, Congdon P. Psychological distress among adolescents, and its relationship to individual, family and area characteristics in East London. *Soc Sci Med* 2006; 63(3):636–648.

768. Auxemery Y. Posttraumatic stress disorder (PTSD) as a consequence of the interaction between an individual genetic susceptibility, a traumatogenic event and a social context. *Encephale* 2012; 38(5):373–380.

769. Kvarstein EH, Karterud S. Large variation of severity and longitudinal change of symptom distress among patients with personality disorders. *Personal Ment Health* 2013; 7(4):265–276.

770. Pollmann L. Circadian variation of potency of placebo as analgesic. *Funct Neurol* 1987; 2(1):99–103.

771. Gobel H, Cordes P. Circadian variation of pain sensitivity in pericranial musculature. *Headache* 1990; 30(7):418–422.

772. Teepker M, Peters M, Vedder H, Schepelmann K, Lautenbacher S. Menstrual variation in experimental pain: correlation with gonadal hormones. *Neuropsychobiology* 2010; 61(3):131–140.

773. Lees-Haley PR, Brown RS. Neuropsychological complaint base rates of 170 personal injury claimants. *Arch Clin Neuropsychol* 1993; 8(3):203–209.

774. Rumpf, Horn, editors. Sechste Jahresversammulung der Gessellschaft, deutscher Nervenarzte. *Z Nervenh* 1912: 358. As cited in Schaller WF. Diagnosis in traumatic neurosis. *JAMA* 1918; 71:338–344.

775. Regler J. *Uber die Folgen der Verletzung auf Eisenbahnen insbesonder der Verletzungen des Ruchenmarks.* Berlin: G. Reimer, 1879.

776. Pearce JM. Psychosocial factors in chronic disability. *Med Sci Monit* 2002; 8(12):RA275–RA281.

777. Cartlidge NEF, Shaw DA. *Head injury.* London: WB Saunders, 1981.

778. Gould R, Miller BL, Goldberg MA, Benson DF. The validity of hysterical signs and symptoms. *J Nerv Ment Dis* 1986; 174(10):593–597.

779. Camfield L, Skevington SM. On subjective well-being and quality of life. *J Health Psychol* 2008; 13(6):764–775.

780. Kondo N, Sembajwe G, Kawachi I, van Dam RM, Subramanian SV, Yamagata Z. Income inequality, mortality, and self rated health: meta-analysis of multilevel studies. *BMJ* 2009; 339:b4471.

781. Haikin M. Is it better to be poor in a high-income or a low-income country? Counter-intuitive reflections, measuring well-being and the impact of inequality. [Internet]; hiiDunia.com. March 21, 2013 [cited 2016 July 16]. Available from: www.hiidunia.com/2013/03/is-it-better-to-be-poor-in-a-high-income-or-a-low-income-country-counter-intuitive-reflections-measuring-well-being-and-the-impact-of-inequality/.

782. Cheung F, Lucas RE. Income inequality is associated with stronger social comparison effects: the effect of relative income on life satisfaction. *J Pers Soc Psychol* 2016; 110(2):332–341.

783. Arango-Lasprilla JC, Rosenthal M, Deluca J, Komaroff E, Sherer M, Cifu D, et al. Traumatic brain injury and functional outcomes: does minority status matter? *Brain Inj* 2007; 21(7):701–708.

784. Haider AH, Efron DT, Haut ER, DiRusso SM, Sullivan T, Cornwell EE, 3rd. Black children experience worse clinical and functional outcomes after traumatic brain injury: an analysis of the National Pediatric Trauma Registry. *J Trauma* 2007; 62(5):1259–1262; discussion 1262–1263.

785. Shafi S, Marquez de la Plata C, Diaz-Arrastia R, Shipman K, Carlile M, Frankel H, et al. Racial disparities in long-term functional outcome after traumatic brain injury. *J Trauma* 2007; 63(6):1263–1268; discussion 1268–1270.

786. Shafi S, de la Plata CM, Diaz-Arrastia R, Bransky A, Frankel H, Elliott AC, et al. Ethnic disparities exist in trauma care. *J Trauma* 2007; 63(5):1138–1142.

787. Jimenez N, Osorio M, Ramos JL, Apkon S, Ebel BE, Rivara FP. Functional independence after inpatient rehabilitation for traumatic brain injury among minority children and adolescents. *Arch Phys Med Rehabil* 2015; 96(7):1255–1261.

788. Arango-Lasprilla JC, Ketchum JM, Williams K, Kreutzer JS, Marquez de la Plata CD, O'Neil-Pirozzi TM, et al. Racial differences in employment outcomes after traumatic brain injury. *Arch Phys Med Rehabil* 2008; 89(5):988–995.

789. Gary KW, Arango-Lasprilla JC, Ketchum JM, Kreutzer JS, Copolillo A, Novack TA, et al. Racial differences in employment outcome after traumatic brain injury at 1, 2, and 5 years postinjury. *Arch Phys Med Rehabil* 2009; 90(10):1699–1707.

790. Krellman JW, Kolakowsky-Hayner SA, Spielman L, Dijkers M, Hammond FM, Bogner J, et al. Predictors of follow-up completeness in longitudinal research on traumatic brain injury: findings from the National Institute on Disability and Rehabilitation Research traumatic brain injury model systems program. *Arch Phys Med Rehabil* 2014; 95(4):633–641.

791. Perrin PB, Krch D, Sutter M, Snipes DJ, Arango-Lasprilla JC, Kolakowsky-Hayner SA, et al. Racial/ethnic disparities in mental health over the first 2 years after traumatic brain injury: a model systems study. *Arch Phys Med Rehabil* 2014; 95(12):2288–2295.

792. Saltapidas H, Ponsford J. The influence of cultural background on motivation for and participation in rehabilitation and outcome following traumatic brain injury. *J Head Trauma Rehabil* 2007; 22(2):132–139.

793. Vanderploeg RD, Curtiss G, Duchnick JJ, Luis CA. Demographic, medical, and psychiatric factors in work and marital status after mild head injury. *J Head Trauma Rehabil* 2003; 18(2):148–163.

794. Max JE, Pardo D, Hanten G, Schachar RJ, Saunders AE, Ewing-Cobbs L, et al. Psychiatric disorders in children and adolescents six-to-twelve months after mild traumatic brain injury. *J Neuropsychiatry Clin Neurosci* 2013; 25(4):272–282.

795. Cancelliere C, Kristman VL, Cassidy JD, Hincapie CA, Cote P, Boyle E, et al. Systematic review of return to work after mild traumatic brain injury: results of the iternational collaboration on mild traumatic brain injury prognosis. *Arch Phys Med Rehabil* 2014; 95(3 Suppl):S201–S209.

796. MacMillan PJ, Hart RP, Martelli MF, Zasler ND. Pre-injury status and adaptation following traumatic brain injury. *Brain Inj* 2002; 16(1):41–49.

797. Forslund MV, Arango-Lasprilla JC, Roe C, Perrin PB, Sigurdardottir S, Andelic N. Multi-level modelling of employment probability trajectories and employment stability at 1, 2 and 5 years after traumatic brain injury. *Brain Inj* 2014; 28(7):980–986.

798. Schalen W, Hansson L, Nordstrom G, Nordstrom CH. Psychosocial outcome 5–8 years after severe traumatic brain lesions and the impact of rehabilitation services. *Brain Inj* 1994; 8(1):49–64.

799. Bakey L, Glasauer F. *Head injury.* Boston: Little Brown, 1980.

800. Rutherford WH. Sequelae of concussion caused by minor head injuries. *Lancet* 1977; 1(8001):1–4.

801. Ruffolo CF, Friedland JF, Dawson DR, Colantonio A, Lindsay PH. Mild traumatic brain injury from motor vehicle accidents: factors associated with return to work. *Arch Phys Med Rehabil* 1999; 80(4):392–398.

802. Walker WC, Marwitz JH, Kreutzer JS, Hart T, Novack TA. Occupational categories and return to work after traumatic brain injury: a multicenter study. *Arch Phys Med Rehabil* 2006; 87(12):1576–1582.

803. Shames J, Treger I, Ring H, Giaquinto S. Return to work following traumatic brain injury: trends and challenges. *Disabil Rehabil* 2007; 29(17):1387–1395.

804. Federici S, Meloni F. WHODAS II: Disability self-evaluation in the ICF conceptual frame. In: Stone J, Blouin M, editors. *International encyclopedia of rehabilitation*. University of Buffalo, Department of Rehabilitation Science: Center for International Rehabilitation Research Information and Exchange, 2010, pp. 1–22. Available at http://bbi.syr.edu/publications/blanck_docs/2010/employment_people_with_disabilities.pdf.

805. Haddon W, Jr. Options for the prevention of motor vehicle crash injury. *Isr J Med Sci* 1980; 16(1):45–65.

806. Runyan CW. Using the Haddon matrix: introducing the third dimension. *Inj Prev* 1998; 4(4):302–307.

807. Hippocrates. *Aphorisms*. Translated by W.H.S. Jones. Cambridge, MA: Harvard University Press, 1931.

808. Penfield W. The significance of the Montreal Neurological Institute. In: *Neurological biographies and addresses (foundation volume, published for the staff, to commemorate the opening of the Montreal Neurological Institute of McGill University)*. London: Humphrey Milford/Oxford University Press, 1936.

8

Emotional Disturbances Following Traumatic Brain Injury

Ricardo E. Jorge and Helen Lee Lin

Introduction

This chapter discusses a vital component of post-concussive neurobehavioral change: the emotional changes that most profoundly impact the quality of life of concussion survivors. The goals of this chapter and those of the complementary chapter titled *Persistent Post-concussive Psychiatric Problems* (Chapter 10) are in harmony: the neuroscientific and medical community is beginning to understand the nature and consequences of biological change after concussive brain injury (CBI). Prior to quite recent times, the community has been slow to realize that persistent post-CBI brain change is common. It is partly our responsibility to aid the paradigm shift under way – a shift that will acknowledge and validate the distress of hundreds of thousands of CBI survivors and catalyze scholarly enterprise on behalf of their well-being. The present chapter, however, has a unique emphasis: emotion itself is the subject of a renaissance of investigation. New techniques and ideas are illuminating – some might say revolutionizing – the understanding of normal versus dysregulated human feelings. The result of this shift is that the more conventional diagnostic taxonomies are being reconsidered in favor of a biological framework that is both more sensitive to the subtle – but common and deeply distressing – effects of concussion and more respectful of human individuality. The authors hope this brief commentary will guide the next generation of scholars and serve future generations of concussion survivors in a meaningful way.

Emotions may be understood as a specific way of interacting with the world and determining the salience and value of its constituents in relation to the subject's personal history and future goals. As such, emotions influence perception, cognition, and decision making. As opposed to other animals, human beings possess highly developed cognitive and linguistic abilities that contribute to the richness of their emotional repertoire. Consequently, any analysis of human emotion, and of its alterations, should incorporate the complexity that results from this unique existential experience.

It is important to emphasize that the pathophysiology of the emotional alterations associated with traumatic brain injury (TBI) or its most common clinical form, CBI, involves an interplay of factors that are related to the injury per se, such as the severity, number, and timing of injuries; factors that precede trauma (e.g., genetic vulnerability, previous psychiatric history); and factors that affect the recovery process (e.g., family and social support, pharmacological and non-pharmacological treatment). Overall, these factors contribute to the structural and functional changes in the neural circuits that link the brain areas specializing in emotional processing, such as the prefrontal cortex, the basal ganglia, and the amygdala.

In this chapter, we describe the emotional changes that may result from single and repeated concussions, with a special emphasis on those that meet the current diagnostic criteria for a mental illness.

Post-Concussive Symptoms

It is traditionally accepted that post-concussive symptoms comprise cognitive, somatic, and emotional components [1]. The latter include depressive and anxiety symptoms, irritability, restlessness, and sleep disturbance [2]. Usually, these symptoms resolve within days or weeks after a concussion, and only a few subjects experience a more protracted and debilitating course. There is also agreement that persistent symptoms in the emotional domain overlap with those observed in another frequent complication of trauma: the collection of seven or more symptoms, occurring alone or in conjunction, referred to by the American Psychiatric Association as post-traumatic stress disorder (PTSD) [3].

Many survivors of CBI suffer persistent symptoms. However, because concussion is not marked by one symptom or a cluster of symptoms, we cannot label any particular phenomenon as "post-concussive syndrome." Though several symptoms may be more commonly attributable to concussion than to other neurologic or psychiatric disorders (such as dizziness or diplopia), the overlap between common clinical phenomenology after a concussion and that after non-brain traumatic injury, or due to depression or "PTSD," is so distinct that we cannot conceive of this as a syndrome. For example, Lagarde and colleagues [4] conducted a prospective study of 534 patients with mild TBI (mTBI) and 827 control patients with other injuries and observed that three months after the trauma the incidence of complaints fulfilling some criteria for "post-concussive syndrome" was not significantly different between subjects with mTBI and injured controls (21.2% and 16.3%, respectively). Their symptoms did not show any pattern of clustering, and there was no significant association with mTBI. Additionally, mTBI was a predictor of PTSD, but not of any collection of complaints that could constitute a syndrome [4]. Epidemiological data also indicate that the symptoms that are the most common at one time point after concussion, e.g., at six weeks, are quite different from the symptoms that are most common at six months or a year post injury – evidence that may not bolster the idea of a discrete syndrome.

These results are consistent with the conclusions of a systematic review undertaken by the International Collaboration on Mild Traumatic Brain Injury Prognosis, which cast doubt on how specific "post-concussive syndrome" is to concussion [5]. Currently, there is no consensus regarding the best replacement for the misleading phrase "post-concussive syndrome." Two options worth considering are: *non-cognitive behavioral complications of CBI* (to parallel similar usage in the dementia literature) or *persistent post-concussive psychiatric problems*, as suggested by Victoroff. (See the chapter by that title in this volume, Chapter 10.)

The emotional consequences of concussions are related to the characteristics of the event in which they occur. The latter may range from relatively minor stressors to life-threatening events. For instance, the level of stress associated with concussions occurring in the context of contact sports, domestic violence, or warfare is different and varies along this dimension. The circumstances under which a concussion occurs influence the structure, severity, and chronicity of emotional symptoms. For instance, intrusive symptoms such as nightmares or flashbacks are rare after sport-related concussions but very frequent in combat-related CBI. As there are also differences in the pathophysiology of these concussions (e.g., blast exposures involve brain alterations produced by the blast wave), it is reasonable to hypothesize that different causes may be associated with specific patterns of structural and functional brain changes that, ultimately, might be associated with a particular set of symptoms. Unfortunately, there has been little research comparing the constellation of emotional symptoms resulting from concussions experienced in combat, motor vehicle accidents, falls, and contact sports.

Emotional Dysregulation

The phylogenetic evolution of the nervous system culminates with the development of the complex prefrontal areas found in the *Homo sapiens* brain. These structures constitute the neurological substrate of refined emotional regulation processes. In this way, emotional responses mediated by phylogenetic older limbic and paralimbic areas of the brain can be reduced, enhanced, initiated, or suppressed [6].

TBI/CBI is known to disrupt prefrontal circuits in multiple ways, ranging from direct damage to areas of the prefrontal cortex, disruption of the white-matter pathways that connect these areas, or alterations in ascending aminergic and cholinergic systems that modulate the function of these networks. Thus, it is not surprising that these changes might be reflected in alterations in emotional regulation and, consequently, in affective disturbances.

Subjects who have experienced single or multiple concussions have a tendency to display rapidly changing emotions, many times incongruent with or disproportionate to the situation. When the frequency and intensity of these emotional outbursts increase to the point that they have a recognizable impact on interpersonal functioning, they constitute a clinical disorder [7–9]. Below, we focus on two conditions akin to emotional deregulation: emotional lability (EL) and irritability/aggression (I/A), which are frequently observed in the post-concussive period and that occasionally have a protracted course.

Emotional Lability

EL refers to a general disposition to experience intense emotions in response to situations in which this type of response is not usually expected. The emotions are short-lived and vary with respect to their affective valence (positive or negative). They also vary in the characteristics of their behavioral expression (e.g., they tend to be more stereotypical than normal emotional displays). However, the emotional displays are congruent with the subject's emotional state (e.g., sadness, anxiety, anger, elation, excitement), and are subject to voluntary control or interruption by distractors [10].

An essential feature of this syndrome is the oscillation between emotional states ("switch"); for instance, from depression to elation or from depression to anger or anxiety. The fact that these emotional perturbations have a limited duration and an identifiable trigger allows us to distinguish them from mood disorders, which have a less definite antecedent and a more characteristic prolonged course. However, EL is nevertheless a change in the individual's personality pattern and impacts interpersonal function and quality of life. According to DSM-5 nomenclature, EL might be categorized as "personality change due to TBI, labile type" ([11], p. 682).

The prevalence of EL following concussions is difficult to determine. It has been reported that, among persons with "mild TBI," it may be as high as 28% in the first three months post injury, usually occurring and resolving in the first couple of weeks [12]. However, most concussion symptom inventories do not assess EL per se, instead registering ill-defined symptoms, such as nervousness, irritability, depression, and anxiety [2, 13]. As a result, the actual frequency of this problem in the early and late post-concussive periods is unclear.

EL can be assessed using the Affective Lability Scale [14], which is also available in an 18-item short form that has been shown to have adequate psychometric properties [15]. The Affective Lability Scale scores subjects' agreement with 18 statements describing the tendency of their emotions to shift between the affective domains of anger, depression, elation, and anxiety.

It is important to emphasize that EL is not specific to the post-concussive state and is also observed following other traumatic experiences and among persons with a broad range of psychiatric conditions [7]. For instance, EL also occurs during depressive episodes [16, 17], the euthymic period of bipolar disorder [18–22], addictive disorders [10], attention deficit-hyperactivity disorder [23], and among persons with maladaptive personality traits [15]. Additionally, there is a significant degree of overlap between EL and the occurrence of mood and anxiety disorders due to TBI, something that needs to be addressed when formulating the diagnosis of these patients and deciding the most appropriate treatment.

When EL does not resolve shortly after a concussion, the treatment of EL comprises non-pharmacologic and pharmacologic options. Cognitive and behavioral psychotherapy focused on improving self-efficacy and self-regulation is a reasonable initial intervention [24, 25]. There is some evidence that more comprehensive and structured rehabilitation programs that combine interventions to foster emotional regulation and improve executive dysfunction might be beneficial for optimizing the cognitive and behavioral outcomes of mTBI [26].

Although there is limited empirical support for possible pharmacotherapies for post-traumatic EL, experts suggest that selective serotonin reuptake inhibitors (SSRIs) might be effective and well tolerated [27]. Sertraline, citalopram, and escitalopram are preferred because of their limited drug–drug interactions and limited side-effect profiles [28]. If an SSRI proves to be ineffective, other potential options include stimulants like methylphenidate (especially among patients with attentional deficits) and amantadine (especially among patients with poor anger control and aggressive behavior), and anticonvulsants such as valproate, carbamazepine, or lamotrigine (especially when there is evidence of coexistent impulsivity, aggressive behaviors, or post-traumatic seizures). Note that these are not clinical recommendations. One must acknowledge: (1) the lack of results from randomized controlled trials; (2) the level at which pre-morbid stressors and psychological predispositions, current life circumstances, and co-morbidities affect drug efficacy; and (3) the near-certainty that pharmacological responses in individuals differ greatly due to genetic variation.

Irritability and Aggression

Irritability is a common experience of sentient organisms that manifests along a continuum that includes diverse affective states, such as impatience, exasperation, anger, and rage. It is useful to distinguish between the subjective aspects of irritation and its overt behavioral expressions. The latter may range from subtle gestural clues to verbal and physical aggression, and these manifestations may differ in severity, frequency, and duration.

Shortly after experiencing trauma, subjects may become irritable when facing minor frustration, a problem that generally resolves in a short period of time [29]. Irritability is also a common and transient symptom in the early period following a concussion [13, 30]. However, as irritability is also frequently observed after other traumatic experiences, it cannot be taken as unequivocal evidence of TBI.

In a modest proportion of individuals, however, irritability may progress to a more complex and chronic condition characterized by recurrent outbursts that are triggered by relatively trivial symptoms. This may represent a change in the way that this person normally responds to a challenging situation. Typically, the emotional state between episodes of irritation is euthymic or neutral, which helps differentiate it from mood disorders. According to DSM-5 nomenclature, I/A might be categorized as personality change due to TBI, aggressive type.

As mentioned above, irritability is a frequent complication of TBI. In a convenience sample of 55 subjects with moderate to severe injuries, McKinlay and colleagues identified irritability among 63%, 69%, and 71% of the subjects, respectively, when assessed at three, six, and 12 months [31]. In addition, Deb and colleagues reported that, at a one-year follow-up, irritability was the most common symptom reported in a cohort of 196 patients hospitalized for TBI. Overall, irritability was observed in 35% of these subjects [32]. It is important to consider that, among persons with more severe injuries, the presence of cognitive and self-awareness deficits affects the validity of self-report measures, and a more accurate estimation of the frequency of this condition should be obtained from collateral sources, such as caregivers [33, 34]. In fact, different methods of neuropsychiatric evaluation may be required to characterize and monitor changes in post-traumatic irritability in persons with mild, rather than moderate and severe, TBI.

Irritability and aggressive behavior may be a feature of coexistent psychiatric conditions, such as mood and anxiety disorders, substance misuse, or chronic pain syndromes. In addition, a comprehensive evaluation of I/A should consider the effect of temperamental aspects that influence the emotional regulation processes of a given individual. Furthermore, pre-injury psychiatric conditions and personality traits may be risk factors for the development of I/A following a concussion.

Among persons with preserved self-awareness after TBI, self-report measures like the Neurobehavioral Symptom Inventory [13, 35] constitute an adequate screening instrument for I/A. In addition, the Irritability Questionnaire [36] or the National Taiwan University Irritability Scale [37] may provide a better characterization of the clinical problem and estimate its severity. In persons who have awareness deficits, the Neuropsychiatry Inventory provides informant-based ratings of irritability among persons with TBI. Its use is recommended for assessing the longitudinal course of this condition and identifying changes related to treatment interventions [38].

Non-pharmacologic interventions constitute the first choice of treatment. These include cognitive behavioral psychotherapy [39, 40] and an anger self-management program validated for persons with TBI [41]. Additionally, structured rehabilitation interventions targeting emotional self-regulation and executive skills are beneficial [26]. Severe cases may require pharmacotherapy to facilitate participation in psychotherapy or behavioral therapies. Previous uncontrolled studies suggest that sertraline [42], valproate [43], methylphenidate [44], carbamazepine [45], quetiapine [46], aripiprazole [47], buspirone [48], and propranolol [49] might be efficacious in treating post-traumatic irritability. An initial parallel-group, randomized double-blind, placebo-controlled trial of amantadine on chronic post-traumatic irritability and aggression in 76 persons more than six months post injury demonstrated a significant decrease in I/A among subjects receiving amantadine [8]. However, a more recent and larger multicenter study of the efficacy of amantadine in treating I/A in similar clinical settings failed to replicate the earlier promising findings [50].

Mood Disorders

Clinical Presentation and Diagnosis

Mood disturbances, especially depressive disorders, are the most frequent neuropsychiatric complication of TBI. Mood disorders have a complex clinical presentation and are highly co-morbid with anxiety, substance misuse, and other behavioral alterations, like emotional deregulation, impulsivity, and aggression. Furthermore, mood disorders have a chronic and refractory course in a significant proportion of the subjects who develop them. Consequently, their functional impact is huge, affecting the recovery and long-term outcome of TBI patients.

Mood disorders are pervasive alterations of human experience that affect a variety of areas, ranging from cognition to occupational performance and quality of life. Although the duration of the mood disturbance may vary in these diverse mood disorders, the relatively long-lasting and recurrent nature of this alteration is at the core of current classification schemes. This nature also helps to differentiate these disorders from other common emotional disorders observed after TBI that are mainly related to the characteristics of emotional responses to external and internal emotionally laden stimuli (e.g., emotional lability, anger outbursts).

The DSM-5 diagnostic nomenclature groups these disorders under the category of "mood disorder due to another medical condition." This category presents the following depressive subtypes: (1) with major depressive-like episode (if the full criteria for a major depressive episode are met); (2) with depressive features (prominent depressed mood but full criteria for a major depressive episode are not met); and (3) with mixed features (e.g., associated with significant expansive or irritable mood, pressured speech, formal thought disorder). However, manic and hypomanic syndromes are categorized as bipolar and related disorders due to TBI. These are subdivided into: (1) with manic or hypomanic-like episode; (2) with manic features; and (3) with mixed features.

Pre-existing mood disorders are frequent in the general population and also among persons who have experienced a concussion. To propose a pathophysiological link between a CBI and the mood disturbance that follows it, the latter should either have a new onset, or there must be a significant change in its clinical features (e.g., the presence of prominent cognitive deficits) or in its clinical course (e.g., depression occurring after a prolonged period of full symptomatic remission). Generally, however, it is not possible to determine degree of causality. Clinically, it is not realistic to attribute the causality of a mood disorder to genetic/epigenetic variation, early-life stress, pre-morbid adversity, baseline temperament and resilience, external force on the brain, or the presence or absence of supportive or therapeutic interventions post injury. Any variety of interactions between these possible causes may exist, thus requiring careful attention to each distinct clinical case. Current knowledge does not allow us to weigh one factor over another.

Mood Disorders with Depressive Features

Post-TBI depression is a complex condition with symptoms and signs that vary along different dimensions. Principal component analyses of symptoms elicited by a structured interview suggest the presence of three major factors [51].

The first factor is related to a negative appraisal of the environment, the self, and the future (e.g., depressed mood, feelings of worthlessness and helplessness, inappropriate guilt, hopelessness, suicidal ideation). These might be clinically expressed by a negative attentional bias or may take the form of automatic thoughts, distorted core beliefs, and dysphoric ruminations.

The second factor is related to alterations in the initiation and consummation of goal-directed activity (i.e., lack of motivation, anhedonia), vegetative symptoms (e.g., lack of energy, sleep or appetite disturbance), as well as subjective complaints of cognitive inefficiency.

Finally, the third factor includes symptoms related to behavioral control and the regulation of emotional responses (e.g., affective instability, expansive or irritable mood, increased goal-directed activity, anger outbursts, poor impulse control, psychomotor agitation, aggression).

Anxiety symptoms (e.g., worrying, anxious foreboding, anxiety expressed as physical concomitants) are frequent and disturbing elements of the clinical picture, and they show increased loadings in both the first and the third factors. Overall, the clinical presentation of depressive disorders due to TBI is quite heterogeneous. In some patients, one of these factors may be predominant, whereas in others, there may be extensive overlap between the three dimensions.

Mood Disorders With Manic, Hypomanic, or Mixed Features

Manic and hypomanic syndromes are characterized by a distinct period (i.e., lasting more than four days) of persistently expansive and/or irritable mood, as well as other symptoms, such as increased energy levels, increased goal-directed activity, decreased need for sleep, pressured speech, formal thought disorder, distractibility, and excessive engagement in pleasurable activities that may be associated with negative consequences (e.g., hyper-sexuality, spending sprees). Paranoia, grandiose delusions, and hallucinatory experiences may also be present in the clinical profile.

A diagnosis of mood disorder with manic or mixed features should not be made if the mood disturbance occurs during the course of delirium or as a consequence of intoxication or withdrawal from different substances, including medications such as stimulants, dopaminergic agents, or amantadine, that are used during the rehabilitation period. Personality changes due to TBI may include irritability, paranoia, aggression, or disinhibited behavior, but the distinction is that these patients do not exhibit the pervasive alteration of mood that characterizes secondary manic and hypomanic syndromes.

Epidemiology – A General Comment

Before we discuss the epidemiology of specific forms of traumatic emotional change, a general comment is necessary. The incidence and prevalence of emotional dysregulation after concussion are unknown. At least three barriers prevent accurate accounting:

1. Most concussions do not come to medical attention.

2. Among patients in the subgroup of typical concussions that come to medical attention – the subject of this textbook – few are ever assessed by a concussion expert and followed for long enough to assess outcome.

3. Among the very few concussion survivors assessed by experts during the year following injury, the methods of diagnosing and measuring emotional dysregulation vary greatly.

Nevertheless, one can state with some confidence that most textbook claims are not supported empirically. Most follow-up studies focus on paper-and-pencil psychological tests of cognition, i.e., "neuro"-psychological tests, even though they cannot reliably identify the neurobiological cause, cerebral location, volume, or tissue type of related brain changes. Meta-analyses of such psychological testing has resulted in claims that only 10–15% of concussion survivors exhibit dysfunction more than three months post injury. Such a claim is misleading because (1) as shown repeatedly elsewhere in this volume, those tests do not detect neurobehavioral changes produced by typical CBI, such as axonal disruption, inflammation, and deposition of neurodegeneration-related proteins, and (2) cognitive changes have far less importance to functional outcome (i.e., reintegration into work and social spheres and quality of life) than do emotional changes. Based on the available empirical data, the best estimate of the prevalence of persistent post-concussive behavioral dysfunction reported or observed at one year or longer after a typical, clinically-attended CBI is more than 40%. (See Chapter 5.)

Mood Disorders With Depressive Features

As mentioned previously, it is difficult to determine the incidence and prevalence of symptoms or disorders specifically associated with typical concussion (i.e., without prolonged coma or intracerebral hemorrhage) because only a minority of the epidemiological literature accurately stratifies results by severity. The data presented here were derived from studies of TBI not otherwise specified, and may not reflect findings from the subset of typical concussions. Depressive disorders are frequently observed among persons with TBI, with estimated frequencies in the range of 25–50% [52, 53] during the first year after TBI, and lifetime rates of 26–64% [54, 55]. Evidence for the incidence and prevalence of manic, hypomanic, and mixed mood disorders after TBI (including typical concussion) is inconsistent. Some consider these disorders to be uncommon consequences of TBI [56]. For example, approximately 1.7–9% of persons with TBI experience secondary mania [56, 57], and, if secondary mania manifests, it tends to happen within the first few months post injury [58]. However, one study reported that

secondary mania was 15 times as common among survivors of head injury compared with those in the general population [59]. Additionally, in a meta-analysis of three studies, Perry et al. [60] reported that prior TBI was associated with an odds ratio of 1.85 for bipolar disorder. Large prospective studies with stratification by injury severity and validated measurement methodology are necessary to resolve these discrepancies between reports on post-concussive mania or bipolar symptoms.

The risk factors for depressive disorders after TBI include genetic factors, pre-injury personal and psychosocial factors, and post-injury psychosocial factors, as well as their interactions.

The role of genetics in the development of post-TBI neuropsychiatric disorders, including depression, is an active area of investigation. Polymorphisms of the serotonin transporter (5HTT) do not appear to influence the occurrence or severity of depression after TBI [61], but they may influence the response to treatment with antidepressants. For instance, adverse effects to citalopram appear to be more frequent among persons with specific 5HTT polymorphisms (including rs25531). Both the C-(677)T polymorphism of the methylenetetrahydrofolate reductase (MTHFR) gene and the Val66Met polymorphism of the brain-derived neurotrophic factor (BDNF) gene have been associated with a favorable treatment response [62].

The development and chronicity of depressive disorders after TBI are also modified by psychosocial factors that precede the injury. These include, among others, poor pre-morbid social functioning or poverty, previous history of psychiatric diagnosis, alcohol abuse, and a history of maladaptive personality traits.

The onset and severity of depressive disorders following TBI are influenced by psychosocial factors that are effective during the period of recovery from the injury. These include the lack of an intimate partner or close friend, and/or dysfunctional interpersonal relationships. Occupational stress, including post-injury job loss, lower income levels, and financial problems also are risk factors for depression after TBI.

Mood Disorders with Manic, Hypomanic, and Mixed Features

The limited evidence pertaining to bipolar-related disorders due to TBI preclude drawing definitive conclusions about risk factors for these conditions. Past studies of manic and hypomanic states associated with TBI did not find a clear relationship between mania and TBI severity, post-traumatic epilepsy, post-TBI physical or cognitive impairments, level of social functioning, or the presence of family or personal history of psychiatric disorders [58]. Shukla and colleagues [63] also observed no relationship between post-traumatic mania and family history of bipolar disorder, but did note associations between post-TBI mania and injury severity, as well as post-traumatic epilepsy. However, note that the incidence of TBI may be elevated among unaffected family members of persons with bipolar disorder [64], suggesting the possibility that some features of the bipolar phenotype (e.g., increased novelty seeking, reduced harm avoidance, cognition) may increase the risk for TBI.

Pathophysiologic Aspects of Mood Disorders Due to TBI

The pathophysiology of post-TBI mood disorders involves not only the etiological factors that are related to structural and functional brain changes brought by the injury, but also other factors that either precede the injury (e.g., genetic variants, developmental history, pre-existent psychiatric disorders), or those that take effect after the brain injury has occurred (e.g., the subject's expectations about the recovery process, quality of social support received).

Injury-related factors include the mechanism of TBI, the context in which the injury took place, and the type, severity, and localization of traumatic brain lesions. The importance of the structural and functional changes produced by TBI in the brain is highlighted by the fact that mood disorders are more common among TBI subjects than in patients with comparable background characteristics and traumatic experiences who did not have a TBI (e.g., subjects with orthopedic injuries caused by a motor vehicle accident). Based on the current knowledge on emotional regulation, it is reasonable to expect that a pathological condition that selectively affects prefrontal and anterior temporal structures and that produces widespread axonal injury is associated with an increased prevalence of mood disorders.

Although, to a certain degree, traumatic axonal injury is present in all TBI patients, it plays a more relevant etiological role among patients on the extremes of the severity spectrum (i.e., mild and severe injuries). Overall, injury severity is not a determining factor for the onset of mood disorders in the aftermath of TBI. Mood disorders are still frequently observed among TBI patients with milder injuries [65–67].

Localization of brain damage might also determine the behavioral consequences of TBI. Establishing brain–behavior correlations, however, requires an accurate description of the behavior that is examined, as well as reliable *in vivo* diagnostic techniques to assess brain damage at cellular, synaptic, and neural circuitry levels. Although there have been significant advances in neurophysiological and neuroimaging techniques over the past few years, the functional anatomy of mood disorders due to TBI has not been elucidated and requires further study. Progress within this field of research requires, first, the formulation of more meaningful models of the circuits involved in emotional processing and, second, the dissection of mood disorders into critical components, whose relationship with a particular neural substrate has been empirically validated. For instance, apathetic states can entail alterations of the brain reward system.

There is some consensus about the neural systems involved in mood regulation and how they might be affected by psychopathology. Over the past two decades, a host of mechanistic studies in experimental animals and humans have clarified the characteristics of different prefrontal circuits, which, although richly interconnected, show some consistent specialization of function.

The orbital–ventromedial prefrontal circuit constitutes a predominantly efferent system modulating visceral function and mood generation [68]. This network includes the ventral and pre-genual aspects of the anterior cingulate cortex, the gyrus rectus, the amygdala and extended amygdala, the hypothalamus, and the periaqueductal gray matter, as well as reciprocal connections of these structures with the ventral and medial striatum, ventral regions of the globus pallidus, and the dorsomedian thalamic nucleus.

However, a more lateral orbital prefrontal circuit (LOPFC) is predominantly a sensory integration system that integrates the information received from secondary and tertiary sensory areas to appraise rewarding and aversive stimuli and their contextual circumstances [69]. The LOPFC consists of the more lateral parts of the orbitofrontal cortex, the ventrolateral prefrontal cortex, and the anterior insula, along with their connections to the striatum and the thalamus.

While the OMPFC is functionally related to the dorsal cingulate cortex and the "default mode network," i.e., a group of interconnected brain areas whose activity characterizes a state in which the subject is not involved in intentional acts or in processing environmental stimuli [70], the LOPFC has important connections with the dorsolateral prefrontal cortex and the "task-positive network," a neural system that is activated while the subject is engaged in sensory discrimination and goal-directed activity [71]. Changes in the orbital–ventromedial prefrontal circuit system have been associated with the intense dysphoria and anxiety experienced by some depressed subjects, as well as with the obsessive, self-referential ruminations that are characteristic of melancholic states [72]. Furthermore, deep-brain stimulation of these ventromedial regions might reduce the severity of these symptoms [73]. However, alterations in the LOPFC are more closely related to other cardinal symptoms of depressive disorders, such as loss of interest and lack of motivation [68, 71].

It is accepted that the predominant cognitive abnormalities observed in TBI patients are related to prefrontal dysfunction. In addition, the prefrontal cortex is a key regulatory region of emotional responses [74, 75]. Following Mayberg's cortical-limbic disconnection model [76], mood disorders could result from decreased function of the dorsolateral prefrontal cortex and abnormal activation of ventral limbic structures, including the ventral anterior cingulate cortex and the amygdala [77–79]. Thus, while deactivation of the lateral prefrontal cortex might be related to apathy and executive dysfunction, high levels of amygdala activation may be associated with an increased prevalence of anxiety symptoms and negative affect [80], a pattern of symptoms that is frequently observed in TBI patients with mood disturbance. Furthermore, defective prefrontal modulation of medial limbic structures might be related to the impulsive and aggressive behavior observed in these patients [81, 82].

TBI patients with major depressive disorder exhibit the presence of structural abnormalities in the left ventrolateral prefrontal cortex and the hippocampus [83, 84]. For subjects who experienced single or multiple concussions, it has been shown that those suffering from depression have reduced activation of the dorsolateral prefrontal cortex and striatum, in addition to gray-matter loss in these brain regions [85]. Furthermore, a preliminary study comparing 11 veterans with major depression following blast-related mTBI with 11 veterans without a history of major depression observed increased amygdala activity and decreased prefrontal activity during a facial emotion-processing functional magnetic resonance imaging (fMRI) task. In addition, the fractional anisotropy of the superior longitudinal fasciculus was significantly decreased in the depressed group [86].

Little is known about the pathogenesis of bipolar-related disorders associated with TBI. Right-hemisphere lesions, particularly those involving the ventral aspects of the right anterior temporal, orbitofrontal, caudate, and thalamic areas, have been related to the development of mania due to TBI [87]. Although the association with right-hemispheric injuries is a common observation across many studies and often cited in the neurobehavioral literature, the cerebral injuries with which secondary manic states are most commonly associated are usually bilateral.

Treatment of Mood Disorders

Mood Disorders With Depressive Features

The treatment of post-TBI depressive disorders includes psychotherapeutic and pharmacological interventions. Education regarding TBI and recovery expectations, reassurance, and frequent support are recommended as part of all treatment plans for persons with these disorders [88]. Cognitive behavioral therapy may decrease depressive, anxious, and anger symptoms, as well as improve problem-solving skills, self-esteem, and psychosocial functioning, following TBI [89].

Peer support programs for persons with TBI and their families increase their knowledge about TBI, foster the development of adaptive coping skills, and improve quality of life [90]. Attending to the psychological needs of caregivers of persons with TBI is also important because depression is common among caregivers of persons with TBI, and enhancing problem-solving and behavioral coping strategies in caregivers reduces the severity of depressive symptoms in the family member with TBI [91]. Thus, engaging both patients and their family members is essential in the treatment of depression following TBI.

There is a surprising lack of adequate randomized controlled trials examining the efficacy of pharmacological agents in treating depressive disorders associated with TBI. As a work-around for this empirical limitation, the U.S. Veterans Administration and Department of Defense have suggested that clinicians prescribe interventions for behavioral symptoms (e.g., PTSD) without regard to the brain injury [92]. This approach is ethically acceptable as a stop-gap measure, although one hopes that pathophysiological assays eventually facilitate the individualization of care.

One example of this practical, albeit relatively untried, approach: antidepressant medication is used extensively in clinical settings. SSRIs and tricyclic antidepressants (TCAs) may improve depression following TBI [93]. Effective treatment of post-TBI depression with SSRIs also reduces co-morbid I/A [94] and might have an effect on cognitive symptoms [95, 96].

Given the frequency of adverse events following the use of TCAs in this population (particularly cognitive deficits associated with their anticholinergic effects), most experts regard them as second-line medications for depression following TBI and recommend SSRIs as the first-line agents in this situation. Among the SSRIs, sertraline and citalopram are favored in light of their beneficial effects, relatively limited side-effects, and short half-lives. The use of other SSRIs, especially fluoxetine and paroxetine, is limited by their relatively greater potential for adverse effects and drug–drug interactions.

Methylphenidate would be an uncommon first-line intervention for depression after TBI in an outpatient clinic. However, stimulants may be useful in acute rehabilitation settings when rapidity of treatment response is essential. Methylphenidate and other stimulants, including dextroamphetamine, are also used commonly to augment partial responses to SSRIs, especially when cognitive impairments or fatigue are residual symptoms during treatment with conventional antidepressants.

The efficacy and tolerability of other antidepressants, including the serotonin–norepinephrine reuptake inhibitors, bupropion, and the monoamine oxidase inhibitors (MAOIs) for the treatment of depression among persons with TBI, are not well established. The use of MAOIs is discouraged among persons with cognitive or other neurobehavioral impairments likely to reduce adherence to their dietary restrictions. Bupropion is also of concern, in light of its propensity for lowering seizure threshold. This risk is greatest with the immediate-release form of bupropion [97]. Using the sustained-release form of bupropion might be considered in the occasional refractory case, provided that close monitoring for treatment-related seizures is in place.

Electroconvulsive therapy (ECT) may be used to treat severe cases of depression among persons with TBI who fail to respond to other interventions. ECT should be administered with the lowest energy levels that would generate a seizure of adequate duration, using pulsatile currents, increased spacing of treatments (i.e., two to five days between treatments), and fewer treatments over an entire course (i.e., four to six) Nondominant unilateral ECT is the preferred technique.

Mood Disorders with Manic, Hypomanic, and Mixed Features

There is no clear guidance regarding the psychotherapeutic approach for persons with mania or mixed mood states after TBI. Psychotherapeutic interventions are modeled after those used in the management of persons with idiopathic bipolar disorders, as described in the current practice guidelines for the treatment of patients with bipolar disorder. Similarly, the literature describing pharmacotherapy of mania among persons with TBI is insufficient to support formal treatment standards

[93]. Therapeutic options used in clinical practice are inspired by what we know about the use of mood stabilizers and other agents in treating bipolar disorder.

Valproate is a plausible option on theoretical grounds. The efficacy of this agent in treating non-TBI-associated mood disorder has been established, and in rodent models, valproate seems to have anti-apoptotic/neuroprotective effects after TBI [98–100]. Limited findings from case reports and small, retrospective, uncontrolled studies suggest that this agent may mitigate chronic post-traumatic agitation/impulsivity [101] or destructive/aggressive behaviors [43]. Despite the fact that no randomized controlled trials support the use of this agent, one recent review stated: "Mood regulating anticonvulsants are the Gold Standard for agitation or aggressiveness after severe TBI if there is an associated epilepsy or bipolar disorders" [102]. Less evidence suggests a possible benefit in cases of post-traumatic bipolar disorder [103, 104], and evidence is insufficient regarding unipolar depression.

Moreover, the use of valproate requires careful and continuous assessment for the development of treatment-related motor (e.g., tremor, incoordination, ataxia, gait disturbances) and cognitive impairments, as well as other adverse somatic side-effects (e.g., weight gain, gastrointestinal problems/diarrhea, hematologic abnormalities, hepatotoxicity, alopecia). Additionally, the risk of polycystic ovarian syndrome requires consideration of alternate treatments in females.

Lithium carbonate is more likely to produce nausea, tremor, ataxia, and lethargy in persons with neurological disorders than in the general psychiatric population. Its effect of lowering seizure threshold represents an additional concern in the TBI population. Several of the newer anticonvulsants (e.g., lamotrigine, oxcarbazepine) and the atypical antipsychotics (e.g., risperidone, olanzapine, ziprasidone, aripiprazole) may be useful in the treatment of post-traumatic mania. However, there is no rigorous empirical evidence supporting their use.

Post-Traumatic Stress Disorder

Both TBI and PTSD are always related to a discrete event that is essential to their definition. Furthermore, there are instances in which TBI occurs in the context of threatened death or serious injury (e.g., TBI from combat, assaults, or motor vehicle accidents) that constitutes a required characteristic of the type of stressors that elicit PTSD. Thus, it is not surprising that symptoms of both conditions overlap over time.

There has been a renewed interest in the clinical correlates and pathophysiological aspects of coexistent PTSD and mild TBI. This is related to the fact that mTBI is considered to be the signature wound of the recent armed conflicts in Iraq and Afghanistan.

Mental health disorders are highly frequent among military personnel returning from these conflicts [105, 106].

An epidemiological study of 103,788 veterans first seen in the Veterans Administration system following active duty in Iraq and Afghanistan reported that approximately 25% of all veterans received a mental health diagnosis, and that the most frequent diagnoses were PTSD (13%) and mood disorders (11%) [107]. Mild TBI is also frequent in this population. It has been estimated that 28% of all injured individuals in these conflicts experienced a TBI, with blast being the wounding etiology in the majority (88%) of cases [108]. A study of 3973 soldiers from a brigade combat team, who had a health assessment immediately after completing their deployment, found that 907 soldiers (22.9%) had experienced a TBI [109]. This underscores the impact of TBI among Operation Enduring Freedom/Operation Iraqi Freedom/Operation New Dawn (OEF/OIF/OND) veterans and questions whether its occurrence would modify the course of the psychiatric disorders observed in this group. For instance, it has been reported that the frequency of PTSD and major depression is significantly higher among veterans who suffered a TBI, compared with non-injured veterans or veterans with other types of injuries [110]. Some investigators have described a triad of TBI, PTSD, and chronic pain in trauma-exposed veterans of recent Middle East military operations. An analysis of diagnostic records of all Veterans Administration patients who served in OEF/OIF/OND found that almost two-thirds of veterans with TBI had experienced this triad; less than 10% of veterans with TBI were free of a co-morbid pain disorder or PTSD [111].

Discriminating mTBI from PTSD is an arduous task because of the lack of reliable biological markers for the two conditions, the symptomatic overlap of PTSD and post-concussive syndrome, and also because patients with PTSD tend to report more traumatic exposures and more symptoms compared with patients without PTSD [112]. Nonetheless, coexisting blast injuries and severe combat-related stress define a unique population of veterans with PTSD. The way TBI modifies the clinical presentation and prognosis of the psychopathological disorders developed by OEF/OIF/OND veterans is not yet clear and requires further study.

Definition and Phenomenological Presentation of PTSD[1]

The current psychiatric nomenclature defines PTSD along eight distinct criteria and four symptomatic dimensions. The DSM-5 classification system identifies four symptom clusters that characterize PTSD. The first symptom cluster relates to intrusive symptoms, including distressing memories of the traumatic event, nightmares, and dissociative experiences in which the subject appears to be re-experiencing the event (i.e., flashbacks). PTSD patients may also have intense physiological responses to trauma-related reminders that could be categorized as intrusive experiences.

[1] Editor's note: As explained in Chapter 10, addressing *Persistent Post-Concussive Psychiatric Problems*, modern scholarship does not support the existence of a unitary entity that comports with the American Psychiatric Association's politically based invention "post-traumatic stress disorder (PTSD)." That unscientific phrase and its abbreviation, however, are familiar to many and will be used in this chapter – with the caveat that at least seven different clinical problems are probably conflated by the American Psychiatric Association's purported mental disorder.

The second symptom cluster involves the active avoidance of distressing memories of either the traumatic event itself or environmental cues reminiscent of its circumstances. According to the DSM-5, at least one form of avoidant behavior must be present to substantiate a PTSD diagnosis.

The third symptom cluster consists of disturbed emotional states. Disturbed emotional states include pervasive negative cognitions and beliefs about the self and the world (e.g., feelings of worthlessness, hopelessness, shame, guilt), a sense of estrangement and detachment in interpersonal relationships (e.g., emotional numbing), and the inability to experience positive emotions and derive gratification from enjoyable activities (i.e., anhedonia). In the DSM-IV, these symptoms were included in the avoidance dimension, but in the DSM-5, they form part of a distinct domain. Furthermore, at least two of these symptoms need to be present to substantiate a PTSD diagnosis.

Finally, the fourth symptom cluster involves alterations of arousal and reactivity, a complex psychopathological construct that includes physiological responses, such as an exaggerated startle response, irritability, angry outbursts, aggressive behavior directed at the self or others, hypervigilance, and sleep disturbance.

Intrusive and hyper-arousal symptoms tend to predominate in the initial phases of PTSD, while avoidance and negative emotional states are more prominent in the chronic phases of the disorder. In fact, there is some evidence that alterations in arousal and reactivity are strong predictors of the severity of symptoms corresponding to other domains.

PTSD and mild TBI independently influence the scope and severity of symptoms that might be observed following a concussion [113]. However, there is evidence suggesting a synergistic effect by which subjects with coexistent PTSD and mild TBI have more frequent and severe symptoms than those observed in persons with either PTSD or mild TBI [3]. Furthermore, suicidal behavior appears to be more frequent in veterans with multiple TBI exposures than in veterans with severe stress-related psychopathology, but without a history of TBI [114].

Diagnosis

PTSD is diagnosed using DSM-5 criteria. A clinical evaluation by a knowledgeable psychiatrist remains the cornerstone of a reliable assessment.

Several structured interviews have been developed to facilitate an accurate diagnosis in both clinical and research settings, with the gold standard being the Clinician-Administered PTSD Scale for the DSM-5 (CAPS-5), developed at the National Center for PTSD [115]. The CAPS-5 is a structured interview that assesses the 20 PTSD symptoms listed in the DSM-5 and obtains information regarding symptom onset, duration, and functional impact. The severity of PTSD symptoms can also be assessed using the PTSD Checklist for the DSM-5. This is a 20-item self-report questionnaire that measures the severity of a particular DSM-5-defined PTSD symptom on a four-point ordinal scale ranging from 0 (not at all) to 4 (extremely) [116].

Epidemiology of PTSD Following TBI

There has been controversy regarding the appropriateness of making a PTSD diagnosis among subjects who, in some cases (e.g., when recovering from a moderate to severe TBI), cannot recall the specific events associated with the trauma. Although initially some researchers speculated that TBI was incompatible with the development of PTSD, theorizing that amnesia for the traumatic event could potentially protect against PTSD, more recent studies have not borne this out. TBI patients can still encode and retrieve trauma memories at an implicit level, and these memories can influence ongoing emotions and behaviors. Limbic structures mediate fear conditioning to traumatic experiences independent of higher cortical processes, and this mechanism might elicit PTSD symptoms among TBI patients with a loss of consciousness or severe post-traumatic amnesia. Overall, there is now support for the idea that PTSD may indeed coexist with TBI [117].

The reported frequency of PTSD following TBI shows a great degree of variability that is related, among other things, to the heterogeneity of the study samples and the way PTSD and TBI were measured. In civilians, the frequency of PTSD ranges from 12 to 30%, 15 to 27%, and 3 to 23% for mild, moderate, and severe TBI, respectively. Among military groups with TBI, the frequency of PTSD has been reported to vary from 12 to 89% [118]. The increased variability observed in military samples might be related to the frequent use of self-report symptom severity scales (e.g., Posttraumatic Checklist, Military form (PCL-M)) for the diagnosis of PTSD. In addition, a clinical diagnosis of mild TBI is hindered by retrospective bias in recalling the mental status changes experienced during an event that occurred months or years before the diagnostic evaluation [118].

Risk Factors

The neurobiology of resilience and vulnerability of developing PTSD has not been studied extensively among individuals with coexistent TBI. However, it is reasonable to expect that factors associated with PTSD in a non-injured population would also be relevant in brain-injured groups.

Childhood abuse produces long-lasting changes in stress reactivity, as measured by hypothalamic–pituitary–adrenal (HPA) axis response and autonomic nervous system activation [119]. Furthermore, a history of childhood abuse is an established risk factor for developing PTSD after adulthood trauma.

Women may be at higher risk for PTSD because of variations in hormonal levels. In this sense, testosterone and dehydroepiandrosterone levels are correlated positively with resilient behavior [120–122], while fluctuating levels of ovarian hormones are correlated positively with anxious responses to stress [123]. In addition, subjects who had lower fluid intelligence scores were reported to be more vulnerable to developing PTSD following trauma [124, 125]. This finding should be interpreted in the light of the known modulating role of the prefrontal cortex over the limbic structures, where emotions and stress responses are integrated. Thus, prefrontal dysfunction resulting from TBI may independently contribute to the onset of stress-related psychopathology.

During the past few years, there has also been progress in understanding genetic factors associated with PTSD. For instance, the short allele (s) of the SLC6A4L gene has been proposed as a vulnerability factor for developing mood and anxiety disorders, while the long allele (l) may have a protective effect [126]. In addition, single-nucleotide polymorphisms in diverse genes, such as the BDNF and FBPK5 genes, have been shown to influence the likelihood of developing PTSD [127]. However, the long-form variant of the neuropeptide Y (NPY) gene has been associated with a decreased risk of developing PTSD [128].

The risk of developing PTSD after exposure to a traumatic event is greater in the presence of physical injury [129]. This might be even greater in the presence of TBI [130]. Furthermore, even when there is no conclusive clinical diagnosis of concussion, the risk of developing PTSD symptoms might be influenced by the presence of subtle structural and functional brain alterations occurring after trauma exposure, e.g., combat-related blasts or contact sports [131].

Pathophysiological Aspects

There is extensive literature on the presence of HPA axis and autonomic changes in subjects with PTSD. This is not surprising, considering both the HPA axis and the autonomic nervous system play a critical role in coordinating stress responses. Although lower basal cortisol levels were once considered a biomarker of PTSD [132], recent experimental findings using more complex hormonal stimulation and suppression paradigms have challenged this notion. Overall, these studies suggest that there is increased HPA axis feedback suppression in PTSD.

PTSD has also been associated with increased autonomic responses to stimuli that are related to trauma (e.g., increased heart rate, increased systolic blood pressure). Overly sensitized sympathetic responses are associated significantly with the severity of general and dysphoric arousal symptoms [133]. In addition, these autonomic changes increase risk of cardiovascular illness, promote significant sleep disturbance, and produce biological changes akin to the metabolic syndrome.

TBI can disrupt the limbic, hypothalamic, and brainstem circuits responsible for a balanced output of the autonomic nervous system. It is well known that severe TBI may be associated with significant dysautonomia complicating the course of acute critical care, i.e., paroxysmal sympathetic hyperactivity [134]. Autonomic alterations at the chronic stage, and among patients with milder forms of TBI, have not been studied sufficiently. However, it is known that cortical lesions affecting the medial frontal and the insular cortices (implicated in sensory and motor visceral functions) are associated with altered cardiovascular control [135, 136]. These prefrontal areas, along with the amygdala, the dorsomedial thalamus, the hypothalamus, and output brainstem nuclei (e.g., nucleus of the solitary tract, dorsal nucleus of the vagus nerve), contribute to the central control of autonomic function [137]. Interestingly, both animal

and clinical studies of blast-related neurotrauma point to a selective disruption of the white-matter pathways connecting these areas of the prefrontal cortex and the brainstem [138]. Therefore, it is conceivable that subjects with a history of repetitive mTBI might be more vulnerable to deregulation of autonomic nervous system function.

The processing of aversive stimuli has been also a subject of intensive psychopathological research. PTSD patients have difficulty discriminating danger from safety cues and have problems suppressing fear in the presence of safety cues [139]. It is generally assumed that increased amygdala activation resulting from faulty modulatory input from the ventromedial prefrontal cortex and, to a lesser extent, the hippocampus, is the biological substrate of the characteristic responses to threatening stimuli observed among subjects with PTSD [140, 141]. The amygdala encodes the salience of aversive cues and integrates a reflex response mediated by effector nuclei in the diencephalon and the brainstem. Animal experiments in rodents indicate that different regions within the ventromedial prefrontal cortex modulate amygdala function, with the infralimbic cortex inhibiting amygdala output, and the prelimbic area facilitating output [142].

The hippocampus also modulates amygdala function through its role in contextual fear conditioning and consolidation of extinction memory [143, 144]. Although PTSD patients show normal extinction of conditioned cues, they exhibit altered retention of the memories generated during the extinction process [145], and their extinction recall is associated with decreased ventromedial prefrontal cortex activation [146]. Once again, the hippocampus and prefrontal circuits are selectively affected by traumatic injury, and it is conceivable that patients with repetitive mTBI might be vulnerable to developing abnormal fear processing.

Overlap of Structural Brain Changes Due to PTSD and TBI

PTSD has been associated with structural changes in the brain, particularly in the prefrontal cortex and the hippocampus. It is unclear whether these changes precede trauma, making the subject more vulnerable to developing psychopathological conditions, or whether they occur as a consequence of the pathophysiological changes that result from the disorder.

Reduced hippocampal volumes have been reported consistently among subjects with PTSD of different etiologies [147–149]. The volumetric changes are most significant in the subfields of the hippocampus that contain the greatest concentration of glucocorticoid receptors (i.e., CA3, dentate gyrus). Corticosteroids may impair neurogenesis, decrease dendritic branching, and potentiate the toxicity of deregulated glutamate neurotransmission, which suggests that they play an etiological role in these atrophic changes [150]. More importantly, the reduction in hippocampal volume is associated with memory deficits, which is the most frequent cognitive alteration observed among PTSD patients [151].

Chronic stress also has a deleterious effect on the prefrontal cortex, and cortical atrophy can also be observed in patients with chronic PTSD [152]. Furthermore, recent diffusion tensor imaging (DTI) studies indicate that, even in the absence of mTBI, PTSD is associated with decreased fractional anisotropy in selective white-matter tracts [153], the latter being a sensitive marker of the structural damage that is also associated with mTBI.

The hippocampus and the prefrontal cortex are areas of the brain that frequently show structural abnormalities as a result of traumatic injury. There is not only overlap between the symptoms associated with mTBI and PTSD; these conditions may both contribute to the disruption of the neural networks involved in the processing of aversive stimuli and the integration of stress responses. A recent study of OEF/OIF veterans showed that, compared with subjects with mTBI reporting only a transient alteration of consciousness, veterans with loss of consciousness exhibited changes in white-matter pathways involved in emotional regulation. In addition, evidence of axonal disruption was associated with more severe PTSD and depressive symptoms. However, Vietnam veterans with penetrating injuries showed that lesions involving the ventromedial prefrontal cortex and the amygdala were significantly related to a decreased prevalence of PTSD [154].

Bazarian and colleagues examined the relationship between combat-related stress, blast exposure, DTI findings, and the severity of PTSD symptoms among 52 OEF/OIF/OND veterans. In this study, PTSD was not only associated with combat exposure (including blast exposure), but there was a significant correlation between white-matter abnormalities observed in DTI and PTSD severity. Of note, they reported abnormal DTI findings in veterans with blast exposure but without a clinical diagnosis of mild TBI [131].

Functional Studies

fMRI, using both resting-state and task-related paradigms, may reveal slight changes or fluctuation in activation patterns and functional connectivity, which may help clarify the effects of TBI and PTSD. Past fMRI studies have indicated that the middle frontal gyrus, the orbital frontal cortex, and the hippocampus are areas that may be commonly affected in TBI and PTSD [155, 156].

Scheibel and colleagues used a simple cognitive control task to compare a group of OEF/OIF veterans with a history of blast-related mTBI with a control group of deployed veterans without this history. Veterans with TBI showed increased brain activation in the anterior cingulate gyrus and medial frontal cortex while performing the task. The differences between the two groups remained significant even when controlling for differences in the severity of PTSD and depressive symptoms, similar to results from previous fMRI studies of subjects with moderate to severe TBI [157].

Despite some of the consistent findings mentioned above, there remains great variability in fMRI findings across past studies, possibly due to the study samples and methodology used. Overall, results in this domain have not indicated any consensus about functional abnormalities that are particular to either PTSD or concussions.

Treatment of PTSD

Currently, there are no evidence-based strategies for treating PTSD that is associated with TBI, though the guidelines for PTSD treatment in the general population provide, at minimum, a pragmatic framework for therapeutic options in working with concussion-related PTSD, an approach that has been endorsed by the Veterans Administration/Department of Defense. Psychotherapeutic interventions appear to be effective in reducing the severity of PTSD symptoms [158]. Although there is variation in psychotherapeutic techniques and in their clinical implementation, both controlled exposure to aversive memories and cognitive processing form the cornerstone of successful approaches. However, meta-analysis of past randomized clinical trials suggests that a significant number of patients with PTSD either drop out or fail to respond to psychotherapy [159].

Regarding pharmacological agents, a meta-analysis of pharmacological interventions used to reduce the severity of PTSD symptoms suggests that they are more effective than a placebo [160]. However, the effect sizes observed in the more rigorous controlled trials were modest and generally smaller than those observed in controlled trials of psychotherapeutic options. Additionally, as of this writing, there are no effectiveness studies that compare medications with psychotherapy. There is little evidence supporting a synergistic effect from combining medications with psychotherapeutic treatment.

It is unlikely that one particular medication would be equally effective in treating all PTSD symptomatic clusters (e.g., intrusive symptoms, avoidance, increased arousal). It is also possible that a pharmacologic agent could prove more effective in the early stages of the disorder than in the more refractory, chronic period.

If pharmacotherapy is an option, SSRIs are often the preferred choice because of their safety profiles. Past work has shown that sertraline, paroxetine, and fluoxetine are significantly more efficacious than a placebo in reducing the severity of PTSD symptoms [161]. This effect is small, however, and varies according to differences in gender, refractoriness of PTSD, type of traumatic event, and symptomatic presentation. Friedman and colleagues found that PTSD in military samples appeared to be less responsive to SSRI treatment [162]. An international multicenter study showed that serotonin norepinephrine reuptake inhibitors, such as venlafaxine, may be more effective for treating PTSD. Patients with PTSD ($n = 329$) were randomized to receive either extended-release venlafaxine or a placebo for 24 weeks. The treatment group had significantly lower CAPS scores. The extended-release venlafaxine was well tolerated by the patients, and drop-out rates resulting from side-effects were similar in the active and placebo groups [163].

Additionally, antiadrenergic agents may have an effect on select PTSD symptoms. The α_1-antagonist prazosin, for example, is efficacious in reducing the frequency and severity of nightmares [164]. However, the α_2-agonist guanfacine was no more effective than placebo in reducing the severity of combat PTSD [165].

Mood stabilizers, such as valproate, lithium, and carbamazepine, have been mostly ineffective in treating PTSD, but may prove efficacious for patients who also have bipolar disorder. The use of topiramate is discouraged in patients with TBI because it may aggravate existing cognitive deficits. Finally, although treatment with antipsychotics is also discouraged in these patients, atypical neuroleptics may be a last-resort solution for controlling disturbing psychotic symptoms.

Anticholinergic medications and benzodiazepines should be avoided, as adverse cognitive side-effects and subsequent addiction are possible.

The goal of exposure therapy is to facilitate the consolidation of new, more adaptive memories of traumatic events, and glutamate transmission through N-methyl-D-aspartate (NMDA) receptors mediates this reconsolidation process. D-cycloserine, which modulates the glycine site of NMDA receptors, was studied in conjunction with exposure therapy to optimize treatment response. Although initial studies were promising, a larger follow-up trial yielded negative results [166].

Overall, although several different medications have proven to be more efficacious than a placebo in reducing the severity of PTSD symptoms, a significant number of patients with PTSD exhibit only a mild response to these medications. There is a need to develop new pharmacological options and integrate them into a comprehensive program that should include established psychotherapies, such as prolonged exposure or cognitive behavioral therapy.

References

1. Laborey M, Masson F, Ribereau-Gayon R, Zongo D, Salmi LR, Lagarde E. Specificity of postconcussion symptoms at 3 months after mild traumatic brain injury: Results from a comparative cohort study. *J Head Trauma Rehabil* 2014; 29(1): E28–E36.
2. King NS, Crawford S, Wenden FJ, Moss NE, Wade DT. The Rivermead Post Concussion Symptoms Questionnaire: A measure of symptoms commonly experienced after head injury and its reliability. *J Neurol* 1995; 242(9): 587–592.
3. Schneiderman AI, Braver ER, Kang HK. Understanding sequelae of injury mechanisms and mild traumatic brain injury incurred during the conflicts in Iraq and Afghanistan: Persistent postconcussive symptoms and posttraumatic stress disorder. *Am J Epidemiol* 2008; 167(12): 1446–1452.
4. Lagarde E, Salmi LR, Holm LW, Contrand B, Masson F, Ribereau-Gayon R, et al. Association of symptoms following mild traumatic brain injury with posttraumatic stress disorder vs. postconcussion syndrome. *JAMA Psychiatry* 2014; 71(9): 1032–1040.
5. Cassidy JD, Cancelliere C, Carroll LJ, Cote P, Hincapie CA, Holm LW, et al. Systematic review of self-reported prognosis in adults after mild traumatic brain injury: Results of the International Collaboration on Mild Traumatic Brain Injury Prognosis. *Arch Phys Med Rehabil* 2014; 95(3 Suppl): S132–S151.
6. Ochsner KN, Silvers JA, Buhle JT. Functional imaging studies of emotion regulation: A synthetic review and evolving model of the cognitive control of emotion. *Ann N Y Acad Sci* 2012; 1251: E1–E24.
7. Arciniegas DB, Topkoff J, Silver JM. Neuropsychiatric aspects of traumatic brain injury. *Curr Treat Options Neurol* 2000; 2(2): 169–186.
8. Hammond FM, Bickett AK, Norton JH, Pershad R. Effectiveness of amantadine hydrochloride in the reduction of chronic traumatic brain injury irritability and aggression. *J Head Trauma Rehabil* 2014; 29(5): 391–399.
9. Tateno A, Jorge RE, Robinson RG. Clinical correlates of aggressive behavior after traumatic brain injury. *J Neuropsychiatry Clin Neurosci* 2003; 15(2): 155–160.
10. Beresford TP, Arciniegas D, Clapp L, Martin B, Alfers J. Reduction of affective lability and alcohol use following traumatic brain injury: A clinical pilot study of anti-convulsant medications. *Brain Inj* 2005; 19(4): 309–313.
11. American Psychiatric Association. *Diagnostic and statistical manual of mental disorders, fifth edition (DSM-5)*. Washington, DC: American Psychiatric Association Press, 2013.
12. Villemure R, Nolin P, Le Sage N. Self-reported symptoms during post-mild traumatic brain injury in acute phase: Influence of interviewing method. *Brain Inj* 2011; 25(1): 53–64.
13. Meterko M, Baker E, Stolzmann KL, Hendricks AM, Cicerone KD, Lew HL. Psychometric assessment of the Neurobehavioral Symptom Inventory-22: The structure of persistent postconcussive symptoms following deployment-related mild traumatic brain injury among veterans. *J Head Trauma Rehabil* 2012; 27(1): 55–62.
14. Harvey PD, Greenberg BR, Serper MR. The affective lability scales: Development, reliability, and validity. *J Clin Psychol* 1989; 45(5): 786–793.
15. Look AE, Flory JD, Harvey PD, Siever LJ. Psychometric properties of a short form of the Affective Lability Scale (ALS-18). *Pers Individ Dif* 2010; 49(3): 187–191.
16. Solhan MB, Trull TJ, Jahng S, Wood PK. Clinical assessment of affective instability: comparing EMA indices, questionnaire reports, and retrospective recall. *Psychol Assess* 2009; 21(3): 425–436.
17. Bowen RC, Balbuena L, Baetz M. Lamotrigine reduces affective instability in depressed patients with mixed mood and anxiety disorders. *J Clin Psychopharmacol* 2014; 34(6): 747–749.
18. Henry C, Van den Bulke D, Bellivier F, Roy I, Swendsen J, M'Bailara K, et al. Affective lability and affect intensity as core dimensions of bipolar disorders during euthymic period. *Psychiatry Res* 2008; 159(1–2): 1–6.
19. Mackinnon DF, Pies R. Affective instability as rapid cycling: Theoretical and clinical implications for borderline personality and bipolar spectrum disorders. *Bipolar Disord* 2006; 8(1): 1–14.
20. Parmentier C, Etain B, Yon L, Misson H, Mathieu F, Lajnef M, et al. Clinical and dimensional characteristics of euthymic bipolar patients with or without suicidal behavior. *Eur Psychiatry* 2012; 27(8): 570–576.
21. Henry C, Mitropoulou V, New AS, Koenigsberg HW, Silverman J, Siever LJ. Affective instability and impulsivity in borderline personality and bipolar II disorders: Similarities and differences. *J Psychiatr Res* 2001; 35(6): 307–312.
22. Aas M, Pedersen G, Henry C, Bjella T, Bellivier F, Leboyer M, et al. Psychometric properties of the Affective Lability Scale (54 and 18-item version) in patients with bipolar disorder, first-degree relatives, and healthy controls. *J Affect Disord* 2014; 172: 375–380.
23. Skirrow C, Ebner-Priemer U, Reinhard I, Malliaris Y, Kuntsi J, Asherson P. Everyday emotional experience of adults with attention deficit hyperactivity disorder: Evidence for reactive and endogenous emotional lability. *Psychol Med* 2014; 44(16): 3571–3583.
24. Block SH. Psychotherapy of the individual with brain injury. *Brain Inj* 1987; 1(2): 203–206.
25. Wilson BA. Neuropsychological rehabilitation. *Annu Rev Clin Psychol* 2008; 4: 141–162.
26. Cattelani R, Zettin M, Zoccolotti P. Rehabilitation treatments for adults with behavioral and psychosocial disorders following

acquired brain injury: A systematic review. *Neuropsychol Rev* 2010; 20(1): 52–85.

27. Arciniegas DB, Topkoff J. The neuropsychiatry of pathologic affect: An approach to evaluation and treatment. *Semin Clin Neuropsychiatry* 2000; 5(4): 290–306.

28. Wortzel HS, Oster TJ, Anderson CA, Arciniegas DB. Pathological laughing and crying: Epidemiology, pathophysiology and treatment. *CNS Drugs* 2008; 22(7): 531–545.

29. Eames PG. Disintinguishing the neuropsychiatric, psychiatric, and psychological consequences of acquired brain injury. In: Wood RL, McMillan T, editors. *Neurobehavioral disability and social handicap following traumatic brain injury.* Hove, UK: Psychology Press; 2001, pp. 29–46.

30. Dikmen S, McLean A, Temkin N. Neuropsychological and psychosocial consequences of minor head injury. *J Neurol Neurosurg Psychiatry* 1986; 49(11): 1227–1232.

31. McKinlay WW, Brooks DN, Bond MR, Martinage DP, Marshall MM. The short-term outcome of severe blunt head injury as reported by relatives of the injured persons. *J Neurol Neurosurg Psychiatry* 1981; 44(6): 527–533.

32. Deb S, Lyons I, Koutzoukis C. Neurobehavioural symptoms one year after a head injury. *Br J Psychiatry* 1999; 174: 360–365.

33. Yang CC, Hua MS, Lin WC, Tsai YH, Huang SJ. Irritability following traumatic brain injury: Divergent manifestations of annoyance and verbal aggression. *Brain Inj* 2012; 26(10): 1185–1191.

34. Yang CC, Huang SJ, Lin WC, Tsai YH, Hua MS. Divergent manifestations of irritability in patients with mild and moderate-to-severe traumatic brain injury: Perspectives of awareness and neurocognitive correlates. *Brain Inj* 2013; 27(9): 1008–1015.

35. Cicerone K, Kalmar K. Peristent postconcussion syndrome: The structure of subjective complaints after mild traumatic brain injury. *J Head Trauma Rehabil* 1995; 10: 1–17.

36. Craig KJ, Hietanen H, Markova IS, Berrios GE. The Irritability Questionnaire: A new scale for the measurement of irritability. *Psychiatry Res* 2008; 159(3): 367–375.

37. Yang CC, Huang SJ, Lin WC, Tsai YH, Hua MS. Evaluating irritability in patients with traumatic brain injury: Development of the National Taiwan University Irritability Scale. *Brain Impair* 2011; 12: 200–209.

38. Cummings JL, Mega M, Gray K, Rosenberg-Thompson S, Carusi DA, Gornbein J. The Neuropsychiatric Inventory: Comprehensive assessment of psychopathology in dementia. *Neurology* 1994; 44(12): 2308–2314.

39. Rees L, Marshall S, Hartridge C, Mackie D, Weiser M. Cognitive interventions post acquired brain injury. *Brain Inj* 2007; 21(2): 161–200.

40. Walker AJ, Nott MT, Doyle M, Onus M, McCarthy K, Baguley IJ. Effectiveness of a group anger management programme after severe traumatic brain injury. *Brain Inj* 2010; 24(3): 517–524.

41. Hart T, Vaccaro MJ, Hays C, Maiuro RD. Anger self-management training for people with traumatic brain injury: A preliminary investigation. *J Head Trauma Rehabil* 2012; 27(2): 113–122.

42. Kant R, Smith-Seemiller L, Zeiler D. Treatment of aggression and irritability after head injury. *Brain Inj* 1998; 12(8): 661–666.

43. Wroblewski BA, Joseph AB, Kupfer J, Kalliel K. Effectiveness of valproic acid on destructive and aggressive behaviours in patients with acquired brain injury. *Brain Inj* 1997; 11(1): 37–47.

44. Evans RW, Gualtieri CT, Patterson D. Treatment of chronic closed head injury with psychostimulant drugs: A controlled case study and an appropriate evaluation procedure. *J Nerv Ment Dis* 1987; 175(2): 106–110.

45. Azouvi P, Jokic C, Attal N, Denys P, Markabi S, Bussel B. Carbamazepine in agitation and aggressive behaviour following

severe closed-head injury: Results of an open trial. *Brain Inj* 1999; 13(10): 797–804.

46. Kim E, Bijlani M. A pilot study of quetiapine treatment of aggression due to traumatic brain injury. *J Neuropsychiatry Clin Neurosci* 2006; 18(4): 547–549.

47. Umene-Nakano W, Yoshimura R, Okamoto T, Hori H, Nakamura J. Aripiprazole improves various cognitive and behavioral impairments after traumatic brain injury: A case report. *Gen Hosp Psychiatry* 2013; 35(1): 103 e107–109.

48. Gualtieri CT. Buspirone: Neuropsychiatric effects. *J Head Trauma Rehabil* 1991; 6: 90–92.

49. Elliott FA. Propranolol for the control of belligerent behavior following acute brain damage. *Ann Neurol* 1977; 1(5): 489–491.

50. Hammond FM, Sherer M, Malec JF, Zafonte RD, Whitney M, Bell K, et al. Amantadine effect on perceptions of irritability after traumatic brain injury: Results of the Amantadine Irritability Multisite Study. *J Neurotrauma* 2015; 32(16): 1230–1238.

51. Jorge RE, Starkstein SE. Pathophysiologic aspects of major depression following traumatic brain injury. *J Head Trauma Rehabil* 2005; 20(6): 475–487.

52. Seel RT, Macciocchi S, Kreutzer JS. Clinical considerations for the diagnosis of major depression after moderate to severe TBI. *J Head Trauma Rehabil* 2010; 25(2): 99–112.

53. Choi-Kwon S, Choi J, Kwon SU, Kang DW, Kim JS. Fluoxetine is not effective in the treatment of post-stroke fatigue: A double-blind, placebo-controlled study. *Cerebrovasc Dis* 2007; 23(2–3): 103–108.

54. Koponen S, Taiminen T, Portin R, Himanen L, Isoniemi H, Heinonen H, et al. Axis I and II psychiatric disorders after traumatic brain injury: A 30-year follow-up study. *Am J Psychiatry* 2002; 159(8): 1315–1321.

55. Hibbard MR, Uysal S, Kepler K, Bogdany J, Silver J. Axis I psychopathology in individuals with traumatic brain injury. *J Head Trauma Rehabil* 1998; 13(4): 24–39.

56. Silver JM, Kramer R, Greenwald S, Weissman M. The association between head injuries and psychiatric disorders: Findings from the New Haven NIMH Epidemiologic Catchment Area Study. *Brain Inj* 2001; 15(11): 935–945.

57. van Reekum R, Cohen T, Wong J. Can traumatic brain injury cause psychiatric disorders? *J Neuropsychiatry Clin Neurosci* 2000; 12(3): 316–327.

58. Jorge RE, Robinson RG, Starkstein SE, Arndt SV, Forrester AW, Geisler FH. Secondary mania following traumatic brain injury. *Am J Psychiatry* 1993; 150(6): 916–921.

59. Evans DL, Byerly MJ, Greer RA. Secondary mania: diagnosis and treatment. *J Clin Psychiatry* 1995; 56 (Suppl 3): 31–37.

60. Perry DC, Sturm VE, Peterson MJ, Pieper CF, Bullock T, Boeve BF, et al. Association of traumatic brain injury with subsequent neurological and psychiatric disease: A meta-analysis. *J Neurosurg* 2016; 124(2): 511–526.

61. Chan F, Lanctot KL, Feinstein A, Herrmann N, Strauss J, Sicard T, et al. The serotonin transporter polymorphisms and major depression following traumatic brain injury. *Brain Inj* 2008; 22(6): 471–479.

62. Lanctot KL, Rapoport MJ, Chan F, Rajaram RD, Strauss J, Sicard T, et al. Genetic predictors of response to treatment with citalopram in depression secondary to traumatic brain injury. *Brain Inj* 2010; 24(7–8): 959–969.

63. Shukla S, Cook BL, Mukherjee S, Godwin C, Miller MG. Mania following head trauma. *Am J Psychiatry* 1987; 144(1): 93–96.

64. Malaspina D, Goetz RR, Friedman JH, Kaufmann CA, Faraone SV, Tsuang M, et al. Traumatic brain injury and schizophrenia in members of schizophrenia and bipolar disorder pedigrees. *Am J Psychiatry* 2001; 158(3): 440–446.

65. Fann JR, Burington B, Leonetti A, Jaffe K, Katon WJ, Thompson RS. Psychiatric illness following traumatic brain injury in an adult health maintenance organization population. *Arch Gen Psychiatry* 2004; 61(1): 53–61.

66. Jorge RE. Neuropsychiatric consequences of traumatic brain injury: A review of recent findings. *Curr Opin Psychiatry* 2005; 18(3): 289–299.

67. Rapoport M, McCauley S, Levin H, Song J, Feinstein A. The role of injury severity in neurobehavioral outcome 3 months after traumatic brain injury. *Neuropsychiatry Neuropsychol Behav Neurol* 2002; 15(2): 123–132.

68. Price JL, Drevets WC. Neural circuits underlying the pathophysiology of mood disorders. *Trends Cogn Sci* 2012; 16(1): 61–71.

69. Ongur D, Price JL. The organization of networks within the orbital and medial prefrontal cortex of rats, monkeys and humans. *Cereb Cortex* 2000; 10(3): 206–219.

70. Raichle ME, MacLeod AM, Snyder AZ, Powers WJ, Gusnard DA, Shulman GL. A default mode of brain function. *Proc Natl Acad Sci U S A* 2001; 98(2): 676–682.

71. Hamilton JP, Furman DJ, Chang C, Thomason ME, Dennis E, Gotlib IH. Default-mode and task-positive network activity in major depressive disorder: Implications for adaptive and maladaptive rumination. *Biol Psychiatry* 2011; 70(4): 327–333.

72. Berman MG, Nee DE, Casement M, Kim HS, Deldin P, Kross E, et al. Neural and behavioral effects of interference resolution in depression and rumination. *Cogn Affect Behav Neurosci* 2011; 11(1): 85–96.

73. Mayberg HS, Lozano AM, Voon V, McNeely HE, Seminowicz D, Hamani C, et al. Deep brain stimulation for treatment-resistant depression. *Neuron* 2005; 45(5): 651–660.

74. Hariri AR, Mattay VS, Tessitore A, Fera F, Weinberger DR. Neocortical modulation of the amygdala response to fearful stimuli. *Biol Psychiatry* 2003; 53(6): 494–501.

75. Hariri AR, Mattay VS, Tessitore A, Kolachana B, Fera F, Goldman D, et al. Serotonin transporter genetic variation and the response of the human amygdala. *Science* 2002; 297(5580): 400–403.

76. Mayberg HS. Defining the neural circuitry of depression: Toward a new nosology with therapeutic implications. *Biol Psychiatry* 2007; 61(6): 729–730.

77. Mayberg HS, Liotti M, Brannan SK, McGinnis S, Mahurin RK, Jerabek PA, et al. Reciprocal limbic-cortical function and negative mood: Converging PET findings in depression and normal sadness. *Am J Psychiatry* 1999; 156(5): 675–682.

78. Drevets WC, Videen TO, Price JL, Preskorn SH, Carmichael ST, Raichle ME. A functional anatomical study of unipolar depression. *J Neurosci* 1992; 12(9): 3628–3641.

79. Drevets WC. Prefrontal cortical-amygdalar metabolism in major depression. *Ann N Y Acad Sci* 1999; 877: 614–637.

80. Davidson RJ, Lewis DA, Alloy LB, Amaral DG, Bush G, Cohen JD, et al. Neural and behavioral substrates of mood and mood regulation. *Biol Psychiatry* 2002; 52(6): 478–502.

81. Parsey RV, Oquendo MA, Simpson NR, Ogden RT, Van Heertum R, Arango V, et al. Effects of sex, age, and aggressive traits in man on brain serotonin 5-HT(1A) receptor binding potential measured by PET using [C-11]WAY-100635. *Brain Res* 2002; 954(2): 173–182.

82. Fava M. Depression with anger attacks. *J Clin Psychiatry* 1998; 59 (Suppl 18): 18–22.

83. Jorge RE, Robinson RG, Moser D, Tateno A, Crespo-Facorro B, Arndt S. Major depression following traumatic brain injury. *Arch Gen Psychiatry* 2004; 61(1): 42–50.

84. Jorge RE, Acion L, Starkstein SE, Magnotta V. Hippocampal volume and mood disorders after traumatic brain injury. *Biol Psychiatry* 2007; 62(4): 332–338.

85. Chen JK, Johnston KM, Petrides M, Ptito A. Neural substrates of symptoms of depression following concussion in male athletes with persisting postconcussion symptoms. *Arch Gen Psychiatry* 2008; 65(1): 81–89.

86. Matthews SC, Strigo IA, Simmons AN, O'Connell RM, Reinhardt LE, Moseley SA. A multimodal imaging study in U.S. veterans of Operations Iraqi and Enduring Freedom with and without major depression after blast-related concussion. *NeuroImage* 2011; 54: S69–S75.

87. Oster TJ, Anderson CA, Filley CM, Wortzel HS, Arciniegas DB. Quetiapine for mania due to traumatic brain injury. *CNS Spectrum* 2007; 12(10): 764–769.

88. Snell DL, Surgenor LJ, Hay-Smith EJ, Siegert RJ. A systematic review of psychological treatments for mild traumatic brain injury: An update on the evidence. *J Clin Exp Neuropsychol* 2009; 31(1): 20–38.

89. Anson K, Ponsford J. Coping and emotional adjustment following traumatic brain injury. *J Head Trauma Rehabil* 2006; 21(3): 248–259.

90. Hibbard MR, Cantor J, Charatz H, Rosenthal R, Ashman T, Gundersen N, et al. Peer support in the community: Initial findings of a mentoring program for individuals with traumatic brain injury and their families. *J Head Trauma Rehabil* 2002; 17(2): 112–131.

91. Leach LR, Frank RG, Bouman DE, Farmer J. Family functioning, social support and depression after traumatic brain injury. *Brain Inj* 1994; 8(7): 599–606.

92. VA/DoD. The Management of Concussion-mild Traumatic Brain Injury Working Group. VA/DoD clinical practice guideline for the management of concussion-mild traumatic brain injury: Department of Veterans Affairs; Department of Defense; 2016 [updated February 2017; cited 07 August 2017]. Available from: www.healthquality.va.gov/guidelines/Rehab/mtbi/mTBICPGFullCPG50821816.pdf.

93. Warden DL, Gordon B, McAllister TW, Silver JM, Barth JT, Bruns J, et al. Guidelines for the pharmacologic treatment of neurobehavioral sequelae of traumatic brain injury. *J Neurotrauma* 2006; 23(10): 1468–1501.

94. Kant R, Duffy JD, Pivovarnik A. Prevalence of apathy following head injury. *Brain Inj* 1998; 12(1): 87–92.

95. Fann JR, Uomoto JM, Katon WJ. Sertraline in the treatment of major depression following mild traumatic brain injury. *J Neuropsychiatry Clin Neurosci* 2000; 12(2): 226–232.

96. Fann JR, Uomoto JM, Katon WJ. Cognitive improvement with treatment of depression following mild traumatic brain injury. *Psychosomatics* 2001; 42(1): 48–54.

97. Alper K, Schwartz KA, Kolts RL, Khan A. Seizure incidence in psychopharmacological clinical trials: An analysis of Food and Drug Administration (FDA) summary basis of approval reports. *Biol Psychiatry* 2007; 62(4): 345–354.

98. Chuang DM. The antiapoptotic actions of mood stabilizers: Molecular mechanisms and therapeutic potentials. *Ann N Y Acad Sci* 2005; 1053: 195–204.

99. Yu F, Wang Z, Tanaka M, Chiu CT, Leeds P, Zhang Y, et al. Posttrauma cotreatment with lithium and valproate: Reduction of lesion volume, attenuation of blood–brain barrier disruption, and improvement in motor coordination in mice with traumatic brain injury. *J Neurosurg* 2013; 119(3): 766–773.

100. Dash PK, Orsi SA, Zhang M, Grill RJ, Pati S, Zhao J, et al. Valproate administered after traumatic brain injury provides neuroprotection and improves cognitive function in rats. *PLoS One* 2010; 5(6): e11383.

101. Chatham Showalter PE, Kimmel DN. Agitated symptom response to divalproex following acute brain injury. *J Neuropsychiatry Clin Neurosci* 2000; 12(3): 395–397.

102. Luaute J, Plantier D, Wiart L, Tell L. Care management of the agitation or aggressiveness crisis in patients with TBI. Systematic review of the literature and practice recommendations. *Ann Phys Rehabil Med* 2016; 59(1): 58–67.

103. Kim E, Humaran TJ. Divalproex in the management of neuropsychiatric complications of remote acquired brain injury. *J Neuropsychiatry Clin Neurosci* 2002; 14(2): 202–205.

104. Murai T, Fujimoto S. Rapid cycling bipolar disorder after left temporal polar damage. *Brain Inj* 2003; 17(4): 355–358.

105. Hoge CW, Castro CA, Messer SC, McGurk D, Cotting DI, Koffman RL. Combat duty in Iraq and Afghanistan, mental health problems, and barriers to care. *N Engl J Med* 2004; 351(1): 13–22.

106. Hoge CW, Auchterlonie JL, Milliken CS. Mental health problems, use of mental health services, and attrition from military service after returning from deployment to Iraq or Afghanistan. *JAMA* 2006; 295(9): 1023–1032.

107. Seal KH, Bertenthal D, Miner CR, Sen S, Marmar C. Bringing the war back home: Mental health disorders among 103,788 US veterans returning from Iraq and Afghanistan seen at Department of Veterans Affairs facilities. *Arch Intern Med* 2007; 167(5): 476–482.

108. Warden D. Military TBI during the Iraq and Afghanistan wars. *J Head Trauma Rehabil* 2006; 21(5): 398–402.

109. Terrio H, Brenner LA, Ivins BJ, Cho JM, Helmick K, Schwab K, et al. Traumatic brain injury screening: Preliminary findings in a US Army Brigade Combat Team. *J Head Trauma Rehabil* 2009; 24(1): 14–23.

110. Hoge CW, McGurk D, Thomas JL, Cox AL, Engel CC, Castro CA. Mild traumatic brain injury in U.S. soldiers returning from Iraq. *N Engl J Med* 2008; 358(5): 453–463.

111. Cifu DX, Taylor BC, Carne WF, Bidelspach D, Sayer NA, Scholten J, et al. Traumatic brain injury, posttraumatic stress disorder, and pain diagnoses in OIF/OEF/OND veterans. *J Rehabil Res Dev* 2013; 50(9): 1169–1176.

112. Hill JJ, 3rd, Mobo BH, Jr., Cullen MR. Separating deployment-related traumatic brain injury and posttraumatic stress disorder in veterans: Preliminary findings from the Veterans Affairs traumatic brain injury screening program. *Am J Phys Med Rehabil* 2009; 88(8): 605–614.

113. Vanderploeg RD, Belanger HG, Curtiss G. Mild traumatic brain injury and posttraumatic stress disorder and their associations with health symptoms. *Arch Phys Med Rehabil* 2009; 90(7): 1084–1093.

114. Bryan CJ, Clemans TA. Repetitive traumatic brain injury, psychological symptoms, and suicide risk in a clinical sample of deployed military personnel. *JAMA Psychiatry* 2013; 70(7): 686–691.

115. Blake DD, Weathers FW, Nagy LM, Kaloupek DG, Gusman FD, Charney DS, et al. The development of a clinician-administered PTSD scale. *J Trauma Stress* 1995; 8(1): 75–90.

116. Weathers FW, Litz BT, Keane TM, Palmieri PA, Marx BP, Schnurr PP. The PTSD Checklist for DMS-5 (PCL-5). National Center for PTSD. 2013. Available at wwwptsdvagov.

117. Carlson KF, Kehle SM, Meis LA, Greer N, Macdonald R, Rutks I, et al. Prevalence, assessment, and treatment of mild traumatic brain injury and posttraumatic stress disorder: A systematic review of the evidence. *J Head Trauma Rehabil* 2011; 26(2): 103–115.

118. Bahraini NH, Breshears RE, Hernandez TD, Schneider AL, Forster JE, Brenner LA. Traumatic brain injury and posttraumatic stress disorder. *Psychiatr Clin North Am* 2014; 37(1): 55–75.

119. Heim C, Newport DJ, Mletzko T, Miller AH, Nemeroff CB. The link between childhood trauma and depression: Insights from HPA axis studies in humans. *Psychoneuroendocrinology* 2008; 33(6): 693–710.

120. Mulchahey JJ, Ekhator NN, Zhang H, Kasckow JW, Baker DG, Geracioti TD, Jr. Cerebrospinal fluid and plasma testosterone levels in post-traumatic stress disorder and tobacco dependence. *Psychoneuroendocrinology* 2001; 26(3): 273–285.

121. Olff M, de Vries GJ, Guzelcan Y, Assies J, Gersons BP. Changes in cortisol and DHEA plasma levels after psychotherapy for PTSD. *Psychoneuroendocrinology* 2007; 32(6): 619–626.

122. Yehuda R, Brand SR, Golier JA, Yang RK. Clinical correlates of DHEA associated with post-traumatic stress disorder. *Acta Psychiatr Scand* 2006; 114(3): 187–193.

123. Lebron-Milad K, Graham BM, Milad MR. Low estradiol levels: A vulnerability factor for the development of posttraumatic stress disorder. *Biol Psychiatry* 2012; 72(1): 6–7.

124. Breslau N, Chen Q, Luo Z. The role of intelligence in posttraumatic stress disorder: Does it vary by trauma severity? *PLoS One* 2013; 8(6): e65391.

125. Macklin ML, Metzger LJ, Litz BT, McNally RJ, Lasko NB, Orr SP, et al. Lower precombat intelligence is a risk factor for posttraumatic stress disorder. *J Consult Clin Psychol* 1998; 66(2): 323–326.

126. Murrough JW, Charney DS. The serotonin transporter and emotionality: Risk, resilience, and new therapeutic opportunities. *Biol Psychiatry* 2011; 69(6): 510–512.

127. Soliman F, Glatt CE, Bath KG, Levita L, Jones RM, Pattwell SS, et al. A genetic variant BDNF polymorphism alters extinction learning in both mouse and human. *Science* 2010; 327(5967): 863–866.

128. Zhou Z, Zhu G, Hariri AR, Enoch MA, Scott D, Sinha R, et al. Genetic variation in human NPY expression affects stress response and emotion. *Nature* 2008; 452(7190): 997–1001.

129. Koren D, Norman D, Cohen A, Berman J, Klein EM. Increased PTSD risk with combat-related injury: A matched comparison study of injured and uninjured soldiers experiencing the same combat events. *Am J Psychiatry* 2005; 162(2): 276–282.

130. Bryant RA, O'Donnell ML, Creamer M, McFarlane AC, Clark CR, Silove D. The psychiatric sequelae of traumatic injury. *Am J Psychiatry* 2010; 167(3): 312–320.

131. Bazarian JJ, Donnelly K, Peterson DR, Warner GC, Zhu T, Zhong J. The relation between posttraumatic stress disorder and mild traumatic brain injury acquired during Operations Enduring Freedom and Iraqi Freedom. *J Head Trauma Rehabil* 2013; 28(1): 1–12.

132. Yehuda R. Biology of posttraumatic stress disorder. *J Clin Psychiatry* 2001; 62 (Suppl 17): 41–46.

133. Liberzon I, Abelson JL, Flagel SB, Raz J, Young EA. Neuroendocrine and psychophysiologic responses in PTSD: A symptom provocation study. *Neuropsychopharmacology* 1999; 21(1): 40–50.

134. Perkes I, Baguley IJ, Nott MT, Menon DK. A review of paroxysmal sympathetic hyperactivity after acquired brain injury. *Ann Neurol* 2010; 68(2): 126–135.

135. Colivicchi F, Bassi A, Santini M, Caltagirone C. Prognostic implications of right-sided insular damage, cardiac autonomic derangement, and arrhythmias after acute ischemic stroke. *Stroke* 2005; 36(8): 1710–1715.

136. Buchanan TW, Driscoll D, Mowrer SM, Sollers JJ, 3rd, Thayer JF, Kirschbaum C, et al. Medial prefrontal cortex damage affects physiological and psychological stress responses differently in men and women. *Psychoneuroendocrinology* 2010; 35(1): 56–66.

137. Williamson JB, Heilman KM, Porges EC, Lamb DG, Porges SW. A possible mechanism for PTSD symptoms in patients with traumatic brain injury: Central autonomic network disruption. *Front Neuroeng* 2013; 6: 13.

138. Mac Donald CL, Johnson AM, Cooper D, Nelson EC, Werner NJ, Shimony JS, et al. Detection of blast-related traumatic brain injury in U.S. military personnel. *N Engl J Med* 2011; 364(22): 2091–2100.

139. Jovanovic T, Norrholm SD. Neural mechanisms of impaired fear inhibition in posttraumatic stress disorder. *Front Behav Neurosci* 2011; 5: 44.

140. Rauch SL, Shin LM, Phelps EA. Neurocircuitry models of posttraumatic stress disorder and extinction: human neuroimaging research – past, present, and future. *Biol Psychiatry* 2006; 60(4): 376–382.

141. Shin LM, Liberzon I. The neurocircuitry of fear, stress, and anxiety disorders. *Neuropsychopharmacology* 2010; 35(1): 169–191.

142. Milad MR, Quirk GJ. Fear extinction as a model for translational neuroscience: Ten years of progress. *Annu Rev Psychol* 2016; 63: 129–151.

143. Schiller D, Phelps EA. Does reconsolidation occur in humans? *Front Behav Neurosci* 2011; 5: 24.

144. Delgado MR, Nearing KI, Ledoux JE, Phelps EA. Neural circuitry underlying the regulation of conditioned fear and its relation to extinction. *Neuron* 2008; 59(5): 829–838.

145. Milad MR, Orr SP, Lasko NB, Chang Y, Rauch SL, Pitman RK. Presence and acquired origin of reduced recall for fear extinction in PTSD: Results of a twin study. *J Psychiatr Res* 2008; 42(7): 515–520.

146. Rougemont-Bucking A, Linnman C, Zeffiro TA, Zeidan MA, Lebron-Milad K, Rodriguez-Romaguera J, et al. Altered processing of contextual information during fear extinction in PTSD: an fMRI study. *CNS Neurosci Ther* 2011; 17(4): 227–236.

147. Bremner JD, Randall P, Scott TM, Bronen RA, Seibyl JP, Southwick SM, et al. MRI-based measurement of hippocampal volume in patients with combat-related posttraumatic stress disorder. *Am J Psychiatry* 1995; 152(7): 973–981.

148. Bremner JD, Randall P, Vermetten E, Staib L, Bronen RA, Mazure C, et al. Magnetic resonance imaging-based measurement of hippocampal volume in posttraumatic stress disorder related to childhood physical and sexual abuse – A preliminary report. *Biol Psychiatry* 1997; 41(1): 23–32.

149. Smith ME. Bilateral hippocampal volume reduction in adults with post-traumatic stress disorder: A meta-analysis of structural MRI studies. *Hippocampus* 2005; 15(6): 798–807.

150. Wang Z, Neylan TC, Mueller SG, Lenoci M, Truran D, Marmar CR, et al. Magnetic resonance imaging of hippocampal subfields in posttraumatic stress disorder. *Arch Gen Psychiatry* 2010; 67(3): 296–303.

151. Johnsen GE, Asbjornsen AE. Consistent impaired verbal memory in PTSD: A meta-analysis. *J Affect Disord* 2008; 111(1): 74–82.

152. McEwen BS, Morrison JH. The brain on stress: Vulnerability and plasticity of the prefrontal cortex over the life course. *Neuron* 2013; 79(1): 16–29.

153. Schuff N, Zhang Y, Zhan W, Lenoci M, Ching C, Boreta L, et al. Patterns of altered cortical perfusion and diminished subcortical integrity in posttraumatic stress disorder: An MRI study. *NeuroImage* 2011; 54 (Suppl 1): S62–S68.

154. Koenigs M, Huey ED, Raymont V, Cheon B, Solomon J, Wassermann EM, et al. Focal brain damage protects against posttraumatic stress disorder in combat veterans. *Nat Neurosci* 2008; 11(2): 232–237.

155. Stein MB, McAllister TW. Exploring the convergence of posttraumatic stress disorder and mild traumatic brain injury. *Am J Psychiatry* 2009; 166(7): 768–776.

156. Vasterling JJ, Verfaellie M, Sullivan KD. Mild traumatic brain injury and posttraumatic stress disorder in returning veterans: Perspectives from cognitive neuroscience. *Clin Psychol Rev* 2009; 29(8): 674–684.

157. Scheibel RS, Newsome MR, Troyanskaya M, Lin X, Steinberg JL, Radaideh M, et al. Altered brain activation in military personnel with one or more traumatic brain injuries following blast. *J Int Neuropsychol Soc* 2012; 18(1): 89–100.

158. Foa EB. Prolonged exposure therapy: Past, present, and future. *Depress Anxiety* 2011; 28(12): 1043–1047.

159. Bisson J, Andrew M. Psychological treatment of post-traumatic stress disorder (PTSD). *Cochrane Database Syst Rev* 2007; (3): CD003388.

160. Stein DJ, Ipser JC, Seedat S. Pharmacotherapy for post traumatic stress disorder (PTSD). *Cochrane Database Syst Rev* 2006; (1): CD002795.

161. Ravindran LN, Stein MB. Pharmacotherapy of post-traumatic stress disorder. *Curr Top Behav Neurosci* 2010; 2: 505–525.

162. Friedman MJ, Marmar CR, Baker DG, Sikes CR, Farfel GM. Randomized, double-blind comparison of sertraline and placebo for posttraumatic stress disorder in a Department of Veterans Affairs setting. *J Clin Psychiatry* 2007; 68(5): 711–720.

163. Davidson J, Baldwin D, Stein DJ, Kuper E, Benattia I, Ahmed S, et al. Treatment of posttraumatic stress disorder with venlafaxine extended release: A 6-month randomized controlled trial. *Arch Gen Psychiatry* 2006; 63(10): 1158–1165.

164. Raskind MA, Peterson K, Williams T, Hoff DJ, Hart K, Holmes H, et al. A trial of prazosin for combat trauma PTSD with nightmares in active-duty soldiers returned from Iraq and Afghanistan. *Am J Psychiatry* 2013; 170(9): 1003–1010.

165. Neylan TC, Lenoci M, Samuelson KW, Metzler TJ, Henn-Haase C, Hierholzer RW, et al. No improvement of posttraumatic stress disorder symptoms with guanfacine treatment. *Am J Psychiatry* 2006; 163(12): 2186–2188.

166. Rothbaum BO, Price M, Jovanovic T, Norrholm SD, Gerardi M, Dunlop B, et al. A randomized, double-blind evaluation of D-cycloserine or alprazolam combined with virtual reality exposure therapy for posttraumatic stress disorder in Iraq and Afghanistan War veterans. *Am J Psychiatry* 2014; 171(6): 640–648.

Chapter

9

Concussion and the 21st-Century Renaissance of Neuropsychology

Jeff Victoroff and Erin D. Bigler

Introduction

This little volume began with a simple observation: history does not record, and may long debate, the moment when it was first discovered that typical clinically attended concussive brain injury (CBI) often leads to lasting neurobehavioral dysfunction. The editors of this text and authors of this chapter hope that, at this point in the narrative, readers have become experts in that history – from the challenge of conceptualizing and defining the most common *natural kind* (Mills's meaning) of traumatic brain injury (TBI) (and tracing a dry path through the mire of semantic laxity), to the challenge of characterizing a dynamic and heterogeneous neurobiological phenomenon based on dubious comparisons to rodent neurology (and making inferences about recently rattled human brains when open caskets are rare as blue moons), to the inescapable, often overlooked challenge of making practical medicine and applied psychology in the face of the infinite variety of human nature. This odyssey through some aery domains of intellectual enterprise is perhaps idiosyncratic in a textbook (some would say iconoclastic) but (we intend) represents a sincere bow to the reader's mind and (we hope) accomplishes a refreshing diversion from the dogmatism that haunts academic medicine.

The recent discovery that typical CBI is often followed by persistent distress and lasting brain change has profound implications for neuropsychology. As this text has summarized:

- More than 40% of concussion survivors experience or exhibit cognitive and/or non-cognitive behavioral problems for one or more years after injury.
- Experimental animal studies report concussive brain changes that persist for at least half of the lifetime of the animal.
- Human neuroimaging studies confirm brain change one or more years after injury.
- Most human studies using conventional neuropsychological testing reveal that those tests lose sensitivity to the effects of concussion by three months after injury. In fact, one study found that the sensitivity of paper-and-pencil test batteries had dropped to 23% by two days post injury [2].

The conclusion is self-evident (and hopefully non-controversial): conventional desktop neuropsychological testing is not sensitive to, and *never* specific for, many types of brain change.

So what? Neither is the neurological examination. Or the 1.5-T magnetic resonance imaging (MRI). Or the 400-power optical microscope. This is not a unique problem for neuropsychology. This is vital, useful news – a foundational truth required for neuropsychology to assume a robust new role in 21st-century clinical neuroscience – and is likely to significantly improve the prevention and clinical management of brain injury.

The authors of this chapter are a neurologist and a neuropsychologist. We are not only on the same page; we are in the same boat. The neurological examination attempts to infer information about the human nervous system by observing responses to stimuli. The neuropsychological examination employs exactly the same approach. Neither neurologists nor neuropsychologists can accurately detect the presence, or absence, or etiology, or location, or severity, or prognosis of most forms of brain dysfunction. Neuropsychologists, however, enjoy two great advantages.

One: although neither of the authors claims empirical proof, we share the impression that the proportion of accomplished psychotherapists may be higher among neuropsychologists than among neurologists, perhaps because the initial training of psychologists specifically emphasizes listening and interpersonal contact.

Two: unlike neurology, neuropsychology has a legitimate chance of improving its examination. Development of the neurological examination plateaued about a century ago and is rarely subjected to serious study. Few neurologists, professors included, have a strong grasp of the daunting intricacies of neuroanatomy. Few are aware of the limitations of the bedside examination, the statistical data regarding the neuroanatomical and biological significance of a given sign, or the frequency with which the examination misguides clinicians. Neuropsychologists, in contrast, seem more aware of the fact that neither a test nor a battery of tests is diagnostic of any particular brain dysfunction. A movement is afoot within neuropsychology to discover and exploit new and improved methods of behavior–brain correlation. While there are diminishing returns to refining observations based on paper-and-pencil desktop quizzes for diagnosing brain dysfunction, reasons exist to expect that several innovations are arming the 21st-century neuropsychologist with significantly enhanced capabilities. These include computerized assessment (which can enhance the precision of both presentation of stimuli and

Eye movement abnormalities demonstrate persistent cerebral dysfunction three to five months after injury despite normalization of neuropsychological tests

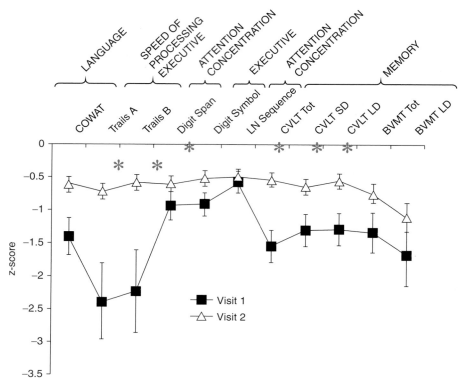

Fig. 9.1 The post-concussive symptom (PCS) group performed worse on anti-saccades, self-paced saccades, memory-guided sequences, and smooth pursuit, suggesting problems in response inhibition, short-term spatial memory, motor sequence programming, visuospatial processing, and visual attention. This poorer oculomotor performance included several measures beyond conscious control, indicating that subcortical functionality in the PCS group was poorer than expected after mild closed head injury. Eye movements provided additional evidence of dysfunction in areas such as decision making under time pressure, response inhibition, short-term spatial memory, motor sequence programming and execution, visuospatial processing and integration, visual attention and subcortical brain function. Indications of poorer subcortical/subconscious oculomotor function in the PCS group support the notion that PCS is not merely a psychological entity but also has a biological substrate. BVMT LD: Brief Visuospatial Memory Test, long delay; BVMT Tot: Brief Visuospatial Memory Test, total recall; COWAT: Controlled Oral Word Association Test; CVLT: California Verbal Learning Test; CVLT SD: California Verbal Learning Test, Short Delay Recall; LN Sequence: Letter and Number Sequencing.

Source: Derived by Bigler using data from Heitger et al., 2009 ([1], pp. 2850, 2868)

observation of responses), potential adoption of other sensitive non-invasive methods (e.g., eye movement analysis (Figure 9.1) or facial expression analysis), and virtual reality-based testing. Ultimately, since the goal is to assess the brain, the integration of neuropsychology with imaging (for instance, monitoring responses to neurocognitive probes with functional neuroimaging techniques) seems certain to increase the biological validity of assessments.

No gold standard exists for the assay of human brain function. No psychologist, psychiatrist, physiatrist, neurologist, neurosurgeon, or neuropathologist has ever achieved such insight. In the clinical realm, the closest approach to a gold standard is a cerebral blood flow study performed to determine brain death. Such studies seem reasonably accurate for distinguishing between the presence and absence of brain function. Beyond that yes-or-no determination, definitively assaying the present state of the brain – which may involve detecting more potential states than the estimated number of elemental particles in the universe – is beyond our most fantastic ambitions. Using observations such as neurological examinations, psychological

tests, imaging, or neuropathological examination cannot possibly unveil the detailed actuality of cerebration. Neuroscience, therefore, does not seek accurate correlations between those crude conventional observations and the truth of function. Human scholars are confined to seeking correlations between such observations and clinically meaningful aspects of function (e.g., dead or alive; conscious or unconscious, able or unable to learn). That inescapable fact trivializes debate about the relative value of observations made by different disciplines. Many approaches may help. None are ideal. Credit is due to every earnest effort.

Biological investigation turned its attention to molecular analysis many decades ago. Pathologists did not fret or abandon weighing the heart. Orthopedists did not fume and convert their tools for gardening. There is no threat, no harm, no loss to neuropsychology in discovering the limits of conventional testing. As the authors will review in this chapter, the architects of neuropsychology never claimed or likely expected that desktop testing would be perfectly sensitive and precise. Revealing subtleties of human biology beyond the resolution

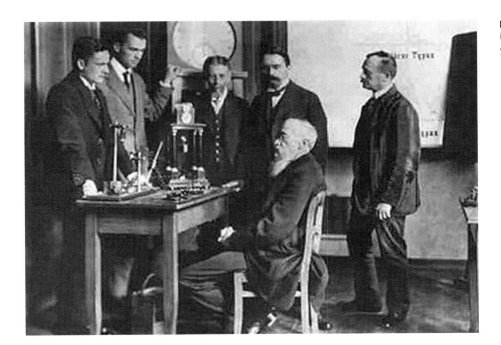

Fig. 9.2 Wilhelm Wundt (seated) with colleagues in his psychological laboratory, the first of its kind.
Source: unknown

of old technologies has been a noble and inevitable enterprise at least since Vesalius. Neuropsychologists are reinventing their field. Humans will benefit.

In this chapter we will:

1. briefly review the history of the neuropsychological assessment of CBI
2. discuss a transient moment of darkness in that history, when early scholars attempted to validate testing without biological standards
3. show how the discovery that concussion often leads to lasting neurobehavioral dysfunction helped to clarify those temporary errors and how a new generation is rapidly constructing a long-awaited, scientifically muscular neuropsychology.

A Brief History of Neuropsychological Assessment of Brain Injury

In order to put today's dramatic and gratifying reboot of neuropsychology in perspective, it will be helpful to briefly consider the history of the job title "neuropsychologist."

The historical origin of scientific psychology, like the purview and virtue of scientific psychology, may not be agreed upon any time soon. The physician Wilhelm Wundt (1832–1920)

arguably organized the first laboratory and graduate school for experimental psychology in 1879 (Figure 9.2) [3].

Wundt famously was among the first who explicitly sought to identify mind/brain relationships [4].[1,2] The philosopher Hermann Ebbinghaus (1850–1909) was also an early scientific empirical psychologist, yet for all his sophisticated observations of memory, he never investigated the cerebral bases of the behaviors he so carefully recorded, either by means of animal experiments or human clinicopathological correlation. The French neurologist Dax, French anthropologist Broca (who is typically given credit for Dax's discovery) and the German neurologist Wernicke are commonly credited with launching neuropsychological discovery in the sense of determining how focal brain damage impacts behavior. That work comports with Hallet's [8] definition: "Neuropsychology can be defined as the study of the relationship between brain structure and behavior" (p. 151). Yet it was not until his paper read before the Boston Society of Psychiatry and Neurology in 1936 [9] that Lashley used the term "neuropsychology" in reference to a discipline[3]:

Nearly a century of psychologizing concerning the cerebral cortex has added practically nothing to knowledge of its fundamental activities … It has been assumed that the properties of experience are represented at the level of some simple nervous activity or in single loci: sensations in

---

1 Unfortunately, Wundt abandoned his empiricist commitment when he championed introspection as if it were a scientific method – a conceptual derailment that resulted in the largely discredited approach called *structuralism* [3, 5].

2 Osler used the very same term in his address on the occasion of opening the Phipps Clinic at Johns Hopkins in 1913, but provided no definition or context [6, 7].

3 "When James B. Conant succeeded Lowell as president of Harvard University one of his early acts … was to appoint his first ad hoc committee to find the 'best psychologist in the world' to elect to a Chair at Harvard" [10]. Lashley was chosen. His 1937 publication reproduced his address to the Boston Society of Psychiatry and Neurology on March 19, 1936 on the occasion of his forthcoming ascendancy to Harvard Research Professor of Neuropsychology.

the sensory areas, volitional patterns in the motor regions or particular forms of intelligent behavior in restricted coordinating centers. Such conceptions of localization are oversimplified and must be abandoned. Nothing is known of the physiologic basis of conscious states, but there is some reason to believe that these states can be correlated only with the summated activity of all centers simultaneously excited. The position of Goldstein, that the functions of every center are dependent on its relations to the rest of the intact nervous system, cannot be too strongly emphasized in considering problems of neuropsychology.

([9], p. 386)

Lashley was clear: the incipient business of correlating gross structural brain lesions with behaviors was simple-minded. In this respect, he echoed Hughlings Jackson, who had long since remarked that finding that damage to a brain part correlates with behavior change is *not finding the part of the brain that mediates that behavior.* Lashley's illustrious Boston lecture was even more categorical in its dismissal of the simplistic notion that a given piece of cortex is responsible for a given behavior. Instead, like Jackson, he asserted that behavior is the product of the whole brain's integrated function.

Conceptions of the organization of mind or of behavior are based on a logical analysis of the activities of the total organism, and the final synthesis of nervous states which constitute these activities must transcend the excitation of any single center.

([9], p. 386)

Lashley, moreover, was wary of the then-creeping tendency of psychologists to dice up cognition into ostensibly differentiable "domains," such as memory, attention, and concentration. He did not so much reject the heuristic value of thus parcellating mind into abstract constructs as warn against attributing any of these parcels of mind to a place in the head, the injury of which deprived the patient of that moiety of mentation:

Thus, one must expect to find fractionings of behavior following organic lesions which cannot be expressed or understood in the current psychologic terminology. Indeed, psychologists are in scarcely better case than neurologists when it comes to interpreting the fundamental variables of behavior.

[9]

After Lashley's lecture in 1936 (but during the 44 subsequent years before neuropsychology became an accredited profession in North America) came Luria. Luria too rejected the "one site–one behavior" fallacy. As Hallet described the approach: "Luria envisaged that complex processes arise from the concerted and integrated action of separate and autonomous cortical and subcortical processing sites" [8]. For that reason, Luria also rejected what has come to be standard operating procedure in professional neuropsychology: the standardized administration of a battery of tests across subjects and examiners, followed by interpretation by reference to statistical analysis against norms derived from cohorts of "controls" and of persons who were labeled "brain-damaged" because they had been clinically diagnosed with a variety of unspecified neurological

disorders. Instead of attending to scores or percentile rankings, Luria was interested in *how* a patient dealt with a test challenge and *why* a patient responded as he or she did [8, 11].

Lashley's admonitions were not universally observed, perhaps because some clinicopathological aphasia studies and Penfield's intraoperative experiments lent credence to the notion that a given brain part did a given job [8, 11, 12]. Victoroff has called this paradigm the *Swiss Watch Fallacy of Behavioral Neurology* – the misguided notion that brains operate like mechanical devices (or, as Freud would have it, like Helmholtzian hydraulic machines) in which circumscribed pieces of tissue have fixed, assigned duties. As Hallet [8] put it: "Where, perhaps, such an approach has its limitations is in its attempt to 'locate' complex cognitions, such as reasoning and abstraction, to single sites of action while ignoring the possibility that such complexity is likely to reflect integrated function across separate processing sites." Yes, of course it represents an advance to discover the manifold aspects of behavior at risk when the medial temporal lobe dysfunctions. But one must never document a behavior and pronounce that a geometrically defined cluster of neurons and glia has been damaged, or point to a brain place and pronounce, for example, "these cells do emotional regulation."

As shown in Chapter 7, *Why Outcomes Vary*, evidence exists that cortical and subcortical localizations of functions are both highly individualized and genome-dependent [13, 14]. Moreover, in the case of TBI, even in animal experimentation no two injuries are biomechanically identical. Coupling this with the uniqueness of each individual's brain, one cannot expect all individuals with concussion to exhibit a biologically uniform brain change. Leaping ahead slightly, these discoveries help to explain not only why conventional neuropsychological tests cannot reliably localize brain change and also why a new neuropsychology, informed by the realization of brain individuality, will leverage knowledge of human cerebral variability to correlate test results not with tissue geometry, or fixed networks, or artificially delineated domains of cognition but with ever-dynamic function.

World War II

Although some soldiers with TBI survived during World War I, medical advances in the years from the early to mid 20th century led to a dramatic increase in the survivability of TBI during World War II. This in turn created a need to assess the mental consequences of those injuries. The first attempts at doing this employed popular methods of the day such as the Rorschach Ink Blot Test [15] and standardized intellectual, perceptual-motor, and ability tests [16–20]. Goldstein was among the pioneers who sought to correlate test results with both focal lesions and aspects of cognition [21, 22]. The beginnings of clinical neuropsychology can be traced to those utilitarian circumstances. Indeed, from the 1940s through the early 1970s, the term *neuropsychological* was usually used to refer to testing subjects thought to have some kind of "brain damage" and assessing how that *brain-damaged* group differed from either healthy, non-injured controls or from patients suffering from disorders that were – at that time – not regarded as neurological [23]. An assumption was made that certain patterns of psychological test performance reliably distinguished between those with and without "brain damage." Therefore, psychological test interpretation from the 1940s through the 1970s routinely included statements about "organicity" and "brain damage," as if an atypical response on a putative test of a psychological construct was proof of brain pathology. Indeed, tests like the Bender Visual Motor Gestalt test [24] were explicitly intended to make the "brain damage" versus "no brain damage" distinction – ostensibly differentiating organicity from normalcy. As this chapter will discuss below, classification of subjects into one of these two purportedly different groups was not always credible.

One consequence of Hitler's rise to power and World War II was the migration of Freudian psychoanalysts from Europe to North America. Hans Sachs (arrived 1932), Ernst Kris (1940), Heinz Hartmann (1941), and Rudolph Lowenstein (1942) became influential advocates. Frequent visits by Otto Rank and Anna Freud enhanced that influence. The American Psychiatric Association established a section on psychoanalysis in 1933. Some medical schools elevated analysts to positions of authority, because psychoanalysis was considered more scientific than alternatives such as mesmerism. In 1946 Menninger founded the Group for the Advancement of Psychiatry. In short, during the 1940s and 1950s, psychoanalysis was taken seriously in the United States [25–28]. So was its unwavering certainty that psychiatric disorders were not brain disorders. The relevance of that error to the history of neuropsychology, and specifically to the neuropsychological assessment of concussive brain injury, will become apparent momentarily.

The Beginnings of Professional Neuropsychology

In the same timeframe, psychoanalytic forces were also influencing North American psychology departments. Successful efforts had already been made to standardize and validate psychological tests, for instance, the IQ test of Alfred Binet and David Wechsler. The new attention to psychodynamic constructs inspired a search for tests – including projective tests – that would better plumb the depths of the human psyche. The assumption was that objectivity could be applied to measures like the Rorschach Inkblot Test, Thematic Apperception Test, draw-a-person test, incomplete sentences test, and others. In fact, some of the leaders who became key players in the development of neuropsychology, such as Arthur Benton [29] and Ralph Reitan [30], published their first papers on how to detect what was then referred to as "organicity" using the Rorschach.

For example, in 1955 Reitan [31] published "Evaluation of the postconcussion syndrome with the Rorschach test." Oliver Zangwill, considered by some to be a founder of the emerging field of neuropsychology in the United Kingdom, also investigated the use of the Rorschach in World War II patients with head injuries. But he concluded the following:

Among more specific psychodiagnostic methods which we have explored I shall mention only the Rorschach method

… Our experience with this procedure has been rather less happy than that of some of its more zealous advocates. In rare cases this method has provided important data bearing on post-traumatic deterioration or has given us evidence of an abnormal personality make-up complicating the organic reaction. In the majority of posttraumatic cases, however, the test findings have added little of real value to expert psychiatric assessment.

([32], p. 248)

It was 1951 when Donald Hebb published "The role of neurological ideas in psychology" in the *Journal of Personality* [33]. As odd as that title may seem to us today, in the psychodynamic world the brain did not play a central role in anything emotional, until it became "organic," a term associated with unequivocal evidence of a structural brain problem, such as epilepsy or hemiplegia. The common attitude regarding brain damage and behavior during that era is captured by the following statement from a 1947 abnormal psychology textbook by James D. Page [34]: "Head injuries and gunshot wounds involving damage to the brain occasionally produce mental disturbances, but such injuries are not an important cause of mental disease."

This was also the era during which frontal lobotomy and leucotomy were hailed as effective treatments for a variety of mental illnesses. Indeed, those cases were among the first in which IQ testing, personality testing, and the Rorschach were administered in a pre–post-operative experiment [35, 36]. The observation that in some cases there was no change in IQ, or even "improvement," was a factor that led to the continued use of these neurosurgical techniques for two more decades. Tragically, it was assumed that these psychological tests "proved" that brain damage was not occurring.

What is interesting about this history is that Zangwill [37, 38], Benton [39], Leonard Diller [40], and Ralph Reitan [30] – who would become key players in the emerging field of neuropsychology in the 1960s and 1970s – soon recognized the limitations of tests like the Rorschach and began their initiatives to develop more effective measures to assess cognitive function.

Part of the impetus to investigate the validity of psychological tests in head-injured patients in this mid-20th-century era was the influence of returning soldiers from World War II, the Korean War and the Vietnam War. The soldiers complained of impaired "thinking," "memory," not being able to work – symptoms that fell into the domain of "psychology." This led Zangwill [20] to write in 1945:

It is not uncommonly supposed that the psychologist is the fortunate possessor of an esoteric tool which in deference to current fashion I shall call a *mental test*. Now, a mental test is often conceived to measure in a. more or less accurate way some specific ability, aptitude, or trait. It is apt to be regarded as the exclusive property of the psychologist, who alone is held competent to wield and interpret it. An attitude of this kind to psychological work is both unfortunate and misleading. Strictly speaking, nothing psychological is truly measurable, and a so-called mental test is nothing more than a device for eliciting some specific psychological response under controlled conditions of examination.

([20], p. 248)

Zangwill went on:

When we turn to functions such as memory, intelligence, and thought, and the immensely complicated repertoire of habits and skills to which they give rise in the educated individual, it is plain not only that the normal limits of individual variation are very wide but also that the potential directions of breakdown are many and varied. Simple clinical tests are in consequence seldom sufficient in assessing the psychological sequelae of cerebral lesion, and the demand for more highly controlled methods is easy to understand.

([20], p. 248)

Although written over 70 years ago, this statement remains true today.

Hence, psychologists initially applied their newly devised tests to patients with known neurological abnormalities. Recall that this was prior to neuroimaging with resolution higher than that afforded by skull X-ray, pneumoencephalography, or technetium-99m scintigraphy, and therefore the neurological groups had to be identified based on coarse criteria (e.g., a lateralized stroke based on motor, language, and perceptual testing by a neurologist, or clinical diagnosis of a degenerative disease like Alzheimer's, or electroencephalogram (EEG)-confirmed epilepsy, or head trauma with obvious neurological findings). None of these conditions are subtle but none produce discrete, uniform focal lesions. In the light of this problem – the imprecision of antemortem neurological tissue diagnosis combined with the realization that specific facets of mind do not necessarily spring from specific pieces of brain – the reader can anticipate the trouble to come: how might the new profession of neuropsychology ever validate its tests?

A Shadow Passed

The basic question has been the validity of the inferences made from these measures of external behavior to central nervous system functioning in the classification of patients with cerebral pathology. Closely connected with this problem is the practical question of the use of these measures, if the results are merely a redundant formulation of that which is medically known.

Stuss, 1973 [41], p. viii

Figure 9.3 illustrates a phenomenon that every neurologist and neuropsychologist encounters routinely: a patient presents with neurological and cognitive complaints. "Her comprehensive neuropsychological evaluation was normal" ([42], p. 2161). Yet imaging indisputably demonstrates multiple types of gross anatomical and marked functional brain abnormalities. We use this non-TBI case merely to illustrate a point. There is but one objective interpretation – this patient has structural damage and normal psychological test results, so those tests are insensitive to such damage. It is important that the new generations of clinicians accept and embrace the implications of such data.

Like pneumoencephalography, and 7-T MRI, and Hitachi's seven-ton scanning transmission electron holography microscope, neuropsychological assessment does not detect all brain dysfunction. This is no mark of shame or obsolescence. Overt behavior, but not thought or subjective feeling, is accessible to observation. Some aspects of brain structure and function are accessible to observation. Different methods are better for these two very different but complementary purposes, neither of which may ever fully account for the essence of human mentation. So we choose the phenomenon we most wish to characterize and choose the method best suited to that goal. Which is more specific for the assessment of structural brain abnormality: 18 h of neuropsychological testing or five minutes of brain imaging? Imaging is almost always superior. Which of those two is more specific for assessing behavioral idiosyncrasy? Desktop testing is always superior. These conclusions should not be a topic of quarrel. Yet quarrel arose. Ironically, the quest to establish a solid scientific footing for neuropsychology derailed it for a generation.

When the late, great behavioral neurologist D. Frank Benson visited Dr. Luria, he inquired, "May I please see your laboratory?"

Luria responded, "This is my laboratory." He gestured modestly toward a wooden table (Benson, personal communication, 1988).

Luria was not a scientist. He spoke eloquently about the patterns of interacting brain areas that constitute functional systems, and how such systems are engaged to respond to a cognitive challenge. He presciently recognized that brain parts do not have assigned roles. The brain, instead, is a complex of networks. A given locus might belong to many such networks; thus, damage to a brain place is likely to impact multiple functional systems and impair multiple behaviors. He posited one might isolate a locus of brain dysfunction by detecting distinctive patterns of qualitative changes in performance that would logically narrow localization to a node where the relevant functional systems converge. He made little effort to confirm that his putative functional systems existed or represented differentiable elements of cerebral processing. He made no effort to systematize his test administration procedure or to determine whether any given test results reflected any given brain change. His theory-driven, seat-of-the-pants approach could surely inspire hypothesis testing but could not possibly serve as the foundation for a scientific discipline. The founders of Western neuropsychology knew this. They sought to forge a steely science from Luria's pig iron materials. Unfortunately, the early attempts to contrive a scientific neuropsychology probably did the field more harm than good.

Four historical phenomena virtually coincided as neuropsychology came of age in the late 1970s:

1. an effort to legitimize the discipline
2. an effort to validate desktop testing
3. the implosion of the organic/functional dichotomy
4. the invention of computed tomography.

The synchronism of these phenomena perhaps explains the delay in securing a solid footing for this important new

Magnetic resonance imaging (MRI) and fluorodeoxyglucose positron emission tomography (FDG-PET) in a 71-year-old woman evaluated for persistent and non-progressive memory difficulties for several years

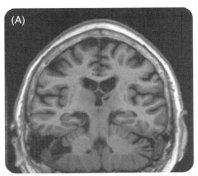

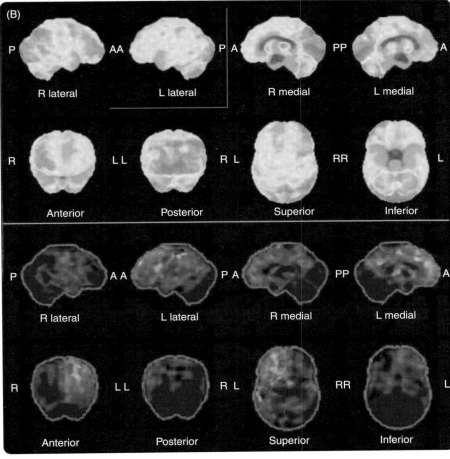

Fig. 9.3 (A) Head MRI shows a chronic left medial thalamic infarct, as well as chronic right caudate head and left corona radiata infarcts. (B) Top, three-dimensional stereotactic surface projection of the patient's FDG-PET scan shows hypometabolism in the left medial thalamus, in addition to the left medial prefrontal, lateral frontal, and posterior cingulate regions. Bottom, statistical map showing regions of significant hypometabolism relative to age-matched controls with green and yellow regions indicating FDG-PET magnitude being 3 and 4 s d, respectively, lower than control subjects. A: anterior; L: left; P: posterior; R: right. [A black and white version of this figure will appear in some formats. For the color version, please refer to the plate section.]

Source: Golden et al., 2016 [42] with permission from Wolters Kluwer Health

sub-specialty. The establishment of several boards to certify new neuropsychologists served the first need. Validating the tests remains a work in progress. The realization that no organic/functional dichotomy exists hamstrung most of the early validation efforts. The invention of the computed tomography (CT) scan, which should have accelerated validation, failed to meet those sanguine expectations. As a result, a shadow passed over the land. The first decades of neuropsychology were compromised by controversy because two simple errors temporarily derailed this vital enterprise: (1) a clinical diagnosis of neurological disease is evidence of brain damage,

and (2) disabling psychiatric disease is evidence of a biologically normal brain.

The Well-Intentioned, Doomed Quest for Validation

Consider the foundational studies cited as evidence for the validity of neuropsychological tests and batteries. In the 1950s and 1960s, some attention was given to demonstrating that single tests revealed brain damage. The Trail Making tests were among the first to be studied. In a seminal 1958 publication

[43], Reitan compared the performance of subjects with "brain damage" to that of healthy control subjects. His damaged cohort was diverse.[4] That paper reported that testing identified 89% of "brain damaged" persons.

However, as Stuss hinted in his 1973 Master's thesis [41], little is gained if a test redundantly reports that which is already known. A better research approach, it was thought, was to determine whether Trails could correctly differentiate "organic" from "functional" disease. To that end, Goldstein and Neuringer [44] compared the performance of persons with brain damage to those with schizophrenia. "The 30 brain-damaged Ss represented a wide range of diagnoses including cases of cerebral vascular accident, cerebral arteriosclerosis, multiple sclerosis, etc. … they were carefully screened for the absence of schizophrenic conditions" ([44], p. 348). The pattern of response was somewhat different – regarded as evidence of discriminatory success. Other studies followed suit, comparing the results of either healthy controls or "functionally" disordered persons with those persons alleged to have "brain damage" [45–48].

Another approach was to employ batteries of tests and serious efforts were made to find a set of tests that could be administered in a practical time frame and would better detect the presence of brain damage than any single test. Halstead [49, 50], for example, published promising results from studies of 27 tests with 237 brain-damaged subjects. Studies of Halstead's battery were replicated and advanced by others such as Reitan [51], Matthews et al. [52], and Vega and Parsons [53]. Again, "brain damage" did not refer to a particular medical problem and could not be confirmed in many cases beyond the best guesses of neurologists and neurosurgeons. Brain damage referred to a mix of conditions. The Vega and Parsons cohort, for instance, included subjects with cerebrovascular disease, trauma, tumor, degenerative disease, neuro-infections, prefrontal lobotomy, and seizures.

By the late 1970s two batteries were competing for pre-eminence: the Halstead–Reitan Neuropsychological Battery [54] and the Luria–Nebraska Neuropsychological Battery [55, 56]. Golden and his colleagues [56] became among the most-cited authorities on the validation of neuropsychological batteries, although their process of doing so was excoriated by Adams in a review [57]. Golden was attempting to do what Christensen, who had studied with Luria, did not believe was proper: to distill Luria's approach down to a standardized, lock-step psychometric test protocol, rather than supporting the flexible, individualized, qualitative assessment that Luria and Christensen advocated. That concern did not impede Golden. In a 1978 paper [58], he and his colleagues stated, "The intention of the present study was to use the material presented by Luria … and Christensen … to form a standardized, objectively

scored version of Luria's neuropsychological procedures" (p. 1259). A total of 285 tests were administered, of which 253 were judged to discriminate between the neurological and control groups. What medically differentiated those groups?

> Fifty subjects had confirmed neurological diagnosis made on the basis of medical exams alone by a qualified physician, usually a neurologist or neurosurgeon. The control subjects had a variety of medical problems including back injuries, infectious diseases, and chronic cases of pain.
>
> ([58], p. 1263)

The standard for confirming a neurological disorder was thus some sort of medical examination. Neurological examinations lack the sensitivity or reliability to detect or diagnose neurological disorders [59–64]. Hence, literally none of the subjects with "confirmed neurological diagnosis" had confirmed neurological diagnoses. The control subjects were also selected without regard to normal versus abnormal brain function. Febrile infectious disease and chronic pain are routinely associated with brain dysfunction and cognitive impairment. Although infection itself does not predict neurobehavioral disorders, infection with fever is known to produce cognitive deficits, delirium, or psychosis, apparently due to the central nervous system effects of inflammatory cytokines [65–68]. Similarly, chronic pain is well known to impact cerebral function and cause multiple cognitive impairments [69–72]. A battery that fails to detect such patients fails as both a test of brain dysfunction and as a test of cognition.

In another paper Golden investigated the Halstead–Reitan battery [73]. He examined 116 patients referred for neuropsychological testing "to differentiate between a possible organic or psychotic condition." Subjects were classified as brain-damaged on the basis of "such evidence as a neurological exam, medical tests such as electroencephalogram, brain scan, and pneumoencephalogram, surgical results, history, and other information" ([73], p. 1045). Although no neurological diagnoses were reported, this method was perhaps superior for classifying brain damage than the method in the previously described study. However, the control group consisted of subjects with "schizophrenia or mixed psychosis" diagnosed on the basis of examination by "a physician, usually a psychiatrist" ([73], p. 1045). The report indicates successful differentiation between "organic" and "nonorganic" conditions – a false distinction.

As mentioned above, the early validation of neuropsychological tests was conducted during the swan song of the functional/organic dichotomy. Although biological psychiatry had been advancing since about 1950, some in the late 1970s maintained the belief that major mental disorders were not brain disorders. That belief apparently misled several well-intentioned neuropsychologists to use psychiatric patients

---

[4]   "The brain-damaged group was heterogeneous with respect to the types of lesions involved, including the following: multiple sclerosis, 39; traumatic head injury, 33; diffuse cerebrovascular disease, 25; cerebrovascular accident, 20; intrinsic brain tumor, 20; cerebral atrophy, 11; epilepsy following head trauma, 8; extrinsic brain tumor, 7; cerebral abscess, 7; epilepsy (idiopathic), 6; epilepsy (surgically treated), 5; subdural hematoma, 5; two each with congenital brain anomaly, cerebellar degenerative disease, dementia paralytica, encephalitis, and acoustic neuroma; and one each with porencephalic cyst, optic nerve adhesions, barbiturate intoxication, and thalamic tumor" (Reitan, 1958 [43] , p. 271).

as "control" subjects. We know now that schizophrenia is an organic condition, often associated with disabling cognitive deficits [74–78]. A test battery that miscategorizes such a serious organic disorder cannot be regarded as sensitive to either brain dysfunction or to cognitive impairment.

What's more, those early studies of neuropsychological test validation employed research protocols that would likely be rejected in this century. The tests were administered and scored by people who knew the presumptive diagnoses and classification of each subject and who were motivated to find a difference between groups. Bias seems likely. Slightly more recent literature sought to correlate psychological test results with CT scans. This failed to rescue the validation project, since, as we now know, CT scans are insensitive to many types of disabling or fatal brain disease.

In briefest summary, early neuropsychology was at the mercy of insensitive neurological diagnostic techniques, insensitive imaging technologies, and fallacious nosology. Their test batteries were validated by comparing persons diagnosed with a wide variety of unconfirmed neurological disorders with persons diagnosed with other (also unconfirmed) disorders that also often cause central nervous system dysfunction and impair cognition. Those empirical efforts were doomed from the outset.

One must be sympathetic. Twentieth-century innovators were eager to establish neuropsychology on a scientific footing, but were hampered by dependence on neurologists and neurosurgeons whose diagnoses of "brain injury" often rested on educated guesswork. Moreover, neuropsychology's early years corresponded with the last gasp of psychodynamic psychiatry and the lingering influence of the false dichotomy between organic and functional illness. Imagine the challenge of validating a desktop test to detect organic brain change when (1) the only credible confirmation of that change was autopsy and (2) many clinicians assumed psychiatric illness equaled biologically normal brain. Of course those tests and batteries do not reliably distinguish between the presence and absence of organic brain damage! Of course they are insensitive to all but the most gross changes! Of course they are unreliable for localization! The tests we inherited were carefully selected to distinguish between:

1. persons with randomly lumped mixtures of unconfirmed, often unspecified, suspected brain dysfunctions of inconsistent type, size, location, and severity versus
2. persons with mixtures of other serious, also unconfirmed, brain dysfunctions that, at that time in history, were not recognized as brain dysfunctions.

Psychological tests selected half a century ago to distinguish between cohorts with one wide array of brain problems and another wide array of brain problems could not possibly be expected to detect the presence or absence of brain problems, especially if those problems were subtle or heterogeneous. That would be equivalent to stating, "I selected my test to tell me whether there is a fish or a crab on the line. Therefore (although I have yet to test this with any rigor), it tells me whether there is anything on the line, or nothing."

Despite these limitations, both the Halstead–Reitan and the Luria–Nebraska were used to investigate "neurocognitive" sequelae from mild TBI [79–82]. Two shortcomings predictably hamstrung this effort. First, given the above limitations, a battery of neuropsychological measures designed to assess the most coarse aspects of cognition and behavior in a controlled laboratory setting would not be expected to detect the cognitive effects of concussion. Second, tests focused on cognition – e.g., memory, attention, or language – would not be expected to detect the most disabling post-concussive problems – psychiatric disorders.

Damage Versus Dysfunction

Semantics drove a less momentous detour from credibility.

Sometimes one still encounters a written report that summarizes test results with a comment about the presence or absence of "brain damage." Testing is valuable, but not for that. Throughout this text, the present authors and editors have strived, trudging through the sucking mire of convention, for semantic rigor. Terms of art (e.g., "concussion") are used without universal consensus in clinical medicine. This delays progress. Another such term is "damage." Neuropsychologists need not concern themselves with brain damage. It is largely irrelevant to clinical practice. However, for two decades, apprentice neuropsychologists were taught to phrase their findings in terms of likelihood of *damage* [45, 83–85].

An analogy might help. You are stuck in a blinding snowstorm 64 miles from the nearest habitation. The temperature has dropped below 0°F, the wolves are howling, and your car will not start due to an inopportune change in state from liquid to solid somewhere in the fuel line. Tragically, you are soon to die. Is your car damaged? Of course not. It is dysfunctional.

In the third edition of her classic text, *Neuropsychological Assessment*, Lezak stated that "Clinical neuropsychology is an applied science concerned with the behavioral expression of brain dysfunction" ([86], p. 7). The present authors heartily support that terminology and urge abandonment of the bootless colloquialism, *damage*. Even in the heady domain of advanced brain imaging, assessing *damage* may not be the most meaningful goal or the best predictor of outcome. Dysfunction, rapidly becoming easier to visualize, better correlates with clinical disorder and human distress.

To Every Thing There is a Season

CBI is dynamic. The brain undergoes constant remodeling for an unknown and variable period of time after visitation by external force. Previous chapters have attempted to summarize what is known about the ensuing battle between hurtful and helpful biology. In most cases, functional impairment with clinically obvious deviation from baseline activities peaks early. This dynamism has implications for neuropsychology. Assessment methods suitable for detecting early change – such as non-invasive observations of behavior in response to given stimuli – must not be assumed to be sensitive to residual change in the fast-healing brain. The same principle applies to the neurological examination, the neuropsychological examination, and many forms of neuroimaging.

For example, the Glasgow Coma Scale (GCS) is sometimes useful in the hyperacute stage of concussion, seconds to hours, because it distinguishes between coma and not-coma. As previously explained in this volume, the GCS does not diagnose. It does not measure brain damage. It does not predict outcome. But it systematizes bedside observation of the crudest sort, perhaps increasing interrater reliability regarding the most obvious differences between levels of consciousness. This can be life-saving. Documented declines on the GCS are often the canary in the mine that alerts hospital staff to scan and operate. Typical concussions cause symptoms lasting for more than 24 h. But, by then, the GCS has almost always exhausted its utility.

Similarly, a CT scan is especially useful in the emergency ward after a concussion. It helps to triage patients to the appropriate level of care, sometime detects changes that require neurosurgical intervention, and is often reassuring when negative. Should the patient deteriorate during the first week, the CT can also be life-saving. Typical concussions cause brain changes that can be detected long after the first week, but by then the CT scan has almost always exhausted its utility. The bedside neurological examination often detects suboptimal mentation, disequilibrium, or eye movement changes for hours to weeks after concussion. It infrequently detects ongoing brain dysfunction beyond three to six months. By then, it too has exhausted its utility.

In the same way, neuropsychological testing is sometimes useful in the subacute stage of concussion – perhaps during the first several weeks. It confirms the patient's subjective reports of cognitive difficulty. It helps to guide interactions with the patient, assessing the level of understanding and capacity to consent. It may help focus the earliest stages of therapy (although change is so rapid that a rehabilitation program designed on the basis of testing at three weeks may be inapplicable three weeks later). Like the GCS and the neurological examination, neuropsychological testing does not diagnosis brain damage, localize brain damage, or predict functional outcome. It infrequently detects "abnormal" cognition beyond three months (in part because few patients have baseline testing with which to compare, such that average scores are misinterpreted as recovery in above-average patients, testing is always done in a laboratory setting with one-on-one test administration, sheltered from wind, rain, and society, so that it never approximates real-world environments).

Yet retesting at that point can be clinically helpful in many ways. It may identify the minority with persistent marked cognitive impairments. It may guide rehabilitation, family adjustment, and community reintegration, if those are still needed. It may reveal hints of somatization or even malingering. However, in the experience of the present authors, the greatest value of neuropsychological testing at the three- to 12-month point may be this: the neurologist, family doctor, pediatrician, and physiatrist have grinned and pronounced, "You are all better!" At that point, the neuropsychologist may step in, detecting and responding to the most commonly disabling and commonly overlooked long-term problem: emotional distress whether or not it is associated with cognitive complaints.

The point is not to fault this approach but simply to clarify the limits of resolution and the season of most fruitful data harvesting. Just as no one is well served by inflating the sensitivity and specificity of the CT or scalp EEG, no one is well served by efforts to inflate the sensitivity and specificity of neuropsychological testing. And just as CT and EEG remain irreplaceable for some purposes, so does neuropsychological testing. Each assessment tool has its season of greatest utility. None are very useful outside of that season. Heitger's study, shown in Figure 9.1 of this chapter, is helpful for illustrating in a readily accessible way the difference between the value of conventional neuropsychological testing of cognitive capacity during the first several weeks post CBI and thereafter. As suggested by a host of previously reviewed meta-analyses, by three months post injury, desktop testing has exhausted its contribution to assessment of cognitive issues in most cases of CBI.

This cannot possibly be considered a failure of neuropsychology! No more would one condemn the neurologist whose patellar tapping missed neuro-brucellosis. The only failure would be unscientifically inflating the specificity and sensitivity or exaggerating the season of utility of our respective methods. In a sense, encounters with concussion were paradigm shifting for neuropsychology. If the strengths and weaknesses of this approach had not been obvious before, if the research priorities for the next two decades had not been apparent, they have now become more clear.

Neuropsychology Tackles, and is Tackled By, Concussion

In a tale of unintended consequences, studies of concussion may prove critical to reorienting neuropsychology. Paradoxically, the discovery that conventional testing is blind to the long-term effects of concussion seems likely to liberate the discipline's heretofore unrealized potential.

In the 1970s, at roughly the same point in history when neuropsychology was seeking authority and validation, some members of this new fraternity began studying CBI. This was, perhaps, a uniquely awkward choice of research focus. Having failed to establish that desktop testing sensitively detects or reliably distinguishes between either the presence or absence of brain lesions or between ablative brain disease, mass brain disease, or neuropsychiatric brain disease, a higher priority might have been finding evidence that single tests or batteries reliably detected at least *some* type of autopsy-confirmed brain disease before tackling subtle forms of dysfunction that remain, to this day, beyond the reach of any *in vivo* confirmatory method.

This volume has already described one unfortunate consequence of the early validation studies: some neuropsychologists interpreted the results as evidence that desktop testing could detect brain damage. The data were available from the beginning. It is not clear why they were sometimes misinterpreted in this way, except (in the memorable phraseology of Alan Greenspan) perhaps due to irrational exuberance. Nonetheless, some studies suggested authentic utility. As previously reviewed, in 1974 Gronwall and Wrightson [87] used psychological tests designed to assess attention and memory in concussion survivors. Arguably, that was the first time it was demonstrated that psychometrically derived test scores were differentially lower in those with histories of CBI when compared to those without such histories. For more than a decade, subsequent studies employed desktop testing in the hope of assessing the trajectory of recovery after CBI. The results were admittedly highly inconsistent, and it is no surprise that few scholars succeeded in detecting significant functional abnormalities beyond several months post injury. Again, no fault attends these earnest efforts. The only issue is interpretation. For committed defenders of the sensitivity of the old tests, absence of abnormal test results was satisfactory proof of absence of brain damage. A crisis of sorts ensued. Contention arose between those who insisted that testing was perfectly sensitive and that no brain damage could escape its piercing gaze and those who adopted more moderate views informed by both knowledge of the flaws in the validation process and evidence of persistent brain dysfunction using other assessment methods.

The ensuing debates and back-and-forth commentary as to whether symptoms/deficits persist and can be detected by neuropsychological techniques have been addressed in the Introduction and in Chapters 1, 5, and 6. Even today, neuropsychologists do not share a firm consensus position on this matter. Many acknowledge the limitations of conventional desktop testing and are eager to transcend the old actuarial/ localizationist paradigm in favor of more sophisticated concepts informed by neuroimaging. Some hew to the premise – never supported by founding figures such as Jackson, Lashley, or Luria – that test scores correlate with brain injuries. And a few actually express what is, by implication, a strong and vocal sentiment against pursuing neuropsychological testing in the assessment of the CBI patient. For example, as late as 2013 Greiffenstein [88] declared that mild traumatic brain injury "is a self-contained condition that resolves quickly without special treatment, a generally accepted conclusion by fair-minded neuropsychologists" (p. xiii). In addition to being factually erroneous, that position implies there is no need for neuropsychological assessment, other than to prove the tester's personal opinion that no deficit has occurred or that the patient is malingering.

Extremism aside, a sober analysis helps explain the strengths and weaknesses of conventional testing for CBI.

The textbook by Lezak et al. [89] provides a comprehensive review of the major neuropsychological measures currently in use, including neuropsychological measures commonly employed in the assessment of TBI. Unfortunately, none of the standard, traditional clinical neuropsychological tests were developed to specifically assess CBI. For example, the Rey Auditory Verbal Learning Test, comprised of 15 different words given to the patient at a rate of approximately one per second, is one of the most commonly used measures for assessing short-term verbal learning and memory. The problem in using this measure and others like it in CBI is illustrated by the study by Heitger et al. [1]. This is arguably one of the best-designed studies examining neuropsychological outcome in CBI using traditional neuropsychological measures. The reasons: (1) the study was conducted in New Zealand, which has a uniform health care system with equal access to services, such that the cohort is more likely to be representative; (2) the investigators controlled for depression and symptom/performance validity (and participants were not in litigation); and (3) the "control" sample comprised individuals who had initially sustained a CBI, but who were asymptomatic and presumed to have "recovered." The main dependent variable in the study was eye tracking, which was found to be distinctly abnormal in the symptomatic CBI group; nonetheless a comprehensive battery of neuropsychological measures was administered.

In the 15 Rey Auditory Verbal Learning Test, words are administered over five trials, with an open, free-recall format after each trial, although the words are always administered in the same order. At the conclusion of the fifth trial, a distractor list is administered and recall of the distractor items queried, followed by a delayed recall and recognition trial. Only retention of the distractor list differed significantly between the two groups. However, despite being statistically significant, the overall group mean difference was miniscule – about one less word recalled by the CBI residual group compared to the CBI recovered group.

When one factors in test–retest variability of the measure, which may be one to two words, and the fact that depression or pain may suppress verbal memory performance, such subtle differences in a neuropsychological measure would make it impossible for the clinician to use that information in a meaningful manner with CBI patients. Far less would one be able to offer any meaningful commentary on the size, location, or prognosis of the dysfunction! Figure 9.1, which introduced this chapter, vividly illustrates the critical point that testing has real but limited sensitivity. While this example focused on a memory task, similar criticisms can be raised with other traditional tasks and domains.

The problem is even greater when one considers the implications of physiological and advanced neuroimaging metrics. For example, Prichep et al. [90] and Gay et al. [91] have both shown that quantitative EEG differences existed in individuals with sport-related concussion when compared to matched non-concussed athletes, even though none of the neuropsychological measures differed. In another controlled EEG study, Sponheim et al. [92] examined nine soldiers who had survived mild blast-related concussions. At an average of 2.7 years after injury, neuropsychological testing failed to detect differences compared with healthy controls. In contrast, electrophysiological measures revealed evidence of persistent discoordination of lateral frontal lobe interhemispheric function.

Similar findings have been made with magnetoencephalography [93] and with advanced MRI techniques [94].[5] For example, Westfall et al. [95] performed functional MRI (fMRI) scanning during a working-memory

---

[5]   Readers will find a wealth of relevant and somewhat worrisome imaging data in the chapters in this volume on structural and functional neuroimaging of human concussive brain injury: Chapters 6, 12, 15, 16, and 22.

Task-related functional magnetic resonance imaging shows significant abnormalities up to five years post concussion

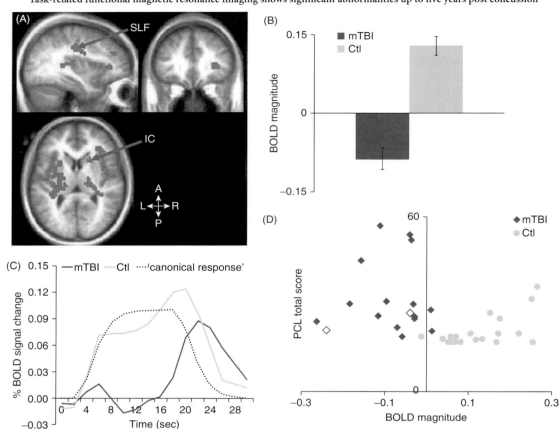

Fig. 9.4 Magnitudes and time courses from large region of interest (ROI). Magnitudes and time courses extracted from voxels demonstrating significant differences between patients and controls. (A) Selected brain slices showing voxels with a significantly reduced blood oxygen level-dependent (BOLD) signal in mild traumatic brain injury (mTBI) patients relative to controls. The set of all voxels showing significant differences formed an "abnormal" ROI. A: anterior; I: internal capsule; L: left; P: posterior; R: right; SLF: superior longitudinal fasciculus. (B) BOLD magnitudes from the abnormal ROI, averaged across tasks. Error bars represent standard error of the mean. (C) The time course of the BOLD signal in the abnormal ROI. The canonical hemodynamic response function used in the analysis to compute the BOLD magnitudes also is shown (labeled "canonical response"). (D) Scatterplot of BOLD magnitude values from the abnormal ROI for mTBI patients (red diamond) and controls (blue circles) vs. Post-traumatic Stress Disorder Checklist (PCL-C) total score. "Complex mTBI" (mTBI patients with positive radiological findings and/or antegrade post-traumatic amnesia longer than 24 h) are indicated by open diamonds. [A black and white version of this figure will appear in some formats. For the color version, please refer to the plate section.]

Source: Astafiev et al., 2015 [96]. Reproduced with permission from Mary Ann Liebert, Inc.

task in 19 adolescents who had suffered "mTBI" three to 12 months before (average = 7.5 months) and 19 matched healthy controls. There were no cognitive differences between the groups, yet activation was abnormal in the concussed subjects up to one year post injury. Those authors concluded: "Differences in brain activation in the mTBI group so long after injury may indicate residual alterations in brain function much later than would be expected based on the typical pattern of natural recovery, which could have important clinical implications."

Even more strikingly, in a study with much longer follow-up, Astafiev et al. [96] studied 45 victims of "mTBI" from three months to five years post injury. fRMI was obtained during an ocular pursuit task. Although neuropsychological measures could not distinguish patients from controls, CBI survivors reliably exhibited abnormal blood oxygen level-dependent signals. Figure 9.4 illustrates those results. As the authors remarked regarding the scatterplot (4d): "A remarkable separation was observed between mTBI and healthy controls" (p. 1263).[6]

Note that, in each of these imaging studies conducted months to years post concussion, neuropsychological testing failed to detect abnormalities, yet imaging revealed persistent brain changes. Sinopoli et al. [97] are among many neuropsychologists who have concluded, "it may be that neuropsychological tests, which typically target isolated areas of functioning, are not sensitive enough to detect long-term impairments following mTBI." As those authors discussed the logical implications of this research:

If mTBI is truly a transient "minor" neurological
disturbance, then the injured children should perform

---

[6] Readers seeking an overview of MR findings long after CBI may look to Chapters 12, 16, and 22.

similarly to non-injured controls with no observable group differences in brain activation. Conversely, if mTBI causes persistent neural dysfunction, then abnormalities should be measurable in behavioral performance, brain imaging, or both, with any group differences in fMRI signaling potentially reflecting differences in the recruitment of processing resources, compensatory mechanisms, or changes in cognitive effort/control required to complete the tasks.

([97], p. 1844)

Sporting a Facade of Consensus

One more historical development unfortunately delayed the passing of the shadow over the credibility of neuropsychology: the emergence of the sub-sub-specialty of sports neuropsychology.

The need for attention to athletic brain injury is indisputable. The goal of understanding such injuries is important to public health and social well-being. Evidence suggests that the repetitive concussions suffered by athletes in many sports (whether or not the activity is formally designated as a "contact" sport) creates special circumstances. Experimental research strongly suggests that a neurometabolic window of vulnerability exists for up to a week after a typical concussion. A second or third injury during that period catches neurons at an apogee of defenselessness. Ionic perturbation, membrane disruption, and an energy crisis tend to provoke apoptosis. Neurodegenerative change apparently seeds the brain in ways that may cause later dementia. One must strive to figure this out and inform rational policies. That, however, requires scientifically based consensus.

In the 1990s, as outlined earlier in this volume, several authorities began organizing "consensus" conferences focusing on sports-related concussions. The resulting group publications tend to include reviews regarding neuropsychological assessment and practice, but only for sports-related CBI. Whether the participants have been authentically representative of experts in concussion, and whether the reports emerging from these events, authored by a small subset of individuals, accurately reflect the sentiments of the whole body are questions that compel caution in interpreting the published conclusions. Similarly, statements on this topic have been generated by several major neuropsychological organizations [98], various medical organizations [99–101], and the recently founded Sports Neuropsychology Society. Despite the well-known flaws of the validation process, despite the burgeoning literature demonstrating that desktop testing often fails to detect lesions that are instantly apparent on imaging, despite the multiplicity of reports that post-concussive symptoms commonly persist long after testing has normalized, all of these publications and organizations support neuropsychological assessment without qualification. The rhetoric typically implies that testing confirms acute impairment and prompt, complete recovery – with the exception of "difficult" cases. *Difficult* is used for those who continue to complain, a phenomenon often attributed in these reports to pre-morbid emotional frailty. However, such opinions are based on the false assumption that traditional testing is sensitive in the chronic phase. It is not.

Table 9.1 Paper-and-pencil neuropsychological tests used to assess National Football League football players [102, 103]

Domain of function	Tests
Intelligence tests	• Wechsler Adult Intelligence Scale, 4th edition (WAIS-IV) • Wechsler Intelligence Scale for Children, 4th edition (WISC-IV)
Neurocognitive batteries	• Repeatable Battery for the Assessment of Neuropsychological Status (RBANS)
Learning and memory	• Brief Visuospatial Memory Test, revised (BVMT-R) • California Verbal Learning Test, 2nd edition (CVLT-II) • Hopkins Verbal Learning Test, revised (HVLT-R) • Rey–Osterrieth Complex Figure Test (RCFT) • Wechsler Memory Scale, 4th edition (WMS-IV)
Attention/concentration	• Connors Continuous Performance Test, 2nd edition (CPT-II) • Trail Making Test – part A
Processing speed	• Paced Auditory Symbol Addition Test (PASAT) • Symbol Digit Modalities Test (SDMT)
Language	• Animal Naming Test • Boston Naming Test • Controlled Oral Word Association Test
Executive function	• Delis Kaplan Executive Function System (DKEFS) • Trail Making Test – part B • Wisconsin Card Sorting Test (WCST)
Effort	• Dot Counting Test • Rey-15 Item Test (Rey-15) • Test of Memory Malingering (TOMM) • Word Memory Test (WMT)
Mood	• Beck Depression Inventory, 2nd edition (BDI–II) • Beck Anxiety Inventory (BAI) • Minnesota Multiphasic Personality Inventory, 2nd edition, restructured form (MMPI–II RF) • Personality Assessment Inventory (PAI)
Self-report	• Behavior Rating Inventory of Executive Function (BRIEF)

Table 9.1, for instance, lists a compilation of paper-and-pencil tests administered to National Football League players in 13 studies [102] These tests, on the whole, were devised after 1920 but before the invention of the CT scan. None were devised to detect CBI. None have been validated by correlation with modern neuroimaging methods. None have demonstrable sensitivity after the acute phase.

Again, long-lasting diffuse and disabling molecular damage seems to be common after concussion, but desktop psychological tests were developed to detect lesions many thousands of times larger. Therefore, whether a CBI survivor scores at the level expected for a healthy person or below that level does not pertain to the question of whether a brain injury occurred. Indeed, in their review of the day-of-injury assessment of sport-related concussion, McCrea and colleagues [104] state, regarding the applicability of neuropsychological tests, that they "do not diagnose whether a concussion has occurred." Rather, neuropsychological and other measures "provide data on the physiological, cognitive, psychological and behavioral changes associated with the injury that can aid the clinician" ([104], p. 280) with test findings to be used for decision making and treatment.

In fairness, the community of sports concussion psychologists deserves credit for promoting important advances. One is the institution of universal pre-season testing. This helps overcome the concern that psychological tests fail to measure individual change. Another is the advocacy for computerized testing. For instance, in the previously mentioned day-of-injury review, McCrea et al. noted, "there has been a proliferation in recent years of computerized neurocognitive tests proposed for concussion assessment" [104]. As discussed earlier in this chapter, that technology potentially enhances the precision and uniformity of stimulus presentation and response recording. It may also make a huge contribution to cost efficiency and possibly enhances sensitivity [105]. The question, as always, is whether these theoretical benefits are reaped in the real world. Unfortunately, as demonstrated by Nelson et al. [106] and Alsalaheen et al. [107], even with widely used computerized neurocognitive assessment tools in current use, there is no consensus or unanimity as to which measure should be used, its validity across different CBI types, and how and when it should be administered.

On the Cusp of a Renaissance

To summarize the relevance of the passing shadow to the urgent global project of understanding concussion: traditional neuropsychological testing methods are mostly insensitive to any but the grossest initial effects of CBI. In fact, psychological testing is inapplicable to the localization or measurement of any kind of brain injury. The slow realization that its methods are limited for understanding brain injury temporarily limited progress in the field. Indeed, one wonders why it was ever imagined that desktop tests that do not involve bone saws are brain assays, or that they might detect and characterize the most subtle of brain changes?

Thankfully, that shadow has largely passed. The new attention to CBI represents a tremendous opportunity to overcome a credibility deficit that haunted neuropsychology since the 1970s. To identify subjects with and without brain dysfunction one is no longer beholden to the best guesses of medical doctors who tapped reflexes and recorded scalp electricity. Better imaging has revolutionized antemortem diagnosis. Neuropsychiatry has buried the functional/organic split. It was no surprise and no shame to discover that those old tests fail to detect persistent brain changes after concussion. They were not selected for any such propose. If Trails B requires 274 s, what can be said with confidence about the brain? Which mitochondria exhibit what degree of energy bottleneck at the Q cycle? What axolemmal change dominates in the uncinate fasciculus? What five inflammatory cytokine genes exhibit the greatest increase in transcription? Assuming little pesticide exposure, by what percent has the patient's risk of Parkinson's disease at age 74 changed?

This is by no means to suggest that psychological assessments lack utility! Far from it.

For all the celebration of new technologies, no biomarkers – no matter how precisely they measure brain change – can translate focal, circuit, or network alterations in metabolism, axonal transport, gene expression into a meaningful assessment of the human condition, including cognitive struggle, emotional distress, and threat to identity. The authors merely wish to examine which approaches, at what stage, best address which elements of concussion. Perceived differences in the contribution of complementary information should not be permitted to distract from the collaborative spirit. A relatively modest conceptual adjustment will enhance that spirit by reframing the division of labor between the members of the interdisciplinary team that is obviously needed to address this widespread medical and social problem. It is the authors' belief that the discovery that conventional testing is insensitive to many of the long-term effects of CBI is not, in any way, a loss for neuropsychology. It is a much-needed clarification of brain–behavior relationships, a provocative stimulus for research, and a likely occasion for rapid evolution in neuropsychological assessment. The clinical neurological examination has stalled. The clinical neuropsychological examination, in contrast, is amenable to agile progress. Pending the availability of the Star Trek tricorder, non-invasive tests that do not require large machines will always have value.

Chen and D'Esposito [108], in outlining how to achieve a better understanding of TBI outcome, emphasize the need for cognitive and behavioral assessments that tap "ecologically relevant, real life contexts." Traditional neuropsychological tests are mostly based on test development and conceptualizations that are more than half a century old. Chen and D'Esposito go on to make the following analogy in regard to traditional neuropsychological testing:

> Unfortunately, most tests of cognitive functioning, including neuropsychological tests and most cognitive neuroscience measures, are not designed to reflect the complexities and low structure of settings in the "real world." Quite the opposite, these tests are typically designed to isolate the processes of interest. This is like trying to judge how accurate a basketball player is at shooting foul shots using measurements of isolated biceps strength. On the other hand, the few functional assessment measures available tend to be quite removed from understanding the underlying neural-cognitive component processes affected by concussion. The field will make a major breakthrough when these two extremes are brought together to measure cognitive control processes in real world settings.
>
> ([108], p. 13)

What Tests to Administer?

Readers may reasonably ask, "Given the fact that conventional tests from two generations past are insensitive to the persistent brain changes often produced by concussion, given the fact that neuropsychology is rapidly recovering from a temporary diversion from scientific principles but has yet to discover the optimum application of behavioral observation to clinical assessment, what tests should we give?" Neuropsychology does not have a "white" paper standard that can be reviewed in this book. That is entirely understandable and, indeed, an inevitable and useful pause in certainty at this time of transition. In the light of their lack of biological validation and insensitivity after the acute phase of injury, one would be hard pressed to interpret scores from the tests listed in Table 9.1. As reviewed by Wilde and Ware in Chapter 21 in this text on the application of the National Institutes of Health's Common Data Elements (CDE) to the assessment of TBI, including CBI (Chapter 21), until there are CDE-accepted and promulgated metrics for concussion, their sensitivity and specificity known, the field is essentially guided by clinicians doing with they feel to be reasonable, not by some universally accepted or scientifically credible standard. This is an important, pragmatic development. But unless and until there exists an accepted, uniform standard, it would be premature to compose a chapter summarizing the findings from this initiative or recommending a particular suite of psychological assessment procedures.

Rather than a list of the most sensitive and prognostically accurate conventional tests, perhaps the most important advice from the present authors might be a simple clarification: like the GCS, the neurological examination, and the CT scan, conventional behavioral testing is most useful at the acute and subacute stage. It was never intended to measure all brain dysfunction. It has poor sensitivity beyond three months post injury. The emphasis should not be on exaggerating the perfection of tests and redefining brain dysfunction as "that which our tests detect." In the near future, one expects a new neuropsychology, informed by the best available biomarkers of brain change. Pending that natural evolutionary development, the tail should not wag the dog.

Ethics: A Plea

Surveys from 2007 and 2015 reveal a trend: "Together with the present broader survey data, both strongly suggest that forensic practice is increasingly prominent and important to U.S. neuropsychology practitioners" ([109], p. 1130). Ethics deserves its own book (or, more importantly, its impregnable ensconcement in professional culture). The present authors merely urge that forensic practice incorporate the knowledge advances discussed in this book.

Medical ethics and jurisprudence require that neurologists and neuropsychologists do our best to provide the triers of fact – judges and juries – with the most scientifically accurate information currently available. Our testimony must, at a minimum, comply with the Daubert standard for scientific credibility [110]. In many cases the most accurate statement would be a candid acknowledgment of the limits of our knowledge. Although the present authors do not expect our professional boards to dictate consensus or police testimony, ideally, forensic practice parameters would facilitate agreement that certain factors are indisputable. For instance:

- Although one might opine that a case meets one of the many published criteria for "mild" TBI, the candid expert would add a qualification such as: "Please understand that 'mild' is not a biological measure. It has an operational definition composed by a committee. At present, no biomarker permits us to scientifically classify the severity of TBI."

- Traditional paper-and-pencil testing often detects impaired cognitive function in the first weeks after concussion. More sensitive tests often detect brain changes long after that. The question remains whether objectively detectable persistent "changes" (e.g., on advanced neuroimaging) represent persistent "injuries" [111]. Literally no one knows for how long a CBI may harm brain function. Pending better understanding of the biology, normal scores on standardized desktop testing cannot be interpreted as "recovery."

- Some concussion survivors have symptoms that persist for more than three months. As discussed in Chapter 7 of this text, pre-morbid factors, injury factors, and reaction-to-injury factors may underlie each symptom. One may reasonably opine that, in this case, the expert suspects pre-morbid traits and/or psychological reaction to traumatic stress have contributed to the presentation. But we must not claim to read minds. Apportionment of cause would require understanding the effects of external force on the brain across all human genomes, understanding the relationship between every instance of brain change and behavior, as well as the ability to measure motives – both conscious and unconscious. Pending dramatic new discoveries, one can certainly opine that persistent symptoms are *possibly* due to pre-morbid factors or post-injury imagination. But one cannot express that opinion to a reasonable degree of medical probability. Candid experts will admit that the relative contribution of different causes to each symptom is beyond the ken of humankind.

- Exaggeration of symptoms seems to be common in clinical medicine – whether or not there is brain injury and whether or not there is litigation. Some evidence suggests that litigation increases the risk of exaggeration, and some observations support a diagnosis of conscious malingering. However, many biopsychosocial factors other than deliberate feigning may inflate or deflate symptom reporting [107]. Pending advancements in mind reading, in the vast majority of cases, neither the patient nor the doctor knows the degree of exaggeration, the degree of consciousness of exaggeration, or how litigation influenced symptom reporting.

- Most recovery from CBI occurs during the first two years. Some evidence suggests that symptoms that persist beyond that point tend to become permanent. Yet evidence also suggests some potential for later recovery, for instance, with the discovery of a treatable somatic problem (e.g., a neuroendocrine deficiency) or with delayed comprehensive neurorehabilitation. Therefore, one may reasonably opine that a concussion survivor *seems* to have reached a state of permanent and stationary disability. But the honest expert will add a comment admitting that our ability to predict lifelong outcomes, needs, and potential for functional reintegration is limited.

In summary, the principle that defends our honor is simple: with the hearts of lions, we must resist the pressure to say more than we know.

Whither Neuropsychology?

Clinical neuroscience, as conventionally practiced, has rubbed up against its terminal limit. As mentioned previously, neuro-biological discovery has revealed such astonishing complexity and unplumbed depths that no gold standard for normal brain function exists, especially from measures developed in the late 19th and early 20th centuries. Hence, neurologists and neuropsychologists cannot perform studies expecting to find correlations between observed responses to stimuli – our common method – and what exactly is happening in the head. Nor should we expect the most facile technology to ever prove that a given behavior correlates with a given cerebral phenom-enon, since, as discussed in the chapter *Why Outcomes Vary* (Chapter 7), new evidence shows that no two cortices process information in the same way.

This does not completely moot the ambition of valid-ation. In fact, the emergence of functional neuroimaging raises hopes that, soon, one might identify nodes of the kind envisioned by Luria that commonly (if not universally) play a role in a specific suite of functions.[7] Acknowledging that: (1) no truly accurate assessment of brain is possible; (2) the most popular current methods are flawed; and (3) "localization" of a psychological construct in the cortex across humans is con-ceptually dubious, the future of neuropsychology may not be primarily a matter of finding desktop cognitive tests the results of which correlate with a brain change. Instead, like neurologists, neuropsychologists seem likely to expand their vision, collaborating with scientists from multiple discip-lines and inventing new and better non-invasive observation methods. When combining such methods with their inter-personal psychological sensitivity, it is the neuropsychologist and neuropsychiatrist who seem most likely to understand the survivor of a concussion and engage with that patient through the trajectory of post-concussive change.

The present authors cannot predict and hardly expect to move the needle. We can, however, urge and hope. We do not envision neuropsychology remaining yoked to the 1950's model of desktop testing. Its intellect is too ambitious to accept those limits. Its practitioners are too restless to hunker in that niche. Its thinkers are too independent to become handmaidens of attorneys. And its potential is almost limitless. Four aspects of the neuropsychological enterprise are poised for revolution:

1. administering stimuli
2. observing responses
3. prioritizing emotions
4. treating: who cares?

How to Administer Stimuli

As previously remarked, the neurological and neuropsycho-logical examinations employ the same model. We stimulate. We observe the response. Computer-administered stimula-tion enhances uniformity. Computer monitoring of responses permits millisecond resolution. These, however, are refinements of a creaky old method. No matter how we present our artificial quizzes and challenges, it is something of a stretch to assume that those bedside or desktop interactions illuminate life as it is lived. Chen and D'Esposito [108] are not the only psychologists to demand ecologically valid testing. Many have commented that desktop tests are bizarrely divorced from real-world tests of adaptation.

How might that demand be satisfied? One obvious and increasingly practical approach is virtual reality.

About a decade ago, laboratories began to experiment with virtual environments for treatment of anxiety disorders and phobias [115–117]. The reasoning was that, "When a user is immersed in a VE [virtual environment], they can be systematically exposed to specific feared stimuli within a contextually relevant setting" ([117, p. 251]). At about the same time, investigators began to test the feasibility of a new approach to neuropsychological testing – presenting cognitive challenges in an immersive, naturalistic, virtual environment and monitoring responses [118]. That approach has now been applied to testing of memory [117, 119, 120], attention [121, 122], spatial functions [119, 122, 123], executive functions [122, 124, 125], and even early detection of dementia [126, 127]. Combined with physiological monitoring, virtual reality has also been used to test up-regulated stress responsiveness [128, 129] – an emotional change often reported by concussion survivors, even without PTSD.

The present authors know too little to recommend this approach. Common sense suggests that predictive validity for activities of daily living would be superior with stimuli that better emulate activities of daily living, but demon-strable superiority to desktop stimulation has yet to be proven. Nonetheless, virtual reality-based functional challenges are an exciting development that may soon revolutionize the input stage of psychological testing.[8]

How to Observe Response

Luria's disciples such as Christensen and Golden sought to systematize his elaborate, individualized methods. In the

---

[7] The authors must wave a red flag. Several laboratories have reported that fMRI methods are often, if not always, misleading with respect to localization of function [112, 113]. For instance, the brain of a dead Atlantic salmon has been shown to display focal social cognitions [114]. As those authors stated, "Across the 130,000 voxels in a typical fMRI volume the probability of a false positive is almost certain." One hesitates to take the whole of the current literature at face value.

[8] One might also mention, in passing, that virtual reality-based neurorehabilitation was proposed as early as 1998 [130]. The recent availability of low-cost, high-resolution headsets might soon help actualize that potential.

process, they felt obliged to strip out individuality. All the subtleties and nuances of the patient's response to a cognitive challenge, from grins and grimaces to tremors and sweating to fluttering eyelids or lost upward gazes to clearing the throat and rocking in the chair – these and scores of other behaviors are important to the observant psychologist but dismissed in the standardization of the neuropsychological battery. The advent of computerized testing further enhances efficiency but threatens a further remove between the patient and the attentive psychologist. By 2014, more than 68% of secondary school athletic trainers had adopted computerized testing [131] and this technique possibly increases sensitivity compared with paper-and-pencil testing [105]. Yet some authorities caution that this approach reduces flexibility and blinds the tester to potentially important behavioral observations [103].

Of course, not every examiner is equally attentive to subtle behaviors or adept at interpreting them. Micro-expressions, for instance, possibly communicate useful data but analysis of those may be challenging to master [132–134]. Eye movement measurement – as illustrated in the example of Heitger et al.'s study shown in Figure 9.1 – seems to be revealing about both cortical and subcortical function but has not become routine in assessments by neurologists or neuropsychologists. The body as a whole, in fact, is an engine of revelation about the brain, but most of its semaphores pass without being analyzed in a sophisticated way. From facial emotion recognition, to voice stress analysis, to pupillary response measurement, to measures of vestibular integrity, and balance, and autonomic function, and whole-body activity monitoring, technology is rapidly enabling systematic and biologically meaningful analysis of this wealth of data streaming across the room from the patient to the doctor. The time has come to capitalize on *all* of the non-invasive observations available to the examiner. Neuropsychologists could potentially integrate many such measures into a comprehensive post-concussive assessment. For instance, eye movement analysis and balance testing have already been combined with cognitive testing for sport-related concussion [135–137]. The tricorder is not so distant: the combination of sensory sensitivity and computational power in a typical cellular telephone may already be sufficient to deeply analyze that data stream.

The present authors are not expert in technology. We are not health care economists and do not know the most cost-efficient path to incorporating these new potentialities into everyday practice. We do believe, however, that a treasure trove of insights about the brain is routinely discarded by both neurologists and neuropsychologists who ignore their own highly evolved sensitivities to innumerable patient behaviors largely because no powerful, valid, and reliable system has standardized the observations we have all been making of one another since infancy, and correlated them with everything we know about the brain. Neuropsychologists, we predict, will be at the leading edge of research to hugely enhance the sensitivity of behavioral observations – *behavior* writ large – and discover exciting new ways of detecting the state of the nervous system.

Prioritizing Emotions

Throughout this little book about concussion the collaborating authors have tried to draw attention to the main reason that CBI often causes persistent life dysfunction: emotional distress. As previously discussed, it is scientifically impossible to determine the matrix of neuroanatomical connectivity and precise pathophysiological sequence that manifests as lasting subjective distress. Multiple exquisitely individual factors converge. One must forcefully reject the popular sophistry that, since pre-injury traits and injury-related stress are definitely among those factors, concussion did not *cause* that lasting distress. Of course it did. But for an external force that rattled the brain, the distress cannot be explained.

Three facts are clear: (1) neuropsychology was originally focused on cognition, not emotion; (2) concussion survivors most need help with matters of emotion, not cognition; and (3) psychologists are savvy about emotion. Without attempting to predict a particular pathway of disciplinary evolution, the present authors hope that, in the course of the current renaissance of neuropsychology, emotions will be accorded a higher priority than has heretofore been the case.

Treating: Who Cares?

The present authors chose that section title self-consciously. Treatment in Western medicine has been homogenized, monetized, and – at least in the minds of its paymasters – reduced to a game of minimizing services played with numerical codes. Doctors are bodies in health maintenance organization cubicles, whipped to burnout by gray-faced administrators who tap their watches at examining room doors. Disenchantment, disenfranchisement, loss of autonomy, and imposition of puppet strings threaten the doctor–patient relationship at every turn. Mental health care has been especially hard hit. Few psychiatrists can pay off their educational debts administering psychotherapy. The resulting default system, largely imposed by insurers, involves psychologist- or other-therapist-administered psychotherapy plus rare physician-administered medication management – a poor excuse for coherent care.

Treating, which guerdons the heart, is not for the faint of heart. Like teaching school, it is unappreciated and under-compensated and desperately needed. The present authors do not see an immediate corrective for the difference in hourly compensation for testing versus treating. In typical inpatient rehabilitation practice, front-line providers include rehabilitation psychologists, therapists, nurses, social workers, and vocational experts, usually collaborating with physiatrists. But few concussion survivors are admitted. They are left largely to their own devices. Based on the estimates presented in this volume's chapter on epidemiology (Chapter 2), several million persons in the United States alone probably survive CBIs each year. Some may require no attention after a month. A few may continue to require treatment for more than a decade. According to the best available empirically based estimate, more than 40% of these concussion survivors will experience persistent distress and therefore might benefit from care. Although there is a remarkable paucity of controlled research investigating the type, timing, and efficacy of post-concussive intervention [138–140], the authors speculate that many would have a better chance of the fullest possible restoration of eudaimonic happiness and reintegration into family, social life, and work with perhaps, on average, three to 18 months of expert follow-up.

Yet the Western health care system has no standard approach to identifying and treating this subgroup, and no designated responsible authority. Who will care for the persistently distressed? Who has the requisite combination of neuroscientific knowledge, cognitive neurorehabilitation knowledge, psychotherapeutic knowledge, and empathy to render this care? Apart from spouses, ministers, and bartenders – those to whom this task typically falls – eight options come to mind:

1. neurologists
2. psychiatrists
3. behavioral neurologists/neuropsychiatrists
4. physiatrists
5. brain injury medicine specialists
6. clinical psychologists
7. rehabilitation psychologists
8. neuropsychologists.

Neurologists are still learning that dismissing concussion survivors after a single follow-up visit may be counterproductive. Some evidence suggests that, without a clinician's support, those who remain symptomatic might recover more slowly or not recover. A potentially counterproductive instruction appears in some neurological practice guidelines: to "reassure" the patient, on the day of injury, that he or she will promptly and completely recover. Often, this does not occur. A patient thus reassured has been primed to perceive failure. And, when confronted by persistence of symptoms, some neurologists suspect a health issue outside their zone of clinical comfort. They are often right. What many concussion survivors most need in the phase of recovery between about three months and 18 months is a brain-savvy mental health care provider. Only a subset of neurologists can or wish to do that job.

Psychiatrists are perhaps more likely to be skilled and empathic psychotherapists. And they are expert psychopharmacologists. Those combined skills equip psychiatrists to provide the coordinated mental health care that probably makes the biggest difference in quality of life during recovery from concussion. Their medical training is also valuable for diagnosing and treating neuroendocrine and sleep disorders. At present, however, psychiatry residency tends to skimp on exposure to TBI and may not provide all the training required to expertly manage CBI. In addition, like desktop testers, psychiatrists are understandably attracted by the larger number of dollars per hour they get from medication management compared to the lower reimbursement rate for cognitive care.

Neuropsychiatry is an old profession that only became a certified subspecialty in the 21st century. The United Council for Neurologic Subspecialties, founded in 2003, accepted its first membership application from the Society for Behavioral and Cognitive Neurology and the American Neuropsychiatric Association [141]. The first examination for certification in Behavioral Neurology and Neuropsychiatry (BNNP) was offered in September of 2006. Although a large number of psychiatrists refer to themselves as "neuropsychiatrists," one should make a distinction between those with self-awarded credentials and those with certification. Physicians certified in BNNP tend to have a great deal of knowledge and skill relevant to care for concussion survivors. There exists a body of highly specialized knowledge about TBI and one guesses that persons with BNNP training are uniquely prepared to readily acquire that knowledge. A subset surely has the wherewithal for compassionate psychotherapy. But will they perceive the reimbursement as satisfactory for educational loan repayment and other aspirations?

Physiatrists are experts in TBI. Some are skilled and empathic psychotherapists. And some have outpatient practices suitable for following survivors of CBI. However, management of the sequelae of concussion, which largely occurs in persons who were never admitted to a hospital, is not the most common practice focus: "Outpatient physiatrists manage nonsurgical conditions including orthopaedic injuries, spine-related pain and dysfunction, occupational injuries and overuse syndromes, neurogenic bowel/bladder, pressure sore management, spasticity management, and chronic pain" [142]. Moreover, the profession focuses on adaptation to disability, whereas, thankfully, even concussion survivors with persistent impairments tend to exhibit an improving course. Adaptations laboriously nurtured at month two may not be useful at month three. The authors believe that physiatrists could contribute a great deal to the treatment of CBI. That might, however, require a slight shift in training emphasis.

The historic eruption of scientific and clinical interest in TBI – perhaps a watershed moment in the history of Western medicine – as well as clamor from multiple potential stakeholders pressed toward a recent foreseeable occurrence: the American Board of Psychiatry and Neurology and the American Board of Physical Medicine and Rehabilitation jointly sponsored an application to the American Board of Medical Specialties to establish a process for certification in brain injury medicine [143, 144]. That petition was accepted in 2011. According to the American Board of Psychiatry and Neurology, "Brain injury medicine is a subspecialty that involves having expertise in the prevention, evaluation, treatment, and rehabilitation of individuals with acquired brain injury" [143]. Applications are being accepted from physicians currently certified in neurology, child neurology, physical medicine and rehabilitation, psychiatry, or those possessing "subspecialty certification in sports medicine through the American Board of Internal Medicine (ABIM), the American Board of Family Medicine (ABFM), the American Board of Pediatrics (ABP), or the American Board of Emergency Medicine (ABEM)" ([144], pp. 32–33).

One declared purpose is "to provide a means of identifying properly trained and experienced physicians in brain injury medicine" [143]. But that requires a prior condition: the existence of such persons. In an ingenious sequence, first the examination was written; then the training programs were devised. Certification requires completion of one or more of the residencies listed above, plus completion of a one-year brain injury medicine fellowship accredited by the Accreditation Council for Graduate Medical Education, plus success on the certifying examination.

Until the very recent invention of the brain injury specialist, the relevant knowledge was scattered across professions with no clear single path leading to enlightenment. This welcome development promises to raise the bar for the average knowledge base among those treating survivors of TBI. However, it remains to be seen whether it impacts the majority of such survivors. Typical CBI accounts for the overwhelming majority of clinically-attended human TBI. Brain injury medicine doctors who assume leadership of inpatient facilities may be funneled away from concussed patients – the subjects, and hopefully beneficiaries, of this textbook. And a gap remains: only a subset of brain injury physicians will be expert in psychotherapy, and few may be expert in cognitive rehabilitation.

Clinical psychologists do the lion's share of expert, empathic psychotherapy in some countries. Like psychiatrists, however, they tend to lack advanced knowledge of TBI. In many cases, that fact may not be a critical limitation. As much as one hopes that persons who treat concussion survivors will be familiar with the commonplace blend of cognitive and non-cognitive behavioral symptoms, with the complexity of the interplay between pre-morbid, injury-related, and post-injury factors, and with the spectrum of trajectories of recovery, frankly, a caring and supportive professional has the most important qualification to help. The clinical psychologist's main handicap is the lack of training and licensure in medicine, given that so many forms of psychic distress are due to medical complications of TBI and perhaps respond best to a combination of psychotherapy and medical treatment.

The foundational principles of rehabilitation psychology were articulated by Wright in 1983 [145]. These repeatedly refer to adjusting to chronic or permanent disability, and even emphasize the "insider–outsider distinction" that separates the mental orientation of the disabled from those of others [146]. Due to the brain's adaptive plasticity and potential for neuronal regeneration, few concussion survivors develop a disabling static encephalopathy. They are often impaired by comparison with their pre-morbid state, but not necessarily "abnormal," and their impairments are often temporary. An unknown proportion is suspected to harbor lifelong residual brain changes, but those changes tend to be subtle and may sometimes be amenable to work-arounds. Hence, the rhetorical and conceptual framework of rehabilitation psychology seems somewhat oblique to the needs of most CBI survivors. This volume intends to alert readers to the neglected reality of post-concussive problems. However, nothing is gained by conflating those problems with all-encompassing, profoundly limiting disabilities that imply isolation from the mainstream of life. Most rehabilitation psychologists practice in the inpatient setting. Pending a study, one does not know what proportion of rehabilitation psychologists address the unique and highly dynamic challenges of outpatient CBI survivors.

In point of fact, it was only recently recognized (and not by all authorities) that these problems exist and are worthy of attention. It seems likely that a very large number of people in the world are living less than optimal lives due to untreated effects of concussion. It seems reasonable that such people qualify for the health care investments urged by the 2005 World Health Assembly Resolution (WHA58.23) "Disability, including prevention, management and rehabilitation" [147] and by the World Health Organization's 2006–2011 action plan [148]. The American Psychological Association has supported this global role for rehabilitation psychology [149, 150]. Therefore, despite the fact that rehabilitation psychology has not previously played a major part in shepherding concussion survivors toward their best possible recoveries, if this vital subdiscipline were to modestly adjust its sights, the CBI population might come sharply into their focus.

Which brings us to consider the possibility that the renaissance of neuropsychology might include a revival of interest in treatment. Most discussions mention two roles for a neuropsychologist on the TBI team: testing to guide treatment and testing to monitor treatment. Effectuating treatment is almost always assumed to be someone else's job [151–153]. When intervention is mentioned, the typical focus is not cognitive rehabilitation or psychotherapy but didactic inculcation of an expectation of recovery, e.g., "Education is the centerpiece of mTBI treatment" [154]. At the same time, some neuropsychologists have long called for a closer embrace of the therapeutic role. As Ruff stated in his "friendly critique of neuropsychology," "Patients' needs are not met by merely diagnosing cognitive deficits … the time has come for neuropsychologists to identify as caretakers for cognitive health" ([155], p. 847).

The present authors appreciate that neuropsychologists represent a small, elite professional group. We understand and respect the choice of testing as a lifestyle. We do not expect many certified neuropsychologists to refocus on management of the ill any more than we expect neurologists to become effective psychotherapists. Moreover, the need for somatic medical care will remain pressing in many cases, meaning that even the most dedicated neuropsychologist cannot do it all. However, relatively few professionals on Earth possess the neuropsychologist's extraordinary combination of pertinent skills. Who else could simultaneously assess cognitive strengths and weaknesses, assess emotional symptoms, rule out response bias, appraise behavior changes informed by the vast body of literature on the neuroscience of concussion, then pick from his or her quiver the best bolts of intervention, for instance, rehabilitation of executive functions, plus cognitive behavior therapy, plus relaxation training, plus family counseling? The sequestering of these polymaths in the testing closet deprives CBI victims of exceptional multidimensional care, and deprives those who are gratified by healing from that matchless reward.

Treatment of patients with persistent post-concussive problems is, thus, something of a calling. It requires more than expertise. It requires devotion. The authors implore the devout to leap into the breach. Western medicine is realizing, but too slowly, that so-called "cognitive" care pays huge dividends via prevention of chronicity, reduced future use of health care and social services, family stability, and productivity. As a result, multiple initiatives have been introduced to enhance reimbursement for expert cognitive care and reduce it for procedures. Awaiting parity, we need devotees.

Do we know what to do? Not really. For an ApoE-e4-negative teenaged boy with his second sports-related concussion, which is most effective for accelerating recovery of dentate gyrus-dependent learning: amantadine, virtual reality-based cognitive rehabilitation, or aerobic exercise? For a woman after menarche and before menopause with a common intron 2 mutation in the gene for 5-hydroxytryptamine receptor 2A and post-concussive mixed depression/anxiety, which is most helpful: escitalopram, mindfulness meditation, or psilocybin? For a 55-year-old man without testosterone deficiency but with Val/Val homozygosity at codon 158 of the COMT gene and post-concussive irritability, which is most likely to reduce the risk of intimate-partner violence: propranolol, relaxation therapy, or the cannabinoid 1 receptor agonist ACEA [156]? The treatment book cannot be written until the research is done. Yet listening, validation, and compassion will never lose their sublimity. As the saying goes, one can rarely cure; one can sometimes ameliorate; but one can always comfort.

References

1. Heitger MH, Jones RD, Macleod AD, Snell DL, Frampton CM, Anderson TJ. Impaired eye movements in post-concussion syndrome indicate suboptimal brain function beyond the influence of depression, malingering or intellectual ability. *Brain* 2009; 132: 2850–2870.
2. McCrea M, Barr WB, Guskiewicz K, Randolph C, Marshall SW, Cantu R, et al. Standard regression-based methods for measuring recovery after sport-related concussion. *J Int Neuropsychol Soc* 2005; 11: 58–69.
3. Carpenter SK. Some neglected contributions of Wilhelm Wundt to the psychology of memory. *Psychol Rep* 2005; 97: 63–73.
4. Wundt W. *Grundzüge der physiologischen Psychologie*. Engelmann: Leipzig, 1874.
5. Ziche P. Neuroscience in its context. Neuroscience and psychology in the work of Wilhelm Wundt. *Physis Riv Int Stor Sci* 1999; 36: 407–429.
6. Bruce D. On the origin of the term "neuropsychology." *Neuropsychologia* 1985; 23: 813–814.
7. Osler W. Specialism in the general hospital. *Bull Johns Hopkins Hosp* 1913; 24: 167–171.
8. Hallet S. Neuropsychology. In: Morgan G, Butler S, editors. *Seminars in basic neurosciences*. London: Gaskel, 1993, pp. 151–185.
9. Lashley KS. Functional determinants of cerebral localization. *Arch Neurol Psychiatry* 1937; 38: 371–387.
10. Beach FA. *Karl Spencer Lashley: A biographical memoir*. Washington, D.C.: National Academy of Sciences, 1961.
11. Benton AL, Adams KM. *Exploring the history of neuropsychology: Selected papers*. London: Oxford University Press, 2000.
12. Richards G. *Putting psychology in its place: Critical historical perspectives*. Hove, East Sussex: Routledge, 2009.
13. Hibar DP, Stein JL, Renteria ME, Arias-Vasquez A, Desrivieres S, Jahanshad N, et al. Common genetic variants influence human subcortical brain structures. *Nature* 2015; 520: 224–229.
14. Tavor I, Parker Jones O, Mars RB, Smith SM, Behrens TE, Jbabdi S. Task-free MRI predicts individual differences in brain activity during task performance. *Science* 2016; 352: 216–220.
15. Koff SA. The Rorschach test in the differential diagnosis of cerebral concussion and psychoneurosis. *Bull U S Army Med Dep* 1946; 5: 170–173.
16. Aita JA, Armitage SG, Reitan RM, Rabinovitz A. The use of certain psychological tests in the evaluation of brain injury. *J Gen Psychol* 1947; 37: 25–44.
17. Goldman R, Greenblatt M, Coon GP. Use of the Bellevue-Wechsler scale in clinical psychiatry; with particular reference to cases with brain damage. *J Nerv Ment Dis* 1946; 104: 144–179.
18. Graham FK, Kendall BS. Performance of brain-damaged cases on a memory-for-designs test. *J Abnorm Psychol* 1946; 41: 303–314.
19. Malamud RF. Validity of the Hunt-Minnesota test for organic brain damage. *J Appl Psychol* 1946; 30: 271–275.
20. Zangwill OL. Psychological work at the Edinburgh Brain Injuries Unit. *Br Med J* 1945; 2: 248–251.
21. Goldstein K. *Aftereffects of brain injury in war*. New York: Grune and Stratton, 1942.
22. Goldstein K, Scheerer M. Abstract and concrete behavior: An experimental study with special tests. *Psychol Monogr* 1941; 53: i.
23. Cipolotti L, Warrington EK. Neuropsychological assessment. *J Neurol Neurosurg Psychiatry* 1995; 58: 655–664.
24. Bender L. Psychological principles of the visual motor gestalt test. *Trans N Y Acad Sci* 1949; 11: 164–170.
25. Hale Jr NG. *The rise and crisis of psychoanalysis in the United States: Freud and the Americans, 1917–1985*. Oxford: Oxford University Press, 1995.
26. Oberndorf CP. *A history of psychoanalysis in America*. New York: Grune & Stratton, 1953.
27. Samuel LR. *Shrink: A cultural history of psychoanalysis in America*. Lincoln, NE: University of Nebraska Press, 2013.
28. Hale NJ. *Freud and the Americans: The beginnings of psychoanalysis in the United States, 1876–1917. Freud in America, vol. 1*. Oxford: Oxford University Press, 1971.
29. Benton AL. The experimental validation of the Rorschach test. *Br J Med Psychol* 1950; 23: 45–58.
30. Aita JA, Reitan RM, Ruth JM. Rorschach's test as a diagnostic aid in brain injury. *Am J Psychiatry* 1947; 103: 770–779.
31. Reitan RM. Evaluation of the postconcussion syndrome with the Rorschach test. *J Nerv Ment Dis* 1955; 121: 463–467.
32. Zangwill OL. A review of psychological work at the brain injuries unit, Edinburgh, 1941–5. *Br Med J* 1945; 2: 248–251.
33. Hebb DO. The role of neurological ideas in psychology. *J Pers* 1951; 20: 39–55.
34. Page JD. *Abnormal psychology*. New York: McGraw Hill, 1947.
35. Hoyt R, Elliott H, Hebb DO. The intelligence of schizophrenic patients following lobotomy. *Treat Serv Bull* 1951; 6: 553–557.
36. McFie J, Piercy MF, Zangwill OL. The Rorschach test in obsessional neurosis with special reference to the effects of pre-frontal leucotomy. *Br J Med Psychol* 1951; 24: 162–179.
37. Paterson A, Zangwill OL. A case of topographical disorientation associated with a unilateral cerebral lesion. *Brain* 1945; 68: 188–212.
38. Zangwill OL. Clinical tests of memory impairment. *Proc R Soc Med* 1943; 36: 576–580.
39. Benton AL. The Rorschach test and the diagnosis of cerebral pathology in children. *Am J Orthopsychiatry* 1956; 26: 783–791.
40. Birch HG, Diller L. Rorschach signs of organicity: A physiological basis for perceptual disturbances. *J Proj Tech* 1959; 23: 184–197.
41. Stuss DT. *Use of behavioral measures in discriminating neurological status*. Ottawa: University of Ottawa (Canada), 1973.
42. Golden EC, Graff-Radford J, Jones DT, Benarroch EE. Mediodorsal nucleus and its multiple cognitive functions. *Neurology* 2016; 87: 2161–2168.
43. Reitan R. The validity of the trail making test as an indicator of organic brain damage. *Percept Motor Skills* 1958; 8: 271–276.

44. Goldstein G, Neuringer C. Schizophrenic and organic signs on the Trail Making Test. *Percept Motor Skills* 1966; 22: 347–350.

45. Boll TJ. Psychological differentiation of patients with schizophrenia versus lateralized cerebrovascular, neoplastic, or traumatic brain damage. *J Abnorm Psychol* 1974; 83: 456–458.

46. Watson CG, Thomas RW, Felling J, Andersen D. Differentiation of organics from schizophrenics with the trail making, dynamometer, critical flicker fusion, and light-intensity matching tests. *J Clin Psychol* 1969; 25: 130–133.

47. Watson CG, Thomas RW, Andersen D, Felling J. Differentiation of organics from schizophrenics at two chronicity levels by use of the Reitan-Halstead organic test battery. *J Consult Clin Psychol* 1968; 32: 679–684.

48. Watson CG. The separation of NP hospital organics from schizophrenics with three visual motor screening tests. *J Clin Psychol* 1968; 24: 412–414.

49. Halstead WC. *Brain and intelligence; a quantitative study of the frontal lobes.* Chicago: University of Chicago Press, 1947.

50. Halstead WC. Biological intelligence. *J Pers* 1951; 20: 118–130.

51. Reitan RM. Investigation of the validity of Halstead's measures of biological intelligence. *AMA Arch Neurol Psychiatry* 1955; 73: 28–35.

52. Matthews CG, Shaw D, Kløve H. Psychological test performances in neurologic and "pseudo-neurologic" subjects. *Cortex* 1966; 2: 244–253.

53. Vega A, Jr., Parsons OA. Cross-validation of the Halstead-Reitan tests for brain damage. *J Consult Psychol* 1967; 31: 619–625.

54. Reitan RM. *The effects of brain lesions on adaptive abilities in human beings.* Seattle, WA: University of Washington, 1959.

55. Christensen AL. *Luria's neuropsychological investigation: Manual.* New York: Spectrum, 1975.

56. Golden CJ, Hammeke TA, Purisch AD. *Manual for the Luria-Nebraska neuropsychological battery.* Lincoln, NE: University of Nebraska Press, 1979.

57. Adams KM. Luria left in the lurch: Unfulfilled promises are not valid tests. *J Clin Neuropsychol* 1984; 6: 455–458.

58. Golden CJ, Hammeke TA, Purisch AD. Diagnostic validity of a standardized neuropsychological battery derived from Luria's neuropsychological tests. *J Consult Clin Psychol* 1978; 46: 1258–1265.

59. Al Nezari NH, Schneiders AG, Hendrick PA. Neurological examination of the peripheral nervous system to diagnose lumbar spinal disc herniation with suspected radiculopathy: A systematic review and meta-analysis. *Spine J* 2013; 13: 657–674.

60. Anderson NE, Mason DF, Fink JN, Bergin PS, Charleston AJ, Gamble GD. Detection of focal cerebral hemisphere lesions using the neurological examination. *J Neurol Neurosurg Psychiatry* 2005; 76: 545–549.

61. Bouwes A, Binnekade JM, Verbaan BW, Zandbergen EG, Koelman JH, Weinstein HC, et al. Predictive value of neurological examination for early cortical responses to somatosensory evoked potentials in patients with postanoxic coma. *J Neurol* 2012; 259: 537–541.

62. Galanis E, Buckner JC, Novotny P, Morton RF, McGinnis WL, Dinapoli R, et al. Efficacy of neuroradiological imaging, neurological examination, and symptom status in follow-up assessment of patients with high-grade gliomas. *J Neurosurg* 2000; 93: 201–207.

63. Vilke GM, Chan TC, Guss DA. Use of a complete neurological examination to screen for significant intracranial abnormalities in minor head injury. *Am J Emerg Med* 2000; 18: 159–163.

64. Werry JS, Aman MG. The reliability and diagnostic validity of the Physical and Neurological Examination for Soft Signs (PANESS). *J Autism Child Schizophr* 1976; 6: 253–262.

65. Cvejic E, Lemon J, Hickie IB, Lloyd AR, Vollmer-Conna U. Neurocognitive disturbances associated with acute infectious mononucleosis, Ross River fever and Q fever: A preliminary investigation of inflammatory and genetic correlates. *Brain Behav Immun* 2014; 36: 207–214.

66. Han JH, Wilber ST. Altered mental status in older patients in the emergency department. *Clin Geriatr Med* 2013; 29: 101–136.

67. Maier SF, Watkins LR. Cytokines for psychologists: Implications of bidirectional immune-to-brain communication for understanding behavior, mood, and cognition. *Psychol Rev* 1998; 105: 83–107.

68. White PD, Dash AR, Thomas JM. Poor concentration and the ability to process information after glandular fever. *J Psychosom Res* 1998; 44: 269–278.

69. Berryman C, Stanton TR, Bowering KJ, Tabor A, McFarlane A, Moseley GL. Do people with chronic pain have impaired executive function? A meta-analytical review. *Clin Psychol Rev* 2014; 34: 563–579.

70. Oosterman JM, Derksen LC, Van Wijck AJ, Veldhuijzen DS, Kessels RP. Memory functions in chronic pain: Examining contributions of attention and age to test performance. *Clin J Pain* 2011; 27: 70–75.

71. Oosterman JM, Veldhuijzen DS. On the interplay between chronic pain and age with regard to neurocognitive integrity: Two interacting conditions? *Neurosci Biobehav Rev* 2016; 69: 174–192.

72. Rathbone M, Parkinson W, Rehman Y, Jiang S, Bhandari M, Kumbhare D. Magnitude and variability of effect sizes for the associations between chronic pain and cognitive test performances: A meta-analysis. *Br J Pain* 2016; 10: 141–155.

73. Golden CJ. Validity of the Halstead-Reitan neuropsychological battery in a mixed psychiatric and brain-injured population. *J Consult Clin Psychol* 1977; 45: 1043–1051.

74. Harvey PD. What is the evidence for changes in cognition and functioning over the lifespan in patients with schizophrenia? *J Clin Psychiatry* 2014; 75 (Suppl 2): 34–38.

75. Kar SK, Jain M. Current understandings about cognition and the neurobiological correlates in schizophrenia. *J Neurosci Rural Pract* 2016; 7: 412–418.

76. Kraus MS, Keefe RS. Cognition as an outcome measure in schizophrenia. *Br J Psychiatry Suppl* 2007; 50: s46–s51.

77. Sheffield JM, Barch DM. Cognition and resting-state functional connectivity in schizophrenia. *Neurosci Biobehav Rev* 2016; 61: 108–120.

78. Szoke A, Trandafir A, Dupont ME, Meary A, Schurhoff F, Leboyer M. Longitudinal studies of cognition in schizophrenia: Meta-analysis. *Br J Psychiatry* 2008; 192: 248–257.

79. Tiller SG, Persinger MA. Test–retest scores for patients who display neuropsychological impairment following "mild head injuries" from mechanical impacts. *Percept Motor Skills* 1998; 86: 1240–1242.

80. Stewart DP, Kaylor J, Koutanis E. Cognitive deficits in presumed minor head-injured patients. *Acad Emerg Med* 1996; 3: 21–26.

81. Rojas DC, Bennett TL. Single versus composite score discriminative validity with the Halstead-Reitan Battery and the Stroop Test in mild brain injury. *Arch Clin Neuropsychol* 1995; 10: 101–110.

82. Makatura TJ, Lam CS, Leahy BJ, Castillo MT, Kalpakjian CZ. Standardized memory tests and the appraisal of everyday memory. *Brain Inj* 1999; 13: 355–367.

83. Hartlage L. Common psychological tests applied to the assessment of brain damage. *J Proj Tech Pers Assess* 1966; 30: 317–338.

84. Schepers JM. The assessment of brain damage from a psychometric point of view. *Forensic Sci* 1972; 1: 269–311.

85. Silverstein ML, Morrison HL, Weinberg J. Relevance of modern neuropsychology to psychiatry. *J Nerv Ment Dis* 1980; 168: 673–678.

86. Lezak MD. *Neuropsychological assessment.* New York: Oxford University Press, 1995.

87. Gronwall D, Wrightson P. Delayed recovery of intellectual function after minor head injury. *Lancet* 1974; 2: 605–609.

88. Greiffenstein MF. Foreword. In: Carone DA, Bush SS, editors. *Mild traumatic brain injury: Symptom validity assessment and malingering.* New York: Springer, 2013, pp. xiii–xiv.

89. Lezak MD, Howieson D, Bigler ED, Tranel D. *Neuropsychological assessment,* 5th edition. New York: Oxford University Press, 2012.

90. Prichep LS, McCrea M, Barr W, Powell M, Chabot RJ. Time course of clinical and electrophysiological recovery after sport-related concussion. *J Head Trauma Rehabil* 2013; 28: 266–273.

91. Gay M, Ray W, Johnson B, Teel E, Geronimo A, Slobounov S. Feasibility of EEG measures in conjunction with light exercise for return-to-play evaluation after sports-related concussion. *Dev Neuropsychol* 2015; 40: 248–253.

92. Sponheim SR, McGuire KA, Kang SS, Davenport ND, Aviyente S, Bernat EM, Lim KO. Evidence of disrupted functional connectivity in the brain after combat-related blast injury. *NeuroImage* 2011; 54: S21–S29

93. Lee RR, Huang M. Magnetoencephalography in the diagnosis of concussion. *Prog Neurol Surg* 2014; 28: 94–111.

94. Mayer AR, Ling JM, Dodd AB, Meier TB, Hanlon FM, Klimaj SD. A prospective microstructure imaging study in mixed-martial artists using geometric measures and diffusion tensor imaging: methods and findings. *Brain Imaging Behav* 2016; 11(3): 698–711.

95. Westfall DR, West JD, Bailey JN, Arnold TW, Kersey PA, Saykin AJ, McDonald BC. Increased brain activation during working memory processing after pediatric mild traumatic brain injury (mTBI). *J Pediatr Rehabil Med* 2015; 8: 297–308.

96. Astafiev SV, Shulman GL, Metcalf NV, Rengachary J, Mac Donald CL, Harrington DL, et al. Abnormal white matter blood-oxygen-level–dependent signals in chronic mild traumatic brain injury. *J Neurotrauma* 2015; 32: 1254–1271.

97. Sinopoli KJ, Chen J-K, Wells G, Fait P, Ptito A, Taha T, Keightley M. Imaging "brain strain" in youth athletes with mild traumatic brain injury during dual-task performance *J Neurotrauma* 2014; 31: 1843–1859.

98. Echemendia RJ, Iverson GL, McCrea M, Broshek DK, Gioia GA, Sautter SW, et al. Role of neuropsychologists in the evaluation and management of sport-related concussion: An inter-organization position statement. *Arch Clin Neuropsychol* 2012; 27: 119–122.

99. Gomez JE, Hergenroeder AC. New guidelines for management of concussion in sport: Special concern for youth. *J Adolesc Health* 2013; 53: 311–313.

100. Harmon KG, Drezner JA, Gammons M, Guskiewicz KM, Halstead M, Herring SA, et al. American Medical Society for Sports Medicine position statement: Concussion in sport. *Br J Sports Med* 2013; 47: 15–26.

101. Marshall S, Bayley M, McCullagh S, Velikonja D, Berrigan L, Ouchterlony D, et al. Updated clinical practice guidelines for concussion/mild traumatic brain injury and persistent symptoms. *Brain Inj* 2015; 29: 688–700.

102. Solomon GS, Lovell MR, Casson IR, Viano DC. Normative neurocognitive data for National Football League players: An initial compendium. *Arch Clin Neuropsychol* 2015; 30: 161–173.

103. Kontos AP, Sufrinko A, Womble M, Kegel N. Neuropsychological assessment following concussion: An evidence-based review

104. McCrea M, Iverson GL, Echemendia RJ, Makdissi M, Raftery M. Day of injury assessment of sport-related concussion. *Br J Sports Med* 2013; 47: 272–284.

105. Broglio SP, Macciocchi SN, Ferrara MS. Sensitivity of the concussion assessment battery. *Neurosurgery* 2007; 60: 1050–1057; discussion 1057–1058.

106. Nelson LD, Laroche AA, Pfaller AY, Lerner EB, Hammeke TA, Randolph C, et al. Prospective, head-to-head study of three Computerized Neurocognitive assessment Tools (CNTs): Reliability and validity for the assessment of sport-related concussion. *J Int Neuropsychol Soc* 2016; 22: 24–37.

107. Alsalaheen B, Stockdale K, Pechumer D, Broglio SP. Validity of the Immediate Post Concussion Assessment and Cognitive Testing (ImPACT). *Sports Med* 2016; 46: 1487–1501.

108. Chen AJ, D'Esposito M. Traumatic brain injury: From bench to bedside [corrected] to society. *Neuron* 2010; 66: 11–14.

109. Sweet JJ, Benson LM, Nelson NW, Moberg PJ. The American Academy of Clinical Neuropsychology, National Academy of Neuropsychology, and Society for Clinical Neuropsychology (APA Division 40) 2015 TCN Professional Practice and 'Salary Survey': Professional practices, beliefs, and incomes of U.S. neuropsychologists. *Clin Neuropsychol* 2015; 29: 1069–1162.

110. Daubert v. Merrell Dow Pharmaceuticals. 1993.

111. Silver JM. Effort, exaggeration and malingering after concussion. *J Neurol Neurosurg Psychiatry* 2012; 83: 836–841.

112. Eklund A, Nichols TE, Knutsson H. Cluster failure: Why fMRI inferences for spatial extent have inflated false-positive rates. *Proc Natl Acad Sci U S A* 2016; 113: 7900–7905.

113. Vul E, Harris C, Winkielman P, Pashler H. Puzzlingly high correlations in fMRI studies of emotion, personality, and social cognition. *Perspect Psychol Sci* 2009; 4: 274–290.

114. Bennett CM, Baird AA, Miller MB, Wolford GL. Neural correlates of interspecies perspective taking in the post-mortem Atlantic Salmon: An argument for multiple comparisons correction. 2009. www.wired.com/2009/09/fmrisalmon/.

115. Opris D, Pintea S, Garcia-Palacios A, Botella C, Szamoskozi S, David D. Virtual reality exposure therapy in anxiety disorders: A quantitative meta-analysis. *Depress Anxiety* 2012; 29: 85–93.

116. Parsons TD. Virtual reality exposure therapy for anxiety and specific phobias. 2015. Available at https://pdfs.semanticscholar.org/84d4/8648feef13cf1053bb0490377101c3c8059b.pdf.

117. Parsons TD, Rizzo AA. Affective outcomes of virtual reality exposure therapy for anxiety and specific phobias: A meta-analysis. *J Behav Ther Exp Psychiatry* 2008; 39: 250–261.

118. Parsons TD, Reinebold JL. Adaptive virtual environments for neuropsychological assessment in serious games. *IEEE Transact Consumer Electron* 2012; 58: 197–204.

119. Goodrich-Hunsaker NJ, Hopkins RO. Spatial memory deficits in a virtual radial arm maze in amnesic participants with hippocampal damage. *Behav Neurosci* 2010; 124: 405–413.

120. Knight RG, Titov N. Use of virtual reality tasks to assess prospective memory: Applicability and evidence. *Brain Impair* 2009; 10: 3–13.

121. Parsons TD, Bowerly T, Buckwalter JG, Rizzo AA. A controlled clinical comparison of attention performance in children with ADHD in a virtual reality classroom compared to standard neuropsychological methods. *Child Neuropsychol* 2007; 13: 363–381.

122. Parsons TD, Courtney CG, Dawson ME. Virtual reality Stroop task for assessment of supervisory attentional processing. *J Clin Exp Neuropsychol* 2013; 35: 812–826.

123. Beck L, Wolter M, Mungard NF, Vohn R, Staedtgen M, Kuhlen T, et al. Evaluation of spatial processing in virtual reality using

functional magnetic resonance imaging (fMRI). *Cyberpsychol Behav Soc Network* 2010; 13: 211–215.

124. Cipresso P, Albani G, Serino S, Pedroli E, Pallavicini F, Mauro A, et al. Virtual multiple errands test (VMET): A virtual reality-based tool to detect early executive functions deficit in Parkinson's disease. *Front Behav Neurosci* 2014; 8: 405.

125. Rand D, Basha-Abu Rukan S, Weiss PL, Katz N. Validation of the Virtual MET as an assessment tool for executive functions. *Neuropsychol Rehabil* 2009; 19: 583–602.

126. Tarnanas I, Tsolaki M, Nef T, M Muri R, Mosimann UP. Can a novel computerized cognitive screening test provide additional information for early detection of Alzheimer's disease? *Alzheimers Dement* 2014; 10: 790–798.

127. Tarnanas I, Schlee W, Tsolaki M, Muri R, Mosimann U, Nef T. Ecological validity of virtual reality daily living activities screening for early dementia: Longitudinal study. *JMIR Serious Games* 2013; 1: e1.

128. Macedonio MF, Parsons TD, Digiuseppe RA, Weiderhold BK, Rizzo AA. Immersiveness and physiological arousal within panoramic video-based virtual reality. *Cyberpsychol Behav* 2007; 10: 508–515.

129. Meehan M, Razzaque S, Insko B, Whitton M, Brooks FP, Jr. Review of four studies on the use of physiological reaction as a measure of presence in stressful virtual environments. *Appl Psychophysiol Biofeedback* 2005; 30: 239–258.

130. Johnson DA, Rose FD, Rushton S, Pentland B, Attree EA. Virtual reality: A new prosthesis for brain injury rehabilitation. *Scott Med J* 1998; 43: 81–83.

131. Williams RM, Welch CE, Weber ML, Parsons JT, Valovich Mcleod TC. Athletic trainers' management practices and referral patterns for adolescent athletes after sport-related concussion. *Sports Health* 2014; 6: 434–439.

132. Cohn JF, Ambadar Z, Ekman P. Observer-based measurement of facial expression with the facial action coding system. In: Coan JA, Allen JB, editors. *The handbook of emotion elicitation and assessment.* Oxford: Oxford University Press Series in Affective Science, 2005, pp. 203–221.

133. Ekman P. Facial expression. In: Seigman A, Feldstein L, editors. *Nonverbal behavior and communication.* NJ: Lawrence Erlbaum Association, 1977, pp. 97–116.

134. Ekman P, Friesen WV, Hager JC. *Facial action coding system: Investigator's guide. A human face.* Salt Lake City, UT: Research Nexus, 2002.

135. Alsalaheen BA, Whitney SL, Marchetti GF, Furman JM, Kontos AP, Collins MW, et al. Relationship between cognitive assessment and balance measures in adolescents referred for vestibular physical therapy after concussion. *Clin J Sport Med* 2016; 26: 46–52.

136. Pearce KL, Sufrinko A, Lau BC, Henry L, Collins MW, Kontos AP. Near point of convergence after a sport-related concussion: Measurement reliability and relationship to neurocognitive impairment and symptoms. *Am J Sports Med* 2015; 43: 3055–3061.

137. Vernau BT, Grady MF, Goodman A, Wiebe DJ, Basta L, Park Y, et al. Oculomotor and neurocognitive assessment of youth ice hockey players: Baseline associations and observations after concussion. *Dev Neuropsychol* 2015; 40: 7–11.

138. Borg J, Holm L, Peloso PM, Cassidy JD, Carroll LJ, Von Holst H, et al. Non-surgical intervention and cost for mild traumatic brain injury: Results of the WHO Collaborating Centre Task Force on Mild Traumatic Brain Injury. *J Rehabil Med* 2004; 76–83.

139. Mittenberg W, Tremont G, Zielinski RE, Fichera S, Rayls KR. Cognitive-behavioral prevention of postconcussion syndrome. *Arch Clin Neuropsychol* 1996; 11: 139–145.

140. Ponsford J, Willmott C, Rothwell A, Cameron P, Ayton G, Nelms R, et al. Impact of early intervention on outcome after mild traumatic brain injury in children. *Pediatrics* 2001; 108: 1297–1303.

141. United Council for Neurologic Subspecialties. Background. 2004. www.ucns.org/go/about/background.

142. American Academy of Physical Medicine and Rehabilitation. What is physical medicine and rehabilitation? 2016. www.aapmr.org.

143. American Board of Psychiatry and Neurology. Brain injury medicine: Deadlines, fees and content for initial certification in brain injury medicine. 2016. www.abpn.com/become-certified/taking-a-subspecialty-exam/brain-injury-medicine/.

144. American Board of Physical Medicine and Rehabilitation. Brain injury medicine: Booklet of information; 2016 examinations. 2016. www.abpmr.org/candidates/bim.html.

145. Wright BA. *Physical disability: A psychosocial approach.* New York: HarperCollins Publishers, 1983.

146. Dunn DS, Ehde DM, Wegener ST. The foundational principles as psychological lodestars: Theoretical inspiration and empirical direction in rehabilitation psychology. *Rehabil Psychol* 2016; 61: 1–6.

147. World Health Assembly. Disability, including prevention, management and rehabilitation. Fifty-Eighth World Health Assembly; 16–25 May, 2005. Geneva.

148. World Health Organization. Disability and rehabilitation: WHO action plan 2006–2011. 2006. www.who.int/disabilities/publications/action_plan/en/.

149. Bentley JA, Bruyère SM, Leblanc J, Maclachlan M. Globalizing rehabilitation psychology: Application of foundational principles to global health and rehabilitation challenges. *Rehabil Psychol* 2016; 61: 65–73.

150. Maclachlan M, Mannan H. The world report on disability and its implications for rehabilitation psychology. *Rehabil Psychol* 2014; 59: 117–124.

151. Constantinidou F, Wertheimer JC, Tsanadis J, Evans C, Paul DR. Assessment of executive functioning in brain injury: Collaboration between speech–language pathology and neuropsychology for an integrative neuropsychological perspective. *Brain Inj* 2012; 26: 1549–1563.

152. McCrea M, Pliskin N, Barth J, Cox D, Fink J, French L, et al. Official position of the military TBI task force on the role of neuropsychology and rehabilitation psychology in the evaluation, management, and research of military veterans with traumatic brain injury. *Clin Neuropsychol* 2008; 22: 10–26.

153. Warschausky S, Kaufman J, Stiers W. Training requirements and scope of practice in rehabilitation psychology and neuropsychology. *J Pediatr Rehabil Med* 2008; 1: 61–65.

154. Riechers RG, 2nd, Ruff RL. Rehabilitation in the patient with mild traumatic brain injury. *Continuum (Minneap Minn)* 2010; 16: 128–149.

155. Ruff RM. A friendly critique of neuropsychology: Facing the challenges of our future. *Arch Clin Neuropsychol* 2003; 18: 847–864.

156. Rodriguez-Arias M, Navarrete F, Daza-Losada M, Navarro D, Aguilar MA, Berbel P, et al. CB1 cannabinoid receptor-mediated aggressive behavior. *Neuropharmacology* 2013; 75: 172–180.

421

Chapter

10

Persistent Post-Concussive Psychiatric Problems

Jeff Victoroff

Thus the traumatic factor may be simply predisponent. Or, at the opposite pole of action, it may be the direct excitant of an insanity already about to appear, the particular spark that happens to fire the prepared train; or it may act on a less fully prepared condition, and modify the course and symptoms of the insanity it precipitates; or it may lead to the formation of a neurasthenic or hysterical condition, and coincidentally or thereupon may come psychic disorder; or to the setting up and development of a special traumatic neurosis, and of a morbid psychosis; or there may perhaps be, primarily, coarse brain damage, organic and often progressive destructive brain disease.

Mickle, 1892 [1], p. 77

We conclude that a substantial number of patients encounter anxiety and depressive disorders after TBI [traumatic brain injury], and that these problems persist over time.

Scholten et al., 2016 [2], p. 1969

This chapter is easy to write. Knowing as little as the author does about the subject, the narrative will be brief and simple. In a nutshell, many people who survive a concussive brain injury (CBI) suffer from persistent[1] non-cognitive (otherwise known as psychiatric or neuropsychiatric) behavioral symptoms. No dulcet acronym comes to mind. Perhaps one could abbreviate persistent post-concussive psychiatric problems – "PPCPPs"? The character of those troubles, the timing of their development with respect to the injury, their duration, and their severity all vary greatly, both within and between CBI survivors. Their causes are manifold and uncertain. As William Mickle asserted several years ago, there are many possible relationships between a trauma and a subsequent "insanity." We are little advanced from his 19th-century capacity to sort them out. Crystalizing:

1. These problems occur.
2. We don't know why.
3. We don't know how to treat them.

Perhaps the most ingenuous way to begin the chapter, therefore, is to explain the profundity of our ignorance. The nature of PPCPPs is poorly understood, poorly researched, hotly debated, and conceptually challenging. Readers seeking definitive answers (including the present author) will justifiably yearn for a different book. What follows is merely data and heartfelt guesswork.

Three issues can be clarified immediately. One: PPCPPs often occur even when there are no cognitive complaints. Two: most PPCPPs are not special psychiatric disorders uniquely attributable to the post-concussive metabolic/inflammatory/vascular melee. Three: although there is persuasive evidence that (1) pre-existing psychiatric disorders are risk factors for persistent post-concussive psychiatric disorders, and even that (2) pre-existing psychiatric disorders are risk for *TBI itself*, neither of those facts justifies reflexively blaming these problems on pre-morbid personality. Battered brains are more interesting than that.

---

[1] For the sake of consistency with other discussions in this chapter we will consider persistence technically to mean clinically significant symptoms beyond three months post CBI. However, most of the empirical data cited derive from studies among the estimated 36–37% of concussion survivors with neurobehavioral dysfunction lasting a year or more post injury.

Regarding the first issue: in 2000 Marschark et al. [3] published what might be described as a seminal study. Seminal not because of clever design, large subject pool, or startling result, but simply because it was a rare controlled long-term follow-up of persons reporting childhood mild TBI. Seventy-nine college students who had survived concussions were compared with students who had experienced general anesthesia and with healthy controls. The abstract is sufficiently clear:

> In comparison with the two control groups, the students with a history of mild TBI produced similar scores on the cognitive tests and similar orientations to studying. However, they showed a significantly higher level of emotional distress on the SCL-90-R.
> [Symptom Checklist 90 Revised] ([3], p. 1227)

This report is not proof and not the sum of all data.[2] However, these unequivocal findings complement the many papers tabulated in previous chapters of this chapter reporting follow-ups at three months to one year. As previously documented, behavioral problems are both more common and more disabling than cognitive problems in the years after concussion.

Regarding the second issue – the non-uniqueness of PPCPPs: previous chapters of this chapter noted that if one simply counts complaints without analysis, the total number of persistent complaints among CBI survivors is similar to the total number after orthopedic injury. This supports the righteous pronouncement of a predictable (if not profound) conclusion: "two medical problems may both lead to lasting distress." The observation of similar complaint tallies, however, ignores the nature of those complaints. As previously discussed, it is useful to draw distinctions between complaints that are common to many diseases (e.g., fatigue, reduced productivity, sleep disturbance, sadness) versus those that are special to one chain of biological causality. In the case of CBI, special complaints seem to include headache, dizziness, slowed thought, and multitasking impairment. As also noted in previous chapters, the existence of CBI-specific long-term problems has been buried, in many published and much-cited studies, by misguidedly analyzing outcome based on total symptom scores reported as an indiscriminate agglomeration. If a CBI survivor is wracked with disabling headaches and suicidal depression, given his recital of just two of 16 potential problems, his Rivermead score may be reported as virtually complete recovery.

Yet attention to the specificity of PPCPPs is obviously a red herring. If cough occurs in both chronic obstructive pulmonary disease and tuberculosis, does this justify concluding that tuberculosis does not cause cough? In one 20th-century study, 138 mild TBI subjects were matched with 125 other-trauma comparison subjects. At 12 months, both traumatized groups showed persistence and even worsening of anger, impulsivity, antisocial tendencies, and poor self-monitoring [5]. The authors admitted their ignorance and ours: "It is difficult to know whether this deterioration represents return to preinjury levels, head injury-related impairments, or exacerbation of preinjury tendencies" ([5], p. 995). That essential barrier to knowledge is one provocation for the crisis in academia, with extremists on each side pointing to the same data to prove (1) CBI frequently causes long-lasting psychiatric problems, or (2) CBI is irrelevant to the occurrence of psychiatric problems. The third way is surely apparent to the reader: it is high time to abandon this fruitless debate. Current science cannot quantify the proportional contributions of, nor untrammel the interactions between, the many pre-morbid, injury-related, and post-injury factors that influence outcome.

Regarding the issue of "pre-morbid personality": of course it is important! Disease impacts that which we are. Moreover (for reasons yet to be fully explained), TBI is one of the bad things that tend to happen to people with psychiatric problems.[3] Consider Susanna,[4] a 36-year-old dental hygienist whose family history suggests a genetic predisposition to emotional dysregulation as well as exposure to suboptimal parenting, and who has long seemed unusually sensitive to stress. She has a somewhat dependent personality, low self-esteem, and a low tolerance for pain. She knows enough about head injury to be worried about it, and in fact had a strong pre-injury belief that head injuries always produce lasting harm. She then suffers a concussion. Reconstructions estimate that her head experienced an 84-**g** linear acceleration when her Mini Cooper was intercepted by a Scion XB. She was rather shocked but not profoundly stressed at the time. However, about four months after the accident she realized that she was re-reading the same paragraphs. She had to give up texting while driving because her capacity for productive divided attention had vaporized. Her supervisor noted the same, and the supervisor began shifting complex assignments from Susanna to others. The patient's execrable attorney encouraged her to believe that she had been damaged irrevocably and enabled her attribution of all of her post-concussive emotional distress to the injury. Her former husband first pressured her to exaggerate her symptoms during the medical assessments early after the injury – in his hope of scoring a personal windfall – and then left her for a 22-year-old cocktail waitress six months post CBI, complaining that she had become irritable and (in his troglodyte rhetoric) "frigid." If, at one year post CBI, Susanna is sad, why?

---

2   These results, based on self-report and long-term follow-up, are different from those from a one-year follow-up of children who survived mild TBI, based on parental reports [4]. As always, valid case ascertainment cannot be assumed.

3   In a 41-year Swedish population-based study published in 2014 [6]. the occurrence of subsequent TBI was compared between people with and without psychiatric diagnosis. Among 2,163,190 persons who did *not* develop a TBI, 83,454 (3.9%) had a pre-existing psychiatric diagnosis. Among 218,300 persons who *did* develop a TBI, 20,378 (9.3%) had a pre-existing psychiatric diagnosis. Hence, a psychiatric diagnosis was associated with about 2.4 times the risk of suffering a TBI. The reasons for this association are not known, but substantial evidence suggests that (1) some psychiatric disorders increase risk taking and (2) risk-taking behavior increases the risk of TBI.

4   Susanna's name has been changed. This is the author's best effort to summarize a memorable patient's story without violating her confidentiality.

To reframe the same question in a way that exposes the conceptual poverty of the current literature: Exactly what role did the transmission of the 84-**g** impulse through her skull play in her sadness a year later – and how would one ever know?

This is the best way I can exemplify our gargantuan challenge. Different people arrive at the sorry moment of a concussive injury involving 84 **g** of linear acceleration with absolutely unique genetic and environmental backgrounds. In Symonds's famous 1937 aphorism, "it is not only the kind of injury that matters, but the kind of head" [7]. What if, by chance, Susanna's childhood friend Zainab had the same age, education, socioeconomic status, height, weight, and Elo chess ranking, and suffered a matching injury? It is perhaps more striking and important in the case of CBI than in most medical disorders that – irrespective of the perfect identity of two noxious insults (in this case, two blows to the head of precisely matched force and direction striking Susanna and Zainab) – one cannot expect the same outcome in any two individuals. As noted in Chapter 2, a typical CBI probably triggers up- or down-regulation of about 1000 genes affecting cerebral processing. Many of those genes are known to exhibit polymorphisms or copy number variations. Therefore, the direct and immediate biological effects of the two 84-**g** injuries will virtually never be the same in the first minute after concussion in two different people. Even if those changes were the same, that initial neurobiological response would act in the context of innumerable aspects of human variation, including every genetic, epigenetic, and environmental difference between Susanna and Zainab relevant to their emotions, personalities, and acuities of reality testing – not to mention the fact that their husbands offer different degrees of support.

To slightly complicate matters, people also vary in their awareness of impairments and resilience in the face of illness. Thus, Susanna and Zainab may both develop post-CBI depression, may have identical Beck Depression Inventory scores, may even have virtually identical degrees of change in the brain circuits mediating mood. But factors such as childhood-inculcated stoicism, denial of illness, litigation stress, and grit may all be different, such that Zainab may go to work, while Susanna sometimes spends days in bed.

Why is she in bed? Which of the hundreds or perhaps thousands of cerebral factors that impact mood and behavior is responsible, and to what degree, for her sadness that day? That is the largely unanswerable question that hovers over any discussion of the biopsychosocial genesis of persistent post-concussive change like an attentive drone, ready to vaporize the simplistic accountings of this complex issue that dominate the 20th-century literature. As Kozol concluded in 1945 [8] based on a psychiatric study of 200 subjects:

> From our data it appears that there is little, or no, correlation between pretraumatic personality and the liability to development of post traumatic mental symptoms. A patient with a pretraumatic "neurotic" personality may be free from symptoms. A patient with a pretraumatic "normal" personality may be crippled by mental symptoms.
>
> ([8], p. 364)

To summarize the sorry quarrel: few scholars would debate the observation that a traumatic life experience *without* CBI may lead to lasting behavioral change. Few would debate the observation that a traumatic life experience *with* CBI may do the same. What is debated, in some cases with unseemly hard-heartedness, is the question of whether the sole explanation for lasting post-brain-injury behavior changes is psychic trauma afflicting fragile psyches. One camp of psychologists has professed for decades that (1) psychological trauma (regarded by them as magically dissociable from the physical brain change) wholly explains persistent post-concussive distress and that (2) pre-concussive "personality" explains vulnerability to such distress. In other words, it is argued with righteous zeal (and indignant discounting of neuroscience) that if a person suffers a so-called "mild TBI" and he or she continues to be depressed, or aggressive, or anxious more than three months later, the biological damage to his or her brain played no role. Based on the available science, this contention insults logic and beggars belief. We know little, but we know better than that.

Throughout the present volume, the authorial team has done its utmost to explain why more than 40% of CBI survivors exhibit ongoing symptoms at one year post injury. This paradigm shift will perhaps be met with some resistance from a subgroup of professionals trained in a previous century. It is, for one thing, directly contrary to the Three-Month Myth (the falsehood that the biomedical effects of typical CBIs resolve within three months) promoted by professional concussion deniers. In 2017, Van Meter et al. published results of their biomarker study. Elevations in brain-derived neurotrophic factor (BDNF), glial acidic fibrillary protein, and neuron-specific enolase in blood drawn within several hours of CBIs – <u>all from victims with negative computed tomography imaging</u> – predicted clinically significant depression six months post injury [9]. Findings such as this are completely inconsistent with the claim that persistent post-concussive depression is explainable by premorbid psychological history and/or post-morbid social circumstances. If replicated, acute biomarker studies of this type support the conclusion that prolonged post-concussive depression, at least at the level of population analysis, if not in every case, is incontrovertibly associated with the biological effects of brain trauma.

One commences, therefore, with that which is self-evident: if the brain is damaged, it may affect behavior. If the person is stressed, it may affect the brain and behavior. But if the brain is damaged *while* the person is stressed, and behavior subsequently changes, no one on earth can say exactly why. That is the deep root of our current ignorance. This chapter will not pretend to solve that mystery. Instead, it will briefly summarize the epidemiology of persistent post-concussive psychiatric symptoms and clarify what is known about the causes and management of the three most frequently disabling and disheartening problems: depression, aggression, and – well,

Table 10.1 Reviews, or large empirical studies, of non-cognitive neuropsychiatric changes after concussive brain injury without known coma or intracranial bleeding; follow-up ≥ 3 months

Authorship	Publication type [a]	Population [b]	Persistent post-concussive psychiatric problems noted [c]
Alexander, 1995 [41]	Rev	NS	Irr, Dep, Anx/PTSD, Ang
Arciniegas et al., 2005 [28]	Rev	NS	Dep, Anx/PTSD, SA
Bohnen and Jolles, 1992 [42]	Rev	NS	Irr, Anx/PTSD
Boyle et al., 2014 [43] [d]	Rev	Mil	Irr
Brown et al., 1994 [44]	Rev	NS	Irr, Dep
Carroll et al., 2014 [45]	Rev	Civ	Dep, Psychos, SA
Drag et al., 2012 [46]	Emp	Mil	Anx/PTSD; Dep
Fann et al., 2004 [18]	Emp	Civ	Psychos; Aff; SA
Fayol et al., 2009 [47]	Rev	NS	Irr, Anx/PTSD, Dep, SA
Halbauer et al., 2009 [48]	Rev	NS	Mood, Mania, Anx/PTSD, Psychos, Agg
Iverson, 2005 [49]	Rev	Ath	Irr
Kiraly and Kiraly, 2007 [50]	Rev	NS	PC, Psychos, Dep, Mania, Anx/PTSD; OCD
Konrad et al., 2011 [39]	Emp	Civ	Dep
Kushner, 1998 [51]	Rev	NS	Anx/PTSD, Dep, Irr
Laborey et al., 2014 [52]	Emp	Civ	Intolerance of stress, PC
Mott et al., 2012 [53]	Rev	NS	Anx/PTSD, Dep, Irr
Symonds, 1962 [54]			Anx/PTSD, Irr

[a] Review (Rev), empirical (Emp).
[b] Athlete (Ath), civilian (Civ), military (Mil), or not specified (NS).
[c] In order of prevalence when indicated:
Aff: affective disorder not otherwise specified; Agg: verbal or physical aggression, distinguished from irritability; Ang: anger; Anx/PTSD: anxiety or "post-traumatic stress disorder"; Dep: depression; Irr: irritability; Mania: mania; Mood: mood disorder not otherwise specified; OCD: obsessive compulsive disorder; PC: personality change, with or without further specification; Psychos: psychosis, with or without further specification; SA: substance abuse, with or without further specification.

something else that is attributed to stress by some writers, sometimes involves anxiety, and is sometimes labeled "PTSD."[5]

What are the Most Common PPCPPs?

Many reviews have summarized the evidence regarding the incidence or prevalence of PPCPPs after TBI [2, 8–40]. In most cases those reviews fail to stratify observations according to injury severity. Readers will reasonably ask, "How often is a typical concussion (i.e., a TBI that does not result in coma, a brain hemorrhage, or more than a day at a hospital) followed by persistent depression, or suicidality, or aggression, or the dissociable miscellany of symptoms sometimes called 'PTSD'"? One is hard put to find a credible answer or even a sophisticated discussion of the baffling complexities of this issue in the conventional literature. Although the severity of TBI is poorly conceptualized and impractical to operationalize and there is no biologically defensible definition of *mild* TBI, it is nonetheless plausible

that the frequency of PPCPPs is different in cohorts with different injury severities: survivors of blows associated with overt structural brain damage or prolonged coma appear to exhibit a somewhat different profile of psychiatric complications compared with survivors of "milder" injuries. In fact, in a seeming paradox that will be addressed shortly, some evidence suggests that milder injuries yield more frequent and persistent PPCPPs. It is disappointing that so little writing focuses on the psychiatric consequences of concussion. Still, by reviewing every cited paper in the reviews, one can winnow the universe of papers down to those reporting on survivors of typical CBIs.

The PPCPPs to be discussed in this chapter, therefore, were selected based on a review of reviews. Seventeen articles were identified that explicitly employ the terms *concussion* or *mild* in their titles and describe neuropsychiatric complications or associations of CBI. Table 10.1 summarizes the basic conclusions of those papers.

---

[5] The author apologizes for mumbling. Here is the problem: many CBI survivors have post-concussive distress. In some, their most painful symptom is anxiety. More than 35 years ago (1980) the American Psychiatric Association (APA) proclaimed the existence of a new anxiety disorder that occurred after stress. They called it "posttraumatic stress disorder" ("PTSD"). A profusion of empirical literature reported that victims of TBI often develop that anxiety problem – making the anxiety disorder called "PTSD" the third most common PPCPP. As it happens, there is no anxiety disorder called PTSD in U.S. psychiatry. It has ceased to exist, if it ever did. The APA defenestrated "PTSD" from its list of anxiety disorders in 2013. That change requires discarding all the epidemiological data that counted cases of "PTSD" as anxiety, and leaves it unclear what to call the third most common form of psychiatric distress after concussion – a multifactorial phenomenon with seven or more clusters of symptoms occurring alone or in any of millions of combinations. Readers are invited to participate in the undeclared academic contest to propose a better name.

These studies exhibit a mix of methodologies and degrees of rigor, rarely represent prospective observations, often fail to specify the follow-up period (or name a range so wide as to hobble comparison), and cite one another like echoes in a box canyon. Deriving a defensible average incidence or prevalence for any given psychiatric problem from this assemblage is not possible. Indeed, there is almost no published research that systematically compared the frequency of different persistent problems in concussed adults using normed and validated methods for case ascertainment. That derelict gap could long since have been filled. As the Common Data Elements (CDE) project has demonstrated [55], many psychometrically sound instruments are ready to hand. Yet no large-scale population-based mild TBI studies have employed (1) a single well-regarded psychiatric screening instrument (such as the Brief Psychiatric Rating Scale [56] or the Structured Clinical Interview for DSM-5 Disorders [57], or (2) a comprehensive screen for post-concussion symptoms (such as the Rivermead Post-Concussion Symptoms Questionnaire (RPCSQ) [58], the Neurobehavioral Symptom Inventory [59, 60]) or (3) an *ad hoc* battery of complementary instruments (such as the Beck Depression Inventory II [61, 62] plus the Civilian PTSD checklist [63], plus the Aggression Questionnaire [64]). The best one can take away from this review is that three PPCPPs are mentioned more than any others. Two of the three make nosological sense. In order of the reported frequency, incidence, and prevalence beyond three months post-CBI, these are:

1. post-concussive depression
2. post-concussive aggression
3. post-concussive "PTSD"-associated symptoms.[6]

The latter is the present author's place holder for the unnamable. Older readers may have been raised on a diet of "post-traumatic stress disorder (PTSD)." But "PTSD" was a mistake. It was employed (and, contrary to all available scientific evidence and judgment, is still employed) to refer to seven or more distresses, alone or in combination, that begin after a stressful event. Since one of those seven is depression, some "PTSD" cases are just post-concussive depression. ("Depression and PTSD ... both may be parts of a common general traumatic stress construct" [68].) The pretense of "PTSD" as promulgated in 1980 by an APA committee was well intentioned, but has outlived its political purpose and must be consigned to the curio cabinet of obsolete onomastics. Indeed, fans of nosological rigor hear that four-letter word and recoil. "What on earth do you mean? Stress after

stress? How can you justify giving the same name to a pathological *increase* in response to emotional provocations and to a pathological *decrease* in response to emotional provocations?"[7] The author hopes to recruit the reader for the job ahead: the APA's classification system is profoundly anti-scientific. It does not offer a logical, scientific painting of the landscape of mental disorder. It dictates the opposite [70–84]. Tugging it off the wall, like a counterfeit Picasso, is an overdue corrective. That will leave a gap. What shall we mount in its stead?

Risk factors for PPCPPs have been studied in two ways. One is the result of a search for generalizations: are there demographic, biological, or personality factors that predict persistent psychiatric troubles overall (never mind the type) after concussion? The other is the result of a search for specifics: what factors predict depression, versus aggression, versus a pathological stress response? Subsections below will discuss those specifics. Still, an overview may be useful. Scholten et al. [2] recently published a summary of findings with regard to anxiety and depressive disorders after TBI. That review, like most, failed to stratify the results by severity of injury. Its findings are not quantitatively informative about the outcome after concussion, but introduce the putative risk factors that receive the most attention:

> The most often assessed risk factors were age ...
> sex ... education ... marital or relationship status ... and
> TBI severity ... Other frequently studied factors were
> personal history of psychiatric disorders preceding TBI ...
> employment, ethnicity, duration of PTA [post-traumatic
> amnesia] ... time post-injury ... history of alcohol or
> substance abuse ... and involvement in litigation. Females,
> those without employment, and those with a history of
> psychiatric disorders or substance abuse pre-TBI were at
> higher risk for psychiatric disorders post-TBI ... Location
> of the brain lesion showed to be related to the risk of
> depressive disorders.
>
> ([2], p. 1979)

Other PPCPPs occur, such as personality change or loss of a sense of identity, bipolar symptoms, thought disorder, and altered sexuality. The empirical literature on epidemiology, risk factors, and management is, if anything, less consistent in those cases. Sleep disorder is addressed in a different chapter (Chapter 25). For the sake of concision this chapter focuses on the top three problems. In addition, a fourth entity is addressed, not because it is among the most common but because it is the most dreadful: post-concussive suicide.

---

6   As the author hopes to explain in the forthcoming narrative, compelling reasons exist to seek a more scientifically justifiable label than "PTSD." Yet one cannot label this very real problem with any single symptom such as "anxiety." First: the APA has dictated that PTSD is not an anxiety disorder [65]. Second, the most recent and sophisticated factor analytic work suggests that so-called PTSD really comprises at least seven different clusters of symptoms: re-experiencing, avoidance, negative affect, anhedonia, externalizing behaviors, and anxious and dysphoric arousal symptoms [66, 67]. One pauses, however, at the prospect of accurately calling this disorder "post-traumatic re-experiencing and/or avoidance and/or negative affect and/or anhedonia and/or externalizing behaviors and/or anxious arousal symptoms and/or dysphoric arousal symptoms." Asking clinicians to write this correct and helpful name would risk triggering flexion dystonia. Girding for semantic adversity, we boldly take on the Augean labor of conceptual housecleaning later in this chapter.

7   In the chapter on post-traumatic stress disorder and traumatic brain injury in 2015's *Handbook of Clinical Neurology*, Motzkin and Koenigs [69] joined the chorus expressing astonishment that the APA has enshrined "contradictory symptom profiles" as evidencing a single disease.

I. Post-Concussive Depression

> Depression is more closely associated with persistence and recurrence of TBI-related functional disability than initial injury severity or persisting cognitive impairment.
>
> Cook et al., 2011 [85], p. 818.

Definition of Depression

Depression is a semantically amorphous psychological construct of unknown biological nature. Writers about depression typically discuss this amorphous concept either as a dimension or a category of human behavior. They typically fail to identify which of those two ideas they have elected and they virtually never discuss the profound implications of that difference. It is hard to overstate the consequences: the non-specifiability of *depression* compromises the credibility of every one of the millions of documents that use that term in reference to human emotion.

For the purposes of this chapter one might provisionally define depression as a poorly specified negative emotion that usually involves low positive affect and high negative affect and occurs in an unknown number of species. For practical purposes one must acknowledge that mental health authorities have published statements of purported "consensus" regarding the meaning of *depression* (in fact, opinions of self-nominated elites) such as that advanced by the APA ([65, p. 160). Such statements, though well intentioned and pragmatic, reify arbitrary operational classification, and research has profited by the initiative to invent diagnostic algorithms, since these facilitate comparability of clinical problems across sites. Yet none of those statements describe a scientifically defined phenomenon or objectifiable entity.

The author is concerned, however, that pointing out the scientific impotence of the existing definitions may distract from a much more important message. He opines (based on instinct, not fact) that the feeling referred to as *depression* was apparent to mammals long before the evolution of anatomically modern humans. That feeling, when severe, is awful. That feeling can be devastating, disabling, and deadly. That feeling seems to be associated with an existential crisis in which the normal, healthy Promethean obliviousness to mortality is penetrated by the inevitability of non-existence and the utter fruitlessness of efforts to escape that fate. That painful negative feeling is very common among survivors of TBIs and concussions. Let us please defer quibbling about semantics, shrug at the cavalier use of the term, hope for a biomarker, and move on – devoting ourselves to assuaging the torment of its victims.

Detection and Measurement of Post-Concussive Depression

Any new-onset medical problem may trigger bad feelings. But which concussed persons with bad feelings are depressed? Several writers have pointed out that it is difficult to distinguish between the post-concussive state with and without depression, since "existing criteria have significant overlap with common TBI sequels" [86]. For example, fatigue, distractability,

diminished concentration, slowed thinking, irritability, preoccupation with pain, sleep disturbance, social withdrawal, guilty thoughts, thoughts of death, hopelessness, and somatic complaints such as headache are common in both disorders [87–88]. As Cook et al. [85] cautioned: "These symptoms could be attributable to TBI rather than to MDD [major depressive disorder]" (p. 818). A massive literature describes psychological instruments for detecting the presence versus absence (the categorical issue) or measuring the degree of (the dimensional issue) depression [78, 91–96]. However, some writers have gone so far as to assert these popular methods of detection and measurement of depression are inapplicable after TBI, both due to that overlap in symptoms and due to the possibility that the very nature of post-CBI depression differs from "major depressive disorder" diagnosed in non-brain-injured cohorts. Guillamondegui et al. [97], for instance, declared, "The literature is insufficient to determine whether tools validated in other populations for detecting depression appropriately identify individuals with depression after a TBI."

These reasonable concerns have inspired efforts to test the validity of conventional depression scales among person with TBI. Among recent papers, the most commonly studied measures include the Hamilton Depression Rating Scale (HAM-D) [98], the Beck Depression Inventory (BDI) or its revised edition (BDI-II) [61, 62, 99], the Hospital Anxiety and Depression Scale (HADS) [100], and the Patient Health Questionnaire-9 (PHQ-9) [101, 102].

Complicating the interpretation of this literature for survivors of typical concussions, most published studies report results with subjects of mixed severity or after severe injuries. For example, Schwarzbold et al. [103] compared the HAM-D, BDI, and HADS, concluding "Our findings support a high validity" for all of those instruments after TBI. Unfortunately, that study included only survivors of severe injuries. The HADS has the advantage of excluding questions related to headaches, dizziness, or insomnia, and some evidence supports the validity of the HADS among TBI subjects across levels of severity [104, 105]. However, as Dawkins et al. [106] noted, some HADS items may equivocally reflect either the cognitive effects of brain injury or emotional distress. For example, when a concussed person reports, "I feel slowed down," or reports that he or she has lost the ability to enjoy things, including television programs, such complaints may represent impaired information processing rather than sadness. Driskell et al. [107] expressed two further concerns about the HADS. First, this instrument has inferior sensitivity compared with clinical interview. Second, factor analysis reveals a strong general factor tapping depression and anxiety together, hinting that this instrument may be best regarded as a general measure of distress.

Cook et al. [85] attempted to assess the validity of the PHQ-9 among TBI mild to severe TBI survivors one year post injury. Modeling with item response theory and testing differential item functioning with logistic regression led to the conclusion that no item spuriously inflated the occurrence of depression among TBI subjects. Hence, those authors judged, "The PHQ-9 is a valid screener of major depressive disorder in people with complicated mild to severe TBI, and all symptoms can be counted toward the diagnosis of major depressive disorder without special concern about over-diagnosis or unnecessary treatment."

The present author lacks expertise in psychometrics. He defers to properly educated authorities regarding the strength of the evidence favoring any particular psychological instrument. His sole recommendations in this regard are simply that researchers or clinicians doing their best to determine the presence or degree of post-concussive depression keep in mind that (1) it is premature to claim knowledge of the essential nature of depression and (2) considerable overlap exists between the semiology of distress that clinicians attribute to depression, anxiety, and somatic illness.

Epidemiology of Post-Concussive Depression

Some clever way probably exists – guarded in their fortress of solitude by biostatisticians – that permits valid analysis of the many papers claiming to accurately report the incidence, prevalence, or frequency of depression after concussion. The author has no privileged entrée. He can only repeat a lament: diverse definitions of depression, incompatible measurement methods, clinically incomparable cohorts, and the overlap between depression and all manner of other distressing problems together prohibit any quotable conclusion about how often CBI is followed by depression. Numbers are available in superfluity. *Meaningful* numbers surely shine among them, like marbles buried on a pebble beach. The most earnest scholar, however, is reduced to a babbling recitation of the published range: 6–77%.

Six relatively recent reviews each offer a range:

1. Warden et al., 2006 [108]:
   "Depression after TBI is very common, with best estimates suggesting that 25–60% of individuals with TBI develop a depressive episode within eight years of their injury" (p. 1469).
2. Kim et al., 2007 [31]:
   Incidence = 11.6–33% at three to 12 months
   Prevalence = 18.5–61% at three months to 8 years.
3. Halbauer et al., 2009 [48]:
   "The incidence of post-TBI depression ranges from 15.3 to 33.0 percent … while the prevalence ranges from 18.5 to 61.0 percent" (p. 774).
4. Rapoport, 2012 [109]:
   "Many studies of prevalence of depression following TBI have not used accepted structured criteria for the diagnoses, but those that did found wide ranges of rates, from 17% to 61%."
5. Mauri et al., 2014 [110]:
   "The published rates of axis I disorders in patients with TBI are 14–77% for MDD" (p. 118).
6. Jorge and Arciniegas, 2014 [111]
   "Depressive disorders develop commonly among persons with TBI, with estimated frequencies ranging from 6–77% … most experts on this subject accept an estimated first-year post-TBI depression frequency in the range of 25–50% and lifetime rates of 26–64%" (p. 2).

These reviews do not exhaust the data, yet almost all recent empirical studies report results within the same unworkably broad range [97, 112, 113]. The most accurate available estimate is 6–77%, settling the fact that post-concussive depression is common, or perhaps not.[8]

Readers will probably share the author's concern that this is hardly helpful information. The numbers say more about the challenge of defining and detecting the phenomenon of interest than about the risk of distressing negative affect after concussion.

Another way to analyze the epidemiological impact is to ask whether concussion affects the lifetime risk of depression. Given the paucity of long-term follow-up studies, the sole data come from cross-sectional retrospective studies. Subjects are asked, "Have you been depressed; have you had a concussion?" – an approach that is exquisitely vulnerable to recall bias. The danger from repetitive concussions is reasonably well established: in Guskiewicz's et al.'s 2007 [114] seminal study of 2552 retired professional football players: those with histories of three or more concussions exhibited three times the rate of depression compared with those without concussions. Similar findings were reported with respect to high school athletes: Schatz et al. [115 found that two or more concussions were associated with a significant increase in depression ratings. The same association seems to obtain after single CBIs (although average velocity, force, and mechanism may have been different): Holsinger et al. [116] found a 1.5-times risk of depression among Vietnam veterans with closed head injuries. Fann et al. [18] reported that the relative risk for affective disorder after "mild TBI" was 1.9 at 7–12 months and still 1.6 at 19–24 months. Chrisman and Richardson [117] found that adolescents with a self-reported history of concussion had a 3.3-fold increase in the risk of depression. Therefore, consistent evidence from multiple studies of single or repetitive concussions demonstrates that CBI is definitely associated with an increased risk of subsequent depression. Candidly acknowledging that one cannot specify the magnitude of that risk based on current data, there remain multiple interesting findings worthy of consideration.

For one: perhaps contrary to intuition, depression may be more common after typical "mild" CBIs than after moderate to severe TBIs. That conclusion is tentative and unsettled. First, to the best of the author's knowledge, no long-term study using standardized assessment psychological tools reports higher rates of depression after more severe injuries. That in itself

---

[8] Chapter 5 offered a great deal of data weakly supporting our best estimate that > 40% of concussed persons express or exhibit persistent clinical problems at one year post-injury or beyond. Averaging the averages from these six reviews, one calculates that 41.8% of CBI survivors develop persistent depression. That number, like all the numbers derived from the world concussion literature's embarrassingly low-quality research, is best looked at askance.

seems surprising; one might instead expect a dose–response effect. Second, multiple studies (e.g., [118, 119]) report that the risk of depression is the same regardless of the severity of injury, suggesting that our workaday measures of initial severity such as the Glasgow Coma Scale fail to assay the special type of brain change most likely to yield self-consciously negative affect. Third, U.S. observations published since the 1940s report an inverse association, such that milder injury is – in a seeming paradox – associated with a greater likelihood of depression [18, 120]. As Ansari et al. [120] reported, "Depression was more common in mild TBI cases than those with moderate TBI (53.7% vs. 46.25%, $P = 0.04$)." In a conceptually consistent finding, Bryan and Clemans [121] found that a longer duration of TBI-induced loss of consciousness was associated with a *lower* risk of subsequent suicide among deployed military personnel, also hinting that more severe brain damage (or possibly less vivid recall?) is protective.

One argument from the early 20th century contended that this inverse association proved that survivors with depression were feigning for profit. Intriguingly, however, experimental animal studies arrive at the same inverse results. Bajwa et al. [122] exposed mice to graded controlled cortical impacts (mild, repeated mild, or moderate). At 90 days post impact, T2-weighted magnetic resonance imaging (MRI) revealed no damage after mild or mild repeated injury but visible lesions after moderate injury. The authors conducted multiple behavioral tests considered to elicit depression-equivalent responses. They concluded: "These data suggest that mild concussive injuries lead to … affective disorders that are not observed after moderate TBI." The awkwardness of testing mouse mood restrains confidence in such findings. Yet these results at least support the plausibility of a causal link between mildness and persistent mood disorder. Why? The rodents were not litigants. The findings suggest a biological explanation. One possibility, offered purely as a speculation: the conscious feeling of *depression* requires the integrity of white-matter cortical–subcortical connections that link primitive (allocortical or subcortical) systems that mediate somatic and affective well-being to higher cortical domains that mediate conscious self-awareness and perceived future security. Beyond some threshold of damage, those long white-matter tracts are more likely to be dysfunctional after a more severe injury. If so, both mildly and moderately injured persons suffer potentially disabling loss, but milder injury better preserves perception.

A second issue worth exploring is the temporal course of post-concussive depression. This is difficult to decipher due to inconsistencies in the literature. Some studies reported a *decrease* in prevalence of depression over time, especially over the course of the year post injury (18, 86, 123–125]. Other studies report an *increase* in prevalence over time [37, 126, 127], including a report that 26% developed depression between the first and second years post injury [112]. Duration is also variable, although Hart et al. found that three-quarters of those who were depressed at one year remained depressed at two years.

Further complicating the question of time course: some patients exhibit acute onset, others delayed onset, some recover, and others report persistent depression. Jorge [87], for example, followed a cohort of patients with closed head injuries for one year. Among those who developed depression, the onset was acute in 61% and delayed in 39%. Bombardier et al. [128] recently attempted to bring order to these perplexing data, investigating the commonsense possibility that the published inconsistencies may be due to clinically distinct subgroups. They analyzed the temporal course of depression over one year among 559 mild- to severely injured subjects using latent class growth mixture modeling. This method reportedly enables the identification of clinically homogeneous subgroups within a heterogeneous population. Four distinct groups emerged: 70.1% of subjects never developed significant depression, 13.2% developed delayed-onset depression, 10.4% developed and then recovered from depression, and 6.3% exhibited depression throughout the period of observation.[9]

That novel approach clarifies the heterogeneous course but leaves open the question: why do many depressions have delayed onset? No definitive answer, and certainly no biologically validated answer, is currently available. However, the author posits one factor that conceivably helps explain this phenomenon: awareness often blossoms as brains do their best to recover. Persons who are newly battered may be confused and forgetful, busy relearning the business of day-to-day life at home and work, and not yet altogether conscious of their new limitations. At that stage they may be somewhat immune from the despair caused by self-conscious awareness of loss. (Again, purely speculating, one wonders whether that period of diminished acuity reflects reversible long white-matter tract dysfunction.) In the author's personal experience, many CBI survivors seem to emerge from that protective shell about six months after concussion. Blooming awareness sometimes provokes a paradoxical-seeming ebb in well-being that may take the patient, the family, and the doctor by surprise. Several other writers discuss the return of awareness as a possible factor in late-onset PPCPPs [129, 130]. One gathers that, contrary to some claims [124], there is no single "natural history of depression in TBI." Just as in depression without injury, people vary.

A third issue – or collection of related matters – is the quest for predictive or risk factors. Several have been reported and replicated in independent samples. Abundant evidence supports the conclusion that a pre-injury history of psychiatric diagnosis, psychiatric treatment, or substance abuse increases the likelihood of post-CBI depression [18, 109, 112, 131, 132]. As discussed in previous chapters, that perhaps reflects both lifelong predispositions and diminished cerebral reserves.

The effect of age is not so clear. While *older* age has been reported to be a risk factor in several studies [97, 133, 134],

---

[9] Recalculating: 29.9% of subjects developed depression at some point, of whom 44% had delayed onset – a proportion that closely matches Jorge et al.'s finding from a study reported 23 years earlier.

other reports attribute depressive risk to *younger* age of injury [132, 135, 136]. How might one reconcile this discrepancy? One possibility, as suggested in the chapter on epidemiology (Chapter 2), is that vulnerability to the harm of CBI conforms to a U-shaped curve, such that teens and the elderly are both more cerebrally fragile than adults aged 25–60.

Sex seems to matter. Among the studies that examined that factor, most report that women are more likely to become depressed after concussion than men [37, 132, 137].[10] Hormonal cycling, as discussed earlier in this text, might contribute to this phenomenon by compromising cerebral resistance to affective stress. Several studies report that depression is more likely among survivors with lower levels of education [124, 136]. Both pain [125] and poverty [117] have also been reported to increase the risk of depression.

Finally, many studies report that co-morbid PTSD is a risk factor for post-concussive depression. This brings up an ongoing controversy: what, after all, is PTSD? Is it a biologically discrete disease or just one part of a predictably variable continuum of human post-stress distress that has been arbitrarily defined (and repeatedly redefined) by an APA committee? Readers familiar with the DSM system know that the approved diagnostic criteria for major depression and PTSD overlap to a great extent. If epidemiological scholars reveal that many people with PTSD are depressed and many with depression have PTSD, is this a deep insight into human nature or an inevitability of one popular diagnostic schema? A second question: assuming, for the sake of argument, that PTSD and depression are biologically dissociable but frequently co-morbid, why? Is one a chicken and the other an egg? Does one cause the other or do they share a common genesis? Deferring those questions for the moment, suffice it to say that empirical studies report co-morbidity [94, 138, 139].

Cause(s) of, or Risk Factors for, Post-Concussive Depression

The risk factors for development of depression following TBI are poorly understood, but past psychiatric history, frontal lesions and atrophy, and family dysfunction have been shown in more than one study to play important roles.
Rapoport, 2012 [109]

No one would debate that being hit on the head tends to be distressing. No one is surprised that stressors – cumulatively over a lifetime and collectively at any moment – increase the risk for sadness. The scientific question is: to what degree can the occurrence of post-CBI depression be attributed to CBI being just another environmental life stressor, as opposed to an injury changing the brain circuitry that regulates mood,

either on its own account or in combination with a predisposition? As previously explained in this chapter no one can answer that question in any given individual or group. Many studies have attempted to do so. A typical design is to compare rates of depression among persons with and without TBI. We have previously reviewed that literature as it pertains to post-concussive symptoms (PCS). The same issues bedevil interpretation of depression studies. Counting symptoms is not comparing amounts of distress. A more fruitful approach would be to compare the brain changes in depression after concussion and depression unrelated to brain injury. Technology is on the verge of enabling that investigation.

As the modified Haddon matrix in Chapter 7 hopefully clarified, no post-CBI problem has a single cause and no two survivors with the same problem could possibly suffer due to the same collection of causes. Genetic, early developmental, biology of injury, and post-injury circumstances all contribute. Without claiming anything like a satisfactory answer, one can nonetheless point to recent discoveries that may some day lead to understanding.

With regard to genes, several findings from both experimental and clinical science support the hypothesis that individuals are born with different risks of post-concussive depression. A study of blast-related injury investigated whether concussion triggered epigenetic changes as part of its known profound effect on gene expression. Haghighi et al. [140] reported DNA methylation changes in 458 neuronal genes and 379 glial genes after blasting rats. "In particular, increased methylation and decreased gene expression were observed in the *Aanat* gene, which is … implicated in sleep disturbance and depression associated with traumatic brain injury."

With regard to humans, two studies of the much-studied gene for the serotonin transporter promoter protein came to opposite results. Chan et al. [141] found no association between the rs25531 variant and the risk for post-concussive depression. Yet Failla et al. [142] reported that persons who are homozygotes for the long variant of the allele for the 5-HTTLPR and who had pre-injury mood disorders are at higher risk of depression after severe TBI. It is clearly premature to declare which gene variants play what role in post-concussive depression.[11]

With regard to pre- and post-morbid psychological risk factors (meaning yet-to-be-understood cerebral traits), it has already been mentioned that a history of psychiatric illness and substance abuse are both risk factors. Rapoport et al. [144] published evidence that family dysfunction was a risk factor. Malec et al. [118] point out that survivors with diminished self-appraisal of their abilities are more likely to become depressed. In addition, Elliott et al. [145] opined that "low social support, avoidant coping, and psychological inflexibility

---

[10] At least one study reported a higher rate of depression among men [124]. That is possibly explained by a larger proportion of severely injured subjects.

[11] Polimanti et al. [143] investigated the possibility that a polygenic risk score reflecting risks of psychiatric or neurodegenerative disorders might be associated with PCS among 854 soldiers. The findings were negative. Unfortunately, that study did not examine possible genetic associations with individual symptoms such as depression, suicidality, or aggression, or anxiety. Of possible interest: larger infant head circumference was a protective factor against PCS.

are related to overcontrolled and undercontrolled personality prototypes," which in turn are associated with more depression and PTSD among brain-injured veterans. Resilience seemed to be protective. As posited by the present author, some evidence suggests that self-awareness quasi-paradoxically increases the risk for depression [130].

At least five medical correlates of post-injury depression have recently been reported. According to Sullivan-Singh et al. [125], pain is a risk factor for depression at one year post injury. That is not a surprise. More interestingly, some evidence exists that hypercortisolemia [119], hyperlipidemia [146], dysautonomia [119, 147, 148], and inflammation [149, 150] may all increase the risk of post-CBI depression.

With regard to localization: the author reiterates his plea that notions of localized brain processing of psychological constructs be abandoned. Such constructs are not biological in nature, the brain employs many regions for any task, no two brains employ the same network for any task, and functional neuroimaging, especially in the case of MRI signals, is a misleading approach to localization [151]. With those admonitions in mind, several investigators have claimed that one or another brain part has a special relationship with post-CBI depression based on structural or functional imaging.

Structural Findings

Jorge et al. [152] studied TBI survivors across the spectrum of severity. They reported not only that survivors of moderate or severe TBI have lower hippocampal volumes compared with survivors of "mild" injuries, but also that depressed survivors of moderate to severe injuries have even more hippocampal atrophy. Those authors posit a "double-hit" mechanism, such that the physical trauma of TBI combines with the subsequent physiological damage associated with mood disorder "(e.g., the neurotoxic effects of increased levels of cortisol or excitotoxic damage resulting from overactivation of glutaminergic pathways)"([152], p. 332) to produce these findings.[12] In a sample of male mild TBI subjects, Chen et al. [153] found that increasing depression scores correlated significantly with reduced gray-matter density in the right anterior cingulate gyrus. Rao et al. [133] reported that frontal subdural hemorrhage in mild injury predicted depression.

In a different study, members of the same research group [154] found that depressed survivors had lower right frontal, left occipital, and temporal lobe regional volumes. Hudak et al. [155] reported an association between depression and atrophy in the left rostral anterior cingulate, as well as in the left and right lateral orbitofrontal regions. Maller et al. [156] also found that post-CBI depression was associated with reduced volume in the anterior cingulate region, but also in the temporal lobe and insula. Readers will have noted the repeated findings of reduced cingulate volume, though it remains unclear whether this is lateralized.

Diffusion tensor imaging (DTI) provides a view with both high-resolution structural and functional implications, since changes probably reflect altered axonal flow. There have been reports of abnormally depressed fractional anisotropy (FA)[13] in the superior longitudinal fasciculus [157], in the frontotemporal white matter [158], in the cingulum and uncinate fasciculus [159].

Functional Findings

Since both concussion and depression are heterogeneous, one would not expect imaging research to discover a marker. And since functional MRI (fMRI) localization is dubiously valid when based on group data, one has little faith in the majority of publications. (If one averages peaks and valleys across the Alps, one may discover that Lake Geneva is a mountain.) Still, readers may wish to be familiar with the state of the art. Chen et al. [153] used fMRI to scan their mildly brain-injured male cohort, some of whom were depressed. When subjects responded to a working-memory task, post-CBI depression was associated with "smaller negative BOLD [blood oxygen level-dependent] signals in the rostral anterior cingulate cortex … and medial orbitofrontal cortex." Also, the higher the depression score, the lower the BOLD signal change in the left dorsolateral prefrontal cortex, striatum, and insula, as well as the bilateral rostral cingulate, medial orbitofrontal cortex, and parahippocampal gyri (Figure 10.1). Such findings are difficult to interpret but conceivably mean that depression reduces responsiveness to cognitive work in multiple regions.

A study that is easier to interpret (because it better comports with intuition, not because it is truer): Matthews et al. [160] compared U.S. veterans with blast-related concussion with and without depression. Both resting DTI and fMRI activated by a face-matching fear detection task were performed. DTI showed reduced FA in the superior longitudinal fasciculus – a big white-matter bundle positioned (among other jobs) to help coordinate limbic with cortical responses to emotion. fMRI showed *increased* activity in the amygdala and *decreased* activity in the dorsolateral prefrontal cortex. This was optimistically interpreted as evidence of a pathological combination of overreaction to emotional stimuli with underreaction of regulatory circuitry – like stamping on the accelerator of distress while losing one's brakes.

More than a decade ago, Jorge et al. [161] offered a theory intended to tie together then-available findings regarding depression after brain injury: "The neuropathological changes produced by TBI may lead to deactivation of lateral and dorsal prefrontal cortices and increased activation of ventral limbic

---

[12] Unfortunately, Jorge et al. did not tabulate the MRI findings stratified by severity and it is not possible to determine whether mild cases with depression were structurally different from mild cases without depression.

[13] Anisotropy is the property of being directionally dependent – like spaghetti in a box. Healthy white-matter bundles of axons are anisotropic. When all is well, axonal transport is running proteins straight and unhindered down the railroad tracks of the axon (think of microtubule-associated proteins as the rail ties). FA is a measure of hewing to the straight and narrow. CBI routinely contorts the rails. Reduced FA probably reflects that contortion.

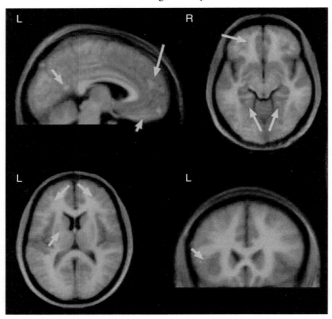

Post-concussive depression alters cerebral reactivity to a working-memory task

Fig. 10.1 Relationship between Beck Depression Inventory II scores and blood oxygenation level-dependent (BOLD) signal changes. The higher the scores, the lower the percentage of BOLD signal changes in the right (R) and left (L) dorsolateral prefrontal cortex, left striatum, and left insula (shown in blue). In addition, the higher the Beck Depression Inventory II scores, the less the negative percentage of BOLD signal changes in the rostral anterior and posterior cingulate, medial orbitofrontal cortex, and left and right parahippocampal gyri (in red) [A black and white version of this figure will appear in some formats. For the color version, please refer to the plate section.]

Source: Chen et al., 2008 [153]. Journal of the American Medical Association

and paralimbic structures including the amygdala." This was, in essence, precisely what Matthews et al. reported (Figure 10.2).

Using a different technology, Rao et al. [154] employed magnetic resonance spectroscopy and found that post-CBI depression was associated with lower choline/creatine and *N*-acetylaspartate/creatine ratios in the right basal ganglia. This (with Chen et al.) is one of the few reports suggesting basal ganglia involvement. They concluded, "The results suggest a possible role of frontotemporal lobe and basal ganglia pathology in depression after TBI" [154].

One reviews these imaging findings, noting their differences with regard to lobe, side, degree, and direction of change, and hesitates to declare understanding. Focal atrophy or altered blood flow does not reveal how neurophysiological processing or molecular biology generates sadness, or how brain changes due to genes, due to past experience, due to brain rattling, and due to all that follows interact to make these pictures. Given today's doubts about the specificity and validity of functional imaging results, a generation may pass before a causal sequence becomes apparent.

Summarizing the subsection on the causes or risk factors for post-concussive depression, one simply refers back to the

Haddon matrix provided in Chapter 7. Claiming one cause in any one case would not satisfy common sense. Quantifying the relative contribution of multiple causes is impossible. Every case involves many causes. No two cases involve the same causes. The best one can do, at this early stage, is to document with care the inconsistent and sometimes opposite statistical associations emerging from the highest-quality empirical work and eagerly await the revelations of our children.

Management of Post-Concussive Depression

No evidence is available to guide treatment choices for depression after head injury.
                                        Guillamondegui et al., 2011 [97]

The introductory quotation from Guillamondegui et al. is refreshingly stark and uncompromising. One might argue that it is rhetorically imprecise. A better summary would be: several treatments have been reported to moderate post-TBI depression but none of those reports satisfy contemporary standards of evidence. One wishes to acknowledge the efforts made. Without the pilot data cited below, one would be altogether at sea when proposing a drug to try or a hypothesis to test. It is nonetheless disheartening that, in even the most technologically advanced societies, caring doctors must still employ trial and error if they wish to help persistently depressed CBI survivors.

Another barrier will limit effective treatment for the foreseeable future even if larger, better studies are done. Management must be individualized. Current so-called "evidence-based therapy" is a misnomer, since it reports results averaged over clinically and genetically heterogeneous cohorts, failing to individualize treatment by subtype of disorder and by premorbid traits, especially but not only genes. Future doctors will justifiably cringe at the recommendations in today's textbooks, recalling the dark days when medications were prescribed blind to personal biology. Ethics perhaps requires both candid acknowledgment of the dangers of our ignorance and, hoping to do more good than harm and not to replicate the popularity of bleeding and clysters, best guesses, identified as such.

Non-Pharmacological Approaches to Post-Concussive Depression

Two major reviews help summarize what is known regarding non-pharmacological approaches to the management of post-concussive depression.[14] Neither stratified findings by severity of injury, but both cite reports that included some mildly injured subjects. Gertler et al.'s [163] Cochrane review identified six randomized controlled trials (RCTs). These authors expressed concern that all six studies exhibited a high risk of bias. Three papers compared cognitive behavior therapy (CBT) or mindfulness-based cognitive therapy with another psychological intervention [164–167]. A meta-analysis found no evidence in favor of any psychological treatment. The other three papers were not more encouraging:

---

[14] A smaller review of the same subject was previously published by Fayol [162], but focused on severe injuries.

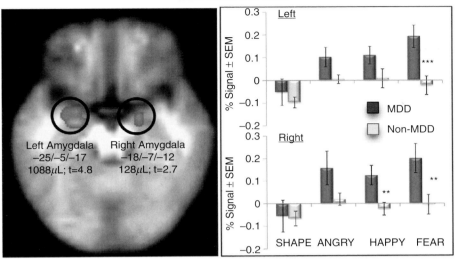

Increased Bilateral Amygdala Activation to Fear in MDD versus Non-MDD

Fig. 10.2 A region-of-interest (ROI) analysis revealed significantly greater fear-related activation in bilateral amygdalae in major depressive disorder (MDD) versus non-MDD subjects (left panel). Mean activation for shape-matching, angry, happy, and fear trials extracted from the amygdalae ROIs is displayed in the right panel. [A black and white version of this figure will appear in some formats. For the color version, please refer to the plate section.]

Source: Matthews et al., 2011 [157] with permission from Elsevier

1. Ashman et al. [168] compared CBT with supportive psychotherapy. There was no evidence of any difference in efficacy (and, without an untreated control group, indeed no evidence of efficacy).

2. Hoffman et al. [169] compared supervised exercise with unsupervised exercise. The severity of the injuries was undocumented and they occurred from six months to five years prior to treatment. No group effect was observed.

3. He et al. [170] compared repetitive transcranial magnetic stimulation (rTMS) plus tricyclic antidepressant versus tricyclic antidepressant alone. No clear treatment effect was observed.[15]

The Cochrane review concluded: "There was very-low quality evidence, small effect sizes and wide variability of results, suggesting that no comparisons showed a reliable effect for any intervention" [163].

The French Society of Physical Medicine and Rehabilitation also published a systematic review of non-pharmacological treatments for behavioral disorders after TBI [174]. This paper instantiates the conundrum faced by readers of the concussion literature: no good evidence is available, yet experts manage to announce official "international recommendations" without choking on chagrin:

Despite the small number of publications and a low level of proof, a number of recommendations for the non-pharmacological approach to psychological and behavioural disorders in TBI is proposed ... It was not possible to reach any scientific grade A recommendation on account of the low levels of proof ... However 37 recommendations were drafted on the basis of expert opinion.

([174], pp. 31, 32)

One supposes that these "buyer beware" disclaimers excuse the publication of opinions under a title that implies knowledge. And our clinical desperation for prescriptive advice will probably perpetuate this kind of work surviving peer review.

Of 458 articles reviewed, most reported management of non-specific "behavioral disorders," but several mentioned depression. Schonberger et al. [175] reported that a good "emotional bond" with therapists reduced depression among patients with various neurological insults. Guetin et al. [176] reported an uncontrolled study in which music therapy was associated with a temporary reduction in depression among a small group of severe TBI survivors. In an uncontrolled study of an unselected clinical sample with adjustment disorder after various types of acquired brain injury, Hofer et al. [177] reported that "psychotherapeutic intervention" reduced depression scores. Bédard et al. [165] reported an uncontrolled trial in which mindfulness-based cognitive therapy reduced depression in a small group of TBI survivors of non-specified severity. The present author tentatively concludes that talking therapy is probably helpful to many patients. It is not clear, however, whether any particular training or approach matters apart from empathy.

Pharmacological Approaches to Post-Concussive Depression

At least six groups published relatively recent reviews, meta-analyses, or guidelines for pharmacological management of

---

[15] Note that other case reports and trials have also explored the efficacy of TMS in post-concussive depression [171]. Baker-Price and Persinger [172] recruited four mild- to moderately concussed persons with depression judged to be resistant to pharmacological treatment. Pulsed magnetic fields firing across the temporal lobes for 30 minutes once a week for five weeks reportedly reduced those depressive symptoms in this uncontrolled trial. George et al. [173] conducted a sham-controlled trial; 24 of 41 subjects had mild TBI and depression. Active treatment was associated with a rapid reduction in suicidal ideation in the whole cohort. However, the effects on the mild TBI subgroup were not reported and the duration of the alleged benefit was only three days.

post-traumatic neurobehavioral disorders [48, 108, 178–181].[16] These reviews primarily summarize reports pertinent to severe injury; none focused on interventions of benefit after typical concussion. Very few of the studies cited across the six reviews report RCTs, of which fewer relate to mood disorders, of which fewer relate to survivors of typical CBI.

Combining and de-duplicating, these reviews included a total of 13 studies of medication trials for depression after TBI. Seven medication trial studies involved depressed survivors of mild or moderate injuries. Saran [184] reported no benefit from amitriptyline. Dinan and Mobayed [185] reported that four of 13 subjects responded to amitriptyline at up to 250 mg/day. Although those authors concluded that post-CBI depression "is relatively resistant to tricyclic therapy" (p. 292), one suspects that any hope of beneficial impact was confounded by the disabling side-effects at that dose.

A study by Fann et al. [186] stands out as encouraging, despite, or perhaps because of, its methodological defects. Fifteen subjects were recruited and treated with sertraline at 25–200 mg/day in a single-blind, non-randomized trial. At eight weeks, 87% were judged to have responded. The lack of a control group or replication limits the credibility of this report. Kanetani et al. [187] reported that milnacipran, a serotonin and norepinephrine reuptake inhibitor, reduced depression in an uncontrolled trial of ten subjects with mild to moderate TBI. Rapoport et al. [188] reported the largest open trial, treating 54 mild- to moderate TBI survivors with citalopram for six weeks and 26 subjects for ten weeks: 46.2% were judged to have responded. Those authors seem to have anticipated comparison with Fann et al.'s astonishing 87% success rate and comment: "The response rate in the present sample was substantially lower than previously reported for patients with TBI, but comparable to the results of the largest effectiveness trial of citalopram" ([188], p. 860). That is, believable.

Several small controlled trials were identified. Lee et al. [189] randomized ten mild to moderate TBI survivors each to treatment with sertraline, methylphenidate, or placebo. Those authors assert that "this study is the first to compare a drug's effectiveness on various neuropsychiatric symptoms following mild to moderate TBI with standardized assessment scales." The results were positive: "When compared with the placebo, methylphenidate and sertraline had significantly better effects on depressive symptoms measured by HAM-D." Of possible interest, subjects receiving methylphenidate fared better in terms of both side-effects and cognitive outcomes.

Rapoport et al. [144] recruited a subgroup from their original citalopram study, treating ten subjects in a small RCT of the same medication. However, the relapse rates were the same in the treatment and placebo groups. Two studies reported sertraline trials, but the cohort were heavily skewed toward moderate to severe TBI. Ashman et al. [190] studied the efficacy of sertraline in a TBI cohort (one-third of whom had mild TBI). Placebo and medication were equally effective. Novack et al. [191] tried to interrupt the development of depression with sertraline during the first year after TBI. There were benefits. They vanished when the drug was stopped. The conclusion: "There is no basis from this study to assume that sertraline administered early in recovery after TBI, when neurotransmitter functioning is often altered, has ongoing effects on the serotonin system after sertraline is discontinued" (p. 1921).

As discussed throughout this chapter one eagerly anticipates the imminent advent of individualized medicine facilitated by pharmacogenomics. In an impressively large study, Lanctôt et al. [192] examined the relationship between six functional single-nucleotide polymorphisms (SNPs) and response to citalopram among 90 survivors of mild to moderate TBI with major depression. Persons with either the C-(677) T variant of the gene for methylene tetrahydrofolate reductase or the Val66Met variant of the gene for BDNF were more likely to benefit from treatment. On the other hand, persons with the rs255531 variant of the gene for the serotonin transporter were more likely to suffer side-effects. Such studies pave the way, one hopes, for heritable-factor-based treatment algorithms.

Recommendations for the Management of Post-Concussive Depression

Limited conclusions are justified. The author retreats to platitudes. For theoretical, empirical, and practical reasons, regular talking with an empathetic professional seems helpful to many psychiatrically distressed persons. After a typical CBI, most survivors retain sufficient sociality to interact fruitfully in psychotherapy. Talk therapy not otherwise specified is probably safe and efficacious. Medication trials also seem worthy of pursuit. Despite legitimate questions about whether the neurobiology of disabling sadness is the same with and without brain concussion, despite the frailty of evidence from RCTs, despite the relatively modest response rate of efficacy of antidepressants among non-TBI patients with major depression, and despite the potential for adverse reactions, the subset of sad CBI survivors who are not disturbed by side-effects might benefit from trials of agents such as low-dose (initially) escitalopram.[17] Methylphenidate may help a subgroup that has yet to be identified. Alternatives are limited. At the time of this writing no evidence supports a meaningful benefit from rTMS.

One research domain receiving escalating attention in both TBI and psychiatric disorders: the previously unexamined role of inflammation. Evidence indeed links inflammatory markers to depression after TBI in both rodents [149] and humans [150]. In 2017, an experimental paper appeared with a provocative title, "Simvastatin therapy in the acute stage of traumatic brain injury attenuates brain trauma-induced depression-like behavior in rats by reducing neuroinflammation in the hippocampus" [195]. Conceivably,

---

[16] Two smaller-scale reviews focused on post-TBI depression [182, 183]. Their conclusions have been incorporated in the forthcoming discussion.

[17] To the best of the author's knowledge, no RCT has tested the efficacy of escitalopram for post-CBI depression. This medication is only suggested (and reservedly so) because of the cumulative evidence that it has somewhat superior efficacy for MDD without TBI [193, 194].

this new focus of inquiry will lead to novel interventions with multiple benefits to survivors of TBI.

II. Post-Concussive Suicidality

In 1971, Achté et al. [196] published a study of suicides among 6498 soldiers who had suffered brain injuries of various severities in the Finnish wars of 1939–1945. The follow-up interval was 27–33 years. Most were "comparatively severely injured" ([196], p. 25). Forty-five percent of the men were described as having an alteration of character:

Those who had previously behaved normally had, as a result of the injury, grown irritable, impulsive, aggressive and egoistic, and the development of such features had made interpersonal relations and social interaction in general difficult for these patients and had led them to isolation.

Anxiety was found in 67%[18]; depression in 75%; aggression in 56% ("33 per cent of the patients in the present series had threatened the life of their relatives": [196], p. 43). Substance abuse was reported in 62%. Post-traumatic psychosis, found in 32% of cases, was a risk factor for suicide. On average, men committed suicide 15 years after brain injury (a vital warning: short-term follow-up, such as a decade, is inadequate for assessment of some PPCPPs). When very mild cases were included, the risk of suicide after TBI was three times the expected rate. When those cases were excluded, the risk ratio was lower but still high: "To sum up, during the 25-year period following injury, the suicide rate for those with definite brain lesions was some 70 to 80 per 100,000 a year; this rate was about twice the rate of those with mild injuries and that for the normal population" ([196], p. 16).

Achté et al.'s historic study makes two points: yes, TBI is a risk factor for completed suicide. But no, "mild TBI" is not necessarily associated with a greater risk than moderate or severe TBI. It is the second point that inspires a pause. The risk of persistent post-concussive distress of many kinds, including anxiety and depression, has repeatedly been shown to be greater among survivors of CBIs. One can guess that this reflects relative preservation of frontolimbic tracts supporting prompt recovery of insight in milder injury, but the true explanation awaits better science. It may therefore come as a surprise that more severe injuries predict suicidality. As we shall demonstrate, that curious fact seems to be frequently (but not always) confirmed by modern research [197–199].

Self-destructive behavior falls between depression and aggression in this chapter and in life. The data just reviewed from the almost 50-year-old report by Achté et al. are consistent with a major point of this chapter: TBI of any severity may trigger both despair and hostility. Both of those behavioral changes are risk factors for suicide. Impulsivity is another risk factor for suicide, also frequently persistent after CBI. That latter point has acquired new importance in the light of one

recent discovery: although some suicides mull and ruminate for years, suicide is shockingly unpredictable because it is *not* a point on a known disease trajectory (like dementia) but often a spur-of-the-moment tragedy. Evidence suggests that about half of suicides consider their act *for less than ten minutes*, and then either proceed or not that one single time [200–206].[19]

The author must again acknowledge that too little is known. In 2007, Simpson and Tate summarized the state of the art: "the literature investigating suicidality among people surviving TBI being sparse and fragmented" ([207], p. 1335). The present author is impressed by recent progress: the literature is no longer sparse; just fragmented. Much of the new writing on this subject has followed upon the U.S. invasions of Afghanistan and Iraq. Thankfully, the U.S. Department of Defense (DoD) and Veterans Administration (VA) have taken more interest in war fighter suicidality than after any previous conflict. Access to care remains abysmal for most veterans. Treatment is rarely in the hands of an expert. Obtaining benefits for the wounds of war requires running a gauntlet of bureaucratic beasts. But research has been funded.

At least three barriers reduce confidence in the published conclusions about suicide after typical concussion. First: very few survivors of typical concussions are engaged in long-term neuropsychiatric follow-up. If anything, they see a primary care doctor four times a decade. Primary care doctors are unlikely to anticipate suicide because they tend not to ask about suicidality [208, 209]. Moreover, given the evidence that TBI survivors may commit suicide an average of 15 years post injury, almost no concussion follow-up studies are sufficiently long to investigate this issue, and – in the clinical setting – when suicide occurs it may not be clear to even the most astute family member or doctor that this final act was influenced by an adolescent brain rattling. Second: the available data are largely confined to reports from retrospective studies in which the injury severity was moderate, severe, mixed, or unspecified. Third: a stigma persists, and life insurance payments are sometimes withheld after suicide. All three factors probably reduce accurate reporting.

A fourth factor potentially adds confusion: medical students often begin with the assumption that suicide and depression are invariably linked. They hopefully learn that that is not so. Suicide is common in schizophrenia and – important in the military setting – PTSD [210]. Suicide is common in complex co-morbidities. For instance, Collett et al. [211] studied 25,546 Iraq and Afghanistan veterans using multiple central nervous system (CNS)-active medications. They reported that "co-morbid traumatic brain injury (TBI), PTSD, and depression had the highest odds of CNS polypharmacy" and that "CNS polypharmacy was significantly associated with drug/alcohol overdose and suicide-related behavior." In other words, concussed veterans with four or five simultaneous problems were most likely to attempt suicide. Such data have cautionary value: even when statistical associations link concussion and

---

[18] "It is interesting to note that anxiety correlated significantly with the mildness of the injury and not with its severity" (p. 38). That is, in contrast to suicide yet consistent with the modern literature, anxiety disorders were more common among the mildly injured men.

[19] This suggests societies receive disproportionate dividends from investing in suicide prevention hotlines. A five-minute empathic de-escalation can preserve a lifetime.

suicide, one must be wary of assuming that concussion is the sole or main explanation for self-destruction.

Detection and Diagnosis of Suicidality

Most primary care clinicians (PCCs) and emergency department (ED) clinicians do not routinely screen for suicide risk.

(Horowitz et al., 2009 [212], p. 620).

Losing a patient to suicide is a heartbreaking reminder of one's clinical fallibility. Little can be done to save impulsive patients who do not themselves realize their risk. Yet a subset of concussion survivors are frank about having self-destructive thoughts. One only needs to ask. For mental health professionals, asking comes automatically. But the burden of detection rests squarely on non-mental health professionals. Targeted screening is helpful for finding a drop in the bucket. Universal screening is needed. Primary care clinicians are far more likely than psychiatrists to encounter new-onset suicidal ideation. Unfortunately, asking about suicidal ideation or planning is not routine in the settings where it would help the most: the annual physical and the emergency department [212, 213]. Should they? U.S. physicians seeking official government recommendations consult the *Recommendations of the U.S. Preventive Services Task Force* [214]. There is no recommendation to perform an annual physical examination. There is no recommendation to screen for suicidality – ever. North American biostatisticians say so.

The present author cannot claim superior knowledge in this regard. He can only trust his instinct that health care would be better, and little harm done, if doctors asked. Family practice and emergency department physicians are ideally situated to help [213, 215–217]. In developed countries other than the United States, primary care givers are strongly urged to assess for suicidality [218, 219]. Exactly contrary to the claims of the U.S. Preventive Services Task Force, screening, especially of adolescents, has been shown to effectively reduce the rate of suicides [220–223]. Formal psychological screening instruments are unlikely to gain traction in the clinical setting, yet several simple questions have been shown to detect suicidality (e.g., "Do you sometimes feel that life is not worth living?" "Do you own a gun?") This is not hard. Respectfully breaking ranks with his federal government on this matter, the author encourages asking.

In research settings, and where mandated by local protocols, screening instruments are used. Although no single instrument seems to have achieved consensus status, several are discussed in the literature. These include the 25-item Suicide Ideation Questionnaire [224, 225]; the 14-item (or abbreviated four-item) Risk of Suicide Questionnaire [216, 226], and the four-item Suicidal Behaviors Questionnaire–Revised [227].[20] A nine-item abbreviation of the Center for Epidemiological Studies-Depression Scale was reported to be as effective as the full instrument [230, 231].

A different approach is to assess suicidality indirectly by inquiring about psychological factors or experiences that impact proneness to suicide attempts. Among these is the Acquired Capability for Suicide Scale [232]. When patients have already made such an attempt, measures are available to judge dangerousness, such as the Lethality of Suicide Attempts Rating Scale [233].

Specifically with regard to suicidality among concussion survivors, the PHQ-9 has been reported to be effective [234, 235]. In fact, question #9 from this instrument is sufficient; it simply asks how frequently the patient had thoughts of hurting him- or herself or would be better off dead. Another recent TBI/suicide study employed the Columbia Suicide Severity Rating Scale [236].

The present author appreciates that too much health care can hurt as badly as too little, and that primary care providers have limited resources of time and psychic energy. He realizes that commonsense caring that statisticians deplore is becoming anathema to health maintenance organizations, and that insufficient evidence exists to support his plea. All that aside: please ask.

Epidemiology of Post-Concussive Suicidality

It has been apparent for decades that moderate or severe injury increases the risk of suicide [237–240]. Perhaps as a result, the overwhelming majority of available data pertains to the long-term prognosis after more severe TBIs. Five early civilian studies focused exclusively on severe injuries [241–245]. A meta-analysis of these five papers reported increased absolute rates of suicide with a risk ratio (compared with non-TBI populations) of 1.43 [246]. A more recent publication [247] determined that a history of TBI (severity not specified) was associated with an odds ratio of 2.09 for suicide attempts. Four studies published between 1979 and 1997 [248–251] reported that between 0.6% and 9% of subjects committed suicide on long-term follow-up. For unclear reasons, more recent studies have reported higher figures, suggesting that both the absolute number and the relative risk of suicide among TBI survivors may have increased over the last 20–30 years. For example, Silver et al. [238] reported that survivors of severe TBI exhibited a significantly increased risk of suicide attempts (odds ratio = 2.39) even after controlling for demographics, alcohol abuse, and any psychiatric disorder. (This last factor, as we will soon comment, is critical, because it supports the conclusions that concussions provoke suicidality even without co-morbid depression.)

Gutierrez et al. [252] reported a 27.3% risk of suicidality among severely injured TBI patients. Harrison-Felix et al. [253] reported that survivors of moderate to severe TBI had three times the normal risk of completed suicide. This change is possibly due to different definitions or methods, or better case ascertainment, which itself may be due to reduced stigma. Yet one cannot rule out the possibility that some systematic social or biological problem has increased the risk over time.

Table 10.2 lists several studies reporting suicide after CBI. (With the exception of Achté et al., the list excludes papers

---

[20] More recent measures, also primarily designed for screening adolescents, include the bullying–insomnia–tobacco–stress test [228] and the Suicidality of Adolescent Screening Scale [229]. These are too new to judge.

Table 10.2 Rates of, and risk factors for, suicidal behavior among survivors of concussive brain injury

Author(s)	Severity	Cohort/n	Clinical problem [a]	No./proportion/risk ratio	Risk factors
Achte et al., 1971 [196]	Severe	Military/6498	CS	85/0.13%/2.0	Psychosis [b]
Teasdale and Engberg, 2001 [197][c]	Mixed	Civilian/ concussion: 126,114 Fx: 7,560 ICH: 11,766	CS	750/0.59%	Male sex Substance misuse TBI severity
Simpson and Tate, 2002 [254]	Mixed	Civilian/172	SI SA	SI = 23% SA = 18%	Hopelessness Post-injury emotional or psychiatric disturbance Suicide attempts Alcohol abuse Other drug abuse Male sex
Oquendo et al., 2004 [255]	Concussion	Civilian/325 [d]	SA	44% of depressed persons had a headache of mild TBI	Male sex Aggression and hostility Cluster B personality disorder
Simpson and Tate, 2005 [256]	NR [e]	Civilian/172	SA	25%	Psychiatric disturbance Substance abuse Loss of friends since the TBI Work difficulties Lack of finances Pressure of multiple stressors
Mainio et al., 2007 [257]	Mixed	Civilian/1877 [f]	CS	5.5% of CS had TBI	TBI severity Male sex Older age Unemployment Psychiatric disorders Alcohol disorders
Brenner et al., 2009 [258]	Mixed	Military/13	SI SA	N/A [g]	Risk factors: Loss of sense of self after TBI Cognitive deficits Emotional/psychiatric disturbances (depression, worthlessness, anger, hopelessness Protective factors: Social support (family, peers, pets) Sense of purpose and hope Religion/spirituality Mental health treatment
Brenner et al., 2011 [259]	Mixed	Military/ Concussion/fx: 12,159 Contusion/ICH: 39,545	CS	Mild: 33/0.03%)/HR 1.98 [h] Severe: 78/0.02%/HR 1.34	Depression
Tsaousides et al., 2011 [260]	Mixed	Civilian/356	SI	23.8–44.9% [i]	NR
Olson-Madden et al., 2012 [261]	Mixed	Military/65	SI SA	NR	Assaultive behavior associated with SI Impulsivity associated with SA
Bryan et al., 2013 [262]	Concussion	Military/158 (135 with mTBI)	SI SA	No TBI: 0% TBI: 16%	Shorter LOC Depression PTSD Severity of insomnia
Bryan and Clemans, 2013 [121]	Concussion	Military/161	SI SA	No TBI: 0% Single TBI: 6.9% Multiple TBIs: 21.7%	Depression Repeated concussion

(continued)

Table 10.2 (Cont.)

Author(s)	Severity	Cohort/n	Clinical problem [a]	No./proportion/risk ratio	Risk factors
Brickell et al., 2014 [263]	Concussion	Military/167	SI	5.6–14.8% "considered suicide or homicide"	NR
Ilie et al., 2014 [264]	Mixed [j]	Civilian/4,685 (882 with lifetime TBI)	SI SA	SI: 15.2% SA: 5.9% OR for SA: 3.39	NR
Mackelprang et al., 2014 [265]	Mixed	Civilian/559	SI	25%	Prior SA Bipolar disorder Less than high school education
Wisco et al., 2014 [266]	Mixed	Military/849	SI	Single TBI: 24.3% Multiple: 32.3%	Depression PTSD Repeated TBI
Finley et al., 2015 [267] [j]	Mixed	Military/211,652 (5653 with suicidality)	SI SA	TBI alone: 1.5 TBI + PTSD: 3.7	Depression
Gradus et al., 2015 [268]	Mixed	Military/1921	SI	Male VA users: OR: 3.64 Male and female VA non-users: OR: 2.65	Depression
Richard et al., 2015 [198]	Mixed	Civilian/135,703 (21,047 with TBI)	CS	0.30 per 1000 person years	Repeated TBI
Kesinger et al., 2016 [199]	Mixed	Civilian/3575	SI SA	SI: 8.2% SA: 3.0%	Extracranial injuries associated with OR of 2.73
Schneider et al., 2016 [269]	NR	Military/1,097 468 with TBI	SA	7/1.5%	NR

[a] CS: completed suicide; SA: suicide attempt; SI: suicidal ideation.

[b] Achte et al. studied 48 risk factors. That detail is not included in the table because their subjects were mostly severe cases. Factors with the largest loadings included anxiety, deviant traits/lack of adaptability, younger age at death, shorter interval between injury and suicide, and threatening toward others.

[c] Re Teasdale and Engberg, 2001: concussion cases were compared with cases with cranial fracture, cerebral contusion, or intracranial hemorrhage. Concussion was regarded as milder in severity.

[d] Re Oquendo et al., 2004: this was a study of depressed persons, seeking the role of mild TBI.

[e] Re Simpson and Tate, 2005: although injury severity was not reported, the paper was included because the subjects were ambulatory outpatients at one year post TBI, implying many less-than-severe injuries.

[f] Re Mainio et al., 2007: this is a retrospective study of TBI among a cohort of completed suicides.

[g] Re Brenner et al., 2009: subjects were preselected for TBI and suicidality.

[h] Re Brenner et al., 2011: the reported HRs are adjusted for demographic and psychiatric variables. When adjusted only for demographics, concussion/fx HR = 2.60; contusion/ICH HR = 1.74.

[i] Re Tsaousides et al., 2011: rates of suicidal ideation were reported by psychiatric diagnosis among a cohort of TBI survivors of mixed severity. The presence of "any DSM-IV diagnosis" was associated with a 23.8% rate. Other diagnoses and rates: major depression: 37.7%; any depressive disorder: 36.1%; anxiety disorder 44.9%; PTSD: 37.8%; alcohol/substance use: 40.5%.

[j] Re Ilie et al., 2014: TBI was ascertained by a questionnaire that required a minimum severity: "19.5% of adolescents in this population based sample reported at least one brain injury in their lifetime that resulted in loss of consciousness for at least 5 minutes or at least one overnight hospitalization" (p. 4). It is not possible to determine the severity of the injuries in this cohort, except by virtue of the fact that about 85% of self-reported TBIs in similar surveys are known to be typical concussion, leading one to guess that the reported results are relevant to CBI.

[k] Re Finley et al., 2015: this is a study of TBI among those with suicidality, rather than a study of suicidality among those with TBI. The proportion of the cohort with TBI was not reported.

Fx: fracture; HR: hazard ratio; ICH: intracranial hemorrhage; LOC: loss of consciousness; mTBI: mild traumatic brain injury; NR: not reported; OR: odds ratio; PTSD: post-traumatic stress disorder; TBI: traumatic brain injury; VA: Veterans Affairs.

solely reporting data about moderate to severe injuries, but includes studies with mixed severities and those that compared mildly injured subjects with more severely injured subjects.) Depending on the data reported, the association between brain injury and suicidality is expressed in terms of a proportion or a risk ratio.

As shown in Table 10.2, many 21st-century studies report that groups with CBI or mixed-severity brain injuries exhibit unequivocally elevated rates of suicidality. In one of the largest available studies that included a substantial proportion of concussed patients, Brenner et al. [259] reported that mild TBI

nearly doubled the hazard ratio for suicidality. One is sorely tempted to have confidence in this much-replicated conclusion. However, two contrary findings raise doubts. Skopp et al. [270] conducted a large retrospective case–control study of U.S. soldiers. Suicide during military service was not associated with mild TBI. However (as those authors acknowledge), the follow-up may have been inadequate since subjects were not followed after military service and evidence suggests a possible 15-year lag between brain injury and suicide.

The second report of contrary results was published by Finley et al. [267], who examined the very large VA database for veterans receiving care from 2009 to 2011. Those authors sought associations between the "polytrauma clinical triad" (TBI, PTSD, pain) and suicidality. This report did not characterize the TBI cohort or describe the incidence of suicidality in TBI subjects. Instead, it calculated the contributions of various health factors to a multivariate model of suicide ideation versus suicide attempts. TBI by itself was not associated with an elevated risk of ideation, but it was associated with a 50% increase in the risk of suicide attempts. That increase was trivial, however, when compared with the effect of co-morbid TBI plus PTSD: an odds ratio of 3.7. Those authors commented:

> In contrast with research reporting that TBI may increase risk of suicide and despite a significant relationship between TBI and SRB [suicide-related behavior] in bivariate analyses, we found no association in the multivariable model once we included demographic and other clinical characteristics.
>
> ([267], p. 384)

That statement requires a response. It reflects not only an observation about the implications of a single study but also a concerning worldview. Just as a cohort of professionals deny that concussions can have consequences beyond three months, an overlapping cohort insists that brain injury does not cause suicide. It is correct to say:

> In a small proportion of studies, the effect of TBI could not be statistically distinguished, with certainty, from the effect of PTSD. Therefore, the cause of suicidality seems to have been one or more of the various forms of human distress that meet APA criteria for "PTSD," and we cannot judge the additional or concurrent contribution of TBI.

That honestly summarizes the limits of current knowledge. But two facts should muffle those who simply and rigidly deny that TBI might provoke suicidal thoughts and actions. First, when "PTSD" follows shortly after TBI – when for the first time in the patient's life, he or she exhibits a constellation of distresses and one intervening variable was brain rattling – it is sensible to consider that the physical effect on the brain was a causal factor in that outcome. In other words, the cause of the psychiatric problem we call "PTSD" may be brain damage. Second, many studies of suicide after TBI reveal strong evidence of a brain injury effect on behavior over and above that of depression or anxiety. For instance, in the study by Brenner et al. [259], injury severity was positively associated with both the risk of psychiatric disorder and the risk of suicide. Those authors make a striking comment:

> The positive associations between concussion/cranial fracture… and suicide were not explained by the presence of psychiatric disorders or demographic factors … The

positive association between history of TBI and suicide risk was not explained by the presence of psychiatric disorders; that is, history of TBI had an independent influence on suicide risk separate from other mental health conditions.
>
> ([259], pp. 261–262)

Readers will recognize the import of that simple observation of statistical fact: throughout this brief collaborative chapter the editors have hoped to explain why attribution of long-term distress after concussion is unknowable, but that mountains of evidence support the conclusion that CBI causes persistent or permanent change in the very brain circuits required for emotional regulation and successful negotiation of the human social milieu. Brenner et al.'s results are illuminating. Suicide, that most perfect distillation of psychic catastrophe, may be caused by TBI, even without depression steering the coracle of Charon.

Among other issues, these findings also raise the question of the relationship between concussion, "PTSD," and suicidality.

Does Concussion Increase the Risk of Suicidality Among Persons with "PTSD"?

It is reasonably well established that persons meeting APA criteria for "PTSD" have elevated risk of suicidality [271–274]. But if the "PTSD" *followed* CBI (the cases of greatest interest, importance, and rarest data), or is comorbid with CBI, does the risk increase? Simpson and Brenner [274] studied veterans with "PTSD" and/or TBI. They report that "PTSD" almost tripled the risk for suicidality, but that TBI added little to that increase. Their conclusion was that psychiatric disorder, rather than TBI, explains most of the risk of suicidality about brain-injured persons. Barnes et al. [275] studied a population of veterans with "PTSD," half of whom also had "mTBI." The combination was associated with suicide risk but brain injury alone was not.

These findings mesh with the observations of Simpson and Tate [256]: in a study of TBI survivors (severity not reported), the risk of suicide was elevated 21 times when there was both substance abuse and another psychiatric diagnosis. What is one to make of these reports? They stand exactly contrary to the reports showing that TBI, without co-morbid psychiatric disorder, is strongly associated with suicidality. The devil, as ever, is in the detail. Readers may wish to examine the narrative account of the factors that provoked the suicides attempts that Simpson and Tate attributed to "psychiatric disorder" rather than to TBI.[21] The symptoms so vividly described – sadness and hopelessness, losing friends since the brain injury, having difficulty at work, impulsivity – are exactly what the universe of literature regarding the impact of TBI on behavior shows to be the impact of TBI on behavior. It is illogical and disingenuous for writers to define away the likelihood of a causal connection by

---

[21] "Respondents identified various antecedent circumstances to the attempts including depression/hopelessness (e.g., 'sick of being the way I was,' 'wish my life had ended at the accident'), relationship breakdown, relationship conflict, social isolation (e.g., loss of friends since the TBI), pressure of multiple stressors, instrumental difficulties (e.g., lack of finances, work difficulties), or more generally, the global impact of the injury. Triggers included arguments, a partner leaving, the availability of means, impulsive responses to an acute stressor (e.g., negative feedback about work performance), or an event (internal or external) that was the end point of an intolerable accumulation of stress (i.e., 'the last straw')" ([256], p. 682).

calling these "psychiatric disorders" and insisting that misery occurring after a brain injury *must* be causally independent of the physical trauma.

Readers will understandably be bemused by the inconsistencies described in the epidemiological data. The present author agrees with Simpson and Tate [234], who opined: "gathering better quality data about the prevalence and clinical features of suicide attempts after TBI is needed, given the wide variability in the findings to date" (p. 1347). Still, conclusions can be made to a reasonable degree of medical probability. In brief,

- Evidence strongly supports the conclusion that CBI is a risk factor for suicidality. The risk is two to four times that of the general population.
- Depressed persons with concussion are more likely to attempt suicide than depressed persons without CBI.
- Persons with suicidality have elevated rates of a history of CBI.
- Evidence suggests that the most worrisome circumstance may be the combination of CBI with "PTSD."

Please let us agree and move on: concussion is a risk factor for suicidality.

Risk Factors for Post-Concussive Suicidality

Accurate prediction of suicidal or homicidal behavior, perhaps more so than prediction of other behaviors, would be a social boon. Risk factor study and algorithm trials hold the promise of enabling that feat. For example, simply inquiring about gun ownership has been shown to increase the accuracy of prediction of fatal completed suicides in U.S. males, but many emergency department personnel fail at this task [276]. It is with some gravity that one approaches the literature on risk factors for post-concussive suicidality. As the quality of the research improves and single findings are replicated, a practical formula to identify those most at risk seems within reach.

In temporal order, the earliest operative risk factor would be *gene variation*. To the best of the author's knowledge, no candidate gene or genome-wide association studies have reported any variant affecting the risk of suicidality after concussion. Nonetheless, XY genotype, male sex, is disproportionately associated with post-CBI suicidality [197, 255, 257]. *Childhood trauma*, adversity, or loss is another potential early risk factor, but few data are available. In one study, Gunter et al. [277] examined the relationship between suicidality and risk factors in a cohort of community-supervised offenders. Although the study did not specifically investigate the effect of childhood stress on the link between TBI and suicide, both brain injury and traumatic experience before age 18 were associated with suicidality.

Regarding injury factors, the first question is whether *TBI severity* is a valid and reliable predictor. As discussed above, Achté et al. [196] reported this to be true, and several other 21st-century publications report that severity is positively correlated with suicidality [197–199]. The evidence, however, is mixed. Brenner et al.'s [259] very large study compared survivors of relatively milder TBIs (concussion/cranial fracture) versus more severe injuries (contusion/intracerebral hemorrhage (ICH). During the observation period 0.03% of

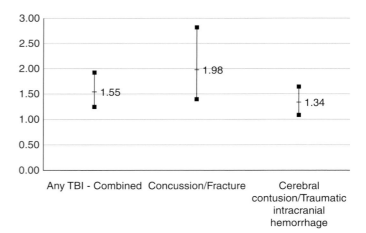

Fig. 10.3 Hazard ratio for suicide by traumatic brain injury (TBI) severity, adjusted for sex, age, and psychiatric conditions.
Source: Brenner et al., 2011 [259] with permission from Wolters Kluwer Health

patients with milder TBIs completed suicide compared with 0.02% with more severe injuries. Figure 10.3 illustrates that comparison. And Bryan et al. [262] found that the longer the loss of consciousness, the lower the risk of suicidality, also suggesting an inverse relationship between severity and risk. It is not clear whether these inconsistencies are better explained by different measures of severity, demographically different cohorts, problems with case ascertainment, or a lack of validity of the hypothesis.

Another potential injury factor is *repeated concussion*. Richard et al. [198] compared the risk of suicide in a cohort of 135,703 children, of whom 21,047 had suffered a TBI during the follow-up period. (Severity ranged from mild to severe, but the analysis did not stratify results by severity.) TBI approximately doubled the incidence of completed suicide and repeated TBIs further increased that risk.

Other studies also report that the number of concussions or TBIs is directly associated with the risk of suicide [266]. The impact of multiplicity of injuries on the risk of suicidality is directly addressed by Bryan and Clemans [121]. In that study, subjects reported from zero to 19 concussions. A larger number of CBIs predicted a higher risk of lifetime suicidal ideation or behaviors: no TBI: 0%; single TBI: 6.9%; multiple TBIs: 21.7%. As shown in Figure 10.4, the risk of both depression and especially "PTSD" was associated with the number of concussions, yet, again, the risk of suicide was still significantly associated with the number of concussions after controlling for both psychiatric disorder and TBI severity. "Results… suggest that the number of TBIs is significantly associated with increased suicide risk *above and beyond* the effects of severity for depression, PTSD, and concussive symptoms" [emphasis added] ([121], p. 689). That finding lends further credence to the conclusion that "psychological reaction to trauma" is an inaccurate explanation for severe emotional distress after concussion. As strongly suggested by the animal literature, physical damage to the emotional regulation circuitry in the head causes persistent emotional distress.

Psychiatric disorders are almost (but not quite) a given in the list of risk factors for suicidality after concussion. Multiple

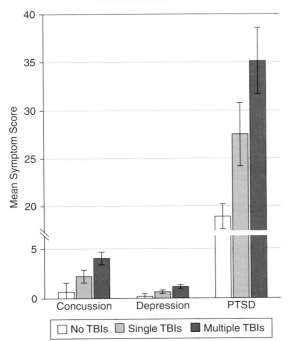

Lifetime risk of suicidal thought and behaviors is associated with number of concussions

Fig. 10.4 Mean symptom scores with 95% confidence intervals by traumatic brain injury (TBI) group. For all scales, pairwise comparisons with Bonferroni corrections revealed significant differences in scores ($p < 0.05$) between the no-TBI and single-TBI groups and between the single- and multiple-TBI groups. PTSD: post-traumatic stress disorder.

Source: Bryan and Clemans, 2013 [121]. Journal of the American Medical Association

reports confirm that association [121, 254, 256–259, 262, 265–268].

The literature is less clear, however, regarding whether pre- or post-morbid onset of psychiatric symptoms is the better predictor. The question of apportioning causality, as always, looms over the scholar's most earnest effort to interpret the crumbs of available data. Interestingly, the limited literature on post-concussive suicide includes some of the best evidence that physical brain change due to external force has effects that are not explained by a psychological reaction to injury. For example, as shown in Figure 10.2, the risks of depression and "PTSD" were associated with the number of concussions, yet the risk of suicide remained significantly associated with the number of concussions after controlling for both psychiatric disorder and TBI severity.

Aggression, anger, and hostility have also been identified repeatedly as risk factors for post-concussive suicidality [255, 258, 261]. That is not surprising, given both the high prevalence of post-concussive aggression (see upcoming section) and the biological overlap between self- and other-destructiveness. *Substance abuse* or dependence also seems to be a risk. Most of the literature simply notes co-morbidity, or the fact that

substance abuse is a risk factor for both TBI and suicide, rather than assaying substance abuse among concussion survivors with later suicidal behavior [278]. However, several papers report data consistent with the conclusion that pre- or post-injury substance abuse/dependence increases the risk of suicide [197, 254, 256, 257].[22]

Several other risk factors have been noted, but not in many studies: older age [257], cognitive deficits [258], insomnia [262], work difficulties/unemployment [256, 257], financial difficulties [256], low level of education [265], and extracranial injuries [199] have all been found to increase the risk.

Anatomical and Physiological Correlates of Post-Concussive Suicidality

Something happens in brains that makes those who host them kill themselves [279]. We do not know what that something is, but we suspect it is different in every case. The question: might there be commonalities – biological factors that occur among suicidal concussion survivors more often than they do among non-suicidal concussion survivors?

Neuroimaging is one potential tactic to explore that possibility. Lopez-Larson et al. [279] used MRI to compare veterans with mild TBI with and without suicidal behavior. Structural imaging showed that concussion with suicidality was associated with larger thalamic volumes. DTI showed that this group also had increased FA of the anterior thalamic radiations. Mechanistically, how might this explain suicide? Those authors pointed to the fact that previous studies have reported associations between thalamic integrity and suicidality [280, 281]. They also note that the anterior thalamic radiation converges with the medial forebrain bundle and, mention scholarship speculating that (1) this convergence mediates the balance between positive and negative emotions and that (2) disruption in either tract would dysregulate that balance [282]. Confirming such hypotheses awaits a great deal of further empirical effort.

Functional imaging studies have also reported possible cerebral correlates of post-concussive suicidality: Matthews et al. [283] scanned 26 veterans, of whom 24 had histories of concussion, administering the stop task, thought to tap self-control. Despite matching performance, the suicidal subjects displayed greater error-related activation in the anterior cingulate gyrus and parts of the prefrontal cortex (Figure 10.5).

This collaborative chapter on concussion began by urging a conceptual shift: external force should not be thought of as triggering a "neurometabolic cascade." The suite of expected brains changes is not a sluice of harm. The concussive blow triggers a to and fro of destructive and reparative happenings. Hours, weeks, and decades after concussion, competing elements are busy in a dynamic theater. Neurodegeneration is our inescapable Act III, although we have yet to figure out how big a role the brain-rattling actor plays in those final scenes.

---

22 The report by Olson-Madden et al. [261] in this respect is hard to interpret; the entire cohort of 65 veterans had both TBI (78% mild) and substance abuse and there were three TBIs, on average, per person. Since all subjects were abusers with repetitive TBIs, one cannot judge whether substance abuse enhances the risk among survivors of single concussions.

Post-concussive suicidality is associated with altered error processing on the stop task

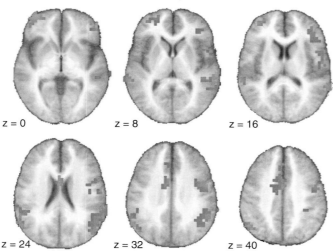

Fig. 10.5 Despite comparable behavioral task performance, the suicidal ideation (SI) relative to the non-SI group showed abnormal hyperactivation of a network of brain structures that includes the dorsal anterior cingulate and several areas of the prefrontal cortex during error processing. [A black and white version of this figure will appear in some formats. For the color version, please refer to the plate section.]

Source: Matthews et al., 2012 [283] with permission from Lippincott Williams & Wilkins, Inc./Wolters Kluwer

But *neurodegeneration* has been used too narrowly. The connotation is toxic protein aggregates. Left aside, as if bit players, are excitatory harm, oxidation, vascular change, and immune/inflammatory processes. Suicide is not reducible to such prime elements. However, an accurate accounting of post-concussive suicide must include basic biology, and inspires questions that would perhaps have been unthinkable a generation ago. Does TBI-related neuroinflammation influence the risk of suicide?

As noted in Chapters 3 and 4, CBI is strongly associated with neuroinflammation and glial activation [284, 285]. Recent evidence suggests that neuroinflammation is also associated with suicidal behavior Two decades of studies have reported intriguing associations between suicidality and inflammatory factors, including interleukin (IL)-1β, 2, 4, 6, 8, and 13, the kynurenine pathway, microgliosis, and perivascular macrophage activity [278, 285–287]. It is therefore natural to speculate that inflammation is one part of whatever occurs in brains that compels their hosts to commit suicide. Juengst et al. [288] studied an inflammatory marker, tumor necrosis factor (TNF)-α, among 48 survivors of moderate to severe TBI with suicidal ideation. At all time points, both serum and cerebrospinal fluid (CSF) TNF-α levels were higher among TBI survivors than controls. More interestingly (although one awaits replication), serum TNF-α at six months predicted disinhibition, which predicted suicidality. Figure 10.6 schematically illustrates the potential pathways connecting TBI inflammation, and suicide.

The present author urges cautious scrutiny of claims regarding the neuroanatomy and physiology of post-concussive suicide. A massive gap divides our astonishing technological *savoir faire* from our understanding of tissue-mediated feelings, ideas, and will. The recent exposure of fallacies in fMRI algorithms and the frequent failure of functional imaging studies to attend to individuality both mandate withholding faith in many "discoveries." Human understanding of humans, like a coral reef, grows at a relaxed pace.

Management of Post-Concussive Suicidality

No RCTs have specifically randomized suicidal concussed persons to two treatments or to active treatment versus placebo or wait list. The published guidelines that touch upon co-morbid concussion and suicidality typically advise: just address the suicidality as best you can without being distracted by the fact that TBI may be responsible. In one of very few empirical trials of management of co-morbid subjects, Simpson et al. [164] randomized subjects, all with both severe TBI and moderate to severe hopelessness, to group CBT or wait list. Hopelessness was reduced, but there was no reduction in suicidal ideation in the active treatment group. One cannot assume similar results in typical (less severe) concussion patients.

The present author has limited experience and no evidence-based knowledge of effective approaches to the problem of suicidality after CBI. One fact may be important: the etiology and pathophysiology of post-concussive suicidality must not be assumed to be depressive. As listed above, many factors might play causal roles. Prescribing an antidepressant may be even less effective than usual if the patient is not only hopeless but also cognitively disabled, paranoid, in pain, aggressive, and abusing alcohol. Cutting to the chase: step one is detecting the problem by making asking the questions routine. Too many suicides shock their doctors, who never suspected the risk. Step two is to care, and let the patient know that you do. What follows, for the time being, is a matter of a best clinical guess.

III. Post-Concussive Aggression

The author convenes, sometimes, with the walking dead (an evocative phrase employed by some San Quentin guards, referring to their East Block companions). To date, only one death row inmate whom the author has assessed reported a life prior to his index offense without at least one concussion. This informal, non-systematic observation jibes with many formal studies of the association between TBI and imprisonment. Evidence is strong that: (1) the frequency of a past history of head injury is disproportionately elevated among prisoners; (2) the likelihood of a child becoming a criminal, especially a violent criminal, is increased if he or she suffers a concussion; and (3) the rate of histories of TBI or concussion among murderers is remarkably high [289–296].

Why?

Defining aggression is as easy as juggling mercury. This slippery concept has no agreed meaning. Therefore, the stack of academic literature boasting to discuss "the neurobiology of aggression" must be treated with indulgence. A great deal of empirical work has recently clarified many phenomenological pieces that seem to fit somewhere in the jigsaw puzzle, but we've misplaced the box top. We are building parts without a vision of the whole – if indeed the various things called aggression comprise a unitary evolutionary function. That caveat in mind,

Traumatic brain injury-related inflammatory factors may play a causal role in post-concussive suicidality

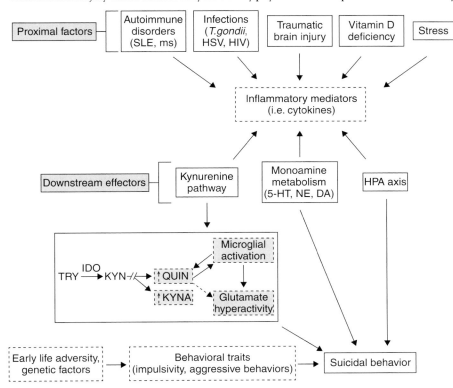

Fig. 10.6 Contributing factors to suicidal behavior etiology. Genetic factors can predispose individuals to behavioral traits that predispose them to exhibit suicidal behavior. Proximal factors with an underlying immune component can induce a sustained immune response, which, then, is known to modulate a variety of downstream effectors including modifying monoamine metabolism, increasing tryptophan metabolism via the kynurenine pathway, and dysregulating the hypothalamic–pituitary axis (HPA). 5-HT: serotonin; DA: dopamine; HIV: human immunodeficiency virus; HSV: herpes simplex virus; IDO: indoleamine; KYN: kynurenine; KYNA: kynurenic acid; MS: multiple sclerosis; NE: norepinephrine; QUIN: quinolinic acid; SLE: systemic lupus erythematosus; TRY: tryptophan..

Source: Brundin et al. (2017) [286] Reprinted by permission from Macmillan

we are beginning to compile a wealth of replicable facts about aggression and the brain [297–301]. The network of implicated brain parts includes the amygdala, ventromedial prefrontal cortex, dorsolateral prefrontal cortex, anterior cingulate gyrus, insula, hypothalamus, and dorsal raphe.[23] Among these, the amygdala and ventromedial prefrontal cortex are often damaged by CBI. Perhaps as a result, irritability and aggression (with or without the added hardship of impulsivity) represent either the most common or the second most common (after depression) persistent non-cognitive behavioral sequelae of CBI. An informative discussion of the likely mechanisms would require another book. This chapter has a more pragmatic focus.

Aggression, Anger, Irritability, Agitation, and "Intermittent Explosive Disorder"

Readers hoping to understand the spectrum of persistent post-concussive behavior changes are served a potpourri of associated concepts, including aggression, irritability, hostility, anger, agitation, and episodic dyscontrol [304–306]. It is common for studies to conflate these diverse phenomena. As a result, literature reporting epidemiology, risk factors, and management is difficult to judge. One must attempt some semantic differentiation, realizing that generations may pass before this suite of problematic behaviors is biologically classified.

There exists no consensus definition of aggression.[24] Without diverting attention to the challenge of homogenizing a heterogeneous behavior, for the purposes of this section, aggression is an approach conflict behavior that includes wishing to, intending to, planning to, or overtly harming a feeling being. This includes fellow humans, certain animals such as dogs, and the self. The limits of aggression are debatable. To what extent is either consciousness or intent required? That depends on what we collectively choose the word to mean. Does aggression include strong emotions such as hatred and hostility? Those emotions are not planned or committed acts of approach, although they imply conflict and seem to share elements of genetics and cerebral processing with aggressive wishes or acts [307–311]. Obviously, aggression varies. A hostile glance, a punch delivered to a victim in non-rapid eye movement sleep, and a Blitzkrieg are different. The question is: at what level of granularity should one classify varieties of post-concussive aggression for the purposes of research and testing interventions?

---

23 Relatively little is known about the functions of the habenula, and isolated injuries are so rare as experiments of nature that behavioral neurology has not arrived at conclusions apart from hints of this region's involvement in reward and aversion [302]. Recently, connectome studies have revealed links between the habenula and multiple other aggression-related areas such as the amygdala, insula, prefrontal cortex, and cingulate [303]. That is, most of the brain parts associated with threat detection versus aggression are the same as or interconnected with one another. The author speculates that post-concussive axonal change perhaps modifies aggressive behavior by interfering with the integrity of this network.

24 The author, who has composed the chapter on human aggression for the successive editions of the *Kaplan and Sadock Comprehensive Textbook of Psychiatry* for more than a decade [301], has yet to discover a characterization that satisfies all experts in animal and human aggression.

Many ethologists and some psychologists urge a strict dichotomy between a proactive, premeditated, offensive form of aggression and a reactive, impulsive, defensive form of aggression [312, 313]. In rodents, stereotyped behaviors labeled in this way are indeed semiologically and biologically differentiable. Theoretically, aggression after CBI might exhibit different forms, with different causes, requiring different treatments. However, making the offensive/defensive distinction is hard in human research. People, whose cerebrations involve juggling of cortical and subcortical processing, almost always exhibit mixed types. As Victoroff explains [301]: "The popular proactive/reactive dichotomy has heuristic virtues but is a flawed description of many real events." Wood and Thomas similarly cautioned [314]: "Aggression can take many forms and there is currently no uniform method of assessment that distinguishes aggressive sub-types in a way that can assist decisions for treatment" (p. 253). Thus, as much as one suspects categorical biological variation and urges consideration of this possibility for future prospective research, the classification of aggression promoted in most 20th-century textbooks is simplistic.

Anger and irritability are related phenomena. Yet neither state necessarily connotes approach or conflict. The angry person might exhibit no external sign or action. The irritable animal might equally be motivated to withdraw from the irritant as to approach. Both of these are commonplace as persistent symptoms after TBI, including concussion [112]. "Even following mild severity of head injuries, irritability has also been recognized as one of the most frequently reported post-concussion symptoms" [315]. Irritability has slightly different connotations than anger; the term is used to refer to two constructs that deserve to be separated: as a mental state – a subjective affect associated with heightened negative responsiveness to stimuli that can be reported by the patient or inferred from his or her behavior – or as a term for diverse objectively observed behaviors. The latter use is exemplified by Kim et al. [316]: "uncooperative, angry, hostile, shouting, or antagonistic language or behavior" (p. 329). Some evidence suggests that irritability is clinically dissociable from both anger and aggression: in one study, post-TBI annoyance occurred in 26.5% while verbal aggression occurred in just 14.7% [315]. For that reason, if one were to propose levels or degrees of aggression, irritability would not fit naturally on that scale. Still, an irritable mental state sometimes precipitates approach conflict behaviors [317] from verbal aggression to impulsive murder. Of interest: among one group of moderate and severe TBI survivors, irritability was not itself associated with aggression, while *attribution of hostile intent to others* was highly correlated with aggression [318]. This suggests the possibility of identifying those circumstances in which irritability/anger is more or less prone to precipitate overt approach. Although depression is subjectively more common, in some studies irritability has been the most commonly observed PCS [20, 319].

Agitation is yet another concept. It is discussed most often in the context of acute and subacute post-TBI behaviors of a person who is not fully aware and sometimes frankly delirious, rather than as a long-term sequela of concussion. In post-acute rehabilitation, delirious agitation is most common during the "agitation crisis in the awakening phase" [320], prior to restoration of orientation, or at Rancho Los Amigos Scale of Cognitive Levels IV or V, during which processing of external stimuli is disorganized [321, 322]. In that acute or subacute phase after moderate or severe TBI, 24–96% of survivors exhibit agitation [14, 323–325]. Agitation cannot be equated with either aggression or irritability. Unlike aggression, there is no connotation of approach and conflict. Unlike irritability, agitation almost always refers to overt behaviors – for instance, the CBI survivor who is combative with emergency medical technicians or hyperactive in a disorganized way during post-acute rehabilitation. Since agitation is rarely, if ever, a persistent behavioral change after CBI, this chapter will not discuss management of agitation. (Interested readers may wish to read recent French evidence-based guidelines for inpatient management of agitation [320].)

Intermittent explosive disorder (IED) refers to a somewhat controversial construct characterized by episodic rage often linked to destructive violence against property or persons. The concept was introduced in modern psychiatry as explosive personality in DSM-II, and relabeled IED for DSM-III and thereafter [326–328]. The essence of the condition is defined in DSM-5: "Recurrent behavioral outbursts represents a failure to control aggressive impulses…grossly out of proportion to the provocation or any precipitating psychosocial stressors" [65]. The term *episodic dyscontrol* evolved in parallel in the 1970s, and came to be favored by neurologists to describe an essentially identical syndrome hypothesized to be due to limbic irritability, for instance, in temporal lobe epilepsy [329–331].[25]

The preceding definitions may have practical implications. Given a cohort of CBI survivors, even though no two will exhibit identical mental states or behaviors, the hope of understanding and effective management depends on discovering plausible discriminators. Three questions seem compelling: (1) How should one assess post-concussive aggression? (2) Why does aggression sometimes occur after CBI? (3) How should one attempt to manage this often disabling problem?

Detection and Measurement of Post-Concussive Aggression

Despite the salmagundi of concepts and phenomena, scholars have devised practical methods of identifying patients with one or more aggressive symptoms and roughly measuring their degree of dysfunction. Studies of post-TBI aggression have employed many such measures. As shown in Table 10.3, those include: (1) normed and validated dedicated aggression measures (these include self-report, other report, or clinician report scales); (2) instruments intended for general health

---

[25] In a sign of persistence of the false dichotomy between "psychological" and "organic," the APA forbids diagnosing IED in epilepsy or after head trauma, even though TBI is probably the most frequent cause of the clinical phenomenology described by their criteria.

Table 10.3 Classification and examples of measures used to document and rate post-concussive aggression

Aggression measures, self-report:
- Hostility and Direction of Hostility Questionnaire, 1967 [332, 333]
- Spielberger State Trait Anger Scale, 1983 [334]
- Multidimensional Anger Inventory (MAI), 1986 [335, 336]
- State-Trait Anger Expression Inventory (STAXI), 1988 [337]
- The Past Feelings and Acts of Violence (PFAV) Scale, 1990 [338]
- Aggression Questionnaire (AQ) [64, 339, 340]

Aggression measures, observer or clinician report
- Conflict Tactics Scales, 1979 [341, 342]
- Overt Aggression Scale, 1986 [343]
- Social Dysfunction and Aggression Scale, 1990 [344]
- Modified Overt Aggression Scale, 1991 [345]
- Global Aggression Scale, 1993 [346]
- Revised Conflict Tactics Scales, 1996 [347]
- Overt Aggression Scale–Modified for Neurorehabiltation–Extended (OAS-MNR-E), 2007 [348]

Instruments intended for general health assessment
- General Health Questionnaire-36 [349, 350]
- Symptom Checklist 90 (SCL-90); SCL-36 [351, 352]

Instruments intended for comprehensive adult behavioral assessment
- Achenbach Adult Self-Report (ASR) (self-report); Achenbach Adult Behavior Checklist (ABCL) (observer report) [353, 354]

Instruments intended to assess psychiatric symptoms
- Brief Psychiatric Rating Scale (BPRS) [56]
- Positive and Negative Syndrome Scale (PANSS) [355, 356]

Instruments intended to assess personality
- Personality Assessment Inventory, 2007 [357]
- Minnesota Multiphasic Personality Inventory II, 2008 [358, 359]
- Millon Clincial Multiaxial Inventory III, 2009 [360]

Instruments intended to assess neurobehavioral symptoms
- Neurobehavioral Functioning Inventory (NFI) [361, 362]
- Neurobehavioral Rating Scale (NBRS) [363, 364]
- Neuropsychiatric Inventory (NPI) [365]
- Neurobehavioral Symptom Inventory (NSI) [366, 367]

Instruments intended to assess post-TBI behavior
- Rivermead Post-Concussion Symptoms Questionnaire (RPCSQ) [58]
- Mayo-Portland Adaptability Inventory (MPAI-4) [368–370]

assessment; (3) instruments intended for comprehensive adult behavioral assessment; (4) instruments intended to assess psychiatric symptoms; (5) instruments intended to assess personality; (6) instruments intended to assess neurobehavioral symptoms; and (7) instruments intended to assess post-TBI behavior.[26]

The dramatic differences in the structure, behavioral constructs assessed, and psychometric properties of these instruments obviate comparison across studies. For instance, a plurality of studies mentioning post-CBI aggression employed only a broad measure of PCSs, typically the Rivermead (RPCSQ) [58]. This instrument, in fact, does not assess aggression. A single item enquires about "Being irritable, easily angered." (By way of comparison, the Neuropsychiatric Inventory [365], originally intended for persons with dementia, assesses the presence, frequency, severity, and caregiver impact of eight agitation/aggression symptoms and seven signs of irritability, and the rarely administered Achenbach Adult Behavior Checklist [353] rates 16 relevant items.[27]) Self-report, caregiver/partner report, and clinician report are complementary and desirable. An example of the utility: Yang et al. [315] compared self- and family-rated post-TBI irritability and found a marked difference: "even though the family-reported post-injury verbal aggression was still remarkably higher than pre-injury verbal aggression…, self-reported post-injury verbal aggression did not differ from pre-injury verbal aggression" (p. 1188).

Unfortunately, the majority of studies that explicitly track post-concussive aggression employ only one source of clinical information. The profusion of non-comparable measures is just one of several barriers to research progress. Epidemiological knowledge of post-CBI aggression is shallow because dedicated aggression scales are rarely employed, even when that research ostensibly investigates clinical correlates of "aggression," and such scales are virtually never completed in clinical practice. No reports, to the best of this author's knowledge, describe a large cohort of clinically comparable CBI survivors, classifying post-CBI aggression in a way that distinguishes between irritability, anger, hostility, verbal and physical aggression, direct and indirect aggression, or proactive and reactive aggression – quantifying each and controlling for age, sex, education, and socioeconomic status. This lack of rigor is one of the major factors limiting the utility of the available data and the sophistication of the published guesswork about why some survivors aggress.

What measure is best? Here the author must express a concern. As previously mentioned, the National Institute of Neurological Disorders and Stroke recommends concussion outcome assessment with CDE instruments. Generally speaking, the author supports that initiative because, even though many CDE instruments assess dubious constructs and are psychometrically suboptimal, they are easy to administer and available in the common domain. Aggression assessment

---

[26] This abbreviated classification excludes a host of alternative measures of possible value that assess impulsivity, conduct, psychopathy, dangerousness, etc.

[27] Argues a lot; cruelty, bullying, meanness to others; deliberately harms self or attempts suicide; damages or destroys his or her own things; damages or destroys things belonging to others; gets in many fights; impulsive or acts without thinking; physically attacks people; screams or yells a lot; stubborn, sullen, or irritable; rushes into things without considering the risks; talks about killing self; does things that may cause trouble with the law; temper tantrums or hot temper; threatens to hurt people; gets upset too easily.

is an exception.[28] No valid and reliable outpatient aggression rating instrument is available in that collection. As a result, one cannot recommend the CDE system wholeheartedly.

Aggression documentation in the real world – among the massive cohort of concussed persons who may or may not go to the emergency room and may or may not receive any follow-up care – is likely to vary in rigor between a family doctor's single scribbled note about a fearful spouse and a computerized medical record from subacute inpatient neurorehabilitation that includes daily quantitative ratings on validated aggression scales. Clearly, no single recommendation for assessment fits all clinical circumstances. Scholars are urged to monitor possible aggression with at least one self-report and one other-report tool. Researchers might compare the Aggression Questionnaire (self-report only) with the Neuropsychiatric Inventory (care-giver report only), with the Achenbach system (combined self- and other report). The author's principal plea is simply that *every clinician encountering a CBI survivor inquire about irritability and aggression*. It takes but a moment – although that moment of inquiry sometimes opens a can of worms urgently requiring intensive intervention. These problems are very common, critically important for quality of life, and potentially treatable (see recommendations for the management of post-concussive aggression, below).

Epidemiology of Post-Concussive Aggression

This subsection will be telegraphically brief because the quality of the data does not lend itself to confident conclusions.

Epidemiology of Irritability

The incidence and prevalence of post-concussive irritability or anger after TBI or CBI are high, on the order of 30–35%, whether assessed by self- or other report and whether assessed as a subacute or persistent problem [20, 306, 317, 319].[29] Unlike agitation, which is most apparent in the acute and subacute period, evidence suggest that irritability is more common at or after six weeks. Of interest, the incidence of persistent irritability seems to be about the same regardless of severity of injury [374, 375]. In a seeming paradox, multiple reports suggest that this symptom tends to increase in the postacute period when other symptoms may be resolving [5, 317, 374, 376, 377]. This observation conceivably hints at the underlying biopsychosocial mediators, since, by the time irritability emerges (possibly peaking at about six months), the metabolic and vascular changes have largely resolved but

the inflammatory and neurodegenerative changes persist, and insight regarding disabilities may be increasing.

Epidemiology of Aggression

The incidence and prevalence of aggression after CBI are difficult to judge, since most studies report this trait in populations of mixed severity. Aggression has been reported in 11–73% of TBI survivors in such studies [291, 378–383]. Readers may share the author's dissatisfaction with such a broad range of findings, and share the impression that lack of consensus regarding definition or measurement of the problem and the heterogeneity of cohorts explains this non-specific and unhelpful conclusion.

Cause(s) of Post-Concussive Aggression

As depicted in the Haddon matrix in Chapter 7, every persistent post-concussive problem is multi-determined. That surely applies to post-CBI irritability and aggression. At this early stage of serious investigation, the best available inference: many risk factors seem relevant to post-CBI aggression, no combination of which is the same in any two patients, and none of which can be assigned a proportional role.

The primary (in the sense of precedent) risk factor is genetic, but genetic research on this subject is in its infancy. Leaping ahead a generation, one expects molecular assessment to greatly enhance the specificity of diagnosis and efficacy of treatments. The only gene variant specifically associated with TBI-related aggression to date is a low-transcriptional-activity polymorphism of the gene for monoamine oxidase-A [385]. Still, based on many recent studies in non-TBI subjects, it seems reasonable (and testable) that carriers of aggression-promoting variations are more prone to irritability or aggression after concussion. Candidate gene studies suggest that variants of possible relevance include those of genes for monoamine oxidase A, the 5-HT transporter promoter (5-HTTLRP), tryptophan hydroxylase, catechol-*O*-methyltransferase (COMT), cyclic adenosine monophosphate (cAMP) response element-binding protein (CREB), neuronal nitric oxide synthase, the androgen receptor, and the ABCG1 transporter [384–392]. Genome-wide association studies (GWAS) have recently suggested additional aggression-promoting gene variants [392–394]. Since some evidence suggests that the APOE e4 allele is a risk factor for post-concussive dementia and for Alzheimer's-related aggression [395], it seems worth exploring (indeed, low-hanging fruit) whether the violence exhibited by some football players is influenced by this gene variant.

---

[28] In 2010 the author was invited to review and comment on the development of those National Institute of Neurological Disorders and Stroke CDEs intended to assess behavioral outcomes. In his presentation to the Advisory Council he pointed out the lack of any aggression assessment instrument among their favored tools, despite the fact that this problem is among the most common and socially disruptive of all post-concussive changes – demonstrably far more important to reintegration than any cognitive deficit. He provided the Council with more than ten validated instruments for consideration. When version 2 of the CDEs was released in 2012, the only instrument included pertaining to aggression was an instrument the faults of which the author demonstrated: the OVERT Aggression scale [343].

[29] Of possible interest, about 40–50% of persons with depressive disorders also exhibit irritability or anger [371, 372], a finding interpreted as "disturbances in the regulation of irritability" ([373, p. 1]). This concept is mentioned because there is a significant overlap between the anatomic circuits associated with mood and aggressive disorders, yet it remains unknown how and why dysfunction in the same regions generates internalized versus externalized behavior change.

Epigenetic changes might also lower the threshold for post-CBI aggression. This has not specifically been investigated. However, multiple non-genetic heritable alterations in genes have been reported to correlate with aggressive behavior in humans [392]. For example, when certain genes for aminergic neurotransmission or inflammatory cytokines undergo post-translational modification of their histones by methylation, the resulting changes in gene expression have been linked to chronic aggression in children and adults [396–398]. Do those same epigenetic factors help explain post-concussive aggression?

As noted in Chapter 7, fetal exposures to toxins, infections or stress, peri-natal complications, early childhood stress or illness, low education, minority status, and many forms of social adversity have been shown – with evidence that varies in persuasiveness – to increase the risk of persistent post-concussive problems. Few empirical studies, however, have explored which of these account for an appreciable amount of the variance in post-concussive aggression.

A completely different question: pre-morbid factors notwithstanding, is there something about typical CBI that increases the risk for aggressive behavior? If so, what basic behavioral functions have been altered (that is, referring to some popular abstract constructs: impulse control, approach versus withdrawal, predation, dominance challenge, threat detection, morality), and are biologically different injuries associated with phenomenologically different forms of aggression?

To the first question, many writers have observed that concussion exhibits a predilection to damage some brain regions or types of cells and tissue more than others. This chapter has previously outlined the wealth of evidence that medial temporal lobe structures such as the hippocampus and amygdala are disproportionately damaged, as are axonal bundles, including those connecting limbic, peri-limbic, and cortical regions thought to mediate emotional regulation and self-control – including the axon avenues between the prefrontal cortex and amygdala. It seems reasonable to postulate that this predilection helps to account for post-concussive irritability and aggression. That thesis, sometimes invoked with cavalier confidence, would be more persuasive if measured cerebral change in specific regions, circuits, or cells reliably predicted aggression. That is not the case. Despite remarkable advances in the resolution of neuroimaging, one is hard put to cite good comparative studies supporting that hypothesis.

There is, however, a growing body of research testing ideas that seem relevant. For example, traumatic events are stressful and, as explained in Chapter 7, there may be reciprocating

neural/mental harm when stress damages the very tissue needed to regulate the stress response.

The Threatened Threat Response

The author tentatively proposes a theory that seems to accommodate the data: trauma (the gestalt of stress independent of a particular cause) represents a threat to well-being. Concussion (the visitation of external force) often damages the circuitry that mediates threat responsiveness. Many survivors of traumatic concussion are consequently obliged to process threat with physiologically dysfunctional threat response circuitry. Threat response is critical both to anxiety and to aggression. Put simply, if one acquires an abnormally sensitive threat response system, more occasions will trigger approach (fight) or withdrawal (flight). The author posits that threat response abnormalities contribute to both post-concussive anxiety and aggression.

Several lines of evidence support this conceptual framework. First, a great deal of evidence demonstrates that brain regions prone to injury in concussion – including the amygdala, prefrontal cortex, cingulate gyrus, and insula – overlap significantly with the regions that mediate the threat response [399–404].[30] Second, acute emotional trauma, anxiety, and PTSD are associated with amplified perception of threat [406–412]. Third, the threat response is thought to be mediated, in part, by serotonin, perhaps explaining why 5HT reuptake inhibitors sometimes reduce threat responsiveness [413–415]. Similarly, cannabinoid reception seems to be involved in the threat response and cannabinoid treatments reportedly reduce threat responsiveness [416, 417]. Fourth, several hormones known to influence aggression moderate the threat response, including testosterone, corticotropin-releasing hormone, and oxytocin [418–420]. Fifth, when attentional resources are compromised (as after concussion), threat responses may increase [421]. Sixth, psychotherapies that reduce anxiety act on the threat detection circuits [422–425].

In addition, it has long been known that injuries to the known threat response regions both alter response to threat and, in some cases, increase aggression [426–428]. However, there are nuances that require attention. Damage to the amygdala can either increase or decrease threat responsiveness. In one experiment [429] ablation of the amygdalae led a mouse to climb on to a cat and nibble its ear. The cat attacked. The mouse climbed up again. This finding of rather bad mouse judgment helped explain the experiments of Klüver and Bucy with monkeys published in 1939 [430]: obliteration of the amygdala usually dramatically reduces aggression – apparently by obliterating threat responsiveness, especially to visual stimuli.[31] The classic result is passivity. *Incomplete* amygdalar injuries, on

---

[30]   Threat responsiveness actually engages an even broader collection of regions. Evidence suggests that the mammalian brain's threat detection and response also involve the periaqueductal gray, superior colliculus, hypothalamus, primary and secondary cortical sensory areas (which perceive and classify data such as worrisome images or sounds), and processing of that information by cortex in the vicinity of the right superior temporal sulcus to extract hints of socially relevant danger [405].

[31]   Note that exceptions occurred. Some lesioned monkeys became inappropriately and maladaptively aggressive, for instance, attacking higher-ranked animals in a social group [431, 432]. The surgical descriptions, unfortunately, were not precise enough to sort out whether this paradox has a simple anatomical explanation.

the other hand, tend to *amplify* the threat response. Damage to the prefrontal cortex has several effects on threat responses. In a normal person the prefrontal cortex restrains and limits the amygdala's response to threat. Some evidence suggests that the prefrontal cortex not only restrains the *behavioral* response but also restrains the *emotional* response – actually inhibiting amygdala reactivity despite the presence of threat [433]. In an anxious person, however, the prefrontal cortex's restraint of the amygdala fails [434]. These findings inspire prudence in attempting to decode post-concussive aggression. One speculates that, if CBI impairs threat responsiveness, the consequent behavioral change will depend not only on the relative degree of injury to various components of the circuit but also on genes and pre-morbid dispositions.

Why, then, does concussion sometimes cause persistent irritability or aggression?

Listing big, complex brain regions such as the amygdala and prefrontal cortex can hardly be regarded as specifying the cause of aggression. As the bedazzling intricacy of the connectome becomes apparent, early behavioral neurology that attributed a function to gigantic clockworks like the amygdala is just embarrassing. Amygdalar injury is very common but aggression may only be observed in about a third of cases. It is natural to inquire, beyond lobe naming, how individual network, connectivity, microscopic, and molecular differences in the anatomy, physiology, and chemistry of the concussion do or do not provoke conflict behavior. One factor (surely oversimplifying) may be the relative damage to prefrontal versus amygdalar tissue. In 1988, Weiger and Bear [435] attempted to summarize the difference in aggression caused by lesions in these two regions. Expanding on Luria [436], they opined that orbitofrontal lesions are more likely to cause impulsive aggression while temporal lobe lesions cause aggression via enhanced emotional responsiveness: "The paranoia (secondary to enhanced fearfulness) experienced by some of these patients may lead them to misinterpret the actions of others as personally threatening to themselves." (This insightful conclusion, by the way, was published about a decade before the neuroanatomy of threat responsiveness was widely known.) Paranoia may not be the right word for the problem in many cases of post-concussive aggression. The issue is not necessarily a cognitive mistake or delusional belief so much as an excessive emotional reaction.

Again, individual differences due to many pre-morbid factors surely moderate the effects of a change in anatomy. In addition, advances in neuroimaging have revealed that people exhibit considerable anatomical differences in the relevant architecture. As a key point eroding the credibility of the last 15 years of functional neuroimaging publications – similar focal lesions have different functional effects. Bonilha et al. [437], for example, studied 35 patients who had undergone anterior temporal lobectomy for epilepsy. The investigators reconstructed the personalized connectomes from MRI data. "Patients were more likely to achieve postsurgical seizure freedom if they exhibited fewer abnormalities within a subnetwork composed of the ipsilateral hippocampus, amygdala, thalamus, superior frontal region, lateral temporal gyri, insula, orbitofrontal cortex, cingulate, and lateral occipital gyrus" (p. 1846). The fact

that the circuit cited is largely identical to the list of regions known to regulate aggression is interesting but not interpretable at this time. The main point is that brains have what might be called (if not sure to cause confusion) personalities.

Short-Circuit: Debunking the Kindling Hypothesis of Post-TBI Aggression

> The pattern of positive and negative predictors of response...tends to support a model of kindling-reinforced reactive/affective/defensive/impulsive aggression.
> Saxena et al., 2005 [438], p. 1541

The published findings raise an old question: might some of the irritability and aggression observed after concussion be due to electrical irritability or abnormal subclinical epileptic brain activity? Might paroxysmal depolarization shifts occur, largely immune from detection by scalp electrodes, that explain untoward violence? The author, candidly, hesitates to even open the door to this discussion. He recalls the 1970s, when many writers achieved publication by shaking the stick of "kindling." It is possible that abnormal brain electrical activity plays a role in an animal's becoming epileptic or aggressive. It is probable (if infrequent) that epilepsy is a risk factor for aggression. It is possible that abnormal brain electrical activity somehow contributes to the phenomenon of post-concussion irritability or aggression. It is profoundly unlikely that kindling has anything to do with these phenomena.

Medicine should long ago have quashed the spread of the illogical speculation, almost never advanced by an epileptologist, that "kindling" explains either the development of seizures (epileptogenesis) or any human behavior. Yet, even into the 21st century, this factual error occasionally sneaks past peer review (see the above quotation from Saxena et al. [438]). Human neurobiology is in its infancy and certainty is a *rara avis*. But kindling has a specific physiological definition – like perfusion or decapitation. Using the term for something else has generated about 50 years of unnecessary confusion.

Again, there are few absolutes. There are many plausible biological factors that contribute to post-concussive aggression. One can say, however, with absolute clarity, that no evidence whatsoever exists that kindling is a contributor. For the sake of black-and-white honor – in the hopes of rescuing students from years of derailment from common sense – please consider the following six differences between kindling and the emergence of increased aggressiveness after a concussion:

1. Unlike kindling, there is no evidence of an initial focal electrical shock to the amygdala.
2. Nothing about the known physiology of concussion, including the neurometabolic cascade or the post-concussive melee, bears the slightest similarity to the physiology of a depth electrode-administered focal shock to the amygdala.
3. Kindled rats and cats all exhibit the same clinical sign: if kindling occurs one witnesses a brief epileptic fit. This hardly ever occurs in typical concussion.

4. Unlike kindling, a typical concussion does not involve repeated once-a-day, one-minute-long externally derived electrical shocks to one small cluster of cells in the amygdala, repeated for weeks or months. Nor does anything currently known about the cerebral events in the weeks or months after a concussion bear the slightest physiological resemblance to a repetitive, focal, once-a-day (and at no other time) shock.

5. Kindling involves an easily observed epileptic fit occurring once a day for many consecutive days. That has, to the best of the author's knowledge, never been reported after CBI.

6. Kindling, by definition, specifically and always involves a measured reduction in the threshold for the electrical current required to trigger a seizure when that current is administered via a depth electrode.

Facts notwithstanding, the kindling hypothesis of post-traumatic aggression survives with roach-like obduracy. Promoters of the kindling hypothesis might reasonably argue that they are not referring to the electrophysiological sequence known as kindling, but chatting metaphorically about a more general phenomenon in which vaguely similar electrical brain changes occur in a different way. For instance, might some neuropsychiatric illnesses involve amygdalar activation *similar* to that produced by a depth electrode, repeated in a pattern somewhat akin to daily one-minute doses, causing the same lowering of seizure threshold not to an external shock but to a subsequent internally brain-generated shock? Such lyrical ruminations have yet to explain data or facilitate scientific progress. The author apologizes for this side bar. He merely hopes to save students from a dead-end detour when so many promising avenues of research lay open for a stroll.

In brief summary of the subsection on causes of post-concussive aggression: like depression, anxiety, personality change, psychosis, or any other new-onset psychiatric problem after an external force visits a human head, no single explanation will suffice. The principal hope for the forthcoming decades is to escape the assumptions of semiological and physiological homogeneity, embrace the truth of individuality, and personalize the response with exquisite care to the unique biology driving each case of this awfully disruptive form of post-CBI life disruption.

Management of Post-Concussive Aggression

Management of persistent post-CBI aggression has rarely been studied in a systematic way. Few of the available reports describe large, double-blind, controlled, prospective studies of comparable patients. Few pertain to typical concussive injuries, focusing instead on severely injured or hospitalized patients. Moreover, since the pathophysiological basis of these behaviors cannot be tested and the contributing factors are probably different in every case, best practices have yet to be discovered. All that is known is what nudged the average on a rating scale for a short time in small cohort that is rarely representative of typical concussion survivors. This is not to dismiss the well-meant efforts of scholars to test the efficacy of treatments, but merely to caution against overconfidence in the credibility of any published recommendations, guidelines, or practice parameters. Pending advances in biomarkers for injury, biomarkers for neuropsychiatric constructs such as irritability, hostility, and aggression, as well as progress in pharmacogenetics, the compassionate clinician remains stuck in the rut of trial and error.

Management approaches to persistent post-CBI aggression are typically classified as environmental/psychotherapeutic/non-pharmacological versus pharmacological. (Another option may be non-pharmacological physiological manipulation such as transcranial magnetic stimulation [439], but no studies to date support efficacy.) Within the non-pharmacological studies one tends to encounter a distinction, in nomenclature if not in practice, between "behavioral" and "psychotherapeutic" approaches. Within the pharmacological studies one finds trials of beta-blockers, neuroleptics, antiepileptic drugs, antidepressants/mood stabilizers, lithium, stimulants, amantadine, and nutriceuticals.

Non-Pharmacological Approaches to Post-Concussive Aggression

Environmental manipulations proposed to treat aggression after moderate to severe TBI include cognitive therapies, behavioral therapies, exposure treatments, cathartic treatments, and multicomponent treatments [174, 306, 440]. Again, no evidence supports efficacy beyond the specific cohorts tested, and none of the interventions have been replicated.

A class of interventions variously referred to as behavioral modification or contingency management therapy, including natural setting behavior management, was popular in the 1980s. Such therapies have been employed for the mitigation of aggression after moderate or severe TBI, with reports of success in individual cases or uncontrolled case series [317, 441, 442]. Research to date does not support its use after concussion. Anger management approaches, sometimes called "psychoeducational programs," usually utilize or build upon "stress inoculation training" – a 20th-century approach originated by Novaco [440, 443]. Several groups have investigated the efficacy of stress inoculation training after moderate to severe TBI, reporting some evidence of efficacy in case reports or series [444–447] and in one small randomized trial [448]. "Anger self-management training," another psychoeducation-based approach, was reportedly efficacious in one small series of survivors of moderate or severe TBI [448]. Psychoeducational approaches have not been reported to reduce persistent aggression after concussion.

CBT, another 20th-century approach popularized by Beck and others [450, 451], has also been used for aggression management after moderate to severe TBI, with success again reported in case reports or uncontrolled open studies [317, 451, 452]. Structured group therapy for TBI, often using elements of the CBT approach, has reportedly been efficacious, again in open studies [453–456]. However, no sham-controlled studies support the efficacy of CBT for post-concussive irritability or aggression. One report encouraged psychoanalytically based interpretation of "projected aggression" and fostering of "reality attunement" for aggressive patients after frontal injury [458]. No evidence was provided.

As noted in the section on depression, the French Society of Physical Medicine and Rehabilitation recently reviewed non-pharmacological treatments for post-TBI behavioral disorders [174]. That review failed to search for treatments for irritability or aggression, failed to stratify findings by injury severity, and again, "No research was classified as level 1 or grade A" ([174], p. 32). Of 458 papers reviewed, only one – a single case report involving violence after severe TBI and temporal lobectomy – explicitly addressed aggression [383]. Lack of data notwithstanding, the authors of the 2016 review summarized their treatment recommendations:

> practice in controlling aggression consists in trying to detect the sensation of increasing tension and knowing how to cut off from other people in these situations. For the family, the training consists in trying to identify the run-up to bouts of aggressiveness, and to analyse and prevent triggering and aggravating factors; there also needs to be a reference person who can soothe bouts of anger, adapt his or her behaviour and style of communication, and use verbal signals to tell the patient he or she is behaving aggressively. This person can also recall pleasant moments.
>
> (EO) [expert opinion] ([174], p. 33)

Readers are justified in questioning the empirical rationale for this "international recommendation." It amounts to a guess. The principal conclusion revealed by reviewing non-pharmacological approaches is that controlled trials have yet to begin.

Pharmacological Approaches to Post-Concussive Aggression

As in the case of depression, multiple classes of medications have been proposed to mitigate aggression after moderate or severe TBI, but very few double-blind RCT studies have been published – almost none relevant to concussion. A fragile case can be made for hoping that some interventions that have transiently worked after more severe TBI will also work after typical concussion.

As noted in the discussion of depression, in the decade prior to this chapter at least six groups published reviews with recommendations for pharmacological management of post-traumatic neurobehavioral disorders. Warden et al.'s 2006 [108] collaborative paper reviewed agents for the management of post-TBI aggression. Those authors did not stratify reports by injury severity, so readers do not know to whom the guidelines apply. The writers arrived at three recommendations:

1. No standard treatment for aggression could be recommended due to insufficient evidence.
2. "Based on well designed class II studies with adequate samples...Beta blockers are recommended as a guideline for the treatment of aggression after TBI."[32]

3. Methylphenidate, cranial electrical stimulation, homeopathic therapy, serotonin reuptake inhibitors, tricyclic antidepressants, valproate, lithium, and buspirone were recommended as "options."

The same year, Fleminger et al. [33] published a systematic review of "Pharmacological management for agitation and aggression in people with acquired brain injury." That paper listed six controlled studies: four reported trials of beta-blockers, one with amantadine, and one with methylphenidate. None were confined to TBI subjects of a particular severity. None of the six studies pertained to persistent aggression or irritability after TBI or concussion. Just as reported by Warden et al., the most promising results came from studies of beta-blockers. The authors of this review were forthright: "However, these studies used relatively small numbers, have not been replicated, used large doses, and did not use a global outcome measure or long-term follow-up" ([33], p. 1).

In a third review, Chew and Zafonte [179] cited the same four low-quality studies of beta-blockers. They also cited a single RCT of sertraline resulting in no benefit [462]. The other reported studies were case reports, case series, or open-label uncontrolled trials of antidepressants, neuroleptics, antiepileptic drugs, stimulants, and lithium.

Halbauer et al.'s 2009 review [48] is unique in that it focuses on mild to moderate TBI among warfighters. As in most manuscripts, those authors failed to discriminate between agitation and aggression. Rather than conducting a novel study these authors simply refer readers to Warden et al. [108], even though that paper did not identify any effective treatments for mild injuries.

The fifth large-scale review was published by Wheaton et al. [180]. These authors cite four clinical trials of treatment for anger/aggression, but only one of those included some subjects with mild or moderate injuries: Mooney and Haas [463] reported a single-blind study in which methylphenidate 30 mg/day reduced aggression among 36 males after various degrees of brain injury.

The sixth and most recent review, as previously described, was published in 2016 by Plantier et al. [181]. Citing the same four papers, the authors declare that propranolol is "effective," without specifying the severity of the cases or type of aggression. They also assert that carbamazepine and valproate "seem effective on agitation and aggression" but do not provide persuasive evidence from controlled studies. Curiously, Plantier et al. explicitly state: "There is no evidence of efficacy for neuroleptics" [181]. Yet they cite Kim and Bijlani [464], who reported a six-week prospective trial among seven closed head injury survivors (mixed severity) that concluded: "the administration of quetiapine in doses of 25mg to 300mg daily was well tolerated and led to significant reductions in aggression

---

[32] Each of the major reviews cites the same four sources in support of the claim that beta-blockers are efficacious: Brooke et al. [378] (21 severely injured patients with acute agitation); Greendyke et al. [459] (four TBI subjects studied up to 30 years post injury); Greendyke et al. [460] (five severely demented patients with TBI and impulsivity); and Greendyke et al. [461] (three inpatient TBI survivors). The present author politely rejects the characterization of these studies by Warden et al. as "well designed." None of these studies are methodologically rigorous and none are relevant to persistent aggression after CBI.

and irritability" ([464], p. 548).[33] In summary, none of these six reviews of post-TBI neurobehavioral disorders offer trustworthy guidance with regard to pharmacological management of irritability or aggression.

Studies of individual agents, or classes of agents, also fail to provide any credible and practical answers for the clinician. However, these reports are worthy of consideration in case researchers are ever funded to conduct the required large-scale RCTs. Lithium was among the first medications administered for post-TBI aggression. Old case reports and case series primarily discuss efficacy after severe injuries. For example, in the review by Deb and Crownshaw [178], only one paper included two cases of mild TBI with dubious efficacy [465], and in the review by Warden et al. [108] none of four papers on lithium pertained to typical CBI. However, some recent evidence suggests that lithium possesses neuroprotective properties relevant to TBI, including inhibition of excitotoxic injury, ischemic injury, inflammation, and amyloid-related neurodegeneration and promotion of neurogenesis [466, 467]. In one animal study, lithium reduced anxiety-like behavior [468]. The author opines that it is premature to dismiss the possible utility of lithium for the management of post-CBI neurobehavioral disorders.

Neuroleptics and atypical antipsychotics have also been administered, again primarily to persons who survived severe injuries. One old case series suggested a benefit from clozapine, but two of nine subjects developed seizures [469]. Other case reports or series discuss possible benefits of quetiapine [464], ziprasidone [470], or olanzapine [471, 472]. No evidence suggests a benefit for post-CBI irritability or aggression. Moreover, these agents are prone to misuse as sedatives and may inhibit recovery [473–475]. Benzodiazepines should also be regarded as ineffective, except as sedatives that are prone to produce cognitive deficits and create a risk of substance dependence and paradoxical agitation [476].

A group of medications has been referred to as "antidepressants" despite evidence that this label perhaps misrepresents the diversity of their potential benefits. Many have been administered in the hope of reducing post-TBI aggression, mostly among survivors of severe injuries. Two reports, however, included or focused on mild cases. Five of 13 cases reported by Kant et al. [477] exhibited reduced aggression (but, interestingly, not depression) after treatment with sertraline. Similarly, Fann et al. [186, 478] reported that sertraline treatment of persistent post-concussive depression also reduced anger and aggression. Multiple case reports and series discuss the effect of agents with antiepileptic properties, such as carbamazepine, oxcarbazine, valproic acid, lamotrigine, and levetiracetam. Although several of these papers mention reduction in agitation or aggression among severely injured persons [479–483], no evidence supports the use of these agents after typical concussion.

Buspirone, for reasons the author has been unable to determine, is routinely mentioned at TBI meetings and even in textbooks as useful for controlling aggression. The evidence supporting this lore is questionable. Case reports [484–487] and a chart review [488] do not satisfy the minimal standards of evidence. At the same time, some evidence suggests that this agent facilitates recovery in experimental TBI [489, 490]. Again, pending a high-quality RCT, no conclusion regarding clinical efficacy is possible.

Apart from the possible benefit of beta-blockers, two agents stand out as slightly promising: amantadine and marijuana.

Amantadine is best known as an influenza-moderating agent that enhances dopaminergic (DA) transmission. Since DA is not known to play a major role in the post-concussive melee of metabolic, inflammatory, and vascular change, it is not clear how such an agent might help after TBI. Yet this medication is also a weak N-methyl-D-aspartate receptor antagonist that perhaps mitigates excitotoxic injury [491]. And experimental studies suggest that amantadine enhances cognitive and motor recovery in rodents [492, 493].[34] In some studies, rodents exhibited not only arousal but also behavioral improvements; for instance, Tan et al. [496] reported a reduction in depression-like behaviors. The hope naturally arose that amantadine would have similar neuropsychiatric benefits in humans. Indeed, case studies and chart reviews suggest that amantadine sometimes reduces irritability or dyscontrol among survivors of severe TBI [491, 497–500]. That data inspired Hammond et al. [501] to conduct a multisite placebo-controlled trial of amantadine 100 mg bid among 76 TBI survivors with persistent (> six months) irritability. There is good news and less good news. Among subjects with baseline aggression, at 28 days there was an average change of −4.56 on the Neuropsychiatry Inventory Aggression subscale in the amantadine group versus −2.46 in the placebo group ($p = 0.046$). Although these subjects mostly survived moderate injuries, it seems plausible that typical, less severely hurt CBI survivors might also benefit. However, when the same research team expanded the number of subjects to 168, improvement was not significantly different between the active and placebo-treated cohorts [502]. This project deserves attention for its rarity in size and rigor. Non-replication of the initial positive results does not detract from those virtues or lead one to abandon hope. The basic science findings are compelling. The present author speculates that some biological difference influences the likelihood of an individual's positive response to amantadine. The authors of the 2012 *New England Journal of Medicine* [494] paper seem reasonable in urging that further research may reveal the traits identifying the survivors most likely to benefit.

Marijuana for Post-Concussive Aggression

On too many occasions to count, adult male CBI survivors have come to the author's clinic requesting a "prescription" or written

---

[33] Perhaps, in France, quetiapine is not a neuroleptic?

[34] Excitement justifiably followed the 2012 *New England Journal of Medicine* publication of a placebo-controlled study reporting that amantadine enhanced human recovery from prolonged arousal deficits after severe TBI [494]. A review, however, points to inconsistencies in the findings with respect to arousal and cognition [495].

recommendation for medical marijuana. "It calms me, doc," is a typical statement. The author has not yet obliged, pending credible scientific evidence of safety and efficacy. However, on three occasions (two involving gang members), the request was memorable because it came from the patients' elderly grandmothers. In Spanish, they reported having observed a marked benefit characterized by reduced irritability and hostility, enhanced self-control, and improved sleep. Smoking marijuana, in these concerned and very conservative grandparents' observations, facilitated a pacific household, dramatically reducing the risk of aggression without producing sedation or apathy. One cannot help being touched and intrigued by these visits.

The relationship between endocannabinoids (metabolites of eicosanoid fatty acids), exogenous marijuana, and post-concussive behavior is unknown. Yet multiple lines of evidence suggest the possibility of beneficial effects in acute TBI. First, there is a significant increase in endocannabinoid levels shortly after TBI that seems to have a neuroprotective effect, perhaps related to vasoregulation [503, 504]. Second, some effects of experimental brain injury appear to be moderated by cannabinoids [505–508]. Third, a large body of evidence suggests involvement of CB2 receptor occupancy with the regulation of post-traumatic inflammation, and manipulation of the cannabinoid-2 receptor reduces inflammation during the inflammatory phase after TBI – a benefit seemingly mediated by inhibition of release of cytokines [509–512]. Fourth, in a mouse model of TBI, a cannabinoid-2 receptor agonist mitigated blood–brain barrier and neurodegenerative change [513]. Fifth, cannabinoid receptor activation has been reported to enhance macrophage clearance of human beta-amyloid [514]. Collectively, these findings suggest that manipulation of cannabinoids has promise in acute TBI intervention. Moreover, since post-CBI degenerative and inflammatory processes may be ongoing for months or years, one wonders whether the informally observed moderation of aggression possibly reflects salubrious effects on these chronic processes. Cannabinoid-1 receptor activation has also been explicitly linked to aggression [515], and two synthetic cannabinoid receptor agonists have reduced aggressive behavior in rodents [516, 517], raising the possibility that optimizing cannabinoid signaling might regulate post-concussive aggression.

How will we ever know? No double-blind RCTs of smoked marijuana to moderate post-concussive aggression have been published. This probably reflects the U.S. federal government's restrictive policies. Sills (2016) [518] recently summarized the problem in *Science*: "The U.S. federal government's Cannabis research policies have blocked externally valid, randomized

clinical trials on the effects of Cannabis" (p. 1182).[35] However, some evidence seems promising: irritability is common in Huntington's disease, and, in one trial of the synthetic 9-keto cannabinoid, nabilone, a reduction was reported in both Unified Huntington's Disease Rating Scale behavioral and Neuropsychiatric Inventory scores [523, 524].

In addition, Celina et al. [525] reviewed six clinical trials of the synthetic cannabinoids nabilone and dronabinol to control aggression and agitation in Alzheimer's disease. That preliminary evidence suggests efficacy. Intriguingly, one study investigated the effects of a mixture of Δ9-tetrahydrocannabinol and cannabidiol (effecting both cannabinoid-1 and cannabinoid-2 receptors) on abnormal behaviors in a murine model of degenerative tauopathy [526]. Treatment reduced aggression against both the self and others. This discovery is potentially important because multiple concussions sometimes trigger a progressive degenerative condition associated with tau, aggression, and suicidality. An aggression-moderating treatment would be valuable for victims of this disease and their families. In summary, although the data are inadequate to support an evidence-based treatment recommendation, cannabinoid intervention appears to be an especially promising area of investigation.

Recommendations for the Management of Post-Concussive Aggression

Any declaration that there exists a safe and efficacious treatment for post-concussive aggression would be inappropriate and probably unethical. The paucity of relevant research precludes a guideline, practice parameter, or specific recommendation. Two forms of variation currently represent insurmountable barriers to painting a management algorithm: first, there is no one phenomenon or symptom to address. The doctor may be asked to help one CBI survivor who curses at his television and his cat, another who becomes embroiled in confrontations in supermarket checkout lines, and a third who has been arrested for intimate-partner abuse. Until the biopsychosocial bases of aggression are better understood, no system permits classification of scientifically valid subtypes, except by reference to arbitrary and largely subjective criteria. Second, imagining some future era when the right questionnaire or large machine identifies those with a biologically specific subtype of aggression, one would not expect that any two persons exhibiting that specific, objectively verifiable PPCPP would respond to the same treatment. It is likely that many genetic and environmental factors influence not only the expression of aggression

---

[35] The author does not advocate any position but the impartial pursuit of science in the interests of humanity, and cannot prescribe based on theory and anecdote. He does, however, regard the current restrictions on research as anti-scientific and historically rooted in racism. Of possible interest: *cannabis* was part of the U.S. formulary until 1937, when "Federal Bureau of Narcotics Commissioner Harry J. Anslinger presented sensationalized newspaper clippings as proof of the harms of marijuana. Congress responded with the Marijuana Tax Act of 1937" [519]. Despite medical testimony to the contrary, marijuana was condemned as invariably harmful by the 1970 Controlled Substances Act [520, 521]. Until very recently, serious researchers had to spend years seeking approval from multiple federal agencies, buy their marijuana exclusively from the National Institute on Drug Abuse's farm at the University of Mississippi, and employ lower doses than are generally used where marijuana is tolerated [518]. Evidence is especially promising that some of the scores of cannabinoids in the marijuana plant are effective antiepileptic drugs. That was one driver of petitions filed in 2009 and 2011 advising the U.S. Drug Enforcement Administration to declassify

but – among those with matching symptoms caused by similar biological changes – the treatment response. As in the case of post-concussive depression or anxiety (or indeed, as in the case of any medical problem), we know enough to realize that individualized treatment is required, but not enough to name the optimum treatment in any case.

The author is therefore obliged to be extremely circumspect. Decades of trial and error have not granted him the skill to reliably guess who will benefit from what. He has routinely prescribed psychotherapy not otherwise specified because contact with a caring person seems helpful. He has suggested trials of sertraline, buspirone, propranolol, and amantadine based more on chatting with patients about co-morbid medical conditions and side-effects than on a concrete anti-aggression rationale. His main recommendation is a plea to scholars: the evidence that heritable variation influences health is so profound that it seems a waste of resources to conduct future clinical trials blind to DNA and its histones. As the cost of sequencing falls, genomic analysis may become an expected element of pharmacological RCTs. Comparing treatment response between persons with similar problems but different genomes will soon revolutionize practice. It cannot happen soon enough.

IV. Post-Concussive Distress of the Types Associated with APA "PTSD"

Because the road curved as it did, Reema saw the school bus first. Her husband tried to fit their old sedan into the man-wide space between the yellow monster and the yellow rocks. "Oh God Oh God," was all the woman said, according to her later shaking narrative in court. She saw the other driver's face loom pale and startled in the massive windshield's frame. Despite her several seconds of unconsciousness, his Munch-like "Oh" came back to visit in many later dreams. She woke to hear the children's screams, too few, she thought, for such a mammoth box. It took a moment more before she recognized the oddness of the world. Because she hung suspended from her seatbelt and the earth was near her head, because her shoulder twisted in an unfamiliar way, she finally grasped that she was upside down. Her husband, so it seemed, had vanished in the crumpled driver's side – a smoking waste of airbag, glass, and steel, unfeasibly spackled in red. The firefighters could not get her out at first. A sparking wire lay across the hood and near the pool of gas. She dangled in her nylon sling, watching as they pulled the bodies of the children,

one by one, up to a waiting van. I read the famous expert's sophistry with no surprise but some despair. "She could not suffer," so he said. "She can't recall the blow."

This case is one that I can't shake. That tends to happen when the patient has been triply harmed: by injury, agony, and cruelty by the well-paid skeptics who invented reasons she must be just fine. When readers whiff the logic of professional concussion deniers, please remember Reema.

Two different questions are at stake. One falls more directly in the province of this book:

1. **"Is a stressful life experience sometimes followed by persistent distress?"** That might, at first, seem broader than the 1970s question: "Is a stressful life experience sometimes followed by post-traumatic stress disorder ('PTSD')?" The author chose the rewording with care and hopes to make his reasons clear within a page or two. As will be shown, "PTSD"[36] is a humanistically inspired but scientifically indefensible concept. No evidence supports its existence as a unitary entity. Readers are invited to join today's global effort to replace "PTSD" with a conceptualization of the spectrum of post-stress distress that is more coherent, scientifically valid, and helpful to patients.

2. **"Is a CBI sometimes followed by persistent distress?"** This is more germane to the present chapter's stated goals. Yet unless one first makes it clear why "PTSD" is a perverse and misleading term, it is hard to discuss an issue of great importance: how stress and brain injury interact. A reflex interrupts the dialogue: despite decades of scholarship patiently explaining that "PTSD" is rooted in political activism, not science [527, 528], textbooks still employ the term. Some older doctors brave the rapids of progress; others cling, shivering defiantly, to the snag of the familiar. All will be revealed.

What, if Anything, is Posttraumatic Stress Disorder ("PTSD")? "The Implications are Vast"[37]

The current challenge in the field of traumatic stress studies is to address the emerging empirical basis of PTSD as central to the validity of the disorder while placing in proper historical perspective that the diagnosis came to be by acceptance of the political and social rights of traumatized groups.

Yehuda and McFarlane, 1995 [529], p. 1710

---

marijuana as a dangerous addictive drug with no medicinal value. Change is afoot. In 2016, the Drug Enforcement Administration liberalized licensure such that more universities will be able to grow marijuana for research [522]. As of 2017, 21 universities have applied. None have been approved. Although non-scientific (or even antiscientific) factors will surely continue to impede this scholarship, perhaps progress will be made in the coming decades.

36 The letter sequence "P-T-S-D" does not refer to any medical problem, but to a periodically reconceived arbitrarily specified combination of symptoms promoted by a professional guild. In order to distinguish between a defensible medical concept and a politically motivated blunder, one is obliged to employ quotation marks.

37 The author wishes to be useful to readers with different life agendas. Some wish to explore the underlying science. Others may be more interested in practical clinical advice. Both are noble enterprises prone to benefit the species. Readers primarily seeking practice advice are

It is the rare moment when most every assumption and theoretical underpinning of a psychiatric disorder comes under attack, or is found to lack empirical support. Yet, this is the situation faced by PTSD. After nearly 25 years of research and clinical experience, there is little about the diagnosis that has gone unchallenged.

Rosen, 2004 [530], p. xi

At least four checkpoints guard the road to a straightforward and sensible account of post-concussive distress of the types rhetorically affiliated under the rubric, "PTSD." First, no evidence suggests that trauma, stress, or tragedy triggers a single human cognitive/emotional syndrome. Of course, stressful events are often followed by distress! A different brain response system would be self-destructive. The concept is, indeed, somewhat circular: stress is stressful (or, more precisely but no more illuminating, a very stressful life experience is often followed by a stress-related change in emotional responsiveness). But some people develop a little distress, others a lot. Some suffer brief distress, others suffer for years. Some become sad, others nervous, others jumpy, others untethered from reality. These problems may occur in any degree and any combination. That variation in symptoms, combined with the variations in onset, severity, and course, means that virtually innumerable tints and flavors of distress are observed after upset.

What should one call that spectrum? Since a change in behavior after a near-death experience may have considerable survival value, since one benefits from vigilance after nearly being eaten, is it more logical to consider the infinite variations of response to a stressor to be sickness or health? Does this phenomenon switch values, at some red line, from the healthy, normal stress response described by Cannon in 1915 [531] to a disease or disorder? As Summerfield [528] warned about "PTSD": "Above all, the diagnosis of post-traumatic stress disorder lacks specificity: it is imprecise in distinguishing between the physiology of normal distress and the physiology of pathological distress" ([528], p. 97). Where is the Goldilocks threshold between too little stress response, just right, and too much? The present author's formulation, "distress after stress," provides a semantically defensible unification. Yet politics rarely chaperones wisdom into authority.

Here one must thread a conceptual needle, hoping to be clear for the sake of those who suffer. There is no "PTSD." There is a great deal of distress after stress.

Political activists in the 1970s themselves became distressed – and justifiably so. The Vietnam Veterans Working Group and its founding advocates – including Leonard Neff, Shaim Shatan, Sharah Haley, and Robert J. Lifton – were moved by the observation that some Vietnam veterans suffered prolonged emotional disability. Some veterans became very sad, even suicidal. That was recognizable and had a name: depression. Yet other veterans suffered mightily from one or more other painful symptoms: becoming preoccupied with bad memories, or suffering from poor sleep and bad nightmares, or struggling to avoid reminders, becoming excessively emotional, easily choked up, easily angered, excessively fearful, jumping at loud sounds, or, quite the contrary, feeling numbed and distanced from their own emotions, unable to feel pleasure, unable to love, withdrawing from the social world. Commonly, the veterans would feel distracted and inattentive, measurably cognitively compromised or dull. Rarely, they would feel as if plunged through a worm hole back through time to the event itself, re-experiencing the horror as they sat safe and sound at home.

Nothing was new about these observations. Many were reported in the *Iliad*. But militaries had long sought to minimize the problem and blame the victims, and psychiatry had never quite gotten around to studying the problem. So the anti-war activists launched a campaign pressing the APA to acknowledge the veterans' distress [528, 530, 532, 533]. The activists deserve credit for their humanistic hearts. They meant well in their aggressive campaign. As Yehuda and McFarlane put it [529], "From a social and political perspective, PTSD as a concept has done much to assist in the recognition of the rights and needs of victims who have been stigmatized, misunderstood, or ignored by the mental health field."

From this ore of heartfelt concern the APA has manufactured absurdity.

Rather than recognizing and studying the broad spectrum of post-traumatic distress, the APA nominated three particular symptoms as the ones worth counting, invented an arbitrary suite of diagnostic criteria, and assigned a label [534].[38] In 1980, a disorder was added to the DSM-III classification system with a rare and special feature: it had a cause.[39] So-called "post-traumatic stress disorder" was explicitly claimed to be the anxiety disorder caused by "a psychologically distressing event that is outside the range of usual human experience"[327]. At the time, "PTSD" was classified as an anxiety disorder and claimed to have three elements: intrusive memories; effortful avoidance of thinking about the event (which, despite the self-evident phenomenological difference, was equated with emotional numbing); and arousal. That notion survived for a decade. More recent "PTSDs", redefined for later manuals, have four elements. But, as explained shortly, persons who meet the approved criteria actually exhibit at least seven clearly

---

of course free to skip the following brief science section. However, the author cannot in good conscience commend any practice suggestions without doing his utmost to plead this caution: so-called "PTSD" does not seem to be anything specific.

[38] Analogies never satisfy, but sometimes clarify: post-stress distress varies. Following the APA's instructions means including some cases and excluding others by applying arbitrary rules that fail in both sensitivity and specificity [528, 535, 536]. The Department of Motor Vehicles might as well define "automobile" as "a black or red steel box with a six-cylinder engine and an average of three to five wheels." No doubt. But what about the other ones?

[39] The APA's classification system is advertised as etiology-agnostic. The diagnostic criteria for APA-approved disorders have mostly been stripped of causal context. Until recently, the two exceptions were conversion disorder and PTSD.

differentiable types of distress. It has yet to be shown that such a disorder exists.

"PTSD" has always been controversial. It has neither a neuroscientific definition nor a fixed diagnostic algorithm. Young [537] summarized the problem:

> The disorder is not timeless, nor does it possess an intrinsic unity. Rather, it is glued together by the practices, technologies, and narratives with which it is diagnosed, studied, treated, and represented and by the various interests, institutions, and moral arguments that mobilised these efforts and resources.

A tsunami of research has subsequently exposed the non-integrity of "PTSD." "[C]ore assumptions… and hypothesized mechanisms… underlying the diagnostic construct have not been supported" ([535], p. 161). The present author has a deeper concern: the APA's classification system insists that, among humans – a species observed to develop infinitely variable responses to stress – and among the subset of humans that meet an imagined threshold of "too much" response to stress – there is a small subset worthy of the label "PTSD." Clinicians who are obedient to the APA's arbitrary rules and regulations are permitted to declare who wins the label and who gets left out.[40] This is not science. This is not evidence-based medicine. This is embracing the political at the expense of the truth.[41]

This is not to debate the question of whether stress can be followed by distress. Of course it can! That has surely been the conclusion based on empathetic human observation since the dawn of humanity, or well before. Scientific descriptions of post-traumatic stress with physiological hyper-reactivity date at least as far back as 1871 [539]. The question is whether trauma is ever followed by a biologically unitary disorder for which the APA deserves credit for having divined a valid diagnostic algorithm or whether, instead, that which the APA calls "PTSD" (periodically changing their minds) is a politically inspired operational definition [540] that, if applied with the utmost care, would identify diverse problems with a wide variety of signs, symptoms, pathophysiologies, prognoses, and responses to attempted management. Let there be no doubt: post-stress distress occurs. But it is essential to clarify the difference between the solid scientific ground of that distress and the quicksand of a misleading phrase.

Many people suffer awful insults to health and peace of mind. Illness and injury are commonly upsetting. Should one expect a single, uniform human response to the billions of potentially upsetting life events? Within limits, the answer is yes. Cannon [531, 541, 542] recognized that some features of stress response are common across events and species. Increased heart rate, for instance, is common among animals with hearts. Creatures equipped with adrenals often exhibit increased levels of glucocorticoids. Thus, at the level of a primitive physiological reflex, one can legitimately expect several uniform bodily changes and even posit a mammalian stress "syndrome" [543–553].

The human mind is something else. Our massive cortex enables heterogeneity in cognitive and emotional responses. Consider, the APA's notorious (and increasingly disreputable) DSM-5 criteria for the diagnosis of PTSD [65]. There are 27 of them. In simple terms, since a patient may or may not exhibit each one of the 27, there are 2^{27} or 134,217,728 possible presentations of these 27 symptoms. The APA declares that many of these 134 million combinations *are PTSD*, so long as they conform with a menu written by a committee.

Compare two cases of APA-approved "PTSD."[42]

Case Number 1

Philomena is a 63-year-old woman who received a phone call reporting that her friend and golf buddy Roseanne had a fall. Roseanne has been hospitalized with a badly broken hip. Philomena, when asked later, has a sharp memory of that upsetting call, although she tries not to think about it. She sleeps well and has not had bad dreams about Roseanne's misfortune; yet, for a month or two, she is less interested in playing golf and feels a bit detached from her husband and his proposals of intimacy. She has not come to the conclusion that the world is a dangerous place. Still, for six weeks she becomes slightly jumpy when that same phone rings. She admits trouble concentrating and feels distracted at work for 17 days – after which those symptoms abate. Her neuroendocrine markers and brain MRI are normal. The APA says Philomena has "PTSD."

Case Number 2

Gregor, a 35-year-old man, survives an airplane crash in the Caucasus in which his wife, mother, and four children were killed. Gregor cannot recall the crash in detail, yet he has frequent nightmares about the plane careening toward the mountain and his failed cardiopulmonary resuscitation on his 12-year-old daughter amid the crash of lightning on a black rocky slope, to the point that his sleep is severely disrupted. He becomes terrified and visibly trembles when his employer asks him to take an airplane flight, so he quits his job and avoids airplane flights for the rest of his life. Gregor has come to feel that the world is a dangerous place and he has little left to live for. Indeed, each waking moment is a torment. Despite all the kindness of his minister and congregation, he withdraws more and more until he becomes incapable of leaving his bedroom for a decade. His neuroendocrine markers are consistent with chronic severe stress and, 18 years after the crash, his brain

---

40 Winning is one oddity of "PTSD." "It is rare to find a psychiatric diagnosis that anyone likes to have, but PTSD seems to be one of them" (Andreasen, 1995 [538], p. 964).

41 Why do many textbooks perpetuate the "PTSD" mistake? One learns in graduate school (and, if sensitive to justice, suffers existential shock) that courage and academic promotion can be antithetical. Many tenure-track professors, feet to the fire, admit having bent to accommodate poor judgments by peer reviewers and editors, selling the illusion of integrity to buy the illusion of success. Collective courage must reach a tipping point before dogma is exorcised by science.

42 Both cases describe the author's clinic patients, altered for protection of unique identifiers.

MRI shows gross atrophy of the medial temporal lobe.[43] The APA says Gregor has "PTSD."

Do Gregor and Philomena have the same problem? The APA says yes. Surely we can devise a more rational approach to classifying human distress.

> Perhaps no other diagnostic category has gone through as many alterations and permutations as has PTSD…It is still not clear whether PTSD, as currently conceptualized, is a distinct and homogeneous category … or whether it would be more accurate to think of PTSD as being part of one or more dimensions or spectra.
>
> (Moreau and Zisook, 2012 [534], p. 776)

Many scholars have noted that symptoms of long-lasting distress following an upsetting life event do not reliably cluster, as claimed by the APA in the various wavering iterations they have published in their DSM. Psychiatrists and psychologists are not oblivious to the parlous logic of the APA's position. Many have tried to determine, in so far as present science permits, whether the APA's successive manifestos make sense. One research strategy has been employed repeatedly in an effort to answer that question: *confirmatory factor analysis* (CFA)[44] [559, 560]. Each time an APA committee published another "now we really understand it" scheme for labeling people with "PTSD," mathematicians investigated whether the new-and-improved menu of allegedly diagnostic symptoms represents one, three, or seven types of distress or dysfunction (never mind whether those symptom clusters occur together in the same person or collectively represent an authentic medical condition. That is a separate question).

Before a quick review of those CFA studies, a caveat may be warranted. CFA does not confirm or disconfirm whether a proposed disorder exists.[45] Nor must a hypothetical disorder be demonstrated, on factor analysis, to be captured by a single factor or symptom for that analysis to support the existence of an entity. Tuberculosis, multiple sclerosis, and beri-beri all commonly present with multiple symptoms or clusters of symptoms. The finding that such disorders are clinically complex (exhibiting multiple dissociable elements) and heterogeneous (exhibiting different combinations of those elements in different patients) does not argue against a common etiological agency.[46] Factor analysis, however, may abet the process of analyzing the validity of a proposed entity by narrowing the search for that common thread. It is easier to

determine whether a disorder is mathematically associated with hypervigilance, numbing, and avoidance than whether it causes (as a guess) 57 million of the 134 million possible combinations of symptoms. In addition – and highly pertinent to the current doubts about treatment efficacy – factor analysis may identify multiple symptoms, each of which has a different cause and deserves a different treatment. That would enable individualization of patient care better than today's one-size-fits-all approach in which persons with vastly disparate forms of misery are lumped together under a single diagnosis and (if a clerical worker at the insurance company is of a mood to approve) funded for a single therapy.

Several early studies reported that a three-factor model distills the essence of DSM-IV PTSD: (1) intrusion; (2) effortful avoidance/emotional numbing; and (3) arousal. However, this tripartite structure is "rarely empirically supported… The implications of this are vast given that PTSD's factor structure is directly related to diagnostic algorithms" ([567], p. 368). That is, stressed and then distressed humans suffer a wide variety of symptoms. The stress response is normal and life preserving. Distress after stress is common. Every reader knows it well. Its character and magnitude may or may not cross the threshold of a disease. Thrashing about in the mud pit of academic committee work to debate how many symptom clusters to acknowledge does not seem productive. But it does support careers. Hence: more papers.

Subsequent CFA publications have reported from two to seven symptom clusters. A four-factor "numbing" model differentiates between the ostensibly unconscious phenomenon of emotional numbing and the conscious avoidance of reminders [568, 569]. A different four-factor model is called the "dysphoria" model [570–572]. That one emphasizes the relationship of "PTSD" to the accepted spectrum of anxiety and mood disorders. A meta-analysis of 40 studies slightly favored the dysphoria model over the numbing model [574]. Yet neither of these models accommodates the observation of symptoms such as sleeping difficulties, concentration difficulties, and irritability. As a result, Elhai and colleagues [575, 576] have more recently published arguments supporting a five-factor "dysphoric arousal" model cleaving human distress after bad events into (1) intrusion; (2) avoidance; (3) numbing; (4) anxious arousal; and (5) dysphoric arousal. To narrate the CFA debate in a comprehensive way transcends the ambitions of this chapter. Suffice it to say that many investigators have

---

[43] The first studies to show an association between a history of PTSD and temporal lobe atrophy reported an average of 18 years from event to scan, suggesting that this anatomical change is delayed (and not necessarily typical) [554–558].

[44] CFA is now a mini-industry within mathematical psychology, sharing publication favor with disciplines called structural analysis, dimensionality analysis, latent class analysis, and taxonometric analysis [559–566]. These approaches, please note, are not investigations of biological disorders. They are quests for little hypothetical constructs that make up big hypothetical constructs.

[45] CFA or latent factor analysis merely helps clarify whether, among people judged to meet the APA's criteria for "PTSD" based on having one of the millions of approved combinations of 27 PTSD symptoms, one or more of those symptoms tends to be found when another one is found; hence, conceivably suggesting that that one, or two, or more symptoms tend to co-occur. For example, if social withdrawal and emotional numbing are found together often enough to satisfy some formula, the mathematician might conclude that there exists a "withdrawal and numbing" factor.

[46] Explaining this concept to medical students, one may discuss a fall from a cliff. The etiology is singular – acute ground deceleration – even if diverse changes are observed from head to toe.

contributed to an exhaustive effort to find the "essential" elements of APA-approved "PTSD" – elements that consistently show up among persons who exhibit persistent distress after exposure to stress [567, 569–580].

DSM-5, published in 2013, again rejigged the definition of "PTSD" and provoked yet another round of investigation. At the time of this writing, the state of the art amounts to a competition, with two-, three-, four-, five-, six-, and seven-factor models of "PTSD" contending for primacy, none validating the APA's politically driven disorder as a medical entity [67, 275, 564, 565, 581–586]. Armour et al. [67] recently asserted:

the 7-factor Hybrid model, which incorporates key features of both 6-factor models and is comprised of re-experiencing, avoidance, negative affect, anhedonia, externalizing behaviors, and anxious and dysphoric arousal symptom clusters, provided superior fit to the data in both samples.

([67], p. 106)

Have we finally unveiled the truth? Is seven the number of types of distress (other than depression) following stress? Two comments by other scholars put the CFA enterprise into perspective:

- "Implications concerning clinical psychopathology and comorbidity of PTSD are discussed, including whether PTSD should be refined by removing its non-specific symptoms" [582].
- "we tested eight PTSD factor structures … CFA revealed that all models provided very good fit … Potential interpretations of these findings include: (1) the indicators (i.e., symptoms) need refinement; or (2) relevant symptoms have yet to be identified" [587].

What can one conclude? Into how many colors must post-traumatic distress be refracted before the academic community recognizes a rainbow?

We demonstrated in an earlier chapter that no credible evidence supports the existence of a "post-concussive syndrome." We will demonstrate in a forthcoming chapter that, although aging is indisputably associated with neurodegeneration, research has yet to discover a unitary and biologically discrete "Alzheimer's disease." Similarly, no credible evidence supports the existence of a unitary "post-traumatic stress disorder." The factor analyses reveal phenomenological Balkanization. No biological marker exists. No two cases are alike. Millions of combinations of symptoms satisfy the APA's criteria – which may change again shortly. One must wholeheartedly sympathize with persons who suffer lasting distress after stressful experiences. But to lop off one piece of the pie and call it by a special name is as logically clever as to rush to the aid of a hundred people who fell from a cliff and, following diagnostic rules in obeisance to an orthopedic committee, label 35 of them with "post-falling-down syndrome."

What Happened in Reema's Head?

"PTSD" does not exist as a unitary entity, but that hardly reduces the number of concussion survivors who face, for months or decades, one of the distresses on the menu. The problem might be named "the occurrence of one or more of the clinically hurtful symptoms, or clusters of symptoms, which are apparently related to the stressful nature of the event, that factor analysis either successfully identifies or should have identified when exploring the persistent distress of hundreds of thousands of concussion survivors." Perhaps that's unwieldy. Call the problem, for convenience, "PTSD"-associated symptoms. Just as we discussed in the section on post-concussive depression and aggression, the genesis of post-concussive "PTSD"-associated symptoms is multifactorial. It is impossible and unnecessary to apportion causality among pre-, and during, and post-morbid factors. Before proceeding, however, one is obliged to address an infamous sophistry.

Several writers have opined that TBI precludes the symptoms of "PTSD" [588–590]. Their argument? TBI is often associated with some amnesia for the event. "PTSD" – according to the mnemonic theory – is due to memories of the event. Those writers ask (in all seriousness): if one cannot recall the blow, how bad could the memory be? If the victim has both retrograde and anterograde amnesia for the event, how can she "experience feelings of fear, helplessness, and horror"? [590]. Superficially, the question seems reasonable. If the essence of "PTSD" is a maladaptive stress response to a perceived and remembered life-threatening stressor, would the problem occur when the trauma is difficult to recall?

Innocent readers may balk at crediting the possibility that editors of peer-reviewed scientific journals would publish such speciousness. They have. One is forced by that embarrassing fact to quickly dispatch this distraction from the serious matter at hand. Dismissing this shallow and unkind position should not absorb more than a moment. Any clinician who treats victims of CBI knows that a trauma includes a period of time far exceeding the millisecond of impact. If an 18-year-old boy from Georgia watches in horror as his platoon comes under attack, runs for his life, trips over the body of a friend and slashes open his arm on the stony road, begins to rise, gets thrown back to the ground and loses consciousness from a blast, regains consciousness to feel blood drip from his scalp into his ear as he listens to screams, smells smoke, then is hustled on to a helicopter, has his clothes snipped off before a crowd of white-clothed strangers in a roasting white tent while needles and tubes are inserted hither and yon, then spends eight weeks in rehabilitation batting flies and trying to recall what those insects are called, he has perhaps been traumatized.

The trauma of TBI is not usefully equated with the blow to the head any more than the trauma of leg amputation by a train is equated with the moment of disconnection. Conscious awareness during the millisecond of impact is not, in any commonsense account, a good discriminator between trauma and not trauma. There is a lot else to remember. Reema may have lost consciousness for a few seconds and truly cannot recall them. Still, she had a bad day. It is traumatic to awaken dangling from one's seatbelt in an inverted sedan on a mountain road, listening to children scream, and seeing blood where one previous saw one's husband.

Common sense aside, the evidence regarding the effect of an amnestic interval on later emotional upset is mixed. Among victims of severe TBIs (not typical concussions), studies that report "PTSD" have sometimes relied on questionnaires to diagnose this condition. Cognitive impairment compromises the validity of such self-report studies and more rigorous studies employing patient interviews have not uniformly reported "PTSD" after severe TBI [590]. On the other hand, in milder cases (CBI without coma or gross intracranial bleeding) the story may be different. Creamer et al. [591], for example, studied the prevalence of "PTSD" among 307 Level 1 trauma admissions. Some had full recall of their brain injuries, others partial recall, and others no recall. Twelve months after injury the rates of "PTSD" were not significantly different between these groups. That is, the completeness of recollection for an event causing a mild TBI does not determine the likelihood of subsequent "PTSD."

The debate has in fact become moot. For clinicians who use the APA's DSM system, the latest edition (number 5) dispenses altogether with the issue of intense fear at the time of the stressor: "Language stipulating an individual's response to the event – intense fear, helplessness or horror, according to DSM-IV – has been deleted because that criterion proved to have no utility in predicting the onset of PTSD" [592, 593]. For the purposes of this chapter one acknowledges that level of awareness at various times before and after a trauma possibly affects the occurrence of persistent symptoms in some way. However, no persuasive evidence settles when or how that might impact "PTSD"-associated symptoms.

That leaves the question open: what happened in Reema's head? Consider the surprise attack by the school bus, her jumbled memories, and her lasting disabilities. Current technology, even autopsy, is inadequate to sort out exactly what is wrong with her brain two years later. No tricorder measures how much of her persistent distress is explained by force-related physiological damage to the circuits that mediate emotion (e.g., due to axon stretch) versus stress-related physiological damage to the circuits that mediate emotion (e.g., due to glucocorticoid toxicity). One can only speculate that a very complex sequence of changes occurred, and – as posited earlier in this chapter – there may have been a reverberant of self-reinforcing phenomenon: First, her brain may have been slightly atypical to begin with due to genes and environment conspiring to make her more than usually vulnerable to stress. Second, external force (having first traversed her hair, scalp skin, galea, skull, dura, and CSF) physically rattled and chemically poisoned cells within and between the circuits of emotions in a neurometabolic/vascular/inflammatory battle between damaging and reparative systems. Third, a stress response kicked in, mediated by biological systems making lazy loops from the adrenal glands to the dorsolateral prefrontal cortex, and interacted with the concussive melee, such that, fourth, the brain she has two years later is the product of all of the above (not to mention the hurt of physical pain and job loss and the mitigating influence of treatment, friends, and family).

The remainder of this chapter, therefore, will attempt to clarify post-concussive "PTSD"-associated distresses. But uppermost in thought remains our certainty that we are not examining a simple matter of cause and effect, like a broken ankle, and our candor in admitting that we are barely able to contemplate the full complexities of change in the heads of our patients.

Detection and Measurement of Post-Concussive Stress-Related Distress Involving the Seven or More Symptoms Associated, Alone or in Combination, With "PTSD," Such as Re-Experiencing and/or Avoidance and/or Negative Affect and/or Anhedonia and/or Externalizing Behaviors and/or Anxious Arousal and/or Dysphoric Arousal

Since the construct called "PTSD" is not unitary, what is caseness and who needs help? Two issues frustrate efforts to detect and measure persistent stress-related distress after concussion. The first is the lack of evidence that this is a discrete disorder. People who meet the APA's criteria for "PTSD" vary tremendously. Some suffer mostly from chronic nervousness, others from hypervigilance, others from depression, others from dissociation, others from withdrawal from social life, others from fear of doing certain things or going certain places, and others from one of literally millions of possible permutations and combination of these symptoms. If the heterogeneity was not clear from the mountain of irreconcilable factor analytic papers, it becomes apparent when biomarkers are sought, for instance, using neuroimaging. Were "PTSD" a specific entity one might legitimately hope for a signature in the CNS. The inconsistencies reported across imaging studies (discussed below) disabuse that hope and helpfully tweak scholars to rethink the construct. Since the construct of PTSD is artificial – arbitrarily including some cases and not others in the approved domain of post-traumatic distress without the support of any biomarker – detection refers to two different duties. Identifying persons meeting APA criteria for "PTSD" is one job. Identifying persons suffering from post-concussive distress, broadly considered, is a different job.

The second issue that frustrates detection is co-morbidity. It has already been mentioned that depression and PTSD present with largely overlapping symptoms. That makes it very challenging (and potentially misleading) to declare with confidence that a given patient suffers from a type of brain change producing just one, just the other, or a mix of symptoms in the domain of the overlap. In the military population especially, persistent post-concussive anxiety seems infrequent as an isolated condition. Instead, such long-term anxiety is frequently accompanied by various degrees of co-morbid cognitive changes [594–597], PCSs [597, 598], depression [274, 599, 600], sleep disturbance [601–604], anger [605, 606], paranoia [607], and pain [608–611], creating a Gordian knot that defies disentangling by the nimblest Linnean.

Still, given the lack of a scientifically valid definition, given the lack of an alternative consensus, one must accept the sour limitations of the current nosology and try to make lemonade.

The three most-cited approaches to detect and measure "PTSD" after concussion are self-report questionnaires, unstructured interviews, and structured clinical interviews. Among the self-report scales the earliest may have been Horowitz's Impact of Event Scale [612–614]. Later came Foa et al.'s Posttraumatic Diagnostic Scale [615] – a 17-item DSM-based instrument available as a self-report questionnaire or interview. Shortly thereafter, Foa et al. [616] published the self-report Posttraumatic Diagnostic Scale. The Stressful Life Events Screening Questionnaire [617] has been employed less commonly; that instrument has a different purpose, screening for life events that might have triggered stress but not diagnosing a disorder. The Neurobehavioral Symptom Inventory, although less narrowly focused on PTSD, has been frequently employed in academic studies of that condition [59, 310, 618–620]. However, by far the most popular screening and diagnostic instrument is the Posttraumatic Checklist (PCL) [621–624]. The PCL was developed at the U.S. National Center for PTSD and is available in several versions, including the Civilian form (PCL-C), the Military form (PCL-M), the "Specific" form, and an abbreviated version [625]. A recent innovation, required due to changes in criteria, is the Posttraumatic Stress Disorder Checklist for DSM-5 (PCL-5) [626, 627].

The gold-standard approach to diagnosis is a structured clinical interview called the Clinician-Administered PTSD Scale (CAPS) [628, 629]; a revision was recently prepared to comport with DSM-5 [630]. However, that instrument has been criticized as an ivory-tower luxury – sensitive, specific, comprehensive, yet far too burdensome on both the patient and the doctor to be of use in the clinic. Foa and Tolin [631] introduced a shorter alternative called the PTSD Symptom Scale – Interview Version. It reportedly offers equally good psychometric qualities in a less burdensome package.

One major reason for the prickly controversy regarding the epidemiology of "PTSD" is the difference in sensitivity and specificity of detection methods. Self-report scales tend to find more disorder. Clinical interviews find less. This discovery arose, in a sense, as an appendix to the argument that TBI victims cannot be stressed due to loss of consciousness. McMillan [632] published a case report describing a 21-year-old man who survived a traffic accident with a TBI. He was diagnosed with PTSD based on questionnaire results. There was no hint of symptom exaggeration. Nonetheless, the overlap between TBI symptoms and PTSD criteria, as well as the subject's confused responses to the self-report questionnaire, were thought to have generated a misdiagnosis. Indeed, Sumpter and McMillan [633, 634] reported that 59% of one cohort could be diagnosed with PTSD based on questionnaire results, while just 2.9% of the same cohort qualified for that diagnosis based on structured clinical interviews. That was a helpful review. But those authors were interested in one subject – how many people develop APA-approved PTSD after TBI? – whereas this chapter is interested in another – how many people develop one or more of the forms of persistent distress considered to belong to the "PTSD" rainbow after concussion? As the next subsection will show, that is unknown.

Epidemiology of Post-Concussive Distress of the Types Associated with "PTSD"

Data across most studies indicate that PTSD is a substantial problem among those with a TBI history…Specific to mTBI, the 3 large US military or veteran studies again had consistent results, reporting probable PTSD in 33–39% of respondents who endorsed have experienced a probable mTBI.

Carlson et al., 2011 [630], p. 111

Setting aside the historical distraction of "PTSD," many people suffer various forms of distress after concussion. How many people? Three issues mandate humility in epidemiology. One: we cannot reliably count APA-approved cases of "PTSD." Published counts based on the CAPS and the PCL have entirely different meanings – both subjective. Rigorous investigators may report a prevalence of 2.9% or 59% in the same group. Any professor who claims to know the incidence or prevalence of "PTSD" after concussion is suffering from pride and prejudice. Pride, because that would be claiming to know the unknowable. Prejudice, because that requires favoring one counting method over another.

Two: if we could count cases of "PTSD," we would not be counting that which matters. A "PTSD" case is one that fulfills an arbitrary diagnostic algorithm that does not seem to identify any unitary disorder. A staggering number of forms of post-traumatic distress meet the criteria. An equally staggering number do not. Thus, even if we overcame the fact that different counting methods lead to equally justifiable numbers more than an order of magnitude apart, perfect counts would only reflect APA-approved persistent misery, not the spectrum of persistent misery observed in humans.

Three: if we are more careful and instead count symptoms (rather than cases of a politically defined syndrome), how would we determine whether each symptom we count is the result of the melee of neurobiological change caused by a forceful bow to the head – a melee that is largely the same in rats and people – or to the human brain's complex and reverberant response to that blow as conditioned by genes, environment, personality, and life circumstances? It would be literally impossible to apportion causality to the first versus the second cause. Both are forks of a false dichotomy.

Please: after reviewing the conventional epidemiology, let us stop counting cases of APA-approved-"PTSD" after concussion. A far more rewarding goal would be determining the incidence and prevalence of what matters: persistent post-concussive distress involving one or more of the many symptoms observed among persons diagnosed with so-called "PTSD."

Having acknowledged that the professional guild-approved diagnostic criteria are shockingly devoid of meaning, and that the hunting and gathering of biomarkers has yet to yield digestible fruit, what is one to make of the available numbers? Carlson et al. [635] published a review of 34 studies of civilian and military TBI and post-traumatic stress. Twenty-four provided epidemiological data regarding the co-morbidity of

TBI and "PTSD." Summarizing that data, those authors stated that, "Frequency of TBI/PTSD ranged from 0% to 70% across all studies" (p. 107). Such a range is not clinically helpful. However, only eight of those 24 studies pertained to mild TBI/concussion [364, 608, 636–643]. Two of those focused on patients requiring hospitalization and do not represent typical CBIs [628, 638]. Two others were confined to burn patients [639, 642]. Considering the remaining four studies:

1. Bryant et al. [637] reported that, "At 6 months post-trauma, PTSD was diagnosed in 20% (N = 9) of MTBI patients."

2. McCauley et al. [364] reported that "11 (12.4%) of the mild TBI group" had PTSD (p. 799).

3. Based on a postal survey of post-deployment subjects, Schneiderman et al. [641] reported that "About 12% of 2,235 respondents reported a history consistent with mild TBI, and 11% screened positive for PTSD." Recalculating the tabulated figures, 39.6% of those with mTBI had PTSD.

4. Hoge et al. [640] surveyed 2525 post-deployment service members and reported that 384 had suspected "mTBIs." Recalculating their data, 32.5% of those with TBI had PTSD. (Contrary to the mnemonic theory of PTSD, the rate was higher among mTBI survivors with loss of consciousness (43.9%) than among those without (27.3%).)

Thus, among the 34 studies in Carlson et al.'s review, four studied relevant populations. None were large studies employing clinical examinations. One credits the authors' effort but cannot have confidence in any of the reported figures.

A more recent review revisited this issue. This shines a brighter Klieg light on the rarity of useful data. Boyle et al. [42] examined 77,914 publications regarding TBI. Sixty-nine full-text papers were reviewed. "[O]nly 3…were found to be at low risk of bias" (p. S232). One of those must be excluded since it focused on burn patients [643]. That brings the total judged worthy of analysis down to two out of 77,914 (0.0026%).

Kennedy et al. [644] studied 130 service members who suffered mTBI secondary to blasts with no other acute injury. Those subjects had an average PCL-C symptom score of 50.14. A common cutoff score for the diagnosis of PTSD is 50 or more [62]. The data, as presented, do not permit determination of the proportion of mTBI subjects with and without PTSD.

The other paper, by Cooper et al. [643], measured PTSD scores among 472 post-deployment service members. A total of 132 (30%) had scores ≤ 30; 232 (49%) had scores between 31 and 59; 108 (22.8%) had PCL-C scores over 60 – at least permitting an estimation of the prevalence of PTSD. Two more studies deserve passing mention: Hill et al. [645] reported that 35% of veterans with mTBI had "PTSD." In a larger study, Kontos et al. [646] reported 28%.

The present author wishes to defend the reader from further data. There is a lot more. It does not get any better. With regard to the epidemiology of "PTSD" among survivors of concussion, 20–35% is a shaky estimate of co-morbidity. That statement comes firmly glued to the disclaimer that counting distress meeting APA criteria for "PTSD" is not a fruitful topic

of study. More useful numbers: what is the frequency of each of the seven or more varieties of persistent post-traumatic distress catalogued in the CFA of "PTSD" after concussion? That has yet to be studied.

A different epidemiological question is: what demographic or other traits predict vulnerability to or diagnosis of post-concussive distress of the types associated with "PTSD"? A large literature reports pre-morbid traits associated with vulnerability to "PTSD" without TBI. Demographic risk factors include female sex, age under 40 (for males), childhood abuse or adversity, prior trauma, prior psychological diagnoses, lower educational achievement, minority status, lower social status, and lack of social supports [647–655]. Personality factors have also been reported, including depression, neuroticism, novelty seeking, trait anger, trait anxiety, disinhibition, and harm avoidance [656–660]. Are these findings relevant to "PTSD" after concussion? That seems to be a reasonable assumption, but it is an assumption. To the best of this author's knowledge, no large study has been published discussing the way that pre-morbid factors specifically influence the risk of persistent "PTSD"-like symptoms after concussion.

Another issue is whether brain injury severity influences the risk of persistent "PTSD"-associated symptoms. Just as in the case of depression, most evidence seems paradoxical: less severe brain injury is associated with a greater risk of persistent "PTSD"-like symptoms. Motzkin and Koenigs [67] reviewed several relevant publications [661–663] and concluded: "Among individuals with documented TBI, there appears to be an inverse relationship between the severity of TBI and the risk of developing PTSD" ([69], p. 637). In fact, some early publications reporting studies of mostly severe TBI asserted that TBI is protective against PTSD [664, 665]. The argument is somewhat similar to the literature claiming that TBI and "PTSD" cannot co-exist because impaired consciousness interferes with establishment of a traumatic memory.

A more biological explanation is supported, to some degree, by a study of penetrating brain injuries. Koenigs et al. [666] specifically found that anterior temporal lobe or medial prefrontal lobe damage reduced the risk. One hypothesis to explain the inverse correlation between injury severity and "PTSD"-associated forms of distress is that conditioned fear requires the integrity of the amygdala and its connections to the ventromedial prefrontal cortex (as well as – though perhaps to a lesser extent – to the hippocampus and anterior cingulate gyrus). That seems entirely plausible.

The present author very tentatively offers an additional explanation. TBI often damages the pituitary gland or stalk. More severe TBI is more likely to produce this effect. This disrupts the hypothalamic–pituitary–adrenal (HPA) axis and causes post-traumatic hypopituitarism in about 27.5% of cases [667–671]. Prolonged stress is mediated by that axis, and the related brain damage (e.g., hippocampal atrophy) may be due to excess production of adrenal glucocorticoids. It seems within the realm of possibility (and would be empirically falsifiable) that traumatic hypopituitarism impairs that process and helps to explain why more severe brain injury is associated with less "PTSD."

We now proceed to summarize the causes and management of that which has no name or number.[47]

Cause(s) of the Various Types of Post-Concussive Distress Associated with "PTSD"

Heritable factors

An exquisitely sensitive question continues to be the role of pre-injury susceptibility to persistent post-concussive emotional distress. Heritable predisposition surely contributes to one's risk of long-term emotional dysfunction, and accumulating evidence suggests that multiple biological pathways are involved. The stress response itself, the many biological impacts of external force, and the interaction between stress and injury are all potentially conditioned by genetic and epigenetic variants. Which variants? Before considering the question of susceptibility genes for "PTSD," one must acknowledge that the project is conceptually misguided and likely doomed. The organizing principal of behavioral genetics is that humans suffer from a number of homogeneous symptoms or distinctive syndromes – behavioral phenotypes. These are mediated by unitary and specific biological abnormalities in the brain – intermediate phenotypes. Those are influenced by genes, epigenes, and gene–epigene–environment interactions. But "PTSD" is a bunch of symptoms. It seems unreasonable to expect that all of them, and every possible combination of them satisfying the APA's criteria, are expressions of a single underlying biological change. Indeed, empirical data strongly suggest that (1) different "PTSD" symptoms are under the influence of different genes, and (2) different "PTSD" symptoms are expressed due to relatively different contributions of heredity and environment. For instance, Wolf et al. [672] reported that the internalizing and externalizing symptoms of "PTSD" have different genetic risk factors and that the heritability of externalizing symptoms is much stronger than that of internalizing symptoms. Be that as it may, and willfully diverting their gaze from the multiplicity of phenotypes, geneticists have pursued "PTSD" susceptibility genes.

One way to find susceptibility genes has been the candidate-gene approach, searching for SNPs or variable number tandem repeat polymorphisms (VNTRs) linked to the diagnosis of "PTSD." Another approach is a GWAS [673, 674]. Such studies tend to inspire more confidence since they are hypothesis-neutral. The present author doubts such work will be very fruitful. One would be surprised if persons satisfying one of "PTSD"'s millions of symptom profiles shared a specific genetic trait.

Still, early twin studies suggested a genetic contribution to the risk of "PTSD" [675, 676]. Other human studies linked stress to alterations in DA function [677, 678]. These two discoveries inspired examination of possible DA-associated gene variation in clinical PTSD. As early as 2002, Segman et al. [679] compared "PTSD" patients with other-trauma survivors. The nine-repeat SLC6A3 3' VNTR polymorphism of the DA transporter gene was found more often among "PTSD" subjects. Since then, multiple studies have used candidate gene research, pursuing the possibility that cerebral DA function influences persistent stress-related distress. Evidence has been reported of links between "PTSD" and variants of the D2 receptor gene [680, 681], the DA transporter gene [682, 683], and – among the most frequently reported associations – with Val158Met polymorphisms of the gene for COMT [684–687]. Some data suggest that these associations are dependent either on race or trauma load.

As many as 20 other gene variants have been reported to influence the risk of PTSD (with or without gene–environment interactions). Most are thought to regulate the physiology of stress. Some mediate serotonin signaling; some are associated with BDNF; many impact the HPA axis. These include: (1) the short allelic variant of SLC64A, the serotonin transporter gene or its promoter, 5-HTTLPR [688–694]; (2) the Val66Met polymorphism of the gene for BDNF [695–697]; and variants of several genes associated with HPA-axis sensitivity, including: (3) the glucocorticoid receptor (GR) gene [701]; (4) the corticotropin-releasing hormone receptor 1 (CRHR1) gene [698, 703]; (5) the FK506-binding protein 5 gene (FKBP5) (which lowers the cortisol-binding affinity of the GR) [698–700]; (6) signal transducer and activator of transcription 5B (STAT5B, an inhibitor of GR) [699, 700]; and (7) ADCYAP1R1 – the gene for the type I receptor of the pituitary adenylate cyclase-activating polypeptide (PAC1) [701–704].

Evidence exists of an intriguing gene–environment interaction: both Binder et al. [706] and Xie et al. [707] found that – although FKBP5 polymorphisms did not, by themselves, correlate with adult PTSD – those polymorphisms combined with a history of childhood abuse or adversity did. Given the genetic evidence that variants in the GR gene increase the risk, it seems plausible that GR and HPA function prior to combat exposure might predict PTSD. Moreover, prior trauma exposure, such as childhood adversity, would be expected to contribute to "PTSD" vulnerability. In other words, consistent with our Haddon matrix, to understand any form of persistent post-concussive distress one needs to know the CBI survivor's genome, life history of trauma, and pre-injury psychological status.

In a conceptually sophisticated study, van Zuiden et al. [710] assessed 448 Dutch soldiers for GR pathway functions, childhood trauma, and PTSD before deployment. Thirty-five soldiers reported more PTSD after deployment. Five

[47] Caveat: virtually none of the research to be cited in the subsections to follow can be trusted to reveal facts about post-concussive distress. The authors admitted that they studied co-morbid "PTSD" and TBI. This is a different subject from "PTSD" *following* TBI. The cohorts probably included many cases of anxiety, or sadness, or jumpiness that predated the visitation of the head by an abrupt external force. Without specifying the temporal sequence, no reason exists to believe that the cited studies describe medical problems caused by, or even coincidentally following, brain injury. Thus, unlike the data regarding post-concussive depression or aggression, little is known about post-concussive troubles like the seven or more beasts in the "PTSD" corral.

461

pre-deployment factors were predictive of membership in that distressed group: (1) more childhood trauma; (2) a higher number of GRs in peripheral blood mononuclear cells; (3) a higher level of expression of glucocorticoid-induced leucine zipper (GILZ, a GR target gene that mediates the anti-inflammatory effects of glucocorticoids); (4) a lower level of expression of FKBP5; and (5) more pre-deployment "PTSD" symptoms. In addition to supporting this chapter's postulate of highly individualized gene, environment, force-related, and stress responsiveness-related multi-determination of concussion outcome, that study hints at the overlooked role of inflammatory/immunomodulatory regulation.

Some evidence also supports associations between "PTSD" and variants of genes for: (1) the GABA receptor gene [709]; (2) the APOE gene [710]; and (3) opioid receptor-like 1 (Oprl1) gene encoding the nociceptin (NOP)/orphanin FQ receptor (NOP-R) [711]. Given the rapidly emerging evidence that psychiatric diseases are linked to immune regulation, it is also intriguing that the ankyrin repeat domain 55 (ANKRD55) protein-coding gene (associated with juvenile arthritis) has been associated with PTSD [712]. This hints at pleiotropy – the influence of a single gene variant on multiple phenotypes.

GWAS have found other potentially influential loci. These include the gene for the RAR-related orphan receptor A (RORA) [673], the RNA gene lincRNA [713], an SNP at chromosome 4p15 near the gene for Tolloid-like 1 (TLL) [674], and a locus near the Cordon-Bleu gene (COBL) [674]. Such findings, candidly, are opaque to interpretation. Yes, the hypothesis-neutral nature of GWAS inspires trust that, unlike candidate gene studies, the findings are not biased by a presumptuous narrowing of the genes examined [714]. But the biological role of these obscure genes in human emotion frustrates intuition. Evidently, we still have a great deal to learn about molecular biology of feelings. Epigenetic variants are also implicated. For instance, in a GWAS, Almli et al. [715] compared combat veterans with and without "PTSD." An SNP called rs717947 seemed to be a risk variant for PTSD, and the number of risk alleles correlated with methylation.[48] This may be the tip of an iceberg of discovery.

The studies reviewed above-investigated genetics and distress, but this chapter's focus is concussion and distress. Very few studies to date have reported gene variants influencing the interaction between TBI and "PTSD." One is Dretsch et al. [717]. In something of a *tour de force* – an act of scholarly chutzpah that considered a model of multi-determination – those authors compiled data on childhood environment, prior trauma, psychological traits, deployment-related stress exposures, and genes among 231 U.S. soldiers. Predictably, many variables, presumably interacting in complex and probably individualized ways, significantly correlated with PCL scores: "being a BDNF Met/Met carrier…sustaining an mTBI… higher levels of combat exposure … and predeployment

traumatic stress … were associated with greater post-PCL-M scores." Still, this collection of risk factors only accounted for 22% of the variance in "PTSD" measures, and most of that – 17% – was due to pre-deployment stress. (A major limitation was that post-deployment data were collected within 30 days, far too soon to test hypotheses regarding persistent distress; follow-up at six to 12 months might have yielded entirely different findings.)

Readers are advised not to memorize the previous several paragraphs. This cornucopia of data may have no more informative value than to credit the hard work of investigators, few of whose discoveries are likely to be replicated or to improve clinical practice. Note that care was rarely taken in any of the reported studies to stratify subsets of "PTSD" patients with comparable symptoms. This undermines the entire enterprise, since the goal is ostensibly a search for behaviorally relevant pieces of human DNA. It remains to be seen, when biologically valid subtypes of stress-related distress are found, whether any of these associations will prove meaningful.

Even if the particulars are untrustworthy, let us assume for the moment that genetic and epigenetic variants influence the risk of PTSD. Genetic variants and pre-morbid psychological traits have both been discussed as risk factors for persistent emotional distress after concussion. What links those two? Ultimately one expects that some intermediate phenotype mediates the effect of genetic variation on both psychological traits and susceptibility to an excessive stress response after TBI [715]. (Of course, the problem with "PTSD" is that one expects at least seven different intermediate phenotypes.) Several findings appear to be relevant. For instance (again, deferring commentary about TBI due to lack of data), evidence suggests that pre-trauma variables in autonomic nervous system or HPA-axis reactivity are associated with an increased risk of PTSD after trauma exposure [718–722]. In a rare prospective study, Orr et al. [723] assessed cognitive and emotional variables and performed two assays of stress reactivity in police and firefighters in training and before trauma exposures: reactivity to startling 95-db tones and fear conditioning to electric shock. Autonomic responses were determined by monitoring heart rate, skin conductance, and facial electromyography. Three factors together predicted the likelihood of developing "PTSD" symptoms after trauma exposure: lower IQ, higher pre-trauma depression scores, and larger facial electromyography responses to psychophysiological stressors. (Genes were not analyzed.) These latter findings may or may not predict post-concussive distress. However, they are consistent with the model proposed throughout this chapter: concussion changes brains, no two of which began with the same baseline, no two of which exhibit the same acute post-concussive changes, and no two of which exhibit the same short- and long-term emotional outcomes.

A recent innovation might help. Neuroimaging is generating intriguing pictures of those mysterious physiological

---

48 This may be the tip of an iceberg of forthcoming discovery. Raabe and Spengler [716] review some of the recent animal literature and comment that, as the impact of childhood adversity on chromatin regulation of DNA expression is investigated, epigenetic mechanisms may prove to be central to the occurrence of persistent anxiety.

Dorsomedial (dm) and dorsolateral (dl) prefrontal cortex (PFC) differentially respond to fearful faces as a function of genotype

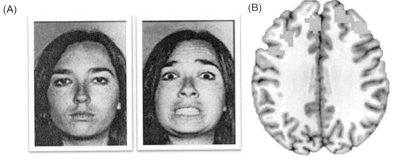

(A)

(B)

33

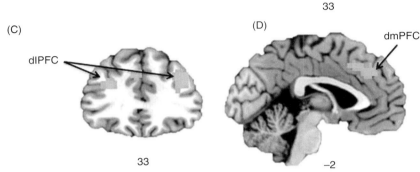

(C)

dlPFC

33

(D)

dmPFC

-2

Fig. 10.7 (A) Example of neutral and fearful face stimuli. (B) Axial section showing medial and lateral prefrontal signal associated with genotype. (C) Dorsolateral and (D) dorsomedial regions surviving whole-brain correction. [A black and white version of this figure will appear in some formats. For the color version, please refer to the plate section.]

Source: Almli et al., 2014 [715] with permission from John Wiley & Sons

effects [724]. That does not show us the steps in the patho-physiological dance, but at least reveals where the feet are.[49] For example, Almli et al. [715] used fMRI determine whether persons with and without a PTSD-associated SNP exhibited different regional activation in response to fear-related stimuli. Figure 10.7 depicts their results. After whole-brain correction, regions within the dorsolateral and dorsomedial prefrontal cortices showed relatively greater oxygenated blood flow among subjects carrying the putative risk allele.[50]

The conundrum for scholars of geno-distress is the inconsistency of results. For example, exactly contrary to other reports, Thakur et al. [725] found that the short allele of the 5-HTTLPR polymorphism was *protective* against PTSD. Also at odds with other claims, Wang's 2015 meta-analysis [726] found no relationship at all between any BDNF Val66Met variant and susceptibility to PTSD. And, in the recently reported New Soldier Study – the largest ever GWAS, which compared 3167 PTSD subjects to 4607 trauma controls – while some evidence emerged of a genetic link between heritable risk for auto-immune disease and PTSD, there was virtually no evidence of association with *any* genetic polymorphism [712].

In summary regarding genes: the author would bet his house – if he had one – that multiple heritable variations combined with multiple developmental influences will prove to significantly condition the risk of the multiple persistent

types of distress observed after concussion and collectively called "PTSD." He does not expect that the correct interactions of genetic, epistatic, epigenetic, pleiotropic, and environmental factors will be discovered in his lifetime. Still, glimmers of hope have flickered: imaging will some day reveal the most-altered circuitry of long-term post-concussive misery, and GWAS combined with rigorous RCTs testing the efficacy of one treatment for one of the multiple distress symptoms will begin to inform management soon.

Neurocircuits

a reasonable estimate is that disruption in neural circuitry of comorbid PTSD/TBI likely involves constituent elements observed within singular diagnosis of PTSD and TBI individually. The most consistent and replicated findings common to both of these populations are anatomical alterations in the vmPFC [ventromedial prefrontal circuit]/sgACC [subgenual anterior cingulate cortex] and amygdalar/hippocampal complex.

Depue et al., 2014 [727], p. 2

Whether the patient's dominant distress is anxiety or numbing or dissociation, tendency to startle or tendency to dream unhappily, whether one calls it "PTSD," "the mis'ries," or existential funk, we know that some concussion survivors

---

49 Readers will soon encounter a helpful schematic illustrating parts of the brain implicated in the regulation of the stress response (Figure 10.8). Referring to that figure may assist in interpreting Figure 10.7.

50 As cautioned in this chapter multiple technical factors bar confidence in today's fMRI results. The main value of such work is to hint at the riches to come when the meaning of differences in functional scans is better understood.

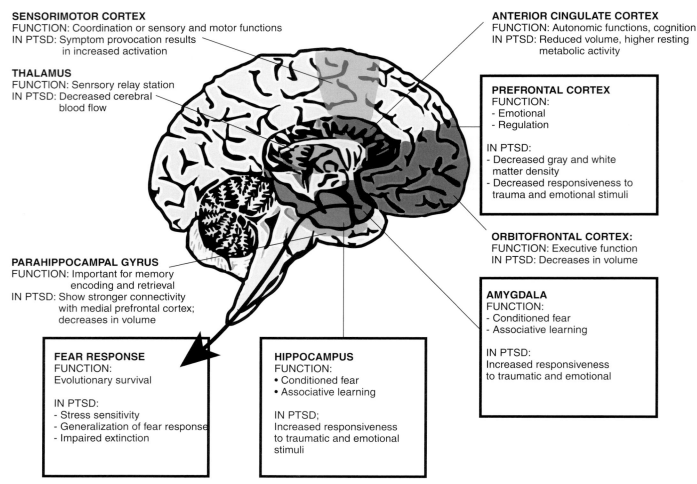

SENSORIMOTOR CORTEX
FUNCTION: Coordination or sensory and motor functions
IN PTSD: Symptom provocation results in increased activation

THALAMUS
FUNCTION: Senrsory relay station
IN PTSD: Decreased cerebral blood flow

PARAHIPPOCAMPAL GYRUS
FUNCTION: Important for memory encoding and retrieval
IN PTSD: Show stronger connectivity with medial prefrontal cortex; decreases in volume

ANTERIOR CINGULATE CORTEX
FUNCTION: Autonomic functions, cognition
IN PTSD: Reduced volume, higher resting metabolic activity

PREFRONTAL CORTEX
FUNCTION:
- Emotional
- Regulation

IN PTSD:
- Decreased gray and white matter density
- Decreased responsiveness to trauma and emotional stimuli

ORBITOFRONTAL CORTEX:
FUNCTION: Executive function
IN PTSD: Decreases in volume

AMYGDALA
FUNCTION:
- Conditioned fear
- Associative learning

IN PTSD:
Increased responsiveness to traumatic and emotional

FEAR RESPONSE
FUNCTION:
Evolutionary survival

IN PTSD:
- Stress sensitivity
- Generalization of fear response
- Impaired extinction

HIPPOCAMPUS
FUNCTION:
• Conditioned fear
• Associative learning

IN PTSD;
Increased responsiveness to traumatic and emotional stimuli

Fig. 10.8 Neuroanatomical regions thought relevant to post-traumatic stress disorder (PTSD)-associated symptoms.
Source: Lebois et al., 2016 [724] with permission from Elsevier

suffer. A concussion rattles every cell in the brain. Which of those rattlings explains the "PTSD"-associated varieties of persistent distress? One must eschew the Swiss Watch Fallacy – the notion that a particular brain part is dedicated to a particular behavior (which jewel makes your watch say 2 o'clock?) Yet different bits and pieces of the head make different contributions to emotion. The deep and presently unanswerable question is how to apportion causality. Is persistent post-concussive distress solely due to brain rattling? Solely due to a physiological stress response? Or – as the author posits – due to both? Please let us shelve that debate and focus on the answerable. What brain parts dysfunction when distress goes on and on?

Long before the invention of "PTSD," Broca (1878 [728]), Bard (1928 [729]), Selye (1936 [543]), Papez (1937 [730]), MacLean (1949 [731]), and others pointed to "*le grand lobe limbique*" and perilimbic regions, including the extended amygdala, anterior cingulate gyrus, ventromedial prefrontal cortex, insula, precuneus, and hypothalamus as centers of emotional processing [732]. On the one hand, since post-traumatic distress is emotional, one would expect some changes in one or more of these regions. On the other hand, since the symptoms

of "PTSD" are diverse, one would not expect any two structural or functional neuroimaging studies to report the same findings unless they imaged genetically matched victims with the same symptom profiles. This concern reduces optimism that even perfect imaging will ever reveal the important intermediate phenotypes. The principal value in reviewing the scanning data is perhaps to confirm that, however variable the behavioral phenomena, emotional circuitry is involved. Hence the quest for the intermediate phenotypes by comparing scans of persons with and without a dubious diagnosis.

Figure 10.8 illustrates some of the regions thought relevant to the "PTSD"-associated symptom clusters. That figure is a pastiche created by synthesizing the results of numerous studies. Structural imaging has, for more than a decade, provided evidence that "PTSD" causes hippocampal atrophy [733–735]. Other studies have reported atrophy in the insula [736, 737], amygdala [735], and anterior cingulate gyrus [735]. The evidence is not entirely consistent, and seems to depend on age, gender, and the type and severity of the trauma – not to mention imaging methodology.

Functional imaging of "PTSD" is a horse of a different color. As mentioned periodically in this chapter, fMRI is not a reliable technique, especially when investigators average results from a group. One is not surprised, therefore, to encounter confusing and sometimes grossly inconsistent results, with the location, degree, laterality, and direction of change of activity varying in almost every report. Generally speaking, the stimuli or tasks imposed on subjects during scanning were either symptom provocation or cognitive challenge. (Please brace yourself and do not become attached to any one report.)

Regarding Provocation Protocols

The early studies employed positron emission tomography (PET) scanning during script-driven imagery. Shin et al. [738] reported increased activity in the orbitofrontal cortex and temporal poles and relatively less increase in anterior cingulate cortex activity compared to controls. Pissiota et al. [739] reported increased activity in the right sensorimotor region, right amygdala, and periaqueductal gray. Britton et al. [740] reported deceased activity in the amygdala and anterior cingulate cortex. More recent studies have used fMRI. Lanius et al. [741] reported that script-driven imagery was associated with subnormal activity in the thalamus and anterior cingulate cortex. Lanius et al. [742] also tested for functional connectivity, seeking simultaneous, correlated changes in linked regions. Symptom provocation led to relatively increased co-variation between the ventrolateral thalamus and the right insula, left parietal lobe, right frontal region, superior temporal gyrus, and right cuneus. Hou et al. [743] compared "PTSD" subjects with healthy controls. On symptom provocation, "PTSD" subjects exhibited relatively decreased right anterior cingulate cortex activity and increased left parahippocampal activity. Morey et al. [744] reported that symptom provocation caused increased activity in the ventral frontolimbic regions, the inferior frontal gyrus, and the anterior cingulate cortex. Mazza et al. [745] reported that affective priming caused supernormal activity in the right insula and left amygdala.

Lanius et al. [746] candidly addressed the inconsistencies among these symptom provocation results. Their conclusion is the same as the present author's: "Grouping all PTSD subjects, regardless of their different symptom patterns, in the same diagnostic category may interfere with our understanding of posttrauma psychopathology" (p. 709).

Regarding the Cognitive Challenge Protocols

Hou et al. [743] reported that a recall task yielded decreased right parahippocampal activity. Chen et al. [737] reported that a recall task produced decreased insular activity. Morey et al. [744] reported that an executive task yielded subnormal activity in the anterior cingulate cortex and middle frontal gyrus. Werner et al.'s [747] memory task triggered increased hippocampal and decreased prefrontal activity. Geuze et al.'s [748] task (retrieval phase) was associated with subnormal activity of the right frontal cortex but supernormal activity of the bilateral middle temporal gyri and left posterior hippocampus/parahippocampal gyri.

The point is not that there is no consistency but that there is a potpourri of findings. Individual hills and valleys might be explained, but no coherent pathophysiological landscape

emerges. Still, students of concussion have surely noted whispers of concordance: as previously explained in this chapter, certain brain parts are disproportionately vulnerable to TBI. Several of the same brain parts tend to be abnormal in "PTSD." That both helps to explain the overlap in symptoms and hints at the possibility that a blow to the head – with or without a psychological collapse – might alter the brain in such a way to generate "PTSD"-associated symptoms.

This chapter has long since reviewed the neuroanatomy of CBI. We have just reviewed the neuroanatomy of "PTSD." Now, what might be said of the neuroanatomy of co-morbid TBI and "PTSD?" It seems plausible that the regions discussed in those separate sections are likely to be involved. Some empirical findings confirm that impression. More meaningfully, the fact that the same brain parts dysfunction in concussion and "PTSD," considered independently, somewhat supports the conclusion – exactly contrary to the dogma of the concussion deniers – that CBI may cause persistent distresses of the type called "PTSD."

Imaging of Post-Concussive Distress of the Types Associated with "PTSD"

> Much of the gossip going back and forth in this area is what we have commonly come to associate with the id, the beast, or sin in man (e.g. gluttony, lechery, etc.). In the light of this it is interesting that through the large uncinate fasciculus, the frontal lobes "stand guard" over this region.
> MacLean, 1949 ([731], p. 347)

Concussion is not post-concussive distress or stress-related distress of the seven or more kinds derived from recent factor analyses of "PTSD." Neither animal studies of "PTSD" nor human neuroimaging studies of "PTSD" are credible, since animals do not fulfill APA criteria and human studies lump together subjects with the grossly different clinical presentations fulfilling APA criteria. The brain does not have a post-concussive multifactorial distress lobe. Yet, if one is tolerant of diagnostic laxity, structural and functional neuroimaging studies support the conclusion that several anatomical regions are consistently affected in both conditions:

- Concussion causes atrophy or dysfunction of the hippocampus in humans [749–753] and PTSD causes hippocampal atrophy or dysfunction in humans [735, 754–759].
- Concussion causes atrophy or dysfunction of the cingulate gyrus in humans [752, 758–761] and PTSD causes atrophy or dysfunction of the cingulate gyrus in humans [762–768].

Caveats abandoned, these imaging data may be interpreted as supporting a potent hypothesis that seemingly settles forever one of the most contentious issues in the history of neuropsychiatry: since concussion by itself produces brain changes highly similar to those repeatedly associated with "PTSD," concussion by itself – without stress or pre-morbid vulnerability to stress – may cause "PTSD"!

On closer inspection of the data, that conclusion is simplistic. "Highly similar" is not "the same." Most imaging studies, even those using advanced technology, only point to vast swaths of cells. They do not consider the cell types affected (for instance, implicating the hippocampus without exploring separate effects on dentate hilus versus cornu ammonis cells), the effect on multi-lobar cortical–subcortical circuits, or, in the case of functional abnormalities, the direction of change in activity from normal. Such considerations are crucial to discussing pathophysiology, rather than replicating the logical errors of 19th-century behavioral neurology and 20th-century neuropsychology. Recent scanning studies therefore must be viewed, respectfully, with reserved enthusiasm.

Structural studies, such as those cited above in the literature on hippocampal and cingulate change, have yielded diverse results. Although it is not possible to apportion the cause of symptoms to TBI versus "PTSD," one can at least compare the amount of brain left in the head of groups with "PTSD" alone versus co-morbid TBI/"PTSD." One review concluded that PTSD causes atrophy, but that CBI has negligible additional impact on brain structure [769]. In contrast, Lindemer et al. [770] studied persons with co-morbid TBI and "PTSD" and found MRI evidence of an interaction: more severe PTSD was associated with frontal cortical atrophy among those with histories of concussion.

Other studies also imaged the structure of co-morbid cases, although it is hard to find two with similar results. Depue et al. [727] employed voxel-based morphometry to analyze MRIs in veterans with both diagnoses. The anterior amygdala was smaller than that of healthy controls, but the relative roles of each diagnosis were not investigated. Davenport et al. [771] employed DTI to scan veterans with PTSD or TBI. Those with PTSD showed increased FA in some regions while (contrary to most other studies) those with TBI did not exhibit FA changes. Isaac et al. [159] scanned triply affected veterans with co-morbid PTSD, TBI, and depression. FA was reduced in two critical fiber bundles: the uncinate fasciculus (thought to coordinate ventromedial prefrontal lobe and limbic response) and cingulum (a bundle with many functions pertaining to assessment of circumstances and coordination of planning) (Figure 10.9). Those results are compatible with the theory of Jorge et al. [161] (mentioned in the section on depression): post-concussive distress may involve damage that simultaneously disrupts emotional reactivity and emotional regulation.

Paul MacLean's 1949 comment on sin and lechery [731], quoted above, reminds us that the uncinate fasciculus has long been thought to police the interplay between the emotional limbic system and the deliberative prefrontal cortex. Jorge's

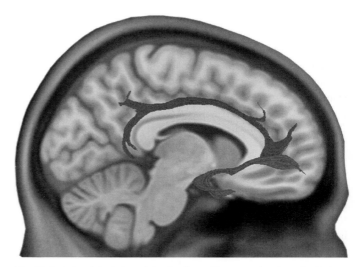

Fig. 10.9 A visual depiction of the significant fiber tracts (uncinate fasciculus (purple) and cingulum (blue)) taken from a male participant in the depression – post-traumatic stress disorder–traumatic brain injury group. [A black and white version of this figure will appear in some formats. For the color version, please refer to the plate section.]

Source: Isaac et al., 2015 [159] with permission from Elsevier

theory and Isaac et al.'s findings extend that narrative; harming the uncinate fasciculus seems to be one mechanism by which CBI could cause "PTSD"-like distress. One team has taken that speculation a step further. Williamson et al. [772] noted that TBI often damages white-matter pathways, including the anterior limb of the internal capsule and the uncinate fasciculus. Those pathways, they suggest, participate in autonomic regulation. This damage hypothetically links concussion with the autonomic dysregulation apparent in many persons diagnosed with "PTSD."[51]

Yeh et al. [777] also employed DTI and focused on fiber tracking in 24 service members with mostly mild brain injuries who had completed a self-report measure of "PTSD." The scans identified diffusion anisotropy deficits. One of the circuits linked by fiber bundles was called a "cortico-striatal-thalamic-cerebellar-cortical (CSTCC) network." Soldiers with more PTSD symptoms showed reduced FA in the nodes of that network. Those authors summarize: "the compromised integrity of white matter fiber connection of this study can be the combination of comorbid PTSD and TBI" (p. 2667). Readers may share the present author's impression that this generalization may be true, but is confusing. How does this extremely complex pattern of changes distributed across essentially the entire subcortex mediate dysphoric arousal?[52]

---

[51] The present author speculates that forceful damage in concussion can trigger "PTSD"-like changes in emotional and somatic reactivity by disrupting axoplasmic flow in other white-matter tracts, the role of which has yet to be identified because they are hard to see with current methods. That is, MacLean and Williamson were referring to the conversation between the limbic tissue of the medial temporal lobe, including the amygdala and hippocampus, and upstream organs of deliberation: the cortex, including prefrontal and precuneus. That limbic tissue also influences downstream organs: corticomedial and basolateral amygdala help regulate both the HPA axis and the sympathetic nervous system via projections within the shorter ventral amygdalofugal pathway and the longer stria terminalis to the medial and lateral hypothalamus and to the rostral nucleus of the solitary tract [773–776]. The author guesses that stretching of those tracts during CBI contributes to some "PTSD"-associated symptoms of post-concussive distress.

[52] A general comment on the perils of progress. A previous generation of structural brain scanners would typically show one or two focal abnormalities – often vascular changes such as bleeds or strokes. A previous generation of behavioral neurologists might see one abnormality in

Functional neuroimaging of TBI/"PTSD" comes closer to exploring pathophysiology. It also illustrated the importance of the crucial admonition stated above: to say that both "PTSD" and concussion affect the same tissue is not informative unless one takes into account the *direction of change in activity*. For example, Simmons and Matthews [778] reported a meta-analysis of fMRI studies seeking overlaps between the effects of TBI and PTSD. Activity was found to be altered in the middle frontal gyrus in both conditions. "However, the differences in middle frontal gyrus activation between PTSD and mTBI individuals appear to be in *opposite directions* (i.e., more activation in PTSD and less activation in mTBI individuals relative to controls) [emphasis added]" (p. 602).

Although Simmons and Matthews were disinclined to believe their own results, attributing them to methodological differences, similar findings were obtained in a very large single-photon emission computed tomography (SPECT) study. Amen et al. [779] studied a multisite cohort in which 11,147 subjects were diagnosed with neither TBI nor PTSD, 7505 diagnosed with TBI (mostly "mild"), 1077 with PTSD, and 1017 with both PTSD and TBI. SPECT imaging was performed in both resting and cognitively activated conditions. If replicated with higher-resolution technology, the findings may be quite illuminating. In essence, PTSD seemed to add activity while TBI took it away: both at rest and with stimulation, the hippocampus, amygdala, cingulum, insula, thalamus, basal ganglia, prefrontal and temporal cortices, and cerebellum all exhibited *hyperactivity* in PTSD subjects and *hypoactivity* in TBI subjects.[53]

In summary, both structural and functional imaging of comorbid cases yield inconsistent results. One cannot infer a particular pattern of cell loss or circuit dysfunction. In light of the many variables in both conditions, and the fact that the functional impact may be exactly opposite, this is no surprise. With misgivings, one can tentatively conclude that survivors of concussion with persistent distress tend to have altered prefrontal-limbic circuits, compromising the capacity to tolerate the combination of emotional insults and physical injury.

Neurobiology

Another tactic for determining the biological bases of persistent post-concussive distress is neurobiology or neurophysiology. Two factors limit the number and value of available publications. First, the animal models of "PTSD" are primitive. Foot shock followed by nervousness when dropped into a maze is not persuasively akin to the broad spectrum of human "PTSD."[54] Second, recall the forbidding caveat above? Almost

no investigators of co-morbid human TBI and "PTSD" have reported their data in a way that permits one to isolate post-concussion: the subset of cases in which the head was rattled first and the upset came later. The following reports at least touch upon possible mechanisms.

In a rare experiment to examine how TBI alters the stress response, Reger et al. [781] first concussed rats and then trained them in a fear-conditioning procedure. Concussion not only increased fear conditioning but also caused overgeneralization of the fear response. Like many animal models of "mild" TBI, there was no cell loss. Yet N-methyl-D-aspartate (NMDA) receptor activity was increased in the basolateral amygdala, suggesting a possibly molecular mediator of the behavioral change.

A human experiment confirms the role of the cingulate region in comorbid TBI/"PTSD": Shu et al. [782] compared evoked potentials in combat veterans with TBI, some of whom also had "PTSD." The Stop Task was performed – a test of inhibitory control. Among the concussed veterans, larger evoked responses when attempting to inhibit their reactions correlated with "PTSD" symptoms. This might be evidence that emotional self-control is more effortful for distressed concussion survivors.

Inflammation, as noted throughout this chapter, is an important pathophysiological factor determining the outcome from CBI, and sleep disorder is an important form of distress associated with both TBI and "PTSD." Barr et al. [602] studied a post-deployment cohort. Among subjects with TBI whose sleep was restored, "PTSD" symptoms were reduced. Of interest, that benefit depended on C-reactive protein levels. In other words, *inflammation may have interfered with the benefit of sleep on PTSD symptoms among concussed veterans*. That (in the present author's opinion) is a rather convoluted observation. Yet attention to the poorly studied role of inflammation is welcome.

Management of Post-Concussive "PTSD"-Associated Symptoms

Some readers will soon find themselves in a clinic in Peru, sitting across from a concussion survivor named Mr. Gage who survived a stagecoach crash (losing his favorite horse) and who presents with one or more of the many symptoms (or clusters of symptoms) that qualify a subset of trauma victims for the "PTSD" label. It is not important whether Mr. Gage meets APA "PTSD" criteria. One cannot trust any empirical literature that claims "this intervention helps people with PTSD" unless the

---

one place thought to have a certain function, and infer the effect on behavior. Advanced imaging now typically depicts multifocal damage – pixelated patchworks of dysfunctional tissue dispersed through the brain. One can name the ten places with the most profound changes. But localization theories that guided interpretation of focal injuries for a century are almost helpless in the face of such pointillist portraits. The paper of Yeh et al. [777] instantiates the revelations of the near future: we will discover much more sophisticated maps, and have much less ability to make head or tail of them.

[53] Interpretation of this study is unclear. Although those authors state that the TBI regions were "hypoactive," the readers will wonder, "hypoactive compared to what?" The report fails to provide data comparing TBI subjects with healthy controls.

[54] "In humans, the diagnosis of PTSD is made only if an individual exhibits a certain number of symptoms…Animal behavioral studies, however, have generally tended to overlook this aspect" [780].

investigators specify which of the seven or more types of post-stress distress were significantly reduced after treatment in a controlled trial. Moreover, no high-quality RCTs have been published reporting efficacy of treatments for any "PTSD"-associated symptoms following concussion, and none of the "PTSD" treatment studies that mention TBI co-morbidity in passing have stratified those cases by the characteristics of the brain injury.[55] It is only important that Mr. Gage is injured, distressed, and your responsibility. What should you do?

Evidence from the 1995 National Comorbidity Survey [783] supported the conclusion that more than one-third of those meeting diagnostic criteria for "PTSD" had persistent symptoms, often lasting for many years, with or without treatment. Those findings, of course, are confounded by the method of case ascertainment and by the limited RCT research published at that time. Increasing public attention to the diagnosis after the publication of DSM-III and, more recently, pressure due to a relative explosion of cases related to Operations Iraqi Freedom and Enduring Freedom stimulated a substantive increase in the size and rigor of management studies. It remains largely unknown whether any treatment shown to mitigate "PTSD" is more, less, or equally effective when the emotional problem seems to have been caused by a concussion.

Still, the peer-reviewed publications reporting RCTs of interventions for "PTSD" alone (without TBI) amount to the main source of guidance. As Capehart and Bass [784] put it:

> Managing comorbid PTSD and TBI remains a challenge for DOD and VA clinicians in mental health, TBI/polytrauma, and primary care because no clear guidance exists on the simultaneous management of these two conditions… As a general rule, neuropsychiatric conditions that appear after TBI are managed similarly to the corresponding idiopathic Axis I condition. …Management of comorbid PTSD and TBI generally should follow the VA/DOD CPG [clinical practice guideline] for each condition.

And what do those VA/DOD guidelines recommend? "Clinicians should not get caught up in debating causation but maintain focus on identifying and treating the symptoms that are contributing to the most impairment" ([598], p. 88). That is, setting aside Mr. Gage's history of concussion, if he is suffering from dysphoric arousal, or having bad dreams about his horse, maybe a "PTSD" treatment will help. Having warned the reader to be wary of the literature that claims to report mitigation

of "PTSD," rather than specific symptoms, the author will review it.

Non-pharmacological treatment options include psychotherapies, behavioral manipulations, and meditation. As always, the present author encourages trials of talking with compassionate professionals – psychotherapy not otherwise specified. Some reviews simply declare that psychotherapy helps persons with "PTSD" [601]. That superficially supports the position that any talk helps more than no talk. However, Capehart and Bass [784] deserve credit for their excellent review emphasizing therapeutic alliance. Evidence from multiple sources supports the view that the quality of the psychotherapy – the patient's confidence that he or she is being cared for – best predicts success [785–787]. Therefore, rather than debating the relative efficacy of one talking treatment versus another, what matters most may be making a human connection.[56]

In the 1980s a treatment called "critical incident stress debriefing" was touted as effective. The advocates of that intervention posited, in essence, that enforced preoccupation with recalling the worst of a painful event cured preoccupation with recalling the worst of a painful event [791]. Empirical work demonstrated that critical incident stress debriefing was not only ineffective but potentially harmful [792–797]. Other early approaches to "PTSD" included multidisciplinary inpatient rehabilitation involving intensive group and individual therapy, behavior manipulations, family counseling, and vocational counseling. In at least one study, that approach was found to have no lasting benefit [798].

Readers might intuit, on theoretical grounds, that it will be challenging to find a single effective "PTSD" treatment: a cohort of distressed persons with heterogeneous and even contradictory symptoms would not, generally speaking, be expected to respond to the same intervention. Still, some psychotherapies seem to help. CBT [451, 799, 800], cognitive processing therapy [801, 802], and prolonged exposure therapy [803–805] have all been reported to show efficacy for "PTSD" [598, 806–808]. The question becomes: "Do these forms of talk therapy also help concussion survivors with "PTSD"-associated symptoms?"

A Cochrane Review [809] examined the evidence that psychotherapy might reduce anxiety in survivors of TBI, considering 23 published trials. Only two small studies were properly randomized and analyzed. One study reported the effects of CBT in mTBI survivors with acute stress reactions

---

[55] For clarification: some day perhaps intermediate phenotypes will be discovered (although the growing awareness of the individuality of disease suggests that the very idea of a disease phenotype may be biologically simplistic). Each of these will be shown to mediate a different symptom, such as post-stress dysphoric arousal, post-stress social withdrawal, or post-stress episodic dissociation. Each will be differently influenced by genes, childhood adversity, age, gender, and perhaps heart rate variability, inflammatory markers, and cortisol receptor occupancy. Each will interact differently with concussion, and that interaction will further vary depending on the individually unique, infinitely diverse characteristics of the post-concussive neurometabolic, inflammatory, vascular, apoptotic, neurogenesis melee. The reader may have, on his or her desk, a print-out of 1000 relevant measures for Mr. Gage. If a study from the early 21st century reported "Clonidine is good for TBI and PTSD" – based on a study that ignored both the subject's main symptoms and every one of those variables – should you prescribe clonidine?

[56] Empirical research on psychotherapy will be hamstrung until ecologically valid placebo treatments and credible markers of lasting efficacy are employed. Therapeutic alliance seems to be a critical variable, yet almost no published studies control for this variable. Some day, science

within two weeks of trauma [810]. The prevalence of PTSD was lower at six months, possibly suggesting a prophylactic effect (but not supporting a benefit for persistent post-concussive anxiety). The other study [811] reported that 11 weeks of CBT combined with "cognitive remediation" reduced anxiety symptoms among survivors of mild to moderate TBI on average about five to six years after injury. This very small study is arguably the best evidence of the efficacy of psychotherapy for persistent post-concussive anxiety.

Chard et al. [812] conduced an uncontrolled observation of 42 TBI/"PTSD" subjects and reported that residential treatment combining cognitive processing therapy with psycho-education helped. More recently, Walter et al. [813] compared two versions of cognitive processing therapy (with and without obliging patients to generate a written account of their trauma) among 86 veterans with TBI/"PTSD." Symptoms declined with time in both treatment groups, with no discernible difference. Since there was no control group, treatment efficacy cannot be assessed.

Sripada et al. [814] conducted an uncontrolled trial of prolonged exposure therapy for veterans with "PTSD," some of whom also had TBI. Brain injury did not influence efficacy (which again cannot be determined since there was no control group). Wolf et al. [815] conducted a retrospective chart review of prolonged exposure therapy for subjects with "PTSD" and mild to severe TBI. The emotional symptoms decreased with time. One case report [816] suggested a possible benefit from transcendental meditation.[57]

Understanding that limited data support the use of psychotherapy for co-morbid TBI/"PTSD," and that even less data support its use for circumstances that are the focus of this chapter – when PTSD-associated symptoms follow and are causally attributed to TBI – the approach promoted by the VA/ DoD in their 2010 guidelines [817] nonetheless seems practical. Treat the PTSD symptoms as best you can with evidence-based therapies. The therapies they call "evidence-based" include CBT, cognitive processing therapy, prolonged exposure therapy, stress inoculation training, and eye movement desensitization and reprocessing (EMDR). Those guidelines specifically advise: "There is no evidence to support withholding PTSD treatments while addressing post-concussive symptoms" (p. 88).

Eye Movement Desensitization and Reprocessing

EMDR perhaps deserves special consideration. Since the late 1990s, randomized studies conducted in both military and civilian settings have reported that EMDR is efficacious for reducing the symptoms of "PTSD." This method consists of a combination of psychotherapy – including talking about the traumatic event and assessing the validity of one's cognitions about the event – with sensory stimulation – typically watching the therapist's finger move from side to side [818–820].[58] The patient is asked to focus attention on a traumatic memory while finger watching, and then "restructure" or "reintegrate" his or her memory.[59] Readers may share the present author's uncertainty about the added value of finger watching. Indeed, although the 2010 VA/DoD guidelines mention the potential value of EMDR, they remark: "Alternating eye-movements are part of the classic EMDR technique… however, comparable effect sizes have been achieved with or without eye movements" (p. 117).

Multiple theories have been published attempting to explain that added value. Shapiro [818] posited that finger watching or some other form of "alternating bilateral stimulation" boosts emotional processing.[60] "It is thought that the bilateral stimulation as a specific element of EMDR facilitates accessing and

---

[ ] might facilitate neurobiological screening to predict psychotherapeutic response [788]. (Might one estimate the quality of therapeutic alliances by monitoring mirror neurons [789, 790]?) For this reason, the author respectfully rejects almost all of the published efficacy literature. To say "psychotherapy works" without controlling for therapeutic alliance is like saying "marriage works" without controlling for assortative mating.

[57] The VA/DoD guidelines [817] state: "Supportive counseling for PTSD has received little study to date and cannot be endorsed as an evidence-based psychotherapeutic strategy. However, it has been shown to be effective compared with no treatment and may be the sole psychotherapeutic option available for the patient with PTSD who is reluctant to seek specialty mental healthcare." The present author would counter that patients with PTSD after concussion may be eager, cooperative, even desperate to comply with referral to evidence-based therapies. Health care funding priorities may be a more formidable barrier than patient reluctance.

[58] The eye movements allegedly provoked by finger watching are called, in the EMDR literature, "saccadic" or "slow saccadic" movements [821]. They are not. An entirely different cerebral mechanism animates following a moving target – called smooth pursuit. Saccadic movement (a sudden jump that involves a momentary loss of vision) does not occur when tracking a moving object with smooth pursuit.

[59] Finger watching is labeled "bilateral stimulation" in the EMDR literature. The phrase is misused. If one follows a target with one's eyes, it remains, like a bull's eye, at the center of vision. It is neurologically nonsensical to call a central stimulus "bilateral." Even more semantically grievous is the phrase "alternating bilateral stimulation." When one is watching something move from side to side, brain stimulation does not "alternate." The image remains fixed in central vision. EMDR promoters emphasize that their intervention works because the patient is instructed to focus on a bilateral sensory stimulus. If the patient is sitting quietly during the therapy, he or she is in fact constantly inundated with bilateral sensory stimuli. The therapist's finger is not such a stimulus. But the patient's buttocks are.

[60] Again, the author confesses a lack of confidence. This use of the phrase "emotional processing" sounds suspiciously like the Freudian analyst's concept of "working through" infantile sexual conflicts. Neurological evidence suggests that one is constantly "processing" emotional information and data, while awake or asleep. The widely distributed brain circuitry thought most relevant to emotion exhibits blood flow and glucose metabolism constantly from early fetal life to death. Increasing the quantity of such metabolism occurs, for instance, during upsetting or exciting events and while ruminating about such events. Encouragement by a caring doctor to either remember stress or see the bright side of life does indeed sound like a stimulus that could enhance limbic blood flow. But a moving-finger stimulus does not represent a plausible mechanism for enhancing that blood flow or for "reintegrating," "reconstructing," or "reprocessing" memories. What, in any case, would "memory

processing of negative stimuli while presumably creating new associative links" [824]. Other psychologists have discussed how finger watching boosts attention to "disintegrated information" [825, 826]. Such theories may not comport with the neurobiology of mammalian emotion, but – as Hippocrates asserted – what works is good. The present author fully supports evidence-based interventions, and EMDR seems to help. He asks, however, that we try to figure out the scientific basis for efficacy, lest we derail the progress toward rational medicine. Therefore, it is important to separate analysis of efficacy from analysis of the reasons for efficacy. Let us consider those two issues in sequence.

Early efficacy rates for EMDR were reported in the range of 77–90% [827–832]. There followed a period of controversy and suspicion. Initially, concerns were raised to the effect that the evidence for this intervention was not rigorous [833] or that the method might only be effective for symptoms following specific types of trauma [834]. However, subsequent reviews make a compelling case for efficacy after a wide spectrum of trauma types among a variety of adult clinical cohorts [835, 836]. Due to this strong track record of efficacy in clinical trials, over the preceding decade there has been growing acceptance of EMDR. Several major organizations have come around to officially recommending EMDR for the management of "PTSD." These include the British National Collaborating Centre for Mental Health [837], the U.S. DoD/VA [817], and the World Health Organization [838].

Thus, not one to stand on ceremony, the author acknowledges the evidence that – despite the fact that there is no specific post-trauma psychological disorder, and despite the fact that there is no telling what is wrong with people who meet the APA's discredited criteria for "PTSD" – whether in terms of etiology, or neurobiology, or symptoms – EMDR probably helps a significant proportion of those people. Why? This is where controversy continues to bedevil the field. Clinicians wish their patient to get better, yet resistance to prescribing EMDR persists. That may be because EMDR promoters have not rested content to say, "Thank goodness it works!" They have insisted on explaining. It seems likely to slow acceptance when the pathophysiological explanations on offer are non-scientifically couched and difficult to believe – *ad hoc* mélanges of psychodynamic theory incompatible with cognitive neuroscience (e.g., vague discussion of "emotional processing," "cognitive reconstruction," or "disintegrated memories") mixed with misapplied neurological terms (e.g., *bilateral*, *alternating*, or *saccade*).

One research domain causes special concern: functional imaging ostensibly proving the efficacy of EMDR. All of us are struggling to make sense of the inconsistent, complex, multifocal patterns of different-than-average blood flow seen among persons with psychiatric conditions at rest or during stimulation. Recent revelations that fMRI software is buggy add to the need for patience and reserve. When one reads a report that, if many scans are lumped together and the results are averaged, a group with APA-approved "PTSD" exhibits a pattern with four regions of increased and six regions of decreased activity, one hardly rushes to the granite with a chisel. Such findings cannot be considered valid, reliable, or interpretable. And when one reads a maceration of logic declaring those findings proof of the investigators' opinions, one politely withdraws.

Lansing et al. [839] employed SPECT. They reported that, after EMDR, police officers with "PTSD" exhibited decreased blood flow in the occipital lobes, the left parietal lobe, and the right precentral frontal lobe and blood flow in the left interior frontal lobe. Those authors concluded, "our findings of the specific increases and decreases seen in SPECT are consistent with many etiological improvements" ([839], p. 530). The present author must gently reject that statement. Scattered foci of altered cerebral blood flow found when averaging across subjects have no specific meaning for health or disease. And the failure to compare interventions with or without finger wagging means that this study offers no evidence that "alternating bilateral stimulation" adds anything to talk therapy.

Herkt et al. [824] published a more recent attempt. Healthy female college students were scanned while looking at disgusting pictures. Some were simultaneously stimulated with sounds to alternating ears (called "bilateral alternating auditory stimulation," despite the fact that each ear is connected to both sides of the brain). With or without noises, the amygdala was activated – hardly a surprise. The authors, however, point to the observation that the alternating sounds caused relatively more right amygdalar and less left dorsolateral prefrontal cortex activation. This study overcomes the problem with Lansing et al. [839], since the impact of stimulation was considered. Nothing in these results suggests a medical benefit of EMDR.

Zantvoord et al. [788] systematically reviewed publications claiming neurobiological treatment effects from CBT or EMDR. CBT reduced blood pressure but had no discernible effect on the brain. The authors concluded: "There is some preliminary evidence that TF-CBT [trauma-focused CBT] influences brain regions involved in fear conditioning, extinction learning and possibly working memory and attention regulation; however, these effects could be nonspecific psychotherapeutic effects." That review found no properly controlled imaging trials of EMDR. Contrary to the claims of promoters, EMDR had no different neurobiological treatment effect compared with non-EMDR psychotherapies. Those results support the VA/DoD's admonition: therapist finger movement or other sensory stimulation has not been shown to explain or enhance EMDR. Zantvoord et al.'s summary regarding CBT could as well be said of EMDR: it seems to have therapeutic benefits; those effects might all be explained by the non-specific benefit of psychotherapy. Reiterating a theme that

---

reconstruction" mean, and how might one test the ability of a stimulus to alter that process? Engrams of fear associations are stored in neuronal ensembles. Allocation of neurons to those engrams appears to involve the lateral amygdala [822]. Events (stimuli) co-occurring within short time windows may be represented in overlapping ensembles, but a much later stimulus (like a finger a year later) has no obvious way to influence the competition for co-allocation that constructed the engram. Nor, based on the current understanding of recall of remote threat memories [823], does there exist any obvious mechanism by which the stimuli used in EMDR could facilitate re-consolidation.

seems worth defending: the author strongly supports the use of compassionate individualized talk therapy. Technique seems less important than heart. Ardito and Rabellino's [788] review says as much in more eloquent words: "The emerging picture suggests that the quality of the client–therapist alliance is a reliable predictor of positive clinical outcome independent of the variety of psychotherapy approaches and outcome measures."

Pharmacological options for the management of co-morbid TBI/"PTSD" were thoughtfully reviewed in 2009 by McAllister [840]. He realistically observed that, not only are there no informative RCTs, but also most doctors tasked with helping TBI/"PTSD" patient have only been trained to treat one problem or the other and find themselves torn between administering a drug considered promising for one disorder versus balking at possibly doing harm. McAllister admonished: "The above discussion presents a treatment dilemma for the clinician treating co-morbid TBI/PTSD: interventions that improve one condition may worsen the other" ([840], p. 1357). Arguments might be made for consideration of antidepressants, anticonvulsants, antipsychotic agents, anxiolytics, alpha-2 agonists, alpha-1 antagonists, beta-blockers, and corticotropin-releasing hormone antagonists. Prudently and laudably, that author made no recommendations except research.[61]

A more recent review by Capehart and Bass [784] cited studies conducted with distressed TBI cohorts but without "PTSD." They concluded that sertraline was a reasonable first-line choice and citalopram a second, but that – given concerns about the cardiac side-effects of citalopram – one might instead consider escitalopram.

A third review was published by Watson et al. [842]. Its principal contribution is a warning: no data are available regarding the efficacy of medications for co-morbid TBI/"PTSD" and the data claiming that any medication helps "PTSD" are insufficiently credible [843, 844]. That review concluded, in essence: just prescribe what reportedly helps for "PTSD," even though that is not likely to help.

Sleep disturbance with or without nightmares is a feature of TBI, "PTSD," and the co-morbid condition. Evidence supports the use of prazosin for controlling nightmares, and (setting aside TBI) the VA/DoD management guidelines for PTSD [817] recommend that agent. One case report [845] found that clonidine also reduced nightmares.

Pharmacogenomics lurks on the horizon, as tantalizing as the end of the rainbow. We will soon routinely pick pills based on genes. However, it would be surprising if studies of persons with concussion and "PTSD" were found to (1) exhibit a consistent association between those diverse diagnoses and a polymorphism or VNTR, or (2) exhibit a reliable differential response to an intervention. The search for gene variants predicting response is nonetheless under way. Lawford et al.

[682] assayed subjects with combat-associated PTSD for TaqI A DRD2 alleles (A1A2 versus A2A2). (The proportion of subjects with co-morbid TBI was not reported.) In this uncontrolled study, subjects with the A1+ allele had higher scores for psychopathology. All were treated with paroxetine. Anxiety and depression were reduced.[62] Of special interest, A1+ subjects had significantly greater improvements with regard to social functioning. Such work previews the future of medicine. Like Canopus, it is bright but distant.

An obvious question is whether psychotherapy should be combined with medications. A Cochrane review addressed that question for "PTSD" alone [848]. Four trials were reviewed. The collective evidence was insufficient to prompt any recommendation except the urgent need for better research.

Recommendations for the Management of Post-Concussive "PTSD"-Associated Symptoms

The brain is full of all sorts of little doors and chambers. Sometimes a knock on the head upsets the whole business. Still, all of it has to do with the soul. Without the soul, the head would be no wiser than the foot.

I. B. Singer, 1970 [849]

One way to conceptualize managing the various "PTSD"-associated distresses after concussion is to set aside the CBI and treat the problem with methods that have good track records for the management of "PTSD." Many people suffer after stressful experiences. It does not matter that "PTSD" is not one thing. The pain is real, and the efforts of a previous generation of mental health professionals to find effective treatments deserve honor and respect.

Two principles help consider what might work to help a person presenting with one or more of the seven or more forms of "PTSD"-associated distress observed after concussion. The first is to acknowledge that seven symptoms might have seven biological underpinnings and require seven treatments. Unless and until evidence emerges of one neurobiological change causing all of these symptoms (some of which are mutually exclusive), it may be useful to disengage from the notion that one is treating "PTSD" and focus on reducing specific types of distress. The second is to acknowledge that the contribution of brain damage from external force may complicate the pathophysiological substrate of distress after stress. In other words: stress can cause the "PTSD" panoply; brain rattling can cause the "PTSD" panoply; stress plus brain rattling can do the same. It is possible that these different etiologies cause different brain changes despite similar symptoms. If so, concussion survivors might have altogether different average profiles of treatment responsiveness. In fact, given the inconsistent

---

[61] Subsequent to that publication, Krystal et al. [841] reported the effects of adjunctive risperidone for PTSD in subjects resistant to antidepressants. No benefit was detected. The effect in co-morbid TBI patients is unknown and no reviews recommend such polypharmacy.

[62] Since most studies of comparative efficacy are industry-funded, current evidence must be cited warily. However, a Cochrane review [846] summarized evidence that paroxetine is inferior to both citalopram and mirtazapine. Paroxetine may also have more adverse effects than other agents. "Escitalopram induced significantly less frequency of adverse effects of weakness … nausea and vomiting … drowsiness … as well as somnolence … than paroxetine" [847]. Having observed too many untoward reactions, the present author does not prescribe paroxetine.

correlation between injury severity and persistent distress, TBI might have either adverse or *protective* effects on each symptom, not to mention that the direction of those effects may be genome-dependent (!)

The author can claim only limited personal success in treating persons with CBI followed by "PTSD." He has only two recommendations.

Practical Recommendation Number One

The author encourages the provision of compassionate talk. Some evidence suggests that this is better delivered by a professional clinician than by a priest or bartender. Beyond that, no persuasive evidence favors an M.D. psychiatrist over a Ph.D. psychologist or another trained and committed professional, and the evidence for relatively greater response rates with one method or another is not altogether credible, since the published studies fail to control for either specific symptoms or therapist compassion. Meditation or relaxation therapy may help those who can do it – which seems to be a subset, membership in which is hard to predict in advance of a trial. Behavioral manipulation (e.g., conditioning, contingency management) seems somewhat Orwellian. Empirical evidence exists of efficacy, but not after typical concussion. This approach might be reserved for persons with severe brain damage who have regressed to a state inaccessible to dialogue.

Practical Recommendation Number Two

The author encourages alert trials of medications. The qualifier "alert" is added because 30 years of observation have convinced the author that few of the millions of patients who receive a prescription for a psychotropic drug also receive sufficient counseling, frequent follow-up, systematic assessment of benefits and side-effects, monitoring of metabolic effects, timely dose adjustment, and timely switch to alternatives. Managed care does not seem to have found cost-efficient ways to assure authentically expert psychopharmacology. VA and community mental health clinics with twice-a-year 12-minute psychiatric visits perhaps explain the diminishing confidence in the utility of antidepressants outside the research setting. Antidepressants can provoke terrible nightmares, suicides, and homicides. More often, they just do nothing because the type or dose is not ideal. Sensitive monitoring is the doctor's sacred duty, even though society declines to pay for the effort. These are big, socially important problems, largely soluble if they ever become political priorities. Although this author is grossly unqualified to orchestrate massive reorganization of global mental health provision, he believes it is sorely needed.

What drugs? For the sake of simplicity, there is a painful, anhedonic, hopeless state that seems – about half the time – to get better with agents that reduce reuptake of serotonin and/ or norepinephrine. There are other painful states that involve more arousal, irritability, and anxiety than hopeless darkness. These too sometimes respond to modern antidepressants. In the author's experience, however, the rate of response is a little less than 50% and the risk of agitated reactions is a little higher in this subgroup. Some evidence hints that escitalopram is slightly more efficacious and better tolerated than other agents. Although the relative efficacy of different agents surely depends on genetic and other factors, a busy clinician can rarely individualize the choice of the first prescription. One might therefore play the odds, start with escitalopram, and revise by trial and error.[63]

Other medications might also help on a symptom-by-symptom, case-by-case basis. Sleep disturbance makes life worse, whatever else is causing mental harm. Good evidence exists that prazosin helps stress-related nightmares. The problem is that some patients have entirely different causes of insomnia, from simple prolonged sleep onset latency to early morning wakening to life-threatening obstructive sleep apnea. Please let us make that distinction before prescribing anything. When resources are available, a formal sleep consultation can help. When nightmares are not the issue or when prazosin does not work, the author has recently seen better response to orexin receptor antagonists. Pain also makes mental life worse. One cannot be optimistic about controlling sadness or anxiety without controlling pain. Young psychiatrists sometimes hesitate to perform a complete physical examination, but that step is necessary to rule out treatable somatic causes of psychic distress. Again, orthopedic or pain consultation is sometimes the most critical step in relieving depression or anxiety.[64] Endocrine disturbances due to pituitary damage are both common and commonly overlooked after concussion [667, 670, 853–856]. It is hard to express how very gratifying it is to discover that a survivor's major symptom, such as fatigue, or anhedonia, or hyposexuality, is due to hypopituitarism and readily treatable. Chapter 26 of this collaborative book will propose an algorithm for testing.

A factory-stamped boilerplate is usually inserted at this point in a review of how to help the ill: more research is needed. The present author cannot condone such puffery. He would propose that more thought is needed – a complete reconceptualization of the problems our patients face, a paradigm shift in the understanding of the dreadful consequences of concussion that dispenses with cognitive test results as the standard of outcome, a rejection of the fallacious convention of "evidence-based" medicine, since publications proudly

---

[63] None of the data regarding who should receive this or any psychotropic agent, at what dose, for how long, is evidence-based. That would require individualized pharmacogenomic and pharmacodynamic information. Modern medicating is like sprinkling salt on a tomato, never tasting to determine the result. Every so often, however, the effect is just right.

[64] The Federal Drug Administration and even the American Academy of Neurology have recently pilloried compassionate pain relief as a slippery slope to opioid death [850]. There is indeed a deadly crisis of opioid abuse in North America. But the AAN's hysterical and unscientific approach seems to be political, not medical. One would need an additional book to expose their cherry-picking of the risk data and the fallacy of their new guidelines. (For instance, anyone who passed high school biology knows that a milligram-per-day limitation is irrational given vast human metabolic differences.) The present author must restrict his concerns to a passing mention. But please review the data for yourself [851, 852].

breasting that label almost never consider human individuality, and a humble embrace of the implications of natural selection: no two humans ever suffer from the same disease.

Consider for a moment how very hard it would be to test the most basic treatment hypotheses in this subset of concussed persons. We work in clinics. We see distress. We try to help. No textbook on this Earth describes the patient we see or predicts the utility of the combination of interventions we end up ordering. So we guess. All day, every day, the honest neurologist or psychiatrist or physiatrist would admit: "just guessin' here." What medication, at what dose and schedule, combined with what form of psychotherapy (applying what minimal standard of therapeutic alliance) helps concussion survivors with which genomes with which of the seven or more types of "PTSD"-associated symptoms? Given the number of variables, a power analysis suggests that a modest effect size could be detected in an experimental population the size of China's.

Still, not to miss a bet: more research is needed.

References

1. Mickle WJ. The traumatic factor in mental disease. *Brain* 1892;15: 76–102.
2. Scholten AC, Haagsma JA, Cnossen MC, Olff M, van Beeck EF, Polinder S. Prevalence of and risk factors for anxiety and depressive disorders after traumatic brain injury: a systematic review. *J Neurotrauma* 2016;33: 1969–1994.
3. Marschark M, Richtsmeier LM, Richardson JT, Crovitz HF, Henry J. Intellectual and emotional functioning in college students following mild traumatic brain injury in childhood and adolescence. *J Head Trauma Rehabil* 2000;15: 1227–1245.
4. Light R, Asarnow R, Satz P, Zaucha K, McCleary C, Lewis R. Mild closed-head injury in children and adolescents: behavior problems and academic outcomes. *J Consult Clin Psychol* 1998;66: 1023–1029.
5. Hanks RA, Temkin N, Machamer J, Dikmen SS. Emotional and behavioural adjustment after traumatic brain injury. *Arch Phys Med Rehabil* 1999;80: 991–997.
6. Fazel S, Wolf A, Pillas D, Lichtenstein P, Långström N. Suicide, fatal injuries, and other causes of premature mortality in patients with traumatic brain injury: a 41-year Swedish population study. *JAMA Psychiatry* 2014;71: 326–333.
7. Symonds CP. Mental disorder following head injury. *Proc R Soc Med* 1937;30: 1081–1094.
8. Kozol HL. Pretraumatic personality and psychiatric sequelae of head injury: categorical pretraumatic personality status correlated with general psychiatric reaction to head injury based on analysis of two hundred cases. *Arch Neurol Psychiatry* 1945;53: 358–364.
9. Van Meter T, Mirshahi N, Peters M, Roy D, Rao V, Diaz-Arrastia R, et al. Machine learning models identify mild traumatic brain injury patients with significant depressive symptoms over six months of recovery using a three biomarker blood test. *Ann Emerg Med* 2017;70: S104–S105.
10. Kozol HL. Pretraumatic personality and psychiatric sequelae of head injury: correlation of multiple, specific factors in the pretraumatic personality and psychiatric reaction to head injury, based on analysis of one hundred and one cases. *Arch Neurol Psychiatry* 1946;56: 245–275.
11. Jacobson SA. *The post-traumatic syndrome following head injury: mechanisms and treatment.* Springfield, IL: Charles C. Thomas, 1963.
12. Lishman WA. Brain damage in relation to psychiatric disability after head injury. *Br J Psychiatry* 1968;114; 373–410.
13. Lishman WA. The psychiatric sequelae of head injury: a review. *Psychol Med* 1973;3: 304–318.
14. Levin HS, Grossman RG. Behavioral sequelae of closed head injury. A quantitative study. *Arch Neurol* 1978;5: 720–727.
15. Keshavan MS, Channabasavanna SM, Narayana Reddy GN. Post-traumatic psychiatric disturbances: patterns and predictors of outcome. *Br J Psychiatry* 1981;138: 157–160.
16. Slagle DA. Psychiatric disorders following closed head injury: an overview of biopsychosocial factors in their etiology and management. *Int J Psychiatry Med* 1990;20: 1–35.
17. Fann JR, Katon WJ, Uomoto JM, Esselman PC. Psychiatric disorders and functional disability in outpatients with traumatic brain injuries. *Am J Psychiatry* 1995;152: 1493–1499.
18. Fann JR, Burington B, Leonetti A, Jaffe K, Katon WJ, Thompson RS. Psychiatric illness following traumatic brain injury in an adult health maintenance organization population. *Arch Gen Psychiatry* 2004;61: 53–61.
19. Hibbard MR, Uysal S, Kepler K, Bogdany J, Silver J. Axis I psychopathology in individuals with traumatic brain injury. *J Head Trauma Rehabil* 1998;13: 24–39.
20. Deb S, Lyons I, Koutzoukis C. Neurobehavioural symptoms one year after a head injury. *Br J Psychiatry* 1999;174: 360–365.
21. Rao V, Constantine Lyketsos C. Neuropsychiatric sequelae of traumatic brain injury. *Psychosom* 2000;41: 95–103.
22. Rao V, Rosenberg P, Bertrand M, Salehinia S, Spiro J, Vaishnavi S, et al. Aggression after traumatic brain injury: prevalence and correlates. *J Neuropsychiatry Clin Neurosci* 2009;21: 420–429.
23. Rao V, Lyketsos CG. Psychiatric aspects of traumatic brain injury. *Psychiatr Clin North Am* 2002;25: 43–69.
24. van Reekum R, Cohen T, Wong J. Can traumatic brain injury cause psychiatric disorders? *J Neuropsychiatry Clin Neurosci* 2000;12: 316–327.
25. Koponen S, Taiminen T, Portin R, Himanen L, Isoniemi H, Heinonen H, et al. *Am J Psychiatry* 2002;159: 1315–1321.
26. Ashman TA, Spielman LA, Hibbard MR, Silver JM, Chandna T, Gordon WA. Psychiatric challenges in the first 6 years after traumatic brain injury: cross-sequential analyses of Axis I disorders. *Arch Phys Med Rehabil* 2004;85 (4 Suppl 2): S36–S42.
27. Ashman TA, Gordon WA, Cantor JB, Hibbard MR. Neurobehavioral consequences of traumatic brain injury. *Mt Sinai J Med* 2006;73: 999–1005.
28. Arciniegas DB, Anderson CA, Topkoff J, McAllister TW. Mild traumatic brain injury: a neuropsychiatric approach to diagnosis, evaluation, and treatment. *Neuropsychiatr Dis Treat* 2005;1: 311–327.
29. Arciniegas DB. Addressing neuropsychiatric disturbances during rehabilitation after traumatic brain injury: current and future methods. *Dialog Clin Neurosci* 2011;13: 325–345.
30. Warriner EM, Velikonja D. Psychiatric disturbances after traumatic brain injury: neurobehavioral and personality changes. *Curr Psychiatry Rep* 2006;8: 73–80.
31. Kim E, Lauterbach EC, Reeve A, Arciniegas DB, Coburn KL, Mendez MF et al. Neuropsychiatric complications of traumatic brain injury: a critical review of the literature (a report by the ANPA Committee on Research). *J Neuropsychiatry Clin Neurosci* 2007;19: 106–127.
32. Rogers JM, Read CA. Psychiatric comorbidity following traumatic brain injury. *Brain Inj* 2007;21: 1321–1333.
33. Fleminger S, Greenwood RRJ, Oliver DL. Pharmacological management for agitation and aggression in people with acquired brain injury. *Cochrane Database Syst Rev* 2006;4:CD003299: 1–27.
34. Schwarzbold M, Diaz A, Martins ET, Rufino A, Amante LN, Thais ME, et al. Psychiatric disorders and traumatic brain injury. *Neuropsychiatr Dis Treat* 2008;4: 797–816.

35. Riggio S, Wong M. Neurobehavioral sequelae of traumatic brain injury. *Mt Sinai J Med* 2009;76: 163–172.

36. Hesdorffer DC, Rauch SL, Tamminga CA. Long-term psychiatric outcomes following traumatic brain injury: a review of the literature. *J Head Trauma Rehabil* 2009;24: 452–459.

37. Whelan-Goodinson R, Ponsford JL, Schonberger M, Johnston L. Predictors of psychiatric disorders following traumatic brain injury. *J Head Trauma Rehabil* 2010;25: 320–329.

38. Gould KR, Ponsford JL, Johnston L, Schönberger M. The nature, frequency and course of psychiatric disorders in the first year after traumatic brain injury: a prospective study. *Psychol Med* 2011;41: 2099–2109.

39. Konrad C, Geburek AJ, Rist F, Blumenroth H, Fischer B, Husstedt I, et al. Long-term cognitive and emotional consequences of mild traumatic brain injury. *Psychol Med* 2011;41: 1197–1211.

40. Max JE, Pardo D, Hanten G, Schachar RJ, Saunders AE, Ewing-Cobbs L, et al. Psychiatric disorders in children and adolescents six-to-twelve months after mild traumatic brain injury. *J Neuropsychiatry Clin Neurosci* 2013;25: 272–282.

41. Alexander MP. Mild traumatic brain injury: pathophysiology, natural history, and clinical management. *Neurology* 1995;45: 1253–1260.

42. Bohnen N, Jolles J. Neurobehavioral aspects of postconcussive symptoms after mild head injury. *J Nerv Mental Dis* 1992;180: 683–692.

43. Boyle E, Cancelliere C, Hartvigsen J, Carroll LJ, Holm LW, Cassidy JD. Systematic review of prognosis after mild traumatic brain injury in the military: results of the international collaboration on mild traumatic brain injury prognosis. *Arch Phys Med Rehabil* 2014;95 (3 Suppl): S230–S237.

44. Brown SJ, Fann JR, Grant I. Postconcussional disorder: time to acknowledge a common source of neurobehavioral morbidity. *J Neuropsychiatry Clin Neurosci* 1994;6: 15–22.

45. Carroll LJ, Cassidy JD, Cancelliere C, Côté P, Hincapié CA, Kristman VL, et al. Systematic review of the prognosis after mild traumatic brain injury in adults: cognitive, psychiatric, and mortality outcomes: results of the international collaboration on mild traumatic brain injury prognosis. *Arch Phys Med Rehabil* 2014;95 (3 Suppl): S152–S173.

46. Drag LL, Spencer RJ, Walker SJ, Pangilinan PH, Bieliauskas LA. The contributions of self-reported injury characteristics and psychiatric symptoms to cognitive functioning in OEF/OIF veterans with mild traumatic brain injury. *J Int Neuropsychol Soc* 2012;18: 576–584.

47. Fayol P, Carrière H, Habonimana D, Dumond JJ. Preliminary questions before studying mild traumatic brain injury outcome. *Ann Phys Rehabil Med* 2009;52: 497–509.

48. Halbauer JD, Ashford JW, Zeitzer JM, Adamson MM, Lew HL, Yesavage JA. Neuropsychiatric diagnosis and management of chronic sequelae of war-related mild to moderate traumatic brain injury. *J Rehabil Res Dev* 2009;46: 757–796.

49. Iverson GL. Outcome from mild traumatic brain injury. *Curr Opin Psychiatry* 2005;18: 301–317.

50. Kiraly MA, Kiraly SJ. Traumatic brain injury and delayed sequelae: a review – traumatic brain injury and mild traumatic brain injury (concussion) are precursors to later-onset brain disorders, including early-onset dementia. *Sci World J* 2007;7: 1768–1776.

51. Kushner D. Mild traumatic brain injury: toward understanding manifestations and treatment. *Arch Intern Med* 1998;158: 1617–1624.

52. Laborey M, Masson F, Ribéreau-Gayon R, Zongo D, Salmi LR, Lagarde E. Specificity of postconcussion symptoms at 3 months after mild traumatic brain injury: results from a comparative cohort study. *J Head Trauma Rehabil* 2014;29: E28–E36.

53. Mott TF, McConnon ML, Rieger BP. Subacute to chronic mild traumatic brain injury. *Am Fam Physician* 2012;86: 1045–1051.

54. Symonds C. Concussion and its sequelae. *Lancet* 1962;279: 1–5.

55. Grinnon ST, Miller K, Marler JR, Lu Y, Stout A, Odenkirchen J, Kunitz S. NINDS common data element project: approach and methods. *Clin Trials* 2012;9: 322–329.

56. Overall JE, Gorham DR. The brief psychiatric rating scale. *Psychol Rep* 1962;10: 799–812.

57. First MB, Williams JBW, Karg RS, Spitzer RL. *Structured Clinical Interview for DSM-5 Disorders, Clinician Version (SCID-5-CV)*. Arlington, VA: American Psychiatric Association, 2015.

58. King NS, Crawford S, Wenden FJ, Moss NE, Wade DT. The Rivermead Post Concussion Symptoms Questionnaire: a measure of symptoms commonly experienced after head injury and its reliability. *J Neurol* 1995;242: 587–592.

59. Cicerone KD, Kalmar K. Persistent postconcussion syndrome: the structure of subjective complaints after mTBI. *J Head Trauma Rehabil* 1995;10: 1–17.

60. King PR, Donnelly KT, Donnelly JP, Dunnam M, Warner G, Kittleson CJ, et al. Psychometric study of the Neurobehavioral Symptom Inventory. *J Rehabil Res Dev* 2012;49: 879–888.

61. Beck AT, Steer RA, Brown GK. *Manual for the Beck Depression Inventory-II*. San Antonio, TX: Psychological Corporation, 1996.

62. Sliwinski M, Gordon WA, Bogdany J. The Beck Depression Inventory: is it a suitable measure of depression for individuals with traumatic brain injury? *J Head Trauma Rehabil* 1998;13: 40–46.

63. Blanchard EB, Jones-Alexander J, Buckley TC, Forneris CA. Psychometric properties of the PTSD checklist (PCL). *Behav Res Ther* 1996;34: 669–673.

64. Buss AH, Warren WL. *Aggression Questionnaire: manual*. Los Angeles, CA: Western Psychological Services, 2000.

65. American Psychiatric Association. *Diagnostic and statistical manual of mental disorders, fifth edition (DSM-5)*. Washington, DC: American Psychiatric Press, 2013.

66. Tsai J, Harpaz-Rotem I, Armour C, Southwick SM, Krystal JH, Pietrzak RH. Dimensional structure of DSM-5 posttraumatic stress symptoms: results from the National Health and Resilience in Veterans Study. *J Clin Psychiatry* 2015;76: 546–553.

67. Armour C, Tsai J, Durham TA, Charak R, Biehn TL, Elhai JD, Pietrzak RH. Dimensional structure of DSM-5 posttraumatic stress symptoms: support for a hybrid anhedonia and externalizing behaviors model. *J Psychiatr Res* 2015;61: 106–113.

68. Dekel S, Solomon Z, Horesh D, Ein-Dor T. Posttraumatic stress disorder and depressive symptoms: joined or independent sequelae of trauma? *J Psychiatr Res* 2014;54: 64–69.

69. Motzkin JC, Koenigs MR. Post traumatic stress disorder and traumatic brain injury. In Grafman J, Salazar AM, editors. *Handbook of clinical neurology. Traumatic brain injury, part II*, vol. 128. Amsterdam, The Netherlands: Elsevier, 2015, pp. 633–648.

70. Haun P. A rational approach to psychiatric nosology. *Psychiatric Q* 1949;308–316.

71. Faraone SV, Tsuang, MT. Measuring diagnostic accuracy in the absence of a "gold standard." *Am J Psychiatry* 1994;151: 650–657.

72. Berganza CE, Mezzich JE, Pouncey C. Concepts of disease: their relevance for psychiatric diagnosis and classification. *Psychopathol* 2005;38: 166–170.

73. Robert JS. Gene maps, brain scans, and psychiatric nosology. *Cambridge Q Healthcare Ethics* 2007;16: 209–218.

74. Insel TR, Wang PS. Rethinking mental illness. *JAMA* 2010;303: 1970–1971.

75. Nesse RM, Stein DJ. Towards a genuinely medical model for psychiatric nosology. *BMC Med* 2012;10: 5.

76. Phillips J, Frances A, Cerullo MA, Chardavoyne J, Decker HS, First MB, et al. The six most essential questions in psychiatric diagnosis: a pluralogue part 2: issues of conservatism and pragmatism in psychiatric diagnosis. *Philos Ethics Humanit Med* 2012;7: 9.

77. de Leon J. Is psychiatry scientific? A letter to a 21st century psychiatry resident. *Psychiatry Investig* 2013;10: 205–217.

78. Keshavan MS. Nosology of psychoses in DSM-5: inches ahead but miles to go. *Schiz Res* 2013;150: 40–41.

79. Stein DJ, Lund C, Nesse RM. Classification systems in psychiatry: diagnosis and global mental health in the era of DSM-5 and ICD-11. *Curr Opin Psychiatry* 2013;26: 493–497.

80. Avasthi A, Sarkar S, Grover S. Approaches to psychiatric nosology: a viewpoint. *Ind J Psychiatry* 2014;56: 301–304.

81. Cuthbert BN. Research domain criteria: toward future psychiatric nosology. *Asian J Psychiatry* 2014;7: 4–5.

82. Goodkind M, Eickhoff SB, Oathes DJ, Jiang Y, Chang A, Jones-Hagata LB, et al. Identification of a common neurobiological substrate for mental illness. *JAMA Psychiatry* 2015;72: 305–315.

83. Walter H, Muller J. Der Beitrag der Neurowissenschaften zum psychiatrischen Krankheitsbegriff [The contribution of neuroscience to the concept of mental disorder]. *Nervenarzt* 2015;86: 22–28.

84. Surís A, Holliday R, North CS. The evolution of the classification of psychiatric disorders. *Behav Sci* 2016;6 (1).

85. Cook KF, Bombardier CH, Bamer AM, Choi SW, Kroenke K, Fann JR. Do somatic and cognitive symptoms of traumatic brain injury confound depression screening? *Arch Phys Med Rehabil* 2011;92: 818–823.

86. Barker-Collo S, Jones A, Jones K, Theadom A, Dowell A, Starkey N, et al. Prevalence, natural course and predictors of depression 1 year following traumatic brain injury from a population-based study in New Zealand. *Brain Inj* 2015;29: 859–865.

87. Jorge RE. Are there symptoms that are specific for depressed mood in patients with traumatic brain injury? *J Nerv Mental Dis* 1993;181: 91–99.

88. Rosenthal M, Christensen BK, Ross TP. Depression following traumatic brain injury. *Arch Phys Med Rehabil* 1998;79: 90–103.

89. Babin PR. Diagnosing depression in persons with brain injuries: a look at theories, the DSM-IV and depression measures, *Brain Inj* 2003;17: 1889–1900.

90. Moldover JE, Goldberg KB, Prout MF. Depression after traumatic brain injury: a review of evidence for clinical heterogeneity. *Neuropsychol Rev* 2004;14: 143–154.

91. Carroll BJ, Fielding JM, Blashki TG. Depression rating scales: a critical review. *Arch Gen Psychiatry* 1973;28: 361–366.

92. Demyttenaere K. Risk factors and predictors of compliance in depression. *Eur Neuropsychopharmacol* 2003;13 (Suppl 3): S69–S75.

93. Löwe B, Spitzer RL, Gräfe K, Kroenke K, Quenter A, Zipfel S, et al. Comparative validity of three screening questionnaires for DSM-IV depressive disorders and physicians' diagnoses. *J Affect Disord* 2004;78: 131–140.

94. O'Connor EA, Whitlock EP, Beil TL, Gaynes BN. Screening for depression in adult patients in primary care settings: a systematic evidence review. *Ann Intern Med* 2009;151: 793–803.

95. US Preventive Services Task Force. Screening and treatment for major depressive disorder in children and adolescents: US Preventive Services Task Force recommendation statement. *Pediatrics* 2009;123: 1223–1228.

96. Lee B-H, Kim Y-K. The roles of BDNF in the pathophysiology of major depression and in antidepressant treatment. *Psychiatry Investig* 2010;7: 231–235.

97. Guillamondegui OD, Montgomery SA, Phibbs FT, McPheeters ML, Alexander PT, Jerome RN, et al. Traumatic brain injury and depression. Comparative effectiveness review no. 25. (Prepared by the Vanderbilt Evidence-based Practice Center under Contract No. 290-2007-10065-I.) AHRQ publication no. 11-EHC017-EF. Rockville, MD: Agency for Healthcare Research and Quality, 2011. Available at: www.effectivehealthcare.ahrq.gov/reports/final.cfm.

98. Hamilton MA. A rating scale for depression. *J Neurol Neurosurg Psychiatry* 1960;23: 56–62.

99. Beck AT, Ward CH, Mendelson M, Mock J, Erbaugh J. An inventory for measuring depression. *Arch Gen Psychiatry* 1961;4: 561–571.

100. Zigmond A, Snaith R. The Hospital Anxiety and Depression Scale. *Acta Psychiatr Scand* 1983;67: 361–370.

101. Kroenke K, Spitzer RL, Williams JBW. The PHQ-9: validity of a brief depression severity measure. *J Gen Intern Med* 2001;16: 606–613.

102. Kroenke K, Spitzer RL, Williams JB, Löwe B. The Patient Health Questionnaire Somatic, Anxiety, and Depressive Symptom Scales: a systematic review. *Gen Hosp Psychiatry* 2010;32: 345–359.

103. Schwarzbold ML, Diaz AP, Nunes JC, Sousa DS, Hohl A, Guarnieri R, et al. Validity and screening properties of three depression rating scales in a prospective sample of patients with severe traumatic brain injury. *Rev Bras Psiquiatr* 2014;36: 206–212.

104. Schönberger M, Ponsford J. The factor structure of the Hospital Anxiety and Depression Scale in individuals with traumatic brain injury. *Psychiatry Res* 2010;179: 342–349.

105. Dahm J, Wong D, Ponsford J. Validity of the Depression Anxiety Stress Scales in assessing depression and anxiety following traumatic brain injury. *J Affect Dis* 2013;151: 392–396.

106. Dawkins N, Cloherty ME, Gracey F, Evans JJ. The factor structure of the Hospital Anxiety and Depression Scale in acquired brain injury. *Brain Inj* 2006;20: 1235–1239.

107. Driskell LD, Starosta AJ, Brenner LA. Clinical utility and measurement characteristics of the Hospital Anxiety and Depression Scale for individuals with traumatic brain injury. *Rehabil Psychol* 2016;61: 112–113.

108. Warden DL, Gordon B, McAllister TW, Silver JM, Barth JT, Bruns J, et al. Neurobehavioral Guidelines Working Group. Guidelines for the pharmacologic treatment of neurobehavioral sequelae of traumatic brain injury. *J Neurotrauma* 2006;23: 1468–1501.

109. Rapoport MJ. Depression following traumatic brain injury: epidemiology, risk factors and management. *CNS Drugs* 2012;26: 111–121.

110. Mauri MC, Paletta S, Colasanti A, Miserocchi G, Altamura AC. Clinical and neuropsychological correlates of major depression following post-traumatic brain injury, a prospective study. *Asian J Psychiatry* 2014;12: 118–124.

111. Jorge RE, Arciniegas DB. Mood disorders after TBI. *Psychiatr Clin North Am* 2014;37: 13–29.

112. Hart T, Hoffman JM, Pretz C, Kennedy R, Clark AN, Brenner LA. A longitudinal study of major and minor depression following traumatic brain injury. *Arch Phys Med Rehabil* 2012;93: 1343–1349.

113. Osborn AJ, Mathias JL, Fairweather-Schmidt AK. Depression following adult, non-penetrating traumatic brain injury: a meta-analysis examining methodological variables and sample characteristics. *Neurosci Biobehav Rev* 2014;47: 1–15.

114. Guskiewicz KM, Marshall SW, Bailes J, McCrea M, Harding HP, Matthews A, et al. Recurrent concussion and risk of depression in retired professional football players. *Med Sci Sports Exerc* 2007;39: 903–909.

115. Schatz P, Moser RS, Covassin T, Karpf R. Early indicators of enduring symptoms in high school athletes with multiple previous concussions. *Neurosurg* 2011;68: 1562–1567.

116. Holsinger T, Steffens DC, Phillips C, Helms MJ, Havlik RJ, Breitner JC, et al. Head injury in early adulthood and the lifetime risk of depression. *Arch Gen Psychiatry* 2002;59: 17–22.

117. Chrisman SPD, Richardson LP. Prevalence of diagnosed depression in adolescents with history of concussion. *J Adolesc Heath* 2014;54: 582–586.

118. Malec JF, Brown AW, Moessner AM, Stump TE, Monahan P. A preliminary model for posttraumatic brain injury depression. *Arch Phys Med Rehabil* 2010;91: 1087–1097.

119. Luo L, Chai Y, Jiang R, Chen X, Yan T. Cortisol supplement combined with psychotherapy and citalopram improves depression outcomes in patients with hypocortisolism after traumatic brain injury. *Aging Dis* 2015;6: 418–425.

120. Ansari A, Jain A, Sharma A, Mittal RS, Gupta ID. Role of sertraline in posttraumatic brain injury depression and quality-of-life in TBI. *Asian J Neurosurg* 2014;9: 182–188.

121. Bryan CJ, Clemans TA. Repetitive traumatic brain injury, psychological symptoms, and suicide risk in a clinical sample of deployed military personnel. *JAMA Psychiatry* 2013;70: 686–691.

122. Bajwa NM, Halavi S, Hamer M, Semple BD, Noble-Haeusslein LJ, Baghchechi M, et al. Mild concussion, but not moderate traumatic brain injury, is associated with long-term depression-like phenotype in mice. *PLoS One* 2016;11: e0146886.

123. Ashman TA, Spielman LA, Hibbard MR, Silver JM, Chandna T, Gordon WA. Psychiatric challenges in the first 6 years after traumatic brain injury: cross-sequential analyses of Axis I disorders. *Arch Phys Med Rehabil* 2004;85 (4 Suppl 2): S36–S42.

124. Dikmen SS, Bombardier CH, Machamer JE, Fann JR, Temkin NR. Natural history of depression in traumatic brain injury. *Arch Phys Med Rehabil* 2004;85: 1457–1464.

125. Sullivan-Singh SJ, Sawyer K, Ehde DM, Bell KR, Temkin N, Dikmen S, et al. Comorbidity of pain and depression among persons with traumatic brain injury. *Arch Phys Med Rehabil* 2014;95: 1100–1105.

126. Hoofien D, Gilboa A, Vakil E, Donovick PJ. Traumatic brain injury (TBI) 10–20 years later: a comprehensive outcome study of psychiatric symptomatology, cognitive abilities and psychosocial functioning. *Brain Inj* 2001;15: 189–209.

127. Lucas S, Smith BM, Temkin N, Bell KR, Dikmen S, Hoffman JM. Comorbidity of headache and depression after mild traumatic brain injury. *Headache* 2016;56: 323–330.

128. Bombardier CH, Hoekstra T, Dikmen S, Fann JR. Depression trajectories during the first year after traumatic brain injury. *J Neurotrauma* 2016;33: 2115–2124.

129. Demakis GJ, Rimland CA. Untreated mild traumatic brain injury in a young adult population. *Arch Clin Neuropsychol* 2010;25: 191–196.

130. Goverover Y, Chiaravalloti N. The impact of self-awareness and depression on subjective reports of memory, quality-of-life and satisfaction with life following TBI. *Brain Inj* 2014;28(2): 174–180.

131. Fedoroff JP, Starkstein SE, Forrester AW, Geisler FH, Jorge RE, Arndt SV, Robinson RG. Depression in acute traumatic brain injury. *Am J Psychiatry* 1992;149: 918–923.

132. Hart T, Brenner L, Clark AN, Bogner JA, Novack TA, Chervoneva I, et al. Major and minor depression after traumatic brain injury. *Arch Phys Med Rehabil* 2011;92: 1211–1219.

133. Rao V, Bertrand M, Rosenberg P, Makley M, Schretlen DJ, Brandt J, et al. Predictors of new-onset depression after mild traumatic brain injury. *J Neuropsychiatry Clin Neurosci* 2010;22: 100–104.

134. Albrecht JS, Kiptanui Z, Tsang Y, Khokhar B, Liu X, Simoni-Wastila L, et al. Depression among older adults after traumatic brain injury: a national analysis. *Am J Geriatr Psychiatry* 2015;23: 607–614.

135. Rapoport MJ, McCullagh S, Streiner D, Feinstein A. Age and major depression after mild traumatic brain injury. *Am J Geriatr Psychiatry* 2003;11: 365–369.

136. Bombardier CH, Fann JR, Temkin NR, Esselman PC, Barber J, Dikmen SS. Rates of major depressive disorder and clinical outcomes following traumatic brain injury. *JAMA* 2010;303: 1938–1945.

137. van der Horn HJ, Spikman JM, Jacobs B, van der Naalt J. Postconcussive complaints, anxiety, and depression related to vocational outcome in minor to severe traumatic brain injury. *Arch Phys Med Rehabil* 2013;94: 867–874.

138. Morissette SB, Woodward M, Kimbrel NA, Meyer EC, Kruse MI, Dolan S, et al. Deployment-related TBI, persistent postconcussive symptoms, PTSD, and depression in OEF/OIF veterans. *Rehabil Psychol* 2011;56: 340–350.

139. Haagsma JA, Scholten AC, Andriessen TM, Vos PE, Van Beeck EF, Polinder S. Impact of depression and post-traumatic stress disorder on functional outcome and health-related quality of life of patients with mild traumatic brain injury. *J Neurotrauma* 2015;32: 853–862.

140. Haghighi F, Ge Y, Chen S, Xin Y, Umali MU, De Gasperi R, et al. Neuronal DNA methylation profiling of blast-related traumatic brain injury. *J Neurotrauma* 2015;32: 1200–1209.

141. Chan F, Lanctôt KL, Feinstein A, Herrmann N, Strauss J, Sicard T, et al. The serotonin transporter polymorphisms and major depression following traumatic brain injury. *Brain Inj* 2008;22: 471–479.

142. Failla MD, Burkhardt JN, Miller MA, Scanlon JM, Conley YP, Ferrell RE, et al. Variants of SLC6A4 in depression risk following severe TBI. *Brain Inj* 2013;27: 696–706.

143. Polimanti R, Chen CY, Ursano RJ, Heeringa SG, Jain S, Kessler RC, et al. Cross-phenotype polygenic risk score analysis of persistent post-concussive symptoms in U.S. army soldiers with deployment-acquired traumatic brain injury. *J Neurotrauma* 2017;34: 781–789.

144. Rapoport MJ, Mitchell RA, McCullagh S, Herrmann N, Chan F, Kiss A, Feinstein A, Lanctôt KL. A randomized controlled trial of antidepressant continuation for major depression following traumatic brain injury. *J Clin Psychiatry* 2010;71: 1125–1130.

145. Elliott TR, Hsiao YY, Kimbrel NA, Meyer EC, DeBeer BB, Gulliver SB, et al. Resilience, traumatic brain injury, depression, and posttraumatic stress among Iraq/Afghanistan war veterans. *Rehabil Psychol* 2015;60: 263–276.

146. Wee HY, Ho CH, Liang FW, Hsieh KY, Wang CC, Wang JJ, et al. Increased risk of new-onset depression in patients with traumatic brain injury and hyperlipidemia: the important role of statin medications. *J Clin Psychiatry* 2016;77: 505–511.

147. Sung CW, Lee HC, Chiang YH, Chiu WT, Chu SF, Ou JC, et al. Early dysautonomia detected by heart rate variability predicts late depression in female patients following mild traumatic brain injury. *Psychophysiol* 2016;53: 455–464.

148. Sung CW, Chen KY, Chiang YH, Chiu WT, Ou JC, Lee HC, et al. Heart rate variability and serum level of insulin-like growth factor-1 are correlated with symptoms of emotional disorders in patients suffering a mild traumatic brain injury. *Clin Neurophysiol* 2016;127: 1629–1638.

149. Fenn AM, Gensel JC, Huang Y, Popovich PG, Lifshitz J, Godbout JP. Immune activation promotes depression one month after diffuse brain injury: a role for primed microglia. *Biol Psychiatry* 2014;76: 575–584.

150. Juengst SB, Kumar RG, Failla MD, Goyal A, Wagner AK. Acute inflammatory biomarker profiles predict depression risk following moderate to severe traumatic brain injury. *J Head Trauma Rehabil* 2015;30: 207–218.

151. Eklund A, Nichols TE, Knutsson H. Cluster failure: why fMRI inferences for spatial extent have inflated false-positive rates. *Proc Natl Acad Sci USA* 2016;113: 7900–7905.

152. Jorge RE, Acion L, Starkstein SE, Magnotta V. Hippocampal volume and mood disorders after traumatic brain injury. *Biol Psychiatry* 2007;62: 332–338.

153. Chen JK, Johnston KM, Petrides M, Ptito A. Neural substrates of symptoms of depression following concussion in male athletes with persisting postconcussion symptoms. *Arch Gen Psychiatry* 2008;65: 81–89.

154. Rao V, Munro CA, Rosenberg P, Ward J, Bertrand M, Degoankar M, et al. Neuroanatomical correlates of depression in post traumatic brain injury: preliminary results of a pilot study. *J Neuropsychiatry Clin Neurosci* 2010;22: 231–235.

155. Hudak A, Warner M, Marquez de la Plata C, Moore C, Harper C, Diaz-Arrastia R. Brain morphometry changes and depressive symptoms after traumatic brain injury. *Psychiatry Res* 2011;191: 160–165.

156. Maller JJ, Thomson RH, Pannek K, Bailey N, Lewis PM, Fitzgerald PB. Volumetrics relate to the development of depression after traumatic brain injury. *Behav Brain Res* 2014;271: 147–153.

157. Matthews SC, Strigo IA, Simmons AN, O'Connell RM, Reinhardt LE, Moseley SA. A multimodal imaging study in U.S. veterans of operations Iraqi and enduring freedom with and without major depression after blast related concussion. *NeuroImage* 2011;54 (Suppl 1): S69–S75.

158. Rao V, Mielke M, Xu X, Smith GS, McCann UD, Bergey A, et al. Diffusion tensor imaging atlas-based analyses in major depression after mild traumatic brain injury. *J Neuropsychiatry Clin Neurosci* 2012;24: 309–315.

159. Isaac L, Main KL, Soman S, Gotlib IH, Furst AJ, Kinoshita LM, et al. The impact of depression on veterans with PTSD and traumatic brain injury: a diffusion tensor imaging study. *Biol Psychol* 2015;105: 20–28.

160. Matthews SC, Simmons AN, Strigo IA. The effects of loss versus alteration of consciousness on inhibition-related brain activity among individuals with a history of blast-related concussion. *Psychiatry Res Neuroimag* 2011;191: 76–79.

161. Jorge RE, Robinson RG, Moser D, Tateno A, Crespo-Facorro B, Arndt S. Major depression following traumatic brain injury. *Arch Gen Psychiatry* 2004;61: 42–50.

162. Fayol PP. Non-pharmacological treatment of neurobehavioural disorders following severe traumatic brain injury. A commented literature review. *Ann Réadapt Méd Phys* 2003;46: 97–103.

163. Gertler P, Tate RL, Cameron ID. Non-pharmacological interventions for depression in adults and children with traumatic brain injury. *Cochrane Database System Rev* 2015;12: CD009871.

164. Simpson GK, Tate RL, Whiting DL, Cotter RE. Suicide prevention after traumatic brain injury: a randomized controlled trial of a program for the psychological treatment of hopelessness. *J Head Trauma Rehabil* 2011;26: 290–300.

165. Bédard M, Felteau M, Marshall S, Dubois S, Gibbons C, Klein R, et al. Mindfulness-based cognitive therapy: benefits in reducing depression following a traumatic brain injury. *Adv Mind Body Med* 2012;26: 14–20.

166. Bédard M, Felteau M, Marshall S, Cullen N, Gibbons C, Dubois S, et al. Mindfulness-based cognitive therapy reduces symptoms of depression in people with a traumatic brain injury: results from a randomized controlled trial. *J Head Trauma Rehabil* 2013;29: E13–E22.

167. Fann JR, Bombardier CH, Vannoy S, Dyer J, Ludman E, Dikmen S, et al. Telephone and in-person cognitive behavioral therapy for major depression after traumatic brain injury: a randomized controlled trial. *J Neurotrauma* 2015;32: 45–57.

168. Ashman T, Cantor J, Tsaousides T, Spielman L, Gordon W. Comparison of cognitive behavioral therapy and supportive psychotherapy for the treatment of depression following traumatic brain injury: a randomized controlled trial. *J Head Trauma Rehabil* 2014;29: 467–478.

169. Hoffman JM, Bell KR, Powell JM, Behr J, Dunn EC, Dikmen S, et al. Randomized controlled trial of exercise to improve mood after traumatic brain injury. *Phys Med Rehabil* 2010;2: 911–919.

170. He CS, Yu Q, Yang DJ, Yang M. Interventional effects of low-frequency repetitive transcranial magnetic stimulation on patients with depression after traumatic brain injury. *Chin J Clin Rehabil* 2004;8: 6044–6045.

171. Reti IM, Schwarz N, Bower A, Tibbs M, Rao V. Transcranial magnetic stimulation: a potential new treatment for depression associated with traumatic brain injury, *Brain Inj* 2015;29: 789–797.

172. Baker-Price LA, Persinger MA. Weak, but complex pulsed magnetic fields may reduce depression following traumatic brain injury. *Percept Motor Skills* 1996;83: 491–498.

173. George MS, Raman R, Benedek DM, Pelic CG, Grammer GG, Stokes KT, et al. A two-site pilot randomized 3 day trial of high dose left prefrontal repetitive transcranial magnetic stimulation (rTMS) for suicidal inpatients. *Brain Stim* 2014;7: 421–431.

174. Wiart L, Luauté J, Stefan A, Plantier D, Hamonet J. Non pharmacological treatments for psychological and behavioural disorders following traumatic brain injury (TBI). A systematic literature review and expert opinion leading to recommendations. *Ann Phys Rehabil Med* 2016;59: 31–41.

175. Schonberger M, Humle F, Zeeman P, Teasdale TW. Patient compliance in brain injury rehabilitation in relation to awareness and cognitive and physical improvement. *Neuropsychol Rehabil* 2006;16: 561–578.

176. Guetin S, Soua B, Voiriot G, Picot MC, Herisson C. The effect of music therapy on mood and anxiety-depression: an observational study in institutionalised patients with traumatic brain injury. *Ann Phys Rehabil Med* 2009;52: 30–40.

177. Hofer H, Holtforth MG, Frischknecht E, Znoj H-J. Fostering adjustment to acquired brain injury by psychotherapeutic interventions: a preliminary study. *Appl Neuropsychol* 2010;17: 18–26.

178. Deb S, Crownshaw T. Review of subject. The role of pharmacotherapy in the management of behaviour disorders in traumatic brain injury patients. *Brain Inj* 2004;18: 1–31.

179. Chew E, Zafonte RD. Pharmacological management of neurobehavioral disorders following traumatic brain injury – a state-of-the-art review. *JRRD* 2009;46: 851–878.

180. Wheaton P, Mathias JL, Vink R. Impact of pharmacological treatments on cognitive and behavioral outcome in the postacute stages of adult traumatic brain injury: a meta-analysis. *J Clin Psychopharmacol* 2011;31: 745–757.

181. Plantier D, Luauté J, the SOFMER group. Drugs for behavior disorders after traumatic brain injury: systematic review and expert consensus leading to French recommendations for good practice. *Ann Phys Rehabil Med* 2016;59: 42–57.

182. Alderfer BS, Arciniegas DB, Silver JM. Treatment of depression following traumatic brain injury. *J Head Trauma Rehabil* 2005;20: 544–562.

183. Silver JM, McAllister TW, Arciniegas DB. Depression and cognitive complaints following mild traumatic brain injury. *Am J Psychiatry* 2009;166: 653–661.

184. Saran AS. Depression after minor closed head injury: role of dexamethasone suppression test and antidepressants. *J Clin Psychiatry* 1985;46: 335–338.

185. Dinan TG, Mobayed M. Treatment resistance of depression after head injury: a preliminary study of amitriptyline response. *Acta Psychiatr Scand* 1992;85: 292–294.

186. Fann JR, Uomoto JM. Katon WJ. Sertraline in the treatment of major depression following mild traumatic brain injury. *J Neuropsychiatry Clin Neurosci* 2000;12: 226–232.

187. Kanetani K, Kimura M, Endo S. Therapeutic effects of milnacipran (serotonin noradrenalin reuptake inhibitor) on depression following mild and moderate traumatic brain injury. *J Nippon Med Sch* 2003;70: 313–320.

188. Rapoport MJ, Chan F, Lanctot K, Herrmann N, McCullagh S, Feinstein A. An open-label study of citalopram for major

477

depression following traumatic brain injury. *J Psychopharmacol* 2008;22: 860–864.

189. Lee H, Kim S-W, Kim, J-M, Shin I-S, Yang S-U, Yoon J-S. Comparing effects of methylphenidate, sertraline and placebo on neuropsychiatric sequelae in patients with traumatic brain injury. *Hum Psychopharmacol Clin Exp* 2005;20: 97–104.

190. Ashman TA, Cantor JB, Gordon WA, Spielman L, Flanagan S, Ginsberg A, et al. A randomized controlled trial of sertraline for the treatment of depression in persons with traumatic brain injury. *Arch Phys Med Rehabil* 2009;90: 733–740.

191. Novack TA, Baños JH, Brunner R, Renfroe S, Meythaler JM. Impact of early administration of sertraline on depressive symptoms in the first year after traumatic brain injury. *J Neurotrauma* 2009;26: 1921–1928.

192. Lanctôt KL, Rapoport MJ, Chan F, Rajaram RD, Strauss J, Sicard T, et al. Genetic predictors of response to treatment with citalopram in depression secondary to traumatic brain injury. *Brain Inj* 2010;24: 959–969.

193. Kennedy SH, Andersen HF, Thase ME. Escitalopram in the treatment of major depressive disorder: a meta-analysis. *Curr Med Res Opin* 2009;25: 161–175.

194. Favré P. [Clinical efficacy and achievement of a complete remission in depression: increasing interest in treatment with escitalopram.] *Encephale* 2012;38: 86–96.

195. Lim SW, Shiue YL, Liao JC, Wee HY, Wang CC, Chio CC, et al. Simvastatin therapy in the acute stage of traumatic brain injury attenuates brain trauma-induced depression-like behavior in rats by reducing neuroinflammation in the hippocampus. *Neurocrit Care* 2017;26: 122–132.

196. Achté KA, Lönnqvist J, Hillbom E. Suicides following war brain-injuries. *Acta Psychiatr Scand Suppl* 1971;225: 1–94.

197. Teasdale TW, Engberg AW. Suicide after traumatic brain injury: a population study. *J Neurol Neurosurg Psychiatry* 2001;71: 436–440.

198. Richard YF, Swaine BR, Sylvestre MP, Lesage A, Zhang X, Feldman DE. The association between traumatic brain injury and suicide: are kids at risk? *Am J Epidemiol* 2015;182: 177–184.

199. Kesinger MR, Juengst SB, Bertisch H, Niemeier JP, Krellman JW, Pugh MJ, et al. Acute trauma factor associations with suicidality across the first 5 years after traumatic brain injury. *Arch Phys Med Rehabil* 2016;97: 1301–1308.

200. Williams CL, Davidson JA, Montgomery I. Impulsive suicidal behavior. *J Clin Psychol* 1980;36: 90–94.

201. Simon TR, Swann AC, Powell KE, Potter LB, Kresnow M-j, O'Carroll PW. Characteristics of impulsive suicide attempts and attempters. *Suicide Life-Threatening Behav* 2001;32(Suppl): 49–59.

202. Eddleston M, Phillips MR. Self poisoning with pesticides. *BMJ* 2004;328: 42–44.

203. Eddleston M, Buckley NA, Gunnell D, Dawson AH, Konradsen F. Identification of strategies to prevent death after pesticide self-poisoning using a Haddon matrix. *Inj Prev* 2006;12: 333–337.

204. Hawton K, Harriss L. Deliberate self-harm in young people: characteristics and subsequent mortality in a 20-year cohort of patients presenting to hospital. *J Clin Psychiatry* 2007;68: 1574–1583.

205. Hawton K, Harriss L. Deliberate self-harm by under-15-year-olds: characteristics, trends and outcome. *J Child Psychol Psychiatry* 2008;49: 441–448.

206. Deisenhammer EA, Hofer S, Schwitzer O, Defrancesco M, Kemmler G, Wildt L, et al. Oxytocin plasma levels in psychiatric patients with and without recent suicide attempt. *Psychiatry Res* 2012;200: 59–62.

207. Simpson G, Tate R. Suicidality in people surviving a traumatic brain injury: prevalence, risk factors and implications for clinical management. *Brain Inj* 2007;21: 1335–1351.

208. Feldman MD, Franks P, Duberstein PR, Vannoy S, Epstein R, Kravitz RL. Let's not talk about it: suicide inquiry in primary care. *Ann Fam Med* 2007;5: 412–418.

209. McDowell AK, Lineberry TW, Bostwick JM. Practical suicide-risk management for the busy primary care physician. *Mayo Clin Proc* 2011;86: 792–800.

210. Panagioti M, Gooding P, Tarrier N. Post-traumatic stress disorder and suicidal behavior: a narrative review. *Clin Psychol Rev* 2009;29: 471–482.

211. Collett GA, Song K, Jaramillo CA, Potter JS, Finley EP. Prevalence of central nervous system polypharmacy and associations with overdose and suicide-related behaviors in Iraq and Afghanistan war veterans in VA Care 2010–2011. *Drugs Real World Outcomes* 2016;3: 45–52.

212. Horowitz LM, Ballard ED, Pao M. Suicide screening in schools, primary care and emergency departments. *Curr Opin Pediatr* 2009;21: 620–627.

213. Mauerhofer A, Berchtold A, Michaud P-A, Suris J-C. GPs' role in the detection of psychological problems of young people: a population-based study. *Br J Gen Pract* 2009;59: e308–e314.

214. U.S. Preventive Services Task Force (USPSTF). The guide to clinical preventive services 2014: recommendations of the U.S. Preventive Services Task Force. Available at www.ahrq.gov/professionals/clinicians-providers/guidelines-recommendations/index.html.

215. Rickwood DJ, Deane FP,Wilson CJ. When and how do young people seek professional help for mental health problems? *Med J Aust* 2007;187: S35–S39.

216. Horowitz L, Ballard E, Teach SJ, Bosk A, Rosenstein DL, Joshi P, et al. Feasibility of screening patients with nonpsychiatric complaints for suicide risk in a pediatric emergency department: a good time to talk? *Pediatr Emerg Care* 2010;26: 787–792.

217. Gold A, Appelbaum PS, Stanley B. Screening for suicidality in the emergency department: when must researchers act to protect subjects' interests? *Arch Suicide Res* 2011;15: 140–150.

218. World Health Organization. *Towards evidence-based suicide prevention programs.* Geneva, Switzerland: WHO, 2010.

219. Haute Autorité de Santé. *Recommandations de bonne pratique. Manifestations dépressives à l'adolescence. Repérage, diagnostic et stratégie des soins de premier recours.* Paris: HAS, 2014.

220. American Academy of Pediatrics Committee on Adolescence. Suicide and suicide attempts in adolescents. Committee on Adolescents. American Academy of Pediatrics. *Pediatrics* 2000;105: 871–874.

221. Pena JB, Caine ED. Screening as an approach for adolescent suicide prevention. *Suicide Life Threat Behav* 2006;36: 614–637.

222. Gould MS, Marrocco FA, Hoagwood K, Kleinman M, Amakawa L, Altschuler E. Service use by at-risk youths after school-based suicide screening. *J Am Acad Child Adolesc Psychiatry* 2009;48: 1193–1201.

223. Hawton K, Saunders KE, O'Connor RC. Self-harm and suicide in adolescents. *Lancet* 2012;379: 2373–2382.

224. Reynolds W. *Suicide Ideation Questionnaire: professional manual.* Odessa: Psychological Assessment Resources, 1988.

225. Reynolds W, Mazza J. Assessment of suicidal ideation in innercity children and young adolescents: reliability and validity of the Suicidal Ideation Questionnaire-JR. *School Psych Rev* 1999;28: 17–30.

226. Horowitz LM, Wang PS, Koocher GP, Burr BH, Smith MF, Klavon S et al. Detecting suicide risk in a pediatric emergency department: development of a brief screening tool. *Pediatrics* 2001;107: 1133–1137.

227. Osman AB. The Suicidal Behaviors Questionnaire Revised: validation with clinical and nonclinical samples. *Assessment* 2001;8: 443–454.

228. Binder P, Heintz A-L, Servant C, Roux M-T, Robin S, Gicque L, et al. Screening for adolescent suicidality in primary care: the bullying–insomnia–tobacco–stress test. A population-based pilot study. *Early Intervent Psychiatry* 2016; doi: 10.1111/eip.12352.

229. Sukhawaha S, Arunpongpaisal S, Cameron Hurst C. Development and psychometric properties of the Suicidality of Adolescent Screening Scale (SASS) using multidimensional item response theory. *Psychiatry Res* 2016;243: 431–438.

230. Radloff LS. The CES-D Scale: a self-report depression scale for research in the general population. *Appl Psychol Measur* 1977;1: 385–401.

231. Cheung YB, Liu KY, Yip PS. Performance of the CES-D and its short forms in screening suicidality and hopelessness in the community. *Suicide Life Threat Behav* 2007;37: 79–88.

232. Van Orden KA, Witte TK, Gordon KH, Bender TW, Joiner TE. Suicidal desire and the capability for suicide: tests of the interpersonal-psychological theory of suicidal behavior among adults. *J Consult Clin Psychol* 2008;76: 72–83.

233. Smith K, Conroy RW, Ehler BD. Lethality of Suicide Attempts Rating Scale. *Suicide Life Threat Behav* 1984;14: 215–242.

234. Fann JR, Bombardier CH, Dikmen S, Esselman P, Warms CA, Pelzer E, et al. Validity of the Patient Health Questionnaire-9 in assessing depression following traumatic brain injury. *J Head Trauma Rehabil* 2005;20: 501–511.

235. Simon GE, Rutter CM, Peterson D, Oliver M, Whiteside U, Operskalski B, et al. Does response on the PHQ-9 Depression Questionnaire predict subsequent suicide attempt or suicide death? *Psychiatr Serv* 2013;64: 1195–1202.

236. Posner K, Brown GK, Stanley B, Brent DA, Yershova KV, Oquendo MA, et al. The Columbia–Suicide Severity Rating Scale: initial validity and internal consistency findings from three multisite studies with adolescents and adults. *Am J Psychiatry* 2011;168: 1266–1277.

237. Shavelle RM, Strauss D, Whyte J, Day SM, Yu YL. Long-term causes of death after traumatic brain injury. *Am J Phys Med Rehabil* 2001;80: 510–516.

238. Silver JM, Kramer R, Greenwald S, Weissman M. The association between head injuries and psychiatric disorders: findings from the New Haven NIMH epidemiologic catchment area study. *Brain Inj* 2001;15: 935–945.

239. Simpson G, Tate R. Suicidality in people surviving a traumatic brain injury: prevalence, risk factors and implications for clinical management. *Brain Inj* 2007;21: 1335–1351.

240. Bahraini NH, Simpson GK, Brenner LA, Hoffberg AS, Schneider AL. Suicidal ideation and behaviours after traumatic brain injury: a systematic review. *Brain Impair* 2013;14 (Special Issue 01): 92–112.

241. Miller H, Stern G. Long-term prognosis of severe head injury. *Lancet* 1965;i: 225–229.

242. Fahy TJ, Irving MH, Millac P. Severe head injuries. *Lancet* 1967;i: 475–479.

243. Wilkinson MIP. The prognosis of severe head injuries in young adults. *Proc R Soc Med* 1969;62: 541–542.

244. Heiskanen O, Sipponen P. Prognosis for severe brain injury. *Acta Neurol Scand* 1970;46: 343–348.

245. Lewin W, Marshal TF, De C, Roberts AH. Long-term outcome after severe head injury. *Br Med J* 1979;ii: 33–38.

246. Harris EC, Barraclough B. Suicide as an outcome for mental disorders. A meta-analysis. *Br J Psychiatry* 1997;170: 205–228.

247. Mann JJ, Waternaux C, Haas GL, Malone KM. Toward a clinical model of suicidal behavior in psychiatric patients. *Am J Psychiatry* 1999;156: 181–189.

248. Roberts AH. *Severe accidental head injury. An assessment of long-term prognosis*. London: MacMillan, 1979.

249. Wilson BA. Life after brain injury: long term outcome of 101 people seen for rehabilitation 5–12 years earlier. In: Fourez J, Page N, eds. *Treatment issues and long term outcomes*. Bowen Hills, Queensland: Australian Academic Press, 1994, pp. 1–6.

250. Klonoff PS, Lage GA. Suicide in patients with traumatic brain injury: risk and prevention. *J Head Trauma Rehabil* 1995;10: 16–24.

251. Tate R, Simpson G, Flanagan S, Coffey M. Completed suicide after traumatic brain injury. *J Head Trauma Rehabil* 1997;12: 16–28.

252. Gutierrez PM, Brenner LA, Huggins JA. A preliminary investigation of suicidality in psychiatrically hospitalized veterans with traumatic brain injury. *Arch Suicide Res* 2008;12: 336–343.

253. Harrison-Felix CL, Whiteneck GG, Jha A, DeVivo MJ, Hammond FM, Hart DM. Mortality over four decades after traumatic brain injury rehabilitation: a retrospective cohort study. *Arch Phys Med Rehabil* 2009;90: 1506–1513.

254. Simpson G, Tate R. Suicidality after traumatic brain injury: demographic, injury, and clinical correlates. *Psychol Med* 2002;32: 687–697.

255. Oquendo MA, Friedman JH, Grunebaum MF, Burke A, Silver JM, Mann JJ. Suicidal behavior and mild traumatic brain injury in major depression. *J Nerv Ment Dis* 2004;192: 430–434.

256. Simpson G, Tate R. Clinical featuresof suicide attempts after traumatic brain injury. *J Nerv Mental Dis* 2005;193: 680–685.

257. Mainio A, Kyllönen T, Viilo K, Hakko H, Särkioja T, Räsänen P. Traumatic brain injury, psychiatric disorders and suicide: a population-based study of suicide victims during the years 1988–2004 in Northern Finland. *Brain Inj* 2007;21: 851–855.

258. Brenner LA, Vanderploeg RD, Terrio H. Assessment and diagnosis of mild traumatic brain injury, posttraumatic stress disorder, and other polytrauma conditions: burden of adversity hypothesis. *Rehabil Psychol* 2009;54: 239–246.

259. Brenner L, Ignacio R, Blow F. Suicide and traumatic brain injury among individuals seeking Veterans Health Administration services. *J Head Trauma Rehab* 2011;26: 257–264.

260. Tsaousides T, Cantor JB, Gordon WA. Suicidal ideation following traumatic brain injury. *J Head Trauma Rehabil* 2011;26: 265–275.

261. Olson-Madden JH, Forster JE, Huggins J, Schneider A. Psychiatric diagnoses, mental health utilization, high-risk behaviors, and self-directed violence among veterans with comorbid history of traumatic brain injury and substance use disorders. *J Head Trauma Rehabil* 2012;27: 370–378.

262. Bryan CJ, Clemans TA, Hernandez AM, Rudd MD. Loss of consciousness, depression, posttraumatic stress disorder, and suicide risk among deployed military personnel with mild traumatic brain injury. *J Head Trauma Rehabil* 2013;28: 13–20.

263. Brickell TA, Lange RT, French LM. Health-related quality of life within the first 5 years following military-related concurrent mild traumatic brain injury and polytrauma. *Mil Med* 2014;179: 827–838.

264. Ilie G, Mann RE, Boak A, Adlaf EM, Hamilton H, Asbridge M, Rehm J, Cusimano MD. Suicidality, bullying and other conduct and mental health correlates of traumatic brain injury in adolescents. *PLoS ONE* 2014;9: e94936.

265. Mackelprang JL, Bombardier CH, Fann JR, Temkin NR, Barber JK, Dikmen SS. Rates and predictors of suicidal ideation during the first year after traumatic brain injury. *Am J Public Health* 2014;104: e100–e107.

266. Wisco BE, Marx BP, Holowka DW, Vasterling JJ, Han SC, Chen MS, et al. Traumatic brain injury, PTSD, and current suicidal ideation among Iraq and Afghanistan U.S. veterans. *J Trauma Stress* 2014;27: 244–248.

267. Finley EP, Bollinger M, Noël PH, Amuan ME, Copeland LA, Pugh JA, et al. A national cohort study of the association between the polytrauma clinical triad and suicide-related behavior

among US veterans who served in Iraq and Afghanistan. *Am J Public Health* 2015;105: 380–387.

268. Gradus JL, Wisco BE, Luciano MT, Iverson KM, Marx BP, Street AE. Traumatic brain injury and suicidal ideation among U.S. Operation Enduring Freedom and Operation Iraqi Freedom veterans. *J Trauma Stress* 2015;28: 361–365.

269. Schneider AL, Hostetter TA, Homaifar BY, Forster JE, Olson-Madden JH, Matarazzo BB, et al. Responses to traumatic brain injury screening questions and suicide attempts among those seeking Veterans Health Administration mental health services. *Front Psychiatry* 2016;7: 59.

270. Skopp NA, Trofimovich L, Grimes J, Oetjen-Gerdes L, Gahm GA. Relations between suicide and traumatic brain injury, psychiatric diagnoses, and relationship problems, active component, U.S. Armed Forces, 2001–2009. *MSMR* 2012;19: 7–11.

271. Bullman TA, Kang HK. Posttraumatic stress disorder and the risk of traumatic deaths among Vietnam veterans. *J Nerv Mental Dis* 1994;182: 604–610.

272. Bell JB, Nye EC. Specific symptoms predict suicidal ideation in Vietnam combat veterans with chronic post-traumatic stress disorder. *Mil Med* 2007;172: 1144–1147.

273. Jakupcak M, Vannoy S, Imel Z, Cook JW, Fontana A, Rosenheck R, et al. Does PTSD moderate the relationship between social support and suicide risk in Iraq and Afghanistan war veterans seeking mental health treatment? *Depress Anxiety* 2010;27: 1001–1005.

274. Simpson GK, Brenner LA. Perspectives on suicide and traumatic brain injury. *J Head Trauma Rehabil* 2011;26: 241–243.

275. Barnes SM, Walter KH, Chard KM. Does a history of mild traumatic brain injury increase suicide risk in veterans with PTSD? *Rehabil Psychol* 2012;57: 18–26.

276. Betz ME, Miller M, Barber C, Betty B, Miller I, Camargo CA, Bourdreaux ED. Lethal means access and assessment among suicidal emergency department patients. *Depress Anxiety* 2016;33: 502–511.

277. Gunter TD, Chibnall JT, Antoniak SK, Philibert RA, Black DW. Childhood trauma, traumatic brain injury, and mental health disorders associated with suicidal ideation and suicide-related behavior in a community corrections sample. *J Am Acad Psychiatry Law* 2013;41: 245–255.

278. Oquendo MA, Sullivan GM, Sudol K, Baca-Garcia E, Stanley BH, Sublette ME, et al. Toward a biosignature for buicide. *Am J Psychiatry* 2014;171: 1259–1277.

279. Lopez-Larson M, King JB, McGlade E, Bueler E, Stoeckel A, Epstein DJ, et al. Enlarged thalamic volumes and increased fractional anisotropy in the thalamic radiations in veterans with suicide behaviors. *Front Psychiatry* 2013;4: 83.

280. Young KA, Bonkale WL, Holcomb LA, Hicks PB, German DC. Major depression, 5HTTLPR genotype, suicide and anti-depressant influences on thalamic volume. *Br J Psychiatry* 2008;192: 285–289.

281. Amen DG, Prunella JR, Fallon JH, Amen B, Hanks C. A comparative analysis of completed suicide using high resolution brain SPECT imaging. *J Neuropsychiatry Clin Neurosci* 2009;21: 430–439.

282. Coenen VA, Panksepp J, Hurwitz TA, Urbach H, Madler B. Human medial forebrain bundle (MFB) and anterior thalamic radiation (ATR): imaging of two major subcortical pathways and the dynamic balance of opposite affects in understanding depression. *J Neuropsychiatry Clin Neurosci* 2012;24: 223–236.

283. Matthews S, Spadoni A, Knox K, Strigo I, Simmons A. Combat-exposed war veterans at risk for suicide show hyperactivation of prefrontal cortex and anterior cingulate during error processing. *Psychosom Med* 2012;74: 471–475.

284. Kumar A, Loane DJ. Neuroinflammation after traumatic brain injury: opportunities for therapeutic intervention. *Brain Behav Immun* 2012;26: 1191–1201.

285. Brundin L, Erhardt S, Bryleva EY, Achtyes ED, Postolache TT. The role of inflammation in suicidal behavior. *Acta Psychiatr Scand* 2015;132: 192–203.

286. Brundin L, Bryleva EY, Rajamani KY. Role of inflammation in suicide: from mechanisms to treatment. *Neuropsychopharmacol* 2017;42: 271–283.

287. Bryleva EY, Brundin L. Kynurenine pathway metabolites and suicidality. *Neuropharmacology* 2017;112: 324–330.

288. Juengst SB, Kumar RG, Arenth PM, Wagner AK. Exploratory associations with tumor necrosis factor alpha, disinhibition and suicidal endorsement after traumatic brain injury. *Brain Behav Immun* 2014;41: 134–143.

289. Timonen M, Miettunen J, Hakko H, Zitting P, Veijola J, von Wendt L, et al. The association of preceding traumatic brain injury with mental disorders, alcoholism and criminality: the Northern Finland 1966 Birth Cohort Study. *Psychiatry Res* 2002;113: 217–226.

290. Baguley IJ, Cooper J, Felmingham K. Aggressive behavior following traumatic brain injury: how common is common? *J Head Trauma Rehabil* 2006;21: 45–56.

291. Rao V, Rosenberg P, Bertrand M, Salehinia S, Spiro J, Vaishnavi S, et al. Aggression after traumatic brain injury: prevalence and correlates. *J Neuropsychiatry Clin Neurosci* 2009;21: 420–429.

292. Farrer TJ, Hedges DW. Prevalence of traumatic brain injury in incarcerated groups compared to the general population: a meta-analysis. *Prog Neuropsychopharmacol Biol Psychiatry* 2011;35: 390–394.

293. Luukkainen S, Riala K, Laukkanen M, Hakko H, Räsänen P. Association of traumatic brain injury with criminality in adolescent psychiatric inpatients from Northern Finland. *Psychiatry Res* 2012;200: 767–772.

294. McKinlay A, Grace RC, McLellan T, Roger D, Clarbour J, MacFarlane MR. Predicting adult offending behavior for individuals who experienced a traumatic brain injury during childhood. *J Head Trauma Rehabil* 2014;29: 507–513.

295. Moore E, Indig D, Haysom L. Traumatic brain injury, mental health, substance use, and offending among incarcerated young people. *J Head Trauma Rehabil* 2014;29: 239–247.

296. O'Rourke C, Linden MA, Lohan M, Bates-Gaston J. Traumatic brain injury and co-occurring problems in prison populations: a systematic review. *Brain Inj* 2016;30: 839–854.

297. Karli P. The neurobiology of aggressive behaviour. *CR Biol* 2006;329: 460–464.

298. Nelson RJ, Trainor BC. Neural mechanisms of aggression. *Nat Rev Neurosci* 2007;8: 536–546.

299. Patrick CJ. Psychophysiological correlates of aggression and violence: an integrative review. *Philos Trans R Soc Lond B Biol Sci* 2008;363: 2543–2555.

300. Rosell DR, Siever LJ. The neurobiology of aggression and violence. *CNS Spectr* 2015;20: 254–279.

301. Victoroff J. The neuropsychiatry of human aggression. In Sadock BJ, Sadock VA, Ruiz P, editors. *Kaplan and Sadock comprehensive textbook of psychiatry*, tenth edition. Philadelphia, PA: Wolters Kluwer, 2017, pp. 2471–2504.

302. Hikosaka O. The habenula: from stress evasion to value based decision-making. *Nat Rev Neurosci* 2010;11: 503–513.

303. Ely BA, Xu J, Goodman WK, Lapidus KA, Gabbay V, Stern ER. Resting-state functional connectivity of the human habenula in

304. Prigatano GP. Personality disturbances associated with traumatic brain injury. *J Counsel Clin Psychol* 1992;60: 360–368.

305. Hanks RA, Temkin N, Machamer J, Dikmen SS. Emotional and behavioral adjustment after traumatic brain injury. *Arch Phys Med Rehabil* 1999;80: 991–997.

306. Demark J, Monica Gemeinhardt M. Anger and its management for survivors of acquired brain injury. *Brain Inj* 2002;16: 91–108.

307. Dougherty DD, Shin LM, Alpert NM, Pitman RK, Orr SP, Lasko M, et al. Anger in healthy men: a PET study using script-driven imagery. *Biol Psychiatry* 1999;46: 466–472.

308. Soliman A, Bagby RM, Wilson AA, Miler L, Clark M, Rusjan P, et al. Relationship of monoamine oxidase A binding to adaptive and maladaptive personality traits. *Psychol Med* 2011;41: 1051–1060.

309. Peper JS, de Reus MA, van den Heuvel MP, Schutter DJ. Short fused? associations between white matter connections, sex steroids, and aggression across adolescence. *Hum Brain Mapp* 2015;36: 1043–1052.

310. Dretsch MN, Silverberg N, Gardner AJ, Panenka WJ, Emmerich T, Crynen G, et al. Genetics and other risk factors for past concussions in active-duty soldiers. *J Neurotrauma* 2017;34: 869–875.

311. Nakagawa S, Takeuchi H, Taki Y, Nouchi R, Sekiguchi A, Kotozaki Y, et al. The anterior midcingulate cortex as a neural node underlying hostility in young adults. *Brain Struct Funct* 2017;222: 61–70.

312. Mathias CW, Stanford MS, Marsh DM, Frick PJ, Moeller FG, Swann AC, et al. Characterizing aggressive behavior with the impulsive/premeditated aggression scale among adolescents with conduct disorder. *Psychiatry Res* 2007;151: 231–242.

313. Fung AL, Raine A, Gao Y. Cross-cultural generalizability of the reactive-proactive aggression questionnaire (RPQ). *J Pers Assess* 2009;91: 473–479.

314. Wood RL, Thomas RH. Impulsive and episodic disorders of aggressive behaviour following traumatic brain injury. *Brain Inj* 2013;27: 253–261.

315. Yang C-C, Hua M-S, Lin W-C, Tsai Y-H, Huang S-J. Irritability following traumatic brain injury: divergent manifestations of annoyance and verbal aggression. *Brain Inj* 2012;26: 1185–1191.

316. Kim SH, Manes F, Kosier T, Baruah S, Robinson RG. Irritability following traumatic brain injury. *J Nerv Ment Dis* 1999;187: 327–335.

317. Alderman N. Contemporary approaches to the management of irritability and aggression following traumatic brain injury. *Neuropsychol Rehabil* 2003;13: 211–240.

318. Neumann D, Malec JF, Hammond FM. The association of negative attributions with irritation and anger after brain injury. *Rehabil Psychol* 2015;60: 155–161.

319. Deb S, Lyons I, Koutzoukis C. Neuropsychiatric sequelae one year after a minor head injury. *J Neurol Neurosurg Psychiatry* 1998;65: 899–902.

320. Luauté J, Plantier D, Wiart L, Tell L, The SOFMER group. Care management of the agitation or aggressiveness crisis in patients with TBI. Systematic review of the literature and practice recommendations. *Ann Phys Med Rehabil Med* 2016;59: 58–67.

321. Herbel K, Schermerhorn L, Howard, J. Management of agitated head-injured patients: a survey of current techniques. *Rehabil Nurs* 1990;15: 66–69.

322. Weir N, Doig EJ, Fleming JM, Wiemers A, Zemljic C. Objective and behavioural assessment of the emergence from post-traumatic amnesia (PTA). *Brain Inj* 2006;20: 927–935.

323. Lombard LA, Zafonte RD. Agitation after traumatic brain injury: considerations and treatment options. *Am J Phys Med Rehabil* 2005;84: 797–812.

324. Nott MT, Chapparo C, Baguley IJ. Agitation following traumatic brain injury: an Australian sample. *Brain Inj* 2006;20: 1175–1182.

325. Phelps TI, Bondi CO, Mattiola VV, Kline AE. Relative to typical antipsychotic drugs, aripiprazole is a safer alternative for alleviating behavioral disturbances after experimental brain trauma. *Neurorehabil Neural Repair* 2017;31: 25–33.

326. American Psychiatric Association. *Diagnostic and statistical manual of mental disorders*, 2nd edition. Washington, DC: American Psychiatric Press, 1968.

327. American Psychiatric Association. *Diagnostic and statistical manual of mental disorders*, 3rd edition. Washington, DC: American Psychiatric Press, 1980.

328. Morrison JR, Minkoff K. Explosive personality as a sequel to the hyperactive-child syndrome. *Compr Psychiatry* 1975;16: 343–348.

329. Bach-y-Rita G, Lion JR, Climent CE, Ervin FR. Episodic dyscontrol: a study of 130 violent patients. *Am J Psychiatry* 1971;127: 49–54.

330. Elliott FA. The episodic dyscontrol syndrome and aggression. *Neurol Clin* 1984;2: 113–125.

331. Lewin J, Sumners D. Successful treatment of episodic dyscontrol with carbamazepine. *Br J Psychiatry* 1992;161: 261–262.

332. Caine TM, Foulds GA, Hope K. *Manual of the Hostility and Direction of Hostility Questionnaire (HDHQ)*. London, UK: University of London Press, 1967.

333. Arrindell WA, Hafkenscheid AJPM, Emmelkamp PMG. The Hostility and Direction of Hostility Questionnaire (HDHQ): a psychometric evaluation in psychiatric outpatients. *Personality Individ Diff* 1984;5: 221–231.

334. Spielberger CD, Jacobs G, Russell S, Crane RS. Assessment of anger: the State-Trait Anger Scale. In Butcher JN, Spielberger CD, editors. *Advances in personality assessment*. Hillsdale, NJ: Lawrence Erlbaum Associates, 1983, pp. 161–189.

335. Siegel JM. The Multidimensional Anger Inventory. *J Personal Social Psychol* 1986;51: 191–200.

336. Kroner DG, Reddon JR, Serin RC. The Multidimensional Anger Inventory: reliability and factor structure in an inmate sample. *Educ Psychol Measur* 1992;52: 687–693.

337. Spielberger CD. *Manual for the State-Trait Anger Expression Inventory (STAXI)*. Odessa, FL: Psychological Assessment Resources, 1988.

338. Plutchik R, van Praag HM. A Self-Report Measure of Violence Risk, II. *Compr Psychiatry* 1990;3: 450–456.

339. Buss AH, Perry M. The Aggression Questionnaire. *J Personal Soc Psychol* 1992;63: 452–459.

340. Bryant FB, Smith BD. Refining the architecture of aggression: a measurement model for the Buss–Perry Aggression Questionnaire. *J Res Personal* 2001;35: 138–167.

341. Straus MA. Measuring intrafamily conflict and violence: the Conflict Tactics Scales. *J Marriage Family* 1979;41: 75–88.

342. Straus MA. *Manual fur the Conflict Tactics Scales*. Durham, NH: Family Research Laboratory, University of New Hampshire, 1995.

343. Yudofsky SC, Silver JM, Jackson W, Endicott J, Williams D. The Overt Aggression Scale for the objective rating of verbal and physical aggression. *Am J Psychiatry* 1986;143: 35–39.

344. Wistedt, B, Rasmussen A, Pedersen L, Malm U, Träskman-Bendz, L, Wakelin J, et al. The development of an observer-scale for measuring social dysfunction and aggression. *Pharmacopsychiatry* 1990;23: 249–252.

345. Sorgi P, Ratey J, Knoedler DW, Markert RJ, Reichman M. Rating aggression in the clinical setting: a retrospective adaptation of the

481

Overt Aggression Scale: preliminary results. *J Neuropsychiatry Clin Neurosci* 1991;3: S52–S56.

346. Bech P. *Rating scales for psychopathology, health status and quality of life: a compendium on documentation in accordance with the DSM-III-R and WHO systems.* Amsterdam: Springer Verlag, 1993.

347. Straus MA, Hamhy SL, Boney-McCoy S, Sugarman DB. The revised Conflict Tactics Scales (CTS2): development and preliminary psychometric data. *J Family Issues* 1996;17: 283–316.

348. Giles GM, Mohr JD. Overview and inter-rater reliability of an incident-based rating scale for aggressive behaviour following traumatic brain injury: the Overt Aggression Scale–Modified for Neurorehabiltation–Extended (OAS-MNR-E). *Brain Inj* 2007;21: 505–511.

349. Goldberg DP. The detection of psychiatric illness by questionnaire; a technique for the identification and assessment of non-psychotic psychiatric illness. In: *Maudsley monographs*, vol. 21. London: Oxford University Press, 1972.

350. Schmitz N, Kruse J, Heckrath C, Alberti L, Tress W. Diagnosing mental disorders in primary care: the General Health Questionnaire (GHQ) and the Symptom Check List (SCL-90-R) as screening instruments. *Soc Psychiatry Psychiatr Epidemiol* 1999;34: 360–366.

351. Derogatis LR, Lipman RS, Covi L. SCL-90: an outpatient psychiatric rating scale – preliminary report. *Psychopharmacol Bull* 1973;9: 13–28.

352. Prinz U, Nutzinger DO, Schulz H, Petermann F, Braukhaus C, Andreas S. Comparative psychometric analyses of the SCL-90-R and its short versions in patients with affective disorders. *BMC Psychiatry* 2013;13: 104.

353. Achenbach TM, Rescorla LA. *Manual for the ASEBA adult forms and profiles.* Burlington, VT: University of Vermont, Research Center for Children, Youth, and Families, 2003.

354. Achenbach TM, Krukowski RA, Dumenci L, Ivanova MY. Assessment of adult psychopathology: meta-analyses and implications of cross-informant correlations. *Psychol Bull* 2005;131: 361–382.

355. Kay SR, Fiszbein A, Opler LA. The Positive and Negative Syndrome Scale (PANSS) for schizophrenia. *Schizophrenia Bull* 1987;13: 261–276.

356. Kay SR, Opler LA, Lindenmayer J-P. Reliability and validity of the positive and negative syndrome scale for schizophrenics. *Psychiatry Res* 1988;23: 99–110.

357. Morey LC. *Personality Assessment Inventory: professional manual (2nd edition).* Tampa, FL: Psychological Assessment Resources, 2007.

358. Tellegen A, Ben-Porath YS. *MMPI-2-RF (Minnesota Multiphasic Personality Inventory-2 Restructured Form): technical manual.* Minneapolis, MN: University of Minnesota Press, 2008/2011.

359. Graham JR. *MMPI-2: assessing personality and psychopathology (5th edition).* New York, NY: Oxford University Press, 2012.

360. Millon T. Millon C, Davis R, Grossman S. *MCMI-III manual (fourth edition).* Minneapolis, MN: Pearson Education, 2009.

361. Kreutzer JS, Leininger BE, Doherty K, Waaland PK. *General health and history questionnaire.* Richmond, VA: Medical College of Virginia, Rehabilitation Research and Training Center on Severe Brain Injury, 1987.

362. Kennedy RE, Livingston L, Riddick A, Marwitz JH, Kreutzer JS, Zasler ND. Evaluation of the Neurobehavioral Functioning Inventory as a depression screening tool after traumatic brain injury. *J Head Trauma Rehabil* 2005;20: 512–526.

363. Levin H, High WM, Goethe KE, Sisson RA, Overall JE, Rhoades HM, et al. The ncurobehavioral rating scale: assessment of the behavioral sequelae of head injury by the clinician. *J Neurol Neurosurg Psychiatry* 1987;50: 183–193.

364. McCauley SR, Boake C, Levin HS, Contant CF, Song JX. Postconcussional disorder following mild to moderate traumatic brain injury: anxiety, depression, and social support as risk factors and comorbidities. *J Clin Exp Neuropsychol* 2001;23: 792–808.

365. Cummings JL, Mega M, Gray K, Rosenberg-Thompson S, Carusi DA, Gornbein J. The neuropsychiatric inventory: comprehensive assessment of psychopathology in dementia. *Neurology* 1994;44: 2308–2314.

366. Cicerone KD, Kalmar K. Persistent postconcussion syndrome: the structure of subjective complaints after mTBI. *J Head Trauma Rehabil* 1995;10: 1–17.

367. King PR, Donnelly KT, Donnelly JP, Dunnam M, Warner G, Kittleson CJ, et al. Psychometric study of the Neurobehavioral Symptom Inventory. *J Rehabil Res Dev* 2012;49: 879–888.

368. Lezak MD. Relationships between personality disorders, social disturbances and physical disability following traumatic brain injury. *J Head Trauma Rehabil* 1987;2: 57–69.

369. Malec JF, Lezak MD. *Manual for the Mayo-Portland Adaptability Inventory (MPAI-4) for adults, children and adolescents.* 2003. Available at: www.tbims.org/mpai/manual.pdf.

370. Malec J. *The Mayo-Portland Adaptability Inventory.* The Center for Outcome Measurement in Brain Injury, 2005. Available at www.tbims.org/combi/mpai.

371. Fava M, Rosenbaum JF, McCarthy M, Pava J, Steingard R, Bless E. Anger attacks in depressed outpatients. *Psychopharmacol Bull* 1991;27: 275–279.

372. Fava M, Hwang I, Rush AJ, Sampson N, Walters EE, Kessler RC. The importance of irritability as a symptom of major depressive disorder: results from the national comorbidity survey replication. *Mol Psychiatry* 2010;15: 856–867.

373. Verhoeven FEA, Booij L, Van derWee NJA, Penninx BWHJ, Van der Does AJW. Clinical and physiological correlates of irritability in depression: results from the Netherlands study of depression and anxiety. *Depress Res Treat* 2010;2011: 126895.

374. Hayes N, Smith A, Berker E. Emergence and persistence of symptoms comprising the post-traumatic syndrome in 322 patients with closed head injury. *Arch Clin Neuropsychol* 1997;12: 333.

375. Van der Naalt J, van Zomeren AH, Sluiter WJ, Minderhoud JM. One year outcome in mild to moderate head injury: the predictive value of acute injury characteristics related to complaints and return to work. *J Neurol Neurosurg Psychiatry* 1999;66: 207–213.

376. van Zomeren AH, van den Burg W. Residual complaints of patients two years after severe head injury. *J Neurol Neurosurg Psychiatry* 1985;48: 21–28.

377. Haboubi NHJ, Long J, Koshy M, Ward AB. Short-term sequelae of minor head injury (6 years experience of minor head injury clinic). *Disabil Rehabil* 2001;23: 635–638.

378. Brooke MM, Questad KA, Patterson DR, Bashak KJ. Agitation and restlessness after closed head injury: a prospective study of 100 consecutive admissions. *Arch Phys Med Rehabil* 1992;73: 320–323.

379. Tateno A, Jorge RE, Robinson RG. Clinical correlates of aggressive behavior after traumatic brain injury. *J Neuropsychiatry Clin Neurosci* 2003;15: 155–160.

380. Kilmer RP, Demakis GJ, Hammond FM, Cook J, Grattan KE, Kornev AA. Use of the Neuropsychiatric Inventory in traumatic brain injury: a pilot investigation. *Rehabil Psychol* 2006;51: 232–238.

381. Ciurli P, Formisano R, Bivona U, Cantagallo A, Angelelli P. Neuropsychiatric disorders in persons with severe traumatic brain injury: prevalence, phenomenology, and relationship with demographic, clinical, and functional features. *J Head Trauma Rehabil* 2011;26: 116–126.

382. Hammond FM, Davis CS, Whiteside YO, Philbrick P, Hirsch MA. Marital adjustment and stability following traumatic brain injury: a pilot qualitative analysis of spouse perspectives. *J Head Trauma Rehabil* 2011;26: 69–78.

383. Saout V, Gambart G, Leguay D, Ferrapie AL, Launay C, Richard I. Aggressive behavior after traumatic brain injury. *Ann Phys Rehabil Med* 2011;54: 259–269.

384. Pardini M, Krueger F, Hodgkinson C, Raymont V, Ferrier C, Goldman D, et al. Prefrontal cortex lesions and MAO-A modulate aggression in penetrating traumatic brain injury. *Neurology* 2011;76: 1038–1045.

385. Craig IW. The importance of stress and genetic variation in human aggression. *Bioessays* 2007;29: 227–236.

386. Gietl A, Giegling I, Hartmann AM, Schneider B, Schnabel A, Maurer K, et al. ABCG1 gene variants in suicidal behavior and aggression-related traits. *Eur Neuropsychopharmacol* 2007;17: 410–416.

387. Rajender S, Pandu G, Sharma JD, Gandhi KPC, Singh L, Thangaraj K. Reduced CAG repeats length in androgen receptor gene is associated with violent criminal behavior. *Int J Legal Med* 2008;122: 367–372.

388. Reif A, Jacob CP, Rujescu D, Herterich S, Lang S, Gutknecht L, et al. Influence of functional variant of neuronal nitric oxide synthase on impulsive behaviors in humans. *Arch Gen Psychiatry* 2009;66: 41–50.

389. Anholt RR, Mackay TF. Genetics of aggression. *Annu Rev Genet* 2012;46: 145–164.

390. Pavlov KA, Chistiakov DA, Chekhonin VP. Genetic determinants of aggression and impulsivity in humans. *J Appl Genet* 2012;53: 61–82.

391. Malki K, Pain O, Du Rietz E, Tosto MG, Paya-Cano J, Sandnabba KN, et al. Genes and gene networks implicated in aggression related behaviour. *Neurogenetics* 2014;15: 255–266.

392. Waltes R, Chiocchetti AG, Freitag CM. The neurobiological basis of human aggression: a review on genetic and epigenetic mechanisms. *Am J Med Genet Part B* 2015;9999: 1–26.

393. Ramírez JM, Andreu JM. Aggression, and some related psychological constructs (anger, hostility, and impulsivity); some comments from a research project. *Neurosci Biobehav Rev* 2006;30: 276–291.

394. Pappa I, St Pourcain B, Benke K, Cavadino A, Hakulinen C, Nivard MG, et al. A genome-wide approach to children's aggressive behavior: the EAGLE consortium. *Am J Med Genet B Neuropsychiatr Genet* 2016;171: 562–572.

395. Craig D, Hart DJ, McCool K, McIlroy SP, Passmore AP. Apolipoprotein E-4 allele influences aggressive behaviour in Alzheimer's disease. *J Neurol Neurosurg Psychiatry* 2004;75: 1327–1330.

396. Beach SR, Brody GH, Todorov AA, Gunter TD, Philibert RA. Methylation at 5HTT mediates the impact of child sex abuse on women's antisocial behavior: an examination of the Iowa adoptee sample. *Psychosom Med* 2011;73: 83–87.

397. Booij L, Tremblay RE, Provençal N, Booij L, Tremblay RE. The developmental origins of chronic physical aggression: biological pathways triggered by early life adversity. *J Exp Biol* 2015;218: 123–133.

398. Provençal N, Binder EB. The neurobiological effects of stress as contributors to psychiatric disorders: focus on epigenetics. *Curr Opin Neurobiol* 2015;30: 31–37.

399. Yang J, Bellgowan PS, Martin A. Threat, domain-specificity and the human amygdala. *Neuropsychologia* 2012;50: 2566–2572.

400. Gold AL, Morey RA, McCarthy G. Amygdala-prefrontal cortex functional connectivity during threat-induced anxiety and goal distraction. *Biol Psychiatry* 2015;77:394–403.

401. Sears RM, Fink AE, Wigestrand MB, Farb CR, de Lecea L, Ledoux JE. Orexin/hypocretin system modulates amygdala-dependent threat learning through the locus coeruleus. *Proc Natl Acad Sci U S A* 2013;110: 20260–20265.

402. Sears RM, Schiff HC, LeDoux JE. Molecular mechanisms of threat learning in the lateral nucleus of the amygdala. *Prog Mol Biol Transl Sci* 2014;122: 263–304.

403. Wheaton MG, Fitzgerald DA, Phan KL, Klumpp H. Perceptual load modulates anterior cingulate cortex response to threat distractors in generalized social anxiety disorder. *Biol Psychol* 2014;101: 13–17.

404. Wheelock MD, Sreenivasan KR, Wood KH, Ver Hoef LW, Deshpande G, Knight DC. Threat-related learning relies on distinct dorsal prefrontal cortex network connectivity. *NeuroImage* 2014;102 (Pt 2): 904–912.

405. Connolly AC, Sha L, Guntupalli JS, Oosterhof N, Halchenko YO, Nastase SA, et al. How the human brain represents perceived dangerousness or "predacity" of animals. *J Neurosci* 2016;36: 5373–5384.

406. Eldar S, Yankelevitch R, Lamy D, Bar-Haim Y. Enhanced neural reactivity and selective attention to threat in anxiety. *Biol Psychol* 2010;85: 252–257.

407. Fani N, Jovanovic T, Ely TD, Bradley B, Gutman D, Tone EB, Ressler KJ. Neural correlates of attention bias to threat in post-traumatic stress disorder. *Biol Psychol* 2012;90: 134–142.

408. Robinson OJ, Charney DR, Overstreet C, Vytal K, Grillon C. The adaptive threat bias in anxiety: amygdala-dorsomedial prefrontal cortex coupling and aversive amplification. *Neuroimage* 2012;60: 523–529.

409. Britton JC, Phan KL, Taylor SF, Fig LM, Liberzon I. Corticolimbic blood flow in posttraumatic stress disorder during script-driven imagery. *Biol Psychiatry* 2005;57: 832–840.

410. Cisler JM, Scott Steele J, Smitherman S, Lenow JK, Kilts CD. Neural processing correlates of assaultive violence exposure and PTSD symptoms during implicit threat processing: a network-level analysis among adolescent girls. *Psychiatry Res* 2013;214: 238–246.

411. Kass MD, Rosenthal MC, Pottackal J, McGann JP. Fear learning enhances neural responses to threat-predictive sensory stimuli. *Science* 2013;342: 1389–1392.

412. MacNamara A, Post D, Kennedy AE, Rabinak CA, Phan KL. Electrocortical processing of social signals of threat in combat-related post-traumatic stress disorder. *Biol Psychol* 2013;94: 441–449.

413. Cools R, Calder AJ, Lawrence AD, Clark L, Bullmore E, Robbins TW. Individual differences in threat sensitivity predict serotonergic modulation of amygdala response to fearful faces. *Psychopharmacol* 2005;180: 670–679.

414. Fisher PM, Hariri AR. Identifying serotonergic mechanisms underlying the corticolimbic response to threat in humans. *Philos Trans R Soc Lond B Biol Sci* 2013;368: 20120192.

415. Phan KL, Coccaro EF, Angstadt M, Kreger KJ, Mayberg HS, Liberzon I, Stein MB. Corticolimbic brain reactivity to social signals of threat before and after sertraline treatment in generalized social phobia. *Biol Psychiatry* 2013;73: 329–336.

416. Campos AC, Ferreira FR, da Silva WA Jr, Guimares FS. Predator threat stress promotes long lasting anxiety-like behaviors and modulates synaptophysin and CB1 receptors expression in brain areas associated with PTSD symptoms. *Neurosci Lett* 2013;533: 34–38.

417. Gunduz-Cinar O, MacPherson KP, Cinar R, Gamble-George J, Sugden K, Williams B, et al. Convergent translational evidence of a role for anandamide in amygdala-mediated fear extinction, threat processing and stress-reactivity. *Mol Psychiatry* 2013;18: 813–823.

418. Roseboom PH, Nanda SA, Bakshi VP, Trentani A, Newman SM, Kalin NH. Predator threat induces behavioral inhibition, pituitary-adrenal activation and changes in amygdala CRF-binding protein gene expression. *Psychoneuroendocrinol* 2007;32: 44–55.

419. Grillon C, Krimsky M, Charney DR, Vytal K, Ernst M, Cornwell B. Oxytocin increases anxiety to unpredictable threat. *Mol Psychiatry* 2013;18: 958–960.

420. Goetz SM, Tang L, Thomason ME, Diamond MP, Hariri AR, Carré JM. Testosterone rapidly increases neural reactivity to threat in healthy men: a novel two-step pharmacological challenge paradigm. *Biol Psychiatry* 2014;76: 324–331.

421. De Martino B, Kalisch R, Rees G, Dolan RJ. Enhanced processing of threat stimuli under limited attentional resources. *Cereb Cortex* 2009;19: 127–133.

422. Fonzo GA, Ramsawh HJ, Flagan TM, Sullivan SG, Simmons AN, Paulus MP, Stein MB. Cognitive-behavioral therapy for generalized anxiety disorder is associated with attenuation of limbic activation to threat-related facial emotions. *J Affect Disord* 2014;169: 76–85.

423. Lipka J, Hoffmann M, Miltner WH, Straube T. Effects of cognitive-behavioral therapy on brain responses to subliminal and supraliminal threat and their functional significance in specific phobia. *Biol Psychiatry* 2014;76: 869–877.

424. Klumpp H, Fitzgerald DA, Phan KL. Neural predictors and mechanisms of cognitive behavioral therapy on threat processing in social anxiety disorder. *Prog Neuropsychopharmacol Biol Psychiatry* 2013;45: 83–91.

425. Reinecke A, Waldenmaier L, Cooper MJ, Harmer CJ. Changes in automatic threat processing precede and predict clinical changes with exposure-based cognitive-behavior therapy for panic disorder. *Biol Psychiatry* 2013;73: 1064–1070.

426. Machado CJ, Bachevalier J. Behavioral and hormonal reactivity to threat: effects of selective amygdala, hippocampal or orbital frontal lesions in monkeys. *Psychoneuroendocrinol* 2008;33: 926–941.

427. Machado CJ, Kazama AM, Bachevalier J. Impact of amygdala, orbital frontal, or hippocampal lesions on threat avoidance and emotional reactivity in nonhuman primates. *Emotion* 2009;9: 147–163.

428. Ahs F, Frans O, Tibblin B, Kumlien E, Fredrikson M. The effects of medial temporal lobe resections on verbal threat and fear conditioning. *Biol Psychol* 2010;83: 41–46.

429. Blanchard DC, Blanchard RJ. Innate and conditioned reactions to threat in rats with amygdaloid lesions. *J Comp Physiol Psychol* 1972;81: 281–290.

430. Klüver H, Bucy P. Preliminary analysis of functions of the temporal lobes in man. *Arch Neurol Psychiatry* 1939;42: 979–1000.

431. Rosvold HE, Mirsky AF, Pribram KH. Influence of amygdalectomy on social behavior I monkeys. *J Comp Physiol Psychol* 1954;47: 173–178.

432. Dicks P, Myers RE, Kling A. Uncus and amygdala lesions: effects on social behavior in the free-ranging rhesus monkey. *Science* 1969;165: 69–71.

433. Eippert F, Veit R, Weiskopf N, Erb M, Birbaumer N, Anders S. Regulation of emotional responses elicited by threat-related stimuli. *Hum Brain Mapp* 2007;28: 409–423.

434. Bishop SJ, Duncan J, Lawrence AD. State anxiety modulation of the amygdala response to unattended threat-related stimuli. *J Neurosci* 2004;24: 10364–10368.

435. Weiger WA, Bear DM. An approach to the neurology of aggression. *J Psychiatr Res* 1988;22: 85–98.

436. Luria AR. *Higher cortical functions in man.* New York: Basic Books, 1980.

437. Bonilha L, Jensen JH, Baker N, Breedlove J, Nesland T, Lin JJ, et al. The brain connectome as a personalized biomarker of seizure outcomes after temporal lobectomy. *Neurology* 2015;84: 1846–1853.

438. Saxena K, Silverman MA, Chang K, Khanzode L, Steiner H. Baseline predictors of response to divalproex in conduct disorder. *J Clin Psychiatry* 2005;66: 1541–1548.

439. Cailhol L, Roussignol B, Klein R, Bousquet B, Simonetta-Moreau M, Schmitt L, et al. Borderline personality disorder and rTMS: a pilot trial. *Psychiatry Res* 2014;216: 155–157.

440. Tafrate RC. Evaluation of treatment strategies for adult anger disorders. In Kassinove H, editor. *Anger disorders: definition, diagnosis, and treatment.* Washington, DC: Taylor & Francis, 1995, pp. 109–129.

441. Burke H, Wesolowski MD, Lane I. A positive approach to the treatment of aggressive brain injured clients. *Int J Rehabil Res* 1988;11: 235–242.

442. Carnevale GJ, Anselmi V, Johnston MV, Kim Busichio K, Walsh V. Natural setting behavior management program for persons with acquired brain injury: a randomized controlled trial. *Arch Phys Med Rehabil* 2006;87: 1289–1297.

443. Novaco RW. *Anger control.* Lexington: D.C. Heath, 1975.

444. Lira FT, Carne W, Masri AM. Treatment of anger and impulsivity in a brain damaged patient: a case study applying stress inoculation. *Clin Neuropsychol* 1983;5: 159–160.

445. Uomoto JM, Brockway JA. Anger management training for brain injured patients and their family members. *Arch Phys Med Rehabil* 1992;73: 674–679.

446. Aeschleman SR, Imes C. Stress inoculation training for impulsive behaviors in adults with traumatic brain injury. *J Rational-Emotive Cognitive-Behav Ther* 1999;17: 51–65.

447. O'Leary CA. Reducing aggression in adults with brain injuries. *Behav Interv* 2000;15: 205–216.

448. Medd J, Tate R. Evaluation of an anger management therapy programme following acquired brain injury: a preliminary study. *Neuropsychol Rehabil* 2000;10: 185–201.

449. Hart T, Vaccaro MJ, Hays C, Maiuro RD. Anger self-management training for people with traumatic brain injury: a preliminary investigation. *J Head Trauma Rehabil* 2012;27: 113–122.

450. Brewin C. Theoretical foundations of cognitive-behavioral therapy for anxiety and depression. *Ann Rev Psychol* 1996;47: 33–57.

451. Beck JS. *Cognitive behavior therapy: basics and beyond (2nd edition).* New York, NY: Guilford Press, 2011.

452. Meichenbaum D. The 'potential' contributions of cognitive behaviour modification to the rehabilitation of individuals with traumatic brain injury. *Sem Speech Lang* 1993;14: 18–31.

453. Whitehouse AM. Applications of cognitive therapy with survivors of head injury. *J Cogn Psychother* 1994;8: 141–160.

454. Prigatano GP. Psychotherapy after brain injury. In: Prigatano GP, editor. *Neuropsychological rehabilitation after brain injury.* Baltimore, MD: Johns Hopkins University Press, 1986, pp. 67–95.

455. Daniels-Zide E, Ben-Yishay Y. Therapeutic milieu day program. In: Christensen AL, Uzzell BP, editors. *International handbook of neuropsychological rehabilitation.* New York: Kluwer Academic/Plenum Publishers, 1989, pp. 183–193.

456. Delmonico RL, Hanley-Peterson P, Englander J. Group psychotherapy for persons with traumatic brain injury: management of frustration and substance abuse. *J Head Trauma Rehabil* 1998;13: 10–22.

457. Walker AJ, Nott MT, Doyle M, Onus M, McCarthy K, Baguley IJ. Effectiveness of a group anger management programme after severe traumatic brain injury. *Brain Inj* 2010;24: 517–524.

458. Lewis L, Athey GI, Eyman J, Saeks S. Psychological treatment of adult psychiatric patients with traumatic frontal lobe injury. *J Neuropsychiatry Clin Neurosci* 1992;4: 323–330.

459. Greendyke RM, Kanter DR, Schuster DB, Verstreate S, Wootton J. Propranolol treatment of assaultive patients with organic brain disease. A double-blind crossover, placebocontrolled study. *J Nerv Mental Dis* 1986;174: 290–294.

460. Greendyke RM, Kanter DR. Therapeutic effects of pindolol on behavioral disturbances associated with organic brain disease: a double-blind study. *J Clin Psychiatry* 1986;47: 423–426.

461. Greendyke RM, Berkner JP, Webster JC,Gulya A. Treatment of behavioral problems with pindolol. *Psychosomatics* 1989;30: 161–165.

462. Meythaler JM, Depalma L, Devivo MJ, Guin Renfroe S, Novack TA. Sertraline to improve arousal and alertness in severe traumatic brain injury secondary to motor vehicle crashes. *Brain Inj* 2001;15: 321–331.

463. Mooney GF, Haas LJ. Effect of methylphenidate on brain injury-related anger. *Arch Phys Med Rehabil* 1993;74: 153–160.

464. Kim E, Bijlani M. A pilot study of quetiapine treatment of aggression due to traumatic brain injury. *J Neuropsychiatry Clin Neurosci* 2006;18: 547–549.

465. Hale MS, Donaldson J. Lithium carbonate in the treatment of organic brain syndrome. *J Nerv Mental Disord* 1982;170: 362–365.

466. Yu F, Zhang Y, Chuang DM. Lithium reduces BACE1 overexpression, β amyloid accumulation, and spatial learning deficits in mice with traumatic brain injury. *J Neurotrauma* 2012;29: 2342–2351.

467. Leeds PR, Yu F, Wang Z, Chiu C-T, Zhang Y, Leng Y, et al. A new avenue for lithium: intervention in traumatic brain injury. *ACS Chem Neurosci* 2014;5: 422–433.

468. Yu F, Wang Z, Tchantchou F, Chiu C-T, Zhang Y, Chuang D-M. Lithium ameliorates neurodegeneration, suppresses neuroinflammation, and improves behavioral performance in a mouse model of traumatic brain injury. *J Neurotrauma* 2012;29: 362–374.

469. Michals ML, Crismon ML, Roberts S, Childs A. Clozapine response and adverse effects in nine brain-injured patients. *J Clin Psychopharmacol* 1993;13: 198–203.

470. Noé E, Ferri J, Trénor C, Chirivella J. Efficacy of ziprasidone in controlling agitation during post-traumatic amnesia. *Behav Neurol* 2007;18: 7–11.

471. Umansky R, Geller V. Olanzapine treatment in an organic hallucinosis patient (letter). *Int J Neuropsychopharmacol* 2000;3: 81–82.

472. Viana Bde M, Prais HA, Nicolato R, Caramelli P. Posttraumatic brain injury psychosis successfully treated with olanzapine. *Prog Neuropsychopharmacol Biol Psychiatry* 2010;34: 233–235.

473. Hoffman AN, Cheng JP, Zafonte RD, Kline AE. Administration of haloperidol and risperidone after neurobehavioral testing hinders the recovery of traumatic brain injury-induced deficits. *Life Sci* 2008;83: 602–607.

474. Tsiouris JA. Pharmacotherapy for aggressive behaviours in persons with intellectual disabilities: treatment or mistreatment? *J Intel Disabil Res* 2010;54: 1–16.

475. Phelps TI, Bondi CO, Ahmed RH, Olugbade YT, Kline AE. Divergent long-term consequences of chronic treatment with haloperidol, risperidone, and bromocriptine on traumatic brain injury-induced cognitive deficits. *J Neurotrauma* 2015;32: 590–597.

476. Barker MJ, Greenwood KM, Jackson M, Crowe SF. Cognitive effects of long-term benzodiazepine use: a meta-analysis. *CNS Drugs* 2004;18: 37–48.

477. Kant R, Smith-Seemiller L, Zeiler D. Treatment of aggression and irritability after head injury. *Brain Inj* 1998;12: 661–666.

478. Fann JR, Hart T, Schomer KG. Treatment for depression after traumatic brain injury: a systematic review. *J Neurotrauma* 2009;26: 2383–2402.

479. Wroblewski BA, Joseph AB, Kepfer J, Kallier K. Effectiveness of valproic acid on destructive and aggressive behaviours in patients with acquired brain injury. *Brain Inj* 1997;11: 37–47.

480. Chatham Showalter PE, Kimmel DN. Agitated symptom response to divalproex following acute brain injury. *J Neuropsychiatry Clin Neurosci* 2000;12: 395–397.

481. Azouvi P, Jokic C, Attal N, Denys P, Markabi S, Bussel B. Carbamazepine in agitation and aggressive behavior following severe closed-head injury: results of an open trial. *Brain Inj* 1999;13: 797–804.

482. Pachet A, Friesen S, Winkelaar D, Gray S. Beneficial behavioural effects of lamotrigine in traumatic brain injury. *Brain Inj* 2003;17: 715–722.

483. Mattes JA. Oxcarbazepine in patients with impulsive aggression: a double-blind, placebo-controlled trial *J Clin Psychopharmacol* 2005;25: 575–579.

484. Levine AM. Buspirone and agitation in head injury. *Brain Inj* 1988;2: 165–167.

485. Gualtieri CT. Buspirone for the behavior problems of patients with organic brain disorders. *J Clin Psychopharmacol* 1991;11: 280–281.

486. Ratey JJ, Leveroni CL, Miller AC, Komry V, Gaffar K. Low-dose buspirone to treat agitation and maladaptive behavior in braininjured patients: two case reports. *J Clin Psychopharmacol* 1992;12: 362–364.

487. Holzer JC. Buspirone and brain injury. *J Neuropsychiatry Clin Neurosci* 1998;10: 113.

488. Stanislav SW, Fabre T, Crismon ML, Childs A. Buspirone's efficacy in organic-induced aggression. *J Clin Psychopharmacol* 1994;14: 126–130.

489. Olsen AS, Sozda CN, Cheng JP, Hoffman AN, Kline AE. Traumatic brain injury-induced cognitive and histological deficits are attenuated by delayed and chronic treatment with the 5-HT1A-receptor agonist buspirone. *J Neurotrauma* 2012;29: 1898–1907.

490. Monaco CM, Gebhardt KM, Chlebowski SM, Shaw KE, Cheng JP, Henchir JJ, Zupa MF, Kline AE. A combined therapeutic regimen of buspirone and environmental enrichment is more efficacious than either alone in enhancing spatial learning in brain-injured pediatric rats. *J Neurotrauma* 2014;31: 1934–1941.

491. Kraus M, Maki P. Case report: the combined use of amantadine and l-dopa/carbidopa in the treatment of chronic brain injury. *Brain Inj* 1997;11: 455–460.

492. Wang T, Huang XJ, Van KC, Went GT, Nguyen JT, Lyeth BG. (2013) Amantadine improves cognitive outcome and increases neuronal survival after fluid percussion TBI in rats. *J Neurotrauma* 2013;31: 370–377.

493. Huang EY-K, Tsui P-F, Kuo T-T, Tsai J-J, Chou Y-C, Ma H-I, et al. Amantadine ameliorates dopamine-releasing deficits and behavioral deficits in rats after fluid percussion injury. *PLoS One* 2014;9: e86354.

494. Giacino JT, Whyte J, Bagiella E, Kalmar K, Childs N, Khademi A, et al. Placebo controlled trial of amantadine for severe traumatic brain injury. *N Engl J Med* 2012;366: 819–826.

495. Sawyer E, Mauro LS, Ohlinger MJ. Amantadine enhancement of arousal and cognition after traumatic brain injury. *Ann Pharmacother* 2008;42: 247–252.

496. Tan L, Ge H, Tang J, Fu C, Duanmu W, Chen Y, et al. Amantadine preserves dopamine level and attenuates depression-like behavior induced by traumatic brain injury in rats. *Behav Brain Res* 2015;279: 274–282.

497. Chandler MC, Barnhill JL, Gualtieri CT. Amantadine for the agitated head-injury patient. *Brain Inj* 1988;2: 309–311.

498. Nickels JL, Schneider WN, Dombovy ML, Wong TM. Clinical use of amantadine in brain injury rehabilitation. *Brain Inj* 1994;8: 709–718.

499. Leone H, Polsonetti BW. Amantadine for traumatic brain injury: does it improve cognition and reduce agitation? *J Clin Pharmacy Ther* 2005;30: 101–104.

500. Gwynette MF, Beck B, VandenBerg A, Stocking N. Under arrest: the use of amantadine for treatment-refractory mood lability and aggression in a patient with traumatic brain injury. *J Clin Psychopharmacol* 2015;35: 102–104.

501. Hammond FM, Bickett AK, Norton JH, Pershad R. Effectiveness of amantadine hydrochloride in the reduction of chronic traumatic brain injury irritability and aggression. *J Head Trauma Rehabil* 2014;29: 391–399.

502. Hammond FM, Sherer M, Malec JF, Zafonte RD, Whitney M, Bell K, et al. Amantadine effect on perceptions of irritability after traumatic brain injury: results of the amantadine irritability multisite study. *J Neurotrauma* 2015;32: 1230–1238.

503. Panikashvili D, Simeonidou C, Ben-Shabat S, Hanus L, Breuer A, Mechoulam R, et al. An endogenous cannabinoid (2-AG) is neuroprotective after brain injury. *Nature* 2001;413: 527–531.

504. Benyó Z, Ruisanchez E, Leszl-Ishiguro M, Sándor P, Pacher P. Endocannabinoids in cerebrovascular regulation. *Am J Physiol – Heart Circ Physiol* 2016;310: H785–H801.

505. Grundy RI. The therapeutic potential of the cannabinoids in neuroprotection. *Exp Opin Invest Drugs* 2002;11: 1365–1374.

506. Mechoulam R, Panikashvili D, Shohami E. Cannabinoids and brain injury: therapeutic implications. *Trends Mol Med* 2002;8: 58–61.

507. Biegon A. Cannabinoids as neuroprotective agents in traumatic brain injury. *Curr Pharm Design* 2004;10: 2177–2183.

508. Shohami E, Cohen-Yeshurun A, Magid L, Algali M, Mechoulam R. Endocannabinoids and traumatic brain injury. *Br J Pharmacol* 2011;163: 1402–1410.

509. Klegeris A, Bissonnette CJ, McGeer PL. Reduction of human monocytic cell neurotoxicity and cytokine secretion by ligands of the cannabinoid-type CB2 receptor. *Br J Pharmacol* 2003;139: 775–786.

510. Sheng WS, Hu S, Min X, Cabral GA, Lokensgard JR, Peterson PK. Synthetic cannabinoid WIN55,212-2 inhibits generation of inflammatory mediators by IL-1beta-stimulated human astrocytes. *Glia* 2005;49: 211–219.

511. Elliott MB, Tuma RF, Amenta PS, Barbe MF, Jallo JI. Acute effects of a selective cannabinoid-2 receptor agonist on neuroinflammation in a model of traumatic brain injury. *J Neurotrauma* 2011;28: 973–981.

512. Amenta PS, Jallo JI, Tuma RF, Hooper DC, Elliott MB. Cannabinoid receptor type-2 stimulation, blockade, and deletion alter the vascular inflammatory responses to traumatic brain injury. *J Neuroinflamm* 2014;11: 191.

513. Amenta PS, Jallo JI, Tuma RF, Elliott MB. A cannabinoid type 2 receptor agonist attenuates blood–brain barrier damage and neurodegeneration in a murine model of traumatic brain injury. *J Neurosci Res* 2012;90: 2293–2305.

514. Tolón RM, Núñez E, Pazos MR, Benito C, Castillo AI, Martínez-Orgado JA, Romero J. The activation of cannabinoid CB2 receptors stimulates in situ and in vitro beta-amyloid removal by human macrophages. *Brain Res* 2009;1283: 148–154.

515. Martin M, Ledent C, Parmentier M, Maldonado R, Valverde O. Involvement of CB1 cannabinoid receptors in emotional behaviour. *Psychopharmacol* 2002;159: 379–387.

516. Rodriguez-Arias M, Navarrete F, Daza-Losada M, Navarro D, Aguilar MA, Berbel P, et al. CB1 cannabinoid receptor-mediated aggressive behavior. *Neuropharmacol* 2013;75: 172–180.

517. Vilela FC, Giusti-Paiva A. Cannabinoid receptor agonist disrupts behavioral and neuroendocrine responses during lactation. *Behav Brain Res* 2014;263: 190–197.

518. Sills, J. Federal barriers to cannabis research. *Science* 2016;352: 1182.

519. Andreae MH, Rhodes E, Bourgoise T, Carter GM, White RS, Indyk D, et al. An ethical exploration of barriers to research on controlled drugs. *Am J Bioeth* 2016;16: 36–47.

520. Earleywine M. *Understanding marijuana: a new look at the scientific evidence.* New York, NY: Oxford University Press, 2005.

521. Aggarwal SK, Carter GT, Sullivan MD, ZumBrunnen C, Morrill R, Mayer JD. Medicinal use of cannabis in the United States: historical perspectives, current trends, and future directions. *J Opioid Manag* 2009;5: 153–168.

522. Saint Loius C, Apuzzo M. Obama administration set to remove barrier to marijuana research. *N Y Times* 2016; August 10.

523. Curtis A, Mitchell I, Patel S, Ives N, Rickards H. A pilot study using nabilone for symptomatic treatment in Huntington's disease. *Mov Disord* 2009;24: 2254–2259.

524. van Duijn E. Treatment of irritability in Huntington's disease. *Curr Treat Options Neurol* 2010;12: 424–433.

525. Liu CS, Chau SA, Ruthirakuhan M, Lanctot KL, Herrmann N. Cannabinoids for the treatment of agitation and aggression in Alzheimer's disease. *CNS Drugs* 2015;29: 615–623.

526. Casarejos MJ, Perucho J, Gomez A, Muñoz MP, Fernandez-Estevez M, Sagredo O, et al. Natural cannabinoids improve dopamine neurotransmission and tau and amyloid pathology in a mouse model of tauopathy. *J Alzheimers Dis* 2013;35: 525–539.

527. Scott W. PTSD in DSM-III: a case in the politics of diagnosis and disease. *Soc Prob* 1990;37: 294–310.

528. Summerfield D. The invention of post-traumatic stress disorder and the social usefulness of a psychiatric category. *BMJ* 2001;322: 95–98.

529. Yehuda R, McFarlane AC. Conflict between current knowledge about posttraumatic stress disorder and its original conceptual basis. *Am J Psychiatry* 1995;152: 1705–1713.

530. Rosen GM. Preface. In: Rosen GM, editor. *Posttraumatic stress disorder: issues and controversies.* Chichester, England: John Wiley, 2004, pp. xi–xii.

531. Cannon WB. *Bodily changes in pain, hunger, fear and rage: an account of recent researches into the function of emotional excitement.* New York: Appleton-Century-Crofts, 1915.

532. Shephard B. *A war of nerves: soldiers and psychiatrists in the twentieth century.* Cambridge, MA: Harvard University Press, 2001.

533. Beall LS. Post-traumatic stress disorder: a bibliographical essay. *Choice* 1997;34: 917–930.

534. Moreau C, Zisook S. Rationale for a posttraumatic stress spectrum disorder. *Psychiatr Clin N Am* 2012;25: 775–790.

535. Rosen GM. Challenges to the PTSD construct and its database: the importance of scientific debate. *J Anxiety Disord* 2007;21: 161–163.

536. Spitzer RL, Rosen GM, Lilienfeld SO. Revisiting the Institute of Medicine report on the validity of posttraumatic stress disorder. *Compr Psychiatry* 2008;49: 319–320.

537. Young A. *The harmony of illusions: inventing posttraumatic stress disorder.* Princeton, NJ: Princeton University Press, 1995.

538. Andreasen NC. Posttraumatic stress disorder: psychology, biology, and the Manichaean warfare between false dichotomies. *Am J Psychiatry* 1995;152: 963–965.

539. Trmble MR. *Post-traumatic neurosis: from railway spine to the whiplash.* New York: John Wiley, 1981.

540. Auxemery Y. [Posttraumatic stress disorder (PTSD) as a consequence of the interaction between an individual

genetic susceptibility, a traumatogenic event and a social context.] *Encephale* 2012;38: 373–380.

541. Cannon WB. Organization for physiological homeostasis. *Physiol Rev* 1929;9: 399–431.
542. Cannon WB. *Wisdom of the body.* New York: W.W. Norton, 1932.
543. Selye H. A syndrome produced by diverse nocuous agents. *Nature* 1936;138: 32.
544. Selye H. Studies on adaptation. *Endocrinol* 1937;21: 169–188.
545. Schachter S, Singer J. Cognitive, social, and physiological determinants of emotional state. *Psychol Rev* 1962;69: 379–399.
546. Cryer PE. Physiology and pathophysiology of the human sympathoadrenal neuroendocrine system. *N Engl J Med* 1980;303: 436–444.
547. Horowitz MJ. Stress-response syndromes: a review of posttraumatic and adjustment disorders. *Hosp Commun Psychiatry* 1986;37: 241–249.
548. Horowitz M: *Stress response syndromes*, 2nd edition. New York: Aronson, 1986.
549. Chrousos GP, Gold PW. The concepts of stress and stress system disorders. Overview of physical and behavioral homeostasis. *JAMA* 1992;267: 1244–1252.
550. Wilson JP, Raphael B. *International handbook of traumatic stress syndromes.* New York: Springer Science+Business Media, 1993.
551. McEwen BS. Stress, adaptation, and disease. Allostasis and allostatic load. *Ann N Y Acad Sci* 1998;840: 33–44.
552. McEwen BS. Allostasis and allostatic load: implications for neuropsychopharmacology. *Neuropsychopharmacol* 2000;22: 108–124.
553. Goldstein DS, McEwen B. Allostasis, homeostats, and the nature of stress. *Stress* 2002;5: 55–58.
554. Bremner JD, Randall P, Scott TM, Bronen RA, Seibyl JP, Southwick SM, et al. MRI-based measurement of hippocampal volume in patients with combat-related posttraumatic stress disorder. *Am J Psychiatry* 1995;152: 973–981.
555. Bremner JD, Staib LH, Kaloupek D, Southwick SM, Soufer R, Charney DS. Neural correlates of exposure to traumatic pictures and sound in Vietnam combat veterans with and without posttraumatic stress disorder: a positron emission tomography study. *Biol Psychiatry* 1999;45:806–816.
556. Bremner JD. Alterations in brain structure and function associated with post-traumatic stress disorder. *Sem Clin Neuropsychiatry* 1999;4: 249–255.
557. Bremner JD. Hypotheses and controversies related to effects of stress on the hippocampus: an argument for stress-induced damage to the hippocampus in patients with posttraumatic stress disorder. *Hippocampus* 2001;11: 75–81.
558. Woon FU, Hedges DW. Hippocampal and amygdala volumes in children and adults with childhood maltreatment related posttraumatic stress disorder: a meta-analysis. *Hippocampus* 2008;18: 729–736.
559. Green BF. A general solution for the latent class model of latent structure analysis. *Psychometrika* 1951;16: 151–166.
560. Breslau N, Reboussin BA, Anthony JC, Storr CL. The structure of posttraumatic stress disorder: latent class analysis in 2 community samples. *Arch Gen Psychiatry* 2005;62: 1343–1351.
561. Dalgleish T, Power MJ. Emotion-specific and emotion-non-specific components of posttraumatic stress disorder (PTSD): implications for a taxonomy of related psychopathology. *Behav Res Ther* 2004;42: 1069–1088.
562. Jackson DL, Gillaspy JA, Purc-Stephenson R. Reporting practices in confirmatory factor analysis: an overview and some recommendations. *Psychol Methods* 2009;14: 6–23.
563. Tsai J, Pietrzak RH, Southwick SM, Harpaz-Rotem I. Examining the dimensionality of combat-related posttraumatic stress and depressive symptoms in treatment-seeking OEF/OIF/OND veterans. *J Affect Disord* 2011;135: 310–314.
564. Marshall GN, Schell TL, Miles JN. A multi-sample confirmatory factor analysis of PTSD symptoms: what exactly is wrong with the DSM-IV structure? *Clin Psychol Rev* 2013;33: 54–66.
565. Harpaz-Rotem I, Tsai J, Pietrzak RH, Hoff S. The dimensional structure of posttraumatic stress symptomatology in 323,903 U.S. veterans. *J Psychiatr Res* 2014;49: 31e6.
566. Frankfurt S, Anders SL, James LM, Engdahl B, Winskowski AM. Evaluating the dimensionality of PTSD in a sample of OIF/OEF veterans. *Psychol Trauma* 2015;7: 430–436.
567. Armour C, Elhai JD, Richardson D, Ractliffe K, Wang Li, Elklit A. Assessing a five factor model of PTSD: is dysphoric arousal a unique PTSD construct showing differential relationships with anxiety and depression? *J Anxiety Disord* 2012;26: 368–376.
568. King DW, Leskin GA, King LA, Weathers FW. Confirmatory factor analysis of the clinician-administered PTSD scale: evidence for the dimensionality of posttraumatic stress disorder. *Psychol Assess* 1998;10: 90–96.
569. Armour C, Layne CM, Naifeh JA, Shevlin M, Durakovic-Belko E, Djapo N. Assessing the factor structure of posttraumatic stress disorder symptoms in participants with and without criterion A2 endorsement. *J Anxiety Disord* 2011;25: 80–87.
570. Simms LJ, Watson D, Doebbeling BN. Confirmatory factor analyses of posttraumatic stress symptoms in deployed and nondeployed veterans of the Gulf War. *J Abnorm Psychol* 2002;111: 637–647.
571. Pietrzak RH, Goldstein MB, Malley JC, Rivers AJ, Southwick SM. Structure of posttraumatic stress disorder symptoms and psychosocial functioning in veterans of Operations Enduring Freedom and Iraqi Freedom. *Psychiatry Res* 2010;178: 323–329.
572. Engdahl RM, Elhai JD, Richardson JD, Frueh BC. Comparing posttraumatic stress disorder's symptom structure between deployed and non-deployed veterans. *Psychol Assess* 2011;23: 1–6.
573. Yufik T, Simms LJ. A meta-analytic investigation of the structure of posttraumatic stress disorder symptoms. *J Abnorm Psychol* 2010;119: 764e76.
574. Elhai JD, Biehn TL, Armour C, Klopper JJ, Frueh BC, Palmieri PA. Evidence for a unique PTSD construct represented by PTSD's D1–D3 symptoms. *J Anxiety Disord* 2011;25: 340–345.
575. Elhai JD, Palmieri PA. Posttraumatic stress disorder's factor structure: an update on the current literature and advancing a research agenda. *J Anxiety Disord* 2011;25: 849–854.
576. Elhai JD, Gray MJ, Docherty AR, Kashdan TB. Kose S. Structural validity of the posttraumatic stress disorder checklist among college students with a trauma history. *J Interpers Violence* 2007;22: 1471–1478.
577. Elhai JD, Grubaugh AL, Kashdan TB, Frueh BC. Empirical examination of a proposed refinement to DSM-IV posttraumatic stress disorder symptom criteria using the National Comorbidity Survey Replication data. *J Clin Psychiatry* 2008;69: 597–602.
578. Elhai JD, Ford JD, Ruggiero KJ, Frueh BC. Diagnostic alterations for posttraumatic stress disorder: examining data from the National Comorbidity Survey Replication and National Survey of Adolescents. *Psychol Med* 2009;39: 1957–1966.
579. Elhai JD, Palmieri PA, Biehn TL, Frueh BC, Magruder KM. Posttraumatic stress disorder's frequency and intensity ratings are associated with factor structure differences in military veterans. *Psychol Assess* 2010;22: 723–728.
580. Elklit A, Armour C, Shevlin M. Testing alternative factor models of PTSD and the robustness of the dysphoria factor. *J Anxiety Disord* 2010;24: 147–154.
581. Elhai JD, Miller ME, Ford JD, Biehn TL, Palmieri PA, Fruehd BC. Posttraumatic stress disorder in DSM-5: estimates of

prevalence and symptom structure in a nonclinical sample of college students. *J Anxiety Disord* 2012;26: 58–64.

582. Elhai JD, Contractor AA, Tamburrino M, Fine TH, Cohen G, Shirley E, et al. Structural relations between DSM-5 PTSD and major depression symptoms in military soldiers. *J Affect Disord* 2015;175: 373–378.

583. Charak C, Armour C, Elklit A, Angmo D, Elhai JD, Koot HM. Factor structure of PTSD, and relation with gender in trauma survivors from India. *Eur J Psychotraumatol* 2014;5: 25547.

584. Contractor AA, Durham TA, Brennan JA, Armour C, Wutrick HR, Frueh BC, et al. DSM-5 PTSD's symptom dimensions and relations with major depression's symptom dimensions in a primary care sample. *PsychiatryRes* 2014;215: 146–153.

585. Gentes EL, Dennis PA, Kimbrel NA, Rissling MB, Beckham JC, VA Mid-Atlantic MIRECC Workgroup, Calhoun PS. DSM-5 posttraumatic stress disorder: factor structure and rates of diagnosis. *J Psychiatr Res* 2014;59: 60–67.

586. Pietrzak RH, Tsai J, Armour C, Mota N, Harpaz-Rotem I, Southwick SM. Functional significance of a novel 7-factor model of DSM-5 PTSD symptoms: results from the National Health and Resilience in Veterans study. *J Affect Disord* 2015;174: 522–526.

587. Ayer LA, Cisler JM, Danielson CK, Amstadter AB, Saunders BE, Kilpatrick DG. Adolescent posttraumatic stress disorder: an examination of factor structure reliability in two national samples. *J Anxiety Disord* 2011;25: 411–421.

588. Price KP. Post-traumatic stress disorder and concussion: are they incompatible? *Defense Law J* 1994;43: 113–120.

589. Sbordone RJ, Liter JC. Mild traumatic brain injury does not produce post-traumatic stress disorder. *Brain Inj* 1995;9: 405–412.

590. Sbordone RJ, Ruff RM. Re-examination of the controversial coexistence of traumatic brain injury and posttraumatic stress disorder: misdiagnosis and self-report measures. *Psychol Inj Law* 2010;3: 63–76.

591. Creamer M, O'Donnell ML, Pattison P. Amnesia, traumatic brain injury, and posttraumatic stress disorder: a methodological inquiry. *Behav Res Ther* 2005;43: 1383–1389.

592. American Psychiatric Association. Posttraumatic stress disorder. Available at www.psychiatry.org/File%20Library/.../Practice/DSM/APA_DSM-5-PTSD.pdf.

593. National Center for PTSD. PTSD. Available at www.ptsd.va.gov/.

594. Aupperle RL, Melrose AJ, Stein MB, Paulus MP. Executive function and PTSD: disengaging from trauma. *Neuropharmacol* 2012;62: 686e694.

595. Troyanskaya M, Pastorek NJ, Scheibel RS, Petersen NJ, McCulloch K, Wilde EA, et al. Combat exposure, PTSD symptoms, and cognition following blast-related traumatic brain injury in OEF/OIF/OND service members and veterans. *Mil Med* 2015;180: 285–289.

596. Clark AL, Sorg SF, Schiehser DM, Luc N, Bondi MW, Sanderson M, et al. Deep white matter hyperintensities affect verbal memory independent of PTSD symptoms in veterans with mild traumatic brain injury. *Brain Inj* 2016;30: 864–871.

597. Defense and Veterans Brain Injury Center. Research review on mild traumatic brain injury and posttraumatic stress disorder. 2016. Available at dvbic.dcoe.mil/.../DVBIC_Research_Research-Review_MildTBI-PTSD_April2016/.

598. Department of Veterans Affairs Department of Defense. VA/DOD clinical practice guideline for the management of concussion-mild traumatic brain injury. Version 2.0 – 2016. Available at www.healthquality.va.gov/guidelines/Rehab/mtbi/mTBICPGFullCPG50821816.pdf.

599. Morissette SB, Woodward M, Kimbrel NA, Meyer EC, Kruse MI, Dolan S, et al. Deployment-related TBI, persistent postconcussive symptoms, PTSD, and depression in OEF/OIF veterans. *Rehabil Psychol* 2011;56: 340–350.

600. Walter KH, Barnes SM, Chard KM. The influence of comorbid MDD on outcome after residential treatment for veterans with PTSD and a history of TBI. *J Trauma Stress* 2012;25: 426–432.

601. Tanev KS, Pentel KZ, Kredlow MA, Charney ME. PTSD and TBI co-morbidity: scope, clinical presentation and treatment options. *Brain Inj* 2014;28: 261–270.

602. Barr T, Livingston W, Guardado P, Baxter T, Mysliwiec V, Gill J. Military personnel with traumatic brain injuries and insomnia have reductions in PTSD and improved perceived health following sleep restoration: a relationship moderated by inflammation. *Annu Rev Nurs Res* 2015;33: 249–266.

603. Gilbert KS, Kark SM, Gehrman P, Bogdanova Y. Sleep disturbances, TBI and PTSD: implications for treatment and recovery. *Clin Psychol Rev* 2015;40: 195–212.

604. Stocker RP, Paul BT, Mammen O, Khan H, Cieply MA, Germain A. Effects of blast exposure on subjective and objective sleep measures in combat veterans with and without PTSD. *J Clin Sleep Med* 2016;12: 49–56.

605. Kulkarnia M, Portera KE, Raucha SAM. Anger, dissociation, and PTSD among male veterans entering into PTSD treatment. *J Anxiety Disord* 2012;26: 271–278.

606. McHugh T, Forbes D, Bates G, Hopwood M, Creamer M, Anger in PTSD: Is there a need for a concept of PTSD-related posttraumatic anger? *Clin Psychol Rev* 2012;32: 93–104.

607. Freeman D, Thompson C, Vorontsova N, Dunn G, Carter LA, Garety P, et al. Paranoia and post-traumatic stress disorder in the months after a physical assault: a longitudinal study examining shared and differential predictors. *Psychol Med* 2013;43: 2673–2684.

608. Bryant RA, Marosszeky JE, Crooks J, Baguley IJ, Gurka JA. Interaction of posttraumatic stress disorder and chronic pain following traumatic brain injury. *J Head Trauma Rehabil* 1999;14: 588–594.

609. Tan G, Fink B, Dao TK, Hebert R, Farmer LS, Sanders A, et al. Associations among pain, PTSD, mTBI, and heart rate variability in veterans of Operation Enduring and Iraqi Freedom: a pilot study. *Pain Med* 2009;10: 1237–1245.

610. Jaramillo CA, Eapen BC, McGeary CA, McGeary DD, Robinson J, Amuan M, et al. A cohort study examining headaches among veterans of Iraq and Afghanistan wars: associations with traumatic brain injury, PTSD, and depression. *Headache* 2016;56: 528–539.

611. Stojanovic MP, Fonda J, Fortier CB, Higgins DM, Rudolph JL, Milberg WP, et al. Influence of mild traumatic brain injury (TBI) and posttraumatic stress disorder (PTSD) on pain intensity levels in OEF/OIF/OND veterans. *Pain Med* 2016;17: 2017–2025.

612. Horowitz M, Wilner N, Alvarez W. Impact of event scale: a measure of subjective stress. *Psychosom Med* 1979;41: 209–218.

613. Zilberg NJ; Weiss DS; Horowitz MJ. A cross-validation study and some empirical evidence supporting a conceptual model of stress response syndromes. *J Consult Clin Psychol* 1982;50: 407–414.

614. Joseph P. Psychometric evaluation of Horowitz's Impact of Event Scale: a review. *J Trauma Stress* 2000;13: 101–113.

615. Foa EB, Riggs DS, Dancu CV, Rothbaum BO. Reliability and validity of a brief instrument for assessing post-traumatic stress disorder. *J Trauma Stress* 1993;6: 459–473.

616. Foa EB, Cashman L, Jaycox L, Perry K. The validation of a self-report measure of posttraumatic stress disorder: the Posttraumatic Diagnostic Scale. *Psychol Assess* 1997;9: 445–451.

617. Goodman L, Corcoran C, Turner K, Yuan N, Green BL. Assessing traumatic event exposure: general issues and preliminary findings for the Stressful Life Events Screening Questionnaire. *Trauma Stress* 1998;11: 521–542.

618. Meterko M, Baker E, Stolzmann KL, Hendricks AM, Cicerone KD, Lew HL. Psychometric assessment of the Neurobehavioral Symptom Inventory-22: the structure of persistent postconcussive symptoms following deployment-related mild traumatic brain injury among veterans. *J Head Trauma Rehabil* 2012;27: 55–62.

619. Vanderploeg RD, Cooper DB, Belanger HG, Donnell AJ, Kennedy JE, Hopewell CA, Scott SG. Screening for postdeployment conditions: development and cross-validation of an embedded validity scale in the neurobehavioral symptom inventory. *J Head Trauma Rehabil* 2014;29: 1–10.

620. Belanger HG, Lange RT, Bailie J, Iverson GL, Arrieux JP, Ivins BJ, et al. Interpreting change on the neurobehavioral symptom inventory and the PTSD checklist in military personnel. *Clin Neuropsychol* 2016;30: 1063–1073.

621. Weathers FW, Litz BT, Herman DS, Huska JA, Keane TM. The PTSD Checklist: reliability, validity, and diagnostic utility. Paper presented at the annual meeting of the International Society for Traumatic Stress Studies, San Antonio, TX, 1993.

622. Ruggiero KJ, Del Ben K, Scotti JR, Rabalais AE. Psychometric properties of the PTSD checklist-civilian version. *J Traum Stress* 2003;16: 495–502.

623. Weathers FW. Posttraumatic Stress Disorder Checklist. In Reyes G, Elhai JD, Ford JD, editors. *Encyclopedia of psychological trauma*. Hoboken, NJ: Wiley, 2008, pp. 491–494.

624. Conybeare D, Behar E, Solomon A, Newman MG, Borkovec TD. The PTSD checklist civilian version: reliability, validity, and factor structure in a nonclinical sample. *J Clin Psychol* 2012;68: 699–713.

625. Lang AJ, Wilkins K, Roy-Byrne PP, Golinelli D, Chavira D, Sherbourne C, et al. Abbreviated PTSD Checklist (PCL) as a guide to clinical response. *Gen Hosp Psychiatry* 2012;34: 332–338.

626. Blevins CA, Weathers FW, Davis MT, Witte TK, Domino JL. The Posttraumatic Stress Disorder Checklist for DSM-5 (PCL-5): development and initial psychometric evaluation. *J Trauma Stress* 2015;28: 489–498.

627. Wortmann JH, Jordan AH, Weathers FW, Resick PA, Dondanville KA, Hall-Clark B, et al. Psychometric analysis of the PTSD Checklist-5 (PCL-5) among treatment-seeking military service members. *Psychol Assess* 2016;28: 1392–1403.

628. Blake DD, Weathers FW, Nagy LM, Kaloupek DG, Gusman FD, Charney DS, et al. The development of a clinician-administered PTSD scale. *J Trauma Stress* 1995;8: 75–90.

629. Weathers FW, Keane TM, Davidson JR. Clinician-administered PTSD scale: a review of the first ten years of research. *Depress Anxiety* 2001;13: 132–156.

630. Weathers FW, Bovin MJ, Lee DJ, Sloan DM, Schnurr PP, Kaloupek DG, et al. The Clinician-Administered PTSD Scale for DSM-5 (CAPS-5): development and initial psychometric evaluation in military veterans. *Psychol Assess* 2017; 13: 383–395 May 11.

631. Foa EB, Tolin DF Comparison of the PTSD Symptom Scale-Interview Version and the Clinician-Administered PTSD scale. *J Trauma Stress* 2000;13: 181–191.

632. McMillan TM. Errors in diagnosing posttraumatic stress disorders after traumatic brain injury. *Brain Inj* 2001;15: 39–46.

633. Sumpter RE, McMillan TM. Misdiagnosis of post-traumatic stress disorder following severe traumatic brain injury. *Br J Psychiatry* 2005;186: 423–426.

634. Sumpter RE, McMillan TM. Errors in self-report of post-traumatic stress disorder after severe traumatic brain injury. *Brain Inj* 2006;20: 93–99.

635. Carlson KF, Kehle SM, Meis LA, Greer N, Macdonald R, Rutks I, et al. Prevalence, assessment, and treatment of mild traumatic brain injury and posttraumatic stress disorder: a systematic review of the evidence. *J Head Trauma Rehabil* 2011;26: 103–115.

636. Middelboe T, Andersen HS, Birket-Smith M, Friis ML. Minor head injury: impact on general health after 1 year. A prospective follow-up study. *Acta Neurol Scand* 1992;85: 5–9.

637. Bryant RA, Harvey AG. Postconcussive symptoms and post-traumatic stress disorder after mild traumatic brain injury. *J Nerv Ment Dis* 1999;187: 302–305.

638. Schwartz I, Tsenter J, Shochina M, Shiri S, Kedary M, Katz-Leurer M, et al. Rehabilitation outcomes of terror victims with multiple traumas. *Arch Phys Med Rehabil* 2007;88: 440–448.

639. Gaylord KM, Cooper DB, Mercado JM, Kennedy JE, Yoder LH, Holcomb JB. Incidence of posttraumatic stress disorder and mild traumatic brain injury in burned service members: preliminary report. *J Trauma* 2008;64: 200–205.

640. Hoge CW, McGurk D, Thomas JL, Cox AL, Engel CC, Castro CA. Mild traumatic brain injury in U.S. soldiers returning from Iraq. *N Engl J Med* 2008;358: 453–463.

641. Schneiderman AI, Braver ER, Kang HK. Understanding sequelae of injury mechanisms and mild traumatic brain injury incurred during the conflicts in Iraq and Afghanistan: persistent postconcussive symptoms and posttraumatic stress disorder. *Am J Epidemiol* 2008;167: 1446–1452.

642. Mora AG, Ritenour AE, Wade CE, Holcomb JB, Blackbourne LH, Gaylord KM. Posttraumatic stress disorder in combat casualties with burns sustaining primary blast and concussive injuries. *J Trauma* 2009;66: S178–S185.

643. Cooper DB, Mercado-Couch JM, Critchfield E, Kennedy J, Vanderploeg RD, DeVillibis C, Gaylord KM. Factors influencing cognitive functioning following mild traumatic brain injury in OIF/OEF burn patients. *NeuroRehabil* 2010;26: 233–238.

644. Kennedy JE, Cullen MA, Amador RR, Huey JC, Leal FO. Symptoms in military service members after blast mTBI with and without associated injuries. *NeuroRehabil* 2010;26: 191–197.

645. Hill JJ, Mobo BH, Cullen MR. Separating deployment-related traumatic brain injury and posttraumatic stress disorder in veterans: preliminary findings from the Veterans Affairs traumatic brain injury screening program. *Am J Phys Med Rehabil* 2009;88: 605–614.

646. Kontos AP, Kotwal RS, Elbin RJ, Lutz RH, Forsten RD, Benson PJ, et al. Residual effects of combat-related mild traumatic brain injury. *J Neurotrauma* 2013;30: 680–686.

647. Davidson JR, Hughes D, Blazer DG, George LK. Post-traumatic stress disorder in the community: an epidemiological study. *Psychol Med* 1991;21: 713–721.

648. Bremner JD, Southwick SM, Johnson DR, Yehuda R, Charney DS. Childhood physical abuse and combat-related posttraumatic stress disorder in Vietnam veterans. *Am J Psychiatry* 1993;150: 235–239.

649. Brewin CR, Andrews B, Valentine JD. Meta-analysis of risk factors for posttraumatic stress disorder in trauma-exposed adults. *J Consult Clin Psychol* 2000;68: 748–766.

650. Breslau N. Epidemiologic studies of trauma, posttraumatic stress disorder, and other psychiatric disorders. *Can J Psychiatry* 2002;47: 923–929.

651. Norris FH, Friedman MJ, Watson PJ, Byrne CM, Diaz E, Kaniasty K. 60,000 disaster victims speak: part I. An empirical review of the empirical literature, 1981–2001. *Psychiatry* 2002;65: 207–239.

652. Ozer EJ, Best SR, Lipsey TL, Weiss DS. Predictors of posttraumatic stress disorder and symptoms in adults: a meta-analysis. *Psychol Bull* 2003;129: 52–73.

653. Jones M, Sundin J, Goodwin L, Hull L, Fear NT, Wessely S, Rona RJ. What explains post-traumatic stress disorder (PTSD) in UK service personnel: deployment or something else? *Psychol Med* 2013;43: 1703–1712.

654. Ramchand R, Rudavsky R, Grant S, Tanielian T, Jaycox L. Prevalence of, risk factors for, and consequences of post-traumatic stress disorder and other mental health problems in military populations deployed to Iraq and Afghanistan. *Curr Psychiatry Rep* 2015;17: 37.

655. Xue C, Ge Y, Tang B, Liu Y, Kang P, Wang M, et al. A meta-analysis of risk factors for combat-related PTSD among military personnel and veterans. *PLoS One* 2015;10:e0120270.

656. Fauerbach JA, Lawrence JW, Schmidt CW, Munster AM, Costa PT. Personality predictors of injury-related posttraumatic stress disorder. *J Nerv Ment Dis* 2000;188: 510–517.

657. Cox BJ, MacPherson PS, Enns MW, McWilliams LA. Neuroticism and self-criticism associated with posttraumatic stress disorder in a nationally representative sample. *Behav Res Ther* 2004;4: 105–114.

658. Gil S. Pre-traumatic personality as a predictor of posttraumatic stress disorder among undergraduate students exposed to a terrorist attack: a prospective study in Israel. *Pers Ind Diff* 2005;39: 819–827.

659. Engelhard IM, van den Hout MA. Preexisting neuroticism, subjective stressor severity, and posttraumatic stress in soldiers deployed to Iraq. *Can J Psychiatry* 2007;52: 505–509.

660. Jakšić N, Brajković L, Ivezić E, Topić R, Jakovljević M. The role of personality traits in posttraumatic stress disorder (PTSD). *Psychiatria Danubina* 2012;24: 256–266.

661. Feinstein A, Hershkop S, Ouchterlony D, Jardine A, McCullagh S. Posttraumatic amnesia and recall of a traumatic event following traumatic brain injury. *J Neuropsychiatry Clin Neurosci* 2002;14: 25–30.

662. Klein E, Caspi Y, Gil S. The relation between memory of the traumatic event and PTSD: evidence from studies of traumatic brain injury. *Can J Psychiatry* 2003;48: 28–33.

663. Vasterling JJ, Verfaellie M, Sullivan KD. Mild traumatic brain injury and posttraumatic stress disorder in returning veterans: perspectives from cognitive neuroscience. *Clin Psychol Rev* 2009;29: 674–684.

664. Mayou R, Bryant B, Duthie R. Psychiatric consequences of road traffic accidents. *BMJ* 1993;307: 647–651.

665. Warden DL, Labbate LA, Salazar AM, Nelson R, Sheley E, Staudenmeir J, Martin E. Posttraumatic stress disorder in patients with traumatic brain injury and amnesia for the event? *J Neuropsychiatry Clin Neurosci* 1997;9: 18–22.

666. Koenigs M, Huey ED, Raymont V, Cheon B, Solomon J, Wassermann EM, Grafman J. Focal brain damage protects against post-traumatic stress disorder in combat veterans. *Nat Neurosci* 2008;11: 232–237.

667. Nourollahi S, Wille J, Weiß V, Wedekind C, Lippert-Grüner M. Quality-of-life in patients with post-traumatic hypopituitarism. *Brain Inj* 2014;28: 1425–1429.

668. Fernandez-Rodriguez E, Bernabeu I, Castro AI, Casanueva FF. Hypopituitarism after traumatic brain injury. *Endocrinol Metab Clin North Am* 2015;44: 151–159.

669. Klose M, Feldt-Rasmussen U. Hypopituitarism in traumatic brain injury – a critical note. *J Clin Med* 2015;4: 1480–1497.

670. Silva PP, Bhatnagar S, Herman SD, Zafonte R, Klibanski A, Miller KK, Tritos NA. Predictors of hypopituitarism in patients with traumatic brain injury. *J Neurotrauma* 2015;32: 1789–1795.

671. Krewer C, Schneider M, Schneider HJ, Kreitschmann-Andermahr I, Buchfelder M, Faust M, et al. Neuroendocrine disturbances one to five or more years after traumatic brain injury and aneurysmal

subarachnoid hemorrhage: data from the German database on hypopituitarism. *J Neurotrauma* 2016;33: 1544–1553.

672. Wolf EJ, Miller MW, Krueger RF, Lyons MJ, Tsuang MT, Koenen KC. Posttraumatic stress disorder and the genetic structure of comorbidity. *J Abnorm Psychol* 2010;119: 320–330.

673. Logue MW, Baldwin C, Guffanti G, Melista E, Wolf EJ, Reardon AF, et al. A genome-wide association study of posttraumatic stress disorder identifies the retinoid-related orphan receptor alpha (RORA) gene as a significant risk locus. *Mol Psychiatry* 2013;18: 937–942.

674. Xie P, Kranzler HR, Yang C, Zhao H, Farrer LA, Gelernter J. Genome-wide association study identifies new susceptibility loci for posttraumatic stress disorder. *Biol Psychiatry* 2013;74: 656–663.

675. True WR, Rice J, Eisen SA, Heath AC, Goldberg J, Lyons MJ, Nowak J. A twin study of genetic and environmental contributions to liability for posttraumatic stress symptoms. *Arch Gen Psychiatry* 1993;50: 257–264.

676. Xian H, Chantarujikapong SI, Scherrer JF, Eisen SA, Lyons MJ, Goldberg J, et al. Genetic and environmental influences on PTSD, alcohol and drug dependence in twin pairs. *Drug Alcohol Depend* 2000;61: 95–102.

677. Yehuda R, Southwick S, Giller EL, Ma X, Mason JW. Urinary catecholamine excretion and severity of PTSD symptoms in Vietnam combat veterans. *J Nerv Ment Dis* 1992;180: 321–325.

678. Hamner MB, Diamond BI. Elevated plasma dopamine in posttraumatic stress disorder: a preliminary report. *Biol Psychiatry* 1993;33: 304–306.

679. Segman RH, Cooper-Kazaz R, Macciardi F, Goltser T, Halfon Y, Dobroborski T, et al. Association between the dopamine transporter gene and posttraumatic stress disorder. *Mol Psychiatry* 2002;7: 903–907.

680. Lawford BR, McD Young R, Noble EP, Kann B, Arnold L, Rowell J, et al. D2 dopamine receptor gene polymorphism: paroxetine and social functioning in posttraumatic stress disorder. *Eur Neuropsychopharmacol* 2003;13: 313–320.

681. Voisey J, Swagell CD, Hughes IP, Morris CP, van Daal A, Noble EP, et al. The DRD2 gene 957C>T polymorphism is associated with posttraumatic stress disorder in war veterans. *Depress Anxiety* 2009;26: 28–33.

682. Valente NL, Vallada H, Cordeiro Q, Miguita K, Bressan RA, Andreoli SB, et al. Candidate-gene approach in posttraumatic stress disorder after urban violence: association analysis of the genes encoding serotonin transporter, dopamine transporter, and BDNF. *J Mol Neurosci* 2011;44: 59–67.

683. Drury SS, Brett ZH, Henry C, Scheeringa M. The association of a novel haplotype in the dopamine transporter with preschool age posttraumatic stress disorder. *J Child Adolesc Psychopharmacol* 2013;23: 236–243.

684. Kolassa I-T, Kolassa S, Ertl V, Papassotiropoulos A, De Quervain DJ-F. The risk of posttraumatic stress disorder after trauma depends on traumatic load and the catechol-*O*-methyltransferase Val(158)Met polymorphism. *Biol Psychiatry* 2010;67: 304–308.

685. Schulz-Heik RJ, Schaer M, Eliez S, Hallmayer JF, Lin X, Kaloupek DG, et al. Catechol-*O*-methyltransferase Val158Met polymorphism moderates anterior cingulate volume in posttraumatic stress disorder. *Biol Psychiatry* 2011;70: 1091–1096.

686. Norrholm SD, Jovanovic T, Smith AK, Binder E, Klengel T, Conneely K, et al. Differential genetic and epigenetic regulation of catechol-*O*-methyltransferase is associated with impaired fear inhibition in posttraumatic stress disorder. *Front Behav Neurosci* 2013;7: 30.

687. Humphreys KL, Scheeringa MS, Drury SS. Race moderates the association of Catechol-*O*-methyltransferase genotype and

posttraumatic stress disorder in preschool children. *J Child Adolesc Psychopharmacol* 2014;24: 454–457.

688. Kilpatrick DG, Koenen KC, Ruggiero KJ, Acierno R, Galea S, Resnick HS, et al. The serotonin transporter genotype and social support and moderation of posttraumatic stress disorder and depression in hurricane-exposed adults. *Am J Psychiatry* 2007;164: 1693–1699.

689. Grabe HJ, Spitzer C, Schwahn C, Marcinek A, Frahnow A, Barnow S, et al. Serotonin transporter gene (SLC6A4) promoter polymorphisms and the susceptibility to posttraumatic stress disorder in the general population. *Am J Psychiatry* 2009;166: 926–933.

690. Xie P, Kranzler HR, Poling J, Stein MB, Anton RF, Brady K, et al. Interactive effect of stressful life events and the serotonin transporter 5-HTTLPR genotype on posttraumatic stress disorder diagnosis in 2 independent populations. *Arch Gen Psychiatry* 2009;66: 1201–1209.

691. Xie P, Kranzler HR, Farrer L, Gelernter J. Serotonin transporter 5-HTTLPR genotype moderates the effects of childhood adversity on posttraumatic stress disorder risk: a replication study. *Am J Med Genet B Neuropsychiatr Genet* 2012;159B: 644–652.

692. Gressier F, Calati R, Balestri M, Marsano A, Alberti S, Antypa N, Serretti A. The 5-HTTLPR polymorphism and posttraumatic stress disorder: a meta-analysis. *J Trauma Stress* 2013;26: 645–653.

693. Kimbrel NA, Morissette SB, Meyer EC, Chrestman R, Jamroz R, Silvia PJ, et al. Effect of the 5-HTTLPR polymorphism on posttraumatic stress disorder, depression, anxiety, and quality of life among Iraq and Afghanistan veterans. *Anxiety Stress Coping* 2015;28: 456–466.

694. Tian Y, Liu H, Guse L, Wong TK, Li J, Bai Y, Jiang X. Association of genetic factors and gene–environment interactions with risk of developing posttraumatic stress disorder in a case–control study. *Biol Res Nurs* 2015;17: 364–372.

695. Pivac N, Kozaric-Kovacic D, Grubisic-Ilic M, Nedic G, Rakos I, Nikolac M, et al. The association between brain-derived neurotrophic factor Val66Met variants and psychotic symptoms in posttraumatic stress disorder. *World J Biol Psychiatry* 2012;13: 306–311.

696. Felmingham KL, Dobson-Stone C, Schofield PR, Quirk GJ, Bryant RA. The brain-derived neurotrophic factor Val66Met polymorphism predicts response to exposure therapy in posttraumatic stress disorder. *Biol Psychiatry* 2013;73: 1059–1063.

697. Li RH, Fan M, Hu MS, Ran MS, Fang DZ. Reduced severity of posttraumatic stress disorder associated with Val allele of Val66Met polymorphism at brain-derived neurotrophic factor gene among Chinese adolescents after Wenchuan earthquake. *Psychophysiol* 2016;53: 705–711.

698. Gillespie CF, Phifer J, Bekh Bradley B, Ressler KJ. Development of the stress response. *Depress Anxiety* 2009;26: 984–992.

699. Yehuda R, Cai G, Golier JA, Sarapas C, Galea S, Ising M, et al. Gene expression patterns associated with posttraumatic stress disorder following exposure to the World Trade Center attacks. *Biol Psychiatry* 2009;66: 708–711.

700. Sarapas C, Cai G, Bierer LM, Golier JA, Galea S, Ising M, et al. Genetic markers for PTSD risk and resilience among survivors of the World Trade Center attacks. *Dis Markers* 2011;30: 101–110.

701. Hauer D, Weis F, Papassotiropoulos A, Schmoeckel M, Beiras-Fernandez A, Lieke J, et al. Relationship of a common polymorphism of the glucocorticoid receptor gene to traumatic memories and posttraumatic stress disorder in patients after intensive care therapy. *Crit Care Med* 2011;39: 643–650.

702. Pohlack ST, Nees F, Ruttorf M, Cacciaglia R, Winkelmann T, Schad LR, Witt SH, et al. Neural mechanism of a sex-specific risk variant for posttraumatic stress disorder in the type I receptor of the pituitary adenylate cyclase activating polypeptide. *Biol Psychiatry* 2015;78: 840–847.

703. Castro-Vale I, van Rossum EF, Machado JC, Mota-Cardoso R, Carvalho D. Genetics of glucocorticoid regulation and posttraumatic stress disorder – what do we know? *Neurosci Biobehav Rev* 2016;63: 143–157.

704. Fani N, King TZ, Shin J, Srivastava A, Brewster RC, Jovanovic T, et al. Structural and functional connectivity in posttraumatic stress disorder: associations with FKBP5. *Depress Anxiety* 2016;33: 300–307.

705. Ressler KJ, Mercer KB, Bradley B, Jovanovic T, Mahan A, Kerley K, et al. Post-traumatic stress disorder is associated with PACAP and the PAC1 receptor. *Nature* 2011;470: 492–497.

706. Binder EB, Bradley RG, Liu W, Epstein MP, Deveau TC, Mercer KB, et al. Association of FKBP5 polymorphisms and childhood abuse with risk of posttraumatic stress disorder symptoms in adults. *JAMA* 2008;299: 1291–1305.

707. Xie P, Kranzler HR, Poling J, Stein MB, Anton RF, Farrer LA, Gelernter J. Interaction of FKBP5 with childhood adversity on risk for post-traumatic stress disorder. *Neuropsychopharmacol* 2010;35: 1684–1692.

708. van Zuiden M, Geuze E, Willemen HLDM, Vermetten E, Maas M, Amarouchi K, et al. Glucocorticoid receptor pathway components predict posttraumatic stress disorder symptom development: a prospective study. *Biol Psychiatry* 2012;71: 309–316.

709. Nelson EC, Agrawal A, Pergadia ML, Lynskey MT, Todorov AA, Wang JC et al. Association of childhood trauma exposure and GABRA2 polymorphisms with risk of posttraumatic stress disorder in adults. *Mol Psychiatry* 2009;14: 234.

710. Freeman T, Roca V, Guggenheim F, Kimbrell T, Griffin WST. Neuropsychiatric associations of apolipoprotein E alleles in subjects with combat-related posttraumatic stress disorder. *J. Neuropsychiatry Clin Neurosci* 2014;17: 541–543.

711. Andero R, Brothers SP, Jovanovic T, Chen YT, Salah-Uddin H, Cameron M, et al. Amygdala-dependent fear is regulated by Oprl1 in mice and humans with PTSD. *Sci Transl Med* 2013;5: 188ra73.

712. Stein MB, Chen CY, Ursano RJ, Cai T, Gelernter J, Heeringa SG, et al. Army Study to Assess Risk and Resilience in Servicemembers (STARRS) collaborators. Genome-wide association studies of posttraumatic stress disorder in 2 cohorts of US Army soldiers. *JAMA Psychiatry* 2016;73: 695–704.

713. Guffanti G, Galea S, Yan L, Roberts AL, Solovieff N, Allison E. Aiello AE, et al. Genome-wide association study implicates a novel RNA gene, the lincRNA AC068718.1, as a risk factor for post-traumatic stress disorder in women. *Psychoneuroendocrinol* 2013;38: 3029–3038.

714. Cornelis MC, Nugent NR, Amstadter AB, Koenen KC. Genetics of post-traumatic stress disorder: review and recommendations for genome-wide association studies. *Curr Psychiatry Rep* 2010;12: 313–326.

715. Almli LM, Duncan R, Feng H, Ghosh D, Binder EB, Bradley B, et al. A genome-wide identified risk variant for PTSD is a methylation quantitative trait locus and confers decreased cortical activation to fearful faces. *JAMA Psychiatry* 2014;71: 1392–1399.

716. Raabe FJ, Spengler D. Epigenetic risk factors in PTSD and depression. *Front Psychiatry* 2013;4: 80.

717. Dretsch MN, Williams K, Emmerich T, Crynen G, Ait-Ghezala G, Chaytow H, et al. Brain-derived neurotropic factor polymorphisms, traumatic stress, mild traumatic brain injury, and combat exposure contribute to postdeployment traumatic stress. *Brain Behav* 2016;6: e00392.

718. Southwick SM, Krystal JH, Morgan CA, Johnson D, Nagy LM, Nicolaou A, et al. Abnormal noradrenergic function in posttraumatic stress disorder. *Arch Gen Psychiatry* 1993;50: 266–274.

719. McFarlane AC, Atchison M, Yehuda R. The acute stress response following motor vehicle accidents and its relation to PTSD. *Ann NY Acad Sci* 1997;821: 437–441.

720. Shalev AY, Sahar T, Freedman S, Peri T, Glick N, Brandes D, Orr SP, Pitman RK. A prospective study of heart rate response following trauma and the subsequent development of posttraumatic stress disorder. *Arch Gen Psychiatry* 1998;55: 553–559.

721. Delahanty DL, Raimonde AJ, Spoonster E. Initial posttraumatic urinary cortisol levels predict subsequent PTSD symptoms in motor vehicle accident victims. *Biol Psychiatry* 2000;48: 940–947.

722. Yehuda R. Risk and resilience in posttraumatic stress disorder. *J ClinPsychiatry* 2004;65 (suppl 1): 29–36.

723. Orr SP, Lasko NB, Macklin ML, Pineles SL, Chang Y, Pitman RK. Predicting post-trauma stress symptoms from pre-trauma psychophysiologic reactivity, personality traits and measures of psychopathology. *Biol Mood Anxiety Disord* 2012;2: 8.

724. Lebois LA, Wolff JD, Ressler KJ. Neuroimaging genetic approaches to posttraumatic stress disorder. *Exp Neurol* 2016;284(B): 141–152.

725. Thakur GA, Joober R, Brunet A. Development and persistence of posttraumatic stress disorder and the 5-HTTLPR polymorphism. *J Trauma Stress* 2009;22: 240–243.

726. Wang T. Does BDNF Val66Met polymorphism confer risk for posttraumatic stress disorder? *Neuropsychobiol* 2015;71: 149–153.

727. Depue BE, Olson-Madden JH, Smolker HR, Rajamani M, Brenner LA, Banich MT. Reduced amygdala volume is associated with deficits in inhibitory control: a voxel- and surface-based morphometric analysis of comorbid PTSD/mild TBI. *Biomed Res Int* 2014;2014: article ID 691505.

728. Broca P. Anatomie comparée des circonvolutions cérébrales: le grand lobe limbique. *Rev Anthropol* 1878;1: 385–498.

729. Bard P. A diencephalic mechanism for the expression of rage with special reference to the central nervous system. *Am J Physiol* 1928;84: 490–513.

730. Papez JW. A proposed mechanism of emotion. *Arch Neurol Psychiatry* 1937;38: 725–743.

731. MacLean P. Psychosomatic disease and the "visceral brain": recent developments bearing on the Papez theory of emotion. *Psychosom Med* 1949;11: 338–353.

732. Lévêque M. The neuroanatomy of emotions. In Lévêque M, editor. *Psychosurgery*. Cham: Springer International Publishing, 2014, pp. 49–106.

733. Brenner LA, Homaifar BY, Adler LE, Wolfman JH, Kemp J. Suicidality and veterans with a history of traumatic brain injury: precipitants, events, protective factors, and prevention strategies. *Rehabil Psychol* 2009;54: 390–397.

734. Brenner LA, Betthauser LM, Homaifar BY, Villarreal E, Harwood JE, Staves PJ, Huggins JA. Posttraumatic stress disorder, traumatic brain injury, and suicide attempt history among veterans receiving mental health services. *Suicide Life Threat Behav* 2011;41: 416–423.

735. Karl A, Schaefer M, Malta LS, Dörfel D, Rohleder N, Werner A. A meta-analysis of structural brain abnormalities in PTSD. *Neurosci Biobehav Rev* 2006;30: 1004–1031.

736. Chen S, Xia W, Li L, Liu J, He Z, Zhang Z, et al. Gray matter density reduction in the insula in fire survivors with posttraumatic stress disorder: a voxel-based morphometric study. *Psychiatry Res* 2006;146: 65–72.

737. Chen S, Li L, Xu B, Liu, J. Insular cortex involvement in declarative memory deficits in patients with post-traumatic stress disorder. *BMC Psychiatry* 2009;9: 39.

738. Shin LM, McNally RJ, Kosslyn SM, Thompson WL, Rauch SL, Alpert NM, et al. Regional cerebral blood flow during script-driven imagery in childhood sexual abuse-related PTSD: a PETinvestigation. *Am J Psychiatry* 1999;156: 575–584.

739. Pissiota A, Frans O, Fernandez M, vonKnorring L, Fischer H, Fredrikson M. Neurofunctional correlates of posttraumatic stress disorder: a PET symptom provocation study. *Eur Arch Psychiatry Clin Neurosci* 2002;252: 68–75.

740. Britton JC, Phan KL, Taylor SF, Fig LM, Liberzon I. Corticolimbic blood flow in posttraumatic stress disorder during script-driven imagery. *Biol Psychiatry* 2005;57: 832–840.

741. Lanius RA, Williamson PC, Boksman K, Densmore M, Gupta M, Neufeld RW, et al. Brain activation during script-driven imagery induced dissociative responses in PTSD: a functional magnetic resonance imaging investigation. *Biol Psychiatry* 2002;52: 305–311.

742. Lanius RA, Williamson PC, Bluhm RL, Densmore, M., Boksman K, Neufeld RW, et al. Functional connectivity of dissociative responses in posttraumatic stress disorder: a functional magnetic resonance imaging investigation. *Biol Psychiatry* 2005;57: 873–884.

743. Hou C, Liu J, Wang K, Li L, Liang M, He Z, et al. Brain responses to symptom provocation and trauma-related short-term memory recall in coal mining accident survivors with acute severe PTSD. *Brain Res* 2007;1144: 165–174.

744. Morey RA, Petty CM, Cooper DA, Labar KS, McCarthy G. Neural systems for executive and emotional processing are modulated by symptoms of posttraumatic stress disorder in Iraq War veterans. *Psychiatry Res* 2008;162: 59–72.

745. Mazza M, Catalucci A, Mariano M, Pino MC, Tripaldi S, Roncone R, Gallucci M. Neural correlates of automatic perceptual sensitivity to facial affect in posttraumatic stress disorder subjects who survived L'Aquila eartquake of April 6, 2009. *Brain Imaging Behav* 2012;6: 374–386.

746. Lanius RA, Bluhm R, Lanius U, Pain C. A review of neuroimaging studies in PTSD: heterogeneity of response to symptom provocation. *J Psychiatr Res* 2006;40: 709–729.

747. Werner NS, Meindl T, Engel RR, Rosner R, Riedel M, Reiser M, et al. Hippocampal function during associative learning in patients with posttraumatic stress disorder. *J Psychiatric Res* 2009;43: 309–318.

748. Geuze E, Vermetten E, Ruf M, de Kloet CS, Westenberg HGM. Neural correlates of associative learning and memory in veterans with posttraumatic stress disorder. *J Psychiatric Res* 2008;42: 659–669.

749. Bigler ED, Blatter DD, Anderson CV, Johnson SC, Gale SD, Hopkins RO, Burnett B. Hippocampal volume in normal aging and traumatic brain injury. *AJNR Am J Neuroradiol* 1997;18: 11–23.

750. Tate DF, Bigler ED. Fornix and hippocampal atrophy in traumatic brain injury. *Learn Memory* 2000;7: 442–446.

751. Himanen L, Portin R, Isoniemi H, Helenius H, Kurki T, Tenovuo O. Cognitive functions in relation to MRI findings 30 years after traumatic brain injury. *Brain Inj* 2005;19: 93–100.

752. Strangman GE, O'Neil-Pirozzi TM, Supelana C, Goldstein R, Katz DI, Glenn MB. Regional brain morphometry predicts memory rehabilitation outcome after traumatic brain injury. *Front Hum Neurosci* 2010;4: 182.

753. Warner MA, Youn TS, Davis T, Chandra A, Marquez de la Plata C, Moore C, et al. Regionally selective atrophy after traumatic axonal injury. *Arch Neurol* 2010;67: 1336–1344.

754. Kitayama N, Vaccarino V, Kutner M, Weiss P, Bremner JD. Magnetic resonance imaging (MRI) measurement of hippocampal volume in posttraumatic stress disorder: a metaanalysis. *J Affective Disord* 2005;88: 79–86.

755. Smith ME. Bilateral hippocampal volume reduction in adults with post-traumatic stress disorder: a meta-analysis of structural MRI studies. *Hippocampus* 2005;15: 798–807.

756. Hughes KC, Shin LM. Functional neuroimaging studies of post-traumatic stress disorder. *Exp Rev Neurother* 2011;11: 275–285.

757. Starcevic A, Postic S, Radojicic Z, Starcevic B, Milovanovic S, Ilankovic A, et al. Volumetric analysis of amygdala, hippocampus, and prefrontal cortex in therapy-naive PTSD participants. *BioMed Res Int* 2014; 968495.

758. Yount R, Raschke KA, Biru M, Tate DF, Miller MJ, Abildskov T, et al. Traumatic brain injury and atrophy of the cingulate gyrus. *J Neuropsychiatry Clin Neurosci* 2002;14: 416–423.

759. Gale SD, Baxter L, Roundy N, Johnson SC. Traumatic brain injury and grey matter concentration: a preliminary voxel based morphometry study. *J Neurol Neurosurg Psychiatry* 2005;76: 984–988.

760. Levine B, Kovacevic N, Nica EI, Cheung G, Gao F, Schwartz ML, Black SE. The Toronto traumatic brain injury study: injury severity and quantified MRI. *Neurology* 2008;70: 771–778.

761. Zhou Y, Kierans A, Kenul D, Ge Y, Rath J, Reaume J, et al. Mild traumatic brain injury: longitudinal regional brain volume changes. *Radiology* 2013;267: 880–890.

762. Yamasue H, Kasai K, Iwanami A, Ohtani T, Yamada H, Abe O, et al. Voxel-based analysisof MRI reveals anterior cingulate gray-matter volume reduction in posttraumatic stress disorder due to terrorism. *Proc Natl Acad Sci U S A* 2003;100: 9039–9043.

763. Corbo V, Clement M-H, Armony JL, Pruessner JC, Brunet A. Size versus shape differences: contrasting voxelbased and volumetric analyses of the anterior cingulate cortex in individuals with acute posttraumatic stress disorder. *Biol Psychiatry* 2005;58: 119–124.

764. Woodward SH, Kaloupek DG, Streeter CC, Martinez C, Schaer M, Eliez S. Decreased anterior cingulate volume in combat-related PTSD. *Biol Psychiatry* 2006;59: 582–587.

765. Sui SG, Wu MX, King ME, Zhang Y, Ling L, Xu JM, et al. Abnormal grey matter in victims of rape with PTSD in mainland China: a voxel-based morphometry study. *Acta Neuropsychiatr* 2010;22: 118–126.

766. Thomaes K, Dorrepaal E, Draijer N, de Ruiter MB, van Balkom AJ, Smit JH, Veltman DJ. Reduced anterior cingulate and orbitofrontal volumes in child abuse-related complex PTSD. *J Clin Psychiatry* 2010;71: 1636–1644.

767. Baldaçara L, Zugman A, Araújo C, Cogo-Moreira H, Lacerda AL, Schoedl A, et al. Reduction of anterior cingulate in adults with urban violence-related PTSD. *J Affect Disord* 2014;168: 13–20.

768. Demers LA, Olson EA, Crowley DJ, Rauch SL, Rosso IM. Dorsal anterior cingulate thickness is related to alexithymia in childhood trauma-related PTSD. *PLoS One* 2015;10: e0139807.

769. Shenton ME, Hamoda HM, Schneiderman JS, Bouix S, Pasternak O, Rathi Y, et al. A review of magnetic resonance imaging and diffusion tensor imaging findings in mild traumatic brain injury. *Brain Imaging Behav* 2012;6: 137–192.

770. Lindemer ER, Salat DH, Leritz EC, McGlinchey RE, Milberg WP. Reduced cortical thickness with increased lifetime burden of PTSD in OEF/OIF veterans and the impact of comorbid TBI. *NeuroImage Clin* 2013;2: 601–611.

771. Davenport ND, Lim KO, Sponheim SR. White matter abnormalities associated with military PTSD in the context of blast TBI. *Hum Brain Mapp* 2015;36: 1053–1064.

772. Williamson JB, Heilman KM, Porges EC, Lamb DG, Porges SW. A possible mechanism for PTSD symptoms in patients with traumatic brain injury: central autonomic network disruption. *Front Neuroeng* 2013;6: 13.

773. Schwaber JS, Kapp BS, Higgins GA, Rapp PR. Amygdaloid and basal forebrain direct connections with the nucleus of the solitary tract and the dorsal motor nucleus. *J Neurosci* 1982;2: 1424–1438.

774. van der Kooy D, Koda LY, McGinty JF, Gerfen CR, Bloom FE. The organization of projections from the cortex, amygdala, and hypothalamus to the nucleus of the solitary tract in rat. *J Comp Neurol* 1984;224: 1–24.

775. Rogers RC, Fryman DL. Direct connections between the central nucleus of the amygdala and the nucleus of the solitary tract: an electrophysiological study in the rat. *J Auton Nerv Syst* 1988;22: 83–87.

776. Reppucci CJ, Petrovich GD. Organization of connections between the amygdala, medial prefrontal cortex, and lateral hypothalamus: a single and double retrograde tracing study in rats. *Brain Struct Funct* 2016;221: 2937–2962.

777. Yeh PH, Wang B, Oakes TR, French LM, Pan H, Graner J, et al. Postconcussional disorder and PTSD symptoms of military-related traumatic brain injury associated with compromised neurocircuitry. *Hum Brain Mapp* 2014;35: 2652–2673.

778. Simmons AN, Matthews SC. Neural circuitry of PTSD with or without mild traumatic brain injury: a meta-analysis. *Neuropharmacol* 2012;62: 598–606.

779. Amen DG, Raji CA, Willeumier K, Taylor D, Tarzwell R, Newberg A, et al. Functional neuroimaging distinguishes posttraumatic stress disorder from traumatic brain injury in focused and large community datasets. *PLoS One* 2015;10: e0129659.

780. Cohen H, Kozlovsky N, Alona C, Matar MA, Joseph Z. Animal model for PTSD: from clinical concept to translational research. *Neuropharmacol* 2012;62: 715–724.

781. Reger ML, Poulos AM, Buen F, Giza CC, Hovda DA, Fanselow MS. Concussive brain injury enhances fear learning and excitatory processes in the amygdala. *Biol Psychiatry* 2012;71: 335–343.

782. Shu IW, Onton JA, O'Connell RM, Simmons AN, Matthews SC. Combat veterans with comorbid PTSD and mild TBI exhibit a greater inhibitory processing ERP from the dorsal anterior cingulate cortex. *Psychiatry Res* 2014;224: 58–66.

783. Kessler RC, Sonnega A, Bromet E, Hughes M, Nelson CB.. Posttraumatic stress disorder in the National Comorbidity Survey. *Arch Gen Psychiatry* 1995;52: 1048–1060.

784. Capehart B, Bass D. Review: managing posttraumatic stress disorder in combat veterans with comorbid traumatic brain injury. *J Rehabil Res Dev* 2012;49(5): 789.

785. Horvath AO, Luborsky L. The role of the therapeutic alliance in psychotherapy. *J Consult Clin Psychol* 1993;61: 561–573.

786. Mueser KT, Rosenberg SD, Xie H, Jankowski MK, Bolton EE, Lu W, et al. A randomized controlled trial of cognitive behavioral treatment for posttraumatic stress disorder in severe mental illness. *J Consult Clin Psychol* 2008;76: 259–271.

787. Ardito RB, Rabellino D. Therapeutic alliance and outcome of psychotherapy: historical excursus, measurements, and prospects for research. *Front Psychol* 2011;2: 270.

788. Zantvoord JB, Diehle J, Lindauer RJ. Using neurobiological measures to predict and assess treatment outcome of psychotherapy in posttraumatic stress disorder: systematic review. *Psychother Psychosom* 2013;82: 142–151.

789. Buccino G, Amore M. Mirror neurons and the understanding of behavioural symptoms in psychiatric disorders. *Curr Opin Psychiatry* 2008;21: 281–285.

790. Schermer VL. Mirror neurons: their implications for group psychotherapy. *Int J Group Psychother* 2010;60: 486–513.

791. Mitchell JT. When disaster strikes: the critical incident stress debriefing process. *J Emerg Med Serv* 1983;13: 49–52.

792. Bisson JI, Jenkins PL, Alexander J, Bannister C. Randomised controlled trial of psychological debriefing for victims of acute burn trauma. *Br J Psychiatry* 1993;171: 78–81.

793. Raphael B, Meldrum L. Does debriefing after psychological trauma work? *Br Med J* 1995;310: 1479–1480.

794. Carlier IVE, Lamberts RD, van Uchelen AJ, Gersons BPR. Disaster-related post-traumatic stress in police officers: a field study of the impact of debriefing. *Stress Med* 1998;14: 143–148.

795. Mayou RA, Ehlers A, Hobbs M. Psychological debriefing for road traffic accident victims. *Br J Psychiatry* 2000;176: 589–593.

796. Rose S, Bisson J, Wessely S. Psychological debriefing for preventing post traumatic stress disorder (PTSD). *Cochrane Database Syst Rev* 2002;(2):CD000560.

797. McNally RJ, Bryant RA, Ehlers A. Does early psychological intervention promote recovery from posttraumatic stress? *Psychol Sci Public Inter* 2003;4: 45–79.

798. Fontana A, Rosenheck R, Horvath T. Social support and psychopathology in the war zone. *J Nerv Ment Dis* 1997;185: 6.

799. Khan-Bourne N, Brown RG. Cognitive behaviour therapy for the treatment of depression in individuals with brain injury. *Neuropsychol Rehabil* 2003;13: 89–107.

800. Lockwood C, Page T, Conroy-Hiller T. Comparing the effectiveness of cognitive behaviour therapy using individual of group therapy in the treatment of depression. *Int J Evid Based Health* 2004;2: 185–206.

801. Resick PA, Schnicke MK. Cognitive processing therapy for sexual assault victims. *J Consult Clin Psychol* 1992;60: 748–756.

802. Monson CM, Schnurr PP, Resick PA, Friedman MJ, Young-Xu Y, Stevens SP. Cognitive processing therapy for veterans with military related posttraumatic stress disorder. *J Consult Clin Psychol* 2006;74: 898–907.

803. Resick PA, Nishith P, Weaver TL, Astin MC, Feuer CA. A comparison of cognitive-processing therapy with prolonged exposure and a waiting condition for the treatment of chronic posttraumatic stress disorder in female rape victims. *J Consult Clin Psychol* 2002;70: 867–879.

804. Creamer M, Forbes D, Phelps A, Humpreys L. Treating traumatic stress: conducting imaginal exposure. 2004. In: PTSD clinician's manual and training video. Australian Centre for Posttraumatic Mental Health, University of Melbourne. Available at: www.acpmh.unilmelb.edu.au.

805. Nacasch N, Foa EB, Huppert JD, Tzur D, Fostick L, Dinstein Y, et al. Prolonged exposure therapy for combat- and terror-related posttraumatic stress disorder: a randomized control comparison with treatment as usual. *J Clin Psychiatry* 2011;72: 1174–1180.

806. Mendes DD, Mello MF, Ventura P, Passarela Cde M, Mari J de J. A systematic review on the effectiveness of cognitive behavioral therapy for posttraumatic stress disorder. *Int J Psychiatry Med* 2008;38: 241–259.

807. Powers MB, Halpern JM, Ferenschak MP, Gillihan SJ, Foa EB. A meta-analytic review of prolonged exposure for posttraumatic stress disorder. *Clin Psychol Rev* 2010;30: 635–641.

808. Steenkamp MM, Litz BT, Hoge CW, Marmar CR. Psychotherapy for military-related PTSD: a review of randomized clinical trials. *JAMA* 2015;314: 489–500.

809. Soo C, Tate R. Psychological treatment for anxiety in people with traumatic brain injury. *Cochrane Database Syst Rev* 2007;(3): CD005239.

810. Bryant RA, Moulds M, Guthrie R, Nixon RD. Treating acute stress disorder following mild traumatic brain injury. *Am J Psychiatry* 2003;160: 585–587.

811. Tiersky LA, Anselmi V, Johnston MV, Kurtyka J, Roosen E, Schwartz T, et al. A trial of neuropsychologic rehabilitation in mild-spectrum traumatic brain injury. *Arch Phys Med Rehabil* 2005;86: 1565–1574.

812. Chard KM, Schumm JA, McIlvain SM, Bailey GW, Parkinson RB. Exploring the efficacy of a residential treatment program incorporating cognitive processing therapy-cognitive for veterans with PTSD and traumatic brain injury. *J Trauma Stress* 2011;24: 347–351.

813. Walter KH, Dickstein BD, Barnes SM, Chard KM. Comparing effectiveness of CPT to CPT-C among U.S. Veterans in an interdisciplinary residential PTSD/TBI treatment program. *J Trauma Stress* 2014;27: 438–445.

814. Sripada RK, Rauch SA, Tuerk PW, Smith E, Defever AM, Mayer RA, et al. Mild traumatic brain injury and treatment response in prolonged exposure for PTSD. *J Trauma Stress* 2013;26: 369–375.

815. Wolf GK, Kretzmer T, Crawford E, Thors C, Wagner R, Strom TQ, et al. Prolonged exposure therapy with veterans and active duty personnel diagnosed with PTSD and traumatic brain injury. *J Trauma Stress* 2015;28: 339–347.

816. Barnes VA, Rigg JL, Williams JJ. Clinical case series: treatment of PTSD with transcendental meditation in active duty military personnel. *Mil Med* 2013;178: e836–e840.

817. Management of Post-Traumatic Stress Working Group. *VA/DoD clinical practice guideline for management of post-traumatic stress.* Washington, DC: Department of Veterans Affairs, Department of Defense, 2010. Available from: www.healthquality.va.gov/ptsd/ptsd full.pdf.

818. Shapiro F. Eye movement desensitization: a new treatment for post- traumatic stress disorder. *J BehavTher Exp Psychiatry* 1989;20: 211–217.

819. Shapiro F. *Eye movement desensitization and reprocessing: basic principles, protocols and procedures.* New York: Guilford Press, 1995.

820. Shapiro F. *Eye movement desensitization and reprocessing: basic principles, protocols and procedures (2nd edition).* New York: Guilford Press, 2001.

821. Samara Z, Elzinga BM, Slagter HA, Nieuwenhuis S. Do horizontal saccadic eye movements increase interhemispheric coherence? Investigation of a hypothesized neural mechanism underlying EMDR. *Front Psychiatry* 2011;2: 4.

822. Rashid AJ, Yan C, Mercaldo V, Hsiang HL, Park S, Cole CJ, et al. Competition between engrams influences fear memory formation and recall. *Science* 2016;353: 383–387.

823. Cambiaghi M, Grosso A, Likhtik E, Mazziotti R, Concina G, Renna A, et al. Higher-order sensory cortex drives basolateral amygdala activity during the recall of remote, but not recently learned fearful memories. *J Neurosci* 2016;36: 1647–1659.

824. Herkt D, Tumani V, Grön G, Kammer, T, Hoffman A, Abler B. Facilitating access to emotions: neural signature of EMDR stimulation. *PLoS One* 2014;9: e106350.

825. Sprang G. The use of eye movement desensitization and reprocessing (EMDR) in the treatment of traumatic stress and complicated mourning: psychological and behavioral outcomes. *Res Soc Work Pract* 2001;11: 300–320.

826. Korn DL, Leeds AM. Preliminary evidence of efficacy for EMDR resource development and installation in the stabilization phase of treatment of complex posttraumatic stress disorder. *J Clin Psychol* 2002;58: 1465–1487.

827. Rothbaum BO. A controlled study of eye movement desensitization and reprocessing in the treatment of post-traumatic stress disordered sexual assault victims. *Bull Menninger Clin* 1997;61: 317–334.

828. Marcus S, Marquis P, Sakai C. Controlled study of treatment of PTSD using EMDR in an HMO setting. *Psychotherapy* 1997;34: 307–315.

829. Marcus S, Marquis P, Sakai C. Three- and 6-month follow-up of EMDR treatment of PTSD in an HMO setting. *Int J Stress Manag* 2004;11: 195–208.

830. Wilson S, Becker LA, Tinker RH. Eye movement desensitization and reprocessing (EMDR): treatment for psychologically traumatized individuals. *J Consult Clin Psychol* 1995;63: 928–937.

831. Wilson S, Becker LA, Tinker RH. Fifteen-month follow-up of eye movement desensitization and reprocessing (EMDR) treatment of post-traumatic stress disorder and psychological trauma. *J Consult Clin Psychol* 1997;65: 1047–1056.

832. Carlson J, Chemtob CM, Rusnak K, Hedlund NL, Muraoka MY. Eye movement desensitization and reprocessing (EMDR): treatment for combat-related post-traumatic stress disorder. *J Trauma Stress* 1998;11: 3–24.

833. Cahill SP, Carrigan MH, Frueh BC. Does EMDR work? And if so, why?: a critical review of controlled outcome and dismantling research. *J Anxiety Disord* 1999;13: 5–33.

834. Ponniah K, Hollon SD. Empirically supported psychological treatments for adult acute stress disorder and posttraumatic stress disorder: a review. *Depress Anxiety* 2009;26: 1086–1109.

835. Bisson JI, Roberts NP, Andrew M, Cooper R, Lewis C. Psychological therapies for chronic post-traumatic stress disorder (PTSD) in adults. *Cochrane Database Syst Rev* 2013;12: CD003388.

836. Boccia M, Piccardi L, Cordellieri P, Guariglia C, Giannini AM. EMDR therapy for PTSD after motor vehicle accidents: meta-analytic evidence for specific treatment. *Front Hum Neurosci* 2015;9: 213.

837. National Collaborating Centre for Mental Health. *Post-traumatic stress disorder. the management of PTSD in adults and children in primary and secondary care.* London: Gaskell, British Psychological Society, 2005.

838. World Health Organization. *Guidelines for the management of conditions that are specifically related to stress.* Geneva: WHO, 2013.

839. Lansing K, Amen DG, Hanks C, Rudy L. High-resolution brain SPECT imaging and eye movement desensitization and reprocessing in police officers with PTSD. *J Neuropsychiatry Clin Neurosci* 2005;17: 526–532.

840. McAllister TW. Psychopharmacological issues in the treatment of TBI and PTSD. *Clin Neuropsychol* 2009;23: 1338–1367.

841. Krystal JH, Rosenheck RA, Cramer JA, Vessicchio JC, Jones KM, Vertrees JE, et al. Adjunctive risperidone treatment for antidepressant-resistant symptoms of chronic military service-related PTSD: a randomized trial. *JAMA* 2011;306: 493–502.

842. Watson HR, Ghani M, Correll T. Treatment options for individuals with PTSD and concurrent TBI: a literature review and case presentation. *Curr Psychiatry Rep* 2016;18: 63.

843. Hoskins M, Pearce J, Bethell A, Dankova L, Barbui C, Tol WA, et al. Pharmacotherapy for post-traumatic stress disorder: systematic review and meta-analysis. *Br J Psychiatry* 2015;206: 93–100.

844. Puetz TW, Youngstedt SD, Herring MP. Effects of pharmacotherapy on combat-related PTSD, anxiety, and depression: a systematic review and meta-regression analysis. *PLoS One* 2015;10: e0126529.

845. Alao A, Selvarajah J, Razi S. The use of clonidine in the treatment of nightmares among patients with co-morbid PTSD and traumatic brain injury. *Int J Psychiatry Med* 2012;44: 165–169.

846. Purgato M, Papola D, Gastaldon C, Trespidi C, Magni LR, Rizzo C, et al. Paroxetine versus other anti-depressive agents for depression. *Cochrane Database Syst Rev* 2014;4: CD006531.

847. Lin HL, Hsu YT, Liu CY, Chen CH, Hsiao MC, Liu YL, et al. Comparison of escitalopram and paroxetine in the treatment of major depressive disorder. *Int Clin Psychopharmacol* 2013;28: 339–345.

848. Hetrick SE, Purcell R, Garner B, Parslow R. Combined pharmacotherapy and psychological therapies for post traumatic stress disorder (PTSD). *Cochrane Database Syst Rev* 2010;7: CD007316.

849. Singer IB. "The Chimney Sweep," in *A friend of Kafka and other stories.* New York: Farrar, Straus & Giroux, 1970.

850. Franklin GM. Opioids for chronic noncancer pain: a position paper of the American Academy of Neurology. *Neurology* 2014;83: 1277–1284.

851. Nadeau SE. Opioids for chronic noncancer pain: to prescribe or not to prescribe – what is the question? *Neurology* 2015;85: 646–651.

852. Argoff CE. Letter to the editor – in response to Franklin GM: evidence misrepresented. *Neurology* 2015;84: 1503–1504.

853. Popovic V, Aimaretti G, Casanueva FF, Ghigo E. Hypopituitarism following traumatic brain injury (TBI): call for attention. *J Endocrinol Invest* 2005;28 (5 Suppl): 61–64.

854. Wilkinson CW, Pagulayan KF, Petrie EC, Mayer CL, Colasurdo EA, Shofer JB, et al. High prevalence of chronic pituitary and target-organ hormone abnormalities after blast-related mild traumatic brain injury. *Front Neurol* 2012;3: 11.

855. Zheng P, He B, Tong WS. Decrease in pituitary apparent diffusion coefficient in normal appearing brain correlates with hypopituitarism following traumatic brain injury. *J Endocrinol Invest* 2014;37: 309–312.

856. Klose M, Stochholm K, Janukonyté J, Christensen LL, Cohen AS, Wagner A, et al. Patient reported outcome in post-traumatic pituitary deficiency: results from the Danish National Study on posttraumatic hypopituitarism. *Eur J Endocrinology* 2015;172: 753–762.

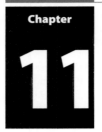

Late Effects

Jeff Victoroff

Introduction

Chani is a 75-year-old Gujjari-American. At age 18, before moving to the United States, he was playing cricket with others in the foothills of Kargil. During a break, the boys engaged in an enthusiastic discussion regarding the 1947 Line of Control. Chani was struck in the head with a cricket bat ("They knocked me stupid!") and was unconscious for less than a minute. He felt entirely better after four months (although his then-girlfriend observed that he remained uncharacteristically irritable for about two years). In his early 20s, before immigrating to the United States, he worked for three years as a high-altitude porter and then a mountain guide. Now he complains of memory loss. Why?

Chani came in for a comprehensive neurobehavioral examination. On history, he acknowledged heavy use of marijuana as a teen and a painful divorce seven years ago. On examination, he seemed somewhat disinhibited. There was a slightly elevated pulse pressure, some subjective lightheadedness on postural blood pressure testing, and questionable left upper-extremity cogwheel rigidity. His verbal memory is subpar. His Dementia Rating Scale score is 0.75. A 3-T magnetic resonance imaging (MRI) shows one subcortical lacune, slight frontotemporal atrophy (questionably in excess of normal aging), and scattered periventricular white-matter changes.

Genomic analysis reveals APOEε 3/3 genotype and a GGGGCC repeat expansion (length about 100) in the non-coding region of Ch9orf72.[1] In addition, there is evidence of up-regulation in the genes for interleukin-1α, 1β, 10, 15, 18, and 1β converting enzyme, C-reactive protein, tumor necrosis factor-α, galectin 3, Sparc/osteonectin, Cwcv and Kazal-like domains proteoglycan (Testican) 3, and the gene for phosphatidylinositol-binding clathrin assembly protein … but (thank goodness!) *not* in the genes for interleukin-1 receptor antagonist, interleukin-6, transforming growth factor-β, complement receptor 1, or clusterin apolipoprotein J. As most readers would predict, Chani carries the A allele for complement C3b/C4b receptor 1 (rs4844609), the clusterin G allele (rs11136000), and a variant close to the heparan sulfate-glucosamine 3-sulfotransferase 4 (HS3ST4) gene[2] – as well as

Table 11.1 Chani's brain

- Hyperphosphorylated tau (p-tau) deposition = 0.61 sd > MM, some allocortical/limbic, some neocortical, but not disproportionately dense in the depths of sulci
- Amyloid β42 deposition = 0.86 sd > MM, primarily in neocortical sulci and amygdala
- Micro-ischemic damage = 1.24 sd > MM
- PrP^C P measure = 0.59 sd > MM
- α-synuclein measure = 1.43 sd > MM
- TDP-43 measure = 0.47 sd > MM
- Neprilysin assay = 0.58 sd < MM
- Microglial migration rate = 1.05 sd < MM
- Basal nucleus of Meynert atrophy = 0.86 sd > MM
- Insulin-degrading enzyme assay = 0.62 sd < MM
- BDNF assay = 0.45 sd < MM
- 15,754,250,315 neocortical neurons.

BDNF: brain-derived neurotrophic factor; MM: mean for age, sex, education, race, socioeconomic status-matched population.

functional polymorphisms of 1267 other minor alleles – not listed to save trees.

With exceptional grace, Chani also volunteered for an antemortem post-mortem. Table 11.1 summarizes his neuropathological results:

By good fortune, Chani had also agreed to a previous pre–post-mortem at age 17 at which time we had counted (by hand) 16,078,634,212 neocortical neurons.

- What is the name of Chani's disease?
- Which of the above findings explains his disinhibition and mild functional impairment?
- Which of these biological parameters was altered, to what degree, by his concussion?

That, in a nutshell, is the problem that has bedeviled neuroscience for decades. The profundity of our ignorance in this regard is unplumbable. The answers to these questions are unknown for at least three reasons. One: science has yet to develop an agreed definition of *natural kinds* that meaningfully distinguishes some biological phenomena from others.

---

[1]   This variable number tandem repeat mutation is associated with a variety of behavioral and neurodegenerative changes. Normal repeat length is in the 20s. Definitely pathological repeat length is probably > 500 [1].

[2]   These genes and variants are thought to mediate or modulate the inflammatory response and perhaps cognition among the elderly [2].

For example, no universally agreed definitions or biological criteria exist for colloquial terms such as *normal, abnormal, health, disease, aging, Alzheimer's disease,* or *dementia.* In fact, the neuroscience community is suffering from the tyranny of terms of art: struggling to discuss vital issues in a common-sensical way while contorting the English language to embrace recently adopted idiosyncratic meanings of otherwise useful terms. Two: due to reason one, science has yet to determine what combination of the 10,000 or 20,000 most important biomarkers of time-passing-related brain change represents "abnormality." Three: no data have been gathered from prospective, controlled, longitudinal research regarding brain change due to concussive brain injury (CBI).

That said, recent discoveries regarding the late effects of CBI are nothing less than revolutionary. Evidence has emerged supporting the conclusion that one – and especially more than one – concussion may trigger or incite at least three classes of disabling neurological disease:

1. demyelinating disease, e.g., multiple sclerosis (MS)
2. motor neuron disease
3. polypathological progressive degenerative encephalopathy.

Let us begin with the knowable. In the modern world, many people continue to live for years or decades after the onset of cerebral somatic maturity (about age 24–25 years). Those who survive decline in cognitive function with the passage of time.[3] This always occurs, with or without CBI. Some people decline to such a marked degree that they are diagnosed with so-called "dementia."[4] Most survivors of typical, clinically attended concussions live for decades after their injuries. Based on advanced neuroimaging research, evidence is rapidly accumulating that a single CBI leads to brain change that not only persists long after conventional cognitive tests normalize, but also long after symptoms resolve. The ultimate duration of those brain changes – or, more realistically given human individuality, the *spectrum* of trajectories of post-concussive brain change – has yet to be determined.

For example: if an adolescent girl suffers two cheerleading-related CBIs, she may be declared "recovered" on the basis of resolution of subjective symptoms and restoration of pre-morbid neuropsychological test scores. As we have noted throughout this volume, those are not evidence of recovery. They provide reassurance to stakeholders, but they fail to consider the rapidly accumulating evidence that concussions, in many cases, change the brain forever. The chain of causality is both vastly complex (as illustrated by the Haddon matrix provided in Chapter 7) and beyond current knowledge. That obliges one to be circumspect about declaring "her two head butts at age 15 first *caused* her MS at age 27 and then *caused* her early-onset dementia at age 71." But the epidemiological evidence is increasingly compelling: entirely apart from subtle neurobiological irregularities that may stress and threaten and prematurely age her brain and reduce her cerebral capacity and emotional resilience in some circumstances, her concussions may increase her risk for developing MS starting about 5–20 years later, and probably increase her risk for a yet-to-be-specified range of other central nervous system deteriorations starting about 10–70 years later.

It is premature to judge the meaning of the long-term changes recently observed with heavy magnets. Have we imaged remarkable and completely successful adaptation? Have we imaged changes that do not, in themselves, guarantee deleterious outcome but represent risk factors for accelerated brain aging? Or have we imaged brain changes that invariably and inevitably create untoward stress – for instance, adaptive cerebral reorganization with the short-term benefit of complete functional recovery at the cost of long-term excess metabolic activity, causing multiple insidious, delayed-onset deleterious effects? And – as the preface of this text inquired – how would one know?

The subject of this chapter is not dementia. "Dementia," as it is conventionally misunderstood, is a late stage in which a person exhibits disabling behavioral consequences of what may be 70 years or more of brain change. As dreaded (and vaguely defined) as "dementia" may be, there are perhaps one or two orders of magnitude more people who are *impaired* (behaviorally less functional than expected) than *disabled*. One does not so much want to answer the trivial question – does one concussion increase the risk of "dementia?" One wants to know whether a typical, clinically attended CBI increases the risk for impairment, meaning any deleterious change in any facet of neurological function, clinically detectable or not – such as inefficient learning, microglial activation, sadness, or an overworked glymphatic pathway. A danger exists in error. If one overestimates the risk of late effects, millions of concussion survivors will be needlessly worried. If one underestimates the risk, there will be less pressure to fund studies of mitigation and millions will go without life-preserving post-traumatic interventions. The stakes are high. The necessary research has never been done. *That is*

---

[3]   The phrase "with the passage of time" is weighty with meaning. *Aging*, as the chapter will discuss, has no agreed definition. The conflation of aging with biological entropy has laden the term with negative value, and generated such logical fallacies as the idea that *development* and *aging* occur at different times in the life history. For instance, at age 65 humans typically exhibit (1) a profound decline in new learning capacity related to polypathological deterioration of the brain and (2) increasing wisdom and eudaimonic happiness, also related to brain change. Is that aging or development? *Time-passing-related brain change* is proposed as an atheoretical, value-neutral, and self-evident biological construct.

[4]   *Dementia* means a decline in mentation. In the last ~40 years, in English-speaking Western medicine, it has been assigned many operational definitions, none convergent with that essential meaning. As discussed in previous chapters, the major source of ambiguity is the fact that change in function can be classified either categorically (e.g., "demented" vs. "normal-aging-related cognitive impairment") or dimensionally (e.g., "Clinical Dementia Rating 0.5 vs. 1.0"). In addition, in some eras *dementia* was used in reference to either psychiatric disorder or combined cognitive and non-cognitive mental dysfunction, while many recent writers have used the term specifically with regard to cognitive deterioration. Readers will find an introduction to the debate regarding the definition of dementia later in this chapter.

the subject of this chapter.[5] And even though concussed persons seem at risk for at least three classes of late effects (demyelinating disease, motor neuron disease, and polypathological degenerative disease), we will focus on the subject about which there exists the most abundant evidence: dementia.

As explained below, dementia does not mean a disabling development of late life. It means a decline from a previous level of mental function. For perspective: a well-known and universal human dementia occurs between age three and about age nine, when individuals loses their previous ability to learn a new language without an accent. Steroid hormones often dement children as they enter puberty, robbing them of previously achieved self-control. Another universal form of dementia is the loss of creative mathematical thinking between age 14 and 24. Does concussion increase the incidence or prevalence of "dementia"? As discussed below, the answer to this pressing question – a question of weighty import to public health – is not currently available. Whether a child rolls off a counter at three months of age or a woman bumps her head on a kitchen cabinet at age 68, no data answer the question, "Is he or she at risk for late effects from that concussion?"

The purpose of this chapter is not to answer that question. Due to a lack of funding to conduct the required long-term prospective research and a global lack of concern about concussed persons (perhaps led down the garden path by the 20th-century misinterpretation of conventional neuropsychological testing's insensitivity to persistent post-CBI deficits), one does not expect an authoritative answer in the foreseeable future. The purpose of this chapter, instead, is to introduce the concepts that deserve attention as we fumble about with our grossly inadequate data and the biologically indefensible terms of art (e.g., "Alzheimer's disease") that stand in for rational classification of neurological disorder, and try to make informed guesses about whether concussions, single or multiple, have late effects.

There is more to it than may be immediately apparent. Philosophy, unfortunately, comes into play.[6] The present author wishes he could think of a way to discuss the evidence for and against the late effects of concussion without wrestling, like Laocoön, with the writhing serpents of nosology. He realizes the awful burden on the reader. Who could be eager to analyze the Aristotelean logic of neurological dogma? He promises, however, that readers will achieve a more profound understanding of why we do not know the long-term effects of concussion after considering that the scholarly uses of terms such as aging, dementia, "Alzheimer's disease," and CTE are not based on science.

It is easy to see why unresolved conceptual conundrums have derailed empirical efforts to determine the late effects of concussion. Imagine a contest to design an informative study. At least three definitional matters instantly torment the contestants: (1) defining subjects with CBI; (2) defining the clinical state of "dementia"; and (3) defining the putative underlying neurological condition (e.g., so-called "Alzheimer's disease" or so-called "frontotemporal dementia," or so-called "CTE").

First, the grant writer would need to specify his or her subjects. Typical clinically attended concussion is the subject of this book. The editors deliberately left that major global health problem in its natural state of naked ambiguity, without the gauzy swaddlings of an operational definition, because – given the lack of a biological marker for TBI severity – any written selection criteria amount to the cavalier invention of a disease. For example, when the American College of Rehabilitation Medicine (ACRM) proposed its 1993 definition for "mild traumatic brain injury"[7] (mTBI), they reified a clinically and biologically heterogeneous phenomenon that is impossible to investigate in a serious way. Subjects would be selected if there was any striking of the head *or* acceleration of the brain that *either* acutely presents with *or* does not acutely present with *either* any alteration in mental state (from being momentarily dazed to 30 minutes of coma) *or* any loss of immediate memory (with recovery of day-to-day new learning within 24 h) *or* any focal neurological deficits, whether or not those deficits are present or absent at presentation and whether their duration is a millisecond or a lifetime. It seems unlikely that all persons who meet these criteria have the same brain changes. Reading the published studies of mTBI and dementia, the experienced clinician therefore sees through the reassurance of "according to ACRM criteria" and realizes that the subjects' actual brain changes are unknowable, and probably diverse.[8]

---

5   The author submits this chapter to readers with hesitation, misgivings, and apologies. Textbooks usually support and explain the status quo. Just as the editors of this little volume could not, in good conscience, perpetuate the illogical current concept of "mild TBI," we cannot impose upon readers the currently popular but scientifically illogical use of phrases such as "Alzheimer's disease" or "chronic traumatic encephalopathy." Our earnest wish to make sense may trigger cognitive dissonance in some readers. Students may become disoriented. Several professors whom I deeply respect may regret their hearty lunches. And, in the end, overthrowing the illogic of neurological nosology may prove impossible – leaving our account a historical outlier. Nonetheless, we both feel ethically compelled to do our best, informed by our rustic faith in basic principles. We dearly hope that – after an awkward period of outrage and adjustment – the result is human benefit.

6   The author means no disrespect to philosophers. He only means that abstract ideas are not typical fare for a medical textbook, and it may not be instantly apparent how attention to them will enhance global health care. He only hopes that his stumbling comments make it easier for readers to see how neurology's illogical nosology has become a barrier to discovery.

7   "1. Any period of loss of consciousness; 2. any loss of memory for events immediately before or after the accident; 3. any alteration in mental state at the time of the accident (e.g., feeling dazed, disoriented, or confused); and 4. focal neurological deficit(s) that may or may not be transient; but where the severity of the injury does not exceed the following: loss of consciousness of approximately 30 minutes or less; after 30 minutes, an initial Glasgow Coma Scale (GCS) of 13–15; and posttraumatic amnesia (PTA) not greater than 24 hours .... some patients may not have the above factors medically documented in the acute stage" [3].

8   The present author recognizes that practical need for diagnostic criteria. Forced to define typical medically attended CBI sufficiently to aid empirical investigation, he might propose provisional research diagnostic criteria such as "deleterious brain change due to an abrupt external

Second, the grant writer would need to define "dementia." As we will see, two thorny tangles impede that path: (1) a controversy exists regarding whether dementia should be defined by cognitive deficits, by psychiatric disorders, by impairment of activities of daily living, or by one of the various combinations of problems promoted by various committees in the most popular competing definitions; and (2) a controversy exists regarding whether "dementia" is truly categorically different from healthy normalcy, or instead a degree of change on a continuous spectrum that can only be diagnosed using an arbitrary operational dividing line. Third, the writer might wish to specify the post-concussive brain disorder that constitutes an abnormality that is definitively different from normal aging. That requires specifying: (1) the boundary line between normal aging and brain disease; (2) the boundaries between many related brain diseases (e.g., "Alzheimer's disease" versus "frontotemporal dementia" versus "vascular dementia")[9]; and (3) whether CBI is a risk factor for disconcerting changes that would not usually be called "disease," or for one or more of the conventionally labeled "diseases" associated with the passage of time that gained popularity in the 20th century, or the cause of a unique kind of post-traumatic neurodegeneration (ND) that some scholars have begun to call "CTE." In fact, fourth, one might wish to determine whether concussion is a risk factor for ND. That, in turn, requires the yet-to-be accomplished scientifically unequivocal definition of "ND."

In short: unless one can answer the questions "What is 'aging'?" "What is 'dementia'?" "What is 'ND'?" "What is 'Alzheimer's disease'?" and "What is 'CTE'?" any late effects of concussion cannot be characterized as a deviation from the normal-and-expected broad spectrum of time-passing-related brain change.

Same and Different[10]

It is true that we instinctively recoil from seeing an object to which our emotions and affections are committed handled by the intellect as any other object is handled. The first thing the intellect does with an object is to class it along with something else. But any object that is infinitely important to us and awakens our devotion feels to us also as if it must be sui generis and unique. Probably a crab would be filled with a sense of personal outrage if it could hear us class it without ado or apology as a crustacean, and thus dispose of it. "I am no such thing, it would say; I am *myself, myself* alone."
William James, Varieties of Religious Experience,
Lecture 1: Religion and Neurology, 1902 [7]

Like Descartes, we will begin with first concepts. (Unlike Descartes, we will not claim privileged access to divine truths.)

The first concept one confronts in attempting to determine whether concussions have late effects is that of same and different. Without a working grasp of this elementary notion, one cannot even attempt to define normal versus abnormal, let alone health versus disease. And without agreeing on what is health versus disease, one can hardly discuss normal brain aging versus abnormal brain aging. The author's motive for retreating to this elementary level is that it helps explain the conceptual barriers that currently hamper agreement about dementia – and the reverence for neurological icons that has delayed progress in understanding and treating so-called "Alzheimer's disease." Unless we can agree what dementia is, we simply cannot investigate whether there is more or less of it among concussion survivors.

The distinction between same and different is arguably the essence of classifying or categorizing natural phenomena. One way to think of sameness was introduced by Plato with his forms and Aristotle with his essences. Both scholars discussed classification by reference to ideal types – somewhat ephemeral dollops of pure thought that did not exist on Earth and could not step on your foot. An example might be "horseness." One cannot point at Platonic horseness. It is an idea.[11] Mill [8] is credited with a more empirical understanding of classification pertinent to biological life. Some things observed on Earth clearly belong to the same category (kind) and the observant mind inductively constructs what is the same about them by comparison. He gives the example of horses. Each horse is an individual, but observation leads to confidence that they are all horses. Mill famously concluded that things the human mind judges to belong to the same category, especially in matter of biology and science, are "natural kinds."[12]

force without gross intracranial bleeding or prolonged coma." But he would readily admit that such criteria are ambiguous and hard to operationalize. Imaging may some day enable more biological specificity. To be avoided, however, is the 20th-century fallacy of inventing categories to classify dimensional differences, for instance, "9–18.7% stretch of the uncinate fasciculus, with a 22–71% increase in axolemmal porosity, and an 11–390% increase in microglial activation, and transsynaptic spread of five kinds of atypically folded protein oligomers, but with no detectable apoptosis."

[9] The forthcoming text explains why one must write the conventional 20th-century labels of putative dementing disease with quotation marks: to date, no credible evidence has emerged that most of them exist as authentically specific and discrete entities, i.e., natural kinds.

[10] It is beyond the author's most fever-driven ambitions to address classification in a serious way. Interested readers – having exhausted Plato, Aristotle, Aquinas, Kant, and Mill – might wish to look at Bird and Tobin's helpful essay on "Natural kinds" [4] or Surján's "The cultural history of medical classifications" [5]. Readers who are not prone to migraine may also consider the psychological equation of *inference* with *mental action required for syllogistic classification of same and different* implied by Lewis Carroll's 1895 essay, "What the tortoise said to Achilles" [6].

[11] While Aristotle equivocated about that which exists, Plato was uncompromising and can therefore be dismissed as a source of insight. With his parable of the cave, he confessed his belief that nothing perceptible is real. Mill, in contrast, explained that perception of real things on Earth (horses, not horseness) enables classification by induction.

[12] Humans have psychological needs to classify, and to agree on classifications. Smith and Medin [9] make the point that concepts gain meaning from categorization. Yet not all classifiable concepts are natural kinds. Consider "cup." Many things labeled by languages and categorized in

Classification and categorization of things on earth are not merely exercises in academic abstraction. It is a matter of life and death. People categorize to keep breathing. So do other mammals and birds. As Smith et al. [10] recently put it: "Categorization – the ability of humans and animals to learn psychological equivalence classes (categories) – is a crucial survival capacity. It lets us differentiate mushrooms from toadstools and garden snakes from rattlesnakes. It has been a vertebrate life preserver for hundreds of millions of years" (p. 266). Thus, neither the classical thinkers nor Mill offered a view of classification compatible with the way it is done or the reasons for doing it in nature. In both cases, these storied philosophers regarded brains as logical. They are not. In so far as a brain does classification, it does so in the interests of fitness. Decision making of such desperate import is not left to the finicky ruminating consciousness of the dorsolateral prefrontal cortex. Important judgments always involve a combination of cortical and subcortical activity. Emotion, in a word, is inseparable from our judgments of natural kinds, since distinguishing a hornet from a fly has more than schoolroom implications.[13]

Moreover, as William James asserted, classifying is rewarding and being unable to classify is unsettling. One is born into a chaos of unfamiliar things. Survival requires sorting them out. Since the ability to stay alive periodically depends on the ability to classify things (e.g., lion from lamb, friend from foe), people feel anxious when faced with uncertainty about the class of a novel stimulus. Feeling (emotionally) that one has figured out the class to which something belongs – feeling that one knows hornet from fly, or kindly from mean, or sick from well – relieves the anxiety of uncertainty. In fact, this feature of human nature seems to explain the heat of many scientific debates.

Why does so much emotion get invested in defense of familiar schemes of classification? Why does so much resistance greet paradigm shifts? Because classification is linked to survival, and hence, to emotion. People all yearn for certainty – meaning strong belief that they know what is correct (which some psychologists call cognitive closure), albeit with different degrees of desperation [11, 12]. People have a limited, but individually variable, tolerance for ambiguity [13]. Once young doctors have firmly embraced a system of classification (e.g., distinguishing black bile from yellow), once that system makes us feel knowledgeable and authoritative, and seem so to patients, and receive rewards for seeming so, it is threatening to be told that what we "know" is wrong. Evidence shows that uncertainty and ambiguity not only cause stress but also trigger rigidity [14].

How does categorization or classification occur? Multiple cognitive functions are involved. Consider that, early in life,

perception is limited. It may be all one can do to perceive black from white, pain from pleasure, and Mom from non-Mom. This implies that: (1) categorizations require perception of difference and (2) initial exposure to novel stimuli perhaps triggers not only anxiety but also innate, non-verbal recognitions of perceptible differences. Infant brains rapidly assign *same* and *different* without didactic instruction or words [15]. But classification has no value without associative memory, so infants combine skills: (1) perception of a trait (e.g., nipple size, shape, texture, and turgor as measured by oral palpation); (2) assignment of value or meaning to that perceptible trait (warmth, comfort, safety, satiety); (3) learning of the association between the percept and the assigned value; (4) perception of sameness of a new percept by comparison with the learned association (e.g., a pacifier is reminiscent of a nipple); and (5) – in ways we have yet to figure out – assignment of new but similar percepts to a temporally stable class (the pacifier is not quite a nipple, but it shares sufficient attributes to trigger similar emotions, so I won't cry). The point is that humans need not translate Aristotle's *Posterior Analytics* [16] or read Mill's *A System of Logic, Ratiocinative and Inductive* [8] to develop instinctive, non-verbal, value- and emotion-weighted classifications of phenomena.

This is inductive learning at the pre-verbal stage. For instance, the infant readily perceives images generating or reflecting light with a wavelength of about 475 nm. He or she does not need words such as *blue* or *red* to perceive that two lights with wavelengths of 464 and 477 nm look similar, whereas a third light with a wavelength 650 nm looks different. The brains of humans and other animals categorize percepts as same or different altogether free of language. A few years on, the cognitive talent of automatic color categorization is supplemented with another cognitive process: socialization to consensus labels. Language and education enable the child to assign socially accepted labels ("Uh … blue?" "Right! Good job, honey!"), yet Tarzan's brain instinctively categorized percepts even if he was raised by gorillas. The take-away message is that categorization is deeply embedded in the mammalian brain, and strongly influenced by instinctive, pre-verbal value judgments.

Progress in scientific knowledge involves a slow march toward agreement on socially acceptable consensus labels. For many years, the socially accepted classification of matter was supplied by the classical elements of Empedocles: earth, air, fire, and water. Over the centuries, careful observations raised questions about whether these were the only natural kinds. Chemical experiments based on the atomic theory suggested a larger number of elements, Mendeleev drew up a periodic table, and Empedocles's four-part classification scheme was

---

brains are more social constructs than natural kinds. Natural kinds, unlike social constructs, have a conceptual integrity that humans discover via science. The same authors make another good point: to fulfill the psychological purpose of classification, a concept must evoke a mental representation. Later in this chapter the author will compare the natural kind tuberculosis with the interloping social construct pleading for recognition as a natural kind, "Alzheimer's disease." In anticipation, readers might compare how readily the mind grasps a mental representation of tuberculosis as "infection by the tubercle bacillus" with how agonized the mind becomes trying to form a mental representation of any of the seven recent competitors for the meaning of "Alzheimer's disease."

[13] The importance of this for explaining the myth of "Alzheimer's disease" will soon be apparent.

disavowed. In that paradigm shift, that which was regarded as *same* and *different* changed dramatically due to better observations and hypothesis testing.[14]

In the same way, health and biological functions were once classified in terms of Galen's four humors: blood, yellow bile, black bile, and phlegm. Same and different were judged by reference to these elemental definers of distinction. That system, in the end, proved to have less explanatory power than other ways of classifying disease, and was abandoned. Due to the empirical labors of centuries, classification of something as a *disease* is now associated with far more sophisticated concepts of biological function. And, with the advent of the microscope, our confidence that we have found natural kinds has been bolstered by that highly persuasive visual evidence. We can see the bug that triggers this kind of misery. We know the etiology. When cholera or tuberculosis were discovered to be caused by specific infectious agents, those diseases could legitimately be categorized as natural kinds. The deadfall intellectual snare of this approach is the assumption that *unfamiliar little things are causes*. One must forgive 20th-century neuropathologists for their embrace of that fallacy. Seeing unfamiliar little things seems to have provoked a cognitive knee-jerk reaction among those who came to believe in so-called "Alzheimer's disease": "We identified the cause!" They did not.

Harriet and Polly

The only difference between man and man all the world over is one of degree, and not of kind, even as there is between trees of the same species. Wherein is the cause for anger, envy or discrimination?

Mahatma Gandhi [18]

and eat and drink until the white thread of dawn appears to you distinct from the black thread, then complete your Sawm till the nightfall.

Quran [19]

During Ramadan, fasting should begin when the white thread of dawn is visibly distinguishable from the black thread of night.[15] Of course, visual acuity differs. Night vision differs. Reasonable people could argue about the moment to forswear the pleasures of the night ("It has been made permissible for you the night preceding fasting to go to your wives [for sexual relations]") for the abstemiousness of the day. It is clear, however, that sometimes day and night are not as categorically different as black and white. Dawn brings a gradual increase in luminance, progressing by infinitesimal steps. Under such circumstances, for practical purposes, one is obliged to make up an arbitrary rule specifying the degree of luminance that distinguishes day from night. That is classification by dimension.

This type of classification is profoundly relevant to determining whether concussions have late effects. In order to determine whether a forceful rattling of the brain causes a later neurological problem, one must first satisfy the fundamental question of whether the neurological problem exists – that is, whether it is a natural kind that is the same or different from the natural kind we call normal. For example, one must know whether dementia is a natural kind that is definitely different from non-dementia, or Alzheimer's disease is a natural kind that is definitely different from non-Alzheimer's disease. Unless that difference in natural kinds can be declared with confidence, it is literally impossible to determine whether concussions are associated with an increased risk of dementia or Alzheimer's disease.

Those medical distinctions superficially seem to be decided and carved in corundum. "Of course Alzheimer's disease is different from non-Alzheimer's disease! Don't you know the heartbreaking story of Auguste Deter!" Yet a sincere consideration of the logic of diagnosis shakes one's faith in that conventional wisdom.

Mrs. Deter was Alzheimer's first patient. By about age 47 she exhibited the kind of mental limitations that were, at that time, associated with "senile dementia." She died at age 51, in 1906. Her brain displayed many plaques and tangles. Perusini reviewed the case at Alzheimer's request. In 1909 that neuropathologist said, "The pathological process recalls main features of senile dementia; however, the alterations in the cases described are *more far reaching*" (emphasis added) [20]. We will return to Perusini's diagnosis shortly. What is vital is that both Alzheimer and Perusini rendered a final diagnosis based on an *amount* (i.e., "more far reaching") – an estimated *degree* of a common brain change, not a black-and-white presence or absence of a specific pathognomonic change. That is, they classified Mrs. Deter's brain by *dimension*. The problem with using a continuous dimension (height, weight, number of plaques, degree of luminance) to classify natural kinds is that it requires drawing a line somewhere along that continuum and declaring that all things below that line are one kind, and all things above are another. Blood pressure of 138/87 mmHg? Healthy. 141/91 mmHg? Diseased.

Therefore, there are at least two different ways of classifying health versus disease. One is by kind or category – for instance, there either is or is not a tumor. The other is by dimension or degree – for instance, there are either an acceptable number of plaques or a few more. Readers instantly see the conundrum. In cases that are distinguished by reference to a natural kind, one has reason for confidence. In cases where an arbitrary dividing line must be drawn somewhere along a continuum based on opinion or consensus, there is less cause for confidence. This raises an essentially philosophical question: when does a difference in degree become a difference in kind?

Darwin is often credited with the most memorable remark regarding classification of differences by kind or by degree. Figure 11.1 is a photograph of Darwin's daughter, Henrietta,

---

[14] The atomic theory and the periodic table may soon be supplanted in their turn: "progress of physics suggests that natural kinds will not feature in the basic (fundamental) laws of nature" [17].

[15] Theological opinions differ regarding whether there must be side-by-side visual comparison of two threads, or whether that language is metaphorical.

501

Polly and Henrietta

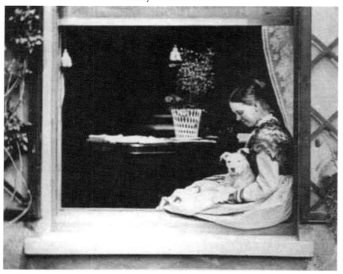

Fig. 11.1 Charles Darwin's daughter, Henrietta and his dog, Polly.
Source: Cambridge University Library

and his dog, Polly. According to Darwin, both had minds. In *The Descent of Man and Selection in Relation to Sex* [21], he posited that humans and certain other animals, such as monkeys and dogs, all have mental powers. Possession of such powers is not a difference of a natural kind that distinguishes Henrietta from Polly; the two are only different by a *matter of degree* (Figure 11.1). As Darwin put it: "Nevertheless the difference in mind between man and the higher animals, great as it is, certainly is *one of degree and not of kind*" [21].

If the mental powers of a dog and a girl are merely different in degree, at what point does a difference in degree of mental power constitute a difference in kind? When does a quantitative change deserve to be called a qualitative change? How much change in brain and behavior exceeds normal variation and becomes abnormal? If the thickness of the frontal lobe cortical normally declines by 0.80% per year [22], is a 0.90% annual decline neurodegenerative disease? If a person's memory progressively worsens over 30 years, on which scientifically valid date and time did he or she switch from *healthy* to *diseased*?

All of these questions simply restate the conceptual challenge of deciding sameness and difference based on a degree, amount, or dimension. In recent years, this question has become central to the struggle to overthrow the ancient regime of Western psychiatry. The American Psychiatric Association's system of classifying disease is enshrined in its *Diagnostic and Statistical Manual* (DSM) [23], a cliquish collaboration with the constancy of Proteus. The present chapter has already introduced the fact that the DSM system has been widely dismissed as unscientific. The goal of the next generation is to replace it with something better. But the quest for biologically valid diagnostic criteria for mental disorders is,

if anything, more difficult in psychiatry than in neurology. At least neurologists have a few biomarkers about which to argue the significance. They can count blobs under the microscope and august committees can proclaim that ten blobs mean health while 11 mean disease.[16]

Psychiatrists rarely have even that dubious evidence of objective differences between normal and abnormal. They are obliged to interpret the same observations as laypersons: everyone gets sad. At what point along that continuous dimension does one reach the category of disease? A large part of this era's effort to advance psychiatry toward science comes down to one question: at what point is a difference in the *amount* or *degree* of a behavioral change justifiably considered a difference in *kind*? Psychiatrists refer to this as the debate regarding categorical versus dimensional diagnosis. Interested readers can access mountains of relevant discussions [24–35]. But we digress.

The point is not that classification by dimension lacks validity. Considering the example of a rainbow, it is obvious that red and blue appear to be different, even though they fall along a continuum of wavelengths. Similarly, no one would disagree that, even though weight is a continuous variable and the precise boundaries of normal are imperceptible, an adult male who weighs either 10 pounds or 1000 pounds would be universally regarded as abnormal. When we come to the issues of dementia and Alzheimer's disease, the fact that diagnosis is dimensional does not automatically invalidate the perception that some persons are profoundly impaired and others are not. Dimensionality and infinite variability do not preclude classification! They simply require candid acknowledgment that we have imposed judgment on nature – an irresistibly comforting procedure to rescue ourselves from the grief of uncertainty in a slightly chaotic and probably unknowable universe.

The point (and this will become glaringly apparent when we try to classify the ever-evolving menu of neurodegenerative diseases) is that classification by dimension typically involves an element of subjectivity. Useful instincts, shared across a species, make animals assign class membership to common phenomena based on subjective judgments. The problem, for medicine, is that phenomena such as dementia are less commonly encountered than colors or weights, and often the exclusive domain of specialist attention. Unlike blue versus red, there is no evolved, natural, and universal perception of the difference between normal aging and abnormal aging. Classifications based on the subjective judgments of a few experts are therefore more likely to provoke debate than the difference between dog and girl.

What, if Anything, is Aging?

There exist no consistent, established values for what constitutes "normal" cognitive impairment and memory loss with advancing years; nor are the neurologic changes, the neurochemical changes, the neurophysiological changes,

---

[16] The term "biomarkers" also seems to be used ill-advisedly. What is the correct conclusion when one sees a good deal of Aβ and tau? The brain is normal. Or not.

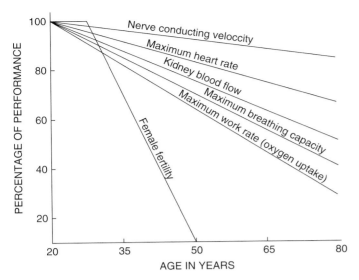

Fig. 11.2 Average human physiological change with the passage of time. Source: Best [37]. Reproduced with permission

or the gross and fine anatomical changes that accompany normal aging well enough understood to provide a firm base for determining "abnormal" changes.

[36]

We perceive changes with the passage of time, such as an increased likelihood of wrinkly skin and fatal disease, and intuit that something must be responsible. Aging is the most popular English name for this phenomenon. But aging turns out to be hard to define.

Is "aging" somatic change with the passage of time? No; not unless we include graduation from pre-school in the concept. Is "aging" change with the passage of time after having achieved the reproductive life stage? No; not unless we call changes from age 13 to 25 aging. Is "aging" deleterious, entropic, fitness-inhibiting change with the passage of time after reaching physiological maturity, roughly after age 25[17] (Figure 11.2)? Perhaps, if that which is *deleterious* were ever agreed upon. But there are gains in function – for instance, in vocabulary, and wisdom, and happiness – during the same time period to which rapid deleterious deterioration is attributed. Are those youthing?

There is no universally accepted definition of aging. There is no universally accepted theory of aging. Yet, in recent years, a tremendous interest has blossomed in answering the question of why we (perhaps) age. This was less of a concern in the ancestral environment. Early modern humans had a life expectancy in the low 20s. Nor was it likely to have been a major concern for Christopher Columbus and his cohort. As shown in Figure 11.3, the average life expectancy at that time was less than 30 years. Note the progression toward the ideal square wave – a life history plan like that of the salmon that preserves survival up until a genetically mandated terminus of life.

Only very recently, when modern sanitation, nutrition, medicine, and peace enabled a few more people to live past age 50, has concern about "aging" arisen. That concern is the natural result of the fact that the normal and expected course of mature life – assuming disease and death by age 45 – has been reconceptualized as *abnormal* (and, to many, undesirable). And only recently has the normal and expected phenomenon of "dementia" at age 77 been reconceptualized as a disease.[18]

Humans are justifiably preoccupied with causality. The cause of death piques particular interest. As in the case of murder, people are eager to know whether time-passing-related death is planned (premeditated or programmed) or not planned (due to random accidents). Setting aside the question of definition, for more than 100 years just two theories of aging have dominated the scholarly tilt. Some writers opine that aging is planned or programmed. Others opine that aging is not programmed.

Many authorities date the onset of this debate to a publication by Weismann et al. [40]. Weismann et al. asserted that aging is programmed.

> To put it briefly, I consider that duration of life is really dependent upon adaptation to external conditions, that its length, whether longer or shorter, is governed by the needs of the species, and that it is determined by precisely the same mechanical process of regulation as that by which the structure and functions of an organism are adapted to its environment.
>
> Weismann et al., 1891 [40], pp. 9–10

As Weismann visualized life in the ancestral environment, he reasonably speculated that old people who do not produce new gene carriers (children) may actually harm their group, since they will compete for resources that could be better invested in healthy young breeders. Hence, it is in the interests of the group that elderly hangers-on age and die.

Weismann's theory has been soundly thrashed for two reasons. One, he failed to provide a mechanism that might account for positive selection of aging and death. Two, he assumed group selection. After the discovery of genes, evolutionary theorists almost uniformly agreed that the unit of selection is the gene. Little evidence supports the hypothesis that traits are selected for the benefit of the species (the group). Far more evidence supports the conclusion that neither the individual organism nor the group is selected by the merciless trial and error of competition for survival. It is the gene. Critics of Weismann and the programmed theory of aging also rightly point out that selection can only act when the raw material is available. Unless there is a substantial cohort of persons living to age 40 or 60 or 80, and unless those persons can influence their own inclusive fitness (either by making more offspring or doing a superior job of helping their offspring survive and reproduce), nature cannot run experiments to see which gene mutations active among 40–80-year-olds favor their gene

---

17 In fact, one concept of aging refers to the force causing the exponential rate of mortality after age 30. This mathematical definition, lacking mechanism or purpose, is hard to accept as an evolved biological process.

18 In a sign of the times, Bulterijs et al. [38] published a paper titled "It is time to classify biological aging as a disease."

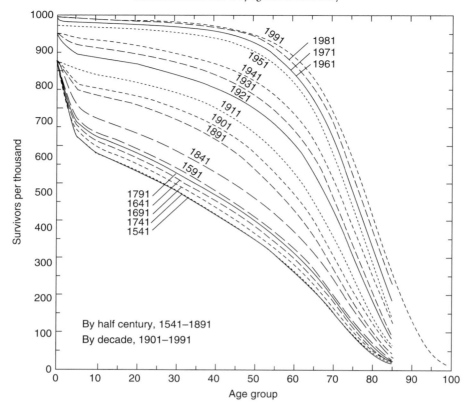

Fig. 11.3 The lower aging plateau is evident in the curves up to that for 1841–1845; here lines are separated by intervals of half a century each. These lines are not only very close together but they change positions with each other in an order that is certainly not chronological. The one for the five-year period 1691–1695, for example, traces a course only just above that for 1541–1545 and well below that for 1591–1595, which in its turn is closest to that for 1841–1845, nearly 250 years later. The run-up to the secular shift is visible in the wide gap between 1841–1845 and 1891, when mortality was evidently falling but at some ages may still not have been below the levels previously reached for an individual year or so on the lower aging plateau. The subsequent course of the secular shift itself shows up vividly in the more and more conspicuous spaces between successive curves, this time temporally successive curves and separated by ten-year and not by 50-year intervals, as is the case for the earlier lines. The approach to the higher aging plateau in our own day is strongly suggested by the marked narrowing of the spaces after 1951.

Source: Kertzer, 1995 [39]. Reproduced with permission from J. Oeppen

replication. In fact, few humans survived beyond age 25 in the ancestral environment and there is a progressive decline in the proportion who survive after that age. That means, with advancing age, natural selection has less and less opportunity for choosing mutations that influence survival. A gene that turns on brain aging at 65 in order to save the neighborhood from dependent old people was unlikely to win a place in the genome. No competition could occur between 65-year-olds with aging- and death-promoting genes and those without such genes because *almost no 65-year-olds ever existed.*

However, it may be premature to dismiss the possibility of programmed aging. If Weismann knew about genes and heard the complaints of his critics, he *might* have proposed a logical refinement in the theory of programmed aging:

I agree. Selection had a reduced chance of preferring old people who age promptly over old people who fail to age, since so few old people survived anyway. However, consider this: woolly mammoths do not always cooperate. If you spear them, they sometimes step on you. That means the longer you live, the greater the chance that you will be

injured or diseased, becoming disabled and dependent. If you are in good health at age 45, you might still do your own genes some good by teaching and supporting and scavenging food for your gene-bearing offspring. But if you are frail and dependent, you may be worth less than nothing to your offspring and your genes. A diseased or disabled 40–80-year-old may literally be taking food from the mouths of his own babes (or grand-babes). Under those circumstances, you do your genes a big favor by aging and dying. And there were enough 40+-year-olds around for a pro-aging and death gene that kicked in at that age to compete for selection into the human genome.

Weismann never wrote that corrective. The objections to his programmed theory of aging stood. And in 1952, Medewar [41] summarized those objections in a persuasive book declaring that aging is not programmed. Medewar could not imagine a scenario in which pro-aging genes might be selected, but he could readily imagine that, after reproducing and rearing off-spring, further survival would have negligible benefit. Beyond that point, two factors would guarantee the decimation of the elderly. First, cells are constantly under threat from mutations. Early in life, when survival is useful, selection favors repair of those mutations. Later, when survival of the organism has little to offer the genes, there would be little selection pressure for a system of continued repair. From that point on, animals are progressively more vulnerable to cell failure and death. Second, even if there were no progressive decline in vitality, a population is forever at risk from accidents. Medewar's famous analogy asked readers to consider a rack of brand-new glass test tubes. Each time an old one is broken in the lab, a new one is purchased. Over time, simply due to chance, there will be an exponential decline in test tubes with age and the lab will have very few old tubes. In the same way, considering tippy boulders, irritable snakes, hungry lions, infectious diseases, and aggressive conspecifics, a human's chance of survival will progressively decline with time. Medewar called this the chance, or stochastic, theory of aging.

Shortly thereafter, in 1957 [42], Williams introduced his new theory of aging, called *antagonist pleiotropy*. Pleiotropy simply refers to a given gene having more than one function. Antagonism occurs, for instance, if a gene is good for survival early in life but bad for survival later. If a gene has beneficial effects up through the age of child rearing, its net effect may be positive even if it has late detrimental effects, so it may be actively selected [43]. This theory skirts the question of programming, even though it implies a life plan design that favors deterioration of the aged.

Recent discoveries have catapulted antagonist pleiotropy into the news. APOE-ε4 is the allelic variant with the greatest known impact on the risk of Alzheimer's disease. Why would it persist in the human population? First, virtually nobody in the ancestral population would have lived long enough to exhibit Alzheimer's disease, so no selective pressure would have acted to reduce the allele's prevalence. More interestingly, multiple lines of evidence suggest that APOE-ε4 confers advantages in youth, including enhanced cognitive function in children, enhanced perinatal survival, and perhaps enhanced fertility in young women [44–50]. It seems fair to say that judgment of the relative benefits and liabilities of this allele is premature.

In 1977 [51], Kirkwood introduced his *disposable soma theory* of aging. He argued that every animal's body has finite resources. The more it invests in maintenance of the cells and body to stay alive, the fewer resources will be available for growth and reproduction. By implication, that theory shares with Weismann's the notion that old animals are not much good for gene replication, such that aging and death are beneficial. Still, despite proposing that aging was selected,[19] Kirkwood dismissed the notion that aging was "programmed."

Over the subsequent decades, the programmed and not-programmed theories of aging have vied for supremacy. Many writers, rehabilitating the instinct of Weismann, now argue that aging is under the control of a biological clock and that phenoptosis (programmed death) benefits the genome [37, 52–66]. Libertini's 2011 paper is sometimes credited as an especially cogent argument in favor of phenoptosis [54]. Yet (at least until very recently) the majority of writers – the mainstream authorities – opined that aging is not programmed, and is simply a matter of accident – the chance result of accumulated deleterious changes, injuries, diseases, and progressive loss of repair capacity [41, 42, 51, 67–77]. Those who opine that aging is a random, stochastic process point to a host of factors that represent threats to longevity. Table 11.2 offers a partial list of biological factors associated with aging-related somatic deterioration – what Gompertz called the force of mortality.

Readers may note with interest that this list overlaps significantly with the mechanisms of brain harm attributed to TBI. That suggests certain deleterious processes associated with "aging" may be triggered in more than one way. Might pro-aging effects be additive – that is, for instance, might time-passing-related brain change reflect the sum of force-of-mortality factors (e.g., oxidation, inflammation, mutation) no matter what triggers their expression? In a moment we will return to the implications of that possibility.

Does the programmed versus not-programmed nature of aging matter? Some authorities believe that this is the critical question for gerontology, arguing that, for the purposes of defeating mortality, it matters very much whether there are pro-aging and death genes. One could presumably find them and turn them off. Other authorities doubt that this theoretical question has much practical import. They regard the two positions as largely a matter of semantics. As Goldsmith recently put it: "The current hair-splitting argument is whether continued survival and reproduction beyond the species-specific age produces only zero evolutionary advantage or at least a minute evolutionary disadvantage in gradually aging mammals" [63].

Toward a Sensible Concept of "*Aging*"

The author very humbly and tentatively proposes his own simple-minded, impressionistic concept of so-called "aging." His goal is only to mention ideas of possible use to answering questions about the late effects of concussion.

Aging seems to overlap – conceptually and perhaps biologically – with *development*. These are two aspects of biological change with the passage of time. In the common run of academics, one often encounters the assumption that these

---

[19] Readers may detect a semantic quibble. Indeed, most champions of the not-programmed theory of aging draw a fierce distinction. They often agree that aging *evolved* by natural selection but disagree that aging is *programmed*. The former, they say, merely refers to the fact that selection failed to positively favor continued DNA repair into old age; hence deterioration occurs by default. To prove the latter, they say, requires discovery of a gene that actively switches on aging and death. Even though both sides agree that aging is partly heritable, and that there seems to be an absolute upper limit to the human lifespan, the not-programmed theorists decline to accept the term "programmed" until a pro-aging gene is isolated. In fact, many genes have been found that influence aging. The demand for discovery of a specific and all-powerful pro-aging gene is not consistent with what is known about multi-determination, epistasis, and epigenetics.

Table 11.2 Agents that contribute to the force of mortality[20]

Cellular senescence and death
- Declining DNA repair
- Apoptosis
- Autophagy
- Telomere shortening
- Declining anti-oxidant defense
- Defective cell cycle control

Metabolic threats
- Glucose intolerance
- Oxidative stress
- Glycation-related stress
- Steroid hormone-mediated cell damage

Cerebrovascular dysfunction and microvascular change

Inflammation

Immunomodulatory dysfunction

Accumulation of noxious humors
- Protein cross-linking and aggregation
- Prion-like dissemination of harmful proteins
- Advanced glycation end-products
- Lipofuscin

two processes occur at different points in the life history, yet the examples previously offered of the simultaneous marked improvement and serious deterioration of brain function, for instance, from age 40 to 75, illustrate the dubiety of that conventional conceptualization. *Aging* and *development* are harder to dichotomize than is generally thought, and are perhaps most readily understood as the coherent expression of a largely adaptive time-passing-related life history process that seems to involve three features.

Time-Passing-Related Life History Feature #1

Development-and-aging is, in the main, an evolved life history plan. Yet the degree to which selective pressures orchestrated the symphony varied greatly with the life stage. Begin with the typical biography of the Neolithic cave painter: a minority survived infancy. Death came at about age 22. It was rare to live beyond 35. For the period of life from conception to full somatic "maturity" (about age 25), the life history plan was composed very much under the strict supervision of competition for survival and reproduction. (Call it one's Bach period.) The result was a rather predictable sequence, similar between conspecifics, controlled by a rhythmic battery of metronome-like biological clocks. For instance, the age of birth hovers around nine months; the age of menarche only varies between about age 9 and 15; the age of complete brain myelination (about age 24) corresponded with the average age of death (about 22). In contrast, in mid-life after the age of rearing one's own children (meaning about age 30–50), there were few survivors

available to exhibit benefits of mutations and their behavior had less and less impact on their fitness. So nature had progressively less need to compulsively compose neat harmonies of biological resilience. Remaining *compos mentis* at age 50–80 was quite unlikely to enhance fitness. Hence, among the handful who made further progress through the life history, nature had neither the opportunity nor the incentive to produce and select – with Baroque compulsion – the mutants whose brains continued to function well. Call this one's aleatoric John Cage period – the stage of life when much gets left to chance.

In the light of such a flickering life expectancy, it seems remarkable that some brain enhancements remained to blossom late, such that wisdom and subjective well-being bloom well into the senium. Can one really attribute that fact to positive selection for inclusive fitness? Are thoughtful, content grandparents so precious to their offsprings' reproductive flourishing? The author guesses that selection played some little role in that happy phenomenon. Yet, in the main, one's late-life biography is much more loosely controlled by the biological clock.

The result? The bottom line of the author's theory of "aging"? *Phenotypes of time-passing-related brain change vary little in childhood but a lot in late adulthood.* That is why doctors have been flummoxed by the question, "What is 'normal aging' and what is 'neurodegenerative disease'?" Please retire this antique dichotomy; those are social constructs, not natural kinds. Nature is not hiding its nature! Time-passing-related brain change is universal and variable.

Time-Passing-Related Life History Feature #2

There are many threats to mortality, such as accidents, diseases, and innate factors eroding the integrity of biomolecules and cells. Although it is popular to refer to these accidental mortal threats as chance, random, or stochastic, that terminology is a perhaps misleading for two reasons. First, out of an infinite number of potential threats, only a few dominate the threat matrix because the environment confronts us with some threats more often than others (e.g., domestic violence versus ball lightning) and because human bodies exhibit much more innate vulnerability to some changes than to others (e.g., stroke versus Abderhalden–Kaufmann–Lignac syndrome). Second, because an interaction occurs between aging feature #1, the development-and-aging life history plan, and feature #2, exposure to accidents. (See aging feature #3.)

Time-Passing-Related Life History Feature #3

There is an interplay between the first two features of development-and-aging: the progressive decline with age of selection pressure on the life history plan is associated with deterioration in the efficacy of rescue tactics on exposure to accidents. During the earlier part of life, selection pressure favored mechanisms to rescue genes from non-replication, such as DNA repair and agile dodging of woolly mammoth

---

[20] Liberally adapted from Best (2016) [37].

tusks. During the post-child-rearing part of life, less selection pressure exists to favor gene rescue tactics. Hence, the development-and-aging life history plan is deeply interwoven with the risk of accidental deterioration.

The author is not sure how many gerontologists will embrace the idea that time-passing-related somatic change is rightly conceptualized as an integrated mammalian trait, a life history plan that capitalizes on the most fitness-promoting facets of gaining and losing functions. Among other things, it perhaps threatens disciplinary identity. This impressionistic paradigm shift might some day be shown to be either a helpful alert to the coherently selected nature of brain life history plans or demonstrably inconsistent with some law of nature. Better concepts are very welcome! This perspective is only offered because it overcomes the simplistic model of life histories according to which development proceeds until day X and aging begins on day $X + 1$. Although human cells share a genome, their biographies are astonishingly divergent. As counterintuitive and even repellent as it sounds, humans are possibly better conceptualized not as organisms but as mosaics of human cells collaborating with one another and with non-human cells,[21] each one and each type following its own life trajectory. An instance of the apparent unitary purpose of development and aging: the acquisition of wisdom after about age 50 or 60 occurs despite the withering of gray matter, the culling of synapses, and a marked decline in the capacity for experience-dependent plasticity. The wise brain is a shrunken shadow of its youthful self. Shall we mourn the split cocoon or cheer the butterfly? One might be forgiven for suspecting that the human life history plan, including the normal biography of the brain, evolved in a meaningful, explainable way. "Development" and "aging" are academic constructs that may obfuscate our biographically brilliant arc. Gene expression choreographs gains and losses such that brain state at each point serves life stage-related needs in an energy-efficient way.

Combining the foregoing concepts with an evolutionary perspective might: (1) clarify the relationship between concussion and aging; (2) explain the heterogeneity of late effects; and (3) explain why it may take decades of further study before we know whether (or how often, or under what circumstances) a single concussion increases the risk of deleterious alteration of time-passing-related brain change or the occurrence of "dementia." First, one notes the overlap between the deleterious biological changes attributed to aging, the agents of the force of mortality, and the changes attributed to TBI. The impact of those agents (e.g., inflammation, microvascular change, seeding and spread of atypically folded proteins) depends on one's genome and environmental exposures. A concussion is one such environmental exposure. Air pollution, immigration stress, and romantic disappointment are others. The relative potency of these deserves study.

What is Neurodegeneration?

Neurodegenerative diseases (NDDs) are characterized by progressive dysfunction and loss of neurons leading to distinct involvement of functional systems defining clinical presentations.

[78]

the manner in which different research groups define neurodegeneration varies considerably.

[79]

A recent paper made the following claim: "These results provide supporting evidence for the evolution not resolution of this brain injury pathology, adding to the growing body of literature describing imaging signatures of chronic neurodegeneration even after mild TBI and concussion" [80]. That study seems to provide further empirical evidence that CBIs cause lasting, deleterious effects on the brain. Yet critical readers – medical students, psychologists, psychiatrists, physiatrists, and neurologists – may have balked upon encountering the freighted term *ND*.

OK, we accept the fact that concussions cause brain changes that may be harmful and long lasting. But why label your results "imaging signatures of ND"? All you saw were false color images estimating fractional anisotropy derived indirectly from bouncing radio waves and liberally interpreted as "white-matter integrity" in 78 regions of interest.[22] Since you did not count neurons or assess net brain function before and after any injury, why use the word *neurodegeneration*?

That critique is perceptive. ND is another term of art, typically typed without pause as if the universe of scholars had settled on a definition. They have not. The term gained favor among 20th-century neuropathologists and remains popular in peer-reviewed publications, but is rarely linked with a specific, let alone validated, biological meaning.

That raises an important question: when scholars discuss "neurodegenerative diseases" or investigate whether concussion provokes "neurodegenerative changes," are any of them discussing the same thing? Jack et al. [79], for instance, explored the impact on diagnosis of subjects when they were classified using five alternate definitions of ND: (1) abnormal adjusted hippocampal volume alone; (2) abnormal Alzheimer's disease signature cortical thickness alone; (3) abnormal fluorodeoxyglucose positron emission tomography (FDG-PET) alone; (4) abnormal adjusted hippocampal volume *or* abnormal FDG-PET; and (5) abnormal Alzheimer's disease signature cortical thickness *or* abnormal FDG-PET. The results are less important than the message. The lack of any shared concept of ND is not conducive to research progress.

Although the present author does not know a "correct" definition of ND, he suspects that recent discoveries make some

---

[21] A human body contains more non-human cells than human cells due to its mutualistic contract with gut bacteria.
[22] Technically inclined readers will want to know that those authors employed a tortoise (tolerably obsessive registration and tensor optimization indolent software ensemble) to conduct their analyses for them.

candidates for defining elements of ND less plausible than others. ND cannot be equated with the presence of atypically conformed proteins. Little evidence links that phenomenon to either loss of function or death of neurons. ND is often diagnosed when there is loss of synapses, but since synaptic pruning identifies healthful experience-dependent plasticity, synaptic loss may not be the best measure of ND. ND should probably not be equated with loss of gray-matter volume. That may also be typical of the normal, healthy life history plan, for instance, in pregnancy. ND certainly cannot be defined by brain atrophy since, without neuron counts, it is not possible to determine whether what's missing is neurons, glia, blood vessels, extracellular space, or water. It cannot have a purely functional definition, since function varies within and between brains from before birth. For instance, metabolism measured by FDG-PET may decline if you lose your dog.

One promising definition might be "a loss of neurons with deleterious consequences for fitness." Yet, as discussed in the section on aging, since death may be beneficial to fitness, who would complain about the mere loss of neurons? "A loss of neurons with deleterious consequences for that organism's functional independence" seems closer to the definition of ND. Yet even that begs the question (in the formal sense of *petitio principii*) because it assumes the yet-to-be-proven hypothesis that changes that discommode an individual organism are always negative in the biological sense.

Even ignoring that problem of logic, to define ND in terms of neuronal loss casts us back into the Sisyphean lifestyle where scholars labor to define categories according to dimensions. Why? Because evidence suggests that *some degree* of neuronal loss with the passing of time is normal and expected. For example, employing modern stereological techniques, Pakkenberg and Gundersen [81] reported that about 10% of cortical neurons are lost between the ages of 20 and 93 in both sexes. How much loss, then, defines the border between health and ND?

In fact, little is agreed about the magnitude of neuron loss in "normal aging." Despite that missing baseline, and despite great uncertainty about how neuron loss impacts behavior, such loss is frequently taken in the peer-reviewed literature to be pathognomonic of ND. Yet (closing our eyes to the weakness of that assumption), in practical terms, how might one determine whether one neuron or 1 million neurons have been lost? The best way would be to somehow label each neuron, count it, await a health event, and repeat the count, listing each neuron that went missing. Such studies have yet to be done. A weak substitute might be to machine-count each neuron in several representative slices from a precisely specified cortical area in 100 80-years-olds, determine the average, and compare that average to the corresponding count in the same place in another 80-year-old's brain. Setting aside the fact that no two humans have the same cellular architecture in any neocortical area, and presuming that averaging counts from comparable pieces of comparable people's brains permits a meaningful estimation of a species-specific trait, one might guess that a smaller total in the subject's brain suggests some cell loss at some point in between gestation and age 80.

Again, our ideals seem to have outpaced the empirical record: even the most vigorous brain bankers have yet to conduct such counts in each architectonically discrete cortical subregion in large post-mortem samples matched for age, sex, and other potentially confounding factors. As Juraska and Lowry summarized the state of the art: "To date, there do not appear to be any studies of cortical subregions that have combined stereological counting techniques with consideration of reference volume … so that the total number of neurons can be calculated during aging" [82]. Instead, what one finds in the literature are partial counts of small fragments of several small regions – such as a thin slice or two of the cornu ammonis, the substantia innominata, the dorsal raphe, the substantia nigra, and other places – derived from small samples of non-comparable people. Thin slicing (in this case, literal) is a cognitive short cut. It is unreliable.

If one does not know the age-adjusted average number of neurons in a specific brain area, or the number of neurons in that area before a patient suffered a change, or the number after that change, how might one claim that there was either loss or deleterious loss? In most cases, loss is not counted but inferred. One sees some shrunken neurons, some pyknotic neurons, signs of suspected apoptosis (e.g., "cell death-associated proteins" such as caspases, or externalization of phosphatidylserine and other phagocytic lures) [83, 84], signs of microgliotic neuronophagia, and/or zones that seem depleted and underpopulated. It seems reasonable to assume loss.

What is harder to tell is whether that is *deleterious* loss – a commonsense criterion for ND. In motor neuron disease or spinal muscular atrophy, a micro-wasteland combined with a devastating clinical change is persuasive and tragic. But when slow, progressive neocortical neuron loss occurs along with mental changes that might have a dozen explanations, cause and effect is harder to argue. And both the most reliable signs of apoptosis and whether signs of apoptosis are common or uncommon in "Alzheimer's disease" are controversial [85]. As a result, the judgment of ND has become a matter of opinion. Alternative biomarkers – such as magnetic resonance spectroscopy (MRS) measures of N-acetyl aspartate (NAA) or its ratio with respect to choline – may eventually be standardized across labs, controlled for confounds such as age and genes, and accepted as evidence of loss [86]. But that *still* does not prove *deleterious* loss.

Perhaps a robust and universally accepted criterion for ND will require an experimentally validated, very strong correlation between a combination of several cell loss or dysfunction markers with discommodious behavior. That finding could reasonably be called "a loss of neurons with deleterious consequences for that organism's functional independence" – the present author's best-guess criterion for ND.

That brings us back around to the challenging issue of what is and is not normal, expected, inevitable species-specific time-passing-related brain change, given that good health means a brilliantly orchestrated symphony of gains and losses. And it requires acceptance of an indisputable biological idea that has yet to become popular in clinical medicine: death is not, by nature, bad.

Death is usually a vital stage in organic development – a completion of the life history plan that fulfills genetic destiny and enhances inclusive fitness by culling creaky, ineffective DNA transporters, reserving limited earthly resources for more fertile and lively transporters of the same messages – for instance, children. Therefore, one must be cautious about attributing "harm" to loss of neurons as one approaches death – or even loss of neurons that *facilitates*-death – unless that also impairs inclusive fitness. The fact that involutional somatic collapse and return to dust are irritating to some does not endow that phenomenon with organic negativity. What is deleterious to one's one-handed jump shot is not necessarily deleterious to one's biological destiny.

That caveat aside, again, one might tentatively, provisionally consider ND a loss of neurons sufficient to have deleterious consequences for functional independence. Scholars more clever than the present author will have to mark the measuring stick.

What do Neuron Counts and Gray-Matter Volume Have to Do With the Passing of Time?

Back in the 20th century, some writers mentioned neuronal loss or loss of gray-matter volume (GMV) in their discussions of human brain aging. The assumption seems to have been that the species-specific evolved life history course involved being born with many neurons, experiencing dramatic synaptic pruning at various stages (with some controversy about whether neurons are routinely lost in that teenaged process), followed by a gradual loss of neurons and GMV with the subsequent passing of time until death. Implied in the lore was that either fewer neurons or loss of GMV is evidence of functional decline. If that were an accurate story, one might claim a relatively straightforward association between aging and brain change. One might even propose that the loss of function with the passing of time has something to do with the loss of neurons or GMV – and attribute the quality of badness to that change, and call the loss "ND."

It is not that simple. First, no one has ever counted the neurons in a human brain. We only estimate. Second, the best guess about the average number of adult human neurons has recently been updated and downgraded. According to Herculano-Houzel [87], based on scaling up from confirmed counts in other primates, human adults have about 16 billion cortical neurons and about the same number of cerebellar neurons. That fits with a range of recent estimates from 10 to 20 billion [88]. Third, whether we refer to that which happens over time as development or aging, the degree of change in counts of cortical neurons, for instance, among neonates and teenagers remains poorly defined and is perhaps *different in every individual* [89–91]. In fact, students are often surprised to learn, "There appears to be a normal biological variation in the number of neocortical neurons by a factor of more than 2; this represents a variance of more than eight times the variance of human body height" [88]. However, it is self-evident that the suspected loss of neurons between age ten and 20 is not a biomarker for functional decline! Quite the opposite. Fourth, the no-new-neurons hypothesis has been disproved. Although

Altman's astonishing 1962 [92] report of new adult human neurons was immediately dismissed with extreme prejudice, abundant evidence now suggests that neurons are added to the brain well into late life by virtue of differentiation from several pools of progenitor cells [93–96].[23] Until the magnitude of that effect is better understood, one hesitates to say neuronal loss parallels aging.

Fifth, there is pregnancy.

That last deserves comment. In a recent study, Hoekzema et al. [98] prospectively measured and followed GMV in women. They reported, "primiparous women were found to undergo a symmetrical pattern of extensive GM volume reductions across pregnancy, primarily affecting the anterior and posterior cortical midline and specific sections of the bilateral lateral prefrontal and temporal cortex" ([98], p. 293). This study confirms similar results long reported in pregnant rodents. Some evidence suggests a fitness advantage for this normal, healthy pregnancy-induced brain atrophy: it is perhaps associated with social bonding. That is, just as socialization and comportment with adult norms accompany the GMV loss of adolescence [99–101], pregnancy might resculpt the brain to focus efficiently on the critical work of parenting. The molecular changes underlying this atrophy are unknown at the time of this writing. Hoekzema et al. cautioned, "Changes in GM signal extracted from MRI images can reflect … changes in the number of synapses, the number of glial cells, the number of neurons, dendritic structure, vasculature, blood volume and circulation, and myelination" ([98], p. 294).

The purpose of this section is merely to disabuse the reader of the simplistic and dated notion that brain atrophy is bad, or that neuronal loss means ND. An automobile's engine might be optimum for some purposes if laden with 100 kg of emission controls. For other purposes, leanness might be preferable.

The present author declines to press onward with the tricky question of defining ND. His impression is that too little is presently known about the relationship between time-passing-related brain change and inclusive fitness to make the required judgments regarding goodness versus badness. For practical purposes, one might declare with confidence, "A theoretical boundary line exists between neuronal loss with the passing of time that does or does not negatively impact inclusive fitness. On the bad side, that is ND." Disabling "Parkinson's disease" at age 14 qualifies. But what about disabling "Parkinson's disease" at age 60?

What is Dementia?

Amazingly, 50 years after the start of modern dementia research, our field lacks clarity on this fundamental question of definition.

(Breitner, 2006 [102])

The best current estimates suggest that between 5% and 15% of current cases of dementia may be TBI related.

(Hay et al., 2016 [103])

---

[23] The role of new neurons in the brain's response to traumatic injury was discussed in Chapter 4 of this volume. Also see Ugoya and Tu [97].

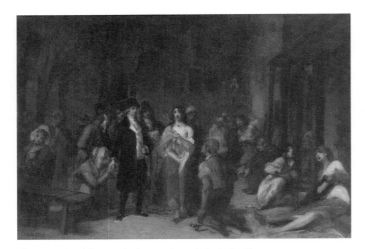

Fig. 11.4 Pinel freeing the insane from their chains: Tony Robert-Fleury, 1876.

The French psychiatrist Phillipe Pinel gained notoriety when he (belatedly) introduced Enlightenment values to European mental health by freeing the insane at the Hôpital de la Salpêtrière from their chains (Figure 11.4).

Pinel is also credited, by most historians of neurology, with the first medical use of the term "dementia." He described *démence sénile* in his 1797 *Nosographie Philosophique* [104], referring to a broad spectrum of changes in behavior, using an adjective to restrict attention to the dementias observed in old age, and giving equal weight to cognitive, mood, and psychotic impairments. That qualifier "*sénile*" was necessary because dementia, standing alone, simply refers to any decline from a previous level of mental function – for instance, the momentary confusion of a seven-year-old who falls from a swing. In fact, tracing the subsequent use of *dementia* in medicine reveals that an association with the elderly is a recent deviation from semantic convention, creating a misleading term of art.

Berrios [105] concisely traced the post-Pinel vagaries in the "dementia" concept through Esquirol, Boisseau, Rostan, Georget, Calmeil, Guislain, Marc, Morel, Prichard, Bucknill and Tuke, Jackson, Maudsley, Crichton Brown, Gombault, Bessière, Toulous, Noetzli, up to Kraepelin [106]. Dementia simply means mental deterioration. For more than a century, a typical adult case report described a 20-year-old woman with catatonic psychosis, or a 33-year-old man with general paralysis of the insane. The contemporary use of the term has been confined in three arbitrary ways and typically refers to (1) progressive (2) cognitive loss in (3) late life. That is very different from the concept discussed by the 19th-century pioneers. Just as our French and German forebears would be baffled by the semantically deviant use of *concussion* to refer to the (1) head and (2) to something mild, so would they be flummoxed by our odd use of "dementia."

Readers may be familiar with the concept that was popularized in the last quartile of the 20th century: dementia as *late-life cognitive incapacitation*. Yet even then consensus remains elusive. One encounters competing definitions from the American Psychiatric Association [23], the American Psychological Association [107], the World Health Organization [108], and the European Dementia Consensus Network [109].

Multiple debates have delayed consensus: whether *dementia* should refer to a clinical state or to expected manifestation of a subset of pathological processes; whether it should be regarded as an all-or-none phenomenon, or something that passes through biologically meaningful stages, or something that progresses insidiously along a continuum from normal aging to decerebration; whether a specific cognitive domain (e.g., memory) must be affected to make the diagnosis; how to diagnose this condition; and how to apply the term among the oldest old – virtually all of whom are afflicted [110–119]. In his 2006 publication, Breitner [102] attempted to crystallize what he believes underlies the contemporary use of the term *dementia*, hoping to derive what he called an "implicit consensus." He identified four factors (abbreviated here for concision):

1. There is a global deficit in cognitive abilities, that is, in several domains of cognitive activity. Other behavioral, ideational, or perceptual disorders occur variably (e.g., agitation or aggression, delusions or overvalued ideas, hallucinations or illusions). Although the last are not a defining feature, they can complicate dementia, adding significantly to the burden or difficulty of its care.

2. The deficit represents a state of decline from a previously established level of abilities.

3. The cognitive deficits or associated features are of sufficient severity to impair accustomed social or occupational functions.

4. The decline in cognition or functional abilities is not attributable to alteration in level of consciousness.

This is not dementia. It is a subtype of dementia. One might better call Breitner's hypothetical disease, "critical cognitive dementia." That confusion of a subtype with the whole problem has probably delayed progress in understanding time-passing-related brain change by granting *cognition* undeserved priority, excluding from *dementia* all cases of devastating psychiatric disorder in the presence of preserved memory. This is an error. It devalues the important and common phenomenon of disabling declines in emotional regulation.[24]

Still, the present author acknowledges that one will have a devil of a time persuading the global community of scholars to abandon an old, familiar term of art in favor of common-sensical terminology. A provisional, place-holder definition of some sort is necessary to interpret the pile of peer-reviewed publications investigating a possible causal relationship between TBI and dementia. Confessing semantic compromise, *dementia* of the sort that dominates that literature might be

---

[24] In addition (and separate from the issue of defining dementia), some late effects of TBI involve motor changes far out of proportion to mental changes. That is not *dementia* by any definition. But it matters.

defined as a *chronic behavioral state sufficiently subnormal to threaten independence.*

Five dissociable research questions have earned attention:

1. *Is a history of TBI associated with an increased risk for later dementia?* Scholars have investigated several questions pertinent to this issue, including: "In a cohort with dementia, is there a higher-than-expected frequency of a history of TBI?" or, "Does a history of TBI increase the likelihood that a person with mild cognitive impairment will progress to dementia?" or, "In a retrospective study, will those with a history of TBI be found more likely to develop dementia?" [103, 120–136]. The present author believes that a better question (if hard to answer) would be: "In a prospective study following TBI survivors until death, will 'dementia' be diagnosed in a larger number of patients than matched controls?"

2. *Is a history of TBI associated with accelerated progression of dementia?* For example, following persons diagnosed with one of the various dementing disorders, such as "Alzheimer's disease," do those with a history of TBI exhibit more rapid decline [137, 138]?

3. *Is a history of TBI associated with reduced adaptability or functional resilience in the face of dementia* [139]?

4. *Is a history of TBI associated with an increased risk for one ore more* of the purportedly distinct neurodegenerative disorders invented by 20th-century neuropathologists? For example, is TBI a risk factor for later "Alzheimer's disease?" "frontotemporal lobe degeneration"? "Parkinson's disease"? "amyotrophic lateral sclerosis (ALS)" [140]?

5. *Are persons with a history of TBI at risk for a form of dementia not seen in persons without a history of TBI?* For example, does TBI trigger a form of CTE that is biologically unitary and specific and distinct from other putative "neurodegenerative diseases" commonly diagnosed by 20th-century neuropathologists [103, 141–148]?

If the answer to any of these questions is "yes," a compelling reason exists to press for safe and effective interventions to mitigate these risks. It is often said that delaying the clinical effects of "Alzheimer's disease" by five years would vastly reduce the global burden of late-life dysfunction. Should the maturing generation of young scholars demonstrate that TBI triggers or magnifies time-passing-related brain change – whether this impacts motor, cognitive, or non-cognitive behavior – it would open the door to focused study of time-passing change in young brains and ought to inspire a worldwide effort to mitigate that insidious chain of causality.

Candidates for contributing biological factors are legion. Inflammatory activity [148–154]? Microvascular dysfunction [151, 155–158]? Blood–brain barrier permeability [158–162]? Metabolic stress (perhaps persistent due to acquired network inefficiency) increasing oxidative injury [149, 163, 164]? Neural transmission dysfunction or excitotoxicity [165–168]? Seeding with atypically folded proteins that spread transsynaptically [169–171]? Insulin-like growth factor signaling change [172,

173]? Pituitary dysfunction [174–177]? Misguided gene expression or epigenetic change [164, 178, 179]? Neurotropic deprivation [180, 181]? Enfeebled glymphatic clearance [160, 182, 183]? Aberrant DNA repair [165, 184]? Lax neurogenesis [179, 185]? Aberrant rewiring of the connectome [186, 187]? Or, most likely (in the author's opinion), do *all of these and more* contribute to the impact of a CBI – to different degrees in different individuals – yielding utterly unique life effects depending on genes, epigenes, and environments?

Readers who have bought a "Here is *the* cascade" model of concussion have been sold a bill of goods. Pieces of a puzzle are important. But one cannot understand Guernica by staring at the flaring left nostril of the central horse.

A worthy goal is to identify, amidst this multifactorial melee of biological change, modifiable risk factors for bad outcome. However, before searching for those modifiable mechanisms by which trauma may influence later-life function, an epidemiological question of profound human importance needs to be resolved. In order to increase risk, need the patient suffer more than one CBI?

What, then, has been discovered in those scores of investigations of a possible link between one or more TBIs and "dementia"? We return to the issue of same and different. If a large and representative sample of the human population had ever been assessed, using identical and valid criteria, reliably applied, for the diagnosis of *concussion* and so-called *dementia*, one might hope to learn something about the association. Due to (1) the inconsistent lumping of brain and/or behavior changes into the artificial dichotomies such as *mild* versus *not mild*, *dementia* versus *not dementia*, as well as (2) the commonplace misrepresentation of cases as pure types (e.g., "Alzheimer's disease") when in fact mixed dementia with polypathology (e.g., Chani's brain) is actually observed at almost every post-mortem, and (3) the unjustifiable priority assigned to *cognitive* decline over equally or more disabling *emotional* or *motor* decline, a comprehensive review of the literature would do the reader a terrible disservice. It is tempting to trust that two laboratories judged the presence, absence, or degree of dementia comparably. In fairness, employment of standardized screening measures such as the Mini Mental State Examination or the Clock-Drawing Test or the Montreal Cognitive Assessment [188–192]: perhaps slightly reduces the confound of incomparable mental states. Yet deep analysis of tabulated published data evokes a shiver. The weight of uncertainty regarding what was actually wrong with each subject in this pile of disappointing literature is, for the purposes of scientific inference, unbearable.

Hence, adding up published reports that are positive and negative regarding the TBI–dementia link will never settle the question. Imagine, for a moment, that a massive and careful review established, "Among 1000 peer-reviewed cross-sectional empirical reports, all titled 'Does TBI increase the risk for dementia?' 900 concluded *yes*; 100 concluded *no*." The reviewers could safely write:

> Given the lack of credible data regarding even one of the 100,000 injuries, the lack of control for the 20 most obvious confounding variables, and the lack of assessment for

ecologically meaningful dysfunction, neither the dependent nor independent variables were properly measured and no conclusion is possible.

These routine deficits in methodological rigor absolutely preclude meta-analysis. (Some scholars have nevertheless tried, charitably overlooking the non-comparability of the data.)

In conclusion regarding "dementia": the term means any mental decline. Mental decline is infinitely variable. In the 20th century, some doctors adopted the habit of classifying patients into two categories, demented or not. The present author wishes to credit an old colleague, John Morris, for his important insistence that dementia is not a categorical but a dimensional concept that varies both in the ways in which it manifests and the degree to which it influences life. One result was the Washington University Clinical Dementia Rating (CDR) scale [114]. That tool rescues dementia from abstraction and provides earthly tethers for behavior.[25] If better research is ever conducted to test the hypothesis that one or more CBIs alters the risk for late-life functional impairment (for instance, either a cross-sectional study of monozygotic (MZ) twins discordant for very-well-documented concussion more than 30 years before, or a prospective longitudinal population-based study with 40–80 years of follow-up) then one might include CDR rating as one outcome variable. However, even the CDR is biased in favor of activities of daily living and ignores both psychiatric distress and quality of life. Since those are, in practical terms, the most important outcome variables, and since Western doctors have yet to redefine dementia in those terms, a definitive answer to the question, "Does one concussion increase the risk for 'dementia'?" is not a definitive answer for the question that matters: "Does one concussion increase the risk for human distress or impairment?"

What, if Anything, is "Alzheimer's Disease"?

there are examples describing instances of head
injury giving rise to a dementia neuropathologically
indistinguishable from AD [Alzheimer's disease] over a long
period (six to 15 years). This raises the possibility that head
injury may be a more important predisposing factor in the
pathogenesis of AD than is presently appreciated.

(Roberts, et al., 1990 [193])

Pooled clinical and neuropathologic data from 3
prospective cohort studies indicate that TBI with LOC
[loss of consciousness] is associated with risk for Lewy
body accumulation, progression of parkinsonism, and
PD [Parkinson's disease], but not dementia, AD, neuritic
plaques, or neurofibrillary tangles.

(Crane et al., 2016 [136])

One very much wants to know whether a single CBI or multiple such injuries increase the risk for deleterious late brain changes. At the time of this writing, many scholars still refer to a large number of differently defined conditions they elect to call "Alzheimer's disease." It is often stated that this collection of somewhat similar conditions is the most common cause of aging-related dementia. If Alzheimer's disease is a natural kind – if some biologically specific neurological problem is ever identified that is distinct from the expected spectrum of time-passing-related brain change in humans and from the classes of brain changes that have been labeled "other ND" (e.g., frontotemporal lobar dementia, corticobasal ganglionic degeneration) – then it behooves researchers to determine whether concussion is a risk factor for "Alzheimer's disease." If no natural kind exists that could rationally be called "Alzheimer's disease," then concussion scholars must refocus and work on a different (and this author would argue, more important) goal: to determine whether and how concussions impact late life.

Many papers have been published reporting epidemiological studies of TBIs of variously defined severities as a possible risk factor for later "Alzheimer's disease," also variously defined [120, 122–124, 128, 194, 195]. The methodologies have not been comparable. The results have been inconsistent. One relatively recent study stands out because of its size. Nordstrom et al. [196] investigated the possibility of a link between TBI and dementia with onset before age 65. A total of 811,622 Swedish male conscripts were followed for a median period of 33 years. In all, 45,249 suffered one or more TBIs. The hazard ratio for Alzheimer's disease among those with "mild TBI" was not significantly different from 1.0. However, the hazard ratio for "other types of dementia" after a single mTBI was 3.8. That ratio dropped to 1.7, but remained significant after adjustment for multiple covariates. That recent and massive study strongly suggests that a single CBI is a risk factor for non-Alzheimer's disease dementia.

One of the quotations that heads this section comes from another recent paper. Crane et al. [136] pooled results from three well-regarded studies. A total of 7130 subjects, whose age averaged 79.9 years, were asked (before becoming demented) if they recalled having suffered a TBI. In all, 618 (8.7%) self-reported a history of TBI with loss of consciousness less than one hour. The subjects were followed for variable periods of time. In one of the three studies, the hazard ratio for dementia among those with TBI was 1.03. In the other two studies, that ratio was 0.87. The hazard ratios for "Alzheimer's disease" in the three studies were similar to those for dementia. One hundred and seventy-six subjects with TBI with LOC < 1 h came to autopsy. No significant differences were found between persons with and without such brain injuries in any feature assessed.[26]

How shall we interpret these two carefully conducted, carefully reported research projects? In essence, they came to opposite

---

[25] For instance, in the domain of home and hobbies, the clinician determines whether the patient is fairly described as having "mild but definite impairment of function at home; more difficult chores abandoned; more complicated hobbies and interests abandoned."

[26] Braak stage V or VI; Consortium to Establish a Registry for Alzheimer's Disease (CERAD) intermediate or frequent; amyloid angiopathy, cystic infarcts, hippocampal sclerosis, or Lewy bodies. Note that the introductory quotation, stating that Lewy bodies and parkinsonian traits were found, refers to those with LOC > 1 h.

conclusions. Two differences can only partially explain that disparity. One: the Swedish study involved longitudinal follow-up. We know that injuries occurred. Although the research did not involve periodic testing, and cannot answer our questions about the trajectory of brain change, Sweden's national patient register, established in 1964, generated the extraordinary database that enabled this unique snapshot. In contrast, the second report was a cross-sectional study with the independent variable of self-reported single head injury some time in the previous 80 years, and the dependent variable of "Alzheimer's disease." Recall bias was surely a confounding factor. This alone gives one more confidence in the Swedish results.

Two: the studies applied a slightly different classification system. The first distinguished "Alzheimer's disease" from "other types of dementia" while the second assessed "Alzheimer's disease" versus "all dementia." It is unclear how that difference in disease labeling affected the assignment of caseness. It is unclear whether any two patients diagnosed with "Alzheimer's disease" in these studies had the same problem. Moreover, there was no assessment of psychiatric status, or quality of life, or subjective well-being – all concussion outcomes that may be more important to the net lifetime impact of TBI than cognitive change.

As the present chapter strives to emphasize, the essential question of whether concussions have late effects lies helpless, tied to the railroad tracks of nosology. Knowing, with the utmost possible certainty, whether or not concussions have late effects has potentially immense consequences for global public health – a fact that will become glaringly practical when CBI treatments are discovered and the question arises, "Is this treatment cost-effective, considering that it may mitigate 70 years of CBI effects?"

Confessing that he literally has no idea if it matters, the author nonetheless proposes to discuss the concept of "Alzheimer's disease." The present section of the chapter may seem to be a detour. And, in fact, one cannot predict whether the detour is worthwhile until more is known about the spectrum of time-passing-related brain change. The author is therefore making a bet: at some future time and place, having a scientifically rational handle on the variations in human brain change – and being able to distinguish the expected from the unexpected – will become important for concussion scholarship.

Perhaps the first agenda item is to expose the shaky foundation that undergirds the popular nosology of ND. Readers will quickly realize: despite a hundred years of semantic fiddling, there is no one accepted "Alzheimer's disease."

The Alzheimer's Disease of Alzheimer

Many readers will have heard the story: a 51-year-old farmer's wife named Auguste Deter became paranoid, lost in her own apartment (topographagnosia), and soon, forgetful. She was hospitalized and examined by Dr. Alzheimer. He describes her as disoriented, agitated, and periodically delirious, with auditory hallucinations, dyslexia, aphasia, lack of understanding of the use of objects (ideational apraxia), and severe memory

disturbance [197]. Mrs. Deter deteriorated over four years and died.

Dr. Alzheimer cut up her brain. Since the slides and tissue were lost, it is unclear what Alzheimer saw – or what he would have seen with superior techniques. But, according to memos written by Alzheimer and others, the brain exhibited gross atrophy and arteriosclerosis of the large vessels. Thus, the obvious and indisputable diagnosis in this case was cerebrovascular disease. Due to curiosity and the then-recently-adopted but naive faith in the meaning of little things, Alzheimer also made thin slices, stained some slices with a few concoctions provided by his colleague, Nissl, and peered at the slices through a stack of lenses. Dr. Alzheimer *suspected* neuronal loss (a phenomenon that remains tough to confirm, since it is impractical (and illegal) to count all the neurons before and after an insult) and he saw some peculiar blobs and swirls. Throughout the patient's cortex, but especially in the upper layers, without any stain Alzheimer saw "miliary foci that were caused by the deposition of a peculiar substance." Looking at the stained brain pieces, microscopic examination allegedly revealed "remarkable changes in the neurofibrils" affecting one-quarter to one-third of the cortical neurons (Figure 11.5). There were also fibrous changes and large fat vesicles in the glia. Although there was endothelial proliferation (typical of cerebrovascular disease), infiltration of the vessels was absent (atypical for cerebrovascular disease).

Alzheimer gave a lecture reporting his observations and later published several descriptive articles [197, 199, 200]. What Alzheimer reported was a case of psychosis with onset in the late 40s, with subsequent progressive loss of a wide range of mental functions in a person with large-vessel cerebrovascular disease. Several smaller-scale brain changes were visible with several then-available techniques.

Alzheimer's drawings of his peculiar lesions

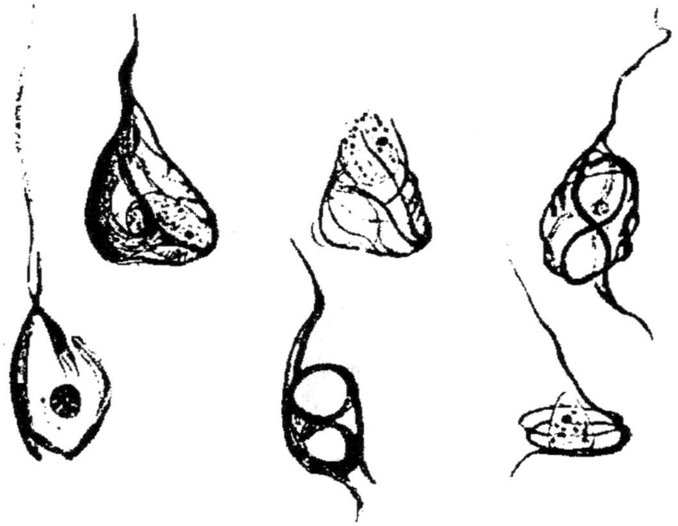

Fig. 11.5 Specimens which were prepared according to Bielschowsky's silver method show very striking changes of the neurofibrils. Inside of a cell which appears to be quite normal, one or several fibrils can be distinguished by their unique thickness and capacity for impregnation. [198]
Source: Alzheimer, 1911 [199]. Reprinted by permission from Springer

513

In fairness to our eagle-eyed predecessor, Alzheimer had no access to scores of techniques now routinely used to examine brains – far less to the scores of techniques to be published by the readers' children. He had no way to rule out lipohyalinosis, advanced glycation end products, activated microglia, prion proteins, α-synuclein, transthyretin. Moreover, a gigantic knowledge gap remains. Even today, evidence suggests that, despite our awareness of a large number of brain changes in late life, those may not be sufficient to fully explain the markedly variable clinical phenomenology. That suggests that we have yet to discover all the brain changes that are most proximally responsible for the growing epidemic of late-life emotional dysregulation and cognitive loss.

The Proliferation of "Alzheimer's Diseases"

If "Alzheimer's disease" were a particular thing – a natural kind – it would have an essence. After more than 100 years, no such essence has been found. In order to pass tests, recent generations of medical students have been obliged to memorize one of various definitive, committee-devised "consensus" diagnostic criteria for "Alzheimer's disease." Each identifies a different population of people. There are overlaps between these competing criteria, to be sure. Yet the emperor is naked: no committee or erudite authority figure has divined that which always and in every case distinguishes "Alzheimer's disease" from non-"Alzheimer's disease."

Little would be gained by a narrative that reviewed the checkered past of this incoherent diagnosis. The simplest fact: if you examine every old brain, you will never find two with the same changes. Chani's brain, described at the beginning of this chapter, is unique. Setting up several pigeon holes and cramming every brain into one or another is intellectually ignominious. The most seriously embarrassing behavior in neurology has been the dogmatic insistence, absent logical scrutiny, that there is normal time-passing-related brain change, and then, there is not-normal time-passing-related brain change. That is: leaning heavily on the pretense that a continuum is a menu of naturally dissociable categories.

That observation in no way diminishes the importance of helping people in distress. Call it what you wish, flail about in committees for as long as you can bear it, but do not expect those earnest deliberations to lead you to a name for Chani's condition. Neurologists – a group with a very high rate of burnout [201, 202] – might slightly reduce their stress if they set aside the contentious babbling that dominates our nosology and acknowledged the truth of uncertainty with grace and aplomb. Of course, there are some conditions that leap from the pack and declare their independent caseness. Bovine

spongiform encephalopathy is possibly a good example. But what is the virtue of taking a patient with some cerebrovascular changes and some Aβ and some p-tau and some α-synuclein and a bunch of activated microglia and an altered blood–brain barrier and some degree of atrophy in 30 different Brodmann areas – and perhaps 1000 other variations from average – who complains of some irritability and anxiety and memory loss and sleep disturbance and unsteadiness and a couple autonomic-sounding symptoms – and slapping the poor guy with a two-word diagnostic label?

Table 11.3 is included with reservations, lest anyone regard it as a source of definitive knowledge. It attempts to summarize the criteria championed by various committees for the one and only true and real "Alzheimer's disease." Older readers may or may not have become attached to one of these mutually exclusive algorithms for definitive diagnosis. Younger readers are cautioned to take the whole idea of "Alzheimer's disease" with a large grain of salt.

Readers need not pore over the table to catch the drift. Studying the similarities and differences between these "Alzheimer's diseases" is the job for a mountain village of silent monks. Finding a bright line between these conditions and normal health is equally tough. One paper inadvertently illustrated this "how many angels on the head of a pin?" problem with the concept of "Alzheimer's disease": "while biomarker abnormalities present in NC [normal control] older people are quite similar to those seen in AD, they are not necessarily identical in degree and topographic specificity" [214]. Not a stirring acclamation for dimensional diagnosis. One thing is apparent: a 51-year-old woman whose prominent presenting symptom is new-onset hallucinations would be unlikely to be diagnosed with one of these "Alzheimer's diseases."[27]

We are faced with a huge population of distressed people and their families. Everyone involved yearns for certainty. That yearning has motivated many efforts to find a bright line between so-called "aging," and so-called "Alzheimer's disease," and an ever-changing menu of alternatives. To date, despite a great deal of evidence that brains change differently with the passing of time, and that some microscopic changes are more common in some brains than in others, no defensible absolute biological criterion has been discovered to justify the label "Alzheimer's disease." As a result, clinicians seeking to render a firm diagnosis may feel a bit lost, realizing that their patient meets two criteria and fails to meet three others.

A detailed account of every logical error published as a rational explanation for why there is so much overlap between the findings in brains of old people with and without given mental symptoms would be dispiriting. Perhaps mentioning a

---

[27] Mrs. Deter's case exemplifies the tension between categorical and dimensional classification. She had an early-onset dementia without prominent amnestic symptoms. Some would call that early-onset Alzheimer's disease. Yet, after 1968, when Blessed et al. reported that the "senile plaques and neurofibrillary tangles" were the same in normal aging, in early-onset Alzheimer's dementia, and in senile dementia [215], and after 1976, when Katzman declared that virtually all cases of dementia are Alzheimer's disease [216], this distinction was abandoned on the grounds that age of onset is an arbitrary dimension. Mendez [217] eloquently makes the point that a *relative* (not absolute) difference in symptoms and pathophysiology might nonetheless identify a *meaningful* difference. He calls cases like Mrs. Deter's early-onset non-amnestic "type 2 AD." Eventually, even if no natural kind of discrete and unitary disease is ever identified, such differences might be critical for the choice of treatment.

Table 11.3 Descriptions of various neurobehavioral conditions or brain findings, all called "Alzheimer's disease" (AD)

Criteria title	Requires dementia?	Clinical diagnosis	Pathological diagnosis	Biomarkers	Levels of certainty
NINCDS-ADRDA[a] [203]	Assumes dementia	**Probable** - Onset 40–90 - Dementia - Deficits in ≥ areas of cognition - Progressively worse memory - Absent alternatives - Other features will increase or decrease certainty **Possible** - Dementia - Absent alternatives - Present second cause	**Definite** - Clinically probable plus "histological evidence"	N/A	Possible "Alzheimer's disease" Probable AD Definite AD
Khachaturian[b] [36]	Not clear	NA	Microscopic × 200 <u>Age < 50</u>: SPs or NPs and NFTs > 2 per field <u>Age 50–65</u>: SPs ≥ 8 <u>Age 66–75</u>: SPs > 10 <u>Age > 75</u>: SPs > 15	NA	"Alzheimer's disease"
CERAD[c] [204, 205]	Assumes dementia based on NINCDS-ADRDA criteria for "probable"	N/A	<u>Definite</u> Age-related plaque score C <u>CERAD NP probable</u> Age-related plaque score B <u>CERAD NP possible</u> Age-related plaque score A	N/A	- Definite "Alzheimer's disease" - CERAD NP probable "Alzheimer's disease" - CERAD NP possible
NIA-Reagan[d] [206, 207]	Assumes dementia without criteria	Assumes dementia	- High: NPs and NFTs in neocortex - Intermediate: moderate NPs + NFTs in limbic areas - Low: limited NPs + NFTs	N/A	- High likelihood of "Alzheimer's disease" - Intermediate likelihood - Low likelihood
Washington University Neuropathological Criteria for AD[e] [208]	Dementia required	CDR ≥ 0.5	Age-adjusted plaque score: < age 50: 2–5/mm² 50–65: ≥ 8/mm² 66–74: ≥ 10/mm² ≥75: ≥ 15/mm2	N/A	"Alzheimer's disease"
IWG-1 New Research Criteria[f] [209]	Dementia not required	Gradual, progressive episodic memory deficit with poor free recall not normalized by cueing	Defer to NIA-Reagan criteria	Supportive features: - volume loss of medial temporal cortex on MRI - low amyloid β_{1-42}, increased total tau, or increased p-tau in CSF - reduced bitemperoparietal glucose metabolism on PET - Autosomal dominant AD mutation in immediate family	"Alzheimer's disease," a clincobiological entity <u>Probable</u> AD = memory loss plus one or more supportive features <u>Definite</u> AD = both memory loss and pathological evidence meeting NIA-Reagan criteria, or both memory loss and familial AD mutations on chromosomes 1, 14, or20

(continued)

Table 11.3 (*Cont.*)

Criteria title	Requires dementia?	Clinical diagnosis	Pathological diagnosis	Biomarkers	Levels of certainty
IWG-2[g] [210]	Dementia not required	<u>Typical</u>: gradual, progressive episodic memory deficit with poor free recall not normalized by cueing <u>Atypical</u>: posterior variant, logopenic variant, frontal variant, Down's syndrome variant <u>Mixed</u>: any of the above <u>Preclinical</u>: none of the above	N/A	"In-vivo evidence" – only for <u>Typical</u> and <u>Atypical</u>: - Decreased amyloid β_{1-42} AND increased total tau, or p-tau in CSF - Increased tracer retention on amyloid PET - AD autosomal dominant mutation <u>Mixed</u>: evidence of Lewy body disease or cerebrovascular disease	<u>Typical AD</u> <u>Atypical AD</u> <u>Mixed AD</u> <u>Asymptomatic at risk for AD</u> = *in vivo* evidence of AD without clinical features <u>Presymptomatic AD</u> = Autosomal-dominant mutation in PSEN1, PSEN2, or APP, or other proven genes, without clinical features

[a] Re the Alzheimer's disease of NINCDS-ADRDA: These are called "clinico pathological" criteria. Clinical dementia is assumed. The criteria are "insidious onset and progressive impairment of memory and other cognitive functions." No criteria are proposed for dementia, and no pathological criteria are specified for Alzheimer's disease.

[b] Re the Alzheimer's disease of Khachaturian:

1. The text is ambiguous regarding whether dementia is a criterion for diagnosis. At one point, the clinical description is "memory loss, confusion, and a variety of cognitive disabilities." At another point, the authors state: "Neuropathologic study may show little or no changes at postmortem examinations of the brain of a patient whose dementia had fulfilled all psychological behavioral requirements for the disease during life." But no behavioral requirements are specified. Thus, the published pathological guidelines were intended only for judging autopsy results in patients with unspecified degree of cognitive change. It is not clear whether persons who meet criteria for "mild cognitive impairment" would qualify for the Alzheimer's disease of Khachaturian.

2. These are the only guidelines that acknowledge uncertainty regarding whether "Alzheimer's disease" is something different from normal aging. "We are still uncertain whether AD is a specific, discrete, qualitative disorder such as an infectious process, endogenous or exogenous toxic disorder, or biochemical deficiency, or whether it is a quantitative disorder, in which an exaggeration and acceleration of the normal aging processes occur and dementia appears when neural reserves are exhausted and compensatory mechanisms fail" (p. 1097).

[c] Re the Alzheimer's disease of CERAD: these criteria were not intended to guide clinical diagnosis but only to report a "practical standardized protocol for the neuropathological evaluation of autopsy brains of demented and control subjects" (p. 479). Age-related scores for NPs are rated by means of a formula: *A* = sparse NPs, age > 75; *B* = sparse NPs, age 50–75 or moderate NPs, age > 75; *C* = any NPs, age < 50; moderate or frequent NPs, age 50–75, or frequent NPs, age > 75. Level of certainty is determined by an algorithm combining NP scores and other data. Definite = *C* + dementia + presence or absence of other causes. Probable = *B* + dementia + presence or absence of other causes. Possible = *A* + dementia + presence or absence of other causes.

[d] Re the Alzheimer's disease of National Institute on Aging-Reagan: Clinical dementia is assumed and the cause of that dementia is expressed in terms of three degrees of certainty. "*High likelihood*" = "Frequent neuritic plaque score according to CERAD [204] … and Stage V/VI according to Braak and Braak [211]." "*Intermediate likelihood*" = "Moderate neocortical neuritic plaques and neurofibrillary tangles in limbic regions (i.e., CERAD moderate, and Braak and Braak Stage III/IV)." "Low likelihood" = "Neuritic plaques and neurofibrillary tangles in a more limited distribution and/or severity (i.e., CERAD infrequent, and Braak and Braak Stage I/II)."

[e] Re the Alzheimer's disease of Washington University: the text is ambiguous. It details methods for counting both NFTs and two types of SPs. It states that the criteria were derived from those of the NIA "and thus utilize both neocortical SPs and NFTs" (p. 1031). Immediately thereafter, however, the text defines neuropathological AD based entirely on SP counts (using the Khachaturian criteria) plus a lower-limit CDR score. Total SP density per mm^2 is defined as the average taken from ten 1-mm^2 microscopic fields in a 6-µm-thick section. Although NFT counts were reported, they seem to have been ignored in making a diagnosis.

[f] Re the Alzheimer's Disease of IWG-1:

1. Some aspects of these criteria are dubious and ambiguous. For instance, the authors regard medial temporal lobe volume loss as indicative of AD, while admitting that this occurs in 29% of normal brains. They require determining "volume loss of hippocampus, entorhinal cortex, amygdala" but never specify whether they meant to say "or amygdala" or "and amygdala." They consider low amyloid β_{1-42}, or increased tau, or p-tau in CSF as supportive, but do not define "low" or "increased."

2. Note that the authors clarified their intentions in a follow-on paper [212]. They urged adoption of a new lexicon: "The cornerstone of this lexicon is to consider AD solely as a clinical and symptomatic entity that encompasses both predementia and dementia phases" (p. 1118). That language, curiously, divorces "AD" from brain change. The lexicon differentiates between "AD," "AD pathology," atypical AD," "mixed AD," "asymptomatic at risk for AD," and "presymptomatic AD." The present authors again suggests cutting this Gordian knot, dismissing such fussy labels, and accepting that time-passing-related brain change varies. The same year, Oksengard et al. [213] published their paper entitled "Lack of accuracy for the proposed 'Dubois criteria' in Alzheimer's disease."

[g] Re the Alzheimer's Disease of IWG-2:

1. The authors define this paper as a refinement and simplification of the IWG-1 criteria. Readers may perceive it as a complication. The clinical picture is expanded to include what they call "atypical" features. The acknowledgment of heterogeneity inspired a completely new nosology differentiating typical AD, atypical AD, mixed AD, and two versions of preclinical AD.

2. Structural imaging has been abandoned in favor of amyloid positron emission tomography.

3. The authors candidly caution: "The proposed refinements will place great demands on the clinical core diagnosis, for which the clinician now needs to identify a range of potential AD phenotypes, including mixed AD phenotypes and focal non-amnestic disease presentations" (p. 622).

4. "Definite AD" is not mentioned as a possible diagnosis.

CDR: Clinical Dementia Rating; NFTs: neurofibrillary tangles; NPs: neuritic plaques; SP: senile plaques.

few errors will be sufficient for the author's modest goal: *gently requesting that scholars of concussion stop trying to determine whether concussion increases the risk of "Alzheimer's disease" and start trying to determine whether there are late effects.*

Error of Logic Number 1: If it's Unfamiliar and Little, it's Harmful

The inescapable fact that irritates some neuropathologists no end: it is literally impossible to know the exact relationship between the brain changes Alzheimer reported and Mrs. Deter's condition, or, for that matter, between any brain changes observed on autopsy and any behavior observed during life. An honorable textbook might begin its Alzheimer's chapter: "Mrs. Deter reportedly suffered tragic behavioral troubles. No one knows why."

Students need to take a deep breath and detect with a probing mind. New discoveries have prompted a dramatic rethinking of the relationship between Dr. Alzheimer's interesting reports and the monumental spectrum of human dementia. Yet the psychology of his age can be reconstructed: the introduction of microscopy to medical pathology was a game changer. Actually seeing the tubercle bacillus must have been astonishing. It is therefore no surprise that doctors with microscopes began to generalize from the success of infectious disease research and attribute causality to little things that only become visible at 50–400 optical power.

First-year medical students will readily detect the fallacy. Many hefty books declare, in essence, "Alzheimer saw blobs and swirls. They were little. Therefore, the blobs and swirls *caused* Mrs. Deter's troubles – and they cause the troubles of almost everyone on Earth who develops – as virtually everyone does who lives long enough – late-life dementia." This is precisely equivalent to saying, "Jakob saw extensive microscopic holes in the brains of his patients. The holes, therefore, cause Jakob–Creutzfeldt disease." Medicine 101: lung cavitations do not *cause* tuberculosis. Glomerular changes in the kidney do not *cause* diabetes. Mees lines do not *cause* arsenic poisoning. A battlefield does not *cause* the death of a heroic legion. Biomarkers can be precious clues to daunting puzzles. But we never, ever assume that biomarkers cause a disease.

Error of Logic Number 2: If we Sequence it, it's Harmful

Time passed. Technology improved. Neuropathologists discovered that the stuff in the blobs seen by Alzheimer had a β-pleated sheet structure. Yet it was not until 1970 (a 64-year wait) that Glenner et al. published the amino acid sequence of those sheets [218]. That discovery was followed by a flurry of investigation attempting to figure out what that amino acid sequence had to do with late-life behavior change. In 1984, Glenner and Wong [219] explicitly proposed that the amyloid protein had a pathophysiological role in Alzheimer's disease and could therefore be used to diagnose Alzheimer's disease.

Again, the medical student will blink with surprise.

Just because one sequences a protein, and finds evidence that that protein occurs in some cases of dementia, why would you damn that protein as a perpetrator of harm? If one finds antibodies at the site of an infection, should we assume that the antibodies *caused* the infection and frantically devise treatments to remove all antibodies from the human body to protect it from infection?

Logic notwithstanding the enthusiasm of people seeking tenure, "Alzheimer's disease" was soon explained by the "amyloid cascade hypothesis." In 1991 Hardy and Allsop opined that amyloid deposition is the "central event in the aetiology of Alzheimer's disease" [220]. That proposition was quickly echoed in complementary contemporaneous publications [221, 222]. This, without having determined why amyloid exists.

In fairness, many early empirical findings could be interpreted as consistent with the conclusion that β-amyloid (Aβ) is neurotoxic. Other evidence suggested that Aβ deposition preceded aggregation and deposition of hyperphosphorylated tau protein (p-tau), which also bolstered the argument that Aβ is the primary disease event. The parsimonious explanation that insoluble extracellular aggregates of fibrillar Aβ *cause* "Alzheimer's disease" was irresistible. However, recent advances suggest a more nuanced appreciation for the role of Aβ in health and disease.

Aβ has a bad reputation. That is unfair. One might as well condemn antibodies. As in the case of many biological phenomena (e.g., immune response, oxidative phosphorylation, neurotransmission, inflammation, or mitosis), the Goldilocks principle applies: a just-right amount favors survival. A little Aβ is essential for health; "too much" – an amount surely different in every human – is harmful. Consider Figure 11.6. This diagram displays some of the suspected physiological and pathological roles of Aβ.

Picomolar amounts of Aβ seem to be necessary to support critical brain functions, including neurogenesis and the plasticity that permits long-term learning and memory [223–225]. Excess, on the other hand, is strongly associated with a wide range of negative consequences. Figure 11.7 illustrates some of those deleterious effects.

Although it is premature today (and may remain premature for a century) to conclude that the molecular biochemistry of ND is understood, some recent evidence reframes the role of Aβ in time-passing-related brain change. It was acknowledged (reluctantly by some) almost two decades ago that counts of Aβ senile plaques (whether diffuse or neuritic) and measures of insoluble Aβ correlate poorly with cognition and degeneration [227–236]. More recent research suggests that no relationship exists between ND and Aβ deposits in presumptive "Alzheimer's disease" [214]. It has also been recognized for more than a decade that Aβ is hardly confined to the extracellular space; it is frequently found in the cytosol. Such observations inspired doubts about the simplest formulation of the amyloid cascade hypothesis.

Physiological and pathological roles of β-amyloid

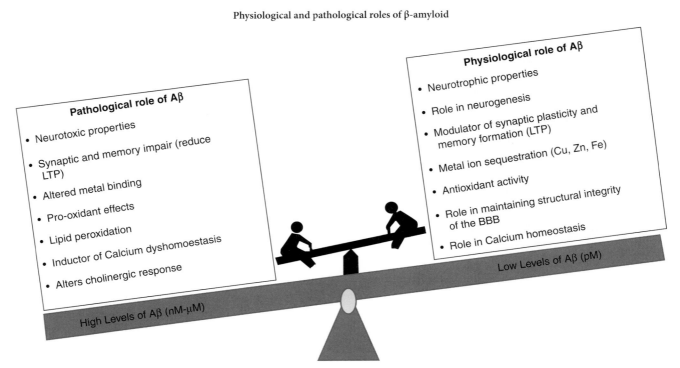

Fig. 11.6 Balance between physiological and pathological effects of Aβ. Like a seesaw in a park, the levels of Aβ change due to environmental factors or genetic background. In normal healthy conditions, Aβ is at lower concentration (pM), and exerts its physiological functions, but in disease conditions the levels of Aβ are elevated (nM to μM) and it switches it functions to pathological effects. BBB: blood–brain barrier; LTP: long-term potentiation.
Source: Cardenas-Aguayo et al., 2014 [223]. Reproduced under the terms of the Creative Commons Attribution licence, CC-BY 3.0

Aβ production may be important, but our gaze has been fixed on the wrong target. It is not the large, insoluble extracellular fibrillar aggregates that cause brain damage. Instead, low-molecular-weight toxic oligomers (varying in size from < 10 kDa to > 100 kDa) are the toxic forms that contribute to dementia largely by impairing synaptic transmission. As summarized by Sakono and Zako (2010) [237]: "It has long been argued that insoluble Aβ fibrillar aggregates found in extracellular amyloid plaques initiate the neurodegenerative cascades of AD. However, recent emerging results indicate that prefibrillar soluble Aβ oligomers are the key intermediates in AD-related synaptic dysfunction" (p. 1354). Gadad et al. [238] echoed that assessment: "The most probable explanation is that inclusions and the aggregates symbolize an end stage of a molecular cascade of several events, and that earlier event in the cascade may be more directly tied up to pathogenesis than the inclusions themselves." The precise mechanism by which Aβ oligomers disrupt synaptic function has yet to be fully elucidated, but some evidence suggests they conspire with complement to provoke a microglial assault.

Second, intriguing results from a sophisticated series of experiments conducted by Sell et al. [239] suggest another way Aβ indirectly targets synapses, finding evidence that the Rho family of GTPases might help mediate the toxic impact. One member of that family is RhoA, which normally participates in the developmental genesis and pruning of synapses. Ephexin5 is a RhoA activator. Little Ephexin5 is found in healthy brains. Its job may be to restrain overgrowth of excitatory synapses. But that can be problematic, since it also inhibits synaptic

development. Importantly, Ephexin5 is known to be elevated in patients with "Alzheimer's disease." Excess Aβ, the scholars showed, triggers a decrease in the protein called EphB2 that normally suppresses the problematic Ephexin5. The cascade: ↑Aβ → ↓ EphB2 → ↑ Ephexin5 → ↑RhoA → synaptic harm in the hippocampus. Might removing Ephexin5 disrupt this chain reaction and save the synapse? Apparently so.

The scholars recruited mice expressing the human amyloid precursor protein – a partial model of familial "Alzheimer's disease" that typically dooms the animal to excess Aβ, plaque formation, and cognitive deficits. When these scientists knocked out Ephexin5, the doomed mice still developed Aβ plaques, but *both their synapses and their cognition were spared*. At the time of this writing, it remains to be seen whether this will be a breakthrough that reveals a new therapeutic target or one more dead end. Yet it adds to the evidence that plaques are not themselves the executioners of the mind.

What, then, is the role of the plaques Alzheimer might have seen? Some scholars propose that these insoluble aggregates serve as reservoirs that enable the generation of toxic intermediate oligomers [238, 240].

And what does Aβ have to do with p-tau? The causal and temporal sequence of accumulation of these two proteins has been a chicken-vs.-egg debate for many years. Evidence from familial Alzheimer's disease favors Aβ-then-tau; evidence from some forms of frontotemporal dementia favors tau-then-Aβ. One proposal [241] is that, in human cases meeting criteria for "Alzheimer's disease," these proteins are parts of a self-reinforcing cycle, such that Aβ facilitates hyperphosphorylated

Some toxic affects of Aβ

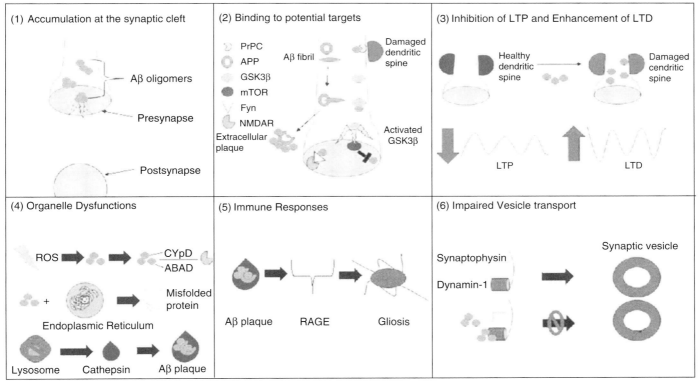

Fig. 11.7 The many sites of neuronal damage by Aβ. (1) Soluble intracellular oligomers of A are cytotoxic (2) Interaction with cellular prion protein (PrPC) leads to dendritic spine damage (top right). A fibril binds to amyloid precursor protein (APP) during formation of extracellular plaques (middle left). Aβ inappropriately activates glycogen synthase kinase 3 (GSK3) (middle right). Aβ synergizes with Fyn to disrupt synaptic receptors (bottom left). Mammalian target of rapamycin (mTOR) may inhibit Aβ (bottom right). (3) Mounting evidence suggests Aβ-mediated destruction of spines and synapses leads to long-term potentiation (LTP) impairment and long-term depression (LTD) enhancement. (4) Mitochondrial distress may lead to production of reactive oxygen species (ROS) that may accelerate Aβ formation. Aβ may then affect N-methyl-d-aspartate receptor (NMDAR) activity by binding to intracellular mitochondrial cyclophilin D or mitochondrial Aβ alcohol dehydrogenase. (Top). Aβ-mediated cytotoxicity may be particularly damaging to the endoplasmic reticulum, affecting its production and modification of crucial proteins (middle). Identification of cathepsins in Aβ plaques suggests protease dysfunctions from lysosomes may play a critical role in advancement of pathology (bottom). (5) Receptor for advanced glycation end products (RAGE) may play a prominent role in the increased microglial activation and proinflammatory markers commonly associated with senile plaques. (6) Aβ interacts with synaptophysin in presynaptic terminals of the hippocampus to impair neurotransmission (top). Aβ also interferes with dynamin-1, allowing synaptic vesicles to re-enter the synaptic pool (bottom). ABAD: mitochondrial Aβ alcohol dehydrogenase; CypD: intracellular mitochondrial cyclophilin D. [A black and white version of this figure will appear in some formats. For the color version, please refer to the plate section.]

Source: Rajmohan and Reddy, 2017 [226] with permission from IOS Press

tau generation and tau, in turn, facilitates Aβ generation. As depicted in Figure 11.8, evidence strongly suggests that Aβ acts in multiple ways to up-regulate tau phosphorylation.

The many roles of Aβ in health and disease have yet to be settled. However, a revision of the amyloid hypothesis, as conceived by Selkoe and Hardy [243], accommodates some of the recent findings and is depicted in Figure 11.9.

Readers, however, may profit by withholding commitment to this scheme. Without doubling the length of this chapter, it deserves note that none of the above brain changes correlates perfectly with behavioral change in old humans. As implied by the case of Chani that introduced this chapter, this neat schematic leaves out the confounding contributions of dozens of possible causes of mental deterioration – not the least of which is the one routinely ignored in discussions of the Alzheimer's disease of Alzheimer: the fact that time-passing-related cerebrovascular disease is virtually universal and harmful. One hesitates to unconditionally accept Selkoe and Hardy's final arrow – the one that says, "Therefore, dementia." It is as logically

valid as noting that competing territorial claims often precede armed conflict and declaring: "Border dispute, therefore, war."

Moreover, perhaps the most important advance reflected in Figure 11.9 is not the role of Aβ oligomers, nor the attribution of primacy to Aβ over tau, but the recently discovered role of neuroinflammation. If every other step were taken along this road, in the absence of inflammation, would there be disability? How does "Alzheimer's disease"-related inflammation compare with "normal" aging-related inflammation? And – given the abundant evidence that the long-term impact of concussion is mediated by inflammation – might that be an important pathway by which TBI increases the risk of deleterious time-passing-related brain change?

Inflammation

it is still to be determined if microglia activation is the cause of neurodegeneration or a secondary reactive (beneficial) process; or if the neurodegeneration is actually secondary

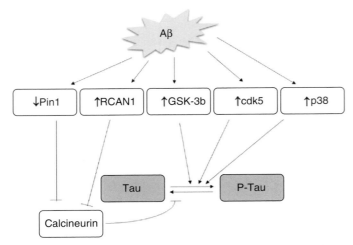

Fig. 11.8 Schematic rendition of proteins affected by Aβ that increase the phosphorylation state of tau. cdk5: cyclin-dependent kinase 5, a serine/threonjine kinase that catalyzes the phosphorylation of neurofilaments and tau. GSK-3b: glycogen synthase kinase 3β, which phosphorylates tau in most of its serine and threonine residues and contributes to Aβ production and Aβ-mediated neuronal death. p38: a mitogen-activated protein kinase that serves as an oxidative stress sensor that also phosphorylates tau. Pin1: prolyl isomerase 1, which catalyzes the conversion of cis/trans protein conformations. RCAN1: regulator of calcineurin 1, involved in the adaptive response to stress.

Source: Lloret et al., 2015 [242] with permission from Elsevier

to microglia senescence and associated loss of microglial protection.

(Taipa et al., 2016 [244])

In the 1980s and 1990s, there was almost no discussion of inflammation as a cause of ND. That has changed. Figure 11.10 shows how activated microglia affiliate with amyloid plaques. However, as explained by Taipa et al. [244], it would be simplistic to conclude "'Alzheimer's disease' provokes damaging pro-inflammatory phenomena." First, inflammation exists to benefit its organismic host. Until more is known about brain change over time, and the brain's response to undesirable contingencies, one cannot presume that the discovery of an inflammatory element to ND is the discovery of a modus of harm. Second, some evidence suggests different effects of the immune–inflammatory response at different ages. It may turn out to be the case that the balance of cytokines (for example) that best promotes brain health is not the same in middle and in old age.

Further speculation regarding the interplay of concussion, inflammation, and so-called "Alzheimer's disease" must await research progress [148]. The point is only to alert the reader to this burgeoning domain of inquiry.

Is "Alzheimer's Disease" Different From Aging?

Having previously declared that aging has yet to be defined, and in the midst of a section demonstrating that "Alzheimer's disease" has no defensible biological definition, the author would be foolhardy to offer a definite answer to this question. It would be like comparing the chemical traits of two undiscovered elements. Unless and until some specific biological phenomenon is indisputably demonstrated to be the essence of aging, no question should be formulated that compares aging

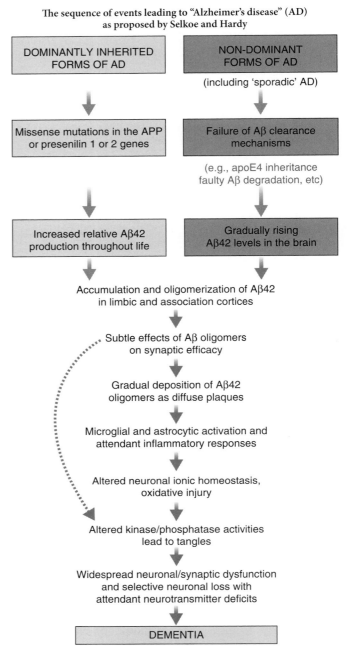

The sequence of events leading to "Alzheimer's disease" (AD) as proposed by Selkoe and Hardy

Fig. 11.9 The curved arrow indicates that Aβ oligomers may directly injure synapses and neurites of brain neurons, in addition to activating microglia and astrocytes.

Source: Selkoe and Hardy, 2016 [243]. Reproduced under the terms of the Creative Commons Attribution license, CC-BY 4.0

(that deep mystery) with anything else. The same caveat applies to "Alzheimer's disease." Still, readers will be exposed to many sources that purport to settle that exact question. In most cases, when writers compare and contrast aging with "Alzheimer's disease," they: (1) pledge allegiance to one of the many concepts of aging; (2) pledge allegiance to one of the many "Alzheimer diseases"; and (3) conduct an empirical study, sometimes decorated with logistic regression, that permits them to report "'Aging' is this but 'Alzheimer's disease' is that."

Activated microglia in "Alzheimer's disease"

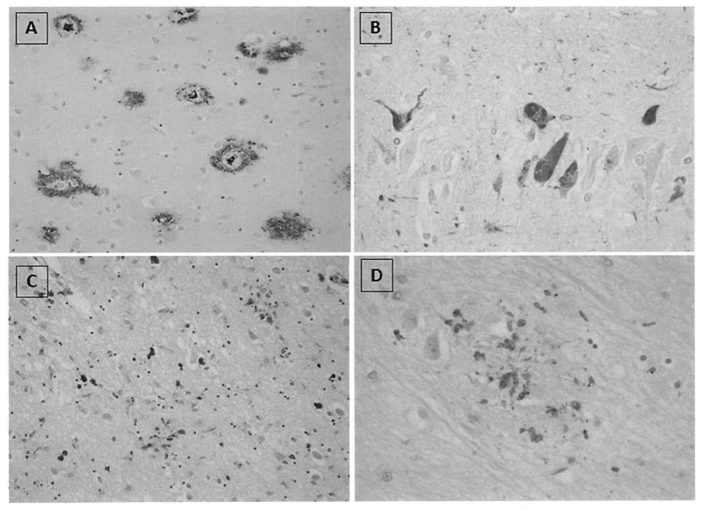

Fig. 11.10 (A) Senile plaques and globose diffuse deposits demonstrated with anti-A antibody (M 0804, Dako). (B) Neurofibrillary tangles demonstrated by phosphorylated tau protein immunohistochemistry (PHF-Tau; AT8, Thermo Scientific). (C) Diffuse distribution of activated microglia in the cortex with clustering within and around amyloid plaques. (D) Higher magnification of amyloid plaque with activated microglial in the CA4 region of the hippocampus (C and D: CD68 immunohistochemistry; PGM1clone, Dako). [A black and white version of this figure will appear in some formats. For the color version, please refer to the plate section.]

Source: Taipa et al., 2016 [244] with permission from IOS Press

A relatively recent example occurred in the 2014 [210] paper in which the International Working Group re-re-defined Alzheimer's disease. Referring back to their 2007 redefinition [209], those authors state:

> The first was a core clinical phenotypic criterion that required evidence of a specific episodic memory profile characterised by a low free recall that is not normalised by cueing. This memory profile differs from that observed in patients with non-AD disorders, such as frontotemporal dementias, progressive supranuclear palsy, Huntington's disease, major depression, or even normal ageing, in which the frontal related retrieval deficit is normalised by the cueing procedure.

([210], p. 614)

Neuropsychologists know that such absolutist statements are misleading. The claim "Cuing helps the aged; cueing does not help those with Alzheimer's disease" is untrue. It is a simplistic reading of papers such as that by Sarazin et al. [245], in which a *difference in the proportion* of those who benefited from cueing was found, not a reliable differentiation. In fact, the effect of cueing on recall is variable among cohorts with aging, mild cognitive impairment, or Alzheimer's disease [246–249].

Another example is the effort to distinguish between aging-related brain atrophy and aging-plus-something-else-related atrophy. Figure 11.11 attempts to differentiate between patterns of volume loss typically found in old people with and without clinically problematic cognitive loss.

Such images are derived from averaging many cases of persons with different degrees of cognitive change. They confirm that atrophy in some places is expected and normal. They imply that atrophy in other places is not. Whether or not any biological measures (e.g., cerebrospinal fluid markers)

Differences in cortical atrophy rates between healthy elderly individuals and those with mild cognitive impairment (MCI)/Alzheimer's disease (AD)

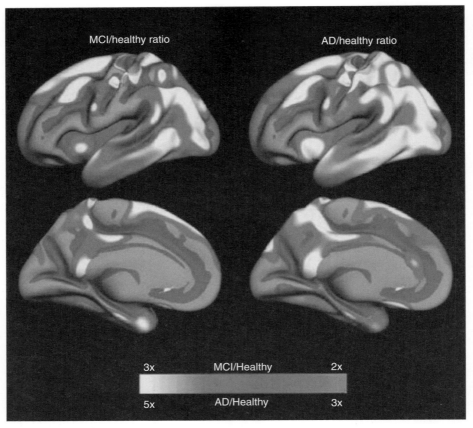

Fig. 11.11 In mild MCI, rates of cortical volumetric reductions are more than double that seen in healthy aging across large areas of the cerebral cortex, and rates more than three times larger are seen in AD. Please note that the scale is different between MCI/healthy and AD/healthy to allow appreciation of the regional patterns of effects across groups. Data from the Alzheimer's Disease Neuroimaging Initiative [A black and white version of this figure will appear in some formats. For the color version, please refer to the plate section.]

Source: Fjell et al., 2014 [250] with permission from Elsevier

suggest "Alzheimer's disease," the interpretation is circular: "If the person exhibits cognitive troubles earlier than he or she would like, the person is diseased. The finding that people with undesirable memory loss have a higher average regional tissue loss in a couple of places confirms the presence of disease." From the author's point of view, one might more readily conclude: "Time-passing-related brain change varies."

Further evidence that so-called "Alzheimer's disease" is debatably unique and completely discrete from either normal aging or from other neurodegenerative diseases comes from plotting Aβ deposition in ostensibly different diseases. Armstrong et al. [251] for instance graphed the first two principal components in an analysis of neuropathological findings from persons with various diagnoses. The authors point out:

A plot of the cases in relation to PC1 and PC2 showed considerable overlap between patient groups with no distinct boundary between the control, DLB [dementia with Lewy bodies], and AD cases. In addition, there was no clear boundary between FAD [familial AD] and sporadic

AD (SAD) … Hence, with reference to the variable "Aβ deposition," control, "pure" DLB, DLB/AD, and "pure" AD cases appear to form a continuum with no abrupt boundaries between the groups of cases.

([251], p. 208)

The author's impression is that neurological nosology with regard to the time-passing-related brain changes popularly labeled "neurodegenerative diseases" is in the midst of a promising but incomplete transition. The 20th-century nosology is rapidly being replaced by a baroquely convoluted schemata, in which the utility of markers for defining "disease" is under debate: molecular biology is sometimes clarifying circumstances in which two patients might be said to have the same problem or a different problem, but sometimes *not*. As shown in Table 11.4 from a recent article by Kovacs [78], a distinction can be drawn between molecular features "currently used for subtyping disease" versus those that are "specific but not (yet) crucial for subtyping." Readers may reasonably ask whether that word "specific" is ideal, in view of the evidence that many patients (such as Chani) exhibit a mix of molecular features (Table 11.4).

Table 11.4 Molecular pathological features that are currently considered for subtyping and those which are disease-specific but not yet implemented for classifications

Disease	Molecular pathological features	
Disease group	**Currently used for subtyping**	**Disease-specific but not (yet) crucial for subtyping**
Alzheimer's disease-related pathology	Anatomical distribution of neuronal tau pathology	Truncated Aβ species
	Anatomical distribution of extracellular Aβ deposits	Pyroglutamate modifications
	Presence and distribution of CAA	Phosphorylation patterns of Aβ and tau
		Subtyping based on predominance of NFT
Prion disease	Morphology of PrP deposition	Oligomer forms
	Glycosylation pattern and electrophoretic mobility of PK-resistant PrP (only WB)	/
	Codon 129 polymorphism	/
	Etiology if known	/
Tauopathies	Morphology of neuronal or glial protein deposits	Detecting phosphorylation epitopes
	Distinguishing 3R and 4R isoforms	Acetylation
	Anatomical distribution of protein deposits	Truncated forms (i.e., C-terminal)
		Trypsin-resistant band patterns
		Oligomer forms
α-Synucleinopathies	Morphology of neuronal or glial protein deposits	Phosphorylation
	Anatomical distribution of protein deposits	Nitration
		Oligomer forms
		Predominance of soluble/insoluble form
		Truncated forms
		Detection of PK-resistant form[a]
TDP-43 proteinopathies	Morphology and subcellular distribution of protein deposits in neurons	Phosphorylation
	Anatomical distribution of protein deposits	C-terminal fragments
		Glial inclusions
FUS proteinopathies	Morphology, subcellular and anatomical distribution of protein deposits	Different immunoreactivity for FET proteins
		Glial inclusions

[a] Depends also on the method (i.e., immunohistochemistry or paraffin-embedded-tissue (PET)-blot method).

CAA: cerebral amyloid angiopathy; FET: FET proteins, a collective name for fused-in sarcoma protein (FUS), Ewing's sarcoma RNA-binding protein 1 (EWSR1), and TATA-binding protein-associated factor 15 (TAF15); NFT: neurofibrillary tangle; PK: proteinase K; PrP: prion protein; WB: Western blot.
Source: Kovacs, 2016 [78]

Readers might conceivably profit by awareness of that which seems to have become the state of the art, as illustrated by the elaborate algorithm shown in Figure 11.12. It is the product of an immense and serious scholarly effort. At the same time, Kovacs's admission that we literally do not know whether given molecular markers do or do not discriminate between "diseases" is a critical step in overthrowing the simplistic classification scheme that has slowed research on the late effects of concussion. What good are molecules for labeling species of human distress? To the general frustration and grumpy dismay of neuroscience, none of Aβ, p-tau, α-synuclein, or TDP-43, or even prion protein distinguishes any disease! One can only repeat the main point: until there exists a scientifically defensible way to discuss the infinite variability of human time-passing-related brain changes, research on the late effects of concussion will be confounded by possibly fruitless efforts to force cases into arbitrary pigeon holes. In the present author's opinion, in the face of uncertainty it is far more virtuous to say: "These are the biological phenomena we can currently detect," rather than "He's got disease *X*."

The resistance to the notion of human heterogeneity, the insistence that there is only one normal trajectory of brain change with time and any other trajectory is disease, does not stand up to logical scrutiny. It is tough to get physicians – who want and need cognitive closure and red lines delineating health from disease – to reconsider the popular (but unstable) nosologies. Yet the fact is indisputable: if a person survives beyond middle adulthood, his or her brain deteriorates, a lot, in many different ways. Consider

Algorithm for the classification of neurodegenerative proteinopathies

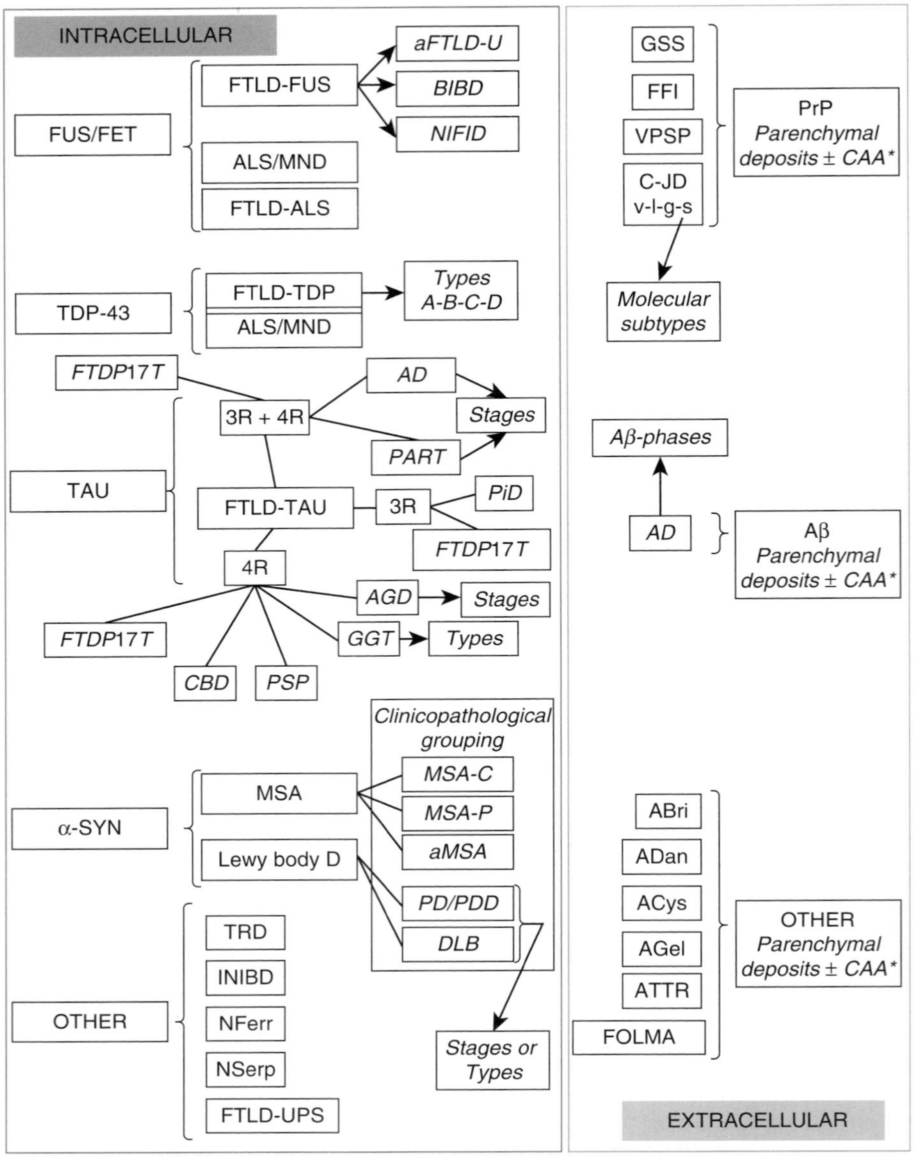

Fig. 11.12 Abri and ADan: amyloidoses related to familial British dementia and familial Danish dementia; ACys: amyloidosis related to cystatin C amyloid; AD: Alzheimer disease; AGD: argyrophilic grain disease; AGel: amyloidosis related to gelsolin amyloid; ALS: amyotrophic lateral sclerosis; ATTR: amyloidosis associated with transthyretin amyloid; BIBD: basophilic inclusion body disease; CAA: sporadic cerebral amyloid angiopathy; CBD: corticobasal degeneration; CJD: Creutzfeldt–Jakob disease; DLB: dementia with Lewy bodies; FTDP-17T: frontotemporal dementia and parkinsonism linked to chromosome 17 caused by mutations in the MAPT (tau) gene; FFI: fatal familial insomnia; FOLMA: familial oculoleptomeningeal amyloidosis; FTLD: frontotemporal lobar degeneration; aFTLD-U: atypical FTLD with ubiquitinated inclusions; FTLD-UPS: FTLD with inclusions immunoreactive only for the components of the ubiquitine proteasome system; GGT: globular glial tauopathies; GSS: Gerstmann–Sträussler–Scheinker disease; INIBD: intranuclear inclusion body diseases; MND: motor neuron disease; MSA: multiple system atrophy (C: cerebellar, P: parkinsonism, aMSA: atypical MSA); NFerr: neuroferritinopathy; NIFID: neurofilament intermediate filament inclusion disease; NSerp: neuroserpinopathy; PART: primary age-related tauopathy; PD: Parkinson disease; PDD: PD with dementia; PiD: Pick disease; PSP: progressive supranuclear palsy; TRD: trinucleotide repeat expansion disorder: refers to genetic disorder and associated with different proteins; VPSP: variably proteinase-sensitive prionopathy. For CJD, v: variant, s: sporadic, i: iatrogenic, and g: genetic. Kuru is not indicated in this figure. Note that overlap between FTLD-TDP and ALS/MND indicates combined phenotypes (FTLD-ALS/MND). *PrP-CAA is very rare; for Aβ, CAA is frequent, for other amyloidoses, CAA is more frequent than parenchymal deposits. Note that FTLD-ni is not indicated here, since no proteinopathy is associated with it. + indicates with or without. Green- and blue-colored box indicates intra-, or extracellular proteins; gray box indicates clinical and/or pathological subtypes; arrows point to subtyping based on pathological aspects.

Source: Kovacs, 2016 [78]. Reproduced under the terms of the Creative Commons Attribution licence, CC-BY 4.0

Figure 11.13. This illustrates the normal (healthy?), expected life history of the human entorhinal cortex.

Readers over age 50 may glance at that figure and pause in thought. Yet the dramatic, expected, normal deterioration of the human brain after age 25, and especially after age 50, is altogether compatible with successful life in the ancestral environment, when few survived to that extremity of senescence. Fjell et al. [250] summarized their inference from the data:

The life history of the thickness of the normal human entorhinal cortex

Annual entorhinal decline

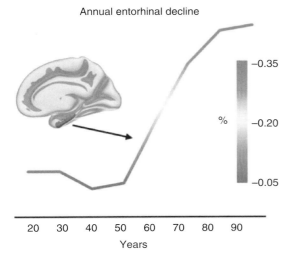

Fig. 11.13 Accelerated entorhinal decline in aging: Cross-sectional estimates of the annual rate of cortical thinning in the entorhinal cortex across the adult life indicate a marked increase in atrophy from 50 years. Age-related acceleration of decline in elderly has been confirmed with longitudinal data. [A black and white version of this figure will appear in some formats. For the color version, please refer to the plate section.]
Source: Fjell et al., 2014 [250] with permission from Elsevier

We suggest that regions characterized by a high degree of lifelong plasticity are vulnerable to detrimental effects of normal aging, and that this age-vulnerability renders them more susceptible to additional, pathological AD-related changes. We conclude that it will be difficult to understand AD without understanding why it preferably affects older brains, and that we need a model that accounts for age-related changes in AD-vulnerable regions independently of AD-pathology.

([250], p. 1)

That is, late-life dementia is probably the result of a grand evolutionary bargain. Build a brain that can change in response to experience and you build a brain that will erode. Expressed another way: the most potent and reliable risk factor for developing one of the various "Alzheimer's diseases" (or one of the other "neurodegenerative diseases") is continuing to live. One defers to semanticists to differentiate between "aging caused these brain changes" and "aging caused these brain changes by making the brain vulnerable to them."

Further defense of the "disease" paradigm of time-passing-related brain change seems imprudent. A less biased approach is needed. In a recent and perhaps visionary paper, Jack et al. [252] recommend that the interpretation of biomarkers associated with "aging" or "Alzheimer's disease" dismisses both labels, remains agnostic to the temporal and causal sequence, and simply documents observations with rigor. While Jack et al. focused on a limited number of molecular suspects, the present author would urge a dramatic expansion. Cut a brain. Please do not desecrate the chart with a two-word diagnosis. Simply report measures of microvascular changes (e.g., lipohyalinosis, foamy macrophages, advanced glycation end products, blood–brain

barrier changes), inflammatory changes, neuroimmunological changes, myelin changes, oxidative changes, insulin signaling changes, glymphatic changes, neurogenesis, gene expression changes, mutations, histone modifications, as well as a host of so-called "ND" phenomena such as prion proteins, α-synuclein, transthyretin, autophagic vacuoles. (Soon, perhaps we will graduate from fussy accounting of these puzzle pieces to systems assessment, such as measures of the connectome [187, 253, 254].) All are *time-passing-related brain changes*. They will remain so no matter how long pathologists bump shoulders while trying to sort them into little black boxes called "aging" versus "ND."

A Quick Summary of the Doubts About the Existence of "Alzheimer's Disease"

Universally accepted neuropathological criteria for differentiating Alzheimer's disease from healthy brain aging do not exist.

(McKeel et al., 2004 [208], p. 1028)

According to one popular 20th-century nosology, "Alzheimer's disease" is a neurodegenerative disorder that is qualitatively distinct both from normal aging and from other neurodegenerative conditions, such as Parkinson's disease, frontotemporal lobar dementia, or vascular dementia [207, 255–257]. According to the most recent iteration in a series of periodic attempts at rehabilitation, three biologically related diagnoses comprise the Alzheimer's spectrum: "Alzheimer's disease," "mild cognitive impairment," and "pre-clinical Alzheimer's disease" [258, 259]. Recently, however, serious doubts have been raised regarding the validity of this classification and, more importantly, regarding the 1980s paradigm of Alzheimer's disease as a unitary disorder whether it is seen among middle-aged or elderly persons, caused by "lesions" referred to as amyloid-associated senile plaques and tau-associated neurofibrillary tangles. Factors that make this logically and biologically implausible include: (1) the failure to identify any phenomenon that categorically distinguishes "Alzheimer's disease" from aging [260–263]; (2) the artificial imposition of discrete "stages" on a continuous process (e.g., the concern expressed by Burns and Bennett [264] regarding "what is obscured when a categorical construct such as mild cognitive impairment (MCI) is applied to what is clearly a continuous process – the gradual progression of MCI to dementia" (p. 1646)); (3) the evidence that, whatever role Aβ plaques play in time-passing-related brain change, they are not reliable measures of degenerative change and not reliable predictors of clinical dementia [227–236]; (4) the overlapping evidence that neither classic "lesions" nor clumps of atypically folded proteins cause any cognitive loss or "ND" (senile plaques and neurofibrillary tangles seem to have roughly the same significance – and are just as harmful – as broken, rusted spears lying half-buried on a battlefield) [214, 235, 264, 265]; (5) the discovery that many of the 21 genetic variants that increase the risk of Alzheimer's disease so far identified via genome-wide association studies have no apparent links to Aβ metabolism

[267–269]. Indeed, multiple non-amyloid pathways to Alzheimer's disease have been discovered involving genes that impact inflammatory functions, cytoskeletal functions, cholesterol metabolism, synaptic membrane integrity, and the immune system – all suggesting that Aβ is not only *insufficient* to cause Alzheimer's disease but perhaps *unnecessary* as well [270, 271]; (6) the overlap between many supposedly unique and dissociable "neurodegenerative diseases" associated with dysfunctional, atypically folded, or aggregated proteins – including β-amyloid, α-synuclein, ubiquitin, cellular prion protein (PrP^C), phosphorylation-dependent transactive response DNA-binding protein 43 (p-TDP-43), neprilysin, and p-tau [272–275]; (7) the evidence that progression may depend less on "lesion" or protein counts than on genetically variant neuroinflammation and immunomodulation [140, 276–278]; (8) the evidence of a causal role of defective insulin signaling and metabolic syndrome [279–281]; and (9) the significant overlap and coincidence of "Alzheimer's disease" (and other supposed forms of ND) with cerebrovascular disease, and evidence that vascular changes in "Alzheimer's disease" correlate better with clinical presentation than do protein deposits; evidence that vascular disease contributes to dementia in a significant number of cases previously diagnosed as "familial Alzheimer's disease"; and evidence that vascular change is currently the most important modifiable risk factor for "Alzheimer's disease" [282–287].

The essay by Whitehouse et al. [261] titled "Describing the dying days of 'Alzheimer's disease'" is a pithy admonition at this historic moment of open-minded reflection:

> Unfortunately, the emperor is not wearing any clothes – and on top of that, he is looking quite feeble and out of shape … We must look beyond the molecular paradigm and understand AD as a multifaceted condition intimately related to aging … what we now call "AD" is in fact a heterogeneous, age-related condition, and that our current disease classifications are as much social markers as they are biological.
>
> ([261], p. 12)

The present-day reconsideration of both neurodegenerative and psychiatric nosology represents a major conundrum for the modern scholar hoping to derive lessons from meticulously reviewing older literature. The weight of the evidence discrediting the 1980s unitary disease hypothesis compels an ethical disclaimer regarding the quality of the data. What can one learn from data collected under the frail assumption that "Alzheimer's disease" is a valid and diagnosable human problem? One lesson is simple: sometimes seeing new little things identifies a natural kind, sometimes not. For example, the tubercle bacillus identified the cause of tuberculosis. Trisomy 21 identified the cause of Down's syndrome. But very few molecules, by themselves, define a disease. Compare the parsimonious phrases that define those two disorders with the tortured paragraph-length algorithms proposed to define "Alzheimer's disease." In the overwhelming majority of cases of time-passing-related brain change, seeing new little things does not nail down a natural kind. A touching faith in "unfamiliar little things are the cause" helps

explain neurology's embarrassing perseveration in the defense of "Alzheimer's disease."

The author acknowledges that the phrase "Alzheimer's disease" remains popular in some circles. Even a few 21st-century journals still accept papers that use it! History will record that many persons of good will and intellectual vitality spent decades in search of a biologically coherent natural kind of Alzheimer's disease. One must honor that effort. It has failed. A hundred years of debate have led to more debate. Laboratory *tours de force* have revealed results that belie the soothing, dogmatic "it's a specific disease!" paradigm.

This is not the time to bemoan the burial of "Alzheimer's disease" as a concept and regret the years wasted trying to pound the round pegs of real-life polypathology into the square holes of yearned-for unity. The time has come to shrug off past errors, sigh with immense relief at the corrected direction of global scientific energy, and revel in the emerging hopes for effective prevention and intervention. One must trust the intentions of investigators who conducted research before the doubts about the existence of "Alzheimer's disease" became inescapable. However, one cannot, in good conscience, recommend any historical works that claim to have determined whether concussion has late effects by testing the hypothesis that a history of CBI is a risk factor for a biologically undefined entity called "Alzheimer's disease."

What is Chronic Traumatic Encephalopathy? Common Sense Rescues Nosology from Terms of Art

Or: *The CTE of Martland, Parker, and Critchley* Does Not Equal *the Tauopathy of Corsellis, Hof, and Geddes.*

> Although generally accepted as a distinct entity, DP [dementia pugilistica] has been controversial since its original description, with absence of prospective data, surprisingly few studies with autopsy correlation, and lack of accounting for comorbidities such as substance abuse, infection, and vascular or neurodegenerative disease.
>
> [288]

> A consensus panel of 7 neuropathologists … described the pathognomonic lesion of CTE as an accumulation of abnormal tau in neurons and astroglia distributed perivascularly at the depths of sulci in the isocortex in an irregular pattern.
>
> McKee et al., 2016 [289]

When Parker introduced the phrase "traumatic encephalopathy" in 1934, he was describing a *clinical* problem suffered by boxers in which repetitive trauma apparently led to a slow "development of disability *during their career*" (emphasis added) [290]. Parker, therefore, was describing an entirely different phenomenon from the so-called brain change labeled "CTE" that has recently become a popular preoccupation for journalists, attorneys, and even some reputable neuropathologists. Parker's cases were living and active, aged 24, 30, and 28. As Parker confessed, "the exact pathological mechanism of these cases is to date unknown" [290]. Still, if a man becomes demented in his 20s and is known to have suffered many blows to the head, unless there is also a history of a co-morbid problem such as child abuse, alcoholism, or neurosyphilis, it is common sense to infer, as did Parker, that his neurological troubles were due to his head traumas. Yes, brain aging (better called species-specific time-passing-related brain change in compliance with an evolved life history plan) is already under way in the 24-year-old. But its influence is small and hard to detect. For that reason, the neurologist attending the 24-year-old boxer is not faced with the conundrum that faces us today: diagnosing single diseases becomes hard to justify when co-morbidities are expected [291]. For instance, when we cut 75-year-old forgetful Chani's brain (a victim of a single CBI) – or the brain of a 63-year-old, sad, angry, retired football player (a victim of repetitive CBIs) – which of the 217,121 Aβ plaques and 166,303 neurofibrillary tangles should be labeled, "due to head trauma," which labeled "due to commonplace time-passing-related brain change," which "due to stress," which "due to insulin resistance," which "due to excess inflammation," which "due to air pollution," which "due to depression"? Using tweezers, can we sort them into piles?

Readers may have paused when, early in this chapter, the author typed the phrase "chronic traumatic encephalopathy" in quotation marks – implying that some doubt exists about the present-day use of this string of words. This is the reason: the contemporary use of that phrase bears little resemblance to its meaning. At the risk of shocking the reader (and certainly those who have embraced a recently popularized nosology), one urges that we step back a pace from terms of art promoted by disciplinary special-interest groups and ask the question: "In English, what does CTE mean?"

The answer is self-evident and should be embraced with the artless endearment one extends to a long-lost friend. A patient who has suffered TBI and who, as a result, exhibits persistent brain dysfunction impacting life function has CTE. Example: a healthy five-year-old child falls from a swing, bumps his head, and loses consciousness for 30 minutes. Imaging confirms axonal changes. He is still behind in school at age nine. Unless a better etiology is found (such as daily carbon monoxide poisoning), that is obviously CTE.

In the light of that simple, straightforward, theoretically agnostic, semantically robust conceptualization, the cases recently published as "CTE" appear to represent a mix:

- *A few* are very sensibly called CTE because the best explanation for all the behavioral symptoms and brain abnormalities is TBI. Whether the insult was a single TBI or repetitive CBIs, a person with traumatically induced persistent brain change affecting behavior has CTE. (This is most readily detected in a young person, since there are not 12 types of brain change to contend with.)
- *Most* of the cases recently labeled "CTE" are actually cases of polypathology. Dying in mid or late life, after having been exposed to TBI and to who knows how many more dementing brain threats (e.g., hypertension, diabetes,

vascular disease, stress, depression, toxins) as well as to time-passing-related brain change, such people's brains almost always exhibit multiple types of abnormalities. Their neurobehavioral symptoms cannot reasonably be attributed solely to TBI.

The myth: repetitive CBI causes dementia associated with a unique tauopathy. One might call that particular tauopathy "CTE pathology" (or perhaps, for enhanced mellifluity, "McKee's disease").

The truth: repetitive CBI is a risk factor for early and late effects. In about one-third of those exposed to sports-related repetitive CBI, that exposure is associated with a variety of clinical problems and some tauopathy. That tauopathy should not be called "CTE pathology" because it also occurs without trauma. Sometimes, clinical problems occur *early* in life near the time of exposure. In such early-onset cases, a tauopathy is sometimes found as the sole pathological change. Other times, clinical problems begin later in life, even decades after the exposure ends. In late-onset cases, a tauopathy is not usually found to be the sole pathological change. It is usually just one element of polypathology.

What is the Independent Variable?

Before providing the scientific basis for these conclusions, a brief but important digression is required. If funding eventually appears, a rigorous effort will finally begin to determine the relationship between repetitive sports-related TBIs and late effects. At that time, investigators will need to agree on the independent (presumably causal) variable. What suspect environmental exposure is worth studying? Remembered number of concussions [292, 293]? Remembered concussions with loss of consciousness [294, 295]? Trainer-documented concussions [296]? Physician-documented concussions [297]? Concussions above a given accelerometer threshold [298]? Concussions repeated within a given temporal window of vulnerability [299, 300]? Age of first exposure [301, 302]? Duration of exposure in years, or seasons, or games [303]? Estimated total lifetime hours of participation [304]? We must do better than some recent reports that quantify the critical independent variable as "multiple past concussions."

Choosing a neuroscientifically justifiable independent variable is crucial for several reasons, not least of which is figuring out what to prevent. If the risky environmental exposure associated with late effects is: (1) the total number of typical concussions of the sort provoking clinical attention, then those should be prevented in so far as possible. But if the risky exposure associated with later mental disability is, instead, (2) the number of times concussions were repeated within one month, or (3) the number of knockouts before the completion of dorsolateral prefrontal cortex myelinization, or (4) the lifetime number of head impacts involving any degree of brain rattling, independent of the victim's awareness of an injury, symptoms, or care – that is a completely different prevention target and a completely different public health campaign will be inspired. In fact, some recent evidence suggests that, to account for the late effects of contact sports, *typical diagnosed concussions may not matter.*

Please recall that the semantically straightforward meaning of CBI is brain rattling due to an abrupt external force. In sports, many brain rattlings do not cause symptoms, do not trigger clinical attention, and are never labeled "concussions." The popular slang for such impacts is "subconcussions." But, as previously explained in this volume, subconcussion is a misleading colloquialism since every so-called "subconcussion" is, in fact, *a brain-rattling concussive impact.*[28] New data will make it clear why this fine linguistic point is important.

Montenigro et al. [306] recently published an alternative metric. Those authors employed a sophisticated quantitative approach to generate an individual severity–weight estimate of cumulative head impact – calculated from self-report of participation among persons who played football in the past and "a measure of estimated head impacts received per season, based on data from published helmet accelerometer studies that report the frequency of head impacts per season by position and level of play" (p. 330). Those authors called their measure the "cumulative head impact index (CHII)." Ninety-three middle-aged persons were recruited who had played high school or college football an average of 26 years before. (Note that these were not "patients" or persons seeking medical help. This was a study of mental effects in volunteering former players, not a test of any hypothesis about "dementia" or "CTE.")

The average number of head impacts was 545 per season for an average of 11 seasons, or 5806 total head impacts. That number, of course, vastly exceeded the average career total of "concussions," which was 20. Subjects were assessed for current cognition, depression, apathy, and behavioral dysregulation. Importantly, late mental effects were better predicted by head impacts than by "concussions." Moreover, the results for each behavioral outcome showed an intriguing and consistent pattern: up to a certain threshold there was no clear correlation between exposure and mental health. Yet above that threshold, which was different for each behavior, the correlation was approximately linear. In other words, the dose–response curves all had an inflection point – an amount of brain rattling beyond which impairment was not only likely but proportionate to exposure. The schematic graph shown in Figure 11.14 illustrates this provocative finding.

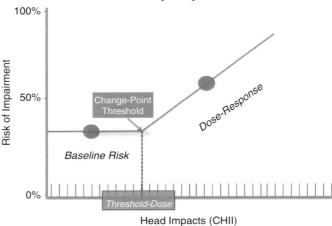

Fig. 11.14 Schematic of the dose–response model with a constant baseline risk of later-life impairment (baseline gradient of slope = 0) below the cumulative head impact threshold dose and with increasing probability of impairment (dose–response gradient of slope > 0) above that threshold dose. CHII: cumulative head impact index.

Source: Montenigro et al., 2017 [306]. Reproduced with permission from Mary Ann Liebert, Inc.

Different impact exposure was required to reach the threshold. Depression required a CHII of 1801. Behavioral dysregulation required 2216. In marked contrast, the threshold for impairment on the Brief Test of Adult cognition was a CHII of 7251.

Until the study by Montenigro et al. is replicated, one must be cautious about its dramatic implications. However, should these data hold up, the finding that one must suffer many thousands of head impacts before that number starts to correlate with impaired cognition suggests that (1) cognition is remarkably resilient in the face of repetitive brain rattling, or that (2) the study was done too soon to detect the awful interactions that perhaps occur between repetitive CBI and time-passing-related brain change, or (3) we are bad at detecting cognitive loss, or (4) all of the above. The finding that emotional dysregulation or disability begins to correlate with exposure at much more modest levels is compatible with the evidence cited earlier in this volume that it is non-cognitive psychiatric problems, not paper-and-pencil-measured cognition, that dominate the clinical disablement of concussed persons. Most important: the finding that asymptomatic brain rattlings (sometimes misleadingly called *subconcussions*) are more predictive than concussions for

---

[28] It is logical to presume that, for every human, there exists some lower limit of external force that must be exceeded for an impact to be risky. One source estimates that force to be 14.4 **g**, as recorded by at least one football helmet accelerometer [298, 305]. At such a modest force, there are no symptoms, yet cognitive and electrophysiological measures suggest an effect. Regarding the discovery that "subconcussive" blows may be harmful, the authors admonished, "These individuals are unlikely to undergo clinical evaluation, and thus may continue to participate in football-related activities, even when changes in brain physiology (and potential brain damage) are present, which will increase the risk of future neurological injury" ([298], p. 327). The present author respectfully disagrees, on principle, with this published measure. It is based on acutely detectable change. The important consequence is not change acutely detectable with today's crude methods, but deleterious life effects.

mental health 26 years after football suggests that we may have been barking up the wrong tree.

What if, for all the frenzied recent discussion of sports-related "concussions," we have overlooked a more important risk? This is another potentially paradigm-shifting discovery: the environmental exposure most closely linked to disabling late effects may not be the injuries that send the athlete to the sideline, but the injuries that don't.

In the light of these findings, for the remainder of this chapter, please understand that the phrase "repetitive concussive brain injuries" refers to the full gamut of brain rattlings due to arrival of abrupt external force. That approach is not only faithful to the simple mechanical definition of concussion we developed in the first chapter, but also respectful of the growing suspicion that brain rattlings, even little ones, may be harmful.

The Birth Pangs of Today's Idiosyncratic Use of the Self-Explanatory Phrase "Chronic Traumatic Encephalopathy"

As summarized in the chapter titled *Traumatic Encephalopathy: Review and Provisional Research Diagnostic Criteria* (Chapter 14), the early contributions to the development of the modern concept of CTE were like Parker's: clinical observations without neuropathological correlation. In 1928 Martland [307] published remarks describing a "parkinsonian syndrome [with] … marked mental deterioration" that appeared in some boxers. He called the syndrome "Punch Drunk." There occurred a two-generation detour during which the more-buttoned-down Latin phrase, *dementia pugilistica* held sway. However, when it became obvious that this condition was not unique to boxers (and also not unique to sports-related concussion), a new terminology gained ground. The first use of *chronic traumatic encephalopathy* seems to have been in an obscure 1942 textbook, but tradition gives primacy to Critchley's 1949 chapter "Punch-drunk syndromes: the chronic traumatic encephalopathy of boxers" [308].

What would be the most commonsense name for the diverse spectrum of chronic clinical encephalopathies so eloquently described by Martland, Parker, and Critchley? How about *"Martland, Parker, and Critchley-type chronic traumatic encephalopathy"*?

Brandenburg and Hallervorden perhaps published the first relevant autopsy findings in 1954 [309]. Yet it was decades before a trickle of publications reported series of cases with post-mortem results, launching the debate that persists to the time of this writing. Does repetitive concussion cause (or serve as a risk factor for) a unique traumatic encephalopathy? Or does it increase the risk of conventionally defined neurodegenerative diseases such as "Alzheimer's disease" and Parkinson's? Or both? And, if there is a special traumatic form of brain degeneration, can a single blow ever trigger that process?

In 1973, Corsellis et al. [310] published their seminal account of neuropathological changes associated with 15 cases of purported "dementia pugilistica." Those authors made multiple errors. First, some of their cases were not clinically impaired; that is, there was no dementia. Second, six of their cases had histories of heavy alcohol abuse and the brain changes could not, in good faith, be attributed solely to boxing. Third, many of their cases exhibited substantial cerebrovascular disease. Fourth, their investigations were incomplete (even by the standards Alzheimer observed in 1907): due to methodological limitations, they could visualize tau tangles but not Aβ plaques. Unfortunately, they concluded that CTE, unlike "Alzheimer's disease," is a disorder of tau. In addition, they neglected to report that these brains were rife with cerebrovascular damage. One wonders to what degree Corsellis et al.'s odd paper is responsible for the persistence of the simplistic claim that CTE is a tauopathy.

In 1990, Roberts et al. [193] published a helpful correction: they obtained the same brain tissue from the same cases that Corsellis et al. had examined, but employed more advanced immunostaining. In addition to revealing that "The cases used in this study showed evidence of significant vascular damage" (p. 377), those authors summarized their findings with regard to amyloid, directly contradicting Corsellis et al.:

> all DP cases with substantial tangle formation showed evidence of extensive β-protein immunoreactive deposits (plaques). The degree of β-protein deposition was comparable to that seen in AD. Our data indicate that the present neuropathological description of DP (tangles but no plaques) should be altered to acknowledge the presence of substantial β protein deposition (plaques).
>
> ([193], p. 373)

Hof et al. published the next classic report in 1991 [311], adding a twist. Three dementia pugilistica cases were examined and compared with eight "Alzheimer's disease" cases. Just one of the three dementia pugilistica cases reportedly exhibited Aβ deposits, and the amyloid plaques were characterized as lacking a core with neuropil threads (a plaque type sometimes called *diffuse* as opposed to *neuritic*). Like Corsellis, these authors emphasized the abundance of tau tangles. But, like Roberts, Hof et al. made a good-faith effort to hunt for amyloid (with not only two conventional stains but also an anti-Aβ antibody). They found little. What impressed them most was that the tau tangles in all their dementia pugilistica cases sat in the superficial cortical layers (II and III), which was dramatically different from the widespread tangles in the deep cortical layers in the "Alzheimer's disease" cases. Three cases? The paper did not settle anything.

Nor did the next batter up. Based on a single case, in 1996 Geddes et al. [312] opined that CTE involved tau but not Aβ. In 1999 [313], those authors expanded their total research to five cases. "Pathological findings in all five cases were of neocortical neurofibrillary tangles (NFTs) and neuropil threads, with groups of tangles consistently situated around blood vessels in the worst affected regions. No Abeta immunoreactivity was detected."

What would be the most commonsense name for the type of tauopathy described by Corsellis, Hof, and Geddes? How about "*Corsellis, Hof, and Geddes-type tauopathy*"?[29]

A major current problem of classification of late effects of concussion can be boiled down to a few simple facts that the author hopes to demonstrate in the next several pages: Corsellis, Hof, and Geddes-type tauopathy (C/H/G tauopathy) does *not* usually occur after exposure to repetitive CBIs. C/H/G tauopathy is *not* the only brain change seen after exposure to rCBIs. C/H/G tauopathy is *not* an indicator of exposure to repetitive CBIs. C/H/G tauopathy is *not* the most common brain change associated with the clinical condition, CTE. In fact, exposure to repetitive CBIs is *not* a common cause of CTE. Most cases of the clinical condition CTE (meaning persistent neurobehavioral problems after TBI) have nothing to do with C/H/G tauopathy. However, a discovery worthy of note is that one unusual clinical subtype of CTE – the Martland, Parker, and Critchley type that sometimes occurs after exposure to repetitive CBIs – is *sometimes* associated with the microscopic findings reported by Corsellis, Hof, and Geddes.

It is hardly the author's intention to review the data in depth. Based on more than 150 published cases of ostensible "CTE" [314], contemporary neuropathologists have hugely advanced the field. Their clinical reports typically lack sufficient information about each injury, or any report of signs and symptoms at the time of and between each injury, to support genuine clinicopathological correlation. That will soon improve with the initiation of widespread pre-exposure and post-traumatic assessments of student and professional athletes. And the microscopic observations are superb and compelling – accepting the limits of today's optical methods.

A Failure to Distinguish Brain Changes Among the Young From Those Among the Old Helps Explain the Failure to Recognize the Fallacy of Equating CTE with Tauopathy

Here the author must, with apologies, impose a categorical distinction on a dimensional measure: as discussed early in this chapter, there exist young people and older people. One admittedly arbitrary way to categorize the dimension of age: young people have yet to reach somatic "maturity" of the sort characterized by the completion of brain myelination at about age 25. Among those youth, selective pressures seem to have discouraged the type of universal, species-specific, time-passing-related brain changes that some doctors elect to call "ND." Older people are those whose brains are completely myelinated and who (due to the diminishing return of selection) have begun to exhibit normal, universal, and disreputable time-passing-related brain changes.

Among the young, a few may develop one relatively discrete and readily identifiable clinical problem, and the pathologist will occasionally encounter one predominant type of atypical change in the brain (for example, the child who becomes deaf and is found to have an acoustic neuroma). Under those circumstances, clinicopathological correlation seems reasonable: it makes sense to attribute a recent and dramatic functional change to a recent and dramatic single atypical brain finding.

Now consider a hypothetical case: an 18–24-year-old athlete suffers many concussions (repetitive CBIs) and *promptly* became persistently demented. If no alternative cause existed, simple English would dictate his clinical diagnosis: like the child who suffered one severe TBI at age five and is still behind in school at age nine, the athlete now has *CTE*. Imagine that our hypothetical teen/young adult athlete died at age 25. One possibility is that the pathologist might find the rather unusual changes described by Corsellis, Hof, and Geddes: excessive deposits of tau (now known to be hyperphosphorylated, or p-tau) characteristically distributed in the depths of the neocortical sulci. In such an extraordinary case – rarely discovered, simply because death before post-age-25 "ND" is rare – it would seem entirely logical and scientific to say: "This is a case of the CTE as described by Martland, Parker, and Critchley. It was probably caused by the tauopathy described by Corsellis, Hof, and Geddes."

Such cases are not merely hypothetical. They are rare, real, and terrible.

Michael Keck began playing tackle football at age six [315]. Michael played throughout high school and he kept playing in college, even after his tenth concussion, an especially violent hit when he was a freshman at the University of Missouri. He reportedly developed headaches, blurred vision, sleep difficulty, and tinnitus. He played only one more game as a sophomore.

Michael's grades plummeted and he withdrew from college without graduating. He subsequently became reclusive, forgetful, and then abusive toward his wife. Having heard about the bad effects of concussions, they sought neuropsychological testing. Findings included impairment of verbal learning, and memory, and attention/executive functions. Unless some other unusual causes were discovered (e.g., cysticercosis), we already know he has a clinical problem: CTE of the Martland, Parker, Critchley type.

Michael died of unrelated causes at age 25. Figure 11.15 shows his brain.

If there still exist any doubters that concussions can cause long-term behavior dysfunction and brain change, Michael's case should put those doubts to rest. If there are any doubters that repetitive CBIs are sometimes followed by a tauopathy, the same is true.

What can one conclude so far?

---

[29] Several recent publications employ the phrase "CTE pathology." The authors in every case seem to be referring to Corsellis, Hof, Geddes-type tauopathy (C/H/G tauopathy). Why make the distinction? The phrase "CTE pathology" assumes, without proof, that *only trauma can cause that type of tauopathy*. As discussed below, evidence raises doubts about that assumption. If more than one problem causes C/H/G tauopathy – if a variety of afflictions produce the same brain changes – calling it "CTE pathology" is as logical as calling a black eye "door pathology."

Neuropathological findings in a 25-year-old man with a history of encephalopathy after repetitive concussions

(A) Multiple perivascular ptau lesions at the sulcal depths

(B) Perivascular ptau neurofibrillary tangles, neurites, and astrocytes

(C) AT8-immunostained paraffin-embedded section

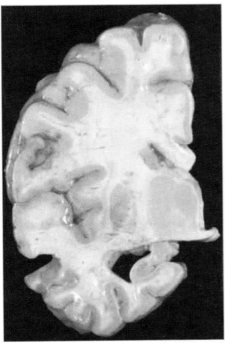 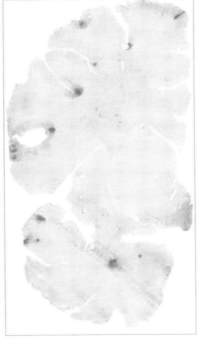 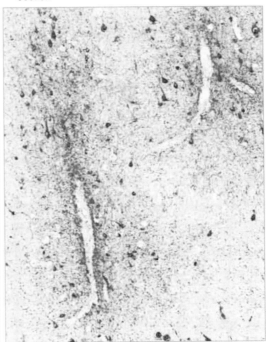

Fig. 11.15 (A) The brain showed mild ventricular dilation and hippocampal atrophy. Pathological lesions of hyperphosphorylated tau (p-tau) consisting of neurofibrillary tangles, neurites, and astrocytes around small blood vessels were found at the sulcal depths of the frontal and temporal lobes. Free-floating 50-μm section immunostained for AT8 (B) and paraffin-embedded 10-μm section immunostained for AT8 (C; original magnification × 200). These p-tau lesions are considered to be pathognomonic for chronic traumatic encephalopathy (CTE) based on the preliminary National Institute of Neurological Disorders and Stroke consensus criteria for the pathological diagnosis of CTE. Characteristic CTE p-tau pathology was also found in the parietal lobes, entorhinal cortex, anterior hippocampus, hypothalamus, nucleus basalis of Meynert, substantia nigra, locus coeruleus, and median raphe. There was no immunopositivity for amyloid-β, TAR DNA-binding protein 43, or α-synuclein. [A black and white version of this figure will appear in some formats. For the color version, please refer to the plate section.]
Source: Mez et al., 2016 [315]. Journal of the American Medical Association

1. Repetitive CBI sometimes causes a prompt and serious persistent encephalopathy.
2. A single TBI sometimes causes a prompt and serious persistent encephalopathy.

Both are CTEs. What is the difference? Possibly: clinical course and brain change. Regarding clinical course after repetitive CBIs, based on experience with multiple retired National Football League (NFL) football players, the author shares exactly the impressions gathered by Martland and Parker:

> It is thus possible that a pugilist may be only mildly affected, and may continue to fight to the end of his career, or he may be so disabled that he ultimately has to quit boxing and yet gets no worse in after life. Lastly, a progressive neurological syndrome may appear.
>
> (Parker, 1934 [290])

That is to say that the course following repetitive CBIs *varies* – and varies considerably. In his study of the historical cases [316], the present author found that the average delay between the end of the career and the onset of dementia was 15 years. But the average is potentially misleading because the range is so broad. Some victims develop a static encephalopathy during exposure, "yet gets no worse in after life." Some develop a progressive encephalopathy during exposure. Some develop a delayed-onset encephalopathy – the course of which also varies, although, in late life, progression is the rule if only because of the coincidence of "aging."[30] In contrast, the occurrence of a clearly progressive dementia following exposure to a single blow is rare and controversial.

The clinically defined CTE of Martland, Parker, and Critchley includes and conflates *all* these variants in course. In that respect, it is hard to countenance as a unitary entity. Why? Because in cases of prompt encephalopathy like that of Mr. Keck, occurring long before normal post-brain-maturity brain "aging," one can confidently attribute the new-onset symptoms entirely to the immediately precedent traumatic brain changes. In cases in which encephalopathy ensues *after* the polypathological assault of "aging" described in the

---

30 A recent report possibly helps to explain that variation in the age of onset of clinical encephalopathy after exposure to repetitive CBI. Alosco et al. reported [317] that, among 25 "autopsy confirmed" NFL football players with CTE, neurobehavioral disorders began later in those who had higher occupational achievement. This supports the cognitive reserve hypothesis.

introductory pages of this chapter, *one cannot plausibly attribute the new-onset symptoms entirely to the long-ago traumatic brain changes.* Therefore, it seems that Corsellis, Hof, and Geddes were on to something: there seems to exist a distinctive, specific pattern of brain change in a small subset of CTE cases that (1) follow exposure to repetitive CBIs and (2) undergo postmortem examination in young adulthood.

What happens to the value and integrity of that concept when a small cadre of modern scholars declares: "Whether the brain shows pure tauopathy at age 25 or a mix of seven pathologies *including* tauopathy at age 75, if the patient had concussions, and tau in the sulcal depths, it's the same disease"?

A Digression on Deviance

Unfortunately, some recently published research on "CTE" has deviated not only from its original concept as a clinical condition, but also from the very essence of clinico pathological correlation. In an embarrassment for neuroscience, very few of the brains that neuropathologists have retrospectively diagnosed with "CTE" in the last decade have been accompanied by meaningful clinical data. A recent publication demonstrates why such retrospective research on late effects of repetitive CBI is virtually certain to be misleading, and again, why using the four-letter word "mild" to label a subset of neurological patients is flirting with absurdity.

In 2017 the exceptional Boston University CBI research group [318] announced results from neuropathological examinations of 202 people who, in life, had reportedly played a mean of 15.1 years of football. Eighty-seven percent of the brains were judged to exhibit "chronic traumatic encephalopathy" – that is, light microscopic changes fulfilling the criteria proposed by McKee (and others) of the same research group and published as consensus criteria in 2016 [289]: "Neuropathological criteria for CTE require at least 1 perivascular ptau lesion consisting of ptau aggregates in neurons, astrocytes, and cell processes around a small blood vessel" ([318], p. 362).[31] Of interest, subjects pathologically diagnosed with "mild CTE" reportedly had about the same proportion of behavioral, mood, or cognitive symptoms (85–96%) as subjects diagnosed with "severe CTE" (89–95%). The difference occurred in the retrospective diagnoses of dementia: 33% among "mild" cases versus 85% among "severe" cases. If the data were reliable, one might infer that an intriguing and perhaps clinically important discovery had been made: cognitive impairment depends on the degree of allegedly pathognomonic "CTE" brain changes. Behavioral disorders, which are more disabling than cognitive disorders, do not.

Yet several issues make it very hard to interpret this study. As the authors readily acknowledge, this was a convenience sample. "Selection" amounted to accepting whatever brains became available when next of kin approached a brain bank near the time of death (81%), referred by a medical examiner (9%), recruited by a Concussion Legacy Foundation representative (6%), or when the subject participated in a Brain Donation Registry during life (4%). Thus, only 4% might have been assessed by the investigators before death, but no self-reported symptoms or clinical examinations were reported, even for that subgroup. "Clinical information" was gathered from "informants" not otherwise specified, either by telephone or via online questionnaires. One hopes that the informants were familiar with the subjects, but the degree of familiarity is not documented. Brains were included whether or not any "symptoms" had been observed during life. (Note: the term "symptoms" is used repeatedly by these authors, but they seem to be referring to signs observed by informants.) Dementia was diagnosed when clinicians who themselves had never met the subjects summarized the history and presented this as hearsay to other clinicians who had not even reviewed the informants' claims.

In fairness, retrospectively obtaining credible clinical information regarding unknown numbers of CBIs at unknown past moments in subjects with unknown pre-morbid and co-morbid disorders is impossible. Even the most sincere detective work might have failed to flesh out a critical minimal database. In essence, zero information was available with regard to pre-CBI exposure neuropsychiatric status. No reliable data describe the occurrence, multiplicity, symptoms, and duration of acute, subacute, or chronic effects of each CBI in any subject. The supposed temporal trajectory of the illness was recorded from the *post hoc* reconstructions from memories of inexpert observers with unknown access to the subject. The investigators did obtain some records regarding years of play. CBI exposure reported in this study, otherwise, largely represents guesswork.

The Boston scholars deserve tremendous credit for pursuing their research initiative in the face of outrageous pressure. Still, absent pre-morbid health assessments and clinical histories of each injury and the intervening periods, the new report cannot technically be called a "clinicopathological correlation study." Moreover, as a result of four almost inevitable limitations, one is obliged to be cautious about assuming a causal relationship between the sketchy concussion histories and the pathological findings. First, this convenience sample was pre-selected (by the player, the family or the investigators) for histories of especially abnormal neurobehavior. Therefore, for example, results from the 44 linemen cannot be regarded as representative of the effects of football on linemen. A different study might have assessed the clinical histories of a randomly selected population of linebackers, examined their brains, and determined whether any relationship existed between documented concussion exposure and any brain change.

Second, the study failed to compare the brains with those of age, sex, education, and socioeconomic status-matched men who had never played contact sports. It would have been informative if the investigators were to have obtained perhaps

---

[31] Readers will immediately see the fallacy of this approach. Should a person become demented due to six major pathophysiological factors, one of which was nine strokes, and he or she is found to have a single perivascular p-tau lesion, he or she could be diagnosed with McKee-type CTE.

three or more non-contact sport comparison subjects' clinical histories and brains for each player.

Third, no control seems to have been attempted for overlapping and co-occurring neurological conditions. No information is provided regarding pre-CBI exposure neuropsychiatric health, such as early-childhood illnesses, learning disabilities, psychiatric treatment, or early non-football TBIs. The results were not stratified according to age of first CBI exposure or years of exposure. Vascular disease risk factors were neither assessed nor reported. Thyroid functions were not tested. Family histories of dementia were not reported. Genetic predispositions to aging-related neurodegenerative diseases were not tested (in so far as currently possible). Adult psychiatric history, substance abuse history, and steroid exposure were not considered.

Fourth (a major theme of this chapter), looking for trauma-related disease in young brains and old brains with the same yardstick fails to consider time-passing-related brain change. These authors found more neurodegenerative change in 71-year-olds than in 44-year-olds. On that basis, they called the purportedly trauma-related disease in old folks more "severe." In what sense is it more severe disease when one waits an extra 30 years before examining the brain, and unsurprisingly finds more degenerative change? Perhaps a more agnostic characterization of these findings would be: "Among persons who were probably exposed to multiple CBIs (actual count unknown) with unknown symptoms, and unknown co-morbidities, those who are, on average, age 71 are more likely than those who are, on average, age 44 to exhibit brain changes of a type that seems to depend on the passing of time."

As a result of these four limitations, it is not possible to determine the likelihood that sport-related repetitive CBI was the primary factor in, or even a major contributor to, the most clinically relevant observed brain changes.

Moreover, "severity" was strictly based on autopsy findings. That leads to counter-intuitive consequences. For instance, among the 44 players who were diagnosed (based on p-tau) with "mild CTE," 12 (27%) reportedly committed suicide, whereas among 133 "severe CTE" cases just six (4.5%) committed suicide. Suicide may be the sole objective clinical fact considered in this study. Since the subjects could not be examined in life and the clinical profile was often derived from lay recollections, the occurrence of suicide may be one of this study's best-documented clinical facts. The rate of suicide was more than five times as high among subjects classified as "mild CTE" versus "severe CTE."[32] It appears that the disorder these investigators called "mild" is the disorder that is most likely to be behaviorally severe. Here, in a manner exactly opposite to that used in classifying TBI severity (e.g., the GCS), the authors imply, "One must not use mere human distress or risk of premature death to rank severity. Severity is judged by the pathologist." In another oddity, "mild CTE" was associated with

a median of 90 alleged concussions while "severe CTE" was associated with a median of 50.5. This seems inconsistent with a dose effect. However, without helmet telemetry and a better understanding of the post-concussive window of vulnerability, "dose" is an ephemeral concept.

Summarizing: the Boston group found that those who suffered almost twice as many concussions and were five times as likely to commit suicide (and died at about age 44 instead of age 71) apparently had a milder disorder. This seems counterintuitive.

Welcome to the state of the art, where non-representative subjects with unknown exposures to many potential causes of brain change and with sparse clinical data have been found to exhibit various brain changes. Proving what? That brain changes are common among the tiny cohort of former contact sport athletes who are either themselves motivated to provide their brains to the Boston group or whose family members are motivated to provide their brains to the Boston group. The observed brain changes are striking. Their discovery may be invaluable in deciphering aspects of concussive pathophysiology. We must, however, defer judgment about the magnitude of the risk of neurodegeneration posed by a given history of concussions in a person with a given genome.

The combined effect of these limitations is that this relatively large, labor-intensive study fails to provide information regarding our nagging questions: who is vulnerable to late effects and what pathophysiological sequence causes them? If any of the clinical data in this study (apart from suicide) were reliable, one might be able to derive some conclusions regarding the statistical (not causal) association between concussion exposure and late brain change. One cannot.

Again, the extraordinary Boston University research team deserves great credit for its persistence and rigor. But brilliantly filleted, cleverly stained, carefully inspected brains tell us frustratingly little – unless we know a lot more about clinical details and about the epidemiology of this grave phenomenon.

Returning to the Implications of Individually Variable Polypathology Among the Old

It is entirely possible that a few brains will be found among older people (with or without quantifiable repetitive CBI exposure) that exhibit the prototypical C/H/G type or the McKee-type change and no other. No atypical focal atrophy or lacunes. No vascular/microvascular change. No microglial infiltration. No Lewy bodies or prion proteins or axolemmal or synaptic or dendritic changes, or neuronal loss. But keen readers know that that is not what pathologists see in old brains. What has emerged in studies of older persons exposed to multiple concussions is exactly what the reader might have predicted, based on all that has come before in this little volume: light microscopic, biochemical, immunological, and molecular

---

[32] As previously documented in this volume, survivors of "mild TBI" are at higher risk for depression. However, it is pure speculation to suggest that the link between mild injury and post-concussive mood disorder and that between "mild CTE" and late mood disorder are related in any biological way.

biological findings are diverse. One of those many findings might be McKee-type tauopathy. But one sees polypathology in almost every case.

This distinction between unipathology and polypathology will hopefully help neurology escape the confusion that has ruffled the feathers of competing camps. *No rationale exists for calling a single pathology and polypathology by the same name.* Answers to four additional questions clarify what CTE is and is not. Please take a quick quiz and check your answers in the footnote[33]:

1. Is repetitive CBI the only thing that causes C/H/G tauopathy?
2. Among men exposed to repetitive CBI, what proportion develop C/H/G tauopathy?
3. Among published cases called "CTE" in the last decade, how common is excessive Aβ?
4. Can a single TBI cause C/H/G tauopathy?

1. Is C/H/G Tauopathy Uniquely Associated with Repetitive CBI? Or, Instead, is it Just One Interesting Way That Brains Change in Response to a Variety of Provocations?

The images of Michael Keck's brain are unforgettable. If you have never seen such a brain you might doubt your eyes. For all the controversy over CTE, for all the caveats about the fact that our microscopic methods are old and weak and questionably relevant to the dynamic biology of life, one cannot question that this is an extraordinary phenomenon. But is this picture – the apotheosis of C/H/G-type tauopathy – uniquely associated with repetitive CBI?

Probably not. In 2016, Puvenna et al. [319] published a report comparing six "CTE" brains (mean age 73.3 years) with 19 surgically resected specimens from the brains of patient with temporal lobe epilepsy (TLE; mean age 27.6 years). The investigators' explicit goal was to determine whether repetitive CBI is "a prerequisite for PT [p-tau] accumulation in the brain" (p. 225). Readers will already be wary. Whatever it is that underlies the clinical syndrome of CTE, it is not going to be clear from looking at the polypathologically afflicted brains of persons in their 70s. In fact, the present author must express reservations about this paper because Puvenna et al. declared, "No age-dependent changes were noted" [319]. Still, in both CTE and TLE, p-tau immunoreactivity was found extensively in cortical neurons and perivascularly. Those authors judged that the degree of immunoreactivity was different between CTE and controls "but not between CTE and TLE." Strikingly, they concluded:

As predicted by the conclusions from McKee's work ... we found in CTE preferential involvement of the superficial cortical layers, irregular, patchy distribution in temporal cortex, propensity for sulcal depths, and prominent

perivascular and sub-pial distribution. However, we found a virtually identical pattern in EPI [epilepsy] brain.

([319], p. 8)

Quibbles might be raised about some technical aspects of that report. And persons with epilepsy may fall and hit their heads. Nonetheless, it raises a vital point practically never mentioned in the CTE literature: rattling the brain over and over may not be the only thing that causes this particular change. Puvenna et al. [319] reasonably speculate that both repetitive concussions and repetitive seizures may have a similar impact on glymphatic clearance and blood–brain barrier integrity, corrupting tau clearance. Pending replication it seems premature to pronounce that C/H/G tauopathy has two causes. Yet the curious confluence of brain findings in two conditions with repetitive altered consciousness punctuating long periods of normal consciousness suggests the possibility of an intriguing convergence of pathophysiologies. Another reasonable inference: the phrase "CTE pathology" should perhaps not be used. If the same pathology arises from non-traumatic causes, that pattern of brain change must not be called "CTE pathology." The phrase "C/H/G tauopathy" is agnostic.

2. Among Men Exposed to Repetitive CBI, About What Proportion Develop C/H/G Tauopathy?

The Mayo Clinic brain bank in Jacksonville, FL, collected 1721 men's brains that exhibited atypical tau pathology and for which a medical history was available [320]. In most cases, the laboratory received left hemibrains fixed and right hemibrains frozen. Sixty-six men had histories of exposure to contact sports – mostly American football. A total of 198 control brains were examined, of which 33 had histories of TBI but not contact sports exposure. Among the 66 athletes, 21 (32%) were found to have "tau pathology consistent with CTE" ([320], p. 5). Sixteen of these had played football; however, *there was no difference in football exposure between the 16 players with "CTE" and the 27 without.* That is, contrary to some other reports, so-called "CTE pathology" (better called C/G/H tauopathy) was not a dose-related phenomenon. Also of interest, among men exposed to contact sports, those with the characteristic tauopathy did not differ from those without that tauopathy with respect to noted clinicopathologic features. "CTE pathology" was not found in any of the 198 control brains, including the 33 with histories of single TBIs. (However, no epilepsy cases were reportedly examined, limiting the value of that observation.)

If replicated, these are very valuable findings. They approach representing a population-based estimate of the risk of C/H/G tauopathy after contact sport exposure. At the same time, they disabuse one from the notions that repetitive CBI reliably leads to C/G/H tauopathy and that more repetitive CBI increases the risk of C/G/H tauopathy. It appears that about one-third of repetitive CBI-exposed persons will develop C/H/G tauopathy. The present author,

---

[33] 1: Probably not. 2: About one-third. 3: About 50%. 4: Unknown.

admittedly speculating, proposes that the occurrence of C/H/G tauopathy is partly independent of trauma dose, reflecting the influence of genetics, cognitive reserve, and other variables that moderate the effects of time-passing-related brain change.

3. Among Cases Called "CTE" in the Last Decade, How Common is Excessive Aβ? Or More Broadly, Among Cases Recently Published with the Diagnosis "CTE" (Most of Which are Actually Cases of Polypathology), What is the Actual Spectrum of Brain Changes?

> Several recent reviews have focused on the various neuropathological findings and the clinical criteria used for the diagnosis of CTE and have drawn attention to the confusion and inconsistency of the diagnosis of CTE. These reviews have highlighted confounding neuropathological findings such as the presence of co-occurring neurodegenerative conditions including Alzheimer's disease, Parkinson's disease and amyotrophic lateral sclerosis (ALS) discovered at the time of death in those reported to have CTE.
>
> (Maroon et al., 2015 [314])

Other chapters in this textbook also address the popular claim: "CTE is a unique tauopathic brain change due to repetitive CBI." Based on the above discussion, the reader knows that CTE is conceivably better regarded not as a definitive post-mortem diagnosis but as a heterogeneous clinical phenomenon due to various environmental exposures associated with various brain changes. Still, respect is due to the efforts of pathologists to explore the broad spectrum of changes found after repetitive CBI. Yes, only cases of youthful unipathology could reasonably be called C/H/G-type tauopathy. Yet it remains important to figure out how repetitive CBI contributes to, interacts with, and (this author suspects) synergizes with time-passing-related brain change.

This section began with two recently published quotations. One comes from a 2016 article auspiciously titled "The first NINDS/NIBIB consensus meeting to define neuropathological criteria for the diagnosis of chronic traumatic encephalopathy" [289]. Those authors state rather uncompromisingly that the "pathognomonic lesion of CTE as an accumulation of abnormal tau in neurons and astroglia distributed perivascularly at the depths of sulci in the isocortex in an irregular pattern" [289]. The other quotation comes from Castellani [288], one of many authorities who question the integrity of the CTE-is-one-disease hypothesis. Here he expresses concerns about the quality of the repeatedly cited "trust me, it's our special disease" research and the failure to control for co-morbidities. In another publication, Castellani et al. [321] conveyed several complementary concerns:

> Much additional research in chronic traumatic encephalopathy is needed to determine if it has unique neuropathology and clinical features, the extent to which the

neuropathologic alterations cause the clinical features, and whether it can be identified accurately in a living person.

> ([321], p. 493)

The present author opines that these well-meaning scholars are talking at cross-purposes. McKee et al. seek the essence. What does repetitive CBI do? Something biologically special? Castellani et al. observe the facts: polypathology is virtually universal in old brains exposed to repetitive CBI. Just to mention one domain of evidence that ought to raise questions about the "CTE-is-tauopathy-due-to-repetitive-concussions" formulation: if that were the case, then one might expect three observations to hold up: (1) survivors of repetitive CBI should exhibit similar clinical conditions; (2) survivors of repetitive CBI who develop dementia should exhibit a uniform and predictable brain change; and (3) survivors of repetitive CBI who exhibit a different (other than tauopathy) brain change should *not* exhibit the same clinical syndrome. None of these is true.

Tauopathy is indeed common in the small number of dementia cases that have been studied to date, but it is not universal and it is not the only brain change in the majority of cases. In fact, a majority of cases that a neuropathologist has labeled "CTE" in the least 15 years exhibit not only abundant deposition of Aβ plaques [322], but a potpourri of alternative protein deposits and other changes. Indeed, neuroinflammation continues to emerge as a major factor in deleterious brains changes called "Alzheimer's disease" or "CTE": Cherry et al. [323] assayed CD68 immunoreactive microglial density in the brains of 66 deceased American football players. Exposure to repetitive CBIs, and both the development and severity of encephalopathic changes, correlated with CD68 counts in the dorsolateral prefrontal cortex. Thus, a more accurate summary was offered by Smith et al. [129]:

> According to current autopsy studies, survival from repetitive mild or single moderate to severe TBI is associated with a range of pathologies, best considered as "polypathology," and including tau and Aβ abnormalities, neuroinflammation, white matter degeneration, and neuronal loss.
>
> (p. 218)

4. Can a Single TBI Produce C/H/G Tauopathy?

> there is a general presumption that CTE is limited to patients exposed to rTBI [repetitive TBI], most often athletes. This misperception may be due in part to a complete absence of comparative research or clinicopathological studies looking at material from both sTBI [single TBI] and rTBI patients in parallel. As such, considering late neurodegenerative outcomes from an sTBI and rTBI as different syndromes is, at best, premature and, arguably, flawed.
>
> (Hay et al., 2016 [103])

Can a single TBI produce CTE? Of course it can! By far the most common cause of CTE (properly defined) is a single TBI. In this case, we refer to a linguistically sensible phrase for the very common medical phenomenon of persistent deleterious post-traumatic brain change, often associated with impairments in behavioral health such as psychiatric symptoms (more important for subjective well-being and social function) or cognitive deficits (less important for well-being and social integration, often missed by conventional neuropsychological testing, but still potentially disabling).

However, the pathophysiological basis of such common-place persistent encephalopathies remains far from under-stood – as does the degree to which force and genes and other pre-morbid factors alter the risk. The previous section of this chapter hopefully raised new doubts about the very concept of ND. Yet, since that term will remain popular for a while, it can be said that the changes typically called "neurodegenerative" are indeed common and expected after a single TBI. Experimental research confirms this. As Uryu et al. put it [324]: "Studies in animal models have shown that traumatic brain injury (TBI) induces the rapid accumula-tion of many of the same key proteins that form pathological aggregates in neurodegenerative diseases" (p. 185).[34] Human studies support the same conclusion. For instance, Johnson et al. [326] commented: "single TBI can induce multiple long-term neurodegenerative changes" (p. 2). It has been known for decades that Aβ appears very quickly after TBI. It was recently demonstrated that even a relatively mild TBI triggers the gen-eration of toxic tau oligomers, with harmful effects on cogni-tion [169]. Tau deposits in fact persist for at least a year after a single TBI [327]. α-Synuclein is the third "degenerative" pro-tein commonly generated after TBI [324].

The pathway from immediate traumatic changes (such as production of multiple "misfolded" or atypically conformed (non-conformist) proteins) to long-term ND remains uncertain [129]. For instance, one piece of evidence that contravenes the myth that a pure tauopathy is a common late effect after repeti-tive CBIs is the observation that about 52% of persons with so-called "CTE pathology" also exhibit excessive Aβ [322] (The fact that the microscopic brain picture is both polypathological and heterogeneous among brains of older persons exposed to repeti-tive CBI is a good reason to shy from the phrase "CTE path-ology.") Yet it has not been proven that late proliferation of Aβ is a direct or necessary effect of the Aβ seen promptly after a TBI.

Hence, the pathway from repeatedly rattling the brain to *sometimes* developing C/H/G tauopathy is unknown. However, an emerging consensus seems to favor three of the previously discussed pathophysiological processes. First, the "seeding" hypothesis: promptly produced non-conformist proteins cata-lyze or serve as nidi for insidious prion-like transsynaptic propa-gation [169–171, 325]. For instance, as Gerson et al. put it: "tau oligomers may be responsible for seeding the spread of path-ology post-TBI" [169]. Second, the vascular hypothesis: some evidence from both animal and human research implicates microvascular changes, microthrombi, and altered blood–brain barrier dynamics in the long-term behavioral effects of con-cussion [150, 155, 156, 158]. Third, the inflammatory hypoth-esis: as Faden and Loane put it: "Nearly lost in the discussions

of post-traumatic neurodegeneration after traumatic brain injury has been the role of sustained neuroinflammation, even though this association has been well established pathologic-ally since the 1950s" ([148], p. 143). Johnson et al. reported empirical evidence of not only acute but also long-lasting post-traumatic inflammation, and concluded: "the identification of active inflammation years after TBI is in a timeframe consistent with epidemiological associations linking TBI with the later onset of dementia" [327].

Smith et al. [129] summarized these interrelated observations boldly: "That TBI represents a major risk factor for the later development of neurodegenerative disease is now accepted." Thus, there is evidence for almost immediate post-traumatic "neurodegenerative" changes, and for dissemination of those changes in the brain over time, and for delayed-onset dementing disease. What is the connection? Is the first a prerequisite for the second? Does the first necessarily cause the second or (as the author speculates) might some humans excel at clearance of non-conformist proteins and be spared late effects?

One must acknowledge that the plurality of both pre-clinical and clinical reports supporting that conclusion refer to "moderate" or more severe TBIs. Why is so little known about the long-term outcome of less severe, typical, clinically attended CBI?

In the case of rodents, the main impediment to determining the long-term effects of single "mild" injuries is that – perhaps astounding to readers – the experiments have yet to be done.[35] In the case of humans – who cannot be experimental subjects and who are almost never followed for long after concus-sion – the research void is probably due to two causally linked factors: (1) the long delay in acknowledging that conventional paper-and-pencil neuropsychological testing is insensitive to the long-term effects of CBI (helping some to deny the lasting effects of CBI for decades); and (2) the lack of funding for lon-gitudinal research. However, as shown below, several human studies shed light on the possibility that single and repeti-tive concussions *both* seem to provoke ND, and there may be something biologically special, but yet to be discovered, about repetitive injuries.

The above paragraphs, though hopefully useful, still do not answer this section's lead-off question: might a single CBI cause C/H/G-type tauopathy? It has long been apparent that a single moderate to severe TBI promptly generates Aβ in about 30% of cases – sometimes within hours [327–331]. (The frequency of this occurrence in a typical CBI is unclear, largely because such brains rarely come to autopsy.) New evidence suggests that a single TBI also promptly generates p-tau. McKee and Robinson [332] reported, "some cases of recent concussion and PCS [post-concussive symptoms] show isolated focal peri-vascular accumulations of hyperphosphorylated tau (p-tau) as neurofibrillary tangles (NFTs) and neurites" (p. S244). Hence,

---

[34] Not every scholar would agree. Brody et al. [325], for instance, reported little tau immunoreactivity in hTau mice, even after repetitive injury. Those authors speculated that perhaps that pathological change requires more time than permitted by the lifespan of a mouse. If they are correct, it represents a tremendous problem for modern concussion research.

[35] At the end of this chapter, the author will promote simple, practical, cost-efficient corrections for this problem.

the brain location of *early* p-tau is similar to the brain location of *late* p-tau immunoreactivity in C/H/G tauopathy. In addition, some types of single injury (e.g., blast) may display pathophysiological elements more similar to those of repetitive CBI: the same paper reported, "detailed kinematic analysis demonstrated that blast winds produce forces similar to multiple, severe concussive impacts occurring over microseconds" (p. S245). Such findings raise suspicion that a single TBI might trigger C/H/G tauopathy, but do not answer that question.

Leaping to the denouement, recent reports *do* in fact support the hypothesis that even exposure to a single moderate to severe TBI may be associated with a late C/H/G-type tauopathy: Johnson et al. [333] reported that, among 39 survivors at one year or more after such a single injury, NFTs were excessive compared with those in the brains of non-TBI controls. Moreover, Smith et al. [129] commented: "Interestingly, as in CTE, in some cases NFTs were found to be *concentrated at the depths of sulci*" (emphasis added). That is: one brain-rattling episode can apparently lead to a late tauopathy that is reasonably typical of the C/H/G type. But can a single, *typical concussion* (e.g., mild brain rattling by an errant baseball) *do the same thing*? Proof remains elusive. The reason: no reason exists to perform a comprehensive post-mortem examination on an elderly person who suffered a little knockout in playing in the Little League 75 years ago. We continue to pace in the dark due to the resistance to funding prospective longitudinal research.

Why Does Repetitive CBI Sometimes, but not Always, Cause a Pure C/H/G Tauopathy in Youth or Contribute to a Polypathological Dementia Including C/H/G Tauopathy Later in Life?

A brief pause to restate the mystery we face today: nothing in the traditional 20th-century theories of CBI explains CTE due to repetitive trauma. Consider three matters:

1. According to the old "neurometabolic cascade" hypothesis, the last and final trivial residual brain effects of a single CBI happily vanish *completely* in days or, at most weeks. *How then, might ten concussions be any worse than one?*

2. *Answer: if they are closely spaced in time.* Strong evidence exists of an infrequent "second-impact syndrome." A person who experiences a new CBI before he or she has lived out the first three to ten days of neurometabolic stress is likely to suffer more than usual cellular damage. *But does that explain CTE due to repetitive concussions?*

3. *Answer: almost never.* Most athletes and soldiers with histories of multiple concussions have never once suffered the second-impact syndrome. They typically have gone weeks, months, or even years between significant brain-rattling blows to the head.

Hence, the conventional theories, the usual suspects, simply do not account for the special threat of C/H/G tauopathy (or any other dementing process) from repetitive CBI. If – as a 20th-century traditionalist might insist – all biological effects of CBI vanish in a few weeks, then there is absolutely no special danger from having 600 concussions – one each month over 50 years!

The present author opines that the traditionalists are wrong and earnestly discourages volunteers for that experiment. If concussive brain change resolved over three to ten days, there would never have been a case of dementia pugilistica and retired NFL players would have no risk of early dementia. That is not the case. Therefore, single CBIs *must* have lasting deleterious effects.

That, of course, does not reduce the possibility that multiple injuries create a risk of exceptional brain changes – changes rarely seen after single injuries – changes that might some day be teased apart from the cornucopia of other brain changes that every injured and uninjured person inescapably and simultaneously experiences as a human naturally destined for multiple time-passing-related brain changes. What might the difference be, then, between ND after one concussion versus neurodegeneration after 600 concussions? Johnson et al. [326] published an intriguing paper that touches upon that very question. An introduction may help frame the findings.

An Introduction to TDP-43

For background: in 2006 it was discovered that sporadic ALS and frontotemporal lobar degeneration with ubiquitinated inclusions (FTLD-U) belong to a spectrum of clinical conditions, both associated with the 43-kDa transactive response (TAR) DNA-binding protein (TDP-43) [334, 335]. "As a result, FTLD-U and ALS are now recognized as representing a clinicopathological spectrum within a new biochemical class of neurodegenerative disease, the TDP-43 proteinopathies" [336]. The normal function of TDP-43 is uncertain, but it perhaps contributes both to DNA regulation and to RNA processing. Subsequent work determined that this protein has a widespread presence across the domain of time-passing-related brain change currently called "neurodegenerative disease"; aggregates of TDP-43 are also present in Parkinson's disease, dementia with Lewy bodies, Huntington's disease, hippocampal sclerosis, corticobasal degeneration, and "Alzheimer's disease" – a finding that starkly illustrates the doubts about employing an atypical molecule (or alternative folding conformation) as a "disease" marker [324, 337–339]. Just as in so-called "Alzheimer's disease," initial suspicion fell on TDP-43 aggregates as the "cause" of neurodegenerative disease. Some evidence, however, suggests aggregates are trivially toxic, and that the harm is instead due to abnormal function of mutant forms of this useful DNA/RNA-binding protein [340].[36] In any case, an emerging consensus suggests that normal TDP-43 is relatively

---

[36] Not wishing to complicate matters: readers may wish to know that TDP-43's toxic effect perhaps depends on its interaction with another protein: fused-in sarcoma/translocation in liposarcoma (FUS/TLS) [341, 342].

benign, whereas hyperphosphorylated and ubiquitinated forms of TDP-43 (p-TDP-43) are neurotoxic.

In 2010, McKee et al. [343] reported that TDP-43 was found in ten of 12 subjects pathologically diagnosed with "CTE," and that three cases involved the clinical features of motor neuron disease. That laboratory has subsequently concluded that more than 85% of "CTE" cases exhibit TDP-43 deposition, sometime co-localized with p-tau [145].

This brings us to Johnson et al's. discovery: those authors examined 62 survivors of single moderate/severe TBIs from ten hours to 47 years post injury [326]. The brains were examined with antibodies that could discriminate between the noxious phosphorylated form of this binding protein (p-TDP-43) and the more conventional phosphorylation-independent form (pi-TPD-43). Unlike demented survivors of repetitive concussion, survivors of single injuries did *not* exhibit much p-TDP-43. Yet – in a dramatic difference from normal controls – survivors of single TBIs *did* exhibit cortical staining for pi-TDP-43. In fact, that curious brain change was seen acutely in 82.6% and it remained one year later in 53.8%.

The meaning of this report may not be clear for a decade. Although methodological challenges of this work remain daunting (and it may take a few more years to quash the lore of single CBI → Alzheimer's disease, while repetitive CBI → CTE), it seems reasonable to expect that reports regarding other authentic biological differences between the late effects of single versus repetitive concussion can be expected.

Seemingly Reasonable Take-Home Messages Thus Far

1. Single TBI or repetitive CBIs can both trigger long-lasting neurodegenerative polypathology.
2. The likelihood of this occurring after a single moderate to severe TBI seems to be higher than the likelihood of this occurring after a single typical clinically attended CBI, and the likelihood of this occurring after greater lifetime repetitive CBI exposure seems to be higher than after a lesser exposure (a plausible dose effect).
3. The likelihood of this occurring almost without question depends on a large number of host-related and environmental factors.
4. Strong evidence has emerged that a subset of persons exposed to at least two known types of repetitive brain insults (TLE and repetitive CBI) may exhibit a distinctive tauopathy characterized by cortical perivascular p-tau deposits, disproportionately dense in the depths of sulci.
5. However, *no evidence suggests that one particular clinical profile is necessary and sufficient to generate this distinctive tauopathy*. Instead, a subset of repetitive CBI patients and of TLE patients (and perhaps patients with other yet-to-be-recognized exposures) develop C/H/G pathology. One recent estimate: about one-third of persons with histories of sports-related repetitive CBI will develop this intriguing brain change.

Why those patients and not the other two-thirds? A dose effect may contribute but seems insufficient to altogether explain this difference. Other factors are probably in play.

Adolescent Concussion Perhaps Triggers Later Multiple Sclerosis

This textbook has striven to politely overthrow the 20th-century credo of a "neurometabolic cascade." A vast horde of new knowledge encourages this reconceptualization. It is hard to account for the changes observed in concussed brains if one yokes oneself to the mental image of a waterfall, when in fact the water is spraying upward from the pool every bit as vigorously. As demonstrated in earlier chapters, CBI sets off a battle between harmful and healthful mechanisms. Inflammation is a key player. It is probable that some aspects of the neuroimmunological–inflammatory response tend to repair the brain, others to harm it, and that genetic/epigenetic differences significantly condition those relative effects.

Given more than a century of experimental research showing that inflammation is common after CBI – and evidence that TBI disrupts the blood–brain barrier, permitting invasion by immunoreactive cells that are otherwise excluded – it is no surprise that epidemiologists have explored the possibility of a link to demyelinating disease and other inflammatory disorders. Given that, for most of the 20th century, even the subset of concussed persons who were clinically attended were ignored after the first 24 h, it is no surprise that those studies have produced ambiguous results.

To begin: in 1999 the Therapeutics and Technology Assessment Subcommittee of the American Academy of Neurology authored a report on this subject [344]. Those authors began with a question: does a neurobiologically plausible mechanism exist by which TBI might precipitate MS? Their answer was yes:

> it is certainly plausible that the peripheral immune system might become activated against certain CNS myelin antigens such as myelin basic protein, proteolipid protein, myelin oligodendrocyte glycoprotein, or myelin-associated glycoprotein and thereby initiate an MS attack. In fact, there is substantial evidence, in other contexts, that trauma can result in demyelinating lesions in the CNS.
>
> [344]

That rationale in mind, the authors first reviewed the historical precedents for this question. They cited papers from 1897 onward, mostly uncontrolled case series, that claimed a trauma–MS association [345–347]. The authors sought more recent data, searching Medline, using the keywords "trauma" and "multiple sclerosis"—and sought to rise above what they called the "often bitter" criticisms inspired by this question. Six reports were reviewed. Only one confined its trauma definition to head trauma. None pertained to concussion. The results were mixed.

This was not a comprehensive systematic review. No effort was made to stratify by methodology, to stratify by demographic variables or duration of follow-up, or to meta-analyze comparable studies. Recall bias was virtually assured by the retrospective designs of five of six reports. "Trauma" was not defined the same way in any two studies (one included dental procedures). Moreover, the conceptual framework of almost all the cited research was close-minded: if "trauma" triggers MS, MS will appear within several months. The authors are to be credited, however, for setting the bar for future scholarship: "[a cohort study] is to demonstrate, prospectively, that the incidence of MS onset or attacks is higher in persons or patients following traumatic injury or stress than in similar persons who have not experienced such antecedent events."

A more recent review and meta-analysis by Warren et al. [348] was more credible. The search was far more comprehensive. But again, "trauma" was defined broadly as "any physical damage inflicted on the body." No neurobiologically plausible rationale was offered for an association between trauma not otherwise specified and CNS demyelination. Of the 16 selected studies, only two were cohort studies of cranial injury [349, 350]. Both, however, were quality studies that cannot be dismissed.

Goldacre et al. [349] compared 110,993 persons (sex ratio not reported) admitted to the hospital with head injury with 534,600 non-injury controls. Their database permitted identification of the subsets of both groups subsequently hospitalized for MS. Follow-up averaged 16.7 years. The rate ratios for MS hospitalization among head trauma and control subjects were not significantly different, leading the authors to conclude: "There was no significant increase in the risk of MS at either short or long time periods after head injury." A total of 12,927 of their head injury subjects fell into the age range of 10–14 years. If four-fifths of those were aged 11–14 years, that makes 10,342. In all, 17,064 were aged 15–19 years. Thus, about 25% (27,406/110,993) of the head injury cohort were injured in adolescence. No stratification by age or accounting for multiplicity of injuries was provided.

An arguably superior cohort report was the prospective study by Pfleger et al. [350]. Those authors identified 150,868 subjects with hospital admission for head injury at under 55 years of age (63% male) and followed them for possible subsequent appearance in the Danish MS Registry. Average follow-up was 14.4 years (range 1–22 years). In all, 182 subjects developed MS. Based on sex, age, and year-specific disease densities, 193 cases would have been expected. The authors firmly concluded, "Head injury of any severity does not affect the risk of acquiring MS later in life." Eyeballing their graph, it appears that about 20,400 subjects were injured at age 10–14. If four-fifths were aged 11–14, that makes 16,320. About 26,100 were injured at age 15–19. Hence, roughly 28% (42,420/ 150,868) of their subjects were adolescents. No stratification by age or accounting for multiplicity of injuries was provided.

A third large cohort study was conducted by Kang et al. [351]. Those authors identified 72,765 TBI patients (age ≥ 18 years; 61.2% male; severity unclear), comparing them with 218,295 non-TBI patients. Over six years of follow-up, 0.055% of TBI patients and 0.037% of comparison subjects developed MS. After stratifying for TBI hospitalization (a proxy for severity) and demographic adjustment, the hazard ratio for head injury subjects was 1.97 compared with controls. Note that two factors compromise interpretation: almost all adolescents were excluded and the follow-up period was relatively short.

A third review paper was also credibly presented: Lunny et al. [352] conducted a meta-analysis of both case–control and cohort studies, but stratified by both age and study quality. Among the high-quality case–control studies, there was a statistically significant association between surviving childhood head trauma and subsequent MS (odds ratio = 1.27). Unfortunately, the childhood studies were not further age-stratified. The pooled odds ratio from the four cohort studies was not significant. Also, unfortunately, these authors included Siva et al. [353] – the study that regarded dental procedures as trauma – making that analysis difficult to interpret.

That was the state of the art in the summer of 2017. Glimmers and hints from both basic and clinical science abounded of a possible association between TBI and later MS, but there was less than a handful of quality cohort studies, and even fewer that considered the question, "If there is an association, perhaps it occurs in a subset?" At least one question might have sparked curiosity: studies that start by identifying TBI patients end up with a predominance of male subjects. MS is more common in females. In addition, as discussed in Chapter 7, some evidence suggests that post-concussive inflammatory change is particularly problematic among menstruating females. What if one started with a typical large cohort of MS patients, likely to be mostly female, and compared their head trauma exposure with that of non-MS patients?

In late August of 2017 the *Annals of Neurology* accepted a paper by Montgomery et al. [354]. That research group employed the Swedish Patient Register and MS Register. A total of 7292 patients diagnosed with MS after age 20 were matched on multiple variables with ten non-MS subjects. In all, 70.3% of the MS patients were female. The authors explained their design: "Rather than examining all head trauma, we focused on a diagnosis of concussion, as this is more likely to identify involvement of the CNS" ([354], p. 555). Persons diagnosed with MS after age 20 and persons without that diagnosis were equally likely to have survived concussion between birth and age 10. However, the adjusted odds ratio for MS among persons concussed at age 11–20 was 1.22 ($p = 0.008$) compared with non-concussed subjects, and the adjusted odds ratio for MS among those with greater than one concussion in that age range was 1.97 ($p = 0.002$). That report became global front-page news. Two statements by Montgomery et al. ([354], p. 558) help summarize the potential significance of the paper:

- "This, coupled with the evidence from sports with a high risk of head trauma such as boxing, indicate the potential role of sports injuries in adolescence as a risk for MS."
- "In theory, it may be possible to reduce the risk of delayed adverse outcomes, such as MS, following a traumatic injury to the CNS through therapies to reduce inflammation."

The present textbook respectfully rejects the dated concept of disease that pervades this literature. As noted in earlier chapters, a tension exists between Osler's pre-1908 theoretical stance – that a disease is a specific biological change, whomever it attacks – and Garrod's post-1908 stance – that a disease is the interaction between an individual and a threat to health. The authors of the old literature on head injury and MS, from 1897 to 2014, largely exhibit loyalty to Osler's model, investigating the possibility of TBI–MS relationship on the assumption that health threat would likely affect all persons in the same way. That concept is rapidly succumbing to the intellectual gravity of precision medicine. Genetics aside, at the very least, one expects demographically different populations to have different responses to the same health threat. By considering the possibility of an age-specific risk, a dose effect, and a late effect, Montgomery et al. [354] have perhaps broken through the traditional conceptual blockade toward a rational test of the hypothesis that concussion can trigger MS. Not in everyone. Not immediately. Just in the gigantic group of adolescents who participate in sports. That discovery, if replicated, has profound implications for medicine – not to mention law.

Earlier chapters discussed a new model of post-concussive brain change as a neurometabolic/inflammatory/vascular melee. The recent observation of a possible causal link with MS may add sophistication to our understanding of concussive effects on neuroimmunomodulation. Speculating about the causal chain of events, Montgomery et al. [354] point out that various injuries to the nervous system expand the pool of myelin antigen-specific T cells, which in turn generate inflammatory cytokines such as interferon-γ, which in turn suppresses remyelination.

Although it is premature to consider the question settled by any means, the possibility of a CBI–MS link may turn out to be as useful as the corner piece of a jigsaw puzzle. A robust international research effort is rapidly growing our knowledge base regarding immune and inflammatory affects of CBI [355–357]. New findings perhaps offer insight into the unresolved question of sex, CBI, and inflammation [358]. And a wide net has been cast seeking safe and effective treatments based on modulating inflammation [359–361]. Only time will tell which observations hold keys to either meaningful biomarkers of brain change or effective intervention.

Toward a Rational Nosology

The early chapters of this introductory textbook demonstrated that long-lasting deleterious changes in brain and behavior are common after a single, typical, clinically attended CBI. The foregoing pages in this chapter represent a very brief introduction to the nosological conundrum posed by that fact. The author tried to demonstrate that the terms of art embraced in neurological nosology tend to be loaded and biased. They make assumptions about biology that sometimes seem inconsistent with neutral scientific observation. The conventional understanding of "development," for instance, implies somatic change with the passing of time in compliance with a life history plan (and driven by a clock) that generates age-appropriate fitness-enhancing phenotypes. At the same time, its use is popularly restricted to a subset of such changes: those preceding "maturity." That restriction seems artificially narrow, in view

of the observation that most people undergo somatic brain changes between ages 40 and 70 that enhance mood, vocabulary, and wisdom – desirable, beneficial, fitness-enhancing changes with time that, in simple English, are *developments*. Similarly, the conventional use of "aging" – typically implying deleterious somatic change after maturity, or the onslaught of entropy, or (circularly) "that which explains increased risk of aging-related diseases with time" – seems vulnerable to concerns about conceptual consistency. Some gains in function, such as those just mentioned, depend on time-passing-related *losses* in the soma, such as a profound depletion of synapses, shrinking of gray matter, and loss of plasticity. As well, some striking and severe functional losses occur in childhood, such as the ability to learn a second language without an accent. Such observations suggest that the essence of aging and the bright line between development and aging remain elusive.[37]

The concept of ND seems yet to be settled in the minds of neurologists. None of the features commonly listed – such as loss of neurons, loss of synapses, loss of gray-matter volume, deposition of non-conformist proteins – are necessarily abnormal or fitness reducing any more than the loss of hefty chunks of marble from a quarried block ruined the statue called David. The popular concept of dementia can be safely dismissed, since doctors have abandoned its root meaning: a decline in mentation from a previous level of function. The conventional concept of "Alzheimer's disease" is simply not supportable based on empirical observations, making "post-traumatic Alzheimer's disease" a non-entity. The presently popular concept of "CTE" as C/H/G-type tauopathy uniquely due to repetitive CBI, associated with a variety of clinical presentations, diagnosable as due to trauma even in the presence of multiple other types of brain change, appears to be a mismatch between English usage and scientific observation.

One term of art has yet to be discussed in this chapter: "pathological change." The author opines that this concept retains worth. One might define as *pathological* those unexpected changes that negatively impact life function – which in turn might be defined as threatening to the organism's inclusive fitness. In the neurobehavioral realm, that tends to include suboptimal emotional, motor, or cognitive function – all seen long after one or more CBIs.

This may be a good time to introduce a novel and (hopefully) logically defensible nosology that respects the data and acknowledges the current limits of human knowledge. We are morally bound to admit that, at this time, a classification of time-passing-related brain change, or of the late effects of concussion, cannot be fully elaborated. Just as psychiatry is duty-bound to replace the American Psychiatric Association's dismal DSM system but has yet to discover a scientifically robust replacement, neurology seems obliged to graduate from misleading labels, even as it awaits the knowledge needed to undergird a more rational approach to biologically same and different. In this transitional phase, one tries to stick with a few

---

[37] The author speculates that aging is the symphony of changes due to the progressively diminishing returns of natural selection with the passing of time after conception. He suspects, however, that that poem will be slow to gain fans.

descriptive concepts that seem easy to support and resilient to future discovery.

So how might one think about (and perhaps even classify) the late effects of one or more CBIs? Pending the discovery of natural kinds (biologically specific and genuinely dissociable "diseases"), the author will tentatively offer a practical research diagnostic classification. Entirely open to ideas that better accommodate the little we currently know, the author proposes that deleterious brain change might be logically divided as follows:

1. pathological brain change negatively impacting cerebral function, probably due to a single primary etiology

2. polypathological brain change negatively impacting cerebral function, with evidence of time-passing-related changes of the type commonly observed in the senium, *without* evidence of a single primary etiology. (Specification of *possible* contributing factors is sometimes justified)

3. polypathological brain change negatively impacting cerebral function, with evidence of time-passing-related changes of the type commonly observed in the senium, *with* evidence of a single primary etiology. (Specification of *possible* additional contributing factors is sometimes justified.)

An example of the first type: infants, young children, teens, and adults normally gain and lose various brain functions over time. Yet the net effect of those changes, prior to about age 25, is enhancement of fitness. In some tragic cases – such as devastating bacterial meningitis, pediatric glioblastoma, intractable TLE, or a single severe childhood TBI with prolonged coma and rapid brain atrophy – the young brain suffers a readily identifiable, discrete, and unitary change that unequivocally detracts from fitness. One can now add a subset of cases of repetitive CBI to that list, for example, the awful case of Michael Keck. That is a good example of the confluence of a *clinical* state justifiably called CTE with a *pathological* state that might respectfully be called *C/H/G-type tauopathy* – a neuropathological pattern that may also be provoked by TLE. Thus, no matter what the initial severity of one or more TBIs was, if brain dysfunction persists and impacts life function (e.g., "She fell from the climbing wall and she's never been the same"), that clinical state is *CTE*. An unknown proportion of clinical CTE cases (perhaps mostly those with a history of repetitive CBI, but possibly also some with a history of a single TBI) have a single dominant pathological change – a tauopathy.

In contrast, rather than having a plausible temporal link (as when a child falls and changes that day), the overwhelming majority of cases published with the label "CTE" in the last decade did *not* exhibit lifelong behavioral change starting milliseconds after a single event, and never exhibit pure tauopathy. Instead, a history of injury is reconstructed by guesswork and the brain exhibits polypathology. The present author implores his colleagues: it is not credible to call a condition "CTE" when many pathological changes are present and when no way exists to sort out traumatic from non-traumatic changes or weigh the relative contribution of either to the clinical status.

Recent data strongly suggest a somewhat different type 1 scenario. As discussed below, the weight of evidence now favors the suspicion that concussions in adolescence (but not necessarily in childhood) significantly increase the risk of developing MS, which usually emerges in one's 20s. If an abrupt force to the hair of the head causes a person's neuroimmunological profile to be altered in a way that favors CNS demyelination five to 20 years later, one might equally classify that phenomenon as *pathological brain change probably due to a single dominant etiology.*

An example of the second type: virtually all cases currently meeting criteria for the arbitrarily defined diagnosis of "dementia" fulfill these criteria for polypathology. Surely, most pathologists report exactly what they see, and would never – for example – diagnose "Alzheimer's disease" if any vascular or inflammatory changes were found. However, early in his career the author was privileged to review slides that clearly exhibited polypathology, which the local pathologist dismissed to push the diagnosis into a single neurodegenerative pigeon hole. If angels stood at the shoulder of neuropathologists, they would encourage unbiased, theoretically agnostic reporting. Perhaps, with that assistance, *every* 20th-century pathologist would have rejected the theoretically driven categories that oversimplified their actual visual observations (which *never* reveal just one kind of brain change in an older person, and which are *never* the same in any two brains) and we would not be faced with today's important but painful duty to overthrow the dated dogmatism that birthed academic inventions like "Alzheimer's disease."

Far from supporting the past century's rigid belief in the existence of a handful of natural kinds of time-passing-related brain change, far from supporting the theory that some people develop brain "disease" in old age and some do not, the empirical data, only touched upon in this chapter, indisputably demonstrate that a comprehensive micro-structural, ultra-structural, molecular biological, and immunological examination of the brain of any old person (even using today's primitive and temporarily popular stains and immunocytochemistry) results in the diagnosis of polypathology. Hence, until we prove that one of the thousands of changes that occur over time is the dominant cause of dysfunction, neurologists would perhaps be prudent to diagnose most patients at a dementia clinic with *polypathological brain change.*

Traditionalists may balk. They should please consider Chani. Or listen when an unspoiled resident cuts the brain.

Note that "cerebral dysfunction" is not always clinically obvious. For instance, the teenaged football player whose brain works harder to get the same test answers is clinically normal, even if excessive reactive oxygen species are busy whittling away at his future. In the vast majority of cases, it is shameful hubris when a doctor claims to know what proportion of functional change is due to what pathological change.

An example of the third type: consider the > 150 cases recently published and labeled "CTE." In how many of those did the pathologist look for, and see, and prove: (1) no cerebrovascular disease except that specifically and solely due to trauma and altogether independent of normally expected time-passing-related brain change; (2) no activated microglia, except those specifically and solely due to trauma; (3) no atypically folded proteins, except those specifically and solely due to trauma; and (4) no evidence of oxidative phosphorylation, except that specifically and solely due to trauma.

The answer is zero. The logical conclusion: it is altogether worth considering, even strongly suspecting, that a person's one or 300 concussions are somehow associated with the polypathological changes later found in his or her brain – even though those changes *always* depend on pre-morbid individual factors and *always* overlap greatly with changes seen in non-concussed brains. Chani is a case in point. Perhaps his single concussion contributed to his behavioral problems 57 years later. But his encephalopathy did not commence the day or week or month after his concussion. His brain (like that of many old, forgetful people) *does* exhibit excessive p-tau. Yet first, its amount and pattern of distribution is not prototypically C/H/G tauopathy and second, no power on Earth can advise us whether his p-tau is causally related to his concussion, or the relative impact of CBI versus altitude exposure on his late-life mentation. Moreover, no pathologist could claim, with a straight face, that Chani's brain at age 75 exhibits persuasive evidence of a single primary etiology. During his rich and colorful life after his brain injury there was undoubtedly an interaction between the thousands of brain changes promptly produced by his CBI, an unknowable number of relevant environmental exposures, and the many time-passing-related brain changes that some attribute to so-called "aging." Even if a measurable harmful effect of Chani's concussion were reported in a divine message, it would be silly to call his clinical condition "CTE" or his polypathology "C/H/G tauopathy." As in most human cases, his primary with polypathology surely has a mixed etiology. Until a biomarker is available that is highly specific and sensitive for the late effects of TBI, his neurologist should diagnose *polypathological brain change with possible contributions from CBI and exposure to high altitude*.

In the same way, a much-beaten-about nose tackle with disabling dementia at age 72 was also a dubious candidate for the "single primary etiology" criterion, especially since he survived 22 years of untreated diabetes and hypertension. A neurologist might sensibly diagnose *polypathological brain change with possible contributions from repetitive CBI, diabetes, and cerebrovascular disease*.

In contrast, the author examined a 36-year-old retired NFL wide receiver. The patient could not name his children or walk without falling. He had attempted suicide four times. He also had hypertension with extensive periventricular white-matter changes. Even though the effect of head impacts was not submerged in a sea of alternatives, one was obliged to acknowledge polypathology. The diagnosis was *polypathological brain change with a probable contribution of repetitive CBIs and hypertension*. That is, even when trauma is a likely suspect, the case is not purely and simply exemplary of "CTE."

"Chronic traumatic encephalopathy" is such a simple phrase! It means persistent deleterious brain change due to one or more brain traumas that cannot be explained by an alternative or concomitant diagnosis. To respect the meaning of those three words and the nearly universal fact of human polypathology, the author would sharply rein in the drive to diagnose all cases affected by concussion as "CTE."

Honest neuropathologists are currently engaged in a great civil war, testing whether that discipline, or any discipline so conceived and so dedicated, can shake off the shackles of terms of art and simply call 'em as they see 'em. Editors will continue to publish articles that indefensibly refer to "Alzheimer's disease" and "CTE" until logic triumphs.

How, then, are we to indicate our suspicions? From the outset of this chapter, the author has tried to emphasize the ultimate goal for public health and human well-being: figuring out whether concussions have late effects that are modifiable by treatment. To candidly acknowledge that *every* retired football player and boxer exhibits polypathology is no retreat from the front line of science. It is a victory for common sense. To quit using the phrase "CTE" when an encephalopathy has three or seven likely causes is not defeat. It is respect for science.

The project that should occupy our attention – the project that (admittedly struggling to estimate cost vs. benefit) perhaps deserves a much larger proportion of National Institutes of Health research dollars is to (1) determine – with utter independence from terms of art, antiquated theories, and political posturing whether (and under what circumstances) concussions cause what class of late effects and (2) if that turns out to be a major contributor to human distress, to plunge wholeheartedly into a well-funded initiative to find safe and effective post-CBI treatments.

In the meantime, and recognizing the strictures of practicality, what more might we be doing to answer our burning question about late effects?

Two Simple Studies

Ideally, the National Institute of Neurological Disorders and Stroke would have initiated large-scale prospective longitudinal studies of concussion when that was proposed in 1969 [362]. They did not. As remarked above, one of the main current projects funded with that ostensible focus is deeply flawed and should perhaps be defunded. Ideally, an angel will step forth and fund a prospective study – knowing that he or she will die long before results are available to save humanity from untold misery. The author of this chapter is not alone in that hope. Maroon et al. [314] put it simply: "We conclude that the incidence of CTE remains unknown due to the lack of large, longitudinal studies" (p. 1). Smith et al. [129] opined, with slightly more elaboration:

> owing to the lack of large-scale controlled studies, our understanding of the pathology of CTE has advanced little since the landmark study by Corsellis et al. in s1973 … a movement towards prospective studies will be important to advance our understanding of TBI-associated

neurodegeneration and, in turn, targeted developments in therapy.

The present author will not live to see the publication of helpful results from such studies. Nor does he expect a timely awakening to the potentially massive importance of this issue and an immediate rebalancing of national research priorities. That does not mean we are helpless. Relatively small investments in several rigorously designed research projects might enable major strides. Two such projects come to mind.

1. Experimental Research to Test the Hypothesis That a Single Typical CBI May Cause Late Effects

Readers may have been shocked to learn, in earlier chapters and this one, that no scholars have yet conducted large, lifelong, longitudinal prospective study of the impact of one concussion on any animal species. Mice just live for a couple years – short enough to practically follow them through a lifetime. Still, as the author has heard from three renowned experimentalists, no one wants to care for a concussed mouse for 24 months. In addition, mice are not ideal creatures for TBI experiments, since their brains do not express the same "neurodegenerative" changes expected in human brains. Even triple transgenics (described earlier in this volume) cannot mimic human traumatic brain change. And relatively few laboratories employ a mouse-hitting technique that is mechanistically comparable to typical human concussions (too many labs stabilize the head, open the skull, squirt something at it, and call that a model for human concussion).

Nonetheless, we will not know the results until the study is done. At a cost that has been variously estimated at $15,000–40,000, a laboratory could: (1) assess behavior; (2) randomize one-half of a genetically matched mice cohort to a *closed* head injury (permitting naturalistic head movement) versus a sham procedure; (3) house them all in an enriched, low-stress environment with access to an exercise wheel; (4) treat them kindly for two years before (5) repeating behavioral tests (including functional MRI) and (6) examining their brains. Note that careful observation of behavioral variables – such as exercise and nutrition and sociality – might reveal lifestyle factors that influence the risk of deleterious late effects.

The transgenic mice (expressing Aβ, p-tau, α-synuclein, and maybe five other suspect proteins) may or may not live long enough to develop changes like those possibly seen in humans. The choice of strain may, by chance, be resistant to injury. Yet someone should start this study now.

2. Cross-Sectional Clinical Research to Test the Hypothesis That a Single Typical CBI May Cause Late Effects

Since monozygotic twins share a common genome and similar socioeconomic, developmental, and psychological backgrounds, the degree to which these factors contribute is greatly reduced.

(Suddath et al., 1990 [363])

As emphasized throughout this volume, it is almost fruitless to compare the long-term effects of identical concussions in two people. Too many pre-injury factors, including genes, epigenes, and environmental exposures, have made their brains different to regard those organs as comparable. Nor do identical brains exist. The chapter addressing *Why Outcomes Vary* (Chapter 7) explained that the phrase "identical twins" is poetic, not scientific. Despite the fact that (contrary to Suddath et al.'s cited assertion [363]) MZ human twins have rather different genomes and quite different brains, MZ twins perhaps represent our best chance of comparing genetically *similar* brains with and without a single CBI.

The Swedish health service has only been collecting universal health care records since 1964. Therefore, since the late effects of a single concussion perhaps require 10–80 years to exert their influence, it may be that too few MZ twins documented in early life to be discordant for concussion have lived long enough after injury for any difference to have appeared.

Again, admitting these limitations, one quick way to test the hypothesis that a single CBI sometimes causes late effects would be to contact Scandinavian MZ twins. One hopes to find a cohort discordant for concussions that occurred more than 30 years ago, and determine whether the concussed MZ twin exhibits the same or a different time-passing-related brain and behavior change compared with the non-concussed twin. A cheap and simple pilot approach: request that subjects complete a psychometrically robust self-rating scale of health and happiness, such as the Short Form 36 [364], or even Deiner's Satisfaction With Life Scale [365].[38] At a higher cost, one might scan the subjects, including structural imaging, immunological imaging (e.g., for tau), and functional imaging at rest and in response to behavioral probes – for instance, to assess the connectome, or the efficiency of information processing, or emotional regulation). The author cannot recommend traditional 20th-century desktop neuropsychological testing, since that is often insensitive to the effects of concussion. Yet some modern cognitive tests, for instance, those that measure response with millisecond temporal resolution, might complement other findings.

Fixing the Problem

Finally, what is the status of efforts to actually treat, or reverse, or at least mitigate the deleterious brain changes discussed in this chapter?

On the one hand, the editors of this volume have striven to retire the pre-1908 notions that first, a disease is the result of a single external cause and second, that any two people ever have the same disease. In a case of clinical CTE (or, for that matter, "Alzheimer's disease") there exists the same kind of melee between harmful and helpful forces as described for acute CBI. Tau oligomers are just part of a river of cascades. For instance, as mentioned above, evidence exists that the harm done by tau is associated with, and perhaps dependent upon, inflammatory change [148, 323, 327]. In addition, new evidence

---

[38] A typical post-concussion self-rating scale (e.g., the Rivermead) [366] may be less informative since it is heavily weighted toward symptoms that tend to vanish in the first year.

suggests that the harmful impact of tau may not be confined to neurotoxicity. Holleran et al. [367] acquired ten brains of persons pathologically diagnosed with "CTE." In 2017, based on 11.74-T high-resolution MRI, those authors reported that p-tau immunoreactivity correlated with axonal microstructural disruption. In other words, one biological cascade may involve p-tau oligomerization, facilitated by activated microglia and spread transsynaptically, both poisoning neurons (risking apoptosis) and degrading axons.

On the other hand, at the risk of implying that there is a single keystone bolstering the pathophysiology of so-called "Alzheimer's disease" and CBI and CTE, let us focus momentarily on tau oligomers.

Gerson et al. [169] helped to confirm that this molecular species is harmful. They found tau oligomers in the brains of patients with "Alzheimer's disease." They found tau oligomers in the brains of animals in two models of TBI. They isolated that TBI-induced tau and injected it into the hippocampi of mice without brain injuries that expressed human tau. The result: not only did this provoke cognitive deficits, but tau oligomers spread through the brain, for instance, to the cerebellum, "suggesting that tau oligomers may be responsible for seeding the spread of pathology post-TBI." They concluded, "Our results suggest that tau oligomers play an important role in the toxicity underlying TBI and may be a viable therapeutic target" (p. 2034).

Flashback to 2015. Castillo-Carranza et al. [368] reported an experiment with aged transgenic $APP_{K670L,M671N}$ Tg 2576 mice – rodents that overproduce and deposit $A\beta$ and produce p-tau but not tangles. Administration of a tau oligomer-specific monoclonal antibody removed tau oligomers and reversed a memory deficit.[39]

Flash forward to 2017. DeVos et al. [369] published a related report titled, "Tau reduction prevents neuronal loss and reverses pathological tau deposition and seeding in mice with tauopathy." Those authors advanced the narrative by injecting tau antisense oligonucleotides into the cerebrospinal fluid of transgenic mice engineered to overexpress human tau. Young mice receiving this novel treatment did not develop tau deposition. Astonishingly, in old mice already peppered with tau clusters, the clusters cleared, the mice lived longer, and their behavior improved. Pilot experiments in *Cynomologus* monkeys suggest equal efficacy in clearing tau from the CNS of primates. The senior author, Timothy Miller, was quoted as saying, "This compound may literally help untangle the brain damage caused by tau" [370].

The present author has seen promising animal models of treatment come and go for 30 years. One learns to curb one's enthusiasm pending stage III human trials. It is, however, impossible not to hope.

Conclusion

Readers need have no fear that the author's proposed nosology will be widely adopted in the foreseeable future. Even the self-evidently neutral and agnostic framework of time-passing-related brain change may piloerect someone's short

hairs. As discussed periodically in this volume, clinical medicine – including faith healing and witch doctoring – is under tremendous pressure to display confidence in the face of uncertainty. Biology keeps getting more complex and astonishing as we progress. Yet lazy eagerness for two-word diagnoses takes no holiday. Honestly stating, "Sorry, there is no way to know what factor had what effect on your brain's current condition, or even if we have discovered the most important post-concussive pathophysiological factors" is not mellifluous. Stating: "The National Institutes of Health could have started the proper studies to determine the late effects of concussion decades ago. They just didn't," does not inspire awe. Patients understandably wish for simple answers and pill-shaped solutions. Doctors understandably wish to project certainty and mastery. Science can shift paradigms – eventually. But (pending the composition of novel germ-line sonatas) not human nature.

All these barriers notwithstanding, the rough beast of precision medicine is slouching toward the National Institutes of Health to be born. At that point, acceptance of individuality and heterogeneity will begin to actualize the sensible concept of "disease" that Archibald Garrod so boldly promulgated in his 1908 Croonian lecture: dis-ease, loss of ease, will always and forever be a unique tapestry woven from the warp of biological change and the weft of a patient's nature [371–373].

A hundred years seems like a reasonable pause before Western medicine accepts the obvious. The author therefore predicts that, by 2118, doctors will be more comfortable with the fact that late effects of concussion are devilishly hard to isolate, are never just due to concussion, and are never the same in any two cases. Satisfying the fancier's plea for pigeon holes is not our first priority. In the final analysis, any agent that mitigates the ravages of time-passing-related brain change, or so-called "Alzheimer's disease," or so-called "CTE" – by any other name – will smell as sweet. Let us please figure out what helps.

References

1. Freibaum BD, Lu Y, Lopez-Gonzalez R, Kim NC, Almeida S, Lee KH, et al. GGGGCC repeat expansion in C9orf72 compromises nucleocytoplasmic transport. *Nature* 2015; 525: 129–33.
2. Stacey D, Ciobanu LG, Baune BT. A systematic review on the association between inflammatory genes and cognitive decline in non-demented elderly individuals. *Eur Neuropsychopharmacol* 2015; 27 (6): 568–88.
3. Mild Traumatic Brain Injury Committee of the Head Injury Interdisciplinary Special Interest Group of the American Congress of Rehabilitation Medicine. Definition of mild traumatic brain injury. *J Head Trauma Rehabil* 1993; 8: 86–87.
4. Bird A, Tobin E. Natural kinds. In: Zalta EN (ed.) *The Stanford encyclopedia of philosophy.* Stanford, CA. Updated 02/17/2017. Available at: https://plato.stanford.edu/entries/natural-kinds/.
5. Surján G. The cultural history of medical classifications. In: *Barriers and challenges of using medical coding systems.* 2011. Available at http://dare.uva.nl
6. Carroll L. What the tortoise said to Achilles. *Mind* 1895; 104: 691–693.

---

[39] At the same time, this therapy *increased* plaque deposition – more evidence that $A\beta$ plaques are hardly the cause of dementia.

7. James W. *Lecture 1: religion and neurology*. New York: Longmans, Green, 1902.

8. Mill JS. *A system of logic, ratiocinative and inductive: being a connected view of the principles of evidence, and the methods of scientific investigation*. London: John W. Parker, 1843.

9. Smith EE, Medin DL. *Categories and concepts*. Cambridge, MA: Harvard University Press, 1981.

10. Smith JD, Zakrzewski AC, Johnson JM, Jeanette C, Valleau JC. Ecology, fitness, evolution: new perspectives on categorization. *Curr Direct Psychol Sci* 2016; 25: 266–274.

11. Kruglanski AW, Webster DM, Klem A. Motivated resistance and openness to persuasion in the presence or absence of prior information. *J Pers Soc Psychol* 1993; 65: 861–76.

12. Webster DM, Kruglanski AW. Individual differences in need for cognitive closure. *J Pers Soc Psychol* 1994; 67: 1049–62.

13. Budner S. Intolerance of ambiguity as a personality variable. *J Pers* 1962; 30: 29–50.

14. Biasi V, Bonaiuto P, Levin JM. Relation between stress conditions, uncertainty and incongruity intolerance, rigidity and mental health: experimental demonstrations. *Health (N Y)* 2015; 7: 71.

15. Hochmann JR, Mody S, Carey S. Infants' representations of same and different in match- and non-match-to-sample. *Cogn Psychol* 2016; 86: 87–111.

16. Aristotle. Posterior analytics. 350 B.C. http://classics.mit.edu/Aristotle/posterior.html.

17. Hawley K, Bird A. What are natural kinds? *Philosoph Perspect* 2011; 25: 205–21.

18. Gandhi M. www.goodreads.com/quotes/31454-the-only-difference-between-man-and-man-all-the-world.

19. Quran. Surah Al-Baqarah [verse 187].

20. Perusini G. Über klinisch und histologisch eigenartige psychische Erkrankungen des späteren Lebensalters. *Histologische und Histopathologische Arbeiten*. Jena: Gustav Fischer Verlag Jena, 1909, pp. 297–351.

21. Darwin C. *The descent of man and selection in relation to sex*. London: John Murray, 1871, p. 6.

22. Freeman SH, Kandel R, Cruz L, Rozkalne A, Newell K, Frosch MP, et al. Preservation of neuronal number despite age-related cortical brain atrophy in elderly subjects without Alzheimer disease. *J Neuropathol Exp Neurol* 2008; 67: 1205–12.

23. American Psychiatric Association. *Diagnostic and statistical manual of mental disorders (DSM-5)*, 5th edition. Washington, DC: American Psychiatric Publishing, 2013.

24. Goldberg D. Plato versus Aristotle: categorical and dimensional models for common mental disorders. *Compr Psychiatry* 2000; 41: 8–13.

25. Schotte CK, Maes M. Descriptive diagnostic assessment of depression: categorical diagnosis, dimensional assessment, and instruments. *Acta Neuropsychiatr* 2001; 13: 2–12.

26. Rosenman S, Korten A, Medway J, Evans M. Dimensional vs. categorical diagnosis in psychosis. *Acta Psychiatr Scand* 2003; 107: 378–84.

27. Kraemer HC, Noda A, O'Hara R. Categorical versus dimensional approaches to diagnosis: methodological challenges. *J Psychiatr Res* 2004; 38: 17–25.

28. Huprich SK, Bornstein RF. Dimensional versus categorical personality disorder diagnosis: implications from and for psychological assessment. *J Pers Assess* 2007; 89: 1–2.

29. Abrams DJ, Rojas DC, Arciniegas DB. Is schizoaffective disorder a distinct categorical diagnosis? A critical review of the literature. *Neuropsychiatr Dis Treat* 2008; 4: 1089–109.

30. McGrath RE, Walters GD. Taxometric analysis as a general strategy for distinguishing categorical from dimensional latent structure. *Psychol Methods* 2012; 17: 284–93.

31. De Beurs E, Barendregt M, Rogmans B, Robbers S, Van Geffen M, Van Aggelen-Gerrits M, et al. Denoting treatment outcome in child and adolescent psychiatry: a comparison of continuous and categorical outcomes. *Eur Child Adolesc Psychiatry* 2015; 24: 553–63.

32. Yee CM, Javitt DC, Miller GA. Replacing DSM categorical analyses with dimensional analyses in psychiatry research: the research domain criteria initiative. *JAMA Psychiatry* 2015; 72: 1159–60.

33. Heinz A, Schlagenhauf F, Beck A, Wackerhagen C. Dimensional psychiatry: mental disorders as dysfunctions of basic learning mechanisms. *J Neural Transm (Vienna)* 2016; 123: 809–21.

34. Hagele C, Schlagenhauf F, Rapp M, Sterzer P, Beck A, Bermpohl F, et al. Dimensional psychiatry: reward dysfunction and depressive mood across psychiatric disorders. *Psychopharmacology (Berl)* 2015; 232: 331–41.

35. Volkmar FR, McPartland JC. Moving beyond a categorical diagnosis of autism. *Lancet Neurol* 2016; 15: 237–8.

36. Khachaturian ZS. Diagnosis of Alzheimer's disease. *Arch Neurol* 1985; 42: 1097–105.

37. Best B. Mechanism of aging. 2016. www.benbest.com/lifeext/aging.html.

38. Bulterijs S, Hull RS, Bjork VC, Roy AG. It is time to classify biological aging as a disease. *Front Genet* 2015; 6: 205.

39. Kertzer DI. *Aging in the past: demography, society, and old age*. Berkeley, CA: University of California Press, 1995.

40. Weismann A, Poulton EB, Schönland S, Shipley AE. *Essays upon heredity and kindred biological problems, 2nd edition*. Oxford: Clarendon Press, 1891.

41. Medawar PB. *An unsolved problem of biology*. London: for the College by H.K. Lewis, 1952.

42. Williams GC. Pleiotropy, natural selection and the evolution of senescence. *Evolution* 1957; 11: 398–411.

43. Ungewitter E, Scrable H. Antagonistic pleiotropy and p53. *Mech Ageing Dev* 2009; 130: 10–17.

44. Alexander DM, Williams LM, Gatt JM, Dobson-Stone C, Kuan SA, Todd EG, et al. The contribution of apolipoprotein E alleles on cognitive performance and dynamic neural activity over six decades. *Biol Psychol* 2007; 75: 229–38.

45. Mondadori CR, De Quervain DJ-F, Buchmann A, Mustovic H, Wollmer MA, Schmidt CF, et al. Better memory and neural efficiency in young apolipoprotein E ε4 carriers. *Cereb Cortex* 2006; 17: 1934–47.

46. Han SD, Bondi MW. Revision of the apolipoprotein E compensatory mechanism recruitment hypothesis. *Alzheimers Dement* 2008; 4: 251–4.

47. Zetterberg H, Alexander DM, Spandidos DA, Blennow K. Additional evidence for antagonistic pleiotropic effects of APOE. *Alzheimers Dement* 2009; 5: 75.

48. Tuminello ER, Han SD. The apolipoprotein E antagonistic pleiotropy hypothesis: review and recommendations. *Int J Alzheimers Dis* 2011; 2011.

49. Jochemsen HM, Muller M, Van Der Graaf Y, Geerlings MI. APOE ε4 differentially influences change in memory performance depending on age. The SMART-MR study. *Neurobiol Aging* 2012; 33 (832): e15–e22.

50. Jasienska G, Ellison PT, Galbarczyk A, Jasienski M, Kalemba-Drozdz M, Kapiszewska M, et al. Apolipoprotein E (ApoE) polymorphism is related to differences in potential fertility in women: a case of antagonistic pleiotropy? *Proc R Soc Lond B: Biol Sci* 2015; 282: 20142395.

51. Kirkwood TB. Evolution of ageing. *Nature* 1977; 270: 301–4.

52. Libertini G. An adaptive theory of increasing mortality with increasing chronological age in populations in the wild. *J Theor Biol* 1988; 132: 145–62.

545

53. Libertini G. Empirical evidence for various evolutionary hypotheses on species demonstrating increasing mortality with increasing chronological age in the wild. *Sci World J* 2008; 8: 182–93.

54. Libertini G. Phylogeny of age-related fitness decline in the wild and of related phenomena. *Evol Interpret Aging, Dis Phenom Sex* 2011; 92.

55. Skulachev VP. Aging is a specific biological function rather than the result of a disorder in complex living systems: biochemical evidence in support of Weismann's hypothesis. *Biochem N Y–Engl Transl Biokhimiya* 1997; 62: 1191–5.

56. Skulachev VP. Phenoptosis: programmed death of an organism. *Biochemistry (Mosc)* 1999; 64: 1418–26.

57. Mitteldorf J. Ageing selected for its own sake. *Evol Ecol Res* 2004; 6: 937–53.

58. Mitteldorf J. Chaotic population dynamics and the evolution of ageing. *Evol Ecol Res* 2006; 8: 561–74.

59. Goldsmith TC. Aging, evolvability, and the individual benefit requirement; medical implications of aging theory controversies. *J Theor Biol* 2008; 252: 764–8.

60. Goldsmith TC. The case for programmed mammal aging. *Russ J Gen Chem* 2010; 80: 1434–46.

61. Goldsmith TC. Arguments against non-programmed aging theories. *Biochemistry (Mosc)* 2013; 78: 971–8.

62. Goldsmith TC. Modern evolutionary mechanics theories and resolving the programmed/non-programmed aging controversy. *Biochemistry (Mosc)* 2014; 79: 1049–55.

63. Goldsmith TC. Is the evolutionary programmed/non-programmed aging argument moot? *Curr Aging Sci* 2015; 8: 41–5.

64. Goldsmith TC. Solving the programmed/non-programmed aging conundrum. *Curr Aging Sci* 2015; 8: 34–40.

65. Mitteldorf J, Pepper J. Senescence as an adaptation to limit the spread of disease. *J Theor Biol* 2009; 260: 186–95.

66. Mitteldorf J, Martins AC. Programmed life span in the context of evolvability. *Am Nat* 2014; 184: 289–302.

67. Kirkwood TB, Holliday R. The evolution of ageing and longevity. *Proc R Soc Lond B Biol Sci* 1979; 205: 531–46.

68. Kirkwood TBL, Holliday R. Ageing as a consequence of natural selection. In Collins AJ, Bittles AH, editors. *The biology of human ageing*, pp. 1–16. Cambridge, UK: Cambridge University Press, 1986.

69. Hayflick L. Theories of biological aging. *Exp Gerontol* 1985; 20: 145–59.

70. Hayflick L, Kirkwood T. How and why we age. *Nature* 1995; 373: 484.

71. Hayflick L. Biological aging is no longer an unsolved problem. *Ann N Y Acad Sci* 2007; 1100: 1–13.

72. Kirkwood TB, Rose MR. Evolution of senescence: late survival sacrificed for reproduction. *Philos Trans R Soc Lond B Biol Sci* 1991; 332: 15–24.

73. Weinert BT, Timiras PS. Invited review: theories of aging. *J Appl Physiol (1985)* 2003; 95: 1706–16.

74. Austad SN. Is aging programed? *Aging Cell* 2004; 3: 249–51.

75. Kirkwood TB, Melov S. On the programmed/non-programmed nature of ageing within the life history. *Curr Biol* 2011; 21: R701–7.

76. De Grey AD. Do we have genes that exist to hasten aging? New data, new arguments, but the answer is still no. *Curr Aging Sci* 2015; 8: 24–33.

77. Kowald A, Kirkwood TB. Can aging be programmed? A critical literature review. *Aging Cell* 2016; doi: 10.1111/acel.12510.

78. Kovacs GG. Molecular pathological classification of neurodegenerative diseases: turning towards precision medicine. *Int J Mol Sci* 2016; 17: 189.

79. Jack Jr CR, Wiste HJ, Weigand SD, Knopman DS, Mielke MM, Vemuri P, et al. Different definitions of neurodegeneration produce similar amyloid/neurodegeneration biomarker group findings. *Brain* 2015; 138: 3747–59.

80. Mac Donald CL, Barber J, Andre J, Evans N, Panks C, Sun S, et al. 5-Year imaging sequelae of concussive blast injury and relation to early clinical outcome. *NeuroImage Clin* 2017; 14: 371–8.

81. Pakkenberg B, Gundersen HJ. Neocortical neuron number in humans: effect of sex and age. *J Comp Neurol* 1997; 384: 312–20.

82. Juraska JM, Lowry NC. Neuroanatomical changes associated with cognitive aging. *Curr Top Behav Neurosci* 2012; 10: 137–62.

83. Stadelmann C, Mews I, Srinivasan A, Deckwerth TL, Lassmann H, Brück W. Expression of cell death-associated proteins in neuronal apoptosis associated with pontosubicular neuron necrosis. *Brain Pathol* 2001; 11: 273–81.

84. Elmore S. Apoptosis: a review of programmed cell death. *Toxicol Pathol* 2007; 35: 495–516.

85. Serrano-Pozo A, Frosch MP, Masliah E, Hyman BT. Neuropathological alterations in Alzheimer disease. *Cold Spring Harb Perspect Med* 2011; 1: a006189.

86. Schuff N, Meyerhoff DJ, Mueller S, Chao L, Sacrey DT, Laxer K, et al. *N*-acetylaspartate as a marker of neuronal injury in neurodegenerative disease. In: Moffett J, Tieman SB, Weinberger DR, Coyle JT, Namboodiri AMA (eds) *N-Acetylaspartate: a unique neuronal molecule in the central nervous system.* New York: Springer; 2006, pp. 241–62.

87. Herculano-Houzel S. The human brain in numbers: a linearly scaled-up primate brain. *Front Hum Neurosci* 2009; 3: 31.

88. Von Bartheld CS, Bahney J, Herculano-Houzel S. The search for true numbers of neurons and glial cells in the human brain: a review of 150 years of cell counting. *J Comp Neurol* 2016; 524: 3865–95.

89. West MJ. New stereological methods for counting neurons. *Neurobiol Aging* 1993; 14: 275–85.

90. Cahalane DJ, Charvet CJ, Finlay BL. Modeling local and cross-species neuron number variations in the cerebral cortex as arising from a common mechanism. *Proc Natl Acad Sci* 2014; 111: 17642–7.

91. Barger N, Sheley MF, Schumann CM. Stereological study of pyramidal neurons in the human superior temporal gyrus from childhood to adulthood. *J Comp Neurol* 2015; 523: 1054–72.

92. Altman J. Are new neurons formed in the brains of adult mammals? *Science* 1962; 135: 1127–8.

93. Goldman SA, Nottebohm F. Neuronal production, migration, and differentiation in a vocal control nucleus of the adult female canary brain. *Proc Natl Acad Sci* 1983; 80: 2390–4.

94. Sohur US, Emsley JG, Mitchell BD, Macklis JD. Adult neurogenesis and cellular brain repair with neural progenitors, precursors and stem cells. *Philos Trans R Soc Lond B: Biol Sci* 2006; 361: 1477–97.

95. Drew MR, Hen R. Adult hippocampal neurogenesis as target for the treatment of depression. *CNS Neurol Disord Drug Targets* 2007; 6: 205–18.

96. Sierra A, Encinas JM, Maletic-Savatic M. Adult human neurogenesis: from microscopy to magnetic resonance imaging. *Front Neurosci* 2011; 5: 47.

97. Ugoya SO, Tu J. Bench to bedside of neural stem cell in traumatic brain injury. *Stem Cells Int* 2012; 2012.

98. Hoekzema E, Barba-Muller E, Pozzobon C, Picado M, Lucco F, Garcia-Garcia D, et al. Pregnancy leads to long-lasting changes in human brain structure. *Nat Neurosci* 2017; 20: 287–96.

99. Simerly RB. Wired for reproduction: organization and development of sexually dimorphic circuits in the mammalian forebrain. *Annu Rev Neurosci* 2002; 25: 507–36.

100. Sisk CL, Zehr JL. Pubertal hormones organize the adolescent brain and behavior. *Front Neuroendocrinol* 2005; 26: 163–74.

101. Peper J, Pol HH, Crone E, Van Honk J. Sex steroids and brain structure in pubertal boys and girls: a mini-review of neuroimaging studies. *Neuroscience* 2011; 191: 28–37.

102. Breitner JC. Dementia – epidemiological considerations, nomenclature, and a tacit consensus definition. *J Geriatr Psychiatry Neurol* 2006; 19: 129–36.

103. Hay J, Johnson VE, Smith DH, Stewart W. Chronic traumatic encephalopathy: The neuropathological legacy of traumatic brain injury. *Annu Rev Pathol* 2016; 11: 21–45.

104. Pinel P. *Nosographie philosophique, ou, La méthode de l'analyse appliquée à la médecine.* Paris: Chez JA Brosson, 1818.

105. Berrios GE. *The history of mental symptoms: descriptive psychopathology since the nineteenth century.* Cambridge, UK: Cambridge University Press, 1996.

106. Kraepelin E. *Psychiatrie – ein Lehrbuch für Studierende und Ärzte,* 8. Aufl I–IV. Leipzig: Barth1909, 1910, 1915.

107. American Psychological Association. Guidelines for the evaluation of dementia and age-related cognitive change. *Am Psychologist* 2012; 67: 1.

108. World Health Organization(WHO). *International statistical classification of diseases and related health problems,* vol. 10th revision. Geneva: WHO, 2011. Available at http://apps.who.int/classifications/icd10/browse/2016/en.

109. The European Dementia Consensus Network (EDCON). For whom and for what the definition of severe dementia is useful: an Edcon consensus. *J Nutrition Health Aging* 2008; 12: 714–719.

110. Wells CE. Dementia: definition and description. *Contemp Neurol Ser* 1977; 15: 1–14.

111. Feigenson JS. Definition of dementia. *Stroke* 1978; 9: 523.

112. Mesulam M-M. Dementia: its definition, differential diagnosis, and subtypes. *JAMA* 1985; 253: 2559–61.

113. Loo H, Plas J. Dementia – a semantic definition. *Gerontology* 1986; 32 (Suppl 1): 64–6.

114. Morris JC. The Clinical Dementia Rating (CDR): current version and scoring rules. *Neurology* 1993; 43: 2412–14.

115. Wallin A. Current definition and classification of dementia diseases. *Acta Neurol Scand Suppl* 1996; 168: 39–44.

116. Mitchell AJ, Malladi S. Screening and case finding tools for the detection of dementia. Part I: evidence-based meta-analysis of multidomain tests. *Am J Geriatr Psychiatry* 2010; 18: 759–82.

117. Walters GD. Dementia: continuum or distinct entity? *Psychol Aging* 2010; 25: 534.

118. Olde Rikkert MG, Tona KD, Janssen L, Burns A, Lobo A, Robert P, et al. Validity, reliability, and feasibility of clinical staging scales in dementia: a systematic review. *Am J Alzheimers Dis Other Dementias* 2011; 26: 357–65.

119. Slavin MJ, Brodaty H, Sachdev PS. Challenges of diagnosing dementia in the oldest old population. *J Gerontol A Biol Sci Med Sci* 2013; 68: 1103–11.

120. Katzman R, Aronson M, Fuld P, Kawas C, Brown T, Morgenstern H, et al. Development of dementing illnesses in an 80-year-old volunteer cohort. *Ann Neurol* 1989; 25: 317–24.

121. Graves AB, White E, Koepsell TD, Reifler BV, Van Belle G, Larson EB, et al. The association between head trauma and Alzheimer's disease. *Am J Epidemiol* 1990; 131: 491–501.

122. Williams D, Annegers J, Kokmen E, O'Brien P, Kurland L. Brain injury and neurologic sequelae: a cohort study of dementia, parkinsonism, and amyotrophic lateral sclerosis. *Neurology* 1991; 41: 1554.

123. Mehta KM, Ott A, Kalmijn S, Slooter AJ, Van Duijn CM, Hofman A, et al. Head trauma and risk of dementia and Alzheimer's disease: the Rotterdam Study. *Neurology* 1999; 53: 1959–62.

124. Plassman BL, Havlik RJ, Steffens DC, Helms MJ, Newman TN, Drosdick D, et al. Documented head injury in early adulthood and risk of Alzheimer's disease and other dementias. *Neurology* 2000; 55: 1158–66.

125. Starkstein SE, Jorge R. Dementia after traumatic brain injury. *Int Psychogeriatr* 2005; 17 (Suppl 1): S93–107.

126. Kiraly MA, Kiraly SJ. Traumatic brain injury and delayed sequelae: a review – traumatic brain injury and mild traumatic brain injury (concussion) are precursors to later-onset brain disorders, including early-onset dementia. *Sci World J* 2007; 7: 1768–76.

127. Jawaid A, Rademakers R, Kass JS, Kalkonde Y, Schulz PE. Traumatic brain injury may increase the risk for frontotemporal dementia through reduced progranulin. *Neurodegen Dis* 2009; 6: 219–20.

128. Dams-O'Connor K, Gibbons LE, Bowen JD, McCurry SM, Larson EB, Crane PK. Risk for late-life re-injury, dementia and death among individuals with traumatic brain injury: a population-based study. *J Neurol Neurosurg Psychiatry* 2013; 84: 177–82.

129. Smith DH, Johnson VE, Stewart W. Chronic neuropathologies of single and repetitive TBI: substrates of dementia? *Nat Rev Neurol* 2013; 9: 211.

130. Barnes DE, Kaup A, Kirby KA, Byers AL, Diaz-Arrastia R, Yaffe K. Traumatic brain injury and risk of dementia in older veterans. *Neurology* 2014; 83: 312–19.

131. Gardner RC, Burke JF, Nettiksimmons J, Kaup A, Barnes DE, Yaffe K. Dementia risk after traumatic brain injury vs nonbrain trauma: the role of age and severity. *JAMA Neurol* 2014; 71: 1490–7.

132. Vincent AS, Roebuck-Spencer TM, Cernich A. Cognitive changes and dementia risk after traumatic brain injury: implications for aging military personnel. *Alzheimers Dement* 2014; 10: S174–87.

133. Gardner RC, Yaffe K. Traumatic brain injury may increase risk of young onset dementia. *Ann Neurol* 2014; 75: 339–341.

134. Johnson VE, Stewart W. Traumatic brain injury: age at injury influences dementia risk after TBI. *Nat Rev Neurol* 2015; 11: 128–30.

135. Plassman BL, Grafman J. Traumatic brain injury and late-life dementia. *Handb Clin Neurol* 2015; 128: 711–22.

136. Crane PK, Gibbons LE, Dams-O'Connor K, Trittschuh E, Leverenz JB, Keene CD, et al. Association of traumatic brain injury with late-life neurodegenerative conditions and neuropathologic findings. *JAMA Neurol* 2016; 73: 1062–9.

137. Gilbert M, Snyder C, Corcoran C, Norton MC, Lyketsos CG, Tschanz JT. The association of traumatic brain injury with rate of progression of cognitive and functional impairment in a population-based cohort of Alzheimer's disease: the Cache County Dementia Progression Study. *Int Psychogeriatr* 2014; 26: 1593–601.

138. Sharp DJ. The association of traumatic brain injury with rate of progression of cognitive and functional impairment in a population-based cohort of Alzheimer's disease: the Cache County dementia progression study by Gilbert et al. Late effects of traumatic brain injury on dementia progression. *Int Psychogeriatr* 2014; 26: 1591–2.

139. Stoner CR, Orrell M, Spector A. Review of positive psychology outcome measures for chronic illness, traumatic brain injury and older adults: adaptability in dementia? *Dement Geriatr Cogn Disord* 2015; 40: 340–57.

140. Wang HK, Lee YC, Huang CY, Liliang PC, Lu K, Chen HJ, Li YC, Tsai KJ. Traumatic brain injury causes frontotemporal dementia and TDP-43 proteolysis. *Neuroscience* 2015; 300: 94–103.

141. Gavett BE, Stern RA, McKee AC. Chronic traumatic encephalopathy: a potential late effect of sport-related concussive and subconcussive head trauma. *Clin Sports Med* 2011; 30: 179–88.

142. Omalu B, Bailes J, Hamilton RL, Kamboh MI, Hammers J, Case M, et al. Emerging histomorphologic phenotypes of chronic traumatic encephalopathy in American athletes. *Neurosurgery* 2011; 69: 173–83.

143. McKee AC, Stern RA, Nowinski CJ, Stein TD, Alvarez VE, Daneshvar DH, et al. The spectrum of disease in chronic traumatic encephalopathy. *Brain* 2013; 136: 43–64.

144. Mez J, Stern RA, McKee AC. Chronic traumatic encephalopathy: where are we and where are we going? *Curr Neurol Neurosci Rep* 2013; 13: 407.

145. Stein TD, Alvarez VE, McKee AC. Chronic traumatic encephalopathy: a spectrum of neuropathological changes following repetitive brain trauma in athletes and military personnel. *Alzheimers Res Ther* 2014; 6: 4.

146. Castellani RJ. Chronic traumatic encephalopathy: a paradigm in search of evidence? *Lab Invest* 2015; 95: 576–84.

147. Daneshvar DH, Goldstein LE, Kiernan PT, Stein TD, McKee AC. Post-traumatic neurodegeneration and chronic traumatic encephalopathy. *Mol Cell Neurosci* 2015; 66: 81–90.

148. Faden AI, Loane DJ. Chronic neurodegeneration after traumatic brain injury: Alzheimer disease, chronic traumatic encephalopathy, or persistent neuroinflammation? *Neurotherapeutics* 2015; 12: 143–50.

149. Zhang Q-G, Laird MD, Han D, Nguyen K, Scott E, Dong Y, et al. Critical role of NADPH oxidase in neuronal oxidative damage and microglia activation following traumatic brain injury. *PLoS One* 2012; 7: e34504.

150. Elder GA, Gama Sosa MA, De Gasperi R, Stone JR, Dickstein DL, Haghighi F, et al. Vascular and inflammatory factors in the pathophysiology of blast-induced brain injury. *Front Neurol* 2015; 6: 48.

151. Collins-Praino LE, Corrigan F. Does neuroinflammation drive the relationship between tau hyperphosphorylation and dementia development following traumatic brain injury? *Brain Behav Immun* 2017; 60: 369–82.

152. Kumar A, Stoica BA, Loane DJ, Yang M, Abulwerdi G, Khan N, et al. Microglial-derived microparticles mediate neuroinflammation after traumatic brain injury. *J Neuroinflamm* 2017; 14: 47.

153. Lagraoui M, Sukumar G, Latoche JR, Maynard SK, Dalgard CL, Schaefer BC. Salsalate treatment following traumatic brain injury reduces inflammation and promotes a neuroprotective and neurogenic transcriptional response with concomitant functional recovery. *Brain Behav Immun* 2017; 61: 96–109.

154. Simon DW, McGeachy MJ, Bayır H, Clark RS, Loane DJ, Kochanek PM. The far-reaching scope of neuroinflammation after traumatic brain injury. *Nat Rev Neurol* 2017; 13: 171–91.

155. Logsdon AF, Lucke-Wold BP, Turner RC, Huber JD, Rosen CL, Simpkins JW. Role of microvascular disruption in brain damage from traumatic brain injury. *Comp Physiol* 2015; 5: 1147–60.

156. Andrews AM, Lutton EM, Merkel SF, Razmpour R, Ramirez SH. Mechanical injury induces brain endothelial-derived microvesicle release: implications for cerebral vascular injury during traumatic brain injury. *Front Cell Neurosci* 2016; 10.

157. Toth P, Szarka N, Farkas E, Ezer E, Czeiter E, Amrein K, et al. Traumatic brain injury-induced autoregulatory dysfunction and spreading depression-related neurovascular uncoupling: pathomechanisms, perspectives, and therapeutic implications. *Am J Physiol-Heart Circ Physiol* 2016; 311: H1118–31.

158. Salehi A, Zhang JH, Obenaus A. Response of the cerebral vasculature following traumatic brain injury. *J Cereb Blood Flow Metab* 2017; 37: 2320–2339. 271678X17701460.

159. Hay JR, Johnson VE, Young AM, Smith DH, Stewart W. Blood–brain barrier disruption is an early event that may persist for many years after traumatic brain injury in humans. *J Neuropathol Exp Neurol* 2015; 74: 1147–57.

160. Plog BA, Dashnaw ML, Hitomi E, Peng W, Liao Y, Lou N, et al. Biomarkers of traumatic injury are transported from brain to blood via the glymphatic system. *J Neurosci* 2015; 35: 518–26.

161. Nasser M, Bejjani F, Raad M, Abou-El-Hassan H, Mantash S, Nokkari A, et al. Traumatic brain injury and blood–brain barrier cross-talk. *CNS Neurol Disord-Drug Targets* 2016; 15: 1030–44.

162. Li W, Watts L, Long J, Zhou W, Shen Q, Jiang Z, et al. Spatiotemporal changes in blood–brain barrier permeability, cerebral blood flow, T2 and diffusion following mild traumatic brain injury. *Brain Res* 2016; 1646: 53–61.

163. Rodriguez-Rodriguez A, Egea-Guerrero JJ, Murillo-Cabezas F, Carrillo-Vico A. Oxidative stress in traumatic brain injury. *Curr Med Chem* 2014; 21: 1201–11.

164. Amorini AM, Lazzarino G, Di Pietro V, Signoretti S, Lazzarino G, Belli A, et al. Metabolic, enzymatic and gene involvement in cerebral glucose dysmetabolism after traumatic brain injury. *Biochim Biophys Acta* 2016; 1862: 679–87.

165. Besson VC. Drug targets for traumatic brain injury from poly(ADP-ribose)polymerase pathway modulation. *Br J Pharmacol* 2009; 157: 695–704.

166. Pu B, Xue Y, Wang Q, Hua C, Li X. Dextromethorphan provides neuroprotection via anti-inflammatory and anti-excitotoxicity effects in the cortex following traumatic brain injury. *Mol Med Report* 2015; 12: 3704–10.

167. Maneshi MM, Maki B, Gnanasambandam R, Belin S, Popescu GK, Sachs F, et al. Mechanical stress activates NMDA receptors in the absence of agonists. *Sci Rep* 2017; 7: 39610.

168. Sommer JB, Bach A, Mala H, Stromgaard K, Mogensen J, Pickering DS. In vitro and in vivo effects of a novel dimeric inhibitor of PSD-95 on excitotoxicity and functional recovery after experimental traumatic brain injury. *Eur J Neurosci* 2017; 45: 238–48.

169. Gerson J, Castillo-Carranza DL, Sengupta U, Bodani R, Prough DS, Dewitt DS, et al. Tau oligomers derived from traumatic brain injury cause cognitive impairment and accelerate onset of pathology in Htau mice. *J Neurotrauma* 2016; 33: 2034–43.

170. Edwards G, 3rd, Moreno-Gonzalez I, Soto C. Amyloid-beta and tau pathology following repetitive mild traumatic brain injury. *Biochem Biophys Res Commun* 2017; 483; 8: 1137–42.

171. Kriegel J, Papadopoulos Z, Mckee AC. Chronic traumatic encephalopathy: is latency in symptom onset explained by tau propagation? *Cold Spring Harb Perspect Med* 2017: a024059.

172. Madathil SK, Saatman KE. IGF-1/IGF-R signaling in traumatic brain injury: impact on cell survival, neurogenesis, and behavioral outcome. In: Kobeissy FH, editor. *Brain neurotrauma: molecular, neuropsychological, and rehabilitation aspects.* Boca Raton, FL: CRC Press, 2015, pp. 61–78.

173. Zheng P, Tong W. IGF-1: an endogenous link between traumatic brain injury and Alzheimer disease? *J Neurosurg Sci* 2017; 61: 416–21.

174. Rothman MS, Arciniegas DB, Filley CM, Wierman ME. The neuroendocrine effects of traumatic brain injury. *J Neuropsychiatry Clin Neurosci* 2007; 19: 363–72.

175. Simpkins JW, Yang S-H, Sarkar SN, Pearce V. Estrogen actions on mitochondria – physiological and pathological implications. *Mol Cell Endocrinol* 2008; 290: 51–9.

176. Srinivasan L, Roberts B, Bushnik T, Englander J, Spain DA, Steinberg GK, et al. The impact of hypopituitarism on function and performance in subjects with recent history of traumatic brain injury and aneurysmal subarachnoid haemorrhage. *Brain Inj* 2009; 23: 639–48.

177. Wilkinson CW, Pagulayan KF, Petrie EC, Mayer CL, Colasurdo EA, Shofer JB, et al. High prevalence of chronic pituitary and

target-organ hormone abnormalities after blast-related mild traumatic brain injury. *Front Neurol* 2012; 3: 11.

178. Haghighi F, Ge Y, Chen S, Xin Y, Umali MU, De Gasperi R, et al. Neuronal DNA methylation profiling of blast-related traumatic brain injury. *J Neurotrauma* 2015; 32: 1200–9.

179. Wang X, Seekaew P, Gao X, Chen J. Traumatic brain injury stimulates neural stem cell proliferation via mammalian target of rapamycin signaling pathway activation. *eneuro* 2016; 3: ENEURO. 0162-16.2016.

180. Buchman AS, Yu L, Boyle PA, Schneider JA, De Jager PL, Bennett DA. Higher brain BDNF gene expression is associated with slower cognitive decline in older adults. *Neurology* 2016; 86: 735–41.

181. Corrigan F, Arulsamy A, Teng J, Collins-Praino LE. Pumping the brakes: neurotrophic factors for the prevention of cognitive impairment and dementia after traumatic brain injury. *J Neurotrauma* 2017; 34: 971–86.

182. Iliff JJ, Chen MJ, Plog BA, Zeppenfeld DM, Soltero M, Yang L, et al. Impairment of glymphatic pathway function promotes tau pathology after traumatic brain injury. *J Neurosci* 2014; 34: 16180–93.

183. Simon MJ, Iliff JJ. Regulation of cerebrospinal fluid (CSF) flow in neurodegenerative, neurovascular and neuroinflammatory disease. *Biochim Biophys Acta* 2016; 1862: 442–51.

184. Jaarsma D, Van Der Pluijm I, De Waard MC, Haasdijk ED, Brandt R, Vermeij M, et al. Age-related neuronal degeneration: complementary roles of nucleotide excision repair and transcription-coupled repair in preventing neuropathology. *PLoS Genet* 2011; 7: e1002405.

185. Wurzelmann M, Romeika J, Sun D. Therapeutic potential of brain-derived neurotrophic factor (BDNF) and a small molecular mimics of BDNF for traumatic brain injury. *Neural Regener Res* 2017; 12: 7.

186. Bonilha L, Jensen JH, Baker N, Breedlove J, Nesland T, Lin JJ, et al. The brain connectome as a personalized biomarker of seizure outcomes after temporal lobectomy. *Neurology* 2015; 84: 1846–53.

187. Bianciardi M, Toschi N, Eichner C, Polimeni JR, Setsompop K, Brown EN, et al. In vivo functional connectome of human brainstem nuclei of the ascending arousal, autonomic, and motor systems by high spatial resolution 7-Tesla fMRI. *MAGMA* 2016; 29: 451–62.

188. Folstein MF, Folstein SE, Mchugh PR. "Mini-mental state". A practical method for grading the cognitive state of patients for the clinician. *J Psychiatr Res* 1975; 12: 189–98.

189. Wolf-Klein GP, Silverstone FA, Levy AP, Brod MS. Screening for Alzheimer's disease by clock drawing. *J Am Geriatr Soc* 1989; 37: 730–4.

190. Nasreddine ZS, Phillips NA, Bédirian V, Charbonneau S, Whitehead V, Collin I, et al. The Montreal Cognitive Assessment, MoCA: a brief screening tool for mild cognitive impairment. *J Am Geriatr Soc* 2005; 53: 695–9.

191. Sheehan B. Assessment scales in dementia. *Ther Adv Neurol Disord* 2012; 5: 349–58.

192. Lin JS, O'Connor E, Rossom RC, Perdue LA, Eckstrom E. Screening for cognitive impairment in older adults: a systematic review for the US Preventive Services Task Force. *Ann Intern Med* 2013; 159: 601–12.

193. Roberts GW, Allsop D, Bruton C. The occult aftermath of boxing. *J Neurol Neurosurg Psychiatry* 1990; 53: 373–8.

194. Mortimer J, Van Duijn C, Chandra V, Fratiglioni L, Graves A, Heyman A, et al. Head trauma as a risk factor for Alzheimer's disease: a collaborative re-analysis of case-control studies. *Int J Epidemiol* 1991; 20: S28–35.

195. Fleminger S, Oliver DL, Lovestone S, Rabe-Hesketh S, Giora A. Head injury as a risk factor for Alzheimer's disease: the evidence 10 years on; a partial replication. *J Neurol Neurosurg Psychiatry* 2003; 74: 857–62.

196. Nordstrom P, Michaelsson K, Gustafson Y, Nordstrom A. Traumatic brain injury and young onset dementia: a nationwide cohort study. *Ann Neurol* 2014; 75: 374–81.

197. Alzheimer A. Uber eine eigenartige Erkrankung der Hirnrinde. *Allg Z Psychiatrie* 1907; 64: 146–8.

198. Stelzmann RA, Schnitzlein HN, Murllagh FR. An English translation of Alzheimer's 1907 Paper, "Uber eine eigenartige Erlranliung der Hirnrinde". *Clin Anat* 1995; 8: 429–431.

199. Alzheimer A. Über eigenartige Krankheitsfälle des späteren Alters. *Z gesamte Neurol Psychiatrie* 1911; 4: 356–85.

200. Alzheimer A. Ueber den Abbau des Nervengewebes. *Allg Z Psychiatrie* 1906; 63: 568.

201. Shanafelt TD, Boone S, Tan L, Dyrbye LN, Sotile W, Satele D, et al. Burnout and satisfaction with work–life balance among US physicians relative to the general US population. *Arch Intern Med* 2012; 172: 1377–85.

202. Busis NA, Shanafelt TD, Keran CM, Levin KH, Schwarz HB, Molano JR, et al. Burnout, career satisfaction, and well-being among US neurologists in 2016. *Neurology* 2017; 88: 797–808.

203. McKhann G, Drachman D, Folstein M, Katzman R, Price D, Stadlan EM. Clinical diagnosis of Alzheimer's disease: report of the NINCDS-ADRDA Work Group under the auspices of Department of Health and Human Services Task Force on Alzheimer's Disease. *Neurology* 1984; 34: 939.

204. Mirra SS, Heyman A, McKeel D, Sumi S, Crain BJ, Brownlee L, et al. The Consortium to Establish a Registry for Alzheimer's Disease (CERAD): part II. Standardization of the neuropathologic assessment of Alzheimer's disease. *Neurology* 1991; 41: 479.

205. Mirra SS, Hart MN, Terry RD. Making the diagnosis of Alzheimer's disease. A primer for practicing pathologists. *Arch Pathol Lab Med* 1993; 117: 132–44.

206. The National Institute on Aging and Reagan Institute Working Group On Diagnostic Criteria for the Neuropathological Assessment of Alzheimer's Disease. Consensus recommendations for the postmortem diagnosis of Alzheimer's disease. *Neurobiol Aging* 1997; 18: S1–S2.

207. Hyman BT, Phelps CH, Beach TG, Bigio EH, Cairns NJ, Carrillo MC, et al. National Institute on Aging-Alzheimer's Association guidelines for the neuropathologic assessment of Alzheimer's disease. *Alzheimers Dement* 2012; 8: 1–13.

208. McKeel Jr DW, Price JL, Miller JP, Grant EA, Xiong C, Berg L, et al. Neuropathologic criteria for diagnosing Alzheimer disease in persons with pure dementia of Alzheimer type. *J Neuropathol Exp Neurol* 2004; 63: 1028–37.

209. Dubois B, Feldman HH, Jacova C, Dekosky ST, Barberger-Gateau P, Cummings J, et al. Research criteria for the diagnosis of Alzheimer's disease: revising the NINCDS–ADRDA criteria. *Lancet Neurol* 2007; 6: 734–46.

210. Dubois B, Feldman HH, Jacova C, Hampel H, Molinuevo JL, Blennow K, et al. Advancing research diagnostic criteria for Alzheimer's disease: the IWG-2 criteria. *Lancet Neurol* 2014; 13: 614–29.

211. Braak H, Braak E. Neuropathological staging of Alzheimer-related changes. *Acta Neuropathol* 1991; 82: 239–59.

212. Dubois B, Feldman HH, Jacova C, Cummings JL, Dekosky ST, Barberger-Gateau P, et al. Revising the definition of Alzheimer's disease: a new lexicon. *Lancet Neurol* 2010; 9: 1118–27.

213. Oksengard A, Cavallin L, Axelsson R, Andersson C, Nägga K, Winblad B, et al. Lack of accuracy for the proposed 'Dubois criteria' in Alzheimer's disease: a validation study from the Swedish brain power initiative. *Dement Geriatr Cogn Disord* 2010; 30: 374–80.

214. Wirth M, Madison CM, Rabinovici GD, Oh H, Landau SM, Jagust WJ. Alzheimer's disease neurodegenerative biomarkers are associated with decreased cognitive function but not β-amyloid in cognitively normal older individuals. *J Neurosci* 2013; 33: 5553–63.

215. Blessed G, Tomlinson BE, Roth M. The association between quantitative measures of dementia and of senile change in the cerebral grey matter of elderly subjects. *Br J Psychiatry* 1968; 114: 797–811.

216. Katzman R. Editorial: the prevalence and malignancy of Alzheimer disease. A major killer. *Arch Neurol* 1976; 33: 217–18.

217. Mendez MF. Early-onset Alzheimer's disease: nonamnestic subtypes and type 2 AD. *Arch Med Res* 2012; 43: 677–85.

218. Glenner G, Harbaugh J, Ohms J, Harada M, Cuatrecasas P. An amyloid protein: the amino-terminal variable fragment of an immunoglobulin light chain. *Biochem Biophys Res Commun* 1970; 41: 1287–9.

219. Glenner GG, Wong CW. Alzheimer's disease: initial report of the purification and characterization of a novel cerebrovascular amyloid protein. *Biochem Biophys Res Commun* 1984; 120: 885–90.

220. Hardy J, Allsop D. Amyloid deposition as the central event in the aetiology of Alzheimer's disease. *Trends Pharmacol Sci* 1991; 12: 383–8.

221. Selkoe DJ. The molecular pathology of Alzheimer's disease. *Neuron* 1991; 6: 487–98.

222. Hardy JA, Higgins GA. Alzheimer's disease: the amyloid cascade hypothesis. *Science* 1992; 256: 184–5.

223. Cárdenas-Aguayo MDC, Silva-Lucero MDC, Cortes-Ortiz M, Jiménez-Ramos B, Gómez-Virgilio L, Ramírez-Rodríguez G, et al. Physiological role of amyloid beta in neural cells: the cellular trophic activity. *InTech* 2014; 1–24.

224. Morley JE, Farr SA, Banks WA, Johnson SN, Yamada KA, Xu L. A physiological role for amyloid-β protein: enhancement of learning and memory. *J Alzheimers Dis* 2010; 19: 441–9.

225. Dawkins E, Small DH. Insights into the physiological function of the beta-amyloid precursor protein: beyond Alzheimer's disease. *J Neurochem* 2014; 129: 756–69.

226. Rajmohan R, Reddy PH. Amyloid-beta and phosphorylated tau accumulations cause abnormalities at synapses of Alzheimer's disease neurons. *J Alzheimers Dis* 2017; 57: 975–99.

227. Greenberg SM, William Rebeck G, Vonsattel JPG, Gomez-Isla T, Hyman BT. Apolipoprotein E ε4 and cerebral hemorrhage associated with amyloid angiopathy. *Ann Neurol* 1995; 38: 254–9.

228. Terry RD, Masliah E, Hansen LA. The neuropathology of Alzheimer disease and the structural basis of its cognitive alterations. *Alzheimer Dis* 1999; 2: 187–206.

229. Mega MS, Dinov ID, Porter V, Chow G, Reback E, Davoodi P, et al. Metabolic patterns associated with the clinical response to galantamine therapy: a fludeoxyglucose F 18 positron emission tomographic study. *Arch Neurol* 2005; 62: 721–8.

230. Aizenstein HJ, Nebes RD, Saxton JA, Price JC, Mathis CA, Tsopelas ND, et al. Frequent amyloid deposition without significant cognitive impairment among the elderly. *Arch Neurol* 2008; 65: 1509–17.

231. Jack Jr CR, Lowe VJ, Senjem ML, Weigand SD, Kemp BJ, Shiung MM, et al. 11C PiB and structural MRI provide complementary information in imaging of Alzheimer's disease and amnestic mild cognitive impairment. *Brain* 2008; 131: 665–80.

232. Sperling RA, Laviolette PS, O'Keefe K, O'Brien J, Rentz DM, Pihlajamaki M, et al. Amyloid deposition is associated with impaired default network function in older persons without dementia. *Neuron* 2009; 63: 178–88.

233. Forsberg A, Almkvist O, Engler H, Wall A, Langstrom B, Nordberg A. High PIB retention in Alzheimer's disease is an early event with complex relationship with CSF biomarkers and functional parameters. *Curr Alzheimer Res* 2010; 7: 56–66.

234. Hyman BT. Amyloid-dependent and amyloid-independent stages of Alzheimer disease. *Arch Neurol* 2011; 68: 1062–4.

235. Morris GP, Clark IA, Vissel B. Inconsistencies and controversies surrounding the amyloid hypothesis of Alzheimer's disease. *Acta Neuropathol Commun* 2014; 2: 135.

236. Karran E, De Strooper B. The amyloid cascade hypothesis: are we poised for success or failure? *J Neurochem* 2016; 139 (Suppl 2): 237–52.

237. Sakono M, Zako T. Amyloid oligomers: formation and toxicity of Ab oligomers. *FEBS* 2010; 277: 1348–1358.

238. Gadad BS, Britton GB, Rao K. Targeting oligomers in neurodegenerative disorders: lessons from α-synuclein, tau, and amyloid-β peptide. *J Alzheimers Dis* 2011; 24: 223–32.

239. Sell GL, Schaffer TB, Margolis SS. Reducing expression of synapse-restricting protein Ephexin5 ameliorates Alzheimer's-like impairment in mice. *J Clin Invest* 2017; 127: 1646–50.

240. Haass C, Selkoe DJ. Soluble protein oligomers in neurodegeneration: lessons from the Alzheimer's amyloid beta-peptide. *Nat Rev Mol Cell Biol* 2007; 8: 101–12.

241. Maruyama M, Shimada H, Suhara T, Shinotoh H, Ji B, Maeda J, et al. Imaging of tau pathology in a tauopathy mouse model and in Alzheimer patients compared to normal controls. *Neuron* 2013; 79: 1094–108.

242. Lloret A, Fuchsberger T, Giraldo E, Vina J. Molecular mechanisms linking amyloid beta toxicity and Tau hyperphosphorylation in Alzheimer's disease. *Free Radic Biol Med* 2015; 83: 186–91.

243. Selkoe DJ, Hardy J. The amyloid hypothesis of Alzheimer's disease at 25 years. *EMBO Mol Med* 2016; 8: 595–608.

244. Taipa R, Sousa AL, Melo Pires M, Sousa N. Does the interplay between aging and neuroinflammation modulate Alzheimer's disease clinical phenotypes? A clinico-pathological perspective. *J Alzheimers Dis* 2016; 53: 403–17.

245. Sarazin M, Berr C, De Rotrou J, Fabrigoule C, Pasquier F, Legrain S, et al. Amnestic syndrome of the medial temporal type identifies prodromal AD: a longitudinal study. *Neurology* 2007; 69: 1859–67.

246. Stones MJ. Aging and semantic memory: structural age differences. *Exp Aging Res* 1978; 4: 125–32.

247. Barbeau E, Didic M, Tramoni E, Felician O, Joubert S, Sontheimer A, et al. Evaluation of visual recognition memory in MCI patients. *Neurology* 2004; 62: 1317–22.

248. Ribeiro F, Guerreiro M, De Mendonça A. Verbal learning and memory deficits in mild cognitive impairment. *J Clin Exp Neuropsychol* 2007; 29: 187–97.

249. Kessels RP, Meulenbroek O, Fernández G, Olde Rikkert MG. Spatial working memory in aging and mild cognitive impairment: effects of task load and contextual cueing. *Aging Neuropsychol Cogn* 2010; 17: 556–74.

250. Fjell AM, McEvoy L, Holland D, Dale AM, Walhovd KB, Alzheimer's Disease Neuroimaging Initiative. What is normal in normal aging? Effects of aging, amyloid and Alzheimer's disease on the cerebral cortex and the hippocampus. *Prog Neurobiol* 2014; 117: 20–40.

251. Armstrong RA. On the 'classification' of neurodegenerative disorders: discrete entities, overlap or continuum? *Folia Neuropathol* 2012; 50: 201–18.

252. Jack CR, Bennett DA, Blennow K, Carrillo MC, Feldman HH, Frisoni GB, et al. A/T/N: an unbiased descriptive classification scheme for Alzheimer disease biomarkers. *Neurology* 2016; 87: 539–547.

253. Prescott JW, Guidon A, Doraiswamy PM, Roy Choudhury K, Liu C, Petrella JR. The Alzheimer structural connectome: changes

in cortical network topology with increased amyloid plaque burden. *Radiology* 2014; 273: 175–84.

254. Van Den Heuvel MP, De Reus MA. Chasing the dreams of early connectionists. *ACS Chem Neurosci* 2014; 5: 491–3.

255. Jack CR, Albert MS, Knopman DS, McKhann GM, Sperling RA, Carrillo MC, et al. Introduction to the recommendations from the National Institute on Aging-Alzheimer's Association workgroups on diagnostic guidelines for Alzheimer's disease. *Alzheimers Dement* 2011; 7: 257–62.

256. Mckhann GM, Knopman DS, Chertkow H, Hyman BT, Jack CR, Kawas CH, et al. The diagnosis of dementia due to Alzheimer's disease: recommendations from the National Institute on Aging-Alzheimer's Association workgroups on diagnostic guidelines for Alzheimer's disease. *Alzheimers Dement* 2011; 7: 263–9.

257. Visser PJ, Vos S, Van Rossum I, Scheltens P. Comparison of International Working Group criteria and National Institute on Aging–Alzheimer's Association criteria for Alzheimer's disease. *Alzheimers Dement* 2012; 8: 560–3.

258. Albert MS, Dekosky ST, Dickson D, Dubois B, Feldman HH, Fox NC, et al. The diagnosis of mild cognitive impairment due to Alzheimer's disease: recommendations from the National Institute on Aging-Alzheimer's Association workgroups on diagnostic guidelines for Alzheimer's disease. *Alzheimers Dement* 2011; 7: 270–9.

259. Sperling RA, Aisen PS, Beckett LA, Bennett DA, Craft S, Fagan AF et al. Toward defining the preclinical stages of Alzheimer's disease: recommendations from the National Institute on Aging-Alzheimer's Association workgroups on diagnostic guidelines for Alzheimer's disease. *Alzheimer Demen* 2011; 7: 280–292.

260. Chen M, Maleski JJ, Sawmiller DR. Scientific truth or false hope? Understanding Alzheimer's disease from an aging perspective. *J Alzheimers Dis* 2011; 24: 3–10.

261. Whitehouse PJ, George DR, D'alton S. Describing the dying days of "Alzheimer's disease." *J Alzheimers Dis* 2011; 24: 11–13.

262. Ferrer I. Defining Alzheimer as a common age-related neurodegenerative process not inevitably leading to dementia. *Prog Neurobiol* 2012; 97: 38–51.

263. Neill D. Should Alzheimer's disease be equated with human brain ageing? A maladaptive interaction between brain evolution and senescence. *Ageing Res Rev* 2012; 11: 104–22.

264. Burns JM, Bennett DA. Parsing the heterogeneity of mild cognitive impairment: lumpers and splitters. *Neurology* 2015; 85: 1646–7.

265. Mullane K, Williams M. Alzheimer's therapeutics: continued clinical failures question the validity of the amyloid hypothesis – but what lies beyond? *Biochem Pharmacol* 2013; 85: 289–305.

266. Drachman DA. The amyloid hypothesis, time to move on: amyloid is the downstream result, not cause, of Alzheimer's disease. *Alzheimers Dement* 2014; 10: 372–80.

267. Lambert JC, Ibrahim-Verbaas CA, Harold D, Naj AC, Sims R, Bellenguez C, et al. Meta-analysis of 74,046 individuals identifies 11 new susceptibility loci for Alzheimer's disease. *Nat Genet* 2013; 45: 1452–8.

268. Karch CM, Goate AM. Alzheimer's disease risk genes and mechanisms of disease pathogenesis. *Biol Psychiatry* 2015; 77: 43–51.

269. Mormino EC, Sperling RA, Holmes AJ, Buckner RL, De Jager PL, Smoller JW, et al. Polygenic risk of Alzheimer disease is associated with early- and late-life processes. *Neurology* 2016; 87: 481–8.

270. Morgan K. The three new pathways leading to Alzheimer's disease. *Neuropathol Appl Neurobiol* 2011; 37: 353–7.

271. International Genomics of Alzheimer's Disease Consortium. Convergent genetic and expression data implicate immunity in Alzheimer's disease. *Alzheimers Dement* 2015; 11: 658–71.

272. Van Der Zee J, Sleegers K, Van Broeckhoven C. Invited article: the Alzheimer disease–frontotemporal lobar degeneration spectrum. *Neurology* 2008; 71: 1191–7.

273. Duker AP, Espay AJ, Wszolek ZK, Rademakers R, Dickson DW, Kelley BJ. Atypical motor and behavioral presentations of Alzheimer disease: a case-based approach. *Neurologist* 2012; 18: 266–72.

274. Dohler F, Sepulveda-Falla D, Krasemann S, Altmeppen H, Schluter H, Hildebrand D, et al. High molecular mass assemblies of amyloid-beta oligomers bind prion protein in patients with Alzheimer's disease. *Brain* 2014; 137: 873–86.

275. Josephs KA, Murray ME, Whitwell JL, Parisi JE, Petrucelli L, Jack CR, et al. Staging TDP-43 pathology in Alzheimer's disease. *Acta Neuropathol* 2014; 127: 441–50.

276. Bettcher BM, Kramer JH. Longitudinal inflammation, cognitive decline, and Alzheimer's disease: a mini-review. *Clin Pharmacol Ther* 2014; 96: 464–9.

277. Kauwe JS, Bailey MH, Ridge PG, Perry R, Wadsworth ME, Hoyt KL, et al. Genome-wide association study of CSF levels of 59 Alzheimer's disease candidate proteins: significant associations with proteins involved in amyloid processing and inflammation. *PLoS Genet* 2014; 10: e1004758.

278. Nelson L, Gard P, Tabet N. Hypertension and inflammation in Alzheimer's disease: close partners in disease development and progression! *J Alzheimers Dis* 2014; 41: 331–43.

279. Steen E, Terry BM, Rivera EJ, Cannon JL, Neely TR, Tavares R, et al. Impaired insulin and insulin-like growth factor expression and signaling mechanisms in Alzheimer's disease – is this type 3 diabetes? *J Alzheimers Dis* 2005; 7: 63–80.

280. Candeias E, Duarte AI, Carvalho C, Correia SC, Cardoso S, Santos RX, et al. The impairment of insulin signaling in Alzheimer's disease. *IUBMB Life* 2012; 64: 951–7.

281. Ferreira ST, Clarke JR, Bomfim TR, De Felice FG. Inflammation, defective insulin signaling, and neuronal dysfunction in Alzheimer's disease. *Alzheimers Dement* 2014; 10: S76–83.

282. Honjo K, Black SE, Verhoeff NP. Alzheimer's disease, cerebrovascular disease, and the beta-amyloid cascade. *Can J Neurol Sci* 2012; 39: 712–28.

283. Kling MA, Trojanowski JQ, Wolk DA, Lee VM, Arnold SE. Vascular disease and dementias: paradigm shifts to drive research in new directions. *Alzheimers Dement* 2013; 9: 76–92.

284. Toledo JB, Arnold SE, Raible K, Brettschneider J, Xie SX, Grossman M, et al. Contribution of cerebrovascular disease in autopsy confirmed neurodegenerative disease cases in the National Alzheimer's Coordinating Centre. *Brain* 2013; 136: 2697–706.

285. Bangen KJ, Nation DA, Delano-Wood L, Weissberger GH, Hansen LA, Galasko DR, et al. Aggregate effects of vascular risk factors on cerebrovascular changes in autopsy-confirmed Alzheimer's disease. *Alzheimers Dement* 2015; 11: 394–403. e1.

286. Lee CW, Shih YH, Kuo YM. Cerebrovascular pathology and amyloid plaque formation in Alzheimer's disease. *Curr Alzheimer Res* 2014; 11: 4–10.

287. Tosto G, Bird TD, Bennet DA, Boeve BF, Brickman AM, Cruchaga C, et al. The role of cardiovascular risk factors and stroke in familial Alzheimer disease. *JAMA Neurology* 2016; 73: 1231–7.

288. Castellani RJ. Chronic traumatic encephalopathy: a paradigm in search of evidence? *Lab Invest* 2015; 95: 576–84.

289. McKee AC, Cairns NJ, Dickson DW, Folkerth RD, Keene CD, Litvan I, et al. The first NINDS/NIBIB consensus meeting to define neuropathological criteria for the diagnosis of chronic traumatic encephalopathy. *Acta Neuropathol* 2016; 131: 75–86.

290. Parker HL. Traumatic encephalopathy ('punch drunk') of professional pugilists. *J Neurol Psychopathol* 1934; 1: 20–8.

291. Figueira I, Fernandes A, Mladenovic Djordjevic A, Lopez-Contreras A, Henriques CM, Selman C, et al. Interventions for age-related diseases: shifting the paradigm. *Mech Ageing Dev* 2016; 160: 69–92.

292. Guskiewicz KM, Marshall SW, Bailes J, McCrea M, Cantu RC, Randolph C, et al. Association between recurrent concussion and late-life cognitive impairment in retired professional football players. *Neurosurgery* 2005; 57: 719–26.

293. Guskiewicz KM, Marshall SW, Bailes J, McCrea M, Harding HP, Jr., Matthews A, et al. Recurrent concussion and risk of depression in retired professional football players. *Med Sci Sports Exerc* 2007; 39: 903–9.

294. Lovell MR, Iverson GL, Collins MW, McKeag D, Maroon JC. Does loss of consciousness predict neuropsychological decrements after concussion? *LWW*; 1999; 9: 193–8.

295. Kelly JP. Loss of consciousness: pathophysiology and implications in grading and safe return to play. *J Athl Train* 2001; 36: 249–52.

296. Broglio SP, Cantu RC, Gioia GA, Guskiewicz KM, Kutcher J, Palm M, et al. National Athletic Trainers' Association position statement: management of sport concussion. *J Athl Train* 2014; 49: 245–65.

297. Scorza KA, Raleigh MF, O'Connor FG. Current concepts in concussion: evaluation and management. *Am Fam Physician* 2012; 85: 123–32.

298. Talavage TM, Nauman EA, Breedlove EL, Yoruk U, Dye AE, Morigaki KE, et al. Functionally-detected cognitive impairment in high school football players without clinically-diagnosed concussion. *J Neurotrauma* 2014; 31: 327–38.

299. Longhi L, Saatman KE, Fujimoto S, Raghupathi R, Meaney DF, Davis J, et al. Temporal window of vulnerability to repetitive experimental concussive brain injury. *Neurosurgery* 2005; 56: 364–74.

300. Tavazzi B, Lazzarino G, Amorini AM, Vagnozzi R, Signoretti S, Di Pietro V. Temporal window of metabolic brain vulnerability to concussion: a pilot 1H-MRS study in concussed athletes-part III. *Neurosurgery* 2008; 2008: 1286–95.

301. Maroon JC, Bailes J, Collins M, Lovell M, Mathyssek C, Andrikopoulos J, et al. Age of first exposure to football and later-life cognitive impairment in former NFL players. *Neurology* 2015; 85: 1007–10.

302. Stamm JM, Koerte IK, Muehlmann M, Pasternak O, Bourlas AP, Baugh CM, et al. Age at first exposure to football is associated with altered corpus callosum white matter microstructure in former professional football players. *J Neurotrauma* 2015; 32: 1768–1776.

303. Gysland SM, Mihalik JP, Register-Mihalik JK, Trulock SC, Shields EW, Guskiewicz KM. The relationship between subconcussive impacts and concussion history on clinical measures of neurologic function in collegiate football players. *Ann Biomed Eng* 2012; 40: 14–22.

304. Kerr ZY, Littleton AC, Cox LM, Defreese JD, Varangis E, Lynall RC, et al. Estimating contact exposure in football using the head impact exposure estimate. *J Neurotrauma* 2015; 32: 1083–9.

305. Greenwald RM, Gwin JT, Chu JJ, Crisco JJ. Head impact severity measures for evaluating mild traumatic brain injury risk exposure. *Neurosurgery* 2008; 62: 789–98; discussion 798.

306. Montenigro PH, Alosco ML, Martin BM, Daneshvar DH, Mez J, Chaisson CE, et al. Cumulative head impact exposure predicts later-life depression, apathy, executive dysfunction, and cognitive impairment in former high school and college football players. *J Neurotrauma* 2017; 34: 328–40.

307. Martland HS. Punch drunk. *JAMA* 1928; 91: 1103–7.

308. Critchley M. Punch-drunk syndromes: the chronic traumatic encephalopathy of boxers. In: *Hommage à Clovis Vincent*. Paris: Maloine; 1949, pp. 131–41.

309. Brandenburg W, Hallervorden J. [Dementia pugilistica with anatomical findings.] *Virchows Arch Pathol Anat Physiol Klin Med* 1954; 325: 680–709.

310. Corsellis JA, Bruton CJ, Freeman-Browne D. The aftermath of boxing. *Psychol Med* 1973; 3: 270–303.

311. Hof P, Knabe R, Bovier P, Bouras C. Neuropathological observations in a case of autism presenting with self-injury behavior. *Acta Neuropathol* 1991; 82: 321–6.

312. Geddes J, Vowles G, Robinson S, Sutcliffe J. Neurofibrillary tangles, but not Alzheimer-type pathology, in a young boxer. *Neuropathol Appl Neurobiol* 1996; 22: 12–16.

313. Geddes JF, Vowles GH, Nicoll JA, Revesz T. Neuronal cytoskeletal changes are an early consequence of repetitive head injury. *Acta Neuropathol* 1999; 98: 171–8.

314. Maroon JC, Winkelman R, Bost J, Amos A, Mathyssek C, Miele V. Chronic traumatic encephalopathy in contact sports: a systematic review of all reported pathological cases. *PLoS One* 2015; 10: e0117338.

315. Mez J, Solomon TM, Daneshvar DH, Stein TD, McKee AC. Pathologically confirmed chronic traumatic encephalopathy in a 25-year-old former college football player. *JAMA Neurol* 2016; 73: 353–5.

316. Victoroff J. Traumatic encephalopathy: review and provisional research diagnostic criteria. *NeuroRehabilitation* 2013; 32: 211–24.

317. Alosco ML, Mez J, Kowall NW, Stein TD, Goldstein LE, Cantu RC, et al. Cognitive reserve as a modifier of clinical expression in chronic traumatic encephalopathy: a preliminary examination. *J Neuropsychiatry Clin Neurosci* 2016; appi. neuropsych. 16030043.

318. Mez J, Daneshvar DH, Kiernan PT, Abdolmohammadi B, Alvarez VE, Huber BR, et al. Clinicopathological evaluation of chronic traumatic encephalopathy in players of American football. *JAMA* 2017; 318(4): 360–70.

319. Puvenna V, Engeler M, Banjara M, Brennan C, Schreiber P, Dadas A, et al. Is phosphorylated tau unique to chronic traumatic encephalopathy? Phosphorylated tau in epileptic brain and chronic traumatic encephalopathy. *Brain Res* 2016; 1630: 225–40.

320. Bieniek KF, Ross OA, Cormier KA, Walton RL, Soto-Ortolaza A, Johnston AE, et al. Chronic traumatic encephalopathy pathology in a neurodegenerative disorders brain bank. *Acta Neuropathol* 2015; 130: 877–89.

321. Castellani RJ, Perry G, Iverson GL. Chronic effects of mild neurotrauma: putting the cart before the horse? *J Neuropathol Exp Neurol* 2015; 74: 493–9.

322. Stein TD, Montenigro PH, Alvarez VE, Xia W, Crary JF, Tripodis Y, et al. Beta-amyloid deposition in chronic traumatic encephalopathy *Acta Neuropathol* 2015; 130: 21–34.

323. Cherry JD, Tripodis Y, Alvarez VE, Huber B, Kiernan PT, Daneshvar DH, et al. Microglial neuroinflammation contributes to tau accumulation in chronic traumatic encephalopathy. *Acta Neuropathol Commun* 2016; 4: 112.

324. Uryu K, Chen X-H, Martinez D, Browne KD, Johnson VE, Graham DI, et al. Multiple proteins implicated in neurodegenerative diseases accumulate in axons after brain trauma in humans. *Exp Neurol* 2007; 208: 185–92.

325. Brody DL, Benetatos J, Bennett RE, Klemenhagen KC, Mac Donald CL. The pathophysiology of repetitive concussive traumatic brain injury in experimental models; new developments and open questions. *Mol Cell Neurosci* 2015; 66: 91–8.

326. Johnson VE, Stewart W, Trojanowski JQ, Smith DH. Acute and chronically increased immunoreactivity to phosphorylation-independent but not pathological TDP-43 after a single traumatic brain injury in humans. *Acta Neuropathol* 2011; 122: 715–26.

327. Johnson VE, Stewart JE, Begbie FD, Trojanowski JQ, Smith DH, Stewart W. Inflammation and white matter degeneration

persist for years after a single traumatic brain injury. *Brain* 2013; 136: 28–42.

328. Roberts G, Gentleman S, Lynch A, Graham D. βA4 amyloid protein deposition in brain after head trauma. *Lancet* 1991; 338: 1422–3.

329. Huber A, Gabbert K, Kelemen J, Cervos-Navarro J. Density of amyloid plaques in brains after head trauma. *J Neurotrauma* 1993; 10: S180.

330. Roberts G, Gentleman S, Lynch A, Murray L, Landon M, Graham D. Beta amyloid protein deposition in the brain after severe head injury: implications for the pathogenesis of Alzheimer's disease. *J Neurol Neurosurg Psychiatry* 1994; 57: 419–25.

331. Ikonomovic MD, Uryu K, Abrahamson EE, Ciallella JR, Trojanowski JQ, Lee VM, et al. Alzheimer's pathology in human temporal cortex surgically excised after severe brain injury. *Exp Neurol* 2004; 190: 192–203.

332. McKee AC, Robinson ME. Military-related traumatic brain injury and neurodegeneration. *Alzheimers Dement* 2014; 10: S242–53.

333. Johnson VE, Stewart W, Smith DH. Widespread tau and amyloid-beta pathology many years after a single traumatic brain injury in humans. *Brain Pathol* 2012; 22: 142–9.

334. Arai T, Hasegawa M, Akiyama H, Ikeda K, Nonaka T, Mori H, et al. TDP-43 is a component of ubiquitin-positive tau-negative inclusions in frontotemporal lobar degeneration and amyotrophic lateral sclerosis. *Biochem Biophys Res Commun* 2006; 351: 602–11.

335. Neumann M, Sampathu DM, Kwong LK, Truax AC, Micsenyi MC, Chou TT, Bruce J, Schuck T, Grossman M, Clark CM, et al. Ubiquitinated TDP-43 in frontotemporal lobar degeneration and amyotrophic lateral sclerosis. *Science* 2006; 314(5796): 130–3.

336. Mackenzie IR, Rademakers R. The role of TDP-43 in amyotrophic lateral sclerosis and frontotemporal dementia. *Curr Opin Neurol* 2008; 21: 693.

337. Amador-Ortiz C, Lin WL, Ahmed Z, Personett D, Davies P, Duara R, et al. TDP-43 immunoreactivity in hippocampal sclerosis and Alzheimer's disease. *Ann Neurol* 2007; 61: 435–45.

338. Higashi S, Iseki E, Yamamoto R, Minegishi M, Hino H, Fujisawa K, et al. Concurrence of TDP-43, tau and alpha-synuclein pathology in brains of Alzheimer's disease and dementia with Lewy bodies. *Brain Res* 2007; 1184: 284–94.

339. Schwab C, Arai T, Hasegawa M, Yu S, Mcgeer PL. Colocalization of transactivation-responsive DNA-binding protein 43 and huntingtin in inclusions of Huntington disease. *J Neuropathol Exp Neurol* 2008; 67: 1159–65.

340. Wegorzewska I, Bell S, Cairns NJ, Miller TM, Baloh RH. TDP-43 mutant transgenic mice develop features of ALS and frontotemporal lobar degeneration. *Proc Natl Acad Sci* 2009; 106: 18809–14.

341. Lagier-Tourenne C, Cleveland DW. Rethinking ALS: the FUS about TDP-43. *Cell* 2009; 136: 1001–4.

342. Ling S-C, Albuquerque CP, Han JS, Lagier-Tourenne C, Tokunaga S, Zhou H, et al. ALS-associated mutations in TDP-43 increase its stability and promote TDP-43 complexes with FUS/TLS. *Proc Natl Acad Sci* 2010; 107: 13318–23.

343. McKee AC, Gavett BE, Stern RA, Nowinski CJ, Cantu RC, Kowall NW, et al. TDP-43 proteinopathy and motor neuron disease in chronic traumatic encephalopathy. *J Neuropathol Exp Neurol* 2010; 69: 918–29.

344. Goodin DS, Ebers GC, Johnson KP, Rodriguez M, Sibley WA, Wolinsky JS. The relationship of MS to physical trauma and psychological stress: report of the Therapeutics and Technology Assessment Subcommittee of the American Academy of Neurology. *Neurology* 1999; 52: 1737–45.

345. Mendel K. Tabes und multiple Sklerose in ihren Beziehungen zum Trauma. *Neurol Ctrbl* 1897; 16: 140–1.

346. Dana CL. Multiple sclerosis and the methods of ecology. *Res Publ Assoc Nerv Ment Dis* 1922; 2: 43–8.

347. McAlpine D, Compston N. Some aspects of the natural history of disseminated sclerosis. *Q J Med* 1952; 21: 135–67.

348. Warren SA, Olivo SA, Contreras JF, Turpin KVL, Gross DP, Carroll LJ, Warren KG. Traumatic injury and multiple sclerosis: a systematic review and meta-analysis. *Can J Neurol Sci* 2013; 40: 168–76.

349. Goldacre MJ, Abisgold JD, Yeates DG, Seagroatt V. Risk of multiple sclerosis after head injury: record linkage study. *J Neurol Neurosurg Psychiatry* 2006; 77: 351–3.

350. Pfleger CC, Koch-Henriksen N, Stenager E, Flachs EM, Johansen C. Head injury is not a risk factor for multiple sclerosis: a prospective cohort study. *Mult Scler* 2009; 15: 294–8.

351. Kang J-H, Lin H-C. Increased risk of multiple sclerosis after traumatic brain injury: a nationwide population-based study. *J Neurotrauma* 2012; 29: 90–5.

352. Lunny CA, Fraser SN, Knopp-Sihota JA. Physical trauma and risk of multiple sclerosis: a systematic review and meta-analysis of observational studies. *J Neurol Sci* 2014; 336: 13–23.

353. Siva A, Radhakrishnan K, Kurland LT, O'Brien PC, Swanson JW, Rodriguez M. Trauma and multiple sclerosis: a population-based cohort study from Olmsted County, Minnesota. *Neurology* 1993; 43: 1878–82.

354. Montgomery M, Hiyoshi A, Burkill S, Alfredsson L, Shahram Bahmanyar S, Tomas Olsson T. Concussion in adolescence and risk of multiple sclerosis. *Ann Neurol* 2017; 82: 554–61.

355. Lafrenaye AD, Todani M, Walker SA, Povlishock JT. Microglia processes associate with diffusely injured axons following mild traumatic brain injury in the micro pig. *J Neuroinflamm* 2015; 12: 186.

356. Constantine G, Buliga M, Mi Q, Constantine F, Abboud A, Zamora R, et al. Dynamic profiling: modeling the dynamics of inflammation and predicting outcomes in traumatic brain injury patients. *Front Pharmacol* 2016; 7: 383.

357. Corrigan F, Mander KA, Leonard AV, Vink R. Neurogenic inflammation after traumatic brain injury and its potentiation of classical inflammation. *J Neuroinflamm* 2016; 13: 264.

358. Naghibi T, Mohajeri M, Dobakhti F. Inflammation and outcome in traumatic brain injury: does gender effect on survival and prognosis? *J Clin Diagn Res* 2017; 11: PC06–9.

359. Mashkouri S, Crowley MG, Liska MG, Corey S, Borlongan CV. Utilizing pharmacotherapy and mesenchymal stem cell therapy to reduce inflammation following traumatic brain injury. *Neural Regen Res* 2016; 11: 1379–84.

360. Chen X, Wu S, Chen C, Xie B, Fang Z, Hu W, et al. Omega-3 polyunsaturated fatty acid supplementation attenuates microglial-induced inflammation by inhibiting the HMGB1/TLR4/NF-κB pathway following experimental traumatic brain injury. *J Neuroinflamm* 2017; 14: 143.

361. Lagraoui M, Sukumar G, Latoche JR, Maynard SK, Dalgard CL, Schaefer BC. Salsalate treatment following traumatic brain injury reduces inflammation and promotes a neuroprotective and neurogenic transcriptional response with concomitant functional recovery. *Brain Behav Immun* 2017; 61: 96–109.

362. Walker AE, Caveness WF, Critchley M. *The late effects of head injury*. Springfield, IL: CC Thomas, 1969.

363. Suddath RL, Christison GW, Torrey EF, Casanova MF, Weinberger DR. Anatomical abnormalities in the brains of monozygotic twins discordant for schizophrenia. *N Engl J Med* 1990; 322: 789–94.

364. Rand Health. 36-Item Short Form Survey Instrument (SF-36). 2017. Available from: www.rand.org/health/surveys_tools/mos/36-item-short-form/survey-instrument.html.

365. Diener E, Emmons RA, Larsen RJ, Griffin S. The Satisfaction With Life Scale. *J Pers Assess* 1985; 49: 71–5.

366. King N, Crawford S, Wenden F, Moss N, Wade D. The Rivermead Post Concussion Symptoms Questionnaire: a measure of symptoms commonly experienced after head injury and its reliability. *J Neurol* 1995; 242: 587–92.

367. Holleran L, Kim JH, Gangolli M, Stein T, Alvarez V, Mckee A, et al. Axonal disruption in white matter underlying cortical sulcus tau pathology in chronic traumatic encephalopathy. *Acta Neuropathol* 2017; 133: 367–80.

368. Castillo-Carranza DL, Guerrero-Muñoz MJ, Sengupta U, Hernandez C, Barrett AD, Dineley K, et al. Tau immunotherapy modulates both pathological tau and upstream amyloid pathology in an Alzheimer's disease mouse model. *J Neurosci* 2015; 35: 4857–68.

369. Devos SL, Miller RL, Schoch KM, Holmes BB, Kebodeaux CS, Wegener AJ, et al. Tau reduction prevents neuronal loss and reverses pathological tau deposition and seeding in mice with tauopathy. *Sci Transl Med* 2017; 9: eaag0481.

370. National Institutes of Health. Designer compound may untangle damage leading to some dementias. 2017. Available from: www.nih.gov/news-events/news-releases/designer-compound-may-untangle-damage-leading-some-dementias.

371. Garrod AE. The Croonian lectures on inborn errors of metabolism. Delivered before the Royal College of Physicians on June 18th, 23rd, 25th, and 30th. *Lancet* 1908; 172(4427): 1–7; 172(4428): 73–79; 172(4429): 142–148; 172(4430): 214–230.

372. Garrod AE, Harris H. *Inborn errors of metabolism.* London: Oxford University Press, 1909.

373. Scriver CR. Garrod's Croonian lectures (1908) and the charter 'Inborn Errors of Metabolism': albinism, alkaptonuria, cystinuria, and pentosuria at age 100 in 2008. *J Inherit Metab Dis* 2008; 31: 580–98.

Chapter

12

Functional Neuroimaging Markers of Persistent Post-Concussive Brain Change

Brian Johnson, Erin D. Bigler, and Semyon Slobounov

Although millions of individuals suffer a traumatic brain injury (TBI) worldwide each year, it is only recently that TBI has been recognized as a major public health problem. Beyond the acute clinical manifestations, there is growing recognition that a single severe TBI (sTBI) or repeated mild TBIs (rTBI) can also induce insidious neurodegenerative processes, which may be associated with early dementia, in particular chronic traumatic encephalopathy (CTE).

Johnson et al., 2017 [1], p. 383

Introduction[1]

Despite Harrison S. Martland's 1928 paper titled, "Punch Drunk," followed by Harry L. Parker's paper titled, "Traumatic Encephalopathy ('Punch Drunk') of Professional Pugilists" in 1934, as the 2017 quote by Johnson et al. implies, research on the late effects of traumatic brain injury (TBI) and the evolution of long-term sequelae resulting in traumatic encephalopathy is mostly a recent phenomenon. Renewed interest began with the Omalu et al. 2005 publication [2] of a National Football League (NFL) player with late effects of neurocognitive and neurobehavioral decline. Characterizing this as "chronic traumatic encephalopathy" or CTE, the study by Omalu et al. [2] launched an intense interest in studying the late effects of concussive brain injury (CBI) and issues that surround the CTE label [3]. Since the typical late onset of neurobehavioral and neurocognitive symptoms associated with CTE are quite distal from when the brain injury or injuries occurred, as described in Chapter 11, there has been considerable interest in the possibility that various types of neuroimaging may be relevant in the identification and clinical assessment of CTE [4]. Since these late effects from brain injury, including CBI, occur only after a period of time when the individual appears to have returned to some level of normalcy [5], the standard clinical indicia of acute TBI, such as loss of consciousness, duration of post-traumatic amnesia, neuroimaging indicators of edema, contusion, and blood byproducts, are not predictive of late effects. Hence, its association with neurodegeneration

has traditionally characterized CTE long after the TBI, where to date there is no "signature" neuroimaging abnormality that is specific to the condition. As such, there is no antemortem confirmation of CTE.

The "chronic" label begs a definitional statement and is part of the source of controversy associated with CTE [6]. While neuropathologists continue to define and debate CTE, as stated by Daneshvar et al. [7], the general agreed-upon pattern is that

> of progressive brain atrophy and accumulation of hyperphosphorylated tau neurofibrillary and glial tangles, dystrophic neurites, 43 kDa TAR DNA-binding protein (TDP-43) neuronal and glial aggregates, microvasculopathy, myelinated axonopathy, neuroinflammation, and white matter degeneration".
>
> (p. 81)

Complicating the classification issues with CTE are post-traumatic neurodegenerative changes that do not fit the diagnosis of CTE, the potential for what may be an adverse synergistic effect between injury and brain reserve, the fact that there are age-typical atrophic brain changes associated with aging and, the problem to date, that there are no definitive antemortem biomarkers of CTE, including neuroimaging. Nonetheless, given the neuropathological features just mentioned, it is anticipated that neuroimaging studies will indeed find associations that will have not only empirical but clinical relevance. In this chapter, both structural and functional neuroimaging will be overviewed in relation to

---

[1] In this chapter, which reviews numerous neuroimaging studies of concussive brain injury (CBI), terminology of how the original classification of the injured participants is often retained, including the mild traumatic brain injury (mTBI) classification. In the book, we attempted to use more uniformly the CBI term, but in chapters like this, where the term was not originally used, we often retained the original terminology.

Hypothetical network schematic

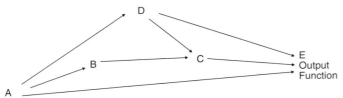

Fig. 12.1 The most simple and direct pathway from A to the location E output function is the direct A–E connection. There are no intermediary points and nothing to impede the connection if the direct pathway is patent. However, if the tracts connecting A to E were damaged or dysfunctional in some way, A remains connected to E, but all of the other connections require intermediate steps that will likely be slower, subject to other influences, and less efficient.

Source: Original

Table 12.1 Asymptomatic persistent brain change – concussive brain injury scenario I

Source	Method	Follow-up
Breedlove et al. [8]	fMRI	Unknown
Abbas K et al. [9]	rs-fMRI	Unknown
Provenzano et al. [10]	PET	Unknown
Coughlin et al. [11]	PET	7 years

fMRI: functional magnetic resonance imaging; PET: positron emission tomography; rs-fMRI: resting-stage functional magnetic resonance imaging.

late effects and CTE. Structural neuroimaging specifically examines anatomy and is therefore constrained by its reliance on detecting structural integrity. An anatomical structure may be "normal" in its size, shape, and overall appearance yet be physiologically impaired and/or not properly connected to other critically important brain regions. Given the limitations of structural neuroimaging, it may be that the combination of both structural and functional neuroimaging provides the best insights into the late effects of CBI. As such, this chapter deals with both types of neuroimaging.

The issue and complexity of this definitional problem, and how neuroimaging may assist in providing answers about CTE, are characterized in the following hypothetical scenarios of a five-year-old who falls from a swing and sustains a CBI. Three different outcomes will be discussed – scenarios I, II, and III. Obviously, there are more potential scenarios but for the sake of brevity, what follows is limited to just these three. To best understand this concept, we return to a network theory of "recovery" in TBI. There are certainly numerous networks at play for any particular cognitive function, where most neural networks that are not specific to a sensory or motor function have redundancies, parallel and back-up systems capable of adaptive responses if some aspect of a network is disrupted through injury. As a simplified example, in Figure 12.1 consider that the single synapse represents the most efficient connection from A to some output response (A–E output function), although other routes are capable of triggering the output function, but never as fast or efficient. However, as the result of a TBI, the single axon link mediating the direct A–E output connection is damaged, the alternate but multi-synaptic A–B–C–E output, A–D–C–E output, or A–D–E output remains to carry out the connection between A and the E output function. Again, assuming the least synaptic connections reflect the most efficient, the two-synapse, A–D–E output likely would be the fastest and most efficient. With just one additional synaptic connection, the A–D–E output connection spontaneously activates and quickly approximates the direct A–E output connection. The now activated A–D–E output connection might even be capable of functioning in a manner where the behavioral or cognitive output is *no* different from the original A–E output function connection.

In such a hypothetical case, even with permanent pathology in the A–E output connection, given the effectiveness of how

the A–D–E output connection has adapted, all neurocognitive and neurobehavioral relations associated with A return to baseline. Thus, with no observable outward change in function after a short recovery period, in this hypothetical scenario the individual goes on to live a life with no known untoward sequelae from TBI, even late in life. Nonetheless, hypothetically there may still be detectable pathology identifiable by neuroimaging, but it no longer adversely influences network functioning and efficiency or influential at the behavioral and cognitive level. As the first scenario, scenario I could be labeled "CBI but asymptomatic persistent brain change." Indeed, as shown in Table 12.1, there are neuroimaging studies that support this notion.

In the second scenario, the five-year-old has residual sequelae and the network does not fully adapt, adjust, or accommodate. Symptoms persist, say, mild inattentiveness. On complex measures of processing speed and attention, this child struggles and the problems become chronic. Returning to the network diagram in Figure 12.1, once the A–E output connection is damaged, none of the backup, secondary multi-synaptic connections are capable of precisely approximating pre-injury level function, but with time, education, maturity, and a supportive environment, effective compensation eventually occurs. The child goes on to live a productive life with no decline later in life. Just as in the first scenario, residual pathology hypothetically would be detectable by neuroimaging studies. In scenario II, the CBI results in symptomatic persistent brain changes, but they remain static and non-progressive, with minimal to no significant disruption in behavioral and cognitive functioning. As with scenario I, there are neuroimaging studies in support of this kind of consequence from CBI, as shown in Table 12.2.

However, the story is quite different for the third child – scenario III. Although the effects of injury may initially result in something very similar to the previous scenarios, after what appears to be recovery or adaptation and being asymptomatic for decades, neurobehavioral problems become evident. Something has interacted with the aging process and/or other genetic or constitutional factors where having experienced a CBI, late-onset post-traumatic neurodegeneration occurs in a manner that would not have happened had the CBI not occurred. What differs in scenario III is that there is delayed onset of symptoms after some period of either stable or symptom-free period. There is now a beginning literature to support this scenario as well, as shown in Table 12.3.

Table 12.2 Symptomatic persistent brain change – concussive brain injury scenario II

Source	Method	Follow-up
Kemp et al. [12]	SPECT	Unknown
Roberts et al. [13]	PET	4 years
Gross et al. [14]	PET	43 months
Peskind et al. [15]	PET	2–5 years
Amen et al. [16]	SPECT	unknown
Mendez et al. [17]	PET	~ 50 months
Tateno et al. [18]	PET	4 years
Chen et al. [19]	fMRI	Two cases: 12 and 14 months
Strigo et al. [20]	fMRI	4 years
Monti et al. [21]	fMRI	Years to decades
Dean et al. [22]	fMRI	> 12 months
Astafiev et al. [23]	fMRI	3 months to 5.5 years
Liu et al. [24]	ASL-fMRI	> 12 months
Astafiev et al. [25]	fMRI	3 months to 5.5 years
Bang et al. [26]	PET	22–30 years
Nathan et al. [27]	fMRI	~ 3 years

ASL-fMRI: arterial spin labeling functional magnetic resonance imaging; fMRI: functional magnetic resonance imaging; PET: positron emission tomography; SPECT: single-photon emission computed tomography.

Table 12.3 Delayed-onset persistent symptoms – concussive brain injury scenario III

Source	Method	Follow-up
Mitsis et al. [28]	PET	Unknown
Dickstein et al. [29]	PET	Unknown
Barrio et al. [30]	PET	Unknown

PET: positron emission tomography.

In each of these scenarios, there may be a meaningful neuroimaging finding. Indeed, Tables 12.1–12.3 highlight some of the recent work involving all three scenarios. Scenario I is that CBI results in detectable neuroimaging findings, which presumably do not relate to neurobehavioral and neurocognitive function and do not progress later in life. Scenario II reflects CBI that results in detectable neuroimaging findings that do relate to impaired neurobehavioral and/or neurocognitive function but stabilize and are non-progressive. Scenario III is that CBI results in detectable neuroimaging findings, which initially may or may not relate to neurobehavioral and/or neurocognitive functioning but later in life progress, where the location and degree of pathological changes do relate to the clinical presentation.

In this chapter we will review some of the neuroimaging findings to date on the late effects of CBI, including what has been published involving CTE, understanding that CTE remains a post-mortem neuropathological diagnosis with considerable heterogeneity of the neurobehavioral and neurocognitive phenotype, along with active debate about the topic [31, 32].

As shown in the Hiploylee et al. [33] investigation, since all participants in that study had negative computed tomography (CT) imaging, yet persisting symptoms that would be defined as chronic, CT is insensitive in detecting any consistent chronic effects from CBI. Later in this chapter we will overview some CT findings in boxers, but for the most part CT imaging will be negative in those meeting criteria for CBI. Likewise, even advanced structural neuroimaging of individuals with a history of CBI may have no findings [34]. Nonetheless, functional neuroimaging holds promise in the study of CTE but, given the three scenarios above, the time post injury, and the interaction effects with the brain's ability for adaptation and accommodation once injured, creates challenges in interpreting functional neuroimaging findings in TBI.

Considering that advanced neuroimaging and processing techniques such as positron emission tomography (PET), functional magnetic resonance imaging (fMRI), and resting-state (rs) functional connectivity fMRI (rs-fMRI) are relatively new, the literature of their use on persistent or progressive traumatic encephalopathy is limited at best. There are few dedicated neuroimaging studies specifically looking at CTE, and none to date that have systematically used fMRI techniques. However, given the speculation that CTE manifests in part due to repetitive brain trauma, whether it be full-blown concussive episodes or subconcussive trauma [35–37], there is functional neuroimaging literature showing detectable changes remote to the initial injury [38, 39]. Additionally, a genetic component or predisposition to chronic effects from CBI, potentially linked to the apolipoprotein E (APOE) gene [40] is an active area of research. In this chapter, we will focus on the structural and functional neuroimaging research associated with CBI as well as repetitive subconcussive head trauma, multiple concussive episodes, and the presence of the APOE ε4 allele.

At present, as already stated, CTE can only be definitively diagnosed postmortem [34] and to date the only information we have on clinical manifestations and symptomology of CTE has been through post-mortem pathological and retrospective studies of patient history [41–43]. These studies have documented a range of cognitive, behavioral, and emotional symptoms along with specific microscopic and gross neuropathological characteristics [44]. As already reviewed, a dominant microscopic feature is the accumulation of hyperphosphorylated tau proteins found in the abundance of neurofibrillary tangles along with global cerebral atrophy, ventricular enlargement, and cavum septum pellucidum [35, 41, 42]. As shown in Figure 12.2, cerebral atrophy, ventricular enlargement, and cavum septum pellucidum can all be identified via neuroimaging in a case of severe TBI, as can cortical thickness. For comparison purposes, a confirmed post-mortem CTE case is shown in coronal view compared to what can be visualized with MRI as well as to a healthy control.

Given what can observed from Figure 12.2, it might be expected that certain patterns of cortical atrophy along with abnormal uptake and distribution of radiotracers might relate to delayed outcome from TBI and the association with age-related degenerative changes. Accordingly, Wang et al. [45] have recently shown that in the open-source Alzheimer's Disease

Neuroimaging of chronic traumatic encephalopathy (CTE)

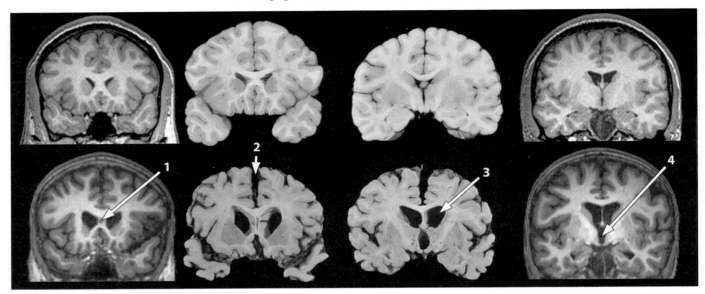

I. Amygdala and Dorsal Midbrain: core regions in (F-18]FDDNP PET

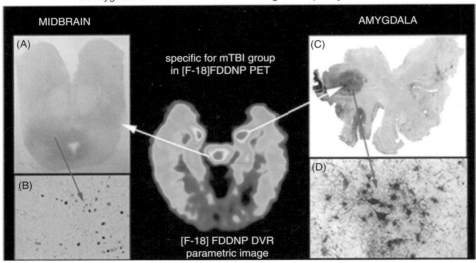

II. Robust tau IHC in amygdala and MTL is consistently present in symptomatic retired football players

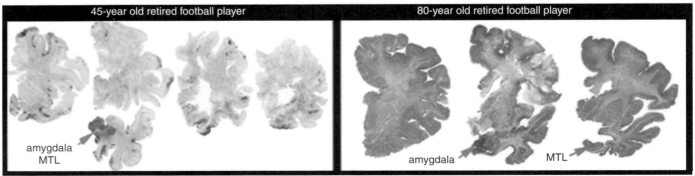

Fig. 12.2 (A) Top row: normal coronal image from magnetic resonance imaging (MRI) of a 14-year-old male (outer images on each side) at a similar level to a post-mortem coronal image of a healthy adult (middle images). Bottom row: similarly, coronal MRI (outer images on each side) at a similar level to a post-mortem severe stage IV CTE is shown, as evidenced by cavum septum pellucidum (1); severe cerebral atrophy (2); dilated lateral ventricles (3); and dilated third ventricle (4). Post-mortem images from Hurley D. Brain bank study of football players finds pervasive CTE, but true prevalence remains unknown. *Neurol Today* 2017; 17 (17): 1–27, reproduced with permission from Wolters Kluwer.
(B) Appearance of hyperphosphorylated tau aggregates within neurons and astrocytes (brown staining in panels A and B) clustered around small cortical vessels (arrows), characteristically in a patchy distribution toward the depths of the cortical sulci, is emerging as the distinctive pathology of CTE. This pathology appears to be virtually exclusive to circumstances in which there has been exposure to brain injury in life, whether as repetitive mild traumatic brain injury (TBI) as shown

Neuroimaging Initiative, wherein CSF tau had been obtained, those with self-reported mild TBI had reduced cortical volume in those considered to be in a "pre-clinical AD [Alzheimer's disease]" group. Since there are now PET-based tau detection techniques [46, 47], how this may relate to a neuroimaging procedure identifying CTE is coming under active investigation. Whether there is a neurobehavioral phenotype related to antemortem *in vivo* neuroimaging remains to be seen, but post-mortem studies to date have provided valuable information regarding the gross and microscopic characteristics of CTE and their accompanying behavioral correlates [42, 43, 48] (Figure 12.2).

Neuroimaging has been performed in a few reported case studies that have positively confirmed CTE by histological examination at autopsy [49, 50]. Utilizing structural MRI and single-photon emission computed tomography (SPECT), Handratta et al. [49] documented periventricular white-matter changes, severe cerebral atrophy, cavum septi pellucidi and cavum vergae, and widespread diffuse hypoperfusion in a 47-year-old male boxer. Raji et al. [51] report on a case of suspect CTE in a 51-year-old former high school football player with a history of multiple concussions that included one associated with loss of consciousness. Prior to neuroimaging studies being initiated in middle age, this former athlete began to display neurobehavioral sequelae, raising the specter of CTE. Sequential MRI studies demonstrated progressive atrophic changes in multiple areas, including brainstem, diencephalon, and frontal lobe. Coughlin et al. [11] examined PET imaging in active and recently retired NFL players using a special ligand ([11C]DPA-713) that is a marker of activated glial cell response [18 kDa (TSPO),], a presumed indicator of injured parenchyma. Two-thirds of the PET regions examined had increased volume of TSPO uptake. These observations suggest active brain injury and repair as part of a neuroinflammatory response. Interestingly, in these NFL players traditional neuropsychological measures were insensitive in detecting any differences between players and controls.

Gardner et al. [32] reported on structural MRI, fluorodeoxyglucose (FDG)-PET and amyloid PET neuroimaging findings in several NFL players who showed a broad spectrum of underlying neuropathologies.

Using [(18)F]-florbetapir PET imaging for amyloid plaque identification along with [(18)F]-T807 PET imaging, a new ligand binding to tau – the main constituent of neurofibrillary tangles, Mitsis et al. [52] compared a retired NFL player with history of multiple concussions to an individual with frontotemporal dementia, demonstrating how functional neuroimaging assists in the differentiation of the late effects of prior brain injury on the clinical diagnosis of dementia. In

this case the [(18)F]-florbetapir PET imaging was negative, essentially excluding Alzheimer's disease as a diagnosis in this 71-year-old retired NFL player. CTE was suspected clinically, and [(18)F]-T807 PET imaging revealed striatal and nigral [(18)F]-T807 retention consistent with the presence of tauopathy. Figure 12.3 shows the comparison of an NFL player with a healthy control in the study by Coughlin et al. [53], highlighting the presence of neuroinflammatory markers in the brain in those who were former NFL players.

Although not confirmed by autopsy when [F-18]FDDNP PET imaging was performed, Barrio et al. [30], who examined 14 American professional football players with suspect CTE, found a different pattern of pathology than observed in Alzheimer's disease. Uptake differences in those with suspect CTE were most notable within brainstem white-matter tracts presumed to undergo early axonal damage in those with CBI and cumulative axonal injuries along subcortical, limbic, and cortical brain circuitries supporting mood, emotions, and behavior. Figure 12.4 depicts various PET imaging findings of different degrees of pathology from an investigation by Barrio et al.

Despite these promising functional neuroimaging advances with CT-based PET imaging, there are many restrictions with this approach, including radiation exposure and cost. Because of the limitations with PET, considerable emphasis has been placed on MRI technology, including fMRI, which will be discussed in the next section.

Using fMRI to Study Chronic Effects of Brain Injury

As one of the more recent advances in neuroscience and neuroimaging, fMRI has grown in popularity and become a common non-invasive research tool to explore the brain [54]. The principle of fMRI is based upon the differences between oxyhemoglobin versus deoxyhemoglobin in the blood, and is known as the blood oxygen level-dependent (BOLD) contrast. This contrast stems from the fact that deoxyhemoglobin produces a larger local magnetic susceptibility. The BOLD signal is used as an index to infer neuronal activity as areas of the brain that require more oxygen due to activation increase their demand for oxyhemoglobin which in turn leads to higher signal intensity and less signal dephasing caused by the local field inhomogeneity's associated with deoxyhemoglobin [55]. The currently accepted notion is that BOLD fMRI most likely detects secondary effects of neuronal firing due to the hemodynamic response, allowing indirect assessment of the neuronal responses to cognitive and/or sensorimotor task demands [56]. A detailed explanation of fMRI principles, applications,

Fig 12. 2 (cont.)
in a 61-year-old male former boxer (A) or a single moderate or severe TBI as shown in a 48-year-old man with three years of survival after a single severe TBI (B). In addition to this distinctive tau pathology, neurodegeneration after TBI is increasingly recognized as a complex pathology, including abnormal amyloid plaque deposition (brown staining in panels C and D). As with tau, aspects of these pathologies can be recognized in brain samples from patients exposed to either repetitive mild TBI as shown in a 59-year-old male former soccer player (C) or a single moderate or severe TBI (D; same patient as in panel B). Phosphorylated tau was stained with antibody CP13 (A) or PHF-1 (B). Amyloid β was stained with antibody 6F3D (C and D). DVR: distribution volume ratio; IHC: immunohistochemistry; MTL: medial temporal lobe; PET: positron emission tomography. Adapted from Barrio et al. [30] (reproduced with permission from PNAS). [A black and white version of this figure will appear in some formats. For the color version, please refer to the plate section.]

Positron emission tomography findings in former American football player

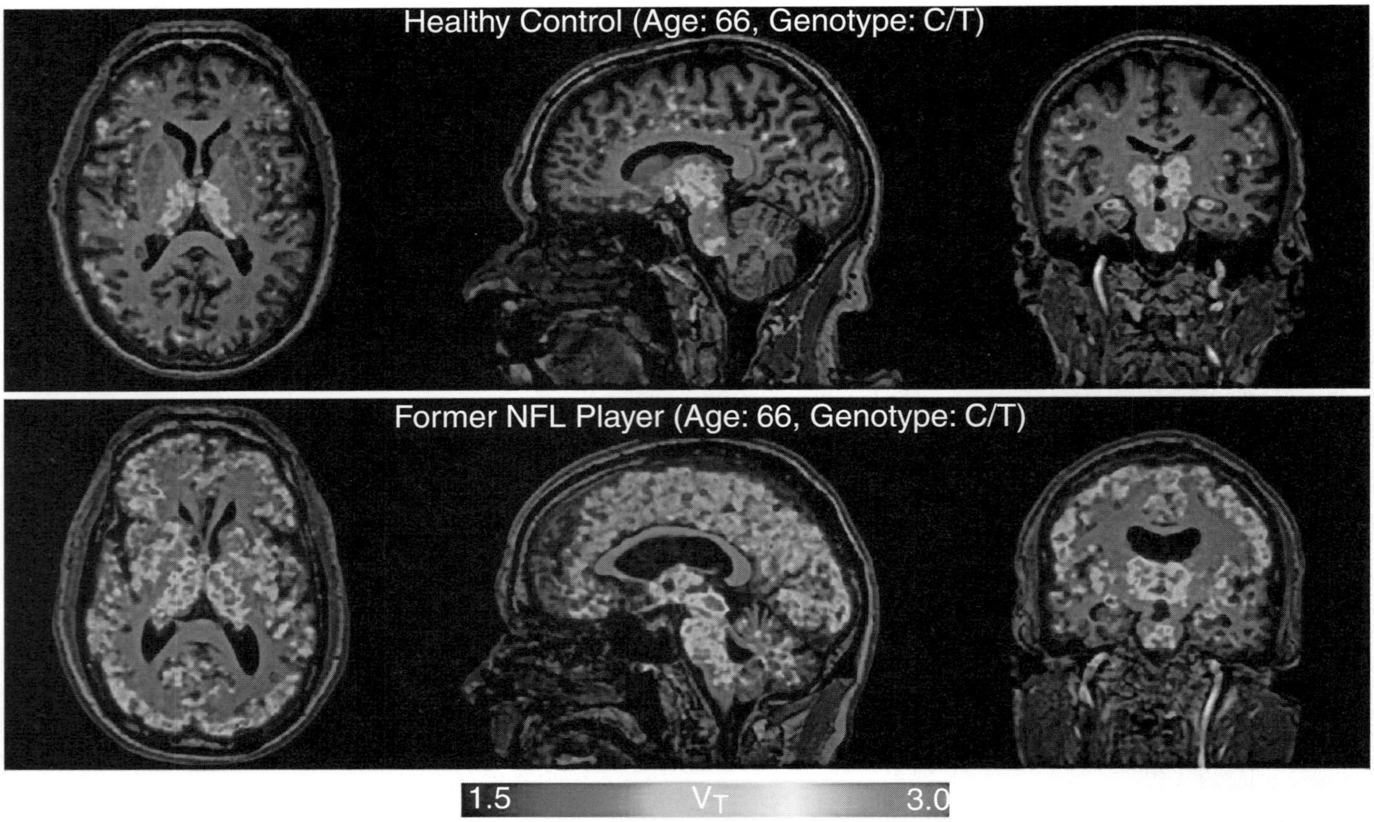

Fig. 12.3 Former National Football League (NFL) players demonstrate increased binding of [^{11}C]DPA-713, reported as total distribution volume (V_T) across many brain regions compared to binding of [11C]DPA-713 in the brains of elderly healthy controls. Parametric [^{11}C]DPA-713 V_T images from one former NFL player and one age- and rs6971 genotype-matched healthy individual are presented for comparison. [A black and white version of this figure will appear in some formats. For the color version, please refer to the plate section.]

Source: Coughlin et al., 2015 [53] with permission from Elsevier

study designs, and analytical methods will not be covered here; for a more in-depth review, the authors refer readers to several well-written comprehensive reviews covering those topics [57, 58].

Although fMRI provides a tool to non-invasively measure functional integrity of neural networks and assess brain function as it relates to specific experimental tasks, a number of factors influence fMRI results. For example, acquisition schemes, event-related versus at-rest paradigms used, methods of analysis, and more, need to be taken into consideration when interpreting findings or comparing studies. fMRI is a powerful tool but, like other imaging techniques, has its advantages and limitations where systematic research is under way for fMRI standardization and harmonization of image acquisition, analysis, and interpretation across the lifespan and clinical condition [59–61].

Functional Neuroimaging of Multiple Concussions

Using fMRI, research has revealed alterations of the BOLD signal in concussed individuals while performing working-memory, attention, sensorimotor, and other neurocognitive

tasks as well as at rest [38, 39]. However, there is still controversy in the concussion literature regarding explanation of fMRI findings due to mixed experimental conditions, time post injury, type of head injury, along with interpretative differences of outcomes and conclusion. Many studies have shown increased and widespread BOLD signal response in concussed subjects successfully performing cognitive tasks, specifically in the prefrontal and dorsolateral prefrontal cortices [62–64], yet other studies have reported a reduction [19, 65]. Whether these contradictory results relate to performance differences, whether more or less activation is required to do the task, time post injury and type of injury, or subject inclusion criteria, or reflect the heterogeneity of injury is still an area of ongoing debate in the concussion literature [66].

Despite these continued controversies, recent fMRI-based functional connectivity studies have shown promise in expanding our understanding of human functional brain networks [67] and support the evidence that structural connectivity and functional connectivity are closely related [68]. Recording temporal oscillation in the BOLD signal permits inferences about which areas are in synchrony and linked, which in turn implies functional connectivity, although probably not one-to-one mapping nor an exclusive ability to

Positron emission tomography imaging findings comparing healthy controls (CTRL) with mild traumatic brain injury
(mTBI) and Alzheimer's disease (AD)

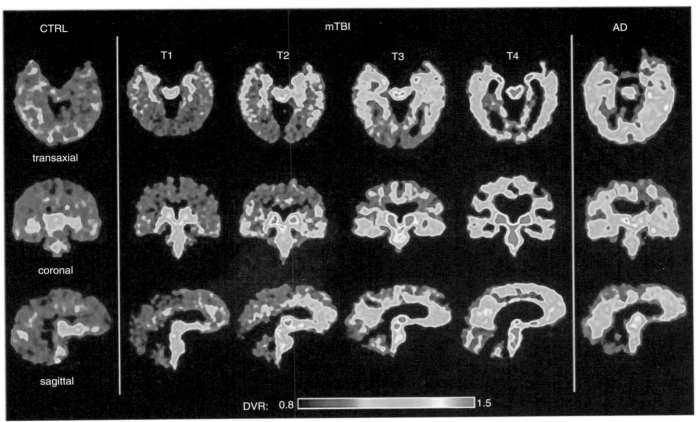

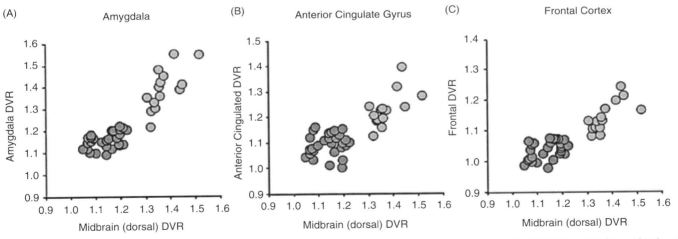

Fig. 12.4 (Upper) [F-18]FDDNP distribution volume ratios (DVR) parametric images showing patterns T1–T4 of increased [F-18]FDDNP signal observed in the mTBI group compared with cognitive control subjects (left). The T1 pattern shows involvement of two core areas which have consistently increased [F-18]FDDNP signal in all four patterns: amygdala (limbic) and dorsal midbrain (subcortical). Patterns T2–T4 are marked by increase of [F-18]FDDNP signal in these two core regions and progressively larger number of subcortical, limbic, and cortical areas. Although more complex patterns (e.g., T4) overlap with AD in the cortex, midbrain and amygdala signals are elevated above the levels in AD. An AD case is shown in the right column for comparison. Lower: A is a two-dimensional scatter plot showing [F-18]FDDNP DVR values in two core areas consistently involved in chronic traumatic encephalopathy (CTE) (subcortical structures (dorsal midbrain) and limbic structures (amygdala)), clearly demonstrating separation of mTBI and CTRL groups. B and C demonstrate similar separation effect when dorsal midbrain is compared with cortical areas typically associated with CTE and its mood disorders, namely the anterior cingulate gyrus (B) and frontal lobe (C). mTBI subjects are represented by green circles, and CTRL subjects are represented by blue circles. [A black and white version of this figure will appear in some formats. For the color version, please refer to the plate section.]

Source: Barrio et al. [30]; reproduced with permission of PNAS.

distinguish direct and indirect pathways involved in a particular function [67].

Biswal et al. [69] were the first to document the spontaneous fluctuations within the motor system and highlight the potential of assessing functional connectivity. Since the discovery of coherent spontaneous fluctuations in the fMRI signal, many studies have shown that several brain regions engaged during various cognitive tasks also form coherent large-scale brain networks, identifiable using fMRI [70]. These intrinsic activity correlations lead to the development of rs-fMRI and offer promise for improving clinical applicability of examining spontaneous modulations in the BOLD signal that occur during resting state [71] and applying these methods in the study of CBI.

Resting state or "rs" refers to the state in which an individual is awake in the scanner lying quietly with eyes closed [72] and does not require a specific experimental task or stimulus [73]. In contrast to the traditional task-related approach, rs-fMRI has provided unique information about brain networks when not engaged in a specific task. A major benefit that rs connectivity provides is the elimination of any bias based upon task performance. Examination of spontaneous activity provides a window into the neural processing that appears to consume the vast majority of brain resources, as there is only a 5% increase associated with task-related changes compared to the high-energy needs of the brain at rest [74].

One of the most studied rs networks is the default-mode network (DMN). The existence of a DMN in the brain was originally reported by Raichle et al. [72], and is also known as a task-negative network. The DMN is comprised of the posterior cingulate cortex/precuneus, medial prefrontal cortex, and medial, lateral, and inferior parietal cortex areas of the brain and some association with medial temporal cortical areas [75, 76]. As part of a task-negative network system, the DMN deactivates during attention or goal-oriented tasks but comes online at rest [72].

Greicius et al. [75] were the first to observe the DMN during rs-fMRI and since then the presence of the DMN has been repeated and validated using rs-fMRI [75, 77–79]. The DMN is identified in the BOLD signal as low-frequency (less than 0.1 Hz) coherent oscillations [75]. Along with the advances in neuroimaging and data analysis techniques, the DMN has become a focus in the neuroscience and psychological community with potential diagnostic implications, where potential clinical applications are being examined involving disorders like Alzheimer's disease, Parkinson's disease, and concussion [70]. To date, rs-fMRI techniques to detect altered network functioning associated with TBI are being established [80, 81].

As with other neurodegenerative diseases like Alzheimer's disease, CTE has a large overlap of clinical symptoms and neuropathology [42, 43]. Work utilizing rs-fMRI in Alzheimer's disease has shown that the underlying preclinical mechanisms of the disease result in distinctive changes in functional connectivity and alterations in large-scale functional networks [82, 83]. All of this has implications for what might be happening to the brain in the individual with a history of CBI, how CBI interacts with the aging process, and the potential for detection

with rs-fMRI technology. Specifically, findings have indicated a predominant loss of long-distance functional connections in the rs pattern in patients presumed to have Alzheimer's disease [84, 85]. DMN studies of Alzheimer's disease have shown a marked reduction in hippocampal connectivity with the rest of the DMN as well as decreases in the posterior hubs of the DMN, while some studies report enhanced functional connectivity in the frontal networks [82, 86]. Given the early success and promise that rs-fMRI has had in being able to detect differences associated with Alzheimer's disease and serve as a potential biomarker for the disease [87], there is hope that changes in brain connectivity patterns due to certain neuropathological changes and altered brain metabolism would be transferable to CBI, and in particular CTE [83]. With the limits of structural MRI in detecting the more subtle pathologies from CBI when present, detecting differences in the individual with CBI using fMRI approaches may be superior in identifying network damage when present [88].

Functional abnormalities of the brain are associated with pathological changes in connectivity and network structures, well documented in psychiatric populations, including attention deficit-hyperactivity disorder, autism, depression, post-traumatic stress disorder, and schizophrenia [89]. If disorder-specific rs-fMRI patterns emerge from clinically oriented research, this has significant implications for improving the sensitivity and specificity of rs-fMRI findings in TBI to be separate and distinct from fMRI signatures associated with these other disorders.

Nakamura et al. [90] examined neural network properties at separate time points during recovery from TBI and reported that the strength of network connections was reduced, but not the number of connections. Slobounov et al. [91], using rs-fMRI, reported reduced interhemispheric functional connectivity in "asymptomatic" mild TBI (mTBI) subjects in the primary visual cortex, hippocampal, and dorsolateral prefrontal cortex networks. Shumskaya et al. [92, 93] also documented altered whole-brain functional connectivity in the sub-acute phase of mTBI in the form of decrease in connectivity in the motor-striatal network. Similarly, Stevens et al. [94] took 30 patients with an mTBI history and scanned them at an average of 61 days post brain injury. Using independent component analysis they comprehensively examined 12 distinct networks and found, compared to matched controls, mTBI patients showed connectivity differences in nearly all networks, whether it be in the form of a deficit or enhancement.

Although the emphasis of CTE research to date has come from individuals who have had a history of repetitive head trauma, including a likely history of subconcussive blows to the head, it seems that these subconcussive and concussive events are an integral component in the initiation of the disease [35]. These forms of repetitive head trauma may act as a catalyst for the formation and progression of CTE [43]. Whether CTE manifests due to subconcussive trauma alone or exposure to full-blown concussive episodes is still unknown [35]. Functional imaging experiments addressing this prolonged and chronic exposure to multiple concussive traumas are limited and have demonstrated contradictory results. Johnson

Functional magnetic resonance imaging-derived default mode network (DMN) activity between pre- and post-game

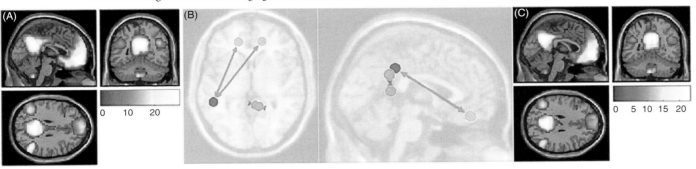

Fig. 12.5A Significant ($p < 0.01$) differences in pre-game and post-game connectivity for all subjects. Left panel: pre-game and (right panel) post-game DMN activation. Middle connectivity diagrams: overall connectivity differences with circles representing seed regions of interest; width of arrow representative of T-scores as well as directionality, with warm colors referring to an increase in connectivity; cool colors represent a decrease in connectivity. [A black and white version of this figure will appear in some formats. For the color version, please refer to the plate section.]

Source: Johnson et al., 2014 [98]; reproduced with permission from Mary Ann Liebert, Inc.

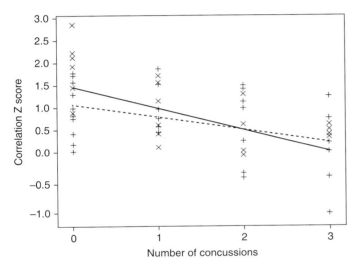

Fig. 12.5B Regression slope indicating the relationship between the number of concussive episodes and magnitude of connectivity. Solid line and x represent connection between left dorsolateral prefrontal cortex (DLPFC) and left lateral parietal, and dashed line and + represent connection between left and right DLPFC.

Source: Johnson et al., 2012 [95]; with permission from Elsevier

et al. [95] used rs-fMRI to evaluate the DMN in individuals meeting mTBI criteria. Through voxel-based correlation analysis, they found disruptions in DMN connections in their sample of mTBI subjects. Concussed individuals showed a reduced number of connections and strength of connections in the posterior cingulate and lateral parietal cortices, and an increased number and strength of connections in the medial prefrontal cortex.

Looking at the effects that multiple concussive episodes have on the functional connectivity of the DMN indicated an overall loss of connectivity as the number of mTBI episodes increased. Specifically, regression analyses revealed a significant reduction in the magnitude of connections between the left dorsolateral prefrontal cortex (DLPFC) and left lateral parietal cortex as a function of number of concussive episodes

(Figure 12.5). Despite not showing any statistically significant connections between the left and right DLPFC and for the left DLPFC and posterior cingulate cortex, the regression analysis showed a downward trend in the number of connections as the number of concussions increased (Figure 12.5B).

Conversely, Terry et al. [96], looking at 20 subjects with a history of two or more concussions, found no significant differences in brain activation patterns when a spatial working-memory task was used during fMRI. This example of differences in fMRI findings highlights potential confounds that need to be taken into consideration when reviewing the literature. First, these two studies used two different paradigms during fMRI acquisition; the first employed an rs approach, while the second used a task-related design. This difference in tasks makes it difficult to make these results transferable across studies. Second, subject population is a major issue when it comes to the fMRI literature on mTBI. Although both studies focused on the effects of multiple concussions on the functional integrity of the brain and had demographically matched controls, the Johnson et al. cohort was in the subacute phase of mTBI, whereas the participants in the study by Terry et al. [96] were, at a minimum, 6 months removed from injury. Both studies did use whole-brain and region of interest analyses.

In a study by Hart et al. [97], 26 retired NFL players with an average of four sustained concussions underwent MRI and neuropsychological testing. As shown in Figure 12.6, an arterial spin labeling (ASL) MRI technique was implemented to measure cerebral perfusion [98], another functional blood flow MRI detection procedure potentially useful in CBI [99]. Compared to healthy controls the players demonstrated altered regional blood flow patterns in the left temporal pole, inferior parietal lobe, and superior temporal gyrus. These differences in blood flow corresponded to brain areas important for memory, naming, and word finding, which may explain why these players performed significantly poorer on similar neuropsychological metrics. More studies that factor in the effects of multiple concussive episodes, or specifically focus on multiple concussions, are needed to help us understand the implications they can have on the brain.

Blood flow differences in athletes with history of concussion

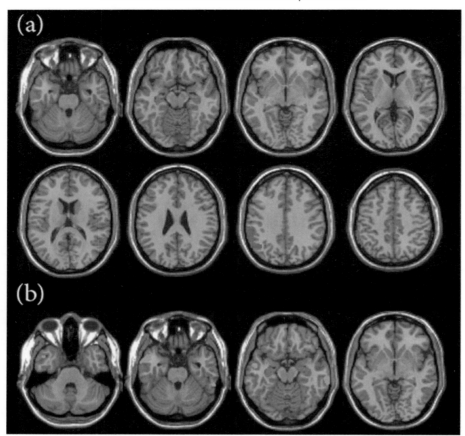

Fig. 12.6 (a) Increases in estimated regional cerebral blood flow for National Football League (NFL) players with cognitive impairment compared to controls ($p < 0.001$). (b) Decrease in estimated regional cerebral blood flow for NFL players with cognitive impairment compared to controls ($p < 0.001$). [A black and white version of this figure will appear in some formats. For the color version, please refer to the plate section.]

Source: Hart et al., 2013 [97]; reproduced with permission from the American Medical Association

Functional Neuroimaging of Subconcussive Head Trauma

Subconcussive blows are below the threshold to cause a concussion [100] and do not elicit clinically identifiable signs or symptoms of a concussion [41, 101, 102]. However, subconcussive blows may not be as harmless as once thought [103, 104]. Subconcussive head blows involving the head have the potential to transfer a high degree of linear and rotational acceleration forces to the brain [105]. Furthermore the sheer number of these hits that players can accumulate over a season can range in the thousands [40] and when you take into account the total number of subconcussive impacts over a career it can be staggering [35, 40]. Despite their inability to produce clinically expressed concussion, animal and human studies have shown potential damage to the central nervous system due to these subconcussive impacts [106, 107]. This has been highlighted by studies utilizing blood serum and cerebrospinal fluid biomarkers that indicate the presence of damage to astroglial cells and axons. Neselius et al. [108, 109] have documented increases of total tau protein, glial fibrillary acidic protein, neurofilament light protein, and S-100β following an Olympic bout of boxing where participants sustained repetitive head trauma, without meeting clinical criteria for concussion. One theory behind the more long-term sequelae associated with subconcussive impacts is that they

may accelerate the cognitive aging process by reducing cognitive and brain reserve, which then leads to altered neuronal biology later in life [110].

Recent research has shown that the accrual of subconcussive blows [111] can cause pathophysiological changes in the brain [112]. Most recently, as part of a large multi-site prospective investigation examining fluid biomarkers across all injury severity levels of TBI [113], it was demonstrated that plasma P-tau levels and P-tau–T-tau ratio outperformed T-tau level as diagnostic and prognostic biomarkers for acute TBI. Compared with T-tau levels alone, P-tau levels and P-tau–T-tau ratios show more robust and sustained elevations among patients with chronic TBI, including those who had sustained what was classified as mTBI.

Given that some recent post-mortem studies of retired professional American football players, who have donated their brains at the time of death, have shown high levels of histologically confirmed CTE [43], concern is growing that subconcussive impacts to the head may adversely affect cerebral functions [41, 101, 102]. Some research has shown that subconcussive head trauma may have minimal impact on cognitive functions [114], although there is mounting evidence that subconcussive blows have detrimental effects on cognitive and cerebral functions [41, 115]. It has been hypothesized that exposure to repeated and multiple subconcussive blows has additive effects throughout an athlete's career, setting the

Regions where repeated head impacts show susceptibility-weighted imaging (SWI) signal changes

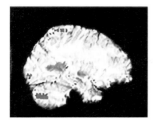 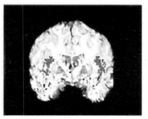 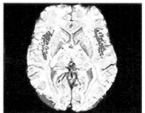

Fig. 12.7 Selected slices for subject 6 (a defensive back) with an overlay highlighting those voxels in which SWI signal decreases were observed at post, relative to pre. Highlighted voxels belong to several of the ten regions in this subject found to be statistically significantly decreased (Wilcoxon rank sum test at the $p_{uncorrected} <$ 0.00005 level, corresponding to $p_{Bonferroni} < 0.05$), with the saturation of the color reflecting the change measure in the given voxel. [A black and white version of this figure will appear in some formats. For the color version, please refer to the plate section.]

Source: Slobounov et al., 2017 [117] with permission from Elsevier

stage for compromised cognitive function, especially later in life [110, 116].

Slobounov and colleagues [117] took a multimodality approach to neuroimaging of repetitive subconcussive blows over a single American football collegiate season, including rs-fMRI findings of the acute effects of subconcussive impacts on the DMN. These studies, combined with earlier findings involving college rugby players, revealed changes in functional connectivity following exposure to a single bout of repetitive head trauma [98]. In the study involving 24 rugby players they underwent pre- and post-game rs-fMRI scanning. Differences between pre-game and post-game scans showed both increased connectivity from the left supramarginal gyrus to bilateral orbitofrontal cortex and decreased connectivity from the retrosplenial cortex and dorsal posterior cingulate cortex. Further analysis was performed by dividing this cohort based upon history of previous diagnosis of a clinically manifested concussive episode. This secondary analysis revealed an interesting finding: those individuals with a prior history exhibited only decreased functional connectivity following exposure to subconcussive blows, while those with no history of concussion displayed increased functional connectivity.

There are few studies utilizing fMRI to investigate the effects of subconcussive head trauma, and the limited research out there focuses more on the acute effects and changes seen over the course of one season. Using a visual working-memory paradigm Talavage et al. [115] scanned 11 high school football players using fMRI. Despite no subjects under study exhibiting any clinical signs to elicit a diagnosable concussion over the course of the season, performance on neuropsychological testing compared to baseline was poorer. They found that the number of collisions was significantly correlated to changes in the subject's fMRI activation. Specifically, subjects who showed no clinical symptoms of concussion, yet showed poorer neuropsychological tests, exhibited a significant reduction of fMRI activation in the DLPFC, middle and superior frontal gyri, and cerebellum.

Expanding on this initial study, Breedlove et al. [118] reported that, despite not sustaining a concussion, a large portion of their cohort under study showed significant neuropsychological changes as assessed by fMRI due to repetitive subconcussive head trauma. Additionally they found a significant relationship between the number of blows and the documented changes in the neuropsychological testing. These two studies reinforced the authors' hypothesis that repetitive subconcussive head trauma may be connected to pathologically altered neurophysiology. Similar neurocognitive vulnerability has also been reported by Shuttleworth-Edwards et al. [119] for rugby players, attributed to years of exposure to subconcussive impacts to the brain.

Returning to the Slobounov et al. [117] study that examined college American football players with subconcussive impact collisions, those athletes were evaluated before and after the season using multiple MRI sequences, including T1-weighted imaging, diffusion tensor imaging (DTI), ASL, rs-fMRI, and susceptibility-weighted imaging (SWI). While no significant differences were found between pre- and post-season for DTI metrics or cortical volumes, seed-based analysis of rs-fMRI revealed significant ($p < 0.05$) changes in functional connections to right isthmus of the cingulate cortex, left isthmus of the cingulate cortex, and left hippocampus. ASL data revealed significant ($p < 0.05$) increases in global cerebral blood flow, with a specific regional increase in right post central gyrus. SWI data revealed that 44% of the players exhibited outlier rates ($p < 0.05$) of regional decreases in SWI signal.

Figure 12.7 is from a single player showing regions of change. A number of these areas are known regions of vulnerability to injury from trauma, and note the bilateral representation where some of these observations were made [34]. Of key interest, athletes in whom changes in rs-fMRI, cerebral blood flow, and SWI were observed were more likely to have experienced high **g**-force impacts on a daily basis.

These findings are indicative of potential pathophysiological changes detected with neuroimaging methods in brain integrity arising from only a single season of participation in college-level football, even in the absence of clinical symptoms or a diagnosis of concussion. Whether these changes reflect compensatory adaptation to cumulative head impacts or more lasting alterations of brain integrity remains to be further explored.

Functional Neuroimaging of APOE ε4

As more and more diseases and pathologies link to certain genetic biomarkers, CTE is no different, and it may be the case there is a genetic predisposition [37]. The APOE gene has received the most attention, not only in Alzheimer's disease but also in TBI and the association between the two [98, 119, 120]. The APOE gene has already been established as a genetic marker linked to assessing the risk and susceptibility of developing Alzheimer's disease [121]. One presumed central nervous system role of APOE is orchestration of movement and distribution of cholesterol, phospholipids, and fatty acids, considered important for brain plasticity and repair [122]. Genetically, the presence of the APOE ε4 allele confers the highest known risk for Alzheimer's disease [123] as well as being linked to prolonged recovery and exacerbating cognitive deficits following TBI, in particular moderate to severe TBI [124]. Therefore, most of the neuroimaging focused on APOE ε4 has been in the Alzheimer's disease population, where there have been documented structural and metabolic differences in those with and without the ε4 allele via MRI and PET imaging [125]. However, there are a few reports looking at the presence of the APOE ε4 allele and its effects on neuroimaging-assessed functional brain activity in younger populations and before any signs or symptoms of Alzheimer's disease are present. While the investigations that have been done were specific to individuals with or at risk for Alzheimer's disease, the relevant functional neuroimaging findings have implications for neuroimaging studies of the late effects of TBI detected via functional neuroimaging studies [120].

Unfortunately, given that this research remains in the preliminary phase of investigation, similar to the research related to concussion, the literature shows that findings from APOE fMRI studies are inconsistent and mixed. There are reports of increases, decreases, or both of the BOLD response in task-based fMRI as well as rs-fMRI. In a study utilizing data from 21 cognitively healthy adults ranging from age 55 to 73 years old, Adamson et al. [121] used a spatial memory task to investigate if there was a difference in carriers of the APOE ε4 compared to non-carriers. Encoding contrast compared to a dot control task revealed significant lower hippocampal activation in ε4 carriers despite similar performance.

Similarly, Filbey et al. [122], using a working-memory paradigm, also reported higher activation in carriers of the APOE ε4 compared to no carriers in the medial frontal and anterior cingulate cortices in young healthy adults. However, these results of greater activation in carriers are not necessarily consistent throughout the literature and also differ as to whether a task-related or rs paradigm was employed. Wishart et al. [123] showed that heterozygous carriers of the ε4 allele had increased activation in the medial frontal, bilateral parietal regions, and right DLPFC performing a working-memory task, although no differences were seen on performance of the task.

Looking at two distinct age groups, Filippini et al. [125] used an encoding memory task during fMRI evaluation to see if age might account for some of the inconsistencies reported on fMRI results between APOE ε4 carriers and non-carriers. The two age groups were split into a younger and older subset with a maximum age of 35 and 78 years old respectively and all subjects under study were cognitively normal. Different activation patterns were found in each age group between carriers

of ε4 and non-carriers. All of these findings suggest that APOE ε4 carriers may possess a different risk for adverse effects from CBI.

In a 2009 study by Filippini et al. [126], 18 subjects below the age of 35 who carried the APOE ε4 allele were compared to non-carrier-matched controls using both rs- and task-based fMRI. The results of their study showed differences in both fMRI activation tasks between APOE ε4 carriers and non-carriers. Specifically, increased DMN activity was found in the medial prefrontal, medial temporal, and retrosplenial cortices, for the APOE ε4 carriers. Significant additional hippocampal activation was also noted in the APOE ε4 carriers during the encoding phase of the memory-based tasked component of the study. Despite most of the literature on fMRI and the influence of APOE gene being done using a task-based approach, rs-fMRI may be a more sensitive marker to identify APOE ε4 carriers from those non-carriers [127, 128].

Trachtenberg and colleagues used rs-fMRI to assess the functional connectivity within eight known rs networks as well as two additional hippocampal networks [128]. This study was conducted on 77 cognitively healthy participants with ages in the range of 32–55 years old and separated into one of four groups based upon APOE genotype. Independent component analysis revealed group differences in the anterior hippocampal, posterior hippocampal, and auditory, lateral visual, and frontal parietal networks. Specifically, ε3 homozygotes showed the most delineated and structured rs networks while ε2 and ε4 allele carriers showed similar widespread diffuse functional connectivity.

These findings led the authors to postulate that another APOE role may be in neurodevelopment to differentiate the functional networks of the brain. In another rs-fMRI, Westlye et al. [129] took 95 cognitively healthy subjects between the ages of 50 and 80 years old to assess the influence that APOE ε4 has on the DMN. Using independent component analysis and dual regression, they found that carriers of the ε4 allele demonstrated increased hippocampal synchronization. In addition, the ε4 allele showed an effect on the posterior cingulate cortex, parietal cortex, and parahippocampal area of the DMN. Furthermore, this increased DMN synchrony was significantly correlated with poorer memory tests.

All of this genetic work in healthy aging and Alzheimer's disease populations has particular relevance to the study of functional neuroimaging using MRI techniques in the study of CBI and their potential role in better understanding the delayed effects of CBI and how adverse effects from remote CBI may play out in relations to CTE.

Other Neuroimaging Studies of Repetitive Subconcussive Impacts, Multiple Concussions, and APOE ε4 Carriers

Despite no current fMRI studies explicitly examining CTE, and the limited research utilizing this technique on the suspected main causes of CTE, other neuroimaging techniques have been used to explore them. One of the current limitations in the literature regarding CBI research is the failure to acknowledge the possible impacts that multiple concussions may have on the brain, and inclusion of a heterogeneous history of concussion population may account for some of the reported inconsistencies. Issues of other health variables, predisposing pre-injury neuropsychiatric history, cognitive and brain reserve issues, along with other factors associated with aging, create a need for complex research designs to study these problems [130, 131]. Using magnetic resonance spectroscopy (MRS), Slobounov and colleagues observed significant reductions in NAA (N-acetyl aspartate)/choline (Cho), and NAA/creatine (Cr) ratios in the genu of the corpus callosum for concussed subjects, regardless of the number of concussions [132, 133].

Subjects recovering from their first concussion showed the largest alteration in NAA/Cho and NAA/Cr ratios. Interestingly, Slobounov et al. noticed that, as the number of concussions increased, so did the length of time for subjects' symptoms to resolve. Additionally, they also observed a trend for increasing NAA/Cho and NAA/Cr ratios as the number of concussions grew. In a pilot study by Tavazzi et al. [134], the authors looked at athletes who were recovering from concussion and who received a second subsequent concussion within 15 days of the initial injury. These individuals showed an early decrease in NAA/Cr ratio following the first concussion and this ratio further decreased acutely after the second concussion and prolonged recovery of symptoms. They also reported that the slowest rate of recovery was within the first 15 days after insult followed by a five-times higher accelerated rate in days 15–30 post-injury. Others have demonstrated similar findings [135, 136].

As already reviewed, neuroimaging studies of subconcussive head trauma have detected changes seen over the season as well as the long-term effects of a career of accumulating these repetitive traumas. Similarly, while conventional neuroimaging techniques have the ability to identify gross anatomical structural changes in the brain, these traditional methods are usually negative for CBI – where it has been assumed the injury is more of a metabolic, physiological reaction to trauma than a structural injury [137]. From a historical perspective, there have been indicators in the literature that even these coarse measures detect some level of pathology in CBI in boxers. For example, one study that looked at boxers longitudinally saw evidence in 13% of the boxers of progressive brain injury, as well as several boxers presenting with cortical atrophy and cavum septum pellucidum [138].

Another CT study evaluating soccer players observed an increase in cerebral atrophy and ventriculomegaly in 27% and 18% of the professional soccer players respectively [139, 140]. However, the general lack of sensitivity of conventional techniques has led to hopes that newer methods of neuroimaging may be beneficial. One study by Bazarian et al. [140] took a cohort of nine high school student athletes and performed DTI pre- and post-season, at an interval of three months apart; subjects sustained 26–399 subconcussive blows! One subject under study was diagnosed with a concussion, and demonstrated the highest number of white-matter voxels with a significant change in fractional anisotropy (FA) and mean diffusivity (MD) values from pre- to post-season. Compared to controls, the cohort that was subject to repetitive subconcussive trauma showed the next highest number of voxels, with a significant FA and MD change, with most subjects displaying an increase in FA and a decrease in MD with these changes correlating to the number of impacts.

In a more recent study by some of these same investigators, Mayinger et al. [141] showed white-matter alterations in 15 college football players after one season of play, with DTI changes returning to baseline after six months of no contact. Chappell et al. [142], reported an increase in the apparent diffusion coefficient and a decrease in FA in the deep white matter of 81 professional boxers. They inferred that the abnormalities reported may reflect the cumulative effects of repetitive subconcussive head trauma. Similarly, using DTI, Koerte et al. [143] reported widespread differences in white-matter integrity between a small cohort of soccer players with no previous concussive episode, compared to swimmers. Specifically they observed significantly increased radial diffusivity in a number of major white-matter tracts, including the corpus callosum, suggestive of compromised myelin integrity. In a pilot MRS study, Lin et al. [144] examined five retired professional athletes with a known exposure to concussions and subconcussive head trauma and revealed a significant increase in Cho and glutamate/glutamine concentrations. Bailey and colleagues [145] demonstrated that cerebral hemodynamic function is compromised in professional boxers assumed to be displaying the effects of chronic TBI using transcranial Doppler ultrasound.

The studies mentioned in the above paragraph, did not examine APOE status. Returning to the APOE issue in CBI, as previously discussed using functional neuroimaging, it is actually the case that most of the neuroimaging studies have focused on the effects of the APOE ε4 allele utilizing volumetric and morphometric analysis, with interesting implications for CBI. As such, there have been numerous reports documenting smaller hippocampal volumes, temporal lobe atrophy, and thinner cortex in the entorhinal region in young and old carriers of APOE ε4 [146–148]. This could suggest vulnerability of these regions to injury in CBI in those who are carriers. As such, the genetic effect may set the stage for vulnerability at the time of initial injury, when some regions are more influenced than others by CBI.

Hua et al. [149] reported that APOE ε4 was associated with increased CSF expansion within the Sylvian fissure, signifying greater levels of frontotemporal atrophy in the presence of APOE. Furthermore, they reported that tensor-based morphometry identified reductions in the hippocampus and temporal lobe correlated with cognitive impairments. Again, these APOE findings point to genetic effects that may lower the resiliency of brain structure and function to the effects of injury, as these are the very regions at high vulnerability for injury in CBI [34].

Additionally, it was reported in an older population of APOE ε4 carriers that cerebral blood flow may be altered at rest [127]. This study brings up another problem when it comes to interpreting fMRI results – the effects of trauma or genetic influence on physiology and vascular functioning, especially if

APOE carriers are at increased risk for any kind of metabolic differences. These changes in neurophysiology can be caused by a single driving factor, modulated by another leading to transient or possible chronic alterations in physiology detected by functional imaging. Therefore, this must be kept in mind when looking at the functional neuroimaging literature, in addition to examining study design, inclusion criteria, and analysis methods. Recently, Hayes et al. [150] examined APOE and genetic risk for Alzheimer's disease in a cohort of individuals meeting criteria for mTBI. They found reduced cortical thickness related to history of mTBI and genetic risk, in a potentially interactive way.

Conclusion

An axiom from studying anatomy is that function determines in part structure and structure underlies function. When a brain injury occurs, even on the mildest end of the spectrum, what are the influences that alter cerebral function and how do these influences affect remodeling of structures in the brain? Likewise, how does structural damage modify function? One has to remember that most of these neuroimaging techniques are adept at investigating one aspect of brain integrity, whether it is from a functional, metabolic, or structural viewpoint. There is a mounting literature indicating that a single CBI as well as repetitive subconcussive impacts, multiple concussions, or the presence of APOE ε4 can have a pathological and adverse influence on brain structure and function. Therefore, multi-modal approaches that go beyond a unidimensional approach to image analysis will undoubtedly offer more information and insights about the role of CBI on the state of the brain over the lifespan of the individual who sustains an injury. It is anticipated that, in the future, neuroimaging will provide reliable methods for *in vivo* detection of CBI and track potential adverse effects over the lifespan, including identification and monitoring what is now referred to as CTE.

References

1. Johnson VE, Stewart W, Arena JD, Smith DH. Traumatic brain injury as a trigger of neurodegeneration. *Adv Neurobiol* 2017; 15: 383–400.
2. Omalu BI, DeKosky ST, Minster RL, Kamboh MI, Hamilton RL, Wecht CH. Chronic traumatic encephalopathy in a National Football League player. *Neurosurgery* 2005; 57(1): 128–134; discussion 128–134.
3. Iacono D, Shively SB, Edlow BL, Perl DP. Chronic traumatic encephalopathy: Known causes, unknown effects. *Phys Med Rehabil Clin N Am* 2017; 28(2): 301–321.
4. Koerte IK, Lin AP, Willems A, Muehlmann M, Hufschmidt J, Coleman MJ, et al. A review of neuroimaging findings in repetitive brain trauma. *Brain Pathol* 2015; 25(3): 318–349.
5. Hay J, Johnson VE, Smith DH, Stewart W. Chronic traumatic encephalopathy: The neuropathological legacy of traumatic brain injury. *Annu Rev Pathol* 2016; 11: 21–45.
6. Carson A. Concussion, dementia and CTE: Are we getting it very wrong? *J Neurol Neurosurg Psychiatry* 2017; 88(6): 462–464.
7. Daneshvar DH, Goldstein LE, Kiernan PT, Stein TD, McKee AC. Post-traumatic neurodegeneration and chronic traumatic encephalopathy. *Mol Cell Neurosci* 2015; 66(Pt B): 81–90.
8. Breedlove EL, Robinson M, Talavage TM, Morigaki KE, Yoruk U, O'Keefe K, et al. Biomechanical correlates of symptomatic and asymptomatic neurophysiological impairment in high school football. *J Biomech* 2012; 45(7): 1265–1272.
9. Abbas K, Shenk TE, Poole VN, Breedlove EL, Leverenz LJ, Nauman EA, et al. Alteration of default mode network in high school football athletes due to repetitive subconcussive mild traumatic brain injury: A resting-state functional magnetic resonance imaging study. *Brain Connect* 2015; 5(2): 91–101.
10. Provenzano FA, Jordan B, Tikofsky RS, Saxena C, Van Heertum RL, Ichise M. F-18 FDG PET imaging of chronic traumatic brain injury in boxers: A statistical parametric analysis. *Nucl Med Commun* 2010; 31(11): 952–957.
11. Coughlin JM, Wang Y, Minn I, Bienko N, Ambinder EB, Xu X, et al. Imaging of glial cell activation and white matter integrity in brains of active and recently retired National Football League players. *JAMA Neurol* 2017; 74(1): 67–74.
12. Kemp PM, Houston AS, Macleod MA, Pethybridge RJ. Cerebral perfusion and psychometric testing in military amateur boxers and controls. *J Neurol Neurosurg Psychiatry* 1995; 59(4): 368–374.
13. Roberts MA, Manshadi F, Bushnell D, Hines M. Neurobehavioural dysfunction following mild traumatic brain injury in childhood: A case report with positive findings on positron emission tomography (PET). *Brain Injury* 1995; 9(5): 427–436.
14. Gross H, Kling A, Henry G, Herndon C, Lavretsky H. Local cerebral glucose metabolism in patients with long-term behavioral and cognitive deficits following mild traumatic brain injury. *J Neuropsychiatry Clin Neurosci* 1996; 8(3): 324–334.
15. Peskind ER, Petrie EC, Cross DJ, Pagulayan K, McCraw K, Hoff D, et al. Cerebrocerebellar hypometabolism associated with repetitive blast exposure mild traumatic brain injury in 12 Iraq war veterans with persistent post-concussive symptoms. *NeuroImage* 2011; 54 (Suppl 1): S76–S82.
16. Amen DG, Newberg A, Thatcher R, Jin Y, Wu J, Keator D, et al. Impact of playing American professional football on long-term brain function. *J Neuropsychiatry Clin Neurosci* 2011; 23(1): 98–106.
17. Mendez MF, Owens EM, Reza Berenji G, Peppers DC, Liang LJ, Licht EA. Mild traumatic brain injury from primary blast vs. blunt forces: Post-concussion consequences and functional neuroimaging. *NeuroRehabilitation* 2013; 32(2): 397–407.
18. Tateno A, Sakayori T, Takizawa Y, Yamamoto K, Minagawa K, Okubo Y. A case of Alzheimer's disease following mild traumatic brain injury. *Gen Hosp Psychiatry* 2015; 37(1): e97–e99.
19. Chen JK, Johnston KM, Frey S, Petrides M, Worsley K, Ptito A. Functional abnormalities in symptomatic concussed athletes: An fMRI study. *NeuroImage* 2004; 22(1): 68–82.
20. Strigo IA, Spadoni AD, Lohr J, Simmons AN. Too hard to control: Compromised pain anticipation and modulation in mild traumatic brain injury. *Transl Psychiatry* 2014; 4: e340.
21. Monti JM, Voss MW, Pence A, McAuley E, Kramer AF, Cohen NJ. History of mild traumatic brain injury is associated with deficits in relational memory, reduced hippocampal volume, and less neural activity later in life. *Front Aging Neurosci* 2013; 5: 41.
22. Dean PJ, Sato JR, Vieira G, McNamara A, Sterr A. Multimodal imaging of mild traumatic brain injury and persistent postconcussion syndrome. *Brain Behav* 2015; 5(1): 45–61.
23. Astafiev SV, Shulman GL, Metcalf NV, Rengachary J, MacDonald CL, Harrington DL, et al. Abnormal white matter blood-oxygen-level-dependent signals in chronic mild traumatic brain injury. *J Neurotrauma* 2015; 32(16): 1254–1271.
24. Liu K, Li B, Qian S, Jiang Q, Li L, Wang W, et al. Mental fatigue after mild traumatic brain injury: A 3D-ASL perfusion study. *Brain Imaging Behav* 2016; 10(3): 857–868.

25. Astafiev SV, Zinn KL, Shulman GL, Corbetta M. Exploring the physiological correlates of chronic mild traumatic brain injury symptoms. *NeuroImage Clin* 2016; 11: 10–19.

26. Bang SA, Song YS, Moon BS, Lee BC, Lee HY, Kim JM, et al. Neuropsychological, metabolic, and GABA$_A$ receptor studies in subjects with repetitive traumatic brain injury. *J Neurotrauma* 2016; 33(11): 1005–1014.

27. Nathan DE, Bellgowan JF, Oakes TR, French LM, Nadar SR, Sham EB, et al. Assessing quantitative changes in intrinsic thalamic networks in blast and nonblast mild traumatic brain injury: Implications for mechanisms of injury. *Brain Connect* 2016; 6(5): 389–402.

28. Mitsis E, Riggio S, Kostakoglu L, Dickstein D, Machac J, Delman B, et al. Tauopathy PET and amyloid PET in the diagnosis of chronic traumatic encephalopathies: Studies of a retired NFL player and of a man with FTD and a severe head injury. *Transl Psychiatry* 2014; 4(9): e441.

29. Dickstein DL, Pullman MY, Fernandez C, Short JA, Kostakoglu L, Knesaurek K, et al. Cerebral [18 F]T807/AV1451 retention pattern in clinically probable CTE resembles pathognomonic distribution of CTE tauopathy. *Transl Psychiatry* 2016; 6(9): e900.

30. Barrio JR, Small GW, Wong KP, Huang SC, Liu J, Merrill DA, et al. In vivo characterization of chronic traumatic encephalopathy using [F-18]FDDNP PET brain imaging. *Proc Natl Acad Sci U S A* 2015; 112(16): E2039–E2047.

31. Shively S, Scher AI, Perl DP, Diaz-Arrastia R. Dementia resulting from traumatic brain injury: What is the pathology? *Arch Neurol* 2012; 69(10): 1245–1251.

32. Gardner RC, Possin KL, Hess CP, Huang EJ, Grinberg LT, Nolan AL, et al. Evaluating and treating neurobehavioral symptoms in professional American football players: Lessons from a case series. *Neurol Clin Pract* 2015; 5(4): 285–295.

33. Hiploylee C, Dufort PA, Davis HS, Wennberg RA, Tartaglia MC, Mikulis D, et al. Longitudinal study of postconcussion syndrome: Not everyone recovers. *J Neurotrauma* 2017; 34(8): 1511–1523.

34. Bigler ED. Neuropathology of mild traumatic brain injury: Correlation to neurocognitive and neurobehavioral findings. In: Kobeissy FH, editor. *Brain neurotrauma: Molecular, neuropsychological, and rehabilitation aspects*. Boca Raton, FL: Frontiers in Neuroengineering, 2015.

35. Baugh CM, Stamm JM, Riley DO, Gavett BE, Shenton ME, Lin A, et al. Chronic traumatic encephalopathy: Neurodegeneration following repetitive concussive and subconcussive brain trauma. *Brain Imaging Behav* 2012; 6(2): 244–254.

36. Smith DH, Johnson VE, Stewart W. Chronic neuropathologies of single and repetitive TBI: Substrates of dementia? *Nature Rev Neurol* 2013; 9(4): 211–221.

37. Blennow K, Hardy J, Zetterberg H. The neuropathology and neurobiology of traumatic brain injury. *Neuron* 2012; 76(5): 886–899.

38. McCrea M, Meier T, Huber D, Ptito A, Bigler E, Debert CT, et al. Role of advanced neuroimaging, fluid biomarkers and genetic testing in the assessment of sport-related concussion: A systematic review. *Br J Sports Med* 2017; 51(12): 919–929.

39. Kamins J, Bigler E, Covassin T, Henry L, Kemp S, Leddy JJ, et al. What is the physiological time to recovery after concussion? A systematic review. *Br J Sports Med* 2017; 51(12): 935–940.

40. McKee AC, Cantu RC, Nowinski CJ, Hedley-Whyte ET, Gavett BE, Budson AE, et al. Chronic traumatic encephalopathy in athletes: Progressive tauopathy after repetitive head injury. *J Neuropathol Exp Neurol* 2009; 68(7):709–735.

41. Gavett BE, Stern RA, McKee AC. Chronic traumatic encephalopathy: A potential late effect of sport-related concussive and subconcussive head trauma. *Clin Sports Med* 2011; 30(1): 179–188.

42. McKee AC, Stern RA, Nowinski CJ, Stein TD, Alvarez VE, Daneshvar DH, et al. The spectrum of disease in chronic traumatic encephalopathy. *Brain* 2013; 136(1): 43–64.

43. Mez J, Daneshvar DH, Kiernan PT, Abdolmohammadi B, Alvarez VE, Huber BR, et al. Clinicopathological evaluation of chronic traumatic encephalopathy in players of American football. *JAMA* 2017; 318(4): 360–370.

44. Sundman M, Doraiswamy PM, Morey RA. Neuroimaging assessment of early and late neurobiological sequelae of traumatic brain injury: implications for CTE. *Front Neurosci* 2015; 9: 334.

45. Wang ML, Wei XE, Yu MM, Li PY, Li WB, Alzheimer's disease neuroimaging I. Self-reported traumatic brain injury and in vivo measure of AD-vulnerable cortical thickness and AD-related biomarkers in the ADNI cohort. *Neurosci Lett* 2017; 655: 115–120.

46. Maass A, Landau S, Baker SL, Horng A, Lockhart SN, La Joie R, et al. Comparison of multiple tau-PET measures as biomarkers in aging and Alzheimer's disease. *NeuroImage* 2017; 157: 448–463.

47. Weiner MW, Veitch DP, Aisen PS, Beckett LA, Cairns NJ, Green RC, et al. Recent publications from the Alzheimer's disease neuroimaging initiative: Reviewing progress toward improved AD clinical trials. *Alzheimers Dement* 2017; 13(4): e1–e85.

48. McKee AC, Gavett BE, Stern RA, Nowinski CJ, Cantu RC, Kowall NW, et al. TDP-43 proteinopathy and motor neuron disease in chronic traumatic encephalopathy. *J Neuropathol Exp Neurol* 2010; 69(9): 918–929.

49. Handratta V, Hsu E, Vento J, Yang C, Tanev K. Neuroimaging findings and brain–behavioral correlates in a former boxer with chronic traumatic brain injury. *Neurocase* 2010; 16(2): 125–134.

50. Saing T, Dick M, Nelson PT, Kim RC, Cribbs DH, Head E. Frontal cortex neuropathology in dementia pugilistica. *J Neurotrauma* 2012; 29(6): 1054–1070.

51. Raji CA, Merrill DA, Barrio JR, Omalu B, Small GW. Progressive focal gray matter volume loss in a former high school football player: A possible magnetic resonance imaging volumetric signature for chronic traumatic encephalopathy. *Am J Geriatr Psychiatry* 2016; 24(10): 784–790.

52. Mitsis EM, Riggio S, Kostakoglu L, Dickstein DL, Machac J, Delman B, et al. Tauopathy PET and amyloid PET in the diagnosis of chronic traumatic encephalopathies: Studies of a retired NFL player and of a man with FTD and a severe head injury. *Transl Psychiatry* 2014; 4: e441.

53. Coughlin JM, Wang Y, Munro CA, Ma S, Yue C, Chen S, et al. Neuroinflammation and brain atrophy in former NFL players: An in vivo multimodal imaging pilot study. *Neurobiol Dis* 2015; 74: 58–65.

54. Logothetis NK. What we can do and what we cannot do with fMRI. *Nature* 2008; 453(7197): 869–878.

55. Ogawa S, Menon RS, Tank DW, Kim SG, Merkle H, Ellermann JM, et al. Functional brain mapping by blood oxygenation level-dependent contrast magnetic resonance imaging. A comparison of signal characteristics with a biophysical model. *Biophys J* 1993; 64(3): 803–812.

56. Jueptner M, Weiller C. Review: Does measurement of regional cerebral blood flow reflect synaptic activity? Implications for PET and fMRI. *NeuroImage* 1995; 2(2): 148–156.

57. Casey BJ, Jones RM, Hare TA. The adolescent brain. *Ann N Y Acad Sci* 2008; 1124: 111–126.

58. Amaro E, Jr., Barker GJ. Study design in fMRI: Basic principles. *Brain Cogn* 2006; 60(3): 220–232.

59. Filippi M, Agosta F. Diffusion tensor imaging and functional MRI. *Handb Clin Neurol* 2016; 136: 1065–1087.

60. Mirzaalian H, Ning L, Savadjiev P, Pasternak O, Bouix S, Michailovich O, et al. Multi-site harmonization of diffusion

MRI data in a registration framework. *Brain Imaging Behav* 2017; doi: 10.1007/s11682-016-9670-y.

61. Mirzaalian H, Ning L, Savadjiev P, Pasternak O, Bouix S, Michailovich O, et al. Inter-site and inter-scanner diffusion MRI data harmonization. *NeuroImage* 2016; 135: 311–323.

62. McAllister TW, Sparling MB, Flashman LA, Guerin SJ, Mamourian AC, Saykin AJ. Differential working memory load effects after mild traumatic brain injury. *NeuroImage* 2001; 14(5): 1004–1012.

63. Jantzen KJ. Functional magnetic resonance imaging of mild traumatic brain injury. *J Head Trauma Rehabil* 2010; 25(4): 256–266.

64. Slobounov SM, Zhang K, Pennell D, Ray W, Johnson B, Sebastianelli W. Functional abnormalities in normally appearing athletes following mild traumatic brain injury: A functional MRI study. *Exp Brain Res* 2010; 202(2): 341–354.

65. Chen JK, Johnston KM, Collie A, McCrory P, Ptito A. A validation of the post concussion symptom scale in the assessment of complex concussion using cognitive testing and functional MRI. *J Neurol Neurosurg Psychiatry* 2007; 78(11): 1231–1238.

66. Hillary FG, Grafman JH. Injured brains and adaptive networks: The benefits and costs of hyperconnectivity. *Trends Cogn Sci* 2017; 21(5): 385–401.

67. Greicius MD, Supekar K, Menon V, Dougherty RF. Resting-state functional connectivity reflects structural connectivity in the default mode network. *Cereb Cortex* 2009; 19(1): 72–78.

68. Honey CJ, Sporns O, Cammoun L, Gigandet X, Thiran JP, Meuli R, et al. Predicting human resting-state functional connectivity from structural connectivity. *Proc Natl Acad Sci U S A* 2009; 106(6): 2035–2040.

69. Biswal B, Yetkin FZ, Haughton VM, Hyde JS. Functional connectivity in the motor cortex of resting human brain using echo-planar MRI. *Magn Reson Med* 1995; 34(4): 537–541.

70. Smith SM, Fox PT, Miller KL, Glahn DC, Fox PM, Mackay CE, et al. Correspondence of the brain's functional architecture during activation and rest. *Proc Natl Acad Sci U S A* 2009; 106(31): 13040–13045.

71. Fox MD, Raichle ME. Spontaneous fluctuations in brain activity observed with functional magnetic resonance imaging. *Nat Rev Neurosci* 2007; 8(9): 700–711.

72. Raichle ME, MacLeod AM, Snyder AZ, Powers WJ, Gusnard DA, Shulman GL. A default mode of brain function. *Proc Natl Acad Sci U S A* 2001; 98(2): 676–682.

73. Wolf RC, Sambataro F, Vasic N, Schmid M, Thomann PA, Bienentreu SD, et al. Aberrant connectivity of resting-state networks in borderline personality disorder. *J Psychiatry Neurosci* 2011; 36(6): 402–411.

74. Raichle ME, Mintun MA. Brain work and brain imaging. *Annu Rev Neurosci* 2006; 29: 449–476.

75. Greicius MD, Krasnow B, Reiss AL, Menon V. Functional connectivity in the resting brain: A network analysis of the default mode hypothesis. *Proc Natl Acad Sci U S A* 2003; 100(1): 253–258.

76. Buckner RL, Andrews-Hanna JR, Schacter DL. The brain's default network: Anatomy, function, and relevance to disease. *Ann N Y Acad Sci* 2008; 1124: 1–38.

77. Beckmann CF, DeLuca M, Devlin JT, Smith SM. Investigations into resting-state connectivity using independent component analysis. *Philos Trans R Soc Lond B Biol Sci* 2005; 360(1457): 1001–1013.

78. De Luca M, Beckmann CF, De Stefano N, Matthews PM, Smith SM. fMRI resting state networks define distinct modes of long-distance interactions in the human brain. *NeuroImage* 2006; 29(4): 1359–1367.

79. Damoiseaux JS, Rombouts SA, Barkhof F, Scheltens P, Stam CJ, Smith SM, et al. Consistent resting-state networks across healthy subjects. *Proc Natl Acad Sci U S A* 2006; 103(37): 13848–13853.

80. Han K, Davis RA, Chapman SB, Krawczyk DC. Strategy-based reasoning training modulates cortical thickness and resting-state functional connectivity in adults with chronic traumatic brain injury. *Brain Behav* 2017; 7(5): e00687.

81. Palacios EM, Yuh EL, Chang YS, Yue JK, Schnyer DM, Okonkwo DO, et al. Resting-state functional connectivity alterations associated with six-month outcomes in mild traumatic brain injury. *J Neurotrauma* 2017; 34(8): 1546–1557.

82. Agosta F, Pievani M, Geroldi C, Copetti M, Frisoni GB, Filippi M. Resting state fMRI in Alzheimer's disease: Beyond the default mode network. *Neurobiol Aging* 2012; 33(8): 1564–1578.

83. Sheline YI, Raichle ME. Resting state functional connectivity in preclinical Alzheimer's disease. *Biol Psychiatry* 2013; 74(5): 340–347.

84. Zhou W, Xu D, Peng X, Zhang Q, Jia J, Crutcher KA. Meta-analysis of APOE4 allele and outcome after traumatic brain injury. *J Neurotrauma* 2008; 25(4): 279–290.

85. Rosenbaum RS, Furey ML, Horwitz B, Grady CL. Altered connectivity among emotion-related brain regions during short-term memory in Alzheimer's disease. *Neurobiol Aging* 2010; 31(5): 780–786.

86. Broyd SJ, Demanuele C, Debener S, Helps SK, James CJ, Sonuga-Barke EJ. Default-mode brain dysfunction in mental disorders: A systematic review. *Neurosci Biobehav Rev* 2009; 33(3): 279–296.

87. Onoda K, Yada N, Ozasa K, Hara S, Yamamoto Y, Kitagaki H, et al. Can a resting-state functional connectivity index identify patients with Alzheimer's disease and mild cognitive impairment across multiple sites? *Brain Connect* 2017; doi: 10.1089/brain.2017.0507.

88. Shin SS, Bales JW, Edward Dixon C, Hwang M. Structural imaging of mild traumatic brain injury may not be enough: Overview of functional and metabolic imaging of mild traumatic brain injury. *Brain Imaging Behav* 2017; 11(2): 591–610.

89. Fox MD, Greicius M. Clinical applications of resting state functional connectivity. *Front Syst Neurosci* 2010; 4: 19.

90. Nakamura T, Hillary FG, Biswal BB. Resting network plasticity following brain injury. *PLoS One* 2009; 4(12): e8220.

91. Slobounov SM, Gay M, Zhang K, Johnson B, Pennell D, Sebastianelli W, et al. Alteration of brain functional network at rest and in response to YMCA physical stress test in concussed athletes: RsFMRI study. *NeuroImage* 2011; 55(4): 1716–1727.

92. Shumskaya E, van Gerven MA, Norris DG, Vos PE, Kessels RP. Abnormal connectivity in the sensorimotor network predicts attention deficits in traumatic brain injury. *Exp Brain Res* 2017; 235(3): 799–807.

93. Shumskaya E, Andriessen TM, Norris DG, Vos PE. Abnormal whole-brain functional networks in homogeneous acute mild traumatic brain injury. *Neurology* 2012; 79(2): 175–182.

94. Stevens MC, Lovejoy D, Kim J, Oakes H, Kureshi I, Witt ST. Multiple resting state network functional connectivity abnormalities in mild traumatic brain injury. *Brain Imaging Behav* 2012; 6(2): 293–318.

95. Johnson B, Zhang K, Gay M, Horovitz S, Hallett M, Sebastianelli W, et al. Alteration of brain default network in subacute phase of injury in concussed individuals: Resting-state fMRI study. *NeuroImage* 2012; 59(1): 511–518.

96. Terry DP, Faraco CC, Smith D, Diddams MJ, Puente AN, Miller LS. Lack of long-term fMRI differences after multiple sports-related concussions. *Brain Inj* 2012; 26(13–14): 1684–1696.

97. Hart J, Jr., Kraut MA, Womack KB, Strain J, Didehbani N, Bartz E, et al. Neuroimaging of cognitive dysfunction and depression in aging retired National Football League players: A cross-sectional study. *JAMA Neurol* 2013; 70(3): 326–335.

98. Johnson B, Neuberger T, Gay M, Hallett M, Slobounov S. Effects of subconcussive head trauma on the default mode network of the brain. *J Neurotrauma* 2014; 31(23): 1907–1913.

99. Clark AL, Bangen KJ, Sorg SF, Schiehser DM, Evangelista ND, McKenna B, et al. Dynamic association between perfusion and white matter integrity across time since injury in veterans with history of TBI. *NeuroImage Clin* 2017; 14: 308–315.

100. Shultz SR, MacFabe DF, Foley KA, Taylor R, Cain DP. Subconcussive brain injury in the Long-Evans rat induces acute neuroinflammation in the absence of behavioral impairments. *Behav Brain Res* 2012; 229(1): 145–152.

101. Martini DN, Sabin MJ, DePesa SA, Leal EW, Negrete TN, Sosnoff JJ, et al. The chronic effects of concussion on gait. *Arch Phys Med Rehabil* 2011; 92(4): 585–589.

102. Witol AD, Webbe FM. Soccer heading frequency predicts neuropsychological deficits. *Arch Clin Neuropsychol* 2003; 18(4): 397–417.

103. Dams-O'Connor K, Tsao JW. Functional decline 5 years after blast traumatic brain injury: Sounding the alarm for a wave of disability? *JAMA Neurol* 2017; 74(7): 763–764.

104. Young GR, Tsao JW. Rate of persistent postconcussive symptoms. *JAMA* 2017; 317(13): 1375.

105. Broglio SP, Eckner JT, Martini D, Sosnoff JJ, Kutcher JS, Randolph C. Cumulative head impact burden in high school football. *J Neurotrauma* 2011; 28(10): 2069–2078.

106. Dashnaw ML, Petraglia AL, Bailes JE. An overview of the basic science of concussion and subconcussion: Where we are and where we are going. *Neurosurg Focus* 2012; 33(6): 1–9.

107. Bauer JA, Thomas TS, Cauraugh JH, Kaminski TW, Hass CJ. Impact forces and neck muscle activity in heading by collegiate female soccer players. *J Sports Sci* 2001; 19(3): 171–179.

108. Neselius S, Zetterberg H, Blennow K, Marcusson J, Brisby H. Increased CSF levels of phosphorylated neurofilament heavy protein following bout in amateur boxers. *PLoS One* 2013; 8(11): e81249.

109. Neselius S, Brisby H, Theodorsson A, Blennow K, Zetterberg H, Marcusson J. CSF-biomarkers in Olympic boxing: Diagnosis and effects of repetitive head trauma. *PLoS One* 2012; 7(4): e33606.

110. Broglio SP, Eckner JT, Paulson HL, Kutcher JS. Cognitive decline and aging: The role of concussive and subconcussive impacts. *Exerc Sport Sci Rev* 2012; 40(3): 138–144.

111. Spiotta AM, Shin JH, Bartsch AJ, Benzel EC. Subconcussive impact in sports: A new era of awareness. *World Neurosurg* 2011; 75(2): 175–178.

112. Talavage TM, Nauman EA, Breedlove EL, Yoruk U, Dye AE, Morigaki KE, et al. Functionally-detected cognitive impairment in high school football players without clinically-diagnosed concussion. *J Neurotrauma* 2014; 31(4): 327–338.

113. Rubenstein R, Chang B, Yue JK, Chiu A, Winkler EA, Puccio AM, et al. Comparing plasma phospho tau, total tau, and phospho tau–total tau ratio as acute and chronic traumatic brain injury biomarkers. *JAMA Neurol* 2017; 74(9): 1063–1072.

114. Miller JR, Adamson GJ, Pink MM, Sweet JC. Comparison of preseason, midseason, and postseason neurocognitive scores in uninjured collegiate football players. *Am J Sports Med* 2007; 35(8): 1284–1288.

115. Talavage TM, Nauman EA, Breedlove EL, Yoruk U, Dye AE, Morigaki KE, et al. Functionally-detected cognitive impairment in high school football players without clinically-diagnosed concussion. *J Neurotrauma* 2014; 31(4): 327–338.

116. Parker TM, Osternig LR, van Donkelaar P, Chou LS. Balance control during gait in athletes and non-athletes following concussion. *Med Eng Phys* 2008; 30(8): 959–967.

117. Slobounov SM, Walter A, Breiter HC, Zhu DC, Bai X, Bream T, et al. The effect of repetitive subconcussive collisions on brain integrity in collegiate football players over a single football season: A multi-modal neuroimaging study. *NeuroImage Clin* 2017; 14: 708–718.

118. Breedlove EL, Robinson M, Talavage TM, Morigaki KE, Yoruk U, O'Keefe K, et al. Biomechanical correlates of symptomatic and asymptomatic neurophysiological impairment in high school football. *J Biomech* 2012; 45(7): 1265–1272.

119. Shuttleworth-Edwards AB, Smith I, Radloff SE. Neurocognitive vulnerability amongst university rugby players versus noncontact sport controls. *J Clin Exp Neuropsychol* 2008; 30(8): 870–884.

120. Pan J, Connolly ID, Dangelmajer S, Kintzing J, Ho AL, Grant G. Sports-related brain injuries: Connecting pathology to diagnosis. *Neurosurg Focus* 2016; 40(4): E14.

121. Adamson MM, Hutchinson JB, Shelton AL, Wagner AD, Taylor JL. Reduced hippocampal activity during encoding in cognitively normal adults carrying the APOE varepsilon4 allele. *Neuropsychologia* 2011; 49(9): 2448–2455.

122. Filbey FM, Slack KJ, Sunderland TP, Cohen RM. Functional magnetic resonance imaging and magnetoencephalography differences associated with APOEepsilon4 in young healthy adults. *Neuroreport* 2006; 17(15): 1585–1590.

123. Wishart HA, Saykin AJ, Rabin LA, Santulli RB, Flashman LA, Guerin SJ, et al. Increased brain activation during working memory in cognitively intact adults with the APOE epsilon4 allele. *Am J Psychiatry* 2006; 163(9): 1603–1610.

124. Echemendia RJ, Iverson GL, McCrea M, Broshek DK, Gioia GA, Sautter SW, et al. Role of neuropsychologists in the evaluation and management of sport-related concussion: An interorganization position statement. *Arch Clin Neuropsychol* 2012; 27(1): 119–122.

125. Filippini N, Ebmeier KP, MacIntosh BJ, Trachtenberg AJ, Frisoni GB, Wilcock GK, et al. Differential effects of the APOE genotype on brain function across the lifespan. *NeuroImage* 2011; 54(1): 602–610.

126. Filippini N, MacIntosh BJ, Hough MG, Goodwin GM, Frisoni GB, Smith SM, et al. Distinct patterns of brain activity in young carriers of the APOE-epsilon4 allele. *Proc Natl Acad Sci U S A* 2009; 106(17): 7209–7214.

127. Fleisher AS, Podraza KM, Bangen KJ, Taylor C, Sherzai A, Sidhar K, et al. Cerebral perfusion and oxygenation differences in Alzheimer's disease risk. *Neurobiol Aging* 2009; 30(11): 1737–1748.

128. Trachtenberg AJ, Filippini N, Mackay CE. The effects of APOE-epsilon4 on the BOLD response. *Neurobiol Aging* 2012; 33(2): 323–334.

129. Westlye ET, Lundervold A, Rootwelt H, Lundervold AJ, Westlye LT. Increased hippocampal default mode synchronization during rest in middle-aged and elderly APOE epsilon4 carriers: Relationships with memory performance. *J Neurosci* 2011; 31(21): 7775–7783.

130. Alosco ML, Mez J, Kowall NW, Stein TD, Goldstein LE, Cantu RC, et al. Cognitive reserve as a modifier of clinical expression in chronic traumatic encephalopathy: A preliminary examination. *J Neuropsychiatry Clin Neurosci* 2017; 29(1): 6–12.

131. Mendez MF. What is the relationship of traumatic brain injury to dementia? *J Alzheimers Dis* 2017; 57(3): 667–681.

132. Johnson B, Gay M, Zhang K, Neuberger T, Horovitz SG, Hallett M, et al. The use of magnetic resonance spectroscopy in the subacute evaluation of athletes recovering from single and multiple mild traumatic brain injury. *J Neurotrauma* 2012; 29(13): 2297–2304.

133. Slobounov S, Gay M, Johnson B, Zhang K. Concussion in athletics: Ongoing clinical and brain imaging research controversies. *Brain Imaging Behav* 2012; 6(2): 224–243.

571

134. Tavazzi B, Vagnozzi R, Signoretti S, Amorini AM, Belli A, Cimatti M, et al. Temporal window of metabolic brain vulnerability to concussions: Oxidative and nitrosative stresses – Part II. *Neurosurgery* 2007; 61(2): 390–395; discussion 395–396.

135. Wilde EA, Bouix S, Tate DF, Lin AP, Newsome MR, Taylor BA, et al. Advanced neuroimaging applied to veterans and service personnel with traumatic brain injury: State of the art and potential benefits. *Brain Imaging Behav* 2015; 9(3): 367–402.

136. Koerte IK, Lin AP, Muehlmann M, Merugumala S, Liao H, Starr T, et al. Altered neurochemistry in former professional soccer players without a history of concussion. *J Neurotrauma* 2015; 32(17): 1287–1293.

137. Lovell MR, Collins MW, Iverson GL, Johnston KM, Bradley JP. Grade 1 or "ding" concussions in high school athletes. *Am J Sports Med* 2004; 32(1): 47–54.

138. McCrory P. Sports concussion and the risk of chronic neurological impairment. *Clin J Sport Med* 2011; 21(1): 6–12.

139. Sortland O, Tysvaer AT. Brain damage in former association football players. An evaluation by cerebral computed tomography. *Neuroradiology* 1989; 31(1): 44–48.

140. Bazarian JJ, Zhu T, Blyth B, Borrino A, Zhong J. Subject-specific changes in brain white matter on diffusion tensor imaging after sports-related concussion. *Magn Reson Imaging* 2012; 30(2): 171–180.

141. Mayinger MC, Merchant-Borna K, Hufschmidt J, Muehlmann M, Weir IR, Rauchmann BS, et al. White matter alterations in college football players: A longitudinal diffusion tensor imaging study. *Brain Imaging Behav* 2017; doi: 10.1007/s11682-017-9672-4.

142. Chappell MH, Ulug AM, Zhang L, Heitger MH, Jordan BD, Zimmerman RD, et al. Distribution of microstructural damage in the brains of professional boxers: A diffusion MRI study. *J Magn Reson Imaging* 2006; 24(3): 537–542.

143. Koerte IK, Ertl-Wagner B, Reiser M, Zafonte R, Shenton ME. White matter integrity in the brains of professional soccer players without a symptomatic concussion. *JAMA* 2012; 308: 1859–1861.

144. Lin AP, Liao HJ, Merugumala SK, Prabhu SP, Meehan WP, 3rd, Ross BD. Metabolic imaging of mild traumatic brain injury. *Brain Imaging Behav* 2012; 6(2): 208–223.

145. Bailey DM, Jones DW, Sinnott A, Brugniaux JV, New KJ, Hodson D, et al. Impaired cerebral haemodynamic function associated with chronic traumatic brain injury in professional boxers. *Clin Sci (Lond)* 2013; 124(3): 177–189.

146. Shaw P, Lerch JP, Pruessner JC, Taylor KN, Rose AB, Greenstein D, et al. Cortical morphology in children and adolescents with different apolipoprotein E gene polymorphisms: An observational study. *Lancet Neurol* 2007; 6(6): 494–500.

147. Wishart HA, Saykin AJ, McAllister TW, Rabin LA, McDonald BC, Flashman LA, et al. Regional brain atrophy in cognitively intact adults with a single APOE epsilon4 allele. *Neurology* 2006; 67(7): 1221–1224.

148. Lemaitre H, Crivello F, Dufouil C, Grassiot B, Tzourio C, Alperovitch A, et al. No epsilon4 gene dose effect on hippocampal atrophy in a large MRI database of healthy elderly subjects. *NeuroImage* 2005; 24(4): 1205–1213.

149. Hua X, Leow AD, Parikshak N, Lee S, Chiang MC, Toga AW, et al. Tensor-based morphometry as a neuroimaging biomarker for Alzheimer's disease: An MRI study of 676 AD, MCI, and normal subjects. *NeuroImage* 2008; 43(3): 458–469.

150. Hayes JP, Logue MW, Sadeh N, Spielberg JM, Verfaellie M, Hayes SM, et al. Mild traumatic brain injury is associated with reduced cortical thickness in those at risk for Alzheimer's disease. *Brain* 2017; 140(3): 813–825.

Chapter 13

Polypathology and Dementia After Brain Trauma: Does Brain Injury Trigger Distinct Neurodegenerative Diseases, or Should They Be Classified Together as Traumatic Encephalopathy?

Patricia M. Washington, Sonia Villapol, and Mark P. Burns

Introduction

Traumatic brain injury (TBI) increases the likelihood of developing dementia later in life, including Alzheimer's disease (AD). Current theories about what drives the development of dementia after TBI are largely based on observations of AD-associated amyloid and tau pathologies in the brain after injury, as the presence of these hallmark pathologies provides a potential pathological link. However, these pathologies are only found in a subset of patients after TBI and there is little clinical or preclinical evidence supporting a direct link between these pathological changes, particularly when observed acutely after TBI, and development of dementia later in life.

In this review we will first summarize epidemiological studies of dementia after TBI to emphasize the current understanding that TBI is associated with increased risk of developing multiple types of dementia, not just AD, and highlight potential factors that may increase an individual's risk of dementia after TBI. Second, we will critically examine previous studies of amyloid and tau pathologies in the brain after TBI in humans and animals in order to identify factors that may explain why these neurodegenerative pathologies are observed in only a subset of patients after injury. As it remains unclear how neuropathological findings of TBI relate to the reported increased risk of dementia and AD, we will speculate on the potential relevance of these pathologies in the brain after TBI and whether there are similarities between factors influencing pathology and dementia development after injury. Finally, we will highlight the emerging hypothesis that, while neuropathological features and clinical symptoms following TBI may overlap those observed in classically defined neurodegenerative disorders, these may be signs of TBI-induced neurodegeneration, or traumatic encephalopathy, as opposed to the development of a specific neurodegenerative disease.

TBI as a Risk Factor for Dementia

While the detrimental effects of repeat mild TBI (mTBI) in sports have been known since the 1920s [1], the association between single TBI and dementia is still an active topic of research. Up to four million TBIs occur annually in the United States [2], with the vast majority being mTBI. The acute and chronic symptoms of head trauma have been historically documented. In 1927 the existence of chronic post-concussion symptoms in a cohort of over 100 clinical cases was termed "traumatic encephalitis" [3]. The "punch-drunk" symptoms of clumsiness, ataxia, and disorientation found in professional boxers were described shortly thereafter in 1928 [1]. While most cases described by Martland were mild, the severe cases were described with what we would now call parkinsonism-type symptoms and dementia [1]. The term "dementia pugilistica" was first used in 1937 to describe these stereotypical symptoms in boxers [4], and "chronic post-traumatic encephalopathy" has been in use since the late 1950s [5]. Chronic traumatic encephalopathy (CTE) is now used by the medical field to describe the neuropathological changes that occur as a result of repeat concussive or subconcussive blows to the head.

To date, there have been approximately 160 pathological descriptions of CTE in the brains of boxers, athletes, soldiers, and civilians with a history of repeat mTBI (reviewed in [6]). While this work has helped describe the neuropathology of CTE, many questions still remain and the clinical presentation of CTE has yet to be fully determined. The patient histories of those with pathologically confirmed CTE show that they can present with a multi-faceted clinical and pathological presentation with aspects of AD, frontotemporal dementia (FTD), Parkinson's disease (PD), and amyotrophic lateral sclerosis (ALS) [7].

The question of whether a single moderate to severe TBI triggers the development of late-onset dementia remains somewhat controversial. AD accounts for 60–80% of all dementias and the focus of most studies on TBI and dementia risk have focused specifically on the development of AD after injury. Several retrospective and prospective studies have been conducted, and a significant number report that there is no effect of TBI on the development of AD [8–12]. Conversely, there are many reports that find a positive interaction between brain trauma and AD, with reported relative risk varying from 2 [13] to 14 [14]. To date, two in-depth meta-analyses have been conducted [15, 16]. The first analyzed 11 case–control studies [15]; the second analyzed 15 case–control studies [16]. Consistent from these studies was the finding that TBI increased the risk of developing AD by 58–82% and that males, but not females, were at increased risk of developing AD after

TBI [15, 16]. More focused studies on gender disparities following TBI are required as it remains unclear why females have a reduced risk of developing AD after TBI, especially given their general increased risk of AD compared to males [17].

Brain injury has also been shown to lead to the development of non-AD dementias. A study of male World War II Navy and Marine veterans, 548 with a medically confirmed record of TBI and 1228 with non-head injury-type wounds or infection, assessed patients for AD and other dementias 50 years after their injuries and found that both moderate and severe TBI significantly increased the risk of developing either late-onset AD or non-AD dementia [18]. The increased risk of AD or non-AD dementia was identical after TBI, clearly showing that a single moderate/severe TBI earlier in life can increase the risk of multiple types of late-onset dementia, and not just AD [18].

This view of TBI as a risk factor for multiple types of dementia is supported by the results of another retrospective cohort study [19]. Gardner and colleagues examined the association between TBI and the development of dementia in 164,661 patients over the age of 55 years old with a history of TBI or non-brain trauma in the prior five to seven years. Their search criteria of the California State Inpatient Databases and State Emergency Department Databases included diagnoses of AD, Pick's disease, or FTD and the authors demonstrate that moderate to severe TBI can increase the risk of dementia for all patients 55 and older with a minimum hazard ratio of 1.3 [19].

Similarly, the view that TBI can increase specific non-AD dementias is enhanced by studies that focus specifically on FTD risk after TBI. A retrospective case–control study of 80 FTD patients and 124 controls demonstrated that TBI increases the risk of developing FTD with an odds ratio of 3.3 [20]. A larger retrospective case–control study of 845 veterans found an association between TBI and FTD with an odds ratio of 4.4 [21] – however, it should be noted that this same study did not find an association between TBI and AD.

Finally, a large retrospective cohort study of 147,510 patients in the Taiwanese Longitudinal Health Insurance Database found that those patients with a fractured skull and intracranial injury had a 4.13-times greater risk of developing FTD in the four years following TBI compared to non-brain-injured controls [22]. This was especially prominent in those under the age of 65, who had at least a sixfold greater risk of developing FTD compared to age-matched controls [22].

Potential Factors Influencing Dementia Risk After TBI

The risk of dementia following TBI is altered by several external and internal factors, including injury severity, survival time, patient age at time of injury, genotype, and cognitive reserve. The World War II Navy andMarine veteran study found an injury severity-dependent association of TBI with dementia. While no risk was associated with mTBI occurring 50 years prior to injury, moderate TBI increased the risk of AD or other dementias by twofold and severe TBI increased the risk by fourfold [18]. Due to the length of time between the recorded injury and dementia

onset in the Plassman study [18], it may be important to striate the patient population when examining the risk of dementia using the patient age at time of injury as a variable.

Indeed, data show that the risk of AD increases as the time between the last brain injury event and the onset of disease symptoms diminishes [23]. This is confirmed in a meta-analysis showing that when TBI occurs more than ten years prior to disease onset the relative risk of AD is 1.63, but when the TBI occurs within ten years of disease onset the relative risk increases to 5.33 [15]. This age discrimination effect is also apparent with mTBI, as Gardner and colleagues report that mTBI did not increase the risk of dementia in patients aged under the age of 65; however there was a 20% increase in the risk of dementia for mTBI patients aged 65 and older [19].

Independent internal risk factors for neurodegenerative disease can also combine with TBI to increase the overall risk of developing dementia. The apolipoprotein E4 (APOE4) gene alone increases the risk of developing AD [24] and the synergistic interaction of TBI and APOE4 together increases the risk of developing AD above predicted levels [25]; however, this remains controversial [13] and more study in this area is required.

A second internal modifier of dementia risk after TBI involves the concept of cognitive reserve. The protective effect of cognitive reserve is seen in the increased risk of AD in those with low levels of education [26] and cognitive reserve may also predict long-term outcome after TBI. In a 30-year follow-up of Vietnam veterans with a history of penetrating injury, a lower pre-injury intelligence was predictive of chronic cognitive decline after trauma [27]. This is an interesting area that requires more exploration.

While TBI is associated with the development of dementia, TBI is also associated with the risk of developing neurodegenerative diseases outside the umbrella of dementia. A meta-analysis of 22 case studies revealed that TBI increased the risk of PD by 57% [28]. This is confirmed in a retrospective cohort study of 165,799 patients aged over 55 with a history of TBI five to seven years prior to disease onset that demonstrated a 44% increase in PD risk after TBI [29]. As this retrospective cohort is essentially the same group used to look for dementia risk [19], we can determine that TBI is a risk factor for a diverse group of neurodegenerative diseases.

In light of the emerging evidence it is apparent that TBI should be viewed as a risk factor for multiple types of neurodegenerative disease. The question becomes whether we should view TBI as a trigger for individual neurodegenerative diseases, or if we should view the chronic clinical symptoms of TBI as an umbrella disease with multiple possible manifestations.

Pathological Protein Accumulation After TBI – Seeds of a Disease or Evidence of Cerebral Dysfunction?

A common factor between different neurodegenerative disorders is abnormal aggregation, misfolding, and/or accumulation of proteins in the brain. Amyloid-beta (Aβ) plaques and phosphorylated tau (p-tau) tangles are the hallmark proteinopathies of AD [30], α-synuclein accumulates in PD [31], and transactive response DNA-binding protein 43 kDa (TDP-43) accumulates in FTD and ALS [32]. While the role of these proteins in the initiation of disease is still under debate, it is clear that this abnormal accumulation is indicative of abnormal cellular processes and cerebral dysfunction. A unifying feature of acute and chronic pathology after TBI or repeat mTBI is the abnormal accumulation of pathological proteins related to neurodegenerative disease. Acutely, TBI brains can present with Aβ, p-tau, and α-synuclein pathology [33]. Chronically, TBI brains can present with Aβ, ptau, TDP-43, and α-synuclein pathology [7, 34]. In this review we will focus on Aβ and tau pathologies after TBI.

Aβ Pathology After TBI

Aβ accumulation and deposition into plaque after TBI have been widely studied in both humans and animal models, providing insight into the common but complex neurodegenerative pathways that can be triggered after TBI. The presence of Aβ plaques in the brain acutely after severe TBI was first reported in a small post-mortem study by Roberts and colleagues [35]. Analysis of 16 TBI cases with survival of 6–18 days post-injury found deposition of diffuse Aβ-positive plaques in 38% of injured brains. While TBI cases ranging in age from 10 to 63 years-old were analyzed, four of the six plaque-positive cases were older than 50 years old [35], an age range at which plaques can occur in the normally aging population [36].

This study was repeated with a much larger cohort of TBI cases in 1994 [37]. In this analysis of 152 post-mortemTBI brains from people aged 8 weeks to 85 years old and surviving 4 h–2.5 years after injury, a total of 46 cases (30%) were positive for Aβ deposition.When teased apart, there was a 20% incidence of amyloid plaque in the brains aged less than 50, and 60% of the TBI brains aged 51–60, compared to 0% of controls. Both control and TBI brains above the age of 60 displayed amyloid deposits, but the TBI brains always had a higher incidence. These data indicate that age at the time of injury increases the incidence of amyloid deposition after TBI [37].

While these post-mortem studies demonstrate the incidence of plaque formation following TBI, a small study on surgically resected tissue from living patients demonstrated just how fast this plaque deposition occurs [38]. Eighteen living TBI patients suffering from severe TBI were examined, and Aβ plaque deposition was found in cortical tissue from six patients (33%). Three of these six patients were in their 30s, again indicating that TBI can reduce the age at which amyloid accumulation is normally observed. Further, with the time between injury and surgery ranging from only 2 to 16 h post TBI in the Aβ-positive cases, this study demonstrates just how rapidly Aβ can accumulate and aggregate after TBI [38].

Aβ pathology has also been detected in long-term survivors of TBI. Post-mortem analysis of brains from patients surviving 1–47 years after a single TBI again identified plaques in approximately 30% of long-term survivors [34]. While Aβ plaques were also found in 30% of control cases, comparison of plaque density and thioflavin-S staining revealed a trend towards greater plaque density in the brains of long-term TBI survivors and the appearance of more fibrillar, thioflavin-S positive Aβ plaques [34].

These neuropathological studies are invaluable to our understanding of Aβ deposition in the brain after TBI and have provided the scientific basis for current studies investigating Aβ as a potential biomarker for brain trauma. However, a major limitation of neuropathological studies is that they can only provide a snapshot of what is occurring in the brain. The development of amyloid imaging tracers for positron emission tomography which have had success in imaging amyloid in AD patients may provide the type of temporal resolution that has been previously impossible in TBI patients. Comparison of an Aβ-binding agent called Pittsburgh compound B [39] in 15 moderate and severe TBI patients and 11 controls revealed increased Pittsburgh compound B binding in the cortical gray matter and striatum of TBI patients when imaged less than one year post injury [40]. Future longitudinal Aβ imaging in TBI patients will be able to address questions about the fate of TBI-induced Aβ plaque – including whether acute plaques are cleared from the brain, and whether TBI patients are more susceptible to early or more aggressive amyloid deposition as they age.

While only approximately 30% of severe TBI brains present with acute amyloid plaques, the study of cortical tissue resected from 18 living TBI patients found increased intracellular staining of Aβ in 80% of cases [38], suggesting that intracellular accumulation of non-plaque species of Aβ is more common than plaque deposition after TBI. This is also true for accumulation of Aβ in axons after TBI, which occurs in a majority of injured brain samples, regardless of the presence or absence of plaque [41, 42]. Prefibrillar, but aggregating, amyloid species have also been detected in TBI patients,with high-molecular-weight Aβ oligomers detected in the cerebrospinal fluid of a subgroup of TBI patients within 72 h of injury [43]. Together, these data suggest that TBI causes increased accumulation of Aβ peptides in the brain, but aggregation and deposition only occur in a subset of patients.

One potential source of abnormal Aβ accumulation after TBI is increased production in the traumatized axon [33, 41, 42]. Amyloid precursor protein accumulates along the lengths of damaged axons in areas of diffuse axonal injury in humans up to three years post injury, and co-localizes with β-secretase (BACE1) and the presenilin subunit (PS1) of γ-secretase, proteins essential for cleavage of amyloid precursor protein into Aβ [42]. Comparison of antibodies recognizing Aβ40 or Aβ42 found that the species accumulating in the axonal bulbs of injured brains is Aβ42 [33]. Aβ accumulation after injury has also been reproduced in animal models of TBI by several groups [44–52] and these studies have proven useful for investigating the source of increased Aβ after TBI. Levels of the proteins involved in Aβ production (BACE1, PS1, and amyloid precursor protein) are increased in the injured cortex after TBI, and follow a timecourse similar to that of Aβ [49, 52]. Preclinical studies confirm that damaged axons are a hotspot of amyloid production after rotational injury in swine [44, 45], and cortical impact in mice [52, 53], and targeting the amyloid precursor protein secretase enzymes can prevent the increase in Aβ after TBI [49, 54], indicating that increased production of Aβ after TBI is the driver of acute amyloid accumulation after injury.

Potential Factors Influencing Aβ Pathology After TBI

Given that human and preclinical evidence points to increased production of Aβ after TBI, it is somewhat confusing that amyloid plaques are not observed in the majority of human TBI post-mortem brains (70%) [35, 37, 38]. This suggests that there are factors influencing Aβ accumulation in the brain after TBI. Two potential factors mentioned earlier are age at time of injury and length of survival, as the incidence of Aβ plaques is higher after acute severe TBI in older patients [37], and longer survival appears to lead to greater extent and more mature Aβ pathology [34].

Another potential factor is genetics. Polymorphisms in the gene for neprilysin, an enzymatic protein associated with degradation of Aβ in the brain [55], have been shown to affect Aβ plaque deposition acutely after TBI, with extended GT repeats in the neprilysin allele associated with increased risk of Aβ plaques, and a separate polymorphism associated with decreased risk of plaques after TBI [56]. In long-term survivors of TBI, neprilysin accumulates in axons and in the same axonal bulbs as amyloid precursor protein and Aβ – indicating that it may be important for the local clearance of TBI-induced Aβ [42]. Furthermore, levels of neprilysin are reduced in patients with traumatic encephalopathy compared to non-demented controls [57].

A second protein known to be involved in Aβ clearance from the brain is APOE. Polymorphisms in the gene encoding this protein result in three common alleles: APOE2, APOE3, and APOE4,with the APOE4 allele associated with impaired Aβ clearance from the brain [58, 59]. Retrospective analysis of cases from the study by Roberts et al. (1994) [37] found increased incidence of Aβ plaque deposition acutely after TBI in APOE4 carriers [60]. This occurred in an APOE4 allele dose-dependent manner, so that, while plaques were found in only 10% of those with no APOE4 allele (five of 50 cases), Aβ plaques were found in 35% of those heterozygous for APOE4 (12 of 34 cases) and 100% of those homozygous for APOE4 (six of six cases) [60]. Similarly, in mice expressing human APOE isoforms there is increased amyloid deposition, including fibrillar Aβ deposits, in PDAPP/APOE4 mice three months after TBI compared to PDAPP/APOE3 mice [61], and greater intracellular Aβ accumulation occurs in PDAPP/APOE4 from one to 12 weeks post injury compared to PDAPP/APOE3 mice [51]. Together these data demonstrate that polymorphisms in two genes associated with Aβ clearance may alter removal of TBI-induced Aβ and predispose certain individuals to greater Aβ accumulation and aggregation in the brain acutely after injury.

Lastly, it is important to note that there are similarities and differences between the plaques described in the brain after TBI and in AD. Similar to the composition of plaques in AD, Aβ42 has been identified as the primary Aβ species in amyloid deposits in TBI brains [38, 62]. However, the plaques found in the brain acutely after TBI are more diffuse than the dense-cored neuritic plaque, or senile plaque, found in advance-stage AD [35, 37, 38] – indicating that the plaques deposited after TBI are a rapidly and recently formed aggregate. While neuritic plaques have been found in a few TBI brains, these were restricted to the oldest cases in the study of acute single TBI [37] and thioflavin-S staining for beta-sheet structure in aggregated plaques was found in only one of 18 acute cases [38]. Again, this may be a factor of time, either from increased age at injury or increased survival time, as more fibrillar, thioflavin-S positive plaques were seen following long-term survival after TBI [34].

Tau Pathology After TBI

Tau pathology has also been studied after acute and chronic survival following single TBI. Evidence of tau phosphorylation at the advanced Ser396/Ser404 epitope is seen in axons and white matter of excised TBI brain tissue within 24 h of injury, but somatodendritic p-tau staining is rare [38], suggesting that hyperphosphorylation, but not tangle formation, occurs acutely after TBI. Sporadic cases of p-tau immunoreactivity have been reported in acute post-mortem TBI brains, but only in 11% of cases [33]. Tau-positive glia also occur in up to 20% of severe TBI post-mortem brains [33, 63].

More recently, the appearance of tau pathology has been examined in 39 severe TBI brains with survival times of 1–47 years after injury, and compared to 47 control brains [34]. In TBI brains aged below 60 years old, 34% of TBI brains presented with tau pathology compared to only 9% of controls. The distribution of tau pathology in TBI brains was different to that seen in control brains with abnormal tau staining in the sulcal depths and superficial layers of the cortex [34]. Tau pathology in TBI brains was widespread and could be observed in the cingulate gyrus, superior frontal gyrus, and insular cortex, but pathology in control brains was limited to the entorhinal cortex and hippocampus [34].

Most reports of tau pathology after TBI have been in repeat mTBI brains with CTE, suggesting that repeated exposure may be a potential factor influencing development of tau pathology after TBI. While the majority of historical reports have focused on boxers [7, 64–76], in the last five years there have been multiple cases of tau pathology in players of impact sports [7, 74, 77, 78]. Recent studies of post-mortem brains of former military personnel with a history of blast- and military-related concussion have also revealed tau pathology [78], suggesting that a variety of injury types can drive tau pathology. While CTE is viewed as primarily a tauopathy, the evidence for polypathology in CTE is highlighted by a recent report where 52% of 114 neuropathologically confirmed CTE brains demonstrated concomitant Aβ plaque deposition [79]. TDP-43 and α-synuclein have also been identified in CTE brains [7].

As occurs with Aβ, there are similarities and differences between the tau pathology observed after TBI compared to AD. The tau-positive somatodendritic inclusions seen in CTE

(A)

APP
after TBI

Axonal bulbs

Ipsilateral
internal capsule

(B)

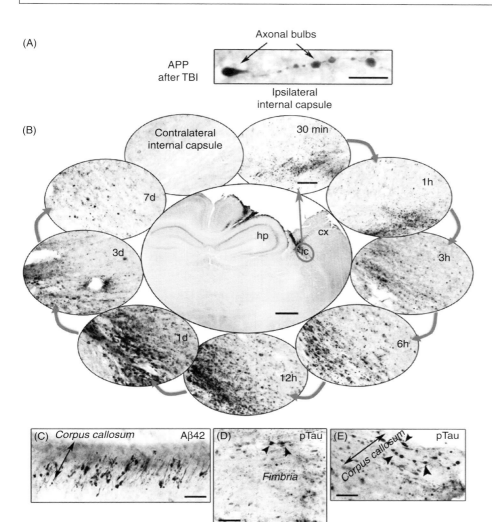

Contralateral
internal capsule

30 min

7d

1h

3d

hp   cx
ic

3h

1d

6h

12h

(C) *Corpus callosum*   Aβ42

(D)   pTau

Fimbria

(E)   pTau

Corpus callosum

Fig. 13.1 Acute polypathology after experimental traumatic brain injury (TBI) in Alzheimer's disease (AD) transgenic mice. 3xTg-AD mice received a unilateral controlled cortical impact injury. (A) Axon injury after TBI is characterized by amyloid precursor protein (APP)-positive axonal bulbs. This abnormal APP staining after TBI reflects damage to the microtubule network and accumulation of proteins trafficked by axonal transport. (B) The timecourse of axonal APP accumulation occurring in the internal capsule of C57/Bl6 mice after cortical impact. APP accumulation can be seen within 30 min of TBI, and is still visible 7 days post injury. (C) Aβ42-positive staining occurs in the white-matter tracts of 3xTg-AD mice 24 h after TBI. (D and E) Intra-axonal accumulation of AT8-positive phosphorylated tau (pTau) occurs in the fimbria and corpus callosum of 3xTg mice 24 h post injury. Scale bar for A, C, D, E = 20 μm, and for B = 500 μm (central image) and 50 μm (surrounding images). cx: cortex; hp: hippocampus; ic: internal capsule. [A black and white version of this figure will appear in some formats. For the color version, please refer to the plate section.]

are morphologically similar to those found in AD; however, there is much more astrocytic tau in CTE compared to AD. Another distinct difference is the distribution of neocortical tangles. As seen in long-term survivors of a single TBI [34], tau immunoreactivity in CTE characteristically presents with preferential deposition in layers II and III of the cortex compared to preferential deposition in layers V and VI in AD [69]. However, there are still many unanswered questions about tau pathology after TBI – we know little about the biochemical profiles of the tau that accumulates after injury, such as the inclusion type (paired helical filaments, straight, or ribbon filaments), the primary phosphorylation sites, or the roles of different tau isoforms. To date, there are only two studies of CTE in the literature that examine the ratio of 4 repeat (4R) to 3 repeat (3R) tau. In the first case, biochemical analysis has revealed that both 3R and 4R tau are hyperphosphorylated in brain extracts from two boxers [72]. In the second case, immunohistological staining demonstrates both 4R and 3R staining in a human CTE case, with 4R tau thought to be predominant in astrocytic tau inclusions [7]. No biochemical analysis has been performed on the chronic tau pathology observed in single TBI brain.

A major obstacle to gaining a better understanding of tau pathology after TBI is the lack of an animal model of repeat mTBI that recapitulates the tau pathology observed in CTE. The acute accumulation of p-tau in more severe TBI models is similar to that described for TBI-induced Aβ, with an acute increase of abnormal p-tau observed in areas of axonal injury. Following cortical impact in the 3xTg AD model mouse (harboring a human P301L tau mutation), the accumulation of p-tau in multiple brain regions was punctate and primarily axonal [51], and was also reportedly increased in the somatodendritic compartments of the contralateral CA1 neuronal cells [51]. Other groups have also demonstrated that endogenous mouse tau can be acutely phosphorylated at multiple sites following blast [78] and closed head injury [50, 80].

However, driving chronic accumulation of p-tau, even in tau transgenic mice, has proven to be difficult. In a study of repeat mTBI using mice overexpressing the shortest tau isoform (T44 mice), mice were exposed to four mTBI/day, once a week for four weeks (16 impacts over four weeks), with a recovery time of nine months, and only one mouse was found to have accelerated tau deposition [81]. A similar study using aged (18-month) human tau mice (hTau mice, which express all six tau

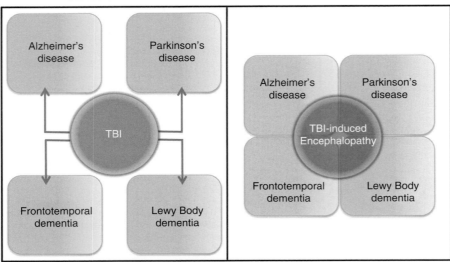

Fig. 13.2 The traditional view of the chronic effects of traumatic brain injury (TBI) classifies brain injury as a risk factor for the precipitation of individual neurodegenerative diseases. The emerging view supported in this review is that TBI-induced neurodegenerative disease, or traumatic encephalopathy, is a spectrum disorder that shares clinical and neuropathological hallmarks with other neurodegenerative disorders.

isoforms) exposed to five mTBIs over a nine-day period showed accelerated tau pathology three weeks after injury compared to sham or single mTBI hTau mice [82].

In general, the mechanisms of action driving this accelerated tau pathology remains unclear and recapitulating the pathology of repeat mTBI in animals remains challenging. It is unclear if a brain injury has to be above a certain velocity, in a specific brain region, or if a certain number of impacts are required to begin the destructive cascade that results in chronic tau accumulation. Other practical issues, such as skin deflection, tissue necrosis, and repeat anesthesia, further complicate the development of repeat mTBI models.

Demonstrating Polypathology After TBI

While there are human studies that examine discrete neurodegenerative pathologies after TBI, and descriptive or smaller studies looking at multiple pathologies in individual cases, the field is lacking a systematic analysis of multiple pathologies in individual cases in a large TBI and control population. Such a comprehensive study could help identify factors that lead to different neuropathological phenotypes after TBI, and help explain the polypathology that has been reported in acute and chronic TBI brains [6, 7, 34, 76, 83, 84]. Such widespread studies may provide a more accurate sense of the actual incidence of neurodegenerative pathology after TBI. Current studies looking for a single pathology report the incidence of amyloid and tau at approximately 30%; however, the incidence of neurodegenerative pathology in the brain after TBI could be considerably higher if all the possible disease-related proteins are studied in the same controlled cohorts.

Animal studies would also benefit from investigating the presence of multiple pathologies simultaneously in individual mice. This could help determine whether different pathologies follow different timecourses after injury, and whether a particular pathology is more associated with injury than others. For example, the studies by Tran et al. investigated both Aβ

and tau pathologies after cortical impact injury in the 3xTg-AD model mouse [51, 53]. An example of acute Aβ and p-tau polypathology after TBI in 3xTg-AD mice is shown in Figure 13.1. Future studies can begin incorporating the factors that appear to influence the phenotype of neurodegenerative pathology after TBI, including injury severity, age at injury, length of survival, and APOE genotype, and look for mixed pathology.

Does Disease Pathology After TBI Relate to Dementia Risk?

Similar to the case in other neurodegenerative diseases we are forced to ask: what does the presence of neurodegenerative disease pathology in a subset of patients after TBI mean? Is it related to dementia risk? Does it drive further neurodegeneration or accelerate brain aging? Indeed, the appearance of neuritic Aβ plaques in CTE brains is associated with advanced CTE disease taging and dementia [79], suggesting that this amyloid may accelerate or drive disease state following repeat mTBI. Looking ahead at potential factors influencing dementia risk after TBI, the appearance of pathology does seem to be the largest associating factor. Other factors include age at the time of injury, duration of survival, repeated exposure or increased severity of injury, and APOE4 genotype. The establishment of large, case-controlled cohorts of TBI brains will be essential for teasing apart the impact of these factors on dementia onset after injury.

Conclusion

As the TBI field continues to grow, a clearer picture is emerging of the array of neuropathological changes and clinical symptoms that can occur. The chronic sequelae of both single TBI and repeat mTBI are as heterogeneous and personalized to the individual patient as other aspects of brain trauma; however they share common neuropathological features and clinical symptoms of classically defined neurodegenerative disorders.While the spectrum of chronic cognitive and neurobehavioral disorders that occur following repeat mTBI is viewed as the symptoms of CTE, the spectrum of chronic cognitive and neurobehavioral symptoms that occur after a single TBI is considered to represent distinct neurodegenerative diseases such as AD. These data support the suggestion that the multiple manifestations of TBI-induced neurodegenerative disorders be classified together as traumatic encephalopathy or trauma-induced neurodegeneration, regardless of the nature or frequency of the precipitating TBI (Figure 13.2).

Acknowledgments

This work was supported by grant number R01 NS067417 from the National Institute of Neurological Disorders and Stroke (MPB). The authors have no conflicts of interest to declare.

References

1. Martland, H.S., 1928. Punch drunk. *J. Am. Med. Assoc.* 91, 1103–1107.
2. Langlois, J.A., Rutland-Brown, W., Wald, M.M., 2006. The epidemiology and impact of traumatic brain injury: a brief overview. *J. Head Trauma Rehabil.* 21, 375–378.
3. Osnato, M., Giliberti, V., 1927. Postconcussion neurosis – traumatic encephalitis: a conception of postconcussion phenomena. *Arch. Neurol. Psychiatry* 18, 181–214.
4. Millspaugh, H.S., 1937. Dementia pugilistica. *U. S. Med. Bull.* 35, 297–303.
5. McCown, I.A., 1959. Boxing injuries. *Am. J. Surg.* 98, 509–516.
6. Smith, D.H., Johnson, V.E., Stewart, W., 2013. Chronic neuropathologies of single and repetitive TBI: substrates of dementia? *Nat. Rev. Neurol.* 9, 211–221.
7. McKee, A.C., Stein, T.D., Nowinski, C.J., Stern, R.A., Daneshvar, D.H., Alvarez, V.E., et al., 2013. The spectrum of disease in chronic traumatic encephalopathy. *Brain* 136, 43–64.
8. Shalat, S.L., Seltzer, B., Pidcock, C., Baker Jr., E.L., 1987. Risk factors for Alzheimer's disease: a case–control study. *Neurology* 37, 1630–1633.
9. Katzman, R., Aronson, M., Fuld, P., Kawas, C., Brown, T., Morgenstern, H., Frishman, W., Gidez, L., Eder, H., Ooi, W.L., 1989. Development of dementing illnesses in an 80-year-old volunteer cohort. *Ann. Neurol.* 25, 317–324.
10. Broe, G.A., Henderson, A.S., Creasey, H., McCusker, E., Korten, A.E., Jorm, A.F., Longley, W., Anthony, J.C., 1990. A case–control study of Alzheimer's disease in Australia. *Neurology* 40, 1698–1707.
11. Fratiglioni, L., Ahlbom, A., Viitanen, M., Winblad, B., 1993. Risk factors for late-onset Alzheimer's disease: a population-based, case–control study. *Ann. Neurol.* 33, 258–266.
12. Tsolaki, M., Fountoulakis, K., Chantzi, E., Kazis, A., 1997. Risk factors for clinically diagnosed Alzheimer's disease: a case–control study of a Greek population. *Int. Psychogeriatr.* 9, 327–341.
13. O'Meara, E.S., Kukull, W.A., Sheppard, L., Bowen, J.D., McCormick, W.C., Teri, L., Pfanschmidt, M., Thompson, J.D., Schellenberg, G.D., Larson, E.B., 1997. Head injury and risk of Alzheimer's disease by apolipoprotein E genotype. *Am. J. Epidemiol.* 146, 373–384.
14. Rasmusson, D.X., Brandt, J., Martin, D.B., Folstein, M.F., 1995. Head injury as a risk factor in Alzheimer's disease. *Brain Inj.* 9, 213–219.
15. Mortimer, J.A., van Duijn, C.M., Chandra, V., Fratiglioni, L., Graves, A.B., Heyman, A., Jorm, A.F., Kokmen, E., Kondo, K., Rocca, W.A., Shalat, S.L., Soininen, H., Hofman, A., 1991. Head trauma as a risk factor for Alzheimer's disease: a collaborative re-analysis of case–control studies. EURODEM Risk Factors Research Group. *Int. J. Epidemiol.* 20 (Suppl. 2), S28–S35.
16. Fleminger, S., Oliver, D.L., Lovestone, S., Rabe-Hesketh, S., Giora, A., 2003. Head injury as a risk factor for Alzheimer's disease: the evidence 10 years on; a partial replication. *J. Neurol. Neurosurg. Psychiatry* 74, 857–862.
17. Bachman, D.L., Wolf, P.A., Linn, R., Knoefel, J.E., Cobb, J., Belanger, A., D'Agostino, R.B., White, L.R., 1992. Prevalence of dementia and probable senile dementia of the Alzheimer type in the Framingham Study. *Neurology* 42, 115–119.
18. Plassman, B.L., Havlik, R.J., Steffens, D.C., Helms, M.J., Newman, T.N., Drosdick, D., Phillips, C., Gau, B.A., Welsh-Bohmer, K.A., Burke, J.R., Guralnik, J.M., Breitner, J.C., 2000. Documented head injury in early adulthood and risk of Alzheimer's disease and other dementias. *Neurology* 55, 1158–1166.
19. Gardner, R.C., Burke, J.F., Nettiksimmons, J., Kaup, A., Barnes, D.E., Yaffe, K., 2014. Dementia risk after traumatic brain injury vs nonbrain trauma: the role of age and severity. *JAMA Neurol.* 71, 1490–1497.
20. Rosso, S.M., Landweer, E.J., Houterman, M., Donker Kaat, L., van Duijn, C.M., van Swieten, J.C., 2003. Medical and environmental risk factors for sporadic frontotemporal dementia: a retrospective case–control study. *J. Neurol. Neurosurg. Psychiatry* 74, 1574–1576.
21. Kalkonde, Y.V., Jawaid, A., Qureshi, S.U., Shirani, P., Wheaton, M., Pinto-Patarroyo, G.P., Schulz, P.E., 2012. Medical and environmental risk factors associated with frontotemporal dementia: a case–control study in a veteran population. *Alzheimers Dement.* 8, 204–210.
22. Wang, H.K., Lee, Y.C., Huang, C.Y., Liliang, P.C., Lu, K., Chen, H.J., Li, Y.C., Tsai, K.J., 2015. Traumatic brain injury causes frontotemporal dementia and TDP-43 proteolysis. *Neuroscience* 14, 94–103.
23. Graves, A.B., White, E., Koepsell, T.D., Reifler, B.V., van Belle, G., Larson, E.B., Raskind, M., 1990. The association between head trauma and Alzheimer's disease. *Am. J. Epidemiol.* 131, 491–501.
24. Corder, E.H., Saunders, A.M., Strittmatter, W.J., Schmechel, D.E., Gaskell, P.C., Small, G.W., Roses, A.D., Haines, J.L., Pericak-Vance, M.A., 1993. Gene dose of apolipoprotein E type 4 allele and the risk of Alzheimer's disease in late onset families. *Science* 261, 921–923.
25. Mayeux, R., Ottman, R., Maestre, G., Ngai, C., Tang, M.X., Ginsberg, H., Chun, M., Tycko, B., Shelanski, M., 1995. Synergistic effects of traumatic head injury and apolipoproteinepsilon 4 in patients with Alzheimer's disease. *Neurology* 45, 555–557.
26. Caamano-Isorna, F., Corral, M., Montes-Martinez, A., Takkouche, B., 2006. Education and dementia: a meta-analytic study. *Neuroepidemiology* 26, 226–232.
27. Raymont, V., Greathouse, A., Reding, K., Lipsky, R., Salazar, A., Grafman, J., 2008. Demographic, structural and genetic predictors of late cognitive decline after penetrating head injury. *Brain* 131, 543–558.
28. Jafari, S., Etminan, M., Aminzadeh, F., Samii, A., 2013. Head injury and risk of Parkinson disease: a systematic review and meta-analysis. *Mov. Disord.* 28, 1222–1229.
29. Gardner, R.C., Burke, J.F., Nettiksimmons, J., Goldman, S., Tanner, C.M., Yaffe, K., 2015. Traumatic brain injury in later life increases risk for Parkinson disease. *Ann. Neurol.* 77, 987–995.
30. Hardy, J., Selkoe, D.J., 2002. The amyloid hypothesis of Alzheimer's disease: progress and problems on the road to therapeutics. *Science* 297, 353–356.

31. Polymeropoulos, M.H., Lavedan, C., Leroy, E., Ide, S.E., Dehejia, A., Dutra, A., Pike, B., Root, H., Rubenstein, J., Boyer, R., Stenroos, E.S., Chandrasekharappa, S., Athanassiadou, A., Papapetropoulos, T., Johnson, W.G., Lazzarini, A.M., Duvoisin, R.C., Di Iorio, G., Golbe, L.I., Nussbaum, R.L., 1997. Mutation in the alpha-synuclein gene identified in families with Parkinson's disease. *Science* 276, 2045–2047.

32. Neumann, M., Sampathu, D.M., Kwong, L.K., Truax, A.C., Micsenyi, M.C., Chou, T.T., Bruce, J., Schuck, T., Grossman, M., Clark, C.M., McCluskey, L.F., Miller, B.L., Masliah, E., Mackenzie, I.R., Feldman, H., Feiden, W., Kretzschmar, H.A., Trojanowski, J.Q., Lee, V.M., 2006. Ubiquitinated TDP-43 in frontotemporal lobar degeneration and amyotrophic lateral sclerosis. *Science* 314, 130–133.

33. Uryu, K., Chen, X.H., Martinez, D., Browne, K.D., Johnson, V.E., Graham, D.I., Lee, V.M., Trojanowski, J.Q., Smith, D.H., 2007. Multiple proteins implicated in neurodegenerative diseases accumulate in axons after brain trauma in humans. *Exp. Neurol.* 208, 185–192.

34. Johnson, V.E., Stewart, W., Smith, D.H., 2012. Widespread tau and amyloid-beta pathology many years after a single traumatic brain injury in humans. *Brain Pathol.* 22, 142–149.

35. Roberts, G.W., Gentleman, S.M., Lynch, A., Graham, D.I., 1991. Beta A4 amyloid protein deposition in brain after head trauma. *Lancet* 338, 1422–1423.

36. Braak, H., Braak, E., 1997. Diagnostic criteria for neuropathologic assessment of Alzheimer's disease. *Neurobiol. Aging* 18, S85–S88.

37. Roberts, G.W., Gentleman, S.M., Lynch, A., Murray, L., Landon, M., Graham, D.I., 1994. Beta amyloid protein deposition in the brain after severe head injury: implications for the pathogenesis of Alzheimer's disease. *J. Neurol. Neurosurg. Psychiatry* 57, 419–425.

38. Ikonomovic, M.D., Uryu, K., Abrahamson, E.E., Ciallella, J.R., Trojanowski, J.Q., Lee, V.M., Clark, R.S., Marion, D.W.,Wisniewski, S.R., Dekosky, S.T., 2004. Alzheimer's pathology in human temporal cortex surgically excised after severe brain injury. *Exp. Neurol.* 190, 192–203.

39. Wu, C., Pike, V.W., Wang, Y., 2005. Amyloid imaging: frombenchtop to bedside. *Curr. Top. Dev. Biol.* 70, 171–213.

40. Hong, Y.T., Veenith, T., Dewar, D., Outtrim, J.G., Mani, V., Williams, C., Pimlott, S., Hutchinson, P.J., Tavares, A., Canales, R., Mathis, C.A., Klunk, W.E., Aigbirhio, F.I., Coles, J.P., Baron, J.C., Pickard, J.D., Fryer, T.D., Stewart,W., Menon, D.K., 2014. Amyloid imaging with carbon 11-labeled Pittsburgh compound B for traumatic brain injury. *JAMA Neurol.* 71, 23–31.

41. Smith, D.H., Chen, X.H., Iwata, A., Graham, D.I., 2003. Amyloid beta accumulation in axons after traumatic brain injury in humans. *J. Neurosurg.* 98, 1072–1077.

42. Chen, X.H., Johnson, V.E., Uryu, K., Trojanowski, J.Q., Smith, D.H., 2009. A lack of amyloid beta plaques despite persistent accumulation of amyloid beta in axons of long-term survivors of traumatic brain injury. *Brain Pathol.* 19, 214–223.

43. Gatson, J.W., Warren, V., Abdelfattah, K., Wolf, S., Hynan, L.S., Moore, C., Diaz-Arrastia, R., Minei, J.P., Madden, C., Wigginton, J.G., 2013. Detection of beta-amyloid oligomers as a predictor of neurological outcome after brain injury. *J. Neurosurg.* 118, 1336–1342.

44. Smith, D.H., Chen, X.H., Nonaka, M., Trojanowski, J.Q., Lee, V.M., Saatman, K.E., Leoni, M.J., Xu, B.N., Wolf, J.A., Meaney, D.F., 1999. Accumulation of amyloid beta and tau and the formation of neurofilament inclusions following diffuse brain injury in the pig. *J. Neuropathol. Exp. Neurol.* 58, 982–992.

45. Chen, X.H., Siman, R., Iwata, A., Meaney, D.F., Trojanowski, J.Q., Smith, D.H., 2004. Longterm accumulation of amyloid-beta, beta-secretase, presenilin-1, and caspase-3 in damaged axons following brain trauma. *Am. J. Pathol.* 165, 357–371.

46. Conte, V., Uryu, K., Fujimoto, S., Yao, Y., Rokach, J., Longhi, L., Trojanowski, J.Q., Lee, V.M., McIntosh, T.K., Pratico, D., 2004. Vitamin E reduces amyloidosis and improves cognitive function in Tg2576 mice following repetitive concussive brain injury. *J. Neurochem.* 90, 758–764.

47. Abrahamson, E.E., Ikonomovic, M.D., Ciallella, J.R., Hope, C.E., Paljug, W.R., Isanski, B.A., Flood, D.G., Clark, R.S., DeKosky, S.T., 2006. Caspase inhibition therapy abolishes brain trauma-induced increases in Abeta peptide: implications for clinical outcome. *Exp. Neurol.* 197, 437–450.

48. Abrahamson, E.E., Ikonomovic, M.D., Dixon, C.E., Dekosky, S.T., 2009. Simvastatin therapy prevents brain trauma-induced increases in beta-amyloid peptide levels. *Ann. Neurol.* 66, 407–414.

49. Loane, D.J., Pocivavsek, A., Moussa, C.E., Thompson, R., Matsuoka, Y., Faden, A.I., Rebeck, G.W., Burns, M.P., 2009. Amyloid precursor protein secretases as therapeutic targets for traumatic brain injury. *Nat. Med.* 15, 377–379.

50. Laskowitz, D.T., Song, P., Wang, H., Mace, B., Sullivan, P.M., Vitek, M.P., Dawson, H.N., 2010. Traumatic brain injury exacerbates neurodegenerative pathology: improvement with an apolipoprotein E-based therapeutic. *J. Neurotrauma* 27, 1983–1995.

51. Tran, H.T., LaFerla, F.M., Holtzman, D.M., Brody, D.L., 2011. Controlled cortical impact traumatic brain injury in 3xTg-AD mice causes acute intra-axonal amyloid-beta accumulation and independently accelerates the development of tau abnormalities. *J. Neurosci. Off. J. Soc. Neurosci.* 31, 9513–9525.

52. Washington, P.M., Morffy, N., Parsadanian, M., Zapple, D.N., Burns, M.P., 2014. Experimental traumatic brain injury induces rapid aggregation and oligomerization of amyloidbeta in an Alzheimer's disease mouse model. *J. Neurotrauma* 31, 125–134.

53. Tran, H.T., Sanchez, L., Esparza, T.J., Brody, D.L., 2011. Distinct temporal and anatomical distributions of amyloid-beta and tau abnormalities following controlled cortical impact in transgenic mice. *PLoS One* 6, e25475.

54. Winston, C.N., Chellappa, D., Wilkins, T., Barton, D.J., Washington, P.M., Loane, D.J., Zapple, D.N., Burns, M.P., 2013. Controlled cortical impact results in an extensive loss of dendritic spines that is not mediated by injury-induced amyloid-beta accumulation. *J. Neurotrauma* 30, 1966–1972.

55. Iwata, N., Tsubuki, S., Takaki, Y., Watanabe, K., Sekiguchi, M., Hosoki, E., Kawashima-Morishima, M., Lee, H.J., Hama, E., Sekine-Aizawa, Y., Saido, T.C., 2000. Identification of the major Abeta1-42-degrading catabolic pathway in brain parenchyma: suppression leads to biochemical and pathological deposition. *Nat. Med.* 6, 143–150.

56. Johnson, V.E., Stewart,W., Graham, D.I., Stewart, J.E., Praestgaard, A.H., Smith, D.H., 2009. A neprilysin polymorphism and amyloid-beta plaques after traumatic brain injury. *J. Neurotrauma* 26, 1197–1202.

57. Kokjohn, T.A., Maarouf, C.L., Daugs, I.D., Hunter, J.M., Whiteside, C.M., Malek-Ahmadi, M., Rodriguez, E., Kalback,W., Jacobson, S.A., Sabbagh, M.N., Beach, T.G., Roher, A.E., 2013. Neurochemical profile of dementia pugilistica. *J. Neurotrauma* 30, 981–997.

58. Deane, R., Sagare, A., Hamm, K., Parisi, M., Lane, S., Finn, M.B., Holtzman, D.M., Zlokovic, B.V., 2008. apoE isoform-specific disruption of amyloid beta peptide clearance from mouse brain. *J. Clin. Invest.* 118, 4002–4013.

59. Jiang, Q., Lee, C.Y., Mandrekar, S., Wilkinson, B., Cramer, P., Zelcer, Richardson, J.C., Smith, J.D., Comery, T.A., Riddell, D., Holtzman, et al., 2008. ApoE promotes the proteolytic degradation of Abeta. *Neuron* 58, 681–693.

60. Nicoll, J.A., Roberts, G.W., Graham, D.I., 1995. Apolipoprotein E epsilon 4 allele is associated with deposition of amyloid beta-protein following head injury. *Nat. Med.* 1, 135–137.

61. Hartman, R.E., Laurer, H., Longhi, L., Bales, K.R., Paul, S.M., McIntosh, T.K., Holtzman, D.M., 2002. Apolipoprotein E4 influences amyloid deposition but not cell loss after traumatic brain injury in a mouse model of Alzheimer's disease. *J. Neurosci.* 22, 10083–10087.

62. Gentleman, S.M., Greenberg, B.D., Savage, M.J., Noori, M., Newman, S.J., Roberts, G.W., Griffin, W.S., et al. 1997. A beta 42 is the predominant form of amyloid beta-protein in the brains of short-term survivors of head injury. *Neuroreport* 8, 1519–1522.

63. Smith, C., Graham, D.I., Murray, L.S., Nicoll, J.A., 2003. Tau immunohistochemistry in acute brain injury. *Neuropathol. Appl. Neurobiol.* 29, 496–502.

64. Constantinidis, J., Tissot, R., 1967. Generalized Alzheimer's neurofibrillary lesions without senile plaques (presentation of one anatomo-clinical case). *Schweiz. Arch. Neurol. Neurochir. Psychiatr.* 100, 117–130.

65. Corsellis, J.A., Bruton, C.J., Freeman-Browne, D., 1973. The aftermath of boxing. *Psychol. Med.* 3, 270–303.

66. Allsop, D., Haga, S., Bruton, C., Ishii, T., Roberts, G.W., 1990. Neurofibrillary tangles in some cases of dementia pugilistica share antigens with amyloid beta-protein of Alzheimer's disease. *Am. J. Pathol.* 136, 255–260.

67. Dale, G.E., Leigh, P.N., Luthert, P., Anderton, B.H., Roberts, G.W., 1991. Neurofibrillary tangles in dementia pugilistica are ubiquitinated. *J. Neurol. Neurosurg. Psychiatry* 54, 116–118.

68. Tokuda, T., Ikeda, S., Yanagisawa, N., Ihara, Y., Glenner, G.G., 1991. Re-examination of exboxers' brains using immunohistochemistry with antibodies to amyloid beta-protein and tau protein. *Acta Neuropathol.* 82, 280–285.

69. Hof, P.R., Bouras, C., Buee, L., Delacourte, A., Perl, D.P., Morrison, J.H., 1992. Differential distribution of neurofibrillary tangles in the cerebral cortex of dementia pugilistica and Alzheimer's disease cases. *Acta Neuropathol.* 85, 23–30.

70. Geddes, J.F., Vowles, G.H., Robinson, S.F., Sutcliffe, J.C., 1996. Neurofibrillary tangles, but not Alzheimer-type pathology, in a young boxer. *Neuropathol. Appl. Neurobiol.* 22, 12–16.

71. Geddes, J.F., Vowles, G.H., Nicoll, J.A., Revesz, T., 1999. Neuronal cytoskeletal changes are an early consequence of repetitive head injury. *Acta Neuropathol.* 98, 171–178.

72. Schmidt, M.L., Zhukareva, V., Newell, K.L., Lee, V.M., Trojanowski, J.Q., 2001. Tau isoform profile and phosphorylation state in dementia pugilistica recapitulate Alzheimer's disease. *Acta Neuropathol.* 101, 518–524.

73. Areza-Fegyveres, R., Rosemberg, S., Castro, R.M., Porto, C.S., Bahia, V.S., Caramelli, P., Nitrini, R., 2007. Dementia pugilistica with clinical features of Alzheimer's disease. *Arq. Neuropsiquiatr.* 65, 830–833.

74. McKee, A.C., Cantu, R.C., Nowinski, C.J., Hedley-Whyte, E.T., Gavett, B.E., Budson, A.E., Santini, V.E., Lee, H.S., Kubilus, C.A., Stern, R.A., 2009. Chronic traumatic encephalopathy in athletes: progressive tauopathy after repetitive head injury. *J. Neuropathol. Exp. Neurol.* 68, 709–735.

75. Saing, T., Dick, M., Nelson, P.T., Kim, R.C., Cribbs, D.H., Head, E., 2012. Frontal cortex neuropathology in dementia pugilistica. *J. Neurotrauma* 29, 1054–1070.

76. McKee, A.C., Stein, T.D., Kiernan, P.T., Alvarez, V.E., 2015. The neuropathology of chronic traumatic encephalopathy. *Brain Pathol.* 25, 350–364.

77. Omalu, B., Bailes, J., Hamilton, R.L., Kamboh, M.I., Hammers, J., Case, M., Fitzsimmons, R., 2011. Emerging histomorphologic phenotypes of chronic traumatic encephalopathy in American athletes. *Neurosurgery* 69, 173–183 (discussion 183).

78. Goldstein, L.E., Fisher, A.M., Tagge, C.A., Zhang, X.-L., Velisek, L., Sullivan, et al., 2012. Chronic traumatic encephalopathy in blast-exposed military veterans and a blast neurotrauma mouse model. *Sci. Transl. Med.* 4, 134ra160.

79. Stein, T.D., Montenigro, P.H., Alvarez, V.E., Xia, W., Crary, J.F., Tripodis, et al., 2015. Beta-amyloid deposition in chronic traumatic encephalopathy. *Acta Neuropathol.* 130, 21–34.

80. Namjoshi, D.R., Cheng, W.H., McInnes, K.A., Martens, K.M., Carr, M., Wilkinson, A., et al., 2014. Merging pathology with biomechanics using CHIMERA (Closed-Head Impact Model of Engineered Rotational Acceleration): a novel, surgery-free model of traumatic brain injury. *Mol. Neurodegener.* 9, 55.

81. Yoshiyama, Y., Uryu, K., Higuchi, M., Longhi, L., Hoover, R., Fujimoto, S., et al., 2005. Enhanced neurofibrillary tangle formation, cerebral atrophy, and cognitive deficits induced by repetitive mild brain injury in a transgenic tauopathy mouse model. *J. Neurotrauma* 22, 1134–1141.

82. Ojo, J.O., Mouzon, B., Greenberg, M.B., Bachmeier, C., Mullan, M., Crawford, F., 2013. Repetitive mild traumatic brain injury augments tau pathology and glial activation in aged hTau mice. *J. Neuropathol. Exp. Neurol.* 72, 137–151.

83. Newell, K.L., Boyer, P., Gomez-Tortosa, E., Hobbs, W., Hedley-Whyte, E.T., Vonsattel, J.P., et al., 1999. Alpha-synuclein immunoreactivity is present in axonal swellings in neuroaxonal dystrophy and acute traumatic brain injury. *J. Neuropathol. Exp. Neurol.* 58, 1263–1268.

84. Johnson, V.E., Stewart, W., Trojanowski, J.Q., Smith, D.H., 2011. Acute and chronically increased immunoreactivity to phosphorylation-independent but not pathological TDP-43 after a single traumatic brain injury in humans. *Acta Neuropathol.* 122, 715–726.

Chapter

14

Traumatic Encephalopathy: Review and Provisional Research Diagnostic Criteria

Jeff Victoroff

The Concept of Traumatic Encephalopathy

Traumatic encephalopathy (TE) has been reported using various nomenclature since Martland's report titled "Punch drunk" in 1928 [1]. For the next 50 years, the TE literature focused on the risk of brain damage among boxers. Reflecting that bias, Millspaugh introduced the term "dementia pugilistica" in 1937 [2]. This phrase gained backing with advances in the study of boxers' brains [3–5]. Other authorities have described a similar or perhaps identical disorder with other names. Parker (1934) may have been the first to publish a peer-reviewed paper referring to TE of pugilists [6]. Similar terminology was employed by Grahmann and Ule (1957) (*traumatischen Boxer-Encephalopathie*) [7], and by La Cava (1963) ("boxer's encephalopathy") [8]. Critchley (1937), noting the striking tendency for gradual worsening in some cases, initially proposed the phrase "chronic progressive traumatic encephalopathy" [9]. Critchley (1949) [10] and Johnson (1969) [11], noting that some cases did not progress, later proposed dropping the qualifier *progressive* and calling this condition *chronic traumatic encephalopathy* (CTE). Critchley's term CTE has recently become popular in the literature, despite many reports suggesting that the course is more often progressive, not persistent, static, or "chronic" [12–16]. For this reason, Victoroff and Baron [17] suggested that the label CTE misleadingly implies a particular, infrequently observed clinical course. It may be more inclusive and accurate to employ Parker's original terminology, TE.

TE is typically described as a persistent or progressive alteration in neurological or neurobehavioral status that follows exposure to head injury, traumatic brain injury, or concussion. Alterations in the primary neurological examination, such as dysarthria, tremor, or gait ataxia, are often combined with alterations in behavior, including memory loss, depression, or aggression [1, 7, 9, 15]. Most reported cases involve exposure to recurrent injuries, although some evidence suggests that a single injury may also generate this condition [5, 15, 18]. Moreover, since this condition has been reported in athletes whose sports involve many collisions or head blows but in whom there is no explicit history of concussion, it has been proposed that multiple subconcussive injuries can similarly harm the brain [15, 19–21].

Neuropathological studies of TE cases have reported a variety of changes in the brainstem and cerebrum, including frequent cavum septum pellucidum, loss of neurons in the substantia nigra, locus coeruleus, and dorsal raphe, loss of Purkinje cells, and deposition of abnormal proteins typically associated with neurodegeneration, especially a patchy distribution of neocortical hyperphosphorylated 4R/3R tau-positive neocortical neurofibrillary tangles and neuropil threads, often perivascular and often found in the depths of sulci, typically out of proportion to diffuse (and less often neuritic) β-amyloid plaques [22–27]. One report raises the possibility that trauma may also activate transactive response DNA-binding protein 43 to produce a motor neuron disease [28]. A putative medical narrative has emerged: exposure to repetitive concussions can cause a clinical disorder, TE, which may progress to tauopathic dementia [15, 29].

Eighty-five years have thus passed since the first clinical description of this putative condition. Yet to date, no clinical diagnostic criteria have been adopted. Like Alzheimer's disease prior to the publication of the National Institute of Neurological and Communicative Disorders and Stroke and the Alzheimer's Disease and Related Disorders Association (NINCDS-ADRDA) Work Group criteria of 1984 [30], TE has been diagnosed for decades without reference to published standards. Absent criteria for the diagnosis of clinically possible or probable TE, it is not possible for neurologists to make this diagnosis reliably, to assess the incidence, prevalence, risk factors, etiology, neuroimaging, biomarkers, or neuropathological correlates of this condition, or to design and conduct clinical trials for promising interventions. In short, diagnostic criteria are required to test hypotheses regarding TE.

In an effort to define the traumatic exposure predictors, clinical symptoms, and neurological/behavioral signs that might comprise TE, a review was conducted of all published cases that have been attributed to TE or to a synonymous condition (e.g., dementia pugilistica). This review identified all pertinent positive symptoms and signs that have been reported in cases that have been accepted in the peer-reviewed literature as exemplary of this condition. Provisional research diagnostic criteria for clinically possible and probable TE were developed based on the results of this review. The hypothesis was then tested that the proposed criteria accurately identify the subset of published cases in which (1) a medical history, a neurological examination, and a behavioral examination were all reported and (2) neuropathological examination of the whole brain ruled out most alternative diagnoses.

Method

A search was conducted using Ovid Medline (1950–July 2010), Ovid OldMedline (1947–1965) and PsycINFO. Search terms included dementia pugilistica (key word: KW), traumatic encephalopathy (brain injuries (KW) or brain injury.mp or traumatic brain injury.mp or craniocerebral trauma (KW) or head injury.mp or brain concussion (KW) or concussion. mp) + encephalopathy (brain injuries (KW) or brain injury.mp or traumatic brain injury.mp or craniocerebral trauma (KW) or head injury.mp or brain concussion (KW) or concussion. mp) + (boxing or football or martial arts or karate or soccer or sports), and (boxing or football or martial arts or karate or soccer or sports) + encephalopathy. All abstracts were reviewed. Articles that discussed persistent or progressive neurological or neurobehavioral changes after one or more traumatic head or brain injuries or concussions were read. Bibliographies of all articles were searched, and all relevant articles in all languages were obtained, translated, and reviewed.

A total of 151 articles and four books were reviewed. Of these, 60 articles and three books were determined to be reviews, 50 articles were scientific reports summarizing neurological, behavioral, laboratory, neuroimaging, or neuropathological findings in populations thought to have been exposed to repetitive head injury (e.g., boxers or football players), and 42 articles and one book reported cases of persons exposed to one or more traumatic brain injuries or concussions followed by the development of persistent or progressive neurological or neurobehavioral dysfunction.

Table 14.1 lists the 43 identified articles and one book, which together report 438 cases.

The completeness of these reports varies. The following criteria were used to select case reports for enumeration of symptoms and signs:

1. Reports document probable exposure to one or more head injuries, traumatic brain injuries, concussions, or multiple subconcussive injuries, with or without documented episodes of loss of consciousness.

2. Reports document onset of persistent or progressive neurological or neurobehavioral symptoms *and* objective signs, both post-dating the traumatic exposure.

3. Cases were excluded: (a) in which an acute focal brain injury (e.g., subdural hematoma) was followed by immediate neurological deterioration, then by coma, death, or recovery; (b) in which a pre-morbid medical condition, e.g., infarct, autism, or progressive supranuclear palsy, was considered possibly to have contributed to the observed neurological condition [25, 43, 49]; or (c) that summed symptoms or signs in a population without identifying which cases exhibited which features [44, 57, 58].

4. Roberts's (1969) case reports received special treatment [54]. His 1969 book was included despite the fact that it was not peer-reviewed because it is the seminal treatise in this field. Roberts provides 11 complete individual case reports. An additional 26 cases are described in less detail, although sufficient information is provided to characterize individuals by symptoms and signs. The enumeration of clinical features distinguished between the totals including Roberts's best-described 11 cases versus all 37 of his case reports.

As shown in Table 14.1, 25 articles and one book reporting 97 cases met inclusion criteria – if one includes *all* those reported by Roberts (1969) [54] – or 82 if one includes only the best described of Roberts's case reports.

Results

Ninety-two of 97 cases were boxers, four were professional American football players, and one was a practitioner of karate. The gender was male in all case reports that specified gender. Descriptive statistics regarding sporting careers versus onset of symptoms are presented in Table 14.2.

Thirty-nine reports included information regarding the occurrence, or lack thereof, of knockouts or episodes of loss of consciousness. A specific number of knockouts or loss of consciousness was reported in 27 cases. Among these, the mean number of episodes was 6.37 (range 0–60; $SD = 14.42$). Concussions were not reported in any of the boxing cases. Among the football cases, the number of concussions was reported as from "3 to 4" to "many."

Age of symptom onset was reported in 44/97 (45.4%) of cases. The mean onset was 36.64 years (range 19–60; $SD = 11.79$). The timing of symptom onset with respect to athletic career was reported only in the best-described 82 cases. Onset occurred during or at the end of the athletic career in 36/82 (44.0%). Onset was delayed after exposure in 21/82 (25.6%). In 20 of those cases the time could be calculated from the end of the sporting career to symptom onset: mean delay was 14.2 years (range 2–42; $SD = 10.52$). Even though 44% presented with symptoms during or at the end of their careers, the mean delay between symptom onset and diagnosis was 15.3 years. The course was described as *progressive* in 47/82 (57.3%), *persistent* or static without progression in 10/82 (12.2%), and *improving* in 3/82 (3.7%) of the best-described cases.

Table 14.3 reports the enumeration of symptoms and signs for all the selected cases. Some clinical descriptors in the case reports were recorded as symptoms, others as signs. For example, "headache" and "dizziness" were always reported as symptoms, while "gaze paresis" and "executive dysfunction" were always reported as signs. There are several exceptions. For instance, "slurred speech," "unsteady gait," and "memory loss" were reported in some cases as symptoms, in others as signs, and in others as both. In so far as practicable, verbatim transcription was employed. For example, different original reports employ the terms "spasticity," "rigidity," or "hypertonia". In the interests of fidelity, the table separately enumerates the occurrence of each term, understanding that these clinicians are perhaps describing similar or identical signs. When the language in the original report was ambiguous, the suffix "not otherwise specified" (NOS) was added. For example, cases described as "mentally off," "mentally deficient," "confused," or "muddled" were all recorded as exhibiting "cognitive disorder NOS."

Table 14.1 Sources and cases in alphabetical order by first author

Report no.	Source	Cases reported (_n_)	Reports meeting inclusion criteria (identification numbers)
1	Aotsuka et al., 1990 [31]	1	1
2	Areza-Fegyveres et al., 2007 [32]	1	1
3	Bouras et al., 1990[a] [33]	1	1
4	Brandenburg and Halloverden, 1954 [3]	1	1
5	Casson et al., 1982 [34]	4	0
6	Casson et al., 1984 [35]	1	0
7	Constantinides and Tissot, 1967[a] [36]	1	1
8	Cordero Junior and de Oliviera, 2001 [37]	1	1
9	Corsellis et al., 1973 [22]	15	10 (cases no. 1–4, 6–10, 13)
10	Courville, 1962 [38]	1	0
11	Critchley, 1949 [10]	7	6 (cases B, C, D, E, F, G)
12	Critchley, 1957[b] [39]	11	6 (cases no. 2, 3, 8–11)
13	Drachman and Newell, 1999 [40]	1	1
14	Geddes et al., 1996 [23]	1	0
15	Geddes et al., [24]	5	0
16	Grahmann and Ule, 1957 [7]	4	4 (cases no. 1–4)
17	Harvey and Newsome Davis, 1974 [41]	1	1
18	Hof et al., 1991 [42]	1	0
19	Hof et al., 1992 [25]	2	2 (cases no. 2, 3)
20	Hof et al., 1992 [43]	6	0
21	Jedlinski et al., 1970 [44]	60	0
22	Johnson, 1969 [11]	17	3 (cases no. 1, 6, 10)
23	Jordan, 1995 [12]	1	0
24	Jordan et al., 1997 [45]	12	2 (cases no. 5, 29)
25	Kaste et al., 1982 [46]	14	1 (case no. 1)
26	Martland, 1928 [1]	1	1 (case no. 2)
27	Mawdsley and Ferguson, 1963 [47]	10	9 (cases no. 2–10)
28	McKee et al., 2009 [15]	3	3 (cases A–C)
29	McKee et al., 2010 [28]	3	3 (cases no. 1–3)
30	Neuberger et al., 1959 [48]	2	2 (cases no. 1, 2)
31	Nowak et al., 2009 [49]	1	0
32	Omalu et al., 2005 [50]	1	0
33	Omalu et al., 2006 [51]	1	1
34	Parker, 1934 [6]	3	3 (cases no. I–III)
35	Payne, 1968 [52]	6	3 (cases no. 2–4)
36	Raevuori-Nallinmaa, 1951 [53]	2	2 (cases no. 1, 2)
37	Roberts, 1969 [54]	37	11 fully described (cases no. 1–11); 26 less fully described (7 cases similar to #7; 7 similar to #8; 5 similar to #9; 4 similar to #10; 3 similar to #11)
38	Roberts et al., 1990 [55]	1	0
39	Rodriguez et al., 1983 [56]	1	0
40	Ross et al., 1983 [57]	40	0
41	Schmidt et al., 2001 [29]	2	0
42	Sercl and Jaros, 1962 [58]	148	0
43	Spillane, 1962 [59]	5	4 (cases no. 1–3, 5)
44	Williams and Tannenberg, 1996 [60]	1	0
	Totals	436	109 (including all of Roberts's cases); 83 (including Roberts's best-described cases)

[a] The same case is reported by Constantinides and Tissot (1967) [36]; Bouras et al. (1990) [33] and Hof et al. (1992) [25].
[b] Critchley's 1949 report [10] includes cases he also reported in 1957 [39]. 1957 cases no. 1 and 5–7 are entered only once and listed among the 1949 reports.

Table 14.2 Demographics and career statistics

Statistic	_n_	_M_ (range)	SD
Age at start of career	54	14.67 (9–21)	2.61
Age at end of career	53	30.51 (22–45)	5.42
Duration of career	51	15.45 (5–32)	6.07
Cases with delayed onset of symptoms	20	36.64 years (19–60 years) Mean = 14.2 years after end of career (2–42 years)	10.52
Age at diagnosis	56	45.38 years (20–69 years) Mean = 15.3 years after end of career	8.04
Age at death	11	61.0 years (45–80 years)	11.61
Estimated number of bouts	38	326.37 (60–1500)	273.68

To facilitate practical analysis, several categories were collapsed. Combining symptoms and signs of "slurred speech" and "dysarthria," speech disturbance was reported in 84/97 (86.6%) cases. Combining the symptoms and signs "tremor NOS," "resting tremor," and "intention tremor," 30/97 (30.9%) of cases exhibited tremor. Combining the symptoms of signs of "spasticity," "rigidity", and "hypertonia," 39/97 (40.2%) of cases exhibited increased muscle tone. Combining the symptoms and signs of "incoordination" "clumsy," "ataxia NOS," and "limb ataxia/dysdiadochokinesis," 45/97 (46.4%) of cases exhibited incoordination. Combining the symptoms and signs of "unsteady gait," "ataxic gait," "spastic gait," "staggering," "slow gait," "shuffling gait," and "wide based gait," 39/97 (40.2%) exhibited gait disturbance.

Memory loss was by far the most frequently reported cognitive problem. Combining symptoms and signs of "memory loss," "cognitive disorder NOS," "mental slowing," "disorientation," "visuospatial dysfunction," "dysphasia," and "dementia," 70/97 (72.2%) of cases exhibited cognitive dysfunction. Anger/aggression was the most commonly reported behavioral disturbance. "Aggressive or violent outbursts," which refers to sudden transient episodes of aggression (and may meet DSM-IV-TR criteria for intermittent explosive disorder) [61], were reported in 13/97 (13.4%) cases. Combining the symptoms or signs of "anger," "aggression NOS," "violence," and "aggressive or violent outbursts" (excluding cases reported only to exhibit irritability or agitation), 32/97 (33.0%) of cases exhibited anger/aggression. Mood disturbance was the second most commonly reported behavioral problem. Nineteen of 97 (19.6%) cases reported depression either as a symptom or a sign. Combining "depression," "euphoria," "mood lability," and "suicide attempts," 28/97 (28.9%) cases reported mood disturbance. Combining "paranoia," "paranoid delusions," "morbid jealousy," and "jealous delusions," and "hallucinations," 21/97 (21.6%) exhibited signs of thought disorder.

In summary, the most commonly reported features of the elementary neurological examination were nystagmus, masked face, speech disturbance, increased tone, hyperreflexia, tremor, limb ataxia, and gait disturbance. The most commonly reported neurobehavioral features were cognitive impairment, aggression, mood disorder, paranoid thought disorder, and sensitivity to alcohol.

Provisional Research Diagnostic Criteria

Provisional research diagnostic criteria for *clinically probable TE* and *clinically possible TE* were developed based on the frequency of clinical symptoms and signs reported in well-described TE case reports published between 1928 and 2010. Signs and symptoms were included that were reportedly present in at least 7% of cases, either in the best-described group of 82 or the well-described group of 97. Criteria for this neuropsychiatric disorder were written to be consistent with the template of the American Psychiatric Association's *Diagnostic and Statistical Manuals* [61]. The proposed provisional criteria are presented in Table 14.4.

Discussion

This review of all published case reports of TE in all languages was undertaken as a step toward consolidating the knowledge regarding the clinical presentation of this putative condition. The resulting enumeration indicates that headache, subjective changes in speech, altered gait, cognitive decline, mood changes, personality changes, and sensitivity to alcohol are the most commonly reported symptoms in historical cases thought to represent TE, probably present in at least 15% of cases. Dysarthria, masked facies, hyperreflexia, tremor, pathological Babinsky reflex, tremor, limb ataxia, gait disturbance, and cognitive impairment are the signs most commonly observed by clinicians who regard their reports as exemplary of TE, probably present in at least 20% of cases. Most cases reported the onset of TE after exposure to multiple head injuries or concussions, although several reports described onset after a single head injury. A delay in onset after the last head trauma was common; among the subgroup whose onset was delayed, that delay typically exceeded a decade. On average, the delay from symptom onset to diagnosis exceeded 15 years. Most cases were *progressive* rather than persistent, static, or "chronic." A small proportion of cases exhibited improvement on follow-up. The provisional research diagnostic criteria that emerge from this review and enumeration are thought to represent the first scientifically based recommendations for the clinical diagnosis of TE.

There are several limitations to this strategy. First, case report literature does not readily lend itself to quantitative analysis. Some otherwise interesting reports had to be excluded due to incomplete clinical information [12, 23, 24, 35, 38, 42, 43]. The evolving conceptualization of this condition and the quality of the reports vary too much to conclude that the proportion of published cases reporting a given feature – e.g., nystagmus – necessarily predicts the statistical likelihood that feature will occur in TE. It also seems likely that most clinicians did not entertain the possibility of an association between trauma and motor neuron disease. The 5.2–6.1% of cases with subjective

Table 14.3 Symptoms and signs of traumatic encephalopathy

Clinical feature	Symptom including the most complete of Roberts's cases _n_ = 82 (%)	Symptom including all of Roberts's cases _n_ = 97 (%)	Sign including the most complete of Roberts's cases _n_ = 82 (%)	Sign including all of Roberts's cases = 97 (%)
Somatic complaints				
Headache	19 (23.2%)	19 (19.6%)		
Dizziness	3 (3.7%)	3 (3.1%)		
Diplopia	3 (3.7%)	3 (3.1%)		
Cranial nerves				
Gaze paresis			9 (11.0%)	9 (9.3%)
Nystagmus			12 (14.6%)	12 (12.4%)
Hearing loss	1 (1.2%)	2 (2.1%)	0	0
Tinnitus (symptoms)	1 (1.2%)	1 (1.0%)		
Dysarthria	9 (11.0%)	9 (9.3%)	44 (53.7%)	70 (72.2%)
Dysphagia	5 (6.1%)	5 (5.2%)		
Slurred speech	22 (26.8%)	25 (25.8)	20 (24.4%)	32 (33.0)
Masked face			22 (26.8%)	34 (35.1%)
Titubation			6 (7.3%)	6 (6.2%)
Frontal release signs			3 (3.7%)	3 (3.1%)
Pseudobulbar affect			3 (3.7%)	3 (3.1%)
Motor				
Weakness	2 (2.4%)	2 (1.8%)	7 (8.5%)	7 (7.2%)
Muscle atrophy			2 (2.4%)	2 (2.1%)
Spasticity			7 (8.5%)	14 (14.4%)
Rigidity/stiffness	3 (3.7%)	3 (2.8%)	13 (15.9%)	13 (13.4%)
Hypertonia			9 (11.0%)	14 (13.4%)
Hemiparesis			9 (11.0%)	9 (9.3%)
Paraparesis			0	0
Drags leg (symptom)	7 (8.5)	7 (7.2%)		
Increased deep tendon reflexes			29 (35.4%)	36 (37.1%)
+Babinsky reflex			18 (22.0%)	18 (18.6%)
Motor slowing	4 (4.9%)	4 (4.1%)	7 (8.5%)	7 (7.2%)
Clumsy	5 (6.1%)	5 (5.2%)	8 (9.8%)	20 (20.6%)
Tremor NOS	10 (12.2%)	10 (10.3%)	17 (20.7%)	17 (17.5%)
Tremor/rest	2 (2.4%)	2 (2.1%)	7 (8.5%)	7 (7.2%)
Tremor/intention			4 (4.9%)	4 (4.1%)
Ataxia NOS			3 (3.7%)	3 (3.1%)
Limb ataxia or dysdiadokokinesis			25 (30.5%)	25 (25.8%)
Unsteadiness NOS	7 (8.5%)	7 (7.2%)	7 (8.5%)	7 (7.2%)
Unsteady stance	3 (3.7%)	3 (3.1%)	6 (7.3%)	6 (6.2%)
Unsteady gait	4 (4.9%)	4 (4.1%)	15 (18.3%)	15 (15.5%)
Disequilibrium/unsteadiness NOS	9 (11.0%)	21 (21.6%)	7 (8.5%)	7 (7.2%)
Imbalance	3 (3.7%)	3 (3.1%)	1 (1.2%)	1 (1.0%)
Falls	10 (12.2%)	10 (10.3%)		
Ataxic gait	3 (3.7%)	3 (3.1%)	16 (19.5%)	24 (24.7%)
Spastic gait			2 (2.4%)	2 (2.1%)
Staggering gait			9 (11.0%)	9 (9.3%)
Slow gait	1 (1.2%)	1 (1.0%)	4 (4.9%)	4 (4.1%)
Shuffling gait	2 (2.4%)	2 (2.1%)	8 (9.8%)	8 (8.2%)
Wide-based gait			3 (3.7%)	3 (3.1%)

Table 14.3 *(Cont.)*

Clinical feature	Symptom including the most complete of Roberts's cases $\underline{n}$ = 82 (%)	Symptom including all of Roberts's cases $\underline{n}$ = 97 (%)	Sign including the most complete of Roberts's cases $\underline{n}$ = 82 (%)	Sign including all of Roberts's cases = 97 (%)
Behavior/cognitive				
Cognitive disorder NOS	3 (3.7%)	3 (3.1%)	9 (11.0%)	9 (9.3%)
Memory loss	32 (39.0%)	32 (33.0%)	47 (51.3%)	47 (48.4%)
Mental slowing	4 (4.9%)	4 (4.1%)	18 (22.0%)	19 (19.6%)
Disorientation	2 (2.4%)	2 (2.1%)	6 (7.3%)	6 (6.2%)
Visuo-spatial dysfunction/"gets lost"	5 (6.1%)	5 (5.2%)	8 (9.8%)	8 (8.2%)
Inattention	2 (2.4%)	2 (2.1%)	1 (1.2%)	1 (1.0%)
Decreased concentration	6 (7.3%)	6 (6.2%)	4 (4.9%)	4 (4.1%)
"Dementia"	6 (7.3%)	6 (6.2%)	13 (15.9%)	16 (16.5%)
Dysphasia			3 (3.7%)	3 (3.1%)
Dyspraxia	1 (1.2%)	1 (1.0%)	5 (6.1%)	5 (5.2%)
Hypomimia			4 (4.9%)	4 (4.1%)
Executive dysfunction (sign only)			4 (4.9%)	4 (4.1%)
Behavior/non-cognitive				
Depression	10 (12.2%)	10 (10.3%)	12 (14.6%)	12 (12.4%)
Suicidal behavior	1 (1.2%)	1 (1.0%)		
Anxiety	6 (7.3%)	6 (6.2%)	3 (3.7%)	3 (3.1%)
Apathy	3 (3.7%)	4 (4.1%)	5 (6.1%)	7 (7.2%)
Euphoria	3 (3.7%)	3 (3.1%)	7 (8.5%)	7 (7.2%)
Hypomania	0	0	0	0
Mood lability	7 (8.5%)	7 (7.2%)	3 (3.7%)	3 (3.1%)
Lethargy	2 (2.4%)	2 (2.1%)		
Paranoia	6 (7.3%)	6 (6.2%)	7 (8.5%)	7 (7.2%)
Paranoid delusions	1 (1.2%)	2 (2.1%)	2 (2.4%)	3 (3.1%)
Jealous delusions	4 (4.9%)	4 (4.1%)	3 (3.7%)	3 (3.1%)
Persecutory delusions	0	0	1 (1.2%)	1 (1.0%)
Grandiose delusions	0	0	1 (1.2%))	1 (1.0%))
Hallucinations NOS	1 (1.2%)	1 (1.0%)		
Visual hallucinations	0	0	0	0
Auditory hallucinations	1 (1.2%)	1 (1.0%)	0	0
Disinhibition/socially inappropriate behavior	3 (3.7%)	3 (3.1%)	2 (2.4%)	2 (2.1%)
Impulsivity	3 (3.7%)	3 (3.1%)	2 (2.4%)	2 (2.1%)
Irritability	9 (11.0%)	9 (9.3%)	4 (4.9%)	4 (4.1%)
Anger/temper	4 (4.9%)	4 (4.1%)	2 (2.4%)	2 (2.1%)
Agitation NOS	3 (3.7%)	3 (23.1%)	4 (4.9%)	4 (4.1%)
Aggression NOS	4 (4.9%)	4 (4.1%)	3 (3.7%)	3 (3.1%)
Violence	13 (15.9%)	13 (13.4%)	3 (3.7%)	3 (3.1%)
Aggressive or violent outbursts	12 (14.6%)	13 (13.4%)	0	0
Childish	2 (2.4%)	2 (2.1%)	3 (3.7%)	3 (3.1%)
ETOH abuse or dependence	8 (9.8%)	9 (9.3%)		
ETOH sensitivity	13 (15.9%)	13 (13.4%)		
Hypersexuality	2 (2.4%)	2 (2.1%)	0	0
Epilepsy	7 (8.5%)	7 (7.2%)		
Rule out epilepsy	2 (2.4%)	2 (2.1%)		

ETOH: ethyl alcohol; NOS: not otherwise specified; R/O epilepsy.

Table 14.4 Provisional research diagnostic criteria for the diagnosis of clinically probable and clinically possible traumatic encephalopathy (TE)

A.	Criterion: history	History of probable or definite exposure to one or more head injuries, traumatic brain injuries, concussions, or subconcussive brain injuries, with or without known loss of consciousness
B.	Criterion: symptoms	Onset of persistent or progressive neurological or neurobehavioral symptoms post-dating the traumatic exposure: a. Headache b. Speech changes (e.g., slurring, slowing) c. Tremor d. Deterioration in stance or gait, or falls e. Cognitive decline (e.g., memory loss, getting lost) f. Mood changes (e.g., depression, lability, or euphoria) g. Anxiety h. Paranoia i. Personality change (e.g., irritability, apathy, impulsivity, agitation, childishness, poor judgment) j. ETOH abuse or dependence k. ETOH sensitivity l. Anger or aggression (e.g., short fuse, uncharacteristic violence)
C.	Criterion: signs	Presence of objective neurological or behavioral signs: C1. Neurological signs: a. Nystagmus b. Dysarthria c. Reduced facial expression d. Hypertonia or rigidity e. Hyperreflexia f. Hemiparesis g. Tremor h. Limb ataxia (e.g., dysmetria or dysdiadokokinesis) i. Disorders of stance or gait (e.g., +Romberg, slowing, shuffling, ataxia, observed falls) C2. Neurobehavioral signs: a. Memory loss b. Other cognitive impairment (e.g., disorientation, mental slowing, confusion, visuospatial impairment, frank dementia) c. Mood disturbance (e.g., depression, lability, euphoria) d. Thought disorder (e.g., paranoia) e. Pathological personality traits (e.g., irritability, apathy, impulsivity, agitation, childishness) f. Anger or aggression
D.	Criterion: persistence	Persistence of both symptoms and signs for at least two years after the traumatic exposure
E.	Criterion: no alternative diagnosis	No alternative medical or psychiatric disorder that might better account for the observed syndrome

Notes:
1. The diagnosis of *clinically probable TE* requires meeting the A, D, and E criteria, as well as at least two symptoms (B criteria), and three signs (C criteria). The diagnosis of *clinically possible TE* requires meeting the A, D, and E criteria, as well as at least one symptom (B criteria), and two signs (C criteria).
2. Cases should be identified as either *acute onset* (no clear period of recovery in the 6–12-month post-concussive phase) or *delayed onset* (evidence of a functional decline after a history of recovery in the post-traumatic phase).
3. Cases should be identified as either *apparently persistent* (signs and symptoms lasting more than 24 months), *apparently progressive* (signs and symptoms for at least two years and unequivocally progressing), or *apparently improving*.

ETOH: ethyl alcohol.

dysphagia, the 7.2–8.5% of cases with objective weakness, and the 2.1–2.4% of cases with objective atrophy conceivably represent undetected cases of this suspected atypical presentation. Moreover, one faces the dilemma that the absence of data is not data supporting the absence of signs and symptoms. That is, some case reports fail to describe complaints often elicited from traumatic brain injury patients on a modern review of systems, and/or fail to document cranial nerve findings, motor status, and cognitive or non-cognitive behavioral disorders often found on examinations of such patients. This lack of history and examination data cannot be interpreted as evidence that those persons did not complain of, for example, dizziness, tinnitus, sleep disorder, anxiety, or suicidality; nor can it be interpreted as evidence that a comprehensive neurological examination would have failed to find, for example, saccadic break-up of smooth-pursuit eye movements, diminished gag reflex, fasciculations, or impulsivity.

The quality of the reported evaluations has profound implications for the diagnostic validity of the proposed provisional research criteria. Clinicians seeking to determine whether patients fulfill such criteria will presumably perform complete examinations. The proposed provisional criteria are merely a starting point. As more evaluations of presumed TE cases are published by independent scholars at different centers – and once sufficient consensus has been achieved to begin clinico pathological correlation studies – the signs and symptoms with the greatest predictive validity for the diagnosis of clinically possible, clinically probably, and pathologically definite TE will gradually evolve.

A related limitation is the emphasis, in many historical cases, on the primary neurological examination. Neuropsychiatric features frequently reported in the modern TBI literature – such as executive dysfunction, disinhibition, impulsivity, personality change, apathy, sleep disorder, anxiety, and post-traumatic stress disorder [62–65] – were infrequently reported in these historical reports. For example, the author has examined a number of retired National Football League players who meet these criteria for persistent or progressive TE. In addition to the behavioral problems noted above, I have noted a very high prevalence of a sleep disorder associated with vigorous physical activity or acting-out of dreams (possibly a rapid eye movement sleep disorder), and a surprisingly high prevalence of suicidal ideation. It is possible that the training and disciplinary orientation of the clinicians who have published most of these reports decreased the likelihood of detecting such co-morbid neuropsychiatric conditions.

The fact that some features that modern clinicians associate with TBI have been infrequently reported in the published cases of TE may be due to: (1) reporting bias related to the disciplinary training and clinical orientation of the authors; (2) lack of resources to conduct comprehensive evaluations at some reporting centers, including neuropsychological testing or psychiatric assessment; (3) evolution in the understanding of TBI, such that the clinical community is becoming more attuned to neuropsychiatric manifestations; and (4) the unresolved nosology of brain injury.

This last factor represents a third challenge to the development of diagnostic criteria. At present, the neurological literature describes a suite of conceptually overlapping conditions, syndromes, or disorders, including concussion, repetitive concussion, mild traumatic brain injury, post-concussion syndrome, TE, persistent sequelae of traumatic brain injury, and post-traumatic dementia. These disorders are addressed in parallel literatures that emphasize different aspects of this spectrum of post-traumatic neurobehavioral dysfunction.

Many of the clinical traits of TE identified in this review are also reported in persistent post-concussion syndrome. The present state of the science of post-traumatic neurological dysfunction does not reveal a definitive pathophysiological difference between TE and persistent post-concussion syndrome. A question yet to be resolved is what operational definition should distinguish the boundaries of TE. A splitter might urge that, whether due to injury variables, innate differences in persons who are injured, or gene–environment interactions, a subset of mild traumatic brain injury cases exhibit an elevated risk of persistence or progression, and only such cases should be called TE. One might propose that some traumatic brain injuries – whether single or recurrent, with or without loss of consciousness – precipitate a neurodegenerative cascade and others do not. Ultimately, TE may be the clinico-physiopathological explanation for the miserable minority who suffer persistent and often progressive effects. A lumper might counter that *every* brain is different after mild traumatic brain injury, and that observed clinical differences are a matter of type and degree within the broad spectrum of post-traumatic neurobehavioral change, all of which might reasonably be called TE.

One potential advantage of employing Parker's original term, *traumatic encephalopathy*, may be to encourage a paradigm shift toward a coherent understanding of these overlapping entities. From the moment of impact to death, victims of brain injury may exhibit neurological and psychiatric changes. TE is a useful umbrella. Seven-year-old Pop Warner football players who suffer a momentary alteration in awareness, 14-year-old hockey players knocked out for five minutes, and claiming no sequelae after a week, 22-year-old college soccer players whose heads have collided with those of others several times, and note a diminution in their grade point averages, 30-year-old victims of motor vehicle accidents who remain in a fog eight months after the evacuation of a small subdural hematoma, and 41-year-old professional boxers or football players who were never aware of any symptoms from their multiple subconcussive injuries but who, a decade after retiring, develop early-onset dementia might all be said to suffer from an encephalopathy due to trauma. It remains to be seen whether the consensus that eventually emerges declares that all these clinical phenomena belong to a common pathophysiological spectrum, or that there are meaningfully dissociable conditions.

One acknowledges the complication of an evolving nosology. One acknowledges the fact that a given symptom or sign that has been reported in a large proportion of peer-reviewed case reports cannot be regarded as evidence that symptom or sign is pathognomonic of TE. Yet a preliminary attempt such as this to enumerate the symptoms or signs most frequently reported as pertinent positives in a systematic review of published cases is a necessary first step in the development of research diagnostic criteria.

A fourth limitation of this strategy for the development of clinical diagnostic criteria – by far the greatest barrier – is the lack of gold-standard neuropathological criteria for TE. Absent such a standard, one can identify cases in which there is no obvious alternative diagnosis (e.g., infarction, neoplasm, or neuroinfection), but one cannot assume that the manifold neuropathological findings published as exemplary of TE all represent a unitary diagnostic entity.

Reports of an association between cases of presumptive TE and neocortical tau suggest that, in some cases and due to yet-to-be-identified genetic risk, environmental risk, and pathophysiological processes, one or more brain injuries may initiate a cascade of events culminating in a biologically distinct progressive neurodegenerative process [4, 15, 22–25, 27, 29, 66]. Yet the frequent observation of hyperphosphorylated tau must be balanced against other frequently observed pathological findings, including cavum septum pellucidum, substantia nigra and Purkinje cell loss, cerebrovascular changes, and deposition of amyloid-β protein – primarily in diffuse rather than in neuritic plaques – in approximately 40% of cases [3, 15, 22–27, 29]. Pending further research, it may be premature to assume that valid neuropathological criteria for a distinct entity have been identified. Given the diversity of precipitating injuries, clinical presentations, courses, and pathological findings, it remains to be seen whether TE is best classified as a unitary environmentally precipitated neurodegenerative tauopathy.

Thus, the neurobehavioral community faces the same Catch-22 addressed by investigators of Alzheimer's disease in decades past: until neuropathologists reach a consensus on caseness – what macro- or microscopic and/or immunocytochemical criteria distinguish TE from not TE – it will not be possible to determine the predictive validity of clinical signs and symptoms. Yet until clinicians reach a consensus regarding caseness – what combination of history, subjective complaints, and atypicalities on objective examination or testing should be regarding as inside versus outside the spectrum of TE – neuropathologists can only speculate that the cases they elect to label TE are diagnosable in life. One predicts an iterative process (and a certain amount of academic drama) in which dialogue between clinicians and pathologists will eventually achieve a common understanding of what is and what is not TE, and whether meaningfully distinct variants occur. Simply put, until *definite* TE can be diagnosed, the sensitivity, specificity, and predictive validity of diagnostic criteria for clinically *probable* and *possible* TE cannot be tested and such criteria will remain provisional.

A fifth limitation arises from the unresolved question whether TE necessarily requires exposure to multiple brain injuries. TE is often discussed as if it were invariably a consequence of repetitive or recurrent head trauma [15, 18, 24, 38, 67]. In fact, several lines of evidence support the notion that repetitive mild injuries produce unique neurobiological effects. Animal studies show that when the brain is recovering from one impulsive injury, viscoelastic changes, ion shifts, and transient neurometabolic crises make axons and cell bodies more vulnerable to damage from a second injury, and that repetitive injuries produce more lasting cognitive effects than single injuries [68–70]. However, no *a priori* logic dictates that multiple small injuries need to produce different persistent brain effects than one large injury, and, although rodent percussion research indeed suggests the additive or synergistic effect of repetitive injuries, no persuasive preclinical neurobiological evidence to date demonstrates that repetitive injuries produce a clinical or pathological condition that cannot be produced by single injuries. Moreover, many animal models of repetitive brain injury do not appear to parallel the experience of contact athletes, who may suffer one concussion in childhood and

three over the course of the next 25 years, and then exhibit symptoms a decade later.

Nor can most animal studies examine subtle changes that might only have functional significance for humans. For example, rodent experiments will fail to detect persistent changes in verbal memory, executive function, or mood.

Preclinical studies of repetitive brain injury are usually designed to test a very different part of the temporal sequence, for instance, determining whether a window of vulnerability to second impact occurs during the period of measurably reduced cerebral blood flow or glucose metabolic rate – about three to ten days [71]. Moreover, as Roberts et al. (1991) stated, "Previous reports suggested that both repetitive head trauma and a single injury can be associated with the presence of diffuse beta A4 amyloid protein plaques in long-term survivors" [72]. The same paper reported that extensive deposition of amyloid-β can occur within days of injury. Other reports have been published in which TE has apparently resulted from a single bout of boxing [9, 73] and in which progressive neurodegeneration has followed a single TBI [5]. Therefore, at this early stage in the evolution of diagnostic criteria, it seems prudent to include cases in which neurological and behavioral problems persist or progress after single injuries.

It is not important that the provisional research diagnostic criteria proposed here gain broad acceptance. It is, however, important that *some* operational clinical criteria gain acceptance, or (1) no two clinicians diagnosing TE will necessarily be referring to comparable cases; (2) little progress can be made in determining the correlation between what pathologists call TE and the various syndromes clinicians encounter; and (3) more important than nosological debates or even advancement in understanding of the molecular pathology of neurodegeneration, one does not have a scientific basis for advising the hundreds of millions of people who participate in contact sports.

While American football is the most common cause of concussion among U.S. athletes, the game that North Americans call soccer probably creates a much greater global risk, since an estimated 100 million people play. Whatever the sport, players, coaches, athletic trainers, and parents are routinely confronted with decisions regarding whether to play (primary prevention) or "return to play" (RTP) (secondary prevention). Should seven-year-olds ever play tackle football? Should headgear be obligatory in high school soccer? For how long should a given person who suffers a concussion avoid participating in the game that caused that concussion?

Numerous RTP guidelines have been advanced by various well-meaning groups, such as the Consensus Statement on Concussion in Sport from the 3rd International Conference on Concussion in Sport [74], or the American Academy of Neurology [75, 76]. The proposals for type of assessment, testing protocol, period of rest, and readiness to return are derived by inference from preclinical investigations and from a very small body of human concussion research with short-term follow-up. In terms of mitigating the risk of persistent or progressive TE (that is, a post-concussion syndrome present more than two years after the last concussion), no prospective longitudinal controlled study comparing RTP protocols has ever demonstrated either that one such protocol is better than another or, in fact, that any protocol is better than no protocol. Moreover, most of the proposed periods of rest before return to play are expressed in days or weeks, or tied to a "neurological examination." Evidence suggests that amateur boxers, even without specific histories of concussion, exhibit elevated neuron-specific enolase two months after their last bout [77]. Moreover, persons who suffer a concussion yet exhibit normal cognitive performance have been shown to have impaired cerebral efficiency a year later, detectable with cognitive testing monitored with functional magnetic resonance imaging [78]. Thus, after a concussion, many people may have both persistent brain damage and persistent vulnerability to repeat injury, neither of which is detectable by the most rigorous combined neurological and neuropsychological examination.

The persistence and progression of this disease may be occult. If so, what is the value of current RTP testing protocols? Indeed, given the accumulating evidence that repetitive injuries have an insidious effect on the brain, inapparent to the athlete and to those who examine him or her in the days, months, and years following injury, RTP is perhaps better conceptualized as return to risk. Clinical diagnostic criteria for TE are an essential first step toward conducting the studies required to generate evidence-based rationale for return to risk, non-return, or primary prevention, because, for the first time, investigators will have an outcome variable – the presence or absence of a diagnosable clinical condition.

Provisional research diagnostic criteria for TE should allow clinicians to focus on this significant subset of TBI victims, and hopefully accelerate the understanding of this important condition.

Declaration of Interest

The author is one of six U.S. neurologists to whom the National Football League (NFL) refers patients in the NFL Neurological Care Program. This program is unfunded. Otherwise, the author has no interest in any enterprise related to the subject matter of this paper.

Acknowledgments

The author wishes to express thanks to Akira Kugaya, M.D. for his kind help in translating Aotsuka et al. (1990) [31]. This work was supported, in part, by a grant from the Freya Foundation for Brain, Behavior, and Society.

References

1. Martland, H.S. (1928). Punch drunk. *Journal of the American Medical Association*, 91, 1103–1107.
2. Millspaugh, J.A. (1937). Dementia pugilistica. *U.S. Naval Medicine Bulletin*, 35, 297–303.
3. Brandenburg, W., & Hallervorden, I. (1954). Dementia pugilistica mit anatomischen Befund [Dementia pugilistica with anatomical findings]. *Virchows Archiv [B]*, 325, 680–709.
4. Roberts, G.W. (1988). Immunocytochemistry of neurofibrillary tangles in dementia pugilistica and Alzheimer's disease: evidence for common genesis. *Lancet*, 2, 1456–1458.
5. Rudelli, R., Strom, J.O., Welch, P.T., & Ambler, M.W. (1982). Post traumatic premature Alzheimer's disease: neuropathological findings and pathogenetic considerations. *Archives of Neurology*, 39, 570–575.
6. Parker, H.L. (1934). Traumatic encephalopathy ('punch drunk') of professional pugilists. *Journal of Neurology and Psychopathology*, 15, 20–28.
7. Grahmann, H., & Ule, G. (1957). Beitrag zur Kenntnis der chronischen cerebralen Krankheitsbilder bei Boxern (Dementia pugilistica und traumatische Boxer-Encephalopathie). [Diagnosis of chronic cerebral symptoms in boxers (dementia pugilistica and traumatic encephalopathy of boxers)]. *Psychiatrie und Neurologie*, 134, 261–283.
8. La Cava, G. (1963). Boxer's encephalopathy. *Journal of Sports Medicine*, 3, 87–92.
9. Critchley, M. (1937). Nervous disorders in boxers. *Medical Annual*, 318–320.
10. Critchley, M. (1949). Punch-drunk syndromes: the chronic traumatic encephalopathy of boxers. In: *Hommage à Clovis Vincent*. Paris: Maloine, pp. 131–145.
11. Johnson, J. (1969). Organic psychosyndromes due to boxing. *British Journal of Psychiatry*, 115, 45–53.
12. Jordan, B.D. (1994). Neurologic aspects of boxing. *Archives of Neurology*, 44, 453–459.
13. Haglund, Y., & Bergstrand, G. (1990). Does Swedish amateur boxing lead to chronic brain damage? Part 2: a retrospective study with CT and MRI. *Acta Neurologica Scandinavica*, 82, 297–302.
14. McCrory, P. (2002). Punch drunk: too many hits or bad genes? *Sport Health*, 20, 2–3.
15. McKee, A.C., Cantu, R.C., Nowinski, C.J., Hedley-Whyte, E.T., Gavett, B.E., Budson, A.E., et al. (2009). Chronic traumatic encephalopathy in athletes: progressive tauopathy after repetitive head injury. *Journal of Neuropathology and Experimental Neurology*, 68, 709–735.
16. Mendez, M.F. (1995). The neuropsychiatric aspects of boxing. *International Journal of Psychiatry and Medicine*, 25, 249–262.
17. Victoroff, J., & Baron, D. (2012). Diagnosis and treatment of sportsrelated traumatic brain injury. *Psychiatric Annals*, 42, 365–370.
18. McCrory, P., Zazryn, T., Cameron, P. (2007). The evidence for chronic traumatic encephalopathy in boxing. *Sports Med*, 37, 467–476.
19. Guskiewicz, K.M., Mihalik, J.P., Shankar, V., Marshall, S.W., Crowell, D.H., Oliaro, S.M., et al. (2007). Measurement of head impacts in collegiate football players: relationship between head impact biomechanics and acute clinical outcome after concussion. *Neurosurgery*, 61, 1244–1252.
20. Miller, J.R., Adamson, G.J., Pink, M.M., & Sweet, J.C. (2007). Comparison of preseason, midseason, and postseason neurocognitive scores in uninjured collegiate football players. *American Journal of Sports Medicine*, 35, 1284–1288.
21. Shaw, N.A. (2003). The neurophysiology of concussion. *Progress in Neurobiology*, 67, 281–344.
22. Corsellis, J.A., Bruton, C.J., & Freeman-Browne, D. (1973). The aftermath of boxing. *Psychological Medicine*, 3, 270–303.
23. Geddes, J.F., Vowles, G.H., Robinson, S.F., & Sutcliffe, J.C. (1996). Neurofibrillary tangles, but not Alzheimer-type pathology, in a young boxer. *Neuropathology and Applied Neurobiology*, 22, 12–16.
24. Geddes, J.F., Vowles, G.H., Nicoll, J.A., & Revesz, T. (1999). Neuronal cytoskeletal changes are an early consequence of repetitive head injury. *Acta Neuropatholologica*, 98, 171–178.
25. Hof, P.R., Bouras, C., Buee, L., Delacourte, A., Perl, D.P., & Morrison, J.H. (1992). Differential distribution of neurofibrillary

tangles in the cerebral cortex of dementia pugilistica and Alzheimer's disease cases. *Acta Neuropathologica*, 85, 23–30.

26. Lampert, P.W., & Hardman, J.M. (1984). Morphological changes in brains of boxers. *Journal of the American Medical Association*, 251, 2676–2679.

27. Tokuda, T., Ikeda, S., Yanagisaw, N., Ihara, Y., & Glenner, G.G. (1991). Re-examination of ex-boxers' brains using immunohistochemistry with antibodies to amyloid betaprotein and tau protein. *Acta Neuropathologica*, 82, 280–285.

28. McKee, A.C., Gavett, B.E., Stern, R.A., Nowinski, C.J., Cantu, R.C., Kowall, N.W., et al. (2010). TDP-43 proteinopathy and motor neuron disease in chronic traumatic encephalopathy. *Journal of Neuropathology and Experimental Neurology*, 69, 918–929.

29. Schmidt, M.L., Zhukareva, V., Newell, K.L., Lee, VM-Y., & Trojanowski, J.Q. (2001). Tau isoform profile and phosphorylation state in dementia pugilistica recapitulate Alzheimer's disease. *Acta Neuropathologica*, 101, 518–524.

30. McKhann, G., Drachman, D., Folstein, M., Katzman, R., Price, D., & Stadlan, E. (1984). Clinical diagnosis of Alzheimer's disease: report of the NINCDS-ADRDA work group under the auspices of Department of Health and Human Services Task Force on Alzheimer's disease. *Neurology*, 34, 939–944.

31. Aotsuka, A.M., Kojima, S.M., Furumoto, H.M., Hattori, T., & Hirayama, K. (1990). Punch drunk syndrome due to repeated karate kicks and punches [in Japanese]. *Rinsho Shinkeigaku*, 30, 1243–1246.

32. Areza-Fegyveres, R., Rosemberg, S., Castro, R.M., Porto, C.S., Bahia, V.S., Caramelli, P., et al. (2007). Dementia pugilistica with clinical features of Alzheimer's disease. *Arquivos de Neuro-Psiquiatria*, 65(3B), 830–833.

33. Bouras, C., Hof, P.R., Guntern, R., & Morrison, J.H. (1990). Down's syndrome (DS), dementia pugilistica (DP), and Alzheimer's disease (AD): a quantitative neuropathological comparison. *Proceedings of the Society of Neuroscience*, 16, 1264.

34. Casson, I.R., Sham, R., Campbell, E.A., Tarlau, M., & DiDomenico, A. (1982). Neurological and CT evaluation of knocked-out boxers. *Journal of Neurology, Neurosurgery and Psychiatry*, 45, 170–174.

35. Casson, I.R., Siegel, O., Sham, R., Campbell, E.A., Tarlau, M., & DiDomenico, A. (1984). Brain damage in modern boxers. *Journal of the American Medical Association*, 251, 2663–2667.

36. Constantinidis, J., & Tissot, R. (1967). Lesions neurofibrillaires d'Alzheimer généralisées sans plaques séniles (Présentation d'une observation anatomo-clinique) [Generalized Alzheimer's neurofibrillary lesions without senile plaques (Presentation of one anatomo-clinical case)]. *Schweizer Archiv für Neurologie, Neurochirurgie und Psychiatrie*, 100, 117–130.

37. Cordero Junior, Q., & de Oliviera, A.M. (2001). Sintomas parkinsonianos, cerebelares, psicóticos e demenciais em ex-pugilista: Relato de caso [Parkinsonian, cerebellar, psychotic and dementia symptoms in an ex-boxer: case report]. *Arquivos de Neuro-Psiquiatria*, 59(2-A), 283–285.

38. Courville, C.B. (1962). Punch drunk. Its pathogenesis and pathology on the basis of a verified case. *Bulletin of the Los Angeles Neurological Society*, 27, 160–168.

39. Critchley, M. (1957). Medical aspects of boxing, particularly from a neurological standpoint. *British Medical Journal*, 1, 357–362.

40. Drachman, D.A., & Newell, K.L. (1999). Weekly clinico-pathological exercises, case 12–1999. A 67 year old man with three years of dementia. *New England Journal of Medicine*, 340, 1269–1277.

41. Harvey, P.K.P., & Newsom Davis , J. (1974). Traumatic encephalopathy in a young boxer. *Lancet*, 19, 928–929.

42. Hof, P.R., Knabe, R., Bovier, P., & Bouras, C. (1991). Neuropathological observations in a case of autism presenting with self-injury behavior. *Acta Neuropathologica*, 82, 321–326.

43. Hof, P.R., Delacourte, A., & Bouras, C. (1992). Distribution of cortical neurofibrillary tangles in progressive supranuclear palsy: a quantitative analysis of six cases. *Acta Neuropathologica*, 84, 45–51.

44. Jedlinski, J., Gatarski, J., & Szymusik, A. (1970). Chronic post-traumatic changes in the central nervous system in pugilists. *Polish Medical Journal*, 9, 743–752.

45. Jordan, B.D., Relkin, N.R., Ravdin, L.D., Jacobs, A.R., Bennett, A., & Gandy, S. (1997). Apolipoprotein E epsilon4 associated with chronic traumatic brain injury in boxing. *Journal of the American Medical Association*, 278, 136–140.

46. Kaste, M., Vilkki, J., Sainio, K., Kuurne, T., Katevuo, K., & Meurala, H. (1982). Is chronic brain damage in boxing a hazard of the past? *Lancet*, 27, 1186–1188.

47. Mawdsley, C., & Ferguson, F.R. (1963). Neurological disease in boxers. *Lancet*, 2, 799–801.

48. Neuberger, K.T., Sinton, D.W., & Denst, J. (1959). Cerebral atrophy associated with boxing. *Archives of Neurology and Psychiatry*, 81, 403–408.

49. Nowak, L.A., Smith, G.G., & Reyes, P.F. (2009). Dementia in a retired world boxing champion: case report and literature review. *Clinics in Neuropathology*, 28, 275–280.

50. Omalu, B.I., DeKosky, S.T., Minster, R.L., Kamboh, M.I., Hamilton, R.L., Wecht, C.H., et al. (2005). Chronic traumatic encephalopathy in a national football league player. *Neurosurgery*, 57, 128–134.

51. Omalu, B.I., DeKosky, S.T., Hamilton, R.L., Minster, R.L., Kamboh, M.I., Shalir, A.M., et al. (2006). Chronic traumatic encephalopathy in a national football league player: part II. *Neurosurgery*, 59, 1086–1092.

52. Payne, E.E. (1968). Brains of boxers. *Neurochirurgia*, 11, 173–188.

53. Raevuori-Nallinmaa, S. (1950). Brain injuries attributable to boxing. *Acta Psychiatrica Scandinavica*, 25, 51–56.

54. Roberts, A.H. (1969). *Brain damage in boxers: a study of the prevalence of traumatic encephalopathy among ex-professional boxers.* London: Pitman Medical & Scientific.

55. Roberts, G.W., Allsop, D., & Bruten, C. (1990). The occult aftermath of boxing. *Journal of Neurology, Neurosurgery and Psychiatry*, 53, 373–378.

56. Rodriguez, R., Ferrillo, F., Montano, V., Rosadini, G., & Sannita, W.G. (1983). Regional cerebral blood flow in boxers. *Lancet*, 322, 858.

57. Ross, R.J., Cole, M., Thompson, J.S., & Kim, K.H. (1983). Boxers – computed tomography, EEG, and neurological evaluation. *Journal of the American Medical Asssociation*, 249, 211–213.

58. Sercl, M., & Jaros, O. (1962). The mechanisms of cerebral concussion in boxing and their consequences. *World Neurology*, 3, 351–358.

59. Spillane, J.D. (1962). Five boxers. *British Medical Journal*, 2, 1205–1210.

60. Williams, D.J., & Tannenberg, A.E. (1996). Dementia pugilistica in an alcoholic achondroplastic dwarf. *Pathology*, 28, 102–104.

61. American Psychiatric Association (2004). *Diagnostic and statistical manual of mental disorders, 4th edition, text revision.* Arlington, VA: American Psychiatric Association.

62. Ashman, T.A., Gordon,W.A., Cantor, J.B., & Hibbard, M.R. (2006). Neurobehavioral consequences of traumatic brain injury. *Mount Sinai Journal of Medicine*, 73, 999–1005.

63. Kim, E., Lauterbach, E.C., Reeve, A., Arciniegas, D.B., Coburn, K.L., Mendez, M., et al. (2007). Neuropsychiatric complications of traumatic brain injury: a critical review of the literature

(a report by the ANPA Committee on Research). *Journal of Neuropsychiatry and Clinical Neurosciences*, 19, 106–127.

64. Rogers, J.M., & Read, C.A. (2007). Psychiatric comorbidity following traumatic brain injury. *Brain Injury*, 21, 1321–1333.

65. Vaishnavi, S., Rao, V., & Fann, J.R. (2009). Neuropsychiatric problems after traumatic brain injury: unraveling the silent epidemic. *Psychosomatics*, 50, 198–205.

66. Allsop, D., Haga, S-I., Bruton, C., Ishii, T., & Roberts, G.W. (1990). Neurofibrillary tangles in some cases of dementia pugilistica share antigens with amyloid β-protein of Alzheimer's disease. *American Journal of Pathology*, 136, 255–260.

67. Rabadi, M.H., & Jordan, B.D. (2001). The cumulative effect of repetitive concussion in sports. *Clinical Journal of Sports Medicine*, 11, 194–198.

68. Friess, S.H., Ichord, R.N., Ralston, J., Ryall, K., Helfaer, M.A., Smith, C., et al. (2009). Repeated traumatic brain injury affects composite cognitive function in piglets. *Journal of Neurotrauma*, 26, 1111–1121.

69. Uryu, K., Laurer, H., McIntosh, T., Pratico, D., Martinez, D., Leight, S., et al. (2002). Repetitive mild brain trauma accelerates Abeta deposition, lipid peroxidation, and cognitive impairment in a transgenic mouse model of Alzheimer amyloidosis. *Journal of Neuroscience*, 22, 446–454.

70. Yoshiyama,Y., Uryu, K., Higuchi, M., Longhi, L., Hoover, R., Fujimoto, S., et al. (2005). Enhanced neurofibrillary tangle formation, cerebral atrophy, and cognitive deficits induced by repetitive mild brain injury in a transgenic tauopathy mouse model. *Journal of Neurotrauma*, 22, 1134–1141.

71. Longhi, L., Saatman, K.E., Fujimoto, S., Raghupathi, R., Meaney, D.F., Davis, J., et al. (2005). Temporal window of vulnerability to repetitive experimental concussive brain injury. *Neurosurgery*, 56, 364–374.

72. Roberts, G.W., Gentleman, S.M., Lynch, A., & Graham, D.I. (1991). Beta A4 amyloid deposition in brain after head trauma. *Lancet*, 338, 1422–1423.

73. Kremer, M., Russell, W., & Ge, S. (1947). A midbrain syndrome following head injury. *Journal of Neurology, Neurosurgery and Psychiatry*, 10, 49–60.

74. McCrory, P., Meeuwisse, W., Johnston, K., Dvorak, J., Aubry, M., Molloy, M., et al. (2009). Consensus statement on concussion in sport – the 3rd International Conference on Concussion in Sport, held in Zurich, November 2008. *Journal of Clinical Neuroscience*, 16, 755–763.

75. American Academy of Neurology (2010). Position statement on sports concussion, October 2010. Retrieved October 29, 2012 from www.sportsconcussions.org/AANguidelines.html.

76. Quality Standards Subcommittee of the American Academy of Neurology (1997). Practice parameter: the management of concussion in sports. *Neurology*, 48, 581–585.

77. Zetterberg, H., Tanriverdi, F., Unluhizarci, K., Selcuklu, A., Kelestimur, F., & Blennow, K. (2009). Sustained release of neuron-specific enolase to serum in amateur boxers. *Brain Injury*, 23, 723–726.

78. Chen, J-K., Johnston, K.M., Frey, S., Petrides, M., Worsley, K., & Ptitoa, A. (2004). Functional abnormalities in symptomatic concussed athletes: an fMRI study. *NeuroImage*, 22, 68–82.

Chapter

15

The Great CT Debate

Jeff Victoroff

Our data do not support attempts to limit the use of cranial CT [computed tomography] scan only for patients with a constellation of certain findings, and this practice would most likely increase the death and complication rates from undiagnosed intracranial injuries.

Livingston et al., 2000 [1]

For the evaluation of patients with minor head injury, the use of CT can be safely limited to those who have certain clinical findings.

Haydel et al., 2000 [2]

you've gotta ask yourself one question: "Do I feel lucky?" Well, do ya, punk?

Malick et al., 1970 [3]

Preface

On February 14, 2018 the U.S. Food and Drug Administration (FDA) approved a blood test marketed by Banyan Biomarkers [4]. That day, the *New York Times* stated, "Concussions can be detected with new blood test approved by F.D.A." [5]. What went wrong at that exceptional newspaper? As explained in the Introduction and in Chapter 17 of this volume, the Banyan test *almost never* detects a typical concussion! It only detects those rare complications of concussion that make a CT scan positive. That, in itself, deserves high praise. If post-marketing research eventually supports the test's sensitivity for those rare complications, it would spare many patients from the necessity of an emergency CT scan – and the present chapter would become largely obsolete. However, although the discovery of a "concussion test" remains an urgent goal, we are simply not there.

Introduction

This chapter addresses a single question: among people over age 15 who come to an emergency department (ED) or doctor's office within 24 h of a suspected concussion, who should be sent for a non-contrast computed tomography (CT) scan of the head?

Boiling down the arguments and conclusions to their essence: doctors seek firm, unambiguous guidelines because they have feelings. They prefer to help. They hate to make dreadful mistakes. They must steel themselves for less-than-soothing facts: one can review the empirical data until the cows come home. No algorithm for selecting which concussed patients to scan will always save us from error. For the foreseeable future, no science

or magic allows a doctor to slip the shackles of uncertainty. Those chain us to a cost–benefit estimate based on five factors:

1. There is a finite, but small, risk that a doctor will harm a concussed patient who seeks medical attention if the doctor fails to order an emergency CT scan (perhaps < 1%).
2. Getting a CT costs time, effort, and money. However, universal scanning usually produces a net saving because watchful observation usually costs more than scanning.
3. Radiation risk from a head CT in teens and adults is immeasurably small, hence, irrelevant.
4. The patient has feelings. (An astonishingly low proportion of writings on this topic consider patient preference.) His or her feelings about management options are important and individual.
5. The doctor has feelings. His or her tolerance for risk and tolerance for having harmed a patient are personal and imponderable.

The solution is simple. If your institution grants (or tolerates) physician discretion, you have two scientifically defensible, cost-efficient, and ethically virtuous options:

1. Discuss the risks of missing intracranial lesions with the patient. If the patient agrees to take the risk of missing some lesions by skipping the scan, then – after consulting the Canadian CT Head Rule (CCHR) [6] recommendations for this type of case – engage with the patient (or with another person with health care decision-making authority) in shared decision making about whether or not to order the scan.
2. Scan everybody.

This conclusion requires some explanation. Hence, this chapter has several more pages.

If the options were cost-neutral, one could blithely follow tradition: comply with local culture and gut instinct. ED expectations would be more accommodating of clinician whim. This chapter could be foregone. However, since occasional clinical catastrophe, widespread radiation exposure, and many millions of dollars are at stake, it seems worth a forthright effort to sort out best practices. The present author confesses his own rough road to these conclusions. Before conducting an extensive review and discussing the data with authorities in emergency medicine, imaging, radiation, and medical ethics, he did not appreciate the complexity of the risk–benefit math, the emotional role of physician risk tolerance, or the ultimate flavor of the preponderance of evidence.[1] He hopes to bake two years of dialogues into a manageable pie.

The Decision Matters

Most investigators agree that a major goal of caring for minor head injuries is to detect and treat appropriately those few patients who deteriorate neurologically after a period of relative alertness. The controversy in this regard centers on the relative importance of clinical versus radiological findings in determining which patients should receive neurological observation under medical supervision.

Dacey et al., 1986, p. 209[8]

The decision regarding whether or not to order a head CT scan is arguably the most important (some would say the sole) ED decision likely to meaningfully impact outcome after concussion. If *no* patients were scanned, how many treatable lesions would be missed? How would that impact human health (whether or not an economist quantifies that in terms of "quality-adjusted life years" (QALYs))? How would that impact the health care economy when balancing the cost of avoidable future care and litigation against the cost of routine scanning? If *all* patients were scanned, how many would suffer radiation side-effects, and to what extent would that impact QALYs? How many abnormal scans are misread as normal, and how many patients with truly normal scans go on to deteriorate and nonetheless require neurosurgical intervention? Is there a valid and reliable algorithm for identifying the subset of patients who really need a scan? The considerations are dauntingly complex, and only some questions have been addressed by high-quality research. This chapter compacts a great deal of information and attempts to explain the ferocious, distracting debate about whom to scan. The solution is simple, once one recognizes that the debate is driven by misunderstanding of radiation risks, faulty cost–benefit analyses, psychological heterogeneity, and

ethical obliviousness. If a single patient is saved from a missed diagnosis, it will have been worth the effort.

Consider Mark – an ebullient, jokey 16-year-old boy who was slow to get up after a play in Junior Varsity football. In the pileup, it was hard to know if there was a head impact. No one, including Mark, is sure if he "lost consciousness." Mark staggered for a minute, dry-retched once (maybe twice?), seemed a bit confused for a few minutes (nobody counted), and then seemed to recover. He said he had a little headache. He asked the same question twice when his coach suggested a quick trip to the ED. His neurological examination seems normal. Scan?

CT scanning has been widely available in developed nations since late 1980. By 1991, authorities were exchanging strong opinions about whether to scan concussed patients. Livingston et al. [9] reported that 14% of scanned mild head injury patients had intracranial injuries. Given the high proportion of abnormal scans, they reasonably opined that routine CT should be used as part of the triage process (the CT-for-triage approach). Their argument: "CT can reliably triage patients who can be discharged … Hospital admission can be avoided in more than 80% of patients sustaining MHI [minor head injury], better utilizing scarce hospital resources" [9]. Hence, economic prudence has been an issue from the outset. Mohanty et al. [10] reported that same year that only 12 of 348 (3.4%) of their mild traumatic brain injury (mTBI) patients had abnormal CT scans, and opined, "routine CT scan for minimal head injury patients is an inefficient use of personnel and equipment."

Readers will instantly ask the appropriate questions: "Why did Livingston et al. find 420% as many CT abnormalities as Mohanty et al.? Was that difference due to subject selection? Differences in the definition of injury? Timing of scans with respect to injuries? Differences in the sensitivities of the machines or the readers?" No certain answer is available, but the contrast between comparable studies illustrates one reason for the ongoing debate: concussive brain injury (CBI) is not a unitary entity but comprises a broad spectrum of neurobiological insults. As Yuh et al. [11] put it: "There is also growing recognition that current classification schemes for TBI based on GCS [Glasgow Coma Scale] are severely limited, with small mean effect sizes in long-term impairment potentially obscuring differences among diverse subgroups of TBI patients with very different prognoses."

Readers might also inquire: "Might clinical risk factors help us determine who is most likely to have an abnormal scan, so that we may limit CT scanning to high-risk patients?" Perhaps. And that question will be carefully considered below. In fact, some findings on clinical assessment are somewhat predictive of intracranial changes (although not necessarily predictive of those changes that would benefit from surgical intervention). And in fact the more such risk factors, the higher the likelihood

---

[1] One tries to resist being swayed by anecdotes. It is therefore not to be taken as more than lore, but the present author's one serious prediction error, denying a CT in the old days of strict limits, involved a concussed teenaged girl. Recently hearing two remarkably similar stories from pediatric ED physicians left an impression that is hard to shake with mere rationality. The author wonders whether this demographic subgroup is especially prone to delayed but rapidly enlarging subdural hematoma. Delayed and undetected bleeds are not rare [7]. Whether teenaged girls are disproportionately vulnerable would be difficult to detect, even with a large study, if that phenomenon is hormone cycle-dependent.

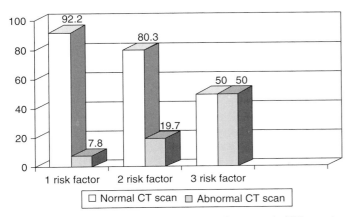

Fig. 15.1 Rate of normal and abnormal computed tomography (CT) scans in concussed patients with different numbers of risk factors.

Source: Saboori et al., 2007 [12] with permission from Elsevier

of an abnormal scan. Figure 15.1 illustrates the findings from one of many studies that sought a formula to predict CT results. Three risk factors? The odds become about 50:50.

But often forgotten in the discussion is the fact that post-concussive brain change: (1) has no single pathological character; (2) has no single natural history; and (3) is not associated with reliable clinical-pathological correlations. It comprises a broad spectrum of symptoms that are unpredictably associated with a broad spectrum of acute brain changes – not to mention unpredictable trajectories of subsequent further brain and behavior change. Miller et al. [13] cautioned:

> Some researchers have attempted to circumvent this debate: by seeking clinical parameters that would identify patients at high risk for brain injury and limiting CT to this group. Unfortunately, no single clinical factor or combination of such factors has been found that can reliably predict who will have an abnormal CT finding.
>
> ([13], p. 291)

In other words, since no demographic or clinical risk factor has high predictive validity for either CT results or clinical outcome, and since only a few CT findings prompt a change in management, all rules sometimes fail. And although one can certainly stir the data pot and dredge up four or nine factors that, considered together across a population, greatly increase the likelihood of an abnormal CT, *no rule predicts that outcome for any individual patient.* As Dacey et al. admonished in 1986 [8], "it may be impossible to predict accurately an individual patient's risk of deteriorating after minor head injury."

The great CT debate has raged for decades. Some clinicians would be more personally inclined to scan Mark, others less so. Some work in settings that impose a rigid protocol, others in settings that defer to physician discretion. Some work in litigious societies (among whom some are more or less vulnerable to liability); others work in lower-legal-risk milieus. In some settings, a CT is readily available and relatively low in cost; in others, a CT is a luxury; in still others, a CT is a dream. The debate has been egregiously oversimplified to "scan everybody and save lives" versus "scan a subset and save money." It's time for some clarity about what's really at stake.

Three facts are indisputable: (1) CTs cost money, but so does watchful waiting; (2) any protocol that withholds CTs risks harming some patients; and (3) both patients and doctors have emotionally influenced preferences.

So whom should we scan? Many authorities would answer, "That's a question to be answered by cost–benefit research." This chapter will summarize the state of the art. The inescapable truth: a great deal of such research has been done and the debate rages on. Yes, of course, the research is imperfect and the quality of studies (as will be described below) varies greatly. Hence, optimists might hope that one more big, well-designed study would finally reveal the best practice. In the present author's opinion, although he strongly advocates for desperately needed research about concussion, in this case waiting for more data is like waiting for Godot. The science is reasonably well understood. Ten more studies would probably confirm the consensus: if you scan everybody, you obtain some clinical information about everybody. The precise value of that information varies from case to case. If you scan selectively, you will doom a small number of patients to bad outcomes that a scan would have averted. This is not a story about the need for more studies. This is a story about clinical culture, medical ethics, and the human heart.

There are two obvious reasons for the ongoing debate about whether to scan everybody or not: First, clinicians naturally vary in the degree to which they personally value obtaining more knowledge about their patient versus fear of radiation and saving money for "society" (a false premise, since the alternative to CT, relief of uncertainty, and prompt discharge is often continued uncertainty plus 12–24 h of pricey observation). Second, some clinicians who withhold CTs rarely inform patients of the risk involved, instead imposing their own judgment that – in Mark's case or your own son's case, for instance – cost savings is a higher good than more clinical knowledge.

It is indisputable that we must ration health care. It is also indisputable that we must weigh the resulting sacrifices. In this chapter, the author will review the bases for these statements and recommend a solution hoping to balance the goods of clinical care, economics, and ethics.

The Research Provides Limited Knowledge About a Small Subset of Patients

From the outset, it is important to make several things clear. First, there is no definitive research on the rate of intracranial abnormalities after human concussion ("mTBI") or, more accurately, CBI. The available literature is almost completely limited to the modest subgroup of concussed persons who present at the ED. Two factors reduce the proportion of total CBIs represented in this literature. First, only a small proportion of concussed persons ever see a clinician [14–18]. (Note, however, that the proportion of concussions coming to medical attention has recently increased due to the concussion awareness revolution: in one study, the rate of ED visits for sport-related concussion increased by a factor of five in recent decades; and one Cincinnati hospital reported a 92% increase in ED visits by concussed youth between 2002 and 2011 [19].) Second, for every 100 concussed patients who seek help at the ED, about

60 instead go to their general practitioner [20]. In addition, every published study of the sensitivity of CT scans restricts its attention to some subset of the subset of CBI patients who present in the ED – for instance, those with a GCS of 15 plus either loss of consciousness (LOC) or amnesia.

Therefore, the available literature about the incidence of CT-visible intracranial abnormalities derived from ED studies only applies to a subset of a subset of cases. Luoto et al. [21] examined the downside of this kind of limited research. For example, if you limit your study of mTBI to those meeting World Health Organization criteria who did not have pre-existing conditions, your study might exclude 95.1% of mTBI patients (!). Those authors concluded, "Studying carefully selected samples is often necessary to address specific research questions, but such studies have serious limitations in terms of translating research findings into clinical practice" [21].

CT Does Not Show CBI

Second, CT is not a definitive diagnostic test for CBI. It is, under ideal circumstances, a dated technology that provides reasonably good visualization of gross hemorrhagic changes and mass effects. Put succinctly: CT is reasonably fast, cheap, safe, and revealing. Assume, for the sake of argument, that the CT readings were accurate in the published studies (an assumption that cannot be confirmed since studies rarely tested inter-reader reliability). What could the readers have seen? CT is excellent at detecting bleeds such as subdural, epidural, intracerebral, and subarachnoid hemorrhages (though not so good at visualizing subacute bleeds, since these can be isodense), as well as skull fractures, pneumocranium, and midline shifts. CT is reasonably helpful in detecting diffuse brain swelling and some types of impending herniation. But it has been known for almost 30 years that CT is blind to most of the clinically important damage produced by CBI – axonal dysfunction, the neurometabolic/vascular/inflammatory/degenerative vs. regenerative melee, and hippocampal compromise [11, 22–25].

Figure 15.2, for example, compares CT on the day of injury with magnetic resonance imaging (MRI) within 2 weeks. It is not an ideal comparison, in the sense that the scans occurred at different times. But it offers a reasonably good contrast between the sensitivities of these two technologies.

In a recent review Toth [25] reported that acute CTs are negative in 90% of cases fulfilling the 1993 American College of Rehabilitation Medicine (ACRM) criteria for "mTBI." Conventional MRI is more sensitive, detecting damage in about 30% of cases with normal CT scans. [11, 23, 24, 26]. Susceptibility-weighted imaging is even more sensitive, especially to traumatic microbleeds [25, 27]. Diffusion tensor imaging is even more sensitive and may show persistent axonal abnormalities long after a concussion [25].[2] Therefore, the goal of CT scanning is never to determine whether a CBI has occurred. It is never to determine how bad the damage was. It cannot predict with confidence what lies ahead. It can,

Sensitivity of acute computed tomography (CT) versus subacute magnetic resonance imaging (MRI)

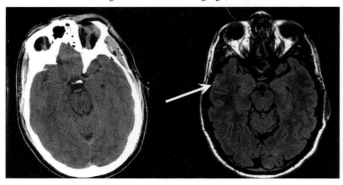

Fig. 15.2 Left: CT of a mild traumatic brain injury patient on emergency department admission (< 24 h of injury) showing no intraparenchymal lesions. Right: 3-T MR fluid-attenuated inversion recovery T2-weighted image showing a small non-hemorrhagic right temporal cortical surface contusion not detected on the CT (arrow).

Source: Lee et al., 2008 [23]. Reproduced with permission from Mary Ann Liebert, Inc.

however, detect those lesions most amenable to the only dramatically effective treatment for CBI: neurosurgery.

Realizing the limitations of this 40-year-old technology, outcomes from CT studies of a subset of a subset of concussed persons are typically classified using a four-tiered system:

1. "normal" (meaning someone opined that the scan showed no untoward changes)
2. "positive" (meaning one or more non-incidental lesions were visualized)
3. "clinically important" (meaning the visualized lesions were judged by the authors as important to know about – a judgment based on criteria that vary between studies)
4. "neurosurgical" (meaning that, according to the local opinion, the visualized lesion(s) mandated surgical intervention).

The literature is remarkably uniform in its bias: it's nice to know when there are lesions, but it is only clinically important to know if there are "clinically important" lesions (a classification that's debated), and the only indisputably useful scans are those that show that the patient needs surgery. A normal scan is universally called "unnecessary."

Unnecessary? It is unclear what proportion of clinicians and patients agree with this value system. Anyone with ED experience has witnessed this moving scenario unfold scores of times: the palpable sense of relief that floods the curtained-off gurney bay when someone in white announces, "It was normal." A normal CT helps guide clinical decision making regarding, for instance, the need for hospital admission, and reassures patients/families (whether it should or not). Knowing that virtually all published analyses of the costs and benefits of CT dismiss a normal scan as an "unnecessary" event and a waste of scarce resources will help readers to understand the ultimate futility of this long-running debate: some will agree with that judgment, others will not, and no dollar figure can be assigned to the human relief and reassurance generated by a negative scan.

---

[2]   However, the significance of observed changes in diffusivity and fractional anisotropy remains open to interpretation.

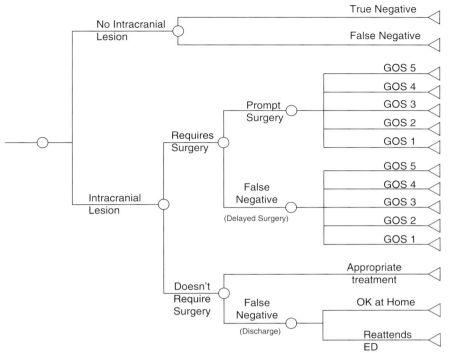

Fig. 15.3 Decision tree: the possible outcomes of following a given management strategy. GOS: Glasgow Outcome Scale score (5 = good outcome; 4 = moderate disability; 3 = severe disability; 2 = vegetative state; 1 = dead).

Explanation: patients presenting at the emergency department (ED) with apparently minor traumatic brain injury may or may not have intracranial lesions. Those who *do not* have lesions may be correctly diagnosed (true negative) and discharged or they may be incorrectly diagnosed (false positive) and subjected to unnecessary workup and/or admission to the hospital. Those who *do* have lesions have intracranial hematomas, subarachnoid hemorrhage, cerebral edema, or contusions. Surgical lesions are intracranial hematomas that require evacuation. Patients with lesions requiring surgery may be correctly diagnosed and receive prompt surgery (true positive for surgical lesions) or they may be incorrectly diagnosed (false negative for surgical lesions) and, by assumption, receive delayed surgery. Outcomes of surgery are described by GOS scores.

Source: Stein et al., 2006 [28] with permission from Lippincott Williams & Wilkins, Inc./Wolters Kluwer

Clinicians are different. Patients are different. Medical systems and societies are different. No single "rule," guideline, or protocol will ever accommodate the infinitude of circumstances or satisfy every stakeholder. This chapter will weigh the possibility that best practice is not compliance with any published rule, nor with physician discretion untethered from patient autonomy. Reviewing the available facts can certainly inform the discussion. Weighing costs and benefits are urgently necessary in any finite economy. But data are weak arbiters, unlikely to resolve the tension between pragmatism and benevolence.

Before comparing the published proposals for granting or withholding CTs, one might consider Figure 15.3. This figure has less value as a guide than as a warning. It depicts the extraordinary heterogeneity and unpredictability of possible clinical courses followed by concussed persons managed in various ways. It helps show why selection algorithms are somewhat beside the point. Yes, a computer could calculate the odds of making dangerous errors of commission or omission. But it would never be an accurate predictor of concussion outcome, it would never eliminate fatal errors, and it would never consider the feelings of the patient and the doctor about making the bet to skip the CT.

Part 1: Proposed CT Protocols

The relatively low incidence of significant complications requiring neurosurgery after minor head injury and the high cost of radiological evaluation and hospital admission for neurological observation have led to the proposal of a variety of alternatives to current management methods.

Dacey et al., 1986, p. 209 [8]

Table 15.1 lists some of the published rules for deciding whether or not to order a CT scan in cases of concussion

(CBI/mTBI/minor head injury/mild head injury). *Rule* is probably a misnomer. Even authors who vigorously champion their own approach caution against prioritizing rigid compliance with a favorite algorithm over clinical judgment. *Protocol* is a better word. Every research group has stated pretty much the same goal: to figure out what clinical factor or factors predict virtually all abnormal CTs. The practical significance of this goal is supported by research: Graham et al. [29] reported a survey showing that 85% of 232 emergency physicians in Canada did not agree with scanning every case of minor head injury. At the same time, 52% required that a decision rule be 100% sensitive. The question: does Miller's 20th-century statement that no such factors have been found remain true today?

Two Dominant Players: The Canadian CT Head Rule and the New Orleans Criteria

Although a profusion of recommendations have been disseminated and will be described later in this chapter, two CT protocols dominate the literature: the CCHR [6, 39, 40] and the New Orleans Criteria (NOC) [2, 39]. The CCHR was originally derived from a study by Stiell et al. [6]. A total of 3121 patients were followed prospectively after "minor head injury," 96.5% of whom had a GCS of 14 or 15 (Table 15.2). Although 8% were judged to have "clinically important" lesions, only 1% required neurosurgical intervention. Five factors identified 100% of patients judged to be at *high risk* for requiring neurosurgical intervention: GCS less than 15 at two hours, suspected open or depressed skull fracture, any sign of basal skull fracture, vomiting two or more times, and age 65 or older. Two additional factors identified those judged to be at *medium risk*: retrograde amnesia of more than 30 minutes and a "dangerous mechanism

Table 15.1 Protocols for computed tomography (CT) scan decision making in the emergency department

- Miller Rule [13, 30]
- New Orleans Criteria (NOC) [2]
- Canadian CT Head Rule (CCHR [6])
- World Federation of Neurosurgical Societies (WFNS [31])
- National Emergency X-Radiography Utilization Study II (NEXUS II) [32]
- American College of Emergency Physicians rule [33]
- Scottish Intercollegiate Guidelines Network [34]
- Advanced Trauma Life Support/American College of Surgeons Guideline [35]
- Scandinavian Neurotrauma Committee (SNC) Guidelines [36, 37]
- National Collaborating Centre for Acute Care Guideline [38]

Table 15.2 The Canadian CT Head Rule (CCHR) [6]

Clinical factors that identify patients aged ≥16 with "minor head injury," a Glasgow Coma Scale (GCS) of 13–15, *plus* either loss of consciousness or amnesia, who should undergo computed tomography (CT)

High risk for neurosurgery:

- GCS < 15 at 2 h post injury
- Suspected open or depressed skull fracture
- Any sign of basilar skull fracture
- ≥ 2 episodes of vomiting
- Age ≥ 65 years

Medium risk for neurosurgery:

- Retrograde amnesia to the event ≥ 30 minutes
- "Dangerous" mechanism (pedestrian struck by motor vehicle, occupant ejected from motor vehicle, or fall from > 3 feet or > 5 stairs)

Table 15.3 The New Orleans Criteria (NOC) [2]

Clinical factors that identify patients aged ≥3 years with "minor head injury," a Glasgow Coma Scale of 15, *plus* either loss of consciousness or amnesia, who should undergo computed tomography

- Headache
- Vomiting
- Age over 60 years
- Drug or alcohol intoxication
- Deficits in short-term memory,
- Physical evidence of trauma above the clavicles
- Seizure

of injury." When combined, these seven *high- and medium-risk* factors had a sensitivity of 98.4% and a negative predictive value of 99.7%. Applying this rule led to missing just four of 254 CT lesions, none of which required surgical intervention. Unfortunately, the sensitivity figures published in the original CCHR paper are not altogether credible: they were based on the authors' assumption that a reassuring telephone interview with a nurse 14 days after the injury was a good proxy for a normal CT scan, even though that method missed 13% of clinically important lesions ([6], p. 1392).

The NOC was derived from a study by Haydel et al. [2, 41]. In all, 1429 patients with "minor head injury" and GCS of 15 were studied, spanning an age range of 3–97 years (Table 15.3). In the first exploratory phase of the study, factors were identified that seemed likely to predict positive findings on a CT scan. In the second validation phase that hypothesis was tested with 909 subjects. In the second phase 6.3% of patients had a positive scan. Based on their subjective responses on non-psychometrically validated questionnaires, patients with a positive CT scan claimed one or more of seven symptoms: headache, vomiting, age over 60 years, drug or alcohol intoxication, deficits in short-term memory, evidence of trauma above the level of the clavicles, or a seizure. These seven symptoms yielded a sensitivity of

100% and a negative predictive value of 100%. In all, 0.4% required neurosurgery.

CT Protocols Recommended in General Guidelines for Clinical Management of Acute Concussive Brain Injury

Multiple guidelines have been published for the management of acute CBI [33–35, 38, 42–49]. Each includes a recommendation regarding CT scanning. In some cases, those guidelines adopt existing CT rules, such as the CCHR or NOC (with or without idiosyncratic revisions). In other cases (e.g., [35, 38, 49]), CT protocols were developed *de novo*. Before analyzing the strengths and weaknesses of the competing CT protocols and before discussing the ethical issue that lurks behind the decision-making process, it might be useful to examine the recommendations regarding CT scanning recommended in the pre-existing guidelines. (The profusion – one might say viscous superfluity – of CT protocols would make it daunting to plow through a detailed narrative reviewing each one. In the interest of efficiency, most protocols are displayed in tabular form.)

American College of Emergency Physicians Guideline

The American College of Emergency Physicians (ACEP) guideline [33] distinguished between when a CT should be done and when a CT should be considered. CT is indicated:

> in head trauma patients with loss of consciousness or posttraumatic amnesia only if one or more of the following is present: headache, vomiting, age greater than 60 years, drug or alcohol intoxication, deficits in short-term memory, physical evidence of trauma above the clavicle, posttraumatic seizure, GCS score less than 15, focal neurologic deficit, or coagulopathy.
>
> [33]

Hence, the ACEP revised the NOC criteria, adding coagulopathy as an indicator and expanding to accommodate cases with GCS 13 and 14. ACEP states CT should be "considered":

> in head trauma patients with no loss of consciousness or posttraumatic amnesia if there is a focal neurologic deficit,

vomiting, severe headache, age 65 years or greater, physical signs of a basilar skull fracture, GCS score less than 15, coagulopathy, or a dangerous mechanism of injury.

[33]

In this case, ACEP expanded the protocol to accommodate the large subset of patients excluded from the NOC study (those without LOC or amnesia), added the indicator "focal deficit," and adopted other indicators from the competing CCHR. To the best of this writer's knowledge, no study has validated the hybrid conglomerate rule assembled by the ACEP.

Scottish Intercollegiate Guides Network Guideline

The Scottish Intercollegiate Guides Network (SIGN) guideline for early management of patients with head injuries [34] includes a CT protocol (Table 15.4). It grades its own recommendation at level B (essentially, based on well-conducted case–control or cohort studies). Of interest, it uses "confusion" as a risk factor. (This writer speculates that sensitivity to confusion is human nature and is perhaps assessed more reliably than GCS score.) The SIGN protocol is problematic in that it lists skull fracture as a decision point for CT, but skull fracture is best assessed with CT. It appends advice to also perform

Table 15.4 Scottish Intercollegiate Guidelines Network (SIGN) computed tomography (CT) protocol ([34], pp. 3–4)

I. Immediate CT scanning should be done in an adult patient who has any of the following features:

- Eye opening only to pain or not conversing (GCS 12/15 or less)
- Confusion or drowsiness (GCS 13/15 or 14/15) followed by failure to improve within at most 1 hour of clinical observation or within 2 h of injury (whether or not intoxication from drugs or alcohol is a possible contributory factor)
- Base of skull or depressed skull fracture and/or suspected penetrating injuries
- A deteriorating level of consciousness or new focal neurological signs
- Full consciousness (GCS 15/15) with no fracture but other features, e.g.
    - Severe and persistent headache
    - Two distinct episodes of vomiting
- A history of coagulopathy (e.g., warfarin use) and loss of consciousness, amnesia, or any neurological feature

II. CT scanning should be performed within 8 h in an adult patient who is otherwise well but has any of the following features:

- Age > 65 years (with loss of consciousness or amnesia)
- Clinical evidence of a skull fracture (e.g., boggy scalp hematoma) but no clinical features indicative of an immediate CT scan
- Features indicative of an immediate CT scan
- Any seizure activity
- Significant retrograde amnesia (> 30 minutes)
- Dangerous mechanism of injury (pedestrian struck by motor vehicle, occupant ejected from motor vehicle, significant fall from height) or significant assault (e.g., blunt trauma with a weapon)

III. In adult patients who are GCS<15 with indications for a CT head scan, scanning should include the cervical spine

GCS: Glasgow Coma Scale.

cervical spine CT in patients with GCS < 15. Otherwise, it is a hybrid of the CCHR and the NOC.

U.S. Veterans Administration/Department of Defense Guideline

The U.S. Veterans Administration/Department of Defense (VA/DoD) guideline [45] is much less specific: "A patient who presents with any signs or symptoms that may indicate an acute neurologic condition that requires urgent intervention should be referred for evaluation that may include neuroimaging studies" (p. CP26). Remember, however, that this guideline is meant for use more than seven days post injury. And "may" is not a prescriptive word.

New South Wales Protocol

The New South Wales (NSW) CT protocol [46] is something of a *tour de force* (or perhaps a *coup de trop?*). Early in the text, the authors initially recommend two indications for CT: (1) "Persistent abnormal mental status manifested by either abnormal GCS or abnormal alertness, behaviour or cognition" and (2) "Known coagulopathy and particularly supratherapeutic anticoagulation" (p. 7). Had they quit there, one could imagine ED physicians learning and complying with the NSW recommendations. However, the authors go on to distinguish three levels of risk and to link each with different scanning recommendation. The authors then add yet another list of criteria to identify patients with no indication for a CT – depending on the time point at which the observation is made. Table 15.5 summarizes the NSW CT protocol. To the best of this writer's knowledge, no study has validated this remarkably convoluted (not to say Baroque) recommendation.

Eastern Association for the Surgery of Trauma Guideline

The Eastern Association for the Surgery of Trauma (EAST) guideline [42] is among the most straightforward: if resources permit, scan everybody. If not, use standardized criteria such as the CCHR or NOC. However, in an insightful commentary, the authors debunk the assumption that use of standardized criteria necessarily leads to standardized practice. For example, when the CHALICE protocol [50–52] (for children) was applied in the United Kingdom, its use led to a CT rate of 14%. When the same protocol was applied in Australia, the scan rate was 46% (see section on compliance, below). The authors also summarize two poignant conundrums: (1) that scanning any subset smaller than everybody means missing some cases; and (2) that values and priorities differ in different places:

published CT scan guidelines all demonstrate a tradeoff between sensitivity and specificity. Efforts to achieve an overall reduction on CT use will inevitably lead to a higher missed injury rate, although whether these injuries are clinically significant is debatable. These differences have

Table 15.5 New South Wales computed tomography (CT) protocol

I. No indication for CT in cases with:
- GCS 15 at 2 h post injury
- No focal neurological deficit
- No clinical suspicion of skull fracture
- No vomiting
- No known coagulopathy or bleeding disorder
- Age <65 years
- No seizure
- Brief loss of consciousness (<5 minutes)
- Brief post-traumatic amnesia (<30 minutes)
- No severe headache
- No large scalp hematoma or laceration
- Isolated head injury
- No dangerous mechanism
- No known neurosurgery / neurological impairment
- No delayed presentation or representation

II. Relative indication for CT in cases with:
- Large scalp hematoma or laceration
- Multi-system trauma
- Dangerous mechanism
- Known neurosurgery / neurological impairment
- Delayed presentation or representation

III. Strong indication for CT in cases with:
- GCS <15 at 2 h post injury
- Deterioration in GCS
- Focal neurological deficit
- Clinical suspicion of skull fracture
- Vomiting (especially if recurrent)
- Known coagulopathy or bleeding disorder
- Age > 65 years
- Seizure
- Prolonged loss of consciousness (> 5 minutes)
- Persistent post traumatic amnesia at 4 h post injury
- Persistent abnormal alertness / behavior / cognition
- Persistent severe headache

IV. Patients should not routinely have CT scanning if they have all of the following features:

On initial assessment
- GCS 15 at 2 h post injury
- No focal neurological deficit
- No clinical suspicion of skull fracture
- No vomiting
- No known coagulopathy or bleeding disorder
- Age <65 years
- No post-traumatic seizure
- Nil or brief loss of consciousness (<5 minutes)
- Nil or brief post-traumatic amnesia (<30 minutes)
- No severe headache
- No large scalp hematoma
- Isolated head injury

- No dangerous mechanism
- No known neurosurgery / neurological impairment
- No delayed presentation or representation

After a period of observation (until at least 4 h post time of injury)
- GCS 15/15
- No post-traumatic amnesia
- Normal mental status including alertness, behavior, and cognition
- No clinical deterioration during observation
- Clinically returning to normal

GCS: Glasgow Coma Scale.

significant implications that may influence the degree to which an algorithm is adopted in different areas. It may not be realistic to expect that a set of criteria that is generated in a given location with its own unique medicolegal environment can be easily transferred to another area with the same degree of acceptance.

([42], p. S309)

Advanced Trauma Life Support/American College of Cardiology Surgeons Guidelines

The Advanced Trauma Life Support/American College of Cardiology Surgeons guidelines (ATLS/ACS) guideline [53] is telegraphic. The authors advise "CT scanning as determined by head CT rules" (p. 164). These surgeons favor the CCHR. When no CT is available, they advise hospital admission. The Ontario Neurotrauma Foundation (ONF) guideline also recommends the CCHR.

Ontario Neurotrauma Foundation Guidelines

The ONF [48] guidelines refer readers to the CCHR.

Scandinavian Neurotrauma Committee Guidelines

The original Scandinavian Neurotrauma Committee (SNC) guideline derived its CT scanning recommendations from a substantive review paper [36]. At that time, the SNC was one of the few developers of guidelines to recommend scanning every case of mild TBI: "The SNC Guidelines strongly recommend routine use of CT scanning in both children and adults with head injuries classified as mild or moderate." (They excluded what they called "minimal" cases, with GCS 15 and no LOC.) The revised SNC guideline [49] is quite different. The authors distinguish four classifications they refer to as: (1) "mild high risk"; (2) "mild medium risk"; (3) "mild low risk"; and (4) "minimal head injury." The new SNC guideline also stands apart as the only one to put faith in, and grant clinical decision-making authority to, the results of a measure of serum S100B. As discussed before, the evidence is weak that S100B is a valid or reliable correlate of severity or a useful predictor of outcome. For that reason, although the theoretical value of a biomarker is indisputable, the present author cannot defend the SNC approach. Unplugging the S100B node eliminates

Table 15.6 Scandinavian Neurotrauma Committee (SNC) computed tomography protocol [49]

"Mild high risk" head injury

- GCS 14–15 plus either:
- Seizure
- Sign of depressed or basal skull fracture
- Focal neurological deficit,
- Therapeutic anticoagulation or coagulation disorders
- Shunt-treated hydrocephalus

"Mild medium risk" cases

- Age ≥ 65 *and* antiplatelet therapy

"Mild low risk" cases

Minimal head injury: no CT required if:

- No loss of consciousness
- No repeated vomiting
- No therapeutic anticoagulation or coagulation disorders
- No seizure
- No sign of depressed or basal skull fracture
- No focal neurological deficits

GCS: Glasgow Coma Scale.

that caveat. Table 15.6 lists the elements of the updated SNC protocol. Figure 15.4 illustrates the SNC clinical flowsheet.

American Academy of Neurology Guideline

The American Academy of Neurology (AAN) guideline [44] recommends using a simplified version of the CCHR. However, the strength of their recommendation is Level C, meaning "possibly useful/predictive or not":

> CT imaging should not be used to diagnose SRC [sport-related concussion] but might be obtained to rule out more serious TBI such as an intracranial hemorrhage in athletes with a suspected concussion who have LOC, posttraumatic amnesia, persistently altered mental status (Glasgow Coma Scale <15), focal neurologic deficit, evidence of skull fracture on examination, or signs of clinical deterioration.

([44], p. 2254)

National Institute for Health and Care Excellence Guideline

Finally, the updated 2014 National Institute for Health and Care Excellence (NICE) adult CT protocol is illustrated in Figure 15.5 [38]. On first glance, this protocol looks like the CCHR. Closer inspection reveals a curious reconfiguration of the decision-making pathway: rather than starting with the inclusion factor "loss of consciousness or amnesia," the protocol begins with selection of the patients to be scanned using a combination of the "high-risk" factors from the CCHR, plus focal neurological deficits, seizure, and warfarin treatment. "Loss of consciousness or amnesia" only becomes a decision node after warfarin-treated patients have been excluded, and the CCHR medium-risk factors are subsidiary to that selection. To the best of this writer's knowledge, no study has validated the new NICE CT protocol.

Part 2: The Available Facts

At this point, the reader knows that multiple protocols have been recommended with the goal of identifying concussed patients with focal lesions while reducing the use of CT. The CCHR is the most popular, and a plurality of pre-existing guidelines for the management of concussion either recommend use of the CCHR or the use of some favored, non-validated revision.

This hardly scrapes the surface of the universe of available data. Nor does it examine the quality of the data, compare the strengths and weaknesses of alternative approaches, provide a cost–benefit analysis, explore the likelihood of any protocol being followed, or consider the ethical implications. The pre-existing concussion guidelines never touch upon the fact that different doctors favor different decision-making approaches, let alone consider that patients have feelings about scans. This section of the chapter addresses those deeper questions left unanswered in the guidelines. It still comes down to this: scan some or scan everybody? There is no right answer, since human values vary. Every reader will decide for him- or herself the "right thing to do." Still, certain factual observations may help when one considers the best answer to the question, "Should we scan everybody?" In this writer's opinion, a glance at the facts makes it clear that the debate over the most robust protocol is secondary. The real issue – the tough issue – is "what matters to you and your patient?"

How Many Adults With Concussion Have Intracranial Lesions Visible on CT?

The answer to this question is (1) unknown or (2) 10%. As mentioned above, Toth's 2015 review [25] claimed that 90% of patients who meet ACRM criteria for "mTBI" have negative CT scans; 10% are positive. That is a reasonable estimate combining data from multiple sources. However, it applies only to the modest subset of concussions that ever receive medical attention, and only to the subset of that subset that seeks ED evaluation, and only to the subset of that subset of that subset meeting the inclusion and exclusion criteria devised by one or another collaborative cadre – such as concussion survivors who visit the ED with GCS 15, loss of consciousness, no anticoagulants, and no seizures. No study has ever scanned a complete and unselected cohort of concussed persons. Moreover, meta-analysis would be fruitless since no two groups of investigators have employed the same selection criteria.

In the interest of at least documenting some sources that account for Toth's estimate: based on 11 studies, Livingston et al. [1] reported that, among the subset with GCS 15 and LOC or amnesia, 3–19% have positive CT scans. Based on ten studies, Ibanez et al. [54] reported that, among the subset with GCS 14 or 15 plus LOC, 3.7–15.3% have post-traumatic intracranial lesions. Based on six studies, Smits et al. [39] reported that 6–21% of persons with minor head injuries suffer intracranial complications. Toth's 10% figure falls neatly in this ballpark. That is about as good as the empirical record gets.

Of course, "lesion" does not mean either "important lesion" or "treatable lesion." Figure 15.6 puts these classifications into

Clinical algorithm for Scandinavian Neurotrauma Committee (SNC) computed tomography (CT) guideline

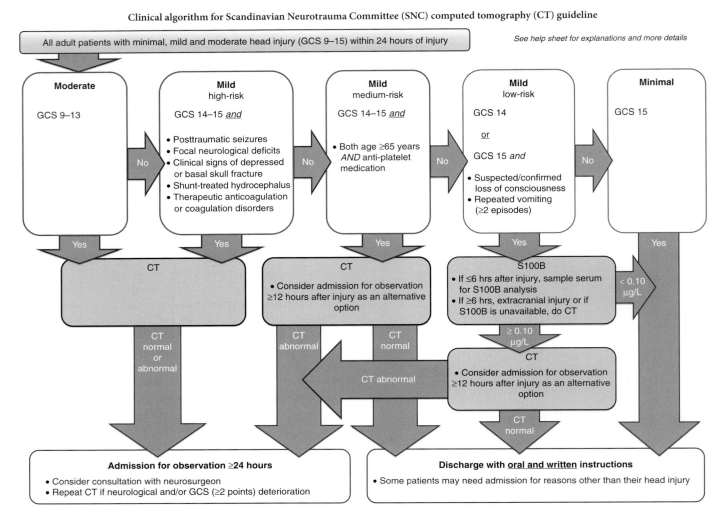

Fig. 15.4 CT is strongly recommended as the primary management routine. If CT is unavailable or logistically difficult, some patients may be admitted for close neurological observation for at least 12 h after injury. Patients with high-risk mild and moderate head injury should be admitted, irrespective of CT findings, for at least 24 h. Observation including Glasgow Coma Scale (GCS), pupil size/reactivity, a simplified neurological exam, blood pressure, pulse rate, oxygen saturation, and respiration rate should be performed every 15 minutes for the first 4 h *after injury*, every 30 minutes for the following 4 h, and at least every hour thereafter. Some patients with minimal head injury or normal CT/serum S100B following mild head injury, where discharge is recommended, may need admission for other reasons than head injury (such as elderly patients without sufficient help at home, patients with other injuries, or patients with heavy intoxication). Since these patients have a very low risk of intracranial injury, they do not need the extensive observation routine mentioned above.

Source: Unden et al., 2013 [49]. Reproduced under the terms of the Creative Commons Attribution licence, CC-BY 2.0.

clinical perspective: it illustrates typical proportions of a very mildly injured cohort that: (1) exhibit CT lesions; (2) exhibit CT lesions judged clinically important; and (3) exhibit CT lesions judged to require neurosurgical intervention.

In partial summary, understanding that we are merely discussing a subset of a subset of a subset of adults with concussion, the best available data suggest that 3–21% develop post-traumatic intracranial lesions visible on non-contrast CT. Whether it is important to know about those lesions is another matter.

Do Intracranial Lesions Matter?

Pathology on acute CT scan examination had no effect on self reported symptoms or global function at 3 months after MTBI.

(Lannsjo et al., 2013 [56])

CT evidence of subarachnoid hemorrhage was associated with a multivariate odds ratio of 3.5 ($p = 0.01$) for poorer 3-month outcome.

(Yuh et al., 2013 [11])

The two introductory quotations tell the tale: studies vary with regard to the clinical significance of intracranial lesions that do not require neurosurgery. Any blanket statement would be false. Moreover, since CT shows very little of the harm produced by CBI, one would not expect a consistent finding with regard to the predictive value of the limited information provided by this hoary old technology. The practical question might be restated: "Is there a potential clinical value to knowing whether or not there are intracranial lesions visible on CT?" That depends on what's seen – and what matters to this particular clinician/patient dyad. As a result, the upside of enhanced knowledge is almost impossible to quantify.

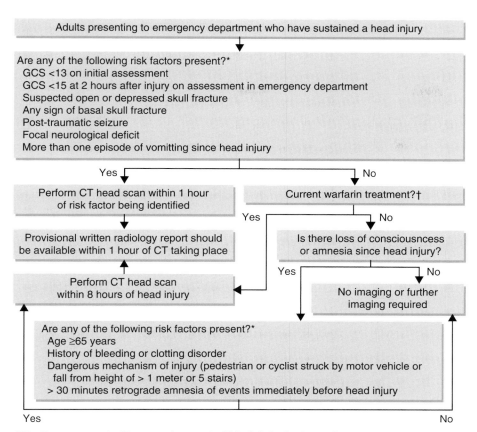

Fig. 15.5 Selection of adults for computed tomography (CT) head scan: National Institute for Health and Care Excellence.

Source: Hodgkinson et al., 2014 [38]. Reproduced with permission from BMJ.

Consider two hypothetical results:

1. Perhaps Mark, our teenaged concussion patient, has a "normal" scan ("normal," in such cases, meaning "a scan employing antiquated technology that notoriously fails to detect a large proportion of disabling pathology"). Might that information spare everyone the trouble and expense of inpatient observation, reassure the family, and help inform follow-up planning?

2. Perhaps his scan shows a 0.6-cm left dorsolateral prefrontal subdural hematoma (SDH) and 1.2-cm right mesial temporal hemorrhagic contusion. Might that information help guide the admission decision – as well as help the patient, family, primary care doctor, neurologist, physiatrist, and psychologist to understand late symptoms and plan follow-up?

Some evidence suggests that non-operable lesions, including subarachnoid hemorrhage, SDH, epidural hemorrhage, microhemorrhages, hemorrhagic contusions, and punctate hemorrhages are predictive of or associated with a higher risk for persistent post-concussive problems [57]. Then the question is whether either the doctor or the patient wants to know. If the only benefit of enhanced knowledge about your patient was more accurate prognosis, it would still seem worthwhile to have this information. More importantly, non-surgical

lesions sometimes serve as the canary in the mine: although post-scan deterioration is rare among those with "normal" CTs, the risk of deterioration after a positive but "non-surgical" CT varies greatly. One retrospective study of 3088 mTBI patients reported that 4.8% had intracranial bleeding but none of these deteriorated in the first 24 h [58]. In another study of 292 mTBI patients, 62.3% had acute traumatic findings; 2.2% deteriorated after that first scan. Yet another study reported that 13.5% of patients with mild to moderate TBI and "non-surgical" lesions on CT subsequently deteriorated and required neurosurgery [59].

One possible explanation for the broad spectrum of findings may be that few studies rescan all patients. White et al. [60] rescanned 46 patients with initial CTs showing intracerebral contusions. Sixty-five percent exhibited progression in the size of the contusion over 24 h (Figure 15.7).

Given these data, the presence of "non-surgical" head CT lesions may be one reason to admit for observation. In fact, a recent cost–benefit analysis demonstrates the value of using non-surgical CT lesions to guide the admissions decision. Holmes et al. reported [61]: "A deterministic analysis indicates that the admission strategy for those with a non-neurosurgical lesion costs approximately £340 less and gains 0.004 QALYs compared to discharge home and therefore dominates discharge home."

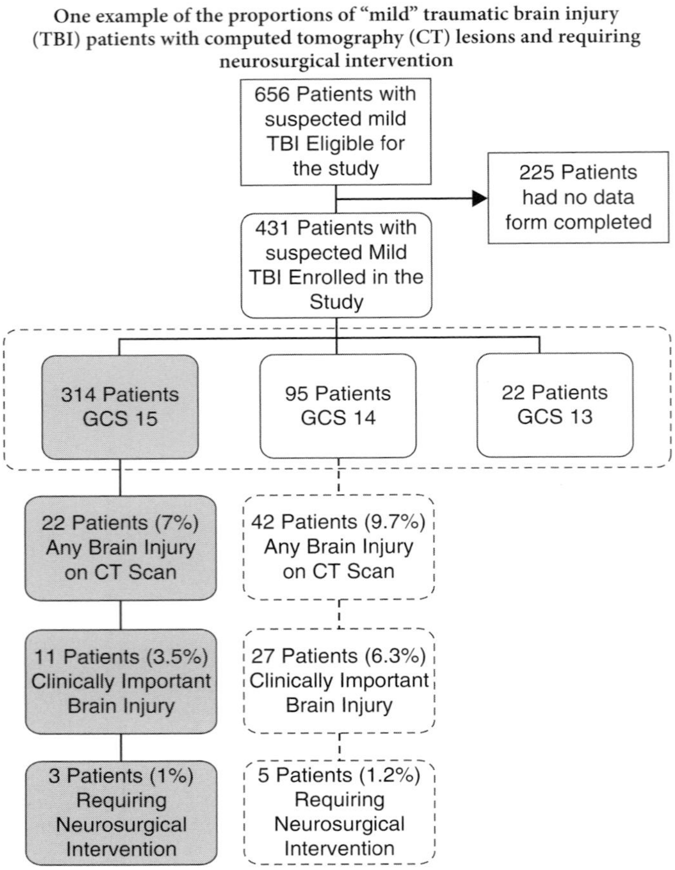

One example of the proportions of "mild" traumatic brain injury (TBI) patients with computed tomography (CT) lesions and requiring neurosurgical intervention

Fig. 15.6 Enrollment flow chart. GCS: Glasgow Coma Scale.
Source: Papa et al., 2012 [55] with permission from John Wiley & Sons

What Studies Have Been Done in the Hopes of Figuring Out a Protocol That Might Reduce the Use of CT Without Missing Too Many Lesions?

The original studies for the popular protocols are hardly the totality of the evidence. At least 42 peer-reviewed studies have reported findings relevant to the question of whether one or more risk factors might predict which concussed persons need a CT scan (Table 15.7). Some of the studies were attempts to replicate the original validation studies, for instance, of the CCHR or the NOC. Others propose alternative protocols. Diagnoses included minimal head injury, minor head injury, mild head injury, mild TBI, minor head trauma, and blunt head trauma. Some studies are confined to patients with GCS 15, others to patients with GCS 13–15. Most studies excluded patients with penetrating head injuries, although one included that group [62]. Most studies excluded patients who presented with neither LOC nor amnesia, but other studies included those patients. The delay in scanning with respect to either the injury or the arrival at the hospital was typically reported as < 24 h, but varied and was not always reported. Few studies included patients with seizures, and fewer included patients

with coagulopathies. The mathematical approach to finding risk factors with predictive validity varied considerably, from trial and error with sequential calculations of sensitivities to contingency analysis, logistic regression, or recursive partitioning – a method of creating a decision tree for dichotomous classification using multiple variables.

Thirty studies were prospective. Among these the n ranged from 58 to 13,507, and the proportion of subjects scanned ranged from 46.8% to 100%. Twelve studies were retrospective. Among these the n ranged from 66 to 105,469 and the proportion scanned from 7.5% to 100%.

To determine the likelihood that a patient with a concussion who goes to the ED will have a positive CT scan, or a scan with "clinically important findings," or a scan triggering neurosurgery, the only unbiased methodology is a prospective study of consecutive patients, 100% of whom are scanned. Eighteen studies met these minimal criteria (if one bends to include Uchino et al. (2001) [89] (97.8%) and Papa et al. (2012) [55] (99.3%)). Findings from the 18 prospective studies that reported results on all subjects are tabulated in Table 15.8. Most of these studies tested clinical risk factors thought to be potentially predictive of a positive scan, such as age, GCS, LOC, amnesia, age, signs of skull fracture, vomiting, headache, dizziness, extracranial injuries, neurological deficits, mechanism of injury, seizure, or coagulopathy. Although few studies tested the exact same catalog of factors, significant overlap is apparent in the risk factors reported to be predictive.

The take-home messages from the prospective studies with virtually universal scanning are as follows. First, the proportion of concussed patients attending an ED whose CT scan will reveal intracranial abnormalities varies from 3.1% to 19%. The unweighted average is 6.83%. Second, the predictive risk factors most often identified were age (especially over 60 years), amnesia, GCS (especially 13), LOC, physical evidence of head trauma, and vomiting – although it is not clear whether multiple vomiting is a better predictor than a single emesis. Note that a meta-analysis of 93 papers came to slightly different conclusions. The United Kingdom's impressive Health Technology Assessment [93] reported that some risk factors are more influential than others, and that two clinical factors commonly reported to be predictive were not:

> In adults, the presence of depressed, basal or radiological skull fracture and post-traumatic seizure (PTS) each substantially increased the likelihood of ICI [intracranial injury] (point estimate for positive likelihood ratio (PLR) > 10). Focal neurological deficit, persistent vomiting, decrease in GCS and previous neurosurgery markedly increased the likelihood (PLR 5–10). Fall from a height, coagulopathy, chronic alcohol use, age over 60 years, pedestrian motor vehicle accident (MVA), any seizure, undefined vomiting, amnesia, GCS < 14 and GCS < 15 moderately increased the likelihood (PLR 2–5). *Loss of consciousness (LOC) or headache had little diagnostic value.* [emphasis added]
>
> [93]

Third, the vaunted 100% sensitivities of the CCHR and NOC are not confirmed. Different populations of concussed persons

Representative case of intracerebral hemorrhagic progression on serial computed tomography (CT) scans

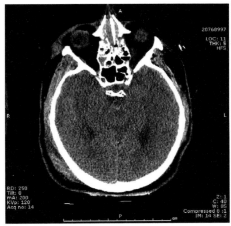 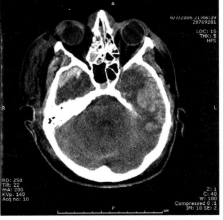

1 hour post-injury   6 hours post-injury

Fig. 15.7

Comparison between first and second CT scans demonstrated progression in absolute size of the contusion in 30 of the total sample (65%). Defining progression by an increase in volume of at least 33% over baseline, two-thirds of the group progressed and for almost 50% of the sample, there was > 100% increase in size of hemorrhage from the initial scan.

Source: White et al., 2009 [60] with permission from Lippincott Williams & Wilkins, Inc./Wolters Kluwer

Table 15.7 Studies reporting computed tomography scanning in concussive brain injury (mild head injury, mild traumatic brain injury) (listed alphabetically)

	Study	Design	*n*	% scanned
1	Atzema et al., 2004 [63]	P	8374 studied (MN)	NR
2	Borczuk, 1995 [64]	R	1448 scanned (MD)	NR
3	Bouida et al., 2013 [65]	P	1582	70.9%
4	Brown et al., 2011 [66]	R	66 scanned (MD)	NR
5	Clement et al., 2006 [67]	Pa	4551	66.3%
6	Culotta et al., 1996 [68]	R	3370	92.2%
7	Fabbri et al., 2005 [69]	P	5578	46.8%
8	Feuerman et al., 1988 [70]	R	373 scanned (MD)	NR
9	Gomez et al., 1996 [71]	R	2484	7.5%
10	Harad and Kerstein, 1992 [72]	R	1875	26.5%
11	Haydel et al., 2000 [2]	P	Phase 1 = 502 Phase 2 = 909	100%
12	Hsiang et al., 1997 [73]	P	1360	62%
13	Holmes et al., 1997 [74]	P	264 scanned (MD)	NR
14	Ibanez et al, 2004 [54]	P	1101	100%
15	Jeret et al., 1993 [75]	P	712	100%
16	Kavalci et al., 2014 [76]	P	175	100%
17	Kisat et al., 2012 [77]	R	105,469	79%
18	Korley et al., 2013 [78]	P	169	76.9%
19	Livingston et al., 1991 [9]	P	111	100%
20	Livingston et al., 2000 [1]	P	2152	100%
21	Miller et al., 1996 [13]	P	1382	100%b
22	Miller et al., 1997 [30]	P	2143	100%
23	Mower et al., 2002 [32]	P	2082c	15.8%
24	Murshid,1998 [92]	R	633	20.7%
25	Nagy et al., 1999 [91]	P	1170	100%
26	Papa et al., 2012 [55]	P	431	99.3%
27	Reinus et al., 1993 [62]	R	373 (MD)	NR

(continued)

Table 15.7 (Cont.)

	Study	Design	n	% scanned
28	Ro et al., 2011 [79]	P	Cohort 1: 6808 Cohort 2: 6699	Cohort 1: 8.6 Cohort 2: 9.8%
29	Rosengren et al., 2004 [80]	R	240	100%
30	Saadat et al., 2009 [81]	P	318	100%
31	Saboori et al., 2007 [12]	P	682	100%
32	Shackford et al, 1992 [82]	R	2766	78.3%
33	Sharif-Alhoseini et al., 2011 [83]	P	642	100%
34	Smits et al., 2005, 2007 [39, 84]	P	3181	100%
35	Stein and Ross, 1990 [85]	P	658	100%
36	Stein and Ross, 1992 [86]	R	1538	100%
37	Stein et al., 2009 [87]	P[1]	7955	52.5%
38	Stiell et al, 2001 [6]	P	3121	67%
39	Stiell et al., 2005 [40]	P	2707 (GCS 13–15) 1822 (GCS 15)	80.2% of 2707 75.6% of 1822
40	Turedi et al., 2008 [88]	P	240: 120 "high risk" 120 "lo risk"	100%
41	Uchino et al., 2001 [89]	P	90	97.8%
42	Vilke et al., 2000 [90]	P (MD)	58	NR

[a] Reanalysis of previous prospective study.
[b] The text is ambiguous regarding proportion scanned.
[c] Mower et al. reported that 13,728 patients with "blunt head injury" were scanned, but failed to report the severities. They mention that 2397 patients were not scanned but do not report if the total studied was the sum (16,125). The figures for minor head injury are inferred from the text.

GCS: Glasgow Coma Scale; MD: missing denominator: the study reports the number of subjects scanned but not the total enrolled; MN: missing numerator: the study reports the total subjects enrolled but not the number scanned; NR: not reported; P: prospective; R: retrospective.

seem more or less likely to include individuals whose clinical presentations would lead protocol followers into skipping a scan that would prove positive. Using the CCHR to select patients for scanning will lead to failure to scan as many as 23.6% of patients whose CTs would reveal intracranial lesions.

How Good is the Research?

a large number of different clinical guidelines and recommendations tailored to this management approach have appeared in the literature during the last years. Unfortunately, the majority of these recommendations and clinical guidelines lack solid scientific basis.

(Ibanez et al., 2004 [54])

The quest for a protocol that will facilitate detection of all the important intracranial lesions and reduce scanning has been inspired not only by theoretical benefits but also by empirical data. As previously noted, most Canadian ED physicians required that a decision rule be 100% sensitive [29]. The original validation studies for the NOC and CCHR (and other protocols) indeed claimed 100% sensitivity. Can one rely on this research?

There are many reasons to question the generalizability (and even the credibility) of the 42 studies listed in Table 15.7. Consider, for instance, the 2001 CCHR study [6]: an unknown

number of adults aged 16 or over suffered "minor head injury" (GCS of 13–15). A subset of these patients, probably a minority, presented to the participating EDs. Of course the authors cannot know how many injuries occurred in the community, but they do not even report the number of minor head injury patients who came to their hospitals. A subset of the subset that came to the ED fulfilled the authors' selection criteria, exhibiting blunt trauma with witnessed LOC, definite amnesia, or witnessed disorientation, but excluding everyone with a depressed fracture, a seizure, a focal neurological deficit, unstable vital signs, or a bleeding disorder or use of anticoagulants, and all those who returned for reassessment. The resulting group – a subset of a subset of a subset of minor head injury patients – numbered 3121. The investigators scanned 67% – a subset of a subset of a subset of a subset. How could they report 100% sensitivity when the test was only applied to this fraction of minor head injury patients? The authors rationalized their declaration of 100% sensitivity, guessing that the missing scans were all negative because the unscanned patients seemed OK when a nurse called them on the telephone two weeks later. CT is a very old technology and detects only some intracranial abnormalities. Telephone is an even older technology, and detects none. Two subsequent CCHR validation studies [40, 94] use the same method (considering a reassuring phone call as equivalent

Table 15.8 Prospective studies employing systematic scanning, in chronological order

Study	Diagnosis inclusion criteria	Age (years)	n	Protocol tested[a]	Risk factors found predictive[b]	Positive scans	CILs	NS	Sensitivity for any lesions (95% CI)	Sensitivity for CILs	Sensitivity for NS	Potential reduction in scanning
Stein and Ross, 1990 [85]	Mild HI GCS 13–15	NR	658	N/A	GCS	17.6%	NR	5%	N/A	N/A	N/A	N/A
Livingston et al., 1991 [9]	Minimal HI GCS 14/15	17–79	111	N/A	None	14%	NR	0%	N/A	N/A	N/A	N/A
Jeret et al., 1993 [75]	BHT GCS 15 + LOC or Amn	18–90	712	N/A	A, BSF, Mol, race	NR	9.4%	0.2%	NR	< 95%	NR	NR
Miller et al., 1996 [13]	Minor HT GCS 15 + LOC or Amn	"All"	1382	N/A	HT, N, V	6.1	NR	0.2%	NR	NR	NR	NR
Miller et al., 1997 [30]	Minor HT GCS 15 + LOC or Amn	NR	2143	HA, N, V, DS	DS, HA, N, V	6.4%	NR	0.2%	65%	NR	100%	61%
Nagy et al., 1999 [91]	Minimal HI GCS 15 +LOC or Amn	33.8 +/- 12.9	1170	N/A	D, N, S, V	3.3%	NR	0.3%	NR	NR	NR	NR
Haydel et al., 2000 [2]	Minor HI GCS 15 +LOC or Amn	3–94	Phase I =-502 Phase II = 909	NOC	A, HA, I, V	Phase I= 6.9% Phase II = 6.3%	NR	0.4%	100 (95–100	100	100	22%
Livingston et al., 2000 [1]	Minimal HI GCS 14/14 +LOC or Amn	≥16	2152	N/A	GCS, Mol	10.1%	NR	NR	NR	NR	NR	NR
Uchino et al., 2001 [89]	Mild HI GCS 13–15	13–80	90	N/A	A, GCS	8.9%	NR	NR	NR	NR	NR	NR
Ibanez et al., 2004 [54]	Mild HI GCS 14/15	15–99	1101	N/A	A, BSF, Coag, ECI, GCS, HA, Hy, LOC	7.5%	6.3%	1%	8 factors = 94%	8 factors = 100%	NR	NR
Smits et al., 2005 [39]	Minor HI GCS 13/14; or 15 + risk factor	> 16	3181	CCHR NOC	Per protocols	9.8%	7.6%	0.5%	CCHR = 83.4% NOC = 97.7%	CCHR = 87.2% NOC = 99.4%	CCHR = 100% NOC = 100%	CCHR = 37.3% NOC = 3%
Smits et al., 2007 [84]	Minor HI GCS 13/14; or 15 + risk factor	≥ 16	3181	CHIP	A, Amn, Coag, GCS, HT, LOC, Mol, ND, S	7.6%	NR	0.5%	Simple model = 96% Complex = 94%	NR	Simple model = 100% Complex = 100%	23–30%

(continued)

Table 15.8 (Cont.)

Study	Diagnosis inclusion criteria	Age (years)	n	Protocol tested[a]	Risk factors found predictive[b]	Positive scans	CILs	NS	Sensitivity for any lesions (95% CI)	Sensitivity for CILs	Sensitivity for NS	Potential reduction in scanning
Saboori et al., 2007 [12]	Minor HI GCS 15	6–85	682	N/A	A, Amn, Conf, HA, LOC, ND, S, V	6.7%	6.7%	0.6%	78%	78%	NR	NR
Turedi et al., 2008 [88]	Minor HI GCS 13–15	0 – >60	240	High-risk criteria: Amn, Coag, GCS, HA, LOC, ND, S, V	SF, V	19%	NR	NR	87%	NR	NR	50%
Saadat et al., 2009 [81]	BHT GCS 13–15	15–70	318	N/A	A, Amn, GCS, HT, V	6.3%	NR	NR	100%	NR	NR	43%
Sharif-Alhoseini et al., 2011 [83]	Minor HI GCS 13–15	3–90	642	NOC	Amn, HA, I, LOC	3.1%	NR	NR	95%	NR	NR	46%
Papa et al., 2012 [55]	Mild HI GCS 15	18–103	314	CCHR NOC	N/A	7%	3.5%	1.0%	CCHR = 100% NOC = 100%	CCHR = 100% NOC = 100%	CCHR = 100% NOC = 100%	NR
Papa et al., 2012 [55]	Mild HI GCS 13–15	18–103	431	CCHR	N/A	9.7%	6.3%	1.2%	100%	NR	100%	NR
Kavalci et al., 2014 [76]	Mild HI GCS 13–15	≥ 18	175	CCHR NOC	Per protocols	9.7%	NR	NR	CCHR = 76.4% NOC = 88.2%	NR	NR	NR

[a] A priori criteria or presumptive risk factors to be tested.
[b] Risk factors found to predict + computed tomography.

A: older age; Amn: amnesia; BHT: blunt head trauma; BSF: suspected basilar skull fracture; CCHR: Canadian CT Head Rule; CHIP: CT in Head Injury Patients; CI: confidence interval; CIL: clinically important lesion; Coag: coagulopathy; Conf: confusion; D: dizziness; DS: depressed skull; ECI: extra-cranial injuries; GCS: Glasgow Coma Scale; HA: headache; HI: head injury; HT: signs of head trauma; Hy: hydrocephalus; I: intoxication; LOC: loss of consciousness; MoI: mechanism of injury; N: nausea; N/A: not applicable; ND: deficits on neurological examination; NOC: New Orleans Criteria; NR: not reported; NS: findings mandating neurosurgery; S: seizure; SF: suspected skull fracture; STM: short-term memory deficits; V: vomiting.

to a scan that was actually performed and read as negative). Setting aside the fact that the CCHR findings would only be applicable to an unmeasured minority of concussed patients, these observations about methodology reveal that the reported "100% sensitivity" was not derived scientifically.

Moreover, as Reynolds [95] pointed out, the sensitivities reported in the validation manuscripts may be unique to certain places or populations. For example: the CCHR's sensitivity for any intracranial lesion and for "clinically important" lesions was originally reported as 100%. However, when replications were attempted abroad, the CCHR's sensitivity for lesions was 85.5% in Spain [54] and 83.4% in the Netherlands [39]. Its sensitivity for "important" lesions was 95% in Tunisia [65], 84.5% in the Netherlands [39], and only 80% in Australia [80]. Similarly, the NOC's original report claimed a sensitivity of 100% for clinically important lesions. While its sensitivity was reported as 97.7% in the Netherlands it was only 86% in Tunisia. If the issue were systematic regional variation, one might still trust these protocols in North America. Yet evidence suggests significant variability in patients selected using the same rules both within institutions and between physicians in the same institution.

Insensitivity aside, it is reasonable to ask whether protocols such as the NOC and CCHR derived from studying the subset of patients with LOC could be predictive of CT results in the larger group – including those who remained conscious. The assumption seems to have been that patients who remained conscious were very unlikely to have positive CT scans. That assumption was debunked when Smits et al. [39] attempted to replicate the CCHR and NOC. As Haydel [96] gracefully acknowledged, "patients without loss of consciousness were excluded from both of the original studies, but Smits et al. (2005) reported that 30% of patients requiring neurosurgical intervention reportedly had no documented or observed loss of consciousness" (p. 1553). Moreover, a meta-analysis of data from 93 papers revealed that LOC does not predict intracranial lesions [93]. Therefore, perhaps contrary to intuition, presence or absence of LOC would be a poor choice of risk factors to select patients for scanning.

Multiple authorities have identified other methodological flaws in the body of literature that claims to have found clinical predictors of positive CTs. For instance, in a review of 22 studies describing a CT rule for mTBI, Harnan et al. [97] stated, "No study scored well on all quality assessment criteria." The authors of the previously mentioned meta-analysis of 93 papers concluded, "The quality of the studies was generally poor" ([93], p. iii). With a few exceptions [75, 76, 81] the CT reading was performed by one or more radiologists, all aware of the clinical findings, without either independent confirmation or tests of interrater reliability. Eng and Chanmugam [98] investigated the quality of the studies and pointed to other common design weaknesses: "none of the studies employed independent observers in the clinical evaluation of participants. The lack of multiple independent clinical and imaging observers was primarily responsible for the uniformly lower quality scores for bias." As Ibanez et al. [54] summarized this large literature:

Clinical guidelines were based on the supposed existence of certain factors that can detect patients at risk. Although many researchers have proposed a large number of theoretical risk factors, few have analyzed their significance from a statistical point of view. Results of those studies on the significance of clinical risk factors are frequently contradictory.

[54]

Therefore, in addition to the paucity of prospective studies with systematic scanning, in addition to the fact that the available studies are only applicable to some fraction of concussed patients, in addition to the fact that different selection criteria make different studies non-comparable, the research methods of seminal reports are not altogether credible.

There is no complete agreement concerning the importance of LOC, PTA [post-traumatic amnesia], headache, nausea and vomiting, cranial soft tissue injury, epilepsy and posttraumatic seizure, acute drug or alcohol intoxication, particular mechanism of injury, coagulopathy, previous intracranial operations, or alcoholism.

([54], p. 831)

How Reliably are Risk Factors Assessed?

Some of the risk factors empirically shown to help predict positive scans are surely assessed with a high degree of accuracy and reliability. Age is the safest example. Presence or absence of headache also seems likely to be assessed reliably (although assessment of "severe headache" is perhaps less reliable). Other risk factors, however, are highly prone to reporting error, clinician subjectivity, and disappointing interrater reliability.

For instance, multiple prospective studies reported that a lower GCS (13 or 14) is a clinical risk factor that contributes to the likelihood of a positive CT. Yet in previous chapters we demonstrated why high GCS scores do not validly discriminate levels of severity and that the GCS is not assessed reliably. Similarly, many studies reported that "amnesia" contributes to the likelihood of a positive CT. Unfortunately, that term is used inconsistently: in the CCHR validation study, amnesia referred to > 30 minutes of retrograde amnesia, or loss of memories from before the accident. In the NOC validation study, the term is used to mean "amnesia for the traumatic event." In still other studies, *amnesia* meant that persistent PTA was detected at the time of examination. Again, we previously demonstrated that PTA (deficient orientation or ability to lay down day-to-day memories) is not assessed reliably by clinicians. One would surmise that a patient's failure to recall his or her accident (NOC amnesia) can be assessed with reasonable reliability, whereas either precise duration of retrograde amnesia (CCHR amnesia) or persistence of PTA is a much tougher call. This problem not only makes the studies non-comparable but also leaves open the question of how "amnesia" bears upon the likelihood of a positive scan.

Several protocols recommend that clinical signs of either a skull fracture or basilar skull fracture be used to select patients for CT. However, the predictive value of clinically suspected skull fracture requires critique. It is true that suspected basilar skull fracture was associated with an increased risk of intracranial lesions in the study reported by Stiell et al. [6]. Moreover, Munoz-Sanchez et al. [99] reported that skull fractures in patients with GCS 14–15 were five times as likely to require neurosurgery. In another study, 49% of children with skull fracture had intracranial lesions and 85% of those with surgically drainable lesions had skull fractures [100]. Such findings would seem to support the protocols' advice to use clinically suspected fracture as a decision point regarding ordering a CT.

Yet that thinking ignores a major point: how useful is clinical examination for detecting the presence of skull fracture? Goh et al. [101] reported on 500 mTBI patients, of whom 144 had clinical signs of basilar skull fracture. Seventy-five were indeed found to have basilar fractures. But 22 patients with no clinical signs also had fractures (4.4%). It is a matter of opinion whether the risk of failing to scan those 22 patients is acceptable, and to whom. In the 2009 Munoz-Sanchez et al. [99] study, "Of mTBI patients with skull fracture and [intracranial lesions], 63.2% showed no clinical signs of bone injury." Hence, *getting the CT is usually necessary to detect the fracture that would trigger getting a CT*. Given the low bedside detection rate, it would seem imprudent to depend on clinical judgment of suspected skull fracture to make the CT decision.

LOC? Setting aside the fact that the evidence regarding the predictive validity of LOC is weak [31, 102], how reliable are ED assessments of a patient's state of mind at the time of the injury? In some cases a reliable witness can provide a credible history. Yet in a large proportion of cases (as in the hypothetical case of Mark, introduced early in this chapter) the occurrence of LOC is altogether ambiguous.

How shall we operationalize history of vomiting? Are we 45% confident in the history of "no vomiting" reported by our concussed 16-year-old patient, or 75% confident? Given the question of source-dependent historical accuracy, shall we restrict the application of this criterion to patients whose histories are provided by a reliable adult who continuously observed the patient from impact until clinical interview? Do vomiting episodes separated by 20 seconds count as one or two? Do dry heaves count? Does vomiting in the setting of dizziness (hence, likely related to vestibulopathy) or intoxication (hence, confounded by a non-injury factor) have the same predictive validity as vomiting without dizziness or intoxication (hence, perhaps related to medullary torsion or increased intracranial pressure)? Since some rules state that vomiting more than once is the predictor and others that *any* vomiting is the predictor, which rule should the ED physician apply?

The point is not to dismiss the potential value of the risk factors for a positive CT identified in the empirical literature. One must be grateful for the major effort of many scholars who have earnestly searched for symptoms or signs that might predict intracranial lesions. The point is merely to candidly acknowledge that some of those predictive symptoms and signs are more likely than others to be assessed and documented accurately.

Do Doctors Follow Guidelines?

Guidelines for the assessment and treatment of minimal and mild head injuries may not have the intended degree of influence on clinical practice.

(Hekestad et al., 2008 [103])

Besides guidelines, fear of missing a traumatic intracranial lesion played a role in ordering head CTs. Although the physicians had been instructed in the use of guidelines, including validated clinical decision rules, this did not prevent them from ordering unnecessary CTs.

(Rohacek et al., 2012 [104])

Clinical practice guidelines always face the "if you build it, will they come?" question. There is frequently a gap between recommendation and implementation. The NOC was published in 2000, the CCHR in 2001, and the first SCN in 2002. Shortly after the publication of the SCN guidelines, which recommend routine CT scanning for all patients with mild head injury, just 25% of hospitals followed that advice [105]. Research on the implementation of the CCHR conducted in 2008 (seven years after dissemination) reported that 86% of Canadian physicians were aware of the protocol and 57% used it. In the United States, 31% were aware of the protocol but only 12% used it [106]. In a survey of more than 1000 emergency physicians and residents published in 2010, only 25% were aware of the protocols [94]. In fact, when the CCHR was implemented at the same centers where it was validated, CT use *increased* rather than decreased [94]. In a study published in 2012, the proportion of CTs ordered that complied with various protocols (CCHR, ACEP, NICE, NOC) ranged from 64.7% to 90.5%, suggesting that up to 35% of scans were not recommended [107]. In a Scandinavian study of 1325 CT examinations for mTBI, compliance with SCN recommendations occurred in just 31.2% of cases and 54.2% of scans were regarded as unnecessary [108]. A 2013 study in China reported that 41.7% of responding emergency physicians were aware of the CCHR but only 24.7% used it [109]. Jones et al. [110] surveyed two academic emergency medicine departments using vignettes and found that compliance with ACEP guidelines was 62.8%. A 2014 review concluded that compliance with these protocols (or any CT protocols) is generally low and highly variable [111]. The most commonly cited reason for declining to use the protocol was fear of malpractice, followed by ignorance of radiation risks.

These findings expose not only a significant variation in compliance rates but also a striking gap between recommendations and implementation. Moreover, in the Canadian study published eight years after dissemination of the CCHR, physician decisions about whether to order a CT were influenced not only by reported risk factors but also by unproven (in essence, irrational) factors, including the mode of arrival at the hospital (i.e., ambulance) and geography (i.e., urban setting). Figure 15.8 illustrates findings from one study that attempted to catalog clinician motivations. Since the findings reflect self-report one cannot necessarily take them at face value. It nonetheless seems credible that emotional factors such as fear and perceived pressure were common priorities. Of interest, motive for scanning was not related to the likelihood of a positive or negative outcome. Evidence also shows that many physicians do not understand statistical concepts [112]. Such findings add to our understanding that ordering CTs will continue to be influenced by non-protocol-based preferences.

Yet ignorance is not the main, or even an important, factor in explaining widespread non-compliance with

Clinicians' self-reported reasons for ordering a computed tomography (CT) scan for concussion: proportions of answers for each reason,
applying the Canadian CT Head Rule

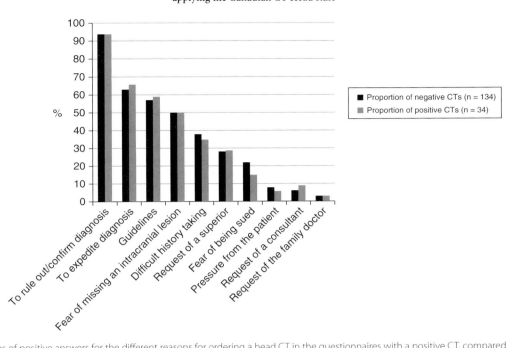

Fig. 15.8 Proportions of positive answers for the different reasons for ordering a head CT in the questionnaires with a positive CT, compared to questionnaires with a negative CT. Differences in proportions were investigated using two-group proportion z-tests. No significant differences were found in the proportions of positive answers. Guidelines specify the following practice: each patient with a minor brain injury should receive a CT of the head if the patient is being treated with anticoagulants or has coagulopathy, is intoxicated, or a seizure is suspected. In the remaining cases, the Canadian CT Head Rule should be used to decide whether a CT is required. If there is no great risk of neurosurgical intervention (Glasgow Coma Scale GCS < 15 2 h after injury, suspected skull fracture, sign of skull fracture, vomiting < 2 episodes, age < 65 years) or intermediate risk of brain injury (amnesia before impact > 30 min, dangerous mechanism), no CT is required.

Source: Rohacek et al., 2012 [104] with permission from Elsevier

carefully elaborated, mathematically rigorous clinical protocols. A deeper and less tractable issue lurks. As hinted at the beginning of this chapter, unconscious biases due to personality and emotions may trump the most apodictic analyses. Poses et al. put it: "teaching physicians to make better judgments of disease probability may not alter their treatment decisions" ([113], p. 65). In other words, even after two decades of hard work to identify promising predictive factors to guide CT decision making, worldwide compliance with scanning recommendations is somewhat akin to the worldwide compliance with the recommendation to stop smoking: variable, and – from the recommenders' point of view – a bit dispiriting.

What might help? Assume for the moment that the best practice is compliance with, rather than abandonment of, published protocols. Automated clinical decision-making advice is a fast-spreading technology. In the United States, the Health Information Technology for Economic and Clinical Health Act mandates the use of computerized "clinical decision support" (CDS). A CDS system links to ordering, such that physicians requesting a CT must input information that the program checks against favored guidelines. Protocol-compliant orders are approved; off-protocol orders trigger a recommendation not to order the scan (though most programs allow physicians to override the robot). How do physicians feel about having a robot tell them whether to order a head CT? Ballard et al. [114] surveyed 339 physicians in a health care system that employs

CDS to guide CT decisions after pediatric head trauma. There was 75–93% agreement with positive statements about the CDS and 60–93% support for its implementation in the ED. Gupta et al. [111] reported a 56% increase in compliance over the two years after CDS was implemented at one Level 1 trauma center.

Psychosocial Factors

The above-cited research on implementation only reports the proportion of compliant physicians. Although it touches upon the role of recency of training and level of experience, it does not provide a compelling answer to the question: why do some physicians order scans when others do not? In some cases, legal, social, or economic factors trump physician discretion. As Ibanez et al. put it:

> In technologically well-developed countries with high-quality medical resources and in which the medicolegal climate shows zero tolerance for misdiagnoses, systematic CT scan indication would probably be the best diagnostic approach.
>
> ([54, p. 832)

Local culture probably influences CT decision making. For instance, among the clinician-deciders, some are working in national health services that both restrain physician autonomy and defend them from liability, while others have more decision-making leeway but work in societies supporting the gainful employment of trial lawyers. Local values also influence whether a positive CT is regarded as "clinically important." As Reynolds ([95, p. 529) admonished, "Although Stiell et al. clearly specify their "consensus-based" criteria down to the millimeter thickness of the lesions that count, most authors don't, and words such as 'generally,' 'normally,' and 'consensus' are the very definition of culture."

Of concern, there is also some evidence that prejudice influences the CT decision. In Australia, for instance, Indigenous patients waited longer for care and were somewhat less likely to get a head CT when it was clinically indicated [115]. And in a large Scandinavian study, suspicion of patient alcohol intoxication was associated with a lower frequency of scanning [108].

Another influential factor may be disciplinary identity. Doctors charged with assessing acute concussion do not all belong to the same specialty and even those in the same department have different training. In the United States, most concussions are initially assessed by emergency medicine doctors. In academic centers, that ED doctor is a resident – a beginner who does his or her best; in community hospitals, that ED physician is more likely to be experienced. Neurosurgeons primarily consult on moderate to severe TBIs, unless a mild case exhibits an intracranial hemorrhage. In contrast, in Norway, 81% of minor head injury patients are managed by general surgeons [116]. It is not known how specialty impacts compliance. And, as hinted above, even within specialties, physicians vary in tenure and experience. A young emergency physician working in a medium-sized suburban hospital may have independently assessed 20–40 concussed persons in his career. An older doctor at an urban trauma center may have assessed several thousand. Should both be given the same instructions? Perhaps a simple, rigid protocol might be more valuable when the decision maker has less expertise, since its outcomes have at least some predictive validity. A rigid rule might be less valuable when the decision maker has more expertise, because it can never accommodate the infinitude of circumstances that an expert would weigh – from patient credibility to patient imbalance to patient claustrophobia to parental anxiety to knowledge of the nurse's skill at neurochecks and, most importantly, to that ineffable discriminator so familiar to experienced doctors: does the patient look sick?

At least some evidence suggests that physician emotions and temperament are the wild cards in the decision-making process. Even with identical training, doctors are human. It only makes sense that some are more comfortable than others at taking risks or acting on incomplete information. For instance, in a Swiss study [104], 94% of physicians reported that they ordered head CTs to rule out an intracranial lesion, but 50% of physicians acknowledged that they ordered the scan because of "fear of missing a traumatic lesion." (Twenty-two percent did so because of "fear of being sued" and 8% due to perceived pressure from the patient.) Fear is not discussed in the published protocols, but it plays a potent role in clinical life – to different degrees in different individuals. Rosengren et al. [80] neatly summarized the emotional underpinnings of the great debate: "Fear of failing to diagnose a significant

intracranial injury has led to the widespread and excessive use of CT scans, exposing some patients to unnecessary radiation and increasing health care expenses" (p. 198).

Perhaps the opposite of fear is enthusiasm for risk taking. Some physicians are simply more willing to take risks, ordering fewer imaging studies based on personal risk tolerance rather than any authoritative guidance or rational choice. For instance, one U.S. study of physician risk behavior assessed decision making among doctors managing ED patients with acute abdominal pain [117]. The likelihood that the doctor would withhold CT scanning was directly related to a measure of risk taking but not to measures of stress due to uncertainty or fear of malpractice.

In another study, U.S. and U.K. doctors were compared. Presented with identical vignettes, the U.S. physicians were (paradoxically?) more likely to expect adverse outcomes from the treatments they prescribed and less likely to be concerned when confronted with the obligation to make a decision under conditions of uncertainty. In essence, U.S. physicians scored higher on risk seeking and lower on stress. (Reassuringly, both U.S. and U.K. doctors reported regret when learning their decision led to harm [113].) Stein et al. ([87, p. 180) crystallized this issue: "choosing which of the two clinical decision instruments to use must be based on decision maker attitudes toward risk."

Even this inventory of decision-making pitfalls barely scratches the surface of the problem. A veritable labyrinth of leaks drains energy away from patient benefit on the route from an evidence-based protocol to real-world care. Figure 15.9 is a light-hearted schematic of the lossy path between advice and health care, depicting that tortuous route as a network of pipes jiggered to deliver at least a little evidence-based medicine.

Clinicians will sigh in recognition of these truths. One can invest many dollars in devising optimum algorithms, and more dollars in teaching them to resident physicians or doctors via continuing medical education. Insurance companies can employ knobby fiscal sticks to force obedience with ostensibly useful clinical policies. But one should never expect that best practices will be followed. Morton and Korley [119] commented:

> findings from a 2008 national survey of US emergency physicians found that only 30% reported awareness of the Canadian CT Head Rule, with significantly fewer (12%) reporting using it. In another survey, 32% of emergency physicians anticipated that they would forget the details of the Canadian CT Head rule in routine practice.
>
> (p. 362)

More broadly, as Glasziou and Haynes [120] put it: "While bedside evidence-based medicine has focused on clinicians becoming aware of and accepting the best-quality research, it is clearly important but insufficient." Perhaps equally important is a factor emphasized in this chapter on concussion: "best" practices will never be good practices until they are individualized – a phenomenon that awaits routine application of not only psychological sensitivity but also genomics.

These observations challenge the hope that research will deliver a protocol acceptable to all physicians, and help explain the previously discussed recommendation – implementation

You can lead a horse to water

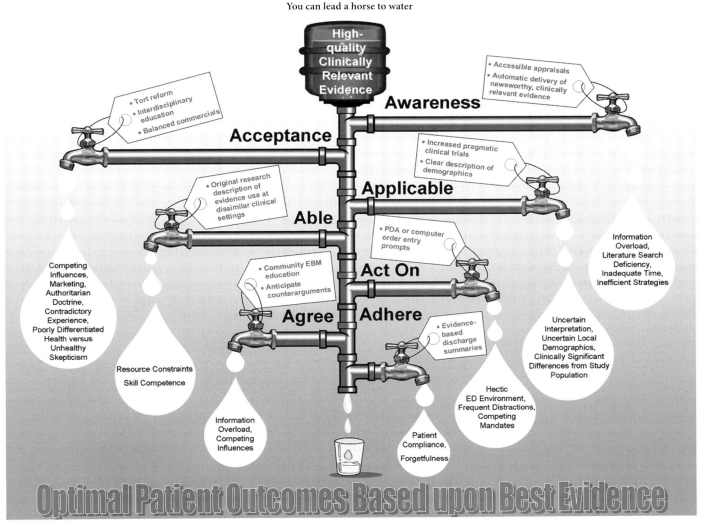

Fig. 15.9 Pathman's pipeline. This illustration depicts the flow of high-quality evidence to optimal patient outcomes. Each water spout represents the preventable leak of information according to unique barriers, with ideas to slow the leaks depicted by the tags around the water handles. The droplets of water provide illustrative examples of information loss, misuse, or inapplicability at each level. The first five leaks deal with the physician and health care team, whereas the last two leaks are specific to the patient's environment. (The authors made modifications to the original Pathman model in this diagram, according to their perception of the model's most relevant factors to emergency medicine graduate medical education.) EBM: evidence-based medicine; ED: emergency department; PDA: personal digital assistant;.

Source: Diner et al., 2007 [118] with permission from John Wiley & Sons

gap. Again, there is no right answer. Who gets scanned will surely continue to be conditioned by multiple factors other than the statistical likelihood of an intracranial lesion, the optimum pecuniary calculus, or what's best for the individual patient. Still, might an institution, a health care network, or a nation select and advocate the use of a protocol superior to "scan everybody"? That depends on one's take on the objections to the CT-for-all approach.

The "It's Too Early" Objection

The major finding of this study is that 3% of patients who sustain a minor head injury severe enough to cause a cerebral concussion will subsequently deteriorate to the point where they require neurosurgical treatment … However, it did not appear possible on the basis of clinically available data

to predict with confidence which of these patients would subsequently deteriorate.

Dacey et al., 1986 [8]

Some authorities recommend universal, routine, early CT scanning when patients arrive at the ED with suspected concussion. In fact, "CT-for-triage," meaning early CT as the first step in the evaluation, has been recommended [9, 85, 121]. CT-for-triage is favored by some authorities not only because this policy would avoid the grim consequences of missing a treatable lesion by withholding CT, but also because it would eliminate the costs of observation and admissions for patients who are extremely unlikely to deteriorate, and accelerate intervention for the ~ 7% who will have abnormal scans.

There is resistance to that algorithm. It is absolutely justifiable. One counterargument is the concern that CT-for-triage

Fatal subacute deterioration after "mild traumatic brain injury"

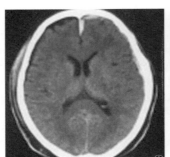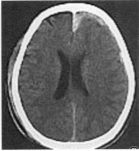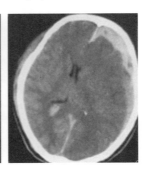

Fig. 15.10 Progression of subdural hematoma and subarachnoid hemorrhage from day 3 (left image), day 8 (middle image), and day 9 (right image) after admission

Source: Shiwen et al., 2014 [122] with permission from Elsevier

would lead to scanning too many patients too soon. Some patients will surely deteriorate *after* that early CT. Consider Figure 15.7 (earlier in this chapter), which depicts the dramatic evolution of an intracerebral contusion/hemorrhage over a few hours between a hyper-acute and an acute scan. Judging by the first image alone, the clinicians might well have discharged the patient before the threat of potential herniation became apparent. Even though very few patients are scanned hyper-acutely (within 60 minutes of injury), a universal *scan-on-triage* rule could sometimes defeat its own purpose, misleading the medical team to a premature conclusion that a patient with an early benign scan was safe from increased intracranial pressure. Given the pressure on trauma room resources, one can well imagine a patient such as this being discharged based on that early scan.

Such cases argue for a delay. But what delay? For optimum life-saving, brain-saving care, how many minutes after injury should the doctor wheel the gurney to the CT suite? Now consider Figure 15.10.

Even three days post admission, this patient's left frontotemporal SDH appeared benign. The rapidity of the deterioration from day 8 to day 9 is astonishing. This is atypical. Yet Figures 15.7 and 15.10 together illustrate the point made early in this chapter and many times in this collaborative book CBIs vary. Virtually any stiff-necked rule will lead to fatal errors.

Might one adopt a rule to delay the scan unless and until the clinical course suggests worrisome developments in the head? Dacey et al. [8], for example, applied the rule, "Only scan those patients who clinically deteriorated over 12 hours." In their study, clinical deterioration occurred in 11.1% of 610 concussed patients. And indeed, more than one-third of those had abnormal scans, suggesting (as the reader could have predicted) that denying scans until things go south will lead to a high proportion of positive scans. But what is the clinical value of such a protocol? As those authors cautioned, "it did not appear possible on the basis of clinically available data to predict with confidence which of these patients would subsequently deteriorate" ([8], p. 208). Presumably, one wishes to know *before* the patent is on the verge of herniation. Using Dacey et al.'s rule, no lesions would be discovered and no surgical interventions would be initiated until *after* the brain had lost function. That might undermine the value of scanning.

At the risk of redundancy: there is no natural history of concussion. One can cite averages and then manufacture algorithms that treat averages as predictions. If so, one will design some bad clinical outcomes into our algorithms.

Admitting that physicians are shackled to uncertainty and no algorithm rescues them from all errors, now reconsider the CCHR. If that rule were adopted throughout the developed world, about 77% of patents would be scanned at some point during their ED visit, sometimes sooner, sometimes later. If a patient arrives at a CT-for-triage hospital at noon and is scanned at 12:15–12:30 pm, after a nurse's or physician assistant's quick assessment to confirm a likely head injury and to rule out contraindications, the emergency physician may know the head CT results by about 12:45 pm. At another hospital, the policy may be to only scan *after* the attending physician completes his or her assessment (with even longer delays in scanning if a neurological consult is sought). So the scan might occur several hours later. How many patients would be expected to deteriorate such that their 12:30 pm scan is normal and the 3:30 pm scan is not? It depends on many clinical factors, including minutes since the injury. Af Geijerstam and Britton [121] offered pertinent data: among 62,000 patients with a GCS of 15 and an early normal CT scan, three suffered adverse outcomes due to later deterioration. The "too early" argument against CT-for-triage is legitimate, but the risk is low.

The principal arguments advanced against routine scanning come down to just two: radiation and cost. For example, the United Kingdom's Health Technology Assessment program opined: "Management involves a potential trade-off between underinvestigation, which risks missed opportunities to provide early effective treatment for ICI, and overinvestigation, which risks unnecessary radiation exposure and waste of NHS [National Health Service] resources" [93]. Do these objections stand up to scientific scrutiny?

The "But it Exposes my Patient to Radiation" Objection

Given the striking increase in the rates of CT imaging in the United States, the known deleterious effects of overexposure to radiation from CT imaging, and the spiraling costs of health care in the United States, it is critical that emergency medicine residents consider improving their implementation of CT guidelines for mild TBI into their daily practice.

(Morton & Korley, 2012 [119, p. 366)

A second conclusion follows from the fact that the estimated CT-related cancer risks are very small: It follows that if a CT examination is clinically justified, there is no doubt that its benefits will by far exceed its risks; there is no need for complicated benefit–risk calculations.

[123]

In the previous section, physician temperament was identified as a probable factor in decision making about head CT for concussed patients. Whether or not study authors frame their objections to scanning in terms of physician fear, almost all of the proposed protocols emphasize saving patients from this perceived threat. Again, local culture influences clinical values. European centers, on the whole, are less enthusiastic about scanning, frequently citing their concern that radiation exposure during head CT will increase the lifetime risk of cancer. North American centers are generally more sanguine about that threat, sometimes pointing to the risk of missing an opportunity for a life-saving intervention. A conservative rule designed to reduce radiation exposure and the use of resources will miss more cases that might have benefited from a scan. A liberal rule designed to maximize detection of lesions will add cost and expose larger numbers of individuals to radiation.

Is fear of radiation exposure from head CT rational? Empirical facts might help and recent research has slightly advanced the understanding of the long-term risks of CT-level radiation.

Radiation exposure is measured in several ways. A gray (Gy, or rad) is a unit of the absorbed dose, while a sievert (Sv) is the "equivalent" dose for potential biological damage. X-rays and gamma-rays have weighting factors of 1.0, which means that the absorbed dose in grays equals the equivalent dose in sieverts. Natural background radiation exposure ranges from 0.4 to 4 mSv per year, largely depending on radon levels. A typical non-contrast CT scan exposes the typical adult human to 2.0 mSv of radiation. Does any evidence exist that one head CT, or ten, or 50, can cause cancer?

The Life Span Study of the survivors of atomic bombings in Hiroshima and Nagasaki remains the most-cited evidence of a relationship been radiation dose and risk of later cancer [124, 125]. (Another source of data is a 15-country study showing a slight increase in cancer risk among radiation workers and has been cited as supporting this theory [126].) Yet the cancer risk attributable to lower doses of radiation of the magnitudes received in clinical imaging (< 100 mSv) remains quite controversial, since there is almost no applicable evidence [127]. The argument about whether or not to order a head CT scan has been especially warm with regard to pediatric mTBI, since toddlers may be as much as an order of magnitude more vulnerable than adults. The temperature of that debate rose in 2001 when Brenner et al. [128] published an estimate that 500 children exposed to head or abdominal CTs each year might ultimately die from radiation exposure (see also [129]). Yet that study rests on the hotly debated assumption that one can extrapolate down from the effects of very much higher doses – atomic bomb doses – to estimate the effects of very much lower doses. The theory that extrapolation is meaningful is called the *linear no-threshold* model. The linear no-threshold model predicts that even the smallest dose – a dose that has never been reported to cause a single human cancer – will increase the risk of cancer.

Several groups have subsequently published their own estimates of the risk of low-dose exposure (e.g., the United Nations Scientific Committee on the Effects of Atomic Radiation, the Biological Effects on Ionizing Radiation Committee's VIIth report [130], and the International Commission on Radiological Protection [131]). However, those estimates are all based on the linear no-threshold assumption [130–133]. A conflict continues to roil the radiological community regarding the validity of the linear no-threshold model and whether the real risk to humans of a single scan can be predicted from the high-dose data. Hendree and O'Connor [134] caution that generating risk estimates with the linear no-threshold is shaky science: "To extrapolate cancer incidence to doses of a few millisieverts from data greater than 100 mSv, a linear no-threshold model is used, even though substantial radiobiological and human exposure data imply that it is not an appropriate model."

What is the basis for published claims that X-radiation, in the low doses used in clinical imaging, presents any risk of cancer? About 75% of survivors in the atomic blast Life Span Study were estimated to have experienced exposures in the range of 5–200 mSv – equivalent to about 2.5–100 head CTs delivered at the same moment, assuming that X- and gamma-rays are biologically equal and discounting any effect of neutrons in the A-bomb blast. Preston et al. [125] reported that 60,792 A-bomb survivors in the Life Span Study cohort were exposed to doses < 5 mSv. Making a number of physical and epidemiological assumptions, they report that the 9597 people who developed cancers included a total of three excess cases ([125], p. 14). That is, accepting all the assumptions of the Life Span Study, 2½ head CTs at the same moment might eventually cause cancer in three of 60,792 people – about one in 20,000. If instead one administered 50 head CTs at the same moment (100 mSv), the risk would be higher: 1.8% of the cancers that eventually occurred over the course of a lifetime might be attributable to those CT scans. Note that these are theoretical risks extrapolated from atomic bomb survivors. No report has ever shown that one head CT (or 50) has ever caused an adult human case of cancer.

The debate was reinvigorated when Pearce et al. published a paper in *The Lancet* in 2012 [135]. Even applying the linear no-threshold model and considering worst-case scenarios, the risk of cancer due to CT is very low: "in the 10 years after the first scan for patients younger than 10 years, one excess case of leukaemia and one excess case of brain tumour per 10,000 head CT scans is estimated to occur." Nonetheless, academics citing the same data continue to argue about whether to emphasize the risks or the benefits of head CT, and both primary care doctors and the public remain ill at ease [136]. The result of this dis-ease may be that fear about the hypothetical, impossible-to-measure, never-demonstrated risk of cancer from CT is interfering with clinical decisions involving the very real risk of missing intracranial lesions. As Hendee and O'Connor [134] admonished:

The predictions of cancers and cancer deaths are sensationalized in electronic and print public media, resulting in anxiety and fear about medical imaging among patients and parents. Not infrequently, patients are anxious about a scheduled imaging procedure because of articles they have read in the public media.

(Brenner & Hall, 2012 [134], p. 312)

Even authorities who previously warned of the danger of CT now warn of the greater danger of skipping a CT out of exaggerated fear. Brenner himself – a strong advocate of the linear no-threshold theory – wrote: "In some cases, medical imaging examinations may be delayed or deferred as a consequence, resulting in a much greater risk to patients than that associated with imaging examinations" [123].

Without getting into radiation physics, another issue is whether perfectly good scans can be acquired at lower radiation doses. A movement is afoot to press for routine use of such techniques [137, 138]. Raman et al. summarized the developing advice, identifying:

8 fundamental CT scan parameters that can be altered or optimized to reduce patient radiation dose, including detector configuration, tube current, tube potential, reconstruction algorithm, patient positioning, scan range, reconstructed slice thickness, and pitch.

[137]

In another development, ultrasound imaging is making strides toward a capability to detect the intracranial lesions most likely to trigger neurosurgical intervention.

The bottom line is that, to date, no human has been shown to develop cancer due to a head CT – or 50 head CTs. The "But it will expose my patient to radiation" objection to routine scanning of persons with concussion is based primarily on guesswork and emotion, not science.

The "It Costs Too Much" Objection

The use of four simple clinical criteria in minor head trauma patients would allow a 61% reduction in the number of head CT scans performed and still identify all patients who require neurosurgical intervention ... This method could lead to a large savings in patient charges nationwide.

(Miller et al., 1997 [30], p. 453)

This ... confirms the fact that patients with MHI must undergo mandatory CT scanning ... Implementation of this practice could result in a potential decrease of more than 500,000 hospital admissions annually.

(Livingston et al., 2000 [1])

Economists and actuaries blithely value human lives and their presumed "quality" in dollars. Several national systems of health care are firmly yoked to this mind-blind system, with standards of clinical care based on the use of computers to judge the worth of better, longer human lives. Unfortunately, such fuzzy math is here to stay. Societies simply cannot afford to deliver all the health care that modern technology has devised. Harsh though it may sound, rationing is inevitable. One must respect the arguments of those who object to routine head CT after concussion on the grounds of fiscal prudence.

However, what does the math actually say?

In a Norwegian study from the mid-1990s [139], 88 minor head injury patients all received early CT scans followed by 24 h of observation. Nine percent of patients had intracranial lesions – a typical result. The authors calculated that promptly discharging patients with negative CTs would have saved 43%. This result highlights the challenge of a real-world cost–benefit analysis. The conclusion surely depends on the dollar cost of the scan, the dollar cost of patient observation, the reliability of nursing neurochecks, the worth in dollars, to patient and family, of hearing the good news that the scan is normal, the dollar costs of neurosurgical procedures, intensive care unit beds, and medications, the frequency of missed lesions, the frequency of late deterioration, the local traditions for compensating injured patients with dollars, the method of assessing outcome, and the dollar quantification of a change in duration or quality of life. A single case of avoidable lifelong disability or a single multi-million-dollar verdict might dramatically change the math. Moreover, the dubious assumption is made that patients with normal scans have no sequelae.

Every cost-effectiveness study of CT for concussion faces similar challenges. For that reason, like so many other faces of the CT decision question, a conclusion depends on one's values. Larger and better studies have been published. Despite the dilemma of how to value human well-being in dollars, it may be worthwhile reviewing some more recent calculations.

Stein et al. [28] calculated the cost-effectiveness of six management strategies, including both selective scanning and scanning for all, considering a hypothetical 20-year-old patient with minor TBI and a GCS of 14 or 15. They considered the effect of missing intracranial lesions on both longevity and quality of life, expressed as QALYs. In such models, when a given approach is shown to be both more effective and less costly than others, it is said to "dominate" the alternatives [140]. The resulting model revealed that:

With regard to effectiveness (QALYs saved), the Selective CT and CT All are significantly better than the other strategies. This is largely a consequence of averting delayed surgery. The number of QALYs saved by applying the Selective CT (or CT All) to the average 20-year-old patient is small (0.05–0.1). However, this is well within the 0.03 to 0.12 range of QALYs saved by mammography and screening procedures for other cancers in high risk individuals.

([140], pp. 563–564)

Hence, this analysis found an insignificant difference in cost-effectiveness whether the ED selected concussed patients for scanning or scanned them all.

Smits et al.'s cost-effectiveness study [141] is one of the most sophisticated currently available. The authors compared routine CT scanning versus selective scanning versus no scanning of 3181 patients with minor head injury. Unlike several previous cost–benefit analyses (e.g., [28, 84]), her team took into account estimates of the lasting disability and decreased quality of life harming a patient whose neurosurgical lesions are missed. Understanding that any such study depends on assumptions made about both patients and costs, the mathematical results were straightforward: if your protocol has extremely high sensitivity for neurosurgical lesions (better than 91–99%), then selective scanning using either the CCHR or CT in Head Injury Protocol (CHIP) is cost-effective. If your protocol is less sensitive, then "performing CT in all patients with MHI is more cost-effective than missing even a small proportion of these patients, because a delayed diagnosis in patients who require neurosurgery presumably leads to poorer outcome and associated higher costs due to disability and lost quality of life" ([141], p. 538).

Holmes et al. [61] devised a mathematical model to test hypotheses about the effect of different CT scanning protocols on QALYs. The authors examined the effect of routine scanning versus scanning selectively using the CCHR high- and medium-risk clinical predictors. Unlike the Norwegian study, which employed observation, these U.K. clinicians achieved considerable cost savings by discharging patients home if the scan was normal. (Like other studies, this one rests on the completely untenable assumption: "We assumed that patients without an intracranial lesion remained well" ([61], p. 1425).) The manuscript makes a critical point: any calculation of cost–benefit depends on assumptions (guesses) about the financial impact of missing a neurosurgical lesion. Yet the authors admit, "Our estimates of the effect of delayed treatment upon intracranial pathology in particular are based on very limited observational data" ([61], p. 1429). Under all of its assumptions, the model suggested that selective scanning using the CCHR is cost-effective. In addition, admitting patients with non-surgical intracranial lesions seemed more than worth the cost in local currency: "A deterministic analysis indicates that the admission strategy for those with a non-neurosurgical lesion costs approximately £340 less and gains 0.004 QALYs compared to discharge home and therefore dominates discharge home" [61],

Arguably the most ambitious review of the cost-effectiveness of CTs for concussion was a product of the United Kingdom's Health Technology Assessment program: Pandor et al. [93] undertook a laborious meta-analysis of then-available data to inform recommendations for the National Health Service. Upon completing their yeomanly effort, these authors concluded:

> Selective CT use was cheaper than discharging without investigation because of the substantial costs of care for patients with worse outcomes due to delayed treatment. It was more effective than CT for all because of the QALY loss through radiation-induced malignancy associated with additional CT scanning.
>
> [93]

Oh? As noted in the previous section, the only source of risk estimates of CT-related malignancy is hypothetical – an extrapolation using an unproven linear model guessing at the harm done by 2.0 mSv based on the harm done by an atomic bomb – according to a theoretical extrapolation from epidemiological reports. No empirical evidence exists that adult humans experience an increased risk of cancers from CT. Therefore, half of the Health Technology Assessment's justification for favoring selective scanning over CT-for-all is scientifically unjustifiable.

Given the variations in the data used for analysis, the analytic models, and the scientific validity of the assumptions, these studies collectively fail to answer the question, "Which is most cost-effective: selective scanning or scanning everybody?" It seems to be a near thing. Again, further study might add a little information, and give comfort to actuaries. Further study will not, however, change the fact that different physicians and different patients feel differently about the dollar-equivalent of the risk of missing lesions and the benefit of enhanced knowledge.

This brings up a factor altogether absent from the guidelines, protocols, and cost-effectiveness analyses: what is an unnecessary scan?

What is an Unnecessary Scan?

> decision making in minor head injury involves a trade-off between unnecessary CT scanning and missed intracranial injury, as reflected in the sensitivity and specificity estimates reported. The substantial benefit of neurosurgical interventions for certain lesions means that specificity should be sacrificed to optimize sensitivity … However, the benefit of identifying and treating injuries that do not require surgical intervention is less certain.
>
> (Harnan et al., 2011 [97], p. 250)

Scan 100 concussed adults. On average, 93 scans will be read as normal; seven will reveal one or more of the trauma-related abnormalities that are visible using this old technology; about half of those will be judged "clinically important" and the other half not; one scan will provoke neurosurgical intervention. What matters? The rhetoric found in studies of CT protocols is revealing. For many authorities, the 93 normal scans are called "unnecessary." Three or four of the seven abnormal scans will be called "therapeutically inconsequential." How fitting are the terms *unnecessary* and *therapeutically inconsequential* to the presumed goal of patient well-being? Several observations suggest that popular value judgments be reconsidered.

First, the term *therapeutically inconsequential* fails to recognize two facts. One is that cost-effectiveness analysis has repeatedly shown that all patients with positive CTs ought to be admitted to the hospital. Some of these patients will deteriorate, requiring prompt and often life-saving inpatient interventions. It has not been shown that this number depends on the classification "clinically important." Therefore, the differentiation between the 93 normal and seven abnormal results directly impacts clinical management. One might, of course, substitute a CT decision protocol for an actual CT, for instance, employing the CCHR to select a subset of patients for scanning. But if one does selective scanning, even accepting the often-claimed figure of 99% sensitivity (which we know to be different in different cohorts), one is going to miss some lesions.

Two, some patients with benign-appearing scans need neurosurgery: in one study of 8374 subjects with CTs after blunt head trauma, 155 (1.85%) had lesions judged to be "therapeutically inconsequential" but 12% of those patients went on to require neurosurgery [63]. The black-and-white dichotomy reported in many studies between *clinically important* and *therapeutically inconsequential* is not a scientific distinction.

That leaves the question of whether normal scans are unnecessary.

The phrase "unnecessary scan" is popular in both the pre-existing concussion management guidelines and the CT protocol literature. Harnan et al.'s excellent review [97], for example, concluded that the CCHR was the best-validated and most practical protocol, since its sensitivity was high enough to catch "most" injuries requiring neurosurgical intervention, and its specificity was high enough to reduce the rate of "unnecessary" scans. In another paper, Lee et al. [142] judged that CTs are "unnecessary" for concussed children with isolated LOC because only 0.5% have "clinically important" TBIs. The authors defined clinically important as "resulting in death, neurosurgery, intubation for > 24 hours, or hospitalization for > 2 nights."

Assuming that Lee et al.'s figure of 0.5% is exactly right in all world cohorts, does that mean 99.5 out of 100 scans are worthless? These authorities have concluded, for example, that there is no value in knowing whether your concussed child has a normal scan, or instead a scan revealing a 6-cm linear skull fracture, plus a little subarachnoid hemorrhage, plus two small hemorrhagic contusions, plus nine petechial hemorrhages, plus a small SDH. Worthless? Some people would want to know.

Many authors of the large and growing collection of concussion recommendations seem to have comfortably bought into the judgment that, if a doctor does a test and the results are normal, the test was unnecessary. That judgment violates common sense. It reckons the value of knowledge about patients at zero without having demonstrated that worthlessness. Until it is shown that a negative test result has no value in clinical medicine, it is presumptuous to discount that value out of hand. The typical physician has innumerable experiences of circumstances when a negative test result guided patient care.

Consider blood tests. These are ordered routinely on the vast majority of the millions of persons attending EDs and a large proportion of patients visiting general practitioners. In one study, 6829 tests of serum electrolytes were ordered for 6401 ED patients [143]. The authors concluded that these tests influenced clinical management in just 2.6% of cases. But how many disorders were ruled out by those 6829 negative tests, and is ruling out a disorder a useful thing to do?

In the United Kingdom's reassuringly titled Vague Medical Problems In Research (VAMPIRE*)* trial, 59% of general practitioners ordered blood tests in cases of unexplained complaints. Ninety-two percent of those blood tests were negative for somatic disease [144, 145]. Given the many millions of blood tests done, the cost of the normal tests is hard to estimate but almost beyond reckoning. If normal results (at an average cost of about $175) are considered worthless information and 92% are "unnecessary," one suspects we might save vastly more health care dollars by ordering blood tests more selectively than we would by outlawing all CT scans (about $450 each). But doctors and patients would not be as well informed.

Is a normal scan an "unnecessary" scan? No clinical study or mathematical model can answer this question. *Unnecessary*

in whose opinion, and considering what outcomes? This is a matter of human values. And doctors are not the only ones with values.

Part 3: What Do Patients Want?

Any human being of adult years and sound mind has the right to determine what should be done with his own body. Justice Benjamin Cardozo: Schloendorff *v.* The Society of New York Hospital, 1914.

[146]

Physicians surely care about what patients want. A substantial empirical literature has tested hypotheses about patient preferences. However, with the exception of a few cheering passages in the VA/DoD manuscript [45], none of the many pre-existing guidelines for the management of concussion and none of the published protocols for head CT consider the fact that patients have wishes, questions, and free will. That is an understandable oversight. Not only is the notion of patient preference relatively new to academic medicine, but also the answer to what patients want and whether that is "best" for the patient is not self-evident. However, consideration of what patients want may be a valid finger on the scale for the doctor torn between ordering or not ordering a CT scan.

Information

One facet of the patient preference question is: "what does the patent wish to know before a scan?" Studies of imaging for cancer suggest more or less what any doctor might predict:

Patients would like to obtain clear explanations so that they can understand why the examination is being performed, what we are looking for, why a CT scan is performed rather that MRI and vice versa, what are the respective advantages of the two techniques, what are the dangers and risks associated with the examinations.

([147], p. S95)

One suspects that patients' wishes are similar in the case of head CT after concussion. A careful reading of the literature suggests that doctors will be surprised and patients may be comforted to know that no human adult has ever been reported to develop cancer from one CT, or ten. The benefits of head CT are harder to quantify, both because the sensitivity number for the protocols are debatable (e.g., results with the CCHR vary from 80% to 100%) and the value of learning that a scan is normal is not considered in the cost-effectiveness literature. Nonetheless, one might reasonably explain to patients:

1. A CT scanner is roughly 98–99% successful in visualizing bleeding in the head (e.g., subarachnoid hemorrhage, SDH, epidural hemorrhage, hemorrhagic contusion).
2. About 7% of concussed people have such a CT-visible lesion.
3. About 0.5% of concussed people will be found to have a lesion that mandates neurosurgery.
4. However, CT scanners are incapable of showing much of the brain damage done by a concussion.

Another facet of the patient preference question pertains to test results. Doctors and patients have overlapping, but not identical, agendas and priorities. Physicians value learning the results of an imaging study, including when that result is normal, yet they have a rather different stake in the process compared with that of patients, whose short- and long-term future may depend on these results. Patients have expressed a strong preference for prompt and direct communication of test results, whether those results are positive *or negative*.

In research on mammography, for instance, it has been reported that the least-preferred outcome of all was failure of the physician to inform the patient of a normal test result [148]. In a study of 888 patients at the Mayo Clinic, a majority was anxious to learn their test results and 67% preferred direct notification by a physician or nurse practitioner. Specifically with respect to negative test results in the ED, among patients tested for group A streptococcus, 85% preferred to receive both positive and negative test results. In another study of notification of normal test results, 65% of patients preferred to be notified directly by their health care provider, and 90% wanted to be notified of all test results, not just abnormal findings [149].

Thus, whatever value the clinician attaches to ordering a test and receiving a result, most patients clearly want the information, "your test was normal," whether or not that fact has the least bearing on management. That is, patients attach their own values to clinical information – a consideration often overlooked in cost-effectiveness studies. At least one component of that value is reassurance.

Reassurance?

Do normal head CT scans reassure, and is that reassurance clinically beneficial?

Hints that normal test results are valuable because they reassure the patient have been reported in research on a variety of laboratory procedures. In a trial of 92 patients referred for exercise stress testing, some subjects were randomized to have a pre-test discussion about the meaning of a normal test result, the others not. Not only was the level of reassurance higher among those who were talked to, but also their chest pain symptoms over the next month were decreased [150]. Thus, communication and reassurance are inextricable. Whether reassurance adds to QALYs or not, and whether it might actually reduce symptoms or not, it can only happen when there is good communication between the doctor and patient.

Specifically in regard to neuroimaging, evidence suggests the potentially high value of negative scans: "Undergoing an imaging examination was of benefit to the patient and improved their sense of well-being mainly by the reassurance they experienced, as reported by 91% of the patients" ([151], p. 444). Make no mistake: almost all patients want you to order the scan.

However, the estimated short- and long-term value of reassurance to the patient, and the impact of that value on cost-effectiveness calculations, has received little attention. For instance, in a review of 141 studies of the cost-effectiveness of laboratory testing, Fang et al. [152] found that just six of those studies attended to the reassurance value of normal test results.

But the *value* of that reassurance was only incorporated into the calculation of QALYs in two of the 141 papers. (In the other cases, reassurance was relegated to the discussion section.) Hence, even though almost every patient wants the scan, limited information is currently available about the economic value of reassurance associated with normal head CT results.

Again, patients vary. Some are more anxious than others. Some are more knowledgeable about technology, or more impressed with technology, or more afraid of technology than others. Other research suggests that reassurance is not a universal or a complete effect of receiving a negative test result; perhaps half of patients will have residual anxiety in spite of hearing that the result was normal [153]. Still, empirical data show that some patients who get a brain scan with a "normal" result are indeed reassured. Mushlin et al. [154] compared the dollar cost of saving an entire QALY achieved with different methods of scanning for equivocal neurological disease.

> MRI use has an incremental cost of $101,670 for each additional quality-adjusted life-year saved compared with $20,290 for CT use. … If a negative MRI result provides reassurance, the incremental costs of immediate MRI use decreases and falls below $25,000 for each quality-adjusted life-year saved no matter the likelihood of disease.
>
> ([154], p. 21)

In other words, it depends on the patient. Some will be reassured by a negative scan. For those, there may be a striking enhancement of cost-effectiveness. But again, virtually none of the CT cost-effectiveness studies estimated the value of reassurance by a normal scan. One is struck by this gap in the literature. It makes the previous discussion of cost versus benefit tenuously meaningful. Until studies are done with attention to the value of a normal scan, one cannot put full faith in the available results. The best summary of the cost-effectiveness literature: equivocal and faulty.

Participation in Decision Making

A spectrum exists between four models of care: (1) paternalism, in which the doctor hijacks decision making for his own; (2) delegated agency, in which the patient agrees to turn decision making entirely over to the doctor; (3) shared decision making, in which the doctor tries to inform the patient about the risk and benefits of the option and then they decide together; and (4) strict informed consent, in which the doctor also tries to educate the patient about the risks and benefits and then leaves the decision entirely to the patient. That fourth option is a misnomer. There will almost always be an asymmetry of knowledge, such that even weeks of discussion and provision of reams of information are unlikely to bring the patient up to the doctor's level of awareness of all the relevant medical considerations. *Informed*, in this case, means provided with a scanty collop and left to guess about the hog.

Although there is an international movement in the direction of enhanced patient autonomy, two problems prevent incorporation of that ideal into everyday medical practice. First, patients vary. Some ethicists rail against the old paternalistic model, but research shows that some patients in fact fear having any role in decision making and are grateful for substituted judgment. Other patients are more eager to share decision making or to make the decisions themselves [155–158]. The reasons for the variation have yet to be fully elucidated. For instance, evidence suggests that older patients tend to be happier to let the doctor decide for them, but the question remains whether that is because of aging effects or because of a cohort effect – having been raised within a culture of deference to doctors [159]. Similarly, younger, more educated patients and women apparently want more input into decision making, but that seems to depend on the severity of the illness [160].

The second problem is the more serious: doctors are bad at figuring out what patients want [157]. In one study, for example, even after substantial discussion and explicit written statements of patient wishes, 45% of primary care doctors remained ignorant of women's preference for treatment [161]. No fault is implied. Human desires are private. Even the patient may be less than fully aware of his or her dearest wishes. So the most compassionate, liberal-minded physician may nonetheless have a devil of a time intuiting what model of care will be most helpful for the frightened stranger on the gurney.

This combination of problems presents a barrier to divining a good answer to the question, "how shall the ED physician or primary care doctors figure out a way to include what the patient wants into the decision about whether or not to do a head CT after concussion?" The difficulty of the job notwithstanding, there is an ethical duty to discuss the risks and benefits of tests and procedures with patients. That includes head CT for concussion.

Informed Consent

Informed consent with regard to performing a diagnostic CT scan has two meanings. The most common refers to discussing the theoretical risk of radiation-related cancer. The second and relatively neglected use is discussing the real risk of forgoing an examination. Both are relevant to whether and how to obtain informed consent before head CT for concussion, although only the latter is associated with a clinically proven risk. It is understood, of course, that emergency management involves special pressures and exceptions, and that some concussed persons cannot fully participate in decision making. However, ethicists point out that the less stringent requirements for informed consent claimed by ED physicians are primarily for doctor convenience. "The same rights to informed consent … should apply in the ED as in any other treatment setting" ([161], p. 49).

How good is so-called informed consent at accomplishing its ostensible intended purpose? A discussion of this subject would be incomplete if it assumes that the typical institutional review board-approved process has utility. Evidence exists that a majority of patients do not understand the procedures or the risks when they read and sign informed consent forms. Whether they understand the words or not, patients tend to be influenced by illogical biases [163]. Moreover, the needs and desires for information vary widely between patients [164]. The

problem is, in part, that it is simply hard to explain matters such as the risk of radiation from CT. As Goske and Bulas put it:

The theoretical risk from radiation-induced cancer is projected onto a background of a frequent disease (nonfatal cancer) in the general population with a life-time risk of almost 40% in both men and women. To further complicate the discussion, the risk of radiation-induced cancer is based on population risk, not risk to individual patients. Yet the question asked by families is "does the CT scan ordered for my child cause cancer?".

([164], p. 902)

The authors further noted: "We are asking parents to navigate a very complex and emotional topic." It seems that both physician and patient emotions factor into the head CT decision-making process.

No national or worldwide consensus exists specifying whether ordering a head CT requires informed consent administered by the ordering physician, the radiologist, or the radiology technician. In one survey of U.S. academic medical centers, 52% proved verbal information and 5% written information to patients before CT. Just 15% explained the possibility of a radiation risk [165]. A survey of 75 physicians at a Level 1 trauma center revealed that 76% did not believe informed consent for a CT ordered in the ED was required and another 13% did not know one way of the other. Some U.S. radiologists have urged routine informed consent for CTs; others disagree. In 2004, for instance, Cascade [166] submitted a resolution to the American College of Radiology arguing for formal consent before screening CTs. Cancer, he noted, is not the only risk. Doubtful efficacy, false positives, and false negatives deserve frank discussion. Citing Hippocrates, Maimonides, the Declaration of Helsinki, and the American Medical Association Code of Medical Ethics, the author opines that radiologists "respect the rights of patients by providing comprehensive and unbiased information about the tests" ([166], p. 83).

In contrast, Berlin [167] published a discussion of a possible legal or ethical duty of radiologists to inform patients of the (theoretical) risk of CT-related radiation. He cites a Wisconsin Supreme Court decision: "The standard to which a physician is held is determined … by what a reasonable person in the patient's position would want to know" [168]. Some data speak to this issue: a survey of parents who had brought their children to the ED reported that 90% wanted to be informed of the possibility of cancer risk before agreeing to the scan [169]. In a study of 941 ED patients with intact mental status, 73.5% preferred to discuss the costs and risks before CT [170]. Although it is clear that patients want to know about possible risks, Berlin opined that – since there are insufficient data to declare that any risk of cancer exists – there is no legal or moral duty to obtain informed consent for CT.

That conclusion will satisfy hair-splitting ethicists. But the problem with this approach is that it dismisses a theoretical risk without considering a real risk. The risk-taking ED physician might elect to follow a protocol such as the CCHR. Any such protocol is associated with a higher risk of missed lesions than the CT-for-triage or CT-for-all protocol. Just as the available literature on cost-effectiveness has limited value since it ignores the possible benefits of a normal scan, the literature on informed consent for CT focuses on the wrong issue. There is no known risk of cancer. The risk that needs discussion – especially when physicians are itching to withhold the scan – is missed lesions. The emergency physician typically chooses between taking a risk with the patient's life or scanning everybody. Missing from the informed consent literature is consideration of the physician's duty to alert patient that the doctor is quietly making that choice. That is, banished from the great CT debate, up to now, is Justice Cardozo's reminder of human autonomy. Doctors type orders. Some may be confused into thinking that the question is what matters to them, what with all their knowledge, experience, and wisdom? But what matters to them must be informed by what matters to the patient.

The Ethics of Withholding a CT Scan

Two observations help settle the issue. One concerns the ethics of cost containment. The other concerns the ethics of emergency circumstances.

With regard to cost containment, it is undeniable that we must collectively reduce the use of tests. The question is where to cut and who gets to decide. The individual doctor confronting the individual patient? Different physicians, of course, will feel more or less compunction about taking the cost containment initiative into their own hands. But that is not ethical.

> An examination of the role that physicians play in the control of health care costs suggests that unilateral rationing decisions by individual physicians at the bedside are morally unacceptable. Such decisions are arbitrary, ineffective in distributing health care resources, and formally unjust.
>
> [171]

With regard to ethics in emergencies: ED patients rarely choose their hospital or doctor. They tend to be under emotional stress. Unlike calm shared decision making with a trusted primary medical doctor ally, the nature of the doctor–patient relationship in the ED demands a more formal protection of patients' rights. As Ladd [172] pointed out, "Although the standards of informed consent apply in emergency care, there seems to be discrepancies between theory and practice, and emergency physicians may be more guilty than others of unjustified paternalism" ([172, p. 149). If a doctor is leaning towards withholding a CT, the risk of missing an operable brain lesion is about 0.5%. If a doctor is leaning toward ordering a cerebral angiogram, the risk of generating a permanent neurological complication (according to one meta-analysis [173]) is only 0.07%. By what logic do we *always* discuss that risk of an angiogram and *never* discuss the risk of withholding CT? If you withhold a head CT to save the patient from radiation, it is unscientific. If you withhold a head CT to save money, it is not only scientifically debatable but also unethical. ED physicians concerned about cost savings for society should feel free to forgo their salaries. They must not paternalistically impose their own guesswork

calculations regarding the cost-effectiveness of CT upon innocent strangers with concussions.

Conclusion

> Had we discharged all of our alert asymptomatic patients with a GCS score of 15, we would have failed to detect intracranial hematomas in Cases 5 and 6.
>
> Dacey et al., 1986, p. 209 [8]

> Policy makers and clinicians must decide on their underlying priorities.
>
> (Harnan et al., 2011 [97], p. 250)

This brief review suggests that many authorities have been worried about the wrong things. Some literature frets about cancer risk. Cancer risk for adults has not been shown. Some literature frets about cost. The most cost-effective protocol is a toss-up between the CCHR and scanning everybody – and the cost-effectiveness of scanning everybody perhaps dominates when one considers the many benefits of normal scans. What we should perhaps be more worried about is missing lesions and deafness to the patient's voice. Some doctors are risk takers and will use the red herrings of cost and radiation to justify their personal preference to withhold CT. Medicine will always employ some risk-taking physicians. Medical ethics requires that patients be protected from them. Most doctors, thankfully, wish to do the right thing, if only that were clarified.

Taking into account the incidence of abnormal CTs after concussion (reasonably approximated at 7%), the clinical importance of knowing whether the CT is abnormal, the flaws in the selective scanning research, the inconsistent sensitivity of selective scanning protocols in different cohorts, the potentially catastrophic consequences of missing surgical lesions, and the fact that most patients value scans and we value patient autonomy, a simple and practical plan would seem to balance the virtues of quality of care, economics, and ethics. If your institution grants (or tolerates) physician discretion, you have two scientifically defensible, cost-efficient, and ethically virtuous options:

1. Discuss the risks of missing intracranial lesions with the patient. If the patient agrees to take the risk of missing some lesions by skipping the scan, then – after consulting the CCHR recommendations for this type of case – engage in shared decision making with the patient (or with another person with health care decision-making authority) about whether or not to order the scan.
2. Otherwise, scan everybody.

References

1. Livingston DH, Lavery RF, Passannante MR, Skurnick JH, Baker S, Fabian TC, et al. Emergency department discharge of patients with a negative cranial computed tomography scan after minimal head injury. *Ann Surg* 2000; 232: 126–132.
2. Haydel MJ, Preston CA, Mills TJ, Luber S, Blaudeau E, Deblieux PM. Indications for computed tomography in patients with minor head injury. *N Engl J Med* 2000; 343: 100–105.

3. Malick T, Milius J, Fink HJ. Dirty Harry: Screenplay. Hollywood, CA: Script City, 1970.

4. U.S. Food and Drug Administration. FDA authorizes marketing of first blood test to aid in the evaluation of concussion in adults. July 14, 2018. Available at: www.fda.gov/NewsEvents/Newsroom/PressAnnouncements/ucm596531.htm.

5. Kaplan S, Belson K. Concussions can be detected with new blood test approved by F.D.A. July 14, 2018. Available at: www.nytimes.com/2018/02/14/health/concussion-fda-bloodtest.html.

6. Stiell IG, Wells GA, Vandemheen K, Clement C, Lesiuk H, Laupacis A, et al. The Canadian CT head rule for patients with minor head injury. Lancet 2001; 357: 1391–1396.

7. Poon WS, Rehman SU, Poon CY, Li AK. Traumatic extradural hematoma of delayed onset is not a rarity. Neurosurgery 1992; 30: 681–686.

8. Dacey RG, Jr., Alves WM, Rimel RW, Winn HR, Jane JA. Neurosurgical complications after apparently minor head injury. Assessment of risk in a series of 610 patients. J Neurosurg 1986; 65: 203–210.

9. Livingston DH, Loder PA, Koziol J, Hunt CD. The use of CT scanning to triage patients requiring admission following minimal head injury. J Trauma 1991; 31: 483–487; discussion 487–489.

10. Mohanty SK, Thompson W, Rakower S. Are CT scans for head injury patients always necessary? J Trauma 1991; 31: 801–804; discussion 804–805.

11. Yuh EL, Mukherjee P, Lingsma HF, Yue JK, Ferguson AR, Gordon WA, et al. Magnetic resonance imaging improves 3-month outcome prediction in mild traumatic brain injury. Ann Neurol 2013; 73: 224–235.

12. Saboori M, Ahmadi J, Farajzadegan Z. Indications for brain CT scan in patients with minor head injury. Clin Neurol Neurosurg 2007; 109: 399–405.

13. Miller EC, Derlet RW, Kinser D. Minor head trauma: Is computed tomography always necessary? Ann Emerg Med 1996; 27: 290–294.

14. Bazarian JJ, McClung J, Shah MN, Cheng YT, Flesher W, Kraus J. Mild traumatic brain injury in the United States, 1998–2000. Brain Inj 2005; 19: 85–91.

15. Cassidy JD, Carroll LJ, Peloso PM, Borg J, Von Holst H, Holm L, et al. Incidence, risk factors and prevention of mild traumatic brain injury: Results of the WHO Collaborating Centre Task Force on Mild Traumatic Brain Injury. J Rehabil Med 2004; 28–60.

16. Faul M, Xu L, Wald MM, Coronado V. Traumatic brain injury in the United States: Emergency department vists, hospitalizations and deaths 2002–2006. Atlanta, GA: Centers for Disease Control and Prevention, 2010.

17. Feigin VL, Theadom A, Barker-Collo S, Starkey NJ, Mcpherson K, Kahan M, et al. Incidence of traumatic brain injury in New Zealand: A population-based study. Lancet Neurol 2013; 12: 53–64.

18. Langlois JA, Kegler SR, Butler JA, Gotsch KE, Johnson RL, Reichard AA, et al. Traumatic brain injury-related hospital discharges. Results from a 14-state surveillance system, 1997. MMWR Surveill Summ 2003; 52: 1–20.

19. Hanson HR, Pomerantz WJ, Gittelman M. ED utilization trends in sports-related traumatic brain injury. Pediatrics 2013; 132: e859–e864.

20. New Zealand Guidelines roup. Traumatic brain injury: Diagnosis, acute management and rehabilitation. Wellington, NZ: New Zealand Guidelines Group, 2006.

21. Luoto TM, Tenovuo O, Kataja A, Brander A, Ohman J, Iverson GL. Who gets recruited in mild traumatic brain injury research? J Neurotrauma 2013; 30: 11–16.

22. Gentry LR, Godersky JC, Thompson B, Dunn VD. Prospective comparative study of intermediate-field MR and CT in the evaluation of closed head trauma. AJR Am J Roentgenol 1988; 150: 673–682.

23. Lee H, Wintermark M, Gean AD, Ghajar J, Manley GT, Mukherjee P. Focal lesions in acute mild traumatic brain injury and neurocognitive outcome: CT versus 3T MRI. J Neurotrauma 2008; 25: 1049–1056.

24. Mittl RL, Grossman RI, Hiehle JF, Hurst RW, Kauder DR, Gennarelli TA, et al. Prevalence of MR evidence of diffuse axonal injury in patients with mild head injury and normal head CT findings. AJNR Am J Neuroradiol 1994; 15: 1583–1589.

25. Toth A. Magnetic resonance imaging application in the area of mild and acute traumatic brain injury: Implications for diagnostic markers? In: Kobeissy FH, editor. Brain neurotrauma: Molecular, neuropsychological, and rehabilitation aspects. Boca Raton, FL: CRC Press/Taylor & Francis, 2015.

26. Hughes DG, Jackson A, Mason DL, Berry E, Hollis S, Yates DW. Abnormalities on magnetic resonance imaging seen acutely following mild traumatic brain injury: Correlation with neuropsychological tests and delayed recovery. Neuroradiology 2004; 46: 550–558.

27. Park JH, Park SW, Kang SH, Nam TK, Min BK, Hwang SN. Detection of traumatic cerebral microbleeds by susceptibility-weighted image of MRI. J Korean Neurosurg Soc 2009; 46: 365–369.

28. Stein SC, Burnett MG, Glick HA. Indications for CT scanning in mild traumatic brain injury: A cost-effectiveness study. J Trauma 2006; 61: 558–566.

29. Graham ID, Stiell IG, Laupacis A, O'connor AM, Wells GA. Emergency physicians' attitudes toward and use of clinical decision rules for radiography. Acad Emerg Med 1998; 5: 134–140.

30. Miller EC, Holmes JF, Derlet RW. Utilizing clinical factors to reduce head CT scan ordering for minor head trauma patients. J Emerg Med 1997; 15: 453–457.

31. Servadei F, Teasdale G, Merry G, Neurotraumatology Committee of the World Federation of Neurosurgical Societies. Defining acute mild head injury in adults: A proposal based on prognostic factors, diagnosis, and management. J Neurotrauma 2001; 18: 657–664.

32. Mower WR, Hoffman JR, Herbert M, Wolfson AB, Pollack CV, Jr., Zucker MI, et al. Developing a clinical decision instrument to rule out intracranial injuries in patients with minor head trauma: Methodology of the NEXUS II investigation. Ann Emerg Med 2002; 40: 505–514.

33. Jagoda AS, Bazarian JJ, Bruns JJ, Jr., Cantrill SV, Gean AD, Howard PK, et al. Clinical policy: Neuroimaging and decision making in adult mild traumatic brain injury in the acute setting. Ann Emerg Med 2008; 52: 714–748.

34. SIGN. Early management of patients with a head injury: A national clinical guideline. Edinburgh, Scotland: Scottish Intercollegiate Guidelines Network, 2009.

35. ATLS Subcommittee, American College of Surgeons' Committee On Trauma, International ATLS Working Group. Advanced trauma life support (ATLS): the ninth edition. J Trauma Acute Care Surg 2013; 74: 1363–1366.

36. Ingebrigtsen T, Romner B, Kock-Jensen C. Scandinavian guidelines for initial management of minimal, mild, and moderate head injuries. The Scandinavian Neurotrauma Committee. J Trauma 2000; 48: 760–766.

37. Sundstrom T, Wester K, Enger M, Melhuus K, Ingebrigtsen T, Romner B, et al. [Scandinavian guidelines for the acute management of adult patients with minimal, mild, or moderate head injuries.] Tidsskr Nor Laegeforen 2013; 133: E1–E6.

38. Hodgkinson S, Pollit V, Sharpin C, Lecky F, National Institute for Health and Care Excellence (NICE) Guideline Development

Group. Early management of head injury: Summary of updated NICE guidance. *BMJ* 2014; 348: g104.

39. Smits M, Dippel DW, De Haan GG, Dekker HM, Vos PE, Kool DR, et al. External validation of the Canadian CT head rule and the New Orleans criteria for CT scanning in patients with minor head injury. *JAMA* 2005; 294: 1519–1525.

40. Stiell IG, Clement CM, Rowe BH, Schull MJ, Brison R, Cass D, et al. Comparison of the Canadian CT head rule and the New Orleans criteria in patients with minor head injury. *JAMA* 2005; 294: 1511–1518.

41. Jagoda AS, Cantrill SV, Wears RL, Valadka A, Gallagher EJ, Gottesfeld SH, et al. Clinical policy: Neuroimaging and decision making in adult mild traumatic brain injury in the acute setting. *Ann Emerg Med* 2002; 40: 231–249.

42. Barbosa RR, Jawa R, Watters JM, Knight JC, Kerwin AJ, Winston ES, et al. Evaluation and management of mild traumatic brain injury: An Eastern Association for the Surgery of Trauma practice management guideline. *J Trauma Acute Care Surg* 2012; 73: S307–S314.

43. Employment Department of Local Affairs. *Traumatic brain injury: Medical treatment guidelines.* State of Colorado: Division of Workers' Compensation; 2012.

44. Giza CC, Kutcher JS, Ashwal S, Barth J, Getchius TS, Gioia GA, et al. Summary of evidence-based guideline update: Evaluation and management of concussion in sports: Report of the Guideline Development Subcommittee of the American Academy of Neurology. *Neurology* 2013; 80: 2250–2257.

45. Management of Concussion/mTBI Working Group. VA/DoD clinical practice guideline for management of concussion/mild traumatic brain injury. *J Rehabil Res Dev* 2009; 46: CP1–CP68.

46. NSW Ministry of Health. *Adult trauma clinical practice guideline: Initial management of closed head injury in adults,* 2nd edition. North Sydney: NSW Ministry of Health, 2011.

47. McCrory P, Meeuwisse WH, Aubry M, Cantu B, Dvorak J, Echemendia RJ, et al. Consensus statement on concussion in sport: The 4th International Conference on Concussion in Sport held in Zurich, November 2012. *Br J Sports Med* 2013; 47: 250–258.

48. Anonymous. Guidelines for concussion/mTBI & persistent symptoms: second edition. 2013. http://onf.org/documents/guidelines-for-concussion-mtbi-persistent-symptoms-second-edition.

49. Unden J, Ingebrigtsen T, Romner B, Scandinavian Neurotrauma Committee. Scandinavian guidelines for initial management of minimal, mild and moderate head injuries in adults: An evidence and consensus-based update. *BMC Med* 2013; 11: 50.

50. Dunning J, Daly JP, Lomas JP, Lecky F, Batchelor J, Mackway-Jones K, et al. Derivation of the children's head injury algorithm for the prediction of important clinical events decision rule for head injury in children. *Arch Dis Child* 2006; 91: 885–891.

51. Harty E, Bellis F. CHALICE head injury rule: An implementation study. *Emerg Med J* 2010; 27: 750–752.

52. National Institute for Health and Care Excellence. Head injury guideline. 2007. www.nice.org.uk/CG56 (accessed 20 Dec 2008).

53. American College of Cardiology Surgeons. *ATLS student course manual: Advanced trauma life support,* 9th edition. Chicago, IL: Advanced Trauma Life Support (ATLS), American College of Cardiology (ACS), 2012.

54. Ibanez J, Arikan F, Pedraza S, Sanchez E, Poca MA, Rodriguez D, et al. Reliability of clinical guidelines in the detection of patients at risk following mild head injury: Results of a prospective study. *J Neurosurg* 2004; 100: 825–834.

55. Papa L, Stiell IG, Clement CM, Pawlowicz A, Wolfram A, Braga C, et al. Performance of the Canadian CT head rule and the New Orleans criteria for predicting any traumatic intracranial injury on computed tomography in a United States level I trauma center. *Acad Emerg Med* 2012; 19: 2–10.

56. Lannsjo M, Backheden M, Johansson U, Af Geijerstam JL, Borg J. Does head CT scan pathology predict outcome after mild traumatic brain injury? *Eur J Neurol* 2013; 20: 124–129.

57. Jacobs B, Beems T, Stulemeijer M, Van Vugt AB, Van Der Vliet TM, Borm GF, et al. Outcome prediction in mild traumatic brain injury: Age and clinical variables are stronger predictors than CT abnormalities. *J Neurotrauma* 2010; 27: 655–668.

58. Albers CE, Von Allmen M, Evangelopoulos DS, Zisakis AK, Zimmermann H, Exadaktylos AK. What is the incidence of intracranial bleeding in patients with mild traumatic brain injury? A retrospective study in 3088 Canadian CT head rule patients. *Biomed Res Int* 2013; 2013: 453978.

59. Fabbri A, Servadei F, Marchesini G, Stein SC, Vandelli A. Observational approach to subjects with mild-to-moderate head injury and initial non-neurosurgical lesions. *J Neurol Neurosurg Psychiatry* 2008; 79: 1180–1185.

60. White CL, Griffith S, Caron JL. Early progression of traumatic cerebral contusions: Characterization and risk factors. *J Trauma* 2009; 67: 508–514; discussion 514–515.

61. Holmes MW, Goodacre S, Stevenson MD, Pandor A, Pickering A. The cost-effectiveness of diagnostic management strategies for adults with minor head injury. *Injury* 2012; 43: 1423–1431.

62. Reinus WR, Wippold FJ, 2nd, Erickson KK. Practical selection criteria for noncontrast cranial computed tomography in patients with head trauma. *Ann Emerg Med* 1993; 22: 1148–1155.

63. Atzema C, Mower WR, Hoffman JR, Holmes JF, Killian AJ, Oman JA, et al. Defining "therapeutically inconsequential" head computed tomographic findings in patients with blunt head trauma. *Ann Emerg Med* 2004; 44: 47–56.

64. Borczuk P. Predictors of intracranial injury in patients with mild head trauma. *Ann Emerg Med* 1995; 25: 731–736.

65. Bouida W, Marghli S, Souissi S, Ksibi H, Methammem M, Haguiga H, et al. Prediction value of the Canadian CT head rule and the New Orleans criteria for positive head CT scan and acute neurosurgical procedures in minor head trauma: A multicenter external validation study. *Ann Emerg Med* 2013; 61: 521–527.

66. Brown AJ, Witham MD, George J. Development of a risk score to guide brain imaging in older patients admitted with falls and confusion. *Br J Radiol* 2011; 84: 756–757.

67. Clement CM, Stiell IG, Schull MJ, Rowe BH, Brison R, Lee JS, et al. Clinical features of head injury patients presenting with a Glasgow Coma Scale score of 15 and who require neurosurgical intervention. *Ann Emerg Med* 2006; 48: 245–251.

68. Culotta VP, Sementilli ME, Gerold K, Watts CC. Clinicopathological heterogeneity in the classification of mild head injury. *Neurosurgery* 1996; 38: 245–250.

69. Fabbri A, Servadei F, Marchesini G, Dente M, Iervese T, Spada M, et al. Clinical performance of NICE recommendations versus NCWFNS proposal in patients with mild head injury. *J Neurotrauma* 2005; 22: 1419–1427.

70. Feuerman T, Wackym PA, Gade GF, Becker DP. Value of skull radiography, head computed tomographic scanning, and admission for observation in cases of minor head injury. *Neurosurgery* 1988; 22: 449–453.

71. Gomez PA, Lobato RD, Ortega JM, De La Cruz J. Mild head injury: Differences in prognosis among patients with a Glasgow Coma Scale score of 13 to 15 and analysis of factors associated with abnormal CT findings. *Br J Neurosurg* 1996; 10: 453–460.

72. Harad FT, Kerstein MD. Inadequacy of bedside clinical indicators in identifying significant intracranial injury in trauma patients. *J Trauma* 1992; 32: 359–361; discussion 361–363.

73. Hsiang JN, Yeung T, Yu AL, Poon WS. High-risk mild head injury. *J Neurosurg* 1997; 87: 234–238.

74. Holmes JF, Baier ME, Derlet RW. Failure of the Miller criteria to predict significant intracranial injury in patients with a Glasgow Coma Scale score of 14 after minor head trauma. *Acad Emerg Med* 1997; 4: 788–792.

75. Jeret JS, Mandell M, Anziska B, Lipitz M, Vilceus AP, Ware JA, et al. Clinical predictors of abnormality disclosed by computed tomography after mild head trauma. *Neurosurgery* 1993; 32: 9–15; discussion 15–16.

76. Kavalci C, Aksel G, Salt O, Yilmaz MS, Demir A, Kavalci G, et al. Comparison of the Canadian CT head rule and the New Orleans criteria in patients with minor head injury. *World J Emerg Surg* 2014; 9: 31.

77. Kisat M, Zafar SN, Latif A, Villegas CV, Efron DT, Stevens KA, et al. Predictors of positive head CT scan and neurosurgical procedures after minor head trauma. *J Surg Res* 2012; 173: 31–37.

78. Korley FK, Morton MJ, Hill PM, Mundangepfupfu T, Zhou T, Mohareb AM, et al. Agreement between routine emergency department care and clinical decision support recommended care in patients evaluated for mild traumatic brain injury. *Acad Emerg Med* 2013; 20: 463–469.

79. Ro YS, Shin SD, Holmes JF, Song KJ, Park JO, Cho JS, et al. Comparison of clinical performance of cranial computed tomography rules in patients with minor head injury: A multicenter prospective study. *Acad Emerg Med* 2011; 18: 597–604.

80. Rosengren D, Rothwell S, Brown AF, Chu K. The application of North American CT scan criteria to an Australian population with minor head injury. *Emerg Med Australas* 2004; 16: 195–200.

81. Saadat S, Ghodsi SM, Naieni KH, Firouznia K, Hosseini M, Kadkhodaie HR, et al. Prediction of intracranial computed tomography findings in patients with minor head injury by using logistic regression. *J Neurosurg* 2009; 111: 688–694.

82. Shackford SR, Wald SL, Ross SE, Cogbill TH, Hoyt DB, Morris JA, et al. The clinical utility of computed tomographic scanning and neurologic examination in the management of patients with minor head injuries. *J Trauma* 1992; 33: 385–394.

83. Sharif-Alhoseini M, Khodadadi H, Chardoli M, Rahimi-Movaghar V. Indications for brain computed tomography scan after minor head injury. *J Emerg Trauma Shock* 2011; 4: 472–476.

84. Smits M, Dippel DW, Steyerberg EW, De Haan GG, Dekker HM, Vos PE, et al. Predicting intracranial traumatic findings on computed tomography in patients with minor head injury: The CHIP prediction rule. *Ann Intern Med* 2007; 146: 397–405.

85. Stein SC, Ross SE. The value of computed tomographic scans in patients with low-risk head injuries. *Neurosurgery* 1990; 26: 638–640.

86. Stein SC, Ross SE. Moderate head injury: A guide to initial management. *J Neurosurg* 1992; 77: 562–564.

87. Stein SC, Fabbri A, Servadei F, Glick HA. A critical comparison of clinical decision instruments for computed tomographic scanning in mild closed traumatic brain injury in adolescents and adults. *Ann Emerg Med* 2009; 53: 180–188.

88. Turedi S, Hasanbasoglu A, Gunduz A, Yandi M. Clinical decision instruments for CT scan in minor head trauma. *J Emerg Med* 2008; 34: 253–259.

89. Uchino Y, Okimura Y, Tanaka M, Saeki N, Yamaura A. Computed tomography and magnetic resonance imaging of mild head injury – Is it appropriate to classify patients with Glasgow Coma Scale score of 13 to 15 as "mild injury"? *Acta Neurochir (Wien)* 2001; 143: 1031–1037.

90. Vilke GM, Chan TC, Guss DA. Use of a complete neurological examination to screen for significant intracranial abnormalities in minor head injury. *Am J Emerg Med* 2000; 18: 159–163.

91. Nagy KK, Joseph KT, Krosner SM, Roberts RR, Leslie CL, Dufty K, et al. The utility of head computed tomography after minimal head injury. *J Trauma* 1999; 46: 268–270.

92. Murshid WR. Management of minor head injuries: Admission criteria, radiological evaluation and treatment of complications. *Acta Neurochir (Wien)* 1998; 140: 56–64.

93. Pandor A, Goodacre S, Harnan S, Holmes M, Pickering A, Fitzgerald P, et al. Diagnostic management strategies for adults and children with minor head injury: A systematic review and an economic evaluation. *Health Technol Assess* 2011; 15 (27):1–202.

94. Stiell IG, Clement CM, Grimshaw JM, Brison RJ, Rowe BH, Lee JS, et al. A prospective cluster-randomized trial to implement the Canadian CT head rule in emergency departments. *CMAJ* 2010; 182: 1527–1532.

95. Reynolds TA. A Tunisian, a Canadian, and an American walk into a bar (sustaining mild head injury). *Ann Emerg Med* 2013; 61: 528–529.

96. Haydel MJ. Clinical decision instruments for CT scanning in minor head injury. *JAMA* 2005; 294: 1551–1553.

97. Harnan SE, Pickering A, Pandor A, Goodacre SW. Clinical decision rules for adults with minor head injury: A systematic review. *J Trauma* 2011; 71: 245–251.

98. Eng J, Chanmugam A. Examining the role of cranial CT in the evaluation of patients with minor head injury: A systematic review. *Neuroimaging Clin N Am* 2003; 13: 273–282.

99. Munoz-Sanchez MA, Murillo-Cabezas F, Cayuela-Dominguez A, Rincon-Ferrari MD, Amaya-Villar R, Leon-Carrion J. Skull fracture, with or without clinical signs, in mTBI is an independent risk marker for neurosurgically relevant intracranial lesion: A cohort study. *Brain Inj* 2009; 23: 39–44.

100. Andronikou S, Kilborn T, Patel M, Fieggen AG. Skull fracture as a herald of intracranial abnormality in children with mild head injury: Is there a role for skull radiographs? *Australas Radiol* 2003; 47: 381–385.

101. Goh KY, Ahuja A, Walkden SB, Poon WS. Is routine computed tomographic (CT) scanning necessary in suspected basal skull fractures? *Injury* 1997; 28: 353–357.

102. Palchak MJ, Holmes JF, Vance CW, Gelber RE, Schauer BA, Harrison MJ, et al. A decision rule for identifying children at low risk for brain injuries after blunt head trauma. *Ann Emerg Med* 2003; 42: 492–506.

103. Heskestad B, Baardsen R, Helseth E, Ingebrigtsen T. Guideline compliance in management of minimal, mild, and moderate head injury: High frequency of noncompliance among individual physicians despite strong guideline support from clinical leaders. *J Trauma Acute Care Surg* 2008; 65: 1309–1313.

104. Rohacek M, Albrecht M, Kleim B, Zimmermann H, Exadaktylos A. Reasons for ordering computed tomography scans of the head in patients with minor brain injury. *Injury* 2012; 43: 1415–1418.

105. Muller K, Waterloo K, Romner B, Wester K, Ingebrigtsen T, Scandinavian Neurotrauma Committee. Mild head injuries: Impact of a national strategy for implementation of management guidelines. *J Trauma* 2003; 55: 1029–1034.

106. Eagles D, Stiell IG, Clement CM, Brehaut J, Taljaard M, Kelly AM, et al. International survey of emergency physicians' awareness and use of the Canadian cervical-spine rule and the Canadian computed tomography head rule. *Acad Emerg Med* 2008; 15: 1256–1261.

107. Melnick ER, Szlezak CM, Bentley SK, Dziura JD, Kotlyar S, Post LA. CT overuse for mild traumatic brain injury. *Jt Comm J Qual Patient Saf* 2012; 38: 483–489.

108. Strand IH, Solheim O, Moen KG, Vik A. Evaluation of the Scandinavian guidelines for head injuries based on a consecutive series with computed tomography from a Norwegian university hospital. *Scand J Trauma Resusc Emerg Med* 2012; 20: 62.

109. Huang X, Zhou JC, Pan KH, Zhao HC. Awareness and use of the Canadian computed tomography head rule for mild head injury patients among Chinese emergency physicians. *Pak J Med Sci* 2013; 29: 951–956.

110. Jones LA, Morley EJ, Grant WD, Wojcik SM, Paolo WF. Adherence to head computed tomography guidelines for mild traumatic brain injury. *West J Emerg Med* 2014; 15: 459–464.

111. Gupta A, Ip IK, Raja AS, Andruchow JE, Sodickson A, Khorasani R. Effect of clinical decision support on documented guideline adherence for head CT in emergency department patients with mild traumatic brain injury. *J Am Med Inform Assoc* 2014; 21: e347–e351.

112. Msaouel P, Kappos T, Tasoulis A, Apostolopoulos AP, Lekkas I, Tripodaki ES, et al. Assessment of cognitive biases and bio-statistics knowledge of medical residents: A multicenter, cross-sectional questionnaire study. *Med Educ Online* 2014; 19: 23646.

113. Poses RM, Cebul RD, Wigton RS. You can lead a horse to water – Improving physicians' knowledge of probabilities may not affect their decisions. *Med Decis Making* 1995; 15: 65–75.

114. Ballard DW, Rauchwerger AS, Reed ME, Vinson DR, Mark DG, Offerman SR, et al. Emergency physicians' knowledge and attitudes of clinical decision support in the electronic health record: A survey-based study. *Acad Emerg Med* 2013; 20: 352–360.

115. Brown R, Furyk J. Racial disparities in health care-emergency department management of minor head injury. *Int J Emerg Med* 2009; 2: 161–166.

116. Ingebrigtsen T, Romner B. Management of minor head injuries in hospitals in Norway. *Acta Neurol Scand* 1997; 95: 51–55.

117. Pines JM, Hollander JE, Isserman JA, Chen EH, Dean AJ, Shofer FS, et al. The association between physician risk tolerance and imaging use in abdominal pain. *Am J Emerg Med* 2009; 27: 552–557.

118. Diner BM, Carpenter CR, O'Connell T, Pang P, Brown MD, Seupaul RA, et al. Graduate medical education and knowledge translation: Role models, information pipelines, and practice change thresholds. *Acad Emerg Med* 2007; 14: 1008–1014.

119. Morton MJ, Korley FK. Head computed tomography use in the emergency department for mild traumatic brain injury: Integrating evidence into practice for the resident physician. *Ann Emerg Med* 2012; 60: 361–367.

120. Glasziou P, Haynes B. The paths from research to improved health outcomes. *ACP J Club* 2005; 142: A8–A10.

121. Af Geijerstam JL, Britton M. Mild head injury: Reliability of early computed tomographic findings in triage for admission. *Emerg Med J* 2005; 22: 103–107.

122. Shiwen C, Chen X, Lutao Y, Hengli T, Heli C, Yan G. Fatal deterioration of delayed acute subdural hematoma after mild traumatic brain injury: Two cases with brief review. *Chin J Traumatol* 2014; 17: 115–117.

123. Brenner DJ, Hall EJ. Cancer risks from CT scans: Now we have data, what next? *Radiology* 2012; 265: 330–331.

124. Pierce DA, Preston DL. Radiation-related cancer risks at low doses among atomic bomb survivors. *Radiat Res* 2000; 154: 178–186.

125. Preston DL, Ron E, Tokuoka S, Funamoto S, Nishi N, Soda M, et al. Solid cancer incidence in atomic bomb survivors: 1958–1998. *Radiat Res* 2007; 168: 1–64.

126. Cardis E, Vrijheid M, Blettner M, Gilbert E, Hakama M, Hill C, et al. Risk of cancer after low doses of ionising radiation: Retrospective cohort study in 15 countries. *BMJ* 2005; 331: 77.

127. Brix G, Nekolla EA, Borowski M, Nosske D. Radiation risk and protection of patients in clinical SPECT/CT. *Eur J Nucl Med Mol Imaging* 2014; 41 (Suppl 1): S125–S136.

128. Brenner DJ, Elliston CD, Hall EJ, Berdon WE. Estimated risks of radiation-induced fatal cancer from pediatric CT. *AJR Am J Roentgenol* 2001; 176: 289–296.

129. Brenner DJ, Hall EJ. Computed tomography – An increasing source of radiation exposure. *N Engl J Med* 2007; 357: 2277–2284.

130. Committee to Assess Health Risks from Exposure to Low Levels of Ionizing Radiation; Board on Radiation Effects Research; Division on Earth and Life Studies; National Research Council of the National Academies. *Health risks from exposure to low levels of ionizing radiation: BEIR VII phase 2*. Washington, D.C.: National Academies Press, 2006.

131. ICRP. ICRP publication 105. Radiation protection in medicine. *Ann ICRP* 2007; 37: 1–63.

132. United Nations Scientific Committee on the Effects of Atomic Radiation. *Effects of ionizing radiation: 2006 Report to the General Assembly, with scientific annexes*. New York: United Nations Publications, 2008. Available at www.unscear.org/docs/publications/2006/UNSCEAR_2006_GA-Report.pdf.

133. Shah DJ, Sachs RK, Wilson DJ. Radiation-induced cancer: A modern view. *Br J Radiol* 2012; 85: e1166–e1173.

134. Hendee WR, O'Connor MK. Radiation risks of medical imaging: Separating fact from fantasy. *Radiology* 2012; 264: 312–321.

135. Pearce MS, Salotti JA, Little MP, McHugh K, Lee C, Kim KP, et al. Radiation exposure from CT scans in childhood and subsequent risk of leukaemia and brain tumours: A retrospective cohort study. *Lancet* 2012; 380: 499–505.

136. Cohen M. Cancer risks from CT radiation: Is there a dose threshold? *J Am Coll Radiol* 2013; 10: 817–819.

137. Raman SP, Mahesh M, Blasko RV, Fishman EK. CT scan parameters and radiation dose: Practical advice for radiologists. *J Am Coll Radiol* 2013; 10: 840–846.

138. Lambert J, Mackenzie JD, Cody DD, Gould R. Techniques and tactics for optimizing CT dose in adults and children: State of the art and future advances. *J Am Coll Radiol* 2014; 11: 262–266.

139. Ingebrigtsen T, Romner B. Routine early CT-scan is cost saving after minor head injury. *Acta Neurol Scand* 1996; 93: 207–210.

140. Gold MR, Siegel JE, Russel LB, Weinstein. MC. *Cost-effectiveness in health and medicine*. New York: Oxford University Press, 1996.

141. Smits M, Dippel DW, Nederkoorn PJ, Dekker HM, Vos PE, Kool DR, et al. Minor head injury: CT-based strategies for management – A cost-effectiveness analysis. *Radiology* 2010; 254: 532–540.

142. Lee LK, Monroe D, Bachman MC, Glass TF, Mahajan PV, Cooper A, et al. Isolated loss of consciousness in children with minor blunt head trauma. *JAMA Pediatr* 2014; 168: 837–843.

143. Rehmani R, Amanullah S. Analysis of blood tests in the emergency department of a tertiary care hospital. *Postgrad Med J* 1999; 75: 662–666.

144. Koch H, Van Bokhoven MA, Ter Riet G, Van Alphen-Jager JT, Van Der Weijden T, Dinant GJ, et al. Ordering blood tests for patients with unexplained fatigue in general practice: What does it yield? Results of the VAMPIRE trial. *Br J Gen Pract* 2009; 59: e93–e100.

145. Koch H, Van Bokhoven MA, Ter Riet G, Hessels KM, Van Der Weijden T, Dinant GJ, et al. What makes general practitioners order blood tests for patients with unexplained complaints? A cross-sectional study. *Eur J Gen Pract* 2009; 15: 22–28.

146. Schloendorff *v*. The Society of New York Hospital (1914).

147. Ollivier L, Apiou F, Leclere J, Sevellec M, Asselain B, Bredart A, et al. Patient experiences and preferences: Development of practice guidelines in a cancer imaging department. *Cancer Imaging* 2009; 9 (Spec No A): S92–S97.

148. Lind SE, Kopans D, Good MJ. Patients' preferences for learning the results of mammographic examinations. *Breast Cancer Res Treat* 1992; 23: 223–232.

149. Baldwin DM, Quintela J, Duclos C, Staton EW, Pace WD. Patient preferences for notification of normal laboratory test results: A report from the ASIPS Collaborative. *BMC Fam Pract* 2005; 6: 11.

150. Petrie KJ, Muller JT, Schirmbeck F, Donkin L, Broadbent E, Ellis CJ, et al. Effect of providing information about normal test results on patients' reassurance: Randomised controlled trial. *BMJ* 2007; 334: 352.

151. Demaerel P, Béatse E, Roels K, Thijs V. Intermediate short-term outcomes after brain computed tomography and magnetic resonance imaging in neurology outpatients. *Med Decis Making* 2001; 21: 444–450.

152. Fang C, Otero HJ, Greenberg D, Neumann PJ. Cost–utility analyses of diagnostic laboratory tests: A systematic review. *Value Health* 2011; 14: 1010–1018.

153. McDonald IG, Daly J, Jelinek VM, Panetta F, Gutman JM. Opening Pandora's box: The unpredictability of reassurance by a normal test result. *BMJ* 1996; 313: 329–332.

154. Mushlin AI, Mooney C, Holloway RG, Detsky AS, Mattson DH, Phelps CE. The cost-effectiveness of magnetic resonance imaging for patients with equivocal neurological symptoms. *Int J Technol Assess Health Care* 1997; 13: 21–34.

155. Coulter A. Partnerships with patients: The pros and cons of shared clinical decision-making. *J Health Serv Res Policy* 1997; 2: 112–121.

156. Ende J, Kazis L, Ash A, Moskowitz MA. Measuring patients' desire for autonomy: Decision making and information-seeking preferences among medical patients. *J Gen Intern Med* 1989; 4: 23–30.

157. Robinson A, Thomson R. Variability in patient preferences for participating in medical decision making: Implication for the use of decision support tools. *Qual Health Care* 2001; 10 (Suppl 1): i34–i38.

158. Strull WM, Lo B, Charles G. Do patients want to participate in medical decision making? *JAMA* 1984; 252: 2990–2994.

159. Beisecker AE. Aging and the desire for information and input in medical decisions: Patient consumerism in medical encounters. *Gerontologist* 1988; 28: 330–335.

160. Vick S, Scott A. Agency in health care. Examining patients' preferences for attributes of the doctor–patient relationship. *J Health Econ* 1998; 17: 587–605.

161. Coulter A, Peto V, Doll H. Patients' preferences and general practitioners' decisions in the treatment of menstrual disorders. *Fam Pract* 1994; 11: 67–74.

162. Moskop JC. Information disclosure and consent: Patient preferences and provider responsibilities. *Am J Bioeth* 2007; 7: 47–49; discussion W3–W4.

163. Lloyd AJ. The extent of patients' understanding of the risk of treatments. *Qual Health Care* 2001; 10 (Suppl 1): i14–i18.

164. Goske MJ, Bulas D. Improving health literacy: Informed decision-making rather than informed consent for CT scans in children. *Pediatr Radiol* 2009; 39: 901–903.

165. Lee CI, Flaster HV, Haims AH, Monico EP, Forman HP. Diagnostic CT scans: institutional informed consent guidelines and practices at academic medical centers. *AJR Am J Roentgenol* 2006; 187: 282–287.

166. Cascade PN. Resolved: That informed consent be obtained before screening CT. *J Am Coll Radiol* 2004; 1: 82–84.

167. Berlin L. Shared decision-making: Is it time to obtain informed consent before radiologic examinations utilizing ionizing radiation? Legal and ethical implications. *J Am Coll Radiol* 2014; 11: 246–251.

168. Johnson *v.* Kokemoor, Supreme Court of Wisconsin (1996).

169. Phend C. Parents want CT cancer risk info in ED. MedPage Today [Internet]. 2013 July 12, 2013. Available from: www.medpagetoday.com/EmergencyMedicine/EmergencyMedicine/40313.

170. Rodriguez RM, Henderson TM, Ritchie AM, Langdorf MI, Raja AS, Silverman E, et al. Patient preferences and acceptable risk for computed tomography in trauma. *Injury* 2014; 45: 1345–1349.

171. Sulmasy DP. Physicians, cost control, and ethics. *Ann Intern Med* 1992; 116: 920–926.

172. Ladd RE. Patients without choices: The ethics of decision-making in emergency medicine. *J Emerg Med* 1985; 3: 149–156.

173. Cloft HJ, Joseph GJ, Dion JE. Risk of cerebral angiography in patients with subarachnoid hemorrhage, cerebral aneurysm, and arteriovenous malformation: A meta-analysis. *Stroke* 1999; 30: 317–320.

Chapter

16

Structural Neuroimaging of Persistent or Delayed-Onset Encephalopathy Following Repetitive Concussive Brain Injuries

Katherine H. Taber and Robin A. Hurley

Editorial Introduction

As demonstrated in the previous chapters of this volume, no rational nosology is available to classify the varieties of long-term changes in brain and neurobehavior that follow one or many CBIs. As a result, it is difficult to answer the basic question, "Neuroimaging of *what*?" It may be helpful to review the options.

More than 40% of survivors of typical, clinically attended CBIs either complain of (subjective) or exhibit (objective) neurobehavioral disorders (psychiatric, cognitive, or somatic) at one year post injury. One might call that cohort, "survivors of single, typical, clinically attended CBI who have exhibited persistent sequelae, apparently due to that brain injury." The prevalence of ongoing problems in that cohort declines over subsequent years. That alone makes the cohort diverse, since some remain symptomatic for two years, others for 20 years. In addition, a few of those with persistent post-concussive symptoms at one year may become free of symptoms, for instance, at 18 months, only to suffer a recrudescence later in life. (Example: a person who was concussed at age 12, who seemed fine by age 13, but who experienced another cerebral threat at age 18 such as another concussion or an episode of stress, and whose initial symptoms re-emerged.) Thus, one imaging goal might be to scan survivors of single, typical, clinically attended CBIs perhaps two to 60 years post injury. Yet even the cohort simply labeled "survivors of single, typical, clinically attended CBI who have exhibited persistent sequelae, apparently due to that brain injury" is a highly diverse population.

Then there is a cohort one might call, "survivors of single, typical, clinically attended CBI who apparently did *not* exhibit persistent sequelae." Most youth who experienced a single sport-related CBI would probably fit in that class. Many feel fine in a week. That, of course, is no indication that their brains are intact. So, another neuroimaging project might focus on that cohort at perhaps one to 60 years post injury.

Then there is the gigantic population of persons who never reported their CBIs. The prevalence of long-term symptoms in that group is unknown, but probably lower than 40% at one year. Again, the little evidence available suggests that the clinical courses of persons in this cohort are highly variable. One imaging goal might be to scan such a cohort. But the size of that study would be large because – in addition to the need to compare scans with those of a demographically matched control group – one would presumably need to stratify for presence or absence, degree, type, and duration of symptoms.

Then there are persons exposed to more than one CBI – the subject of this chapter.

As discussed in Chapter 11, there exists a spectrum of post-concussive cerebral dysfunction and distress among persons who are assumed to have experienced multiple or "repetitive" CBIs.[1] Authors of studies on this topic seem to be referring to subjects with a history of more than one concussion (sometimes hundreds) that have allegedly occurred in one of an infinite number of possible temporal patterns. "Repetitive concussion," therefore, is neither a specifiable environmental exposure nor a medical entity. Some cases conform to the early-20th-century concept of dementia pugilistica – a disorder described in male boxers at a mean of about 28 years old, most of whom were still busy boxing. Other cases conform to a curious late-20th-century concept of "chronic traumatic encephalopathy," or CTE, another condition suspected of association with many past CBIs. That more contemporary concept of post-many-CBIs encephalopathy has been described in case reports primarily discussing persons in mid to late life who had enjoyed an average of 15 years symptom-free after exposure and before the onset of dementia [1]. Although atypically folded proteins seem to occur in both groups, the degree to which these two cohorts are neurobiologically related is unclear, since virtually all members of the latter group exhibit polypathology. Collectively, one might refer to these two as exhibiting "persistent or delayed-onset encephalopathy following repetitive CBIs."

Now add to that rough dichotomy of clinical presentations and symptom trajectories the fact that "neurobehavioral

---

1   Editor's note: in the North American neurological tradition of cavalier English, the term "repetitive" has been widely adopted without being defined. This makes it difficult to synthesize results from studies that use the term differently. *Repetition* bears a somewhat horological connotation, characterizing events separated by equal time intervals such as the ticking of a clock, or a metronome, or the beeps of an orbiting satellite. Practically no humans experience repetitive concussions in that sense. Yet the time-honored term "multiple" has been largely rejected in the concussion literature. A small but worthy project might be to operationalize a term for "more than one CBI occurring in an infinitely variable temporal pattern."

disorders not otherwise specified" does not specify any clinical condition. Every reader can list a dozen commonly encountered problems in the menu. No one dares claim that there exists a "syndrome." Late effects suspected of being causally related to more than one past CBIs are different in every case.

A third point that mandates extreme caution in reviewing publications in this field: almost no high-quality clinico-pathological correlation research has been done. Several brain banks have collected convenience samples of brains from persons (mostly contact sport athletes and soldiers) alleged to have experienced more than one past CBI. Several detailed pathological case reports have been disseminated. However, it stretches credulity when authors call these *clinico pathological correlation studies*, since the poverty of clinical description is profound.

Consider, for a moment, the clinical descriptions typically provided in a comparable study of multiple sclerosis. One expects to read about family history, fetal exposures, birth trauma, childhood illnesses, perhaps school performance and social life, along with a detailed account of the sequence of symptoms, functional independence levels, imaging findings, cerebrospinal fluid (CSF) findings, and treatment exposures documented over a decade. That is a clinical history. Now read one of the recently published compilations of case reports purporting to be "clinico pathological studies" of "CTE" (e.g., [2]). Even the most well-meaning authors are at a tremendous disadvantage, since prospective observations were rarely made. For instance, a supplied clinical history might read: "linebacker for four years in college and two years in professional football. Surviving niece – who lived in a different city – estimates 'a lot of' concussions, and states, 'He seemed to change.'" Yet one would definitely want to know: "What was the average duration of the seizures he suffered at age 1.5 during his bout of aseptic meningitis? For how many months was he hypomanic after his romantic disaster in high school? What was his working-memory index at six months after his 11th concussion 14 years ago?"

This brief review of the remarkable heterogeneity of late effects after human concussive injury has one purpose: to put the immediately forthcoming chapter in perspective. In view of the above introduction, *neuroimaging of late effects after more than one CBI must not be considered neuroimaging of any one mammalian disorder.*

Structural Neuroimaging of Persistent or Delayed-Onset Encephalopathy Following Repetitive Concussive Brain Injuries

Neuroimaging research of the long-term effects of concussive brain injury (CBI) is in its infancy. At present, the prevalence of persistent post-CBI is unknown and the incidence of late effects (delay post-injury development of deleterious changes in brain and behavior such as neurodegenerative dementias) has yet to be determined. Investigation of this spectrum of neurobehavioral impairments is compromised because no validated in vivo

biomarkers exist for CBI and because the vast majority of concussion survivors live for years or decades after their injuries, such that little neuropathological data is available regarding cases in which injury promptly triggers a life-long encephalopathy. There clearly exists a subset of survivors of one or more CBI that develop a disabling encephalopathy. There are late effects – meaning that after a period of apparent recovery (or at least apparent functionality), perhaps ten to 40 years after exposure to one or more CBIs, neurobehavioral symptoms and signs become overt and disabling [1–6] no single clinical picture or trajectory describes this subset of patients, no subtypes have been validated, and no uniform neuropathological profile has been discovered. Some seem to suffer static encephalopathies that emerge years after injury, plateau, and persist as neurobehavioral impairments. In other cases, functional impairments emerge and inexorably progress in the manner of degenerative dementias. And, in virtually all cases, aging-related brain changes common among people without CBI complicate whatever late effects occur. It is especially clear that a history of multiple "mild traumatic brain injuries" "mTBIs" and/or subconcussive events is an important risk factor [4–6]. Understanding that no unitary entity is implied, one way to refer to these cases collectively is *persistent or delayed-onset encephalopathy following repetitive CBIs* (PDEFrCBI).

Several barriers make investigation of this often conflated congeries of post-concussive encephalopathies challenging. First, no widely accepted clinical criteria have been established to classify or diagnose the spectrum of late effects [1–6]. As a result, definitive diagnosis of such a condition as "post-TBI neurodegeneration" or "CTE" is currently based on neuropathological criteria. The limited available clinico pathological studies of CBI published over the last decade raise a fundamental question: does repetitive CBI primarily serve as a risk factor for conventional neurodegenerative diseases popularly classified as "Alzheimer's disease (AD),"[2] Parkinson's disease (PD), or motor neuron disease, or does CBI trigger atypical conditions that are unique to the post-traumatic state and biologically distinct from those in the conventional catalog (i.e., "CTE")? To add another level of complexity: it is increasingly clear that mixed or combined pathologies are more common than pure instances of classic 20th-century neurodegenerative diseases. In fact, neuropathological studies indicate that co-occurrence of post-concussive change with other neurodegenerative conditions (e.g., AD or vascular disease) is common. Together, these barriers hugely complicate both antemortem diagnosis based on history of trauma and/or clinical symptoms and postmortem diagnosis based on brain cutting [7–10].

How, then, might one apply the robust new armamentarium of neuroimaging technology to this still-to-be-classified potpourri of deleterious post-concussive encephalopathies? Neuropathological studies of PDEFrCBI have identified several structural changes that can either be detected using current clinical neuroimaging methods or have the potential to be detected

---

[2] Editor's note: as explained in Chapter 11, multiple competing concepts and operational definitions have been promoted as identifiers of a variety of ostensibly "neurodegenerative" conditions (which are conceivably better characterized as the expected, if variable, results of the passing of time), all called "Alzheimer's disease." To date, little evidence supports the hypothesis that "Alzheimer's disease" is a distinct and unitary biologically entity.

Companion axial images from a patient illustrate the four types of magnetic resonance imaging (MRI) commonly used for clinical neuroimaging of traumatic brain injury

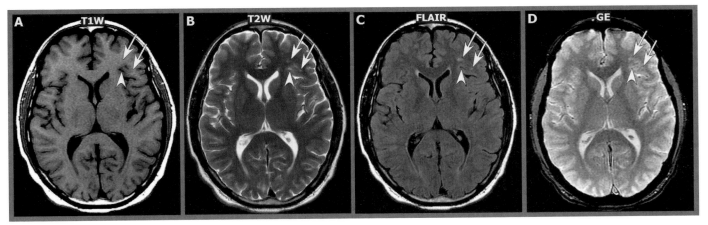

Fig. 16.1 (A) T1-weighted (T1W) MRI provides good delineation of anatomy, but not of most types of pathology. (B) T2-weighted (T2W) MRI is very sensitive to many types of pathology, which can be identified by their high signal intensity compared to surrounding brain. (C) Fluid-attenuated inversion recovery (FLAIR) MRI, a T2W image in which the signal of CSF is nulled, provides much better visualization of pathology in the vicinity of cerebrospinal fluid. (D) Gradient echo (GE) MRI is sensitive to presence of anything that changes the magnetic susceptibility of tissue, and may allow detection of small hemorrhagic lesions that are not visible on T2W or FLAIR MRI. In this set of example images there are multiple areas of diffuse axonal injury. The locations of two are marked with arrows and a nearby cerebrospinal fluid-containing space is marked with an arrowhead. Note that the cerebrospinal fluid-containing space that might be mistaken for an area of diffuse axonal injury in the T2W image (B) is easily distinguished on the FLAIR image (C). [A black and white version of this figure will appear in some formats. For the color version, please refer to the plate section.]

Source: used with permission of the Mid Atlantic Mental Illness Research, Education and Clinical Center

in the near future. Thus, setting aside nosological classification, structural neuroimaging studies of individuals with a history of multiple concussive and/or subconcussive events may be able to detect brain changes that herald the development of PDEFrCBI, even prior to the emergence of overt symptoms. As preventive interventions improve and pre-morbid management of neurodegenerative change becomes routine, non-invasive imaging should help enable early mitigation of disabling late post-concussive brain change. Just as biomarkers are urgently needed to accelerate the understanding of acute and post-acute CBI, biomarkers are also needed to identify persons whose late adulthood is at risk from early concussions. Imaging is likely to serve both vital purposes.

Present

The higher resolution provided by magnetic resonance imaging (MRI) makes it the generally preferred modality for identifying pathologic changes in the brain [11, 12]. There are multiple types of MRI commonly used in clinical neuroimaging that allow visualization of different aspects of tissue structure (Figure 16.1). T1-weighted (T1W) MRI provides the best view of anatomy, but is not particularly sensitive to most types of pathology. T2-weighted (T2W) MRI is very sensitive to many types of pathology, most of which are easily identified by their high signal intensity compared to surrounding brain. CSF also has high signal intensity on T2W MRI, making identification of abnormalities adjacent to CSF-filled spaces difficult. Fluid-attenuated inversion recovery (FLAIR) MRI, a T2W image in which the signal of CSF is nulled, provides much better visualization of pathology in the vicinity of CSF. Gradient echo (GE) MRI is sensitive to the presence of anything that changes the magnetic susceptibility of tissue (e.g., deoxygenated blood,

iron, calcium). Areas of resolved hemorrhage often contain residual hemosiderin, a breakdown product of hemoglobin. GE MRI allows detection of small hemorrhagic lesions that are not visible on T2W or FLAIR MRI [13]. Susceptibility-weighted imaging (SWI), which combines phase and magnitude information into a single image, is even more sensitive than standard GE MRI, especially to microhemorrhages [13–15].

As noted above, at the present time structural neuroimaging studies of individuals with a history of exposure to chronic repetitive concussive/subconcussive events may be the most fruitful source for identifying findings that might indicate early-stage PDEFrCBI. A review of the neuroimaging literature indicated 11 imaging findings that might be biomarkers of chronic repetitive concussive/subconcussive events [16]. These were tested in a retrospective study of clinical MRI (T1W, T2W, FLAIR, GE) obtained from active professional fighters ($n = 100$, boxing and mixed martial arts) [16]. A checklist approach was implemented to facilitate systematic visual assessment. Only seven findings were present in more than 5% of the group. Four involved brain atrophy in some manner: hippocampal atrophy (59%), cerebral atrophy (24%), pituitary gland atrophy (14%), and lateral ventricle enlargement (19%). The remaining three were: cavum septi pellucidi (CSP, 43%), dilated perivascular (Virchow–Robin) spaces (PVS: 32%) that surround penetrating arterioles and venules, and shearing/diffuse axonal injury (DAI: 29%). No DAIs were hemorrhagic (i.e., no evidence of hemosiderin), and almost all were in frontal cortex (89/94). The dilated PVS, in contrast, were in parietal cortex. Weaknesses of this study were its cross-sectional nature and the absence of comparison to other groups. Although a new prospective longitudinal study of professional fighters (boxers, mixed martial arts) has been designed to avoid some of these methodological limitations, the initial publications have focused on other aspects of the baseline data [17, 18].

Two smaller prospective studies of boxers included comparison to control groups. A study comparing amateur boxers ($n = 21$) to healthy controls ($n = 21$) reported a significantly higher incidence of CSP (57%) and dilated PVS (90%) in the boxers, but not of cerebral atrophy or ventricular dilation [19]. This study reported that microhemorrhages were identified in two boxers by SWI that were not visible on conventional GE imaging. A study comparing professional boxers ($n = 164$) to healthy controls ($n = 43$) reported similar prevalence of CSP (49% versus 40%), with a trend toward larger CSP in boxers [20]. In addition, serial imaging demonstrated new-onset CSP in eight boxers, and increased size in three.

Another study compared neuroimaging of retired professional football players with a remote history of at least one concussion with and without cognitive impairment and/or depression to matched (age, education, IQ) healthy controls [21]. The cognitively impaired retired players ($n = 10$) had a significantly greater volume of white-matter lesions on FLAIR imaging than their matched controls ($n = 20$), but were not significantly different from unimpaired retired players ($n = 12$). Microhemorrhages were present on SWI in three retired players and three healthy controls, none in the vicinity of the FLAIR lesions [21]. A small study compared neuroimaging and functional measures between former (time elapsed > two decades) college athletes (ice hockey, football) with ($n = 15$) and without ($n = 15$) a history of at least one sports-related concussion [22]. Subjects were screened for a wide range of potentially confounding conditions (no history of alcohol or substance misuse, no medical condition requiring daily medication, no history of psychiatric or neurological conditions, no TBI unrelated to college sports, regular physical activity). Ventricular volume was significantly greater and multiple areas of cortex were thinner in the group with a remote history of concussion [22].

In summary, several gross neuropathological findings that are commonly reported in cases considered to fall within the spectrum of persistent or progressive post-concussive encephalopathy (PPPCE) can be identified by clinical MRI in groups with a history of repetitive head trauma. The most common findings were presence of CSP and evidence of some type of brain atrophy. A commonly used visual rating scale for CSP (Figure 16.2) categorizes the degree of separation between the septa pellucida [16, 23, 24]. Although quantitative volumetric measurements are preferred in research studies, these are not easily implemented in clinical practice, whereas linear measurements and visual rating scales can be both quick and reliable [25, 26]. While not validated for the study of PPPCE, studies in other neurodegenerative conditions (e.g., "AD," mild cognitive impairment, multiple sclerosis, amyotrophic lateral sclerosis (ALS), frontotemporal dementia) indicate that these approaches can provide valid measures of brain atrophy.

Linear measures of lateral ventricle expansion (Figure 16.3A–C) have been utilized successfully in longitudinal studies of patients with multiple sclerosis [27, 28]. Several visual rating scales have been developed to capture atrophy in the hippocampal region. A simple approach is based on the size of

the temporal horn adjacent to the hippocampus (Figure 16.3D–H) [16]. A more complex visual rating system of medial temporal atrophy that also incorporates assessment of the adjacent cortical regions has been validated as a biomarker for differentiating AD and mild cognitive impairment [29–31]. Recent studies demonstrating the development of visual atrophy rating scales tailored to specific degenerative conditions, such as differentiating ALS from frontotemporal dementia, indicate the strength and flexibility of this approach [32, 33].

It is important to bear in mind that the current resolution of clinical neuroimaging limits sensitivity to several neuropathological findings that are frequently caused by mTBI and so may be associated with PDEFrCBI. For example, DAI commonly involves only a small portion of the axons in an affected area, making it unlikely to increase the signal intensity of an imaging voxel (usually at least a 1-mm cube) sufficiently to be clearly recognized (Figure 16.4). In order to be identified by visual inspection, areas of DAI must be large enough to affect the signal intensity of several contiguous voxels. Another relatively common occurrence is microvascular injury, which may result in small areas of hemorrhage (i.e., microbleed, petechial hemorrhage) with or without associated DAI. Like DAI, such areas will be visible only if occupying sufficient tissue volume to clearly alter the signal intensity of several voxels.

Near Future

Newer methods of MRI show promise for improving identification of small areas of brain injury as they are sensitive to different aspects of tissue microstructure [11, 12, 34]. The one that has been studied the most is diffusion tensor imaging (DTI), which provides metrics of the direction and speed of water diffusion within each voxel. A measure of the average directionality of water diffusion is provided by fractional anisotropy (FA). In gray matter the speed of diffusion is similar in all directions, so gray-matter areas have low FA. In white-matter presence of multiple microstructural barriers (e.g., myelin, axon cell membranes) makes diffusion faster parallel to the major direction of the fibers, so white matter has high FA. A voxel will have the highest FA in areas in which myelinated axons are tightly packed and parallel (coherent). Any loss of structural integrity is expected to reduce FA, although the nature of the change (e.g., shearing injury, demyelination) cannot be determined. A growing number of studies have reported the presence of multiple small areas of reduced FA in the chronic stage (> three months post injury) of TBI [35–37]. Of most relevance to PDEFrCBI are studies of repetitive brain injury in sports. Altered DTI metrics have been associated with higher number of headings in soccer, and with subconcussive events in young athletes (high school, college) participating in contact sports (soccer, hockey, football) [38–41]. An analysis of the baseline imaging from participants in the Professional Fighters' Brain Health Study with no abnormalities on clinical MRI ($n = 155$) found that the number of prior knockouts in boxers predicted presence of altered DTI metrics in multiple brain regions [42].

A variant on DTI is diffusion kurtosis imaging (DKI), which shows promise as a complementary technique as it appears

Cavum septi pellucidi may be biomarkers of chronic repetitive concussive/subconcussive events

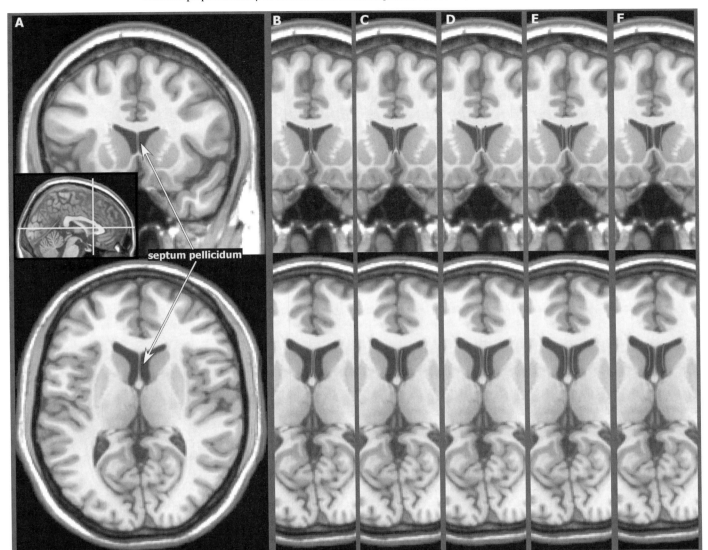

Fig. 16.2 The two bodies of the lateral ventricle are separated by a paired set of clear (pellucid) membranes, the septa pellucida [23]. (A) In most individuals the two membranes fuse during development to form the septum pellucidum. A separation between the two septa pellucida (red lines) forms the cavum (cavity) septi pellucidi. A simple visual grading system categorizes cavum septi pellucidi as: (B) absent, (C) questionable, (D) mild, (E) moderate, or (F) severe [16, 24]. [A black and white version of this figure will appear in some formats. For the color version, please refer to the plate section.]

Source: used with permission of the Mid Atlantic Mental Illness Research, Education and Clinical Center

to be more sensitive than DTI to some types of microstructural changes, including reactive gliosis [34, 43, 44]. Although diffusion-based MRI methods are very promising in research studies, further development and standardization of both acquisition and analysis protocols are required for clinical translation [45–47]. Research studies rely on group-based comparisons that are difficult to adapt for clinical assessment of individual patients. For DTI and DKI to become clinically useful techniques, they must be validated for use on an individual basis [12].

On the Horizon

Current clinical neuroimaging is insensitive to several neuropathological findings that are associated with

PDEFrCBI, such as presence of diffuse neurofibrillary tangles, deposition of abnormal proteins (e.g., tau, amyloid beta), and neuronal loss with reduced pigmentation of the substantia nigra and locus coeruleus [8, 9]. There are several types of MRI that may be sensitive to these neuropathological changes [12, 34].

Magnetization transfer (MT) imaging is a way to estimate the fraction of protons that are bound within macromolecules (i.e., bound pool) and thus may provide a way to assess changes in the concentration of relevant macromolecules (e.g., myelin, tau, amyloid beta) [12, 34]. The bound pool is normally invisible on MRI, which gets its signal from protons in the free pool. MT takes advantage of the fact that the protons in the two pools are in fast exchange.

Linear measures of the lateral ventricles have been shown to correlate well with volumetric measures of atrophy in studies of patients with multiple sclerosis [27, 28]

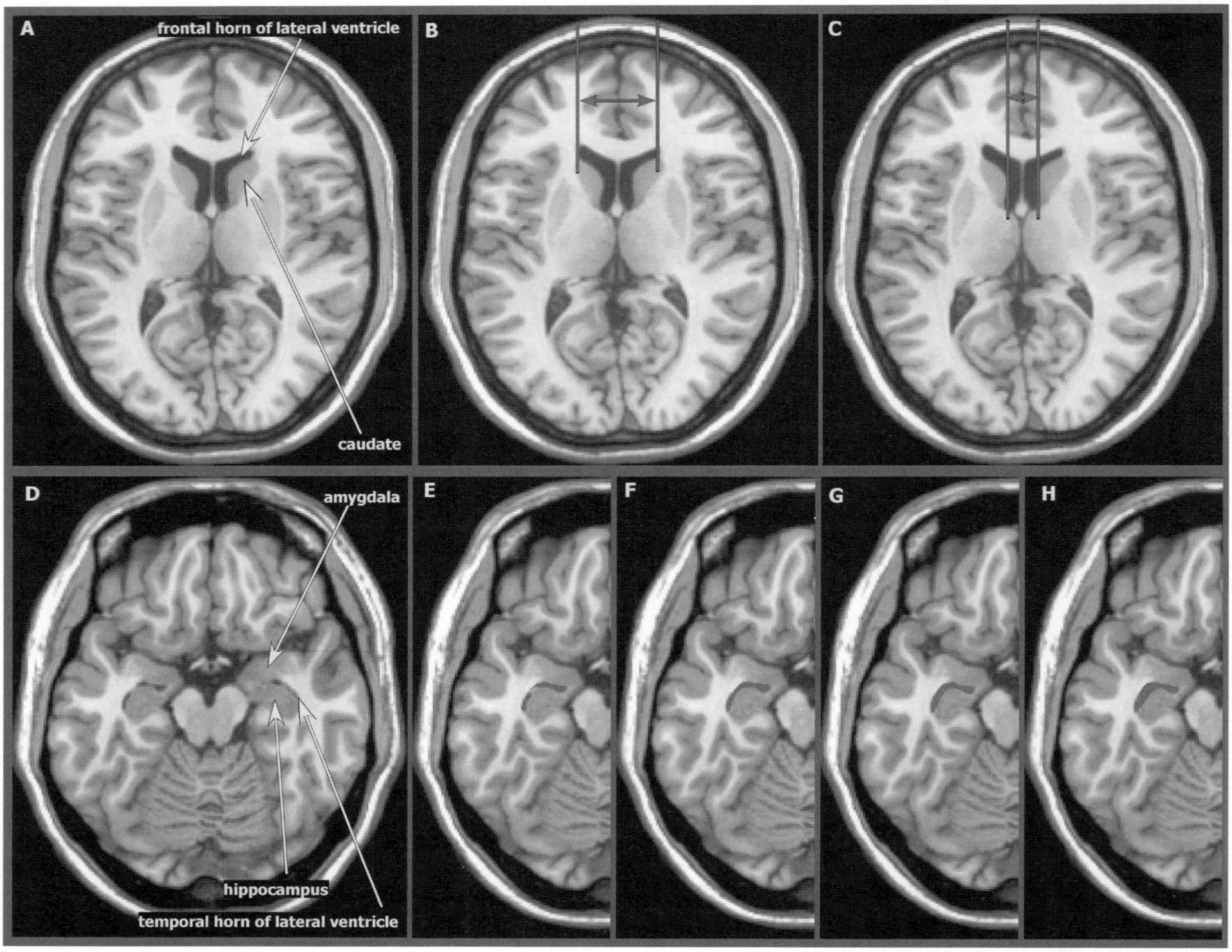

Fig. 16.3 (A) The location of the frontal horns of the lateral ventricle and the adjacent head of caudate is indicated on an axial magnetic resonance imaging (MRI). Both the width of the frontal horns (B, red arrows) and the distance between the caudate heads (C, red arrows) correlated well with volumetric measures. (D) The locations of important structures in the medial temporal lobe are indicated on an axial MRI. A simple visual grading system for assessing medial temporal atrophy categorizes hippocampal atrophy by the size of the temporal horn (red area) adjacent to the hippocampus: (E) absent, (F) mild, (G) moderate, or (H) severe [16]. [A black and white version of this figure will appear in some formats. For the color version, please refer to the plate section.]
Source: used with permission of the Mid Atlantic Mental Illness Research, Education and Clinical Center

A pulse is applied that saturates magnetization of the bound pool protons. As protons exchange between the bound and free pools, the free pool becomes partially saturated, which decreases the observed MRI signal intensity. The simplest metric is to calculate the relative change in intensity between the images acquired without and with the saturation pulse, the MT ratio (MTR).

Multiple studies have reported decreased MTR associated with demyelination and increased MTR associated with re-myelination in conditions such as multiple sclerosis [34, 48]. Decreased MTR in areas of white matter that appeared normal on conventional MRI has been reported in patients with mild TBI who were impaired on neuropsychological testing [49].

Recent studies utilizing animal models of AD have reported increased MTR in areas of abnormal protein deposition (e.g., tau, amyloid beta, amyloid plaques), suggesting that MT imaging may provide a non-invasive method for identifying and perhaps tracking such changes [50, 51]. Although the MTR is relatively easy to measure, it is greatly influenced by multiple factors related to both hardware (e.g., scanner, coils, magnetic field strength) and software (e.g., pulse sequence parameters, saturation pulse parameters), which limits clinical utility [34].

Quantitative MT methods have been developed that improve the stability of the metrics and also increase sensitivity to specific aspects of tissue structure [34, 52]. Two quantitative

Current resolution of magnetic resonance imaging (MRI)

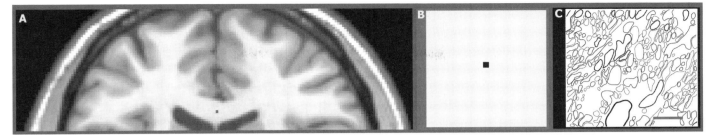

Fig. 16.4 While MRI is the best method currently available for identifying structural changes in the brain, it is important to understand the resolution limitations. Each image is made up of many small cubes (voxels) that are seldom less than 1 mm on a side. (A) A single voxel in the corpus callosum is colored red on MRI. The signal intensity of each voxel is the average of the signals from all the tissue types within the cube. (B) The single voxel in (A) is expanded to illustrate the averaging of signal. Although 1 mm seems like a tiny distance, it is very large compared to the size of cellular structures within the brain. A voxel in a white-matter area such as the corpus callosum will contain many thousands of axons. (C) A small section (black square) of the voxel in B is expanded to show the actual complexity of the tissue (red scale bar = 10 μm). The illustration in (C) is a simplification of an electron microscopy image. In order to be identified by visual inspection, an area of brain injury must be large enough to affect the signal intensity of several contiguous voxels. [A black and white version of this figure will appear in some formats. For the color version, please refer to the plate section.]

Source: used with permission of the Mid Atlantic Mental Illness Research, Education and Clinical Center

MT studies in animal models (multiple sclerosis, myelin mutant *shaking* pup) reported strong correlations between MT metrics and myelin content [53, 54]. A recent study of combat veterans using a quantitative approach (macromolecular proton fraction imaging) reported multiple areas of decreased signal in veterans ($n = 34$) with military blast-related mild TBI (range 1–100 events) compared to veterans ($n = 18$) without a history of TBI [55]. As noted by the authors, further studies are required to determine the neuropathologic changes underlying signal loss. Overall, these studies indicate that MT imaging may be useful for identifying several types of neuropathology that are considered markers of PDEFrCBI as this condition is associated with both focal increases (e.g., deposition of tau) and decreases (e.g., demyelination) in concentration of specific macromolecules.

The reduced pigmentation (pallor) of the substantia nigra and locus coeruleus that has been reported in some cases of PDEFrCBI is due to loss of neuromelanin, which is normally found within neuronal cytoplasm of catecholamine (dopamine, norepinephrine) neurons in these brainstem nuclei [56, 57]. Although long considered an inert byproduct of synthesis of dopamine, studies now suggest important cellular functions [56, 57]. Two groups have demonstrated direct visualization of both substantia nigra and locus coeruleus using multi-slice T1W fast spin echo acquisitions [58–60]. Another approach that has proven successful is use of a three-dimensional GE acquisition with addition of an off-resonance saturation pulse [61–63]. This adds MT contrast that preferentially decreases the signal from tissue that does not contain neuromelanin, increasing the signal to noise for areas that are rich in this substance. Compared to healthy individuals, signal intensity in these brainstem nuclei has been shown to be reduced in patients with neurodegenerative diseases involving these areas (e.g., "AD," PD," dementia with Lewy bodies, multiple system atrophy) [58–60, 63, 64]. Thus, neuromelanin-sensitive MRI may provide a non-invasive method for monitoring changes in these areas.

Conclusion

Although no structural neuroimaging studies of PDEFrCBI are available at this time, studies in TBI and in other neurodegenerative conditions indicate that several types of MRI have considerable potential to contribute to diagnosis and – eventually – clinical management. Most exciting is the possibility that newer modalities may be able to characterize changes in tissue that presently can only be assessed post mortem, such as protein deposition. The actualization of this potential seems likely to facilitate the impending revolution in the treatment of CBI and its long-term sequelae.

References for Editorial Introduction

1. Victoroff J. Traumatic encephalopathy: Review and provisional research diagnostic criteria. *NeuroRehabilitation* 2013;32: 211–224.
2. Mez J, Daneshvar DH, Kiernan PT, Abdolmohammadi B, Alvarez VE, Huber BR et al. Clinicopathological evaluation of chronic traumatic encephalopathy in players of American football. *JAMA* 2017;318(4):360–370.

References for Main Chapter

1. Gardner A, Iverson GL, McCrory P. Chronic traumatic encephalopathy in sport: A systematic review. *Br J Sports Med* 2014;48:84–90.
2. Karantzoulis S, Randolph C. Modern chronic traumatic encephalopathy in retired athletes: What is the evidence? *Neuropsychol Rev* 2013;23:350–360.
3. Mez J, Stern RA, McKee AC. Chronic traumatic encephalopathy: Where are we and where are we going? *Curr Neurol Neurosci Rep* 2013;13:407.
4. Smith DH, Johnson VE, Stewart W. Chronic neuropathologies of single and repetitive TBI: Substrates of dementia? *Nat Rev Neurol* 2013;9:211–221.
5. Turner RC, Lucke-Wold BP, Robson MJ, Omalu BI, Petraglia AL, Bailes JE. Repetitive traumatic brain injury and development of chronic traumatic encephalopathy: A potential role for biomarkers in diagnosis, prognosis, and treatment? *Front Neurol* 2013;3:186.

6. Victoroff J. Traumatic encephalopathy: Review and provisional research diagnostic criteria. *NeuroRehabilitation* 2013;32:211–224.

7. Omula B, Bailes J, Hamilton RL, Kamboh MI, Hammers J, Case M, et al. Emerging histomorphologic phenotypes of chronic traumatic encephalopathy in American athletes. *Neurosurgery* 2011;69:173–183.

8. Hazrati LN, Tartaglia MC, Diamandis P, Davis KD, Green RE, Wennberg R, et al. Absence of chronic traumatic encephalopathy in retired football players with multiple concussions and neurological symptomatology. *Front Hum Neurosci* 2013;7:222.

9. McKee AC, Stein TD, Nowinski CJ, Stern RA, Daneshvar DH, Alvarez VE, et al. The spectrum of disease in chronic traumatic encephalopathy. *Brain* 2013;136:43–64.

10. Tartaglia MC, Hazrati LN, Davis KD, Green REA, Wennberg R, Mikulis D, et al. Chronic traumatic encephalopathy and other neurodegenerative proteinopathies. *Front Hum Neurosci* 2014;8:30.

11. Bigler ED. Neuroimaging biomarkers in mild traumatic brain injury. *Neuropsychol Rev* 2013;23:169–209.

12. Mechtler LL, Shastri KK, Crutchfield KE. Advanced neuroimaging of mild traumatic brain injury. *Neurol Clin* 2014;32:31–58.

13. Geurts BHJ, Andriessen TMJC, Goraj BM, Vos PE. The reliability of magnetic resonance imaging in traumatic brain injury lesion detection. *Brain Inj* 2012;26:1439–1450.

14. Haacke EM, Mittal S, Wu Z, Neelavalli J, Cheng Y-CN. Susceptibility-weighted imaging: Technical aspects and clincal applications, part 1. *Am J Neuroradiol* 2009;30:19–30.

15. Benson RR, Gattu R, Sewick B, Kou Z, Zakariah N, Cavanaugh JM, et al. Detection of hemorrhagic and axonal pathology in mild traumatic brain injury using advanced MRI: Implications for neurorehabilitation. *NeuroRehabilitation* 2012;31:261–279.

16. Orrison WW, Hanson EH, Alamo T, Watson D, Sharma M, Perkins TG, et al. Traumatic brain injury: A review and high-field MRI findings in 100 unarmed combatants using a literature-based checklist approach. *J Neurotrauma* 2009;26:1–13.

17. Bernick C, Banks S, Phillips M, Lowe M, Shin W, Obuchowski N, et al. Professional Fighters Brain Health Study: Rationale and methods. *Am J Epidemiol* 2013;178:280–286.

18. Bernick C, Banks S. What boxing tells us about repetitive head trauma and the brain. *Alzheimer's Res Ther* 2013;5:23.

19. Hasiloglu ZI, Albayram S, Selcuk H, Ceyhan E, Delil S, Arkan B, et al. Cerebral microhemorrhages detected by susceptibility-weighted imaging in amatuer boxers. *Am J Neuroradiol* 2011;32:99–102.

20. Aviv RI, Tomlinson G, Kendall B, Thakkar C, Valentine A. Cavum septi pellucidi in boxers. *Can Assoc Radiol J* 2010;61:29–32.

21. Hart JJ, Kraut MA, Womack KB, Strain J, Didehbani N, Bartz E, et al. Neuroimaging of cognitive dysfunction and depression in aging retired National Football League players. *JAMA Neurol* 2013;70:326–335.

22. Tremblay S, De Beaumont L, Henry LC, Boulanger Y, Evans AC, Bourgouin P, et al. Sports concussions and aging: A neuroimaging investigation. *Cereb Cortex* 2013;23:1159–1166.

23. Winter T, Toscano MM. Proper latin terminology for the cavum septi pellucidi. *Am J Roentgenol* 2011;197:W1170.

24. Silk T, Beare R, Crossley L, Rogers K, Emsell L, Catroppa C, et al. Cavum septum pellucidum in pediatric traumatic brain injury. *Psychiatry Res* 2013;213:186–192.

25. Zhang Y, Londos E, Minthon L, Wattmo C, Liu H, Aspelin P, et al. Usefulness of computed tomography linear measurements in diagnosing Alzheimer's disease. *Acta Radiol* 2008;49:91–97.

26. Hampstead BM, Brown GS. Using neuroimaging to inform clincal practice for the diagnosis and treatment of mild cognitive impairment. *Clin Geriatr Med* 2013;29:829–845.

27. Butzkueven H, Kolbe SC, Jolley DJ, Brown JY, Cook MJ, van der Mei IA, et al. Validation of linear cerebral atrophy markers in multiple sclerosis. *J Clin Neurosci* 2008;15:130–137.

28. Martola J, Bergstrom J, Fredrikson S, Stawiarz L, Hillert J, Zhang Y, et al. A longitudinal observational study of brain atrophy rate reflecting four decades of multiple sclerosis: A comparison of serial 1D, 2D, and volumetric measurements from MRI images. *Neuroradiology* 2010;52:109–117.

29. Urs R, Potter E, Barker W, Appel J, Loewenstein DA, Zhao W, et al. Visual rating system for assessing magnetic resonance images: A tool in the diagnosis of mild cognitive impairment and Alzheimer disease. *J Comput Assist Tomogr* 2009;33:73–78.

30. Becker JT, Duara R, Lee CW, Teverovsky L, Snitz BE, Chang CC, et al. Cross-validation of brain structural biomarkers and cognitive aging in a community-based study. *Int Psychogeriatr* 2012;24:1065–1075.

31. Duara R, Loewenstein DA, Shen Q, Barker W, Varon D, Greig MT, et al. The utility of age-specific cut-offs for visual rating of medial temporal atrophy in classifying Alzheimer's disease, MCI and cognitively normal elderly subjects. *Front Aging Neurosci* 2013;5:47.

32. Ambikairajah A, Devenney E, Flanagan E, Yew B, Moishi E, Kiernan MC, et al. A visual MRI atrophy reating scale for the amyotrophic lateral sclerosis-frontotemporal dementia continuum. *Amyotroph Lateral Scler Frontotemporal Degener* 2014;15(3–4):226–234.

33. Moller C, van der Flier WM, Versteeg A, Benedictus MR, Wattjes MP, Koedam ELGM, et al. Quantitative regional validation of the visual rating scale for posterior cortical atrophy. *Eur Radiol* 2014;24:397–404.

34. Alexander AL, Hurley SA, Samsonov AA, Adluru N, Hosseinbor AP, Mossahebi P, et al. Characterization of cerebral white matter properties using quantitative magnetic resonance imaging stains. *Brain Connect* 2011;1:423–446.

35. Aoki Y, Inokuchi R, Gunshin M, Yahagi N, Suwa H. Diffusion tensor imaging studies of mild traumatic brain injury: A meta-analysis. *J Neurol Neurosurg Psychiatry* 2012;83:870–876.

36. Hulkower MB, Poliak DB, Rosenbaum SB, Zimmerman ME, Lipton ML. A decade of DTI in traumatic brain injury: 10 years and 100 articles later. *Am J Neuroradiol* 2013;34:2064–2074.

37. Xiong KL, Zhu YS, Zhang WG. Diffusion tensor imaging and magnetic resonance spectroscopy in traumatic brain injury: A review of recent literature. *Brain Imaging Behav* 2014;8(4):487–496.

38. Bazarian JJ, Zhu T, Blyth B, Borrino A, Zhong J. Subject-specific changes in brain white matter on diffusion tensor imaging after sports-related concussion. *Magn Reson Imaging* 2012;30:171–180.

39. Koerte IK, Kaufmann D, Hartl E, Bouix S, Pasternak O, Kubicki M, et al. A prospective study of physician-observed concussion during a varsity university hockey season: White matter integrity in ice hockey players. Part 3 of 4. *Neurosurg Focus* 2012;33:E3.

40. Koerte IK, Ertl-Wagner B, Reiser M, Zafonte R, Shenton ME. White matter integrity in the brains of professional soccer players without a symptomatic concussion. *JAMA* 2012;308:1859–1861.

41. Lipton ML, Kim N, Zimmerman ME, Kim M, Stewart WF, Branch CA, et al. Soccer heading is associated with white matter microstructural and cognitive abnormalities. *Radiology* 2013;268:850–857.

42. Shin W, Mahmoud SY, Sakaie K, Banks SJ, Lowe MJ, Phillips M, et al. Diffusion measures indicate fight exposure-related damage to cerebral white matter in boxers and mixed martial arts fighters. *Am J Neuroradiol* 2014;35:285–290.

43. Grossman EJ, Ge Y, Jensen JH, Babb JS, Miles L, Reaume J, et al. Thalamus and cognitive impairment in mild traumatic brain injury: A diffusional kurtosis imaging study. *J Neurotrauma* 2012;29:2318–2327.

44. Hori M, Fukunaga I, Masutani Y, Taoka T, Kamagata K, Suzuki Y, et al. Visualizing non-gaussian diffusion: Clinical application of q-space imaging and diffusional kurtosis imaging of the brain and spine. *Magn Reson Med Sci* 2012;11:221–233.

45. Duhaime AC, Gean AD, Haacke EM, Hicks R, Wintermark M, Mukherjee P, et al. Common data elements in radiologic imaging of traumatic brain imaging. *Arch Phys Med Rehabil* 2010;91:1661–1666.

46. Haacke EM, Duhaime AC, Gean AD, Riedy G, Wintermark M, Mukherjee P, et al. Common data elements in radiologic imaging of traumatic brain injury. *J Magn Reson Imaging* 2010;32:516–543.

47. Maas AIR, Harrison-Felix CL, Menon D, Adelson PD, Balkin T, Bullock R, et al. Standardizing data collection in traumatic brain injury. *J Neurotrauma* 2011;28:177–187.

48. Brown RA, Narayanan S, Arnold DL. Segmentation of magnetization transfer ratio lesions for longitudinal analysis of demyelination and remyelination in multiple sclerosis. *NeuroImage* 2013;66:103–109.

49. McGowan JC, Yang JH, Plotkin RC, Grossman RI, Umile EM, Cecil KM, et al. Magnetization transfer imaging in the detection of injury associated with mild head trauma. *Am J Neuroradiol* 2000;21:875–880.

50. Perez-Torres CJ, Reynolds JO, Pautler RG. Use of magnetization transfer contrast MRI to detect early molecular pathology in Alzheimer's disease. *Magn Reson Med* 2014;71:333–338.

51. Bigot C, Vanhoutte G, Verhoye M, Van Der Linden A. Magnetization transfer contract imaging reveals amyloid pathology in Alzheimer's disease transgenic mice. *NeuroImage* 2014;87:111–119.

52. Garcia M, Gloor M, Radue EW, Stippich C, Wetzel SG, Scheffler K, et al. Fast high-resolution brain imaging with balanced SSFP: Interpretation of quantitative magnetization transfer toward simple MTR. *NeuroImage* 2012;59:202–211.

53. Samsonov A, Alexander AL, Mossahebi P, Wu YC, Duncan ID, Field AS. Quantitative MR imaging of two-pool magnetization transfer model parameters in myelin mutant shaking pup. *NeuroImage* 2012;62:1390–1398.

54. Janve VA, Zu Z, Yao SY, Li K, Zhang FL, Wilson KJ, et al. The radial diffusivity and magnetization transfer pool size ratio are sensitive markers for demyelination in a rat model of type III multiple sclerosis (MS) lesions. *NeuroImage* 2013;74:298–305.

55. Petrie EC, Cross DJ, Yarnykh VL, Richards T, Martin NM, Pagulayan K, et al. Neuroimaging, behavioral, and psychological sequelae of repetitive combined blast/impact mild traumatic brain injury in Iraq and Afghanistan war veterans. *J Neurotrauma* 2014;31:425–436.

56. Double KL, Dedov VN, Fedorow H, Kettle E, Halliday GM, Garner B, et al. The comparative biology of neuromelanin and lipofuscin in the human brain. *Cell Mol Life Sci* 2008;65:1669–1682.

57. Double KL. Neuronal vulnerability in Parkinson's disease. *Parkinsonism Relat Disord* 2012;18:s52–s54.

58. Sasaki M, Shibata E, Tohyama K, Takahashi J, Otsuka K, Tsuchiya S, et al. Neuromelanin magnetic resonance imaging of locus ceruleus and substantia nigra in Parkinson's disease. *Neuroreport* 2006;17:1215–1218.

59. Matsuura K, Maeda M, Yata K, Ichiba Y, Yamaguchi T, Kanamaru K, et al. Neuromelanin magnetic resonance imaging in Parkinson's disease and multiple system atrophy. *Eur Neurol* 2013;70:70–77.

60. Ohtsuka C, Sasaki M, Konno K, Koide M, Kato K, Takahashi J, et al. Changes in substantia migra and locus coeruleus in patients with early-stage Parkinson's disease using neuromelanin-sensitive MR imaging. *Neurosci Lett* 2013;541:93–98.

61. Nakane T, Nihashi T, Kawai H, Naganawa S. Visualization of neuromelanin in the substantia nigra and locus ceruleus at 1.5T using a 3D-gradient echo sequence with magnetization transfer contrast. *Magn Reson Med Sci* 2008;7:205–210.

62. Ogisu K, Kudo K, Sasaki M, Sakushima K, Yabe I, Sasaki H, et al. 3D neuromelanin-sensitive magnetic resonance imaging with semi-automated volume measurement of the substantia nigra pars compacta for diagnosis of Parkinson's disease. *Neuroradiology* 2013;55:719–724.

63. Kitao S, Matsusue E, Fujii S, Miyoshi F, Kaminou T, Kato S, et al. Correlation between pathology and neuromelanin MR imaging in Parkinson's disease and dementia with Lewy bodies. *Neuroradiology* 2013;55:947–953.

64. Takahashi J, Shibata T, Sasaki M, Kudo M, Yanezawa H, Obara S, et al. Detection of changes in the locus coeruleus in patients with mild cognitive impairment and Alzheimer's disease: High-resolution fast spin-echo T1-weighted imaging. *Geriatr Gerontol Int* 2015;15(3):334–340.

Chapter

17

Biomarkers for Concussion: The Need and the Prospects for the Near Future

Henrik Zetterberg and Kaj Blennow

Editorial Introduction

What would a biomarker mark? Readers are invited to take this quick and easy quiz:

1. the untoward apoptotic death of one neuron?
2. a 1% increase in microporation of the axolemma of 1% of axons, as inferred from electron microscopy, lasting ten minutes?
3. a 0.1% decrease in the net efficiency of synaptic connectivity, as inferred from diffusion kurtosis imaging, lasting 24 hours?
4. a 2.5% increase in the likelihood of a 5% decrease in new learning plasticity, as inferred from functional magnetic resonance imaging, measured 60 years post injury?
5. any deleterious brain change?

The answer is obviously (5). The question is: since humans will never be able to detect (5), what should suffice for clinical and research purposes?

On February 14th, 2018, the U.S. Food and Drug Administration announced approval of a two-element blood test for "concussion" [1]. The U.S. Department of Defense and the Army Medical Research and Materiel Command reportedly spent more than $100 million developing this test via the ALERT-TBI Multicenter Study. The test is currently marketed by the for-profit entity, Banyan Biomarkers.

The test draws inferences from circulating levels of ubiquitin carboxy-terminal hydrolase-L1 (UCHL1) and glial fibrillary acidic protein (GFAP). A total of 2011 subjects alleged to have "mild to moderate" traumatic brain injuries were enrolled at 24 centers. Although the investigators had not released their data when this volume went to press, they claimed their test has high sensitivity and high negative predictive value [2]. Banyan published the statement that their test has "99.5% accuracy." Accuracy for what? Certainly not for concussion!

Biomarker experts were quick to issue caveats and disclaimers [3]. As the reader will immediately infer, the Banyan test is not relevant for typical concussive brain injury (CBI). By definition, persons with typical CBI have no gross bleeding visible on computed tomography (CT). Almost all typical CBI survivors, therefore, will have negative Banyan test results. Hence, no evidence exists that the Banyan test will detect typical CBIs.

Moreover, as reported in Chapter 10 of this volume, prompt post-concussive blood testing of GFAP (along with other markers) predicts prolonged depression – but those elevated levels, in every case, were associated with negative CT scans [4]. Welch et al. [5] studied the utility of blood biomarkers among 167 subjects with "mild-to-moderate" traumatic brain injuries and reported, "There was no significant increase in either UCH-L1 or S100 B in CT-positive patients." Both findings support the conclusion that the Banyan test is not a concussion test and perhaps not a trustworthy test of CT positivity.

The editors of this brief volume applaud this advance. It may reduce the number of negative CT scans and spare patients exposure to radiation. Someday, perhaps within a decade, it may be more apparent whether the new test provides any demonstrable clinical benefit for the tens of millions of persons concussed every year. Yet we must firmly express several concerns regarding this new test:

- Its for-profit promoters have apparently misrepresented it as a "concussion test." This test cannot detect typical, clinically attended CBIs by any stretch of the imagination.
- Some laboratory findings suggest that neither GFAP nor UCH-L1 is sensitive to CT scan positivity. Forgoing an emergency CT due to a negative Banyan test could result in missed opportunities for life-saving neurosurgical intervention.
- The Department of Defense has a strong incentive to press survivors of CBI to return to duty. Test results might be inappropriately used as a factor in fitness-for-duty determinations.

The marketing of this test might tempt at least two forms of duplicity. One: some persons are incentivized, by money, training, or temperament, to doubt, minimize, or deny the long-term suffering of concussion survivors. Those persons might be tempted to misapply this new test, pretending that it is a marker for concussion and that negative test results decrease the odds that there will be permanent traumatic brain damage. Hopefully, such ruthless sophistry will be promptly exposed. Two: some employers – including the U.S. military – may be sorely tempted to misuse this test to judge disability, or worthiness for disability benefits.

The authors of the present chapter are world authorities on the issue of biomarkers. They summarize the actual state of the art. Readers must, however, arrive at their own personal judgment regarding the "what" question. What would you require a good concussion test to mark? One predicts a vast difference in opinions, associated with the natural variation in clinical empathy. For the editors, what a test should sensitively detect, at a minimum, would be a subjective sense of difference at a year post-injury or any change in the risk of late effects.

Introduction

Concussion or mild traumatic brain injury (mTBI) is defined by the American Congress of Rehabilitation Medicine as a head trauma resulting in any or a combination of the following: loss of consciousness for less than 30 min, alteration of mental state for up to 24 h (being dazed, confused, disoriented), or loss of memory for events immediately before or after the trauma [6]. Most often, concussions are benign, with symptoms disappearing within a few days up to a couple of weeks and the treatment is simple: rest. However, emerging evidence shows that repeated mTBIs, particularly before the brain has fully recovered, may cause chronic and sometimes progressive neurological or psychiatric symptoms and neuropathological changes [7]. This problem has attracted considerable media attention lately, as several athletes active in contact sports in which concussion is common have had to end their careers prematurely due to persisting symptoms following repeated concussions. This condition has been known for a long time in boxing, where it is called dementia pugilistica or punch-drunk syndrome, but has recently been given the more general, descriptive term chronic traumatic encephalopathy (CTE) [8].

Concussion (or mTBI) is a complex pathophysiological process in the brain induced by external mechanical forces on the head. The process involves diffuse axonal injury, i.e., tearing and stretching of the neuronal axons, which is regarded as the central mechanism for the damage, together with tau hyperphosphorylation and aggregation, de-regulated amyloid precursor protein (APP) metabolism with amyloid β (Aβ) aggregation and formation of diffuse Aβ plaques in close proximity to injured axons, microglial activation, and also frank neuronal death [8]. Although clinical practice has assumed that the course of concussion is reversed within one to two weeks [9], magnetic resonance spectroscopy, electrophysiological data, and neuropsychological assessments suggest a more prolonged timeline, with physiological metrics returning to baseline after 30–45 days as measured by magnetic resonance spectroscopy [10, 11]. We recently presented a case report on a knocked-out amateur boxer in whom the cerebrospinal fluid (CSF) levels of neurofilament light (NF-L: for details on this axonal injury marker, see below) remained abnormally elevated for more than half a year following the knockout punch [12]. These data suggest that mTBI results in a pathophysiological cascade that is much more extended in time than previously thought.

Repeated concussions may in unfortunate cases cause CTE. Symptoms of CTE include chronic or progressive changes in cognition, mood, personality, and behavior, as well as movement disorders (in particular parkinsonism and signs of motor neuron disease) [13]. Neuropathologically, brains of patients with CTE may display hallmark pathologies of Alzheimer's disease, neurofibrillary pathology composed of hyperphosphorylated tau and Aβ plaques [14, 15], which may be consequences of the neuroaxonal trauma [16]. Risk factors for CTE have been delineated in professional boxers and include a long boxing career, many bouts, high sparring exposure, many knockouts, poor performance as a boxer, and being able to tolerate many blows without being knocked out, all more or less directly associated with accumulated exposure to repetitive brain trauma [17]. These risk factors are most likely identical to what athletes in other sports in which concussion is common, such as American football, ice hockey, rugby, as well as military personnel, may be exposed to.

Fluid Biomarkers for Brain Injury

Accurate biochemical tests for axonal, neuronal. and astroglial injury would reveal: (1) whether a person exposed to head trauma also suffered from injury to brain neurons or glial cells; (2) the degree and nature of the injury; and (3) when the brain has recovered from the injury. In sports-related concussion, an objective "return-to-play" test would be highly desirable. This reasoning may also be applicable to other high-risk groups, such as military personnel. In addition to the acute and subacute settings after concussion, it would also be important to develop biomarkers to enable clinical studies of potential ongoing neurochemical changes and neuropathological cascades in persons at risk or with symptoms of CTE.

A biomarker is an objective measure of a biological or pathogenic process that can be used to evaluate prognosis, guide clinical diagnosis, and/or monitor the disease course and therapeutic interventions. The CSF is in direct contact with the extracellular space of the brain and can reflect biochemical changes that occur in the latter [18]. For these reasons, CSF may be considered an optimal fluid for the discovery of biomarkers for brain injury. The best-established CSF biomarkers for brain injury to date include proteins that reflect blood–brain barrier function (CSF/serum albumin ratio), neuroinflammation (interleukins (ILs) and cytokines), axonal (total tau protein, T-tau, and NF-L), neuronal (neuron-specific enolase, NSE) and astroglial (S-100B and glial fibrillary acidic protein, GFAp) integrity, and amyloid-related proteins (soluble APP and Aβ fragments). Some proteins that are highly expressed within the central nervous system (CNS), e.g., tau proteins, are detectable at very low concentrations also in the peripheral blood [19, 20]. This list is getting longer as the analytical tools become more sensitive [21, 22]. As blood is more accessible than CSF in clinical routine work, we end this overview by discussing peripheral blood biomarkers for mTBI.

CSF Biomarkers for Acute Brain Injury

CSF/Serum Albumin Ratio

The blood–brain barrier (BBB), which is formed by the endothelial cells that line cerebral microvessels, has an important role in maintaining a regulated microenvironment for reliable neuronal signaling in the brain [23]. The CSF/serum albumin ratio is a standard fluid biomarker for BBB function. Albumin is mainly synthesized in the liver and for this reason most albumin in the CSF is derived from the blood through passage across the BBB. An increase in this ratio indicates impaired BBB function, or BBB damage, and is found in a variety of CNS disorders, such as infections, inflammatory diseases, brain tumors, and cerebrovascular disease [18]. Two studies detected increased CSF/serum albumin ratio in the context of a neuroinflammatory response in patients with severe TBI [24, 25], but in studies of mTBI in boxers and blast exposure in military personnel no such changes have been seen [26, 27], suggesting that the BBB remains rather intact in mTBI or that the albumin ratio is not sensitive enough to identify subtle BBB damage that may occur in concussion.

CSF Biomarkers for Neuroinflammation

A large number of studies report increased CSF levels of acute-phase response proteins following severe TBI [28]. In general, inflammatory proteins, such as IL-6, IL-8, and IL-10, increase in the CSF in response to brain trauma and the magnitude of the rise correlates with outcome and in some studies also with the degree of BBB dysfunction, which is an important confounder. However, studies on mTBI are lacking. Many of the studies listed above were performed on ventricular CSF, which limits their relevance to mTBI in which samples will consist of lumbar CSF.

CSF Biomarkers for Axonal Injury

The best-established CSF biomarkers for axonal injury are T-tau and neurofilaments (NF-L or neurofilament heavy (NF-H)). These proteins have distinct regional distributions in the brain, which may be helpful to determine which areas of the brain were mainly affected. Tau is highly expressed in thin, unmyelinated axons of cortical interneurons, whereas neurofilaments are more abundant in large-caliber myelinated axons of long tracts that project into deeper brain layers and the spinal cord [18].

T-tau levels in ventricular CSF correlate with lesion size and outcome in TBI, so that high levels indicate worse injury [29–31]. Studies on mTBI, as approximated by amateur boxing, show elevated lumbar CSF levels of T-tau 4–10 days after a bout, also in boxers not having been knocked out, with normalizing levels during the following 8–12 weeks, provided the boxer has not participated in new bouts [27, 32]. This release pattern is similar to what has been reported in regard to T-tau levels in CSF following stroke [33]. T-tau may thus serve as a sensitive marker of axonal damage in gray-matter neurons following mTBI.

Studies have been performed on ventricular CSF levels of phosphorylated forms of NF-H in severe TBI [34], and lumbar CSF levels of NF-L in mTBI [27, 32]. High levels are seen in severely injured patients [34] and also in amateur boxers after a bout [27, 32] The magnitude of the rise is larger than for T-tau, suggesting that blows to the head most often impact long tracts

in the white matter more than short axons in the cortex [27, 32]. CSF NF-L appears to be the most sensitive fluid biomarker for diffuse axonal injury to date and, interestingly, its levels in amateur boxers correlate positively with exposure data, such as the number of received hits to the head and subjective and objective estimates of how hard the fight was [27, 32].

CSF Biomarkers for Neuronal Injury

NSE is a glycolytic enzyme enriched in neuronal cell bodies [35]. It was first analyzed in serum and CSF by Scarna et al., who could demonstrate that NSE levels in CSF were increased in severe head trauma cases with coma, suggesting that it was a promising marker of neuronal damage [36]. NSE levels are higher in ventricular CSF of non-survivors following severe TBI than in survivors and correlate with other TBI severity scores [37, 38]. Lumbar CSF levels of NSE have been suggested as a possible screening tool for inflicted TBI in children [39], but apart from this investigation, studies on lumbar CSF levels and mTBI are lacking. The major limitation of CSF NSE as a biomarker for neuronal injury is its high sensitivity to *in vitro* lysis of erythrocytes from blood contamination of the sample [40], which may occur in around 10% of lumbar punctures.

CSF Biomarkers for Astroglial Injury

S100 proteins are Ca^{2+}-binding proteins that help regulate the intracellular levels of calcium. There are two different subunits of S100, α and β. Homodimers of S100 α are referred to as S100A1, whereas αβ heterodimers and ββ homodimers are called S100B. Previously, S100B was thought to be specific for astrocytes but has now been detected in maturing oligodendrocytes and various extracerebral cell types, e.g., chondrocytes and adipocytes [35]. Thus, multi-trauma also involving peripheral tissues may confound the interpretation of S100B as a marker of mTBI severity.

S100B has been examined extensively in relation to TBI in the peripheral blood, but studies on CSF are not that common. Amateur boxers have slightly elevated CSF levels after a bout, but the changes are not as pronounced as those for the axonal markers T-tau and NF-L [32]. Similar results have been reported for GFAp [27, 32], which is an intermediate filament that is almost exclusively expressed in astrocytes [35]. However, CSF GFAp has also been evaluated in the context of severe TBI and ventricular levels have been shown to improve outcome prediction models in conjunction with clinical data [41].

CSF Biomarkers for Amyloid-Related Processes

Studies in both animals and humans have demonstrated that APP and Aβ (Alzheimer-associated, aggregation-prone Aβ42, in particular) accumulate in neurons and axons after brain trauma with axonal damage [8]. Ventricular CSF levels of the 40- and 42-amino-acid isoforms of Aβ increase during the first week of brain injury in severe TBI [42, 43]. Similar results were obtained for soluble isoforms of APP [43]. Prolonged elevations of Aβ in brain interstitial fluid for more than six days have been reported in patients with intracranial pressure-monitoring catheters and moderate to severe TBI [44]. However, in studies of mTBI performed on lumbar CSF samples, no amyloid-related changes have been seen [27, 32]. It is possible that CSF APP and Aβ are less sensitive, or have a faster turnover, than NF-L and T-tau, and thus do not change in mTBI in any detectable manner.

Upcoming CSF Biomarkers for Acute Brain Injury

αII-Spectrin breakdown products (SBDPs) have been described as potential biomarkers for brain injury in rats and humans [45, 46]. αII-Spectrin is primarily found in neurons, and is abundant in axons and presynaptic terminals [47]. The protein is processed to breakdown products by calpain and caspase-3, which are up-regulated in necrosis and apoptosis, respectively, in TBI.

SBDPs have been analyzed in ventricular CSF from patients with severe TBI and the levels correlate with clinical correlates of the severity of the injury and predict outcome [41, 48, 49]. In one of these studies, CSF SBDPs were evaluated together with another upcoming marker, ubiquitin C-terminal hydrolase-L1 (UCHL1) [41], which is a de-ubiquitinating enzyme highly expressed in neurons [50]. The two markers were found to contribute clinically relevant information in addition to routine assessments. Exploratory proteomics work to identify new CSF biomarkers has not yet produced any clinically useful tests [51]. In short, there are a number of CSF biomarkers for TBI that show an increase that correlates with the severity of the brain injury and predicts outcome. Longitudinal clinical studies in the context of mTBI are now needed to learn how these biomarkers could be employed in clinical practice and to establish whether such biomarker changes can elucidate how concussions may translate into CTE.

Peripheral Blood Biomarkers for Acute Brain Injury

Peripheral blood biomarkers for brain injury would be easier to implement in routine clinical work but a number of factors, e.g., proteolytic degradation, clearance in the liver or kidney, dilution in the large plasma volume or extracellular space of peripheral tissues, other matrix effects, such as binding to carrier proteins, and extracerebral biomarker release, may confound the results, making the diagnostic precision lower. Further, the BBB makes it difficult to assess biochemical changes in the brain using biomarkers in the blood. As a consequence, it has been extremely difficult to find reliable blood biomarkers for neurodegenerative processes, such as Alzheimer's disease, also in the presence of advanced neuropathology [18]. Nevertheless, the literature on peripheral blood biomarkers for brain injury in severe TBI is abundant [52].

S100B and GFAp have received considerable attention as potential peripheral blood markers of astroglial injury. Studies have shown that both S100B and GFAp levels in serum are increased in TBI patients and correlate with scores on the Glasgow Coma Scale and neuroradiological findings at hospital admission, helping to differentiate mild from severe injury and correlating with outcome [52, 53]. A recent consensus statement from the Scandinavian Neurotrauma Committee recommends the use of serum levels of S100B to determine which of the patients with mild head injury (Glasgow Coma

Scale 14 or 15) need a computed tomography scan of the brain to detect injuries requiring neurosurgical intervention [54]. However, before implementation these guidelines require extensive external validation. Further, less observable mTBI consequences were not discussed in this paper. In fact, a recent study on concussion in professional ice hockey showed that only five out of 28 concussed players reached above the S100B cut-off point suggested by Unden et al. [54] suggesting that it is a quite insensitive biomarker for mTBI [54].

S100B is also expressed in extracerebral cell types, including adipocytes and chondrocytes [35]. For this reason, there is a concern that an increase in serum S100B in trauma patients may come from peripheral tissues, such as fractured bones or injured skeletal muscles. Indeed, elevated serum levels have been observed in multiple trauma patients and sportsmen without head injuries [56–60]. From that perspective, GFAp may be considered more promising, as extracerebral expression has not yet been detected for this protein.

Promising results in mTBI were recently reported; serum levels of GFAp were found to be elevated in mTBI patients with abnormal computed tomography or magnetic resonance imaging (MRI) of the brain [61]. However, the marker did not predict outcome six months post injury. Other peripheral blood biomarker candidates for brain injury are NSE, myelin basic protein (MBP), hyperphosphorylated NF-H, and SBDPs. Elevated plasma levels of SBDPs have been reported in a subset of mTBI patients with persistent cognitive dysfunction following trauma, which suggests that the levels may relate to injury severity [62]. As mentioned above regarding measurements of NSE in CSF, its levels increase in response to lysis of erythrocytes, which is a major limitation of this biomarker. MBP may be more specific but its sensitivity for brain injury seems suboptimal [63]. Serum levels of NF-H in consecutive samples from severe TBI patients during six days were found to grow higher in patients who eventually died from their injury, but in all, the marker did not perform better than S100B and had a slower response [64]. There may, however, be clinically important differences in biomarker release profiles. For example, NF-H levels in serum remained elevated two to four days post injury in children with TBI with poor prognosis, whereas an early drop predicted good outcome [65].

A challenge with peripheral blood biomarkers for brain injury is that BBB integrity may influence the levels of brain-derived proteins in the blood. This has been reported for both S100B and UCHL1, whereas serum levels of NF-H appear to be more resistant [66]. UCHL1 and SBDPs are two more recent candidate biomarkers for TBI that have been studied in both CSF and blood [41]. They behave in a manner similar to S100B and GFAp in regard to correlations with other measures of TBI severity, as well as clinical outcome [52]. There are as yet no conclusive studies on the diagnostic performance of these peripheral blood biomarkers in the context of mTBI, but one prospective cohort study of 96 patients with mild to moderate TBI showed that UCHL1 is detectable in serum within an hour of injury and is associated with measures of injury severity, including the Glasgow Coma Scale score, lesions on brain imaging, and the need for neurosurgical intervention [67].

A number of explorative studies on peripheral blood biomarkers for TBI have been published but apart from replicating findings from more targeted analyses of candidate markers, novel biomarker patterns that have been validated in independent studies using independent techniques are yet to be described [52].

A common problem with peripheral blood biomarkers for TBI is that the levels of CNS-derived proteins are very low in the blood, challenging the technical limitations of most standard immunoassays. An ultra-sensitive digital immunoassay for the quantification of tau, one of the most CNS-specific proteins, in serum has been developed [20]. Provided the antibodies are of high quality, the technique may be around 1000 times as sensitive as standard enzyme-linked immunosorbent assays for the same molecule.

In a proof-of-principle pilot study to test tau in serum as a biomarker for brain injury in patients resuscitated after cardiac arrest, which results in severe brain ischemia, a marked and bi-modal increase was found that correlated with clinical outcome [68]. In the first study examining plasma tau as a biomarker for mTBI, the release pattern of tau into the blood stream in concussed ice hockey players in the Swedish professional hockey league was highly predictive of symptom severity and when the players could return to play following concussion, which contrasted with the mostly negative results for S100B and NSE [55].

Biomarkers for Chronic Brain Changes Following TBI

Neuropathological characteristics of CTE were described in boxers in the 1970s, with the most prominent feature being neurofibrillary tangle pathology in cortical areas [69]. The best-established biomarker to date for tangle pathology, at least as it appears in Alzheimer's disease, is CSF phospho-tau [18], which has not yet been examined in CTE patients.

Recently, another pathological feature of CTE was described at the molecular level: inclusions of TDP-43 [70–72], which is otherwise typical of frontotemporal dementia and amyotrophic lateral sclerosis [73]. TDP-43 accumulation in CTE may be widespread and found in several gray-matter structures, the brainstem and basal ganglia cortical areas, as well as in subcortical white-matter tissue [71, 72]. Assays for CSF TDP-43 have been published [74], but studies on CTE are lacking.

Chronic pituitary dysfunction caused by tearing of axons in the pituitary stalk is highly prevalent following TBI [75]. mTBI-related chronic pituitary dysfunction is highly prevalent (around 40%) in retired American football players [76] and has also been reported in boxers and kick boxers. In a pilot study, 45% of professional boxers were growth hormone (GH)-deficient [77]. In a larger study of active and retired boxers, 18% had pituitary hormone deficiencies in one or more axes [78]. An investigation of pituitary dysfunction in amateur kick boxers revealed GH and/or adrenocorticotropin deficiencies in 27% of the athletes [79].

More recently, Wilkinson and colleagues measured concentrations of 12 pituitary and target organ hormones in two groups of male U.S. veterans of combat in Iraq or Afghanistan and found abnormal levels in 11 out of 26 study participants with a history of blast-induced concussion [80]. Such abnormalities correlate with lasting cognitive symptoms following the TBI [75]. As these hormone disturbances are treatable, it is important to identify them.

Conclusions

A large number of CSF and peripheral blood biomarkers for the detection of injury to different cell types and structures within the CNS are at hand. Several of these have been investigated in relation to severe TBI and been found to produce clinically relevant results, often in relation to outcome prediction, but more studies on concussion in clinically relevant settings are needed. Apart from S100B and NSE, only research grade assays exist for which there are no certified reference materials or methods for assay calibration. A reliable biomarker signature of mTBI, preferably in blood, would reduce the number of unnecessary computed tomography scans and would also be a valuable diagnostic and "return-to-play" test in concussed individuals. In the absence of detailed studies on mTBI with repeated biomarker testing, it is difficult to suggest more detailed diagnostic algorithms incorporating fluid biomarkers at this stage. The lack of standardized methods also precludes the use of globally standardized biomarker cut-off points to guide clinical decision making. Achieving this is an important goal of current mTBI biomarker research.

This review has identified a number of additional areas in which more research is needed. Axons appear to be the most vulnerable structure within the CNS and we need reliable peripheral blood biomarkers for axonal damage. Tau and neurofilament proteins appear promising in this regard, but for this class of biomarkers the analytical techniques need to improve in sensitivity, beyond what can be normally reached using conventional enzyme-linked immunosorbent assay methods. The instruments should preferably be automated and not too large or expensive to allow for implementation in general clinical care. We also need better animal models that recapitulate the relevant pathophysiological processes in mTBI in humans in which new biomarker candidates can be discovered and evaluated. Important advances in this regard were recently made in the development of a mouse model of blast-induced neurotrauma, which appears to present key features of the neuropathology seen in humans [81]. A critical step in the research on CTE is the ability to diagnose CTE in living patients. Hopefully, biomarkers for neuropathological characteristics of CTE will prove as useful as the plaque and tangle markers have been in research on Alzheimer's disease.

Future research needs to address if individuals exposed to repetitive head trauma indeed are at increased risk of CTE as determined by biomarkers. Large prospective clinical multicenter longitudinal studies combining clinical evaluations with biomarker examinations have proven highly important to elucidate the interrelation between clinical symptoms, disease onset, and the temporal evolutions of the pathogenic mechanisms in chronic brain diseases such as Alzheimer's disease. This type of longitudinal study also on individuals exposed to repetitive head trauma or with early symptoms of CTE also examining both fluid (CSF/blood) and imaging (MRI and amyloid/tau PET) markers are highly warranted. Such studies will likely provide answers to a number of important questions on pathogenic mechanisms and their clinical relevance. Is there a certain threshold with regard to exposure or is CTE risk mainly attributable to individual vulnerability? Is the degree of brain damage stable after repeated mTBI, with age-related changes determining if and when symptoms will appear, or do repeated mTBIs initiate a self-propagating brain disorder? Can biomarkers help to identify preclinical CTE and can the process be halted?

Acknowledgments

Work in the authors' laboratory is supported by the Swedish Research Council, Swedish State Support for Clinical Research, the Knut and Alice Wallenberg Foundation, and the Wolfson Foundation.

References

1. U.S. Food and Drug Administration. FDA authorizes marketing of first blood test to aid in the evaluation of concussion in adults. July 14, 2018. Available at: www.fda.gov/NewsEvents/Newsroom/PressAnnouncements/ucm596531.htm.

2. Bazarian JJ. Serum GFAP and UCH1-L1 predict traumatic injuries on head CT scan after mild-moderate traumatic brain injury: Results of the ALERT-TBI multicenter study. *Ann Emerg Med* 2017; 70:S2.

3. Costandi M. FDA okays first concussion blood test – but some experts are wary. *Scientific American* 02/18/18. Available at: www.scientificamerican.com/article/fda-okays-first-concussion-blood-test-but-some-experts-are-wary/.

4. Van Meter T, Mirshahi N, Peters M, Roy D, Rao V, Diaz-Arrastia R, et al. Machine learning models identify mild traumatic brain injury patients with significant depressive symptoms over six months of recovery using a three biomarker blood test. *Ann Emerg Med* 2017; 70:S104–S105.

5. Welch RD, Ellis M, Lewis LM, Ayaz SI, Mika VH, Millis S, et al. Modeling the kinetics of serum glial fibrillary acidic protein, ubiquitin carboxyl-terminal hydrolase-L1, and S100B concentrations in patients with traumatic brain injury. *J Neurotrauma* 2017;34:1957–1971.

6. American Congress of Rehabilitation Medicine. Definition of mild traumatic brain injury. *J Head Trauma Rehabil* 1993;8:86–87.

7. Baugh CM, Stamm JM, Riley DO, Gavett BE, Shenton ME, Lin A, Nowinski CJ, Cantu RC, McKee AC, Stern RA. Chronic traumatic encephalopathy: Neurodegeneration following repetitive concussive and subconcussive brain trauma. *Brain Imaging Behav* 2012;6(2):244–254.

8. Blennow K, Hardy J, Zetterberg H. The neuropathology and neurobiology of traumatic brain injury. *Neuron* 2012;76(5):886–899.

9. New Zealand Guidelines Group. *Traumatic brain injury: Diagnosis, acute management and rehabilitation.* Wellington, NZ: New Zealand Guidelines Group, 2006.

10. Iverson GL, Gaetz M, Lovell MR, Collins MW. Cumulative effects of concussion in amateur athletes. *Brain Inj* 2004;18(5):433–443.

11. Brooks WM, Stidley CA, Petropoulos H, Jung RE, Weers DC, Friedman SD, Barlow MA, Sibbitt WL, Jr., Yeo RA. Metabolic and cognitive response to human traumatic brain injury: A quantitative proton magnetic resonance study. *J Neurotrauma* 2000;17(8):629–640.

12. Neselius S, Brisby H, Granholm F, Zetterberg H, Blennow K. Monitoring severity of brain damage and recovery after boxing knockout by CSF biomarkers for axonal damage. *Knee Surg Sports Traumatol Arthrosc* 2015; 23:2536–2539.

13. Stern RA, Riley DO, Daneshvar DH, Nowinski CJ, Cantu RC, McKee AC. Long-term consequences of repetitive brain trauma: Chronic traumatic encephalopathy. *PM R* 2011; 3(10 Suppl 2):S460–S467.

14. Roberts GW, Allsop D, Bruton C. The occult aftermath of boxing. *J Neurol Neurosurg Psychiatry* 1990;53(5):373–378.

15. Tokuda T, Ikeda S, Yanagisawa N, Ihara Y, Glenner GG. Re-examination of ex-boxers' brains using immunohistochemistry with antibodies to amyloid beta-protein and tau protein. *Acta Neuropathol* 1991;82(4):280–285.

16. Johnson VE, Stewart W, Smith DH. Traumatic brain injury and amyloid-beta pathology: A link to Alzheimer's disease? *Nat Rev Neurosci* 2010;11(5):361–370.

17. Jordan BD. Chronic traumatic brain injury associated with boxing. *Semin Neurol* 2000;20(2):179–185.

18. Blennow K, Hampel H, Weiner M, Zetterberg H. Cerebrospinal fluid and plasma biomarkers in Alzheimer disease. *Nat Rev Neurol* 2010;6(3):131–144.

19. Mortberg E, Zetterberg H, Nordmark J, Blennow K, Catry C, Decraemer H, Vanmechelen E, Rubertsson S. Plasma tau protein in comatose patients after cardiac arrest treated with therapeutic hypothermia. *Acta Anaesthesiol Scand* 2011;55(9):1132–1138.

20. Randall J, Mortberg E, Provuncher GK, Fournier DR, Duffy DC, Rubertsson S, Blennow K, Zetterberg H, Wilson DH. Tau proteins in serum predict neurological outcome after hypoxic brain injury from cardiac arrest: Results of a pilot study. *Resuscitation* 2013; 84: 351–356.

21. Rissin DM, Kan CW, Campbell TG, Howes SC, Fournier DR, Song L, Piech T, Patel PP, Chang L, Rivnak AJ, et al. Single-molecule enzyme-linked immunosorbent assay detects serum proteins at subfemtomolar concentrations. *Nat Biotechnol* 2010;28(6):595–599.

22. Savage MJ, Kalinina J, Wolfe A, Tugusheva K, Korn R, Cash-Mason T, Maxwell JW, Hatcher NG, Haugabook SJ, Wu G, et al. A sensitive abeta oligomer assay discriminates Alzheimer's and aged control cerebrospinal fluid. *J Neurosci* 2014;34(8):2884–2897.

23. Abbott NJ, Ronnback L, Hansson E. Astrocyte–endothelial interactions at the blood–brain barrier. *Nat Rev Neurosci* 2006;7(1):41–53.

24. Csuka E, Morganti-Kossmann MC, Lenzlinger PM, Joller H, Trentz O, Kossmann T. IL-10 levels in cerebrospinal fluid and serum of patients with severe traumatic brain injury: Relationship to IL-6, TNF-alpha, TGF-beta1 and blood–brain barrier function. *J Neuroimmunol* 1999;101(2):211–221.

25. Kossmann T, Hans VH, Imhof HG, Stocker R, Grob P, Trentz O, Morganti-Kossmann C. Intrathecal and serum interleukin-6 and the acute-phase response in patients with severe traumatic brain injuries. *Shock* 1995;4(5):311–317.

26. Blennow K, Jonsson M, Andreasen N, Rosengren L, Wallin A, Hellstrom PA, Zetterberg H. No neurochemical evidence of brain injury after blast overpressure by repeated explosions or firing heavy weapons. *Acta Neurol Scand* 2011;123(4):245–251.

27. Zetterberg H, Hietala MA, Jonsson M, Andreasen N, Styrud E, Karlsson I, Edman A, Popa C, Rasulzada A, Wahlund LO, et al. Neurochemical aftermath of amateur boxing. *Arch Neurol* 2006;63(9):1277–1280.

28. Zetterberg H, Smith DH, Blennow K. Biomarkers of mild traumatic brain injury in cerebrospinal fluid and blood. *Nat Rev Neurol* 2013;9(4):201–210.

29. Ost M, Nylen K, Csajbok L, Ohrfelt AO, Tullberg M, Wikkelso C, Nellgard P, Rosengren L, Blennow K, Nellgard B. Initial CSF total tau correlates with 1-year outcome in patients with traumatic brain injury. *Neurology* 2006;67(9):1600–1604.

30. Franz G, Beer R, Kampfl A, Engelhardt K, Schmutzhard E, Ulmer H, Deisenhammer F. Amyloid beta 1–42 and tau in cerebrospinal fluid after severe traumatic brain injury. *Neurology* 2003;60(9):1457–1461.

31. Zemlan FP, Jauch EC, Mulchahey JJ, Gabbita SP, Rosenberg WS, Speciale SG, Zuccarello M. C-tau biomarker of neuronal damage in severe brain injured patients: Association with elevated intracranial pressure and clinical outcome. *Brain Res* 2002;947(1):131–139.

32. Neselius S, Brisby H, Theodorsson A, Blennow K, Zetterberg H, Marcusson J. CSF-biomarkers in Olympic boxing: Diagnosis and effects of repetitive head trauma. *PLoS One* 2012;7(4):e33606.

33. Hesse C, Rosengren L, Andreasen N, Davidsson P, Vanderstichele H, Vanmechelen E, Blennow K. Transient increase in total tau but not phospho-tau in human cerebrospinal fluid after acute stroke. *Neurosci Lett* 2001;297(3):187–190.

34. Siman R, Toraskar N, Dang A, McNeil E, McGarvey M, Plaum J, Maloney E, Grady MS. A panel of neuron-enriched proteins as markers for traumatic brain injury in humans. *J Neurotrauma* 2009;26(11):1867–1877.

35. Olsson B, Zetterberg H, Hampel H, Blennow K. Biomarker-based dissection of neurodegenerative diseases. *Prog Neurobiol* 2011;95(4):520–534.

36. Scarna H, Delafosse B, Steinberg R, Debilly G, Mandrand B, Keller A, Pujol JF. Neuron-specific enolase as a marker of neuronal lesions during various comas in man. *Neurochem Int* 1982;4(5):405–411.

37. Bohmer AE, Oses JP, Schmidt AP, Peron CS, Krebs CL, Oppitz PP, D'Avila TT, Souza DO, Portela LV, Stefani MA. Neuron-specific enolase, S100B, and glial fibrillary acidic protein levels as outcome predictors in patients with severe traumatic brain injury. *Neurosurgery* 2011;68(6):1624–1630; discussion 1630-1631.

38. Chiaretti A, Barone G, Riccardi R, Antonelli A, Pezzotti P, Genovese O, Tortorolo L, Conti G. NGF, DCX, and NSE upregulation correlates with severity and outcome of head trauma in children. *Neurology* 2009;72(7):609–616.

39. Berger RP, Dulani T, Adelson PD, Leventhal JM, Richichi R, Kochanek PM. Identification of inflicted traumatic brain injury in well-appearing infants using serum and cerebrospinal markers: A possible screening tool. *Pediatrics* 2006;117(2):325–332.

40. Ramont L, Thoannes H, Volondat A, Chastang F, Millet MC, Maquart FX. Effects of hemolysis and storage condition on neuron-specific enolase (NSE) in cerebrospinal fluid and serum: Implications in clinical practice. *Clin Chem Lab Med* 2005;43(11):1215–1217.

41. Czeiter E, Mondello S, Kovacs N, Sandor J, Gabrielli A, Schmid K, Tortella F, Wang KK, Hayes RL, Barzo P, et al. Brain injury biomarkers may improve the predictive power of the IMPACT outcome calculator. *J Neurotrauma* 2012;29(9):1770–1778.

42. Raby CA, Morganti-Kossmann MC, Kossmann T, Stahel PF, Watson MD, Evans LM, Mehta PD, Spiegel K, Kuo YM, Roher AE, et al. Traumatic brain injury increases beta-amyloid peptide 1–42 in cerebrospinal fluid. *J Neurochem* 1998;71(6):2505–2509.

43. Olsson A, Csajbok L, Ost M, Hoglund K, Nylen K, Rosengren L, Nellgard B, Blennow K. Marked increase of beta-amyloid(1–42) and amyloid precursor protein in ventricular cerebrospinal fluid after severe traumatic brain injury. *J Neurol* 2004;251(7):870–876.

44. Marklund N, Farrokhnia N, Hanell A, Vanmechelen E, Enblad P, Zetterberg H, Blennow K, Hillered L. Monitoring of beta-amyloid dynamics after human traumatic brain injury. *J Neurotrauma* 2014;31(1):42–55.

45. Pike BR, Flint J, Dutta S, Johnson E, Wang KK, Hayes RL. Accumulation of non-erythroid alpha II-spectrin and calpain-cleaved alpha II-spectrin breakdown products in cerebrospinal fluid after traumatic brain injury in rats. *J Neurochem* 2001;78(6):1297–1306.

46. Pineda JA, Lewis SB, Valadka AB, Papa L, Hannay HJ, Heaton SC, Demery JA, Liu MC, Aikman JM, Akle V, et al. Clinical significance of alphaII-spectrin breakdown products in cerebrospinal fluid after severe traumatic brain injury. *J Neurotrauma* 2007;24(2):354–366.

47. Riederer BM, Zagon IS, Goodman SR. Brain spectrin(240/235) and brain spectrin(240/235E): Two distinct spectrin subtypes with different locations within mammalian neural cells. *J Cell Biol* 1986;102(6):2088–2097.

48. Farkas O, Polgar B, Szekeres-Bartho J, Doczi T, Povlishock JT, Buki A. Spectrin breakdown products in the cerebrospinal fluid in severe head injury – Preliminary observations. *Acta Neurochir (Wien)* 2005;147(8):855–861.

49. Mondello S, Robicsek SA, Gabrielli A, Brophy GM, Papa L, Tepas J, Robertson C, Buki A, Scharf D, Jixiang M, et al. AlphaII-spectrin breakdown products (SBDPs): Diagnosis and outcome in severe traumatic brain injury patients. *J Neurotrauma* 2010;27(7):1203–1213.

50. Wilkinson KD, Lee KM, Deshpande S, Duerksen-Hughes P, Boss JM, Pohl J. The neuron-specific protein PGP 9.5 is a ubiquitin carboxyl-terminal hydrolase. *Science* 1989;246(4930):670–673.

51. Ottens AK, Kobeissy FH, Golden EC, Zhang Z, Haskins WE, Chen SS, Hayes RL, Wang KK, Denslow ND. Neuroproteomics in neurotrauma. *Mass Spectrom Rev* 2006;25(3):380–408.

52. Mondello S, Muller U, Jeromin A, Streeter J, Hayes RL, Wang KK. Blood-based diagnostics of traumatic brain injuries. *Expert Rev Mol Diagn* 2011;11(1):65–78.

53. Kovesdi E, Luckl J, Bukovics P, Farkas O, Pal J, Czeiter E, Szellar D, Doczi T, Komoly S, Buki A. Update on protein biomarkers in traumatic brain injury with emphasis on clinical use in adults and pediatrics. *Acta Neurochir (Wien)* 2010;152(1):1–17.

54. Unden J, Ingebrigtsen T, Romner B. Scandinavian guidelines for initial management of minimal, mild and moderate head injuries in adults: An evidence and consensus-based update. *BMC Med* 2013;11:50.

55. Shahim P, Tegner Y, Wilson DH, Randall J, Skillback T, Pazooki D, Kallberg B, Blennow K, Zetterberg H. Blood biomarkers for brain injury in concussed professional ice hockey players. *JAMA Neurol* 2014;71(6):684–692.

56. Mussack T, Kirchhoff C, Buhmann S, Biberthaler P, Ladurner R, Gippner-Steppert C, Mutschler W, Jochum M. Significance of Elecsys S100 immunoassay for real-time assessment of traumatic brain damage in multiple trauma patients. *Clin Chem Lab Med* 2006;44(9):1140–1145.

57. Rothoerl RD, Woertgen C. High serum S100B levels for trauma patients without head injuries. *Neurosurgery* 2001;49(6):1490–1491; author reply 1492–1493.

58. Anderson RE, Hansson LO, Nilsson O, Dijlai-Merzoug R, Settergren G. High serum S100B levels for trauma patients without head injuries. *Neurosurgery* 2001;48(6):1255–1258; discussion 1258–1260.

59. Romner B, Ingebrigtsen T. High serum S100B levels for trauma patients without head injuries. *Neurosurgery* 2001;49(6):1490; author reply 1492–1493.

60. Stalnacke BM, Ohlsson A, Tegner Y, Sojka P. Serum concentrations of two biochemical markers of brain tissue damage S-100B and neurone specific enolase are increased in elite female soccer players after a competitive game. *Br J Sports Med* 2006;40(4):313–316.

61. Metting Z, Wilczak N, Rodiger LA, Schaaf JM, van der Naalt J. GFAP and S100B in the acute phase of mild traumatic brain injury. *Neurology* 2012;78(18):1428–1433.

62. Siman R, Giovannone N, Hanten G, Wilde EA, McCauley SR, Hunter JV, Li X, Levin HS, Smith DH. Evidence that the blood biomarker SNTF predicts brain imaging changes and persistent cognitive dysfunction in mild TBI patients. *Front Neurol* 2013;4:190.

63. Berger RP, Adelson PD, Pierce MC, Dulani T, Cassidy LD, Kochanek PM. Serum neuron-specific enolase, S100B, and myelin basic protein concentrations after inflicted and noninflicted traumatic brain injury in children. *J Neurosurg* 2005;103 (1 Suppl):61–68.

64. Zurek J, Fedora M. The usefulness of S100B, NSE, GFAP, NF-H, secretagogin and Hsp70 as a predictive biomarker of outcome in children with traumatic brain injury. *Acta Neurochir (Wien)* 2012;154(1):93–103; discussion 103.

65. Zurek J, Bartlova L, Fedora M. Hyperphosphorylated neurofilament NF-H as a predictor of mortality after brain injury in children. *Brain Inj* 2011;25(2):221–226.

66. Blyth BJ, Farahvar A, He H, Nayak A, Yang C, Shaw G, Bazarian JJ. Elevated serum ubiquitin carboxy-terminal hydrolase L1 is associated with abnormal blood–brain barrier function after traumatic brain injury. *J Neurotrauma* 2011;28(12):2453–2462.

67. Papa L, Lewis LM, Silvestri S, Falk JL, Giordano P, Brophy GM, Demery JA, Liu MC, Mo J, Akinyi L, et al. Serum levels of ubiquitin C-terminal hydrolase distinguish mild traumatic brain injury from trauma controls and are elevated in mild and moderate traumatic brain injury patients with intracranial lesions and neurosurgical intervention. *J Trauma Acute Care Surg* 2012;72(5):1335–1344.

68. Randall J, Mortberg E, Provuncher GK, Fournier DR, Duffy DC, Rubertsson S, Blennow K, Zetterberg H, Wilson DH. Tau proteins in serum predict neurological outcome after hypoxic brain injury from cardiac arrest: Results of a pilot study. *Resuscitation* 2013;84(3):351–356.

69. Corsellis JA, Bruton CJ, Freeman-Browne D. The aftermath of boxing. *Psychol Med* 1973;3(3):270–303.

70. King A, Sweeney F, Bodi I, Troakes C, Maekawa S, Al-Sarraj S. Abnormal TDP-43 expression is identified in the neocortex in cases of dementia pugilistica, but is mainly confined to the limbic system when identified in high and moderate stages of Alzheimer's disease. *Neuropathology* 2010;30(4):408–419.

71. McKee AC, Gavett BE, Stern RA, Nowinski CJ, Cantu RC, Kowall NW, Perl DP, Hedley-Whyte ET, Price B, Sullivan C, et al. TDP-43 proteinopathy and motor neuron disease in chronic traumatic encephalopathy. *J Neuropathol Exp Neurol* 2010;69(9): 918–929.

72. Johnson VE, Stewart W, Trojanowski JQ, Smith DH. Acute and chronically increased immunoreactivity to phosphorylation-independent but not pathological TDP-43 after a single traumatic brain injury in humans. *Acta Neuropathol* 2011;122(6): 715–726.

73. Neumann M, Sampathu DM, Kwong LK, Truax AC, Micsenyi MC, Chou TT, Bruce J, Schuck T, Grossman M, Clark CM, et al. Ubiquitinated TDP-43 in frontotemporal lobar degeneration and amyotrophic lateral sclerosis. *Science* 2006;314(5796):130–133.

74. Geser F, Prvulovic D, O'Dwyer L, Hardiman O, Bede P, Bokde AL, Trojanowski JQ, Hampel H. On the development of markers for pathological TDP-43 in amyotrophic lateral sclerosis with and without dementia. *Prog Neurobiol* 2011;95(4):649–662.

75. Kozlowski Moreau O, Yollin E, Merlen E, Daveluy W, Rousseaux M. Lasting pituitary hormone deficiency after traumatic brain injury. *J Neurotrauma* 2012;29(1):81–89.

76. Kelly DF, Chaloner C, Evans D, Matthews A, Cohan P, Wang C, Swerdloff R, Sim MS, Lee J, Wright MJ, et al. Prevalence of pituitary hormone dysfunction, metabolic syndrome and impaired quality of life in retired professional football players: A prospective study. *J Neurotrauma* 2014;31(13):1161–1171.

77. Kelestimur F, Tanriverdi F, Atmaca H, Unluhizarci K, Selcuklu A, Casanueva FF. Boxing as a sport activity associated with isolated GH deficiency. *J Endocrinol Invest* 2004;27(11):RC28–RC32.

78. Tanriverdi F, Unluhizarci K, Kocyigit I, Tuna IS, Karaca Z, Durak AC, Selcuklu A, Casanueva FF, Kelestimur F. Brief communication: pituitary volume and function in competing and retired male boxers. *Ann Intern Med* 2008;148(11):827–831.

79. Tanriverdi F, Unluhizarci K, Coksevim B, Selcuklu A, Casanueva FF, Kelestimur F. Kickboxing sport as a new cause of traumatic brain injury-mediated hypopituitarism. *Clin Endocrinol (Oxf)* 2007;66(3):360–366.

80. Wilkinson CW, Pagulayan KF, Petrie EC, Mayer CL, Colasurdo EA, Shofer JB, Hart KL, Hoff D, Tarabochia MA, Peskind ER. High prevalence of chronic pituitary and target-organ hormone abnormalities after blast-related mild traumatic brain injury. *Front Neurol* 2012;3:11.

81. Goldstein LE, Fisher AM, Tagge CA, Zhang XL, Velisek L, Sullivan JA, Upreti C, Kracht JM, Ericsson M, Wojnarowicz MW, et al. Chronic traumatic encephalopathy in blast-exposed military veterans and a blast neurotrauma mouse model. *Sci Transl Med* 2012;4(134):134ra160.

18 Pediatric Concussion: Understanding, Assessment, and Management, with Special Attention to Sports-Related Brain Injury

Adam Darby, Jeff Victoroff, and Christopher C. Giza

Most of the individuals participating in organized sports are pediatric athletes and, although there is an increasing amount of published work in high school athlete groups offering some insight into this distinct population, there is not nearly such breadth of study in younger children. An estimated two million concussions were treated in U.S. emergency departments from January 2007 to December 2011 according to a retrospective analysis using the National Electronic Injury Surveillance System-All Injury Program, with approximately 40% occurring in patients aged 12–24 years [1]. During this period the number of concussions was seen to increase by more than 30% with attribution to sports-related injuries. The question of this representing a true increase in the annual incidence versus it being a function of heightened concussion awareness is up for debate with many favoring the latter.

As shocking as these numbers are, they likely remain a significant underestimation of the true burden of pediatric concussive brain injury (CBI),[1] given that many patients may seek care in non-emergency settings (such as physicians' offices or on the sidelines from an athletic trainer) and are not routinely captured in systematic databases. The American College of Sports Medicine has estimated that 85% of sport-related concussions (SRCs) go undiagnosed. In fact, as discussed in this volume's Chapter 2 on *Epidemiology of Concussive Brain Injury*, it is impossible to meaningfully estimate the true incidence of SRC in youth, because most youth sports are not organized and most concussions do not present for medical attention. Moreover, even when clinically significant CBIs occur in organized sports in first-world countries, a minority of those injuries may come to medical attention.

Nor can one assume that symptoms reliably alert the player that he or she suffered a clinically significant SRC. Talavage et al. [2], for instance, studied high school football players by comparing head impacts monitored by helmet telemetry with neurocognitive testing and functional magnetic resonance imaging (fMRI). As expected, athletes with known, diagnosed concussion exhibited both cognitive and imaging abnormalities. Other players with recorded head impacts had no reported or observable concussion symptoms – yet they exhibited visual working-memory deficits and imaging abnormalities. As illustrated in Figure 18.1, some players assessed as "controls" due to being asymptomatic had demonstrable cognitive impairment and brain change.

Acknowledging the small size of this study, the authors nonetheless expressed a legitimate concern:

> The discovery of this new category suggests that more players are suffering neurological injury than are currently being detected using traditional concussion-assessment tools. These individuals are unlikely to undergo clinical evaluation, and thus may continue to participate in football-related activities, even when changes in brain physiology (and potential brain damage) are present.
>
> [2]

This study was far too small to permit meaningful estimation of the frequency of this category of injury. Pending cost-effective sideline tools that validly and reliably detect CBI, one can only guess the seasonal incidence of overlooked athletes with asymptomatic yet significant SRC.

Another study from the same group [3] measured resting-state fMRI connectivity in the default-mode network (DMN) and reported football players exhibited altered connectivity compared with controls. Of interest, these cerebral changes were detected *before* the season and in *asymptomatic* athletes. While the overall significance of this finding is not clear, the authors concluded:

> Football athletes exhibited hyperconnectivity in the DMN compared to controls for most of the sessions, which indicates that, despite the absence of symptoms typically associated with concussion, the repetitive trauma accrued produced long-term brain changes compared to their healthy peers.
>
> ([3], p. 91)

Findings of brain change in concussion-exposed athletes without symptoms highlights one of the important themes of this text: clinical recovery is important and desirable, but one must not assume that it indicates return to neurobiological normality.

---

[1] The topic of this chapter is typical, clinically attended concussive brain injury (CBI) – meaning a brain-rattling injury due to an abrupt external force that is assessed by some clinician and typically does not cause prolonged coma or gross intracranial bleeding. Some sources cited in this chapter employed the unscientific 20th-century term "mild traumatic brain injury (mTBI)." Although that phrase does not identify a specific, biologically defined degree of brain damage, the terminology is occasionally preserved for fidelity with those sources.

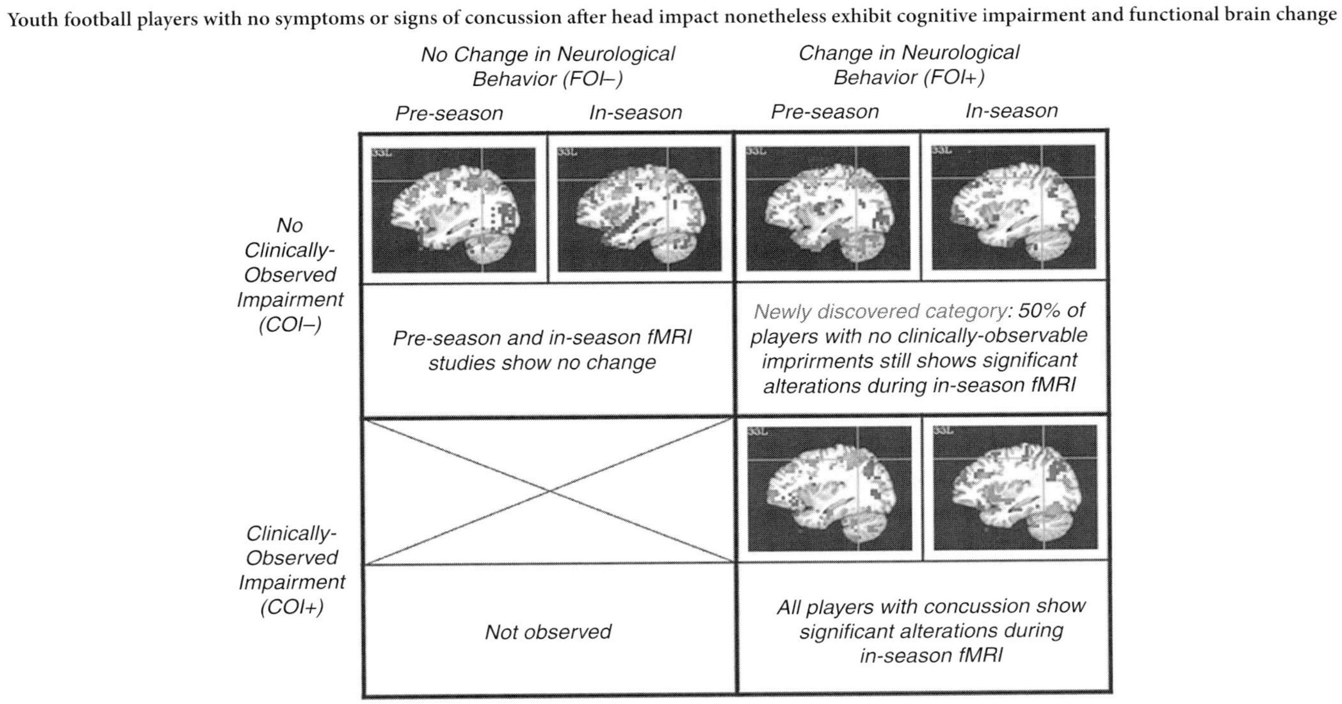

Youth football players with no symptoms or signs of concussion after head impact nonetheless exhibit cognitive impairment and functional brain change

Fig. 18.1 Summary of observed player categories, with representative functional magnetic resonance imaging (fMRI) observations. Categories are based on both clinical observation by the team physician of impairment associated with concussion (clinically observed impairment: COI+ or COI–), and the presence or absence of significant neurocognitive impairment via Immediate Post-Concussion Assessment and Cognitive Testing (ImPACT) (functionally observed impairment; FOI+ or FOI–). fMRI activations are depicted for all players using a sagittal slice through the left inferior parietal lobule, to illustrate the presence of many changes, relative to pre-season assessment, for FOI+ players. As expected, all (3/3) players who were diagnosed by the team physician as having experienced a concussion (COI+) were also found to exhibit significantly reduced ImPACT scores (FOI+), and are categorized as COI+ /FOI+(top left). Half (4/8) of players brought in for assessment ostensibly for control purposes (i.e., presenting with no clinically observable impairments, COI–) were found to be neurocognitively consistent with pre-season assessment (FOI–), and are categorized as COI– /FOI– (top right). The other half (4/8) of the intended control group, studied in the absence of diagnosed concussion (COI–), were found to exhibit significantly impaired ImPACT performance (FOI+), and are categorized as COI–/FOI+. This group represents a newly observed category of possible neurological injury (bottom left). No players who were diagnosed with a concussion (COI+) were found to exhibit ImPACT scores consistent with pre-season assessments (FOI–). [A black and white version of this figure will appear in some formats. For the color version, please refer to the plate section.]

Source: Talavage et al., 2014 [2]. Reproduced with permission from Mary Ann Liebert, Inc.

There is both scientific and clinical evidence that traumatic brain injury (TBI) in children differs from that in adults. To date there has been much inference as to symptoms, assessment, and management of this group from studies in older individuals. This overall lack of published data, particularly in pre-high school-aged children, is concerning given the continued brain growth and development during this life stage.

The life of a child is very different to that of an adult, from the differing expectations for daily knowledge acquisition and frequent learning assessment to the very different social dynamic and challenges. The role played by sports participation in their lives is also very different and, as such, the recommendations for managing young athletes with concussion can differ significantly.

Initial signs and symptoms of concussion in children as in adults can cross multiple domains of functioning, typically across four categories: physical (headache, neck pain, nausea, dizziness, and balance dysfunction), cognitive (memory, concentration), emotional (sadness, irritability), and sleep (drowsiness, difficulty falling asleep). Again, as with adults, severe or worsening signs or symptoms may indicate a devastating injury and features such as seizure, abnormal neurological exam, repeated vomiting, and worsening headaches would certainly warrant a prompt emergency department evaluation for imaging and possible intervention.

Immediate Assessment

Given similar signs and symptoms to adult concussion, a similar symptom checklist is often used in assessment. There is a younger child version of the often used Sports Concussion Assessment Tool (SCAT) [4, 5] that includes both a parent and child symptom checklist with modified language that is felt to be more child-friendly.

The sideline and/or locker room health care providers are charged with making decisions regarding whether it is appropriate for an individual to return to play (RTP). Essentially, these concussion clinicians rely on four key principles: symptom/history evaluation, balance assessment, cognitive/memory evaluation, and aspects of the neurological examination. The SCAT, now in its third version (SCAT-3), has become one of the more commonly used tools for immediate concussion assessment in athletes, employed in collegiate and high school athletic settings as well as many professional and international athletic groups.

SCAT-3 has a pretest section that highlights the indications for seeking emergency care and states that any athlete with any signs/symptoms of concussion after any blow to the head should be immediately removed from competition and referred to a concussion specialist. The body of the test includes the Glasgow Coma Scale (GCS) score and orientation questions followed by a symptom assessment. This is followed by Maddock's questions (five well-established questions used to assess short-term memory and cognitive function ((1) Where are we? (2) What quarter is it right now? (3) Who scored last in the game/practice? (4) Who did we play in the last game? (5) Did we win the last game?), then the Standardized Assessment of Concussion (SAC: a tool to assess orientation, immediate memory. and concentration), a balance assessment test (Balance Error Scoring System: BESS) [6], and coordination testing. SCAT-3 also incorporates an examination of the neck/cervical spine, which is a modification from prior versions.

As spoken to above, there is a Child SCAT [5] test recommended for athletes 5–12 years of age aimed at addressing the difficulties with self-reporting in this age group, whether it be a result of misinterpretation of symptoms or a lack of appreciation. In addition there are child-friendly modifications to the Maddock's questions and SAC portion. SCAT-3 is used for children 13 years and older. The precursor, SCAT-2, had been standardized as an easy-to-use tool with adequate psychometric properties for identifying concussions within the first seven days. Normative data for Child SCAT and SCAT-3 are not yet available.

Pediatric Vulnerability

One difference that should be considered as a contributor to an increased vulnerability to concussion in pediatric patients is the relative size of the head compared to the rest of the body. The heads of most children reach 90% that of an adult between the ages of three and six years; however, the cervical strength and tone are not even close to that of an adult. In certain sports this mismatch is further added to by additional helmet weight and so it is not difficult to appreciate a problem with head stability and amplified brain acceleration/deceleration following an impact to a child's head or body.

Another thing to consider with regard to the question of increased pediatric vulnerability is the degree of myelination. It is well known that white-matter myelination is incomplete throughout much of childhood and adolescence, with the frontal lobes representing some of the last regions to develop. Reeves et al. [7] demonstrated the vulnerability of unmyelinated axons in animal models to experimental TBI. Diffusion tensor imaging (DTI) has indicated white-matter changes after TBI and studies by Wilde et al. in 2008 [8] and Mayer et al. in 2012 [9] showed early and persistent changes in fractional anisotropy in children and adolescents after mild TBI (mTBI).

Acute Symptom Onset and Recovery

Although a rapid onset of neurological and cognitive sequelae is more common, acute post-concussive signs and symptoms are delayed in some cases and may take minutes to hours to emerge. Numerous, somewhat arbitrary, cut-offs have been assigned, after which new symptom onset is thought not to be directly related to the initial trauma. Here a distinction should be made between what is typical and what is biologically possible: pending the availability of valid and reliable biomarkers for human CBI, the spectrum of post-impact brain change in humans cannot be assessed with confidence.

It is known that some survivors of a single CBI will experience trivial symptoms in the immediate aftermath and decline to seek medical attention, only to subjectively experience injury-related symptoms after a delay of days. As previously discussed in this volume, it is also known that different symptoms tend to emerge at different times post CBI. For instance, a study by Eisenberg et al. [10] looked at questionnaires from 235 individuals aged 11–22 years presenting to the emergency room at Boston Children's Hospital. They found that, while headache, dizziness, and blurry vision often appear right after a concussion, emotional and mental symptoms such as irritability and frustration show up much later. In fact, numerous studies have shown that, when compared to adults, children appear more likely to experience a longer delay in the onset of symptoms.

For both practical and research purposes, however, it is useful to focus on the typical presentation of acute CBI so that one is discussing a relatively homogeneous condition. To that end, a stance has been adopted at UCLA based on much of the previously published animal data, in addition to a wealth of concussion clinic data, to assign a 24-hour cut-off for symptoms one can confidently attribute to the direct effects of the abrupt impact of a brain-rattling force. Thus, one criterion employed in estimating the degree of certainty of a concussion diagnosis in the UCLA clinic is "onset of symptoms within the first 24 hours." The point to be emphasized here is the importance of holding an athlete from RTP in the event of a suspected concussion.

The average time from injury to recovery and the proportion of concussion survivors with delayed recovery are topics of considerable controversy. As discussed in the chapters in this volume on epidemiology (Chapter 2) and on post-concussive brain change (Chapter 12), some evidence suggests that victims of SRC tend to recover more rapidly than victims of other injury types. The reason for this is unclear. Some evidence supports the hypothesis that the lower velocity of SRC permits quicker recovery. Some evidence suggests that athletes are more prone to deny symptoms than, for instance, victims of motor vehicle collisions due to their incentive to RTP. While the consensus statement from the 2012 International Conference on Concussion in Sport [11] reports that 80–90% of SRC recover within ten days, this is a generalized statement across all age groups. Varying rates of recovery, particularly in children and adolescents, have been reported, with multiple studies supporting a longer recovery timeframe, particularly in pediatric/teenage patients compared to adults.

Eisenberg et al.'s 2014 study [10] followed that same 11–22-year-old cohort through recovery; note was made that most recovered within two weeks of injury. However, 25% still suffered headaches, 20% noted continued fatigue, and 20% reported school work difficulties at the one-month mark.

Field et al. [12] looked at neurocognitive recovery patterns in 183 high school and 371 college athletes with a finding of prolonged memory dysfunction in the high school athletes. In an investigation of high school football players by Collins et al. [13] at least 25% of the group took up to four weeks to reach recovery criteria. Zuckerman et al. showed in a 2012 paper [14] that 13–16-year-olds showed a significantly longer time to return to baseline compared to 18–22-year-olds in three out of four neurocognitive measures (verbal memory, visual memory, and reaction time) and on the total symptom score following an SRC. Williams et al. [15] reported that neurocognitive recovery rates are similar among high school and college athletes, while symptom reporting shows longer recovery time points in high school than in college athletes.

Some data suggest that younger rodents exhibit a *shorter* post-injury hypometabolic period compared to adults [16]. That hypometabolic period has been attributed to a metabolic "mismatch" in which cellular needs exceed available energy due to a combination of compromised energy production and compromised substrate delivery. Yet other data suggest that the juvenile brain requires longer to recover – perhaps due to decreases in cerebral blood flow. The challenge has been in trying to identify this period of metabolic vulnerability on a reproducible basis in a clinical setting given the concerns surrounding premature repeat injuries.[2] There is evidence that even relatively asymptomatic (GCS 13–15) patients may demonstrate depressed glucose metabolism on positron emission tomography (PET) imaging following TBI [17]. In pediatric studies, cerebral blood flow (CBF) has been seen to increase during the first day following mild TBI, followed by decreased CBF for many days after [18]. fMRI studies have begun to examine blood oxygen level dependent brain activity following head impacts. Data comparing CBF in pediatric TBI patients have shown impaired autoregulation in 17% of mild injuries [19].

A more recent study by Maugans et al. in 2012 [20] reported that, in the early adolescent population, the decrease in normal CBF following a concussion is significantly prolonged as compared to adults. Chambers et al. [21] studied cerebral perfusion pressures following severe head injuries in children and reported critical threshold values below which secondary brain injury has a significant impact on the injured child's outcome for children aged 2–6, 7–10, and 11–15 years of 48, 54, and 58 mmHg respectively. This suggests that younger children may be better able to tolerate lower cerebral perfusion pressures and therefore suggests the possibility of better resistance to such dysregulation compared with older children and adults.

As described in the chapter on the neuroendocrinology of CBI (Chapter 26), acute activation of the hypothalamic–pituitary–adrenal axis has been shown to occur initially after brain injury. That activation has mixed effects. On the one hand, it seems to serve as a protective response that modulates the immune/inflammatory response and increases metabolic substrate availability, even with mild injuries [22]. On the other hand, the resulting generation of excess adrenal cortisol represents a potential threat to neurons, especially in hippocampus, and perhaps helps to account for both post-concussive depression and insomnia [23, 24]. (See Chapter 8 in this volume, titled *Emotional Disturbances Following Traumatic Brain Injury*.) Niederland et al. [25] reported a high risk for hypopituitarism in children hospitalized with TBI independent of severity and in the absence of obvious clinical symptoms. Recently, Zhou [26] employed fMRI and diffusion kurtosis imaging (DKI) to study hypothalamic connectivity after mild TBI in young adults. Both structural and functional abnormalities were reported, which may contribute to the elevated prevalence of hypopituitarism. As discussed in this volume's chapter *Neuroendocrine Dysfunction Following Concussion: A Missed Opportunity for Enhancing Recovery?* (Chapter 26), the risk of the two most common resulting persistent endocrinopathies – growth hormone deficiency and hypogonadism – are both age- and body mass-dependent.

Repeat Injury Risk

Multiple studies have shown that there is an increased risk of a repeat concussion after an initial injury. For instance, Gessel et al. [27] reported that high school athletes who have been concussed are three times more likely to suffer another concussion in the same season. Marar et al. [28] reported that between 11.5% and 13.2% of concussions among high school athletes are recurrent. Schulz et al. [29] reported that a history of head injury is an independent risk factor for concussion, with a relative risk between 2.04 and 2.28 in athletes who have sustained a previous concussion. And a seminal, prospective cohort study of 2905 college football players published in 2003 by Guskiewicz et al. [30] suggested that players with a history of previous concussions are more likely to have future concussive injuries.

The reasons for this phenomenon are not entirely clear. However, examining some of the proposed consequences of multiple concussions may offer some insight. For example, Schatz et al. [31] reported that high school students with a history of two or more concussions continue to report significantly more physical, cognitive, and sleep-related symptoms at "baseline" than students with a history of one or no concussions.[3] Brooks et al. [32] found that male adolescent football players with three or more prior concussions reported more symptoms than did athletes with no or one prior injury. New evidence also suggests that hypothalamic injury caused

---

[2] The term *premature* is used in reference to a subsequent CBI early in the course of neurometabolic recovery after the first concussion – a time during which neurons seem to be exquisitely vulnerable to synergistic effects leading to persistent dysfunction. That period is sometimes referred to as the *window of vulnerability*.

[3] One might quibble with the meaning of "baseline" in the Schatz study, given the clear presence of symptoms. But that raises a larger question: since many student athletes have played sports for a decade prior to their first high school concussion, and many have probably suffered childhood closed head injuries, it may be more accurate to refer to "baseline" testing as pre-season testing.

by concussion is associated with increased daytime sleepiness [33]. Such findings suggest the possibility of increased vulnerability on the field, perhaps due to impaired attention or slowed reaction time.

It also deserves consideration whether the published epidemiological data regarding repeat concussions is accurate. A major problem in the study of SRC is that no good way exists to confirm self-reported history of prior concussions. Many studies suggest that underreporting of concussion symptoms by youth athletes is common. There has recently been a focus on identifying the reasons behind non-reporting in hopes of overcoming this behavior – especially in view of the mounting evidence that repeat concussions during a period of neurobiological vulnerability are associated with worse outcome.

The systematic underreporting of post-concussion symptoms has been thought to be primarily a function of motivated behavior on the part of the athletes. Yet a lack of understanding of the injury and differences in self-reporting data acquisition may also be factors.

McCrea et al. [34] conducted a retrospective confidential survey on 1532 varsity football players at the end of a season. They found a higher prevalence of concussion than previously reported in the literature and, of those reporting a history of concussion, only 47.3% had reported their injury. The most common reasons put forth for not reporting included a player not thinking the injury was serious enough to warrant medical attention, motivation not to be withheld from competition, and lack of awareness of probable concussion. Work by Williamson and Goodman [35] found that concussions were considerably underreported to the British Columbia Amateur Hockey Association by youth hockey players and team personnel. A study by Bramley et al. [36] evaluated the likelihood that high school soccer players would identify themselves as having concussion-related symptoms during game situations with a questionnaire inquiring about past concussion education and the likelihood of notifying their coach of concussion symptoms: 72% of players who reported having previously received concussion training stated they would always alert their coach to CBI symptoms, whereas only 36% of players without such training stated they would do so.

Register-Mihalik et al. [37] also examined the influence of knowledge and attitude on concussion-reporting behaviors in a cross-sectional study of 167 high school male and female athletes participating in football, soccer, lacrosse, or cheerleading. Only 40% of concussion events and 13% of "bell-ringer"-recalled events in the sample were disclosed after possible concussive injury. Increased athlete knowledge of concussion topics (assessed with a series of 35 questions concerning symptom recognition, complications related to multiple concussions, and general knowledge of concussion) was associated with increased reporting prevalence occurring in practice. Studies such as these further highlight the importance of concussion education, which is now mandated in many states.

In addition to the number of concussions an individual has sustained, the time interval between concussions and progressively less impact force needed to cause a clinically significant injury are likely important factors to be considered in the risk

for and resulting severity of subsequent concussions. In prospective studies, the risk of repeat concussion appears greatest in the first ten days post injury [30, 38]. That finding is of particular concern because, as animal models have highlighted, a repeat injury within the window of cerebral vulnerability after a prior concussion compounds the negative effects. Prins et al., for example, reported in their 2013 study [39] of a closed head impact model in juvenile rats that, when a second injury occurred within the period of impaired glucose metabolism, the severity of hypometabolism and memory impairment was greater. However, if the injury occurred after full metabolic recovery from the first injury, the second impact acted like a single separate injury with a similar recovery time.

Second Impact Syndrome

The idea that a devastating head injury may occur after repetitive head traumas within a short temporal window was reported as early as 1973. Richard Schneider [40] reported that two young athletes died after sustaining a concussive head injury followed by a second minor head injury. Following the publication of further reports of possible examples, in 1984 Saunders and Harbaugh [41] called that phenomenon *second impact syndrome* (SIS). It has been hypothesized that the syndrome results from a loss of autoregulation of CBF causing vascular engorgement and brain herniation as a result of repeat concussion occurring while the person is still symptomatic from – or still experiencing significant metabolic compromise from – an initial concussion. Catecholamine and glutamate surges have been suggested as critical components driving the rapid cerebral edema. Although abundant evidence from rodent studies confirms that early re-injury is associated with worse outcome, the existence of SIS in humans has been repeatedly questioned because evidence has relied on case reports and the risk factors have not been consistently supported or established. Despite these questions, most concussion specialists acknowledge the rare risk of cerebral edema after CBI and consider this when making RTP recommendations. A recent systematic review addresses aspects of the definition of SIS and suggests it should be limited to cases with catastrophic brain injury and not simply worsened symptoms after repeated CBI [42].

Prolonged Recovery

Certain initial symptom profiles have been put forward as being predictive of longer recovery times. For instance, Meehan et al. [43] reported that severity of acute symptoms better predicted prolonged recovery than did either age or duration of amnesia. Lau et al. [44, 45] showed that athletes who had more symptoms in the cognitive or migraine symptom clusters often required more recovery time. Makdissi et al. [46] showed that prolonged headaches (> 60 h), three or more symptoms at initial presentation, and the presence of fatigue/fogginess were associated with a longer recovery. A study by Iverson et al. [47] looking at concussion in high school athletes found that subjective "fogginess" was related to increased symptom scores, lower memory functioning, slower processing and reaction time as compared with those who did not experience this symptom.

Lovell et al. [48] reported that the duration of on-field mental status changes such as retrograde amnesia and post-traumatic confusion was related to the presence of memory impairment at 36 h, four days, and seven days post injury and was also related to slower resolution of self-reported symptoms in high school athletes. Collins et al. [49] found that the presence of retrograde amnesia in adolescent athletes was associated with higher overall symptom score and decreased neurocognitive data acutely post injury. Others have reported that anterograde amnesia may be an important indicator of more serious injury in pediatric athletes.

Yet the previously cited studies by Meehan et al. [43] and Lau et al. [45] found that amnesia was not predictive of protracted recovery. The study by Meehan et al. [43] found that only the total post-concussive symptom score was independently associated with symptoms lasting longer than 28 days.

Amnesia does, however, remain a "modifying" factor for predicting the potential prolonged symptoms, according to the 4th International Conference on Concussion in Sport, 2012 [11]. Likewise, the 2013 American Academy of Neurology's evidence-based guidelines for the evaluation and management of concussion in sports include early amnesia among the probable risk factors for persistent neurocognitive problems or prolonged RTP [50].

Perhaps the most reliable predictor of prolonged recovery or persistent symptoms is a history of previous CBI (for review, see [50]; also see [30, 51, 52]. Slobounov et al. [53], for example, studied recovery of symptoms and balance in a cohort of 160 collegiate athletes. Thirty-eight suffered CBI, of whom nine suffered a second concussion. All concussed athletes had resolution of their symptoms within ten days, but imbalance persisted for at least 30 days (more evidence that resolution of symptoms is not a valid indicator of brain recovery). Moreover, athletes who had suffered a second injury exhibited reduced restoration of balance. Those authors concluded: "athletes with a history of previous concussion demonstrate significantly slower rates of recovery of neurological functions after the second episode of MTBI" [53].

As with adult patients, pre-morbid mood disorders, migraine, and learning and attention disorders have been proposed to predispose to an increased chance of concussion and also increase the likelihood of persistent symptoms. Such conditions can share common features, with concussions making diagnosis and management in these individuals more challenging. When evaluating an athlete it is often difficult to determine which symptoms preceded the concussion, which have been caused by the concussion, and which symptoms are worsened after the concussion, highlighting a benefit of baseline testing.

As discussed in the chapter on persistent post-concussive psychiatric problems (Chapter 10), depression is by far the most common non-cognitive behavioral complication of CBI. Symptoms of anxiety, depression, or irritability occur in 17–46% of high school and college athletes [54]. Although no evidence has been published to date suggesting that pre-existing mood disorder predisposes athletes to concussion, it is not difficult to see how such symptoms could complicate the recovery process. Retrospective studies have shown an increased incidence of depression to be associated with a history of concussion among retired boxers and professional football players. Chrisman and Richardson [55] showed in a large nationally representative adolescent data set that a history of concussion was associated with a higher prevalence of diagnosed depression. Vargas et al. [56] found several predictors of post-concussion depression symptoms in concussed athletes over those without a history of recent concussion, including baseline post-concussion symptoms, estimated pre-morbid intelligence, and age of first participation in organized sport. Baseline depression symptoms and number of previous concussions were predictors in both groups. Covassin et al. [57] reported that high school and college athletes with severe depression report more concussion symptoms than athletes with minimal and moderate depression scores, and Chamelian and Feinstein [58] found that mild to moderate TBI patients had persisting cognitive dysfunction that was linked to co-morbid major depression. Clinicians should be routinely screening for depression in their adolescent patients with concussion.

Studies suggest that up to 5% of the pediatric population in the United States experience migraine, with a mean age of onset for boys of seven years and 11 years for girls. The prevalence of migraine increases during the adolescent and young-adult years and, following menarche, a female predominance occurs, continuing to increase until middle age [59]. Gordon et al. [60] showed an association between a concussion and pre-existing migraine in a retrospective population study; however, such association is not clear and has not been reproduced. Studies looking at pre-existing migraine have not shown an association with prolonged course of concussion recovery; however, migrainous symptoms as part of the post-concussion symptom set are associated with a prolonged recovery period.

Lau and colleagues [61] reported that patients with higher somatic symptom scores that include migraine-like symptoms in the first days following a concussion were more likely to have a protracted recovery. Heyer et al. [62] reported that post-traumatic headache correlates strongly with other migraine symptoms among youth with concussion, regardless of pre-morbid headaches. This clustering of migraine symptoms supports the existence of post-traumatic migraine as a distinct clinical entity in some patients.

Akinbami et al. [63] reported the prevalence of attention deficit-hyperactivity disorder (ADHD) among children aged five to 17 years in the United States to be about 9.0% as of 2009. The increased prevalence in boys is well established. Numerous older studies reported that children with ADHD are more likely to be injured than children without ADHD in free-play activities, attributing this to them anticipating fewer negative consequences, expecting less severe injury, and reporting greater likelihood of participating in risky behavior. DiScala et al. [64] reported that five- to 14-year-old children with ADHD were more likely to have severe head injuries than children without ADHD.

There are some more recent studies looking at the association with milder head injuries. A study by Alosco et al. [65] on 139 National Collegiate Athletic Association (NCAA) Division

I athletes showed that athletes with ADHD were more likely to report a past history of concussions than those without ADHD. A large-scale retrospective survey published in 2016 by Iverson et al. [66] showed that high school-aged boys and girls with ADHD were significantly more likely to report a history of concussion. Such data are not too surprising given that individuals with low attention levels may be more prone to participate in fast-paced, unpredictable sports, therefore increasing the opportunity for head injury, including concussions.

Although Lau et al. [61] found no association between learning disability or attention deficit disorder and protracted recovery in 108 concussed athletes, Bonfield et al. did in their 2013 study [67]. They reviewed the charts of all patients with diagnosis of mTBI as a result of closed head injury and ADHD admitted to the hospital between 2003 and 2010, and compared them to a control group of patients admitted with a diagnosis of closed head injury without ADHD. Patients with ADHD were statistically significantly more disabled after mild TBI than were control patients without ADHD, even when controlling for age, sex, initial GCS score, hospital length of stay, length of follow-up, mechanism of injury, and presence of other (extracranial) injury.

Sex Differences

Sex differences in the age-related incidence of SRC were introduced in this volume's chapter on epidemiology (Chapter 2). However, several observations deserve clarification and expansion. A 2009 review by Dick [68] looking at sport concussion by sex suggested that in sports with similar rules female athletes sustain more concussions than their male counterparts. A particular concern pertains to ice hockey – the sport associated with the greatest risk of SRC for high school girls. The relatively weaker neck of female athletes compared to male athletes may contribute in part, although other factors for higher concussion rates in females may include hormonal differences, symptom reporting, higher rates of co-morbidities (i.e., migraine, anxiety) and possibly even implicit bias in health care providers.

As previously discussed, there also is mixed evidence that sex differences exist in outcomes of concussions, such that female athletes tend to report a higher number and severity of symptoms with a longer duration of recovery. Again, reports of higher incidence among menstruating girls and women suggest that hormones play a role, but which hormones? As explained in this volume's chapter on *Why Outcomes Vary* (Chapter 7), there exists a mysterious inconsistency between the rodent and human literature. Estrogen and progesterone may be neuroprotective in experimental models of TBI, although even in animals these effects are complex. One clinical study found cycling women at higher risk for persistent post-concussive symptoms than non-cycling women and – reflecting the challenging interactions between hormones and mTBI – they are most vulnerable during the luteal phase when progesterone is *higher*. As noted in the epidemiology chapter (Chapter 2), Wunderle et al. [69] found that women (aged 16–60 years) suffering mTBI during the luteal phase of their menstrual cycle

had lower quality-of-life and worse neurologic outcomes at one month compared with women injured during the follicular phase of their cycle or women taking oral contraceptives. Women injured in the two weeks following their period fared better, as well as women taking birth control pills. Another suggestion that hormones may explain the apparent gender difference in recovery from concussion is that persons with early migraine symptoms tend to have a protracted recovery and there is a known female predominance of migraine in adolescent and young adults.

One possible clue to excess female morbidity pertains to sex differences in the relative rates of different post-concussive symptoms. For instance, a recent study by Ono et al. [70] evaluated sex-based differences as a predictor of recovery trajectories using baseline and post-concussion Immediate Post-Concussion Assessment and Cognitive Testing (ImPACT) assessment in 135 male and 41 female high-impact sport athletes (10–18 years in age). Results revealed that male and female adolescent athletes recover to baseline at the same rate and exhibit similar recovery patterns. However, results indicated that female athletes experience higher rates of symptoms at baseline and throughout return to baseline (i.e., recovery), particularly for somatic and emotional symptoms. As previously discussed, one possible explanation for the higher rate of emotional post-concussive symptoms among females is increased sensitivity to the trauma-related surge in cortisol. Also during adolescence, the baseline rates of depression are greater among females than among males [71]. Further study is needed to understand how gender and hormone status affect the risk of CBI, the neurobiological effects of CBI, the rate of symptom reporting, and the possibility of late effects.

Post-Concussion Symptoms (PCS)

The understanding of the natural history of concussion is rapidly evolving. During the 20th century it was often stated that typical concussions (then often called "mild traumatic brain injuries") resolved within three months. That claim was largely based on self-report and meta-analyses of neuropsychological studies. More recently, it has become clear that neuropsychological testing alone has limitations when examining effects of concussion, and many advanced neuroimaging studies have demonstrated that longer-persisting brain changes – of unclear significance – are common. Similarly, older published estimates of the proportion of individuals with persistent symptoms from a concussion in the range of 10–15% have been overthrown by systematic reviews suggesting the true rate is more than 40% (although the prevalence of persistent neurobehavioral problems is suspected to be lower after SRC, possibly due to the lower average velocity, not just athletes' notorious tendency to underreport. See this volume's Chapters 5 and 7 regarding human post-concussive brain change).

What might cause confusion is the fact that, historically, both the DSM system [72] and the ICD system [73] promoted the notion of a "post-concussive syndrome" despite the lack of evidence supporting that nosological concept. As explained in this volume's chapters *What Happens to Concussed Humans?*

and *Why Outcomes Vary* (Chapters 5 and 7), analysis of the available data demonstrates that no unitary "post-concussive syndrome" occurs. Instead, each PCS seems to follow its own natural history, and each patient seems to express his or her own dynamic symptom clusters, such that the precise combination and degree of symptoms are heterogeneous, ever-changing, and infinitely variable during the months after injury. The dated term "syndrome" is long overdue for abandonment.

PCS are often subtle and difficult to link directly to the head trauma. In the 20th century, some researchers hypothesized that early PCS were more likely to be "organic," whereas symptoms that persist for months were described as having a "non-organic" or "psychological" basis. As previously discussed in this volume, the organic/functional distinction is a false dichotomy. It is impossible to determine to what extent a given persistent symptom reflects persistent brain change directly or secondarily attributable to the rattling impact of external force, pre-morbid genetic or psychological vulnerabilities, psychological reaction to injury (which also changes the brain), or – most likely – the interaction of all these factors. In any case, the observable behavior is always the product of organic processes. And, in fact, many recent studies have demonstrated that individuals complaining of PCS may show neurological differences from controls, as demonstrated by abnormal functional neuroimaging, neurochemical imbalances, and/or electrophysiological indices of impairment.

In a dubious advance, the American Psychiatric Association's *Diagnostic and Statistical Manual of Mental Disorders*, Fifth Edition (DSM-V) [74] now refers to a condition called "neurocognitive disorder due to traumatic brain injury." The good news is that this revision abandons the misleading term *syndrome* and acknowledges the biological etiology. The bad news is the unjustifiable focus on "cognitive" troubles rather than on the authentic spectrum of behavioral and somatic symptoms that are more likely to be disabling after CBI.[4] The newly proposed putative disorder no longer requires the presence of three symptoms or the three-month symptom persistence of DSM-IV. To meet criteria, there must be evidence of a TBI with one or more of the following: loss of consciousness, post-traumatic amnesia, disorientation and confusion, or neurological signs. The so-called "neurocognitive disorder" must present immediately after the occurrence of the TBI or immediately after recovery of consciousness and persist past the acute post-injury period. ICD-10, in contrast, continues to refer to a "post-concussional syndrome" [75]. That supposed entity has no temporal specification.

Whatever the underlying biopsychosocial processes, a substantial number of concussion survivors exhibit long-term cognitive and non-cognitive neurobehavioral problems. A consensus seems to have emerged to the effect that patients whose symptoms remain problematic for more than three months might be characterized as having prolonged recovery or persistent PCS (PPCS). Barlow et al. [76], for example, investigated the epidemiology and natural history of PCS in a large cohort of children with mTBI. In a 2016 review, that author reported that between 14% and 29% of children with mTBI will continue to have PCS at three months. Despite such high numbers progressing to this syndrome, the long-term outcome in most children is good [77].

Not surprisingly, many of the things thought to result in a worsened or more prolonged concussion recovery are thought to be risk factors for PPCS. Chapter 7 in this volume, titled *Why Outcomes Vary*, summarizes the strength of the published evidence for a large number of potential risk factors. For instance, increasing age (all comers) has been suggested as a risk factor for PPCS after sport-related concussion. As a group, individuals who have sustained SRCs are less likely to progress to PPCS than other concussion groups. Again, it remains unclear to what extent this reflects a biological difference versus a difference in incentives for reporting related to sports.

To date, no firm consensus has emerged regarding which of the various PCS measures has the best predictive validity after pediatric SRC [78]. By far the most widely employed self-report scale is the Rivermead Post Concussion Symptoms Questionnaire [79]. However, that instrument was not designed for children or for SRC. A graded symptom checklist is included as a stand-alone component of the SAC [30, 80, 81] and intended for the assessment of SRC in the emergency department. A factorial analysis concluded that nine common symptoms could be explained by three factors: somatic symptoms, neurobehavioral symptoms, and "cognitive" symptoms [82]. Evidence suggests that this checklist is reliable in pediatric patients presenting to emergency departments [83]. However, that instrument is intended as an acute survey and does not seem appropriate for persistent problems.

Lovell et al. [84, 85] developed a sport-concussion-oriented instrument called the Post-Concussion Scale (PC Scale) based on responses from young men and women athletes. Evidence suggesting the validity of that scale was found in a study by Chen et al. [86], who reported correlations between PC Scale results, persistent cognitive impairment, and abnormalities of CBF. The PC Scale, however, is not directly applicable to pediatric cases.

When Gioia et al. reviewed the utility of five measures for pediatric concussion symptoms in 2009 [87], those authors reported disappointing validity and reliability. Some progress seems to have been made. The Child SCAT-3 [5, 88, 89] is a new instrument and limited data are available regarding its use [90, 91].

In another recent review, Gioia [92] discussed the challenge of assessing PCS in children and the utility of two instruments: the Acute Concussion Evaluation (ACE) [93] and the Post-Concussion Symptom Inventory (PCSI) [94].

---

[4] Editor's note: as addressed in this volume's Chapter 9 (*Concussion and the 21st Century Renaissance of Neuropsychology*), TBI scholarship is still suffering in the throes of a 20th-century error that narrowly characterized the effects of concussions as "cognitive" and mistakenly claimed that the relevant brain changes could be detected via desktop paper-and-pencil tests. That error plausibly originated, in part, in a professional guild's effort to monopolize reimbursable assessment. Modern neuropsychologists deserve praise for having forthrightly discredited that dated dogma.

The PCSI is a revision of Lovell et al.'s. PC Scale, but explicitly designed to offer age-appropriate probes. A five-symptom PCSI is available for five- to seven-year-old children, a 17-item PCSI is available for eight- to 12-year-olds, and a 20-item adolescent PCSI is available for 13–18-year-olds – in addition to a 21-item form for parents. The combination of these two instruments permits assessment over the course of recovery. Further research is needed to clarify the optimum approach to assessment and to determine the biological significance and predictive validity of individual items and overall scores.

Multiple studies have attempted to identify early predictors of PPCS. Sheedy et al. [95], for example, reported that a simple test in the emergency department of immediate and delayed memory for five words and a visual analog scale for acute headache yielded an 80% sensitivity and 76% specificity for the subsequent development of PPCS. Other studies have found that higher educational levels, along with mild symptoms and no extracranial symptoms, predict a low likelihood of significant dysfunction from PPCS. Peterson et al. [96] reported that parent psychiatric symptoms predicted internalizing symptoms in children with brain injuries, and Raj et al. [97] reported that parental psychological functioning and communication factors have explained externalizing behaviors after pediatric TBI, independent of injury severity.

Zemek et al. [98] recently conducted a prospective observational study attempting to derive and validate a clinical risk score for PPCS among children presenting to the emergency department within 48 h of concussion. They identified nine factors that are easily obtainable from the history and physical examination that were highly associated with PPCS. The strongest risk factors were female sex, age of 13 years or older, migraine history, previous concussion with symptoms lasting longer than one week, headache, sensitivity to noise, fatigue, answering questions slowly, and four or more errors on the BESS balance assessment. The primary outcome was PPCS risk score at 28 days defined by three or more new or worsening symptoms using the patient PCS inventory. Among the 3063 patients included in the study, 801 (31%) had PPCS, which was comparable with the estimate of 33% given by most pediatric emergency departments. Their nine-factor model was found to have fair ability to predict PPCS and the authors generated a 12-point scoring regimen with three proposed levels of risk that could help guide the emergency department physician in a discussion of possible expectations with a patient and his or her family.

A study by Ayr et al. [99] looking at parent/child agreement regarding the dimensions of PPCS found that the symptoms reported by parents and children were similar when ratings involve cognitive and somatic symptoms but are somewhat less consistent for emotional symptoms and not similar for behavioral symptoms.

It is clear that many factors affect the trajectory of recovery. The main difficulty in predicting PPCS stems from the fact that recovery and impact on later development of a child are highly individualized. That is, the course of recovery is uniquely shaped not only by injury-related factors (nature of injury and developmental status of child), but by many personal and family variables (e.g., pre-injury genetic, cognitive, and psychological status of the child, family functioning and resources, and coping style) [100].

Concussion and Cognitive Development

In the 20th century many authorities opined that having a younger brain at the time of injury was a protective factor with regard to long-term recovery. That belief derived, in part, from work by Margaret Kennard, who in 1936 [101] articulated the observation from her studies in primates that young brains reorganize more effectively than adult brains. This supported the then-popular notion that the brain develops during a critical period in early childhood and remains relatively static thereafter. Numerous studies have subsequently been conducted investigating developmental neuroplasticity. Towards the end of the 20th century, research revealed that many aspects of the brain remain dynamic and changeable even into adulthood [102, 103]. Contrary to late-20th-century opinions, numerous studies have indicated that brain injuries acquired in early childhood exhibit a pattern of poorer functional outcomes. In contrast to the chronic effects in adults, TBI in young children impacts development of cognitive abilities with impairments of attention, memory, processing speed, and executive functions that may not become apparent until a child has reached certain developmental milestones.

Brain maturation is not a linear process. Periods of increased brain development activity have been reported. Crowe et al. [104] reported that an injury in middle childhood (ages seven to nine years) may be associated with the worst cognitive outcomes compared with children of other ages – a finding that perhaps suggests a critical period of brain and cognitive development around this age. Spencer-Smith and Anderson [105] reported a peak in myelination between age seven and nine and another peak between the ages of ten and 12. The possibility of a peri-pubertal critical period has been supported by more recent studies of rodent brain development reporting that the onset of puberty corresponds with marked cortical reorganization [106] – findings that may conceivably help to account for both the vulnerability and the resilience of adolescent athletes.

A childhood TBI can not only affect the level of previously achieved function but can potentially impact the course and rate of future cognitive development. Attention deficits may interfere with learning and acquisition of new knowledge, both within the school environment as well as outside it, which could contribute to global cognitive deficits in the long term following childhood TBI. The question is how often and to what degree a typical concussion triggers such deleterious effects.

Catroppa and Anderson [107] described a dose–response relationship such that those sustaining mild TBI only exhibited minimal attentional changes, and a meta-analysis by Babikian and Asarnow. [108] reported that children with mild head injuries showed negligible attention deficits and small effects for processing speed post-injury initially, with considerable improvement in processing speed by two years. Findings from Catroppa et al. [109] indicated that attentional skills that were in process of development at the time of injury were more vulnerable and that following injury these skills might not develop at a rate comparable to that of typically developing children.

There also appears to be a relationship between memory impairments and severity of brain injury, with numerous studies, including the meta-analysis by Babikian and Asarnow [108], reporting that children with mild head injuries showed minimal memory deficits post injury and this plus time post injury are significant predictors of memory performance. Earlier age has been reported to relate to relatively poorer memory performance in the chronic stage of TBI recovery after severe TBI; however such a relation has not been observed in milder TBI.

Babikian et al. [110] reported that children with mild head injuries showed negligible to small deficits in working memory and problem solving post injury compared to those with more severe head trauma. As a group, children with mild head injuries show greater improvement in problem solving and working-memory performance at two years post injury and beyond which may reflect relative retained ability to make gains from practice effects.

One of the main brain regions concerned with executive functions is the prefrontal cortex. It is known to be one of the last cortical regions to mature during normal development and many believe that the prefrontal cortex is not fully developed until the early to mid-20s. Anderson et al. [111] reported evidence that pre-injury ability is a significant predictor of executive functioning and functional skills in the wake of a brain injury with poorer outcomes for children who did not develop certain cognitive skills prior to injury. Ewing-Cobbs et al. [112] reported evidence that skills that are in a rapid stage of development are relatively more vulnerable to the effects of TBI, which would suggest greater vulnerability for executive function and attention problems in childhood compared to such an injury in adults.

When the cognitive functions discussed above are undermined for an extended period for any reason it is not surprising that there are often co-morbid learning and behavioral changes. Those might be expected to increase throughout childhood, given the escalation of academic and social challenges. Numerous studies have shown that emotion and cognition are profoundly interrelated processes. Cacioppo and Gardner [113] reported that emotion and cognition work together, jointly informing the child's impressions of situations and influencing behavior and together, emotion and cognition contribute to attentional processes, decision making, and learning.

Persistent Post-Concussive Psychiatric Symptoms

Many studies have investigated chronic psychiatric symptoms following pediatric concussion. For example, Massagli et al. [114] conducted a cohort study of 490 children who experienced an mTBI before age 14 and who had no prior history of psychiatric illness. The authors reported that these children were significantly more likely to have psychiatric issues in

the three years following injury than were uninjured controls. It has been proposed however that children more likely to experience concussions are also more likely to have undiagnosed psychiatric issues, an observation that complicates this finding. In the Massagli study the children most commonly presented with attentional problems in the first year following injury. However, no difference was observed in children who had a history of psychiatric illness in the year preceding the injury.

McKinlay et al. [115] studied 1265 children from a longitudinal birth cohort and found that those with a history of hospital admission for mTBI before age five were significantly more likely to show symptoms of ADHD, conduct disorder/oppositional defiant disorder, substance abuse, and mood disorder at age 14–16 years. Taylor et al. [114] reported that children aged eight to 15 years with mTBI are at risk for persistent symptoms of behavior problems, especially if mTBI is more severe or occurs at a younger age.

Social relationships are particularly important during adolescence and this is also a time when individuals are developing a "sense of self." Traumatic disruption of regions, including the prefrontal cortex and posterior cingulate, may interrupt the development of these functional domains and can cause chronic problems in overall quality of life that may continue into adulthood. Again, the timing of an injury in the child's developmental history may be a critical factor in determining the outcome. Given the growing evidence that, contrary to the 20th-century paradigm of concussion as a temporary problem, a CBI may trigger a cascade of biological and psychosocial changes, which, particularly if repetitive, may have profound long-term consequences, it behooves us to improve prevention, prompt diagnosis, and development of efficacious interventions.

Office Assessment and Neuropsychological Evaluation

As discussed in this volume's chapter titled *Concussion and the 21st Century Renaissance of Neuropsychology* (Chapter 9), in the late 20th century, neuropsychological assessment came to be regarded as an important aspect of the diagnosis and management of persistent PCS. Multiple consensus guidelines have advised that neuropsychological testing be part of the multidisciplinary approach to concussion.

Neuropsychological tests comprise a heterogeneous suite of desktop psychological assessments, originally administered with paper and pencil and now often including computerized administration and scoring. Although they were originally developed in the hope of non-invasively detecting brain lesions, validation studies have had mixed results. Nevertheless, decades of refinement and clinical pathological correlation have clarified what such tests can and cannot achieve. By standardizing the stimuli or cognitive challenges presented to patients and comparing results with those of large databases, the neuropsychologist may expertly measure multiple domains of cerebral/cognitive activity from the most basic – such as motor coordination and reaction time – to complex aspects of higher cortical function such as language, reasoning, and executive function. Evidence suggests that such formal testing is more reliable and sensitive than the typical bedside examination in the detection of cognitive strengths and weaknesses. Abundant evidence suggests that typical concussion patients will exhibit measurable abnormalities on such testing, especially within the first days or weeks post injury. In addition to assessing current cognitive status and generating scores to serve as a reference point or baseline against which to compare future scores post concussion, test results are also helpful in identifying pre-existing conditions that may complicate the interpretation of post-concussion test scores. For instance, a background of attention deficit disorder, depression, or anxiety disorders may conflate or significantly skew test results. Detecting such conditions may help explain prolonged recovery and help individualize rehabilitation.

Testing should be used only as part of a comprehensive concussion management strategy and not in isolation. The ideal time for testing has yet to be determined. For example, testing in the first few days will predictably be abnormal, but may not be the best guide to neurorehabilitation because the identified deficits may vanish shortly thereafter. Testing at three months will usually result in "normal" scores, but that sometimes leads to a false sense of resolution since traditional tests may fail to detect subtle ongoing cerebral problems responsible for the patient's complaints. In view of the heterogeneity of CBI effects and recovery, the best time and need for testing probably vary on a case-by-case basis. Clinical judgment helps estimate when detailed information about the patient's cognitive status is most likely to assist in decisions regarding return to activities or treatment planning.

Traditional paper-and-pencil neuropsychological tests are designed to assess various domains of cognitive functioning and can assist clinicians in estimating the severity of the injury and eliminating some of the guesswork regarding the underlying cause of observed functional impairments. Tests sometimes used include the Hopkins Verbal Learning Test, Trail Making: Parts A and B, the Wechsler Letter Number Sequencing Test, the Wechsler Digit Span, and the Stroop Color Word Test. Symptom validity or response bias testing helps to confirm whether patients are giving their best effort. Instruments such as the Test of Memory Malingering have become popular for this purpose, but validity measures are also embedded in certain standard tests.

More recently, computer-generated neuropsychological test programs have been developed, and some are currently being validated in the sports setting. The rapid scoring, ease of administration, and greater accessibility are considered advantages over more traditional neuropsychological tests. Many have significant variety of test questions aimed at increasing the test–retest reliability and reducing practice effects. They include the now fairly widely used ImPACT [117]. This was developed at the University of Pittsburgh Medical Center. Other tests include the CogStat Brief Battery [118], the Computerized Cognitive Assessment Tool [119], the Concussion Resolution Index [120], the Automated Neuropsychological Assessment Metrics [121], and Concussion Vital Signs [122].

ImPACT has become a commonly used tool for baseline assessment and to track recovery following a concussion. Schatz et al. [123] explored the diagnostic utility of the composite scores of ImPACT in recently concussed high school athletes within 72 h of sustaining a concussion compared to non-concussed high school athletes with no history of concussion. They found the sensitivity to be 81.9%, and the specificity 89.4%. They concluded that ImPACT is a useful tool as part of a formal concussion management program and can provide post-injury cognitive and symptom data that can assist a practitioner in making safer RTP decisions. In a 2013 paper [124] Schatz and Sandel revisited this, looking at sensitivity and specificity of the online version in high school and collegiate athletes, and reported high levels of sensitivity and specificity, even when athletes appear to be denying PCS. The test–retest reliability has been shown to be somewhat inconsistent and Lichtenstein et al. [125] reported that younger athletes tend to exhibit a greater prevalence of invalid baseline results on ImPACT than older youth athletes.

Iverson et al. [126] examined the test–retest reliability over a seven-day time span using a sample of 56 non-concussed children (average age of 17.6 years). There was a significant difference between the first and seven-day retest on the processing speed composite, with 68% of the sample performing better on the seven-day retest than at the first test session.

Miller et al. [127] conducted a test–retest study over a longer time period (four months) with 58 Division III college football players. The results indicated no significant differences in verbal memory or in processing speed but significant improvements for visual memory and reaction time over three testing occasions (pre-, mid-, and post-season).

Elbin et al. [128] investigated a one-year test–retest reliability of the online version of ImPACT using baseline data from 369 high school varsity athletes with results indicating that motor processing speed was actually the most stable composite score and Post-Concussion Symptom Scale (PCSS) was least stable. Nakayama et al. [129] examined the test–retest reliability of ImPACT in 85 physically active college students using baseline, 45-day, and 50-day scores with findings that suggest that the ImPACT is a reliable neurocognitive test battery for this timeframe after the baseline assessment. Such findings agree with those of other studies that have reported acceptable intra-class correlation coefficients across 30-day to one-year testing intervals. Nonetheless, a recent systematic review supported convergent validity of this test; however, many other factors were found to influence not only validity but utility of ImPACT scores [130].

An intuitive key to any successful concussion testing program is having valid results from pre-season baseline testing for comparison to post-injury results. Baseline testing is becoming more commonplace. While a decade ago it was only seen at the professional and college level, it is becoming more common in high school-level sports. Such testing, however, has yet to be widely adopted or validated for younger athletes.

Numerous studies have shown that baseline neuropsychological testing scores can be negatively affected by post-concussive migraine symptoms, or by anxiety and depression, and are often lower in those with learning and attention disabilities independent of the concussion history. There is a strong recommendation for baseline SCAT testing supported by a study by Schneider et al. [131], who tested more than 4000 youth hockey players with the original SCAT and reported baseline scores showing absolute differences with age and sex. Jinguji et al. [132], in their effort to establish baseline SCAT-2 scores in normal male and female high school athletes, found a high error rate on the concentration portion of the assessment in non-concussed athletes. The study also showed significant sex differences, with females scoring higher on the balance, immediate memory, and concentration components of the assessment. In addition, McLeod et al. [133] assessed 1134 high school students. Male high school athletes had significantly lower scores than female athletes and ninth graders were found to have significantly lower total scores than upperclassmen. They also found that a self-reported history of previous concussion affected the symptom and total SCAT-2 scores.

Although the practice of RTP protocol baseline testing has now been voluntarily implemented by hundreds of districts across the country, only four state laws actually require baseline testing. Some studies have attempted to determine how often to conduct baseline testing. Findings from Schatz [134] suggest that stretching the time between baseline assessments from one to two years may have little effect on the clinical management of concussions in collegiate athletes (football players not included in the sample). Given the lack of prospective study looking at the same in youth athletes, some recommend annually updated baseline assessments.

An important and often overlooked problem is that of the appropriate test setting. The 2014 study by Lichtenstein et al. [125] evaluated this and found that the prevalence of invalid baseline results increases when testing is conducted in a large group and non-clinical setting.

Three limitations of neuropsychological testing bear consideration. First, most CBI symptoms and signs resolve within the first three months. Advanced psychological methods, neurophysiological methods, and functional neuroimaging detect subtle objective impairments that may persist for a year or longer, but evidence shows that traditional desktop testing is often insensitive to such deficits. For that reasons, test results within normal limits cannot be regarded as proof of a normal brain. Second, given that many cognitive functions are not yet fully developed in pediatric populations, cognitive assessment tools designed for adults may have significant limitations when applied to young athletes. Third, athletes have learned to game the testing, deliberately underperforming on the baseline examination to try to conceal later concussion-related impairments. Again, individual supervised administration may reduce the risk of invalid results found on group testing.

Symptom Assessment

There are numerous different symptom checklists. The PCSS [86] has the strongest pediatric data behind it, at least for adolescent populations. The PCSS is a 21-item self-report measure that records symptom severity using a seven-point Likert scale. Iverson et al. [126] reported evidence of moderate test–retest reliability to detect reliable change in contrast to other symptom measures. Numerous studies have demonstrated that the PCSS is able to identify concussed athletes. Of interest, its findings have been validated with measures of neurocognitive performance and regional hyperactivation on fMRI during a working-memory task. The PCSI has also been evaluated in younger athletes. This has both a child report and a parent/teacher report. Interrater reliability on the child forms was moderate to high and there was evidence of predictive and discriminant validity [135].

The SAC evaluation is often employed in the office setting independent of the SCAT [80]. Studies have found the SAC to have good sensitivity and specificity but significant differences in scores have been reported for males and females in healthy young athletes (nine to 14 years of age), and in high school athletes, suggesting the need for separate norms for males and females in these age groups.

Other Neurobehavioral Tests of Possible Value

Other testing often employed in the post-concussion evaluation acutely and beyond includes the King–Devick (K-D) test [136], designed to assess reading-related saccadic eye movements by requiring the patient to rapidly read aloud a series of single-digit numbers from left to right and line to line. This test measures the speed of number naming as well as errors made by the athlete, with the goal of detecting impairments of eye movement, attention, and language, as well as impairments in other functional domains that would suggest suboptimal brain function. Deficits do not localize to a single anatomical region. Instead, the generation and regulation of saccades require coordination of a distributed cortical/subcortical network, including the frontal and supplementary eye fields, dorsolateral prefrontal cortex, parietal cortex, and brainstem [137]. Thus, concussion (or any other factors) impacting any part of this network may slow number reading.

One question has been how best to validate the K-D test, confirm its reliability, and determine thresholds diagnostic of CBI. A large cross-sectional study was recently completed by Weise et al. [138] on school-aged athletes during preseason physicals for a variety of sports to determine the repeatability of the K-D. They showed that scores in junior high and high school athletes are variable but get faster and more repeatable with increasing age. Based on grouped data, a slowing of ten seconds for younger athletes and six seconds for older athletes on a second administration represents a true difference in testing speed. Such data suggest that the test might be uniquely sensitive as a sideline test to detect the acute effects of concussion, and some research supports that conclusion. For instance, adult studies have shown that times increase significantly immediately after a match both in boxers and in mixed martial arts fighters who sustained head trauma.

Galetta et al. [136] showed that, among 219 collegiate athletes tested at baseline, post-season K-D scores were improved over the best pre-season scores, reflecting mild learning effects in the absence of concussion. For the ten athletes who had concussions, K-D testing on the sidelines showed significant worsening from baseline. However, due to the small sample size, this study lacked sufficient power to determine whether the test was effective in diagnosing a concussion.

Somewhat more persuasive evidence comes from the study by King et al. [137] who studied 104 amateur rugby union and rugby league players before and after each match. Employment of the K-D test detected six times as many unwitnessed as witnessed concussions. The K-D results also correlated with symptoms on the SAC. This finding, if replicated, raises hope that the K-D test could help mitigate a serious problem in a cost-efficient way: detecting injuries that are asymptomatic yet cause objective behavior and brain dysfunction.

Given the importance of reaction time in sport, particularly in the avoidance of injury, tests aimed at assessing this sport-related protective response seem highly appropriate. A simple tool for measuring clinical reaction time was developed by Eckner and colleagues [139]. The test involves a systematic approach to dropping a weighted stick that is calibrated to reflect speed of reaction for catching it. The initial test of reliability at one-year intervals is promising, and the diagnostic statistics indicate adequate utility for use as part of a concussion evaluation. Early reports suggest that this test is a valid measure of baseline reaction time when compared to previously validated computerized tests in college athletes, but age and sex standardization and replication are required.

The BESS [6] is a quantifiable version of a modified Romberg test for balance. It measures postural stability or balance and consists of six stances: three on a firm surface and the same three stances on an unstable (medium-density foam) surface with eyes closed and with hands on hips for 20 seconds. For every error made one point is added, with a higher score indicating a worse performance. The test has very good test–retest reliability.

A number of studies have utilized the BESS to assist in the diagnosis of concussion with consistent demonstration of elevated BESS scores (i.e., worse balance performance) at the time of injury and within the initial 24 h post injury relative to the athletes' individualized baseline scores or those of matched control subjects. For most, BESS performance returned to pre-season baseline levels by three to seven days post injury.

A 2005 study by McCrea et al. [140] of collegiate football players reported BESS scores signaling impairment in 36% of injured subjects immediately following concussion, relative to 5% in the control group. Although quite specific, the BESS is not highly sensitive in detecting concussion. That observation may simply reflect the fact that CBIs vary – some impacting the cervical spine/brainstem/cerebellar/subcortical/cortical network of balance more than others – as does pre-morbid balance function between individuals.

Multiple studies have shown that such a combination of diagnostic tests, as compared with individual tests, is likely to improve diagnostic accuracy of concussion. The most sensitive, specific, and cost-effective combination of measures has yet to be determined.

Imaging

Relatively few published studies focus specifically on imaging in pediatric sports-related concussion –to guide either the critical decision regarding the possible benefit of an acute CT scan or the utility of imaging in post-acute and chronic stages of CBI. Readers can review the evidence regarding acute CT decision making in this volume's Chapter 15, titled *The Great CT Debate*. Here we focus on imaging in the post-acute or chronic phase. Those seeking a more detailed discussion of methods and findings may refer to this volume's three chapters on the state of the art of concussion imaging by Johnson, Bigler, and Slobounov (Chapter 12), Taber and Hurley (Chapter 16), and Mayer and Bellgowan (Chapter 22).

Traditional structural imaging methods such as anatomical T1, T2, and even susceptibility-weighted MRI have not revealed abnormalities in brain structure following pediatric concussion/mTBI. Ellis et al. [141] conducted a review to summarize the results of clinical neuroimaging studies performed in patients with SRC who were referred to a multidisciplinary pediatric concussion program. They found that in the majority of pediatric cases of SRC results of clinical neuroimaging studies are normal. Advanced neuroimaging, predominantly useful in research studies and more sensitive than standard anatomical imaging, shows promise for future clinical utility.

For example, a study by Lovell et al. [142] found that, as a group, high school athletes who demonstrated frontal cortex hyperactivation at the time of their first fMRI scan following an SRC demonstrated a more prolonged clinical recovery (as measured by brief computerized neuropsychological testing) than did athletes without such hyperactivation. A study by Keightley et al. [143] of slightly younger teens (average age 14.5 years) after concussion showed worse working memory associated with significantly reduced task-related blood oxygen level dependent (BOLD) signal. Work by Maugans et al. [144] highlighted the utility of phase-contrast angiography in the post-concussive period in a pediatric population aged 11–15 years. Statistically significant alterations in CBF were documented in the SRC group despite a lack of abnormalities on either structural MRI (T1 and susceptibility-weighted image, diffusion tensor imaging) or proton magnetic resonance spectroscopy. It must be noted that there were only 12 subjects in this study.

More recent studies have enhanced the understanding of the trajectory of recovery and the relationship between CBF and persistent symptoms. For instance, Meier et al. [145] compared the time course of CBF recovery with that of cognitive and behavioral symptoms in a sample of concussed collegiate athletes. Using arterial spin labeling MRI, a neuropsychiatric evaluation and a brief cognitive screen conducted at one day, one week, and one month post injury, they were able to show reduced CBF in human concussion and a resolution pattern similar to that previously described in animal models. Interestingly, CBF in the dorsal mid-insular cortex was decreased at one month in slower-to-recover athletes and was inversely related to the magnitude of initial psychiatric symptoms, suggesting a potential prognostic indication for CBF as a biomarker for PPCS.

Mutch et al. [146] reviewed brain CO_2 stress testing in adolescents with "post-concussion syndrome" (ICD-10 criteria) compared to healthy controls and found that adolescent ICD-10-defined "PC Syndrome" is associated with patient-specific abnormalities in regional mean CBF and BOLD cerebrovascular responsiveness that occur in the setting of normal global resting CBF. As discussed in this book's neuroimaging chapters, Mutch et al.'s [146] study exemplifies a research problem that has perhaps delayed progress in understanding the typical outcome after typical concussion: many laboratories have detected long-lived post-concussive brain changes in studies selectively scanning patients with PPCS. An important but unanswered question is the prevalence of post-CBI brain changes, for example, at two years post injury, across a large cohort of pediatric SRC patients, many of whom will have subjectively recovered in a matter of seven to ten days.

Physical and Cognitive Rest

Most physicians are now familiar with the hypothesis that physical and cognitive rest may be beneficial in the immediate post-injury period. As reviewed in this volume's Chapter 27 on *Evidence-Based Rehabilitation*, accumulating empirical data support the beneficial effects of a relatively brief period of rest (i.e., < seven days). The benefit of rest was promoted by the International Concussion in Sport Group at the International Conference on Concussion in Sport [147], with the addition that such rest should continue until the acute symptoms resolve and then a graded program of exertion should be followed prior to medical clearance and RTP. The rationale behind the statement is the above-described metabolic mismatch and the suspected period of vulnerability to repeat injury and protracted recovery. Given the individual nature of CBIs and the lack of agreed-upon definition for what constitutes rest, no consistent practice has arisen. However, in the light of some evidence that both cognition and brain function may remain abnormal in completely asymptomatic athletes, it is not clear that "symptom resolution" is the ideal flag for RTP.

The existing data supporting the efficacy of rest have come largely from observational studies. Gioia et al. [148] reported that more than 80% of students with concussion have a significant increase in symptom severity at school during the first two weeks post injury. The implication that premature neuronal activation in the absence of re-injury could in and of itself have a negative effect on recovery has been supported by numerous studies. A study by Moser et al. [149] suggested that one week of complete cognitive rest during either the acute or a subacute healing phase has benefits in decreasing symptoms and improving cognitive performance. More recently, Asken et al. [150] showed in a sample of 97 NCAA Division I athletes that those who do not immediately report symptoms of a

concussion and continue to participate in athletic activity are at risk for longer recoveries than athletes who immediately report symptoms and are removed from play.

The statement regarding cognitive and physical rest from the International Concussion in Sport Group [147] has resulted in many clinicians instructing athletes to avoid any physical and cognitive activity until symptoms completely resolve. Fallout observations from such practice have included protracted recovery and other complications. DiFazio et al. [151] put forward Williamson's Activity Restriction Model of Depression as being central to the potential harms of prolonged activity restriction and how an "activity restriction cascade" can unfold. According to this model, psychological consequences of removal from validating life activities, combined with physical deconditioning, contribute to the development and persistence of PCS after mTBI in some youth. It is not difficult to appreciate that student athletes, who for the majority are team players, many with strong social connections, may begin to experience emotional distress caused by physical and social activity restriction. In addition, the possibility has been raised that more restrictive post-concussion instructions may influence a patient's perception of illness, possibly leading to more symptom reporting.

Thomas et al. [152] looked at a group aged 11–22 years presenting to the emergency department within 24 h of sustaining a concussion. There was a slower resolution of symptoms in the group advised to rest for five days at home without cognitive challenge compared to the group instructed to rest for one or two days and then return to school. Those authors did not appreciate a clinically significant difference in neurocognitive or balance outcomes between groups. Questions were raised following this study regarding the compliance of the stricter-restrictions group given that many in that group had reported mental activity adding up to hours per day.

That finding brings up a basic question: in an awake child whose brain has evolved to constantly sponge up observations and make new associations, what constitutes cognitive rest? No definitive definition for cognitive rest exists and there is no obvious way (short of biomarkers such as electroencephalogram telemetry) to measure the delivered dose of this prescription. In practical terms, rest could include the reduction of brain-stimulating activities such as television, video games, school work, computer use, cell phone use, reading, and writing.

Brown et al. [153] studied 335 patients with a mean age of 15 years and evaluated their recovery from SRC in the setting of different intensities of cognitive activity. Those engaged in the lower three quartiles of activity had similar trajectories of symptom duration. So while it is appreciated that limitation of cognitive activity is associated with shorter symptom duration, this study suggests that complete abstinence may be unnecessary. The 2012 study by Moser et al. [149] also showed significantly improved performance in 49 high school and collegiate athletes on Immediate Post-Concussion Assessment and Cognitive Testing, as well as decreased symptom reporting following prescribed cognitive and physical rest. Interestingly, the latter finding was independent of the time between concussion and onset of rest. That flies in the face of the hypothesis that rest helps because it reduces cerebral energy demands during the initial time-limited decoupling of metabolism (~ ten days), but a major limitation of this study is absence of any control group. Hence, the biological mechanism explaining the benefit of rest has yet to be determined.

Ultimately, the goal is to keep disruptions to the student's life to a minimum and to return the recovering student to school as soon as possible. Informal targeted accommodations can be implemented to address specific school demands that have the potential for increasing symptoms. These can include reduced school day length, reduced class length, reduced homework burden, frequent rest breaks, and no class testing.

Halstead et al. [154] opine that the student should return to school when able to tolerate cognitive activity or stimulation for approximately 30–45 minutes. This arbitrary cutoff is based on the observation that a good amount of learning takes place in 30–45-minute increments. Upon return, observation by teachers, nurses, and counselors may identify the classes or circumstances that exacerbate symptoms (e.g., the noisy bustle of the lunch break). Those observations can inform ongoing adjustments to help reduce symptom provocation.

This raises the issue of negotiating school accommodations. Districts and individual school administrations vary in their knowledge, flexibility, and tolerance of the need for graded return to activity after CBI. The U.S. Centers for Disease Control and Prevention (CDC) Heads Up program recently published a suite of documents – freely available online and specifically tailored for school nurses, teachers, counselors, and administrators – containing practical facts about concussion and recommendations for school accommodation [155, 156]. Sady et al. [157] published explicit recommendations that every school develop a concussion response policy that includes three elements:

1. Preparing a statement of policies and procedures compatible with CDC guidelines. That statement should include: (a) the school's commitment to safety; (b) a brief description of CBI; (c) a plan to help students gradually return to the full spectrum of school life (i.e., learning, social activity, sports); and (d) information to guide safe return to physical activity. There needs to be a school-wide or system-wide "concussion management program" that assures school personnel are educated about (a) the effects of concussion, and (b) each professional's role in the management program, with written guidelines specifying staff responsibilities. *All* school staff should be expected to understand the guiding principles of supporting the concussed student's return in collaboration with health professionals. The concussion management program should define the roles of the student, the parents, the school nurse, administrators, counselors, teachers, school psychologist, physical education instructors, and athletic trainers. In essence, in addition to staff-wide education, each school with an athletic program should have an identified *school concussion resource team* prepared to devise individually appropriate accommodations (which sometimes requires a formal process such as a 504

plan: see below), to continuously monitor the student's progress, and to adjust the plan as recovery permits.

2. Developing a concussion education program. Ideally, all staff with direct student contact should be engaged in a formal process of learning about concussion and its typical effects. That education should be conducted before the start of each school year.

3. Initiating a policy that guarantees that the school-wide management program is implemented and updated before the start of school each year.

Sady et al. [157] included a useful table summarizing the elements of an effective concussion management policy (Table 18.1).

In spite of those recommendations, parents and brain injury advocates report mixed success in persuading school authorities to adopt published recommendations and adapt curricula to the needs of concussed student athletes. There appears to by a yawning gap between expert advice and school acquiescence.

That problem is understandable. Public schools, in particular, typically regard enrollment as an all-or-none proposition. The idea of graded return to activity does not comport with that concept. Few school systems have implemented the kind of staff-wide education promoted by Sady et al. [157], Halstead et al. [154], Ransom et al. [158], or Gioia [92]. Who among the staff has the time and skill to "continuously monitor the student's progress, and to adjust the plan as recovery permits"? Collaborations between medical professionals and school administrators are sometimes awkward [92]. Moreover, protocols originally developed to assure individualized school accommodations for those with permanent disabilities may not always translate smoothly to the unique needs of the concussed student athlete. For instance, in some districts curricular accommodation requires a 504 plan (referring to the Rehabilitation Act that provides medical need accommodations) often combined with an Individualized Education Plan. Either plan requires extensive medical documentation and psychological testing. Yet, due to the typically rapid recovery from concussion, test results obtained one week may be outdated the next, and plans developed to optimize learning in the first month after concussion may no longer be applicable the next. Paradoxically perhaps, it may be easier for schools to accommodate the unfortunate minority with severe PPCS because their chronic, somewhat stable symptoms better lend themselves to measurements of abilities and design of interventions that may still be relevant months later.

The increased awareness of SRC and the publication of CDC recommendations will hopefully encourage schools to adopt common-sense graded return to the academic milieu. It is debatable whether legislation will be required to assist that change. (Halstead et al. [154], for instance, cited the recent proliferation of state laws intended to protect concussed student athletes, but opined that new laws are not necessary, given the flexibility of existing protections for persons with disabilities.) With or without legislation, advocacy and pro-active education may be required to increase the proportion of schools that are prepared to facilitate graduated return.

Table 18.1 School concussion management: activities and responsibilities

Activity	Responsible parties	Completion date	Evidence of completion
Prior to school year			
1. Concussion management policies and procedures (P & P)	School administration (school nurse, counselor, psychologist)	Prior to start of school year	Written policy in school manual; copy provided to all school staff
2. Development of school concussion resource team	School administration; school nurse, counselor, psychologist, designated teacher, athletic trainer	Prior to start of school year	Written policy in school manual
3. Examine teaching/support methods to support recovery, maximize learning/performance, reduce symptom exacerbation	School administration; school nurse, counselor, psychologist	Prior to start of school year	Written policies on teaching methods
4. Teacher/staff education and training (online video training, CDC school professional fact sheet)	Teacher, school counselor, school nurse, administrators	Prior to start of school year	Verification of completion provided to school administration
5. Develop list of concussion resources for education, consultation, and referral (medical, school, state/local Brain Injury Association)	School administration	Prior to school year	List of resources provided in P & P; available to school staff and families
During school year (pre-injury)			
1. Review/reinforce concussion policy and procedures	School administration, school nurse/counselor	First faculty meeting, parent back-to-school night	Verbal report
2. Monitoring for injury; parent informed of injury	Coach, athletic trainer, school health personnel	Day of injury	Concussion Symptom Checklist; parent-provided ACE; post-concussion home/school instructions
School management (post-injury)			
1. Medical evaluation and school treatment planning	Licensed health care professional with concussion training, school concussion resource team	Early post-injury	Plan for school return/activity
2. Gradual return-to-school program	Licensed health care professional with concussion training, school concussion resource team	When medically determined to tolerate 30+ minutes of cognitive activity	Medical documentation
2. In-school observation, monitoring, and support	School concussion resource team	Ongoing	Concussion Symptom Checklist[a]
4. Clearance for full return to school	Licensed health care professional with concussion training, school concussion resource team	Asymptomatic with full cognitive and physical exertion	Medical documentation (provided to family and school)

[a] Concussion Symptom Checklist = Post Concussion Symptom Checklist (PCSC). ACE: acute concussion evaluation [93].

Source: Sady et al., 2011 [157]

Despite the consensus favoring some cognitive rest, it is important to note that prolonged cognitive rest and reduction of school engagement have the potential to exacerbate symptoms or cause negative mental health issues. This may occur not only because of reduced social interaction but also because the student experiences anxiety due to awareness that he or she is not completing school assignments and falling behind friends and peers. The more rigorous the academic setting and schedule, the greater the potential for such anxiety. The stress seems to be greater among high school compared with middle school students, especially in the critical junior year, and especially in more competitive school districts. Students whose personal and family expectations from childhood involved attending a good college perhaps feel this the most.

The negative effects of removing student athletes from play for prolonged periods after non-concussive injuries have been repeatedly shown with reports of depression, anxiety, and lower self-esteem thought to be the result of high levels of athletic identity. Manuel et al. [159] reported that injured (non-concussed) high school athletes missing a minimum of three weeks of athletic participation showed higher rates of depression than non-injured athletes.

This raises the issue of exercise as rehabilitation. Detailed evidence supporting the efficacy of aerobic exercise for rehabilitation after adult concussion is reviewed in this volume's Chapter 27 on *Evidence-Based Rehabilitation*. Multiple experimental studies support the conclusion that exercise may hasten recovery or reduce symptoms after concussion. Mild voluntary aerobic exercise reportedly enhances regulation of CBF and promotes expression of potentially beneficial peptides, including brain-derived neurotrophic factor [160–162].

The unresolved questions for pediatric rehabilitation are how to optimize the type, the timing, and the exertion level of this intervention. Majerske et al. [163] retrospectively evaluated activity shortly after concussion in 95 student-athletes using self-reported physical and cognitive measures in the 30 days following injury and compared the findings to a neurocognitive assessment. Results showed that athletes engaging in a medium level of physical and cognitive activity performed better on the neurocognitive test than those with no physical and cognitive activity and those with the highest levels of physical and cognitive activity.

A recent randomized pilot study by Maerlender et al. [164] that studied "Programmed physical exertion in recovery from sports-related concussion" in college-age athletes reported that programmed physical exertion during recovery produced no significant differences in recovery time between groups of participants. However, high levels of exertion were deleterious, providing more evidence that mild to moderate physical activity, but not high-level exertion, seems to facilitate recovery. In an observational study of 3063 children and adolescents presenting to emergency departments after mTBI, Grool et al. [165] found a lower rate of PPCS at four weeks associated with beginning activity in the first week.

Howell et al. [166] suggested a possible age-dependent component to the benefit of returning to physical activity with their examination of the association between physical activity and symptom duration in patients seen initially within three weeks of a concussion. They found that, for participants aged between 13 and 18 years, higher levels of self-reported physical activity after the injury were associated with shorter symptom duration (PPCS) compared with older and younger groups. The benefit of controlled physical activity for more persistent symptoms following an SRC has been shown in numerous studies.

Leddy et al. [167] implemented a graded return to activity as part of an exercise protocol on concussed athletes who had been symptomatic for a minimum of six weeks following a concussive event. The athletes had a significant decrease in their symptom reports and were able to return to sport. However, for reasons that are unclear, the same improvement was not seen in a concussed non-athlete group completing the same protocol.

Although aerobic exercise therapy may be helpful even later in recovery, the current evidence suggests a temporal window of opportunity: (1) mild to moderate aerobic exercise may be beneficial to the recovery process once the athlete has moved beyond the acute injury stage (the first few days); (2) unrestricted exercise in the immediate acute phase of concussion recovery may increase the risk of symptom exacerbation and/or delay recovery; yet (3) no exercise in the first week may actually increase the risk of persistent symptoms.

Gagnon et al. [168] examined the effectiveness of a multidisciplinary active rehabilitation intervention for ten adolescents who were slow to recover (> four weeks) after an SRC. The rehabilitation program included gradual, closely monitored light aerobic exercise, general coordination exercises, mental imagery, as well as reassurance, normalization of recovery, and stress/anxiety reduction strategies. After the six-week intervention, PCS significantly decreased for participants with an additional decrease in fatigue and improvement in mood. Unfortunately, this study was confined to a group pre-selected for atypical outcome and did not employ a control intervention or group. Since spontaneous recovery is expected, the reported findings cannot be interpreted as evidence of efficacy. Large controlled prospective studies with longitudinal follow-up are eagerly awaited to clarify the optimal kinds and combinations of post-SRC interventions – ultimately supporting evidence-based algorithms that permit individualization of rehabilitation.

Concussion Safety Laws and Sports-Specific Rule Changes

Beginning in 2009, the state of Washington passed the first concussion in sports law, called the Zackery Lystedt Law [169]. One month later, Max's law passed in Oregon [170] and now 49 states and the District of Columbia have enacted strong youth sports concussion safety laws [171].

These laws had three action steps at their core: first, to educate coaches, athletes, and their parents/guardians about concussion through training and/or a concussion information sheet. Second, an athlete who is believed to have a concussion is to be removed from play right away and thirdly, return to practice or play is only permitted after at least 24 h and with permission from a licensed health care professional. However, some states have made modifications to these requirements [172]. For example, California and New Mexico have mandated a seven-day minimum waiting period before RTP following a diagnosed concussion.

Forty of the state laws require student athletes and parents to sign concussion information forms. However, given a lack of a consensus concussion document, this does not necessarily translate to the parents and athletes of these states all receiving the same meaningful education. Some states do require signed acknowledgment of receipt of a Department of Education educational fact sheet about sports-related concussion and other head injuries from parents or guardians of student athletes annually. States such as Oregon and Colorado, along with others, have expanded coverage to younger age groups and to intramural sports and club sports. Private schools have also been included in some states. Vermont recently enacted into law a requirement that school athletic coaches and referees receive training on how to prevent and appropriately manage concussions. In addition, the home team is required to ensure that a licensed athletic trainer or health care provider is present at any athletic event involving a contact sport. Virginia signed into law a bill requiring the Commonwealth's Board of Education to include in its policies a "Return to Learn Protocol" [173].

Given the growing concern about the long-term outcome of repetitive head impacts, California introduced a 2014 mandate that limited full-contact football practices to three hours per week during the pre-season and regular season, and banned off-season contact practices altogether. The University Interscholastic League, Texas's state association, now limits full-contact practice to 90 minutes per week.

The Arizona Interscholastic Association limits full-pads pre-season practices to half or less of all practices. Some in the high school football community have voiced the concern that restrictions of this kind create an offensive advantage early in the season, since defensive linemen will have little experience in their roles. That concern may be particularly applicable at the freshman level, given that for many student athletes this may be the first exposure to contact game situations. Others have speculated about unintended consequences: to compensate for time limits, coaches may escalate the intensity of the contact practice sessions, paradoxically creating the potential for *more* repetitive head impact exposure.

A recent study by McGuine [174] examined sports-related concussion rates among Wisconsin high school football players after their state's interscholastic athletic association mandated new limits on the amount and duration of full-contact activities during team practices. The rule prohibits full contact during the first week of practice, limits full contact to 75 minutes per week during week 2, and caps it at 60 minutes thereafter. Findings show that the rate of concussions sustained during practice was more than twice as high in the two seasons prior to the rule change as compared to the 2014 season following the change.

In 2017, Ivy League football coaches finally came to a unanimous decision to eliminate all full-contact hitting from practices during the regular season. This is in addition to the Ivy League's existing limits on the amount of full contact in practice during the spring and pre-season, which are among the most stringent in collegiate football. The decision was inspired by Dartmouth, where full-contact practices throughout the year had been eliminated since 2010. Instead of hitting other players in practice, Dartmouth players hit pads and tackling dummies, including a specially designed mobile virtual player.

Mirroring a similar move by the National Football League (NFL) that had reduced the number of concussions reported on kickoffs by over 40% reported by some sources, the NCAA playing rules oversight panel voted to move kickoffs 5 yards forward, to the 35-yard line, in 2012. This was the result of data that suggested injuries occur more during kickoffs than other plays in a football game and shortening the distance between opposing teams would reduce potential for high-velocity impacts.

Increasingly, authorities stress the importance of appropriate equipment. Guidelines include making sure the equipment fits the athletes well, is in good condition, is stored properly, and is repaired and replaced based on instructions from the equipment companies. To encourage players and teams to adhere to equipment checks, various sanctions are being established. The National Federation of State High School Associations Football Rules Committee requires players to sit out one play if their helmet comes off while the ball is live. A helmet-less player is not allowed to block, tackle, or otherwise participate beyond the immediate action in which he was engaged when the helmet came completely off.

The recent increase in attention to SRC has raised a biotechnology issue that is far from resolved: what good are helmets? Several studies have shown that headgear in rugby probably reduces the incidence of concussion. A parallel study has yet to be conducted in American football, perhaps due to the long-standing tradition of using helmets and reluctance to experiment with a helmetless control group. Data are also limited to support or refute the superiority of one type of football helmet over another in preventing concussions.

Although Virginia Tech developed a helmet rating system based on a series of impact tests, the group acknowledges that no helmet is concussion-proof and that any athlete can sustain a head injury, even with the best head protection. That initiative's stated goal is simply to identify the helmets that best reduce the chance of players sustaining a concussion.

Results from the first year of a two-year study testing helmetless tackling drills by Swartz et al. [175], released in 2015, have been encouraging. The randomized controlled trial divided 50 athletes into two groups: an intervention group and a control group. Before each workout session, an X-Patch head impact sensor was placed on the skin just behind the right ear of each athlete which monitored the frequency, location, and acceleration of all the head impacts. Football players in the intervention group performed five-minute tackling drills without their helmets and shoulder pads twice a week in pre-season and once a week during football season. The intervention drills consisted of repetitions of proper tackling technique while the control group performed non-contact football skills at the same time, rate, and duration. At the end of one football season, the intervention group that had performed the helmetless-tackling training program had experienced 30% fewer head impacts per exposure than the control group. Other newer guidelines include restrictions on blocking below the waist and blocking on punt returns. Players are also prohibited from leaping over blockers when trying to block punts.

Such rule changes have taken place at the youth level in other sports such as ice hockey. As far back as 2000 the American Academy of Pediatrics recommended that checking not be allowed in hockey leagues for children ages 15 and younger, though some felt that rule was poorly substantiated at that time [176]. A 2006 analysis of data by Macpherson et al. [177] on 4736 hockey injuries from Canadian Hospitals Injury Reporting and Prevention Program (CHIRPP) injury surveillance system between 1995 and 2002 found that the majority of the injuries in younger divisions (10–13 years of age) occurred in Ontario, where body checking was allowed at those ages, and nearly half of those injuries were related to checking.

Another analysis of CHIRPP data by Cusimano et al. [178] on 8552 hockey-related injuries from 1994 to 2004 found that 52.2% were attributable to body checking. Following a rule change in 1998 that lowered the age for body checking from 12–13 years to 10–11 years, the odds of a body checking-related injury increased twofold in the newly allowed checking divisions.

Two systematic reviews of the literature published in 2009 and 2010 [179, 180] examined the association between body checking and injury in boys' ice hockey. All but one of their included studies demonstrated that body checking increases the risk of all injuries. Body checking can also be associated with more aggressive play that further increases the risk of serious injury. In the 2011–2012 season, USA Hockey raised the age of legalized checking from 11 to 13 years, with many pushing for a further increase to age 15. Checking is not allowed in girls' hockey at this time.

In November 2015, following a 15-month lawsuit in United States District Court in California charging U.S. Soccer with negligence in treating and monitoring head injuries, U.S. Soccer announced a new series of initiatives. The initiatives are intended to reduce the number of concussions suffered by youth soccer players, including the elimination of heading for children aged ten and under and the limiting of heading in practice for children between the ages of 11 and 13 years.

Comstock et al. [181] conducted a retrospective analysis of longitudinal surveillance data collected from 2005–2006 through 2013–2014 in a large, nationally representative sample of U.S. high school soccer players. Although heading was found to be the most common activity associated with concussions, the most frequent mechanism was athlete–athlete contact, with resultant concussions coming from direct player-to-player impact (most often when competing for a header) or player-to-ground impact as a result of the player-to-player contact. Another common cause of concussion was a direct blow from a kicked ball.

While the emerging data from soccer-related concussions are somewhat in tune with the larger body of sport concussion literature, the long-term effects of soccer participation and the influence of heading are less well understood. Although biomechanical experiments demonstrate that a simple resilient headband markedly reduces the force of impacts, insufficient studies of soccer protective headgear have been conducted to estimate the effectiveness of this device for preventing concussion.

Impact Quantification

Efforts have been made to try to quantify the head impact exposure in youth and collegiate athletes by instrumenting the helmets with mounted accelerometers. Also in recent years, researchers have come to suspect that head rotation may play an important role in concussions and so direct measurement of rotational acceleration could prove valuable. The hope is that such technology can serve as another set of eyes to alert coaches and trainers to potentially harmful hits. A study using telemetry in high school football players by Urban et al. [182] found a wide variability in the force of impacts: the median impact ranged for each player from 15.2 to 27.0 **g**, and the average value was 21.7 **g**. The impact frequency was shown to be greater during games (15.5 **g**) than during practices (9.4 **g**). However, overall exposure over the course of the season was greater during practices.

Cobb et al. [183] sought to quantify the head impact exposure of 50 youth football players, age 9–12 years, for all practices and games over the course of a single season. While the acceleration magnitudes tended to be lower than those reported for older players, some recorded high-magnitude impacts similar to those seen at the high school and college level. Those authors remarked that exposure may be appreciably reduced by limiting contact in practices.

Two popular head impact monitoring systems are Riddell's Head Impact Telemetry System and the newer X2 Biosystems X-Patch (a small behind-the-ear device). Other sensor types under investigation include mouth guards, oral retainers, and earpieces. Beyond research, these systems have the potential to identify "big hits" that might be missed visually or players with dangerous tackling styles who may be coachable to less risky techniques.

One problem that has been repeatedly raised with respect to such sensor systems is individual data privacy. Many have cautioned that such data might be employed in recruitment and selection decisions. That prospect would be particularly concerning to those seeking college admission and scholarships. Another concern is that of a player getting marked by opponents as a potential on-field target following a flagged hit. This has been a particular concern with respect to helmet light sensor technology activated following a hit exceeding a certain threshold. A further concern has been raised regarding the reliance on such data as a marker for concussion. Given the highly variable nature of concussion, and evidence of significant individual differences in vulnerability to brain injury at similar force levels, no numerical force threshold can be used as a cutoff. However, having age bracket cutoffs above which a brief evaluation is prompted has been suggested. Data to inform such a protocol are being collected at the time of writing.

This brings up the question of device accuracy. The sensitivity to impact, specificity to the linear and rotational accelerations most relevant to brain change, reliability, and precision of measurements of the commercially marketed products have been shown to be highly variable. In view of the likelihood that the majority of SRCs are unwitnessed, many go unreported, and many seem to be asymptomatic, one cannot rely on either athletic trainers or players to detect clinically significant hits. That fact strongly suggests a place for helmet telemetry. However, technology of this type needs to be integrated into a comprehensive surveillance plan that also involves well-trained concussion personnel.

Subconcussions

An increasing concern that is gaining more attention of late is that of "subconcussive" impacts. Post-mortem evidence suggests that accrual of damage to the brain may occur with repeated blows to the head, even when the individual blows fail to produce clinical symptoms. The absence of symptoms with these impacts will result in a lack of medical attention, premature return to play, and increased risk of further neurological injury. Abnormal white-matter integrity related to head impact exposure was demonstrated by Davenport et al. [184] in a high school football cohort free of clinical concussions. They reported a strong correlation between MRI DTI measures and change in the Verbal Memory subscore of the ImPACT. This was offered as evidence that a single season of football can produce brain MRI changes in the absence of clinical concussion.

As discussed early in this chapter, Talavage et al. [2] used neurocognitive testing (ImPACT), and fMRI to show neurocognitive (primarily visual working memory) and neurophysiological (altered activation in the dorsolateral prefrontal cortex) impairments in asymptomatic high school football players – even before the start of the season. The observation from both experimental and clinical studies that brain injury may occur without subjective symptoms is one of the discoveries that raises questions about the traditional lore that removal from play and RTP can be guided by symptoms.

Late Effects

As discussed in depth in this volume's Chapter 11 on *Late Effects,* three conceptually dissociable phenomena have been observed and all await biological explanation:

1. After a single "mild TBI" or typical concussion, a subset of individuals exhibit persistent symptoms or prolonged recovery but virtually none develop static or ongoing encephalopathy.

2. It is well established that high levels of repetitive exposure to CBI – as in professional boxers or football players – can be associated with both neurocognitive impairment and delayed but early-onset dementia. That is, after a relatively asymptomatic period that usually ranges from five to 20 years post career, some sports professionals develop a striking dementia syndrome. (For details, see the chapter in this volume titled *Traumatic Encephalopathy*: Chapter 14.) Several neuropathologists have advanced the opinion that this is a unitary entity with a distinct profile of symptoms and with predictable brain changes dominated by tau deposition. That entity, formerly called dementia pugilistica, has recently been relabeled "chronic traumatic encephalopathy." However, other neuropathologists have remarked that autopsy evidence in fact reveals significant heterogeneity, with widely varying counts and distributions of β amyloid, tau, Lewy bodies, TDP43, and vascular changes – and have proposed a more agnostic approach to classification (see Chapter 13 in this volume on *Polypathology and Dementia After Brain Trauma*). Pending larger-scale and especially prospective research, it may be premature to expect closure regarding the nosology of the broad spectrum of changes found after repetitive concussion.

3. Moderate to severe TBI has long been known to be the most common environmental risk factor for the development of Alzheimer's-type dementia. Evidence has emerged that, with the exception of pesticides, TBI is also the most common environmental risk factor for Parkinson's disease. And – a rather surprising observation – new evidence suggests that brain trauma is a risk factor for non-familial amyotrophic lateral sclerosis. Thus, abundant evidence supports the conclusion that TBI is a risk factor for later development of multiple conventional neurodegenerative diseases (as opposed to chronic traumatic encephalopathy (CTE).

What remains controversial – and is exquisitely difficult to study – is whether a single concussion is a risk factor for late effects.

With respect to SRC, almost all of the peer-reviewed publications in the last decade that refer to late effects discuss repetitive rather than single concussions. Some of that evidence is derived from epidemiological studies. For example, an NFL Player Care Foundation study of retired NFL players conducted by Weir et al. [185] found that the number of NFL retirees with a diagnosis of dementia was significantly higher than that in the general population, particularly in the 50+ age group (6.1% vs. 1.2%).

Although neurodegenerative changes clearly occur in persons who played only high school or college football (see below), epidemiological evidence remains to be published showing that a systematic increased risk of dementia occurs among players who did not progress beyond collegiate or high school level of play. Savica et al. [186], for example, studied 438 high school students who played American football from 1946 to 1956 and found no increased risk of later developing dementia, Parkinson's disease, or amyotrophic lateral sclerosis compared with 140 non-football-playing high school males.

A second study compared football players with non-football athletes from 1956 to 1970 and also showed no higher risk for neurodegeneration among football players [187]. However, the generalizability of these studies to players today is questioned. Although some speak to poorer equipment and less regard for concussions at that time, many would argue that the increased quality of equipment may be partly responsible for the false sense of invincibility. This, combined with the higher velocity of hits in today's game, may be one factor behind an apparent increase in prevalence of head trauma in the sport.

Other evidence that repetitive CBI leads to dementia comes from a rapidly growing pool of case reports. Strong evidence suggests that persons with known or presumed histories of repetitive concussions and subconcussions may develop delayed-onset traumatic encephalopathies detectable on post-mortem diagnosis. For instance, "CTE," originally described in boxers, has more recently been reported in football players and participants in other sports, including ice hockey, rugby, professional wrestling, and several other martial arts. In contrast (with the exception of rare case reports from the mid 20th century), single concussions have not been reported to provoke this disorder.

According to numbers shared from the Boston University brain bank in 2015 with the U.S. Public Broadcasting System's investigative program, *FRONTLINE*, CTE was found in the brain tissue of 131 out of 165 individuals (79%) who, before their deaths, played football at some level from high school to professional level. Ninety-six percent of the NFL players they examined had evidence of CTE. This led McKee to make the statement that: "The higher the level you play football and the longer you play football, the higher your risk" [188].

The major barrier to scientific interpretation of these case reports is that large-scale population-based case ascertainment has yet to be done. Concerns have been raised regarding sample bias skewing the data set, given that families of symptomatic individuals with a history of concussions are much more likely to participate in brain donation. A study by Bieniek et al. [189] looking at brains from a Mayo Clinic neurodegenerative brain bank was suggested to be more representative of the extent of the problem. Twenty-one of 66 men (32%) with exposure to contact sports had pathology consistent with CTE. Interestingly, only two of these had played a professional sport. In addition, those authors reported examinations of 198 brains of individuals without documentation of participation in contact sports, including 66 women. No evidence of CTE pathology was found.

A small case series brain autopsy study was carried out by Hazrati et al. [190] on six retired professional football players from the Canadian Football League with histories of multiple concussions and significant neurological decline: only 50% had neuropathological findings consistent with CTE. All three cases showed co-morbid pathology.

While most cases have been described in professional athletes years after their playing careers have ended, cases have also been described in amateur athletes. Yet perhaps the biggest surprises have come from reports of CTE in several young athletes. At the time of this writing, the youngest of these was a 17-year-old male. One of the most concerning cases was that of a 25-year-old former college football player who was reported with widespread tau deposition suggestive of a rather advanced stage of CTE. He had begun playing tackle football at age six and was noted to have a significant concussion history.

The risk of cumulative damage is probably linked to duration of exposure, which is logically greater when exposure to concussions begins at a younger age. However, cases such as this raise the question of the possibility that early-life concussive/subconcussive exposure may be especially problematic. A 2015 National Institutes of Health-funded Boston University study by Stamm et al. [191] found that former NFL players who participated in tackle football before the age of 12 were more likely to have greater impairment in mental flexibility, memory, and intelligence as adults, even after controlling for total number of years played. Early head trauma exposure together with a lengthy career in collision sports is suggested as a particularly risky combination for potential long-term cognitive problems.

Concluding Remarks

No two concussions are alike, regardless of age. Some student athletes only experience symptoms for a few days immediately after concussion, whereas others have delayed and/or more chronic symptoms. New discoveries raise another concern: reliance on symptoms alone to detect clinically significant brain injury or confirm recovery must not be considered a reliable approach. Moreover, since repetitive concussions are suspected to cause chronic neurocognitive impairment and potentially delayed-onset early dementia, there is also a growing concern about the risks for late effects. Thus, there is a need to elevate the index of suspicion for the occurrence of concussion, to consider each concussion individually, and to adopt flexible management approaches. Although one cannot definitively predict who will take which recovery path – especially at this transitional moment in history as we await advances in precision medicine based on genomics and epigenomics – there are several known risk factors. Documenting those factors in a baseline assessment and adequate post-injury evaluations is a vital part of proper management.

The long-held belief of younger being better (more protective) can no longer be assumed. In fact, some evidence suggests that participation in contact/collision sports from early childhood not only exposes individuals to a potentially longer exposure period (which, in itself, may or may not be a risk factor), but also that there may be an increased vulnerability to poorer outcome, particularly if those early injuries are not detected and managed properly. Concussion and injury prevention education is critical for all involved parties, especially the student athlete and parent. In addition, a major initiative is under way to prepare schools to create a safer sporting environment, to assure universal staff education, and to organize dedicated concussion response teams skilled at orchestrating a graded return to learning and playing.

In closing this introductory discussion, it is important to highlight the importance of physical activity on the brain. For all the discussion of the risks of sports, it may be forgotten that a large body of recent research supports the conclusion that regular physical activity not only optimizes cerebral function but may help preserve the brain against the threats of aging.

Dik et al. [192], for instance, conducted a prospective population-based study looking at early-life physical activity (retrospectively recalled) and cognition at old age. Those authors reported a positive association between such early activity and speed of information processing in older men that could not be explained by current physical activity or other lifestyle factors.

Similarly, a 2010 study by Middleton et al. [193] found that women who reported being physically active at any point in their life, but especially as teenagers, had a lower likelihood of cognitive impairment in late life. Whether early activity is directly related to long-term cognitive health or there is a more indirect association (for instance, that early-adopted behaviors promote lifelong healthful habits), a common theme appears to be that regular physical activity is good for the brain. Ultimately, prospective longitudinal research is required for society to discover the best balance between strong encouragement of activity and robust defense against injury.

References

1. Gaw CE, Zonfrillo MR. Emergency department visits for head trauma in the United States. *BMC Emerg Med* 2016; 16: 5.
2. Talavage TM, Nauman EA, Breedlove EL, Yoruk U, Dye AE, Morigaki KE, et al. Functionally-detected cognitive impairment in high school football players without clinically-diagnosed concussion. *J Neurotrauma* 2014; 31: 327–338.
3. Abbas K, Shenk TE, Poole VN, Breedlove EL, Leverenz LJ, Nauman EA, et al. Alteration of default mode network in high school football athletes due to repetitive subconcussive mild traumatic brain injury: A resting-state functional magnetic resonance imaging study. *Brain Connect* 2015; 5: 91–101.
4. Concussion in Sport Group. Sport Concussion Assessment Tool – 3rd edition. 2013. Available at http://bjsm.bmj.com.
5. Concussion in Sport Group. Sport Concussion Assessment Tool for children ages 5 to 12 years. 2013. Available at http://bjsm.bmj.com.
6. Bell DR, Guskiewicz KM, Clark MA, Padua DA. Systematic review of the Balance Error Scoring System. *Sports Health* 2011; 3: 287–295.
7. Reeves TM, Smith TL, Williamson JC, Phillips LL. Unmyelinated axons show selective rostrocaudal pathology in the corpus

callosum following traumatic brain injury. *J Neuropathol Exp Neurol* 2012; 71: 198–210.

8. Wilde EA, McCauley SR, Hunter JV, Bigler ED, Chu Z, Wang ZJ, et al. Diffusion tensor imaging of acute mild traumatic brain injury in adolescents. *Neurology* 2008; 70: 948–955.

9. Mayer AR, Ling JM, Yang Z, Pena A, Yeo RA, Klimaj S. Diffusion abnormalities in pediatric mild traumatic brain injury. *J Neurosci* 2012; 32: 17961–17969.

10. Eisenberg MA, Meehan WP, Mannix R. Duration and course of post-concussive symptoms. *Pediatrics* 2014; 133: 999–1006.

11. McCrory P, Meeuwisse WH, Aubry M, Cantu B, Dvořák J, Echemendia RJ, et al. Consensus statement on concussion in sport: The 4th International Conference on Concussion in Sport held in Zurich, November 2012. *Br J Sports Med* 2013; 47: 250–258.

12. Field M, Collins MW, Lovell MR, Maroon J. Does age play a role in recovery from sports-related concussion? A comparison of high school and collegiate athletes. *J Pediatr* 2003; 142: 546–553.

13. Coll+ins MC, Lovell MR, Iverson GL. Examining concussion rates and return to play in high school football players wearing newer helmet technology: A three year prospective cohort study. *Neurosurg* 2005; 58: 275–286.

14. Zuckerman SL, Lee YM, Odom MJ, Solomon GS, Forbes JA, Sills AK. Recovery from sports-related concussion: Days to return to neurocognitive baseline in adolescents versus young adults. *Surg Neurol Int* 2012; 3: 130.

15. Williams RM, Puetz TW, Giza CC, Broglio SP. Concussion recovery time among high school and collegiate athletes: A systematic review and meta-analysis. *Sports Med* 2015; 45: 893–903.

16. Thomas S, Prins ML, Samii M, Hovda DA. Cerebral metabolic response to traumatic brain injury sustained early in development: A 2-deoxy-D-glucose autoradiographic study. *J Neurotrauma* 2000; 17: 649–665.

17. Giza CC, Hovda DA. The neurometabolic cascade of concussion. *J Athletic Train* 2001; 36(3): 228–235.

18. Mandera M, Larysz D, Wojtacha M. Changes in cerebral hemodynamics assessed by transcranial Doppler ultrasonography in children after head injury. *Child's Nerv Syst* 2002; 18(3–4): 124–128.

19. Vavilala MS, Lee LA, Boddu K, Visco E, Newell DW, Zimmerman JJ, Lam AM. Cerebral autoregulation in pediatric traumatic brain injury. *Pediatr Crit Care Med* 2004; 5(3): 257–263.

20. Maugans TA, Farley C, Altaye M, Leach J, Cecil KM. Pediatric sports-related concussion produces cerebral blood flow alterations. *Pediatrics* 2012; 129(1): 28–37.

21. Chambers IR, Stobbart L, Jones PA, Kirkham FJ, Marsh M, Mendelow AD, et al. Age-related differences in intracranial pressure and cerebral perfusion pressure in the first 6 hours of monitoring after children's head injury: Association with outcome; *Childs Nerv Syst* 2005; 21: 195–199.

22. Dong T, Zhi L, Bhayana B, Wu MX. Cortisol-induced immune suppression by a blockade of lymphocyte egress in traumatic brain injury. *J Neuroinflamm* 2016; 13(197): 1–13.

23. Jorge RE, Acion L, Starkstein SE, Magnotta V. Hippocampal volume and mood disorders after traumatic brain injury. *Biol Psychiatry* 2007; 62: 332–338.

24. Zhou D, Zhao Y, Wan Y, Wang Y, Xie D, Qin Lu Q, et al. Neuroendocrine dysfunction and insomnia in mild traumatic brain injury patients. *Neurosci Lett* 2016; 610: 154–159.

25. Niederland T, Makovi H, Gál V, Andréka B, Ábrahám CS, Kovács J. Abnormalities of pituitary function after traumatic brain injury in children. *J Neurotrauma* 2007; 24(1): 119–127.

26. Zhou Y. Abnormal structural and functional hypothalamic connectivity in mild traumatic brain injury. *J Magn Reson Imaging* 2017; 45(4): 1105–1112.

27. Gessel LM, Fields SK, Collins CL, Dick RW, Comstock RD. Concussions among United States high school and collegiate athletes. *J Athl Train* 2007; 42(4): 495–503.

28. Marar M, McIlvain N, Fields S, Comstock R. Epidemiology of concussions among United States high school athletes in 20 sports. *Am J Sports Med* 2012; 40(4): 747–755.

29. Schulz MR, Marshall SW, Mueller FO, Yang J, Weaver NL, Kalsbeek WD, et al. Incidence and risk factors for concussion in high school athletes, North Carolina, 1996–1999. *Am J Epidemiol* 2004; 160(10): 937–944.

30. Guskiewicz KM, McCrea M, Marshall SW, Cantu RC, Randolph C, Onate JA, et al. Cumulative effects associated with recurrent concussion in collegiate football players: The NCAA Concussion Study. *JAMA* 2003; 290: 2549–2555.

31. Schatz P, ScolaroMoser R, Covassin T, Karpf R. Early indicators of enduring symptoms in high school athletes with multiple previous concussions. *Neurosurgery* 2011; 68: 1562–1567.

32. Brooks BL, Mannix R, Maxwell B, Zafonte R, Berkner PD, Iverson GL. Multiple past concussions in high school football players: Are there differences in cognitive functioning and symptom reporting? *Am J Sports Med* 2016; 44 (12): 3243–3251.

33. Jang SH, Yi JH, Kim SH, Kwon HG. Relation between injury of the hypothalamus and subjective excessive daytime sleepiness in patients with mild traumatic brain injury. *J Neurol Neurosurg Psychiatry* 2016; 87: 1260–1261.

34. McCrea M, Hammeke T, Olsen G, Leo P, Guskiewicz K. Unreported concussion in high school football players: Implications for prevention. *Clin J Sport Med* 2004; 14: 13–17.

35. Williamson IJS, Goodman D. Converging evidence for the under-reporting of concussions in youth ice hockey. *Br J Sports Med* 2006; 40(2): 128–132.

36. Bramley H, Patrick K, Lehman E, Silvis M. High school soccer players with concussion education are more likely to notify their coach of a suspected concussion. *Clin Pediatr* 2012; 51(4): 332–336.

37. Register-Mihalik JK, Guskiewicz KM, McLeod TC, Linnan LA, Mueller FO, Marshall SW. Knowledge, attitude, and concussion-reporting behaviors among high school athletes: A preliminary study. *J Athl Train* 2013; 48(5): 645–653.

38. McCrea M, Guskiewicz K, Randolph C, Barr WB, Hammeke TA, Marshal SW, Kelly JP. Effects of a symptom-free waiting period on clinical outcome and risk of reinjury after sport-related concussion. *Neurosurg* 2009; 65: 876–882.

39. Prins ML, Alexander D, Giza CC, Hovda DA. Repeated mild traumatic brain injury: Mechanisms of cerebral vulnerability. *J Neurotrauma* 2013; 30: 30–38.

40. Schneider R. Mechanisms of injury. In Schneider R. *Head and neck injuries in football: Mechanisms, treatment, and prevention.* Baltimore, MD: Williams & Wilkins, 1973, pp. 77–126.

41. Saunders RL, Harbaugh RE. The second impact in catastrophic contact-sports head trauma. *JAMA* 1984; 252: 538–539.

42. Stovitz SD, Weseman JD, Hooks MC, Schmidt RJ, Koffel JB, Patricios JS. What definition is used to describe second impact syndrome in sports? A systematic and critical review. *Curr Sports Med Rep* 2017; 16: 50–55.

43. Meehan WP, Mannix RC, Stracciolini A, Elbin RJ, Collins MW. Symptom severity predicts prolonged recovery after sport-related concussion: Age and amnesia do not. *J Pediatr* 2013; 163: 721–725.

44. Lau B, Lovell MR, Collins MW, Pardini J. Neurocognitive and symptom predictors of recovery in high school athletes. *Clin J Sport Med* 2009; 19: 216–221.

45. Lau BC, Kontos AP, Collins MW, Mucha A, Lovell MR. Which on-field signs/symptoms predict protracted recovery from sport-related concussion among high school football players? *Am J Sports Med* 2011; 39: 2311–2318.

46. Makdissi M, Darby D, Maruff P, Ugoni A, Brukner P, McCrory PR. Natural history of concussion in sport. *Am J Sports Med* 2010; 38: 464–471.

47. Iverson GL, Gaetz M, Lovell MR, Collins MW. Relation between subjective fogginess and neuropsychological testing following concussion. *J Int Neuropsychol Soc* 2004; 10: 904–906.

48. Lovell MR, Collins MW, Iverson GL, Field M, Maroon JC, Cantu R, Podell K, et al. Recovery from mild concussion in high school athletes; *J Neurosurg* 2003; 98: 296–301.

49. Collins MW, Lovell MR, Iverson GL, Cantu RC, Maroon JC, Field M. Cumulative effects of concussion in high school athletes. *Neurosurg* 2002; 51: 1175–1179.

50. Giza CC, Kutcher JS, Ashwal S, Barth J, Getchius TS, Gioia GA, Gronseth GS, et al. Summary of evidence-based guideline update: Evaluation and management of concussion in sports. Report of the Guideline Development Subcommittee of the American Academy of Neurology. *Neurology* 2013; 80: 2250–2257.

51. Emery CA, Kang J, Shrier I, Goulet C, Hagel BE, Benson BW, Nettel-Aguirre A, et al. Risk of injury associated with body checking among youth ice hockey players. *JAMA* 2010; 303: 2265–2272.

52. Morgan CD, Zuckerman SL, Lee YM, King L, Beaird S, Sills AK, Solomon GS. Predictors of postconcussion syndrome after sports-related concussion in young athletes: A matched case-control study. *J Neurosurg Pediatr* 2015; 15: 589–598.

53. Slobounov S, Slobounov E, Sebastianelli W, Cheng C, Newell K. Differential rate of recovery in athletes after first and second concussion episodes. *Neurosurg* 2007; 61: 338–344.

54. Kontos AP, Covassin T, Elbin RJ, Parker T. Depression and neurocognitive performance after concussion among male and female high school and collegiate athletes. *Arch Phys Med Rehabil* 2012; 93: 1751–1756.

55. Chrisman SPD, Richardson LP. Prevalence of diagnosed depression in adolescents with history of concussion. *J Adolesc Health* 2014; 54: 582–586.

56. Vargas GA, Rabinowitz A, Meyer J, Arnett PA. Predictors and prevalence of postconcussion depression symptoms in collegiate athletes; *J Athl Train* 2015; 50: 250–255.

57. Covassin T, Elbin RJ, Larson E, Kontos AP. Sex and age differences in depression and baseline sport-related concussion neurocognitive performance and symptoms. *Clin J Sport Med* 2012; 22: 98–104.

58. Chamelian L, Feinstein A. The effect of major depression on subjective and objective cognitive deficits in mild to moderate traumatic brain injury. *J Neuropsychiatry Clin Neurosci* 2006; 18: 33–38.

59. Lewis DW. Pediatric migraine. *Neurol Clin* 2009; 27: 481–501.

60. Gordon KE, Dooley JM, Wood EP. Is migraine a risk factor for the development of concussion? *Br J Sports Med* 2006; 40: 184–185.

61. Lau BC, Collins MW, Lovell MR. Cutoff scores in neurocognitive testing and symptom clusters that predict protracted recovery from concussions in high school athletes. *Neurosurgery* 2012; 70(2): 371–379.

62. Heyer G, Young JA, Young SC, Rose K, McNally A, Fischer AN. Post-traumatic headaches correlate with migraine symptoms in youth with concussion. *Cephalgia* 2015; 36: 309–316.

63. Akinbami LJ, Liu X, Pastor PN, Reuben CA. *Attention deficit hyperactivity disorder among children aged 5–17 years in the United States, 1998–2009. NCHS data brief.* Number 70. Atlanta, GA: Centers for Disease Control and Prevention, 2011.

64. DiScala C, Lescohier I, Barthel M, Li G. Injuries to children with attention deficit hyperactivity disorder. *Pediatrics* 1998; 102: 1415–1421.

65. Alosco ML, Fedor AF, Gunstad J. Attention deficit hyperactivity disorder as a risk factor for concussions in NCAA Division-I athletes. *Brain Inj* 2014; 28: 472–474.

66. Iverson GL, Wojtowicz M, Brooks BL, Maxwell BA, Atkins JE, Zafonte R, et al. High school athletes with ADHD and learning difficulties have a greater lifetime concussion history. *J Attent Disord* 2016; pii: 1087054716657410.

67. Bonfield C, Lam S, Lin Y, Greene S. The impact of attention deficit hyperactivity disorder on recovery from mild traumatic brain injury. *J Neurosurg: Pediatr* 2013; 12: 97–102.

68. Dick RW. Is there a gender difference in concussion incidence and outcomes? *Br J Sports Med* 2009; 43(Suppl 1): i46–i50.

69. Wunderle K, Hoeger KM, Wasserman E, Bazarian JJ. Menstrual phase as predictor of outcome after mild traumatic brain injury in women. *J Head Trauma Rehabil* 2014; 29: E1–E8.

70. Ono KE, Burns TG, Bearden DJ, McManus SM, King H, Reisner A. Sex-based differences as a predictor of recovery trajectories in young athletes after a sports-related concussion. *Am J Sports Med* 2016; 44: 748–752.

71. Cohen P, Cohen J, Kasen S, Velez CN, Hartmark C, Johnson J, Rojas M, et al. An epidemiological study of disorders in late childhood and adolescence – I. Age- and gender-specific prevalence. *J Child Psychol Psychiatry* 1993; 34: 851–867.

72. American Psychiatric Association. DSM history. Available at www.psychiatry.org/psychiatrists/practice/dsm/history-of-the-dsm.

73. World Health Organization. International statistical classification of diseases and related health problems. Available at: www.who.int/classifications/icd/en/.

74. American Psychiatric Association. *Diagnostic and statistical manual of mental disorders, fifth edition (DSM-V).* Washington, DC: American Psychiatric Association Press, 2013.

75. World Health Organization. International statistical classification of diseases and related health problems, 10th revision. Available at: http://apps.who.int/classifications/icd10/browse/2016/en.

76. Barlow KM, Crawford S, Stevenson A, Sandhu SS, Belanger F, Dewey D. Epidemiology of postconcussion syndrome in pediatric mild traumatic brain injury. *Pediatrics* 2010; 126: e374–e381.

77. Barlow KM. Postconcussion syndrome: A review. *J Child Neurol* 2016; 31: 57.

78. Graham R, Rivara FP, Ford MA, Spicer CM (editors). Committee on Sports-Related Concussions in Youth. Board on Children, Youth, and Families; Institute of Medicine. National Research Council Sports-Related Concussions in Youth. *Improving the science, changing the culture.* Washington, DC: National Academies Press, 2014.

79. King NS, Crawford S, Wenden FJ, Moss NEG, Wade DT. The Rivermead Post Concussion Symptoms Questionnaire: A measure of symptoms commonly experienced after head injury and its reliability. *J Neurol* 1995; 242: 587–592.

80. McCrea M, Kelly JP, Randolph C, Kluge J, Bartolic E, Finn G, Baxter B. Standardized assessment of concussion (SAC): On-site mental status evaluation of the athlete. *J Head Trauma Rehabil* 1998; 13: 27–35.

81. McCrea M, Guskiewicz KM, Marshall SW, Barr W, Randolph C, Cantu RC, et al. Acute effects and recovery time following concussion in collegiate football players: The NCAA Concussion Study. *JAMA* 2003; 290: 2556–2563.

82. Piland SG, Motl RW, Guskiewicz KM, McCrea M, Ferrara MS. Structural validity of a self-report concussion-related symptom scale. *Med Sci Sports Exerc* 2006; 38(1): 278–232.

83. Grubenhoff JA, Kirkwood M, Gao D, Deakyne S, Wathen J. Evaluation of the standardized assessment of concussion in a pediatric emergency department. *Pediatrics* 2010; 126: 688–695.

84. Lovell MR, Collins MW. Neuropsychological assessment of the college football player. *J Head Trauma Rehabil* 1998; 13: 9–26.

85. Lovell MR, Iverson GL, Collins MW, Podell K, Johnston KM, Pardini D, et al. Measurement of symptoms following sports-related concussion: Reliability and normative data for the post-concussion scale. *Appl Neuropsychol* 2006; 13: 166–174.

86. Chen J-K, Johnston KM, Collie A, McCrory P, Ptito A. A validation of the post concussion symptom scale in the assessment of complex concussion using cognitive testing and functional MRI. *J Neurol Neurosurg Psychiatry* 2007; 78: 1231–1238.

87. Gioia GA, Schneider JC, Vaughan CG, Isquith PK. Which symptom assessments and approaches are uniquely appropriate for paediatric concussion? *Br J Sports Med* 2009; 43 (Suppl I): i13–i22.

88. Anonymous. Child SCAT3. Sport Concussion Assessment Tool for children ages 5 to 12 years. *Br J Sports Med* 2013; 47 (5): 263. Available at: http://bjsm.bmj.com/content/bjsports/47/5/263.full.pdf.

89. Guskiewicz KM, Register-Mihalik J, McCrory P, McCrea M, Johnston K, Makdissi M, et al. Evidence-based approach to revising the SCAT2: Introducing the SCAT3. *Br J Sports Med* 2013; 47: 289–293.

90. Nelson LD, Loman MM, LaRoche AA, Furger RE, McCrea MA. Baseline performance and psychometric properties of the child Sport Concussion Assessment Tool 3 (Child-SCAT3) in 5- to 13-year-old athletes. *Clin J Sport Med* 2017; 27 (4): 381–387.

91. Porter S, Smith-Forrester J, Alhajri N, Kusch C, Sun J, Barrable B, William J, et al. The Child Sport Concussion Assessment Tool (Child SCAT3): Normative values and correspondence between child and parent symptom scores in male child athletes. *BMJ Open Sport Exerc Med* 2015; 1 (1): e000029.

92. Gioia GA. Multimodal evaluation and management of children with concussion: Using our heads and available evidence. *Brain Inj* 2015; 29: 195–206.

93. Gioia GA, Collins MW. Acute concussion evaluation (ACE): Physician/clinician version. 2006. Available at: www.cdc.gov/ncipc/tbi/PhysiciansTool Kit.htm.

94. Sady MD, Vaughan CG, Gioia GA. Psychometric characteristics of the postconcussion symptom inventory in children and adolescents. *Arch Clin Neuropsychol* 2014; 29: 348–363.

95. Sheedy J, Harvey E, Faux S, Geffen G, Shores EA. Emergency department assessment of mild traumatic brain injury and the prediction of postconcussive symptoms: A 3-month prospective study. *J Head Trauma Rehabil* 2009; 24: 333–343.

96. Peterson RL, Kirkwood MW, Taylor HG, Stancin T, Brown TM, Wade SL. Adolescents' internalizing problems following traumatic brain injury are related to parents' psychiatric symptoms. *J Head Trauma Rehabil* 2013; 28: E1.

97. Raj SP, Wade SL, Cassedy A, Taylor G, Stancin T, Brown TM, et al. Parent psychological functioning and communication predict externalizing behavior problems after pediatric traumatic brain injury. *J Pediatr Psychol* 2014; 39 (1): 84–95.

98. Zemek R, Barrowman N, Freedman SB, Grave J, Gagnon I, McGahern C, et al. Clinical risk score for persistent postconcussion symptoms among children with acute concussion in the ED. *JAMA* 2016; 315: 1014–1025.

99. Ayr LK, Yeates KO, Taylor HG, Browne M. Dimensions of postconcussive symptoms in children with mild traumatic brain injuries. *J Int Neuropsychol Soc* 2009; 15: 19–30.

100. Babikian T, Merkley T, Savage RC, Giza CC, Levin H. Chronic aspects of pediatric traumatic brain injury: Review of the literature. *J Neurotrauma* 2015; 32: 1849–1860.

101. Kennard MA. Age and other factors in motor recovery from precentral lesions in monkeys. *Am J Physiol-Legacy Content* 1936; 115: 138–146.

102. Stiles J, Jernigan TL. The basics of brain development. *Neuropsychol Rev* 2010; 20: 327–348.

103. Juraska JM, Lowry NC. Neuroanatomical changes associated with cognitive aging. *Curr Top Behav Neurosci* 2012; 10: 137–162.

104. Crowe LM, Catroppa C, Babl FE, Rosenfeld JV, Anderson V. Timing of traumatic brain injury in childhood and intellectual outcome. *J Pediatr Psychol* 2012; 37: 745–754.

105. Spencer-Smith M, Anderson V. Healthy and abnormal development of the prefrontal cortex. *Dev Neurorehabil* 2009; 12: 279–297.

106. Juraska JM, Willing J. Pubertal onset as a critical transition for neural development and cognition. *Brain Res* 2017; 1654: 87–94.

107. Catroppa C, Anderson V. A prospective study of the recovery of attention from acute to 2 years following pediatric traumatic brain injury. *J Int Neuropsychol Soc* 2005; 11: 84–98.

108. Babikian T, Asarnow R. Neurocognitive outcomes and recovery after pediatric TBI: Meta-analytic review of the literature. *Neuropsychology* 2009; 23(3): 283–296.

109. Catroppa C, Anderson VA, Morse SA, Haritou F, Rosenfeld JV. Children's attentional skills 5 years post-TBI. *J Pediatr Psychol* 2007; 32: 354–369.

110. Babikian T, Satz P, Zaucha K, Light R, Lewis RS, Asarnow RF. The UCLA longitudinal study of neurocognitive outcomes following mild pediatric traumatic brain injury. *J Int Neuropsychol Soc* 2011; 17: 886–895.

111. Anderson V, Catroppa C, Morse S, Haritou F, Rosenfeld J. Attentional and processing skills following traumatic brain injury in early childhood. *Brain Inj* 2005; 19: 699–710.

112. Ewing-Cobbs L, Prasad MR, Landry SH, Kramer L, DeLeon R. Executive functions following traumatic brain injury in young children: A preliminary analysis. *Dev Neuropsychol* 2004; 26: 487–512.

113. Cacioppo JT, Gardner WL. Emotion. *Annu Rev Psychol* 1999; 50: 191–214.

114. Massagli TL, Fann JR, Burington BE, Jaffe KM, Katon WJ, Thompson RS. Psychiatric illness after mild traumatic brain injury in children. *Arch Phys Med Rehabili* 2004; 85: 1428–1434.

115. McKinlay A, Grace R, Horwood J, Fergusson D, MacFarlane M. Adolescent psychiatric symptoms following preschool childhood mild traumatic brain injury: Evidence from a birth cohort. *J Head Trauma Rehabil* 2009; 24: 221–227.

116. Taylor HG. Orchinik LJ, Minich N, Dietrich A, Nuss K, Wright M, et al. Symptoms of persistent behavior problems in children with mild traumatic brain injury. *J Head Trauma Rehabil* 2015; 30: 302–310.

117. Lovell MR, Collins MW, Podell K, Powell J, Maroon J. *ImPACT: Immediate Post-Concussion Assessment and cognitive Testing*. Pittsburgh, PA: NeuroHealth Systems, 2000.

118. Maruff P, Thomas E, Cysique L, Bre B, Collie A, Snyder P, Pietrzak RH. Validity of the CogState brief battery: Relationship to standardized tests and sensitivity to cognitive impairment in mild traumatic brain injury, schizophrenia, and AIDS dementia complex. *Arch Clin Neuropsychol* 2009; 24: 165–178.

119. Moriarity J. Cogstate Computerized Cognitive Assessment Tool (CCAT). Available at: www.axonsports.ca/index.cfm?pid=65.

120. Erlanger D, Saliba E, Barth J, Almquist J. Monitoring resolution of postconcussion symptoms in athletes: Preliminary results of a web-based neuropsychological test protocol. *J Athl Train* 2001; 36: 280–287.

121. Levinson D, Reeves D. Monitoring recovery from traumatic brain injury using Automated Neuropsychological Assessment Metrics (ANAM V1.0). *Arch Clin Neuropsychol* 1997; 12 (2): 155–166.

122. Gualtieri CT, Johnson LG. Reliability and validity of a computerized neurocognitive test battery, CNS Vital Signs. *Arch Clin Neuropsychol* 2006; 21: 623–643.

123. Schatz P, Pardini JE, Lovell MR, Collins MW, Podell K. Sensitivity and specificity of the ImPACT test battery for concussion in athletes. *Arch Clin Neuropsychol* 2006; 21: 91–99.

124. Schatz P, Sandel N. Sensitivity and specificity of the online version of ImPACT in high school and collegiate athletes. *Am J Sports Med* 2013; 41: 321–326.

125. Lichtenstein JD, Moser RS, Schatz P. Age and test setting affect the prevalence of invalid baseline scores on neurocognitive tests. *Am J Sports Med* 2014; 42: 479–484.

126. Iverson GL, Lovell MR, Collins MW. Interpreting change on ImPACT following sport concussion. *Clin Neuropsychol* 2003; 17: 460–467.

127. Miller JR, Adamson GJ, Pink MM, Sweet JC. Comparison of preseason, midseason, and postseason neurocognitive scores in uninjured collegiate football players. *Am J Sports Med* 2007; 35: 1284–1288.

128. Elbin RJ, Schatz P, Covassin T. One-year test–retest reliability of the online version of ImPACT in high school athletes. *Am J Sports Med* 2011; 39: 2319–2324.

129. Nakayama Y, Covassin T, Schatz P, Nogle S, Kovan J. Examination of the test–retest reliability of a computerized neurocognitive test battery. *Am J Sports Med* 2014; 42: 2000–2005.

130. Alsalaheen BA, Whitney SL, Marchetti GF, Furman JM, Kontos AP, Collins MW, Sparto PJ. Relationship between cognitive assessment and balance measures in adolescents referred for vestibular physical therapy after concussion *Clin J Sport Med* 2016; 26: 46–52.

131. Schneider KJ, Emery CA, Kang J, Schneider GM, Meeuwisse WH. Examining Sport Concussion Assessment Tool ratings for male and female youth hockey players with and without a history of concussion. *Br J Sports Med* 2010; 44: 1112–1117.

132. Jinguji TM, Bompadre V, Harmon KG, Satchell EK, Gilbert K, Wild J, Eary JF. Sport Concussion Assessment Tool-2: Baseline values for high school athletes. *Br J Sports Med* 2012; 46: 365–370.

133. McLeod TCV, Bay RC, Lam KC, Chhabra A. Representative baseline values on the Sport Concussion Assessment Tool 2 (SCAT2) in adolescent athletes vary by gender, grade, and concussion history. *Am J Sports Med* 2012; 40: 927–933.

134. Schatz P. Long-term test–retest reliability of baseline cognitive assessments using ImPACT. *Am J Sports Med* 2010; 38: 47–53.

135. Vaughan CG, Gioia G, Vincent D. Initial examination of self-reported post-concussion symptoms in normal and mTBI children ages 5 to 12. *J Int Neuropsych Soc* 2008; 14(Suppl 1): 207.

136. Galetta KM, Brandes LE, Maki K, Dziemianowicz MS, Laudano E, Allen M, et al. The King–Devick test and sports-related concussion: study of a rapid visual screening tool in a collegiate cohort. *J Neurol Sci* 2011; 309: 34–39.

137. King D, Gissane C, Hume PA, Flaws M. The King-Devick Test was useful in management of concussion in amateur rugby union and rugby league in New Zealand. *J Neurol Sci* 2015; 351: 58–64.

138. Weise KK, Swanson MW, Penix K, Hale MH, Ferguson D. King-Devick and pre-season visual function in adolescent athletes. *Optom Vision Sci* 2017; 94: 89–95.

139. Eckner JT, Kutcher JS, Richardson JK. Between-seasons test–retest reliability of clinically measured reaction time in National Collegiate Athletic Association Division I athletes. *J Athl Train* 2011; 46: 409–414.

140. McCrea M, Barr WB, Guskiewicz K, Randolph C, Marshall S, Cantu R, et al. Standard regression-based methods for measuring recovery after sport-related concussion. *J Int Neuropsychol Soc* 2005; 11: 58–69.

141. Ellis MJ, Leiter J, Hall T, McDonald PJ, Sawyer S, Silver N, et al. Neuroimaging findings in pediatric sports-related concussion. *J Neurosurg Pediatr* 2015; 16: 241–247.

142. Lovell MR, Pardini JE, Welling J, Collins MW, Bakal J, Lazar N, et al. Functional brain abnormalities are related to clinical recovery and time to return-to-play in athletes. *Neurosurg* 2007; 61: 352–360.

143. Keightley ML, Singh Saluja R, Chen JK, Gagnon I, Leonard G, Petrides M, et al. A functional magnetic resonance imaging study of working memory in youth after sports-related concussion: Is it still working? *J Neurotrauma* 2014; 31: 437–451.

144. Maugans TA, Farley C, Altaye M, Leach J, Cecil KM. Pediatric sports-related concussion produces cerebral blood flow alterations. *Pediatrics* 2012; 129: 28–37.

145. Meier TB, Bellgowan PS, Singh R, Kuplicki R, Polanski DW, Mayer AR. Recovery of cerebral blood flow following sports-related concussion. *JAMA Neurol* 2015; 72: 530–538.

146. Mutch WAC, Ellis MJ, Ryner LN, Ruth Graham M, Dufault B, et al. Brain magnetic resonance imaging CO_2 stress testing in adolescent postconcussion syndrome. *J Neurosurg* 2015; 125: 1–13.

147. McCrory P, Meeuwisse W, Dvorak J, Aubry M, Bailes J, Broglio S, et al. Consensus statement on concussion in sport – the 5th International Conference on Concussion in Sport held in Berlin, October 2016. *Br J Sports Med* 2017; 51: 1–10.

148. Gioia G, Vaughan C, Reesman J, McGuire E, Gathercole L, Padia H, et al. Characterizing post-concussion exertional effects in the child and adolescent. *J Int Neuropsychol Soc* 2010; 16: 178.

149. Moser RS, Glatts C, Schatz P. Efficacy of immediate and delayed cognitive and physical rest for treatment of sports-related concussion. *J Pediatr* 2012; 161: 922–926.

150. Asken BM, McCrea MA, Clugston JR, Snyder AR, Houck ZM, Bauer RM. "Playing Through It": Delayed reporting and removal from athletic activity after concussion predicts prolonged recovery. *J Athl Train* 2016; 51: 329–335.

151. DiFazio M, Silverberg ND, Kirkwood MW, Bernier R, Iverson GL. Prolonged activity restriction after concussion: Are we worsening outcomes? *Clin Pediatr* 2016; 55: 443–451.

152. Thomas DG, Apps JN, Hoffmann RG, McCrea M, Hammeke T. Benefits of strict rest after acute concussion: a randomized controlled trial. *Pediatrics* 2015; 135: 213–223.

153. Brown NJ, Mannix RC, O'Brien MJ, Gostine D, Collins MW, Meehan WP. Effect of cognitive activity level on duration of post-concussion symptoms. *Pediatrics* 2014; 133: e299–e304.

154. Halstead ME, McAvoy K, Devore CD, Carl R, Lee M, Logan K, et al. Returning to learning following a concussion. *Pediatrics* 2013; 132: 948–957.

155. Centers for Disease Control and Prevention; U.S. Department of Health and Human Services. Returning to school after a concussion: A fact sheet for school professionals. 2016. Available at: www.cdc.gov/headsup/highschoolsports/index.html.

156. Centers for Disease Control and Prevention; U.S. Department of Health and Human Services. Helping students recover from a concussion: Classroom tips for teachers. 2016. Available at: www.cdc.gov/headsup/highschoolsports/index.html.

157. Sady MD, Vaughan CG, Gioia GA. School and the concussed youth: Recommendations for concussion education and management. *Phys Med Rehabil Clin N Am* 2011; 22: 701–719.

158. Ransom DM, Vaughan CG, Pratson L, Sady MD, McGill CA, Gioia GA. Academic effects of concussion in children and adolescents. *Pediatrics* 2015; 135: 1043–1050.

159. Manuel JC, Shilt JS, Curl WW, Smith JA, Durant R, Lester L, Sinal SH. Coping with sports injuries: An examination of the adolescent athlete. *J Adolesc Health* 2002; 31: 391–393.

160. Griesbach GS, Hovda DA, Gomez-Pinilla F. Exercise-induced improvement in cognitive performance after traumatic brain injury in rats is dependent on BDNF activation. *Brain Res* 2009; 1288: 105–115.

161. Griesbach GS, Tio DL, Nair S, Hovda A. Recovery of stress response coincides with responsiveness to voluntary exercise after traumatic brain injury. *J Neurotrauma* 2014; 31: 674–682.

162. Tan CO, Meehan WP 3rd, Iverson GL, Taylor JA. Cerebrovascular regulation, exercise, and mild traumatic brain injury. *Neurology* 2014; 83: 1665–1672.

163. Majerske CW, Mihalik JP, Ren D, Collins MW, Reddy CC, Lovell MR, Wagner AK. Concussion in sports: Postconcussive activity levels, symptoms, and neurocognitive performance. *J Athl Training* 2008; 43: 265–274.

164. Maerlender A, Rieman W, Lichtenstein J, Condiracci C. Programmed physical exertion in recovery from sports-related concussion: A randomized pilot study. *Develop Neuropsychol* 2015; 40: 273–278.

165. Grool AM, Aglipay M, Momoli F, Meehan WP, Freedman SB, Yeates KO, Gravel J, et al. for the Pediatric Emergency Research Canada (PERC) Concussion Team. Association between early participation in physical activity following acute concussion and persistent postconcussive symptoms in children and adolescents. *JAMA* 2016; 316(23): 2504–2514.

166. Howell DR, Mannix RC, Quinn B, Taylor JA, Tan CO, Meehan WP. Physical activity level and symptom duration are not associated after concussion. *Am J Sports Med* 2016; 44(4): 1040–1046.

167. Leddy JJ, Kowslowski K, Donnelly JP, Pendergast DR, Epstein LH, Willer B. A preliminary study of subsystem threshold exercise training for refractory postconcussion syndrome. *Clin J Sport Med* 2010; 20(1): 21–27.

168. Gagnon I, Grilli L, Friedman D, Iverson GL. A pilot study of active rehabilitation for adolescents who are slow to recover from sport-related concussion. *Scand J Med Sci Sports* 2016; 26: 299–306.

169. Adler RH. Youth sports and concussions: Preventing preventable brain injuries. One client, one cause, and a new law. *Phys Med Rehabil Clin N Am* 2011; 22: 721–728.

170. Oregon Concussion Awareness and Management Program. Max's law: Concussion management implementation guide. Available at: www.ode.state.or.us/teachlearn/subjects/pe/ocampguide.pdf.

171. Chrisman SP, Schiff MA, Chung SK, Herring SA, Rivara FP. Implementation of concussion legislation and extent of concussion education for athletes, parents, and coaches in Washington state. *Am J Sports Med* 2014; 42: 1190–1196.

172. Ellenbogen RG. Concussion advocacy and legislation: A neurological surgeon's view from the epicenter. *Neurosurg* 2014; 75: S122–S130.

173. Code of Virginia § 22.1–271.5. Guidelines and policies and procedures on concussions in student-athletes. Available at: http://law.lis.virginia.gov/vacode/title22.1/chapter14/section22.1–271.5/.

174. McGuine TA. Effect of new rule limiting full contact practice on incidence of sport related concussion in high school football players. In 2015 AAP National Conference and Exhibition, American Academy of Pediatrics.

175. Swartz EE, Broglio SP, Cook SB, Cantu RC, Ferrara MS, Guskiewicz KM, Myers JL. Early results of a helmetless-tackling intervention to decrease head impacts in football players. *J Athl Train* 2015; 50: 1219–1222.

176. American Academy of Pediatrics Committee on Sports Medicine and Fitness Safety in Youth Ice Hockey. The effects of body checking. *Pediatrics* 2000; 105: 657–658.

177. Macpherson A, Rothman L, Howard A. Body-checking rules and childhood injuries in ice hockey. *Pediatrics* 2006; 117: e143–e147.

178. Cusimano M, Taback N, McFaull S, Hodgins R, Bekele T, Elfeki N. Effect of bodychecking on rate of injuries among minor hockey players. *Open Med* 2011; 5: 57–64.

179. Warsh JM, Constantin SA, Howard A, Macpherson A. A systematic review of the association between body checking and injury in youth ice hockey. *Clin J Sport Med* 2009; 19: 134–144.

180. Emery CA, Kang J, Shrier I, Goulet C, Hagel B, Benson BW, et al. Risk of injury associated with body checking among youth ice hockey players. *JAMA* 2010; 303: 2265–2272.

181. Comstock RD, Currie DW, Pierpoint LA, Grubenhoff JA, Fields SK. An evidence-based discussion of heading the ball and concussions in high school soccer. *JAMA Pediatr* 2015; 169: 830–837.

182. Urban JE, Davenport EM, Golman AJ, Maldjian JA, Whitlow CT, Powers AK, et al. Head impact exposure in youth football: High school ages 14 to 18 years and cumulative impact analysis. *Ann Biomed Eng* 2013; 41: 2474–2487.

183. Cobb BR, Urban JE, Davenport EM, Rowson S, Duma SM, Maldjian JA, et al. Head impact exposure in youth football: Elementary school ages 9–12 years and the effect of practice structure. *Ann Biomed Eng* 2013; 41: 2463–2473.

184. Davenport EM, Whitlow CT, Urban JE, Espeland MA, Jung Y, Rosenbaum DA, et al. Abnormal white matter integrity related to head impact exposure in a season of high school varsity football. *J Neurotrauma* 2014; 31: 1617–1624.

185. Weir DR, Jackson JS, Sonnega A. *National Football League Player Care Foundation study of retired NFL players*. Ann Arbor, MI: University of Michigan Institute for Social Research, 2009.

186. Savica R, Parisi JE, Wold LE, Josephs KA, Ahlskog JE. High school football and risk of neurodegeneration: A community-based study. *Mayo Clin Proc* 2012; 87(4): 335–340.

187. Janssen PH, Mandrekar J, Mielke MM, Ahlskog JE, Boeve BF, Josephs K, Savica R. High school football and late-life risk of neurodegenerative syndromes, 1956–1970. *Mayo Clin Proc* 2017; 92(1): 66–71.

188. McKee A. Interview, Public Broadcasting Service. FRONTLINE interviews; league of denial: the NFL's concussion crisis. May 20, 2013. Available at: www.pbs.org/wgbh/pages/frontline/sports/league-of-denial/the-frontline-interview-ann-mckee/.

189. Bieniek KF, Ross OA, Cormier KA, Walton RL, Soto-Ortolaza A, Johnston AE, et al. Chronic traumatic encephalopathy pathology in a neurodegenerative disorders brain bank. *Acta Neuropathol* 2015; 130(6): 877–889.

190. Hazrati LN, Tartaglia MC, Diamandis P, Davis K, Green, RE, Wennberg R et al. Absence of chronic traumatic encephalopathy in retired football players with multiple concussions and neurological symptomatology. *Front Hum Neurosci* 2103; 7: 222.

191. Stamm JM, Bourlas AP, Baugh CM, Fritts NG, Daneshvar DH, Martin BM, et al. Age of first exposure to football and later-life cognitive impairment in former NFL players. *Neurology* 2015; 84(11): 1114–1120.

192. Dik MG, Deeg DJ, Visser M, Jonker C. Early life physical activity and cognition at old age. *J Clin Exper Neuropsychol* 2003; 25(5): 643–653.

193. Middleton LE, Barnes DE, Lui LY, Yaffe K. Physical activity over the life course and its association with cognitive performance and impairment in old age. *J Am Geriatr Soc* 2010; 58: 1322–1326.

Contribution of Objective Tests to the Diagnosis of Sport-Related Concussion

Elizabeth Teel and Kevin Guskiewicz

Introduction

Despite common belief, *cerebral concussion* is an injury that occurs in nearly all competitive sports, as well as a host of work and recreational activities. Whether on the sideline, in the athletic training room, in theater (warfare), or in a clinical/hospital environment, a thorough and consistent approach to evaluating individuals suspected of a concussion will aid in improving clinical diagnoses and return-to-activity decisions. However, when traumatic brain injury (TBI) is suspected the nature and severity of the injury must first be determined in order to develop an appropriate management plan. An injury that at first appears to be a concussion could actually involve more serious pathology such as a subdural hematoma, epidural hematoma, or diffuse cerebral edema. The clinician managing these injuries should be skilled in the early detection, diagnosis, and follow-up evaluation procedures of brain-related injuries. The focus of this chapter is to introduce a systematic approach to acute diagnosis and management of concussion, with an emphasis on the psychometric properties of the various tools utilized in a multifaceted assessment battery.

On-Field Evaluation

The first step in management is to determine whether a concussion has occurred, as well as to determine if the athlete is at risk for more serious or catastrophic progressions. On-field and sideline assessments largely serve as triage, in order to ascertain the extent of the injury and the best course of care for the athlete. Clinicians, such as athletic trainers or physicians, should first perform a primary assessment to rule out any life-threatening injuries. Although loss of consciousness (LOC) occurs infrequently with sport-related concussion – less than 10% of all concussions [1, 2]. An athlete who does present with LOC should also be carefully evaluated for a cervical spine injury [3]. Along with assessing level of consciousness, the primary survey should also include establishing an airway and checking pulse and breathing rates [3]. If no significant clinical findings are observed, the athlete can be moved to the sideline for further evaluation.

Once moved to the sideline, the clinician can begin taking a history of the incident, including the specific mechanism of injury if not observed. By asking the athlete to recall events associated with the injury and shortly thereafter, the clinician can establish if the athlete is suffering from anterograde amnesia. Anterograde amnesia can be quickly assessed during this period, by providing the athlete with three unrelated words and asking the athlete to recall these words after 10–15-minutes. The clinician should also assess the athlete for retrograde amnesia by asking the athlete to recall events from earlier in the day, or earlier in the week preceding the injury. Establishing a general duration of the amnesia if present is also helpful in determining the severity of the concussion, although duration of overall symptoms is equally important.

Following the history, observation and palpation of the athlete can begin. This includes checking pupil size, reactivity to light, fluidity of eye movement, monitoring for aphasia (difficulty finding words), and checking pulse and blood pressure. Abnormalities on any of these measures may be indicative of more serious injury than concussion and warrants immediate transportation to a medical facility. Should the athlete complete the primary and secondary surveys with no significant clinical findings, a variety of special tests can be used to more definitively diagnosis a concussive episode [3].

Sideline Tools

There are a variety of assessment tools designed for use on the sideline immediately after a suspected injury that have been shown to be sensitive to the effects of concussion. As other conditions have been shown to mimic the signs and symptoms of concussion, such as dehydration [3], it is important to have valid and sensitive assessment tools that can accurately differentiate between concussed and non-concussed participants. Since concussive episodes are highly variable in nature, it is important that each athlete receive an individualized approach to injury management [4]. Therefore, baseline measures of normal symptomology, cognitive functioning, and postural control are recommended whenever possible. If baseline values are not available, most clinically used concussion assessment tools have normative values that can be used for comparison.

Symptom Checklists

One of the simplest and most important tools for assessing possible concussive injuries is a graded symptom checklist (GSC). Traditionally, these lists offer a number of common concussion symptoms, whereby the athlete is asked to rate the severity of each symptom on a Likert scale (0 represents "not experiencing" the symptom, 1 represents "mild", and

6 represents a "severe" presentation of the symptom). A variety of different symptom rating scales are employed in clinical use, though a number of studies have used scales which range between 14 and 22 listed symptoms [5–9]. A review by the American Academy of Neurology found that, on average, composite symptom scores increased by 23–25 points after a concussion, which is approximately three to five times higher than reported baseline symptoms [10]. Following a concussive episode, the most commonly reported symptoms include headache, balance problems, and mental slowing [1, 11].

McCrea et al. [6] investigated the sensitivity and specificity of the 17-item GSC. Changes were deemed clinically meaningful between baseline and post-injury measures if the difference between observed and predicted scores, divided by the standard error of prediction, was larger than a specific criterion value (which translated into a 90% confidence interval). Using this cutoff, the GSC was found to have a sensitivity of 0.89 and a specificity of 1.00. A similar study by Van Kampen et al. [12] evaluated the sensitivity of the post-concussion symptoms (PCS) scale. Changes between testing sessions were considered clinically meaningful if the scores exceeded the reliable change index calculated for the PCS. Using this method, the PCS scale had a sensitivity of 64% and a specificity of 91%.

Overall, symptom checklists are valuable diagnostic tools. The large increase in reported symptoms after concussive episodes provides a clear way to distinguish between concussed and non-concussed athletes with moderate to high sensitivity and a high specificity.

Standardized Assessment of Concussion (SAC)

While not as extensive as computer-based or traditional paper-and-pencil neuropsychological exams, the SAC is a brief mental status exam designed primarily as a sideline tool, which takes approximately six to eight minutes to administer. If the administrator is properly trained, the SAC can be interpreted without the help of a neuropsychologist [13]. The SAC consists of five different sections that evaluate orientation, immediate memory, concentration, and delayed recall. These sections, when added together, are worth a total of 30 points. Higher scores are indicative of better performance on the SAC. Multiple versions of the SAC are available, to reduce the risk of practice effects from multiple iterations. Additionally, there is a portion of the SAC that is used to rule out gross neurological dysfunction, but this portion does not contribute to the total score.

Several studies have shown a decrease in total SAC score immediately following a concussive event compared to both pre-season baselines and/or a control group [5, 13, 14]. Although the average decline in total SAC score is four points after concussion, a 2001 study by Barr et al. [15] identified that a decrease of one point from baseline values could be indicative of a concussive injury. Using this cutoff, the SAC was found to have a sensitivity of 94% and a specificity of 76% when administered immediately after injury.

In a 2005 study by McCrea et al. [6] applying standard regression-based methods, the SAC was 80% sensitive and 91% specific when compared to controls over the first seven days post injury. While the SAC is a useful sideline tool, it is important to note that it is only valid for the first 48 h post injury [5, 6]. Therefore, while it is a useful diagnostic tool within the first two days post injury, it is not suggested for long-term injury tracking.

In general, the SAC appears to be a valuable diagnostic tool, capable of being administered and interpreted quickly on the sideline. The SAC has been shown to be highly sensitive and specific, with more than even a one-point drop in total score suggestive of possible concussive injury.

Military Acute Concussion Evaluation (MACE)

The MACE is a tool designed to acutely diagnose concussions in theater. It is designed to be a quickly administered tool that can be easily interpreted by trained military medical personnel during training or warfare. The MACE has the SAC embedded within the assessment, testing the same domains of orientation, immediate memory, concentration, and delayed recall [16]. Scoring for the MACE is identical to the SAC, with a total possible score of 30 points, with higher scores indicating better performance. Additionally, there is a neurologic screening portion of the MACE which does not contribute to the total score but is designed to rule out more catastrophic brain injury.

The MACE has previously been shown to be a valid tool for concussion diagnosis in a military population [17]. A study by Coldren et al. [18] tested military personnel 12–72 h post concussive injury. Using a cutoff score of below 27, the MACE was found to have a sensitivity of 51% and a specificity of 64%. However, this study was limited by a lack of baseline scores for comparison and long time (+48 h) between injury and testing. Without these limitations, the sensitivity and specificity of the MACE would likely improve.

Overall, the MACE is a validated and useful tool for concussion diagnosis in the immediate period after injury, specifically for military service members. When testing soldiers more than 12 h after injury, caution should be used as it appears there is a rapid return to baseline utilizing this tool.

Balance Error Scoring System (BESS)

Sideline concussion assessments should also include an evaluation of balance, as postural sway is known to increase after concussion, particularly when the eyes are closed and visual referencing has been removed. While there are a number of balance assessments available, the BESS is one of the most widely used as it is designed to be clinic-friendly, fast, and easily administered on the sideline or in locker rooms [19].

The BESS consists of six different conditions: double-leg, single-leg, and tandem stances completed first on firm surfaces than repeated on a foam pad. Individuals hold each stance for 20 s each, with their eyes closed and hands on hips, while the test administrator counts the number of errors throughout each trial. The six conditions and list of errors are found in Figure 19.1 and Table 19.1. A maximum score of ten can be given for each condition, with the highest possible score on the BESS being 60. Importantly, higher scores on the BESS represent poorer balance, and therefore, individuals should be striving for the lowest possible scores.

The six Balance Error Scoring System (BESS) conditions

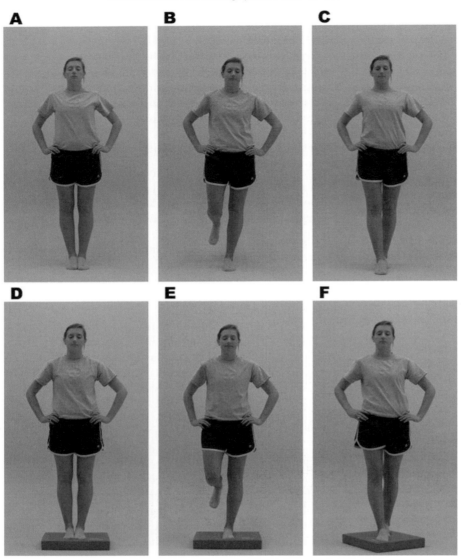

Fig. 19.1 (A) Double-leg, firm condition. (B) Single-leg (non-dominant foot), firm condition. (C) Tandem stance (non-dominant foot in back), firm condition. (D) Double-leg, foam condition. (E) Single-leg (non-dominant foot), foam condition. (F) Tandem stance (non-dominant leg in back), foam condition.

Source: Balance Error Scoring System (BESS) Manual [20]

Table 19.1 List of errors for Balance Error Scoring System (BESS)

An error is credited to the subject when any of the following occur:

- Moving the hands off the iliac crests
- Opening the eyes
- Step, stumble, or fall
- Abduction or flexion of the hip beyond 30°
- Lifting the forefoot or heel off the testing surface
- Remaining out of the proper testing position for greater than 5 seconds

The maximum total number of errors for any single condition is ten.

Several studies have found the BESS capable of detecting postural stability deficits in concussed individuals compared to control groups [21–23] or to healthy (pre-season) baselines [5]. Typically, BESS scores are highest immediately after injury and return to baseline over a three- to five-day period [5, 23].

A change in BESS scores of three points or more has been considered the benchmark for clinically meaningful changes [24]. Due to the variability in balance performance in general, baseline balance testing is very important for an accurate interpretation of post-injury performance. McCrea et al. [6] found that the BESS had a relatively low sensitivity (34%); however, impairments were observed in 36% of the concussed subjects immediately following the injury, compared to 5% of the control group. Twenty-four percent of injured subjects remained impaired on the BESS on day 2, compared to 9% by day 7 post injury. Additionally, the BESS has relatively high specificity (91%). As with most balance assessments, the BESS can be influenced by several factors, including the use of braces, taping, or fatigue. It is suggested that the clinicians wait 13–20 minutes after physical activity to administer the BESS [25, 26].

The BESS is a balance assessment tool that can be easily administered on the sidelines by clinicians in a timely manner.

BESS scores usually increase immediately after injury and decrease after three to five days post injury, which make it a useful diagnostic tool with especially high specificity.

Sport Concussion Assessment Tool – 3rd Edition (SCAT-3)

The SCAT-3 [27] is a sideline concussion assessment comprising a battery of several different concussion assessment components. The SCAT-3 includes the ability to evaluate for the possibility of catastrophic injury (Glasgow Coma Scale, Maddock's Scores), symptoms (Post-Concussion Symptom Scale), neuropsychological measures (SAC), balance (modified BESS), and functional deficits (neck and coordination exams). Currently, the recommendation is to score and analyze each component of the SCAT-3 individually [28], so as to have separate scores for each section (GSC, SAC, BESS, etc.) opposed to a composite score of all subtests, which was previously recommended with the SCAT-2. The SCAT-3 was created after the 4th International Conference on Concussions in Sports with the intent of providing clinicians with a more sensitive and user-friendly upgrade of the SCAT-2 [28]. In addition to minor changes in administering the test and the aforementioned scoring changes, a timed tandem gait assessment was added to the balance testing in situations where the foam pad is not available for the BESS.

A recent study by Putukian et al. [29] concluded that the SCAT-2 (and thus SCAT-3) was a useful tool in the acute assessment of concussion. In a sample of collegiate athletes, the SCAT-2 and SCAT-3 found significant differences between baseline and post-injury scores. The study also found that lower SCAT-2 scores were not associated with self-reported concussion history and LOC. Additionally, although pre-injury measures of depression and anxiety were correlated with higher baseline symptom scores, these factors were not associated with lower SCAT-2 scores or worse clinical outcomes. Resolution of symptoms and return to activity were not influenced by factors such as gender or history of concussion.

Using a 3.5-drop from total baseline SCAT-2 score, the test has a 96% sensitivity and 83% specificity in identifying athletes with concussion. When baseline data were not available, a cutoff score of 74.5 was used, and the SCAT-2 has a sensitivity of 83% and a specificity of 91%. Together, this study supports the clinically recommended concept of using a baseline and post-injury assessment model, but shows that there is still test utility in situations where baseline SCAT-2 scores are not available (but group normative data exist).

In general, all of the aforementioned sideline tools discussed can be quickly and easily administered by clinicians in a variety of sport settings and require little to no equipment. These assessment tools are able to distinguish concussive injuries with moderate to high sensitivity and moderate to high specificity, making them useful concussion diagnostic tools. While sideline tools have the benefit of immediate administration and help to quickly identify injury and severity, many of the sideline tools are limited in their sensitivity over several days. Clinicians utilizing these tools should keep this information

in mind when making return-to-play decisions for athletes returning from concussion.

Clinical/Laboratory Tools

While sideline tools do a considerable job in injury identification, they are designed to recognize gross deficits. Therefore, some of the more subtle deficits experienced post concussion can be missed if only using sideline tools. In order to combat this issue, a large number of clinical or laboratory-based concussion diagnostic tools have been developed. Although often not as quickly administered or, in some cases, easily interpreted, laboratory tools delve into the finer aspects of cognition, balance, and gait after concussion and serve as sensitive tools for more extended periods of time.

Neuropsychological Testing

Neuropsychological assessments have become an important fixture of concussion diagnosis and management. There are several commercially available computerized batteries, such as the Immediate Post-Concussion Assessment and Cognitive Testing (ImPACT [30, 31]), Concussion Vitals Signs [32], Automated Neuropsychological Assessment Metrics (ANAM [33]), HeadMinder Concussion Resolution Index (CRI [34]), and CogState [35].

In addition to computerized batteries, a number of more traditional paper-and-pencil neuropsychological tests have high utility in concussion diagnosis. In general, most of the neuropsychological assessments used in concussion care assess domains such as immediate and delayed memory (verbal and/or visual), attention, cognitive flexibility, response speed, executive functioning, concentration, and information processing. These types of assessments often require a trained neuropsychologist for interpretation, but other clinicians can administer many of the specific tests.

A number of studies have shown neuropsychological assessments to be a useful diagnostic tool in concussion care, with neuropsychological batteries capable of differentiating concussed individuals in within-subjects (baseline scores) or between-subjects (control groups) settings. The domains of memory and response speed seem to be particularly valuable diagnostic markers [36–39]. Neuropsychological testing has been shown as a useful diagnostic tool seven days post injury [9, 40] with resolution typically occurring by day 10 post injury [41].

Several studies have investigated the sensitivity and specificity of neuropsychological tests. As each testing platform is slightly different, discussing psychometric properties of each neuropsychological tool is beyond the scope of this work. A review by Randolph et al. [42] details the sensitivity, reliability, and utility of several different neuropsychological tools mentioned here, including information on many paper-and-pencil neuropsychological tests. In general, most neuropsychological tests have reported sensitivity and/or specificity scores above 80% [31, 33, 43]. However, it is important to investigate the psychometric properties of a specific neuropsychological battery before implementing the test into a concussion care protocol.

In summary, neuropsychological testing is an important diagnostic tool in acute concussion care. It is highly likely that neuropsychological testing batteries can differentiate between concussed and non-concussed individuals, with memory and response speed domains being particularly useful. Although there are many different types of neuropsychological batteries available for commercial use, they are generally comparable in terms of their psychometric properties. As noted throughout this volume, the main limitation of traditional neuropsychological testing is its insensitivity to the persistent effects of concussion. That discovery has inspired a search for tests that better detect the neurobiological changes that perhaps underlie persistence of symptoms beyond three months post injury.

Sensory Organization Test (SOT)

The SOT [44] is an assessment of dynamic posturography utilizing a computerized force plate and moving visual surround. Similar to the BESS, the SOT tests athletes during six different conditions, each lasting for 20 s (Figure 19.2). Athletes performing the SOT remain in a double-leg stance position on a force plate throughout the test. Testing conditions include the combination of having the athlete open or close the eyes, referencing a fixed or swaying surround, and referencing a fixed or swaying floor. By altering these components, the SOT is not only capable of detecting balance deficits after concussion, but can also parcel out the components of balance to determine whether visual, somatosensory, and/or vestibular deficits are contributing to the larger balance issues.

SOT scores have been shown to decrease immediately after concussive injury [21, 23, 45], with deficits typically lasting for the first three days post injury [21, 23]. When tested within the first 24 h post injury, athletes' SOT scores typically dropped

The six conditions of the Sensory Organization Test (SOT)

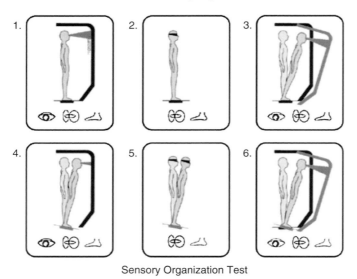

Sensory Organization Test

Fig. 19.2 (1) Fixed floor/fixed surround, eyes open. (2) Fixed floor, eyes closed. (3) Sway surround/fixed floor, eyes open. (4) Fixed surround/sway floor, eyes open. (5) Sway floor, eyes closed. (6) Sway surround/sway floor, eyes open. Source: Broglio et al., 2008 [44] with permission from Lippincott Williams & Wilkins, Inc./Wolters Kluwer

8–12 points [10]. A 2008 study by Broglio et al. [44], using a 1-standard deviation cutoff (approximately four-point composite score drop), found the SOT to have a sensitivity of 61%. A later study, using reliable change scores, found that the SOT had a sensitivity of 57% and a specificity of 80% [45].

Overall, the SOT displays similar findings compared to other balance assessment tools, with slightly higher sensitivity compared to sideline balance tools. The SOT can detect balance deficits immediately after injury, with deficits typically subsiding within three days post injury. The SOT is capable of distinguishing between concussed and non-concussed individuals with moderate sensitivity and moderate to high specificity. Most importantly, it can identify visual or vestibular deficits that can then be addressed through specialized rehabilitation strategies.

Virtual Reality (VR)

Virtual reality is designed to be an interactive, three-dimensional (3D) environment generated by a computer that mimics the real world and causes participants to be fully immersed in the environment. Compared to more traditional and clinically used balance tests, a benefit of VR is the 3D nature of the tests, which can assess depth perception. Unlike the aforementioned diagnostic tools, there is no standard platform from VR assessments, which means that there is a high degree of variability between the equipment, set-up, assessments, and psychometric properties across the different studies.

VR environments, while not readily available to most clinicians, produce egomotion (actual motion in the participant) and vection (illusionary effect of self-motion due to the movement of the VR environment) [46] as part of the assessment. In a VR balance assessment utilized at the Pennsylvania State University, participants are asked to stand as motionless as possible while the VR environment remains still or sways in a yaw, pitch, or roll direction. Using this VR paradigm, multiple studies have found that concussed individuals display poorer balance (compared to controls or their own baseline) up to 30 days post injury [47–49].

In addition to postural control assessment, VR paradigms can assess cognitive domains. Few studies have examined the usefulness of spatial navigation tasks in a VR environment, which is thought to have high ecological validity. In these paradigms, participants are passively led down a virtual hallway, making three or four turns before reaching a doorway. Participants are then given a joystick and asked to actively navigate through the route as quickly as possible. Several studies have found that concussed participants display significantly different brain activation patterns when actively navigating the route compared to non-concussed controls up to 30 days post injury [48, 50, 51].

A benefit to VR technology is that the postural control and cognitive domains, some of which are mentioned above, can be easily combined into a dual-task condition. The possibilities of dual-task assessments and training provided in a VR environment have garnered the technology much attention as a novel and useful modality for the future. Additionally, VR technology has proven useful as a rehabilitation mechanism in more severely brain-injured patients (see Rose et al. [52] for a review).

Overall, VR balance and spatial navigation have been shown to differentiate between concussed and non-concussed controls. While there are early studies suggesting that VR technology is promising and that VR has high sensitivity and specificity, there are no published data available. Future studies must address the feasibility and utility of these tests in the sports medicine setting.

Gait Measures

Along with static postural control tools, more dynamic balance assessments, such as gait analysis, have been utilized in concussion care. Similar to the VR assessments, there are a wide variety of procedures used and variables studied in gait analysis studies. It is believed that these assessments hold potential for added benefits to the traditional sideline and laboratory postural control and balance tests. Since gait assessments can simultaneously assess dynamic motor function with the ability to add in a cognitive task, these types of assessment can more closely mimic the dual-task nature of sport and can be considered more applicable to real sporting situations.

Several studies have found differences between concussed and control individuals in center-of-mass sway [53, 54], decreased gait velocity [53, 54], increased sway velocity [55, 56], and generally more conservative gait patterns [54]. These findings were observed under both single- and dual-task conditions and were present up to 28 days post injury [55, 56]. Although there is increasing evidence to suggest that gait analysis can identify deficits in concussed individuals, the measures utilized have limited sensitivity and specificity. While gait assessments can include dual-task components and may be considered more consistent to real sporting situations, the lack of information regarding the sensitivity and specificity limits the utility of the assessment as a diagnostic tool.

In general, the available scientific evidence suggests that *neuropsychological testing* and *balance/postural stability testing* are clearly critical pieces of the concussion assessment puzzle. These tools (in their various forms) are widely utilized in concussion diagnosis and management, and when used in combination are capable of distinguishing concussed from non-injured athletes. Balance deficits found using the SOT appear to resolve along a similar timeline to those found using the BESS (three to five days). Computerized neurocognitive tests appear to identify more deficits than found using sideline tools, making such testing a more sensitive diagnostic tool over time and useful when making return-to-play decisions.

Although less utilized clinically, VR and gait measures have also been shown to detect deficits following concussion. It is important to note that there are currently no universally accepted VR and gait measures for concussion diagnosis, so there may be a large amount of variation in the psychometric properties of different batteries. Regardless, research using both of these tools found deficits lasting upwards of 30 days post injury. The importance of these subtle deficits and their role in sport performance, re-injury risk, and long-term outcomes have yet to be established.

Overall, clinical and laboratory testing tools are useful in concussion diagnosis. While laboratory tools are generally more expensive, require additional equipment, and are more time-intensive, they can provide information beyond that which is attained using sideline tools alone. Neuropsychological testing and the SOT are extensively used in concussion diagnosis and deliver useful information regarding return-to-play activities. The psychometric properties of these tools slightly vary based on the specific battery, but have generally been well established. VR and gait testing are more novel laboratory tests, with psychometric properties still being investigated. However, these diagnostic tools have been shown to be sensitive to deficits far beyond the typical seven- to ten-day recovery window. While more research needs to be conducted, both VR and gait measures hold promise as potentially useful tools in concussion diagnosis.

Multimodal Concussion Assessment Battery

Although the aforementioned tools may have diagnostic utility as stand-alone assessments, standard of care for concussion management utilizes a multi-modal battery of assessment tools. Both the National Athletic Trainer's Association [57] and the 4th International Conference on Concussion [4] recommend a battery of tests, including symptom checklists, neuropsychological evaluations, and postural stability assessments. As concussion signs and symptoms are highly variable and individualized, using a multi-faceted concussion battery maximizes the chances of an appropriate diagnosis.

A 2008 study by Broglio et al. [44] examined the sensitivity of a variety of assessments as stand-alone tools and as part of a larger battery in the same sample of participants. When assessing the tools as stand-alone, computerized neuropsychological batteries (ImPACT and CRI) had the highest sensitivity, at 79.2% and 78.6%, respectively. The symptom checklist was the next most useful diagnostic tool, with a sensitivity of 68%, following by postural control (SOT) evaluations, with a sensitivity of 61.9%. Paper-and-pencil neuropsychological tests had the lowest diagnostic value in this study, with a reported sensitivity of only 43.5%. When the entire battery was evaluated, 95.7% of concussed individuals were correctly identified. When using only one of the neuropsychological assessments, in combination with the symptom checklist and balance assessments, the most sensitive battery included ImPACT with a correct identification rate of 91.7%.

Although each assessment tool has diagnostic value alone, there is a clear increase in sensitivity to concussive injury when a multi-faceted battery is utilized. A concussion assessment protocol that combines symptom checklists, neuropsychological evaluations, and postural control assessments provides the most sensitive battery of testing for diagnosing concussive injuries.

Neurophysiological Assessment Tools

Sideline and laboratory tests are important tools for clinicians and physicians to diagnose and manage concussions. However, all of the diagnostic tools mentioned throughout the chapter only measure the functional deficits associated with concussion. More contemporary diagnostic and assessment tools have been proposed for detecting concussion. Studies examining the utility of neuroimaging and neurophysiological changes following concussion have been inconclusive. This section describes diagnostic tools that more directly assess the structure and function of the brain and can begin to establish connections between the physiological damage and the functional deficits of concussions.

Electroencephalography (EEG)

EEG is a technique that measures the summed current flow of extracellular electrical activity of a large number of neurons [58]. Compared to other neuroimaging techniques, EEGs are relatively low-cost, have non-invasive procedures, have high reliability, and are characteristically stable [58, 59]. Conventionally, EEGs can be understood as a raw recording of the brain's electrical activity, detected by scalp electrodes and amplified, and presented as electrical waveforms. More traditionally, these electrical waveforms were inspected visually. However, visual inspection of raw EEG signals often shows a lack of clear deficits and is not currently recommended as a diagnostic tool in concussion care [60].

While most studies conclude that conventional EEGs lack the sensitivity to detect changes following concussion, there is a growing body of literature that suggests that more complex EEG paradigms, including quantitative EEG (qEEG), may be used to assess changes in mental status after concussive injuries [58]. Where conventional EEGs call for the visual inspection of raw EEG signals, qEEG transforms raw EEG signals into numerical values via software-assisted data analysis.

More recent studies, using discriminant function analyses, have investigated the utility of qEEG analysis in concussion diagnosis. A study by Thatcher et al. [61], using 608 patients with mild TBI and 108 age-matched normal controls, showed that a qEEG discriminant function alone had a sensitivity of 94.8%. The injury classification in this study was based on three different neurophysiological variables: (1) frontal, and frontotemporal, regions displayed decreased phase and increased coherence; (2) anterior and posterior cortical regions showed decreased differences in overall power values; and (3) posterior regions showed decreased alpha power. Three independent cross-validations of this function were conducted, with the discriminant function having a sensitivity ranging from 92.8% to 96.2%.

While qEEG may be highly sensitive to concussive injuries as a stand-alone tool, there are inconsistencies among researchers as to the appropriate parameters for using EEG as a concussion diagnosis tool (e.g., number of electrodes to use, which neurophysiological variables to analyze). While EEGs are cheaper than most other neuroimaging devices, they are still expensive, especially compared to traditional clinical diagnostic tools. While EEGs have advantages over clinical tools, including lack of practice/learning effects, their immunity to malingering, and their ability to provide objective physiological data about the brain, the interpretation of results and overall utility following concussion are still questionable.

Event-Related Potentials (ERPs)

Along with whole-brain or resting-state brain analyses, another aspect of EEG analysis is ERP analysis. Unlike general EEG analysis, ERPs are time-locked responses to specific mental or physical events. The voltage changes noticed in response to the stimuli are indicative of the reception and processing of sensory information, as well as higher-order cognitive processing. ERP components are defined by a number of factors, including their polarity (positive or negative), latency, and distribution of the signal over the scalp. The two main variables associated with ERP analysis are the latency and amplitude of the neuroelectric signal. The latency of the signal details the time course of the cognitive processing in milliseconds, whereas the amplitude delineates the allocation of neural resources to a particular cognitive process [62].

Unlike qEEG, there have been no formal studies evaluating the sensitivity and specificity of ERP components in concussed individuals. However, concussed individuals have displayed several differences, in both latency and amplitude, compared to non-concussed controls. Interestingly, concussed individuals often display these abnormal ERP results in spite of achieving normal cognitive functioning on clinical neuropsychological exams. Broglio et al. [63] provided a review of several studies incorporating ERP analysis on concussed individuals.

ERPs offer additional advantages over EEG and qEEG analyses, including a specific look at the information-processing deficits that underlie the cognitive dysfunction seen in concussed individuals. However, the methodological nature behind ERP analysis often requires longer testing sessions, making ERP analysis less clinically useful as a diagnostic tool. While ERPs are a useful research tool, the lack of information regarding the psychometric properties and the methodological considerations behind this type of analysis currently prevent it from being a clinically useful diagnostic tool following sport-related concussion.

Functional Magnetic Resonance Imaging (fMRI) and Diffusion Tensor Imaging (DTI)

Neuroimaging tools are useful in distinguishing moderate and severe TBI. However, traditional neuroimaging tools, such as computed tomography (CT) and magnetic resonance imaging (MRI) scans, often show an absence of significant findings in concussed patients [64–67]. This is likely due to the fact that concussions are a form of diffuse axonal injury, which CT and MRI scans are not sensitive enough to detect [68]. However, more recent neuroimaging tools, such as fMRI and DTI, have been shown useful in detecting abnormalities in concussed individuals [69, 70].

fMRI uses the blood oxygen level-dependent (BOLD) signal as an index of neuronal activity [71]. When using the BOLD signal in fMRI research, the assumption is made that an increase in neural activity is accompanied by an increased local blood flow, resulting in reduced concentrations of deoxyhemoglobin in nearby vessels [72]. Through the BOLD signal, it is believed that the fMRI is measuring the firing of the neurons due to the hemodynamic response, which is a secondary and indirect assessment of neural responses due to cognitive and/or sensorimotor demands [73–75].

A more contemporary and advanced imaging technique, DTI, utilizes the Brownian motion of water due to thermal energy in order to map white-matter tracks of the brain [76]. Diffuse axonal injury, which occur after concussion, can result in myelin loss, microscopic lesions, and axonal degeneration and swelling [77]. All of these deficits alter the diffusivity of water in the white matter, making DTI a sensitive tool for assessing the neurophysiological deficits of concussions [78].

There are several studies that utilize one or both of these neuroimaging techniques to investigate the neurophysiological deficits seen after concussion. A 2012 publication by Shenton et al. [68] provides a thorough, although not all-encompassing, review of the fMRI and DTI findings as related to mild TBI. While many studies using these technologies have shown changes after concussion, there is little clinical utility in fMRI or DTI in concussion diagnosis. Issues surrounding fMRI and DTI in clinical care revolve around a large number of issues, including the high cost, expertise needed to run and analyze scans, and availability of these technologies. While they currently have little clinical use in concussion diagnosis, neuroimaging does remain important in ruling out more severe and life-threatening brain injuries. Additionally, fMRI and DTI can serve as useful research tools to understand the neural underpinnings that cause clinically seen deficits and abnormalities post concussion.

Debate still exists as to whether cerebral concussion (mild TBI) is only a *functional* injury due to the inability of neuroimaging techniques to consistently identify structural damage. While neuroimaging tools can present challenges for clinical use, including cost, availability, lack of mobility, and length of testing, there are still benefits to their use. The ability to potentially understand the neural underpinning creating the functional deficits following concussion may prove to provide great value (i.e., white-matter connectivity as measured by DTI). EEG discriminant functions have been shown to be highly sensitive and specific as stand-alone tools; however, there is no universally accepted EEG concussion diagnostic battery. Current ERP, fMRI, and DTI protocols are not used specifically for concussion diagnosis, and no sensitivity and specificity properties have been reported in the literature.

Results from a combination of these assessments may have important value in implementing rehabilitation paradigms and understanding the long-term effects of concussion. Although none of the tools discussed in this section are currently considered a necessary part of the clinical concussion diagnosis battery, many have proven to be excellent research tools which are helping to advance our understanding of these complex neurological injuries.

Conclusions

Concussions are highly variable injuries that have many different clinical presentations. In order to help diagnose with the highest sensitivity, current recommendations for diagnosis and management include a thorough clinical exam by a trained professional and a combination of objective tests, specifically symptom checklists, neuropsychological testing, and postural control evaluation. There are many validated tools that are capable of assessing these domains, each with its own advantages and drawbacks. The tools described throughout this chapter are summarized in Tables 19.2–19.4.

In general, there are a variety of cost-effective sideline tools that can be quickly administered, and are relatively easy to interpret. Sideline tools tend to have moderate to high sensitivity and specificity, but are only valid for short periods of time after injury. Clinical and laboratory tools are often more time-intensive, require more equipment, and the results are often more difficult to interpret. However, clinical and laboratory tools have generally been shown to have higher sensitivity and specificity than sideline tools. Additionally, the improved sensitivity of laboratory tools has been observed further out from injury, with some modalities capable of detecting subtle deficits over 30 days post injury, compared to sideline assessment tools.

Table 19.2 Summary of the potential contribution of the sideline tools discussed in this chapter to concussion diagnosis

Sideline tools						
Diagnostic tool	**Studies**	**Method**	**Effect**		**Diagnostic utility**	**Clinical utility**
			Sensitivity	**Specificity**		
Symptom checklists	McCrea et al. [6]	90% confidence interval	89%	100%	High	High
	Van Kampen et al. [12]	Reliable change scores	64%	91%		
SAC	Barr et al. [15]	+1-point decline	94%	76%	High	High
	McCrea et al. [6]	Regression-based method	80%	91%		
MACE	Coldren et al. [18]	Score < 27	51%	64%	Moderate	High
BESS	McCrea et al. [6]	+3-point decline	34%	91%	Moderate	High
SCAT-3	No psychometric data available				Unknown[a]	High

[a] No studies have formally evaluated the psychometric properties of the SCAT-3. However, psychometric properties of several of the components of the SCAT-3 (symptom checklists, SAC, BESS) have been evaluated and found to have high diagnostic and clinical utility in concussion diagnosis.

BESS: Balance Error Scoring System; MACE: Military Acute Concussion Evaluation; SAC, Standardized Assessment of Concussion; SCAT-3: Sport Concussion Assessment Tool – 3rd Edition.

Table 19.3 Summary of the potential contribution of the clinical and laboratory tools discussed in this chapter to concussion diagnosis

Clinical/laboratory tools						
Diagnostic tool	**Studies**	**Method**	**Effect**		**Diagnostic utility**	**Clinical utility**
			Sensitivity	**Specificity**		
Neuropsychological tests	Several	Each battery has different cutoff indicators	+80%	+80%	High	High
SOT	Broglio et al. [63]	1-standard deviation cutoff	61%	Not reported	Moderate	Moderate
	Broglio et al. [63]	Reliable change scores	57%	80%		
VR	Teel et al. [48]	8.25-point cutoff	86%	88%	High	Moderate
	Unpublished data	Receiver operating characteristic curve	86%	77%		
Gait	Several	No psychometric data available			Unknown	Moderate

SOT: Sensory Organization Test; VR: virtual reality.

Table 19.4 Summary of the potential contribution of the neurophysiological assessment tools discussed in this chapter to concussion diagnosis

Neuropsychological assessment tools						
Diagnostic tool	**Studies**	**Method**	**Effect**		**Diagnostic utility**	**Clinical utility**
			Sensitivity	**Specificity**		
EEG	Thatcher et al. [61]	Discriminant function	94.8%	Not reported	High	Low
ERP	Several	No psychometric data available			Unknown	Low
fMRI	Several	No psychometric data available			Unknown	Low
DTI	Several	No psychometric data available			Unknown	Low

DTI: diffusion tensor imaging; EEG: electroencephalogram; ERP: event-related potential; fMRI: functional magnetic resonance imaging.

Lastly, neuroimaging tools have few psychometric data available and are currently not useful as diagnostic tools but are showing promise. Neuroimaging remains an important diagnostic tool for ruling out more severe neurologic conditions, such as skull fractures, intracranial hemorrhages, or diffuse cerebral edema.

References

1. Guskiewicz KM, McCrea M, Marshall SW, et al. Cumulative effects associated with recurrent concussion in collegiate football players: The NCAA Concussion Study. *JAMA* 2003;290(19):2549–2555.

2. Delaney JS, Lacroix VJ, Leclerc S, Johnston KM. Concussions among university football and soccer players. *Clin J Sport Med* 2002;12(6):331–338.

3. Patel AV, Mihalik JP, Notebaert AJ, Guskiewicz KM, Prentice WE. Neuropsychological performance, postural stability, and symptoms after dehydration. *J Athl Train* 2007;42(1):66.

4. McCrory P, Meeuwisse WH, Aubry M, et al. Consensus statement on concussion in sport: the 4th International Conference on Concussion in Sport held in Zurich, November 2012. *J Am Coll Surg* 2013;216(5):11.

5. McCrea M, Guskiewicz KM, Marshall SW, et al. Acute effects and recovery time following concussion in collegiate football players: The NCAA Concussion Study. *JAMA* 2003;290(19):2556–2563.

6. McCrea M, Barr WB, Guskiewicz K, et al. Standard regression-based methods for measuring recovery after sport-related concussion. *J Int Neuropsychol Soc* 2005;11(01):58–69.

7. Piland SG, Motl RW, Ferrara MS, Peterson CL. Evidence for the factorial and construct validity of a self-report concussion symptoms scale. *J Athl Train* 2003;38(2):104.

8. Collins MW, Iverson GL, Lovell MR, McKeag DB, Norwig J, Maroon J. On-field predictors of neuropsychological and symptom deficit following sports-related concussion. *Clin J Sport Med* 2003;13(4):222–229.

9. Lovell MR, Collins MW, Iverson GL, et al. Recovery from mild concussion in high school athletes. *J Neurosurg* 2003;98(2):296–301.

10. Giza CC, Kutcher JS, Ashwal S, et al. Summary of evidence-based guideline update: Evaluation and management of concussion in sports. Report of the Guideline Development Subcommittee of the American Academy of Neurology. *Neurology* 2013; 80(24):2250–2257.

11. Mansell JL, Tierney RT, Higgins M, McDevitt J, Toone N, Glutting J. Concussive signs and symptoms following head impacts in collegiate athletes. *Brain Inj* 2010;24(9):1070–1074.

12. Van Kampen DA, Lovell MR, Pardini JE, Collins MW, Fu FH. The "value added" of neurocognitive testing after sports-related concussion. *Am J Sports Med* 2006;34(10):1630–1635.

13. McCrea M. Standardized mental status testing on the sideline after sport-related concussion. *J Athl Train* 2001;36(3):274–279.

14. McCrea M, Kelly JP, Randolph C, et al. Standardized assessment of concussion (SAC): On-site mental status evaluation of the athlete. *J Head Trauma Rehabil* 1998;13(2):27–35.

15. Barr WB, McCrea M. Sensitivity and specificity of standardized neurocognitive testing immediately following sports concussion. *J Int Neuropsychol Soc* 2001;7(6):693–702.

16. French L, McCrea M, Baggett M. The Military Acute Concussion Evaluation (MACE). *J Special Ops Med* 2008;8(1):68–77.

17. McCrea M, Jaffee M, Helmick K, Guskiewicz K, Doncevic S. Validation of the Military Acute Concussion Evaluation (MACE) for in-theater evaluation of combat-related traumatic brain injury. DTIC document; 2009. Defense Technical Information Center document. Available at www.dtic.mil/dtic/tr/fulltext/u2/a515492.pdf.

18. Coldren RL, Kelly MP, Parish RV, Dretsch M, Russell ML. Evaluation of the Military Acute Concussion Evaluation for use in combat operations more than 12 hours after injury. *Milit Med* 2010;175(7):477–481.

19. Riemann BL, Guskiewicz KM, Shields EW. Relationship between clinical and forceplate measures of postural stability. *J Sport Rehabil* 1999;8:71–82.

20. *Balance Error Scoring System (BESS) manual.* Developed by researchers and clinicians at the University of North Carolina's Sports Medicine Research Laboratory. Available at www.carolinashealthcare.org/documents/carolinasrehab/bess_manual_.pdf.

21. Riemann BL, Guskiewicz KM. Effects of mild head injury on postural stability as measured through clinical balance testing. *J Athl Train* 2000;35(1):19–25.

22. McCrea M, Guskiewicz K, Randolph C, et al. Incidence, clinical course, and predictors of prolonged recovery time following sport-related concussion in high school and college athletes. *J Int Neuropsychol Soc* 2013;19(1):22–33.

23. Guskiewicz KM. Postural stability assessment following concussion: One piece of the puzzle. *Clin J Sport Med* 2001;11(3):182–189.

24. Valovich McLeod TC, Perrin DH, Guskiewicz KM, Shultz SJ, Diamond R, Gansneder BM. Serial administration of clinical concussion assessments and learning effects in healthy young athletes. *Clin J Sport Med* 2004;14(5):287–295.

25. Susco TM, McLeod TCV, Gansneder BM, Shultz SJ. Balance recovers within 20 minutes after exertion as measured by the Balance Error Scoring System. *J Athl Train* 2004;39(3):241.

26. Fox ZG, Mihalik JP, Blackburn JT, Battaglini CL, Guskiewicz KM. Return of postural control to baseline after anaerobic and aerobic exercise protocols. *J Athl Train* 2008;43(5):456–463.

27. Sport Concussion Assessment Tool, 3rd edition. Available at: http://bjsm.bmj.com/content/47/5/259.full.pdf.

28. Guskiewicz KM, Register-Mihalik J, McCrory P, et al. Evidence-based approach to revising the SCAT2: Introducing the SCAT3. *Br J Sports Med* 2013;47(5):289–293.

29. Putukian M, Echemendia R, Dettwiler-Danspeckgruber A, Duliba T, Bruce J, Furtado JL, et al. Prospective clinical assessment using Sideline Concussion Assessment Tool-2 testing in the evaluation of sport-related concussion in college athletes. *Clin J Sport Med* 2015;25:36–42.

30. Iverson GL, Lovell MR, Collins MW. Interpreting change on ImPACT following sport concussion. *Clin Neuropsychol* 2003;17(4):460–467.

31. Schatz P, Pardini JE, Lovell MR, Collins MW, Podell K. Sensitivity and specificity of the ImPACT test battery for concussion in athletes. *Arch Clin Neuropsychol* 2006;21:91–99.

32. Gualtieri CT, Johnson LG, Reliability and validity of a computerized neurocognitive test battery, CNS Vital Signs. *Arch Clin Neuropsychol* 2006;21:623–643.

33. Levinson D, Reeves D. Monitoring recovery from traumatic brain injury using Automated Neuropsychological Assessment Metrics (ANAM V1.0). *Arch Clin Neuropsychol* 1997;12(2):155–166.

34. Erlanger D, Saliba E, Barth J, Almquist J. Monitoring resolution of postconcussion symptoms in athletes: Preliminary results of a web-based neuropsychological test protocol. *J Athl Train* 2001;36:280–287.

35. Louey AG, Cromer JA, Schembri A., Darby DG, Maruff P, Makdissi M, McCrory P. Detecting cognitive impairment after concussion: Sensitivity of change from baseline and normative data methods using the CogSport/Axon cognitive test battery. *Arch Clin Neuropsychol* 2014;29(5):432–441.

36. Erlanger D, Feldman D, Kutner K, et al. Development and validation of a web-based neuropsychological test protocol for sports-related return-to-play decision-making. *Arch Clin Neuropsychol* 2003;18(3):293–316.

37. Erlanger D, Kaushik T, Cantu R, et al. Symptom-based assessment of the severity of a concussion. *J Neurosurg* 2003;98(3):477–484.

38. Collie A, Makdissi M, Maruff P, Bennell K, McCrory P. Cognition in the days following concussion: Comparison of symptomatic versus asymptomatic athletes. *J Neurol Neurosurg Psychiatry* 2006;77(2):241–245.

39. Broglio SP, Macciocchi SN, Ferrara MS. Sensitivity of the concussion assessment battery. *Neurosurgery* 2007;60(6):1050–1057.

40. McClincy MP, Lovell MR, Pardini J, Collins MW, Spore MK. Recovery from sports concussion in high school and collegiate athletes. *Brain Inj* 2006;20(1):33–39.

41. Macciocchi SN, Barth JT, Alves W, Rimel RW, Jane JA. Neuropsychological functioning and recovery after mild head injury in collegiate athletes. *Neurosurg* 1996;39(3):510–514.

42. Randolph C, McCrea M, Barr WB. Is neuropsychological testing useful in the management of sport-related concussion? *J Athl Train* 2005;40(3):139–152.

43. Collins MW, Grindel SH, Lovell MR, et al. Relationship between concussion and neuropsychological performance in college football players. *JAMA* 1999;282(10):964–970.

44. Broglio SP, Ferrara MS, Sopiarz K, Kelly MS. Reliable change of the sensory organization test. *Clin J Sport Med* 2008;18(2):148–154.

45. Peterson CL, Ferrara MS, Mrazik M, Piland S, Elliott R. Evaluation of neuropsychological domain scores and postural stability following cerebral concussion in sports. *Clin J Sport Med* 2003;13(4):230–237.

46. Slobounov S, Slobounov E, Newell K. Application of virtual reality graphics in assessment of concussion. *Cyberpsychol Behav* 2006;9(2):188–191.

47. Slobounov S, Tutwiler R, Sebastianelli W, Slobounov E. Alteration of postural responses to visual field motion in mild traumatic brain injury. *Neurosurg* 2006;59(1):134–139.

48. Teel EF, Ray WJ, Geronimo AM, Slobounov SM. Residual alterations of brain electrical activity in clinically asymptomatic concussed individuals: An EEG study. *Clin Neurophysiol* 2014;125(4):703–707.

49. Slobounov S, Wu T, Hallett M, Shibasaki H, Slobounov E, Newell K. Neural underpinning of postural responses to visual field motion. *Biol Psychol* 2006;72(2):188–197.

50. Slobounov SM, Zhang K, Pennell D, Ray W, Johnson B, Sebastianelli W. Functional abnormalities in normally appearing athletes following mild traumatic brain injury: A functional MRI study. *Exp Brain Res* 2010;202(2):341–354.

51. Jaiswal N, Ray W, Slobounov S. Encoding of visual-spatial information in working memory requires more cerebral efforts than retrieval: Evidence from an EEG and virtual reality study. *Brain Res* 2010;6:80–89.

52. Rose FD, Brooks BM, Rizzo AA. Virtual reality in brain damage rehabilitation: Review. *CyberPsychol Behav* 2005;8(3):241–262.

53. Parker TM, Osternig LR, Lee H-J, Donkelaar Pv, Chou L-S. The effect of divided attention on gait stability following concussion. *Clin Biomech* 2005;20(4):389–395.

54. Catena RD, van Donkelaar P, Chou L-S. Cognitive task effects on gait stability following concussion. *Exp Brain Res* 2007; 176(1):23–31.

55. Parker TM, Osternig LR, van Donkelaar P, Chou L-S. Balance control during gait in athletes and non-athletes following concussion. *Med Engineer Physics* 2008;30(8):959–967.

56. Parker TM, Osternig LR, P VAND, Chou LS. Gait stability following concussion. *Med Sci Sports Exerc* 2006;38(6):1032–1040.

57. Guskiewicz K, Bruce S, Cantu R, Ferrara MS, Kelly JP, McCrea M, et al. Research based recommendations on management of sport related concussion: Summary of the National Athletic Trainers' Association position statement. *Br J Sports Med* 2006;40(1):6–10.

58. Gaetz M, Bernstein DM. The current status of electrophysiologic procedures for the assessment of mild traumatic brain injury. *J Head Trauma Rehabil* 2001;16(4):386–405.

59. Leon-Carrion J, Martin-Rodriguez JF, Damas-Lopez J, Martin JMB, Dominguez-Morales MDR. A QEEG index of level of functional dependence for people sustaining acquired brain injury: The Seville Independence Index (SINDI). *Brain Inj* 2008;22(1):61–74.

60. Arciniegas DB. Clinical electrophysiologic assessments and mild traumatic brain injury: State-of-the-science and implications for clinical practice. *Int J Psychophysiol* 2011;82(1):41–52.

61. Thatcher RW, Walker R, Gerson I, Geisler F. EEG discriminant analyses of mild head trauma. *Electroencephalogr Clin Neurophysiol* 1989;73(2):94–106.

62. Duncan CC, Barry RJ, Connolly JF, et al. Event-related potentials in clinical research: Guidelines for eliciting, recording, and quantifying mismatch negativity, P300, and N400. *Clin Neurophysiol* 2009;120(11):1883–1908.

63. Broglio SP, Pontifex MB, O'Connor P, Hillman CH. The persistent effects of concussion on neuroelectric indices of attention. *J Neurotrauma* 2009;26(9):1463–1470.

64. Bazarian JJ, Zhong J, Blyth B, Zhu T, Kavcic V, Peterson D. Diffusion tensor imaging detects clinically important axonal damage after mild traumatic brain injury: A pilot study. *J Neurotrauma* 2007;24(9):1447–1459.

65. Miller L. Neuropsychology and pathophysiology of mild head injury and the postconcussion syndrome: Clinical and forensic considerations. *J Cogn Rehabil* 1996;15:8–23.

66. Mittl R, Grossman R, Hiehle J, et al. Prevalence of MR evidence of diffuse axonal injury in patients with mild head injury and normal head CT findings. *Am J Neuroradiol* 1994;15(8):1583–1589.

67. Povlishock JT, Coburn TH. Morphopathological change associated with mild head injury. *Mild Head Inj* 1989;37–53.

68. Shenton M, Hamoda H, Schneiderman J, et al. A review of magnetic resonance imaging and diffusion tensor imaging findings in mild traumatic brain injury. *Brain Imaging Behav* 2012;6(2):137–192.

69. Bazarian JJ, Zhu T, Blyth B, Borrino A, Zhong J. Subject-specific changes in brain white matter on diffusion tensor imaging after sports-related concussion. *Magnet Res Imag* 2012;30(2):171–180.

70. Hammeke TA, McCrea M, Coats SM, et al. Acute and subacute changes in neural activation during the recovery from sport-related concussion. *J Int Neuropsychol Soc* 2013;19(8):863–872.

71. Ogawa S, Lee T, Kay A, Tank D. Brain magnetic resonance imaging with contrast dependent on blood oxygenation. *Proc Natl Acad Sci* 1990;87(24):9868–9872.

72. Ogawa S, Menon R, Tank D, et al. Functional brain mapping by blood oxygenation level-dependent contrast magnetic resonance imaging. A comparison of signal characteristics with a biophysical model. *Biophys J* 1993;64(3):803–812.

73. Jueptner M, Weiller C. Review: Does measurement of regional cerebral blood flow reflect synaptic activity? Implications for PET and fMRI. *NeuroImage* 1995;2(2PA):148–156.

74. Hillary FG, Steffener J, Biswal BB, Lange G, DeLuca J, Ashburner J. Functional magnetic resonance imaging technology and traumatic brain injury rehabilitation: Guidelines for methodological and conceptual pitfalls. *J Head Trauma Rehabil* 2002;17(5):411–430.

75. Heeger DJ, Ress D. What does fMRI tell us about neuronal activity? *Nature Rev Neurosci* 2002;3(2):142–151.

76. Slobounov S, Gay M, Johnson B, Zhang K. Concussion in athletics: Ongoing clinical and brain imaging research controversies. *Brain Imaging Behav* 2012;6(2):224–243.

77. Maruta J, Lee SW, Jacobs EF, Ghajar J. A unified science of concussion. *Ann NY Acad Sci* 2010;1208(1):58–66.

78. Chu Z, Wilde E, Hunter J, et al. Voxel-based analysis of diffusion tensor imaging in mild traumatic brain injury in adolescents. *Am J Neuroradiol* 2010;31(2):340–346.

Fig. 1.10 A modern photomicrograph of one of Betz's original slides.

Source: Kushchayev et al., 2011 [105]. By permission of Oxford University Press

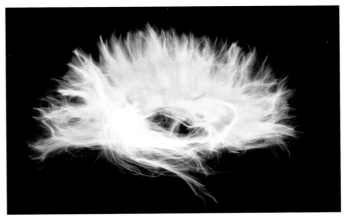

Fig. 1.23a Sagittal view of the corpus callosum white-matter tracts on diffusion tensor imaging.

Source: Shenton et al., 2012 [227]. Reprinted by permission from Springer

Fiber tractography of commonly damaged tracts in mild traumatic brain injury

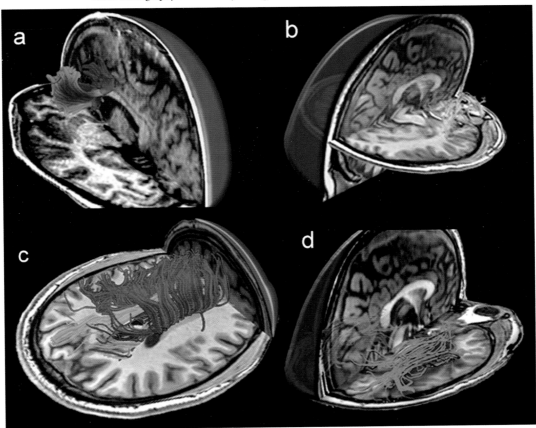

Fig. 1.23b (a) Anterior corona radiata and the genu of corpus callosum; (b) uncinate fasciculus; (c) cingulum bundle in green and the body of corpus callosum in red; (d) inferior longitudinal fasciculus.

Source: Niogi and Mukherjee, 2010 [228] with permission from Lippincott Williams & Wilkins, Inc./Wolters Kluwer

Localization and interaction of genes that were differentially expressed following mild experimental traumatic brain injury

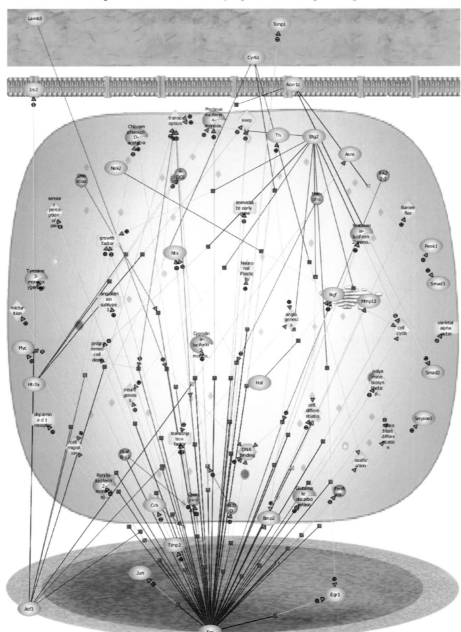

Fig. 1.31 "One hour after trauma (first experimental group), 35 genes were down-regulated, and 32 genes were up-regulated…We observed that most of the genes with altered expression levels after trauma normally function in cell signalling pathways, cell proliferation, cell differentiation and the regulation of transcription…The expression levels of Bdnf, C1ql2, Cbnl, Cd47, Mmp9, Sdc1, Slc27a2, and Tnnt3 were higher in the first hour of trauma than either the control group or at other experimental time points …In contrast, the expression levels of Dmkn, F2rl2, Hal, Htr2a, Pilra, and Slc22a25 were decreased in the first hour of trauma, increasing gradually after 1-h." The classification of affected genes is color-coded. The authors state: "For interpretation of the references to color in this figure, the reader is referred to the web version of the article."

Source: Colak et al., 2012 [276] with permission from Elsevier

Pathway analysis following mild traumatic brain injury (10% stretch)

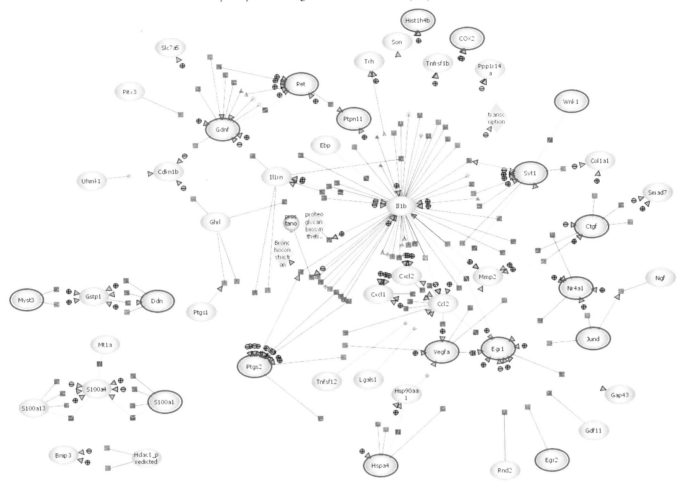

Fig. 1.32 "Most of the genes expressed following 10% stretch are involved in signal transducer activity, regulation of transcription, and cell communication… Additionally, we have found that following 10% stretch, certain genes involved in the apoptotic process, such as Vdac1 (voltage-dependent anion-selective channel protein 1), Sh3glb1 (SH3-domain GRB2-like endophilin B1), Phlda1 (leckstrin homology-like domain, family A, member 1), Rock1 (Rho-associated coiled-coil containing protein kinase 1), and Eif4g2-predicted (eukaryotic translation initiation factor 4 gamma, 2) were downregulated. Further, an upregulation was seen in genes involved in the anti-apoptotic process, such as Ccl2 (chemokine [C-C motif] ligand 2), Vegfa (vascular endothelial growth factor A), BIRC3 (baculoviral IAP repeat-containing 3), Tsc22d3 (TSC22 domain family, member 3), Bnip3 (BCL2=adenovirus E1B 19-kDa interacting protein 3), and Nr4a1 (nuclear receptor subfamily 4, group A, member 1)."

Source: Di Pietro et al., 2010 [278]. Reproduced with permission from Mary Ann Liebert, Inc.

A proposed chain of causality linking concussive brain injury to neurodegeneration

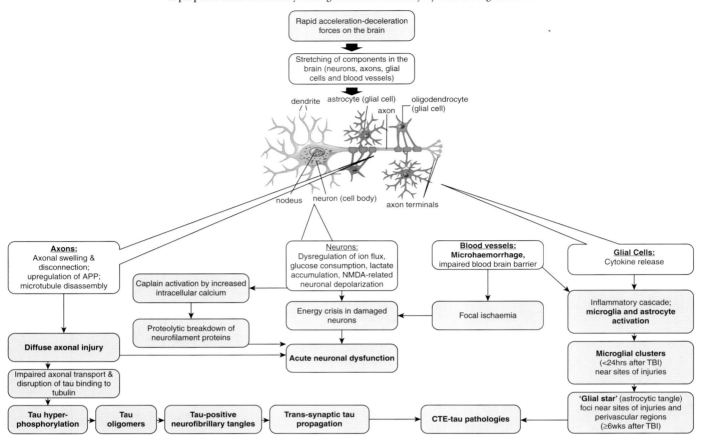

Fig. 1.35 Schematic illustration of the proposed cascade of events triggered by acute traumatic brain injuries (TBIs) and its possible mechanistic links with the development of chronic traumatic encephalopathy (CTE) pathology. APP: amyloid precursor protein; NMDA: N-methyl-d-aspartate.

Source: Ling et al., 2015 [290] with permission from Elsevier

Altered cerebral activation in survivors of mild traumatic brain injury (TBI) due to blast at 964 days (M) after injury

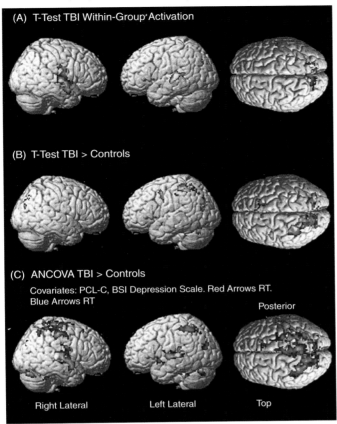

Fig. 1.37 Brain surface images displaying cortical areas with significant *t*-test and analysis of covariance (ANCOVA) results: (A) significant activation in subjects with TBI; (B) areas where the TBI group had greater activation than the control group; and (C) areas where the TBI group had greater activation than the control group after controlling for blue arrows reaction time (RT), red arrows RT, and scores on the Brief Symptom Inventory (BSI) Depression Scale and Post-traumatic Stress Disorder Checklist (PCL-C).

Source: Scheibel et al., 2012 [307, p. 96] by permission of Cambridge University Press

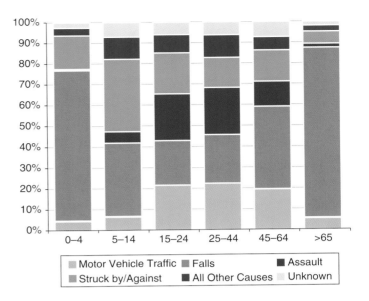

Fig. 2.4 Emergency department visits by age group and injury mechanism: United States, 2006–2010.

Source: Centers for Disease Control and Prevention [65]. CDC, 2016. www.cdc.gov/traumaticbraininjury/data/dist_ed.html

Diffusion tensor imaging reveals persistent white-matter microstructural abnormalities among concussed hockey players

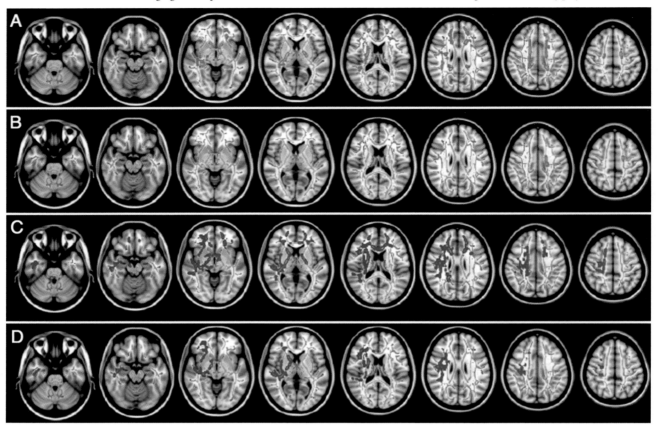

Fig. 2.17 Results of the tract-based spatial statistics analysis showing the clusters of significantly increased fractional anisotropy (A) and axial diffusivity (B) (red to yellow), and decreased radial diffusivity (C) and trace (D) (blue to light blue) for concussed players compared with non-concussed players ($p < 0.05$). Voxels are thickened into local tracts on the fractional anisotropy skeleton (green) and a T1-weighted template image. The left side in each image corresponds to the right hemisphere.

Source: Sasaki et al., 2014 [256] with permission from the American Association of Neurological Surgeons

Exposure to heading over 12 months is associated with scattered foci of altered fractional anisotropy on diffusion tensor imaging

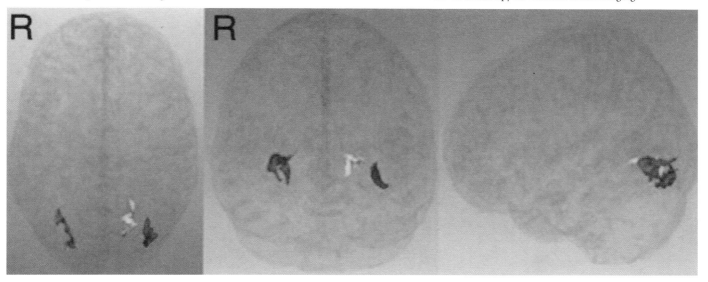

Fig. 2.20 Three regions of interest in the temporo-occipital white matter detected by the initial voxelwise linear regression of estimated prior 12 months of heading on fractional anisotropy, shown as color regions rendered in three-dimensional images and superimposed on T1-weighted axial (left), coronal (middle), and sagittal (right) images from the Montreal Neurological Institute template.

Source: Lipton et al., 2013 [279] with permission by the Radiological Society of North America

Apparatus for experimental open-field blast injury

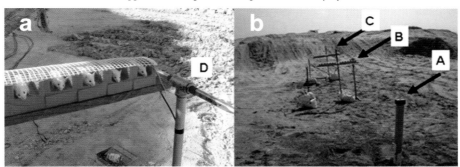

Fig. 4.9 (a) The anesthetized mice were placed in a loose restraint device on a platform, which was covered with white plastic mesh. Each platform had space for 12 anesthetized mice. (b) Photograph of the explosive charge (A) and mice immediately prior to detonation. A cast of 500 g TNT (A) was placed on a pedestal 1 meter above the ground. The 1-meter-high platforms constraining the anesthetized mice were situated 4 meters (B) and 7 meters (C) from the TNT charge. Two pressure gauges were mounted at the ends of each platform (D).

Source: Rubovitch et al., 2011 [53] with permission from Elsevier

Membrane-less organelles formed by ribonucleoproteins host assembly of stress granules that promote fibrillization

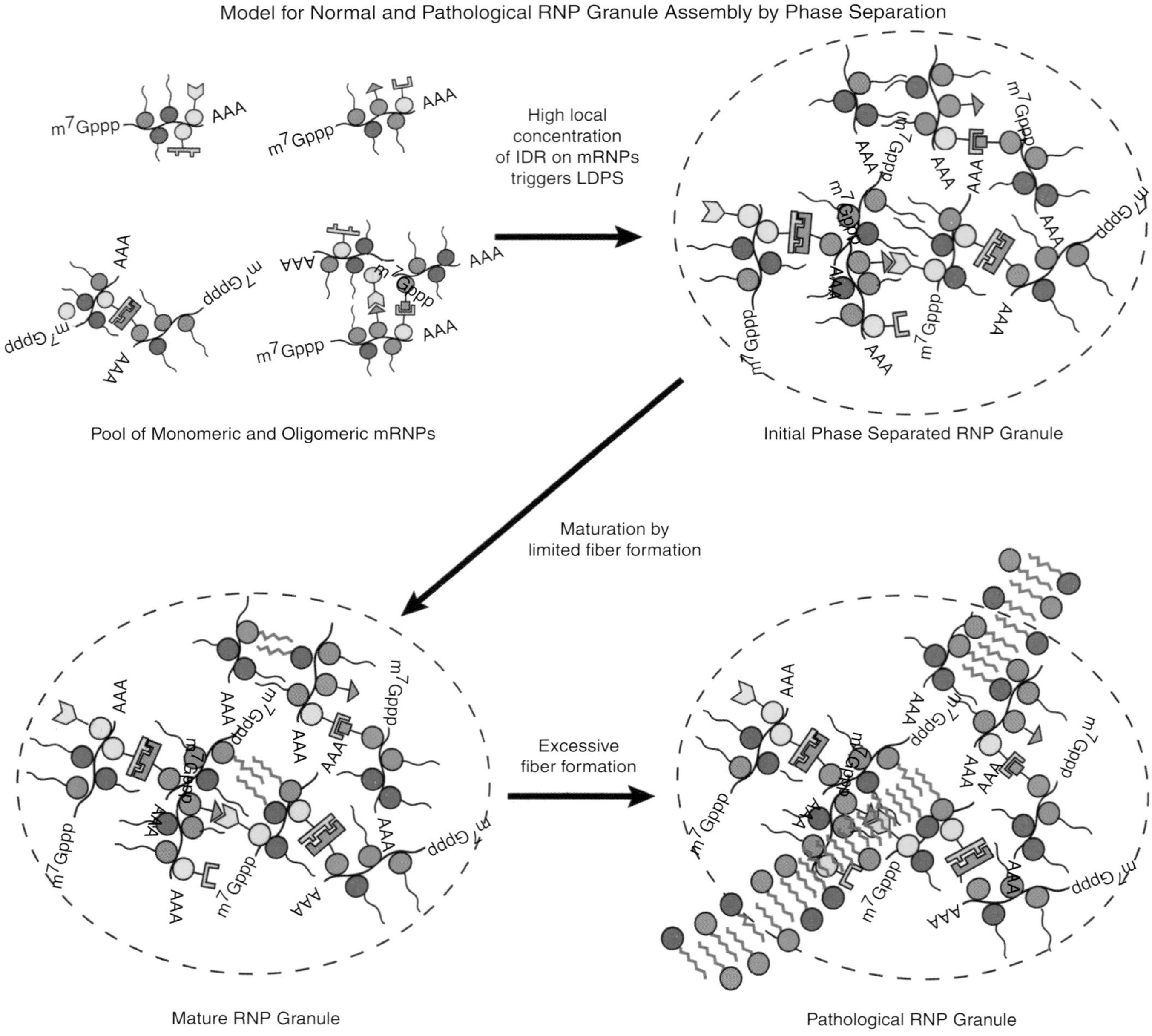

Model for Normal and Pathological RNP Granule Assembly by Phase Separation

High local concentration of IDR on mRNPs triggers LDPS

Pool of Monomeric and Oligomeric mRNPs

Initial Phase Separated RNP Granule

Maturation by limited fiber formation

Mature RNP Granule

Excessive fiber formation

Pathological RNP Granule

Fig. 4.15 Liquid–liquid phase separation by RNA-binding proteins (RNPs) harboring low-complexity sequence domains is the molecular basis for stress granule assembly, and persistent stress granules promote pathological protein fibrillization. IDR: innate defense regulator; LDPS: phospholipids and associated proteins; mRNPs: messenger ribonucleoprotein complexes.

Source: Molliex et al., 2015 [118] with permission from Elsevier

Adult neurogenesis in the hippocampus

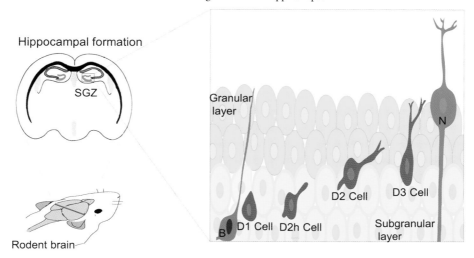

Fig. 4.16 Schematic drawing that represents the cytoarchitecture of the subgranular zone SGZ of the adult hippocampus. The neural progenitor cells (in blue), also known as type-1 cells or type-B cells, give rise to type-2 cells (in red), also known as type-D cells. Intermediate progenitors migrate locally and undergo different maturation stages (D2h, D2, D3 cells) to finally differentiate into functional granular neurons (N).

Source: Gonzalez et al., 2012 [132] with permission from Elsevier

Post-concussive functional incorporation of new neurons

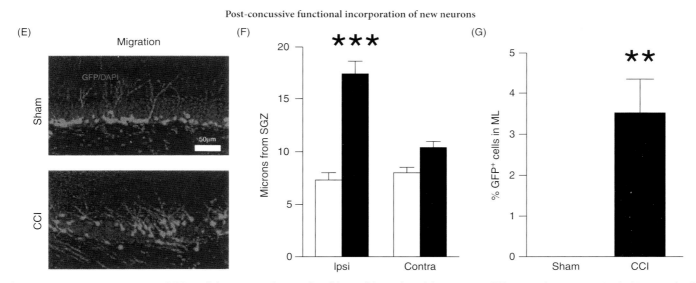

Fig. 4.17 E: Representative images of GFP+ cell dispersion in the granule cell layer of the ipsilateral dentate gyrus. F: Traumatic brain injury mice had increased cell migration away from the subgranular zone on the injured hemisphere compared with sham mice. G: A greater percentage of GFP+ cells from traumatized mice migrated into the molecular layer (ML) of the ipsilateral dentate gyrus. CCI: controlled cortical impact; DAPI: 4'6-diamidino-2-phenylindole; GFP: green fluorescent protein.

Source: Villasana et al., 2015 [154]. Reproduced under the terms of the Creative Commons Attribution licence, CC-BY.

Post-concussive neurogenesis

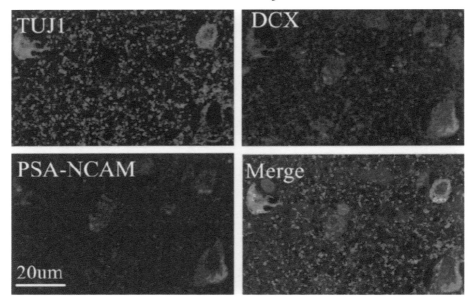

Fig. 4.18 Triple immunostaining shows that TUJ1 (green) is expressed in the DCX (red)- and PSA-NCAM (purple)-positive cells in the cortical regions of adult human brain after traumatic brain injury.

Source: Zheng et al., 2013 [189]. Reproduced with permission from Mary Ann Liebert, Inc.

"Mild" traumatic brain injury may cause extensive neurodegeneration

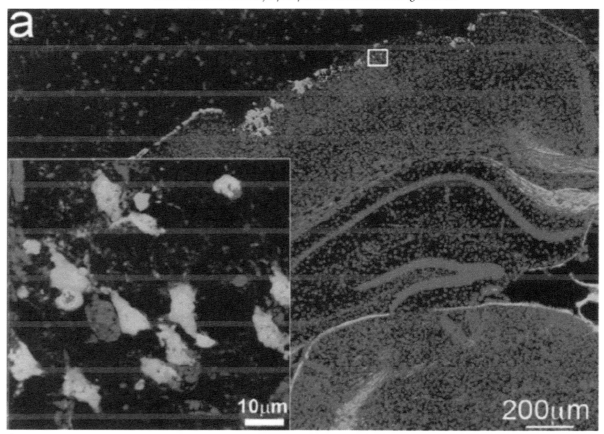

Fig. 4.19 Cell death in the neocortex of mice with mild traumatic brain injury (mTBI). (a) Fluoro-Jade B (FJB)-positive cells are green in the epicenter on the ipsilateral side of the neocortex.

Source: Gao and Chen, 2011 [194], by permission of Oxford University Press

A horizontal section through the hippocampus

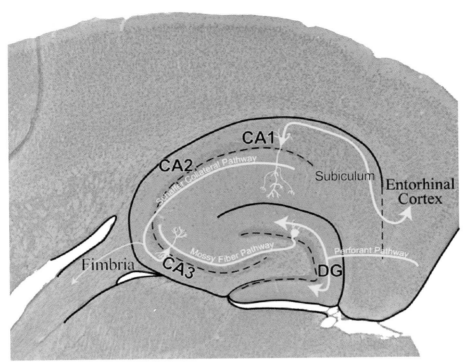

Fig. 4.22 The major pathways are in yellow. Axons from neurons in the entorhinal cortex project via the perforant pathway to synapse on dentate granular cells. The dentate hilus is the area embraced within the crook of the dentate gyrus (DG). These project via mossy fibers to synapse with CA3 pyramidal neurons, which, in turn, project via Schaffer collaterals to CA1 pyramidal neurons.

Source: Smith et al., 2012 [218]. Reproduced with permission from A. Cohen

Luminescent TUNEL-staining neurons in the hippocampus after
mild traumatic brain injury

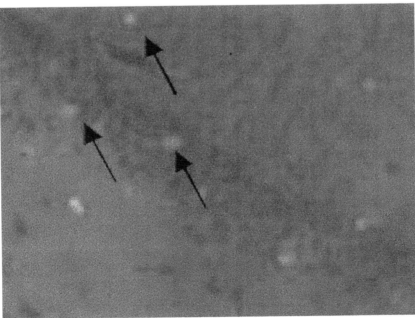

Fig. 4.24 Arrows identify TUNEL-staining neurons in the CA3 hippocampus after mild TBI.

Source: Tashlykov et al., 2007 [29] with permission from Elsevier

Impact of low-intensity blast injury on brain microvessels

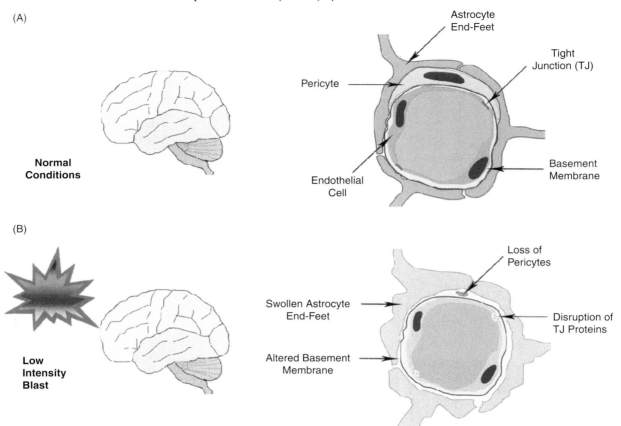

Fig. 4.26 In brain microvessels, low-intensity blast swells astrocyte end-feet, eliminates pericytes, damages the basement membrane, and disrupts tight junctions (TJ). (A) Normal conditions; (B) low-intensity blast.

Computed tomography (CT) and magnetic resonance imaging (MRI) images of two child survivors of "mild TBI" (traumatic brain injury)

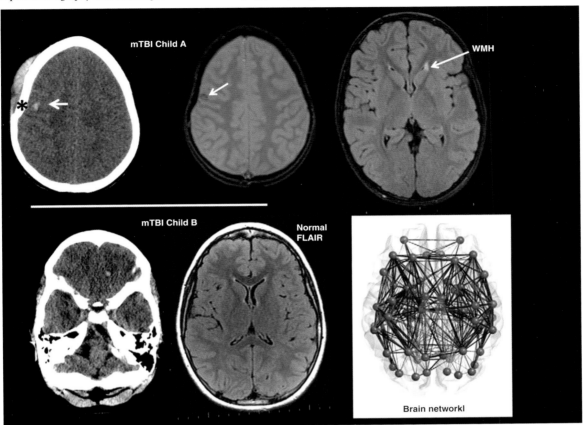

Fig. 6.1 Top: Child A had a Glasgow Coma Scale of 14, but sustained a skull fracture on the day-of-injury CT (black asterisk). The top middle scan is gradient-recalled echo that shows residual blood by-product in the same region on MRI done two years post injury. Just as importantly, the fluid-attenuated inversion recovery (FLAIR: top right) shows prominent white-matter hyperintensities (WMH) in the contralateral frontal white matter adjacent to the anterior horn of the lateral ventricle, plausibly part of a contrecoup injury. Child B's case is illustrated by the images on the bottom left. The leftmost image is the day-of-injury CT scan (Glasgow Coma Scale =15). It shows multiple petechial hemorrhages in the inferior frontal region. However, on the MRI 2.5 years post injury there was no detectable hemosiderin on the gradient-recalled echo sequence, and no discernible WMHs, although the overall volume of FLAIR frontal white matter was reduced. The diagram on the lower right depicts a network of tracts and nodes derived from streamline tractography. Note that actual tracts cannot be visualized. The presumed space path of a tract can be estimated as a curve derived from regressing information from multiple adjacent voxels. Technically, the black lines represent mathematically derived "edges" of linkage, where the weight of an edge stands for the number of "streamlines" (lines created by connecting pixels sharing a preferred direction of diffusivity) linking nodes. In informal terms, black lines depict connectivity and red circles depict nodes and hubs.

Sources: CTs and MRIs are original images from E.D. Bigler's research program. The brain connectivity diagram is from Qiu et al., 2015 [69]

How diffusion-weighted imaging data can be used to map the connectome

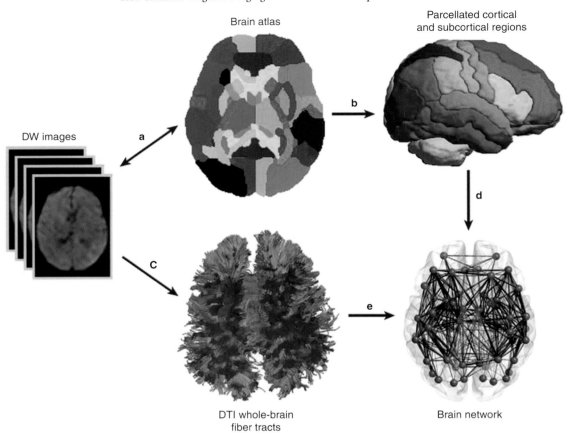

Brain atlas

Parcellated cortical
and subcortical regions

DW images

DTI whole-brain
fiber tracts

Brain network

Fig. 6.2 The major processes involved in structural network analysis using diffusion tensor imaging (DTI). (a) Diffusion-weighted (DW) images of each subject are aligned to those of the brain atlas. (b) The parcellation of cortical and subcortical regions using the brain atlas. (c) The whole-brain tractography using DTI deterministic tractography. (d) Nodes (red spheres) representing cortical and subcortical regions. (e) Weighted edges (black lines) obtained using the tract information. (Figure adapted with permission from Ratnarajah et al. (2013) [72].)

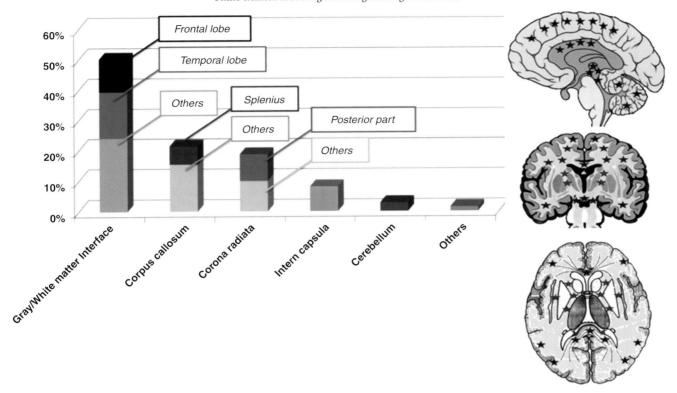

Fig. 6.4 Main diffuse axonal injury (DAI) locations in human brain. Data summarize results from various epidemiological studies. The most common locations of DAI are represented by stars.

Source: Chatelin et al., 2011 [81] with permission from Elsevier

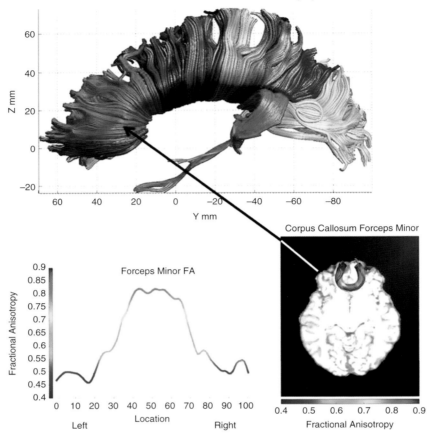

Diffusion tensor imaging (DTI) tractography shows decreased fractional anisotropy (FA) in the forceps minor of the corpus callosum after frontal traumatic brain injury

Fig. 6.6 The upper colorized tractography image depicts the projection territory of aggregated corpus callosum fiber tracts (anterior projection in red and green, with posterior projections in yellow, temporal projections in violet, with posterior frontal in purple to orange and parietal projections in orange to aquamarine blue). This child sustained a concussive brain injury which involved a documented frontal contusion. Plotting the tractography results across the forceps minor shows that FA significantly drops in the region where the contusion appeared, whereas normal values were observed in other regions of the tract. The combination of tractography and advanced methods in DTI analysis may revolutionize how microstructural abnormalities are defined in concussive brain injury.

Source: original image adapted from Bigler et al., 2016 [101]

White-matter regions colored to indicate the number of publications reporting abnormalities

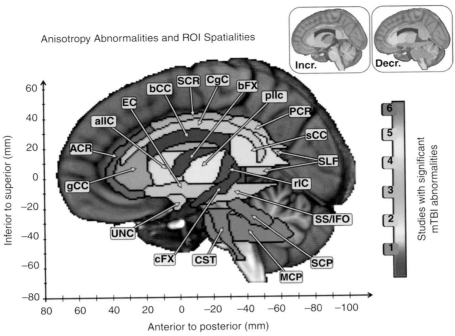

Fig. 6.7 Shown are the International Consortium of Brain Mapping (ICBM-81) white-matter regions, colored to indicate the number of publications reporting white-matter abnormalities (regions with no abnormal findings in the literature are not shown). The Montreal Neurological Institute (MNI-152) template is added for anatomical reference. Using the center of mass for each ICBM-81 structure, we determined that a significant anterior-to-posterior relationship exists between frequency in the literature and anatomical location. Note that since more lateral structures are only partially visible, the anatomical labels point to a convenient, visible location and do not necessarily reflect a structure's center of mass. For example, SLF is mostly covered by more medial structures, and is only visible at its most posterior-inferior part. Coordinates are displayed in MNI-152 space. ACR: anterior corona radiata; aIC: anterior limb of internal capsule; bCC: body of corpus callosum; bFX: body of fornix; cFX: fornix crus; CgC: cingulate cortex; CST: corticospinal tract; EC: entorhinal cortex; gCC: genu of corpus callosum; MCP: middle cerebellar peduncle; PCR: posterior corona radiata; pIIC: posterior limb of internal capsule; rIC: retrolenticular part of internal capsule; ROI: region of interest; SCC: splenium of corpus callosum; SCP: superior cerebellar peduncle; SCR: superior corona radiata; SLF: superior longitudinal fasciculus; SS/IFO: superior stratum/inferior fronto-occipital fasciculus; UNC: uncinate fasciculi.

Source: Eierud et al., 2014 [35] with permission from Elsevier

Atlas-based region-of-interest placement and group comparisons of fractional anisotropy values

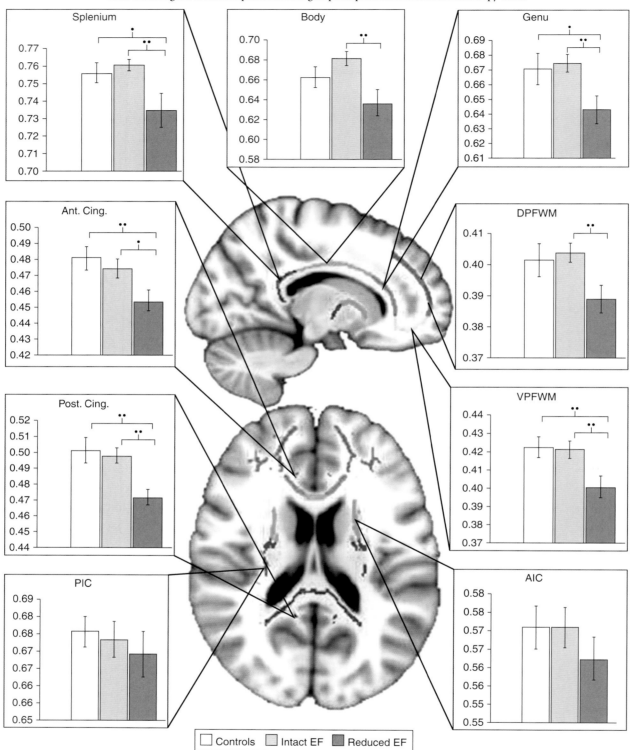

Fig. 6.8 Placement of the TBSS-derived white-matter skeleton regions of interest in standard space on a T1 image. AIC: anterior internal capsule; Ant. Cing.: anterior cingulum bundle; DPFWM: dorsal prefrontal white matter; EF: executive functions; PIC: posterior internal capsule; Post. Cing.: posterior cingulum bundle; TBSS, tract-based spatial statistics; VPFWM: ventral prefrontal white matter. Error bars represent s e m . a: corrected $p < 0.10$; b: corrected $p < 0.05$.

Source: Sorg et al., 2014 [128] with permission from Lippincott Williams & Wilkins, Inc./Wolters Kluwer

Magnetic resonance imaging changes at 3 T in three survivors of pediatric traumatic brain injury

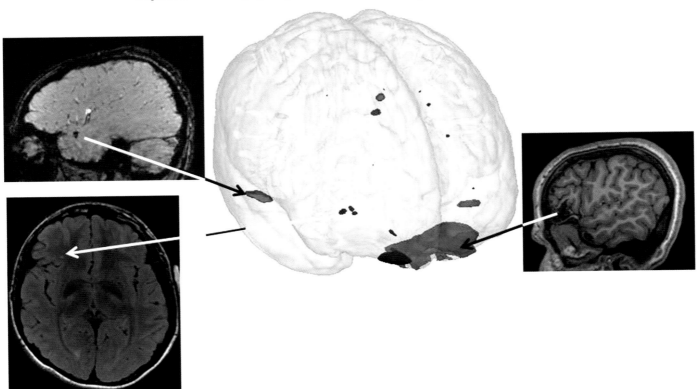

Fig. 6.11 Three cases from the Pediatric mTBI study highlight the independently identified magnetic resonance imaging abnormalities (blinded to group) observed in the first 251 patients screened for participant inclusion. Research magnetic resonance imaging studies were obtained all from the same GE 3-T scanner and included a sagittal-plane volume acquisition T1 IR-SPGR sequence (TR: 7.15 ms, TE: 2.90 ms, 1.2 mm slice thickness), T2-fluid-attenuated inversion recovery sequence (TR: 8000 ms, TE: 140.58 ms, 3.0 mm slice thickness) and a three-dimensional susceptibility-weighted imaging sequence (TR: 30 ms, TE: 23 ms, 1.0 mm slice thickness). Each abnormality was neuroradiologically defined as a region of interest generated by hand tracing the lesion boundaries on to a template image using Mango (http://ric.uthscsa.edu/mango/). Then, a surface model was generated to represent each lesion area in three-dimensional space. The regions of interest represent the relative location where lesions were located. Small white-matter hyperintensities and regions of hemosiderin deposition were slightly enlarged to improve visualization.

Source: Bigler et al., 2016 [101] with permission from Lippincott Williams & Wilkins, Inc./Wolters Kluwer

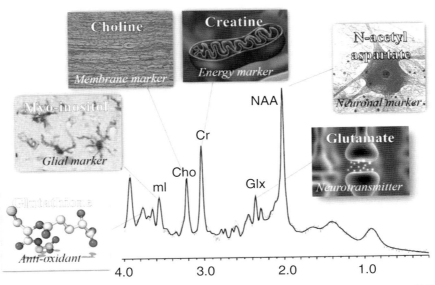

Fig. 6.12 The six MRS spectroscopic peaks most commonly measured. Cho: choline; Cr: creatine; Glx: glutamate; ml: myoinositol; NAA: N-acetyl aspartate.

Source: Koerte et al., 2015 [166] © Georg Thieme Verlag KG. Reproduced with permission

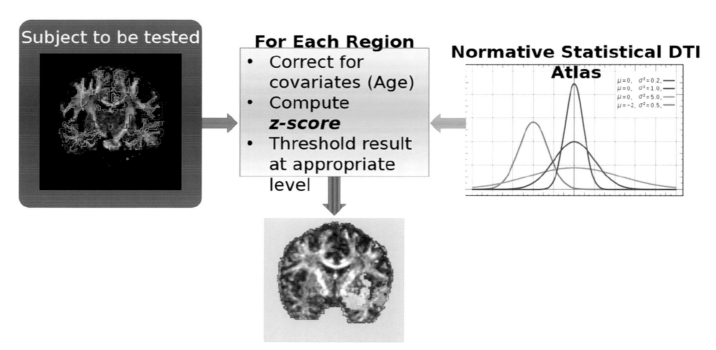

A schematic showing how individuals can be compared with norms

Individual Subject Testing

Subject to be tested

For Each Region
- Correct for covariates (Age)
- Compute **z-score**
- Threshold result at appropriate level

Normative Statistical DTI Atlas

$\mu=0, \sigma^2=0.2,$ ——
$\mu=0, \sigma^2=1.0,$ ——
$\mu=0, \sigma^2=5.0,$ ——
$\mu=-2, \sigma^2=0.5,$ ——

Subject-specific abnormality map

Fig. 6.14 A coronal diffusion tensor imaging (DTI) color map depicting the raw fractional anisotropy data for an individual subject is depicted in the upper left. A voxel-by-voxel comparison is made with a normative statistical DTI atlas where various demographic variables are taken into consideration, as shown in the middle box. The subject-specific output is displayed as a "heat map," showing where the most significant statistical deviations occur in the individual patient with concussive brain injury compared to the healthy, typically developing normative sample.

Source: illustration courtesy of Sylvain Bouix, Ph.D. and Martha E. Shenton, Ph.D., Psychiatry Neuroimaging Lab, Brigham and Women's Hospital and Harvard Medical School

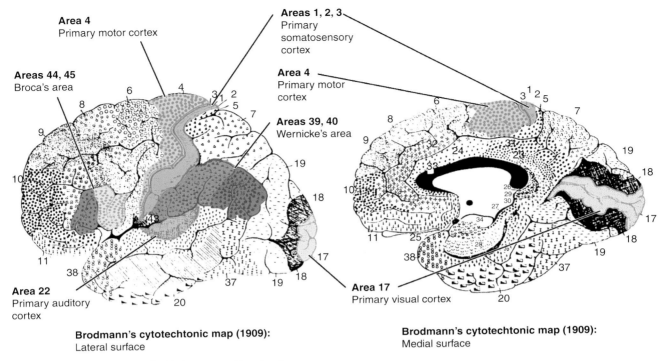

Area 4
Primary motor cortex

Areas 1, 2, 3
Primary somatosensory cortex

Areas 44, 45
Broca's area

Area 4
Primary motor cortex

Areas 39, 40
Wernicke's area

Area 22
Primary auditory cortex

Area 17
Primary visual cortex

Brodmann's cytotechtonic map (1909):
Lateral surface

Brodmann's cytotechtonic map (1909):
Medial surface

Fig. 7.6 Brodmann's map, colored to highlight purported functional areas

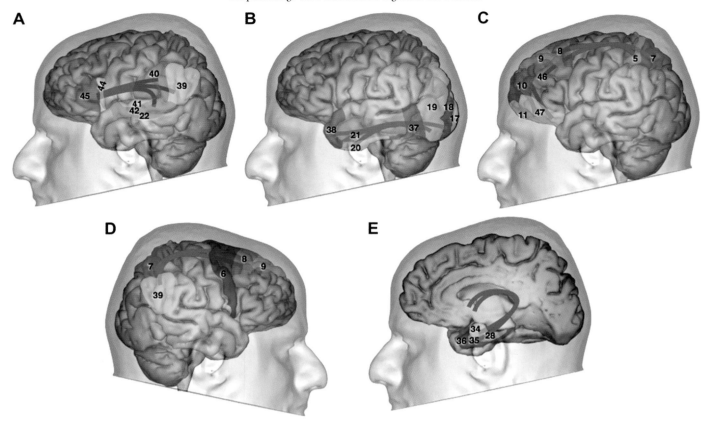

Fig. 7.8 (A) A left-hemisphere-dominant language network with epicenters in Wernicke's and Broca's areas. (B) A face object identification network with epicenters in occipitotemporal and temporopolar cortex. (C) An executive function comportment network with epicenters in lateral prefrontal cortex, orbitofrontal cortex, and posterior parietal cortex. (D) A right-hemisphere-dominant spatial attention network with epicenters in dorsal posterior parietal cortex, the frontal eye fields, and the cingulate gyrus. (E) A memory emotion network with epicenters in the hippocampal-entorhinal regions and the amygdaloid complex.

Source: Catani et al., 2012 [111] with permission from Elsevier

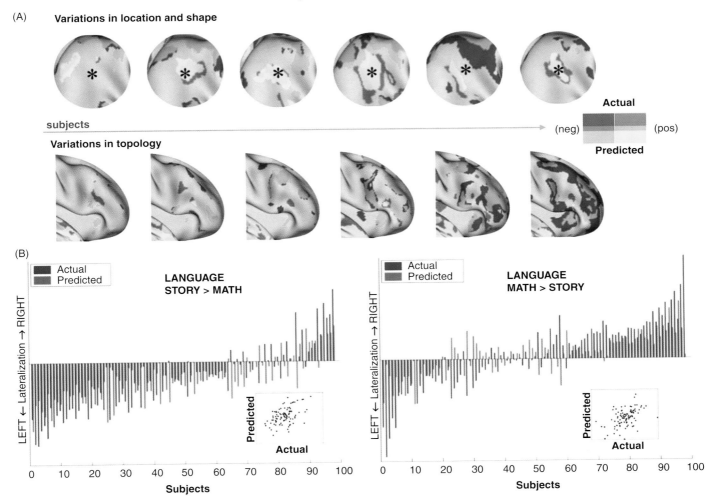

Fig. 7.9 (A) Variations in location, shape, and topology are predicted by the model (contrast: language math > story). (B) Peak *Z* scores were calculated for each hemisphere to examine how well the model can predict the amount of activation for each subject. A lateralization index (difference between right and left peak activation levels) is then calculated for each subject for both predicted and actual data and is shown as red and blue bars, respectively (language task). The model is able to predict individual subjects' lateralization index for both contrasts, including the case where the majority of the subjects are left-lateralized. Statistical tests: math > story (correlation coefficient (r) = 0.47, $p < 10-5$), story > math ($r = 0.48$, $p < 10-6$).

Source: Tavor et al., 2016 [116]. Reprinted with permission from AAAS.

Genetically influenced individual variation in the human putamen

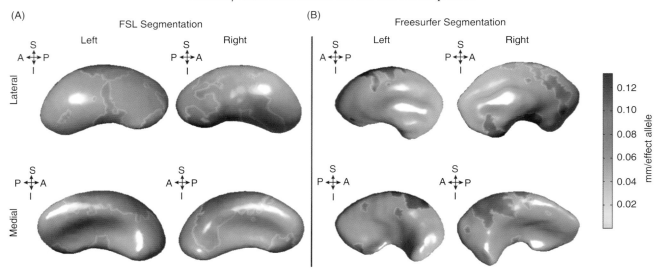

Fig. 7.10 Shape analysis in 1541 young healthy subjects shows consistent deformations of the putamen regardless of segmentation protocol. (a, b) The distance from a medial core to surfaces derived from FSL FIRST (a) or FreeSurfer (b) segmentations was derived in the same 1541 subjects. Each copy of the rs945270-C allele was significantly associated with an increased width in colored areas (false discovery rate corrected at q50.05) and the degree of deformation is labeled by color. The orientation is indicated by arrows. A: anterior; I: inferior; P: posterior; S: superior. Shape analysis in both software suites gives statistically significant associations in the same direction. Although the effects are more widespread in the FSL segmentations, FreeSurfer segmentations also show overlapping regions of effect, which appears strongest in anterior and superior sections.

Source: Hibar et al. [117]. Reprinted by permission from Macmillan

Finite-element modeling of traumatic brain injury

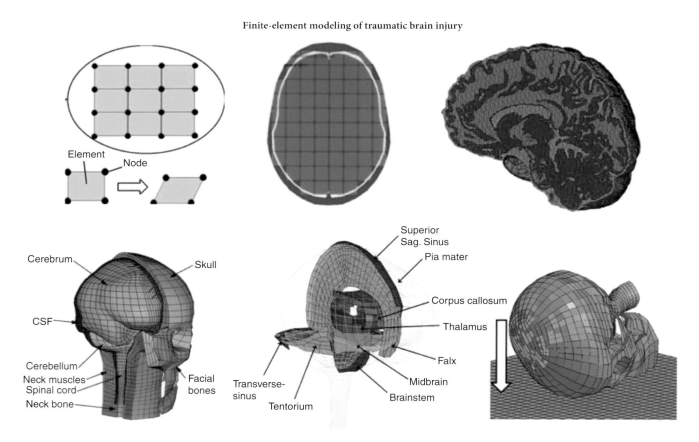

Fig. 7.11 The continuum of a tissue mass is approximated by many finite elements connected at nodes. The two pictures on the lower left illustrate the model's division into tissue types. The image on the right depicts a simulated right frontal head injury. CSF: cerebrospinal fluid.

Source: von Holst and Li [123]. Reproduced under the terms of the Creative Commons Attribution licence, CC-BY.

The geography of the transcriptome: regional gene expression in three dimensions

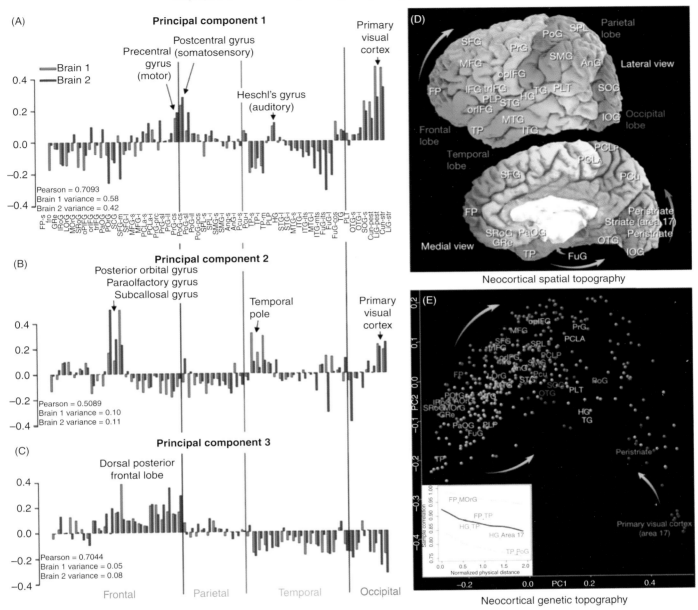

Fig. 7.14 The neocortical transcriptome reflects primary sensorimotor specialization and *in vivo* spatial topography. (a–c) First three neocortical principal components, plotted across 57 cortical divisions ordered roughly from rostral to caudal (frontal to occipital pole), are highly reproducible between brains. PC1 (Pearson $r = 0.71$) is selective for primary sensory and motor areas (a). PC2 (Pearson $r = 0.51$) is differential for specific subdivisions of the frontal, temporal, and occipital poles (b), whereas PC3 (Pearson $r = 0.70$) is selective for the caudal portion of the frontal lobe (c). (d, e) Relationship between the (x, y, z) location of sampled cortical gyri and their transcriptional similarities. Native brain 1 magnetic resonance imaging is shown in (d) with major gyri labeled. (e) Multidimensional scaling (MDS) applied to the same cortical samples, where distance between points reflects similarity in gene expression profiles. Median samples for major gyri are labeled. Samples cluster by lobe, and both lobe positions and gyral positions generally mirror the native spatial topography, emphasized by arrows in (d) and (e). Inset panel in (e) plots the relationship (mean ± 1 s d) between three-dimensional (3D) MDS-based similarity and 3D *in vivo* sample distance, demonstrating correlations that are stronger between proximal samples and multi-dimensional scaling applied to cortical samples, where distance between points reflects similarity in gene expression profiles. Median samples for major gyri are labeled. Samples cluster by lobe, and both lobe positions and gyral positions generally mirror the native spatial topography, emphasized by arrows in d and e. Inset panel in e plots the relationship (mean ± 1 s d) between 3D MDS-based similarity and 3D in vivo sample distance, demonstrating correlations that are stronger between proximal samples and decrease with distance. Selected gyral pairs are labeled.

Source: Hawrylycz et al., 2012 [194]. Reprinted by permission from Macmillan

Structural variation in gene expression, comparing two human brains

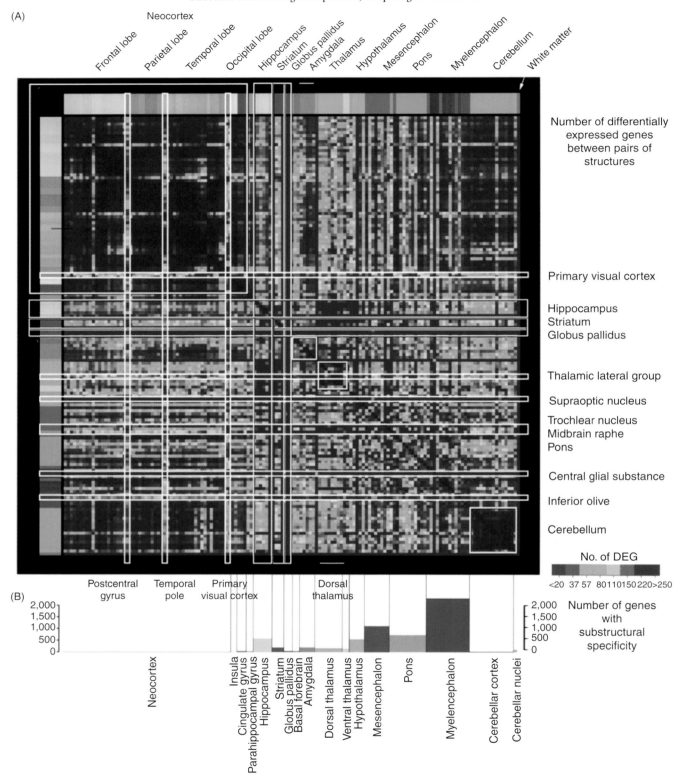

Fig. 7.15 (a) Matrix of differential expression between 146 regions in both brains. Each point represents the number of common genes enriched in one structure over another in both brains (Benjamini–Hochberg-corrected *p* < 0.01, log2(fold change) > 1.5). DEG: differentially expressed genes. Several major regions exhibit relatively low internal variation (blue), including the neocortex, cerebellum, dorsal thalamus, and amygdala. Subcortical regions show highly complex differential patterns between specific nuclei. (b) Frequency of marker genes with selective expression in specific subdivisions of major brain regions (greater than twofold enrichment in a particular subdivision compared to the remaining subdivisions).

Source: Hawrylycz et al., 2012 [194]. Reprinted by permission from Macmillan

Neurofibrillary tangles in the fusiform gyrus of a 27-year-old man 1.5 years after traumatic brain injury (TBI): comparison with similar lesions in other conditions

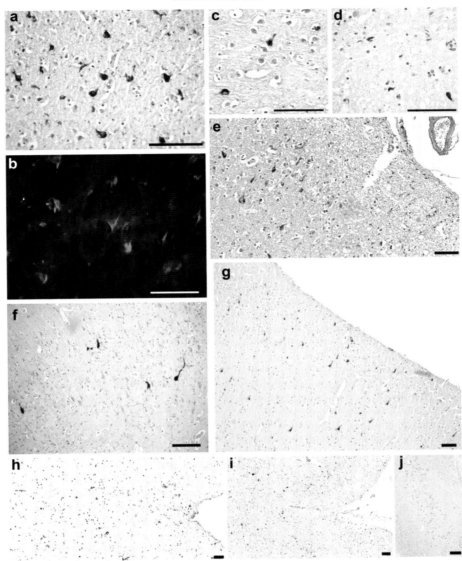

Fig. 7.16 Representative immunohistochemical and thioflavine-S staining for neurofibrillary tangles (NFTs). (A) NFTs in the parahippocampal gyrus of a 49-year-old male 1 year post-TBI. (B) Representative thioflavine-S positive staining in the same case as a. (C) NFTs in the fusiform gyrus of a 27-year-old male 1.5 years after TBI. (D) NFTs in the frontal lobe of a case of advanced Alzheimer's disease (positive control). (E, G) Representative images showing prevalent NFTs in the superficial layers of the cortex of the medial temporal lobe. (F) Extensive neuropil threads and occasional NFTS in a 53-year-old individual who died 8 years following TBI. (H-I) representative images showing Isolated clusters of NFTs within the depth of sulci. (J) Uninjured control case displaying no neurons positive for tau immunostaining in the hippocampal region CA1. All scale bars approx. 100 µm.

Source: Johnson et al., 2012 [247] with permission from John Wiley & Sons

Nodes of functional connectivity exhibiting sex differences on diffusion
tensor imaging

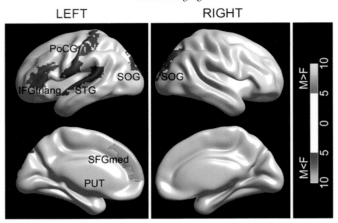

Fig. 7.18 The spatial distribution of cortical regions showing significant
gender effect. The color bar represents F values of group comparison. Left
and right represent left and right hemispheres, respectively. IFGtriang: inferior
frontal gyrus (triangular); PoCG: post-central gyrus; PUT: putamen;
SFGmed: superior frontal gyrus (medial); SOG: superior occipital gyrus;
STG: superior temporal gyrus.

Source: Sun et al., 2015 [568]. Reproduced under the terms of the Creative
Commons Attribution licence, CC-BY.

Sex differences in connectivity

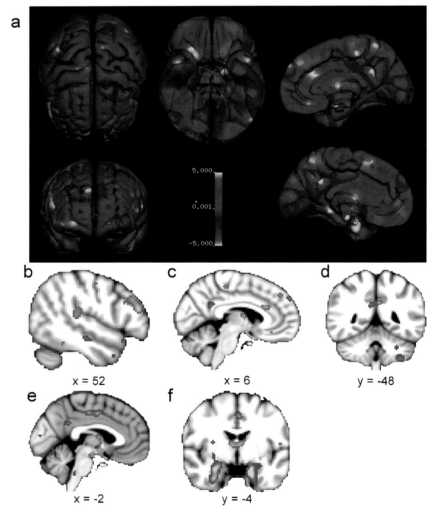

Fig. 7.19 Female > Male in red, and Male > Female is in
blue. Panel a, rendered overview of uncorrected regional
sex differences in grey matter volume. All other panels are
thresholded at FDR q < 0.01. Panels b–f display areas of larger
volume in females (red) including (b) the right inferior and
middle frontal gyri, pars triangularis and planum temporale;
(c) thalamus and right anterior cingulate gyrus; and (f) left
and right thalamus; and areas of larger volume in males
(blue), including (c) the anterior cingulate gyrus; (d) bilateral
posterior cingulate gyrus and precuneus and left cerebellum;
(e) anterior and posterior cingulate gyri; and (f) left and right
amygdalae, hippocampi and parahippocampal gyri.

Source: Ruigrok et al., Elsevier 2014 [561]. Reproduced under
the terms of the Creative Commons Attribution licence,
CC-BY.

Magnetic resonance imaging (MRI) and fluorodeoxyglucose positron emission tomography (FDG-PET) in a 71-year-old woman evaluated for persistent and non-progressive memory difficulties for several years

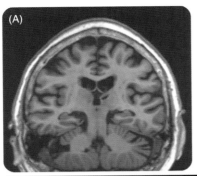

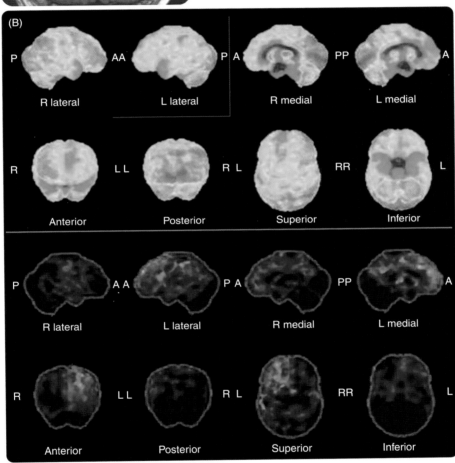

Fig. 9.3 (A) Head MRI shows a chronic left medial thalamic infarct, as well as chronic right caudate head and left corona radiata infarcts. (B) Top, three-dimensional stereotactic surface projection of the patient's FDG-PET scan shows hypometabolism in the left medial thalamus, in addition to the left medial prefrontal, lateral frontal, and posterior cingulate regions. Bottom, statistical map showing regions of significant hypometabolism relative to age-matched controls with green and yellow regions indicating FDG-PET magnitude being 3 and 4 s d, respectively, lower than control subjects. A: anterior; L: left; P: posterior; R: right.

Source: Golden et al., 2016 [42] with permission from Wolters Kluwer Health

Task-related functional magnetic resonance imaging shows significant abnormalities up to five years post concussion

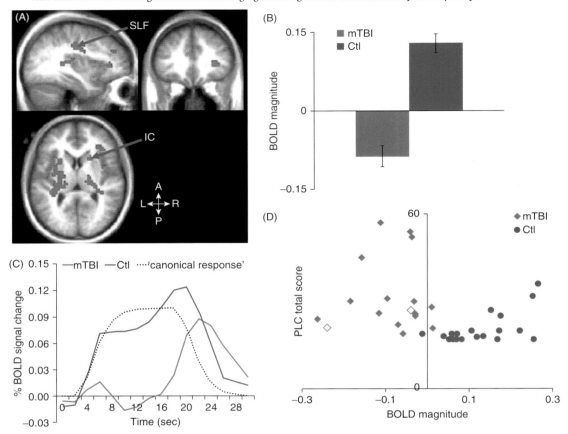

Fig. 9.4 Magnitudes and time courses from large region of interest (ROI). Magnitudes and time courses extracted from voxels demonstrating significant differences between patients and controls. (A) Selected brain slices showing voxels with a significantly reduced blood oxygen level-dependent (BOLD) signal in mild traumatic brain injury (mTBI) patients relative to controls. The set of all voxels showing significant differences formed an "abnormal" ROI. A: anterior; I: internal capsule; L: left; P: posterior; R: right; SLF: superior longitudinal fasciculus. (B) BOLD magnitudes from the abnormal ROI, averaged across tasks. Error bars represent standard error of the mean. (C) The time course of the BOLD signal in the abnormal ROI. The canonical hemodynamic response function used in the analysis to compute the BOLD magnitudes also is shown (labeled "canonical response"). (D) Scatterplot of BOLD magnitude values from the abnormal ROI for mTBI patients (red diamond) and controls (blue circles) vs. Post-traumatic Stress Disorder Checklist (PCL-C) total score. "Complex mTBI" (mTBI patients with positive radiological findings and/or antegrade post-traumatic amnesia longer than 24 h) are indicated by open diamonds.

Source: Astafiev et al., 2015 [96]. Reproduced with permission from Mary Ann Liebert, Inc.

Post-concussive depression alters cerebral reactivity to a working-memory task

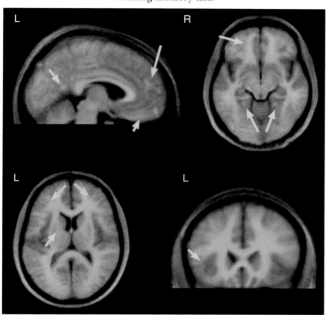

Fig. 10.1 Relationship between Beck Depression Inventory II scores and blood oxygenation level-dependent (BOLD) signal changes. The higher the scores, the lower the percentage of BOLD signal changes in the right (R) and left (L) dorsolateral prefrontal cortex, left striatum, and left insula (shown in blue). In addition, the higher the Beck Depression Inventory II scores, the less the negative percentage of BOLD signal changes in the rostral anterior and posterior cingulate, medial orbitofrontal cortex, and left and right parahippocampal gyri (in red).

Source: Chen et al., 2008 [153]. Journal of the American Medical Association

Increased Bilateral Amygdala Activation to Fear in MDD versus Non-MDD

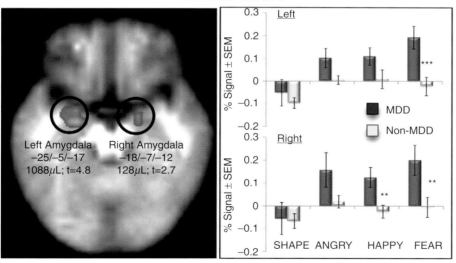

Fig. 10.2 A region-of-interest (ROI) analysis revealed significantly greater fear-related activation in bilateral amygdalae in major depressive disorder (MDD) versus non-MDD subjects (left panel). Mean activation for shape-matching, angry, happy, and fear trials extracted from the amygdalae ROIs is displayed in the right panel.

Source: Matthews et al., 2011 [157] with permission from Elsevier

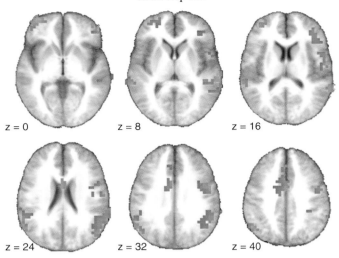

Post-concussive suicidality is associated with altered error processing on the stop task

z = 0   z = 8   z = 16

z = 24   z = 32   z = 40

Fig. 10.5 Despite comparable behavioral task performance, the suicidal ideation (SI) relative to the non-SI group showed abnormal hyperactivation of a network of brain structures that includes the dorsal anterior cingulate and several areas of the prefrontal cortex during error processing.

Source: Matthews et al., 2012 [283] with permission from Lippincott Williams & Wilkins, Inc./Wolters Kluwer

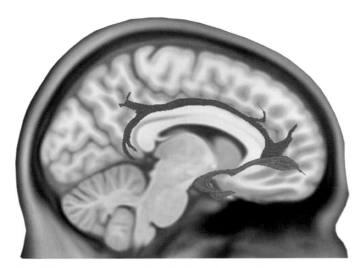

Fig. 10.9 A visual depiction of the significant fiber tracts (uncinate fasciculus (purple) and cingulum (blue)) taken from a male participant in the depression – post-traumatic stress disorder–traumatic brain injury group.

Source: Isaac et al., 2015 [159] with permission from Elsevier

Dorsomedial (dm) and dorsolateral (dl) prefrontal cortex (PFC) differentially respond to fearful faces as a function of genotype

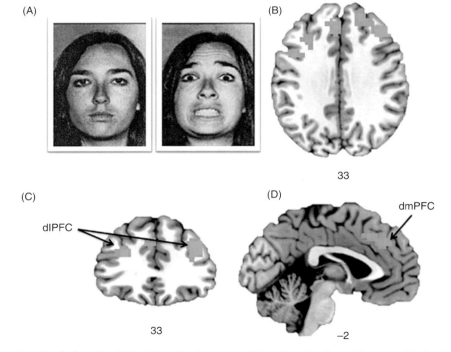

(A)   (B)

33

(C)   (D)

dlPFC   dmPFC

33   −2

Fig. 10.7 (A) Example of neutral and fearful face stimuli. (B) Axial section showing medial and lateral prefrontal signal associated with genotype. (C) Dorsolateral and (D) dorsomedial regions surviving whole-brain correction.

Source: Almli et al., 2014 [715] with permission from John Wiley & Sons

Some toxic affects of Aβ

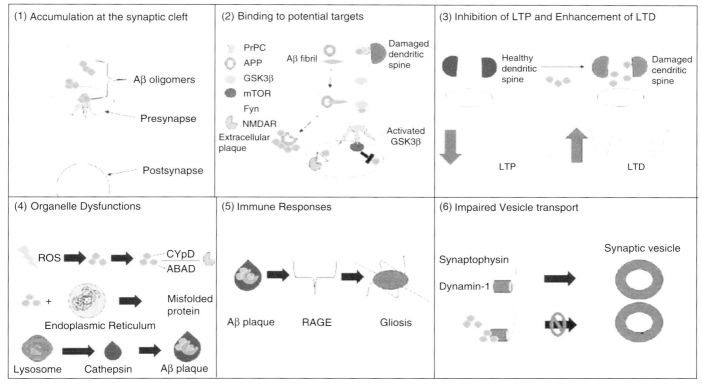

Fig. 11.7 The many sites of neuronal damage by Aβ. (1) Soluble intracellular oligomers of A are cytotoxic (2) Interaction with cellular prion protein (PrPC) leads to dendritic spine damage (top right). A fibril binds to amyloid precursor protein (APP) during formation of extracellular plaques (middle left). Aβ inappropriately activates glycogen synthase kinase 3 (GSK3) (middle right). Aβ synergizes with Fyn to disrupt synaptic receptors (bottom left). Mammalian target of rapamycin (mTOR) may inhibit Aβ (bottom right). (3) Mounting evidence suggests Aβ-mediated destruction of spines and synapses leads to long-term potentiation (LTP) impairment and long-term depression (LTD) enhancement. (4) Mitochondrial distress may lead to production of reactive oxygen species (ROS) that may accelerate Aβ formation. Aβ may then affect N-methyl-d-aspartate receptor (NMDAR) activity by binding to intracellular mitochondrial cyclophilin D or mitochondrial Aβ alcohol dehydrogenase. (Top). Aβ -mediated cytotoxicity may be particularly damaging to the endoplasmic reticulum, affecting its production and modification of crucial proteins (middle). Identification of cathepsins in Aβ plaques suggests protease dysfunctions from lysosomes may play a critical role in advancement of pathology (bottom). (5) Receptor for advanced glycation end products (RAGE) may play a prominent role in the increased microglial activation and proinflammatory markers commonly associated with senile plaques. (6) Aβ interacts with synaptophysin in presynaptic terminals of the hippocampus to impair neurotransmission (top). Aβ also interferes with dynamin-1, allowing synaptic vesicles to re-enter the synaptic pool (bottom). ABAD: mitochondrial Aβ alcohol dehydrogenase; CypD: intracellular mitochondrial cyclophilin D.

Source: Rajmohan and Reddy, 2017 [226] with permission from IOS Press

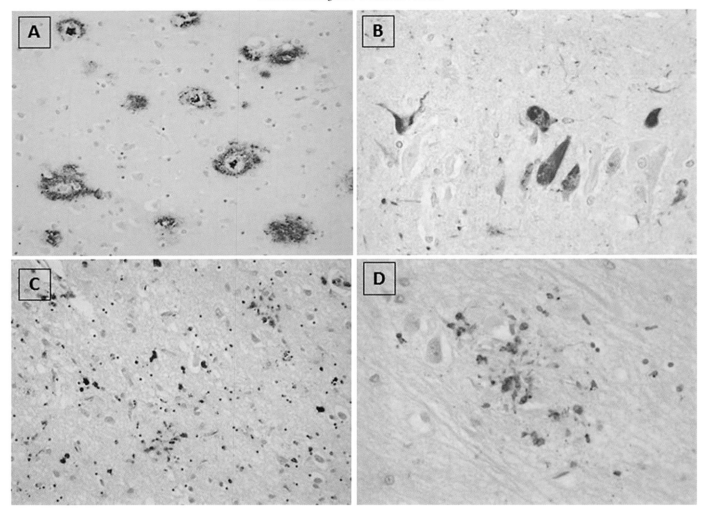

Fig. 11.10 (A) Senile plaques and globose diffuse deposits demonstrated with anti-A antibody (M 0804, Dako). (B) Neurofibrillary tangles demonstrated by phosphorylated tau protein immunohistochemistry (PHF-Tau; AT8, Thermo Scientific). (C) Diffuse distribution of activated microglia in the cortex with clustering within and around amyloid plaques. (D) Higher magnification of amyloid plaque with activated microglial in the CA4 region of the hippocampus (C and D: CD68 immunohistochemistry; PGM1clone, Dako).

Source: Taipa et al., 2016 [244] with permission from IOS Press

Differences in cortical atrophy rates between healthy elderly individuals and those with mild cognitive impairment (MCI)/Alzheimer's disease (AD)

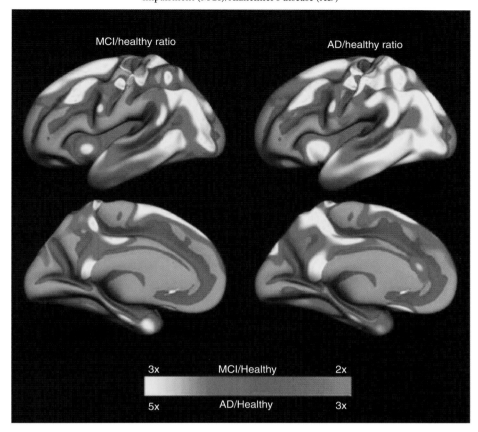

Fig. 11.11 In mild MCI, rates of cortical volumetric reductions are more than double that seen in healthy aging across large areas of the cerebral cortex, and rates more than three times larger are seen in AD. Please note that the scale is different between MCI/healthy and AD/healthy to allow appreciation of the regional patterns of effects across groups. Data from the Alzheimer's Disease Neuroimaging Initiative.

Source: Fjell et al., 2014 [250] with permission from Elsevier

The life history of the thickness of the normal human entorhinal cortex

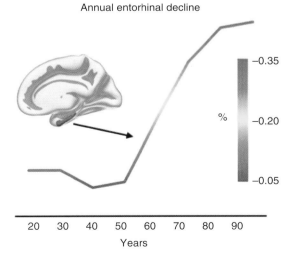

Fig. 11.13 Accelerated entorhinal decline in aging: Cross-sectional estimates of the annual rate of cortical thinning in the entorhinal cortex across the adult life indicate a marked increase in atrophy from 50 years. Age-related acceleration of decline in elderly has been confirmed with longitudinal data.

Source: Fjell et al., 2014 [250] with permission from Elsevier

Neuropathological findings in a 25-year-old man with a history of encephalopathy after repetitive concussions

(A) Multiple perivascular ptau lesions at the sulcal depths

(B) Perivascular ptau neurofibrillary tangles, neurites, and astrocytes

(C) AT8-immunostained paraffin-embedded section

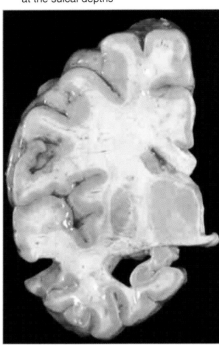 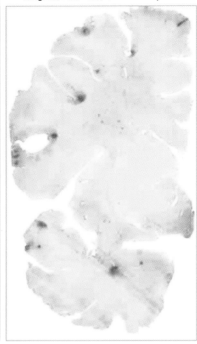 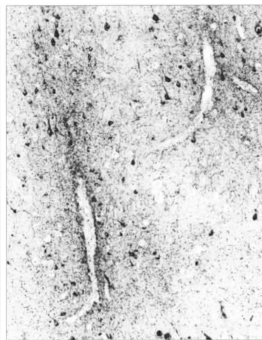

Fig. 11.15 (A) The brain showed mild ventricular dilation and hippocampal atrophy. Pathological lesions of hyperphosphorylated tau (p-tau) consisting of neurofibrillary tangles, neurites, and astrocytes around small blood vessels were found at the sulcal depths of the frontal and temporal lobes. Free-floating 50-μm section immunostained for AT8 (B) and paraffin-embedded 10-μm section immunostained for AT8 (C; original magnification × 200). These p-tau lesions are considered to be pathognomonic for chronic traumatic encephalopathy (CTE) based on the preliminary National Institute of Neurological Disorders and Stroke consensus criteria for the pathological diagnosis of CTE. Characteristic CTE p-tau pathology was also found in the parietal lobes, entorhinal cortex, anterior hippocampus, hypothalamus, nucleus basalis of Meynert, substantia nigra, locus coeruleus, and median raphe. There was no immunopositivity for amyloid-β, TAR DNA-binding protein 43, or α-synuclein.

Source: Mez et al., 2016 [315]. Journal of the American Medical Association

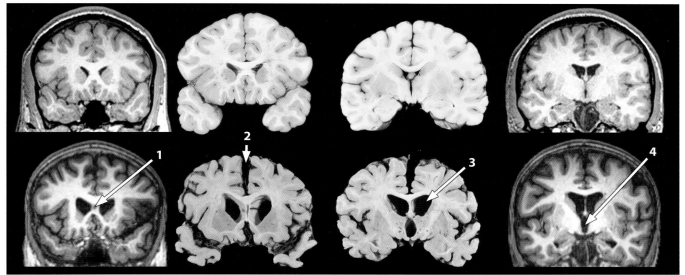

I. Amygdala and Dorsal Midbrain: core regions in (F-18)FDDNP PET

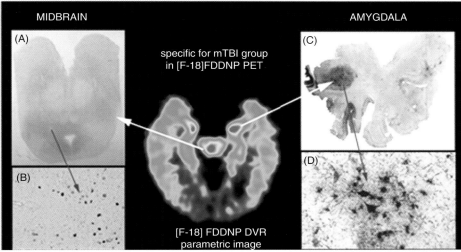

II. Robust tau IHC in amygdala and MTL is consistently present in symptomatic retired football players

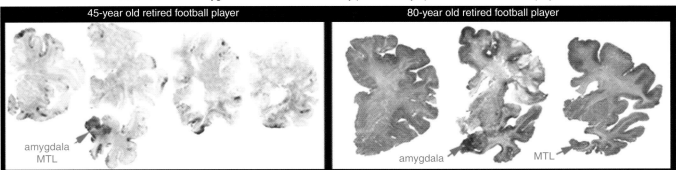

Fig. 12.2 (A) Top row: normal coronal image from magnetic resonance imaging (MRI) of a 14-year-old male (outer images on each side) at a similar level to a post-mortem coronal image of a healthy adult (middle images). Bottom row: similarly, coronal MRI (outer images on each side) at a similar level to a post-mortem severe stage IV CTE is shown, as evidenced by cavum septum pellucidum (1); severe cerebral atrophy (2); dilated lateral ventricles (3); and dilated third ventricle (4). Post-mortem images from Hurley D. Brain bank study of football players finds pervasive CTE, but true prevalence remains unknown. *Neurol Today* 2017; 17 (17): 1–27, reproduced with permission from Wolters Kluwer. (B) Appearance of hyperphosphorylated tau aggregates within neurons and astrocytes (brown staining in panels A and B) clustered around small cortical vessels (arrows), characteristically in a patchy distribution toward the depths of the cortical sulci, is emerging as the distinctive pathology of CTE. This pathology appears to be virtually exclusive to circumstances in which there has been exposure to brain injury in life, whether as repetitive mild traumatic brain injury (TBI) as shown in a 61-year-old male former boxer (A) or a single moderate or severe TBI as shown in a 48-year-old man with three years of survival after a single severe TBI (B). In addition to this distinctive tau pathology, neurodegeneration after TBI is increasingly recognized as a complex pathology, including abnormal amyloid plaque deposition (brown staining in panels C and D). As with tau, aspects of these pathologies can be recognized in brain samples from patients exposed to either repetitive mild TBI as shown in a 59-year-old male former soccer player (C) or a single moderate or severe TBI (D; same patient as in panel B). Phosphorylated tau was stained with antibody CP13 (A) or PHF-1 (B). Amyloid β was stained with antibody 6F3D (C and D). DVR: distribution volume ratio; IHC: immunohistochemistry; MTL: medial temporal lobe; PET: positron emission tomography. Adapted from Barrio et al. [30] (reproduced with permission from PNAS).

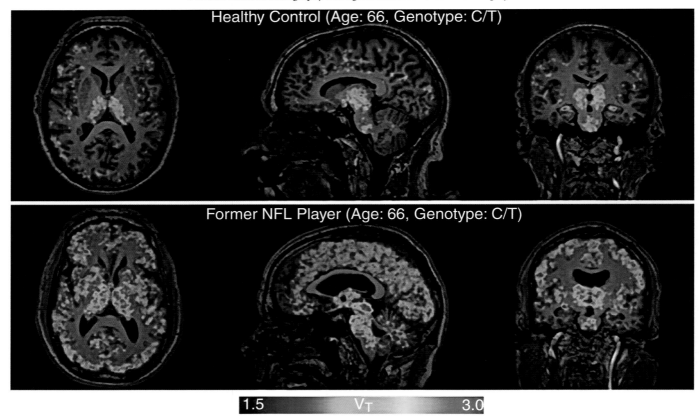

Fig. 12.3 Former National Football League (NFL) players demonstrate increased binding of [^{11}C]DPA-713, reported as total distribution volume (V$_T$) across many brain regions compared to binding of [11C]DPA-713 in the brains of elderly healthy controls. Parametric [^{11}C]DPA-713 V$_T$ images from one former NFL player and one age- and rs6971 genotype-matched healthy individual are presented for comparison.

Source: Coughlin et al., 2015 [53]; reproduced with permission from Elsevier

Positron emission tomography imaging findings comparing healthy controls (CTRL) with mild traumatic brain injury (mTBI) and Alzheimer's disease (AD)

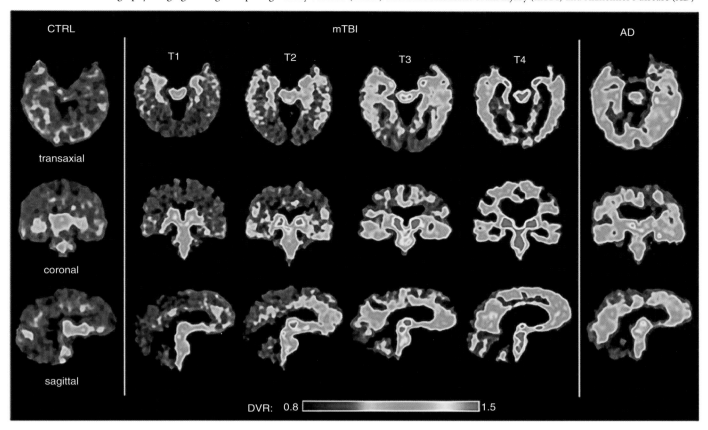

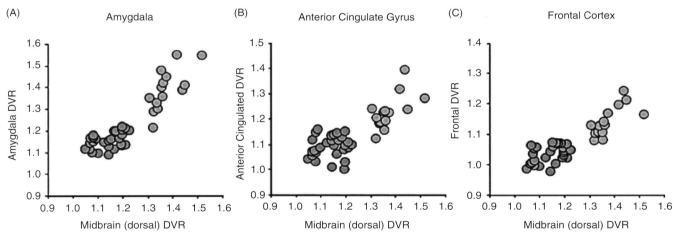

Fig. 12.4 (Upper) [F-18]FDDNP distribution volume ratios (DVR) parametric images showing patterns T1–T4 of increased [F-18]FDDNP signal observed in the mTBI group compared with cognitive control subjects (left). The T1 pattern shows involvement of two core areas which have consistently increased [F-18]FDDNP signal in all four patterns: amygdala (limbic) and dorsal midbrain (subcortical). Patterns T2–T4 are marked by increase of [F-18]FDDNP signal in these two core regions and progressively larger number of subcortical, limbic, and cortical areas. Although more complex patterns (e.g., T4) overlap with AD in the cortex, midbrain and amygdala signals are elevated above the levels in AD. An AD case is shown in the right column for comparison. Lower: A is a two-dimensional scatter plot showing [F-18]FDDNP DVR values in two core areas consistently involved in chronic traumatic encephalopathy (CTE) (subcortical structures (dorsal midbrain) and limbic structures (amygdala)), clearly demonstrating separation of mTBI and CTRL groups. B and C demonstrate similar separation effect when dorsal midbrain is compared with cortical areas typically associated with CTE and its mood disorders, namely the anterior cingulate gyrus (B) and frontal lobe (C). mTBI subjects are represented by green circles, and CTRL subjects are represented by blue circles.

Source: Barrio et al. [30]; reproduced with permission of PNAS.

Functional magnetic resonance imaging-derived default mode network (DMN) activity between pre- and post-game

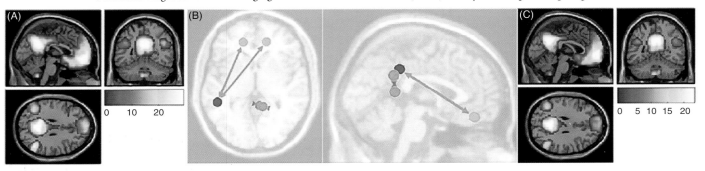

Fig. 12.5A Significant (*p* < 0.01) differences in pre-game and post-game connectivity for all subjects. Left panel: pre-game and (right panel) post-game DMN activation. Middle connectivity diagrams: overall connectivity differences with circles representing seed regions of interest; width of arrow representative of T-scores as well as directionality, with warm colors referring to an increase in connectivity; cool colors represent a decrease in connectivity.

Source: Johnson et al., 2014 [98]; reproduced with permission from Mary Ann Liebert, Inc.

Blood flow differences in athletes with history of concussion

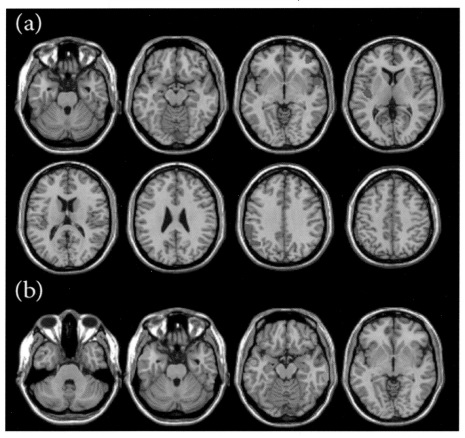

Fig. 12.6 (a) Increases in estimated regional cerebral blood flow for National Football League (NFL) players with cognitive impairment compared to controls (*p* < 0.001). (b) Decrease in estimated regional cerebral blood flow for NFL players with cognitive impairment compared to controls (*p* < 0.001).

Source: Hart et al., 2013 [97]; reproduced with permission from the American Medical Association

Regions where repeated head impacts show susceptibility-weighted imaging (SWI) signal changes

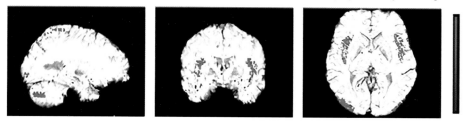

Fig. 12.7 Selected slices for subject 6 (a defensive back) with an overlay highlighting those voxels in which SWI signal decreases were observed at post, relative to pre. Highlighted voxels belong to several of the ten regions in this subject found to be statistically significantly decreased (Wilcoxon rank sum test at the $p_{uncorrected} <$ 0.00005 level, corresponding to $p_{Bonferroni} < 0.05$), with the saturation of the color reflecting the change measure in the given voxel.

Source: Slobounov et al., 2017 [117]; reproduced with permission from Elsevier

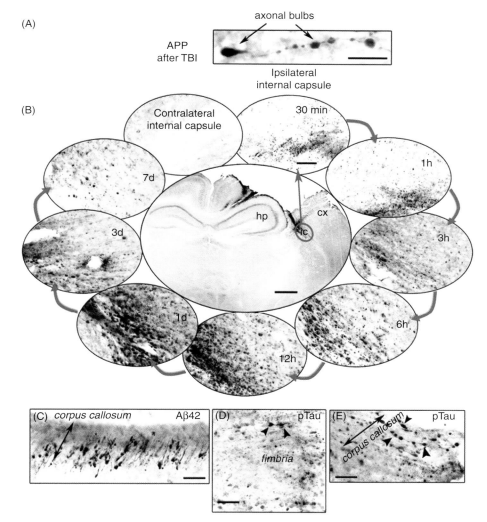

Fig. 13.1. Acute polypathology after experimental traumatic brain injury (TBI) in Alzheimer's disease (AD) transgenic mice. 3xTg-AD mice received a unilateral controlled cortical impact injury. (A) Axon injury after TBI is characterized by amyloid precursor protein (APP)-positive axonal bulbs. This abnormal APP staining after TBI reflects damage to the microtubule network and accumulation of proteins trafficked by axonal transport. (B) The timecourse of axonal APP accumulation occurring in the internal capsule of C57/Bl6 mice after cortical impact. APP accumulation can be seen within 30 min of TBI, and is still visible 7 days post injury. (C) Aβ42-positive staining occurs in the white-matter tracts of 3xTg-AD mice 24 h after TBI. (D and E) Intra-axonal accumulation of AT8-positive phosphorylated tau (pTau) occurs in the fimbria and corpus callosum of 3xTg mice 24 h post injury. Scale bar for A, C, D, E = 20 μm, and for B = 500 μm (central image) and 50 μm (surrounding images). cx: cortex; hp: hippocampus; ic: internal capsule.

Companion axial images from a patient illustrate the four types of magnetic resonance imaging (MRI) commonly used for clinical neuroimaging of traumatic brain injury

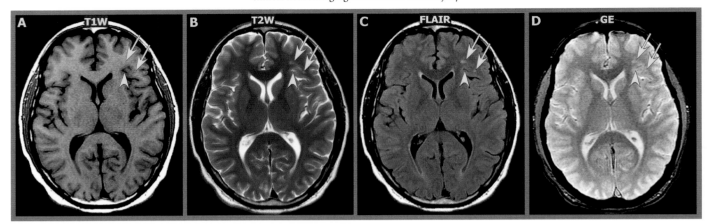

Fig. 16.1 (A) T1-weighted (T1W) MRI provides good delineation of anatomy, but not of most types of pathology. (B) T2-weighted (T2W) MRI is very sensitive to many types of pathology, which can be identified by their high signal intensity compared to surrounding brain. (C) Fluid-attenuated inversion recovery (FLAIR) MRI, a T2W image in which the signal of CSF is nulled, provides much better visualization of pathology in the vicinity of cerebrospinal fluid. (D) Gradient echo (GE) MRI is sensitive to presence of anything that changes the magnetic susceptibility of tissue, and may allow detection of small hemorrhagic lesions that are not visible on T2W or FLAIR MRI. In this set of example images there are multiple areas of diffuse axonal injury. The locations of two are marked with arrows and a nearby cerebrospinal fluid-containing space is marked with an arrowhead. Note that the cerebrospinal fluid-containing space that might be mistaken for an area of diffuse axonal injury in the T2W image (B) is easily distinguished on the FLAIR image (C).

Source: used with permission of the Mid Atlantic Mental Illness Research, Education and Clinical Center

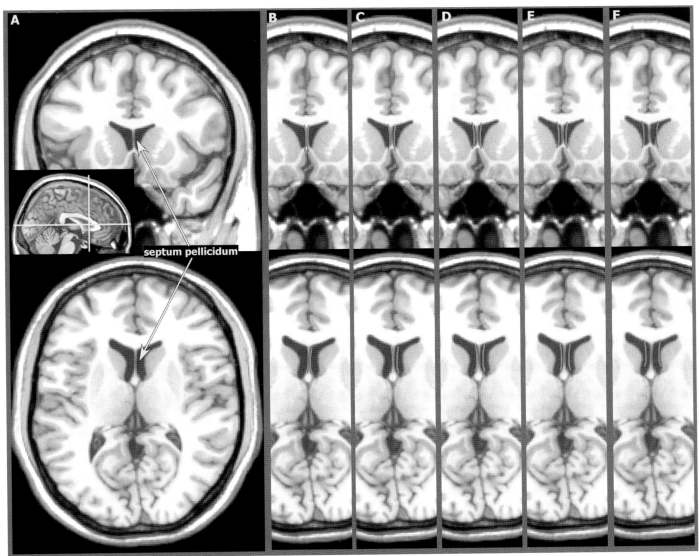

septum pellicidum

Fig. 16.2 The two bodies of the lateral ventricle are separated by a paired set of clear (pellucid) membranes, the septa pellucida [23]. (A) In most individuals the two membranes fuse during development to form the septum pellucidum. A separation between the two septa pellucida (red lines) forms the cavum (cavity) septi pellucidi. A simple visual grading system categorizes cavum septi pellucidi as: (B) absent, (C) questionable, (D) mild, (E) moderate, or (F) severe [16, 24].

Source: used with permission of the Mid Atlantic Mental Illness Research, Education and Clinical Center

Linear measures of the lateral ventricles have been shown to correlate well with volumetric measures of atrophy in studies of patients with multiple sclerosis [27, 28]

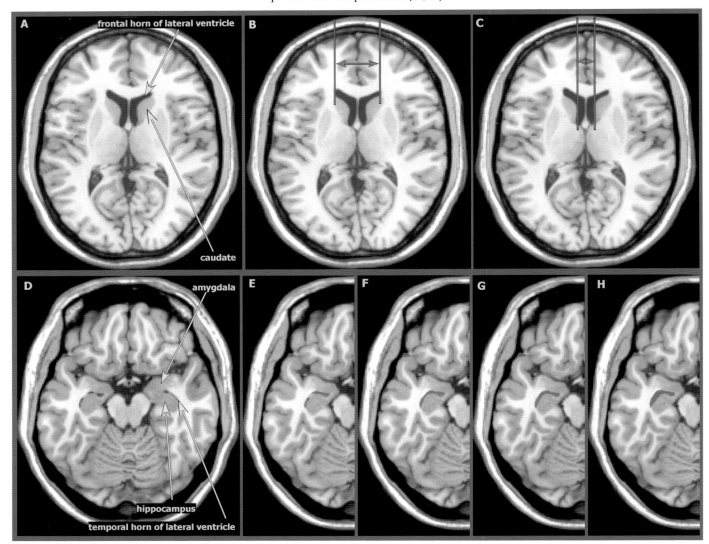

Fig. 16.3 (A) The location of the frontal horns of the lateral ventricle and the adjacent head of caudate is indicated on an axial magnetic resonance imaging (MRI). Both the width of the frontal horns (B, red arrows) and the distance between the caudate heads (C, red arrows) correlated well with volumetric measures. (D) The locations of important structures in the medial temporal lobe are indicated on an axial MRI. A simple visual grading system for assessing medial temporal atrophy categorizes hippocampal atrophy by the size of the temporal horn (red area) adjacent to the hippocampus: (E) absent, (F) mild, (G) moderate, or (H) severe [16].

Source: used with permission of the Mid Atlantic Mental Illness Research, Education and Clinical Center

Current resolution of magnetic resonance imaging (MRI)

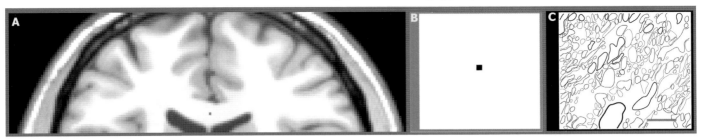

Fig. 16.4 While MRI is the best method currently available for identifying structural changes in the brain, it is important to understand the resolution limitations. Each image is made up of many small cubes (voxels) that are seldom less than 1 mm on a side. (A) A single voxel in the corpus callosum is colored red on MRI. The signal intensity of each voxel is the average of the signals from all the tissue types within the cube. (B) The single voxel in (A) is expanded to illustrate the averaging of signal. Although 1 mm seems like a tiny distance, it is very large compared to the size of cellular structures within the brain. A voxel in a white-matter area such as the corpus callosum will contain many thousands of axons. (C) A small section (black square) of the voxel in B is expanded to show the actual complexity of the tissue (red scale bar = 10 μm). The illustration in (C) is a simplification of an electron microscopy image. In order to be identified by visual inspection, an area of brain injury must be large enough to affect the signal intensity of several contiguous voxels.

Source: used with permission of the Mid Atlantic Mental Illness Research, Education and Clinical Center

Youth football players with no symptoms or signs of concussion after head impact nonetheless exhibit cognitive impairment and functional brain change

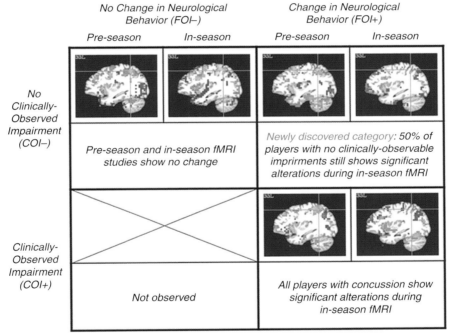

Fig. 18.1 Summary of observed player categories, with representative functional magnetic resonance imaging (fMRI) observations. Categories are based on both clinical observation by the team physician of impairment associated with concussion (clinically observed impairment: COI+ or COI–), and the presence or absence of significant neurocognitive impairment via Immediate Post-Concussion Assessment and Cognitive Testing (ImPACT) (functionally observed impairment; FOI+ or FOI–). fMRI activations are depicted for all players using a sagittal slice through the left inferior parietal lobule, to illustrate the presence of many changes, relative to pre-season assessment, for FOI+ players. As expected, all (3/3) players who were diagnosed by the team physician as having experienced a concussion (COI+) were also found to exhibit significantly reduced ImPACT scores (FOI+), and are categorized as COI+ /FOI+(top left). Half (4/8) of players brought in for assessment ostensibly for control purposes (i.e., presenting with no clinically observable impairments, COI–) were found to be neurocognitively consistent with pre-season assessment (FOI–), and are categorized as COI– /FOI– (top right). The other half (4/8) of the intended control group, studied in the absence of diagnosed concussion (COI–), were found to exhibit significantly impaired ImPACT performance (FOI+), and are categorized as COI–/FOI+. This group represents a newly observed category of possible neurological injury (bottom left). No players who were diagnosed with a concussion (COI+) were found to exhibit ImPACT scores consistent with pre-season assessments (FOI–).

Source: Talavage et al., 2014 [2]. Reproduced with permission from Mary Ann Liebert, Inc.

"Mild traumatic brain injury" ("mTBI") is associated with multi-focal hypoactivation on functional magnetic resonance imaging (fMRI) of auditory orienting in both adults and children

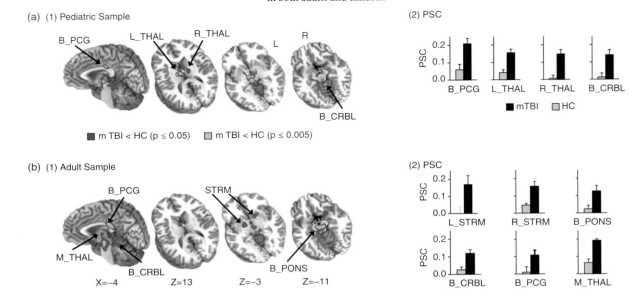

Fig. 22.1 Regions of hypoactivation during an auditory orienting task across independent samples of pediatric and adult mTBI patients relative to age- and education-matched healthy controls (HC). (A.1) Regions showing significantly reduced activity for pediatric mTBI patients, with the magnitude of *p*-values denoted by either blue or cyan coloring. Locations of the sagittal (X) and axial (Z) slices are given according to the Talairach atlas (L: left; R: right) and are identical across both pediatric and adult samples. (A.2) Percent signal change (PSC) data for selected regions for both patient (black bars) and control (gray bars) groups. Decreased activation for pediatric mTBI patients was observed within bilateral posterior cingulate gyrus (B_PCG), left and right thalamus (L_THAL, R_THAL) extending into the basal ganglia, and bilateral cerebellum (B_CRBL). Data from adult mTBI patients and matched HC are presented in an identical scheme in B.1 and B.2. Clusters of decreased activation for the adult mTBI sample included the posterior cingulate gyrus (PCG), right and left striatum (STRM), pons and midbrain nuclei (PONS), cerebellum (CRBL), and thalamus (THAL). Error bars correspond to the standard error of mean.

Source: Yang et al., 2012 [47]. Reproduced with permission from Mary Ann Liebert, Inc.

Deactivation within default-mode network and decreased cortical activation in "mild traumatic brain injury" ("mTBI") patients during Stroop

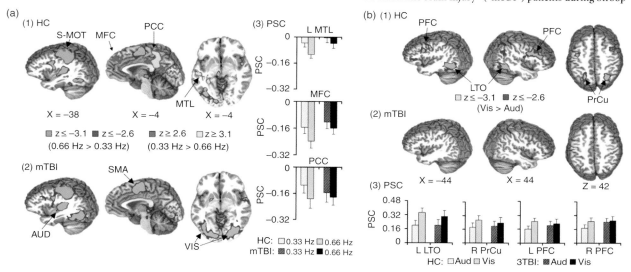

Fig. 22.2 Regions showing differential within-group activation between low- (0.33 Hz) and high- (0.66 Hz) frequency trials and between attend-visual (VIS) and attend-auditory (AUD) conditions for healthy controls (HC: panels A.1 and B.1, respectively) and adult mTBI patients (panels A.2 and B.2, respectively). The overall task involved a multisensory Stroop task during which congruent and incongruent stimuli (auditory and visual numbers) were presented at low or high frequencies. The main effect of frequency (panels A.1 and A.2) indicated increased activation during high-frequency (blue/cyan coloring) trials for both groups within the bilateral primary and secondary auditory cortex (AUD), visual cortex (VIS), bilateral supplemental motor area (SMA), and bilateral sensorimotor cortex (S-MOT). In contrast, only HC demonstrated significantly greater deactivation within the default-mode network for high- compared to low-frequency (red/yellow coloring) trials. The regions included the left medial temporal lobes (L MTL), bilateral medial frontal cortex (MFC), and bilateral posterior cingulate gyrus (PCC), with percent signal change data (PSC) presented in panel A.3 (mTBI patients (black bars) and HC (gray bars) during low-(striped bars) and high- (solid bars) frequency trials). Importantly, PSC for regions of interest were determined solely based on the unique areas of deactivation from HC in statistical parametric maps (panel A.1 red/yellow regions). Increased activation for HC (panel B.1) but not mTBI patients (panel B.2) was observed in the bilateral prefrontal cortex (PFC), "what" (lateral temporal-occipital cortex; LTO) and "where" (precuneus/cuneus; PrCu) pathways during the VIS relative to AUD conditions. PSC values for selected regions are presented in panel B.3 for both mTBI (black bars) and HC (gray bars) during AUD (striped bars) and VIS (solid bars) conditions based on selected regions from panel B.1 (HC group only). The magnitudes of z-scores are color-coded for all comparisons across all maps, with the locations of sagittal (X) and axial (Z) slices provided according to the Talairach atlas. Error bars in panels A.3 and B.3 correspond to the standard error of the mean.

Source: Mayer et al., 2012 [48]. Reprinted by permission from Springer

Evidence that mental performance more quickly fatigues and requires greater expense of cerebral resources at ≥12 months post-concussion

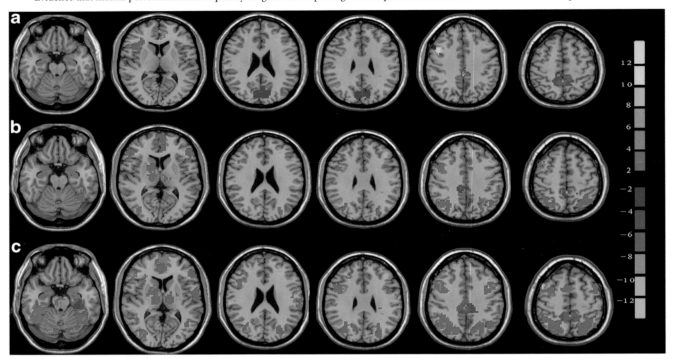

Fig. 24.2 Brain areas associated with the second 5-min psychomotor vigilance test (PVT) vs. the first 5-min PVT (a), comparison of the third 5-min PVT vs. the first 5-min PVT (b), and comparison of the last 5-min PVT vs. the first 5-min PVT (c) for mild traumatic brain injury patients in the chronic phase.

Deployment Stress and Concussive Brain Injury: Diagnostic Challenges in Polytrauma Care

Colleen E. Jackson, Rebecca L. Wilken, and Jennifer J. Vasterling

Introduction

Over 2.6 million members of the U.S. military have been deployed to Iraq and/or Afghanistan in support of Operations Enduring Freedom (OEF), Iraqi Freedom (OIF), and New Dawn (OND) [1]. Compared with prior military conflicts, more deployed military personnel are surviving now due to advanced protective gear and medical treatment. However, those surviving battlefield injuries frequently return with multiple significant physical and, in some cases, psychological injuries [2]. Injuries sustained from encounters with improvised explosive devices have been particularly common and may include traumatic brain injury (TBI), orthopedic injury, sensory impairment, and stress-related mental disorders, among other injury types.

Often labeled a "signature" injury of the wars in Iraq and Afghanistan [3], an estimated 12–20% of OEF/OIF veterans have sustained a TBI [2, 4–6]. Just as in the civilian population, the overwhelming majority of those TBIs are typical concussive brain injuries (CBIs), meaning TBI without prolonged coma, brain penetration, or damage due to mass effects [7]. In addition to improvised explosive devices, other deployment-related sources of CBI include, but are not limited to, blasts related to rocket-propelled grenades, motor vehicle accidents, falls, and other accidents. The U.S. Veterans Health

Administration defines polytrauma as "two or more injuries to physical regions or organ systems, one of which may be life threatening, resulting in physical, cognitive, psychological, or psychosocial impairments and functional disability" [8]; however, because of the frequency of concussion among returning veterans, the common usage of the term often implies that one of the multiple injuries involves CBI [9, 10].

Due to the psychologically traumatic nature of many warzone events, including those leading to CBI, post-traumatic stress disorder (PTSD) has likewise been labeled a signature injury of OEF/OIF [11] and occurs in 5–20% of returning veterans, with prevalence estimates varying according to sample attributes (e.g., the entire deployed population versus operational infantry units deployment location, when the sample was assessed within the continuing OEF/OIF engagements) and assessment methodology [12, 13]. Rates of PTSD increase in the context of military CBI. One review reported PTSD prevalence to range from 33% to 39% among U.S. warzone returnees with "probable TBI" [14]. Because the largely overlapping presentation of PTSD and persistent post-concussive symptoms (PPCS) following some CBIs often presents a particular diagnostic quandary, the co-morbidity of CBI and PTSD has received particular attention in polytrauma contexts and will be a focus of this chapter.

The chapter begins with a brief historical overview of post-deployment multi-symptom disorders, followed by descriptions of common psychological and physical co-morbidities accompanying deployment-related polytrauma. The chapter next addresses challenges associated with the diagnosis of possible TBI and psychological trauma in the context of polytrauma, and concludes by providing potential approaches to addressing these challenges.

Deployment-Related Polytraumatic Health Concerns: A Historical Perspective

Multi-symptom deployment-related health concerns and the challenges of determining their etiology within a context of polytraumatic injury are not unique to the current military operations in Iraq and Afghanistan. Military reports from the American Civil War through the Gulf War indicate that military service members commonly described post-deployment symptoms, such as persistent headache, amnesia, poor concentration, impaired sleep, and mood problems [15]. Potential

Table 20.1 Abbreviations commonly employed in the discussion of concussive brain injury (CBI) in the military context

Abbreviation	Full text description
CAPS	Clinician-Administered PTSD Scale
DoD	Department of Defense
DSM-5	*Diagnostic and Statistical Manual of Mental Disorders*, 5th Edition
LOC	loss of consciousness
OEF	Operation Enduring Freedom
OIF	Operation Iraqi Freedom
OND	Operation New Dawn
(P)PCS	(persistent) post-concussive symptoms
PTA	post-traumatic amnesia
PTSD	post-traumatic stress disorder
TBI	traumatic brain injury
VA	Department of Veterans Affairs

etiologies were hypothesized at various points in history to include the effects of training and faulty equipment, bacterial infection, microscopic brain hemorrhage, and "psychic exhaustion." Such etiologic considerations were arguably influenced by the cultural forces behind physicians' and patients' views of the presenting symptoms and possible medical explanations for such symptoms [15].

During World War I, there was a notable lack of clarity regarding the etiology of post-deployment non-specific symptoms, evident in the variable labeling of these symptoms [16]. "Shell shock" most commonly reflected the attribution of non-specific symptoms to microscopic brain lesions as a result of compression and decompression associated with proximity to an explosion [17] or, more generally, changes to the brain or meninges [16]. However, the terms "shell shock," "war neurosis," and "war neurasthenia" were also used to capture the experience of psychological trauma by combat veterans [16, 18], creating etiological ambiguity for non-specific symptoms.

Troops returning from World War II and the Korean War reported similar symptoms, including neuropsychiatric symptoms, sleep disturbance, substance abuse, and suicide [19]. The presumed etiology of such symptoms was both somatic and psychological in nature, with terms such as "post-concussion syndrome" and "post-concussion neurosis" used to describe similar sets of symptoms [16, 18]. Service members returning from the 1991 Gulf War likewise reported multi-symptom complaints, sometimes labeled "Gulf War syndrome," with many of these individuals reporting high rates of fatigue, changes in mood and cognition, and musculoskeletal pain [20]. There remains ongoing debate about the relative contributions of biological (e.g., toxin exposure) and physical environmental exposures (e.g., oil fires) versus psychological stress on the expression of these symptoms among Gulf War veterans.

Etiological Considerations in Contemporary Polytrauma Contexts

As in previous wars, health care providers caring for veterans of the wars in Afghanistan and Iraq are challenged with determining the etiology of a range of somatic and emotional health complaints, many of which are non-specific. The challenge in determining the etiology of non-specific symptoms becomes particularly difficult when symptoms endure beyond the acute phases of recovery. In patients with CBI, post-concussive symptoms (PCS), including headache, dizziness, balance problems, irritability, and memory problems, typically return to baseline in the days and weeks following the injury [21]. However, 10–20% of individuals with a history of CBI continue to report PCS following this time period [22, 23]. Dikmen and colleagues [24] reported even higher rates of PPCS at one year post injury, the prevalence ranging between 14% and 42% depending on the symptom.

Although there is evidence of lasting pathophysiological alterations (see Bigler [25] for review), including post-mortem evidence of brain changes [26] following CBI, psychological factors, such as PTSD, may also influence PPCS. The relative contributions of these factors to PCS and PPCS are unclear. For example, Brenner et al. [27] found that co-morbid PTSD and "mild TBI" were more strongly associated with experiencing PPCS compared with PTSD or mild TBI alone.

A more recent prospective study of civilian patients presenting for emergency care compared the three-month prevalence of post-concussive syndrome (according to four diagnostic taxonomies) and PTSD in 534 head-injured patients with 827 patients with injuries not involving the head [28]. The results suggested that so-called "mild TBI" was more closely related to subsequent development of PTSD than to the development of post-concussive syndrome, suggesting that PPCS in this sample was not strongly related to concussive brain change. Correspondence analyses examining symptom clustering and associations suggested that PPCS behaved similarly to PTSD hyperarousal symptoms, raising the possibility that they were etiologically related to PTSD and calling into question the utility of conceptualizing persistent non-specific symptoms following mild TBI as a diagnostic entity. It is important to note, however, that TBI classification was based on reported injury characteristics (e.g., loss of consciousness (LOC), altered mental status, post-traumatic amnesia (PTA), transient neurological signs), and it is unclear how integration of advanced imaging findings might have altered that classification had they been available.

The findings from Lagarde et al. [28] nonetheless underscore the importance of considering the evidence for shared biological pathways between PTSD hyperarousal symptoms and those brain areas most susceptible to mild TBI (e.g., dorsolateral prefrontal cortex, orbitofrontal cortex, temporal cortex, limbic system, cerebellum, ventral brainstem). The role of these brain regions in emotion, attention, executive functioning, memory, and physiologic arousal [29] suggests that damage to these areas may increase risk for, or exacerbate, hyperarousal symptoms. Early hyperarousal symptoms following trauma exposure have been found to predict subsequent development and exacerbation of PTSD symptoms [30], suggesting that individuals experiencing hyperarousal symptoms, regardless of their etiology, may be at increased risk for experiencing more severe PTSD symptoms.

Within this context of etiological complexity, clinicians often face pressure to attribute symptoms to single etiologies. However, the complicated clinical and functional presentation of patients with polytraumatic injuries may necessitate a more integrated perspective. Biopsychosocial conceptualizations of CBI that recognize pre-injury, biological, psychosocial, and contextual factors may prove informative in understanding the development, expression, and recovery of symptoms following polytraumatic injury. Iverson (personal communication, August 2014), for example, has proposed a comprehensive model, depicted in Figure 20.1.

It is also likely that certain etiologies drive symptoms to lesser or greater extents at different times in the course and recovery from CBI. For example, in a study of 123 mild TBI patients and 100 patients with non-TBI physical trauma recruited from a civilian emergency care setting, Ponsford et al. [31] found that mild TBI, pre-morbid psychiatric history, and

A biopsychosocial conceptualization of poor outcome after typical concussive brain injury (CBI)

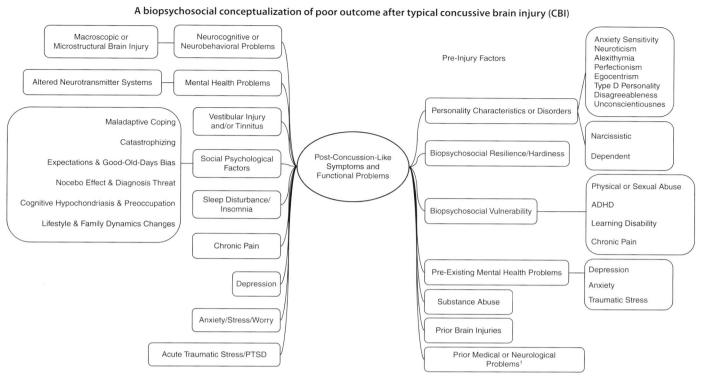

Fig. 20.1 Structural and/or microstructural damage to the brain is not necessary to cause or to maintain the symptoms comprising a post-concussion syndrome. Moreover, structural and/or microstructural damage, if present, is likely insufficient to causally maintain a *persistent* post-concussion syndrome. Assuming that a constellation of persistent symptoms are present (i.e., not exaggerated), there are many factors that could, singly or in combination, be the underlying cause of these symptoms.[1] Notably, patients with chronic pain frequently report a constellation of symptoms that are post-concussion-like, and patients with depression are virtually guaranteed to report symptoms that mimic a post-concussion syndrome (in the absence of a history of head trauma). ADHD: attention deficit-hyperactivity disorder; PTSD, post-traumatic stress disorder.

[1] For example, hypertension, heart disease, cardiac surgery, diabetes, thyroid problems, and small-vessel ischemic disease.

Source: Grant L. Iverson, used with permission

current anxiety predicted PCS one week post injury; however, pre-injury physical or psychiatric problems but not TBI most strongly predicted continuing symptoms three months later. Within the mild TBI group, early and concurrent anxiety, concurrent PTSD symptoms, and life stressors were also associated with enduring PCS. Finally, the relative contribution of etiological factors likely varies across patients.

The studies reviewed in this section examined civilian samples. To appreciate the full complexity of potential etiological contributions in patients with polytraumatic warzone injuries, it is first helpful to understand the scope of comorbidities in occurring survivors of CBI.

Comorbidities of Deployment-Related TBI

PTSD and Other Psychological Co-Morbidities

Deployment-related TBI, the vast majority of which are typical CBIs, is often associated with other psychological disorders, particularly PTSD (see O'Neill et al. [32] and Vasterling et al. [33] for reviews). As discussed within the Diagnostic Considerations and Challenges section below, these co-morbidities may not only lead to more complex clinical presentations, but they also overlap in symptoms (Table 20.2).

High rates of co-morbid CBI and PTSD are not surprising, given that deployment-related events leading to CBI (e.g., explosions, motor vehicle accidents) are often psychologically traumatic, occur within high-stress contexts (e.g., combat), and are associated with injuries significant enough to lead to functional losses (e.g., occupational interruption, loss of mobility) that may be sufficiently stressful such that they exacerbate trauma-related emotional symptoms.

Depression is also frequently associated with CBI and PTSD. Carlson et al. [34] found that OEF/OIF veterans with positive TBI screens were three times more likely to have co-morbid PTSD and two times more likely to have additional depression diagnoses. Maguen and colleagues [35] similarly found that veterans with positive TBI screens were approximately twice as likely to also screen positive for depression and PTSD. Finally, in comparing veterans returning from Iraq with "mild TBI," non-TBI injuries, and no injuries, Hoge et al. [5] found that mild TBI increased risk of PTSD and depression diagnoses, especially if the head injury was associated with LOC, as opposed to alteration of consciousness.

Rates of post-TBI substance use disorders are high among civilians and military personnel [36, 37]. Excessive use of substances may be particularly problematic in patients with polytraumatic injuries given the potential for: (1) an individual with a history of TBI to experience greater cognitive impairment while under the influence of substances [38]; and (2) increased risk for medical and psychiatric co-morbidity among substance users [36]. Carlson and colleagues [34] found that OEF/OIF veterans with positive TBI screens were twice as likely to have additional substance use diagnoses compared with veterans with negative TBI screens. In a sample of veterans seeking outpatient substance use treatment, 55% screened positive for TBI [39]. Of the 55% of the sample screening positive for TBI, 40% had been diagnosed with alcohol-related disorders, 20% with drug abuse/dependence, and 37% with both drug- and alcohol-related disorders. There is also evidence that veterans with a history of substance use disorder are more likely to be psychiatrically hospitalized after TBI compared to veterans without history of substance misuse [40].

Physical Co-Morbidities

In addition to psychiatric co-morbidities, physical injuries and disorders accompany deployment-related TBI. For example, sensory (e.g., hearing and vision) loss occurs commonly among returning veterans, especially veterans exposed to blast [41]. In addition to the over-1500 battle injury limb amputations among OEF/OIF/OND veterans [7], there are high rates of orthopedic injuries, open wounds, burns, and systemic (e.g., cardiovascular, pulmonary) disorders [42]. Such injuries are significant in that they not only contribute to possible physical limitations and functional impairment in and of themselves, but they may also result in chronic pain, which may further adversely affect functional abilities.

Pain is one of the most frequently reported problems in OEF/OIF veterans. Medical record review of 529 OEF/OIF veterans with a possible history of TBI presenting to a Department of Veterans Affairs (VA) polytrauma clinic revealed that over 80% reported pain, with 20–30% reporting severe or extreme pain interference in daily life [43]. In an examination of all returning veterans accessing inpatient or outpatient VA health care between 2009 and 2013, Cifu et al. [44] found that 246,883 (40.2%) veterans were diagnosed with head, neck, or back pain. Pain also constitutes a significant concern for veterans presenting with symptoms of PTSD. One study reported that, of the 85 veteran participants seeking treatment for PTSD, 66% also carried chronic pain diagnoses [45]. Another indicated that veterans with PTSD, with and without depression, were more likely to endorse back, muscle, or headache pain, compared to individuals without PTSD [46].

The triad of chronic pain, PPCS, and PTSD (the "polytrauma triad") following polytraumatic injuries occurs commonly among OEF/OIF veterans [44]. In a review of medical records from 340 VA polytrauma patients referred to a Level 2 polytrauma network site providing specialized, post-acute rehabilitation services, Lew et al. reported prevalence rates of 66.8%, 68.2%, and 81.5% of PPCS, PTSD, and chronic pain, respectively [47]. Moreover, 42.1% of the patient sample met diagnostic criteria for all three conditions simultaneously [47]. A separate study of 62 veterans also evaluated at a Level

2 polytrauma network site found that 97% of patients reported three or more PPCS, 97% reported chronic pain, and 71% met criteria for PTSD [48].

Given the high rates of reported pain in polytrauma settings, it is important to consider the role of pain on brain functioning. There is evidence that chronic pain is associated with gray-matter changes in the default-mode network, thalamus-basal ganglia circuit, and attention networks, with more specific gray-matter changes associated with particular pain syndromes [49]. White-matter connectivity changes in brain areas related to pain have also been identified in individuals experiencing chronic pain [50, 51]. These brain changes, in concert with prefrontal cortical and limbic dysfunction in CBI and PTSD, may lead to impairments in cognition, and particularly executive dysfunction, when the conditions are co-morbid, as is frequently the case in polytrauma contexts [52].

The extent of both physical and psychological co-morbidity associated with polytraumatic injuries can make establishing diagnoses in polytrauma contexts challenging. We discuss in the next section some of the considerations in establishing working diagnoses.

Diagnostic Considerations and Challenges: Concussive Brain Injury and Psychological Trauma

For both PCS/PPCS and PTSD, an initial exposure and enduring symptoms must be established. Because neither CBI nor psychological trauma exposure necessarily leads to lasting symptoms, a historical injury or exposure alone is not sufficient to make a determination of PCS/PPCS or PTSD, respectively. Current symptoms are likewise insufficient for a determination of these conditions unless they occur in the context of a brain injury or psychologically traumatic exposure. We discuss establishing historical injuries/exposures and assessing symptoms in the following sections.

Challenges in Establishing Injury Events and Psychological Trauma Exposure

Establishing that a history of an event leading to brain injury and/or psychological trauma occurred during deployment may prove particularly challenging in post-acute settings. Unlike civilian TBI, which may have been witnessed and for which care may have been sought immediately, in combat settings documentation may not be present and clinicians may be in the position of establishing and characterizing the event weeks or months after it occurred. The lack of documentation regarding loss or alteration of consciousness, as well as physical and/or cognitive symptoms immediately following the injury, forces clinicians to rely on the veteran's self-report of the event, which may be subject to variability over time [53]. Similarly, psychologically traumatic events have been found to be vulnerable to retrospective reporting biases [54], especially in the context of current PTSD symptoms [55, 56].

For TBI events, the extraordinary psychological stress of the injury context may make it difficult for warzone veterans to distinguish between alterations in consciousness related to a neural event versus altered mental states related to psychophysiological (e.g., rapid changes in autonomic response), sensory (e.g., confusion associated with extreme noise and/or vision changes), and emotional (e.g., changes in focus) responses associated with extreme stress. Many veterans also report experiencing multiple physically traumatic (e.g., blunt-force head trauma, blast exposure), as well as psychologically stressful, events during their deployment. It is not uncommon, under such circumstances, for the details of one specific event to become difficult to separate from other, similarly stressful events [9], which further complicates the process of obtaining a report of the target event.

Establishing the TBI Event

Recognizing that clinicians may need to rely on self-report in addition to drawing on available documentation, U.S. VA and Department of Defense (DoD) guidelines [57, 58] suggest that clinicians, to the extent possible, evaluate: (1) injury characteristics (e.g., direct or indirect blow to the head, location of impact); (2) circumstances surrounding the injury (e.g., cause of injury); and (3) the veteran's mental state (i.e., loss or alterations in consciousness) at the time of the injury and/or shortly after the injury (e.g., PTA, confusion).

The use of a structured or semi-structured interview (e.g., Ohio State University TBI Identification Method [59]; Boston Assessment of TBI-Lifetime [60]; Structured Interview for TBI Diagnosis [61]) may assist clinicians by providing a framework to ensure that details regarding the nature of the injury event (e.g., blunt-force trauma, blast) and changes in consciousness or cognition are fully assessed. Ulloa et al. [62] recommend that clinicians initially gather the veteran's spontaneous description of his/her injury event, followed by the use of open-ended questions to reduce the potential for bias, an approach adopted by the VA TBI Identification Clinical Interview [63].

Ulloa et al. [62] further underscore the importance of distinguishing between LOC and PTA, although this is a notably difficult challenge when assessing for TBI without the benefit of witness reports. However, clinicians should consider querying for this type of information, as the veteran may be able to report on details that he or she was told about his or her injury, including duration of alterations in consciousness or LOC, or behavior following the injury, by others who witnessed it or interacted with the individual shortly thereafter.

The clinical interview should also assess other factors that may affect injury type or severity following a concussion, including the individual's proximity to the blast, location of other objects (e.g., buildings, trucks) between the individual and the blast, existence of other objects that may have become airborne during the course of the event, and the use of a helmet and/or Kevlar body armor (or other types of protective clothing). Clinicians may additionally find it helpful to obtain information about the veteran's emotional and psychological functioning immediately before and after the injury

event, as well as query whether the individual experienced changes in sensory functioning, particularly hearing and vision impairment, following the injury event. This information can be considered when determining whether the veteran experienced alterations in mental state secondary to a physiological disruption of brain functioning, as opposed to a psychological response (e.g., fear, dissociation), or response secondary to sensory changes (e.g., loud noise, bright flash).

Establishing the Psychological Trauma

The diagnosis of PTSD requires the establishment of a psychological trauma exposure that involves personally experiencing, witnessing, or learning about actual or threatened death, serious injury, or sexual violence occurring to someone close to the patient, or repeated or extreme exposure to aversive details of traumatic events (i.e., *Diagnostic and Statistical Manual of Mental Disorders, 5th edition (DSM-5)* [64] PTSD Criterion A). Evaluation of sub-syndromal post-traumatic stress responses similarly requires the establishment of a trauma event. To establish the Criterion A event, Ulloa and colleagues [62] recommend gathering information from multiple sources (e.g., military, medical, or occupational records; collateral reports) when possible. Weathers et al. [65] note the importance of both identifying the type of trauma exposure (i.e., personally experiencing, witnessing, or learning about the event, repeated or extreme exposure to aversive details of the event and determining that the event involved life threat, serious injury, or sexual violence.

Use of semi-structured interviews such as the Evaluation of Lifetime Stressors [66] may be particularly helpful in obtaining a detailed narrative of possible psychological trauma experiences while reducing the chance of asking leading questions that may bias the veteran's responses. Self-report checklists, such as the Life Events Checklist [67] or Traumatic Life Events Questionnaire [68], may also be used to elicit one or more potential traumatic events, which may then be further clarified and evaluated as a potential Criterion A event prior to assessing PTSD symptoms.

Challenges in Assessing Current Symptoms and Functioning

Symptom and Measurement Overlap

There is extensive overlap between PCS/PPCS and symptoms frequently associated with, or inherent to, PTSD. As shown in Table 20.2, PCS/PPCS overlaps with PTSD symptoms, including sleep and cognitive difficulties, mood changes, anhedonia, and incomplete recall of the injury event (i.e., TBI-related PTA versus psychogenic amnesia for PTSD). Such symptom overlap complicates determining the etiology of specific symptoms, as well as the interpretation of self-report measures, given the potential for an individual to endorse the same symptom across self-report measures containing similar items. In addition, although this chapter focuses primarily on PPCS and PTSD as a common polytrauma dyad, symptom overlap exists between PPCS and other stress-related psychiatric conditions, including anxiety disorders and depression. Chronic pain, another common co-morbid condition within the polytrauma context, may likewise be associated with symptoms such as headaches, irritability, sleep disturbance, cognitive impairment, social isolation, and mood disturbance, which overlap with PPCS [69].

The problem of potential symptom overlap between enduring symptoms of CBI and post-traumatic stress sequelae is highlighted in the findings of Hoge et al. [5], which indicated that, in a sample of 2714 OIF veterans with a history of "mild TBI," headache was the only symptom complaint that remained significantly associated with LOC after controlling for PTSD and depression. However, such notable symptom overlap is not consistent across studies. For example, in a sample of over 1500 OEF/OIF veterans who completed post-deployment TBI, PTSD, and depression screens, Maguen et al. [35] identified several symptoms unique to TBI (dizziness/balance problems, headache, memory problems, light sensitivity) in addition to symptoms common to both TBI and PTSD (irritability) and to TBI and depression (sleep problems).

Table 20.2 Examples of overlap and non-overlap between potential post-concussive and post-traumatic stress disorder (PTSD) symptoms[a]

	Post-concussive symptoms	PTSD symptoms
Cognitive symptoms		
Amnesia for the event	X	X
Attention/memory difficulties	X	X
Physical symptoms		
Sleep problems	X	X
Fatigue	X	
Headache	X	
Vertigo/dizziness	X	
Sensitivity to light/sound	X	
Behavioral and emotional symptoms		
Anxiety/depressed mood	X	X
Irritability/anger/aggression	X	X
Apathy/anhedonia	X	X
Personality changes (e.g., social or sexual inappropriateness)	X	
Guilt/Blame		X
Recklessness		X
Hypervigilance		X
Other symptoms		
Re-experiencing (e.g., intrusive memories, nightmares, flashbacks, emotional/physiological reactions to reminders)		X
Avoidance of internal or external reminders		X

[a] List is not inclusive of all potential symptoms/associated symptoms.

Overlapping symptoms across disorders are mirrored in the item content of scales meant to measure PCS/PPCS (e.g., Neurobehavioral Symptom Inventory [70, 71]), PTSD symptoms (e.g., PTSD Checklist for DSM-5 [72]), and depression (e.g., Beck Depression Inventory-II [73]) symptoms. Thus, endorsement of shared symptoms may artificially inflate scores across all measures. For this reason, it is critical to consider not just the total score on a psychometric instrument but also whether symptoms unique to the construct being measured are endorsed. For example, on the PTSD Checklist, to establish linkage to PTSD, specific symptoms such as re-experiencing of the trauma and avoidance of reminders of the trauma should be endorsed in addition to less specific symptoms such sleep disturbance or concentration problems.

Contextual and Motivational Factors Influencing Symptom Report

A number of factors may contribute to a patient's symptom report, which ultimately affects diagnostic accuracy. Secondary gain factors, including receiving attention/positive reinforcement from family, physicians, or society for symptoms, use of symptoms to explain difficulties readjusting from deployment, avoidance of employment or duties due to symptomatology [74], and potential for financial gain through compensation processes may contribute to possible post-concussive, psychiatric, and/or other polytraumatic symptom enhancement [75, 76]. It should be noted, however, that symptom enhancement is not synonymous with symptom generation. Individuals demonstrating evidence of symptom enhancement during clinical interview or psychological assessment should not necessarily be presumed to be "malingering" but may instead over-emphasize symptoms as a reflection of acute distress, attempts to draw attention to valid concerns, or as a result of other psychological and contextual factors, highlighting the benefit of integrating symptom validity measures with the broader psychosocial context in which the patient is functioning.

Conversely, incentives and other factors may also lead to the minimization of symptoms. Milliken and colleagues [77] found that, compared to the initial Post-Deployment Health Assessment administered immediately after deployment, reported rates of depression and PTSD in service members returning from Iraq were 1.5–2 times greater on the Post-Deployment Health Re-Assessment (a DoD-administered mental health screening occurring three to six months after the initial Post-Deployment Health Assessment). Brenner and colleagues [9] hypothesized that this notable increase in symptom reporting may have been attributable to beliefs among service members that their symptoms would reduce in frequency and/or severity after they return home, the concern of service members that the leave normally provided following return from deployment would be delayed if they reported symptoms, and/or difficulty by service members recognizing symptoms until they returned to relatively less structured civilian or garrison contexts.

Concern about public stigma related to seeking mental health treatment may also affect symptom reporting and treatment utilization, particularly for military personnel experiencing symptoms of PTSD, depression, or other mental health disorders (see Vogt [78] for a review). Hoge and colleagues [79] found that veterans who met screening criteria for a mental health condition were approximately twice as likely to report feeling concerned about stigma and other barriers to mental health services compared to individuals who did not meet screening criteria. In fact, results from one study of OEF/OIF veterans revealed that fear of being labeled as having a mental disorder was concerning for 70% of participants [80].

Assessment Approaches: Post-Concussive Symptoms/Persistent Post-Concussive Symptoms

There is evidence that interviewing method (patient spontaneous report vs. clinician-suggested symptoms) may influence patient PCS report, such that higher rates of PCS are reported when clinicians provide patients with a proposed list of possible symptoms [81]. Therefore, it is often beneficial to first ask open-ended questions to obtain information about PCS/PPCS, functional abilities, emotional well-being, and attitudes about reported PCS/PPCS [57, 58]. However, after eliciting the veteran's description of his or her PCS/PPCS, clinicians may consider using structured or semi-structured diagnostic interviews such as the Boston Assessment of TBI – Lifetime [60] or Structured Interview for TBI Diagnosis [61] that include questions assessing PCS, or administering standard self-report PCS checklists (e.g., Neurobehavioral Symptom Inventory [70]) to assess for specific PCS/PPCS. Given the potential for response biases and memory failures [82–83, 84], psychometric self-report questionnaires are often considered to be best used for screening and not as stand-alone diagnostic assessments.

In relation specifically to neurocognitive impairment, neuropsychological assessment provides a performance-based index of cognitive functioning following a CBI that is less dependent on subjective self-appraisal. (See Chapter 9 of this volume, *Concussion and the 21st-Century Renaissance of Neuropsychology*, for a more complete review of the utility of neuropsychological assessment following CBI.) Neuropsychological evaluation is often useful to capture neurocognitive deficits that may be of significant functional relevance, inform treatment, educational, and vocational planning, contribute to diagnosis of moderate to severe TBI, and rule out other significant neural disorders that may require medical attention. However, due to the relatively mild level of enduring neurocognitive impairment typically observed after CBI, as well as the non-specificity of the neurocognitive performance deficits identified in individuals with polytraumatic conditions, neuropsychological testing is often less useful in differentiating post-acute TBI at the milder end of the severity spectrum from psychiatric co-morbidities and other common polytraumatic conditions such as chronic pain. For example, in a study that assessed 760 U.S. Army soldiers before and after deployment to Iraq, Vasterling et al. [85] found that, after controlling for pre-deployment cognitive performance, post-deployment cognitive performance was predicted by PTSD and depression but not by mild TBI incurred in the interim period.

Assessment Approaches: PTSD

Once a psychologically traumatic event has been identified, clinician-administered structured or semi-structured diagnostic interviews (e.g., Clinician-Administered PTSD Scale for DSM-5 (CAPS-5) [86]) are highly valuable in comprehensively assessing PTSD diagnostic symptom criteria, resulting in improved diagnostic accuracy compared to non-standardized interview approaches [87]. Structured or semi-structured diagnostic interviews allow clinicians to obtain more detailed information about symptoms (e.g., frequency, intensity) and make necessary linkages of symptoms to the trauma event. These types of diagnostic interview may also yield similarly valuable information about subsyndromal PTSD symptoms.

Like TBI symptom checklists, self-report questionnaires assessing PTSD symptoms are best used as screening tools or as components of more comprehensive evaluations. Using the *Diagnostic and Statistical Manual, IVth edition* [88] versions of PTSD assessment measures, one study comparing self-rated PTSD symptoms measured by the PTSD Checklist [89] with clinician diagnostic interview (CAPS [90]) in 97 Vietnam veterans before and after PTSD treatment found that the PTSD Checklist demonstrated strong overall diagnostic accuracy. However, this study also identified variable symptom diagnostic accuracy between the PTSD Checklist and CAPS, as well as reduced diagnostic accuracy as symptoms approached threshold criteria [91], providing support against the sole use of self-report questionnaires for diagnostic use, particularly within a polytrauma context, where high rates of non-specific symptom endorsement are common.

Self-report questionnaires are limited as stand-alone PTSD symptom assessments due to their fixed content and dependence on patients accurately interpreting, and responding to, items as they are worded [65]. However, self-report questionnaires also often serve as useful complements to structured diagnostic interviews, as they have the potential to provide further support for the presence or absence of a PTSD symptom, provide a continuous measure of symptom severity as perceived by the patient, and in some cases (e.g., Minnesota Multiphasic Personality Inventory-2-RF [92]) provide information about response validity, which may assist clinicians in assessing for over- or underreporting [93].

Summary and Conclusions

Polytraumatic injuries occur in many veterans returning from Iraq and Afghanistan. Veterans with polytraumatic injuries frequently report persisting physical, emotional, and behavioral symptoms that cannot be readily attributed to any single condition or disorder. The etiology of these non-specific symptoms, whether somatic or psychological, stands as a source of uncertainty for health care providers.

Given the high rates of symptom overlap between conditions such as PPCS and PTSD that are commonly co-morbid in individuals with polytraumatic injuries, attempting in post-acute settings to differentiate the origin of all symptoms can be useful in certain circumstances but will not uniformly yield clinically useful information. Making etiological attributions is most beneficial when the etiology influences treatment choices. For returning veterans who have a history of both mild TBI and psychological trauma, identifying symptoms specific to PTSD (e.g., re-experiencing symptoms) is important to initiate treatment of PTSD, for which several evidence-based interventions have proven to be effective (see Koucky et al. [94] for a review). It is likewise clinically useful to establish when there has been a CBI, especially soon after the event, given that psychoeducation around symptom course and recovery appears to be perhaps the most effective intervention in preventing PPCS following CBI [95].

Etiological attribution may be less valuable in relation to non-specific symptoms that can be treated independently of etiology. For example, treating attention and memory dysfunction or other cognitive impairments with cognitive rehabilitation strategies may prove helpful for a warzone veteran with cognitive complaints, regardless of whether his or her cognitive difficulties are due to concussion, PTSD, and/or pain (see Wortzel and Arciniegas [96] for a review of treatment of posttraumatic cognitive impairment). Similarly, treating sleep difficulties with empirically supported sleep interventions, such as cognitive behavioral therapy for insomnia [97], may improve the quantity and quality of the individual's sleep without the need for identifying the cause(s) of such sleep problems, such as psychiatric conditions (see Taylor and Pruiksma [98] for a review) or pain [99].

In conclusion, warzone participation may be associated with polytraumatic injuries resulting in an array of both specific and non-specific symptoms. The challenge of assessing PCS/PPCS following a warzone TBI, and in particular a typical CBI (comprising the vast majority of TBIs occurring in the milder part of the severity spectrum), is complex, especially in regard to determining the etiology of non-specific symptoms. In this chapter, we have conceptualized the clinical problem from a biopsychosocial perspective, recognizing the interplay between somatic, emotional, and contextual factors. We anticipate that clinicians may have greater confidence in differentiating potential etiologies as advanced imaging techniques become more refined and accessible.

For further discussion, see the pertinent chapters in this volume including:

- Chapter 6: *Neuroimaging Biomarkers for the Neuropsychological Investigation of Concussive Brain Injury (CBI) Outcome*
- Chapter 12: *Functional Neuroimaging Markers of Persistent Post-Concussive Brain Change*
- Chapter 15: *The Great CT Debate*
- Chapter 16: *Structural Neuroimaging of Persistent or Delayed-Onset Encephalopathy Following Repetitive Concussive Brain Injuries*
- Chapter 22: *Functional Neuroimaging of Concussion.*

The community of scholars and clinicians devoted to understanding and treating CBI is still anxiously awaiting sufficient progress in experimental neuroscience to begin clinical trials of treatments that will mitigate the specific underlying biological causes of persistent post-concussive impairments.

We are reassured, however, that treatable conditions such as PTSD can be identified even in the context of polytraumatic injury and that interventions are continually being developed and refined for treatment of non-specific symptoms, including neurocognitive impairment.

References

1. Department of Veterans Affairs. Analysis of VA health care utilization among Operation Enduring Freedom (OEF), Operation Iraqi Freedom (OIF), and Operation New Dawn (OND) veterans. 2014 [updated 2014 June 25; cited 2014 Sept 10]. Available at: www.publichealth.va.gov/epidemiology/reports/oefoifond/health-care-utilization/index.asp.
2. Tanielian TL, Jaycox LH. *Invisible wounds of war: Psychological and cognitive injuries, their consequences, and services to assist recovery.* Santa Monica, CA: RAND Corporation, 2008.
3. Hayward P. Traumatic brain injury: The signature of modern conflicts. *Lancet Neurol* 2008; 7: 200–201.
4. Hendricks AM, Amara J, Baker E, Charns MP, Gardner JA, Iverson KM, et al. Screening for mild traumatic brain injury in OEF-OIF deployed US military: An empirical assessment of VHA's experience. *Brain Inj* 2013; 27: 125–134.
5. Hoge CW, McGurk D, Thomas JL, Cox AL, Engel CC, Castro CA. Mild traumatic brain injury in U.S. soldiers returning from Iraq. *N Engl J Med* 2008; 358: 453–463.
6. Schneiderman AI, Braver ER, Kang HK. Understanding sequelae of injury mechanisms and mild traumatic brain injury incurred during the conflicts in Iraq and Afghanistan: Persistent postconcussive symptoms and posttraumatic stress disorder. *Am J Epidemiol* 2008; 167: 1446–1452.
7. Fischer H. A guide to U.S. military casualty statistics: Operation New Dawn, Operation Iraqi Freedom, and Operation Enduring Freedom. Congressional Research Service. [updated 2014 Feb 19; cited 2014 Sept 10]. 2014. Available at: www.fas.org/sgp/crs/natsec/RS22452.pdf.
8. Veterans Health Administration. Polytrauma/TBI system of care. 2014 [updated 2014 Aug 18; cited 2014 Sept 10]. Available at: www.polytrauma.va.gov/.
9. Brenner LA, Vanderploeg RD, Terrio H. Assessment and diagnosis of mild traumatic brain injury, posttraumatic stress disorder, and other polytrauma conditions: Burden of adversity hypothesis. *Rehabil Psychol* 2009; 54: 239–246.
10. Geiling J, Rosen JM, Edwards RD. Medical costs of war in 2035: Long-term care challenges for veterans of Iraq and Afghanistan. *Milit Med* 2012; 1777: 1235–1244.
11. Department of Defense Task Force on Mental Health. *An achievable vision: Report of the Department of Defense Task Force on Mental Health.* Falls Church: Defense Health Board, 2007.
12. Kok BC, Herrell RK, Thomas JL, Hoge CW. Posttraumatic stress disorder associated with combat service in Iraq or Afghanistan: Reconciling prevalence differences between studies. *J Nerv Ment Dis* 2013; 200: 444–450.
13. Ramchand R, Schell TL, Karney BR, Osilla KC, Burns RM, Caldarone LB. Disparate prevalence estimates of PTSD among service members who served in Iraq and Afghanistan: Possible explanations. *J Trauma Stress* 2010; 23: 59–68.
14. Carlson KF, Kehle SM, Meis LA, Greer N, MacDonald R, Rutks I, et al. Prevalence, assessment, and treatment of mild traumatic brain injury and posttraumatic stress disorder: A systematic review of the evidence. *J Head Trauma Rehabil* 2011; 26: 103–115.
15. Jones E, Wessely S. War syndromes: The impact of culture on medically unexplained symptoms. *Med Hist* 2005; 49: 55–78.

16. Crocq M-A, Crocq L. From shell shock and war neurosis to posttraumatic stress disorder: A history of psychotraumatology. *Dialogues Clin Neurosci* 2000; 2: 47–55.

17. Mott FW. Special discussion on shell shock without visible signs of injury. *Proc R Med* 1916; 9: i–xxiv.

18. Jones E, Fear NT, Wessely S. Shell shock and mild traumatic brain injury: A historical review. *Am J Psychiatry* 2007; 164: 1641–1645.

19. Shively SB, Perl DP. Traumatic brain injury, shell shock, and posttraumatic stress disorder in the military – Past, present, and future. *J Head Trauma Rehabil* 2012; 27: 234–239.

20. Thomas HV, Stimpson NJ, Weightman AL, Dunstan F, Lewis G. Systematic review of multi-symptom conditions in Gulf War veterans. *Psychol Med* 2006; 36: 735–747.

21. Bigler ED. Neuropsychology and clinical neuroscience of persistent post-concussion syndrome. *J Int Neuropsychol Soc* 2008; 14: 1–22.

22. Ruff RM, Camenzuli L, Mueller J. Miserable minority: emotional risk factors that influence the outcome of a mild traumatic brain injury. *Brain Inj* 1996; 10: 551–565.

23. Wood R. Understanding the 'miserable minority': A diathesis-stress paradigm for post-concussional syndrome. *Brain Inj* 2004; 18: 1135–1153.

24. Dikmen S, Machamer J, Fann JR, Temkin NR. Rates of symptom reporting following traumatic brain injury. *J Int Neuropsychol Soc* 2010; 16: 401–411.

25. Bigler ED. Neuroimaging biomarkers in mild traumatic brain injury (mild TBI). *Neuropsychol Rev* 2013; 23: 169–209.

26. Bigler ED. Neuropsychological results and neuropathological findings at autopsy in a case of mild traumatic brain injury. *J Int Neuropsychol Soc* 2004; 10: 794–806.

27. Brenner LA, Ivins B, Schwab K, Warden D, Nelson LA, Jaffee M, et al. Traumatic brain injury, posttraumatic stress disorder, and postconcussive symptom reporting among troops returning from Iraq. *J Head Trauma Rehabil* 2010; 25: 307–312.

28. Lagarde EM, Salmi LR, Holm LW, Contrand B, Masson F, Ribéreau-Gayon R, et al. Association of symptoms following mild traumatic brain injury with posttraumatic stress disorder vs postconcussion syndrome. *JAMA Psychiatry* 2014; 71: 1032–1040.

29. McAllister TW. Neurobiological consequences of traumatic brain injury. *Dialogues Clin Neurosci* 2011; 13: 287–300.

30. Schell TL, Marshall GN, Jaycox LH. All symptoms are not created equal: The prominent role of hyperarousal in the natural course of posttraumatic psychological distress. *J Abnorm Psychol* 2004; 113: 189–197.

31. Ponsford J, Cameron P, Fitzgerald M, Grant M, Mikocka-Walus A, Schönberger M. Predictors of postconcussive symptoms 3 months after mild traumatic brain injury. *Neuropsychology* 2012; 26: 304–313.

32. O'Neil ME, Carlson KF, Storzbach D, Brenner LA, Freeman M, Quiñones A, et al. Complications of mild traumatic brain injury in veterans and military personnel: A systematic review. *J Int Neuropsychol Soc* 2014; 20: 1–13.

33. Vasterling JJ, Verfaellie M, Sullivan KD. Mild traumatic brain injury and posttraumatic stress disorder in returning veterans: Perspectives from cognitive neuroscience. *Clin Psychol Rev* 2009; 29: 674–684.

34. Carlson KF, Nelson D, Orazem RJ, Nugent S, Cifu DX, Sayer NA. Psychiatric diagnoses among Iraq and Afghanistan war veterans screened for deployment-related traumatic brain injury. *J Trauma Stress* 2010; 23: 17–24.

35. Maguen S, Lau KM, Madden E, Seal K. Relationship of screen-based symptoms for mild traumatic brain injury and mental health problems in Iraq and Afghanistan veterans: Distinct or overlapping symptoms? *J Rehabil Res Devel* 2012; 49: 1115–1126.

36. West SL. Substance use among persons with traumatic brain injury: A review. *Neuro Rehabil* 2011; 29: 1–8.

37. Sirratt D, Ozanian A, Traenkner B. Epidemiology and prevention of substance use disorders in the military. *Milit Med* 2012; 177: 21–28.

38. Halbauer JD, Ashford JW, Zeitzer JM, Adamson MM, Lew HL, Yesavage JA. Neuropsychiatric diagnosis and management of chronic sequelae of war-related mild to moderate traumatic brain injury. *J Rehabil Res Devel* 2009; 46: 757–796.

39. Olson-Madden JH, Brenner L, Harwood JEF, Emrick CD, Corrigan JD, Thompson C. Traumatic brain injury and psychiatric diagnoses in veterans seeking outpatient substance abuse treatment. *J Head Trauma Rehabil* 2010; 25: 470–479.

40. Brenner LA, Harwood JEF, Homaifar BY, Cawthra E, Waldman J, Adler LE. Psychiatric hospitalization and veterans with traumatic brain injury: A retrospective study. *J Head Trauma Rehabil* 2008; 23: 401–406.

41. Lew HL, Pogoda TK, Baker E, Stolzmann KL, Meterko M, Cifu DX, et al. Prevalence of dual sensory impairment and its association with traumatic brain injury and blast exposure in OEF/OIF veterans. *J Head Trauma Rehabil* 2011; 26: 489–496.

42. Sayer NA, Chiros CE, Sigford B, Scott S, Clothier B, Pickett T, et al. Characteristics and rehabilitation outcomes among patients with blast and other injuries sustained during the global war on terror. *Arch Phys Med Rehabil* 2008; 89: 163–170.

43. Romesser J, Booth J, Benge J, Pastorek N, Helmer D. Mild traumatic brain injury and pain in Operation Iraqi Freedom/Operation Enduring Freedom veterans. *J Rehabil Res Dev* 2012; 49: 1127–1136.

44. Cifu DX, Taylor BC, Carne WF, Bidelspach D, Sayer NA, Scholten J, et al. Traumatic brain injury, posttraumatic stress disorder, and pain diagnoses in OIF/OEF/OND veterans. *J Rehabil Res Dev* 2013; 50: 1169–1176.

45. Shipherd JC, Keyes M, Jovanovic T, Ready DJ, Baltzell D, Worley V, et al. Veterans seeking treatment for posttraumatic stress disorder: What about comorbid chronic pain? *J Rehabil Res Dev* 2007; 44: 153–166.

46. Runnals JJ, Van Voorhees E, Robbins AT, Brancu M, Straits-Troster K, Beckham JC, et al. Self-reported pain complaints among Afghanistan/Iraq era men and women veterans with comorbid posttraumatic stress disorder and major depressive disorder. *Pain Med* 2013; 14: 1529–1533.

47. Lew HL, Otis JD, Tun C, Kerns RD, Clark ME, Cifu DX. Prevalence of chronic pain, posttraumatic stress disorder, and persistent postconcussive symptoms in OIF/OEF veterans: Polytrauma clinical triad. *J Rehabil Res Dev* 2009; 46: 697–702.

48. Lew HL, Poole JH, Vanderploeg RD, Goodrich GL, Dekelboum S, Guillory SB, et al. Program development and defining characteristics of returning military in a VA Polytrauma Network Site. *J Rehabil Res Dev* 2007; 44: 1027–1034.

49. Cauda F, Palermo S, Costa T, Torta R, Duca S, Vercelli U, et al. Gray matter alterations in chronic pain: A network-oriented meta-analytic approach. *Neuroimage Clin* 2014; 4: 676–685.

50. Lutz J, Jäger L, de Quervain D, Krauseneck T, Padberg F, Wichnalek M, et al. White and gray matter abnormalities in the brain of patients with fibromyalgia. *Arthritis Rheum* 2008; 58: 3960–3969.

51. Teepker M, Menzler K, Belke M, Heverhagen JT, Voelker M, Mylius V, et al. Diffusion tensor imaging in episodic cluster headache. *Headache* 2011; 52: 274–282.

52. Otis JD, Fortier CB, Keane TM. Chronic pain. In: Vasterling JJ, Bryant RA, Keane TM, editors. *PTSD and mild traumatic brain injury*. New York: Guilford Press, 2012, pp. 105–123.

53. Wessely S, Unwin C, Hotopf M, Hull L, Ismail K, Nicolaou V, et al. Stability of recall of military hazards over time: Evidence from the Persian Gulf War of 1991. *Br J Psychiatry* 2003; 183: 314–322.

54. Candel I, Merckelbach H. Peritraumatic dissociation as a predictor of post-traumatic stress disorder: A critical review. *Compr Psychiatry* 2004; 45: 44–50.

55. Schwartz ED, Kowalski JM, McNally RJ. Malignant memories: Post-traumatic changes in memory in adults after a school shooting. *J Trauma Stress* 1993; 6: 545–553.

56. Southwick SM, Morgan CA III, Nicolaou AL, Charney DS. Consistency of memory for combat-related traumatic events in veterans of Operation Desert Storm. *Am J Psychiatry* 1997; 154: 173–177.

57. Management of Concussion/Mild TBI Workgroup. VA/DoD clinical practice guideline for management of concussion/mild traumatic brain injury. *J Rehabil Res Dev* 2009; 46: CP1–CP58.

58. The Management of Concussion-mild Traumatic Brain Injury Working Group. VA/DoD clinical practice guideline for the management of concussion-mild traumatic brain injury. Version 2.0 – 2016 Available at: www.healthquality.va.gov/guidelines/Rehab/mtbi/mTBICPGFullCPG50821816.pdf.

59. Corrigan JD, Bogner JA. Initial reliability and validity of the OSU TBI identification method. *J Head Trauma Rehabil* 2007; 22: 318–329.

60. Fortier CB, Amick MM, Grande L, McGlynn S, Kenna A, Morra L, et al. The Boston Assessment of Traumatic Brain Injury – Lifetime (BAT-L) semistructured interview: Evidence of research utility and validity. *J Head Trauma Rehabil* 2013; 29: 89–98.

61. Donnelly KT, Donnelly JP, Dunnam M, Warner GC, Kittleson CJ, Constance JE, et al. Reliability, sensitivity, and specificity of the VA Traumatic Brain Injury Screening tool. *J Head Trauma Rehabil* 2011; 26: 439–453.

62. Ulloa EW, Marx BP, Vanderploeg RD, Vasterling JJ. Assessment. In: Vasterling JJ, Bryant RA, Keane TM, editors. *PTSD and mild traumatic brain injury*. New York: Guilford Press, 2012, pp. 149–173.

63. Vanderploeg RD, Groer S, Belanger HG. Initial developmental process of VA semistructured clinical interview for TBI identification. *J Rehabil Res Dev* 2012; 49: 545–556.

64. American Psychiatric Association. *Diagnostic and statistical manual of mental disorders*, 5th edition. Arlington, VA: American Psychiatric Publishing, 2013.

65. Weathers FW, Keane TM, Foa FB. Assessment and diagnosis of adults. In: Foa E, Friedman MJ, Cohen JA, editors. *Effective treatments for PTSD: Practice guidelines from the International Society for Traumatic Stress Studies*. New York: Guilford Press, 2009, pp. 23–61.

66. Krinsley KE. Psychometric review of The Evaluation of Lifetime Stressors Questionnaire and Interview. In: Stamm BH, editor. *Measurement of stress, trauma, and adaptation*. Luberville: Sidran Press, 1996.

67. Gray M, Litz B, Hsu J, Lombardo T. Psychometric properties of the Life Events Checklist. *Assessment* 2004; 11: 330–341.

68. Kubany E, Haynes S, Leisen M, Owens J, Kaplan A, Watson S, et al. Development and preliminary validation of a brief broad-spectrum measure of trauma exposure: The Traumatic Life Events Questionnaire. *Psychol Assess* 2000; 12: 210–224.

69. Otis JD, McGlinchey R, Vasterling JJ, Kerns RD. Complicating factors associated with mild traumatic brain injury: Impact on pain and posttraumatic stress disorder treatment. *J Clin Psychol Med Settings* 2011; 18: 145–154.

70. Cicerone KD, Kalmar K. Persistent post-concussion syndrome: The structure of subjective complaints after mild traumatic brain injury. *J Head Trauma Rehabil* 1995; 10: 1–17.

71. King PR, Donnelly KT, Donnelly JP, Dunnam M, Warner G, Kittleson CJ, et al. Psychometric study of the Neurobehavioral Symptom Inventory. *J Rehabil Res Dev* 2012; 49: 879–888.

72. Weathers FW, Litz BT, Keane TM, Palmieri PA, Marx BP, Schnurr PP. The PTSD Checklist for DSM-5 (PCL-5). 2013 [updated 2014 May 2, cited 2014 Sept 15]. Available at: www.ptsd.va.gov.

73. Beck AT, Steer RA, Brown GK. *Manual for the Beck Depression Inventory-II*. San Antonio, TX: Psychological Corporation, 1996.

74. Howe LLS. Giving context to post-deployment post-concussive-like symptoms: Blast-related potential mild traumatic brain injury and comorbidities. *Clin Neuropsychol* 2009; 23: 1315–1337.

75. Elhai JD, Sweet JJ, Guidotti Breting LM, Kaloupek D. Assessment in contexts that threaten response validity. In: Vasterling JJ, Bryant RA, Keane TM, editors. *PTSD and mild traumatic brain injury*. New York, Guilford Press, 2012, pp. 174–198.

76. Greiffenstein MF, Baker WJ. Validity testing in dually diagnosed post-traumatic stress disorder and mild closed head injury. *Clin Neuropsychol* 2008; 22: 565–582.

77. Milliken CS, Auchterlonie JL, Hoge CW. Longitudinal assessment of mental health problems among active and reserve component soldiers returning from the Iraq war. *JAMA* 2007; 298: 2141–2148.

78. Vogt D. Mental health-related beliefs as a barrier to service use for military personnel and veterans: a review. *Psychiatr Serv* 2011; 62: 135–142.

79. Hoge CW, Castro CA, Messer SC, McGurk D, Cotting DI, Koffman RL. Combat duty in Iraq and Afghanistan, mental health problems, and barriers to care. *N Engl J Med* 2004; 351: 13–22.

80. Stecker T, Fortney JC, Hamilton F, Ajzen I. An assessment of beliefs about mental health care among veterans who served in Iraq. *Psychiatr Serv* 2007; 58: 1358–1361.

81. Villemure R, Nolin P, LeSage N. Self-reported symptoms during post-mild traumatic brain injury in acute phase: Influence of interviewing method. *Brain Inj* 2011; 25: 53–64.

82. Freeman T, Powell M, Kimbrell T. Measuring symptom exaggeration in veterans with chronic posttraumatic stress disorder. *Psychiatry Res* 2008; 158: 374–380.

83. Iverson GL, Brooks BL, Ashton VL, Lange RT. Interview versus questionnaire symptom reporting in people with the postconcussion syndrome. *J Head Trauma Rehabil* 2010; 25: 23–30.

84. Lange RT, Iverson GL, Rose A. Post-concussion symptom reporting and the good-old days bias following mild traumatic brain injury. *Arch Clin Neuropsychol* 2010; 25: 442–450.

85. Vasterling JJ, Brailey K, Proctor SP, Kane R, Heeren T, Franz M. Neuropsychological outcomes of mild traumatic brain injury, post-traumatic stress disorder and depression in Iraq-deployed US Army soldiers. *Br J Psychiatry* 2012; 201: 186–192.

86. Weathers FW, Blake DD, Schnurr PP, Kaloupek DG, Marx BP, Keane TM. The Clinician-Administered PTSD Scale for DSM-5 (CAPS-5). 2013 [updated 2014 May 2, cited 2014 Sept 15]. Available at: www.ptsd.va.gov.

87. Reardon AF, Brief DJ, Miller MW, Keane TM. Assessment of PTSD and its comorbidities in Adults. In: Friedman MJ, Keane TM, Resick PA, editors. *Handbook of PTSD: Science and practice*. New York: Guilford Press, 2014, pp. 369–390.

88. American Psychiatric Association. *Diagnostic and statistical manual of mental disorders*, 4th edition. Washington, DC: American Psychiatric Association, 1994.

89. Weathers F, Litz B, Herman D, Huska J, Keane T. The PTSD Checklist (PCL): Reliability, validity, and diagnostic utility. Paper presented at: The Annual Convention of the International Society for Traumatic Stress Studies; 1993; San Antonio, TX.

90. Blake DD, Weathers F, Nagy LM, Kaloupek DG, Klauminzer G, Charney DS, et al. A clinician rating scale for assessing current and lifetime PTSD: The CAPS-1. *Behav Ther* 1990; 13: 187–188.

91. Forbes D, Creamer M, Biddle D. The validity of the PTSD checklist as a measure of symptomatic change in combat-related PTSD. *Behav Res Ther* 2001; 39: 977–986.

92. Goodwin BE, Sellbom M, Arbisi PA. Posttraumatic stress disorder in veterans: The utility of the MMPI-2-RF validity scales in detecting overreported symptoms. *Psychol Assess* 2013; 25: 671–678.

93. Castro F, Hayes JP, Keane TM. Issues in the assessment of PTSD. In: Moor BA, Penk WE, editors. *Treating PTSD in military personnel: A clinical handbook.* New York: Guilford Press, 2011, pp. 23–41.

94. Koucky EM, Dickstein BD, Chard KM. Cognitive behavioral treatments for posttraumatic stress disorder: Empirical foundation and new directions. *CNS Spectr* 2013; 18: 73–81.

95. Ponsford J. Treatment of mild traumatic brain injury. In: Vasterling JJ, Bryant RA, Keane TM, editors. *PTSD and mild traumatic brain injury.* New York: Guilford Press, 2012, pp. 199–218.

96. Wortzel HS, Arciniegas DB. Treatment of post-traumatic cognitive impairments. *Curr Treat Options Neurol* 2012; 14: 493–508.

97. Mitchell MD, Gehrman P, Perlis M, Umscheid CA. Comparative effectiveness of cognitive behavioral therapy for insomnia: A systematic review. *BMC Fam Pract* 2012; 13: 40–50.

98. Taylor DJ, Pruiksma KE. Cognitive and behavioural therapy for insomnia (CBT-I) in psychiatric populations: A systematic review. *Int Rev Psychiatry* 2014; 26: 205–213.

99. Jungquist CR, O'Brien C, Matteson-Rusby S, Smith MT, Pigeon WR, Xia Y, et al. The efficacy of cognitive-behavioral therapy for insomnia in patients with chronic pain. *Sleep Med* 2010; 11: 302–309.

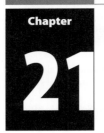

How Should One Measure "Outcome" of Concussion?: An Introduction to the Common Data Elements for Mild TBI and Concussion

Elisabeth A. Wilde and Ashley L. Ware

History and Goals of the Common Data Elements Initiative in Traumatic Brain Injury

The Common Data Elements (CDEs) project was established by the National Institute of Neurological Disorders and Stroke (NINDS) of the National Institutes of Health (NIH) in 2005 to standardize definitions, variables, and protocols in neurological diseases. The CDEs project was intended to promote consistency in data collection and to facilitate data exchange within and between specific disease entities [1]. The project was also intended to hasten data collection and increase comparability of research samples by standardizing data structure. Such efforts could then facilitate data aggregation and formal meta-analyses. Additionally, the CDEs could provide guidance for new investigators (or investigators new to specific areas) regarding the importance of specific measurement domains and the most cost-effective ways of assessing them.

With regard to traumatic brain injury (TBI) specifically, the CDEs initiative began in 2008 in response to recommendations from the October 2007 Workshop for the Classification of TBI for Targeted Therapies co-sponsored by the NINDS, the National Institute on Disability and Rehabilitation Research (NIDRR), the Defense and Veterans Brain Injury Center (DVBIC), and the Brain Injury Association of America [2]. Members of this workshop concluded that a set of CDEs should be developed and instituted in collaboration with the NINDS CDEs initiative described above, and they also recommended that a new databank should be created to enable and enhance data sharing and analysis [3].

The CDE effort for TBI was supported not only by the NINDS, but in collaboration with four other federal agencies with an interest in funding research in TBI: the Department of Veterans Affairs (VA), NIDRR) of the Department of Education, the Defense Centers of Excellence for Psychological Health and Traumatic Brain Injury (DCoE) of the Department of Defense (DoD) and DVBIC of the DoD. Working groups of expert panel members were formed to address four areas of data collection: (1) acute and demographic data; (2) biospecimens; (3) neuroimaging; and (4) outcome measurement. The original (Version 1.0) recommendations for each of these areas in TBI and psychological health were published in November

2010 in a special issue of the *Archives of Physical Medicine and Rehabilitation* [4–10].

Version 1.0 Outcome Measures

Specific to the selection of outcome measures, the outcome measurement expert panel considered the function, activity, and participation levels of the *International Classification of Functioning, Disability, and Health* as well as other outcome domains of importance to consumers, practitioners, and scientists in the field of TBI. The Workgroup considered outcome measures that would collectively cover the spectrum of both injury acuity (i.e., acute to chronic) and severity (i.e., mild to severe TBI). Initial outcome domains included: (1) global outcome; (2) recovery of consciousness; (3) neuropsychological impairment;(4) psychological status; (5) TBI-related symptoms; (6) performance of activities related to behavioral, cognitive, and physical demands; (7) social role participation; (8) perceived health-related quality of life; and (9) health economic measures. Additionally, an area of "patient-reported outcomes," which included several outcome measures under development as part the NIH Blueprint for Neuroscience Research, was identified as a promising multidimensional domain for examining comparisons across studies.

Outcome measures within each of the above domains were selected according to criteria, including: (1) widespread application in TBI research and clinical communities with respect to diagnosis, prediction, or outcome measurement, or treatment effectiveness; (2) evidence of sound psychometric characteristics, including (as applicable) construct validity, internal consistency, sensitivity to change, test–retest reliability, intra-/interrater agreement (such as subject/proxy and telephone/in-person administration); (3) well-established normative data; (4) applicability across a range of injury severity and functional levels; (5) availability in the public domain; (6) ease of administration; and (7) brevity. Other practical characteristics, such as cost, applicability for use in international, non-English-speaking, and different ethnic populations were also taken into account. Considerations emphasized measures of health-related quality of life, activity/participation and psychological function, and maximized flexibility of the administration format (e.g., whether a measure could be administered via telephone interview versus in-person administration only, self-report only versus administration via proxy-respondent as well). Finally, for neuropsychological measures, the existence of alternate forms (to mitigate potential impact of practice effects) was considered. Further information regarding the deliberation process and the psychometric characteristics of each of the measures can be found in Wilde et al.'s summary of the outcome recommendations [9].

Within each domain of outcomes, the Workgroup proposed, reviewed, discussed, and selected outcome measures for a tiered system of "core," "supplemental," and "emerging" variables. Core variables were defined as well-established measures covering outcome domains important to a broad range of studies within TBI. Primary emphasis was placed on selecting a single measure (or limited set of measures) that best represented each outcome domain. For the primary tier, or core measures, established use in individuals with TBI and favorable psychometric characteristics were considered the primary criteria in selection. Brevity and ease of administration also influenced the selection of core measures because the intent was to recommend measures that would be feasible to administer in a reasonable time (i.e., no longer than 90 min) by a range of investigators and staff with varying expertise. Availability of multiple, validated response formats (e.g., self- and other-proxy) was also considered given feasibility and/or reliability concerns for some individuals with TBI. Finally, applicability of each measure across a range of post-injury functional levels was deemed important since one of the primary objectives of the CDEs was to foster comparability of outcome measurement across different studies within the field of TBI [9].

The second tier included "supplemental" data elements, which denoted additional measures in each domain that could be considered for more in-depth outcome assessment within a certain domain or for patients at a specific functional level. For example, in studies in which neuropsychological outcome is of particular interest, investigators may draw on additional outcome measures from the supplemental list that target additional aspects of cognitive functioning not covered by the core measures (e.g., visual memory, verbal fluency, fine motor control). Finally, additional measures of psychological and/or family functioning or substance abuse may be of importance, depending on the study design, functional level, or target population [9].

The third tier of outcome recommendations included "emerging" measures for which more limited psychometric data were available, consensus had not been achieved, or where measured, were considered more exploratory or evolving, or which had not achieved widespread use in the field of TBI. Measures in this category were considered promising measures which, pending additional data, might eventually be added to the core or supplemental CDE lists [9].

Acknowledged Limitations

Several well-recognized limitations of the Version 1.0 recommendations were identified. With respect to outcome assessment, acknowledged gaps included the inadequate consideration of outcome measures that could be used in pediatric TBI populations and that many of the recommended outcome measures were not applicable to populations of patients with

so-called "mild TBI" (an ambiguous 20th-century terminology best replaced by the more clinically concrete phrase, *typical clinically attended concussive brain injury* (CBI), and particularly sports-related and military concussion [11].

Incorporation of Pediatric CDEs

The CDEs were modified to better incorporate assessment domains and measures more compatible with the needs of pediatric TBI research one year later [12–19]. Several domains were added to address concerns specific to pediatric populations, including academic achievement, daily life skills/adaptive functioning, family/environment, language and communication, social cognition, and social competence/role participation. Where possible, the Workgroup attempted to maintain consistency with the original recommendations, either by retaining Version 1.0 measures when the age range extended down to a child or adolescent age range or selecting measures that were most similar in content to those for adults.

Again, for the core measures, the Pediatric CDEs Working Group sought to select a single measure (or a limited set of measures) that best covered each domain. Brevity, ease of administration, and purchase cost influenced measure selection, with the intent to include measures that could feasibly be administered in a variety of settings and across a range of ages and post-injury functional levels. When possible, measures were identified that spanned a wide age range to avoid the need to change measures between childhood and adolescence. Also, a small subset of measures that could be used with infants and toddlers was included, given the unique developmental issues and the lack of suitability of the other measures for younger age ranges. Considerations further included the availability of tests in Spanish or other languages. Measures with established psychometric properties in pediatric populations with TBI were prioritized when available [18].

As before, supplemental and emerging measures were selected to include additional measures within each domain that could be utilized for more in-depth outcome assessment within a certain domain or for patients at a specific functional level. Other reasons for inclusion in this category included a requirement for specialized training, normative data limitations, cost, or the probability of ceiling effects in more chronic or less severe populations [18]. While the additional pediatric outcome measures addressed an important gap and represented an attempt to be comprehensive, the list of measures has also been criticized as being too lengthy.

Version 2.0 Outcome Measures

Following the incorporation of the revised pediatric elements, the TBI CDEs Workgroups were later restructured to further address differences in elements that were relevant within different patient populations and across the spectrum of acuity and severity. New Workgroups were established to better tailor the original recommendations for: (1) epidemiological studies; (2) acute hospitalization studies; (3) rehabilitation studies; and (4) mild TBI/concussion. The Workgroup's recommendations from these efforts were published in Version 2.0 of the TBI

CDEs in 2013 [11] and are publically available at www.commondataelements.ninds.nih.gov/TBI.aspx#tab=Data_Standards.

The most significant changes between Version 1.0 and Version 2.0 of the TBI CDEs were: (1) a marked decrease in the number of core CDEs; (2) an expansion of the *total number* of CDEs to include more items relevant to milder injuries and more chronic phases of TBI; (3) reorganization of the respective categories from "core," "supplemental," and "emerging" to "core," "basic," and "supplemental" (which entailed the addition of a second tier ("basic") for items highly relevant to specific types of studies (e.g., mild TBI) but not to all studies within TBI, and dropping the "emerging" tier); and (4) change in the name of the project to the *International TBI Common Data Elements Project*. Additional minor changes included alignment of demographic data elements with those endorsed by the National Library of Medicine (to increase their generalizability across other disease areas), and separation of the lists of other data elements from outcome measures *per se* [11].

Although many TBI CDEs outcome measures from Version 1.0 were retained, several were added to Version 2.0 to specifically address common research questions specific to mild TBI and concussion. For example, the Workgroup added symptom validity testing, computerized batteries, and telephone follow-up as these were considered important in many studies in this area. As the focus of the chapter is outcome measurement in mild TBI and concussion, those elements will subsequently be elaborated upon.

Mild TBI and Concussion Outcome CDEs

The Workgroup for mild TBI/concussion studies addressed data elements pertinent to the milder end of the severity spectrum. Specifically, considerations emphasized those who either required no hospitalization or acute medical care, only a brief visit to the emergency department or physician without hospital admission, or only a brief hospitalization related to the TBI. The Workgroup considered both acute and chronic phases of mild TBI and concussion. Through additional supplemental measure recommendations, attempts were made to incorporate elements that would be applicable not only in studies of hospital and clinic-based community samples with mild TBI and concussion, but also in studies of sports-related concussion and head injury within military populations [11]. Current measures for mild TBI and concussion studies are summarized below.

Core Measures

Core measures continue to be defined as "a very small set of items relevant to all TBI clinical studies" (across the spectrum of severity and acuity) [11]. The only core TBI CDEs outcome measure for adults is the Glasgow Outcome Scale – Extended (GOS-E). Interestingly, the Pediatric GOS-E was not recommended as a core data element for pediatric TBI, reflecting differences in expert opinion regarding its utility in studying milder forms of TBI in youth, especially in more chronic post-injury intervals.

Basic Measures

Basic measures are defined as "a small set of data elements, beyond the Core, recommended for inclusion in specific types of studies" [11] This category includes CDEs for outcome measures that are highly relevant or essential for specific types of studies (epidemiological, acute hospitalization, rehabilitation, mild TBI/concussion), but not necessarily relevant to all other types of studies. Basic measures selected for mild TBI/concussion are summarized in Table 21.1.

Supplemental Measures

Supplemental outcomes measures for studies in mild TBI and concussion include a wide range of additional CDEs that can be considered for more in-depth assessment within certain domains or for use with certain subpopulations. A comprehensive list of the supplemental measures for mild TBI and concussion (for both pediatric and adult studies) is contained in Table 21.2, with additional information related to the intended age ranges for the measures, availability in various languages, approximate administration times, and other notes related to their use. Note that the selection of measures from this extensive list may vary based upon the study objectives, scope, focus, and population.

While there are advantages to maintaining a consistent set of measures in order to amass a sufficient amount of data, the outcome measurement Working Group acknowledged that CDEs may evolve, and the specific list of measures may evolve over time. Please see the CDEs website (www.commondataelements.ninds.nih.gov/#page=Default) for the most current listing of CDEs, brief description and references, and case report forms, including questionnaires and instruments. Information regarding the use of copyrighted or trademarked instruments or tools is also provided.

Sports-Related Concussion Outcomes CDEs

Although the Workgroup did contain expertise in sports-related concussion and created a domain for sports-related studies (all supplemental measures), the detailed and systematic consideration of CDEs for this domain was recognized as a weakness. Thus, an additional Working Group was formed (in 2016) to specifically address CDEs for sports-related concussion, including CDEs applicable in acute, subacute, and persistent phases of injury. These recommendations were recently released by the NINDS Common Data Elements research group [165].

Implementation of the TBI CDEs

Implementation of Version 2.0 of the TBI CDEs has been facilitated by several organizations and research initiatives.

Federal Interagency TBI Research (FITBIR) Informatics System

Implementation of Version 2 of the TBI CDEs has been facilitated by the FITBIR informatics system, which is a secure, centralized informatics system (database) that serves as a

Table 21.1 Basic measures for mild traumatic brain injury (TBI)/concussion

Domain and measure	Applicable age range	Languages	Estimated administration time	Other notes
Academics				
(None)				
Adaptive and daily living skills				
Pediatric Evaluation of Disability Inventory (PEDI) – Self Care subscales [126]	Pediatric (6 months to 7½ years)	Normed in English Translations in Chinese, Dutch, French (Canada), German, Hebrew, Icelandic, Japanese, Norwegian, Portuguese (Brazil), Slovene, Spanish (United States), Swedish, Turkish	Approximately 45–60 minutes	
Behavioral function				
(None)				
Cognitive activity limitations				
(None)				
Effort/symptom validity				
(None)				
Family and environment				
(None)				
Global outcome				
(None, but see core measures)				
Health-economic measures				
(None)				
Infant and toddler measures				
(None)				
Language and communication				
Wechsler Abbreviated Scale of Intelligence-Second Edition (WASI-II) – Vocabulary subtest [20]	Pediatric (ages 6–90 years)	English, Lithuanian, Norwegian	Approximately 15–25 minutes (including other subtest: Matrix Reasoning)	This subtest is a portion of the *(WASI-II)* – Two-Subtest Form, also recommended in the neuropsychological impairment domain
Military studies				
(None)				
Neuropsychological impairment				
California Verbal Learning Test-Children's Version (CVLT-C) [21]	Pediatric (normative ages 5–16 years; for 4-year-olds, see [22]	English, Spanish [23]	Approximately 15–20 minutes plus a 20-minute delay interval	Alternate forms available
Delis-Kaplan Executive Function System (D-KEFS) – Verbal Fluency [24]	Pediatric (ages 8–89 years)	English, Danish, Dutch, Norwegian, Swedish	Approximately 10–15 minutes	Alternate forms available
Wechsler Abbreviated Scale of Intelligence-Second Edition (WASI-II) – Two-Subtest Form [20]	Pediatric (ages 6–90 years)	Chinese, Czech, Danish, Dutch, English (United States; Australia; Canada; United Kingdom), Finnish, French (France), German, Italian, Japanese, Korean, Norwegian, Spanish (Spain), Swedish	Approximately 20–30 minutes	
Wechsler Intelligence Scale for Children – Fourth Edition (WISC-IV)/Wechsler Preschool and Primary Scale of Intelligence – Third Edition (WPPSI-III) – Processing Speed Index [25, 26]	Pediatric *(WPPSI-III: ages 2½–7 years; WISC-IV: ages 6–16 years)*	WISC-IV: English, Spanish, among other languages WPPSI-III: Spanish, French (France; Canada), German, Italian, Swedish, Korean, Japanese, English (United States; United Kingdom; Australia; Canada), Dutch, Hebrew	Approximately 10–20 minutes	

(continued)

Table 21.1 (Cont.)

Domain and measure	Applicable age range	Languages	Estimated administration time	Other notes
Rey Auditory Verbal Learning Test (RAVLT) [27–29]	Pediatric and adult (ages 5–89 years)	English, Spanish Translations in many languages	Approximately 10–15 minutes	Alternate forms available
Trail Making Test (TMT) [30]	Adult	Arabic, Chinese, Hebrew	Approximately 10–15 minutes	
Wechsler Adult Intelligence Scale – Fourth Edition *(WAIS-IV) – Processing Speed Index Scale* [31]	Adult (ages 16–90 years)	English, Chinese, Danish, Dutch, English (United States; Australia; Canada; United Kingdom), Finnish, French (Canada; France), German, Greek, Hebrew, Hungarian, Icelandic, Italian, Japanese, Korean, Lithuanian, Norwegian, Polish, Portuguese (Brazil), Spanish (Chile; Mexico; Spain), Swedish	Approximately 10–15 minutes	
Patient-reported outcomes (future multidimensional tools)				
(None)				
Perceived generic and disease-specific health-related quality of life				
Pediatric Quality of Life Inventory (PedsQL) – Generic core [32–34]	Pediatric (ages 5–18 years)	English, Spanish Translations in over 48 languages	Approximately 5 minutes	The full PedsQL is also recommended in the Global Outcome domain Child-Self Report and Parent-Proxy Report available for ages 8 to 12 years
Satisfaction with Life Scale (SWLS) [35]	Adult	English; available in several other languages (http://internal.psychology.illinois.edu/~ediener/SWLS.html)	Approximately 1 minute	Copyrighted but can be used with permission
Physical functioning				
Pediatric Evaluation of Disability Inventory (PEDI) – Mobility subscale	Pediatric (6 months to 7½ years)	Normed in English Translations in German, Dutch, Norwegian, Swedish, Spanish (United States), Portuguese (Brazil), Slovene, Turkish, Icelandic, French (Canada), Hebrew, Japanese, and Chinese	Approximately 45–60 minutes	
Post-concussive/TBI-related symptoms				
Health and Behavior Inventory (HBI) [36]	Pediatric (ages 8–15 years)		Approximately 5–10 minutes	
Rivermead Postconcussive Symptom Questionnaire (RPQ) [37]	Adult		Approximately 5 minutes	
Psychiatric and psychological status				
Brief Symptom Inventory – 18 Item (BSI-18) [38]	Adult		Approximately 5–10 minutes	
Recovery of consciousness and memory recovery				
(None)				
Social cognition				
(None)				
Social role participation and social competence				
(None)				
Sports-related studies				
(None)				

Table 21.1 (*Cont.*)

Domain and measure	Applicable age range	Languages	Estimated administration time	Other notes
Academics				
Child Behavior Checklist (CBCL) – School Competence scale [39]	Pediatric (ages 18 months to 5 years; 6–18 years)	English, Spanish	Less than 5 minutes	
Comprehensive Test of Phonological Processing (CTOPP) [40]	Pediatric (ages 5–24 years)	English	Approximately 30 minutes	
Gray Oral Reading Test – Fourth Edition (GORT-4) [41]	Pediatric (ages 6–18 years)		Approximately 20–30 minutes	
KeyMath-3 Diagnostic Assessment (KeyMath-3) [42]	Pediatric (ages 4½–21 years)	English	Approximately 30–90 minutes (depending on the child's age)	
Test of Word Reading Efficiency (TOWRE) [43]	Pediatric (ages 7–24 years)	English	Less than 5 minutes	
Woodcock-Johnson III (WJ-III ACH) Tests of Achievement [44]	Pediatric (ages 2–90 years)		Approximately 60–90 minutes	
Adaptive and daily living skills				
Adaptive Behavior Assessment System, Second Edition (ABAS-II) [45]	Pediatric (ages birth to 89 years)	English, Spanish	Approximately 15–20 per rating form	
Functional Independence Measure for Children (WeeFIM) [46]	Pediatric (ages 6 months to 7 years)	Spanish available from the publisher and others have been tested (e.g., Chinese)	Approximately 20–45 minutes, depending on child's age	
Vineland Adaptive Behavior Scales, Second Edition (VABS-II)	Pediatric (ages birth to 89 years)	English, German, Italian, Dutch, Danish, Norwegian, Spanish (Spain)	Approximately 20–90 minutes (depending on form)	
Mayo-Portland Adaptability Inventory (MPAI-4)[a] [47]	Pediatric and adult (ages 1 year and older)	English, French, German, Danish, and Spanish	Approximately 20–25 minutes	[a]Pediatric: Adaptive and Daily Living Skills; Adult: Global Outcome
Behavioral function				
Frontal Systems Behavior Scale (FrSBe)	Adult (ages 18–95 years)	English, Spanish (United States; Spain), Afrikaans, Portuguese (Brazil), Chinese, Czech, Dutch, French, German, Icelandic, Italian, Japanese, Polish, Romanian, Swedish	Approximately 10 minutes	
Cognitive activity limitations				
Functional Independence Measure – Cognition subscale (Cog-FIM) [48]	Adult (ages 18 years to older adult)	Spanish and others (see above)	Approximately 10–20 minutes	
Brief Test of Adult Cognition by Telephone	Adult	Spanish	Less than 20 minutes	
Effort/symptom validity				
Medical Symptom Validity Test (MSVT) (http://wordmemorytest.com/medical-symptom-validity-test/)	Pediatric and adult	English, German, Portuguese (Brazil), French (Canada), Spanish, Dutch, Norwegian, Swedish, Danish	Approximately 5–10 minutes	
Test of Memory Malingering (TOMM)	Pediatric and adult (ages 16–84 years)	English	Approximately 15–20 minutes	

(continued)

Table 21.1 *(Cont.)*

Domain and measure	Applicable age range	Languages	Estimated administration time	Other notes
Victoria Symptom Validity Test	Pediatric and adult (ages 18–72 years)	Norms in English, Spanish	Approximately 20–25 minutes	
Word Memory Test (http://wordmemorytest.com/word-memory-test/)	Pediatric and adult	English, Spanish, French, German, Dutch, Portuguese, Turkish, Russian, Danish, Hebrew	Approximately 15–20 minutes	
Family and environment				
Child and Adolescent Scale of Environment (CASE) [49, 50]8	Pediatric (ages 5–17 years, although somewhat flexible)	English	Approximately 5 minutes	
Conflict Behavior Questionnaire (CBQ)/Interaction Behavior Questionnaire (IBQ) [51, 52]	Pediatric (ages 3–7 years)	English, Arabic, Catalan, Chinese, Dutch, Finnish, French (France; Canada), German, Greek, Hebrew, Italian, Japanese, Lithuanian, Norwegian, Polish, Portuguese (Brazil; Portugal), Romanian, Spanish, Syrian, Turkish	Approximately 5 minutes	
Family Burden of Injury Interview (FBII) [53]	Pediatric (school-aged children)	English, Danish, Dutch, German	Approximately 20 minutes	Self-report or interview forms available
Family History Research Diagnostic Criteria (FHRDC) [54]	Pediatric		Varies (approximately 10–50 minutes)	
Family Assessment Device (FAD)[b] [55]	Pediatric and adult (ages 12 and older)	English, Arabic Armenian, Chinese, Dutch, French, Hungarian, Italian, Japanese, Spanish, Thai, Turkish	Approximately 15–20 minutes	[b]Pediatric: family and environment; Adult: psychiatric and psychological status
Global outcome				
Glasgow Outcome Scale – Extended Pediatric Revision (GOS-E Peds) [56]	Pediatric (ages birth through 17 years)		Approximately 5–15 minutes	
Pediatric Quality of Life Inventory (PedsQ) [32–34]	Pediatric (ages 2–18 years; normed for ages 5–18 years)	Multiple languages	Approximately 5 minutes	
Pediatric Test of Brain Injury (PTBI) [57]	Pediatric (ages 6–16 years)		Approximately 30 minutes	
Mayo-Portland Adaptability Inventory (MPAI-4)[c] [47]	Pediatric and adult (ages 1 year and older)	English, French, German, Danish, Spanish	Approximately 20–25 minutes	[c]Pediatric: Adaptive and Daily Living Skills; Adult: Global Outcome
Disability Rating Scale (DRS)	Adult	Multiple languages	Approximately 5–15 minutes	
Glasgow Outcome Scale [58, 59]	Adult	Multiple languages	Approximately 5–10 minutes	
Short Form-12 (SF™-12) – Health Survey [60]	Adult (normed 18–65 years)	Multiple languages	Approximately 5–10 minutes	
Short Form-36 (SF™-36 v2) – Medical Outcome Study [60]	Adult (normed 18–65 years)	Translations in more than 50 languages	Approximately 10–15 minutes	
Health-economic measures				
EuroQOL [61]	Adult (ages 16 years and older)	Multiple languages	Approximately 5 minutes	

Table 21.1 *(Cont.)*

Domain and measure	Applicable age range	Languages	Estimated administration time	Other notes
Infant and toddler measures				
Bayley Scales of Infant and Toddler Development, Third Edition (Bayley-III) [62]	Pediatric (ages 1–42 months)	English	Approximately 30–90 minutes depending upon age of child	
Brief Infant Toddler Social Emotional Assessment (BITSEA) [63]	Pediatric (ages 12–36 months)	English, Spanish, among other languages	Approximately 7–10 minutes	
Child Behavior Checklist (CBCL) [39]	Pediatric (ages 18 months to 5 years; 6–18 years)	English, Spanish	Approximately 20 minutes	
Mullen Scales of Early Learning [64]	Pediatric (ages birth to 68 months)	English	Approximately 15–60 minutes depending upon age of child	
Shape School [65]	Pediatric (ages 3–6 years)	English	Variable depending upon age of child	
Trails-Preschool (Trails-P) [66]	Pediatric (ages 3–5 years)	English		
Language and communication				
Caregiver Unintelligible Speech Rating [67, 68]	Pediatric (ages under 60 months)	Translations in more than 60 languages	Approximately 1 minute	
Clinical Evaluation of Language Fundamentals – Fourth Edition (CELF-4) [69]	Pediatric (ages 5–21 years)	English, Spanish	Approximately 30–60 minutes	
Comprehensive Assessment of Spoken Language (CASL) [70]	Pediatric (ages 3–21 years)	English, French, German, Italian, Portuguese, Russian, Spanish	Approximately 30–45 minutes	
Goldman-Fristoe Test of Articulation, Second Edition (GFTA-2) [71]	Pediatric (ages 2–21 years)		Approximately 5–15 minutes	
Language Sample [72]	Pediatric		Approximately 5–10 minutes	
Peabody Picture Vocabulary Test, Fourth Edition (PPVT-4) [73]	Pediatric (ages 2.5–90 years)	English, Spanish (Test de Vocabulario en Imágenes Peabody (TVIP) for children and adolescents [74]	Approximately 15 minutes	
Percentage of Consonants Correct-Revised (PCC) [75]	Pediatric (ages 18 months to 21 years)	English, Spanish, among other languages	Approximately 15–20 minutes to collect conversational speech sample; transcription approximately 60 minutes	
Test of Language Competence-Expanded Edition (TLC-Expanded) [76]	Pediatric (ages 5–9 years; 10–18 years)	English	Approximately 60 minutes	
Verbal Motor Production Assessment for Children (VMPAC) [77]	Pediatric (ages 3–12 years)	English, Spanish, Portuguese	Approximately 30 minutes	
Western Aphasia Battery-Revised, Bedside Tool	Adult (ages 18–89 years)	English	Approximately 15 minutes	

(continued)

Table 21.1 (*Cont.*)

Domain and measure	Applicable age range	Languages	Estimated administration time	Other notes
National Adult Reading Test (NART) [78]; *see also* www.academia.edu/2515150/National_Adult_Reading_Test_NART_test_manual_Part_1)	Adult (ages 18 years and older)	English	Approximately 5–10 minutes	
Wechsler Test of Adult Reading (WTAR)	Adult (ages 16–89 years)	English	Approximately 5–10 minutes	
Military studies				
Combat Exposure Scale (CES) [79] (see also www.ptsd.va.gov/professional/assessment/te-measures/ces.asp)	Adult		Approximately 5–10 minutes	
Military Acute Concussion Evaluation (MACE) [80] (see also www.pdhealth.mil/downloads/mace.pdf)	Adult		Approximately 15 minutes	
Veterans RAND 36 Item Health Survey (VR-36) (www.rand.org/health/surveys_tools/mos/mos_core_36item.html; www.outcomes-trust.org/monitor/0100mntr.pdfadult)	Adult		Approximately 5–10 minutes	
Neuropsychological impairment				
Beery-Buktenica Developmental Test of Visual-Motor Integration, Sixth Edition (Beery VMI) [81]	Pediatric (ages 2–99 years; short form ages 2–8 years)		Approximately 10–15 minutes	
Behavioral Rating Inventory of Executive Function (BRIEF) [82–84]	Pediatric (ages 5–18 years; self-report form: ages 11–22 years)		Approximately 15 minutes	
Wechsler Intelligence Scale for Children – Fourth Edition (WISC-IV)/Wechsler Preschool and Primary Scale of Intelligence – Third Edition (WPPSI-III) – Block Design [25, 26]	Pediatric (*WPPSI-III ages 2.5 to a little over 7 years; WISC-IV ages 6–16 years*)	*WISC-IV*: English, Spanish, among other languages; *WPPSI-III*: Spanish, French (France; Canada), German, Italian, Swedish, Korean, Japanese, Canadian, English (United States; Australia), Dutch, Hebrew	Approximately 10–15 minutes	
Conners' Continuous Performance Test-Revised (CPT-2) [85]	Pediatric (ages 6 to over 55 years)		Approximately 15 minutes	
Contingency Naming Test (CNT) [86]	Pediatric (ages 6–16 years; adolescent and adult norms available)		Approximately 15–20 minutes	
Delis-Kaplan Executive Function System (D-KEFS) – Trail Making Test [87]	Pediatric (ages 8–89 years)	English, Dutch, Danish, Norwegian, Swedish	Approximately 10–15 minutes	
Eriksen Flanker Test [88]	Pediatric			
Functional Assessment of Verbal Reasoning and Executive Strategies – Student Version (S-FAVRES) [89]	Pediatric (ages 12–19 years)		Approximately 50 minutes	

Table 21.1 (Cont.)

Domain and measure	Applicable age range	Languages	Estimated administration time	Other notes
Test of Everyday Attention (Tea-Ch) [90]	Pediatric (ages 6–15 years)	English (UK normative sample)	Approximately 55–60 minutes	
Tasks of Executive Control (TEC) [91]	Pediatric (ages 5–18 years)		Approximately 20–30 minutes	
Test of Memory and Learning, Second Edition (TOMAL-2) [92]	Pediatric (ages 5–60 years)		Core battery: approximately 30 minutes; Core battery plus supplementary: approximately 60 minutes	
Test of Strategic Learning (TOSL) [93]	Pediatric (ages 7–20 years)		Approximately 15–20 minutes	
Wide-Range Assessment of Memory and Learning, Second Edition (WRAML2) [94]	Pediatric (ages 5–90 years)		Approximately 55–60 minutes	
Grooved Pegboard Test [95]	Pediatric and adult (norms available for most ages)		Approximately 5–10 minutes	
NIH Toolbox Cognitive Battery (see www.nihtoolbox.org)	Pediatric and adult (ages 3–85 years)		Less than 5 minutes	
Symbol Digit Modalities Test (SDMT) [96]	Pediatric and adult (ages 8 years and older)			
Automated Neuropsychological Assessment Metrics (ANAM) [97]	Adult			
Brief Visuospatial Memory Test – Revised (BVMT-R)	Adult (ages 18–79 years)		Approximately 45 minutes (with delay)	
Color-Word Interference Test Delis-Kaplan Executive Function System (D-KEFS) – Color Word Interference subtest [24]	Adult (ages 8–89 years)	English, Dutch, Danish, Norwegian, Swedish	Approximately 10 minutes	
Controlled Oral Word Association Test (COWAT)	Adult (normed for ages 20–85 years)	Translations in many languages	Approximately 5–10 minutes	
Wechsler Adult Intelligence Scale – Wechsler Adult Intelligence Scale – Fourth Edition (WAIS-IV) – Digit Span subtest [31]	Adult (ages 16–90 years)	English (United States; Australia; Canada; United Kingdom), Chinese, Danish, Dutch, Finnish, French (Canada; France), German, Greek, Hebrew, Hungarian, Icelandic, Italian, Japanese, Korean, Lithuanian, Norwegian, Polish, Portuguese (Brazil), Spanish (Chile; Mexico; Spain), Swedish	Approximately 10–15 minutes	
Wechsler Adult Intelligence Scale – Fourth Edition (WAIS-IV) – Letter-Number Sequencing subtest [31]	Adult (ages 16–90 years)	English (United States; Australia; Canada; United Kingdom), Chinese, Danish, Dutch, Finnish, French (Canada; France), German, Greek, Hebrew, Hungarian, Icelandic, Italian, Japanese, Korean, Lithuanian, Norwegian, Polish, Portuguese (Brazil), Spanish (Chile; Mexico; Spain), Swedish	Approximately 10–15 minutes	
Wide Range Achievement Test (WRAT-4) – Word Reading subtest	Adult (ages 5–94 years)		Approximately 10–15 minutes	

(continued)

Table 21.1 (*Cont.*)

Domain and measure	Applicable age range	Languages	Estimated administration time	Other notes
Patient-reported outcomes (future multidimensional tools)				
Neuro-QOL [98, 99]	Pediatric and adult (ages 8–17 years; ages 18 years and older)	English, Spanish, among others (www.neuroqol.org)	Approximately five questions per minute answered by respondents	
Patient Reported Outcomes Measurement Information System (PROMIS) [100]	Pediatric and adult (ages 5–17 years; ages 18 years and older)	English translations in many languages (dependent upon subdomain)	Dependent upon domain	
Traumatic brain injury-quality of life (TBI-QOL)	Pediatric and adult			
Perceived generic and disease-specific health-related quality of life				
Quality of Life after Brain Injury (QOLIBRI) (www.qolibrinet.com)	Adult (normed ages 17–68 years)	Validated in two large, multi-language studies	Approximately 7–10 minutes	Free for research use
Physical functioning				
Bruininks–Oseretsky Test of Motor Proficiency, Second Edition (BOT-2) [101]	Pediatric (ages 4–21 years)		Short form approximately 15–20 minutes; complete battery approximately 45–60 minutes	
Functional Independence Measure for Children (WeeFIM) – Motor subscale [46]	Pediatric (ages 6 months to 7 years)		Complete battery approximately 20–30 minutes	The full WeeFIM is also recommended in the Adaptive and Daily Living Skills domain
Gross Motor Function Measure (GMFM-66 and GMFM-88) [102, 103]	Pediatric (ages 5 months to 16 years)	Translations in many languages	Approximately 45–60 minutes depending upon version	
Neuro-QOL mobility/ ambulation domain [98, 99]	Pediatric (ages 8–17 years; ages 18 years and older)	English, Spanish, among others (www.neuroqol.org)	Approximately five questions per minute answered by respondents	Neuro-QOL is also recommended in the Patient Reported Outcomes (Future Multidimensional Tools) domain
Patient Reported Outcomes Measurement Information System (PROMIS) – Mobility and upper extremity domains [104]	Pediatric (ages 5–17 years; ages 18 years and older)	English Translated into many languages (dependent upon subdomain)	Dependent upon domain	PROMIS is also recommended in the Patient Reported Outcomes (Future Multidimensional Tools) domain
Peabody Developmental Motor Scales, 2nd Edition (PMDS-2) [105]	Pediatric (ages birth to 5 years)		Approximately 45–60 minutes	
Balance Error Scoring System (Modified) [106]	Pediatric and adult (norms provided for ages 7–69 years)		Approximately 10–20 minutes	
NIH Toolbox Motor Battery (see www.nihtoolbox.org)	Pediatric and adult (ages 3–85 years)		Dependent upon domains examined; approximately 20–30 minutes	
NIH Toolbox Sensory Battery (see www.nihtoolbox.org)	Pediatric and adult (ages 3–85 years)		Dependent upon domains examined; approximately 20–30 minutes	
Functional Independence Measure (FIM) – Motor Subscale [48]	Adult (ages 18 years and older)		Approximately 30–45 minutes	
Neurological Outcome Scale for Traumatic Brain Injury (NOS-TBI) [107]	Adult		Approximately 15–20 minutes	

Table 21.1 *(Cont.)*

Domain and measure	Applicable age range	Languages	Estimated administration time	Other notes
Post-concussive/TBI-related symptoms				
Post-concussion Symptom Inventory (PCSI) [108]	Pediatric (ages 5–7 years; ages 8–12 years; ages 13–18 years)		Approximately 10–15 minutes	Public domain
Neurobehavioral Symptom Inventory (NSI) [109]	Adult (validated in veterans ages 18 years and older)			
Psychiatric and psychological status				
Child Behavior Checklist (CBCL) Problem Behaviors subscale [39]	Pediatric (ages 6–18 years)		Approximately 20 minutes	
Child Behavior Checklist (CBCL) Teacher Report Form [39]	Pediatric (ages 6–18 years)		Approximately 20 minutes	
Children's Affective Lability Scale (CALS) [110]	Pediatric (ages 6–16 years)		Approximately 5 minutes	
Children's Motivation Scale (CMS) [111]	Pediatric (ages 6–16 years)		Approximately 5 minutes	
Modified Overt Aggression Scale (MOAS) [112]	Pediatric		Approximately 5 minutes	
Neuropsychiatric Rating Schedule (NPRS) [113]	Pediatric (normed ages 6–18 years)			
Schedule for Affective Disorders and Schizophrenia for School-Age Children-Present and Lifetime Version (K-SADS-PL) [114]	Pediatric (ages 6–18 years)		Approximately 75 minutes	
Screen for Child Anxiety Related Emotional Disorders (SCARED) [115–118]	Pediatric (ages 8–18 years)		Approximately 10 minutes	Parent and Child Version
Short Mood and Feelings Questionnaire (SMFQ) [119, 120]	Pediatric (ages 6–17 years)		Approximately 5 minutes	
Strengths and Difficulties Questionnaire (SDQ) [121]	Pediatric (ages 4–16 years; youth self-report ages 11 to 16 years)		Approximately 5–10 minutes	
UCLA PTSD Index for the DSM-IV [[122]	Pediatric (ages 7–12 years; ages 13 years and older)	English, Spanish	Approximately 20 minutes	
Alcohol, Smoking, and Substance Use Involvement Screening Test (ASSIST) [123]	Pediatric and adult		Approximately 5–10 minutes	
Family Assessment Device (FAD)[d] [55]	Pediatric and adult (ages 12 and older)	English, Arabic, Armenian, Chinese, Dutch, French, Hungarian, Italian, Japanese, Spanish, Thai, Turkish	Approximately 15–20 minutes	[d]Pediatric: Family and Environment; Adult: Psychiatric and Psychological Status

(continued)

Table 21.1 (*Cont.*)

Domain and measure	Applicable age range	Languages	Estimated administration time	Other notes
Alcohol Use Disorders Identification Test: Self-Report Version (AUDIT) [124]	Adult			
Beck Depression Inventory – 2 (BDI-2) [125]	Adult (ages 13–80 years)	English, Spanish	Approximately 5 minutes	
Center for Epidemiologic Studies Depression Scale (CES-D) [126]	Adult (validated in wide range of ages)		Approximately 5 minutes	Revised version (CESD-R) now administrable online http://cesd-r.com
Clinician-Administered PTSD Scale (CAPS) [127] Interview available from the National Center for PTSD at www.ptsd.va.gov	Adult (primarily over age 18 years, but some modifications are being made for children)		Approximately 45–60 minutes for complete interview	Clinician-administered; currently revised for compatibility with the DSM-5
Minnesota Multiphasic Personality Inventory – 2 -Restructured Form (MMPI-2-RF) [128]	Adult (ages 18 years and older)		Approximately 35–50 minutes	5th-grade reading level
NIH Toolbox Emotional Battery (see www.nihtoolbox.org)	Adult (ages 3–85 years)		Dependent upon domains examined; approximately 20–30 minutes	
Patient Health Questionnaire (9 Item) (PHQ-9) [129]	Adult, adapted for use in adolescents	Translations in many languages	Approximately 5–10 minutes	
PTSD Checklist –Civilian/Military/Stressor Specific (PCL- C/M/S) [130]	Adult		Approximately 5–10 minutes	The PTSD Checklist for DSM-5 (PCL-5). Scale available from the National Center for PTSD at www.ptsd.va.gov
Substance Abuse Questions from the TBI Model Systems Database (SAQTBIMSD) [131] www.tbims.org/combi/subst/index	Adult		Approximately 10–15 minutes	
Recovery of consciousness and memory recovery				
Children's Orientation and Amnesia Test (COAT) [132]	Pediatric (ages 3–15 years; temporal orientation ages 8–15 years only)		Approximately 5–10 minutes	
Galveston Orientation and Amnesia Test (GOAT) [133]	Pediatric and adult	English, Spanish	Approximately 5–10 minutes	
JFK Coma Recovery Scale – Revised (CRS-R) [134]; *see also* www.tbims.org/combi/crs	Adult		Approximately 5–10 minutes	
Social cognition				
Interpersonal Negotiations Strategies (INS) [135]	Pediatric (ages 6–16 years)		Approximately 30 minutes	
Reading the Mind in the Eyes Test-Child Version [136]	Pediatric (ages under 18 years)		Approximately 20 minutes	

Table 21.1 (*Cont.*)

Domain and measure	Applicable age range	Languages	Estimated administration time	Other notes
Video Social Inference Test (VSIT) [137]	Pediatric		Approximately 20 minutes	
Social role participation and social competence				
Child and Adolescent Scale of Participation (CASP) [48, 138, 139]	Pediatric (ages 5 years and older)		Approximately 5–10 minutes	
Child Behavior Checklist (CBCL) – School Competence scale [39]	Pediatric (6–18 years)	English, Spanish	Less than 5 minutes	
Pediatric Evaluation of Disability Inventory (PEDI) – Social Functioning Scale [140]	Pediatric (6 months to 7½ years)	Normed in English Translations in many languages (e.g., German, Dutch, Norwegian, Swedish, Spanish (United States), Portuguese (Brazil), Slovene, Turkish, Icelandic, French (Canada), Hebrew, Japanese and Chinese	Total administration time approximately 45–60 minutes	
Pediatric Quality of Life Inventory (PedsQL) – Social subscale [32–34]	Pediatric (ages 5–18 years)	English, Spanish Translations in more than 48 languages	Approximately 5 minutes	The full PedsQL is also recommended in the Global Outcome Domain; Child Self-Report and ParentProxy-Report available for ages 8 to 12 years
Social Skills Rating Scale (SSRS) [141]	Pediatric (ages 3–18 years)		Approximately 25 minutes	
Strengths and Difficulties Questionnaire (SDQ) [121] *– Peer Relations and Prosocial Behavior subscales*	Pediatric (ages 4–16 years; youth self-report ages 11–16 years)		Approximately 5–10 minutes	The full SDQ is also recommended in the Psychiatric and Psychological Status domain
Vineland Adaptive Behavior Scales, Second Edition™ (VABS-II) – Socialization scale	Pediatric (ages birth to 89 years)	English, German, Italian, Dutch, Danish, Norwegian, Spanish (Spain)	Approximately 20–90 minutes (depending on form)	The full VABS-II is also recommended in the Adaptive and Daily Living Skills domain
Craig Handicap and Assessment Reporting Technique (CHART-SF) *Participation Assessment with Recombined Tools (PART)* [142] www.tbims.org/combi/chartsf	Adult		Approximately 15–20 minutes	
Participation Assessment with Recombined Tools (PART) [143] (www.tbims.org/combi/parto)	Adult		Approximately 10–15 minutes	
Sports-related studies				
Axon Sports Computerized Cognitive Assessment Tool (CCAT) [144]	Pediatric and adult			Computerized
CNS Vital Signs [145] (*see also* www.cnsvitalsigns.com)	Pediatric and adult (ages 8–90 years)	Translations in many languages	Approximately 25–30 minutes	Computerized; assessment also indicated sensitivity to malingering/symptom invalidity

(*continued*)

Table 21.1 (*Cont.*)

Domain and measure	Applicable age range	Languages	Estimated administration time	Other notes
Headminder Concussion Resolution Index [146]	Pediatric and adult		Approximately 25 minutes	
Immediate Post-Concussion Assessment and Cognitive Testing (imPACT) (www.impacttest.com)	Pediatric and adult (5–59 years)		Approximately 25–30 minutes	
Sport Concussion Assessment Tool (SCAT-2) (https://bjsm.bmj.com)	Pediatric and adult		Approximately 10–15 minutes	
Deafness and other communication disorders				
Auditory Figure-Ground Tests [147]	Pediatric and adult		Approximately 10–15 minutes	
Competing Sentences Test of SCAN-C and SCAN-A [147, 148]	Pediatric and adult		Approximately 10–15 minutes	Distributed through Pearson
Competing Words Test of SCAN-C and SCAN-A [147, 148]	Pediatric (normed for ages 5–11 years) and adult		Approximately 10–15 minutes	Distributed through Pearson
Filtered Words Tests [149, 150]	Pediatric and adult		Varies	
NIH Toolbox Balance Accelerometry Measure (BAM) (see www.nihtoolbox.org)	Pediatric and adult		Dependent upon domains examined; approximately 20–30 minutes	The NIH Toolbox is also recommended in the domain of Physical Function
NIH Toolbox Dynamic Visual Acuity Test (see www.nihtoolbox.org)	Pediatric and adult		Dependent upon domains examined; approximately 20–30 minutes	The NIH Toolbox is also recommended in the domain of Physical Function
NIH Toolbox Odor Identification Test (OIT) (see www.nihtoolbox.org)	Pediatric and adult		Dependent upon domains examined; approximately 20–30 minutes	The NIH Toolbox is also recommended in the domain of Physical Function
NIH Toolbox Taste Test (see www.nihtoolbox.org)	Pediatric and adult		Dependent upon domains examined; approximately 20–30 minutes	The NIH Toolbox is also recommended in the domain of Physical Function
Random-Gap Detection Test [151–153]	Pediatric and adult (typically ages 5 years and older)		Approximately 10 minutes to administer and score	Auditory processing disorder test using non-verbal stimuli
Taste and Smell Questionnaire	Pediatric and adult			
Time-Compressed Sentence Test [154, 155]	Pediatric and adult		8 minutes to administer; 15 to administer and score	
Words in Noise Test	Pediatric and adult			
Dizziness Handicap Inventory (DHI) [156]	Adult		Approximately 10 minutes	The DHI is a 25-item self-assessment scale composed of a nine-item functional subscale, a nine-item emotional subscale, and a seven-item physical subscale.

Table 21.1 (*Cont.*)

Domain and measure	Applicable age range	Languages	Estimated administration time	Other notes
				Possible scores on the DHI range from 0, suggesting no handicap, to 100, indicating significant perceived handicap
Hearing Handicap Inventory [157, 158]	Adult (younger adults and elderly)		Approximately 10–15 minutes	A 25-item self-assessment scale composed of two subscales (emotional and social/situational)
Tinnitus Functional Index (TFI) [159]	Adult	TFI has been formally evaluated recently in the United Kingdom [160] and in New Zealand [161]. Efforts are underway to translate the TFI into at least 13 languages	Approximately 10–15 minutes	25-item TFI is available online, with scoring instructions. Can be downloaded and printed (permission to use the copyrighted TFI is required from Oregon Health and Science University – there is no cost in most cases) at www.formstack.com/forms/?1265642-Ir7f92V4rb)
Tinnitus Handicap Inventory [162]	Adult	Translated into several languages.	Approximately 10–15 minutes	Publically available
Voice Handicap Index (VHI) [163, 164]	Adult		Approximately 5–10 minutes	Publically available. A pediatric version is also available.
NIH resources				
NIH Toolbox (see www.nihtoolbox.org)	Pediatric and adult (ages 3–85 years)		Dependent upon domains examined; approximately 20–30 minutes	
Patient Reported Outcomes Measurement Information System (PROMIS) [100]	Pediatric and adult (ages 5–17 years; ages 18 years and older)	English Translations in many languages (dependent upon subdomain)	Dependent upon domain	
Neuro-QOL [98, 99]	Pediatric and adult (ages 8–17 years; ages 18 years and older)	English, Spanish, with others in progress (www.neuroqol.org)	Approximately five questions per minute answered by respondents	

central repository for new and previously collected data of all types (e.g., text, numeric, image, time series, including outcome CDEs). It has been sponsored by the U.S. Army Medical Research and Materiel Command (funded through the Defense Medical Research and Development Program) and supported by the NIH Center for Information Technology in addition to NINDS. The FITBIR informatics system was developed to promote the objectives of the CDEs initiative as well as to enable interconnectivity with other informatics platforms. FITBIR implements the data dictionary and specific variables developed from the TBI CDEs.

The FITBIR website (http:fitbir.nih.gov) includes information on ongoing training webinars, data sharing and other repository policies, standard operating procedures, and the process of submission of data to FITBIR. The website portal provides access to data that have been contributed by others. Form structures and a data dictionary are also provided, as is a listing of data contributors. Technical support is available to researchers through weekly FITBIR users' conference calls and individual project consultations, though investigators must supply the resources (both financial and personnel) to perform the data entry or extraction. FITBIR does provide a model for cost estimation related to this process (http:fitbir.nih.gov).

In some circumstances, investigators may be required to submit data from TBI-related projects collected using U.S. federal funding to FITBIR, though submission of data from any relevant project is encouraged. Both the DoD (Combat Casualty Care) and NINDS have provided funding for "legacy data" projects to be submitted into FITBIR. The FITBIR website contains information regarding the application process for investigators to contribute or access data from FITBIR, as well as the quality standards required by FITBIR. For investigators with approved projects, data are generally submitted quarterly to FITBIR. Investigators identify which data are considered experimental (i.e., addressing specific study hypotheses). These core and basic CDEs may be available to other researchers contributing data to FITBIR six months following the end of the study funding period and 12 months for all other researchers [2, 166]. In addition to CDEs (for which case forms are available), researchers may enter data for unique data elements, which are also added to the repository.

The FITBIR system utilizes global unique identifiers (GUIDs), which are randomly generated codes, to share data regarding individual subjects without disclosing personally identifiable information and to ensure that subjects who may be enrolled in more than one study can be identified as the same subject. For retrospective studies where required information is not available (i.e., full name at birth; date of birth including month, day, and year; city and country of birth; and sex at birth), pseudo-GUIDs are utilized. An additional tool available from FITBIR is the Protocol and Form Research Management System, which allows for the creation of case report forms linked to the FITBIR data dictionary.

Clinical Data Interchange Standards Consortium (C-DISC)

C-DISC is a global, multidisciplinary, non-profit organization whose goal is to establish well-defined standards to support the acquisition, exchange, submission, and archive of clinical research data and metadata. The U.S. Food and Drug Administration (FDA) has announced that it will develop guidance requiring study data and new drug applications to conform to C-DISC standards [167, 168]. This has reportedly accelerated the rate of review for FDA-regulated treatments and is intended to assist in the integration of data.

C-DISC released the first version (v1) of the TBI Therapeutic Area User Guide (TAUG-TBI) in 2015 [167]. Version 1 of the TAUG-TBI emphasized the most commonly collected data used across TBI trials. C-DISC involved members of the CDEs Steering Committee in clarifying and refining versions and definitions, as necessary, and in enhancing consistency, as appropriate. These standards are intended to further facilitate clinical information, including outcome data, as well as injury characteristics and data, imaging, and physical examination.

The user guide also includes annotated case report forms and examples as well as a set of standardized terminology and clinical outcome assessment supplements for approximately 25 of the most commonly used CDE instruments.

Transforming Research and Clinical Knowledge in TBI (TRACK-TBI)

Under the American Reinvestment and Recovery Act, the NIH-NINDS funded the TRACK-TBI multicenter study in 2009. The aim of the project was to test the feasibility of implementing the TBI CDEs and examine their validity [169]. TRACK-TBI was a multicenter prospective, observational study with participants recruited through four study sites, including both acute care and rehabilitation level settings. The majority of the subjects recruited (83%) had a mild TBI, as defined by a Glasgow Coma Scale (GCS) score of 13–15 upon admission to the emergency department (83%), though the project also included 4% with moderate TBI (GCS 9–12), and 13% with severe TBI (GCS 3–8). The multidisciplinary team established an operational version of TBI CDEs, developed a web-enabled TBI CDEs database and created imaging and biospecimen repositories. With regard to outcome measures, the project prospectively collected core measures as well as a few supplemental measures from Version 1.0 of the TBI CDEs. These measures were collected at three months (via telephone interview) and six months post injury, with significant success. TRACK-TBI investigators worked closely with the FITBIR team, providing the data dictionary that was used in the project, contributing clinical and imaging data, and testing methods for data transfer. This TRACK-TBI pilot data set was the first to populate FITBIR. Additional projects from the TRACK-TBI investigators are currently under way.

Remaining Limitations and Caveats

Investigators have identified several remaining gaps in the outcome measures of the TBI CDEs. There persists a lack of validated outcome measures that can be used with *all TBI/concussion patient populations* to assess patients across the entire continuum of severity and acuity. For example, administration of some of the core outcome measures is not possible in patients with poor outcome (i.e., GOS-E levels 2 (vegetative state), 3 (lower severe disability), and 4 (upper severe disability)).Similarly, other outcome measures frequently used in more severe head trauma are not considered sensitive enough to reflect the nature or degree of certain deficits of interest in individuals with more mild injury. For instance, the use of the GOS-E for the assessment of outcomes in mild TBI is particularly controversial, as previously mentioned.

Limitations of the TBI CDEs outcome measures have also included limited application in non-English-speaking patients [169]. Although the inclusion of fewer verbal measures and greater number of non-verbal tasks has been proposed as a means to overcome this limitation for patients nationally and internationally, a resolution is still under way and the development of robust measures in multiple languages is considered high research priority. Similar concerns for the assessment of patients across heterogeneous ethnic and cultural backgrounds have also been raised.

In-person assessment required by the core outcome battery also may pose difficulties for a number of reasons in some patient populations. Patient cooperation and accessibility can challenge various types of studies (e.g., longitudinal, epidemiological). This is particularly problematic given that the completion of the currently recommended outcome assessment measures may be lengthy. While a very brief battery would be ideal, the inherent heterogeneity of outcomes in TBI has complicated a shorter, universal battery. Concerns regarding the use and application of current outcome measures have been raised, with concerns around rigorous selection of evidence-based procedures on one hand, balanced with practicality, feasibility, and accessibility. For example, newer measures that have not been thoroughly validated in TBI *per se* (e.g., NIH ToolKit, which allows for a two-hour, comprehensive neuropsychological assessment) may offer significant advantages in terms of ease of administration and scoring and time to administer the measure [170]. Additional concerns also involve inconsistencies across studies with regard to measurement administration and scoring, although C-DISC efforts have more explicitly addressed these by obtaining expert consensus regarding administration instructions, record forms, and scoring procedures and providing explicit information in this regard. There have been additional criticisms regarding the specifics of data entry and query procedures as well as concerns about the regulatory approval process necessary for entry of data with and without explicit consent of the subjects, though guidance on these issues has also been provided by FITBIR and the NINDS.

Conclusions

Despite remaining limitations, the CDE effort represents a tremendous advance in our ability to harmonize data collection, share data, and pose questions that can be best addressed by large amounts of data. The CDE initiative laid a necessary foundation for the creation of a large data repository for TBI (i.e., FITBIR), as well as facilitation of explicit standards that can be applied in seeking FDA approval. Furthermore, the standardization via CDEs paves the way for investigators to utilize several "Big Data" analytic methods (e.g., machine learning techniques) to more thoroughly interrogate previously acquired data as well as to more cost-effectively examine prospectively collected data. It facilitates assessment of data collected across numerous sites, projects, and patient populations within TBI. While there are remaining limitations in the existing CDEs, significant efforts to address previously noted shortcomings have been ongoing since the creation and initial application of the CDEs for TBI, and this work continues as the CDEs evolve.

References

1. NINDS. Data Standards. 2016. Available at: www.commondataelements.ninds.nih.gov/tbi.aspx#tab=Data_Standards.
2. Thompson HJ, Vavilala MS, Rivara FP. Common data elements and federal interagency traumatic brain injury research informatics system for TBI Research. *Annu Rev Nurs Res* 2015; 33: 1–11.
3. Saatman KE, Duhaime AC, Bullock R, Maas AI, Valadka A, Manley GT, et al. Classification of traumatic brain injury for targeted therapies. *J Neurotrauma* 2008; 25: 719–738.
4. Thurmond VA, Hicks R, Gleason T, Miller AC, Szuflita N, Orman J, et al. Advancing integrated research in psychological health and traumatic brain injury: Common data elements. *Arch Phys Med Rehabil* 2010; 91: 1633–1636.
5. Duhaime AC, Gean AD, Haacke EM, Hicks R, Wintermark M, Mukherjee P, et al. Common data elements in radiologic imaging of traumatic brain injury. *Arch Phys Med Rehabil* 2010; 91: 1661–1666.
6. Maas AI, Harrison-Felix CL, Menon D, Adelson PD, Balkin T, Bullock R, et al. Common data elements for traumatic brain injury: Recommendations from the interagency working group on demographics and clinical assessment. *Arch Phys Med Rehabil* 2010; 91: 1641–1649.
7. Manley GT, Diaz-Arrastia R, Brophy M, Engel D, Goodman C, Gwinn K, et al. Common data elements for traumatic brain injury: Recommendations from the biospecimens and biomarkers working group. *Arch Phys Med Rehabil* 2010; 91: 1667–1672.
8. Haacke EM, Duhaime AC, Gean AD, Riedy G, Wintermark M, Mukherjee P, et al. Common data elements in radiologic imaging of traumatic brain injury. *J Magn Reson Imaging* 2010; 32: 516–543.
9. Wilde EA, Whiteneck GG, Bogner J, Bushnik T, Cifu DX, Dikmen S, et al. Recommendations for the use of common outcome measures in traumatic brain injury research. *Arch Phys Med Rehabil* 2010; 91: 1650–1660 e17.
10. Whyte J, Vasterling J, Manley GT. Common data elements for research on traumatic brain injury and psychological health: Current status and future development. *Arch Phys Med Rehabil* 2010; 91: 1692–1696.
11. Hicks R, Giacino J, Harrison-Felix C, Manley G, Valadka A, Wilde EA. Progress in developing common data elements for traumatic brain injury research: Version two – The end of the beginning. *J Neurotrauma* 2013; 30: 1852–1861.
12. Adelson PD, Pineda J, Bell MJ, Abend NS, Berger RP, Giza CC, et al. Common data elements for pediatric traumatic brain injury: Recommendations from the working group on demographics and clinical assessment. *J Neurotrauma* 2012; 29: 639–53.
13. Bell MJ, Kochanek PM. Pediatric traumatic brain injury in 2012: The year with new guidelines and common data elements. *Crit Care Clin* 2013; 29: 223–238.
14. Berger RP, Beers SR, Papa L, Bell M. Common data elements for pediatric traumatic brain injury: Recommendations from the biospecimens and biomarkers workgroup. *J Neurotrauma* 2012; 29: 672–677.
15. Duhaime AC, Holshouser B, Hunter JV, Tong K. Common data elements for neuroimaging of traumatic brain injury: Pediatric considerations. *J Neurotrauma* 2012; 29: 629–633.
16. Gerring JP, Wade S. The essential role of psychosocial risk and protective factors in pediatric traumatic brain injury research. *J Neurotrauma* 2012; 29: 621–628.
17. Hunter JV, Wilde EA, Tong KA, Holshouser BA. Emerging imaging tools for use with traumatic brain injury research. *J Neurotrauma* 2012; 29: 654–671.
18. McCauley SR, Wilde EA, Anderson VA, Bedell G, Beers SR, Campbell TF, et al. Recommendations for the use of common outcome measures in pediatric traumatic brain injury research. *J Neurotrauma* 2012; 29: 678–705.
19. Miller AC, Odenkirchen J, Duhaime AC, Hicks R. Common data elements for research on traumatic brain injury: Pediatric considerations. *J Neurotrauma* 2012; 29: 634–638.

20. Wechsler D. *Wechsler Abbreviated Scale of Intelligence* – Second edition. Bloomington, MN: Pearson, 2011.

21. Delis D, Kramar J, Kaplan E, Ober B. California Verbal Learning Test – Children's version. San Antonio, TX: Pearson Assessments, 1994.

22. Goodman A, Delis D, Mattson S. Normative data for four-year old children on the California Verbal Learning Test-Children's version. *Clin Neuropsychol* 1999; 13: 274–282.

23. Rosselli M, Ardila A, Bateman J, Guzman M. Neuropsychological test scorse, academic performance, and developmental disorders in Spanish-speaker children. *Dev Neuropsychol* 2001; 20: 355–373.

24. Delis D, Kaplan E, Kramer J. Delis-Kaplan executive function system examiner's manual. San Antonio, TX: NCS Pearson, 2001.

25. Wechsler D. *WISC-IV administration manual*. San Antonio, TX: Pearson Assessments, 2003.

26. Wechsler D. *WISC-IV technical and interpretive manual*. San Antonio, TX: Pearson Assessments, 2003.

27. Mitrushina M, Boone KB, Razani J, D'elia LF. *Handbook of normative data for neuropsychological assessment*, 2nd edition. New York: Oxford University Press, 2005.

28. Ivnik RJ, Malec JE, Tangalos EG, Peterson RC, Kokmen E, Kurland LT. Mayo's older American's normative studies: Updated AVLT norms for ages 56 to 97. *Clin Neuropsychologist* 1992; 6: 83–104.

29. Schmidt M. *Rey auditory verbal learning test: A handbook*. Los Angeles, CA: Western Psychological Services, 1996.

30. Reitan R, Wolfson D. *Neuropsychological evaluation of older children*. Tucson, AZ: Neuropsychology Press, 1992.

31. Wechsler D. *Wechsler Adult Intelligence Scale – Fourth edition (WAIS-IV)*. San Antonio, TX: Harcourt Assessment, 2008.

32. Varni J, Seid M, Rode C. The PedsQL: Measurement model for the pediatric quality of life inventory. *Med Care* 1999; 37: 126–139.

33. Varni J, Seid M, Kurtin P. PedsQL 4.0: Reliability and validity of the Pediatric Quality of Life Inventory version 4.0 generic core scales in healthy and patient populations. *Med Care* 2001; 39: 800–812.

34. Varni J, Burwinkle T, Seid M, Skarr D. The PedsQL 4.0 as a pediatric population health measure: Feasibility, reliability, and validity. *Ambul Pediatr* 2003; 3: 329–341.

35. Diener E, Emmons RA, Larsen RJ, Griffin S. The Satisfaction With Life Scale. *J Pers Assess* 1985; 49: 71–75.

36. Ayr L, Yeates K, Taylor H, Brown M. Dimensions of post-concussive symptoms in children with mild traumatic brain injuries. *J Int Neuropsychol Soc* 2009; 15: 19–30.

37. King NS, Crawford S, Wenden FJ, Moss NE, Wade DT. The Rivermead Post Concussion Symptoms Questionnaire: A measure of symptoms commonly experienced after head injury and its reliability. *J Neurol* 1995; 242: 587–592.

38. Derogatis LR, Melisaratos N. The Brief Symptom Inventory: An introductory report. *Psychol Med* 1983; 13: 595–605.

39. Achenbach T. *Manual for child behavior checklist/4–18 and 1991 profile*. Burlington, VT: University of Vermont, Department of Psychiatry, 1991.

40. Wagner R, Torgesen J, Rashotte C. *Comprehensive test of phonological processing. Examiner's manual*. San Antonio, TX: Pearson Assessments, 1999.

41. Wiederholt J, Bryant B. *Gray Oral Reading Test(GORT-4) manual*, fourth edition. San Antonio, TX: Pearson Assessments, 2001.

42. Connelly J. *KeyMath 3 diagnostic assessment*. San Antonio, TX: Pearson Education, 2007.

43. Torgesen J, Wagner R, Rashotte C. *Test of word reading efficiency*. Austin, TX: Pro-Ed, 1999.

44. Woodcock R, Mcgrew K, Mather N. *Woodcock-Johnson tests of achievement manual*, 3rd edition. Itasca, IL: Riverside Publishing, 2001.

45. Harrison P, Oakland T. *Adaptive behavior assessment system*, second edition. San Antonio, TX: Harcourt Assessment, 2003.

46. Msall ME, DiGaudio K, Rogers BT, LaForest S, Catanzaro NL, Campbell J, et al. The Functional Independence Measure for Children (WeeFIM): conceptual basis and pilot use in children with developmental disabilities. *Clin Pediatr* 1994; 33: 421–430.

47. Malec JF, Lezak MD. Manual for the Mayo-Portland Adaptability Inventory (MPAI-4) for adults, children and adolescents; revised with adaptations for pediatric version added January 2008. Available at: http://tbims.org/combi/mpai/manual.pdf.

48. Granger C. The emerging science of functional assessment: Our tool for outcomes analysis. *Arch Phys Med Rehabil* 1998; 79: 235–240.

49. Bedell G. Developing a follow-up survey focused on participation of children and youth with acquired brain injuries after inpatient rehabilitation. *NeuroRehabilitation* 2004; 19: 191–205.

50. Bedell G, Dumas H. Social participation of children and youth with acquired brain injuries discharged from inpatient rehabilitation: A follow-up study. *Brain Inj* 2004; 18: 65–82.

51. Prinz R, Foster S, Kent R, Kd OL. Multivariate assessment of conflict in distressed and nondistressed parent-adolescent dyads. *J Appl Behav Anal* 1979; 12: 691–700.

52. Robin A, Foster S. *Negotiating parent adolescent conflict: A behavioral family systems approach*. New York: Guilford, 1989.

53. Burgess ES, Drotar D, Taylor HG, Wade S, Stancin T, Yeates KO. The family burden of injury interview: Reliability and validity studies. *J Head Trauma Rehabil* 1999; 14: 394–405.

54. Andreasen NC, Endicott J, Spitzer RL, Winokur G. The family history method using diagnostic criteria. Reliability and validity. *Arch Gen Psychiatry* 1977; 34: 1229-1235.

55. Epstein N, Baldwin L, Bishop D. The McMaster family assessment device. *J Marital Fam Ther* 1983; 9: 171–180.

56. Beers S, Hahner T, Adelson P. Validity of a pediatric version of the Glasgow Outcome Scale – Extended (GOS-E Peds). *J Neurotrauma* 2005; 22: 1224.

57. Hotz G, Helm-Estabrooks N, Nelson NW, Plante E. *Pediatric Test of Brain Injury (PTBI)*. Baltimore, MD: Paul H. Brookes Publishing, 2010.

58. Jennett B, Bond M. Assessment of outcome after severe brain damage. *Lancet* 1975; 1: 480–484.

59. Teasdale GM, Pettigrew LE, Wilson JT, Murray G, Jennett B. Analyzing outcome of treatment of severe head injury: A review and update on advancing the use of the Glasgow Outcome Scale. *J Neurotrauma* 1998; 15: 587–597.

60. Mackenzie EJ, McCarthy ML, Ditunno JF, Forrester-Staz C, Gruen GS, Marion DW, et al. Using the SF-36 for characterizing outcome after multiple trauma involving head injury. *J Trauma* 2002; 52: 527–534.

61. EuroQol Group. EuroQol – a new facility for the measurement of health-related quality of life. *Health Policy* 1990; 16: 199–208.

62. Bayley N. *Bayley scales of infant and toddler development*, third edition. San Antonio, TX: Psychological Corporation, 2005.

63. Briggs-Gowan M, Carter A. *Brief Infant Toddler Social Emotional Assessment (BITSEA)*. San Antonio, TX: Pearson Education, 2006.

64. Mullen E. *Mullen scales of early learning*. Circle Pines, MN: American Guidance Service, 1995.

65. Espy K. The shape school: Assessing executive function in preschool children. *Dev Neuropsychol* 1997; 13: 495–499.

66. Espy K, Cwik M. The development of a Trail Making Test in young children: The TRAILS-P. *Clin Neuropsychol* 2004; 18: 1–12.

67. Coplan J, Gleason J. Unclear speech: Recognition and significance of unintelligible speech in preschool children. *Pediatrics* 1988; 82: 447–452.

68. Campbell T. Functional treatment outcomes for young children with neurogenic communication disorders. *Semin Speech Lang* 1999; 19: 223–247.

69. Semel W, Wiig E, Secord W. *Clinical evaluation of language fundamentals*, fourth edition. San Antonio, TX: Pearson Assessments, 2003.

70. Carrow-Woolfolk E. *Comprehensive assessment of spoken language*. Circle Pines, MN: American Guidance Service, 1999.

71. Goldman R, Fristoe M. *Goldman-Fristoe test of articulation*, second edition. San Antonio, TX: Pearson Assessments, 2000.

72. Miller J, Chapman J. *The SALT guide*. Standard version, 8th edition. Madison, WI: Language Analysis Laboratory, Waisman Center, University of Wisconsin, 2004.

73. Dunn L, Dunn D. *Peabody picture vocabulary test. Examiner's manual*, fourth edition. San Antonio, TX: Pearson Assessments, 2007.

74. Dunn L, Lugo D, Padilla E, Dunn L. *Test de vocabulario en imágenes Peabody*. San Antonio, TX: Pearson Assessments, 1986.

75. Shriberg L, Austin D, Lewis B, McSweeney J, Wilson D. The percentage of consonants correct (PCC) metric. Extension and reliability data. *J Speech Lang Hear Res* 1997; 40: 708–722.

76. Wiig E, Secord W. *Test of language competence*, expanded edition. San Antonio, TX: Psychological Corporation, 1989.

77. Hayden D, Square P. *Verbal Motor Assessment of Children (VMPAC)*. San Antonio, TX: Pearson, 1999.

78. Nelson HE. *The National Adult Reading Test (NART): Test manual*. Windsor, UK: NFER-Nelson, 1982.

79. Keane TM, Fairbank JA, Caddell JM, Zimering RT, Taylor KL, Mora C. Clinical evaluation of a measure to assess combat exposure. *Psychol Assess* 1989; 1: 53–55.

80. French L, McCrea M, Baggett M. The Military Acute Concussion Evaluation (MACE). *J Special Ops Med* 2008; 8: 68–77.

81. Beery K, Buktenica N, Beery N. *Beery-Buktenica developmental test of visual-motor integration*, sixth edition. San Antonio, TX: Pearson Assessments, 2010.

82. Gioia G, Espy K, Isquith P. *Behavior rating inventory of executive function – Preschool version*. Odessa, FL: Psychological Assessment Resources, 2003.

83. Gioia G, Isquith P, Guy S, Kenworthy L. *BRIEF: Behavior Rating Inventory of Executive Function*. Lutz, FL: Psychological Assessment Resources, 2000.

84. Guy S, Isquith P, Gioia G. *Behavior Rating Inventory of Executive Function – Self report version*. Odessa, FL: Psychological Assessment Resources, 2004.

85. Conners C. *Continuous performance test. Technical guide and software manual,* second edition. North Tonawanda, NY: MultiHealth Systems, 2004.

86. Taylor H, Schatsneider C, Rich D. Sequelae of *Haemophilus influenzae* meningitis: Implications for the study of brain disease and development. In: Tramontana M, Hooper S, editors. *Advances in clinical neuropsychology*. I. New York: Springer-Verlag, 1992, pp. 50–108.

87. Delis D, Kaplan E, Kramar J. *Delis-Kaplan executive function system*. San Antonio, TX: Pearson Assessment, 2001.

88. Eriksen B, Eriksen C. Effects of noise letters upon identification of a target letter in a nonsearch task. *Percept Psychophys* 1974; 16: 143–149.

89. Macdonald S. Assessment of higher level cognitive-communication functions in adolescents with ABI: Standardization of the student version of the functional assessment of verbal reasoning and executive strategies (S-FAVRES). *Brain Inj* 2016; 30: 295–310.

90. Manly T, Robertson I, Anderson V, Nimmo-Smith I. *TEA-Ch: The Test of Everyday Attention for Children*. Bury St. Edmunds, England: Thames Valley Test Company, 1999.

91. Isquith P, Roth R, Gioia G. *Tasks of Executive Control (TEC)*. Odessa, FL: Psychological Assessment Resources, 2010.

92. Reynolds CR, Voress JK. *Test of memory and learning – Second edition*. Austin, TX: PRO-ED, 2007.

93. Gamino JF, Chapman SB, Cook LG. Strategic learning in youth with traumatic brain injury: Evidence for stall in higher-order cognition. *Top Lang Disorders* 2009; 29: 224–235.

94. Sheslow D, Adams W. *Wide Range Assessment of Memory and Learning; second edition (WRAML2)*. Lutz, FL: Psychological Assessment Resources, 2003.

95. Mathews C, Kløve K. *Instruction manual for the adult neuropsychology test battery*. Madison, WI: University of Wisconsin Medical School, 1964.

96. Smith A. *Symbol Digit Modalities Test (SDMT)*. Torrance, CA: Western Psychological Services, 1973.

97. Reeves D, Kane R, Winter K. *Automated Neuropsychological Assessment Metrics (ANAM): Test administrator's guide version 3.11 (report no. NCRF-95-01)*. San Diego, CA: National Cognitive Recovery Foundation, 1995.

98. Miller D, Nowinski C, Victorson D, Peterman A, Perez L. The Neuro-QOL project: Establishing research priorities through qualitative research and consensus development. *Qual Life Res* 2005; 14: 2031.

99. Perez L, Huang J, Jansky L, Nowinski C, Victorson D, Peterman A, et al. Using focus groups to inform the Neuro-QOL measurement tool: Exploring patient-centered, health-related quality of life concepts across neurological conditions. *J Neurosci Nurs* 2007; 39: 342–353.

100. Cella D, Yount S, Rothrock N, Gershon R, Cook K, Reeve B, Ader D, et al. The Patient-Reported Outcomes Measurement Information System (PROMIS): Progress of an NIH Roadmap Cooperative Group during its first two years. *Med Care* 2007; 45(5: Suppl. 1): S3–S11.

101. Bruininks RH, Bruininks BD. *BOT-2, Bruininks-Oseretsky Test of Motor Proficiency, second edition*. Minneapolis, MN: Pearson Assessments, 2005.

102. Russell D, Rosenbaum P, Cadman D, Gowland C, Hardy S, Jarvis S. The Gross Motor Function Measure: A means to evaluate the effects of physical therapy. *Dev Med Child Neurol* 1989; 31: 341–352.

103. Russell D, Avery L, Rosenbaum P, Raina P, Walter S, Palisano R. Improved scaling of the Gross Motor Function Measure for children with cerebral palsy: Evidence of reliability and validity. *Phys Ther* 2000; 80: 873–885.

104. Hays RD, Spritzer KL, Amtmann D, Lai J-S, DeWitt EM, Rothrock N, et al. Upper-extremity and mobility subdomains from the Patient-Reported Outcomes Measurement Information System (PROMIS) Adult Physical Functioning Item Bank. *Arch Phys Med Rehabil* 2013; 94: 2291–2296.

105. Folio MR, Fewell RR. *Peabody Developmental Motor Scales, second edition (PDMS-2)*. San Antonio, TX: Pearson, 2000.

106. Iverson GL, Kaarto ML, Koehle MS. Normative data for the balance error scoring system: Implications for brain injury evaluations. *Brain Inj* 2008; 22: 147–152.

107. Wilde EA, Mccauley SR, Kelly TM, Levin HS, Pedroza C, Clifton GL, et al. Feasibility of the Neurological Outcome Scale for Traumatic Brain Injury (NOS-TBI) in adults. *J Neurotrauma* 2010; 27: 975–981.

108. Gioia G, Schneider J, Vaughan C, Isquith P. Which symptom assessments and approaches are uniquely appropriate for paediatric concussion? *Br J Sports Med* 2009; 43: i13–i22.

109. Meterko M, Baker E, Stolzmann KL, Hendricks AM, Cicerone KD, Lew HL. Psychometric assessment of the Neurobehavioral Symptom Inventory-22: The structure of persistent postconcussive symptoms following deployment-related mild traumatic brain injury among veterans. *J Head Trauma Rehabil* 2012; 27: 55–62.

110. Gerson A, Gerring J, Freund L, Joshi P, Capozzoli J, Brady K, et al. The Children's Affective Lability Scale: A psychometric evaluation of reliability. *Psychiatry Res* 1996; 65: 189–198.

111. Gerring J, Freund L, Gerson A, Joshi P, Capozzoli J, Frosch E, et al. Psychometric characteristics of the Children's Motivation Scale. *Psychiatry Res* 1996; 63: 205–217.

112. Kay S, Wolkenfeld F, Murrill L. Profiles of aggression among psychiatric patients. I. Nature and prevalence. *J Nerv Ment Dis* 1988; 176: 539–546.

113. Max JE, Castillo CS, Lindgren SD, Arndt S. The Neuropsychiatric Rating Schedule: Reliability and validity. *J Am Acad Child Adol Psychiatry* 1998; 37: 297–304.

114. Kaufman J, Birmaher B, Brent D, Rao U, Flynn C, Williamson D, et al. Schedule for Affective Disorders and Schizophrenia for School-Age Children – Present and Lifetime version (K-SADS-PL): Initial reliability and validity data. *J Am Acad Child Adolesc Psychiatry* 1997; 36: 980–988.

115. Monga S, Birmaher B, Chiappetta L, Brent D, Kaufman J, Bridge J, et al. Screen for Child Anxiety-Related Emotional Disorders (SCARED): Convergent and divergent validity. *Depress Anxiety* 2000; 12: 85–91.

116. Hale WR, Raaijmakers Q, Muris P, Meeus W. Psychometric properties of the Screen for Child Anxiety Related Emotional Disorders (SCARED) in the general adolescent population. *J Am Acad Child Adolesc Psychiatry* 2005; 44: 283–290.

117. Birmaher B, Brent D, Chiappetta L, Bridge J, Monga S, Baugher M. Psychometric properties of the Screen for Child Anxiety Related Emotional Disorders (SCARED): A replication study. *J Am Acad Child Adolesc Psychiatry* 1999; 38: 1230–1236.

118. Birmaher B, Khetarpal S, Brent D, Cully M, Balach L, Kaufman J, et al. The Screen for Child Anxiety Related Emotional Disorders (SCARED): Scale construction and psychometric characteristics *J Am Acad Child Adolesc Psychiatry* 1997; 36: 545–553.

119. Angold A, Costello E, Messer S, Pickles A, Winder F, Silver D. Development of a short questionnaire for use in epidemiological studies of depression in children and adolescents. *Int J Methods Psychiatr Res* 1995; 5: 237–249.

120. Costello E, Angold A. Scales to assess child and adolescent depression: Checklists, screens and nets. *J Am Acad Child Adolesc Psychiatry* 1988; 27: 726–737.

121. Goodman R. The Strengths and Difficulties Questionnaire: A research note. *J Child Psychol Psychiatry* 1997; 43: 1159–1167.

122. Steinberg AM, Brymer MJ, Decker KB, Pynoos RS. The University of California at Los Angeles Post-traumatic Stress Disorder Reaction Index. *Curr Psychiatry Rep* 2004; 6: 96–100.

123. WHO ASSIST Working Group. The Alcohol, Smoking and Substance Involvement Screening Test (ASSIST): Development, reliability and feasibility. *Addiction* 2002; 97: 1183–1194.

124. Saunders JB, Aasland OG, Babor TF, De La Fuente JR, Grant M. Development of the Alcohol Use Disorders Identification Test (AUDIT): WHO collaborative project on early detection of persons with harmful alcohol consumption – II. *Addiction* 1993; 88: 791–804.

125. Beck AT, Steer RA, Ball R, Ranieri W. Comparison of Beck Depression Inventories -IA and -II in psychiatric outpatients. *J Pers Assess* 1996; 67: 588–597.

126. Radloff LS. The CES-D scale: A self-report depression scale for research in the general population. *Appl Psychol Measure* 1977; 1: 385–401.

127. Weathers FW, Blake DD, Schnurr PP, Kaloupek DG, Marx BP, Keane TM. The Clinician-Administered PTSD scale for DSM-5 (CAPS-5). 2013. Available at www.ptsd.va.gov.

128. Tellegen A, Ben-Porath YS. *Minnesota Multiphasic Personality Inventory technical manual*. Minneapolis, MN: University of Minneapolis Press, 2008.

129. Kroenke K, Spitzer RL, Williams JB. The PHQ-9: Validity of a brief depression severity measure. *J Gen Intern Med* 2001; 16: 606–613.

130. Weathers FW, Litz BT, Keane TM, Palmieri PA, Marx BP, Schnurr PP. The PTSD Checklist for DSM-5 (PCL-5). 2013. Available at www.ptsd.va.gov.

131. Corrigan JD, Bogner J, Lamb-Hart G, Sivak-Sears N. *Technical report on problematic substance use identified in the TBI Model Systems National Dataset*. Center for Outcome Measurement in Brain Injury. Available at: www.tbims.org/combi/subst/index.

132. Ewing-Cobbs L, Levin H, Fletcher J, Miner M, Eisenberg H. The children's orientation and amnesia test: Relationship to severity of acute head injury and to recovery of memory. *Neurosurg.* 1990; 27: 683–691.

133. Levin HS, O'Donnell VM, Grossman RG. The Galveston Orientation and Amnesia Test. A practical scale to assess cognition after head injury. *J Nerv Mental Dis* 1979; 167: 675–684.

134. Giacino JT, Kalmar K, Whyte J. The JFK Coma Recovery Scale-Revised: Measurement characteristics and diagnostic utility. *Arch Phys Med Rehabil* 2004; 85: 2020–2029.

135. Yeates K, Schultz L, Selman R. Bridging the gaps in child-clinical assessment: Toward the application of social-cognitive development theory. *Clin Psychol Rev* 1990; 10: 567–588.

136. Baron-Cohen S, Wheelwright S, Scahill V, Lawson J, Spong A. Are intuitive physics and intuitive psychology independent? A test with children with Asperger syndrome. *J Dev Learn Disord* 2001; 5: 47–78.

137. Turkstra L. Conversation-based assessment of social cognition in adults with traumatic brain injury. *Brain Inj* 2008; 22: 397–409.

138. Bedell G. Further validation of the Child and Adolescent Scale of Participation (CASP). *Dev Neurorehabil* 2009; 12: 342–351.

139. Ziviani J, Desha L, Feeney R, Boyd R. Measures of participation outcomes and environmental considerations for children with acquired brain injury: A systematic review. *Brain Impair* 2010; 11: 93–112.

140. Haley S, Coster W, Ludlow L, Haltiwanger J, Andrellos P. *Pediatric evaluation of disability inventory: Development, standardization, and administration manual, version 1.0*. Boston, MA: Trustees of Boston University, Health and Disability Research Institute, 1992.

141. Elliott S, Gresham F, Freeman T, Mccloskey G. Teacher and observer ratings of children's social skills: Validation of the Social Skills Rating Scale. *J Psychoeduc Assess* 1988; 6: 152–161.

142. Whiteneck GG, Brooks CA, Charlifue S, Gerhart KA, Mellick M, Overholser D, et al. *Guide for use of the chart: Craig Handicap Assessment and reporting technique*. Englewood, CO: Craig Hospital, 1988, 1992.

143. Bogner J, Bellon K, Kolakowsky-Hayner SA, Whiteneck G. Participation Assessment With Recombined Tools–Objective (PART-O). *J Head Trauma Rehabil* 2013; 28: 337–339.

144. Collie A, Darby D, Maruff P. Computerised cognitive assessment of athletes with sports related head injury. *Br J Sports Med* 2001; 35: 297–302.

145. Gualtieri CT, Johnson LG. Reliability and validity of a computerized neurocognitive test battery, CNS vital signs. *Arch Clin Neuropsychol* 2006; 21: 623–643.

146. Erlanger DM, Feldman D, Kutner KC. *Concussion Resolution Index*. New York, NY: HeadMinder, 1999.

147. Keith RW. Development and standardization of SCAN-C test for auditory processing disorders in children. *J Am Acad Audiol* 2000; 11: 438–445.

148. Keith RW. Development and standardization of SCAN-A: Test of auditory processing disorders in adolescents and adults. *J Am Acad Audiol* 1995; 6: 286–292.

149. Arnott W, Goli T, Bradley A, Smith A, Wilson W. The filtered words test and the influence of lexicality. *J Speech Lang Hear Res* 2014; 57: 1722–1730.

150. O'Beirne GA, Mcgaffin AJ, Rickard NA. Development of an adaptive low-pass filtered speech test for the identification of auditory processing disorders. *Int J Pediatr Otorhinolaryngol* 2012; 76: 777–782.
151. Auditec. Quality auditory test recordings since 1972. https://auditecincorporated.wordpress.com/.
152. Auditec. Random gap detection test (RGDT). 2015. https://auditecincorporated.wordpress.com/2015/09/28/random-gap-detection-test-rgdt/.
153. Keith RW. Random gap detection test [CD; CD-Rom]. Bloomington, MN: NCS Pearson.
154. Keith RW. Standardization of the time compressed sentence test. *J Educ Audiol* 2002; 10: 15–20.
155. Keith RW. *Time compressed sentence test, Examiner's manual.* St. Louis, MO: Auditec, 2002.
156. Jacobson GP, Newman CW. The development of the Dizziness Handicap Inventory. *Arch Otolaryngol Head Neck Surg* 1990; 116: 424–427.
157. Newman CW, Weinstein BE, Jacobson GP, Hug GA. The hearing handicap inventory for adults: Psychometric adequacy and audiometric correlates. *Ear Hear* 1990; 11: 430–433.
158. Ventry IM, Weinstein BE. The hearing handicap inventory for the elderly: A new tool. *Ear Hear* 1982; 3: 128–134.
159. Meikle MB, Henry JA, Griest SE, Stewart BJ, Abrams HB, Mcardle R, et al. The tinnitus functional index: Development of a new clinical measure for chronic, intrusive tinnitus. *Ear Hear* 2012; 33: 153–176.
160. Fackrell K, Hall DA, Barry J, Hoare DJ. Tools for tinnitus measurement: development and validity of questionnaires to assess handicap and treatment effects. In: Signorelli F, Turjman F, editors. *Tinnitus: Causes, Treatment and Short and Long-term Health Effects* (pp. 13–60). New York: Nova Science Publishers, 2014.
161. Chandra N. New Zealand validation of the Tinnitus Functional Index. 2013. Available at www.fmhs.auckland.ac.nz/assets/fmhs/soph/bhsc_hons/docs/presentation-slides/2013/navshika-chandra.pdf.
162. Newman CW, Jacobson GP, Spitzer JB. Development of the tinnitus handicap inventory. *Arch Otolaryngol Head Neck Surg* 1996; 122: 143–148.
163. Jacobson BH, Johnson A, Grywalski C, Silbergleit A, Jacobson G, Benninger MS, et al. The voice handicap index (VHI) development and validation. *Am J Speech-Lang Pathol* 1997; 6: 66–70.
164. Rosen CA, Lee AS, Osborne J, Zullo T, Murry T. Development and validation of the voice handicap index-10. *Laryngoscope* 2004; 114: 1549–1556.
165. NINDS Common Data Elements. Sport-related concussion. 2018. Available at www.commondataelements.ninds.nih.gov/SRC.aspx#tab=Data_Standards.
166. Fitbir. Informatics System. 2015. https://fitbir.nih.gov/.
167. Clinical Data Interchange Standards Consortium. Traumatic brain injury therapeutic area. 2016. www.cdisc.org/traumatic-brain-injury-therapeutic-area.
168. U.S. Food and Drug Administration. FDA study data technical conformance guide; Technical specifications document, 2017. Available at www.fda.gov/downloads/ForIndustry/DataStandards/StudyDataStandards/UCM384744.pdf.
169. Yue JK, Vassar MJ, Lingsma HF, Cooper SR, Okonkwo DO, Valadka AB, et al. Transforming research and clinical knowledge in traumatic brain injury pilot: Multicenter implementation of the common data elements for traumatic brain injury. *J Neurotrauma* 2013; 30: 1831–1844.
170. Gershon RC, Cella D, Fox NA, Havlik RJ, Hendrie HC, Wagster MV. Assessment of neurological and behavioural function: The NIH Toolbox. *Lancet Neurol* 2010; 9: 138–139.

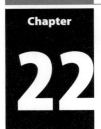

Chapter

Functional Neuroimaging of Concussion

Andrew R. Mayer and Patrick S.F. Bellgowan

Introduction

There can be no doubt of the recent sea change that has occurred in the study of concussion, also commonly referred to as mild traumatic brain injury (mTBI). It was initially believed that concussion resulted in no long-term behavioral or neurological consequences [1], except for a small percentage of patients with pre-existing psychiatric conditions, which predisposed them to long-term emotional sequelae. Standard clinical neuroimaging methods (computed tomography scans; T1- and T2-weighted images) are typically negative for the majority of concussed patients [2, 3], which further helped propagate the view that mTBI did not lead to frank neuronal pathology.

However, more recent studies suggest that the life-long effects of concussion may be greater than initially believed, predominantly a result of the dramatic increase in the diagnoses of chronic traumatic encephalopathy (CTE) amongst recently deceased athletes [4]. Neuroimaging studies of mTBI have also proliferated, with different imaging modalities suggesting that neuronal pathology may be present long after traditional outcome measures (e.g., balance and neuropsychological testing) have returned to pre-morbid levels of functioning [5-7]. As a result of these new lines of evidence, it has been suggested that a single concussion can result in lifetime impairment for some individuals. However, a more realistic assessment of the field suggests a nascent understanding of the neuronal and behavioral consequences of both single and repetitive mTBIs, with several key challenges remaining to be resolved.

The goals of the current chapter are to provide the reader with a more thorough appreciation for the challenges of conducting neuroimaging studies in mTBI.[1] The current chapter focuses on functional magnetic resonanace imaging (fMRI), which can be used to perform non-invasive, *in vivo* measurements during demanding cognitive tasks [8], and more recently to characterize intrinsic (i.e., functional connectivity) neuronal activity [9–11].

We begin with a review of the physiological underpinnings of the fMRI response, how it may be altered by mTBI, and the analytic strategies through which researchers attempt to non-invasively capture the effects of neuronal injury. Next we provide a brief review of mTBI research using both task-based (i.e., evoked) paradigms as well as resting-state measurements that are used to study intrinsic brain activity. Finally, we focus on the methodological challenges of performing fMRI research with brain-injured patients from a clinical perspective.

fMRI Physiology and Putative Effects of Trauma

The relation between neuronal activity and the resultant hemodynamic response (i.e., neurovascular coupling) remains a topic of active investigation. In the absence of evoked activity, the cerebral metabolic rate of glucose (CMR_{glu}), the cerebral metabolic rate of oxygen ($CMRO_2$) and cerebral blood flow (CBF) are tightly coupled. Metabolic demands change following excitatory neuronal transmission, and energy (glucose) is required to reverse the ionic influx that results in depolarization while excess glutamate must be rapidly removed from the synaptic cleft [12, 13]. Astrocytes take up excess glutamate, converting it to glutamine, and release vasoactive agents. Neurons concurrently release nitric oxide [12]. All of these events likely contribute to vasodilation and a concomitant increase in CBF following excitatory neuronal transmission. There is also a decoupling between CBF and oxidative metabolism, leading to an excess of oxygenated blood, a decrease in the ratio of deoxyhemoglobin relative to oxyhemoglobin, and a subsequent increase in MR signal due to differences in magnetic properties between the two forms of hemoglobin. Thus, the blood oxygen level-dependent (BOLD) response during normal neurovascular coupling represents an amalgamation of signals derived primarily from

---

[1] Editor's note (JV): concussive brain injury (CBI) is the broadly defined neurobiological entity about which this volume is written. Increased definitional specificity awaits the discovery of markers distinguishing *biologically* discreete subtypes of TBI. In contrast, "mild traumatic brain injury" ("mTBI") is a popular phrase for a subset of head injuries defined with various *clinical* criteria, even though evidence suggests such criteria do not identify any homogeneous neurobiological entity. Pragmatically, of course, scholars investigating correlations between subsets of TBI (such as those that do not cause immediate death or require emergency neurosurgical intervention) and biomarkers (e.g., neuropathological findings or imaging) are obliged to employ clinical criteria to select subjects. The term "mTBI" will be used sometimes in this chapter because some of the cited empirical sources selected subjects using one of the clinical criteria for so-called "mTBI."

the ratio of oxy- to deoxyhemoglobin, with contributions from CBF and cerebral blood volume (CBV).

The resultant shape of the BOLD response is similarly complex in nature. The canonical hemodynamic response function (HRF) consists of two primary components, a positive signal change that peaks approximately 4–6 s after stimulus onset, and a post-stimulus undershoot (PSU) that reaches maximum 6–10 s after stimulus end. As previously discussed, the positive phase of the BOLD response has been associated with an increase in CBF, and the resultant change in the ratio of oxy- to deoxyhemoglobin intravascularly [14]. The biophysical origins of the PSU are less well established. An early model attributed the PSU to differences in timing of the return of CBF (earlier response) and CBV (delayed response) to baseline levels [12]. However, more recent work suggests that the duration of the PSU extends beyond the time when CBV returns to baseline, leading others to suggest that increased demands for $CMRO_2$ following cellular signaling also contribute to the PSU [15].

Thus, there are several different mechanisms, as well as combinations of mechanisms, through which head trauma can affect the BOLD response. Importantly, non-specific effects of trauma (e.g., pain and fatigue), as well as the presence of prescribed medications (e.g., narcotics or sedatives), can also alter neurovascular coupling. Principally, trauma can cause frank neuronal dysfunction (e.g., alterations in synchronous neuronal activity), resulting in downstream effects on BOLD-based activity through changes in the amount of glutamate in the synaptic cleft and the energetic needs of cells following neurotransmission. Reports of neuronal loss in animal models of fluid percussion injury [16] and abnormal cell signaling [17] directly support this hypothesis. Indirect support comes from magnetic resonance spectroscopy findings of altered glutamate and glutamine concentrations in the semi-acute stage of mTBI, as well as through more invasive measures during severe injury models [18–20].

The structural integrity of the microvasculature can also be directly affected by trauma. Fluid percussion studies in animal models indicate a semi-acute reduction in capillary number and diameter both at the injury site and distally [21], with several other studies indicating a reduction in cerebral vascular reactivity. Similarly, hemosiderin depositions, secondary to microhemorrhages and inflammation, have been noted in human cases of mTBI using both non-invasive neuroimaging as well as at autopsy [6]. TBI also directly affects CBF transit time as well as cerebral perfusion [22]. Arterial spin labeling can be used to directly measure CBF and calibrate the BOLD signal for CBF changes [23], although the measurements must be made in a quantitative fashion.

Third, even in the presence of normal perfusion, metabolic failure may occur after TBI [24]. Specifically, both animal and human models suggest an initial decoupling between CBF and CMR_{glu}, followed by a generally reduced cerebral metabolism after injury [22, 25]. Alterations in CBF and CMR_{glu} may be the most long-lasting effects of concussion [25], providing a physiological basis for a more prolonged impairment (i.e., days to weeks post injury) of the BOLD response following injury. A challenge for reconciling findings from animal studies is the frequent recording of physiological states in the absence of evoked activity and in the presence of anesthesia. As previously noted, resting-state activity is associated with differential dynamics between BOLD constituents (e.g., CBF, $CMRO_2$ and CMR_{glu}) relative to more dynamic states (evoked activity). Anesthesia can also affect both neuronal activity as well as neurovascular coupling. Although there has been an effort to reduce or eliminate anesthesia protocols in animal models [26], this model is only starting to be applied to the trauma field. Additional animal studies that specifically examine how mTBI affects both intrinsic and evoked activity will greatly improve our knowledge of the true bench-to-bedside capabilities of the technique in a more controlled environment.

Methodological Challenges Associated with Analyses

There are several analytic considerations for conducting fMRI research following mTBI given the known complexity of the BOLD response. Foremost, both region of interest and voxel-wise analyses inherently assume that heterogeneous initial injury conditions (e.g., motor vehicle accidents versus a blow to the left temple) result in a homogeneous pattern (i.e., high degree of spatial overlap) of gray-matter abnormalities. Specifically, to survive group-wise statistics, traditional regions of interest (ROIs) and voxel-wise analyses assume that resulting BOLD disruptions occur in the same neuronal regions. Although the diencephalon, mid-brain, limbic circuit, and prefrontal cortex are more commonly injured [6, 27], the basic premise of this spatial homogeneity assumption is likely to be flawed. Novel approaches for classifying heterogeneous lesion locations are increasingly being sought as necessary bases for performing mTBI imaging research, and have been used to identify voxel-wise abnormalities in diffusion tensor imaging (DTI) data on a patient-by-patient basis [28, 29]. However, this approach has not been applied to BOLD imaging data. The appeal of these newer analytic techniques lies in their clearly superior logic. However, the underlying assumptions are likely to be dependent on the statistical properties of the data (e.g., sample size, distribution properties, and normalcy). Thus, methods that are robust across different distributions and account for the smaller sample sizes that typify most imaging studies require development and further validation.

Secondly, the majority of fMRI studies in both mild and more severe forms of TBI have typically estimated only a single parameter (e.g., a beta coefficient) by convolving an assumed canonical hemodynamic response function (HRF) with known experimental conditions (e.g., onset of a particular trial) in order to derive a predictor function (e.g., regressor). fMRI studies typically use either a gamma variate or a double gamma variate function as the canonical HRF shape, with the double gamma variate function having the additional benefit of modeling the PSU. These standard regression analyses assume that the relationship between the positive phase and PSU are largely unaffected by mTBI, and that a single parameter adequately captures resultant alterations in the HRF. However, currently there is scant evidence to verify whether this assumption is actually correct.

To date, only a few studies have explicitly examined the shape of the HRF in mild [30] and more severe TBI [33]. Palmer and colleagues [31] reported no differences in the basic shape of the HRF following more severe TBI, with patients exhibiting an increased volume of activation within the visual cortex during visual stimulation. Mayer and colleagues [30] reported differences in the shape of the HRF in semi-acute mTBI patients and HC within the bilateral primary/secondary visual cortex, right supramarginal gyrus and the right parahippocampal gyrus during a sensorimotor task. In contrast, the HRF within auditory, motor and other heteromodal cortical areas was similar across the two groups. These results suggest the need for additional fMRI studies that explicitly compare the different phases of the HRF in both human and animal models.

Finally, fMRI data is financially costly to accumulate and mTBI patients who meet strict inclusion criteria (homogeneous in both injury severity and scan-time post injury with no pre-existing psychiatric history) are challenging to recruit. Not surprisingly, the combination of these two factors has resulted in the utilization of small sample sizes for most fMRI studies of mTBI, despite the inherently low signal-to-noise ratio of the technique [32]. Specifically, the majority of fMRI studies following mTBI have been conducted with sample sizes that are below commonly accepted recommendations ($n = 24$) for this imaging modality [33]. As a result, the majority of published studies may be underpowered, suffer from low positive predictive power, and/or provide poor estimates of true effect sizes. All of these factors, in conjunction with clinical design, may contribute to the conflicting findings of hypo- and hyperactivation observed across different fMRI studies (reviewed in the following section). To combat this problem of small sample sizes, funding agencies have recently begun to develop standard clinical definitions, common data elements and informational platforms for creating community-wide data-sharing initiatives (e.g., Federal Interagency Traumatic Brain Injury Research; (FITBIR)). These efforts should accelerate research in this critical area by permitting the pooling of fMRI data for use in meta-analyses.

Review of Current Findings from the Literature

As discussed in previous sections, fMRI offers great promise for elucidating the underlying neuropathology associated with neurobehavioral sequelae following mTBI, especially given its adaptability for use in conjunction with tasks that dynamically tap into higher-order cognitive functioning. The reader is also referred to an excellent review of this topic [8]. The seminal fMRI studies of mTBI utilized working-memory paradigms, with results suggesting a complex relationship between cognitive load and functional activation. In a series of studies on semi-acute (within 1 month of injury) mTBI patients, McAllister and colleagues [34, 35] reported hyperactivation in right dorsolateral prefrontal cortex (DLPFC) and lateral parietal regions for mTBI patients compared to healthy controls under moderate processing loads (1-back to 2-back

conditions), with hypoactivation observed for lower processing loads (0- to 1-back conditions). Additional studies by McAllister et al. [35] confirmed that mTBI patients exhibited frontoparietal hyperactivation in the moderate load condition, but also found hypoactivation at higher processing loads (going from 2- to 3-back). Positive correlations between self-report measures of symptom severity and increased activation both within the working-memory network (e.g., dorsolateral and ventrolateral prefrontal cortex) and other regions have been reported by other groups, suggesting potential compensatory activation [36]. In contrast, in a study using both fMRI and event-related potentials, Gosselin et al. [37] reported that mTBI patients had decreased BOLD signal changes in the left and right mid-DLPFC (which correlated with symptom severity), the putamen, the body of the caudate nucleus, and the right thalamus, coupled with a reduced N350 event-related potential amplitude. Additionally, others have observed no significant differences between a relatively large cohort of mTBI patients ($n = 43$) and healthy controls ($n = 20$) on a similar n-back task, instead finding that length of post-traumatic amnesia was related to deactivation of the hippocampus (0-back > 2-back) [38].

Results from fMRI studies of working memory using concussed athletes have also been conflicting, further demonstrating many of the methodological and interpretive challenges involved in functional imaging of mTBI patients. In contrast to McAllister's findings of hyperactivation in the right DLPFC, athletes with persistent post-concussive symptoms (PCS) who were imaged while performing both verbal and visual working-memory tasks showed hypoactivation in this region [39, 40]. Chen et al. [40] also reported that the degree of activation was not related to PCS severity and, in general, more diffuse activation patterns were seen in the PCS athlete group. Evidence for a negative correlation between right DLPFC activation and symptom severity but not between DLPFC activation and symptom duration was found in one patient with persistent symptoms who was imaged at 6 months, and later at 9 months when symptoms had improved. A further study provided support for the correlation between PCS symptom severity and bilateral DLPFC hypoactivation, using a whole-brain analysis to compare 9 low and 9 high PCS severity patients on a verbal working-memory task [41]. Interestingly, a study of asymptomatic high school and college athletes (mean time post recovery = approximately 9 months) found no differences in regional brain activation during the n-back task [42]. The multiple methodological differences between these findings, including auditory versus visual working memory, athletes versus emergency room patients, time post injury and operational definitions of symptom severity, may provide a context for elucidating the basis of these discrepant findings.

Additional examples of hyperactivation measured with fMRI during task-based paradigms have also been reported. Using a pre- vs. post-injury design, Jantzen et al. showed hyperactivation of frontal regions post injury even in the absence of cognitive performance differences on a variety of neurocognitive tests, suggestive of a compensatory mechanism [43].

Another study found that the degree of abnormal hyperactivation may be indicative of a prolonged recovery profile in athletes, particularly when accompanied by more sparse and diffuse activation patterns [44]. It has been proposed that sub-concussive hits also contribute to the development of chronic traumatic encephalopathy (CTE), based on the high frequency of American-rules football offensive linemen in post-mortem neuropathological cases [4]. Similarly, recent fMRI findings suggest that significant neuropathological changes may be missed if studies of sports-related head injuries focus only on diagnosed concussions. To investigate the effects of such sub-concussive hits, high school football athletes were scanned both pre and post season with embedded sensors in their helmets to tally the number of head hits throughout the season. Results in this study by Talavage and colleagues demonstrated that prolonged exposure to sub-concussive hits resulted in hypoactivation within left middle and superior temporal gyri, left middle occipital gyrus, and bilateral cerebellum during an *n*-back working-memory task [45]. Interestingly, they also showed that this pattern of decreased activity correlated with poorer working-memory performance in the non-concussed high school football players.

Several evoked fMRI studies have also examined attentional and memory functioning following mTBI. Increased activation during attention tasks within the anterior cingulate gyrus, inferior frontal gyrus, insula, and posterior parietal areas with an increased incidence of PCS was reported by Smits and colleagues [36]. In contrast, results from our lab (Figure 22.1) have indicated hypoactivation within several deep cortical, cerebellar, and sub-cortical sites during an auditory attention task in independent adult [46] and pediatric mTBI [47] cohorts. Within-group comparisons also indicated decreased frontoparietal activation for mTBI patients during more attentionally demanding conditions [48].

Similarly, we have also observed aberrant task-induced deactivation within the default-mode network (DMN) (Figure 22.2A) [48] in addition to decreased cortical activation (Figure 22.2B) for mTBI patients (within-subject comparisons) during a multimodal numeric Stroop task [48]. During detection of novel stimuli in a three-stimulus (standard, target, and novel stimuli) auditory oddball paradigm with low attentional demand, mTBI patients in another study exhibited decreased activation in the DMN and increased activation in right superior and inferior parietal areas [49]. A ROI analysis also suggested that mTBI patients exhibited less activity in right DLPFC compared to healthy controls during detection of target stimuli. Finally, increased volumes of activity within the DLPFC, parietal cortex, and hippocampus were reported in a spatial memory task for recently concussed athletes relative to non-concussed healthy controls [50].

The effects of various treatments on BOLD activity following mTBI are only beginning to be explored. To investigate whether pharmacological challenges to the dopaminergic system may explain abnormalities in the working-memory circuitry following mTBI, McAllister and colleagues examined performance during the *n*-back task following the administration of bromocriptine (a dopamine agonist) compared

to placebo. The authors reported that, while healthy control performance improved, mTBI patients did not show any behavioral improvement [51]. Moreover, healthy controls had higher activation in areas involved in working memory relative to patients in both drug conditions; in contrast, mTBI patients on bromocriptine instead had higher activation in areas outside this working-memory network. When mTBI patients were placed on guanfacine, which indirectly affects dopamine transmission, a similar complex pattern of activations was observed within the working-memory circuitry [52]. Following cognitive rehabilitation therapy on visually guided saccades and reading comprehension tasks, a relatively small sample of mTBI patients also exhibited both increased and decreased activations [53]. Though in their preliminary stages, these studies suggest that BOLD-based activity may offer a mechanism for non-invasively measuring how treatment affects disrupted neurophysiology following mTBI.

In addition to studies of evoked BOLD activity, researchers are increasingly turning to measures of intrinsic activity, or functional connectivity (fcMRI), to examine neuronal health following mTBI. Connectivity studies are based on neuronal fluctuations that occur synchronously over spatially distributed networks, and are found in both humans and animals. The majority (60–80%) of the brain's energy resources is expended to maintain homeostasis, with intrinsic neuronal activity likely contributing to this heavy metabolic load [54]. Previous research indicates that, following TBI, changes in baseline metabolism occur, as well as abnormal slow-wave electrophysiological activity during passive mental activities [55, 56], providing biological relevance for fcMRI as a biomarker of mTBI.

These intrinsic fluctuations in neuronal activity tend to alias towards lower frequencies (0.01–0.10 Hz) in the BOLD signal, and therefore can be measured on any MRI scanner with a conventional echo-planar sequence. During these "resting-state" scans, participants are asked to either fixate on a visual stimulus or close their eyes for a relatively brief period of time (approximately 5 minutes). As a consequence of the simplicity of these instructions, resting-state paradigms have been criticized based on the general lack of control over participants' mental activities and the inability to specify what cognitive tasks the participant actually performed during data collection. A second criticism of resting-state scans is that by definition mTBI participants are not asked to perform difficult cognitive tasks. Cognitive challenges are typically of greater interest to clinicians given that mTBI patients tend to report more difficulties under conditions of high cognitive load in everyday life. A third critique of resting-state studies is that the various analytic approaches (e.g., seed-based analysis vs. independent component analysis (ICA) vs. graph theory metrics) that are used to parse network activation can result in different findings during data analyses of the same subjects. Finally, noise has a more direct influence on fcMRI relative to evoked studies due to the lack of independent predictor variables [57], resulting in further complications when interpreting group results.

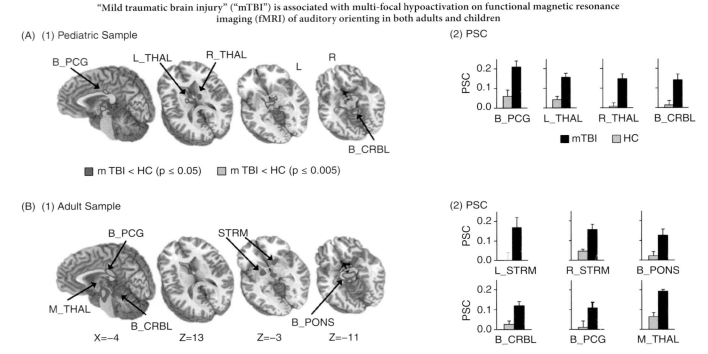

"Mild traumatic brain injury" ("mTBI") is associated with multi-focal hypoactivation on functional magnetic resonance imaging (fMRI) of auditory orienting in both adults and children

Fig. 22.1 Regions of hypoactivation during an auditory orienting task across independent samples of pediatric and adult mTBI patients relative to age- and education-matched healthy controls (HC). (A.1) Regions showing significantly reduced activity for pediatric mTBI patients, with the magnitude of p-values denoted by either blue or cyan coloring. Locations of the sagittal (X) and axial (Z) slices are given according to the Talairach atlas (L: left; R: right) and are identical across both pediatric and adult samples. (A.2) Percent signal change (PSC) data for selected regions for both patient (black bars) and control (gray bars) groups. Decreased activation for pediatric mTBI patients was observed within bilateral posterior cingulate gyrus (B_PCG), left and right thalamus (L_THAL, R_THAL) extending into the basal ganglia, and bilateral cerebellum (B_CRBL). Data from adult mTBI patients and matched HC are presented in an identical scheme in B.1 and B.2. Clusters of decreased activation for the adult mTBI sample included the posterior cingulate gyrus (PCG), right and left striatum (STRM), pons and midbrain nuclei (PONS), cerebellum (CRBL), and thalamus (THAL). Error bars correspond to the standard error of mean. [A black and white version of this figure will appear in some formats. For the color version, please refer to the plate section.]

Source: Yang et al., 2012 [47]. Reproduced with permission from Mary Ann Liebert, Inc.

However, resting-state scans also have several advantages over more traditional evoked activation studies, and may eliminate several potential confounds associated with cognitive tasks. Foremost, by using a relatively simple task (i.e., passively maintaining fixation), the neuronal integrity of multiple sensory, motor, and cognitive networks can be probed. Specifically, Smith and colleagues demonstrated that intrinsic neuronal activity measured in 36 participants was organized into distinct networks that mirrored activity evoked across a variety (30,000 archival data sets) of cognitive tasks [58]. Second, fcMRI can be used across the entire TBI spectrum (e.g., mildest injury to minimally conscious patients), as has already been demonstrated by several research groups [59]. Third, fcMRI eliminates the complex requirements for presenting sensory stimuli and monitoring motor responses (e.g., interfacing with a computer, projecting stimuli, special non-ferrous motor response devices), making it more feasible to perform fcMRI in both clinical and research settings.

Fourth, the passive nature of resting-state scans (eyes closed or maintaining fixation) reduces some of the non-specific effects of trauma (e.g., poor effort, effects of pain, and fatigue) associated with studies of evoked activity. Fifth, differences in task performance can complicate the interpretation of BOLD-related activity. Specifically, it is impossible to disambiguate whether BOLD differences result from trauma-induced alterations in neurophysiology, from task–performance differences (e.g., accuracy or reaction time), or from a combination of these effects. Similarly, interpretation of data from task-based studies is also frequently complicated by learning and/or practice effects, which are minimal during passive rest. Regardless of design (task versus resting-state), recruiting orthopedically injured patients as controls can also reduce several of the non-specific effects associated with trauma (e.g., pain and fatigue), and provide a better control for medication issues.

The majority of connectivity studies conducted in mTBI patients have focused on the DMN. The DMN is characterized by nodes in the rostral anterior cingulate gyrus/ventromedial prefrontal cortex (rACC), posterior cingulate gyrus (PCC), and superior temporal/supramarginal gyrus (SMG), with the rACC and PCC serving as central hubs [60]. This network is believed to mediate a variety of mental activities such as episodic memory review and future-oriented thought processes that occur during periods of unconstrained mental activity. The degree of DMN deactivation varies parametrically with task difficulty during evoked studies [61] and is predictive of attentional lapses during cognitively demanding tasks [62]. Additionally, DMN BOLD signals are negatively correlated (i.e., anti-correlated) with activation in lateral frontal/posterior parietal networks typically associated with a variety of cognitive tasks [63], and both

Deactivation within default-mode network and decreased cortical activation in "mild traumatic brain injury" ("mTBI") patients during Stroop

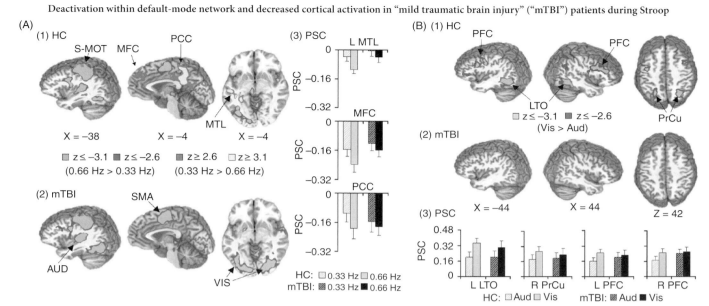

Fig. 22.2 Regions showing differential within-group activation between low- (0.33 Hz) and high- (0.66 Hz) frequency trials and between attend-visual (VIS) and attend-auditory (AUD) conditions for healthy controls (HC: panels A.1 and B.1, respectively) and adult mTBI patients (panels A.2 and B.2, respectively). The overall task involved a multisensory Stroop task during which congruent and incongruent stimuli (auditory and visual numbers) were presented at low or high frequencies. The main effect of frequency (panels A.1 and A.2) indicated increased activation during high-frequency (blue/cyan coloring) trials for both groups within the bilateral primary and secondary auditory cortex (AUD), visual cortex (VIS), bilateral supplemental motor area (SMA), and bilateral sensorimotor cortex (S-MOT). In contrast, only HC demonstrated significantly greater deactivation within the default-mode network for high- compared to low-frequency (red/yellow coloring) trials. The regions included the left medial temporal lobes (L MTL), bilateral medial frontal cortex (MFC), and bilateral posterior cingulate gyrus (PCC), with percent signal change data (PSC) presented in panel A.3 (mTBI patients (black bars) and HC (gray bars) during low-(striped bars) and high- (solid bars) frequency trials). Importantly, PSC for regions of interest were determined solely based on the unique areas of deactivation from HC in statistical parametric maps (panel A.1 red/yellow regions). Increased activation for HC (panel B.1) but not mTBI patients (panel B.2) was observed in the bilateral prefrontal cortex (PFC), "what" (lateral temporal-occipital cortex; LTO) and "where" (precuneus/cuneus; PrCu) pathways during the VIS relative to AUD conditions. PSC values for selected regions are presented in panel B.3 for both mTBI (black bars) and HC (gray bars) during AUD (striped bars) and VIS (solid bars) conditions based on selected regions from panel B.1 (HC group only). The magnitudes of z-scores are color-coded for all comparisons across all maps, with the locations of sagittal (X) and axial (Z) slices provided according to the Talairach atlas. Error bars in panels A.3 and B.3 correspond to the standard error of the mean. [A black and white version of this figure will appear in some formats. For the color version, please refer to the plate section.]

Source: Mayer et al., 2012 [48]. Reprinted by permission from Springer

demonstrate more variable connectivity to other networks [64]. This finding suggests that the DMN and frontoparietal networks may act in conjunction to produce states of high (decreased DMN/increased frontoparietal activity) or low (increased DMN/decreased frontoparietal activity) attentiveness to external events.

In mTBI patients, reduced connectivity has been reported within the DMN in the semi-acute phase using a seed-based approach, with additional findings of increased connectivity between the rACC and ventrolateral prefrontal cortex [10]. These connectivity abnormalities remained relatively stable when retested approximately four months post injury, in spite of normal recovery on neuropsychological evaluations and reduced self-reported symptoms. Another study utilizing ICA reported reduced connectivity in the posterior hubs (PCC and SMG) of the DMN in conjunction with increased connectivity within the ventromedial prefrontal cortex [65]. Similarly, generally reduced connections across multiple nodes of the DMN have been reported in recently concussed athletes relative to healthy controls, as well as a larger departure from typical DMN connectivity as a function of the number of previous concussions [9]. However, a subsequent study by the same group did not find any significant differences within DMN

connectivity unless a physical stress challenge was presented to recently concussed athletes [66].

Functional connectivity studies have revealed abnormalities in other networks aside from the DMN following mTBI. Disrupted interhemispheric fcMRI in the visual cortex, hippocampus, and DLPFC during task-based connectivity analyses [67], as well as decreased symmetry of connectivity based on thalamic seeds [68] has been reported. Another group used ICA to investigate fcMRI following mTBI [69], reporting decreased functional connectivity within the motor-striatal network and increased connectivity in the right frontoparietal network. Finally, disrupted (both increased and decreased) connectivity in 30 semi-acutely injured mTBI patients across 12 different sensory and cognitive networks have been reported in a group of patients with persistent post-concussive syndrome [70]. The variety of target networks investigated and reported on by these authors supports the view that fcMRI is well poised for interrogating connectivity within all major structures and networks of the brain following mTBI.

Multimodal neuroimaging studies, which incorporate various imaging technologies in addition to standard BOLD imaging, have recently been used to examine physiological changes following mTBI. For example, Matthews and colleagues used combined DTI and fMRI to examine differences in amygdala activation in response to emotional faces in concussed veterans of Operations Enduring Freedom and Iraqi Freedom with and without depressive symptoms [71]. fMRI results demonstrated decreased activity in the amygdala in veterans with depressive symptoms, which was associated with lower fractional anisotropy (FA) in several white-matter tracts, suggesting that functional disruption may be the direct result of white-matter pathology. In contrast, we observed increased FA within white-matter tracts connecting the DMN and frontal areas [7]. Unlike fcMRI measures, FA showed some evidence of normalization across a four-month recovery period in our study. Future work incorporating simultaneously acquired electrophysiological measures and fMRI will provide unheralded access to brain functioning following mTBI. The combination of these complementary techniques will afford both high spatial resolution and temporal fidelity, as well as simultaneously measure different aspects of neuronal and vascular response.

Overarching Clinical Challenges in fMRI Research following mTBI

The previous sections briefly introduced several challenges for conducting fMRI studies following mTBI, which are reviewed in greater detail here. Perhaps the largest challenge facing the field of concussion research is the various definitions for diagnosing "mTBI," which are still being actively debated by multiple governing bodies [72, 73]. Under these various nosologies, patients who are only dazed following a blow to the head, patients who are unconscious for up to 30 minutes, and patients with large subdural hematomas can all be currently classified as having experienced a concussion/mTBI. This variety in injury severity complicates direct comparisons across individual studies and the combination of data for meta-analyses. Moreover, the underlying neuropathology, neurobehavioral sequelae, and recovery trajectory are likely to be very different across these three patient types [74]. For all current classification systems, concussions are entirely determined by clinical judgment based self-reported symptoms rather than objective biomarkers. The basis for these classification systems soon becomes circular in nature, as the lack of objective biomarkers directly propagates the use of differential criteria for the diagnosis of mTBI. It also hampers the progression of evidence-based treatment (e.g., did treatment X cause biomarker Y to change?) and confounds the difficult differential diagnosis that characterizes persistent post-concussive syndrome (e.g., are these symptoms the result of a recent fall or from previous history of depression?).

A second major challenge involves the considerable heterogeneity in time post injury during which mTBI patients are recruited both within and across different fMRI studies. The temporal dynamics of TBI has been partially elucidated in animal models, demonstrating a complex, multifaceted, and time-varying pattern of pathologies that occurs in the minutes to weeks following injury [25]. In contrast, human mTBI studies frequently utilize very liberal time post-injury inclusion criteria that can range from days to weeks to years post injury. This naturally increases variability in an already heterogeneous condition, but may also result in an over-sampling of mTBI patients with persistent post-concussive syndrome. Specifically, several meta-analyses (as reviewed in Bigler [75]) and large N studies [76, 77] have documented that the majority of single-episode mTBI patients exhibit a rapid and spontaneous recovery within the first few days to weeks post injury *on traditional measures* (see discussion below), with 80–95% of adult patients fully recovered at 3 to 6 months post injury. Although it is imperative to understand why a minority of single-episode mTBI patients remain chronically symptomatic, it is equally critical to recognize that findings from this patient cohort will likely not generalize to the majority of mTBI patients typically evaluated in the emergency room and sports concussion clinics. Thus, more careful analysis and interpretation about what type of subset of mTBI patients are being evaluated by particular fMRI studies is warranted. Importantly, both heterogeneity in time post injury and patient inclusion criteria can be controlled through more stringent experimental design, resulting in more homogeneous samples (i.e., only persistent post-concussive patients, only typically recovering patients, or direct comparisons of both cohorts). These simple improvements in methodology will greatly facilitate advancement of the field.

Similarly, recent evidence suggests that there are likely to be differences in the neuropathology and course of recovery (short and long-term) between patients who receive a single mTBI (e.g., more typically occurring in an emergency room cohort) and patients who received temporally proximal, repetitive mTBIs (e.g., athletes and military personnel). Athletes with a history of concussion report more baseline symptoms than those with no history of concussion [78]. Repeat concussions within the same sports season increase the risk of long-term cognitive and psychiatric dysregulation by 1.5- to three-fold relative to athletes with a single concussive incident, and an initial concussion dramatically increases player's risk for future concussions [79]. Over the lifespan, the cumulative effects of repetitive mTBIs result in a four-fold increase in neurodegenerative disease [80] and a unique neuropathological syndrome (CTE) involving tauopathies in periventricular spaces and deep cortical sulci [4]. These neuropathies tend to aggregate within frontal and medial temporal lobes, and are frequently associated with behavioral disturbances. Animal studies have also confirmed the increased risks of neuropathological incidence and behavioral decline associated with repeat concussions [81], indicating that a detailed history of previous head trauma is critical for any imaging study.

Due to the current lack of objective bio-markers, a third challenge for the field pertains to the self-reporting of post-concussive symptomatology. This is critical for neuroimaging studies, as imaging-based metrics are frequently expected to correlate with patients' self-report from both diagnostic and prognostic perspectives. However, the veracity of self-report is likely to vary as a function of sample. Sports-related populations may under-report neurobehavioral symptoms following concussion in order to return to play [82], with the rate of under-reporting in high school football estimated to be as high as 53% [83]. Multiple sociological barriers may account for the underreporting of concussive symptoms, ranging from a lack of education regarding the seriousness of concussion (parents, players, and coaches), desire not to be removed from play, hesitancy to report symptoms that do not result in significant pain, and stigmatization of concussion as a non-real injury [84]. The peer-pressure to continue play and not report injury is of particular importance in vulnerable populations such as children who may not comprehend and may underestimate the risks involved in continued participation, and in low-socioeconomic areas where participation is perceived as a path to future benefit [85]. In contrast, chronically symptomatic and litigation-seeking patients tend to over-report symptoms [86], especially if there is the potential for financial gain.

A fourth challenge for the field is to recognize that "recovery" may not represent a unitary concept, as it is currently conceptualized in most studies of concussion. For example, in animal models there are clearly different recovery trajectories for various biomarkers [25]. Based on abnormal glutamate levels secondary to excitotoxicity, an animal would be classified as "recovered" within the first minutes of injury, whereas CBF is still typically abnormal up to one week post injury. Similarly, it is likely that different recovery trajectories may characterize self-report and objective biomarkers in human studies of mTBI. Thus, just because someone demonstrates (e.g., cognitive testing) or self-reports recovery following mTBI, it does not necessarily mean that other biomarkers are expected to have returned to baseline. Intuitively, this concept is similar to other injuries such as second-degree skin burns, during which the physical effects of an injury (e.g., scar tissue) are present long-after the patient ceases to report symptoms (e.g., pain). The possibility that neuronal recovery may lag behind the recovery of behavioral and cognitive symptoms [7], and the potential under-reporting of symptoms, further emphasizes the need for objective biomarkers of injury. Otherwise the field risks premature "return to play" decisions, putting players at risk for exacerbated outcomes related to the occurrence of multiple sports-related mTBI [78, 87].

Emotional Sequelae Following mTBI

Of all of the challenges faced in mTBI research, operationalizing the psychiatric sequelae of injury may be the most challenging. Understanding and assessment of mood dysregulation following mTBI is complicated by the possibility of three potentially coexisting, yet distinct, etiological mechanisms. First, predisposition for mood disorder, including family history of mood disorders, has been shown to be a strong factor in the presence and severity of post-concussive symptoms [88]. As discussed in the introduction, this has helped promote a long-standing belief that only mTBI patients with previous psychiatric histories are likely to remain chronically symptomatic. A second etiological mechanism suggests that psychiatric sequelae are an indirect result of events associated with mTBI. These include secondary psychosocial and psychosomatic consequences of the injury (somatoform depression), including decreased ability to perform at a job, poor social functioning, perceived stigma of a non-visible injury and depression secondary to other injuries or losses (e.g., deceased spouse) sustained during the traumatic incident [88, 89].

A final primary etiological path for psychiatric sequelae is a biologically-based disruption of the emotional processing neural network, leading to a more direct effect on neurovascular coupling. Potential pathologies include damage to the network nodes and/or damage to white-matter connections within emotional-processing networks. Secondary events such as neuroinflammation may also contribute by inducing "sickness behavior" [90], and may be critically involved in CTE and post-concussive disorder [91]. Regardless of etiological mechanism, all result in increased negative affect and/or stress, further compromising the hypothalamic–pituitary–adrenal axis. This ultimately results in further dysregulation of emotional-processing networks [92].

Episodes of major depression are the most commonly diagnosed neuropsychiatric complication of mTBI [88, 93]. The incidence of anxiety, depression, and irritability among concussed high school and collegiate athletes ranges between 17% and 46% [94, 95], while base rates of self-reported mood disorders in collegiate athletes are equal to or slightly less (15–30%) than those of typical college students [96]. Although younger athletes with concussion-induced mood sequelae are more likely to report prolonged depressive episodes [97], affective dysregulation from sports-related concussion can persist for years across all ages [98].

This may be best typified by the increased incidence of mood disturbances observed in retired boxers and professional football players with a history of concussion [4]. Other studies have demonstrated that later-life diagnosis of clinical depression is correlated with concussion history [99]. Suicide rates for concussed persons at risk for mood disorder or with a diagnostic history of mood disorder are also significantly elevated [100], as is the suicide rate for those retrospectively diagnosed with CTE [4]. Evidence of long-term affective changes in retired athletes combined with neuroimaging results demonstrating that young concussed athletes with persistent depressive symptoms show decreased activity in emotional-processing networks [39] provide an impetus for developing objective psychiatric metrics for determining neuropsychiatric recovery from concussion. fcMRI measures within the emotional-processing networks may also be a potential method for assisting clinical judgment regarding neuropsychiatric recovery following concussion.

Conclusions

fMRI provides researchers with a powerful tool for non-invasively measuring the functional integrity and modulation of neuronal circuitry in both animal and human models of injury. Evoked fMRI studies capture dynamic changes in brain function during higher-order cognitive and emotional tasks, mimicking the real-world environments under which patients are more likely to complain of symptoms. Thus, fMRI provides a clear advantage relative to other imaging techniques that are only capable of measuring structural integrity (e.g., susceptibility-weighted imaging, DTI). In addition, unlike other functional imaging techniques (electrophysiological and optical imaging), fMRI can be utilized to probe deep gray structures as well as more superficial cortical structures, a powerful advantage given that shear stresses are more likely to accumulate in these regions [101]. However, the sensitivity of fMRI also represents a weakness, as BOLD signals are also more susceptible to non-specific effects of trauma (e.g., pain and fatigue), behavioral performance, effort on testing, and normal day-to-day variations in human behavior. The BOLD signal also represents an indirect measure of neuronal activity, resulting from a complex mixture of many underlying physiological processes that is temporally sluggish. As most of these physiological processes are affected by trauma, it is simply unfeasible to "isolate" a single biological mechanism that underlies an abnormal BOLD response when fMRI is used in isolation [46, 102].

In summary, fMRI has helped reshape our understanding of the neuropathological effects associated with concussion. Given the heterogeneity and "chaos" inherently associated with mTBI research [103], well-powered studies with more homogeneous inclusion criteria (time post injury, injury severity, and past history) are critically needed for truly understanding the underlying pathophysiology and natural recovery course of the injury.

References

1. Pellman EJ, Powell JW, Viano DC, Casson IR, Tucker AM, Feuer H, et al. Concussion in professional football: Epidemiological features of game injuries and review of the literature – Part 3. *Neurosurgery* 2004; 54: 81–94.

2. Hughes DG, Jackson A, Mason DL, Berry E, Hollis S, Yates DW. Abnormalities on magnetic resonance imaging seen acutely following mild traumatic brain injury: Correlation with neuropsychological tests and delayed recovery. *Neuroradiology* 2004; 46: 550–558.

3. Iverson GL. Complicated vs uncomplicated mild traumatic brain injury: Acute neuropsychological outcome. *Brain Inj* 2006; 20: 1335–1344.

4. McKee AC, Stein TD, Nowinski CJ, Stern RA, Daneshva DH, Alvarez VE. et al. The spectrum of disease in chronic traumatic encephalopathy. *Brain* 2012; 136: 43–64.

5. Belanger HG, Vanderploeg RD, Curtiss G, Warden DL. Recent neuroimaging techniques in mild traumatic brain injury. *J Neuropsychiatry Clin Neurosci* 2007; 19: 5–20.

6. Bigler ED, Maxwell WL. Neuropathology of mild traumatic brain injury: Relationship to neuroimaging findings. *Brain Imaging Behav* 2012; 6: 108–136.

7. Mayer AR, Mannell MV, Ling J, Gasparovic C, Yeo RA. Functional connectivity in mild traumatic brain injury. *Hum Brain Mapp* 2011; 32: 1825–1835.

8. McDonald BC, Saykin AJ, McAllister TW. Functional MRI of mild traumatic brain injury (mTBI): Progress and perspectives from the first decade of studies. *Brain Imaging Behav* 2012; 6: 193–207.

9. Johnson B, Zhang K, Gay M, Horovitz S, Hallett M, Sebastianelli W, et al. Alteration of brain default network in subacute phase of injury in concussed individuals: Resting-state fMRI study. *NeuroImage* 2012; 59: 511–518.

10. Mayer AR, Mannell MV, Ling J, Gasparovic C, Yeo RA. Functional connectivity in mild traumatic brain injury. *Hum Brain Mapp* 2011; 32: 1825–1835.

11. Shumskaya E, Andriessen TM, Norris DG, Vos PE. Abnormal whole-brain functional networks in homogeneous acute mild traumatic brain injury. *Neurology* 2012; 79: 175–182.

12. Attwell D, Buchan AM, Charpak S, Lauritzen M, MacVicar BA, Newman EA. Glial and neuronal control of brain blood flow. *Nature* 2010; 468: 232–243.

13. Logothetis NK. What we can do and what we cannot do with fMRI. *Nature* 2008; 453: 869–878.

14. Buxton RB, Uludag K, Dubowitz DJ, Liu TT. Modeling the hemodynamic response to brain activation. *NeuroImage* 2004; 23 (Suppl 1): S220–S233.

15. Schroeter ML, Kupka T, Mildner T, Uludag K, von Cramon DY. Investigating the post-stimulus undershoot of the BOLD signal – A simultaneous fMRI and fNIRS study. *NeuroImage* 2006; 30: 349–358.

16. Lowenstein DH, Thomas MJ, Smith DH, McIntosh TK. Selective vulnerability of dentate hilar neurons following traumatic brain injury: A potential mechanistic link between head trauma and disorders of the hippocampus. *J Neurosci* 1992; 12: 4846–4853.

17. Alwis DS, Yan EB, Morganti-Kossmann MC, Rajan R. Sensory cortex underpinnings of traumatic brain injury deficits. *PLoS One* 2012; 7: e52169.

18. Hartley CE, Varma M, Fischer JP, Riccardi R, Strauss JA, Shah S. et al. Neuroprotective effects of erythropoietin on acute metabolic and pathological changes in experimentally induced neurotrauma. *J Neurosurg* 2008; 109: 708–714.

19. Henry LC, Tremblay S, Leclerc S, Khiat A, Boulanger Y, Ellemberg D. et al. Metabolic changes in concussed American football players during the acute and chronic post-injury phases. *BMC Neurol* 2011; 11: 105.

20. Yeo RA, Gasparovic C, Merideth F, Ruhl D, Doezema D, Mayer AR. A longitudinal proton magnetic resonance spectroscopy study of mild traumatic brain injury. *J Neurotrauma* 2011; 28: 1–11.

21. Park E, Bell JD, Siddiq IP, Baker AJ. An analysis of regional microvascular loss and recovery following two grades of fluid percussion trauma: A role for hypoxia-inducible factors in traumatic brain injury. *J Cereb Blood Flow Metab* 2009; 29: 575–584.

22. Soustiel JF, Sviri GE. Monitoring of cerebral metabolism: Non-ischemic impairment of oxidative metabolism following severe traumatic brain injury. *Neurol Res* 2007; 29: 654–660.

23. Liau J, Liu TT. Inter-subject variability in hypercapnic normalization of the BOLD fMRI response. *NeuroImage* 2009; 45: 420–430.

24. Vespa PM, O'Phelan K, McArthur D, Miller C, Eliseo, M, Hirt D, et al. Pericontusional brain tissue exhibits persistent elevation of lactate/pyruvate ratio independent of cerebral perfusion pressure. *Crit Care Med* 2007; 35: 1153–1160.

25. Giza CC, Hovda DA. The neurometabolic cascade of concussion. *J Athl Train* 2001; 36: 228–235.

26. Liang Z, King J, Zhang N. Uncovering intrinsic connectional architecture of functional networks in awake rat brain. *J Neurosci* 2011; 31: 3776–3783.

27. McAllister TW, Stein MB. Effects of psychological and biomechanical trauma on brain and behavior. *Ann N Y Acad Sci* 2010; 1208: 46–57.

28. Bazarian JJ, Zhu T, Blyth B, Borrino A, Zhong J. Subject-specific changes in brain white matter on diffusion tensor imaging after sports-related concussion. *Magn Reson Imaging* 2012; 30: 171–180.

29. Kim N, Branch CA, Kim M, Lipton ML. Whole brain approaches for identification of microstructural abnormalities in individual patients: Comparison of techniques applied to mild traumatic brain injury. *PLoS One* 2013; 8: e59382.

30. Mayer A, Toulouse T, Klimaj S, Ling J, Pena A, Bellgowan P. Investigating the properties of the hemodynamic response function following mild traumatic brain injury. *J Neurotrauma* 2014; 31: 189–197.

31. Palmer HS, Garzon B, Xu J, Berntsen EM, Skandsen T, Haberg AK. Reduced fractional anisotropy does not change the shape of the hemodynamic response in survivors of severe traumatic brain injury. *J Neurotrauma* 2010; 27: 853–862.

32. Logothetis NK. What we can do and what we cannot do with fMRI. *Nature* 2008; 453: 869–878.

33. Desmond JE, Glover GH. Estimating sample size in functional MRI (fMRI) neuroimaging studies: Statistical power analyses. *J Neurosci Methods* 2012; 118: 115–128.

34. McAllister TW, Saykin AJ, Flashman LA, Sparling MB, Johnson SC, Guerin SJ, et al. Brain activation during working memory 1 month after mild traumatic brain injury: A functional MRI study. *Neurology* 1999; 53: 1300–1308.

35. McAllister TW, Sparling MB, Flashman LA, Guerin SJ, Mamourian AC, Saykin AJ. Differential working memory load effects after mild traumatic brain injury. *NeuroImage* 2001; 14: 1004–1012.

36. Smits M, Dippel DW, Houston GC, Wielopolski PA, Koudstaal PJ, Hunink MG, et al. Postconcussion syndrome after minor head injury: Brain activation of working memory and attention. *Hum Brain Mapp* 2008; 30: 2789–2803.

37. Gosselin N, Bottari C, Chen JK, Petrides M, Tinawi S, de Guise E, et al. Electrophysiology and functional MRI in post-acute mild traumatic brain injury. *J Neurotrauma* 2011; 28: 329–341.

38. Stulemeijer M, Vos PE, van der Werf S, Van DG, Rijpkema M, Fernandez G. How mild traumatic brain injury may affect declarative memory performance in the post-acute stage. *J Neurotrauma* 2010; 27: 1585–1595.

39. Chen JK, Johnston KM, Frey S, Petrides M, Worsley K, Ptito A. Functional abnormalities in symptomatic concussed athletes: An fMRI study. *NeuroImage* 2004; 22: 68–82.

40. Chen JK, Johnston KM, Collie A, McCrory P, Ptito A. A validation of the post concussion symptom scale in the assessment of complex concussion using cognitive testing and functional MRI. *J Neurol Neurosurg Psychiatry* 2007; 78: 1231–1238.

41. Chen JK, Johnston KM, Petrides M, Ptito A. Neural substrates of symptoms of depression following concussion in male athletes with persisting postconcussion symptoms. *Arch Gen Psychiatry* 2008; 65: 81–89.

42. Elbin RJ, Covassin T, Hakun J, Kontos AP. Berger K, Pfeiffer K, et al. Do brain activation changes persist in athletes with a history of multiple concussions who are asymptomatic? *Brain Inj* 2012; 26: 1217–1225.

43. Jantzen KJ, Anderson B, Steinberg FL, Kelso JA. A prospective functional MR imaging study of mild traumatic brain injury in college football players. *AJNR Am J Neuroradiol* 2004; 25: 738–745.

44. Lovell MR, Pardini JE, Welling J, Collins MW, Bakal J, Lazar N, et al. Functional brain abnormalities are related to clinical recovery and time to return-to-play in athletes. *Neurosurgery* 2007; 61: 352–359.

45. Talavage TM, Nauman E, Breedlove EL, Yoruk U, Dye AE, Morigaki K, et al. Functionally-detected cognitive impairment in high school football players without clinically-diagnosed concussion. *J Neurotrauma* 2014; 31: 327–338.

46. Mayer AR, Mannell MV, Ling J, Elgie R, Gasparovic C, Phillips JP, et al. Auditory orienting and inhibition of return in mild traumatic brain injury: A FMRI study. *Hum Brain Mapp* 2009; 30: 4152–4166.

47. Yang Z, Yeo R, Pena A, Ling J, Klimaj S, Campbell R, et al. A fMRI study of auditory orienting and inhibition of return in pediatric mild traumatic brain injury. *J Neurotrauma* 2012; 26: 2124–2136.

48. Mayer AR, Yang Z, Yeo RA, Pena A, Ling JM, Mannell MV, et al. A functional MRI study of multimodal selective attention following mild traumatic brain injury. *Brain Imaging Behav* 2012; 6: 343–354.

49. Witt ST, Lovejoy DW, Pearlson GD, Stevens MC. Decreased prefrontal cortex activity in mild traumatic brain injury during performance of an auditory oddball task. *Brain Imaging Behav* 2010; 4: 232–247.

50. Slobounov SM, Zhang K, Pennell D, Ray W, Johnson B, Sebastianelli W. Functional abnormalities in normally appearing athletes following mild traumatic brain injury: A functional MRI study. *Exp Brain Res* 2010; 202: 341–354.

51. McAllister TW, Flashman LA, McDonald BC, Ferrell RB, Tosteson TD, Yanofsky NN, et al. Dopaminergic challenge with bromocriptine one month after mild traumatic brain injury: Altered working memory and BOLD response. *J Neuropsychiatry Clin Neurosci* 2011; 23: 277–286.

52. McAllister TW, McDonald BC, Flashman LA, Ferrell RB, Tosteson TD, Yanofsky NN, et al. Alpha-2 adrenergic challenge with guanfacine one month after mild traumatic brain injury: Altered working memory and BOLD response. *Int J Psychophysiol* 2011; 82: 107–114.

53. Laatsch LK, Thulborn KR, Krisky CM, Shobat DM, Sweeney JA. Investigating the neurobiological basis of cognitive rehabilitation therapy with fMRI. *Brain Inj* 2004; 18: 957–974.

54. Raichle ME, Mintun MA. Brain work and brain imaging. *Annu Rev Neurosci* 2006; 29: 449–476.

55. Huang MX, Nichols S, Robb A, Angeles A, Drake A, Holland M, et al. An automatic MEG low-frequency source imaging approach for detecting injuries in mild and moderate TBI patients with blast and non-blast causes. *NeuroImage* 2012; 61: 1067–1082.

56. Lewine JD, Davis JT, Bugler ED, Thoma R, Hill D, Funke M, et al. Objective documentation of traumatic brain injury subsequent to mild head trauma: Multimodal brain imaging with MEG, SPECT, and MRI. *J Head Trauma Rehabil* 2007; 22: 141–155.

57. Saad ZS, Gotts SJ, Murphy K, Chen G, Jo HJ, Martin A, et al. Trouble at rest: How correlation patterns and group differences become distorted after global signal regression. *Brain Connect* 2012; 2: 25–32.

58. Smith SM, Fox PT, Miller KL, Glahn DC, Fox PM, Mackay CE, et al. Correspondence of the brain's functional architecture during activation and rest. *PNAS* 2009; 106: 13040–13045.

59. Bonnelle V, Leech R, Kinnunen KM, Ham TE, Beckmann CF, De Boissezon X, et al. Default mode network connectivity predicts

sustained attention deficits after traumatic brain injury. *J Neurosci* 2011; 31: 13442–13451.

60. Buckner RL, Andrews-Hanna J, Schacter D. The brain's default network: Anatomy, function, and relevance to disease. *Ann NY Acad Sci* 2008; 1124: 1–38.

61. Binder JR, Frost JA, Hammeke TA, Bellgowan PS, Rao SM, Cox RW. Conceptual processing during the conscious resting state: A functional MRI study. *J Cogn Neurosci* 1999; 11: 80–95.

62. Eichele T, Debener S, Calhoun VD, Specht K, Engel AK, Hugdahl K, et al. Prediction of human errors by maladaptive changes in event-related brain networks. *PNAS* 2008; 105: 6173–6178.

63. Fox MD, Snyder AZ, Vincent JL, Corbetta M, Van E, Raichle ME. The human brain is intrinsically organized into dynamic, anticorrelated functional networks. *PNAS* 2005; 102: 9673–9678.

64. Allen EA, Damaraju E, Plis SM, Erhardt EB, Eichele T, Calhoun VD. Tracking whole-brain connectivity dynamics in the resting state. *Cereb Cortex* 2012; 24: 663–676.

65. Zhou Y, Milham MP, Lui YW, Miles L, Reaume J, Sodickson DK, et al. Default-mode network disruption in mild traumatic brain injury. *Radiology* 2012; 265: 882–892.

66. Zhang L, Yang KH, King AI. A proposed injury threshold for mild traumatic brain injury. *J Biomech Eng* 2004; 126: 226–236.

67. Slobounov SM, Gay M, Zhang K, Johnson B, Pennell D, Sebastianelli W, et al. Alteration of brain functional network at rest and in response to YMCA physical stress test in concussed athletes: RsFMRI study. *NeuroImage* 2011; 55: 1716–1727.

68. Tang L, Ge Y, Sodickson DK, Miles L, Zhou Y, Reaume J, et al. Thalamic resting-state functional networks: Disruption in patients with mild traumatic brain injury. *Radiology* 2011; 260: 831–840.

69. Shumskaya E, Andriessen TM, Norris DG, Vos PE. Abnormal whole-brain functional networks in homogeneous acute mild traumatic brain injury. *Neurology* 2012; 79: 175–182.

70. Stevens MC, Lovejoy D, Kim J, Oakes H, Kureshi I, Witt ST. Multiple resting state network functional connectivity abnormalities in mild traumatic brain injury. *Brain Imag Behav* 2012; 6: 293–318.

71. Matthews SC, Strigo IA, Simmons AN, O'Connell RM, Reinhardt LE, Moseley SA. A multimodal imaging study in U.S. veterans of Operations Iraqi and Enduring Freedom with and without major depression after blast-related concussion. *NeuroImage* 2011; 54 (Suppl 1): S69–S79.

72. Ruff RM, Iverson GL, Barth JT, Bush SS, Broshek DK. Recommendations for diagnosing a mild traumatic brain injury: A National Academy of Neuropsychology education paper. *Arch Clin Neuropsychol* 2009; 24: 3–10.

73. West TA, Marion DW. Current recommendations for the diagnosis and treatment of concussion in sport: A comparison of three new guidelines. *J Neurotrauma* 2014; 31: 159–168.

74. Kashluba S, Hanks RA, Casey JE, Millis SR. Neuropsychologic and functional outcome after complicated mild traumatic brain injury. *Arch Phys Med Rehabil* 2008; 89: 904–911.

75. Bigler ED. Neuropsychology and clinical neuroscience of persistent post-concussive syndrome. *J Int Neuropsychol Soc* 2008; 14: 1–22.

76. McCrea M, Guskiewicz KM, Marshall SW, Barr W, Randolph C, Cantu RC, et al. Acute effects and recovery time following concussion in collegiate football players: The NCAA Concussion Study. *JAMA* 2003; 290: 2556–2563.

77. McCrea M, Guskiewicz K, Randolph C, Barr WB, Hammeke TA, Marshall SW, et al. Incidence, clinical course, and predictors of prolonged recovery time following sport-related concussion in high school and college athletes. *J Int Neuropsychol Soc* 2013; 19: 22–33.

78. Harmon KG, Drezner JA, Gammons M, Guskiewicz KM, Halstead M, Herring SA, et al. American Medical Society for Sports Medicine position statement: Concussion in sport. *Br J Sports Med* 2013; 47: 15–26.

79. Guskiewicz KM, McCrea M, Marshall SW, Cantu RC, Randolph C, Barr W, et al. Cumulative effects associated with recurrent concussion in collegiate football players: The NCAA Concussion Study. *JAMA* 2003; 290: 2549–2555.

80. Lehman EJ, Hein MJ, Baron SL, Gersic CM. Neurodegenerative causes of death among retired National Football League players. *Neurology* 2012; 79: 1970–1974.

81. Friess SH, Ichord RN, Ralston J, Ryall K, Helfaer MA, Smith C, et al. Repeated traumatic brain injury affects composite cognitive function in piglets. *J Neurotrauma* 2009; 26: 1111–1121.

82. Greenwald RM, Chu JJ, Beckwith JG, Crisco JJ. A proposed method to reduce underreporting of brain injury in sports. *Clin J Sport Med* 2012; 22: 83–85.

83. McCrea M, Hammeke T, Olsen G, Leo P, Guskiewicz K. Unreported concussion in high school football players: Implications for prevention. *Clin J Sport Med* 2004; 14: 13–17.

84. Chrisman SP, Quitiquit C, Rivara FP. Qualitative study of barriers to concussive symptom reporting in high school athletics. *J Adolesc Health* 2013; 52: 330–335.

85. Gilbert F, Johnson LS. The impact of American tackle football-related concussion in youth athletes. *AJOB Neurosci* 2011; 2: 48–59.

86. Bianchini KJ, Curtis KL, Greve KW. Compensation and malingering in traumatic brain injury: A dose–response relationship? *Clin Neuropsychol* 2006; 20: 831–847.

87. Guskiewicz KM, Marshall SW, Bailes J, McCrea M, Harding HP Jr, Matthews A, et al. Recurrent concussion and risk of depression in retired professional football players. *Med Sci Sports Exerc* 2007; 39: 903–909.

88. Dikmen SS, Bombardier CH, Machamer JE, Fann JR, Temkin NR. Natural history of depression in traumatic brain injury. *Arch Phys Med Rehabil* 2004; 85: 1457–1464.

89. Bay E, Kirsch N, Gillespie B. Chronic stress conditions do explain posttraumatic brain injury depression. *Res Theory Nurs Pract* 2004; 18: 213–228.

90. Dantzer R, O'Connor JC, Lawson MA, Kelley KW. Inflammation-associated depression: From serotonin to kynurenine. *Psychoneuroendocrinol* 2011; 36: 426–436.

91. Blaylock RL, Maroon J. Immunoexcitotoxicity as a central mechanism in chronic traumatic encephalopathy – A unifying hypothesis. *Surg Neurol Int* 2011; 2: 107.

92. Erickson K, Drevets W, Schulkin J. Glucocorticoid regulation of diverse cognitive functions in normal and pathological emotional states. *Neurosci Biobehav Rev* 2003; 27: 233–246.

93. Kreutzer JS, Seel RT, Gourley E. The prevalence and symptom rates of depression after traumatic brain injury: A comprehensive examination. *Brain Inj* 2001; 15: 563–576.

94. Hutchison M, Mainwaring LM, Comper P, Richards DW, Bisschop SM. Differential emotional responses of varsity athletes to concussion and musculoskeletal injuries. *Clin J Sport Med* 2009; 19: 13–19.

95. Schaal K, Tafflet M, Nassif H, Thibault V, Pichard C, Alcotte M, et al. Psychological balance in high level athletes: Gender-based differences and sport-specific patterns. *PLoS One* 2011; 6: e19007.

96. American College of Health Association. *American College Health Association – National college health assessment II: Reference group executive summary fall 2011.* Hanover, MD: American College Health Association, 2012.

97. Field M, Collins MW, Lovell MR, Maroon J. Does age play a role in recovery from sports-related concussion? A comparison of high school and collegiate athletes. *J Pediatr* 2003; 142: 546–553.

98. Konrad C, Geburek AJ, Rist F, Blumenroth H, Fischer B, Husstedt I, et al. Long-term cognitive and emotional consequences of mild traumatic brain injury. *Psychol Med* 2011; 41: 1197–1211.

99. Guskiewicz KM, Marshall SW, Bailes J, McCrea M, Harding HP Jr., Matthews A, et al. Recurrent concussion and risk of depression in retired professional football players. *Med Sci Sports Exerc* 2007; 39: 903–909.

100. Barnes SM, Walter KH, Chard KM. Does a history of mild traumatic brain injury increase suicide risk in veterans with PTSD? *Rehabil Psychol* 2012; 57: 18–26.

101. Zhang L, Yang KH, King AI. A proposed injury threshold for mild traumatic brain injury. *J Biomech Eng* 2004; 126: 226–236.

102. McDonald BC, Saykin AJ, McAllister TW. Functional MRI of mild traumatic brain injury (mTBI): Progress and perspectives from the first decade of studies. *Brain Imaging Behav* 2012; 6: 193–207.

103. Rosenbaum SB, Lipton ML. Embracing chaos: The scope and importance of clinical and pathological heterogeneity in mTBI. *Brain Imaging Behav* 2012; 6: 255–282.

Civilian Post-Concussive Headache

Nathan D. Zasler, Michael F. Martelli, and Barry D. Jordan

Headache … is common as a sequel to head injuries of all grades of severity, and bears no obvious relation to the amount of gross destructive damage … it will simplify the problem if we limit ourselves to headache occurring as the sequel of head injuries of minor severity … It might be thought that these restrictions of our subject have reduced it to insignificance. This is, however, far from being the case, and it is often of the utmost practical importance to recognise that seriously disabling headache is a common sequel to head injuries of an apparently minor kind

Wilfred Trotter, 1924 [1], p. 935

Introduction

Historically, civilian post-concussive headache (PCH) – meaning headache following a concussive brain injury (CBI) – has been viewed as a singular headache disorder with some quoting an incidence of headache occurring in nearly 90% of certain types of CBIs, and of those, approximately 15% went on to develop a more chronic PCH [2, 3]. Current consensus though seems to be shifting away from an Ockham's razor approach to diagnosis and to a greater appreciation of the diverse biopsychosocial factors that may influence symptom presentation and promulgation. There is also a growing understanding of the potential role of a number of post-traumatic pain generators in PCH [4, 5]. PCH is not just migraine headache. If clinicians treat all PCH as migraine then they will be disappointed in the response rates of their patients. Unfortunately, there are still opinions being published in the scientific literature that demonstrate misperceptions of the causes and treatment of PCH [6], and post-traumatic headache (PTHA) in general, even though there has been a burgeoning of our knowledge on PCH genesis, assessment, and treatment. How exactly specific headache phenotypes differ in different types of civilian CBI (i.e., assaults, vehicular, sports, and whiplash), if at all, has yet to be determined. Additionally, the acute, sub-acute, and chronic variants of PCH have not, as of yet, been rigorously studied as far as incidence, prevalence, etiology, evaluation, treatment, and/or prognosis [7, 8].

Similarly, risk factors for PCH and vulnerabilities for developing chronic PCH have received little attention. Some literature suggests that post-traumatic migraine (PTM) is associated with protracted recovery from sports-related CBI, greater level of post-concussive symptom complaints, as well as more impairment on sub-acute neuropsychological testing

[8–12]. Research examining the impact, if any, of PCH on balance testing via such instruments as the Balance Error Scoring System has interestingly shown disparate results [10, 11].

The effect genetic loading risk factors, pre-existing neck pain, and/or headache-associated whiplash injury, "preparedness" for impact, dizziness, sex, anatomic variables across players and males/females, cultural, affective disorders, and/or characterological traits have on influencing PCH incidence, severity, and duration is unknown. There is some literature, however, that suggests that such factors may indeed be predictive of outcome variables [13–18]. For example, studies have shown that pre-season neck pain, dizziness, and/or headaches may, in and of themselves, be risk factors for subsequent CBI in athletes [17]. PCH can be associated with poorer performance on neuropsychological testing [19], altered sleep efficiency, changes in personality (i.e., irritability and decreased frustration tolerance), as well as depression and anxiety [4, 20].

There remains controversy on the best way to classify PCH, and for that matter PTHA more generally. Use of the current International Headache Society (IHS) International Classification of Headache Disorders (ICHD) system [21] will tend to incorrectly classify many PCHs as migrainous headaches. Whether classification systems, such as IHS ICHD or *International Classification of Diseases and Related Health Problems*, 10th edition (ICD-10) [22] can help in refining our assessment or treatment of any type of PTHA remains to be seen. Additionally, and anecdotally, there has been little correlation between these classification systems and clinical exam findings of patients with PCH [23, 24].

One significant concern when examining the extant literature is the rampant nomenclature misuse across studies as related to brain, head, and neck injuries, as well as the lack of definitional criteria consistency in the PTHA literature. Another common misstep is the unfounded focus on CBI as the sole or main underlying pathoetiologic explanation of PCH. Clinicians should also understand that pre-existing headache disorders and/or headaches due to post-injury causes other than trauma sequelae, such as pharmacologically induced headaches and medication overuse headache (MOH), are not uncommon [25, 26].

There has been a historical lack of a "big-picture view" of PCH, as exemplified most recently by three position papers dealing with sports CBI [27–29], as well as a review article comparing the conclusions of the aforementioned article recommendations [30]. All neglected to stipulate any guidelines or recommendations for PCH prevention, classification, determination of pathoetiology, or methodologies for evaluation or treatment, even though headache remains the most commonly reported somatic complaint following sports concussion. The American Medical Society Sports Medicine Position Statement on Concussion and Sports [29] did include a brief mention of migraines as a risk factor for concussion, as well as concussion being a risk factor for triggering migraine. Headache treatment was also briefly mentioned, including actually noting the fact that there were PTHA subtypes, including migraine, tension, and occipital neuralgia, without any elaboration of any other potential causes of PCH. The guidelines also noted general pharmacological and physical modality interventions but did not stipulate what types of headaches might respond to which specific intervention(s). There are no evidence-based guidelines currently available that deal with classification, physical assessment, and/or treatment of PCH and, for that matter, PTHA, in general [31].

Post-Concussive Headache Pathoetiology and Neurobiology

Potential anatomic sources of head pain that may be relevant in the assessment of a patient presenting with PCH include the dura, venous sinuses, and cranial cavities, including sinuses and eye sockets. The skin, nerves, muscles, and periosteum of the cranium are all pain-sensitive. Cervical/cranial joint capsules (including the temporomandibular joint), cervical facets/ zygapophyseal joints, peripheral nerves (supra-orbital, trochlear, greater occipital, lesser occipital, as well as third occipital nerves), and the cervical sympathetic plexus may all be primary nociceptive pain generators that produce local or referred head pain [4].

Given CBI mechanisms, it is possible to incur various types of trauma to the aforementioned structures, including, but not limited to, impact injuries (both long and short impulse), stretch injuries of various tissues (both rotational and linear), penetrating injuries, shearing/tearing injuries, and compression, as well as herniation-related forces [5]. One of the most common, yet often overlooked, sources of head pain following CBI is referred cervical pain typically associated with acceleration deceleration insults or whiplash-associated disorders [32, 33]. Such injuries can produce an array of pain generators, including, but not limited to, myofascial pain emanating from any of the four layers of posterior cervical, as well as anterolateral cervical, musculature, traumatic neuralgias (as noted above), osseous somatic

dysfunction, disc herniation and/or rupture, ligamentous injury, and/or facet joint trauma (with potential for osteoarthropathy and/or traumatic injury to the medial branches of the dorsal ramus). The aforementioned injuries can be seen in the absence of traumatic brain injury (TBI), mild or otherwise, and should always be considered in the context of identifying the specific pain generators contributing to the PCH.

The neurobiology of PCH following a single traumatic insult to the head likely involves cerebral/intracranial, cranial, and/or cervical structures involved with encoding and processing of noxious stimuli. Pain receptors may be activated by tissue injury and inflammation and mediated by bradykinin, serotonin, substance P, histamine, leukotrienes, cytokines, and prostaglandins [4].

There is no consensus on the exact pathophysiology of PTHA generally speaking or, for that matter, PCH. There are likely different mechanisms involved across patients and the potential for multiple pain sources (including psychogenic ones) in the same patient. Some have speculated that central mechanisms involving increased brainstem nociceptive neuropeptides such as calcitonin gene-related peptide and substance P, as well as glial fibrillary acidic protein-positive astrocytes, might be associated with persistent allodynia related to somatosensory cortex injury in a rodent model [34, 35]. Similar to migraine, inducible nitric oxide synthase and calcitonin gene-related peptide have been implicated as at least potentially contributory to mediating allodynia in PCH/PTHA. Others have speculated that the pathophysiology of PTHA is shared with the pathophysiology of brain injury itself relative to inflammatory responses. These could persist beyond timeframes for actual beneficial physiological effect leading to secondary injuries due to alterations in neuronal excitability, axonal integrity, central processing, as well as other changes [36]. That being said, poor correlation between injury severity parameters and type, frequency, severity, and duration of PTHA seemingly begs the question of whether other non-CBI/TBI pain generators and/or mechanisms are involved in both the origin of PCH/PTHA pain and/or its perpetuation.

The pathogenesis of migraine may be secondary to pain-producing structures in the cranium associated with a disturbance or altered function in subcortical aminergic sensory modulatory systems involving the brainstem, hypothalamic and thalamic structures, resulting in an inherited, episodic disorder of sensory sensitivity [37]. It is generally considered that migraine is a complex, multifactorial disorder, caused by a combination of genetic and environmental factors. Potential genes involved in the susceptibility or pathogenesis of migraine include mutations in the methyltetrahydrofolate reductase (MTHFR), the ATP1A2, the SCN1A, and the CACNA1A genes [37]. Of interest, indirect evidence has linked missense mutations in the CACNA1A calcium channel subunit gene to delayed cerebral edema and fatal coma following mild TBI [38].

The frequency and clinical significance of PCH following repetitive concussion/TBI, especially in "chronic traumatic encephalopathy" (CTE) [39, 40], is not yet clearly delineated.[1]

---

[1] Editor's note: as explained in Chapter 11, on *Late Effects*, chronic traumatic encephalopathy (CTE) means deleterious brain function lasting for six months or more after one or more traumatic brain injuries. Early in the 21st century it became popular to use "CTE" to refer to a rare subtype – the dementia seen after repetitive CBIs. In the present chapter, the authors use the term in the latter sense.

Stern and colleagues identified two clinical phenotypes of CTE based on age at post-mortem examination and retrospective clinical presentation [41]. The behavioral phenotype characterized by a younger age of presentation with a predominant psychiatric component appears to have headache as a more consistent symptom compared to the older cognitive phenotype more typically associated with the development of dementia. Headaches were noted among 38% of the behavioral/mood group compared to 27% of those in the older cognitive group. Clinical characteristics of the headache reported in CTE have not been clearly delineated. There exists an additional point of debate relating to the causal relationship of headache in such cases to CTE itself. There are currently ongoing methodological concerns about CTE research relative to the absence of an asymptomatic group of athletes with a history of multiple concussions who have had brain histological studies done post-mortem to compare with the symptomatic group of concussed players. Randolph [42] noted that recent studies of National Football League (NFL) retirees reported that they had an all-cause mortality rate that was approximately half of the expected rate, and even lower suicide rates. How much can be said about headache in this particular group of patients is debatable; however, McKee and co-authors have noted that headaches were commonly reported by the athlete's families in stages I and II, less commonly in stage III, and not at all in stage IV [40, 43]. The reports, however, were from family members and not the athletes with CTE. No one has examined whether these headaches are psychogenic, tension, cervicogenic, migraine, or some combination of the aforementioned, or of some other origin. Why these headaches would be more common in milder forms of CTE neuropathology than more advanced forms remains unknown; if headache is in fact a by-product of the disorder, then why would this seemingly paradoxical phenomenon occur with advancing disease? Another mystery awaiting an answer.

Classification of Post-Concussive Headache

Current classification systems for PTHA, in general, have much to be desired given their general nature, as well as the empirical basis for the definitional criteria. If one examines the ICHD, 3rd edition [21] or ICD-10 [22], it is readily apparent that there are a number of problems with the currently available/proposed systems for PTHA classification.

The ICHD III classification system uses criteria that are primarily concerned with the temporal onset and pathoetiological relationship of the headache to the trauma and not with the clinical features of the headache condition. ICHD III criteria for PTHA require that headache onset occur within seven days of the traumatic event or regaining consciousness. This temporal-onset criterion appears to have been determined only on the basis of empiricism due to a lack of evidence-based medicine to determine same with an acknowledgment by most of many reported cases having longer lag times prior to headache onset [5, 14]. ICHD distinguishes between acute PTHA (those which persist less than three months after injury) and persistent PTHA (persisting longer than three months). It should be noted, however, that this timeframe is inconsistent

Table 23.1 ICD-10 classification of post-traumatic headaches

5.1 Acute headache attributed to traumatic injury to the head

    5.1.1 Acute headache attributed to moderate or severe traumatic injury to the head

    5.1.2 Acute headache attributed to mild traumatic injury to the head

5.2 Persistent headache attributed to traumatic injury to the head

    5.2.1 Persistent headache attributed to moderate or severe traumatic injury to the head

    5.2.2 Persistent headache attributed to mild traumatic injury to the head

5.3 Acute headache attributed to whiplash

5.4 Persistent headache attributed to whiplash

5.5 Acute headache attributed to craniotomy

5.6 Persistent headache attributed to craniotomy

ICD-10: *International Classification of Diseases and Related Health Problems*, 10th edition [22].

with typical historical definitions of chronic pain, which traditionally define "chronic pain" as pain lasting longer than six months. Each of these conditions is further divided into headache following mild versus severe head trauma (note that "head trauma" and not "brain injury" is used as the phraseology, again confounding not only the definitional criteria, but also research based on same). Whiplash-induced headache is also included in the latest version of the ICHD, but the mechanisms and site of pain generation are not stipulated.

It should also be noted that ICHD defines PTHA as a singular disorder and does not distinguish between headache subtypes, i.e., migraine, tension, neuralgic, and/or cervicogenic or other causes under the post-traumatic rubric, although, all these conditions and others exist as separate primary diagnostic entities in the classification system.

ICD-10 divides PTHA into several broad categories: PTHA, unspecified, acute PTHA, and chronic PTHA (Table 23.1).

Each category is further divided into intractable or not intractable. Although there are classifications for other types of headache that may be applicable to causes of headache after trauma, they would not, by definition, fall under "post-traumatic headache" by ICD-10 criteria. Patients with "minor head trauma and no confirmatory signs" are grouped in a separate classification. The continued use of outdated and unclear terminology such as "minor" and "head trauma" simply adds to nomenclature confusion, further compromising both clinical and research work in this area of brain injury medicine.

Common Post-Concussive and Related Headaches

The following is a brief review of headache subtypes that may be confused with PCH, occur together with PCH, or be the cause of PCH.

Exertional Headache

Exertional headaches tend to be the most common type of sports headache [44, 45]. Sports associated with exertional headache include running/jogging, aerobics, weights/gym exercises, cycling, rugby, and hockey [44, 45] These headaches are rapid in onset, short in duration, and tend to occur in response to maximal or excessive activity near the initiation of exercise. These headaches are usually associated with straining and Valsalva-like maneuvers [46] associated with lifting, pulling, pushing, sexual activity, coughing, or sneezing [47]. These headaches tend to be benign, but may be associated with intracranial pathologies such as Arnold–Chiari malformation, platybasia, basilar impression, subdural hematoma, and brain tumor [48]. They must be differentiated from true PCH which require some type of direct-impact blow or a sudden accelerative or decelerative force applied to the head, neck, and/or body.

Effort-Induced Headache

The distinction between effort-induced headaches and exertional headaches is not clearly delineated in the clinical literature and is often utilized to describe similar entities [45]. Effort-induced headache differs from the traditional exertional headache in that the headaches are gradual in onset and are longer lasting [44, 45]. These headaches tend to be associated with aerobic effort and are exacerbated by dehydration, heat, fatigue, and endurance exercise [44, 45]. The majority of effort-induced headaches may present with a migrainous quality characterized by moderate or severe unilateral pain accompanied by nausea, photophobia, and/or phonophobia [45] and could, therefore, be confused with PCH.

Effort-induced headaches have also been described by patients after concussion when tasked with cognitive demands or exercise and typically present as tension-type headache (TTHA) that is bitemporal or holocephalic. The etiology of this phenomenon is still poorly understood, although regularly seen in clinical practice.

Dehydration Headache

Headaches can also be associated with dehydration, especially in the setting of heat over-exposure and/or hyperthermia. Conditions associated with dehydration such as excessive sweating, vomiting, diarrhea, inadequate water intake, and excessive urination may predispose to headache. Signs of dehydration may include increased thirst, dry mouth, dry skin, sunken eyes, and decreased urine output. Athletes, and persons in general, subject to dehydration are at increased risk of reporting symptoms commonly associated with concussion including headache, dizziness, balance problems, difficulty concentrating, impaired memory, fatigue, and feeling in a "fog" compared to hydrated athletes [49]. It is therefore important not only to maintain hydration, particularly in active sports participation, but also to differentiate such headaches and their associated symptoms from true PCH. Obviously, if someone is dehydrated and gets concussed there can be a confluence of symptoms making clinical assessment more challenging.

Musculoskeletal Headache

Musculoskeletal headache is classically characterized as a cap-like discomfort, but varies with the specifics of the pain generator. Any clinician evaluating a patient with headache following concussion should be familiar with myofascial pain and trigger point referral patterns [50, 51]. Sternocleidomastoid trigger points, for example, may refer pain retro- or periorbitally, whereas, trigger points in the clavicular portion of the sternocleidomastoid muscle can refer to the external ear, causing earache. Musculoskeletal pain may be constant or intermittent, relieved by application of heat, cold, massage, and many over-the-counter medications, including non-steroidal anti-inflammatory drugs (NSAIDs). There may be autonomic components such as dizziness or tinnitus due to specific muscle myofascial dysfunction [51].

Within the broad category of musculoskeletal headache, other etiologies beyond myofascial pain include craniomandibular syndrome, cervical zygapophyseal joint disorders (see section below on cervicogenic headache) with referred facet-mediated pain, and craniovertebral somatic dysfunctions. In craniomandibular disorders, there may be internal derangement of the temporomandibular joint (TMJ), and there is almost always a myofascial element associated with this involving the muscles of mastication (temporalis, pterygoids, or masseters) [52]. TMJ dysfunction or craniomandibular syndrome is almost always seen following direct trauma to the craniomandibular complex when traumatic in origin but has also been associated with cervical whiplash-type injuries. This type of trauma can produce focal headache and is also frequently overlooked as a primary or contributory cause of PCH. In TMJ dysfunction, clicking, popping, or malocclusion of the jaw may be noticed [4].

Cervicogenic Headache

These types of headache may be related to dysfunction of the facet joints, occipital neuralgia, post-traumatic myofascial pain, and/or cervical vertebral somatic dysfunction. Others have hypothesized that chronic pain following cervical acceleration–deceleration-type injuries may be due to central sensitization. Obligatory for the diagnosis is unilateral head pain without side shift and symptoms or signs of cervical involvement, the latter of which could include provocation of pain by neck movement or by external pressure to the upper posterior neck, concurrent cervicalgia, or reduced cervical range of motion. Bilateral occurrence may occur on occasion. Most patients present with unilateral sub-occipital pain, as well as secondary oculofrontotemporal discomfort/pain, particularly when the pain generators in question are more flared. This type of headache is commonly mislabeled as migrainous [53, 54].

Dysfunction of the cervical zygapophyseal joints, particularly at C2 and C3, may refer pain to the head. Familiarity with the cervical root sensory dermatomes and sclerotomes is important in the context of differential diagnostic assessment of such patients. Treatment considerations include intra-articular injection of local anesthetic, or block of the medial branches of the dorsal rami supplying the joint. It is important for clinicians to be able to differentiate referred pain that is dermatomal from referred pain of other origins, including sclerotomal, ligamentous/tendinous, and myofascial.

Craniovertebral somatic dysfunction may occur secondary to trauma and cause headache (both primary and referred). These disorders are typically treated with manual, chiropractic, and/or osteopathic manipulative and/or muscle energy techniques designed to realign dysfunctional units. Careful cervical physical examination is paramount in the context of evaluating any patient with PCH [55]. Cervical mobilization and manipulation may be effective in the treatment of PCH, although there is no well-controlled literature specific to this population. Various manipulative techniques may be used, but caution should be exercised with high-velocity procedures due to risk of cervical fracture and/or vertebral artery injury, which are generally avoided by not mobilizing the neck in extension.

Cervicogenic referred pain is quite a common cause of PCH, although, there is a dearth of literature examining headache subtypes in this group of patients. Some have argued that cervicogenic pathology and referred headache pain are likely the most common causes of PTHA [32]. Studies suggest that, in appropriate cases, manual therapy, exercise, postural education, and blocks (diagnostic, as well as therapeutic) may play important roles in modulating cervicogenic headache pain.

Neuritic and Neuralgic Head Pain

Neuritic scalp pain may occur from local blunt trauma, surgical scalp incision, or penetrating scalp injuries. Occasionally, neuromatous lesions may form after scalp nerve injury and serve as a pain nidus. Pain complaints may vary from dysesthetic "numbness"-type discomfort on touching the affected area of scalp to lancinating-type pain that spontaneously occurs without provocative actions. Neuralgic pain may occur secondary to occipital (greater and/or lesser), third-nerve occipital, supra-orbital, and/or infra-orbital neuralgia as the most common clinical post-traumatic cephalic and/or facial neuralgias seen in clinical practice associated with PTHA, although, other post-traumatic neuralgias/neuropathies may occur.

Occipital neuralgia (ON) may occur following cervical acceleration–deceleration-type injuries, as well as direct trauma to the craniocervical junction. ON may be perpetuated by contraction or myodystonia of the splenius muscle, which it penetrates. Pain is typically felt at the craniocervical junction and the sensory distribution of the nerve (e.g., C2 or C3). The affected nerve is tender to palpation, which generally replicates the pain associated with the headache (e.g., stabbing quality) with numbness in the sensory distribution of the nerve. There is frequently referral of pain into the ipsilateral frontotemporal scalp and less frequently retro-orbitally secondary to ephaptic transmission between the proximal part of the C2 origin of the nerve and the ophthalmic branch of the fifth cranial nerve.

Third occipital nerve headache has also been described and has been shown to be a fairly common cause of chronic post-whiplash headache. The posterior division of the third cervical nerve has a medial branch which runs between the semispinalis capitis and cervicis, and pierces the splenius and trapezius, ending in the skin. While under the trapezius, it gives off a branch called the third occipital nerve, which pierces the trapezius and ends

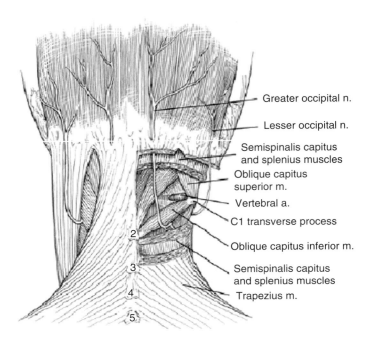

Fig. 23.1 Anatomy of the upper posterior cervical region with specific reference to C2 terminal branches of the greater and lesser occipital nerves.
Source: Zasler et al., 2013 [58]

in the skin of the lower part of the back of the head, lying just medial to the greater occipital nerve and communicating with it.

Whether the etiology is local neuroma formation in scar tissue in the scalp, or a neuralgia, the pharmacological interventions are essentially the same and include NSAIDs, tricyclic antidepressants, and anticonvulsants, particularly gabapentin or pregabalin. Injection of local anesthetic with or without steroid may also be indicated for both diagnostic and therapeutic purposes for neuritic and neuralgic pain disorders [56, 57]. For greater and lesser occipital neuralgia, and in particular, for third occipital nerve headache, clinicians should be familiar with the anatomy of the region given the risk of injection into nearby key vascular structures (Figure 23.1).

In either of the aforementioned situations, myofascial pain may be a secondary or perpetuating pain generator and must be treated concurrently. Another treatment option that has garnered success is the use of topical compounded pain medications, particularly for more diffuse scalp or post-craniotomy or impact injury dysesthetic-type pain.

An exciting treatment option for certain post-traumatic neuralgias is neuromodulation with either implantable units or, more attractively, external units [59–61]. Rarely, surgical decompression or nerve lysis (surgical or via cryotherapy) is necessary for these types of neuralgic cephalalgias, although long-term pain palliation is rarely achieved with surgical intervention.

Tension-Type Headache

TTHA, also known as muscle contraction-type headaches, represent the most common type of headache in the general population. TTHA are typically described as dull, constant, non-throbbing, pressure, or band-like pain originating in the cervical/occipital regions. Unlike migraine, TTHA is not associated with an aura. TTHA does not normally result in nausea or emesis. Uncommonly, TTHA may be associated with increased sensitivity to light and sound.

Per ICHD III, diagnostic categories for TTHA include: infrequent episodic TTHA, frequent episodic TTHA, chronic TTHA, and probable TTHA. Advances in basic pain and clinical research have improved the understanding of the pathophysiologic mechanisms of TTHA. Increased excitability of the central nervous system generated by repetitive and sustained pericranial myofascial input may be responsible for the transformation of episodic TTHA into the chronic form. Muscular and psychogenic factors are believed to be associated with TTHA [4].

Patients with chronic tension headaches have been shown to have a tendency to have lower cortisol levels, postulated to be due to hippocampal atrophy resulting from chronic stress. How such stress might be involved in the pathogenesis of TTHA after TBI is unclear; however, it would certainly seem to be warranted to investigate the interactions of stress post TBI, in its myriad dimensions, with disease pathogenesis and perpetuation. Prior studies have shown that, at least in some series, TTHA is the most common variant of PTHA and was correlated with both physical and psychological (social and/or emotional maladjustment) determinants [62].

The mechanisms by which trauma, whether to the neck, cranium, or cranial adnexal structures or the brain itself, may trigger TTHA are poorly understood. TTHA may result from an interaction between changes in the descending control of second-order trigeminal brainstem nociceptors and interrelated peripheral changes, such as myofascial-mediated pain and/or pericranial muscle nociceptive afferent input. Clearly, stress and negative emotional states (mediated through limbic circuitry) may trigger such headaches through central mechanisms; what role TBI itself has in potentially triggering such headaches in susceptible individuals is less clear. With more frequent episodes of headache, central changes have been theorized to become increasingly more important. With greater duration, long-term sensitization of nociceptive neurons and decreased activity in the anti-nociceptive system gradually leads to chronic TTHA. Current consensus is that peripheral mechanisms are most likely involved in episodic TTHA and central mechanisms play a more important role in chronic TTHA. There is still debate as to whether the pain in TTHA originates from peripheral (e.g., myofascial) versus central origins, with the latter also theorized to occur due to hyperexcitability of the trigeminal caudal nucleus and other structures involved with pain processing [63].

Studies of nitric oxide mechanisms suggest that it may play a key role in the pathophysiology of chronic TTHA by sensitizing pain pathways. Patients with chronic TTHA typically have increased muscle and skin pain sensitivity, demonstrated by decreased mechanical, thermal, and electrical pain thresholds [63]. Abnormal central nervous system pain processing may be linked to hyperexcitability of central nociceptive neurons (both cortically and sub-cortically) and may underlie the pathophysiology of chronic TTHA. Additionally, some have speculated that there may also be a dysfunction in pain-inhibitory systems [64].

Treatment of TTHA should include pharmacotherapy, both acute and prophylactic, as well as non-pharmacologic approaches [62]. The mainstay of acute pharmacotherapy is NSAIDs, sometimes in conjunction with caffeine, sedatives, and/or tranquilizers. Adequate doses of NSAIDs must be utilized prior to labeling a trial as a failure. There is no scientific evidence to support the use of traditional muscle relaxants in TTHA. Prophylactic pharmacotherapy for TTHA is much more diversified, with various drug classes being utilized for treatment, including tricyclic antidepressants, tizanidine, Botulinum toxin, and certain serotonin and norepinephrine reuptake inhibitors such as venlafaxine [65]. Nitric oxide synthase inhibitors may also hold therapeutic promise but are not in clinical use at this time. Non-pharmacological treatments may include relaxation therapy, as well as electromyogram biofeedback, cognitive behavioral therapies, including stress management, limited contact treatment, spinal manipulation [66], physical therapy when appropriate, including postural retraining and muscle trigger point therapies [67], use of modalities such as heat and cold therapies, and lastly, oromandibular treatment in selected patients.

Migraine Headaches

Migraine headaches typically present as unilateral and pounding/throbbing type of pain which may last several hours to days. Although in primary headache there are fairly clear mechanisms established for migraine pathoetiology [37], the same cannot be said for PTM. Classical migraine presents with an aura of a visual and/or sensory disturbance followed by severe headache associated with nausea, vomiting, photophobia, and/or phonophobia. Common migraine presents similarly to the classic migraine; however, without the aura. Complicated migraine may be associated with a persistent neurologic deficit secondary to cerebral infarction.

Migraine headaches can be provoked by a variety of factors, including stress, red wine, light, fumes/heavy scents, hormones, lack of sleep, and physical effort [68]. Effort-induced migraines are typically insidious in onset, usually unilateral, throbbing in nature, and triggered by aerobic exercise. Trauma may also induce migraine headaches; however, the mechanism remains unknown. PTMs exhibit a pounding/throbbing quality and can be associated with a preceding aura followed by severe headache, nausea, and vomiting [47, 48]. The incidence of aura in PCH is unknown. Unlike effort-induced migraine, which is predominantly experienced by women, PTMs appear to be more common in men [47, 48].

PTM or neurovascular headache is well described in the concussion and general TBI literature, although its true incidence remains debated, in part because use of traditional classification systems in the absence of clinical exam may overestimate its occurrence [4]. Patients with PTM may have a genetic predisposition to development of migraine following trauma to either the head/brain and/or neck. There is inadequate information to stipulate how acute PTM may differ mechanistically and otherwise from chronic PTM, if at all. PTM pain is most likely to be described as throbbing. Vascular headache is usually unilateral and is exacerbated by coughing, and bending over. Cold may help but heat usually makes the headache worse. There may be associated nausea, vomiting, or anorexia. Hemicranial allodynia may occur after central sensitization takes place, which is a bad prognostic sign for triptan efficacy moving forward.

Trauma-triggered migraine is typically seen in children, adolescents, and young adults, although there is a substantive literature on its occurrence in professional athletes [5]. Studies assessing the test–retest reliability of migraine outcome instruments in this population are limited [69]. The migraine attack may present variably, including with visual disturbance (i.e., temporary blindness), change in level of consciousness, or hemiparesis or brainstem symptoms (i.e., basilar migraine); however, an aura may be absent. A severe headache, nausea, and vomiting typically follow. Symptoms of acute PTM typically begin within one to ten minutes after a blow to the head, but have not been described secondary to blows to the rest of the body. The attack usually resolves within a few to 24 h. On rare occasion, neurologic deficits may not totally clear. These post-traumatic attacks may be mistaken for cerebral concussions, contusions, or acute epidural or subdural hematoma. Trauma-triggered migraines have been reported with soccer, football, rugby, volleyball, and wrestling [70–75].

Because of the differences in participation level between girls and boys in contact sports, these headaches will be seen more typically in boys and young men. The clinical presentation of PTM is similar to other migraine attacks. The incidence of spontaneous migraine is much higher in children with traumatriggered migraine. A positive family history of migraine is seen in over 70% of children with this variety of headache.

Bennett et al. of the University of Nebraska reviewed three members of a university football team, aged 18–21 years old, who were evaluated because of migraine symptoms precipitated by head trauma. Analysis of the clinical data from these cases, as well as in eight previously reported cases among athletes revealed that the head trauma was usually minor and not associated with amnesia. Visual, motor, sensory, or confusional signs and symptoms began after a short symptom-free interval. Symptoms lasted for 15–30 minutes and were followed by a headache frequently accompanied by nausea and vomiting. In nine of 11 cases, the attacks recurred with subsequent head trauma [76].

Patients with PCH may present with a combination of vascular, tension, neuralgic, and/or musculoskeletal headache pain generators, all of which may require treatment. Sensory nerve fibers in the descending tract of the trigeminal nerve connect with sensory fibers from C1 to C3 and possibly C4 cervical roots. Cervical nociceptive pain generators can promulgate migraine through the trigeminocervical complex and therefore must be addressed as part and parcel of comprehensive migraine assessment and treatment [4] (Figure 23.2).

The aim of treatment of migraine headache is to prevent or reduce the frequency of the onset of headache (prophylactic treatment), abort a headache rapidly should it occur (as

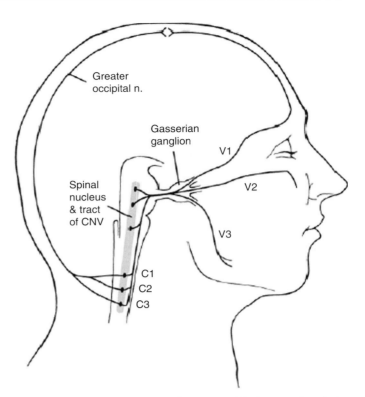

Fig. 23.2 Schematic representation of interconnectivity between the spinal nucleus and tract of cranial nerve V (CNV), upper three cervical roots, and the ophthalmic branch of the fifth cranial nerve through the Gasserian ganglion
Source: Zasler et al., 2013 [58]

well as sustain the headache relief once aborted), and treat the associated symptoms such as nausea and emesis.

Prophylactic migraine medications include some NSAIDs, beta-blockers, calcium channel blockers, tricyclic antidepressants, and antiepileptic drugs (i.e., topiramate, valproic acid, gabapentin) as more traditional treatments. Naturopathic agents such as butterbar and feverfew, as well as therapies such as B-complex vitamins and magnesium supplementation, in addition to complementary treatments may also augment treatment response [65, 77]. Abortive medications may include ergot derivatives, dihydroergotamine derivatives, triptans, parenteral atypical antipsychotics and/or narcotics, or combination medications (i.e., NSAID with triptan), among other drugs, but only a smattering of information is available on their use (triptans specifically) for PCH [78]. Triptans, as a class, may be ineffective if their use is delayed and allodynia develops. Botulinum toxin may be used for treatment of chronic migraine headache, although, there is no specific indication for its use in PCH-related migraine. Neurotoxins may exert a therapeutic effect for this type of headache not only through muscle relaxation but through inhibiting release of sensitizing neurotransmitters such as glutamate and substance P [79]. Behavioral and physical treatments may also have a role in the treatment of migraine [80], as can complementary medicine treatments [77].

If patients experience chronic daily headache and use abortive analgesics, they are at risk for developing rebound or mediMOH (see below). Caffeine over-use may also contribute to patients becoming refractory to abortive migraine medications containing this substance.

Uncommon Headache Variants Following Concussion

Various dysautonomic headaches have been reported and, although rare, should be considered in the differential diagnostic work-up of a patient with PCH [81–83]. Clues to a dysautonomic source of headache pain include a unilateral episodic throbbing pain in association with hyperactive sympathetics involving the ipsilateral face during the attack (miosis, sweating) but between attacks, a mild Horner's syndrome. Post-traumatic trigeminal autonomic headaches have also been reported.

Post-traumatic cluster headache and paroxysmal hemicrania are relatively rare types of PTHA, although case reports have been published on both following trauma [84, 85]. It should be noted, however, that with less common headache variants there is always a question about the causal relationship of the injury to the headache and/or its persistence. The literature is scant in proving a causal link between trauma and these headache sub-types.

Arterial dissections of the carotid, as well as the vertebral, artery may also be seen following trauma, although they are rare [86, 87]. Both can be associated with headache and neck pain [5].

Medication Overuse Headache

Medication overuse may result in chronic headaches. MOH is a common headache disorder with a prevalence of approximately 2% [26], although, its incidence following concussion has not been verified. MOH may be seen from overuse of a variety of analgesic and/or abortive headache agents, including ergotamines, opiates, caffeine, triptans, and/or barbiturates [88]. Overuse of these medications may lead to development of chronic daily headache. Patients may become dependent on these symptomatic headache medications. Drug withdrawal normally results in worsening of the headache, particularly when medications are stopped suddenly as opposed to being slowly weaned with concurrent alternative headache management options prescribed. Headache medication overuse may also make headaches refractory to prophylactic headache medication [4].

Medication-Induced Headache

Headaches can be induced by medications, alcohol, or illicit drugs. Medications capable of causing headache include anabolic steroids, analgesics, antibiotics, anti-hypertensives, corticosteroids, dipyridamole, NSAIDs, nitrazepam, oral contraceptives, sympathomimetics, certain antidepressants and vasodilator agents, among other agents [44]. Other commonly used agents which may also be associated with headache include alcohol, caffeine, and nicotine. It is therefore of critical importance to know what medications (prescription, over-the-counter, and otherwise) a given patient is on and the temporal relationship of any of those medications to headache onset.

Table 23.2 Post-concussive headache/post-traumatic headache headache historical points for inquiry

- Timing of headache onset
- Pattern of progression of pain over time
- Treatment history relative to pharmacologic and non-pharmacologic approaches that have either helped headache pain or made it worse
- Frequency of pain
- Severity of pain, typically rated using some type of pain scale (i.e., pain faces)
- "COLDER" mnemonic – character of pain, onset, location, duration, exacerbation, and relief
- Functional consequences of pain (i.e., how this pain affects ability to perform work and non-work-related activities)
- Determine if the patient had headache of any kind pre-dating the injury and, if so, whether it has been altered in any way post injury
- Review relevant medical records to increase understanding of potential pain generators based on the injury history, including mechanics (if known)
- Check on genetic loading risk factors for post-concussive headache/post-traumatic headache such as migraine
- Interview corroboratory sources, as persons with traumatic brain injury may not have adequate insight into or memory regarding the accident, symptoms evolution, and/or functional consequences of the headache disorder

Evaluation of Post-Concussive Headache

The Post-Concussive Headache History

One of the major challenges in diagnosing PCH is distinguishing it from other types of non-traumatic headache and, once having done so, identifying the specific pain generators involved. Generally, a thorough history in combination with a focused physical exam can diagnose most PCH variants (Table 23.2).

The evaluation of the patient with PCH requires a detailed clinical history outlining the clinical characteristics of the headache, including the onset, character, frequency, location, intensity, and duration of the pain. In addition, all alleviating and aggravating conditions and associated symptoms need to be identified. Clinicians should also inquire as to the time of onset of the PCH, its evolution over time, and response to prior treatments, whether pharmacological or otherwise.

The physical forces involved in PTHA, in general, and PCH, more specifically, include impact and/or acceleration/deceleration (inertial) loading, the latter including whiplash-type injury to the neck. Therefore, inquiries directed at understanding the injury mechanics are considered critical. The more information gathered by the clinician regarding the headache history, the better able the clinician will be in determining the root cause(s) of the headache disorder [4].

The PCH Physical Examination

The physical examination should note any signs of trauma, such as bruising, deformities, tenderness to palpation/trigger points, and cervical range of motion. The general physical examination should also exclude any systemic illnesses that could be associated with a secondary headache.

The physical examination of the patient with PCH should take into consideration central and peripheral neurological, as well as musculoskeletal, clinical findings. The neurological evaluation should include an elemental neurological exam including full cranial nerve assessment (including cranial nerve I for olfactory function and, as relevant, oculovestibular testing), fundoscopic exam (to rule out papilledema), deep tendon reflexes, including pathological reflexes, sensory exam, including visual fields, motor exam, and cerebellar assessment, including measures of postural stability, assessment for meningismus, and mental status evaluation [89]. Appropriate and timely cognitive screening should be performed in conjunction with follow-up cognitive testing as deemed clinically appropriate. Peripheral neurological examination should include the face, head, and craniocervical junction mainly focused on assessment for neuralgic and/or neuritic headache pain generators.

The musculoskeletal evaluation should include inspection for body asymmetries (such as head tilt, shoulder droop, tilted pelvis, leg length discrepancy, or asymmetric gait), postural assessment, including head-forward posture, rounded shoulders stance, pelvic alignment, as well as assessment for cervical and lumbar lordosis, or lack thereof. Jaw range of motion and tracking, as well as spinal range of motion, particularly cervicothoracic, should be addressed in any patient with PCH. Assessment for cervical vertebral somatic dysfunctions should be included in the assessment, particularly those involving C1, C2, or C3. Ligamentous integrity testing of the upper cervical spine assessing the alar and transverse ligaments should also be done, although, the sensitivity and specificity of these techniques are not particularly impressive. Auscultation for bruits should be done as appropriate over the carotids, closed eyes, temporal arteries, and mastoids, as well as over the TMJ, the latter as indicated, for abnormal articular sounds. Palpatory exam should include the face, head (including TMJ and masticatory muscles), as well as the muscles of the shoulder girdle and neck. Palpatory examination must be done in a controlled, layer-by-layer fashion to truly localize pathology [4, 90].

Psychological Assessment

Psychological assessment is often undervalued and underused in the treatment of persons with PCH. Anticipation of pain activates cortical networks similar to pain itself [91]. This highlights the complex, multidimensional, subjective perceptual pain process comprised of behavioral, affective, cognitive, and sensory components that can be seen with PCH. Consequently, a comprehensive, biopsychosocial assessment is considered the standard of care when pain is chronic (i.e., greater than six months in duration) [92]. In addition to the aforementioned neuromedical evaluations, pain assessment should address self-report, via interview of patient and relevant others, and use of appropriate assessment instruments, in the following areas: (1) pain onset, location, intensity level, duration, course, quality/characteristics; (2) affective and autonomic stress-related effects (including psychophysiological

assessment as indicated); (3) pain behaviors, environmental effects/responses, specific effect on mood, activity, cognition, affect, sleep, appetite, irritating/relieving factors; (4) medications and effects; (5) beliefs and expectancies about the pain condition; (6) coping strategies and effectiveness; (7) psychosocial context and social responses to pain; (8) personality and psychoemotional status and adjustment, including general coping, specific pain coping, and how these affect or are affected by pain; and (8) activity, level of function/disability and quality of life, including current activities, pain-related changes [20, 93].

Martelli et al. [20] presented a survey of useful pain assessment instruments (www.villamartelli.com/PainAssess Table.pdf), including ones for special populations. These are intended to be integrated with a thorough history, interview (patient, relevant others), and examination of relevant medical and health care records. Included are measures of response bias or tendency to report or present pain/related disability inaccurately. This is important given the nature of pain (avoidance is a reflexive response), frequent forensic contexts of PCH, frequent pain-related anxieties (fear of re-injury, avoidance of unpleasant situations), and possible dependency or avoidance personality traits, among other factors. Martelli and colleagues [20] also offered a thorough analysis and strategy for this challenging task.

Other PCH Testing

Neuroimaging plays an important role in the evaluation of the individual with PTHA. Any headache associated with focal neurological findings should be evaluated with standard structural neuroimaging to rule out a more significant brain injury or other intracranial process presenting with headache. Acutely, computed tomography (CT) is preferable to magnetic resonance imaging (MRI) in patients meeting imaging criteria to document acute intracranial hemorrhage and/or mass effect and dictate the need for neurosurgical management. In the non-acute setting MRI would be preferable [94].

Clinical tests pertinent to assessment of the patient with PCH may also include cervical imaging and electrophysiological testing, as well as general functional assessment testing. Tests should only be ordered when it is anticipated that the results will have an impact on clarifying a diagnosis and/or treatment plan or facilitating prognostication.

Management of Post-Concussive Headache
Neuromedical and Rehabilitative Management Overview

The treating clinician should establish realistic treatment end points for the patient with PCH and include the patient (and guardian as relevant)/family in this process so that all are on the "same page." Consensus recommendations exist for a period of post-injury rest, both cognitive and physical, until the patient is asymptomatic, with graduated return-to-normal activities including sports participation [43].

There should also be education regarding headache treatment options for PCH, including their risks versus benefits. The simplest, least invasive, lowest-risk, and most cost-effective management approaches that allow for optimization of patient compliance and maximal functional restoration should be used whenever possible.

When pharmacologic agents are used, analgesia should be delivered with minimal adverse effects and inconvenience to the patient, with clearly defined treatment expectations, including education regarding medication side-effects. Proper communication should be maintained between the patient, the caregiver, and treating clinician regarding response to individual pain treatment interventions. The treating clinician should maintain ongoing communication with any other clinicians involved with the patient's health management to adequately coordinate clinical care and avoid risks associated with uncoordinated care, including drug–drug interactions. One should try to avoid use of opiates to modulate pain, particularly as a first-line intervention, unless other options have failed. Opiates do not treat all pain well; that is, not all pain is opiate-sensitive. Additionally, opiates may lead to both physical and psychological dependency, have numerous adverse physiological effects with more chronic use, and may compound other TBI-related impairments, including cognitive difficulties. If opiates are used, they should be used judiciously and with appropriate screening (i.e., Opiate Risk Tool [95]) and monitoring procedures (including use of opiate agreements and random urine screens) [20, 65]. Attempts should also be made to minimize polypharmacy and use drugs that can be dosed one to two times per day (as opposed to more) as both measures will improve compliance, decrease drug–drug interactions, improve quality of life, and likely result in lower expense. Additionally, whenever possible, use of medications whose mechanism of action may impede neural plasticity (e.g., opiates, barbiturates, certain anticonvulsants) should be minimized or avoided [65].

Exercise is an under-prescribed treatment intervention in PCH pain management. Beneficial effects can include pain modulation on both a central and peripheral basis, weight control, positive affective modulation, including stress reduction, benefits to brain function, improvement of general sense of well-being, and improved general state of health [20, 96]. When there are any significant musculoskeletal contributors to PCH, appropriate prescription of adaptive equipment, as well as ergonomically modified study or work environments may also add to overall management of PCH to facilitate greater pain modulation and tolerance.

The role of newer technologies such as neuromodulation (i.e., cranial electrical stimulation, electroencephalogram-based neurotherapies, supra-orbital and occipital nerve stimulation), transcranial magnetic stimulation, transcranial direct current stimulation, and transcranial near infrared laser phototherapy remains to be established.

Psychological Management Overview

Pain management parallels the pain assessment process with treatment evolving over time from (1) acute treatment, where the focus should be on reducing pain, promoting healing and/or correcting underlying pathophysiology, minimizing physical, cognitive, or emotional distress reactions and preventing "chronification," including peripheral or central nervous system sensitization effects, to (2) functional treatment, or improving adaptation and reducing functional disability. Comprehensive biopsychosocial assessment provides the framework for individually tailored treatment interventions and recommendations [92]. Behavioral and psychological treatment interventions in persons with persistent PCH include individualized interventions that follow from the biopsychosocial assessment that provides a treatment framework, defines goals, expectations, and sequences, and provides psychoeducational information about the particular type of chronic pain and rationale for treatment [20].

Specific outcome studies that examine PCH treatments are only recently emerging. These are demonstrating the clear phenomenological similarities in clinical presentation and treatment response of PCH compared to non-traumatic headache disorders. Patient education may assist in improving post-traumatic coping abilities, depression, and anxiety. The earlier such interventions are begun and continue till completion of therapeutic goals, the better the longer-term outcome.

Several authors have systematically reviewed evidence supporting the efficacy of behavioral interventions for chronic pain that includes chronic headache. Campbell et al. [80] offered evidence-based guidelines for behavioral and physical treatments of migraine. Kröner-Herwig [97] reviewed evidence confirming the efficacy of behavioral treatment outcomes for chronic back pain, headache, fibromyalgia, and temporomandibular pain and reported some encouraging results for chronic headache. Lake [98] found that controlled studies of cognitive behavioral therapies for migraine, such as biofeedback and relaxation therapy, had a prophylactic efficacy of about 50%, roughly equivalent to propranolol, while the combination of behavioral therapies greatly increased efficacy. Rains et al. [99] noted that meta-analytic reviews have consistently shown behavioral interventions (relaxation training, biofeedback, cognitive behavioral therapy, and stress management training) to yield 35–55% improvements in subjective symptoms in patients with migraine and TTHA. Thorn et al. [100] offered randomized clinical trial data supporting the efficacy of a brief cognitive behavioral intervention for improving headache status. Notably, in a critical systematic review, Watanabe et al [31] noted that high-quality evidence from studies of interventions for PCH were rare and sorely needed.

Despite the dearth of quality evidence that specifically evaluates treatment of PCH, returning veterans from military conflict areas with a high incidence of PCH are a population that has produced increased interest in PCH/PTHA assessment and treatment, spurring such studies as the one presented by Ruff et al. [101]. They reported on important findings for a combined behavioral (sleep hygiene counseling) and pharmacologic (prazosin) treatment intervention for this population. Sleep was improved and average frequency and intensity of PCH were decreased by 66% with improved cognitive assessment scores. Results were maintained at six months.

Prognosis

There is not much known about headache prognostication in PCH, mainly due to the fact that little has been done to investigate this headache disorder in a blinded, prospective manner over any substantive length of time. Based on the extant PTHA literature, it is known that traumatically triggered headaches may often be persistent and, in general, are not promulgated by ongoing litigation [62, 102], although no one has, as of yet, addressed validity and effort issues in the context of a PCH/PTHA outcome study. That being said, it is unclear from the existing literature, which is both lacking and variable in terms of quality, how well patients with PTHA were actually diagnosed relative to their specific pain generators and therefore it is difficult to know if they were ever really appropriately treated for their headache disorders.

Also, the literature showing a relatively high incidence of inaccurate history reporting in litigating relative to non-litigating patients is often ignored in the context of examining prognosis in PCH [103], as is the propensity for individuals' status post brain injury to not provide accurate histories when comparing their pre-injury to post-injury status [104]. Any study looking at prognosis and longer-term prevalence of PCH must examine not only the validity of symptom reporting and performance but also the presence of response biases (some patients may be stoic and under-report, others may report accurately, and some may amplify complaints). It is also critical to consider base rates of headache in the general population, as well as understand that some studies of PCH have found a pre-injury headache history in approximately 20% of affected patients [105].

Confounding variables, including pre-injury headache history, genetic loading, sex and body morphology, injury biomechanics and forces, cultural issues, pain chronicity, pain coping resources (both internal and external), pre-injury characterological traits, social support, litigation (if any), concurrent affective disorder issues, including depression, as well as anxiety/post-traumatic stress disorder and other factors, may all play a role in the ultimate prognosis for PCH. Delayed recovery may in part, or wholly, be related to multiple factors including, but not limited to, inappropriate diagnosis and/or treatment, iatrogenic promulgation of PCH (i.e., via use of medications that produce MOH or medication-induced headache), patient misuse of prescribed medication, pre-existing characterological traits and/or suboptimal coping resources, pre-injury headache disorders, as well as affective disorders (whether injury-related or not), including depression and anxiety disorders (including post-traumatic stress disorder) [106, 107], stressors associated with financial hardships, loss of primary life role, and/or litigation, among other possible explanations.

Numerous studies are available that demonstrate that a significant percentage of patients after CBI continue to have headache beyond six months post injury and some studies even indicate that beyond 12 months post injury, 18–58% of persons continue to experience headache [105, 108]. The etiology of the headache disorder will have an impact on prognosis, as will a pre-injury history of headache. It has been noted that headache may be an independent symptom of TBI per se and not be causally related to the brain injury but to other injury-related factors.

Impairment Rating in PCH

Impairment rating is controversial in and of itself; however, impairment rating as related to pain is even more controversial. Currently, there are no evidence-based, standardized criteria available for establishing impairment ratings for PTHA, including for PCH. The sixth edition of the American Medical Association's *Guides to the Evaluation of Permanent Impairment* (GEPI) [109] has two potentially relevant sections to rating impairment associated with PTHA. The first is under Chapter 3 or pain-related impairment. In this chapter various controversies regarding the rating of pain are discussed, including inclusion of pain ratings in the first place given that they are based on subjective report rather than objective data. Challenges relating to pain rating, including congruence with established conditions, consistency over time and situation, consistency with anatomy and physiology, agreement between observers and inappropriate illness behavior are appropriately acknowledged and address in this chapter. Pain impairment rating is further divided into ratings involving pain that accompanies objective findings of injury or illness from rating impairment when the pain is not accompanied by objective findings. The Pain Disability Questionnaire is an integral part of pain rating under the sixth edition of the GEPI. Clearly, as with other impairment ratings, the patient must be considered at maximum medical improvement. In order for a pain rating to be performed it must be established that the pain has been determined to have a reasonable medical basis, the patient identifies pain is a major problem, the condition cannot be rated according to principals described in other chapters (i.e., GEPI Chapters 4–17), and the rating is not specifically excluded by relevant jurisdiction. The Pain Disability Questionnaire score is then used to determine the patient's presumptive whole-person impairment from 0 to 3%, with the maximum of 3% being empirically based. Furthermore, the clinician must make a "judgment" about the reliability and credibility of the patient's presentation and modify the impairment rating accordingly within the available range for pain-related impairment. There is no specific guidance given for how one goes about the process of judging reliability and credibility; however, it is noted that ratings may be either decreased or increased depending on case analysis and whether it is felt that the patient is demonstrating negative versus positive response bias with regard to pain reporting [109]. Within the GEPI, there is a separate section (3.11) relating to criteria for rating impairments associated with craniocephalic pain due to migraine headaches (3.11a) via use of the Migraine Disability Assessment questionnaire. The five questions are summed and Tables 13–18 are used to determine an impairment rating for migraine headache.

An alternative to the current American Medical Association GEPI, edition 6, was previously proposed by Drs. Packard and Ham in 1993 [110]. Criteria for PTHA are proposed in the form of an acronym, IMPAIRMENT: intensity, medication use, physical signs/symptoms, adjustment, incapacitation, recreation, miscellaneous activities of daily living, employment, number (frequency), time (attack duration). Each category was scored from 0 to 2 with three additional "physician modifiers," each scored from 0 to –4 points: (1) motivation for treatment; (2) over-exaggeration or overt concern; and (3) degree of legal "interest." In practice, this classification system is rarely, if ever, utilized in part, probably due to the fact that states utilize an edition of the American Medical Association GEPI as the basis for all impairment ratings.

Directions for Future Research

Research on the topic of PCH must use a common nomenclature and definitional criteria. Mechanisms for PTHA need to be elucidated and differentiated from primary headache disorders, assuming they are unique. Increased understanding of factors that increase risk for PCH and persistent PCH (i.e., pain duration greater than six months) are needed, along with efforts at modulating these risk factors to minimize morbidity. An evidence-based medicine approach to classification needs to be developed that incorporates proper nomenclature use, injury, and headache history, as well as headache features (based on both subjective patient report and physical exam findings) into a rational paradigm. Standardized assessment protocols are needed for each of the identified PCH subtypes. Randomized controlled trials examining the natural history, evaluation, treatment, and prognosis of PCH subtypes are crucial to moving the science forward in this area of brain injury medicine.

Conclusions

The assessment and treatment of chronic head pain following CBI are challenging processes. Pain and its concomitants can have a more disabling effect across a wider range of functions than mild brain injury [20, 111, 112]. Available evidence strongly supports the conclusion that resolution of post-concussive symptoms and successful adaptation to residual sequelae frequently relies on successful coping with PCH and associated symptomatology [111].

Early, competent, specialized intervention offers the greatest hope of facilitating adaptation to pain. Complex or persistent pain presentations warrant referral to pain management specialists or specialty interdisciplinary pain programs. Biopsychosocial assessment and treatment strategies have emerged as the standard of care in chronic pain. The most promising current treatment interventions are combination treatments that are holistic in nature and target the patient's reaction to pain within his/her daily life and ability to exercise self-control. Multicomponent treatment packages are currently the preferred treatment choice for chronic pain generally, and especially when it accompanies TBI [20]. Early, competent, specialized intervention, that includes education and combination medical and behavioral treatments directed at simultaneously improving adaption to PCH and improving its associated symptoms of sleep disturbance, emotional distress, and depression, is indicated.

Acknowledgments

We are grateful to Emily R. Joyner, LPN, CMOM, for assistance with manuscript preparation.

References

1. Trotter W. Annual oration on certain minor injuries of the brain. *Lancet* 1924; May 10: 935–939.
2. Conidi FX. Sports-related concussion: The role of the headache specialist. *Headache* 2012; 52(Suppl 1): 15–21.
3. Faux S, Sheedy J. A prospective controlled study in the prevalence of posttraumatic headache following mild traumatic brain injury. *Pain Med* 2008; 9(8): 1001–1011.
4. Horn LJ, Siebert B, Patel N, Zasler N. Post-traumatic headache. In: Zasler N, Katz D, Zafonte R, editors. *Brain injury medicine*, second edition. New York: Demos, 2013, pp. 932–953.
5. Zasler ND. Sports concussion headache: A review. *Brain Inj* 2015; 9(2): 207–220.
6. Tepper D. Headache after sports-related concussion. *Headache J Head Face Pain* 2013; 53(7): 1197–1198.
7. Blume HK, Lucas S, Bell KR. Subacute concussion-related symptoms in youth. *Phys Med Rehabil Clin N Am* 2011; 22(4): 665–681; viii–ix.
8. Kontos AP, Elbin RJ, Lau B, Simensky S, Freund B, French J, et al. Posttraumatic migraine as a predictor of recovery and cognitive impairment after sport-related concussion. *Am J Sports Med* 2013; 41(7): 1497–1504.
9. Mihalik JP, Register-Mihalik J, Kerr ZY, Marshall SW, McCrea MC, Guskiewicz KM. Recovery of posttraumatic migraine characteristics in patients after mild traumatic brain injury. *Am J Sports Med* 2013; 41(7): 1490–1496.
10. Register-Mihalik J, Guskiewicz KM, Mann JD, Shields EW. The effects of headache on clinical measures of neurocognitive function. *Clin J Sport Med* 2007; 17(4): 282–288.
11. Sabin MJ, Van Boxtel BA, Nohren MW, Broglio SP. Presence of headache does not influence sideline neurostatus or balance in high school football athletes. *Clin J Sport Med* 2011; 21(5): 411–415.
12. Walker WC, Marwitz JH, Wilk AR, Ketchum JM, Hoffman JM, Brown AW, et al. Prediction of headache severity (density and functional impact) after traumatic brain injury: A longitudinal multicenter study. *Cephalalgia* 2013; 33(12): 998–1008.
13. Hoffman JM, Lucas S, Dikmen S, Braden CA, Brown AW, Brunner R, et al. Natural history of headache after traumatic brain injury. *J Neurotrauma* 2011; 28(9): 1719–1725.
14. Lucas S. Headache management in concussion and mild traumatic brain injury. *PM R* 2011; 3(10; Suppl 2): S406–S412.
15. Treleaven J. Dizziness, unsteadiness, visual disturbances, and postural control: Implications for the transition to chronic symptoms after a whiplash trauma. *Spine* 2011; 36(25 Suppl): S211–S217.
16. Ahman S, Saveman B-I, Styrke J, Björnstig U, Stålnacke B-M. Long-term follow-up of patients with mild traumatic brain injury: A mixed-method study. *J Rehabil Med* 2013; 45(8): 758–764.
17. Schneider KJ, Meeuwisse WH, Kang J, Schneider GM, Emery CA. Preseason reports of neck pain, dizziness, and headache as risk factors for concussion in male youth ice hockey players. *Clin J Sport Med* 2013; 23(4): 267–272.
18. Walton DM, Macdermid JC, Giorgianni AA, Mascarenhas JC, West SC, Zammit CA. Risk factors for persistent problems following acute whiplash injury: Update of a systematic review and meta-analysis. *J Orthop Sports Phys Ther* 2013; 43(2): 31–43.
19. Collins MW, Field M, Lovell MR, Iverson G, Johnston KM, Maroon J, et al. Relationship between postconcussion headache

and neuropsychological test performance in high school athletes. *Am J Sports Med* 2003; 31(2): 168–173.

20. Martelli M, Nicholson K, Zasler N. Psychological assessment and management of post-traumatic pain. In: Zasler N, Katz D, Zafonte R, editors. *Brain injury medicine*, second edition. New York: Demos, 2013, pp. 974–989.

21. International Headache Society. IHS Classification ICHD-3 beta. 2016. www.ihs-classification.org/_downloads/mixed/International-Headache-Classification-III-ICHD-III-2013-Beta.pdf.

22. World Health Organization. ICD-10. 2010. http://apps.who.int/classifications/icd10/browse/2010/en#/G44.3 (accessed 11/15/13).

23. Zasler ND. Posttraumatic headache: Caveats and controversies. *J Head Trauma Rehabil* 1999; 14(1): 1–8.

24. Formisano R, Bivona U, Catani S, D'Ippolito M, Buzzi MG. Posttraumatic headache: Facts and doubts. *J Headache Pain* 2009; 10(3): 145–152.

25. Seifert TD. Sports concussion and associated post-traumatic headache. *Headache* 2013; 53(5): 726–736.

26. Katsarava Z, Obermann M. Medication-overuse headache. *Curr Opin Neurol* 2013; 26(3): 276–281.

27. McCrory P, Meeuwisse WH, Aubry M, Cantu B, Dvořák J, Echemendia RJ, et al. Consensus statement on concussion in sport: The 4th International Conference on Concussion in Sport held in Zurich, November 2012. *Br J Sports Med* 2013; 47(5): 250–258.

28. Giza CC, Kutcher JS, Ashwal S, Barth J, Getchius TSD, Gioia GA, et al. Summary of evidence-based guideline update: Evaluation and management of concussion in sports. Report of the Guideline Development Subcommittee of the American Academy of Neurology. *Neurology* 2013; 80(24): 2250–2257.

29. Harmon KG, Drezner JA, Gammons M, Guskiewicz KM, Halstead M, Herring SA, et al. American Medical Society for Sports Medicine position statement: Concussion in sport. *Br J Sports Med* 2013; 47(1): 15–26.

30. West TA, Marion DW. Current recommendations for the diagnosis and treatment of concussion in sport: A comparison of three new guidelines. *J Neurotrauma* 2014; 31: 159–168.

31. Watanabe TK, Bell KR, Walker WC, Schomer K. Systematic review of interventions for post-traumatic headache. *PM R* 2012; 4(2): 129–140.

32. Packard R. The relationship of neck injury and post-traumatic headache. *Curr Pain Headache Rep* 2002; 6(4): 301–307.

33. Watson DH, Drummond PD. Head pain referral during examination of the neck in migraine and tension-type headache. *Headache* 2012; 52(8): 1226–1235.

34. Kamins J, Charles A. Posttraumatic headache: basic mechanisms and therapeutic targets. *Headache* 2018; 58: 811–826.

35. Elliott MB, Oshinsky ML, Amenta PS, Awe OO, Jallo JI. Nociceptive neuropeptide increases and periorbital allodynia in a model of traumatic brain injury. *Headache* 2012; 52(6): 966–984.

36. Mayer CL, Huber BR, Peskind E. Traumatic brain injury, neuroinflammation, and post-traumatic headaches. *Headache* 2013; 53(9): 1523–1530.

37. Goadsby PJ. Pathophysiology of migraine. *Neurol Clin* 2009; 27(2): 335–360.

38. Kors EE, Terwindt GM, Vermeulen FL, Fitzsimons RB, Jardine PE, Heywood P, et al. Delayed cerebral edema and fatal coma after minor head trauma: Role of the CACNA1A calcium channel subunit gene and relationship with familial hemiplegic migraine. *Ann Neurol* 2001; 49(6): 753–760.

39. McKee AC, Cantu RC, Nowinski CJ, Hedley-Whyte ET, Gavett BE, Budson AE, et al. Chronic traumatic encephalopathy in athletes: Progressive tauopathy following repetitive head injury. *J Neuropathol Exp Neurol* 2009; 68(7): 709–735.

40. McKee AC, Stern RA, Nowinski CJ, Stein TD, Alvarez VE, Daneshvar DH, et al. The spectrum of disease in chronic traumatic encephalopathy. *Brain* 2013; 136(1):43–64.

41. Stern RA, Daneshvar DH, Baugh CM, Seichepine DR, Montenigro PH, Riley DO, et al. Clinical presentation of chronic traumatic encephalopathy. *Neurology* 2013; 81(13): 1122–1129.

42. Randolph C. Is chronic traumatic encephalopathy a real disease? *Curr Sports Med Rep* 2014; 13(1): 33–37.

43. Jordan BD. The clinical spectrum of sport-related traumatic brain injury. *Nat Rev Neurol* 2013; 9(4): 222–230.

44. Williams SJ, Nukada H. Sport and exercise headache: Part 1. Prevalence among university students. *Br J Sports Med* 1994; 28(2): 90–95.

45. Williams SJ, Nukada H. Sport and exercise headache: Part 2. Diagnosis and classification. *Br J Sports Med* 1994; 28(2): 96–100.

46. McCrory P. Headaches and exercise. *Sports Med* 2000; 30(3): 221–229.

47. Mauskop A. Headaches in sports. New York Headache Center. [cited 2014 Feb 25]. Available at: http://nyheadache.com/scientific-articles/headaches-in-sports/.

48. Rooke ED. Benign exertional headache. *Med Clin North Am* 1968; 52(4): 801–808.

49. Patel AV, Mihalik JP, Notebaert AJ, Guskiewicz KM, Prentice WE. Neuropsychological performance, postural stability, and symptoms after dehydration. *J Athl Train* 2007; 42(1): 66–75.

50. Campbell DG. Referred head pain and its concomitants: – Google Scholar. [cited 2013 Sep 26]. Available at: http://scholar.google.com/scholar?cluster=17952199131180977582&hl=en&oi=scholarr.

51. Travell J, Simons D. *Myofascial pain and dysfunction. The trigger point manual.* Baltimore, MD: Williams & Wilkins, 1992.

52. De Boever JA, Keersmaekers K. Trauma in patients with temporomandibular disorders: Frequency and treatment outcome. *J Oral Rehabil* 1996; 23(2): 91–96.

53. Haldeman S, Dagenais S. Cervicogenic headaches: A critical review. *Spine J* 2001; 1(1): 31–46.

54. Page P. Cervicogenic headaches: An evidence-led approach to clinical management. *Int J Sports Phys Ther* 2011; 6(3): 254–266.

55. Zasler ND, Etheredge S. Post-traumatic headache: Knowledge update. *Pain Pract Summer* 2015; 25(2): 19–22.

56. Levin M. Nerve blocks in the treatment of headache. *Neurotherapeut* 2010; 7(2): 197–203.

57. Ashkenazi A, Blumenfeld A, Napchan U, Narouze S, Grosberg B, Nett R, et al. Peripheral nerve blocks and trigger point injections in headache management – A systematic review and suggestions for future research. *Headache* 2010; 50(6): 943–952.

58. Zasler ND, Katz DI, Zafonte RD (editors) *Brain injury medicine: Principles and practice*, second edition. New York: Demos Medical Publishing, 2013.

59. Magis D, Sava S, D Elia TS, Baschi R, Schoenen J. Safety and patients' satisfaction of transcutaneous supraorbital neurostimulation (tSNS) with the Cefaly device in headache treatment: A survey of 2,313 headache sufferers in the general population. *J Headache Pain* 2013; 14(1): 95.

60. Jürgens TP, Leone M. Pearls and pitfalls: Neurostimulation in headache. *Cephalalgia* 2013; 33(8): 512–525.

61. Martelletti P, Jensen RH, Antal A, Arcioni R, Brighina F, de Tommaso M, et al. Neuromodulation of chronic headaches: Position statement from the European Headache Federation. *J Headache Pain* 2013; 14(1): 86.

62. De Benedittis G, De Santis A. Chronic post-traumatic headache: Clinical, psychopathological features and outcome determinants. *J Neurosurg Sci* 1983; 27(3): 177–186.

63. Bezov D, Ashina S, Jensen R, Bendtsen L. Pain perception studies in tension-type headache. *Headache* 2011; 51(2): 262–271.

64. Singh M. Muscle contraction tension headache. 2013 Aug 29 [cited 2013 Dec 7]. Available at: http://emedicine.medscape.com/article/1142908-overview.

65. Zasler ND. Pharmacotherapy and posttraumatic cephalalgia. *J Head Trauma Rehabil* 2011; 26(5): 397–399.

66. Posadzki P, Ernst E. Spinal manipulations for tension-type headaches: A systematic review of randomized controlled trials. *Complement Ther Med* 2012; 20(4): 232–239.

67. Alonso-Blanco C, de-la-Llave-Rincón AI, Fernández-de-las-Peñas C. Muscle trigger point therapy in tension-type headache. *Expert Rev Neurother* 2012; 12(3): 315–322.

68. Hauge AW, Kirchmann M, Olesen J. Characterization of consistent triggers of migraine with aura. *Cephalalgia* 2011; 31(4): 416–438.

69. Piebes SK, Snyder AR, Bay RC, Valovich McLeod TC. Measurement properties of headache-specific outcomes scales in adolescent athletes. *J Sport Rehabil* 2011; 20(1): 129–142.

70. Kalenak A, Petro DJ, Brennan RW. Migraine secondary to head trauma in wrestling. A case report. *Am J Sports Med* 1978; 6(3): 112–113.

71. McCrory PR, Ariens T, Berkovic SF. The nature and duration of acute concussive symptoms in Australian football. *Clin J Sport Med* 2000; 10(4): 235–238.

72. Hinton-Bayre AD, Geffen G, Friis P. Presentation and mechanisms of concussion in professional rugby league football. *J Sci Med Sport* 2004; 7(3): 400–404.

73. McCrory P, Heywood J, Coffey C. Prevalence of headache in Australian footballers. *Br J Sports Med* 2005; 39(2): e10.

74. Mainardi F, Alicicco E, Maggioni F, Devetag F, Lisotto C, Zanchin G. Headache and soccer: A survey in professional soccer players of the Italian "Series A." *Neurol Sci* 2009; 30(1): 33–36.

75. Sallis RE, Jones K. Prevalence of headaches in football players. *Med Sci Sports Exerc* 2000; 32(11): 1820–1824.

76. Bennett DR, Fuenning SI, Sullivan G, Weber J. Migraine precipitated by head trauma in athletes. *Am J Sports Med* 1980; 8(3): 202–205.

77. Mauskop A. Nonmedication, alternative, and complementary treatments for migraine. *Continuum (MinneapMinn)* 2012; 18(4): 796–806.

78. McCrory P, Heywood J, Ugoni A. Open label study of intranasal sumatriptan (Imigran) for footballer's headache. *Br J Sports Med* 2005; 39(8): 552–554.

79. Aurora SK, Dodick DW, Diener H-C, DeGryse RE, Turkel CC, Lipton RB, et al. OnabotulinumtoxinA for chronic migraine: Efficacy, safety, and tolerability in patients who received all five treatment cycles in the PREEMPT clinical program. *Acta Neurol Scand* 2014; 129(1): 61–70.

80. Campbell J, Penzien D, Wall E. Evidence-based guidelines for migraine headache: behavioral and physical treatments. [cited 2014 Feb 10]. Available at: http://tools.aan.com/professionals/practice/pdfs/gl0089.pdf.

81. Khurana RK, Nirankari VS. Bilateral sympathetic dysfunction in post-traumatic headaches. *Headache* 1986; 26(4): 183–188.

82. Khurana RK. Oculocephalic sympathetic dysfunction in post-traumatic headaches. *Headache* 1995; 35(10): 614–620.

83. Jacob S, Saha A, Rajabally Y. Post-traumatic short-lasting unilateral headache with cranial autonomic symptoms (SUNA). *Cephalalgia* 2008; 28(9): 991–993.

84. Formisano R, Angelini A, DeVuojno G, Calisse P, Fiacco F, Catarci T, et al. Cluster-like headache and head injury: Case report. *Ital J Neurol Sci* 1990; 11(3): 303–305.

85. Lambru G, Castellini P, Manzoni GC, Torelli P. Post-traumatic cluster headache: From the periphery to the central nervous system? *Headache* 2009; 49(7): 1059–1061.

86. Haneline MT, Lewkovich GN. An analysis of the etiology of cervical artery dissections: 1994 to 2003. *J Manipul Physiol Ther* 2005; 28(8): 617–622.

87. Shea K, Stahmer S. Carotid and vertebral arterial dissections in the emergency department. *Emerg Med Pract* 2012; 14(4): 1–23.

88. Srikiatkhachorn A, le Grand SM, Supornsilpchai W, Storer RJ. Pathophysiology of medication overuse headache – An update. *Headache* 2014; 54(1): 204–210.

89. Dimberg EL, Burns TM. Management of common neurologic conditions in sports. *Clin Sports Med* 2005; 24(3): 637–662.

90. Bell KR, Kraus EE, Zasler ND. Medical management of posttraumatic headaches: Pharmacological and physical treatment. *J Head Trauma Rehabil* 1999; 14(1): 34–48.

91. Atlas LY, Bolger N, Lindquist MA, Wager TD. Brain mediators of predictive cue effects on perceived pain. *J Neurosci* 2010; 30(39): 12964–12977.

92. Gatchel R, Peters M, Fuchs P, Turk D. The biopsychosocial approach to chronic pain: Scientific advances and future directions. *Psychol Bull* 2007; 133(4): 581–624.

93. Zasler N, Martelli M, Nicholson K. Chronic pain. In: Silver J, McAllister T, Yudofsky S, editors. *Textbook of traumatic brain injury*, second edition. Washington, D.C.: American Psychiatric Publishing, 2004, pp. 419–436.

94. Mechtler LL, Shastri KK, Crutchfield KE. Advanced neuroimaging of mild traumatic brain injury. *Neurol Clin* 2014; 32(1): 31–58.

95. Webster LR, Webster R. Predicting aberrant behaviors in opioid-treated patients: Preliminary validation of the Opioid Risk Tool. *Pain Med* 2005; 6: 432–442.

96. Martelli MF, Zasler ND, Tiernan P. Community based rehabilitation: Special issues. *NeuroRehabilitation* 2012; 31(1): 3–18.

97. Kröner-Herwig B. Chronic pain syndromes and their treatment by psychological interventions. *Curr Opin Psychiatry* 2009; 22(2): 200–204.

98. Lake AE 3rd. Behavioral and nonpharmacologic treatments of headache. *Med Clin North Am* 2001; 85(4): 1055–1075.

99. Rains JC, Penzien DB, McCrory DC, Gray RN. Behavioral headache treatment: History, review of the empirical literature, and methodological critique. *Headache: J Head Face Pain* 2005; 45: S92–S109.

100. Thorn BE, Pence LB, Ward LC, Kilgo G, Clements KL, Cross TH, et al. A randomized clinical trial of targeted cognitive behavioral treatment to reduce catastrophizing in chronic headache sufferers. *J Pain* 2007; 8(12): 938–949.

101. Ruff RL, Ruff SS, Wang X-F. Improving sleep: Initial headache treatment in OIF/OEF veterans with blast-induced mild traumatic brain injury. *J Rehabil Res Dev* 2009; 46(9): 1071–1084.

102. Packard R. Posttraumatic headache: Permanency and relationship to legal settlement. *Headache* 1992; 32(10): 496–500.

103. Lees-Haley PR, Williams CW, English LT. Response bias in self-reported history of plaintiffs compared with nonlitigating patients. *Psychol Rep* 1996; 79(3): 811–818.

104. Lees-Haley PR, Williams CW, Zasler ND, Marguilies S, English LT, Stevens KB. Response bias in plaintiffs' histories. *Brain Inj* 1997; 11(11): 791–799.

105. Lucas S, Hoffman JM, Bell KR, Dikmen S. A prospective study of prevalence and characterization of headache following mild traumatic brain injury. *Cephalalgia* 2014; 34(2): 93–102.

106. Kjeldgaard D, Forchhammer H, Teasdale T, Jensen RH. Chronic post-traumatic headache after mild head injury: A descriptive study. *Cephalalgia* 2014; 34: 191–200.

107. Sawyer K, Bell KR, Ehde DM, Temkin N, Dikmen S, Williams RM, et al. Longitudinal study of headache trajectories in the year after mild traumatic brain injury: Relation to posttraumatic stress disorder symptoms. *Arch Phys Med Rehabil* 2015; 96(11): 2000–2006.

108. Lew HL, Lin P-H, Fuh J-L, Wang S-J, Clark DJ, Walker WC. Characteristics and treatment of headache after traumatic brain injury: A focused review. *Am J Phys Med Rehabil* 2006; 85(7): 619–627.

109. Rondinelli R. *Guides to the evaluation of permanent impairment,* 6th edition. Chicago, IL: American Medical Association, 2008.

110. Packard RC, Ham LP. Impairment ratings for posttraumatic headache. *Headache* 1993; 33(7): 359–364.

111. Martelli MF, Zasler ND, Bender MC, Nicholson K. Psychological, neuropsychological, and medical considerations in assessment and management of pain. *J Head Trauma Rehabil* 2004; 19(1): 10–28.

112. Nicholson K, Martelli MF. Confounding effects of pain, psychoemotional problems or psychiatric disorder, premorbid ability structure, and motivational or other factors on neuropsychological test performance. In: Young G, Nicholson K, Kane AW, editors. *Psychological knowledge in court.* New York: Springer US, 2006, pp. 335–351.

Chapter

24

Fatigue after Concussion: Epidemiology, Causal Factors, Assessment, and Management

Benton Giap and Jeffrey Englander

Introduction (Epidemiology)

In 2010, 2.5 million traumatic brain injuries (TBIs) occurred either as an isolated injury or along with other injuries [1–3]. TBI presents an ever-growing, serious public health problem that causes a considerable number of fatalities and cases of permanent disability annually. "Mild traumatic brain injury" ("mTBI"), or concussion, comprises about 75–80% of all cases.[1]

Although many individuals with mTBI experience near, if not full, recovery, many live with lingering effects. Much symptomatology can persist as post-concussional syndrome and can be quite disabling in a small subset. The focus of this particular chapter is on post-traumatic brain injury fatigue (PTF).

PTF has been particularly challenging to define and measure. PTF is common in all types of severity of TBI. While there is no universally accepted definition of post-TBI fatigue, it has frequently been conceptualized as a multidimensional construct characterized by "extreme and persistent tiredness, weakness or exhaustion – mental, physical or both" [4]. Aaronson and colleagues [5] describe post-TBI fatigue as: "the awareness of a decreased capacity for physical and/or mental activity due to

an imbalance in the availability, utilization, and/or restoration of resources needed to perform activity." Henrie and Elovic point out that PTF is a symptom and not a diagnosis [6].

Despite strong indications that fatigue is one of the most common and debilitating symptom after TBI, the literature is limited with regard to frequency, natural history, or relation to other factors. The natural recovery process varies between different cohorts with different measurement methodologies. Ouellet and Morin reported no difference in the fatigue severity among the groups of TBI severity [7]. Although this textbook focuses on typical concussive brain injury, the authors will use the terminology "post-traumatic brain injury fatigue" since this symptom affects all severities of brain injury (Table 24.1).

It is consistently noted that the incidence of PTF is generally high. When individuals with TBIs are asked about what affects their ability to maintain independent living, PTF is consistently mentioned as the most important barrier to resuming normalcy of function. Lachappelle and Finlayson note that approximately 50% of patients with TBI identify fatigue as one of their worst or most distressing symptoms [8]. Ouellet and Morin [9] found that PTF ranged between 50% and 77%

Table 24.1 Summary of studies reporting prevalence of fatigue

Study	Design	Measurements	Findings
Lachappelle and Finlayson (1998) [8]	Objective Measure	Fatigue Impact Scale (FIS), Visual Analogue Scale for Fatigue (VAS-F), Fatigue Severity Scale (FSS)	Patients with brain injury were found to experience significant levels of fatigue and the FIS provided the most comprehensive examination of fatigue
Ouellet and Morin (2006) [9]	Survey (all severities)	General Questionnaire (self- and significant other-report), Multidimensional Fatigue Inventory (MFI), Insomnia Severity Index (ISI)	50–77% (10–28% in non-TBI control)
Bushnik et al. (2008) [10]	Prospective	FSS, multidimensional	16–32% at year 1 and 21–34% at year 2
Norrie (2012) [11]	Longitudinal in mTBI	FSS	68%, 38%, 34% (at 1 week, 3 months, and 6 months)
Cantor et al. (2008) [12]	Interviews, questionnaire	Global Fatigue Index, Beck Depression Inventory (BDI-II), McGill Pain Questionnaire (MPQ), Pittsburgh Sleep Quality Inventory (PSQI), Participation Objective Participation Subjective (POPS), Short Form-36, Life-3	Fatigue was more severe and prevalent in individuals with TBI

FSS: Fatigue Severity Scale; mTBI: mild traumatic brain injury; TBI: traumatic brain injury.

---

[1] Editor's note: the authors of this chapter cite articles that employed the phrase "mild traumatic brain injury" ("mTBI"). As previously discussed, "mTBI" has been defined in many ways, none representing a unitary biological condition. For that reason, readers cannot assume either that (a) the cases within each cited study were comparable to one another nor that (b) any two studies assessed authentically comparable pools of subjects.

of individuals with TBI years after their injuries. Englander and colleagues reported that one-third to one-half endorsed PTF on the Fatigue Severity Scale and the Multi-dimensional Fatigue Severity Scale [13].

In a longitudinal study conducted in 159 individuals with concussions, Norrie [11] found that prevalence of 68%, 38%, and 34% at one week, three months, and six months after the onset using the Fatigue Severity Scale and the Rivermead Post-concussion Symptoms Questionnaire. Norrie noted that early fatigue strongly predicts later fatigue. Not surprisingly, depression, but not anxiety, is associated with fatigue [11]. Bay and De-Leon highlighted the variability and frequency of PTF in the comparison studies of mild TBI [14].

Studies showed conflicting results in reported fatigue and resolution [15]. The prevalence of fatigue does not appear to change over time. Fatigue is found to persist months to years after the injury in a number of studies. In a study of individuals with TBI living in the community, 68% reported fatigue at two years post-injury and, when surveyed again at five years post injury, a slightly higher percentage of these individuals, 73%, reported problems with fatigue [12].

Bushnik et al.'s prospective study [10] examines the rate and types of fatigue that are experienced by a cohort of individuals with TBI within the first two years, using a multidimensional fatigue scale. Using two self-reported measures of fatigue, 16–32% at year 1 and 21–34% at year 2 reported significant levels of fatigue. Fatigue did not appear to change between one and two years post TBI [16]. Belmont and colleagues noted in their literature review that fatigue was reported in 43–73% of patients and does not seem to be significantly related to injury severity or to time since injury [17].

Causal Factors

Fatigue is well appreciated in other conditions, such as multiple sclerosis, cardiovascular, pulmonary disease (chronic obstructive pulmonary disease), depression, post-polio syndrome, thyroid disease, obesity, HIV/AIDs, and diabetes mellitus [18].

What makes fatigue challenging to define is the mere fact that there is an array of physical, cognitive, and behavioral changes that could occur after a TBI. How other factors, including depression and sleep disorders, affect post-TBI fatigue is waiting to be better defined. Ouellet and colleagues followed a cohort of 452 individuals with brain injury [19]. With an average time since injury onset of 7.8 years, anxiety symptoms, long-term disability, insomnia severity, and cognitive symptoms were factors associated with PTF. Factors not associated were age, severity, sex, depressive symptoms, irritability symptoms, and perceived pain level. More than 50% reported insomnia symptoms. The insomnia was a severe and chronic condition remaining untreated in almost 60% of cases. The authors explained this high prevalence by clinical characteristics associated with insomnia symptoms such as higher levels of fatigue, depression, and pain.

Englander and associates [13] noted fatigue is present in a high percentage of community-based populations of individuals with TBI. Robust correlates of fatigue were gender, depression, pain, and memory and motor dysfunction. Sleep quality was the most prevalent concomitant disturbance, followed by depression and pain. In this study, there was no correlation between pituitary dysfunction and fatigue; however, the relatively high prevalence of hypothyroidism and adrenal dysfunction suggests screening for these hormone deficiencies [13].

Multiple other studies note that PTF correlates with sleep disorders, perceived stress, somatic symptoms, anxiety, and depression [20, 21]. In their prospective comparative study, Stulemeijer and associates found that fatigue and emotional distress were associated with self-reported cognitive difficulties, suggesting that treatment of distress and fatigue could improve perceived cognitive difficulties [22]. Borgaro and colleagues found that fatigue and somatic symptoms, such as "dizzy," "headaches," or "ringing in the ears," were positively associated [23]. Thus increased somatic complaints and emotional distress are associated with increased fatigue (Figure 24.1).

Anatomical Considerations

The cellular and structural cascades following TBI are complex. Neuroplastic processes occur and continue invariably, dependent on a complex set of factors. It is becoming clear that TBI is the most complex disease process occurring to the most complex human organ. Neurobehavioral changes following TBI are poorly correlated with focal lesions detected by structural neuroimaging techniques such as computed tomography scan or MRI [25]. There is not one set of structures that directly correlate with fatigue symptoms. Damage to the brain's networks results in suboptimal and dysfunctional circuitry and eventually an inefficiently functioning brain. As a result of the slowed processing and inefficient circuitry resulting from many microscopic sites of damage diffusely distributed throughout cerebral white matter and the upper brainstem, activities that were once automatic now may only be accomplished with deliberate effort.

Fatigue is commonly associated with slowed information processing and the need for increased effort in performing tasks. In Ziino and Ponsford's study of 46 individuals with and without a TBI, those without a TBI scored higher on the vigilance task test than those with a TBI. The number of misses recorded on the vigilance task was significantly higher for those with a TBI ($p < 0.001$) [26].

One new report lends support to the observation that mental fatigue, perhaps due to deficits in the efficiency of mental processing, may persist for a year or more post concussion. In a recent study, 21 subjects with "mTBI" were asked about mental fatigue [27]. Their subjective responses did not differ from those of healthy comparison subjects, nor were the reaction times of the concussion survivors significantly longer than those of the controls. However, this performance seemed to come at the cost of significantly greater expense of cerebral resources. Concussion survivors at least one year post injury performed a 20-min psychomotor vigilance test during 3-T fMRI. As depicted in Figure 24.2, chronic patients exhibited dramatically increased blood oxygen level-dependent responses in multiple brain regions compared with controls, especially in the final five minutes of testing. The authors noted

The vicious cycle of fatigue.

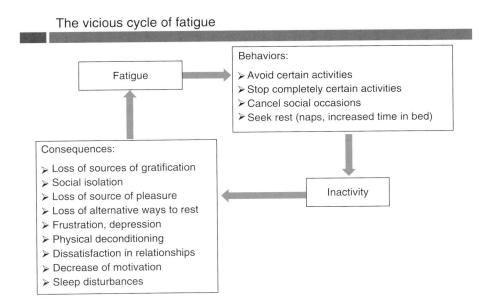

The vicious cycle of fatigue

Fig. 24.1

Source: Ouellet, 2011 [24]. Ouellet, 2011.
Reproduced with permission from Pr M. Ouellet

Evidence that mental performance more quickly fatigues and requires greater expense of cerebral resources at ≥12 months post-concussion

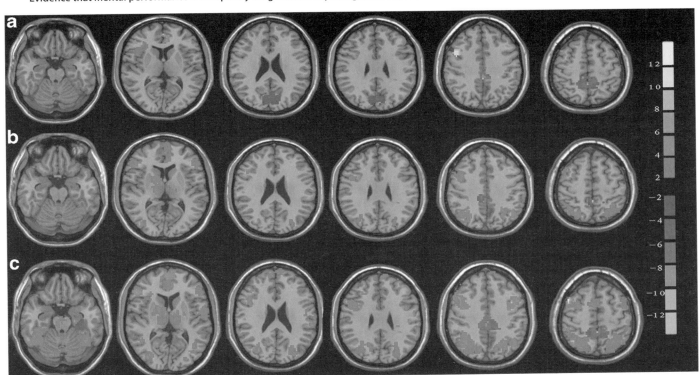

Fig. 24.2 Brain areas associated with the second 5-min psychomotor vigilance test (PVT) vs. the first 5-min PVT (a), comparison of the third 5-min PVT vs. the first 5-min PVT (b), and comparison of the last 5-min PVT vs. the first 5-min PVT (c) for mild traumatic brain injury patients in the chronic phase. [A black and white version of this figure will appear in some formats. For the color version, please refer to the plate section.]

Source: Liu et al., 2016 [27]. Reprinted by permission from Springer

that the chronic patients suffered "aggravated mental fatigue … after PVT for 15 min, which was shorter than in healthy subjects and was longer than in patients in the acute phase." They concluded, "Mental fatigue of MTBI patients persists for more than 12 months … To our knowledge, this is the first study to evaluate mental fatigue in MTBI patients and the underlying neural mechanisms." Findings such as this conceivably help to account for the subjective report of some students that, post concussion, they must expend considerably more mental effort to maintain the same grades.

Lezak identified fatigue as one of the "subtle" sequelae of brain damage, along with distractibility and perplexity. It is also believed that, because fatigue is common with all who sustain a brain injury, it is therefore not related to damage within a specific area of the brain [28]. Cognitive dimensions such as attention, concentration, information processing, learning, memory, and mood/behaviors are often affected. The activities that are normally automatic but become effortful after the injury, particularly during the first weeks or months, include many that are performed frequently throughout normal activities of daily living, such as concentrating, warding off distractions, reading for meaning, doing mental calculations, monitoring ongoing performances, planning the day's activities, attending to two conversations at once, or conversing with background noise. Many individuals with TBI note that by late morning or afternoon, they hit a "brick wall" or are "exhausted," failing to meet the demands of their life. Described as "sensory overload," individuals with TBI could become even more error-prone, distractible, and uncoordinated without cognitive breaks [29].

fMRI is a potentially useful tool for understanding the neural mechanisms and circuitry associated with posttraumatic fatigue. In one study, fMRI was used to track brain activity across time in 11 patients with moderate to severe TBI while they performed a modified Symbol Digit Modalities Task (mSDMT). Cognitive fatigue was operationally defined as a relative increase in cerebral activation across time compared to that seen in 11 age-matched healthy controls. While performing the mSDMT, participants with a TBI showed increased activity, while healthy controls subsequently showed decreased activity in several regions, including the middle frontal gyrus, superior parietal cortex, basal ganglia, and anterior cingulate. The authors concluded that increased brain activity exhibited by participants with a TBI might represent increased cerebral effort which may be manifested as cognitive fatigue.

Although there may be undetectable changes in conventional imaging studies after mTBI, the collective body of work in single- photon emission computed tomography and functional magnetic resonance imaging (fMRI) point to physiological changes during mental tasks suggestive of inefficient neurological processing. It is proposed that widespread brain activation after mTBI contributes to brain fatigue [30]. Christodoulou and colleagues [31] highlighted cerebral alteration during working-memory tasks. fMRI was used to assess brain activation during a working-memory task (a modified version of the paced auditory serial addition test). Participants with TBI were able to perform the task, but made significantly more errors than healthy controls. Cerebral activation in both groups was found in similar regions of the frontal, parietal, and temporal lobes, and resembled patterns of activation found in previous neuroimaging studies of working memory in healthy persons. However, compared with the healthy controls, the TBI group displayed a pattern of cerebral activation that was more regionally dispersed and more lateralized to the right hemisphere.

The study also demonstrates the dose-dependent impact of cognitive demand. Animal models support a model of brain activation in which there is an increased hemodynamic response in relation to increasing task difficulty [31]. The dispersion index analysis showed that the TBI group did display a more dispersed activation in regions immediately surrounding the region of interest (middle frontal gyrus and middle temporal gyrus). This finding may represent an attempt by the brain to engage additional regional cerebral resources to complete the task, similar to the increased cerebral representation seen using motor tasks. The authors conclude that the direct relationship of these altered cognitive pathways to fatigue is unclear [31]. However, the presence of a more dispersed cerebral activation during cognitive tasks points to a neurophysiologic basis for changes after TBI that can contribute to cognitive fatigue.

Genetic Influences and Individual Variation

The more we learn about brain injuries, the more we appreciate the incredible heterogeneity. It is worth remembering that brain injury is the most complex disease process impacting the most complex organ system. As in many areas of medicine and recovery from illness or injury, some individuals have more difficulty with recovery from brain injuries than others. Correlations with location of anatomic injury are not always helpful; pre-injury physical and psychological makeup or personality may be more indicative of gauging an individual's potential to recover from a new insult. The interplay between central nervous system physiological changes with functional and psychological adaptation contributes to the variability in outcomes. The impact of these factors and actual health outcomes are described in the emerging field of epigenetics. There is a strong variability in different individuals' responses to the same impact. It is not uncommon to see different outcomes from individuals who were involved in the same event. One person may sustain a severe brain injury and even death, while others in the same event seem to be minimally affected. It is our understanding that genetic, biomechanical, and other environmental factors help explain variations in why certain individuals with brain injuries complain of fatigue after concussion, and why some people continue to perceive fatigue after a year, and others perceive resolution in a week.

Some empirical research hints at what those moderating factors might be. Several review papers have explored the potential for genetic and epigenetic factors to impact fatigue in general. The authors have remarked on the need to clarify the phenotype of fatigue and standardizing its measurement [32, 33].

Efficacious studies will require large sample sizes and require analysis of both systems biology in combination with environmental influences along with differential gene expression. Phenotypic fatigue measurement after brain injury is an ongoing challenge with the need to measure not only an individual's experience of fatigue but also its impact on physical, mental, and social activities [34].

Neuroendocrine Considerations

Although TBI poses a significant risk of harms to the hypothalamic and pituitary axis, our understanding for prevalence of endocrinological challenges and their impact on cognitive functioning is still incomplete. The prevalence of specific pituitary deficit is quite challenging since there is heterogeneity in severity and type of TBI in the populations studied, the tests applied for endocrine evaluation, and in the definition of normal or impaired hormone secretion. Further complicating the issues is the lack of clinical symptoms even when laboratory abnormalities are detected. The lack of systematic surveillance and registry presents an additional barrier for monitoring and intervention.

Belmont and colleagues found that PTF is common, independent of TBI severity, and may be related to insufficiency in the hypothalamic–pituitary axis [17]. A prospective study with general trauma controls by Kelly and colleagues showed a moderate association of growth hormone insufficiency with fatigue and reduced quality of life in the first nine months post TBI [35]. Prevalence of pituitary dysfunction following moderate or severe head injury or subarachnoid hemorrhage of 25–56% may persist into the chronic phases of recovery [36].

Benvenga and colleagues have estimated the prevalence of hypopituitarism to be 42.7% (range 28–68.5%) in a series of 357 cases [37]. Five major studies on post-traumatic hypopituitarism (PTHP) have been published with 344 patients (258 males, 86 females, with the diagnosis made some time between one month and 23 years). Some of the associated findings for the development of PTHP include diffuse axonal injury as the primary mechanism of brain injury, the presence of coma, especially when prolonged (PTHP found in 93% in cohort) and when associated with basilar skull, facial fractures, and cranial nerve injuries. PTHP was noted to have a higher prevalence in females in a large series published by Benvenga and colleagues.

Schneider and colleagues [38] note that, after TBI, likely changes occur in the brain's ability to regulate the biological stress response (i.e., activation of stress hormones, then deactivation when the threat has subsided). Compounding the physiological changes are the environmental factors leading to chronic stress, further compromising the flexibility of the biological stress system.

Bay and Covassin [39] suggest that chronic stress, previously shown to mediate the relationship between depressive symptoms and psychological function after TBI, may also mediate relationships between pre-injury (age or other demographic variables) or injury-related factors, such as severity of injury, frequency of somatic symptoms or time since injury and fatigue-related quality of life, reflecting the functional impact of fatigue on everyday living.

Bay and colleagues [40] found that nearly 50% of post-TBI fatigue was associated with somatic symptoms and chronic situational stress ($n = 75$). The concept of "allostatic load," proposed by McEwen [41] and reflected by altered flexibility in the biological stress response, increases the likelihood for stress-related disorders or functional alterations. Chronic exposure and deterioration of the body's hypothalamic–pituitary–adrenal stress axis have been associated with both hypo- and hyperhypercortisolemia or dysregulation of the hypothalamic–pituitary–adrenal stress axis [40].

Although endocrine abnormalities were relatively common in this population, particularly growth hormone insufficiency, secondary hypothyroidism, and low testosterone in males, the correlation of neuroendocrine dysfunction with fatigue was not statistically significant [42]. Although there was no correlation between pituitary dysfunction and fatigue, the relatively high prevalence of hypothyroidism and adrenal dysfunction suggests screening for these hormone deficiencies. Growth hormone deficiency diagnosis and replacement are more controversial as few studies have demonstrated its benefit in individuals with brain injuries [43].

Assessment of Post-TBI Fatigue

Although post-traumatic fatigue, like many other post-concussion symptoms, can be difficult to quantify and no particular medication or intervention is known to be curative, listening to patients is crucial to problem solving. In their own words, many individuals report fatigue as "my head is foggy" or "life is too overwhelming!" It is easy to not fully explore these comments during a typical physician or therapy visit due to other lingering issues that require more urgent intervention. A recurring theme that commonly surfaces is that fatigue impacts areas including memory, learning, and effectively returning to previous social roles.

The subjective nature of this particular symptom can make it elusive. A great place to start is a detailed history looking at pre-injury level of physical activity, cognitive function, and mental health to determine the effects of fatigue in relation to the injury. Thorough assessment, including understanding the alleviating and provocative factors, and its impact on everyday cognitive, physical, and psychosocial activities of everyday living, would be more likely to lead to interventions, which is no different than the pragmatic diagnostic approach used in other commonly noted symptoms such as headache or pain.

Providing that sleep architecture has not been disturbed, individuals with TBI start the day with some feeling of energy. Then, fairly suddenly, often they feel like a curtain is falling down; they find they are struggling to keep going; and may have difficulty making sense of what they're doing. PTF is a subjective feeling of weariness and depleted energy with no real objective measure. It can have physical, cognitive and/ or emotional components.

A thorough medication review is a must. Equally important is differentiating fatigue from excessive daytime sleepiness. Excessive daytime sleepiness means that there is a physiological drive to sleep, with measurable behavioral signs (yawning, eyes drooping, reduced alertness) and can be quantified in a sleep laboratory(multiple sleep latency test). This is by no means a comprehensive list, but co-conditions that need to be considered in post-concussive fatigue include:

- depression
- sleep problems, such as sleep apnea
- hypothyroidism or other endocrine gland disorders
- respiratory or cardiac problems
- headaches
- musculoskeletal pain

Table 24.2 Summary of common metrics used in fatigue assessment

Metric	Key features
Multidimensional Assessment of Fatigue (MAF)	Sixteen-item scale that measures severity of fatigue and impact on function
Fatigue Severity Scale (FSS)	Nine-item measure that assesses how fatigue affects a person's functioning in general (rating 1–7)
Barrow Neurological Institute (BNI) Fatigue Scale	Designed specifically for brain-injured patients, a self-report measure on ten fatigue-related items and an additional rating of overall fatigue severity level
Fatigue Impact Scale (FIS)	Forty-item multidimensional instrument designed to measure how fatigue affects specific aspects of physical, cognitive, and psychosocial functioning
Modified Fatigue Impact Scale (MFIS)	Valid multidimensional measure that can be used to evaluate the impact of fatigue on cognitive and physical functioning in individuals with mild to moderate traumatic brain injury
TBI Quality of Life (TBI-QOL) Fatigue Short Form	Collaborative Traumatic Brain Injury Model Systems (TBIMS) project involving five TBIMS centers

- lack of physical exercise
- vitamin deficiency/poor nutrition
- stress
- anemia.

There is no criterion standard for measuring fatigue, but the most prevalent method is by self-report rating instruments (Table 24.2). There are number assessments, including the Global Fatigue Index, the Barrow Neurological Institute Fatigue Scale Overall Severity Index Score, and the Multidimensional Fatigue Inventory. Potempa and colleagues (1986) offered the first model of fatigue as multidimensional and as an outcome associated with many factors [44].

Lachapelle and Finlayson [8] examined three self-report scales and an objective measure for their value in assessing fatigue in patients with brain injury. Individuals with brain injury and healthy controls completed the Fatigue Impact Scale (FIS), Visual Analogue Scale for Fatigue, and Fatigue Severity Scale (FSS). Fatigue was objectively measured via a continuous thumb-pressing task. They found individuals with brain injuries scored higher on all fatigue measures than did participants without brain injury and the FIS provided the most comprehensive examination of fatigue [8].

In a recent review of fatigue scales for individuals with TBIs, the FIS and FSS were identified as two short instruments with demonstrably good psychometric properties [8]. While both the FIS and the FSS have demonstrated utility in TBI, the FIS may be the most comprehensive since it measures various dimensions of fatigue, distinguishes those with brain injury from a control group, and significantly correlates with an objective measure of fatigue, making it particularly useful [8]. It is important to note that the FSS, the FIS, the Visual Analogue Scale-F, the Global Fatigue Index, and the Barroso Fatigue Scale were not designed for people with brain injury,

but rather they were developed for HIV or multiple sclerosis populations [45, 46].

The 40-item FIS has been shortened to 21 items and renamed the Modified Fatigue Impact Scale (MFIS). Schiehser and colleagues [47] validated the MFIS as a multidimensional measure with two subscales (physical/activities and cognitive) that can be used to evaluate the impact of fatigue on cognitive and physical functioning in individuals with mild to moderate TBI. MFIS measures the impact of fatigue on functioning by having participants rate how often fatigue has affected 21 functions during the past four weeks using a zero (never) to four-point (almost always) scale. Scores range from zero to 84, with higher scores indicating greater impact of fatigue [47].

Neuroendocrine Assessment

Because pituitary deficits may affect 20–30% patients in the subacute and chronic phase after TBI, physicians must continuously monitor their patients for signs and symptoms. Consulting with endocrinological specialists can be helpful in diagnostic and hormone replacement therapy decisions.

It is beyond the scope of this chapter to review neuroendocrine dysregulation following TBI; readers are advised to review the recommendations from the TBI Consensus Group for Neuroendocrine workup [48]. Some key recommendations:

- *All* individuals hospitalized for TBI should undergo an adequate evaluation of anterior and posterior pituitary function.
- *All* individuals with moderate to severe TBI and clinical signs or symptoms associated with hypopituitarism should be screened when there is evidence of:
  - unexplained symptoms (hypotension, weight loss, fatigue, loss of libido, depression)
  - suspicious biochemical alterations (hyponatremia, hypoglycemia, reduced blood cell count)
  - the patient not achieving the expected recovery.

The Department of Defense/Department of Veterans Affairs *Clinical Practice Guideline for Management of Concussion/Mild Traumatic Brain Injury* recommends blood count, metabolic panel, vitamin B_{12} and folate levels, thyroid function test, and erythrocyte sedimentation rate as part of the workup [20].

Management of Post-Concussive Fatigue

Interventions for fatigue using both pharmacological and non-pharmacological measures have been trialed. In a systematic review of pharmacological, psychological, and environmental interventions (physical activity, bright blue light, electroencephalographic biofeedback, or electrical stimulation) by Cantor and co-authors [49], two interventions (modafinil and cognitive behavioral therapy with fatigue management) were evaluated in more than one study. They concluded that there is insufficient evidence to recommend or contraindicate any treatments for PTF [49].

Fatigue management

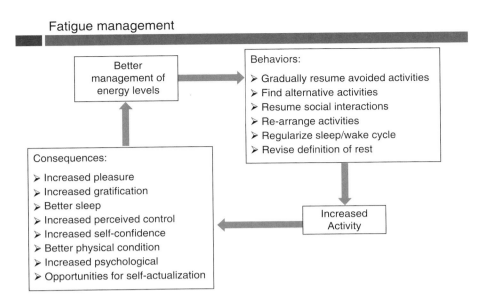

Fig. 24.3 Fatigue management algorithm.
Source: Ouellet, 2011 [24]. Ouellet, 2011.
Reproduced with permission from Pr M. Ouellet

Effective management begins with a thorough diagnostic approach, quantifying the level of dysfunction. Just as important is educating both patients and their caregivers about the occurrence of post-concussive fatigue and expectations following an injury. There is a high variability in how TBI survivors recover from various symptoms over time. This individual variation should be taken into account when a treatment plan is generated (Figure 24.3). What is generally agreed is that with delay for individuals with concussion to access proper evaluation, education, and management of the symptoms, the likelihood is higher that the symptomatology can persist. Despite the current challenges, individuals with concussions can reach and sustain purposeful, goal-directed mental effort. This long-term treatment objective is a key requirement for independent functioning at home and in work settings. Managing expectations will be crucial since post-concussion individuals may have reduced insight and low frustration tolerance.

Bay and De-Leon [14] propose that, rather than focus on fatigue as a single symptom or symptom cluster, the assessment of PTF should shift to reducing its negative impact on quality of life. Just as fatigue is multidimensional, so is its management. The challenging work lies in investing time in activity and behavioral analysis to gain insights into the triggers and alleviating factors.

Management also includes deprogramming and modifying compensation modes. Some of the compensation strategies observed include longer time in bed, more naps, increased intake of caffeine, canceling or reducing activities, and sleep/wake regulation [14]. Per Ouellet and colleagues, fatigue management encompasses self-monitoring of fatigue and energy, identification of signs of fatigue, gradual augmentation of activity levels, and activity planning (rest periods, alternating tasks, task segregation, and realistic goal setting [19].

Timing of interventions can also be a factor with regard to optimizing success. Just like the body, the brain needs time for healing after a traumatic injury. For some individuals with concussion, fatigue gradually lessens over time while stamina and endurance improve. And for others, their endurance is just not what it used to be. In most cases, fatigue is brought on most quickly by cognitive effort, desk work, reading, or any activity that needs attention and concentration. Physical effort does have some effect, particularly in early stages when it may bring on somatic symptoms, but later it is better tolerated. It is important to help individuals understand that it may require multiple visits and working with a team (physicians, therapists, neuropsychologists, rehab psychologists, counselors, and exercise trainer) to identify triggers and treatment interventions, which may take time to show some benefits.

It is crucial to address post-concussion impairments such as vertigo, visuo-perceptual disturbances, pain, and sleep–wake cycle and mood disturbances. These neurocognitive residuals need to be addressed in therapies in a comprehensive program, along the way, being mindful that managing fatigue may be derailed in that treatments for other symptoms can potentially worsen fatigue. One common scenario is that medications to enhance sleep could produce daytime sedation. Psychiatric and psychological services to address changes in mood and behaviors following concussion are not adjunctive, but medically indicated for management of PTF to be effective.

Behavioral/Lifestyle Interventions

Educational efforts should be in the areas of factors contributing to fatigue, importance of well-balanced nutrition, and promotion of sleep hygiene and regular exercise. The following section outlines a number of areas to consider in managing PTF. Clearly, there is no one intervention that will be a stand-alone in addressing fatigue. Individuals have tried some approaches to addressing fatigue by changing routine and other non-pharmacological approaches. Some approaches have been more successful and seem to have emerging evidence to support their role. It is crucial to adapt treatments to the particular needs of the individual with PTF.

Exercise

Aerobic exercise appears to offer some hope in alleviation of fatigue in a host of other medical conditions. Both animal and human studies have validated the role of exercise in enhancing cognitive functioning. In the early phase, exercise appears to influence neuroplasticity via neurogenesis and neurotrophin up-regulation. Itoh and colleagues found that exercise, particularly running, enhances neuronal stem cell proliferation and neurogenesis [50]. This elegant model demonstrates that rats with induced concussion assigned to the exercise group (that ran on a treadmill for 30 min/day at 22 m/min for seven consecutive days) showed increases in the proliferation of neuronal stem cells around the damaged area following TBI even as early as three to seven days after the exercise intervention [50]. Mota and colleagues [51] suggest that previous physical training reduces initial damage and limits long-term secondary degeneration after TBI. In an animal model (subjected to fluid percussion injury), previous running exercise (four weeks) protected against fluid percussion injury-induced inflammatory and secondary impact of the initial injury [51].

The improvements induced by physical exercise regimes in brain plasticity and neurocognitive performance are evident both in healthy individuals and in those afflicted by TBI. It is postulated that physical exercise reinforces the adaptive processes of the brain and facilitates the development of existing networks to compensate for those lost through damage. Exercise intervention induces beneficial changes in cerebral blood flow, angiogenesis, and vascular disease improvement [52]. The area of the brain that seems to benefit the most is the hippocampus, often viewed as the center for memory integration. Fogelman and Zafonte recommend resuming exercise as soon as possible in patients with mTBI. Their review includes human clinical studies of exercise intervention after TBI [53].

Gordon and colleagues note that individuals with TBI who exercised regularly were less depressed and had fewer residual symptoms [54]. Driver and Ede highlight the benefits of an eight-week program of physical activities; various components of mood were enhanced (anxiety, depression, anger, confusion), including a reduction in fatigue and an increase in vigor [55].

Most recently, a randomized control trial of walking to ameliorate fatigue following brain injury was successful in lowering fatigue, as measured by three different fatigue scales, compared to a sham treatment arm in a double crossover study of 123 community-dwelling individuals with TBI [56].

If exercise seems to be a cost-effective and promising intervention, why is it difficult for many individuals with TBI to access this intervention? In the TBI population, adherence to an exercise program may be problematic due to neurocognitive challenges (impaired memory, insight, problem solving, safety awareness, executive dysfunction/follow-through, social interaction challenges) as well as logistical problems (inability to get to a gym, weather conditions, the need for supervision for safety, costs, lack of accommodation).

An effective approach would be to enroll patients in a number of supported programs generally available at community colleges/universities/adult education. Working closely with the Disabled Students Offices, these adaptive physical education programs generally have better retention and success over self-directed exercise programs. Scheduling of exercise may need to be addressed depending upon when the patient is at his or her best. Exercise routines should be individualized to maximize benefit and promote proper ratio of activity/rest.

Barriers to access such as costs may be reduced for students with disabilities through state funding or scholarships. Over the years, these programs have been found to be helpful for individuals with brain injury who have residual neurocognitive impairments to stay motivated and active. Many individuals report the benefits of being in a school or community setting, with staff and peer support at these programs as the main reasons for the sustainability over self-directed exercise programs.

Sleep Hygiene

Sleep–wake dysregulation is a common problem following all severities of TBI. Baumann and colleagues found in a prospective study that sleep–wake disturbances subsequent to TBI were present in three out of four individuals with TBIs and that the most prevalent sleep–wake disturbances were excessive daytime sleepiness/fatigue (55%) and post-traumatic hypersomnia (22%) [57].

Many studies note similar findings. In a retrospective study comprising a heterogeneous population of 184 somnolent subjects suffering from TBI or head and neck trauma (whiplash injury), 45% of patients reported insomnia ("disturbed nocturnal sleep"), mostly due to nocturnal pain. Sleep–wake disorders are frequent among survivors of traumatic brain injury [58], which is consistent with a questionnaire study by Ouellet and colleagues. More than 50% of 452 TBI patients reported insomnia symptoms, and insomnia was a severe and chronic condition that remained untreated in almost 60% of cases [9, 20].

Ouellet et al. noted that, in their large cohorts of 452 individuals with mild to severe TBI at an average of 7.8 years from injury onset, 50% reported insomnia symptoms and about 30% had insomnia syndrome. They found factors associated with insomnia following TBI included severity, depressive symptoms, fatigue, and pain level [19].

Ponsford and colleagues [59] evaluated a cohort of community-based individuals with TBI. Measures of subjective fatigue and sleep disturbances, as well as attentional measures, were gathered. They found fatigue and sleep disturbance to be common and associated with anxiety, depression, and pain. A subgroup of participants completed polysomnography which showed reduced sleep efficiency, increased sleep onset latency, and increased time awake after sleep onset. Depression and pain exacerbate but cannot entirely account for these problems. There is increased slow-wave sleep. Individuals with TBI show lower levels of evening melatonin production, associated with less rapid eye movement sleep [59]. Not surprisingly, sleep disturbances are highly correlated with fatigue.

Ouellet outlined potential causes of sleep–wake disturbance following TBI, including damage to structures important for sleep, hormonal and neurotransmitter alterations, pain, alcohol use/abuse, and medications [60]. Psycho-social factors to consider are environment (e.g., hospital, new home, stimulation load), stress, and unhealthy sleep/wake habits.

The spectrum of most common sleep–wake disturbances seen following TBI includes excessive daytime sleepiness from sleep apnea (obstructive or central), narcolepsy, post-traumatic hypersomnia, and circadian rhythm sleep disorders. Proper laboratory and sleep studies may be diagnostic for delayed sleep onset, multiple awakenings, prolonged awakenings, and early-morning awakenings.

Given what we currently understand about the role of sleep in neurocognitive functioning, mood, and pain, it is crucial that a careful sleep history and investigation should be sought in patients who describe ongoing sleep disturbance. After the appropriate diagnostic interventions, logical steps to optimize sleep–wake cycle start with education of the patients on sleep hygiene. For many individuals with TBI, restoring sleep–wake cycle is the first and most important step in the management of daytime fatigue. Together with exercise, these interventions are generally well accepted by most patients and their families.

Non-pharmacological options such as relaxation-based interventions and cognitive therapy have been shown to be effective and perhaps more durable than pharmacological therapy [61]. In Ouellet and Morin's case study with 11 participants, participants underwent cognitive behavioral therapy for insomnia (eight or ten weekly sessions lasting one hour). Cognitive behavioral therapy included stimulus control, sleep restrictions, cognitive restructuring, sleep hygiene education, and fatigue management. Following the treatment eight of the 11 participants had improved their sleep and these improvements could be seen at follow-up for most of the participants. One caveat to keep in mind is that pharmacologic treatment to ameliorate sleep disturbances or depression can also exacerbate fatigue and memory functioning.

Substance Use

Review of illicit drugs, alcohol, tobacco, and caffeine or other stimulant use or abuse should be routinely discussed. Emphasis on "wellness" components includes education of the impact of many substances that affect individuals differently after a brain injury. Alcohol is a central depressant and is a widely available agent that could contribute to decreasing cognitive stamina and judgment.

According to the Brain Injury Association, people who experience brain injuries often have a prior history of substance use or abuse [62, 63]. Several studies have shown that before their injury people who sustain a TBI are twice as likely (35%) as others in the community (17%) to be either a significant user or abuser of drugs or alcohol – sometimes both [64]. Many different research groups have explored this topic and have found that as many as 25% of the people in their studies have used/abused alcohol and/or marijuana *at some time after* brain injury. However, fewer people say they are *currently* using or abusing.

The specific negative effects of drug and alcohol use after TBI also include interfering with brain recovery and increased frequency of behavioral dyscontrol. Hibbard and colleagues [65] recommend that all individuals with TBI should be screened for prior drug and alcohol use patterns at the time of injury. Second, all individuals, regardless of prior usage, should be educated about the negative consequences of continuing, or starting, to use drugs or alcohol after injury. Third, those with TBI who have drug/alcohol problems need rehabilitation programs that provide dual treatment – not aimed just at TBI or at substance use, but at both. Training in self-monitoring is part of helping individuals with TBIs cope.

Hydration

Certain brain injuries and memory deficits also can prevent people from recognizing when they need to drink. The urge to drink fluids is a natural instinct regulated by a negative-feedback loop between the brain and other organs in the body. Thirst and satiety mechanisms can be altered due to damage to the hypothalamic–pituitary axis and cranial nerve disturbances. To complicate matters, some individuals with TBI may also consume more caffeine to compensate for fatigue or use alcohol to help them sleep. An enhanced response to these substances for variable duration after their injuries is reported by many individuals with TBI. Education about the effects of caffeine (natural stimulant) and alcohol needs to be a part of wellness after a brain injury.

Various models of drinking behavior have been used to identify the site of dysregulation of water consumption. In brain injury survivors, however, that loop is sometimes weakened, putting them at risk for dehydration and it could be a contributing factor to the feeling of being "tired."

The body's primary "thirst center" in the brain is the hypothalamus. When the body gets low on water, the hypothalamus increases the synthesis of an antidiuretic hormone, which is secreted by the posterior pituitary gland and stimulates water reabsorption by the kidneys, thus reducing urine flow and conserving water in the body until more fluids are consumed. Brain injury can dampen the hypothalamic–pituitary axis, affecting regulation of blood sodium concentration, and people can lose their sense of thirst completely. They must be prescribed a fixed amount of fluids daily to keep their body safely hydrated [66].

If the pituitary gland becomes damaged, however, or if the kidneys are unable to respond to antidiuretic hormone, the body is unable to conserve fluids. The result can be diabetes insipidus, a condition marked by excessive urination and extreme, uncontrollable thirst. Dopaminergic, cholinergic, and hippocampal etiologies have been implicated in this abnormality of fluid homeostasis [67].

Energy Conservation

Following concussions, many may find that simple tasks require more concentration and effort and they tire more easily. Principles of energy conservation can be very crucial in addressing symptoms of fatigue. This set of principles has been noted to be beneficial in other medical conditions such as post-polio syndrome and multiple sclerosis. These important behavioral changes often require the input of family members and therapists (occupational, physical, and/or speech) and co-workers who are knowledgeable to help the individuals to be more aware of signs of fatigue, and when they happen.

Comprehensive holistic neuropsychological rehabilitation is centered on the goals of fostering awareness of their functional potential and adapting to the chronic limitations imposed by their injury, in order to alleviate disability in everyday social functioning. Neuropsychologists, rehabilitation psychologists, and therapists are part of the care team to help individuals with TBIs understand their ongoing and evolving challenges. As part of their rehabilitation, individuals may be taught or re-taught how to prioritize their commitments and are encouraged to recognize their abilities and limitations [68]. Formal instruction on concepts of energy conservation to maximize daily productivity is emphasized.

Below are some of the main components of energy conservation [69].

Plan

- Plan days and weeks ahead of time so that activities requiring more energy and less energy are alternated.
- Plan for days when there may be increased pain or fatigue – learn the "warning signs" that your body is telling you and stop an activity before you feel completely exhausted.
- Plan to complete activities that are the most physically demanding at times when you have the most energy, e.g., some people have most energy in the morning and then feel more tired in the afternoon.
- Limit changes in daily routine.

Prioritize

- Recognize that everything may not get done and learn to be OK with that.
- Decide what is most important.
- Ask or allow other people to help you when possible.
- Be sure to include activities you enjoy doing.
- Work to change your perspective on what "productivity" means to you. It may be that you have to learn that it's best to be satisfied with completing fewer tasks more efficiently and without feeling overwhelmed by fatigue.

Pace

- Slow down the pace for completing your daily activities.
- Give yourself plenty of time to do each task For example: every hour take a five- to ten-minute break and use an alarm watch or phone to remind you.
- Perform the tasks that require the most concentration earlier in the day, whenever possible.
- Balance activities with rest breaks. Rest *before* you are tired.
- Break up a large task by doing a little each day.

- Alternate between heavy and light tasks and between physical and cognitive demands.
- Start with familiar tasks at home or work that you can complete without fatigue. Gradually increase the complexity of each task, taking breaks as needed.

Eliminate

- Think about the activities you try to complete each day. Is there anything you would be comfortable eliminating for a while?
- Avoid over-scheduling.
- If visitors make you tired, limit time with them.

Organize

- Minimize clutter. Keep things in easy-to-find places so that little energy is used to locate them.
- Make sure items you use regularly are easily accessible. For example, try labeling boxes and storage containers.
- Make a daily "To Do" list; place it in a readily accessible spot.
- Review the "To Do" list, and check off the tasks as they are completed.
- Use a memory aid regularly, such as an organizer, smart phone, calendar, day planner, sticky notes, or a watch timer.

Restore

- Try to include activities in your day that bring you pleasure and add to your energy bank.
- For example, set aside time to read an interesting book, talk with an upbeat friend or family member on the phone, listen to music, and find a way to be playful or laugh.

Environmental Modification

Alleviating factors such as lighting level, ambient noise level, and complexity of the activities all need to be taken into account. There are many other practical and low-cost interventions to reduce unnecessary stimulation, including the following:

- Remove visual and auditory distractions (TV, radio) whenever possible.
- Reduce clutter and remove things that are not essential for performing day-to-day tasks.
- Build in a strategy for interruptions.
- Build in periodic breaks as fatigue affects memory.
- Educate the family and co-workers about ways they can help, such as providing information and instructions in writing as well as verbally.
- Family and co-workers can also assist by providing cues when they notice help is needed.

Pharmacological Approach

No effective pharmacological option has been identified to decrease PTF. However, some general management approaches could be helpful in caring for individuals with post-concussive fatigue.

Medication Review

Due to the large number of centrally acting medications, ongoing medication review is necessary. In general, when caring for individuals with TBIs, the rule of "less is more" applies. Medications prescribed to treat sleep–wake disturbances, seizures, depression, and pain can be sedating. If a medication appears contributory, performance of an applied behavioral analysis trial is indicated to determine the association. Consideration should be given for removal of the most sedating agents or at least reducing dosage or substitution of less sedating medications. Modifiable factors should be addressed and typical conservative measures taken prior to initiating pharmacotherapy for fatigue.

Neurostimulants

Neurostimulants are used "off-label" to enhance daytime alertness and arousal. Although widely used after brain injury, there is limited evidence in use of these medications for treatment of fatigue in individuals with concussion. Several stimulants have had success in other disease states, such as multiple sclerosis and narcolepsy associated with fatigue. There are potential therapeutic benefits of using methylphenidate, dextroamphetamine, carbidopa, amantadine, and modafinil to treat PTF [70].

A clinical guideline from the Department of Defense/ Department of Veterans Affairs supports a neurostimulant trial if symptoms have persisted for more than four weeks post injury and the fatigue level has not improved with the management of sleep, pain, depression, or lifestyle [20]. In addition, medication trials should persist for at least 3 months and the use of neurostimulant medications is contraindicated if there is a history of substance abuse.

Two randomized controlled trials evaluated the effects of modafinil on fatigue and excessive daytime sleepiness [71, 72]. Modafinil, a wakefulness-promoting agent, was initially approved for use with those who were having difficulty with excessive daytime sleepiness [71].

In the study conducted by Kaiser and colleagues [72], modafinil (100–200 mg daily) was administered to a treatment group of ten patients who had been diagnosed with fatigue or excessive daytime sleepiness. The control group was administered a placebo. Sleepiness and fatigue were assessed using the Epworth Sleepiness Scale (ESS) and the FSS. No significant changes were noted on the FSS between the two groups at the end of the six-week period as a result of taking the modafinil. A decrease in the ESS scores was also noted: the Modafinil group's scores were significantly decreased throughout the treatment period ($p < 0.005$) compared to the placebo group. Overall, modafinil improves sleepiness but not fatigue [72].

Jha and colleagues [71] had 51 participants in their study. Participants were divided into two groups: one group ($n = 27$) received modafinil and the other ($n = 24$) received a placebo. At the end of phase 1, groups were "crossed over." For the intervention group, modafinil was given 100 mg daily for three days, increased to 100 mg BID for 11 days. Eventually a maintenance dose of 200 mg was given BID. The researchers found that modafinil was well tolerated but it was not effective treatment for either daytime sleepiness or fatigue.

Closing Summary and Recommendations

PTF significantly harms recovery, quality of life, and social functioning. With further study, a better understanding of the pathophysiology of TBI and PTF should lead to better therapeutic strategies for these patients.

Fatigue can be challenging to quantify because of its multidimensionality (physical, mental, and psychological). We recommend using a tool such as the MFIS to evaluate the impact of fatigue on cognitive and physical functioning in individuals with mild to moderate TBI.

PTF can be due to a primary effect related to central nervous system dysfunction or a secondary effect such as common co-existing disorders in concussion/mTBI, such as depression or sleep disturbances. Pre-morbid level of functioning, level of stress, and other psychological and environmental factors need to be considered during evaluation. When assessing PTF, consider the influence of co-morbidities of depression, pain, sleep disturbance, and neuroendocrine abnormalities. Its mechanisms are complex and multi-factorial.

Because fatigue is a symptom, the diagnostic assessment includes understanding the alleviating and provocative factors. Patients need to pay attention to what triggers fatigue, and learn to identify the early signs of fatigue, such as becoming more irritable or distracted.

The field of epigenetics contributes to our evolving understanding for the genetic, biochemical, and environmental factors in explaining individual outcome variations.

A multimodal and multidisciplinary management approach should be used.

Potential treatments, including cognitive behavior therapy supporting lifestyle modifications to decrease fatigue level and improve functional performance, pharmacologic treatments, and hormone replacement therapy, may be helpful with posttraumatic fatigue.

Medications, substance use, and lifestyle factors may contribute to fatigue. Alcohol and marijuana will generally make fatigue worse. Caffeine (coffee, cola products) should be avoided after lunch if sleeping is a problem. It is important to screen for drug and alcohol abuse in this population because of their potential effect on brain recovery. With identification, education about the consequences of continued use and abuse post TBI can be provided and individuals can be referred to drug treatment programs.

Aerobic exercise offers one of the most compelling and effective interventions to improve human performance. Exercise therapy (rehabilitation) has the potential to enhance recovery in TBI. Research has shown that people with TBI who exercise have better mental function and alertness. Over time, exercise and being more active help lessen physical and mental fatigue and build stamina. Exercise has been shown to improve fatigue, even years after injury.

Cardiovascular exercise is an important tool and a highly recommended intervention for patients with PTF. Exercise offers one of the most effective interventions to enhance neurocognitive functioning. It also may decrease depression and improve sleep.

Practicing energy conservation principles and prioritizing, planning, and pacing for those important tasks of the day are very often helpful. Focusing on resumption of important daily routines at the opportune time of day, augmenting healthy habits like exercise and sleep hygiene are likely to remain the foundations of treatment for fatigue after brain injury.

References

1. National Center for Health Statistics. National hospital discharge survey (NHDS). 2010. Available at www.cdc.gov/nchs/nhds/.

2. National Center for Health Statistics. National hospital ambulatory medical care survey (NHAMCS). 2010. Available at www.cdc.gov/nchs/data/ahcd/nhamcs_emergency/2010_ed_web_tables.pdf.

3. National Center for Health Statistics. National vital statistics system (NVSS). 2010. Available at www.cdc.gov/nchs/nvss/.

4. Dittner AJ, Wessely SC, Brown RG. The assessment of fatigue: A practical guide for clinicians and researchers. *J Psychosom Res* 2004; 56: 157–170.

5. Aaronson LS, Teel CS, Cassmeyer V, Neuberger GB, Pallikkathayil L, Pierce J, et al. Defining and measuring fatigue. *Image J Nurs Sch* 1999; 31: 45–50.

6. Henrie M, Elovic E. Fatigue: Assessment and treatment. In: Zasler N, Katz D, Zafonte R, editors. *Brain injury medicine: Principles and practice*, 2nd edition. New York: Demos Medical Publishing, 2012, pp. 693–706.

7. Ouellet M-C, Morin CM. Fatigue following traumatic brain injury: Frequency, characteristics, and associated factors. *Rehabil Psychol* 2006; 51: 140.

8. Lachapelle DL, Finlayson MA. An evaluation of subjective and objective measures of fatigue in patients with brain injury and healthy controls. *Brain Inj* 1998; 12: 649–659.

9. Ouellet MC, Morin CM. Subjective and objective measures of insomnia in the context of traumatic brain injury: A preliminary study. *Sleep Med* 2006; 7: 486–497.

10. Bushnik T, Englander J, Wright J. Patterns of fatigue and its correlates over the first 2 years after traumatic brain injury. *J Head Trauma Rehabil* 2008; 23: 25–32.

11. Norrie J. Energy crisis: prevalence, severity, treatment and persistence of fatigue after mild traumatic brain injury: A dissertation presented in partial fulfilment of the requirements for the degree of Doctor of Philosophy in Psychology at Massey University, Palmerston North, New Zealand, 2012.

12. Cantor JB, Ashman T, Gordon W, Ginsberg A, Engmann C, Egan M, et al. Fatigue after traumatic brain injury and its impact on participation and quality of life. *J Head Trauma Rehabil* 2008; 23: 41–51.

13. Englander J, Bushnik T, Oggins J, Katznelson L. Fatigue after traumatic brain injury: Association with neuroendocrine, sleep, depression and other factors. *Brain Inj* 2010; 24: 1379–1388.

14. Bay E, De-Leon MB. Chronic stress and fatigue-related quality of life after mild to moderate traumatic brain injury. *J Head Trauma Rehabil* 2011; 26: 355–363.

15. Ponsford JL, Ziino C, Parcell DL, Shekleton JA, Roper M, Redman JR, et al. Fatigue and sleep disturbance following traumatic brain injury – Their nature, causes, and potential treatments. *J Head Trauma Rehabil* 2012; 27: 224–233.

16. Bushnik T, Englander J, Wright J. The experience of fatigue in the first 2 years after moderate-to-severe traumatic brain injury: A preliminary report. *J Head Trauma Rehabil* 2008; 23: 17–24.

17. Belmont A, Agar N, Hugeron C, Gallais B, Azouvi P. Fatigue and traumatic brain injury. *Ann Readapt Med Phys* 2006; 49: 283–288, 370–374.

18. Levine J, Greenwald BD. Fatigue in Parkinson disease, stroke, and traumatic brain injury. *Phys Med Rehabil Clin N Am* 2009; 20: 347–361.

19. Ouellet MC, Beaulieu-Bonneau S, Morin CM. Insomnia in patients with traumatic brain injury: Frequency, characteristics, and risk factors. *J Head Trauma Rehabil* 2006; 21: 199–212.

20. The Management of Concussion/mTBI Working Group, Department of Veterans Affairs. Department of Defense (VA/DoD). *Clinical practice guideline for management of concussion/mild traumatic brain injury*. Washington, D.C.: Department of Veteran's Affairs/Department of Defense, 2009, p. 112.

21. Juengst S, Skidmore E, Arenth PM, Niyonkuru C, Raina KD. Unique contribution of fatigue to disability in community-dwelling adults with traumatic brain injury. *Arch Phys Med Rehabil* 2013; 94: 74–79.

22. Stulemeijer M, Vos PE, Bleijenberg G, Van Der Werf SP. Cognitive complaints after mild traumatic brain injury: Things are not always what they seem. *J Psychosom Res* 2007; 63: 637–645.

23. Borgaro SR, Gierok S, Caples H, Kwasnica C. Fatigue after brain injury: Initial reliability study of the BNI Fatigue Scale. *Brain Inj* 2004; 18: 685–690.

24. Ouellet MC. *Strategies for managing sleep disturbances and fatigue following traumatic brain injury*. Charlottetown: Brain Injury Association of Canada, 2011, pp. 1–107.

25. Kohl AD, Wylie G, Genova H, Hillary F, Deluca J. The neural correlates of cognitive fatigue in traumatic brain injury using functional MRI. *Brain Inj* 2009; 23: 420–432.

26. Ziino C, Ponsford J. Selective attention deficits and subjective fatigue following traumatic brain injury. *Neuropsychology* 2006; 20: 383–390.

27. Liu K, Li B, Qian S, Jiang Q, Li L, Wang W, et al. Mental fatigue after mild traumatic brain injury: A 3D-ASL perfusion study. *Brain Imaging Behav* 2016; 10: 857–868.

28. Lezak MD. Subtle sequelae of brain damage. Perplexity, distractibility, and fatigue. *Am J Phys Med* 1978; 57: 9–15.

29. Wrightson P, Gronwall D. *Mild head injury: A guide to management*. Oxford: Oxford University Press, 1999.

30. Bigler ED. Structural imaging. In: Silver J, McAllister TW, Yudofsky S, editors. *Textbook of traumatic brain injury*. Washington, D.C.: American Psychiatric Publishing, 2005, pp. 79–105.

31. Christodoulou C, Deluca J, Ricker JH, Madigan NK, Bly BM, Lange G, et al. Functional magnetic resonance imaging of working memory impairment after traumatic brain injury. *J Neurol Neurosurg Psychiatry* 2001; 71: 161–168.

32. Landmark-Hoyvik H, Reinertsen KV, Loge JH, Kristensen VN, Dumeaux V, Fossa SD, et al. The genetics and epigenetics of fatigue. *PMR* 2010; 2: 456–465.

33. Lyon DE, Mccain NL, Pickler RH, Munro C, Elswick RK, Jr. Advancing the biobehavioral research of fatigue with genetics and genomics. *J Nurs Scholarsh* 2011; 43: 274–281.

34. Cella D, Yount S, Rothrock N, Gershon R, Cook K, Reeve B, et al. The Patient-Reported Outcomes Measurement Information System (PROMIS): Progress of an NIH Roadmap cooperative group during its first two years. *Med Care* 2007; 45: S3–S11.

35. Kelly DF, Mcarthur DL, Levin H, Swimmer S, Dusick JR, Cohan P, et al. Neurobehavioral and quality of life changes associated with growth hormone insufficiency after complicated mild, moderate, or severe traumatic brain injury. *J Neurotrauma* 2006; 23: 928–942.

36. Srinivasan L, Roberts B, Bushnik T, Englander J, Spain DA, Steinberg GK, et al. The impact of hypopituitarism on function and performance in subjects with recent history of traumatic brain injury and aneurysmal subarachnoid haemorrhage. *Brain Inj* 2009; 23: 639–648.

37. Benvenga S, Campenni A, Ruggeri RM, Trimarchi F. Clinical review 113: Hypopituitarism secondary to head trauma. *J Clin Endocrinol Metab* 2000; 85: 1353–1361.

38. Schneider HJ, Kreitschmann-Andermahr I, Ghigo E, Stalla GK, Agha A. Hypothalamopituitary dysfunction following traumatic brain injury and aneurysmal subarachnoid hemorrhage: A systematic review. *JAMA* 2007; 298: 1429–1438.

39. Bay E, Covassin T. Chronic stress, somatic and depressive symptoms following mild to moderate traumatic brain injury. *Arch Psychiatric Nurs* 2012; 26: 477–486.

40. Bay E, Sikorskii A, Fuli G. Functional status, chronic stress, and cortisol response after mild-to-moderate traumatic brain injury. *Biol Res Nurs* 2009; 10: 213–225.

41. McEwen BS. Stress, adaptation, and disease. Allostasis and allostatic load. *Ann N Y Acad Sci* 1998; 840: 33–44.

42. Bushnik T, Englander J, Katznelson L. Fatigue after TBI: Association with neuroendocrine abnormalities. *Brain Inj* 2007; 21: 559–566.

43. Zgaljardic DJ, Durham WJ, Mossberg KA, Foreman J, Joshipura K, Masel BE, et al. Neuropsychological and physiological correlates of fatigue following traumatic brain injury. *Brain Inj* 2014; 28: 389–397.

44. Potempa K, Lopez M, Reid C, Lawson L. Chronic fatigue. *Image J Nurs Sch* 1986; 18: 165–169.

45. Armutlu K, Korkmaz NC, Keser I, Sumbuloglu V, Akbiyik DI, Guney Z, et al. The validity and reliability of the Fatigue Severity Scale in Turkish multiple sclerosis patients. *Int J Rehabil Res* 2007; 30: 81–85.

46. Pence BW, Barroso J, Leserman J, Harmon JL, Salahuddin N. Measuring fatigue in people living with HIV/AIDS: Psychometric characteristics of the HIV-related fatigue scale. *AIDS Care* 2008; 20: 829–837.

47. Schiehser DM, Ayers CR, Liu L, Lessig S, Song DS, Filoteo JV. Validation of the Modified Fatigue Impact Scale in Parkinson's disease. *Parkinsonism Relat Disord* 2013; 19: 335–338.

48. Ghigo E, Masel B, Aimaretti G, Léon-Carrión J, Casanueva FF, Dominguez-Morales MR, et al. Consensus guidelines on screening for hypopituitarism following traumatic brain injury. *Brain Inj* 2005; 19: 711–724.

49. Cantor JB, Ashman T, Bushnik T, Cai X, Farrell-Carnahan L, Gumber S, et al. Systematic review of interventions for fatigue after traumatic brain injury: A NIDRR Traumatic Brain Injury Model Systems study. *J Head Trauma Rehabil* 2014; 29: 490–497.

50. Itoh T, Imano M, Nishida S, Tsubaki M, Hashimoto S, Ito A, et al. Exercise increases neural stem cell proliferation surrounding the area of damage following rat traumatic brain injury. *J Neural Transm (Vienna)* 2011; 118: 193–202.

51. Mota BC, Pereira L, Souza MA, Silva LFA, Magni DV, Ferreira APO, et al. Exercise pre-conditioning reduces brain inflammation and protects against toxicity induced by traumatic brain injury: Behavioral and neurochemical approach. *Neurotox Res* 2012; 21: 175–184.

52. Archer T. Influence of physical exercise on traumatic brain injury deficits: Scaffolding effect. *Neurotox Res* 2012; 21: 418–434.

53. Fogelman D, Zafonte R. Exercise to enhance neurocognitive function after traumatic brain injury. *PMR* 2012; 4: 908–913.

54. Gordon WA, Sliwinski M, Echo J, Mcloughlin M, Sheerer MS, Meili TE. The benefits of exercise in individuals with traumatic brain injury: A retrospective study. *J Head Trauma Rehabil* 1998; 13: 58–67.

55. Driver S, Ede A. Impact of physical activity on mood after TBI. *Brain Inj* 2009; 23: 203–212.

56. Kolakowsky-Hayner SA, Bellon K, Toda K, Bushnik T, Wright J, Isaac L, Englander J. A randomised control trial of walking to ameliorate brain injury fatigue: A NIDRR TBI model system centre-based study. *Neuropsychological Rehabilitation* 2016.

57. Baumann CR, Werth E, Stocker R, Ludwig S, Bassetti CL. Sleep–wake disturbances 6 months after traumatic brain injury: A prospective study. *Brain* 2007; 130: 1873–1883.

58. Guilleminault C, Yuen KM, Gulevich MG, Karadeniz D, Leger D, Philip P. Hypersomnia after head–neck trauma: A medicolegal dilemma. *Neurology* 2000; 54: 653–659.

59. Ponsford J, Willmott C, Rothwell A, Cameron P, Kelly AM, Nelms R, et al. Factors influencing outcome following mild traumatic brain injury in adults. *J Int Neuropsychol Soc* 2000; 6: 568–579.

60. Ouellet M-C, Beaulieu-Bonneau S, Morin CM. Sleep–wake disturbances after traumatic brain injury. *Lancet Neurol* 2015; 14: 746–757.

61. Ouellet MC, Morin CM. Efficacy of cognitive-behavioral therapy for insomnia associated with traumatic brain injury: A single-case experimental design. *Arch Phys Med Rehabil* 2007; 88: 1581–1592.

62. Ashman TA, Spielman LA, Hibbard MR, Silver JM, Chandna T, Gordon WA. Psychiatric challenges in the first 6 years after traumatic brain injury: Cross-sequential analyses of Axis I disorders. *Arch Phys Med Rehabil* 2004; 85: S36–S42.

63. Center MSM. TBI consumer report: Coping with substance abuse after TBI. 2004. Available at www.brainline.org/content/2008/07/tbi-consumer-report-coping-substance-abuse-after-tbi_pageall.html.

64. Kreutzer JS, Wehman PH, Harris JA, Burns CT, Young HF. Substance abuse and crime patterns among persons with traumatic brain injury referred for supported employment. *Brain Inj* 1991; 5: 177–187.

65. Hibbard MR, Ashman TA, Spielman LA, Chun D, Charatz HJ, Melvin S. Relationship between depression and psychosocial functioning after traumatic brain injury. *Arch Phys Med Rehabil* 2004; 85 (4 Suppl 2): S43–S53.

66. Mckinley MJ, Johnson AK. The physiological regulation of thirst and fluid intake. *News Physiol Sci* 2004; 19: 1–6.

67. Zafonte RD, Watanabe TK, Mann NR, Ko DH. Psychogenic polydipsia after traumatic brain injury. A case report. *Am J Phys Med Rehabil* 1997; 76: 246–248.

68. Fellus J, Elovic E. Fatigue: Assessment and treatment. In: Zasler N, Katz D, Zafonte R, editors. *Brain injury medicine: Principles and practice*, 2nd edition. New York, NY: Demos Medical Publishing, 2007, pp. 545–555.

69. Decker K. Using energy conservation strategies to treat mild traumatic brain injury. Information fact sheet. 2013. Available at http://gla-rehab.com/using-energy-conservation-strategies-to-treat-mild-traumatic-brain-injury/.

70. Rao V, Rollings P, Spiro J. Fatigue and sleep problems. In: Silver J, McAllister J, Yudofsky S, editors. *Textbook of traumatic brain injury*. Washington, D.C.: American Psychiatric Publishing, 2005, pp. 369–384.

71. Jha A, Weintraub A, Allshouse A, Morey C, Cusick C, Kittelson J, et al. A randomized trial of modafinil for the treatment of fatigue and excessive daytime sleepiness in individuals with chronic traumatic brain injury. *J Head Trauma Rehabil* 2008; 23: 52–63.

72. Kaiser PR, Valko P, Werth E, Thomann J, Meier J, Stocker R, et al. Modafinil ameliorates excessive daytime sleepiness after traumatic brain injury. *Neurology* 2010; 75: 1780–1785.

Sleep Disorders after Typical Concussive Brain Injury: Classification, Diagnosis, and Management

Curtis McKnight and Jeff Victoroff

Introduction

Sleep disorders are one of the most common and disabling among the persistent neurobehavioral sequelae of traumatic brain injury (TBI). This is true of both cases labeled as "mild" and cases labeled as more severe [1]. This chapter will briefly review the epidemiology, pathophysiology, and treatment for this serious and frequently overlooked type of post-concussive problem.

Sleep is an essential homeostatic process. It is characterized by decreased level of arousal and reduced average muscle tone in conjunction with specific neuronal activation patterns. It is demanded, initiated, maintained, and finally terminated by a coordinated group of neuronal, behavioral, and hormonal mechanisms. Sleep has restorative value, promotes memory formation, learning, and tissue growth, and improves immune function. Sleep specifically enables hippocampal neurogenesis – a process that is possibly critical to post-TBI recovery and is blocked by sleep deprivation [2]. Recent evidence suggests that, during sleep, convective fluxes occur between interstitial fluid and cerebrospinal fluid that increase the rate of β-amyloid clearance [3]. Yet in spite of major advances in the understanding of the biology of sleep, and the indisputable deleterious effects of sleep deprivation, it remains unclear why humans sleep.

Although there is a conceptual and phenomenological overlap between post-concussive sleep disorders (PCSDs) – most often insomnia or daytime sleepiness – and post-concussive fatigue, it is important to make a distinction. Sleep disorders exhibit a diverse and complex typology and can be measured objectively; fatigue is a highly subjective construct (although motor or cognitive *fatigability* is measurable). The prevalence of sleep disorders is inversely associated with severity of concussive brain injury (CBI),[1] whereas the association between fatigue and severity is less clear [4]. Both

conditions deserve attention and, in so far as the limited randomized controlled trial literature permits, evidence-based management. This chapter focuses on sleep.

It is also important to acknowledge that the phrase "sleep disorder" misleadingly implies a unitary condition. From difficulty falling asleep, impaired sleep maintenance, and early awakening (these three sometimes regarded as comprising *insomnia*), to sleep inefficiency, hypersomnia, altered proportion of time in different sleep stages, sleep-disordered breathing, nightmares and sleep walking/talking, to excessive daytime sleepiness and circadian rhythm disorders, the universe of sleep disturbances is broad and deep. Indeed, a meta-analysis of sleep disorders after TBI recognized 65 post-concussive sleep problems [5].

Sleep is the result of several coordinated physiologic systems. Disruption in one or more of those systems may result in dysfunction. CBI/mild TBI (mTBI) can disrupt any and all these processes, making post-concussive sleep disorders common, distressing, and sometimes disabling. Evidence exists that poor sleep after mTBI is associated not only with inferior cognitive recovery performance but also with persistent anxiety and depression [6]. As Fakhran et al. expressed the concern,

> These disturbances are among the most disabling symptoms, directly decreasing quality of life and productivity, exacerbating other postconcussion symptoms, aggravating psychiatric disturbances, and magnifying postconcussion memory and social dysfunction.
>
> ([7], p. 250)

CBI/mTBI can also lead or interact with a range of neuropsychiatric syndromes that include insomnia or other disordered sleep as either symptoms or risk factors – such as mood disorders, pain disorders, and cognitive impairment. Since pain, anxiety, and depression may provoke sleep disorders, and since sleep disorders themselves can provoke depression, irritability, and

---

[1]   Clarification of terminology: traumatic brain injury (TBI) means altered brain function or other evidence of brain pathology due to external force. "Mild traumatic brain injury" ("mTBI") is a discredited phrase from a previous century that has dozens of clinical definitions and no biological definition. Concussive brain injury (CBI) has a specific biological meaning: it refers to the major elements of the TBIs that are most likely to come to clinical attention: those that have deleterious effects on brains due to the transmission of external force through the skull. CBIs are diverse. In addition to the effects of force transmitted through the skull, some exhibit additional elements such as skull fracture, intracranial hemorrhage, or parenchymal penetration. However, the overwhelming majority of clinically attended TBIs are CBIs without brain penetration, prolonged coma, or gross intracranial hemorrhage visible on computed tomography. Such injuries overlap with some of those formerly called "mTBIs," but are biologically definable. In this chapter, the term CBI/mTBI is used to refer to that most common form of TBI.

cognitive dysfunction, it is challenging and possibly fruitless to try to determine cause and effect when sleep disorders co-occur with these problems in post-concussive patients in what may sometimes amount to a vicious cycle.

Considering the healthy sleep cycle and its governing mechanisms will inform the discussion of the heterogeneous sleep disorders associated with the heterogeneous phenomena of CBI/mTBI.

Normal Sleep Cycle

Healthy sleep is broadly separated into two types: rapid eye movement (REM) versus non-rapid eye movement (NREM) sleep. NREM is further divided into three stages numerically named stages 1, 2, and 3. Stage 3 sleep is also called slow-wave sleep (SWS) due to its electroencephalogram (EEG) signature of lower-frequency waves. Historically, SWS was composed of sleep stages 3 and 4, which have since been combined.

EEG activity is the most useful way to identify and characterize stages of sleep. During wakefulness, healthy adults display low-voltage fast EEG activities that are designated as the alpha (8–13 Hz) and beta (> 13 Hz) rhythms.

When conditions are right for sleep, a transition from wakefulness to stage 1 occurs as the EEG alpha rhythm slows to the theta rhythm (4–7 Hz). During this time, conscious awareness diminishes while muscle tone decreases and myoclonic jerks can occur. This is also the stage of sleep in which hypnagogic hallucinations are experienced. Stage 1 sleep occupies around 5% of the total night's sleep time. When the EEG demonstrates K complexes, sleep spindles, and theta rhythm (6–7 Hz), stage 2 sleep is occurring. Stage 2 sleep is longer and occupies approximately 50% of total sleep time. Next the delta rhythm (1–4 Hz) predominates, indicating stage 3 sleep has been reached. Stage 3 sleep has the highest arousal threshold and the lowest metabolic activity of the healthy sleep cycle.

REM sleep is characterized by the EEG activity of stage 1 sleep plus REM, sawtooth theta waves, and muscle atonia. Cerebral blood flow and oxygen consumption are similar to wakefulness while dreaming occurs.

A typical sleep cycle from stage 1 to REM lasts 90 min. This cycle repeats several times during a restful period of sleep. NREM sleep predominates at the beginning of the sleep period and transitions to REM being predominant toward the end of the sleep. Infants spend a higher percentage of sleep in REM; this diminishes slowly over the lifespan.

What Controls Sleep

Sleep is a result of multiple interconnected systems of control and regulation. Psychosocially, controlling the sleep environment and daily schedule will have significant effects on the duration and quality of sleep.

Thinking more neuropsychiatrically, the autonomic nervous system, homeostatic sleep drive, and circadian rhythm are the main regulatory mechanisms for sleep. They exert their influence over wakefulness in part via the reticular activating system (RAS). Although necessary, the RAS is not sufficient to sustain healthy sleep and arousal; it is facilitated by several discrete neuronal groups localized within and adjacent to the pontine and midbrain reticular formation and its extension into the hypothalamus [8]. Multiple neurotransmitters are involved. The RAS utilizes monoaminergic and cholinergic projections [9] in coordination with histamine input from the tuberomammillary nucleus (TMN) and orexin from the lateral hypothalamus [10].

Sleep can be conceptualized as inhibition of the RAS and associated nuclei. The ventrolateral preoptic nucleus of the anterior hypothalamus has gamma-aminobutyric acid (GABA) input that inhibits TMN release of histamine to the cortex. Also, during darkness the suprachiasmatic nucleus increases melatonin release from the pineal gland. This is a sleep-promoting mechanism.

Autonomic Nervous System and Arousal

Emotional arousal increases sympathetic nervous system activation and inhibits sleep. This may be due to anxious rumination, physical pain, or dysautonomia.

Homeostatic Sleep Drive

Prolonged wakefulness produces increased need for sleep. The underlying mechanism for this drive is still being defined but current thinking is that the neurotransmitter adenosine is one factor influencing this drive. Adenosine levels in the basal forebrain increase with sustained neuronal activity and decrease with sleep [11]. Additionally, caffeine can act as an adenosine antagonist, which would also support adenosine's role in the homeostatic sleep drive [12].

Circadian Rhythm

The circadian rhythm is a 24-h cycle of physiologic processes typically resulting in sleep at night and wakefulness during the day. The circadian rhythm is influenced by light, social cues, and the environment. Although it is traditionally rounded to 24 h, accurate attempts to characterize the exact length of the average human circadian cycle have found it to be 24.18 h [13]. The length of the circadian cycle shortens slowly with age. The timing of sleep, along with the fluctuation of melatonin, basal body temperature, and cortisol are features of the circadian rhythm.

During sleep states the skin has reliably increased blood flow, which results in heat loss and lower core temperature. This is thought to be the reason we prefer bedding when sleeping, especially in cold environments.

Changes Reported After Traumatic Brain Injury

Setting aside (momentarily) the issues of severity and persistence, multiple laboratories have reported changes in the electrophysiological patterns observed in survivors of TBIs. Like the clinical aspects of PCSDs, these changes in sleep architecture are heterogeneous and, in some cases, inconsistent. For instance, multiple studies report that REM sleep may be persistently altered; although some laboratories find decreased

REM onset latency, others find reduced overall REM, others find increased REM in the latter part of the night, and still others report no change in REM [14–19]. NREM or SWS might also be altered, with reports of increased SWS not only in moderate to severe TBI [17, 20], but also in mTBI [18] – although another study reported relatively *decreased* stage 2 NREM in mTBI [21]. Suffice it to say that no single long-term architectural change is consistently reported after TBI of any severity. This merely supports the observation that TBI is not a unitary brain disorder, but a convenient label for an event associated with diverse intracranial changes.

Prevalence of Sleep Disorders After CBI/mTBI

PCSDs are common. However, it is difficult to assign a single number to their prevalence. In part, this reflects the variety of research approaches that have been employed, included subjective data from interviews and self-report questionnaires and objective measures such as actigraphy or polysomnography. Table 25.1 summarizes reports of prevalence of PCSDs, either reported as a proportion of subjects affected at a given time post injury (with or without a comparison group) or objectively measured at a given time post injury (with or without a comparison group). Note that reports regarding populations with mixed severity were cited when reported results were stratified to permit extraction of the CBI/mTBI data.

Table 25.1 [7, 16, 18, 22–37] demonstrates that PCSDs are prevalent and may persist for as long as the longest available post-injury follow-up data – almost eight years. Among the five studies that reported prevalence at ≥ 12 months, 32–57.5% of CBI/mTBI patients reported persistent sleep disturbances [16, 24, 32, 34, 35]. By way of comparison, the 2009 Behavioral Risk Factor Surveillance System [38] assessed sleep and wake complaints among more than 74,000 persons: 35.3% complained of getting less than seven hours of sleep, on average, in a 24-h period [38]. The high population base rate of sleep complaints inspires caution regarding the relative risk for these problems after concussion – although the studies comparing CBI survivors with healthy persons suggest an authentic elevation of risk.

Other available results show that this elevated frequency of persistent post-concussive sleep complaints is confirmed by objective measures. That is, the three controlled studies that employed actigraphy, polysomnography or multiple sleep latency tests (MSLT) all reported abnormal sleep parameters among concussed persons [28, 29, 37]. In fact, evidence exists that patients with TBI tend to *underreport* their sleep disturbances [28, 39]. Evidence also exists that insomnia is more common after milder injuries – even controlling for pain, depression, and litigation – perhaps because those with milder brain injury have more self-awareness [39, 40].

Several observations help to characterize the most common post-concussive sleep complaints – insomnia and daytime sleepiness. For example, Perlis et al. [34] found that patients with post-concussion syndrome reported more difficulty compared with healthy persons in initiating and maintaining sleep at night and greater difficulty with sleepiness during the day for at least two years after initial injury. Schreiber et al. [18] examined sleep patterns in 26 adults with minor TBI against matched controls by using polysomnography and MSLT. The use of more objective measures was done to characterize the subjective complaint of "sleepy during the day" in patients who sustained an mTBI one to 21 years previously. Polysomnogram showed sleep architecture alterations with more stage 2 sleep and less REM. The mTBI patients had higher number of falling asleep episodes during the MSLT compared to controls (3.4 vs. 1.9), suggesting some degree of excessive daytime sleepiness is common following mTBI and may persist.

Some 20th century writers claimed that post-concussive problems vanish by three months after injury, except in cases of conversion or feigning, or when these complaints represent non-specific symptoms of trauma. These are serious considerations. Those claims, however, are not consistent with the available tests of their hypotheses. One controlled study [26] explicitly excluded litigants and nonetheless found sleep disturbances more frequent among CBI/mTBI survivors. Employment of injured non-TBI comparison subjects is also a useful approach to the question of whether sleep disorders are TBI-specific. The controlled study reported by Perlis et al. [34] suggests that they are.

Atypical Post-Concussive Sleep Disorders
Hypersomnia

Excessive sleep, non-restorative sleep, and daytime sleepiness are all considered elements of hypersomnia. Although this is a common complaint after CBI/mTBI, the exact prevalence is unknown. Hypersomnia is the experience of excessive sleepiness despite adequate time spent devoted to sleeping. In addition to patient history, an MSLT with score < 10 (that is, a tendency to fall asleep within ten minutes) can further aid in diagnosis. And again, hypersomnia should be distinguished from fatigue, which doesn't lead to reduced sleep onset latency.

Since sleepiness can impair cognitive and motor function it has also been shown that excessive daytime sleepiness is a risk factor for CBI/mTBI [41]. In a study of 182 patients and 145 controls, Bradshaw et al. interviewed previously healthy young men shortly after sustaining an mTBI. Overall, 41% of patients versus 31% of controls reported significant daytime sleepiness – another mechanism that helps account for the fact that one concussion significantly increases the risk for another.

Obstructive Sleep Apnea

It is something of a curiosity that obstructive sleep apnea (OSA) is commonly diagnosed after TBI. According to the conventional wisdom, OSA is associated with morphological risk factors such as obesity or variation in oral-pharyngeal architecture. Although CBI is often associated with decreased activity and sometimes with weight gain, one would not expect TBI-related weight gain to produce the observed high prevalence of post-concussive OSA. In one study, for example, OSA was diagnosed in 23% of 57 adult survivors of TBI (mostly moderate to severe) [42]. The problem clearly also occurs

Table 25.1 Sleep disorder (SD) after concussive brain injury: prevalence studies

Author(s)	Subjects	Comparison subjects	Method	Follow-up	Results/prevalence of SD
Baumann et al., 2009 [22]	26 adults with "mTBI"	N/A	Multiple sleep latency test	6 months	MLST < 5 min (excessive daytime sleepiness) in 34.6%
Castriotta et al., 2007 [23]	7 adults with "mTBI"	N/A	Multiple sleep latency test	≥ 3 months	MLST < 10 min (excessive daytime sleepiness) 2/7 (28.5%)
Chan and Feinstein, 2015 [24]	374 adults with "mTBI"	N/A	Questionnaire	12 months	53.7% SD
Chaput et al., 2009 [25]	443 adults with "mTBI"	N/A	Questionnaire	6 weeks	33.5% SD
Dean and Stern, 2013 [26]	36 adults with "mTBI"	36 healthy	Questionnaire	12 months	SD more common among mTBI ($p = 0.001$) (controlling for litigation)
Fakhran et al., 2013 [7]	64 "mTBI"	N/A	Questionnaire	Mean = 71 days	53.1% SD
Haboubi et al., 2001 [27]	179 adults with "minor head injury"	N/A	Interview	6 weeks	45% SD
Imbach et al., 2015 [28]	29 adults with "mTBI"	42 healthy	Actigraph × 2 weeks	6 months	Total sleep time: mTBI > comparison ($p < 0.01$) Sleep onset latency: mTBI < comparison ($p < 0.01$)
Kaufman et al., 2001 [29]	19 adolescents with "minor head injury"	19 healthy	Actigraph × 5 days	36 months	Sleep efficiency: MHI < comparison ($p < 0.05$) Awake time: MHI > comparison ($p < 0.05$)
Kraus et al., 2009 [30]	689 adults with "mTBI"	1318 with non-TBI injuries	Questionnaire	3 months	SD in mTBI: 22.5% SD in comparison: 16.3% SD significantly more common among mTBI
Levitt et al., 1994 [31]	95 adults with "minor head trauma"	N/A	Questionnaire	3–4 weeks	67%
McMahon et al., 2014 [32]	163 "mTBI"	N/A	Questionnaire	12 months	53.5%
Ouelet and Morin, 2006 [16]	90 adults with "mild" or "minor" TBI	N/A	Questionnaire	Mean = 7.85 years	38% insomnia
Parsons and Ver Beek, 1982 [33]	75 adults with "minor head injury"	N/A	Questionnaire	3 months	• Sleep complaints ($p = 0.001$) • Sleep quality ($p = 0.001$)
Perlis et al., 1997 [34]	39 adults with "minor head injury" (MHI)	27 with orthopedic injury	Questionnaire	Mean = 24 months	Sleep initiation diff: MHI = 52.6% (vs. 16%) • Sleep duration: MHI = 53.8% (vs. 20%) Daytime sleepiness: MHI = 20.5% (vs. 0%)
Schreiber et al., 2008 [18]	26 adults with "mTBI"	26 healthy			
Segalowitz and Lawson, 1995 [35]	385 adolescents with "mild head injury"	675 adolescents without	Questionnaire	~ 5 years	Sleep difficulty: 32% in MHI vs. 25% in non-MHI ($p < 0.02$)
Segalowitz and Lawson, 1995 [35]	371 university students with "mild head injury"	565 university students without	Questionnaire	N/A	Disturbed sleep: more common among those with MHI ($p < 0.002$)
Tham et al., 2012 [36]	510 children with "mTBI"	197 with orthopedic injuries	Questionnaire	24 months	Sleep disturbances: more common among those with mTBI ($\beta = -6.3$)
Tham et al., 2015 [37]	50 adolescents "mTBI"	50 healthy	Actigraph × 10 days	3–12 months	SD more common among mTBI ($p = 0.002$) (controlling for depression, age, sex, and pain)

MLST: multiple sleep latency test; mTBI: mild traumatic brain injury.

after mTBI: in one study, 116 consecutive soldiers with mTBI underwent comprehensive sleep evaluations. 97.4% reported sleep problems: 55.2% had insomnia, but 34.5% had demonstrable OSA [43]. In another study, among the 93 U.S. military personnel with mTBI who underwent polysomnography/sleep testing in 2010, 30% had mild OSA and another 21% had moderate to severe OSA [44]. Without a prospective study documenting pre-injury sleep, of course, it is not possible to confirm that mTBI was the principal cause of these disorders.

Narcolepsy

Narcolepsy, a sleep disorder characterized by irresistible sleep attacks and excessive daytime sleepiness, occasionally occurs after CBI/mTBI [45]. Narcolepsy is also associated with *cataplexy* (sudden muscle weakness associated with emotional expression such as laughing, crying, anger, or surprise), *sleep paralysis* (the sensation of being unable to move although conscious, which occurs most often at the beginning or end of a sleep cycle), and *hypnagogic* (on falling asleep) or *hypnopompic* (while awakening) hallucinations. A diagnosis of narcolepsy is typically made when the clinical history of episodically and suddenly falling asleep is associated with abnormalities on the MLST, including rapid onset of sleep and REM periods during brief naps. Most persons with narcolepsy also have a depressed level of hypocretin-1 in their cerebrospinal fluid, and hypocretin-1 (aka orexin) deficiency has been identified as the etiologic agent for narcolepsy. These findings have led to the current view that autoimmune orexin (hypocretin) cell destruction is the presumed etiology for many cases of narcolepsy. In fact, loss of hypocretin cells has been reported after experimental TBI [22]. It is therefore conceivable that hypocretin cell death in the hypothalamus underlies human cases of post-concussive narcolepsy.

This leads naturally to the question: why do some victims of concussion develop sleep disorders, and others not?

Pathophysiology of Post-Concussive Sleep Disorders

We acknowledge: it is rather disingenuous to discuss the pathophysiology of post-concussive sleep disorders. First, it is reasonable to guess that each of the 65 types of sleep disorder is mediated by different cerebral happenings. Second, it is reasonable to guess that individuality – i.e., gene variants, epigenes, and premorbid environments – plays an important role in determining the presence, absence, type, severity, and treatability of PCSDs. Third, there simply has not been adequate quality research investigating TBI, or CBI, or so-called mTBI and their corollary forms of lasting distress. No major research entity has made controlled longitudinal research a priority. Therefore, the best one can offer regarding the neurobiological basis of post-concussive sleep disorders is a handful of preliminary observations.

For instance, although sleep disorders can be identified by certain electrophysiological biomarkers, it is not known whether the most common EEG abnormalities after CBI – or even those EEG abnormalities most commonly found in

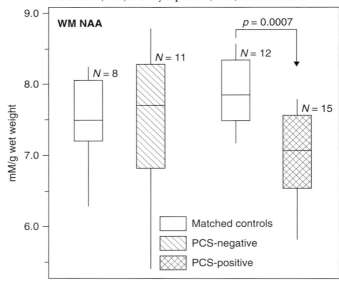

Fig. 25.1 Box plots displaying 25%, median and 75% (box) and 95% (whiskers) of the NAA concentration distributions in the white matter of post-concussive symptoms (PCS)-negative and PCS-positive mild traumatic brain injury patients, compared with their age- and gender-matched controls. Note that a highly significant ($p = 0.0007$) NAA deficit is observed only in the PCS-positive cohort (124 · 105 mm; 300 · 300 DPI).

Source: Kirov et al., 2103 [46]. Reproduced with permission from Mary Ann Liebert, Inc.

cases of post-concussive sleep disorder – have any relationship to the subjective experience of disrupted sleep. In one study [46], for instance, 26 adults diagnosed with mTBI were divided into those with and without one or more post-concussive complaints, including sleep disorder, dizziness, headache, memory deficits, and visual complaints. At a mean of 21 days post injury, these two groups (mTBI with post-concussive symptoms and mTBI without post-concussive symptoms) were compared with healthy comparison subjects. mTBI with post-concussive symptoms was associated with decreased white-matter N-acetyl aspartate (NAA) on magnetic resonance spectroscopy. On such scans, depressed global NAA levels correlate with microstructural axonal dysfunction, while other metabolic markers (e.g., creatine, choline, or myoinositol) reflect cell death. In this study there was almost no overlap between the NAA levels of healthy persons and those of mTBI + post-concussive symptom patients ($p = 0.0007$). In contrast, other metabolites were not significantly different (Figure 25.1).

A tentative conclusion is that white-matter axonal disruption plays some role in post-concussive symptoms, including sleep disorder. Yet another study employed diffusion tensor imaging of 64 mTBI patients [7]. Thirty-four of the 64 subjects reported sleep disturbances. The sleep-disordered subgroup exhibited significantly lower fractional anisotropy in the parahippocampal gyrus compared with mTBI patients without sleep disorder – again hinting that axonal dysfunction plays some role in PCSDs.

Another study reported that survivors of mild to moderate TBIs who had objectively verifiable excessive daytime sleepiness exhibited an increase in the resting motor threshold (decreased cortical excitability) on transcranial magnetic stimulation compared with other TBI patients and with controls [47]. Although the association between sleepiness and hypo-excitability seems logical, such work requires replication.

One report proposes that anatomical variation explains why some CBI survivors do and others do not have post-concussive sleep problems: Yaeger et al. [48] used structural magnetic resonance imaging to compare the brains of 34 TBI patients *with* PCSD with 30 TBI patients *without* PCSD. The groups had similar cognitive function. However, those with PCSDs had significantly flatter and longer tentoria. The authors speculated that this normal anatomical variant causes an increased likelihood of pineal injury during TBI, leading to disruption of melatonin homeostasis. That speculation is consistent with at least one study reporting that, at an average follow-up of 14 months post injury, evening melatonin levels were decreased in TBI survivors – and these hormonal changes correlated with REM sleep markers [20].

Although this collection of results is intriguing, we believe it is premature to interpret these studies as identifying either a focal or biological basis of post-concussive sleep problems. Moreover, these laboratory studies fail to address the likelihood that concussion-associated clinical problems such as pain, anxiety, and depression might play important roles in the genesis of sleep disorders.

Associated Clinical Problems

Since post-concussive sleep disorders comprise a clinically heterogeneous domain, research should ideally investigate what risk factors are associated with this spectrum of problems, stratifying results not only by characteristics of the patient (e.g., demographic factors) and by characteristics of the injury (e.g., impact versus blast, with or without prolonged post-traumatic amnesia or intracranial hemorrhage), but also by the type of sleep disorder (e.g., insomnia versus excessive daytime sleepiness). We are unaware of any published study that undertook that kind of analytic stratification.

Several reports nonetheless suggest associations between PCSDs, broadly defined, and other clinical problems. In some cases, the direction of causality (what caused what) seems self-evident. For instance, in a group of patients selected for continuing neurocognitive complaints, sleep concerns were more prevalent among 127 mTBI subjects than among a matched group of 123 non-TBI neurological comparison subjects. In that study, pain was associated with a near doubling in the frequency of reported insomnia [49]. It seems plausible that pain played a causal role in sleep disruption.

In another study, 443 mTBI patients were followed for six weeks, at which point 33.5% had sleep complaints [25]. Again, subjects attributed their sleep problems to their pain – a causal direction that comports with intuition. However, in the same study, sleep complaints were also associated with three times the likelihood of concomitant headaches (independent of pain) and 6.3 times the likelihood of depression. Similarly, a long-term follow-up study ($\geq$ 29 months) of 98 TBI patients,

of whom 69 (70%) were mild, reported that TBI with insomnia was associated with significantly higher scores for depression and anxiety [50]. A controlled study of 153 TBI patients (mixed severity) found that patient-reported sleep quality was clearly related to anxiety, depression, and pain [51]. And a study of 101 closed head injury patients reported that sleep problems within three months of injury predicted depression, anxiety, and apathy 12 months after injury [52].

Moreover, several studies have reported an association between mTBI plus PTSD and sleep disorders. For instance, in a review of 20 studies, military TBI (mostly CBI/mTBI) plus post-traumatic stress disorder (PTSD) was associated with more post-concussive symptoms [53].

In another study, 29,640 U.S. Navy and Marines were screened for PTSD, TBI, and sleep problems [54]. Controlling for sleep problems led to major shifts in the odds: sleep disorders accounted for 26% of the likelihood that a soldier with TBI would develop PTSD. Similarly, sleep problems accounted for 41% of the risk that soldiers with TBI would develop depression. The conclusion is that sleep problems mediate the effect of TBI on the development of mental health disorders.

Yet what causes what? As suggested at the outset of this chapter, associative data do not permit one to infer whether PCSDs *cause* headaches, anxiety, depression, and PTSD, whether those problems *cause* PCSDs, or whether a self-reinforcing cycle of deleterious symptoms may occur.

Genetics and Sleep Disorders

So far, the discussion has generalized about the neurobiology of sleep as if the nervous system of every individual operates in the same way. Of course, it does not. In-born differences due to heritable variation are likely to impact many aspects of both the normal function of sleep circuitry and the response to injury. It seems reasonable to predict that the pathophysiology and clinical expression of CBI/mTBI will soon be shown to be modulated in part by genetics. Increased efficiency in DNA genotypic analysis has provided better understanding of human sleep genetic pathophysiology. The interdependence of the neurotransmitter pathways with the circadian rhythm and homeostatic controls makes the genetic study of sleep disorders complex and wide ranging. Recent descriptions of allelic polymorphisms affecting sleep may help explain why some concussion survivors have little trouble with sleep and others have serious sleep disorders. Newer lines of investigation focus on the transcriptome after CBI/mTBI and its effects on sleep.

"Clock genes" are integral to timing and circadian rhythm control of sleep. The T/C single polymorphism in position 3111 (3111T/C) of the circadian locomotor output cycles kaput (CLOCK) gene corresponds to altered sleep patterns [55]. This polymorphism has also since been associated with phenotypic expression of mood disorders and metabolic abnormalities. In relation to sleep disturbance, the 3111T/C polymorphism has been linked to the phenomenon of "eveningness" as well as delayed sleep onset [56]. Results have been mixed [57], but those with the 3111C homozygous polymorphism are more likely to have sleep changes following stressful life events

[58]. This "sensitive" genotype is probably more prone to also experience sleep disturbance after CBI/mTBI. Another Clock gene, Tef (polymorphism (TT)) is associated with depression and parkinsonism but not strongly with sleep disturbance [59].

The PERIOD3 (PER3) gene regulates sleep. A variable-number tandem polymorphism is distributed in populations with a 4 or 5 allele repeat [60]. The PER3 5/5 polymorphism has been associated with higher homeostatic sleep drive and a higher drive aids recovery sleep following a sleep deficit. Conversely, the PER3 4/4 polymorphism is associated with a lower homeostatic drive [61]. PER3 4/4 polymorphism is also associated with more severe insomnia in patients with alcohol addiction [62].

The serotonin transporter (5HTT) polymorphism 5HTT short (S) allele, which is more commonly correlated with mood disorders, is also associated with increased insomnia even absent depression [63]. A Val-Met substitution at codon 158 of the catechol-O-methyltransferase enzyme leads to higher dopamine concentrations [64]. Met/Met homozygous subjects have increased homeostatic sleep and drive and a more efficient response, making them less vulnerable to the effects of sleep loss. It is unclear if this extends to CBI/mTBI but it makes for an intriguing hypothesis.

Single-nucleotide polymorphisms of the melatonin receptors have been associated with circadian rhythm dysfunction [65, 66], and may likely be another risk factor for developing a sleep disorder after CBI/mTBI.

The proinflammatory cytokine interleukin-6 (IL-6) shows genotypic variation that predisposes oncology patients to increased fatigue and sleep disturbance [67]. An IL-4 minor allele is predictive of depression, pain, fatigue, and sleep disturbance [68].

A Val-Met substitution of codon 66 polymorphism of the brain-derived neurotrophic factor gene has been shown to increase sleep need and intensity [69].

Although abundant research, as briefly reviewed above, confirms that sleep parameters are influenced by genetic variation, few studies have specifically tested the hypothesis that genetic variation accounts for the observed difference in the occurrence and type of PCSDs. One mouse study, however, found that mild experimental TBI not only altered sleep but also triggered changes in cortical gene expression, impacting the expression of genes involved in inflammation, immunity, and glial function. The investigators went on to determine how sleep deprivation affects brains attempting to recover from mTBI, and concluded: "Sleep loss post-mTBI reprograms the transcriptome in a brain area-specific manner and in a way that could be deleterious to brain recovery" [70]. If so, then PCSD adds injury to injury.

Sleep and Cytokines

CBI/mTBI-mediated release of inflammatory cytokines, including tumor necrosis factor (TNF) and IL-1 is thought to affect sleep. TNF and IL-1 are sleep-regulatory substances in so far as their administration increases the duration of NREM and patients undergoing IL-1 therapy experience excessive daytime sleepiness [71]. IL-1 receptor antagonist and soluble

TNF receptors inhibit sleep and fatigue. Downstream effects include activation of transcription factors, including nuclear factor kappa B and c-Fos.

Adenosine triphosphate (ATP) induces release of TNF and IL-1 from central nervous system glial cells. Disturbance of ATP consumption post CBI/mTBI [71] leads to elevated levels of IL-1 and TNF in the first few hours following brain injury. IL-1 recruits leukocytes and modulates glutamate release and gliosis, which is neuroprotective but disrupts the blood–brain barrier. TNF is neurotoxic initially but neuroprotective during late-stage neuronal repair [72]. All these factors help explain why the acute post-traumatic sleep period is mediated by the early release of cytokines [73].

In addition to cytokine and neuron metabolism disruption, neurometabolic changes result from CBI/mTBI mechanical damage to the brain [74]. Lipid membrane disruption leads to ionic flux and indiscriminate neurotransmitter release. Intracellular potassium efflux and calcium influx lead to diffuse depolarization with resultant phenomenon of "spreading depression": silencing of evoked potentials. Ionic flux also causes an ATP energy crisis as sodium/potassium pumps use more than in homeostasis to restore ionic balance. Cerebral blood flow is reduced too, resulting in deficit of energy substrates. CBI/mTBI can also alter the balance of the transmitters glutamate (excitatory) and GABA (inhibitory), and cause N-methyl-D-aspartate receptors for glutamate to develop subunit changes that lead to excessive influx of calcium [74].

The well-known sleep controls melatonin and orexin are disrupted after CBI/mTBI. Reduced melatonin production in the evenings has been seen in patients following TBI of varying severity, and the same patients displayed altered REM sleep [20]. As with melatonin, low levels of cerebrospinal fluid orexin have been observed in mixed-severity TBI patients, and have persisted for patients complaining of excessive daytime sleepiness [75].

Management of Post-Concussive Sleep Disorders

Since PCSDs are heterogeneous, only two management recommendations might be regarded as useful in virtually every case. First, one is obliged to investigate the problem seriously: a polysomnographic sleep study, including EEG, is indicated for symptoms of insomnia. MSLT is indicated for symptoms of daytime sleepiness. Complaints about the cost, in developed countries, are not worthy of discussion. Setting aside ethics and empathy, even setting aside the likelihood that properly selected interventions will enhance cognitive and emotional recovery, the loss of productivity associated with PCSDs is surely enough of an incentive to mandate testing. Otherwise, one is merely guessing about the choice of an efficacious intervention and exposing the patient to trial-and-error medicine.

Second, sleep hygiene must be explained and exhorted. Sleep complaints are ubiquitous, regardless of other health concerns. Modern life, with its artificial light, unnatural time periods of work and rest, widespread sedentary lifestyles, stimulant drugs, and digital stimulants, is not conducive to the sleep–wake cycle of the hunter-gatherer for which our brains are optimized. For these reasons, too few modern persons follow the simple behavioral patterns most likely to provide sufficient restful sleep. Clinicians, of course, have relatively little power to alter lifelong habits. It is nonetheless ethically required that one spends time with a patient urging that he or she heed the boilerplate recommendations of the National Sleep Foundation [76]:

- Go to bed and arise at the same time every day.
- Get approximately eight hours of sleep each night.
- Avoid stimulants, including caffeine, alcohol, and nicotine, in the evening.
- Exercise prior to the late afternoon.
- Avoid large meals near bedtime.
- Ensure adequate natural light exposure.
- Avoid exposure to media such as screens in bed [77].

(We have excluded one common recommendation: to avoid naps. Recent data suggest that middle-aged napping may be positively associated with human longevity.)

Two studies have reported the benefit of individualized treatment for PCSDs. Both cohorts were dominated by moderate to severe patients, reducing confidence that their findings can be extrapolated to survivors of single concussions. In one study, 57 adults were enrolled ≥ three months after TBI [42]. Twenty-two had PCSDs. Those with post-traumatic OSA were treated with continuous positive airway pressure (a highly effective but notoriously cumbersome method, often rejected by patients, involving all-night attachment of the patient's face to a machine via plastic tubing). Those with post-traumatic hypersomnia/narcolepsy were treated with modafinil 200 mg. Those with post-traumatic periodic limb movements in sleep were treated with pramipexole 0.375 mg. OSA patients exhibited increased REM, but no improvement in daytime sleepiness. Hypersomnia patients exhibited increased MSLT times, but only a minority had resolution of daytime hypersomnia. Those with periodic limb movements in sleep exhibited fewer limb movements. However, cognitive testing did not show improvement in any group.

In another study of mixed-severity patients at 1–22 years post injury, 12 adults underwent polysomnography [78]. Note that two of the subjects had been struggling with post-traumatic sleep disorders for more than 15 years. Treatment was individualized. Cases of OSA were treated with continuous positive airway pressure; cases of hypersomnia were treated with modafinil or an activating antidepressant; cases of restless leg syndrome were treated with gabapentin or pramipexole plus a sleep hygiene program. Follow-up averaged eight months. Ten of 12 reported improved sleep; 11 of 12 reported decreased depression; ten of 12 reported decreased anxiety. Aggregate scores were significantly improved for speed of information processing and language.

Such uncontrolled findings are encouraging but hardly definitive. Even fewer studies have been published regarding the efficacy of interventions for PCSDs after mTBI. One paper reported improved sleep in one patient several years after mTBI in response to hyperbaric oxygen treatment [79]. Yet a multicenter, double-blind, sham-controlled trial of hyperbaric oxygen among 72 soldiers with mTBI and persistent post-concussive symptoms showed that any change in sleep was likely due to placebo effect [80]. One hopes that well-designed randomized controlled trials will eventually reveal an efficacious treatment for one or more of the PCSDs. The major exception to this historical dearth of research: efforts to treat mTBI-plus-PTSD-related nightmares.

Management of mTBI-Plus-PTSD-Related Nightmares

It has been hypothesized that so-called "PTSD" and its association with sleep disorders, especially nightmares, is caused in part by hyper-adrenergic drive. Post-traumatic stress is indeed associated with increased cerebrospinal fluid norepinephrine, which, in turn is associated with decreased REM sleep. These observations prompted the proposal, more than a decade ago, that damping adrenergic function might improve sleep in "PTSD." That idea propelled trials, mostly testing the efficacy of oral prazosin – an alpha-blocker typically used to treat hypertension or benign prostatic hyperplasia. As a result of U.S.-led wars in the Middle-East, a large cohort of young military personnel has recently developed the combination of "mTBI plus PTSD." These victims have been the principal subjects of this research.

For example, Ruff et al. [82] conducted an observational study: among 74 veterans with concussion, headaches, and neurological examination abnormalities (almost all of whom also had "PTSD"), 69 reported sleep problems. Sixty-two of these were treated with sleep hygiene education and 7 mg oral prazosin at bedtime. Treatment was associated with improved sleep in 60 of those subjects (97%), fewer or no nightmares, decreased headaches, and enhanced cognition that persisted for the six months of follow-up. A 2012 review [83] reported that prazosin effectively improved sleep quality in three of four randomized controlled trials with similar patient cohorts. Still off-label at the time of this writing, oral prazosin has become the standard of care for sleep disorders associated with "PTSD" – with or without CBI/mTBI [84]. However, it is currently unknown whether prazosin significantly mitigates PCSDs in survivors of CBI/mTBI without "PTSD."

Alternatives

One recent study reported a double-blind placebo-controlled trial among 13 persons with TBI and sleep complaints [85]. Ramelteon (8 mg) at bedtime was associated with improved sleep and enhanced executive functioning. Another theory of management rests on the observation that mice with nominally "mild" TBI suffer persistent problems maintaining wakefulness, associated with decreased orexin neuron activity. Experimental treatment of mice with a dietary supplement of branched-chain amino acids precursors for glutamate synthesis led to reactivation of those orexin neurons and enhanced wakefulness [86]. It is premature to judge the effectiveness of such a dietary approach in humans.

However, the discovery of the role of orexin/hypocretin in the sleep–wake cycle has inspired a new avenue for the management of insomnia. Evidence suggests that at least some insomniac persons exhibit a combination of decreased GABA and increased orexin/hypocretin levels at night. Blockade of orexin receptors by dual-action receptor antagonists has been shown to promote sleep in rats, dogs, and humans [87]. Recently, such agents have been tested for clinical safety and efficacy [81, 88–89]. In 2014, the agent suvorexant was approved for the management of insomnia in the United States by the Federal Drug Administration. To the best of our knowledge, this novel agent has yet to be tested among those with post-concussive insomnia. Its relatively benign side-effect profile suggests the possibility that it might mitigate insomnia in persons with brain injury without compromising cognition.

Conclusion

Like all persistent post-concussive medical problems, sleep disorders have received inadequate clinical attention and little empirical investigation. Their prevalence after CBI/mTBI may be over 50%. Some evidence suggests that these problems are treatable. It behooves us to assess every CBI survivor for PCSDs and to attempt, in so far as the infant state of the art permits, to intervene.

References

1. Wiseman-Hakes C, Colantonio A, Judith Gargaro J. Sleep and wake disorders following traumatic brain injury: A systematic review of the literature. *Crit Rev Phys Rehabil Med* 2009;21:317–374.
2. Meerlo P, Mistlberger RE, Noiman L, Gould E. Sleep deprivation inhibits adult neurogenesis in the hippocampus by elevating glucocorticoids. *Proc Natl Acad Sci* 2006;103:19170–19175.
3. Xie L, Kang H, Xu Q, Chen MJ, Liao Y, Thiyagarajan M, O'Donnell J, et al. Sleep drives metabolite clearance from the adult brain. *Science* 2013;342:373–377.
4. Cantor JB, Bushnik T, Cicerone C, Dijkers MP, Gordon W, Hammond FM, et al. Insomnia, fatigue, and sleepiness in the first 2 years after traumatic brain injury: An NIDRR TBI Model System Module Study. *J Head Trauma Rehabil* 2012;27: E1–E14.
5. Mathias JL, Alvaro PK. Prevalence of sleep disturbances, disorders, and problems following traumatic brain injury: A meta-analysis. *Sleep Med* 2012;13:898–905.
6. Waldron-Perrine B, McGuire AP, Spencer RJ, Drag LL, Pangilinan PH, Bieliauskas LA. The influence of sleep and mood on cognitive functioning among veterans being evaluated for mild traumatic brain injury. *Milit Med* 2012;177:1293–1301.
7. Fakhran S, Yaeger K, Alhilali L. Symptomatic white matter changes in mild traumatic brain injury resemble pathologic features of early Alzheimer dementia. *Radiol* 2013;269: 249–257.
8. McGinty D, Szymusiak R. Neural control of sleep in mammals. In Kryger MH, Roth T, Dement WC, editors. *Principles and practices of sleep medicine*, 5th edition. St Louis, MO: Elsevier, 2011.
9. Kinomura S, Larsson J, Gulyás B, Roland PE. Activation by attention of the human reticular formation and thalamic intralaminar nuclei. *Science* 1996;271:512–515.
10. Sakurai T, Mieda M. Connectomics of orexin-producing neurons: Interface of systems of emotion, energy homeostasis and arousal. *Trends Pharmacol Sci* 2011;32:451–462.
11. Strecker RE, Morairty S, Thakkar MM, Porkka-Heiskanen T, Basheer R, Dauphin LJ, Rainnie DG, et al. Adenosinergic modulation of basal forebrain and preoptic/anterior hypothalamic neuronal activity in the control of behavioral state. *Behav Brain Res* 2000;115:183–204.
12. Fisone G, Borgkvist A, Usiello A. Caffeine as a psychomotor stimulant: Mechanism of action. *Cell Mol Life Sci* 2004;61:857–872.
13. Czeisler CA, Duffy JF, Shanahan TL, Brown EN, Mitchell JF, Rimmer DW, Ronda JM, et al. Stability, precision, and near-24-hour period of the human circadian pacemaker. *Science* 1999;284:2177–2181.
14. Frieboes RM, Muller U, Murck H, von Cramon DY, Holsboer F, Steiger A. Nocturnal hormone secretion and the sleep EEG in patients several months after traumatic brain injury. *J Neuropsychiatry Clin Neurosci* 1999;11:354–360.
15. Tobe EH, Schneider JS, Mrozik T, Lidsky TI. Persisting insomnia following traumatic brain injury. *J Neuropsychiatry Clin Neurosci* 1999;11:504–506.
16. Ouellet MC, Morin CM. Subjective and objective measures of insomnia in the context of traumatic brain injury: A preliminary study. *Sleep Med* 2006;7:486–497.
17. Parcell DL, Ponsford JL, Redman JR, Rajaratnam SM. Poor sleep quality and changes in objectively recorded sleep after traumatic brain injury: A preliminary study. *Arch Phys Med Rehabil* 2008;89:843–850.
18. Schreiber S, Barkai G, Gur-Hartman T, Peles E, Tov N, Dolberg O, Pick C. Long-lasting sleep patterns of adult patients with minor traumatic brain injury (mTBI) and non-mTBI subjects. *Sleep Med* 2008;9:481–487.
19. Williams BR, Lazic SE, Ogilvie RD. Polysomnographic and quantitative EEG analysis of subjects with long-term insomnia complaints associated with mild traumatic brain injury. *Clin Neurophysiol* 2008;119:429–438.
20. Shekleton JA, Parcell DL, Redman JR, Phipps-Nelson J, Ponsford JL, Rajaratnam SM. Sleep disturbance and melatonin levels following traumatic brain injury. *Neurology* 2010;74:1732–1738.
21. Rao V, Bergey A, Hill H, Efron D, McCann U. Sleep disturbance after mild traumatic brain injury: Indicator of injury? *J Neuropsychiatry Clin Neurosci* 2011;23:201–205.
22. Baumann CR, Bassetti CL, Valko PO, Haybaeck J, Keller M, Clark E, et al. Loss of hypocretin (orexin) neurons with traumatic brain injury. *Ann Neurol* 2009;66:555–559.
23. Castriotta RJ, Wilde MC, Lai JM, Atanasov S, Masel BE, Kuna ST. Prevalence and consequences of sleep disorders in traumatic brain injury. *J Clin Sleep Med* 2007;3:349–356.
24. Chan LG, Feinstein A. Persistent sleep disturbances independently predict poorer functional and social outcomes 1 year after mild traumatic brain injury. *J Head Trauma Rehabil* 2015;30:E67–E75.
25. Chaput G, Giguère JF, Chauny JM, Denis R, Lavigne G. Relationship among subjective sleep complaints, headaches, and mood alterations following a mild traumatic brain injury. *Sleep Med* 2009;7:713–716.
26. Dean PJ, Sterr A. Long-term effects of mild traumatic brain injury on cognitive performance. *Front Hum Neurosci* 2013;12:30.
27. Haboubi NHJ, Long J, Koshy M, Ward AB. Short-term sequelae of minor head injury (6 years experience of minor head injury clinic). *Disabil Rehabil* 2001;23:635–638.

28. Imbach LL, Valko PO, Li T, Maric A, Symeonidou E-R, Stover JF, Bassetti CL, et al. Increased sleep need and daytime sleepiness 6 months after traumatic brain injury: A prospective controlled clinical trial. *Brain* 2015;138;726–735.

29. Kaufman Y, Tzischinsky O, Epstein R, Etzioni A, Lavie P, Pillar G. Long-term sleep disturbances in adolescents after minor head injury. *Pediatr Neurol* 2001;24:129–134.

30. Kraus J, Hsu P, Schaffer K, Vaca F, Ayers K, Kennedy F, Afifi AA. Preinjury factors and 3-month outcomes following emergency department diagnosis of mild traumatic brain injury. *J Head Trauma Rehabil* 2009;24:344–354.

31. Levitt MA, Sutton TM, Goldman J, Mikhail M, Christopher T. Cognitive dysfunction in patients suffering minor head trauma. *Am J Emerg Med* 1994;12:172–175.

32. McMahon P, Hricik A, Yue JK, Puccio AM, Inoue T, Lingsma HF, Beers SR, et al. TRACK-TBI investigators. Symptomatology and functional outcome in mild traumatic brain injury: Results from the prospective TRACK-TBI study. *J Neurotrauma* 2014; 3:26–33.

33. Parsons LC, Ver Beek D. Sleep–awake patterns following cerebral concussion. *Nurs Res* 1982;31:260–264.

34. Perlis ML, Artiola L, Giles DE. Sleep complaints in chronic postconcussion syndrome. *Percept Mot Skills* 1997;84:595–599.

35. Segalowitz SJ, Lawson L. Subtle symptoms associated with self-reported mild head injury. *J Learning Disabil* 1995;28:309–319.

36. Tham SW, Palermo TM, Vavilala MS, Wang J, Jaffe KM, Koepsell TD, Dorsch A, et al. The longitudinal course, risk factors, and impact of sleep disturbances in children with traumatic brain injury *J Neurotrauma* 2012;29:154–161.

37. Tham SW, Fales J, Palermo TM. Subjective and objective assessment of sleep in adolescents with mild traumatic brain injury. *J Neurotrauma* 2015;32:847–852.

38. Centers for Disease Control and Prevention. Behavioral risk factor surveillance system. 2009. Available at www.cdc.gov/brfss/.

39. Ouellet M-C, Beaulieu-Bonneau S, Morin CM, Sleep–wake disturbances after traumatic brain injury. *Lancet Neurol* 2015; 14:746–757.

40. Mahmood O, Rapport LJ, Hanks RA, Fichtenberg NL. Neuropsychological performance and sleep disturbance following traumatic brain injury. *J Head Trauma Rehabil* 2004; 19:378–390.

41. Bradshaw D, Drake A, Magnus N, Gray N, McDonald E. Pre-injury sleep complaints in patients with mild traumatic brain injury. *Sleep* 2001;24(Suppl):A374.

42. Castriotta RJ, Atanasov S, Wilde MC, Masel BE, Lai JM, Kuna ST. Treatment of sleep disorders after traumatic brain injury. *J Clin Sleep Med* 2009;5:137–144.

43. Collen J, Orr N, Lettieri CJ, Carter K, Holley AB. Sleep disturbances among soldiers with combat-related traumatic brain injury. *Chest* 2012;142:622–630.

44. Mysliwiec V, McGraw L, Pierce R, Smith P, Trapp B, Roth BJ. Sleep disorders and associated medical comorbidities in active duty military personnel. *Sleep* 2013;36:167–174.

45. Lankford D, Wellman J, O'Hara C. Posttraumatic narcolepsy in mild to moderate closed head injury. *Sleep* 1994;17:S25–S28.

46. Kirov II, Tal A, Babb JS, Reaume J, Bushnik T, Ashman TA, Flanagan S, et al. Proton MR spectroscopy correlates diffuse axonal abnormalities with post-concussive symptoms in mild traumatic brain injury. *J Neurotrauma* 2013;30:1200–1204.

47. Nardone R, Bergmann J, Kunz A, Caleri F, Seidl M, Tezzon F, Gerstenbrand F, et al. Cortical excitability changes in patients with sleep–wake disturbances after traumatic brain injury. *J Neurotrauma* 2011;28:1165–1171.

48. Yaeger K, Alhilali L, Fakhran S. Evaluation of tentorial length and angle in sleep–wake disturbances after mild traumatic brain injury. *AJR Am J Roentgenol* 2014;202:614–618.

49. Beetar J, Guilmette T, Sparadeo F. Sleep and pain complaints in symptomatic traumatic brain injury and neurologic populations. *Arch Phys Med Rehabil* 1996;77:1298–1302.

50. Hou L, Han X, Sheng P, Tong W, Li Z, Xu D, Yu M, et al. Risk factors associated with sleep disturbance following traumatic brain injury: Clinical findings and questionnaire based study. *PLoS One* 2013;8:e76087.

51. Ponsford JL, Parcell DL, Sinclair KL, Roper M, Rajaratnam SME. Changes in sleep patterns following traumatic brain injury: A controlled study. *Neurorehabil Neural Repair* 2013;27:613–621.

52. Rao V, McCann U, Han D, Bergey A, Smith MT. Does acute TBI-related sleep disturbance predict subsequent neuropsychiatric disturbances? *Brain Inj* 2014;28:20–26.

53. Wall PL. Posttraumatic stress disorder and traumatic brain injury in current military populations: A critical analysis. *J Am Psychiatr Nurses Assoc* 2012;18:278–298.

54. Macera CA, Aralis HJ, Rauh, MJ, MacGregor AJ. Do sleep problems mediate the relationship between traumatic brain injury and development of mental health symptoms after deployment? *Sleep* 2013;36:83–90.

55. Katzenberg D, Young T, Finn L, Lin L, King, DP, Takahashi JS, Mignot E. A CLOCK polymorphism associated with human diurnal preference. *Sleep* 1998;21:569–576.

56. Benedetti F, Dallaspezia S, Fulgosi MC, Lorenzi C, Serretti A, Barbini B, Colombo C, et al. Actimetric evidence that CLOCK 3111 T/C SNP influences sleep and activity patterns in patients affected by bipolar depression. *Am J Med Genet B: Neuropsychiatr Genetics* 2007;144B:631–635.

57. Serretti A, Gaspar-Barba E, Calati R, Cruz-Fuentes CS, Gomez-Sanchez A, Perez-Molina A, De Ronchi D. 3111T/C clock gene polymorphism is not associated with sleep disturbances in untreated depressed patients. *Chronobiol Int* 2010;27:265–277.

58. Antypa N, Mandelli L, Nearchou FA, Vaiopoulos C, Stefanis CN, Serretti A, Stefanis NC. The 3111T/C polymorphism interacts with stressful life events to influence patterns of sleep in females. *Chronobiol Int* 2012;29:891–897.

59. Hua P, Liu W, Zhao Y, Ding H, Wang L, Xiao H. Tef polymorphism is associated with sleep disturbances in patients with Parkinson's disease. *Sleep Med* 2012;13:297–300.

60. Dijk DJ, Archer SN. PERIOD3, circadian phenotypes, and sleep homeostasis. *Sleep Med Rev* 2010;14:151–160.

61. Goel N, Banks S, Mignot E, Dinges DF. PER3 polymorphism predicts cumulative sleep homeostatic but not neurobehavioral changes to chronic partial sleep deprivation. *PLoS One* 2009; 4:e5874.

62. Brower KJ, Wojnar M, Sliwerska E, Armitage R, Burmeister M. PER3 polymorphism and insomnia severity in alcohol dependence. *Sleep* 2012;35:571–577.

63. Deuschle M, Schredl M, Schilling C, Wüst S, Frank J, Witt SH, Rietschel M, et al. Association between a serotonin transporter length polymorphism and primary insomnia. *Sleep* 2010;33:343–347.

64. Goel N, Banks S, Lin L, Mignot E, Dinges DF. Catechol-O-methyltransferase Val158Met polymorphism associates with individual differences in sleep physiologic responses to chronic sleep loss. *PLoS One* 2011;6:e29283.

65. Trbovic SM. Schizophrenia as a possible dysfunction of the suprachiasmatic nucleus. *Med Hypoth* 2010;74:127–131.

66. Park HJ, Park JK, Kim SK, Cho AR, Kim JW, Yim SV, Chung JH. Association of polymorphism in the promoter of the melatonin receptor 1A gene with schizophrenia and with insomnia

symptoms in schizophrenia patients. *J Mol Neurosci* 2011; 45:304–308.

67. Miaskowski C, Dodd M, Lee K, West C, Paul SM, Cooper BA, Wara W, et al. Preliminary evidence of an association between a functional interleukin-6 polymorphism and fatigue and sleep disturbance in oncology patients and their family caregivers. *J Pain Symptom Manage* 2010;40:531–544.

68. Illi J, Miaskowski C, Cooper B, Levine JD, Dunn L, West C, Dodd M, et al. Association between pro- and anti-inflammatory cytokine genes and a symptom cluster of pain, fatigue, sleep disturbance, and depression. *Cytokine* 2012;58:437–447.

69. Bachmann V, Klein C, Bodenmann S, Schäfer N, Berger W, Brugger P, Landolt HP. The BDNF Val66Met polymorphism modulates sleep intensity: EEG frequency- and state-specificity. *Sleep* 2012;35:335–344.

70. Sabir M, Gaudreault P-O, Freyburger M, Massart R. Impact of traumatic brain injury on sleep structure, electrocorticographic activity and transcriptome in mice. *Brain Behav Immun* 2015; 47:118–130.

71. Davis CJ, Krueger JM. Sleep and cytokines. *Sleep Med Clin* 2012;7:517–527.

72. Ziebell JM, Morganti-Kossmann MC. Involvement of pro and antiinflammatory cytokines and chemokines in the pathophysiology of traumatic brain injury. *Neurotherapeutics* 2010;7:22–30.

73. Rowe RK, Striz M, Bachstetter AD, Van Eldik LJ, Donohue KD, O'Hara BF, Lifshitz J. Diffuse brain injury induces acute post-traumatic sleep. *PLoS One* 2014;9(1):e82507.

74. Giza CC, Hovda DA. The neurometabolic cascade of concussion. *J Athletic Train* 2001;36:228–235.

75. Clark IA, Vissel B. Inflammation–sleep interface in brain disease: TNF, insulin, orexin. *J Neuroinflamm* 2014;11:51.

76. National Sleep Foundation. National Sleep Foundation recommends new sleep times. Available at: https://sleepfoundation.org/press-release/national-sleep-foundation-recommends-new-sleep-times/page/0/1.

77. Thorpy M. Sleep hygiene. National Sleep Foundation. Available at: http://sleepfoundation.org/ask-the-expert/sleep-hygiene.

78. Wiseman-Hakes C, Murray B, Moineddin R, Rochon E, Cullen N, Gargaro J, Colantonio A. Evaluating the impact of treatment for sleep/wake disorders on recovery of cognition and communication in adults with chronic TBI, *Brain Inj* 2013;27:1364–1376.

79. Boussi-Gross R, Golan H, Fishlev G, Bechor Y, Volkov O, Bergan J, Friedman M, et al. Hyperbaric oxygen therapy can improve post concussion syndrome years after mild traumatic brain injury – Randomized prospective trial. *PLoS One* 2013;8:e79995.

80. Miller RS, Weaver LK, Bahraini N, Churchill S, Price RC, Skiba V, Caviness J, et al. Effects of hyperbaric oxygen on symptoms and quality of life among service members with persistent postconcussion symptoms: A randomized clinical trial. *JAMA Intern Med* 2015;175:43–52.

81. Winrow CJ, Renger JJ. Discovery and development of orexin receptor antagonists as therapeutics for insomnia. *Br J Pharmacol* 2014;171:283–293.

82. Ruff RL, Ruff SS, Wang XF. Improving sleep: Initial headache treatment in OIF/OEF veterans with blast-induced mild traumatic brain injury. *J Rehabil Res Dev* 2009;46:1071–1084.

83. Kung S, Espinel Z, Lapid MI. Treatment of nightmares with prazosin: A systematic review. *Mayo Clin Proc* 2012; 87:890–900.

84. Writer BW, Meyer EG, Schillerstrom JE. Prazosin for military combat-related PTSD nightmares: A critical review. *J Neuropsychiatry Clin Neurosci* 2014;26:24–33.

85. Lequerica A, Jasey N, Portelli-Tremont JN, Chiaravalloti ND. Pilot study on the effect of Ramelteon on sleep disturbance after traumatic brain injury: preliminary evidence from a clinical trial. *Arch Phys Med Rehabil* 2015; 96(10):1802–9.

86. Lim MM, Elkind J, Xiong G, Galante R, Zhu J, Zhang L, Lian J, et al. Dietary therapy mitigates persistent wake deficits caused by mild traumatic brain injury. *Sci Transl Med* 2013;5:215ra173.

87. Krystal AD, Benca RM, Kilduff TS. Understanding the sleep–wake cycle: Sleep, insomnia, and the orexin system. *J Clin Psychiatry* 2013;74(suppl 1):3–20.

88. Herring WJ, Snyder E, Budd K, Hutzelmann J, Snavely D, Liu K, et al. Orexin receptor antagonism for treatment of insomnia: A randomized clinical trial of suvorexant. *Neurology* 2012;79(23):2265–2274.

89. Pałasz A, Lapray D, Peyron C, Rojczyk-Gołębiewska E, Skowronek R, Markowski G, Czajkowska B, et al. Dual orexin receptor antagonists – Promising agents in the treatment of sleep disorders. *Int J Neuropsychopharmacol* 2014;17:157–168.

Chapter 26

Neuroendocrine Dysfunction Following Concussion: A Missed Opportunity for Enhancing Recovery?

Nigel Glynn and Amar Agha

Introduction

In 1918, Cyran published what may have been the first report of anterior pituitary dysfunction after traumatic cranial injury [1]. However, this entity was thought to be very rare and only in the last 15 years pituitary hormone deficiency has come to be recognized as a frequent complication of traumatic brain injury (TBI). The majority of research has focused on survivors of moderate to severe head injury or repetitive concussion – for example, among boxers, kickboxers, and football players. This is largely due to the fact that mild cases – typical single concussive brain injuries (CBIs) without prolonged coma or intracranial bleeding that briefly come to medical attention in the emergency department – rarely receive long-term medical follow-up. However, a review of the available data supports the conclusion that survivors of single concussions may be at risk of persistent pituitary dysfunction.

The physical and psychological consequences of pituitary hormone deficiency are varied and may be subtle. In addition, there is significant overlap between symptoms of hypopituitarism and common post-concussive symptoms. This leads to a reasonable suspicion that some persistent symptoms after CBI are due to one or more unrecognized hormone deficiencies that, if appropriately treated, could enhance recovery.

The Pituitary Gland

The pituitary gland is located within the bony sella turcica of the skull base. In humans the gland is composed of two distinct parts – the anterior lobe (adenohypophysis) and posterior lobe (neurohypophysis) (Figure 26.1). The anterior lobe is a glandular structure derived from Rathke's pouch, a portion of primitive oral ectoderm. It secretes prolactin, growth hormone (GH), adrenocorticotropic hormone (ACTH), gonadotropins (luteinizing hormone and follicle-stimulating hormone), and thyroid-stimulating hormone (TSH). Secretion of these hormones is controlled by releasing factors which are synthesized by hypothalamic neurons and carried to the anterior pituitary by means of the hypophyseal–portal circulation. Hypothalamic peptides stimulate secretion of anterior pituitary hormones, with the exception of prolactin which is under tonic, inhibitory control by the hypothalamic catecholamine dopamine. Target gland hormones (e.g., thyroid hormone, cortisol) exert a negative feedback on hypothalamic and anterior pituitary hormones, resulting in a finely balanced hypothalamic–pituitary–target organ axis (e.g., the hypothalamic–pituitary–thyroid axis).

The posterior pituitary lobe is composed mainly of dilated nerve endings whose bodies reside in hypothalamic nuclei. These neurons secrete arginine vasopressin (AVP) and oxytocin directly into the systemic circulation in response to physiological and neural stimuli. AVP regulates the body's water balance by promoting renal water reabsorption in response to thirst. Oxytocin stimulates contraction of the uterus during labor and promotes milk ejection during lactation.

Historical Perspective

Damage to the pituitary gland or hypothalamus following head trauma which results in impaired secretion of pituitary hormones is termed post-traumatic hypopituitarism. It remains among the less well-recognized and potentially underdiagnosed complications of head injury. As noted above, Cyran published the first report of pituitary damage following a base-of-skull fracture in 1918 [1]. However, a case series published in 1942 reported post-traumatic hypopituitarism to be a rare cause of hypopituitarism, accounting for only 0.7% of cases [2].

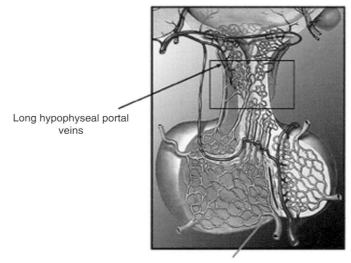

Long hypophyseal portal veins

Short hypophyseal portal veins

Fig. 26.1 Diagrammatic representation of the pituitary gland and its complex blood supply.

Source: Glynn and Agha (authors' own)

Table 26.1 Common clinical consequences of pituitary hormone deficiency

Pituitary hormone	Symptoms of deficiency
Anterior pituitary	
Growth hormone (GH)	Children: short stature Adults: altered body composition (increased fat mass), poor exercise tolerance, impaired quality of life, dyslipidaemia, reduced bone density
Gonadotropins (FSH, LH)	Pre-menopausal women: oligomenorrhea, infertility, low libido, reduced bone density Men: low libido, erectile dysfunction, infertility, reduced muscle mass, decreased bone density
Adrenocorticotropic hormone (ACTH)	Fatigue, lassitude, weight loss, postural dizziness
Thyroid-stimulating hormone (TSH)	Fatigue, cold intolerance, dry skin, brittle hair, weight gain, mood disturbance, constipation
Prolactin	Inability to lactate after parturition
Posterior pituitary	
Arginine vasopressin	Polyuria and polydipsia

FSH: follicle-stimulating hormone; LH: luteinizing hormone.

Subsequently, several post-mortem studies recorded pituitary gland infarction in up to one-third of head trauma victims [3, 4].

Contemporary research has now identified a high prevalence of hypopituitarism among survivors of moderate to severe TBI [5]. Furthermore, emerging evidence suggests that even minor head injury, often suffered repetitively during contact sports, may also result in damage to the hypothalamus or pituitary [6]. There is a growing recognition of the considerable overlap between the sequelae of chronic traumatic encephalopathy and the clinical consequences of hypopituitarism, including lethargy, memory impairment, low libido, and mood disturbance. Table 26.1 summarizes the most common symptoms after anterior and/or posterior pituitary damage. This suggests that post-traumatic hypopituitarism may contribute to persistent post-concussive symptoms and appropriate hormone replacement may attenuate some neurobehavioral symptoms and augment rehabilitation.

Pathophysiology

The vast majority of the blood supply to the anterior pituitary is derived from the long hypophyseal arteries (Figure 26.1). These give rise to hypophyseal portal vessels which traverse the thick diaphragma sella – an extension of dura mater which separates the sella turcica from the suprasellar cistern. It is speculated that interruption of blood flow through these delicate vessels due to edema, shear forces, or raised intracranial pressure may lead to pituitary gland ischemia and infarction. Short hypophyseal portal vessels, arising from the intracavernous portion of the internal carotid artery, supply a small area in the medial portion of the pituitary gland. They are believed to be less susceptible to shear forces or compression as they enter the sella below the diaphragma.

Direct trauma to the hypothalamus, infundibulum, or the pituitary gland itself, within the bony sella turcica, has been reported in severe, often fatal, head trauma. In survivors of TBI, it has been proposed that inflammatory or necrotic processes may expose hypothalamic and/or pituitary antigens and trigger a destructive autoimmune cascade similar to other endocrine glands, such as the thyroid and adrenal glands. High titers of anti-pituitary and anti-hypothalamic antibodies have been reported in boxers who suffered repeated, mild TBI [7]. High titers of the latter are associated with pituitary dysfunction in this cohort. However, it is unclear whether they play a direct role in the pathogenesis of post-traumatic hypopituitarism or simply indicate more severe hypothalamic damage. Damage to the vascular structures of the hypothalamic–pituitary region is a more likely mechanism in survivors of TBI and those suffering chronic, mild head injury.

Numerous lines of clinicopathological evidence support the vascular injury theory. Modern post-mortem studies have demonstrated ischemic necrosis of the anterior pituitary gland in 43% of individuals who died up to one week following a TBI suffered in a motor vehicle accident [8]. Also, ischemic and/or hemorrhagic lesions in the anterior hypothalamus have been reported in a similar percentage of TBI victims [9]. More recently, magnetic resonance imaging (MRI) studies have reported that patients with chronic post-traumatic hypopituitarism had a smaller pituitary volume in comparison to eupituitary controls, consistent with gland infarction and necrosis [10]. This finding has been demonstrated after a single, moderate to severe TBI as well as following repeated mild head injury.

Furthermore, the pattern of hormonal loss also suggests a vascular etiology. Decline in GH and gonadotropin reserve is the most commonly reported pituitary dysfunction following head injury. Somatotorphs (GH-producing cells) and gonadotrophs occupy peripheral portions of the gland, perfused by the long hypophyseal portal vessels. In contrast, corticotrophs (ACTH-producing cells) and thyrotrophs (TSH-producing cells) are found in more medial portions of the gland supplied by the short hypophyseal vessels. This may explain why ACTH and TSH deficiency is relatively less common following TBI.

The posterior pituitary is less susceptible to vascular injury as it is perfused by the inferior hypophyseal vessels which do not traverse the diaphragma sella. Inflammatory edema around the neurons of the paraventricular and supraoptic nuclei in the hypothalamus or compression of their axons due to hemorrhage into the sella is believed to be responsible for diabetes insipidus, seen in up to 26% of victims following moderate to severe TBI. This is typically a transient phenomenon which resolves once the edema subsides. Posterior pituitary dysfunction, however, is extremely rare following mild TBI or concussion.

Anterior Pituitary Dysfunction

The incidence and prevalence of pituitary dysfunction in adults following TBI cannot be stated with confidence. Prospective and retrospective studies have reported such a wide spectrum of findings – from 0 to 80% – that no single report, meta-analysis, or review can be regarded as definitive. In addition, as noted in the introduction, the overwhelming majority of endocrine studies report findings after moderate or severe TBIs, with a smaller number of publications discussing endocrinopathies after repetitive concussions. This textbook is primarily devoted to discussing single, typical CBI – by far the most common form of clinically significant human head trauma. In an effort to better understand the epidemiology of post-concussive hypopituitarism, we reviewed the English-language peer-reviewed empirical studies that reported the incidence or prevalence of post-concussive hormone disorders or deficiencies. In addition to a PubMed search of the terms "traumatic brain injury" and "hormone" or "endocrine," or "pituitary," or "hypopituitarism," we obtained and read all the primary sources cited in 34 reviews and compiled the relevant data[1] [5, 6, 11–43]. In most cases, this involved extracting the subset of data regarding "mild" cases from reports that studied the full spectrum of injury and stratified findings by severity. Several reports were also included because the authors: (1) indicated the number of "mild" cases; (2) reported the prevalence of endocrinopathies across levels of severity; and (3) determined that the occurrence was not associated with severity [44–50]. In such cases, prevalence of disorders in the whole cohort at least provides an estimate of the prevalence among the subset of mild cases.

Some reports were excluded because they failed to report injury severity, or reported severity but failed to stratify endocrine findings by severity despite including mild cases [51–60]. One report was excluded because it was confined to subjects with multiple concussions and poor life quality [61]. One report was excluded because it preselected subjects with persistent neurobehavioral symptoms or deficits [62]. Table 26.2 lists all the studies identified in our searches that met the criteria for selection.

As shown in Table 26.2, confining attention to studies conducted at ≥ one year post concussion, persistent hypopituitarism occurs in 0–76.4% of cases. Since the report with the highest estimate [49] is one of those in which the prevalence among mild cases is estimated from the prevalence across levels of severity, one might exclude that figure. Limiting the review to studies that explicitly stratified results by severity, therefore, the range shrinks to 0–65%.

How is one to interpret such data?

Given that CBI is among the most common causes of human disability, and given the fact that many endocrinopathies are manageable, it is a matter of considerable importance and some urgency to accurately estimate the occurrence of these problems. A range of 0–65% has almost no utility for clinical planning or public health. If anterior pituitary deficiencies are rare after concussion (so-called "mild" TBI), then universal screening is hard to justify due to the cost and effort. If those deficiencies are common, then clinicians around the world may be routinely missing an opportunity to diagnose and initiate safe and effective intervention. Statistical maneuvers

offer little comfort. A weighted average of the reported results would reify a conclusion that credits the validity of all of the sources equally, even if some seem less credible on their faces. A median result is hardly more worthy of confidence. However, for the sake of discussion, if one excludes the highest outlier (76.4%) and confines the analysis to studies with follow-up of ≥ one year, the median prevalence of post-concussive anterior hypopituitarism is 24.6%. The most common problems are GH deficiency (GHD), often severe, and hypogonadism. Evidence suggests that hypopituitarism often has a delayed onset, with the possibility of new deficits occurring at or beyond three years post injury. However, the peak prevalence (reflecting recovery of some early-onset cases and new presentation of some late-onset cases) seems to occur at about one year post injury. Based on the two studies that retested the same cohort at one and three years [70, 71], the prevalence significantly decreases during that interval.

What accounts for this extraordinary diversity of findings? The present authors do not claim to know the answer, or the proportionate contribution of multiple potential confounding factors. However, (1) variations in the classification of cases as "mild" TBIs; (2) variation in demographic and biological traits of cohorts; and (3) variation in endocrine measurement methods all plausibly played a role in the observed discrepancies.

With regard to injury classification: as explained throughout this textbook, the TBI severity label "mild" is neither biologically nor clinically meaningful. In addition to the fact that no marker validly measures severity and no neuroscientific rationale exists for drawing a red line between mild and not mild, the old convention for clinical assessment of severity – initial Glasgow Coma Scale (GCS) – is not valid, reliable, nor stable over passing minutes. For example, Wachter et al. [72] reported pituitary insufficiency in 53 cases of TBI. When those authors employed GCS at the scene, 35 of their subjects (66%) had "mild" TBIs. When they employed GCS at the emergency room, just nine of their subjects (17%) had "mild" TBI. Which of these two subgroups should be analyzed to determine the prevalence of hypopituitarism after "mild" TBI? This is a useful warning. No matter how carefully it is reviewed, the published data about "mild" injuries are riven with the dubiety.

With regard to demographic factors: the two most common problems were GHD and hypogonadism. Both are age- and body mass index-dependent.[2] Without a consistent method of controlling for those factors, no two studies are comparable.

However, methodological differences in the way that pituitary deficiency was ascertained are probably crucial to understanding these variations. Many studies found that GHD is the most common abnormality, yet diagnosis of GHD requires a stimulation test (random baseline GH measurements are of no value) and hence the response is

---

[1] Our review was systematic but not necessarily comprehensive. Still, Table 26.2 should be reasonably representative of the universe of published reports.

[2] Of interest: although sex and age are known to interact in determining the risk of persistent post-concussive symptoms, the available data do not support the conclusion that sex influences the risk of post-traumatic hypopituitarism [74–76].

Table 26.2 Reports of post-concussive hypopituitarism

Authors	Subjects	Follow-up	Prevalence of one or more endocrine abnormalities	Comments
Aimaretti et al., 2004 [44][a]	Total = 100 Mild = 55	3 months	35%	Most common: • GHD • Hypogonadism
Aimaretti et al., 2005 [45][b]	Total = 70 Mild = 33	12 months	22.2%	Most common: • GHD • Hypogonadism
Aimaretti et al., 2005 [63]	Total = 23 Mild = 10	12 months	30%	• One hypogonadism • One hyperPRL • One severe GHD
Bondanelli et al., 2004 [64]	Total = 50 Mild = 16	≥ 5 years	37.5%	Most common: • GHD • Hypogonadism • Hypothyroidism
Englander et al., 2010 [47][c]	Total = 119 Mild = 26	Mean = 9 years	65%	Most common: • GHD • Hypoadrenalism • Hypogonadism
Kelly et al., 2000 [65]	Total = 22 Mild = 3	Mean = 26 months	0%	N/A
Klose et al., 2007 [66]	Total = 104 Mild = 44	13 months	0.45%	Most common: • GHD • Hypoadrenalism
Klose et al., 2007 [67]	Total = 46 Mild = 22	12 months	0%	Most common: • GHD • Hypoadrenalism
Klose et al., 2014 [50][d]	Total = 439 Mild = 306	Mean = 2.5 years	4.5–18.9%	Prevalence of GHD lower by ITT than by GHRH-Arg or GHRH-PD
Kokshoorn et al., 2011 [48]	Total = 112 Mild = 64	Mean = 4 years	3.1%	Hypopituitarism associated with higher BMI
Krewer et al., 2016 [68][e]	Total = 245 Mild = 51	1 to > 5 years	24.1%	Most common: • GHD • Hypogonadism
Moreau et al., 2012 [49][f]	Total = 55 Mild = 9	Mean = 79.2 months	76.4%	GHD associated with cognitive impairment
Silva et al., 2015 [69][g]	Total = 166 Mild = 114	Mean = 40.4 months	29%	Most common: • GHD • ACTH deficiency • LH/FSH deficiency
Tanriverdi et al., 2006 [46]	Total = 52 Mild = 31	12 months	50.9%	Most common: • GHD • ACTH deficiency • Hypogonadism
Tanriverdi et al., 2008 [70][h]	Total = 30 Mild = 19	1 year and 3 years	42.1% (1 year) 15.8% (3 years)	Most common: • GHD • ACTH deficiency
Tanriverdi et al., 2013 [71][i]	Total = 25 Mild = 16	1 yr. & 5 yrs.	43.7% (1 year) 18.7% (5 years)	Most common: • GHD
Wachter et al., 2009 [72][j]	Total = 53 Mild = 9 or 35	12–36 months	25.7%	Most common: • Hypogonadism • Hypothyroidism
Wilkinson et al., 2012 [73]	26 with mild blast concussions	≥ 1 year	42%	Most common: • GHD • Hypogonadism

Table 26.2 (*Cont.*)

a Re Aimaretti et al., 2004: "The occurrence of hypopituitarism was not associated with the GCS [Glasgow Coma Scale]" (p. 324).

b Re Aimaretti et al., 2005: one or more anterior pituitary hormone abnormalities were found in 22.2% across levels of injury severity. Prevalence was not associated with severity.

c Re Englander et al., 2010: the authors report: "This sample contained a relatively even distribution of severities of injury between mild, moderate and severe TBI" (p. 1382). Based on that statement and duration of loss of consciousness, one estimates that 26/119 cases were mild. The authors also report that duration of loss of consciousness was not associated with endocrine abnormalities – on which basis one estimates that the findings across levels of severity approximate those among the mild cases. Sixty-five percent had moderate to severe GHD; 64% had adrenal insufficiency based on low morning cortisol.

d Re Klose et al., 2014: prevalence of GHD ranged from 4.5 to 18.9% across levels of injury severity depending on the standard of measurement. Prevalence was not associated with severity.

e Re Krewer et al., 2016: follow-up occurred at one to > five years post injury: "the severity of TBI [traumatic brain injury] did not correlate with the number of impaired pituitary axes in our cohort of patients" (p. 1548). At one to two years, gonadotropic insufficiency was more common than GHD, while at > five years, GHD was more common than gonadotropic insufficiency. At > five years, 24.1% of TBI subjects had GHD.

f Re Moreau et al., 2012: one or more anterior pituitary hormone abnormalities were found in 76.4% across levels of injury severity. Prevalence was not associated with severity.

g Re Silva et al., 2015: note that the subjects were recruited from an endocrine clinic.

h Re Tanriverdi et al., 2008: at one year, eight of 19 mild subjects had GHD (42.1%). At three years, five of those eight subjects exhibited normalized GH, leaving three of 19 (15.8%) with persistent GHD. Persistence of hypopituitarism was more common among subjects with initially severe injuries.

i Re Tanriverdi et al., 2013: at one year, seven of 16 mild subjects had GHD (43.7%). At three years, four of those seven subjects exhibited normalized GH, leaving three of 16 (18.7%) with persistent GHD.

j Re Wachter et al., 2009: based on GCS at the scene, 35/53 (66%) of cases were mild. Based on GCS at the emergency department, nine of 53 (17%) were mild.

ACTH: adrenocorticotropic hormone; BMI: body mass index; FSH: follicle-stimulating hormone; GHD: growth hormone deficiency; GHRH-ARG: growth hormone-releasing hormone – arginine; GHRH-PD: GHRH – pyridostigmine; ITT: insulin tolerance test; LH: luteinizing hormone; PRL: prolactin.

highly stimulus-dependent. Such stimulation tests include the insulin tolerance test, the glucagon test, the GH-releasing hormone – arginine test, the GHRH-pyridostigmine test, or estimates derived from age-adjusted insulin-like growth factor I (IGF-1) serum levels: the latter lacks sufficient sensitivity. Each approach may yield different results [48, 50, 63, 73]. Although the insulin tolerance test is widely regarded as the gold standard [77], it is labor-intensive and is contraindicated in patients with seizures or heart disease. Therefore many clinicians and investigators avoid it after TBI. In addition, when two stimulation tests are used to define GHD, the prevalence of GHD drops sharply [26].

Three other factors are probably important yet rarely controlled for in the available empirical literature. First: the elapsed time since injury influences the likelihood of hypopituitarism as some abnormalities recover over time while new abnormalities can evolve, particularly in the first six months after injury, and some time later. Figures 26.2 and 26.3 illustrate the change in prevalence over time. While hypogonadism perhaps dominates the acute phase, long-term follow-up suggests that GHD is the most common form of persistent post-concussive hypopituitarism.

Second: mechanism of injury may impact the risk. Blast wave forces, for example, impact brains differently than direct mechanical impacts to the head. One report was included that investigated pituitary dysfunction after mild blast-related injuries [73]. The finding that persistent hypopituitarism is common in such a cohort is supported by a different study of 834 survivors of blast-related TBI [79]. A total of 767 of these (92% of the cohort) were mild cases, and 29% of the total cohort exhibited structural damage to the pituitary gland on 3-T MRI.[3]

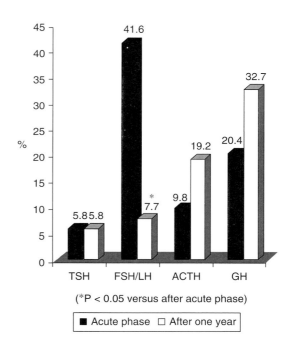

(*P < 0.05 versus after acute phase)

■ Acute phase □ After one year

Fig. 26.2 Percentages of pituitary hormone deficiencies in the acute phase and 12 months after traumatic brain injury. ACTH: adrenocorticotropic hormone; FSH/LH: follicle-stimulating hormone/luteinizing hormone; GH: growth hormone; TSH: thyroid-stimulating hormone.

Source: Tanriverdi et al., 2006 [46] by permission of Oxford University Press/The Endocrine Society

Third: some evidence suggests that genetic variation influences the risk of post-concussive hypopituitarism. Tanriverdi et al. [81] found that persons who are homozygous with the genotype apolipoprotein E e3/e3 were more resistant to hypopituitarism after TBI. It is possible that many

---

3 Another study of pituitary dysfunction after blast was published by Baxter et al. [80] but excluded mild cases.

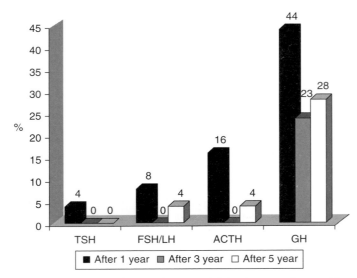

Fig. 26.3 Percentages of pituitary hormone deficiencies at one, three, and five years after traumatic brain injury. ACTH: adrenocorticotropic hormone; FSH/LH: follicle-stimulating hormone/luteinizing hormone; GH: growth hormone; TSH: thyroid-stimulating hormone.

Source: Tanriverdi et al., 2013 [71]. Reproduced with permission from Mary Ann Liebert, Inc.

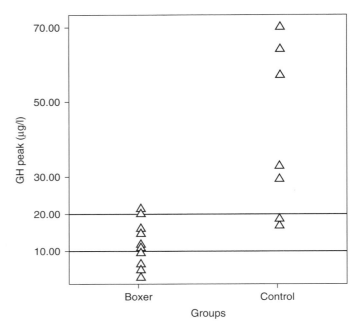

Individual growth hormone-releasing hormone (GHRH) + growth hormone-releasing peptide-6 (GHRP-6)-stimulated growth hormone (GH) peaks in controls and asymptomatic boxers

Fig. 26.4 The cut-off peak GH value for GH deficiency was ≤10 μg/L and peak GH values ≥20 μg/L were considered as normal. The peak GH levels in five (45%) boxers were measured as <10 μg/L and considered as severe GH deficiency, despite absence of traditional endocrine symptoms.

Source: Kelestimur et al., 2004 [84] With kind permission of Springer Science+Business Media

other genetic variations influence vulnerability to brain injury-related hypopituitarism, but further investigation is required in this field.

In summary: based on our systematic review, the median prevalence of persistent (≥ one year) post-concussive anterior hypopituitarism is 24.6%. However, due to failure to standardize the definitions of disorders, methodologies, and stratification of diverse populations, it would be imprudent to fix upon a single number. Broadly speaking, recent reports tend to challenge the old belief that this problem is infrequent. Resolution of the epidemiological question awaits large, rigorous prospective studies.

The Special Case of Repetitive Concussion

Repeated mild head injury, often suffered during contact sports or active military service, appears to pose a significant risk of hypothalamic–pituitary damage. Emerging evidence suggests that boxers, kickboxers, and professional football players who suffer repeated, low-intensity head trauma may suffer from hypopituitarism, with reported rates ranging from 18% to 27% of subjects [82–84].

Kelestimur and colleagues were among the first investigators to demonstrate the risk of hypopituitarism, in particular GHD, among boxers who suffered repeated concussion (Figure 26.4) [84]. They have subsequently elaborated on these findings by reporting hypopituitarism in kickboxers and highlighting the clinical implications of pituitary hormone deficiencies in these athletes [10, 71, 83]. More recently, Kelly et al. robustly

evaluated pituitary function in retired National Football League players [61]. They selected a high-risk cohort who reported a poor quality of life and found pituitary hormone dysfunction in 23.5% of subjects overall.

Isolated hormone deficiency, typically GH, is the most common abnormal finding in all repetitive concussion cohorts. A minority of subjects have multiple pituitary hormone deficiencies. It is unknown whether these findings can be extended to other sports in which concussion is relatively common, including rugby, ice hockey, and skiing. An important confounder, in studies of pituitary function in athletes, is the impact of current or prior use of performance-enhancing drugs such as anabolic steroids. The true prevalence of drug abuse can be difficult to ascertain and steroid use can have a prolonged impact on pituitary function if used at high dose or for a long duration.

Protective head gear is now mandatory in many contact sports and is frequently worn by military personnel in war zones. However, many of the subjects in the currently available studies are now retired and competed in sports before protective head gear was commonly employed. Therefore, it is not known at present whether helmets worn in some sporting activities reduce the risk of pituitary damage.[4]

---

4 The available studies of blast-related post-concussive hypopituitarism did not report whether helmets were worn. However, since blast forces are transmitted to the brain via pressure waves rather than focal impact, it seems plausible that helmets are less efficacious for defending brains against nearby explosions than against direct sporting collisions.

The Special Case of Children

Children and adolescents warrant special attention. Mild, often recurrent head injuries are common during this stage of life. Also, children and adolescents are particularly vulnerable to the consequences of post-traumatic hypopituitarism which may lead to growth failure and/or disturbance of normal pubertal development. Despite evidence of delayed recovery from concussion in childhood, robust research indicates that children under five years of age who survive structural head injury (both accidental and non-accidental) rarely develop long-term hypopituitarism [85]. Concussion is commonly suffered during adolescence in the context of sports and violence. Limited research in this age group suggests a prevalence of hypopituitarism, following moderate to severe trauma, of approximately 35% [63]. In keeping with the data in adult patients, isolated hormone deficiency is the most common finding. It remains unclear whether the data on "mild" TBI in adults can be extrapolated to children and adolescents.

Neurohypophyseal Damage

The patients represented a group of supposedly normal people who suffered head injuries involving slight to severe brain damage, who then, at periods varying from a few hours to three years later, developed disturbances in the use of sugar, water and fat such as those known to occur when the hypothalamus is injured.

Pickles, 1947 [86] (p. 861)

Disturbance of water balance due to neurohypophyseal dysfunction is common and easily recognized following moderate to severe TBI. Impaired secretion of AVP results in a diminished urinary concentrating ability and consequent production of copious amounts of dilute urine. Subjects with preserved thirst can maintain water balance by drinking water to replace urinary losses. However, if the patient has an impaired consciousness level or inability to access water this can lead to intravascular volume contraction, dehydration, and hypernatremia. This is typically a transient phenomenon and most cases resolve within a few days or weeks following injury. Prospective data suggest that the incidence of cranial diabetes insipidus may be as high as 26% in the acute phase following moderate to severe TBI [87]. However, 70% of cases had recovered completely from diabetes insipidus within 12 months.

Hypontremia due to the syndrome of inappropriate antidiuresis (SIAD) can also occur, with a reported incidence ranging from 2.3% to 33% post TBI [88]. Post-traumatic SIAD is caused by damage to the magnocellular neurons in the hypothalamus or their axons as they travel through the pituitary stalk and terminate in the posterior pituitary. The wide incidence range is accounted for by different characteristics of the patient cohorts studied, variable criteria for the diagnosis of SIAD, and variable duration of monitoring following injury. This disorder tends to emerge early following injury and resolve spontaneously after a few days.

In contrast to moderate and severe head injury, posterior pituitary dysfunction is exceptionally rare following concussion or repetitive sports-related head injury. Isolated case reports have described patients with possible partial cranial diabetes insipidus following "mild" TBI [89]. Overall, it seems that a greater degree of injury is required to denervate posterior pituitary tissue or the axons terminating in the posterior pituitary.

Most studies of post-concussive endocrine deficiency address pituitary damage. Despite Pickle's 1947 speculation [86], little is known about the effect of typical CBI on the hypothalamus. However, some recent evidence suggests that "mild" TBI may cause clinically relevant hypothalamic dysfunction and even structural injury. For instance, in a diffusion tensor imaging study of 53 concussion survivors, Jang et al. [90] found that daytime sleepiness was significantly correlated with decreased fractional anisotropy and increased apparent diffusion coefficient in the hypothalamus.

Zhou [91] compared connectivity between concussion survivors and normal controls. CBI subjects displayed abnormal resting-state network hypothalamic connectivity. In the same study post-concussive fatigue negatively correlated with diffusion kurtosis in the hypothalamus. That author speculated:

> disruption of functional and structural hypothalamic connectivity and activity in patients with MTBI [mild TBI] and significant correlation with fatigue symptoms might help to resolve an array of clinical symptoms in MTBI related to sleep disturbance and fatigue due to orexin level changes.
>
> [91]

Orexin is a hypothalamic peptide believed to play an important role in wakefulness and arousal. Evidence also exists of hypothalamic atrophy after repetitive concussion [92]. Advances in imaging may soon facilitate the study of potential causal links between concussion, hypothalamic injury, and, conceivably, orexin-related persistent clinical symptoms. If confirmed, these discoveries may open the door to new options for managing several extremely common and disabling post-concussive symptoms.

Natural History

Prospective, longitudinal studies following TBI have revealed that anterior pituitary dysfunction is a dynamic process. A study of 50 patients following moderate to severe TBI demonstrated recovery of anterior pituitary function in some subjects when re-evaluated six months following injury [93]. Gonadotropin deficiency was the most likely axis to recover. A return to normal GH and cortisol reserve was seen in 66% and 50% of subjects respectively. Conversely, some patients who exhibited normal pituitary function during the acute phase developed late pituitary hormone deficiencies, particularly ACTH deficiency, which was apparent at six months. Notwithstanding methodological differences between different longitudinal studies, other investigators have found similar dynamic changes in pituitary function following moderate and severe TBI. This has obvious implications for the follow-up and screening of these patients. Given that typical concussions ("mild" TBIs) account for up to 90% of head traumas coming to medical attention and may comprise more than two million annual cases in the United States alone, it may be even more important to clarify the natural history of hypopituitarism after less severe injuries.

There is a dearth of prospective research on pituitary dysfunction in the context of repetitive mild head trauma. However, some conclusions can be inferred from anecdotal case reports and available cross-sectional studies. Research conducted on amateur boxers and kickboxers demonstrated a negative correlation between age, number of bouts contested, and stimulated serum level of GH, suggesting a cumulative effect of repetitive injury on the secretory ability of pituitary somatotrophs [82, 83, 84]. Also, a later retirement age was associated with a higher titer of anti-pituitary antibodies which may play a pathogenic role in post-traumatic hypopituitarism [94]. This limited evidence suggests that the more mild head injuries or concussions an individual accumulates, the greater the risk of hypopituitarism. If this can be confirmed, it will be of significant importance for at-risk sportsmen and women as well as active military personnel and veterans.

Future longitudinal studies should define more clearly the natural history of pituitary dysfunction following concussion. It remains to be seen whether the dynamic process observed following moderate to severe TBI also applies to milder, repetitive trauma. Correlation of pituitary dysfunction over time with persistent symptoms after CBI will provide insight into the interaction between post-traumatic hypopituitarism and long-term post-concussive outcomes.

Clinical Consequences

Although the available literature is inconsistent, some studies suggest that persistent post-concussive pituitary dysfunction occurs at a higher frequency than previously thought. Symptoms of chronic hypopituitarism can be subtle and highly variable due to different combinations and severity of hormone deficiencies (Table 26.1). Isolated GH deficiency is the most common hormonal abnormality identified following head injury, but a minority of subjects have multiple pituitary hormone deficiencies. Interestingly, there is significant overlap between the typical symptoms of chronic hypopituitarism and several common persistent post-concussive symptoms, including lethargy, emotional lability, low libido, poor memory, and diminished concentration. This raises the question: to what degree might post-traumatic hypopituitarism be contributing to the post-concussive symptomatology? Again, only large, long-term, prospective studies with universal testing can answer that question.

ACTH deficiency (and consequent glucocorticoid deficiency) is uncommon following repetitive mild head injury, with prevalence rates reported between 5% and 9%. However, untreated glucocorticoid deficiency can be life threatening, particularly during intercurrent illness or in patients undergoing surgery. To date, only a single case report has highlighted the benefits of glucocorticoid replacement in a patient who developed progressive ACTH and cortisol deficiency following repeated sports-related concussion [95].

GHD impairs linear growth in childhood and adolescence. Adult GHD is now an increasingly recognized syndrome associated with several adverse features. Body composition is altered due to increased fat mass and reduced muscle mass. Exercise capacity is reduced and quality of life is impaired.

The plasma lipid profile is unfavorable and cardiovascular morbidity may be increased. In addition, neuropsychiatric manifestations are common among adults with GHD. Poor concentration, fatigue, and irritability are commonly reported and may improve with GH replacement [96]. Current research highlights the impact of GHD following repetitive concussion. Affected individuals have an altered body composition, an adverse lipid profile, and impaired cognitive performance when compared with GH-sufficient individuals [82, 83, 97]. An improvement in these clinical parameters might be expected following replacement of GH. However, robust clinical evidence to support this theory is currently lacking.

Damage to the gonadotroph axis leading to testosterone deficiency in men can result in poor libido, muscle weakness, and impaired exercise performance. Once again, there is considerable cross-over with persistent post-concussive symptoms. Gonadotropin deficiency in women is manifest by oligo-or amenorrhea. In both men and women, long-term sex steroid deficiency can lead to reduced bone density. Thyroid-stimulating hormone and resultant thyroxine deficiency, although rare following TBI, can manifest with fatigue, myalgia, and low mood.

Integrated pituitary hormone replacement is recommended for all patients with hypopituitarism, taking into account the patient's age and co-morbidities. It is generally accepted that in more conventional causes of hypopituitarism (e.g., pituitary tumors, radiotherapy) health-related quality of life may improve substantially with appropriate hormone replacement [98, 99]. However, large-scale prospective clinical trials of hormone replacement in patients with hypopituitarism following chronic, CBI are lacking at present.

Screening Protocols

The common occurrence of CBIs, particularly among athletes, makes it impractical to evaluate all such individuals for post-traumatic hypopituitarism. A rational approach to screening is necessary in order to identify those most likely to suffer hypopituitarism and consequently those who may accrue benefit from treatment.

The symptoms of hypopituitarism, in particular adult GHD, are subtle and commonplace. It would seem sensible, however, to restrict formal pituitary testing to patients with persistent or late-onset post-concussive symptoms whose symptoms do not respond to conventional treatment, those with atypical clinical features, and patients with specific symptoms suggestive of hypothalamic pituitary disease, such as amenorrhea or low libido/erectile dysfunction. Also, children with poor growth, who have suffered concussion, should be screened.

Overall, the available evidence suggests that the number of concussive episodes suffered by an individual often correlates positively with the risk of hypopituitarism. Therefore, patients exposed to numerous mild head injuries constitute a high-risk group. They include children and young adults participating in contact sports and those engaged in active military service. Retired professional athletes who suffered repeated concussion during their career could also be targeted for screening. A careful history should be taken from all patients selected

Proposed algorithm for screening candidates at high risk for hypopituitarism following repetitive, mild head injury

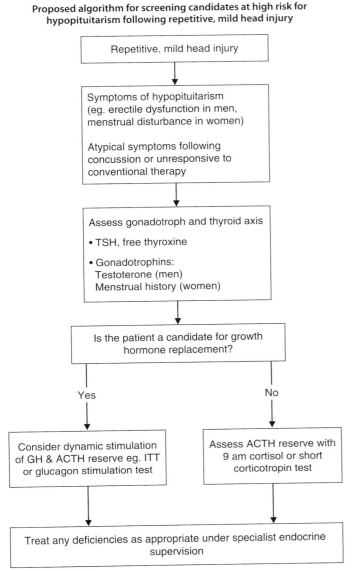

Fig. 26.5 Suggestions for monitoring and evaluation of pituitary function in patients with repetitive, concussive brain injury ACTH: adrenocorticotrophic hormone; CTE: chronic traumatic encephalopathy; GH: growth hormone; ITT: insulin tolerance test; TSH: thyroid-stimulating hormone.

Source: author's own

for screening, particularly in relation to current or prior exposure to performance-enhancing steroids, the effects of which may mimic the biochemical finding of post-traumatic hypopituitarism.

Figure 26.5 outlines a suggested algorithm for the assessment of patients with persistent or late-onset post-concussive symptoms, including those with progressive dementia. All patients selected for screening should undergo assessment of the adrenal, thyroid, and gonadal axes. Basal thyroid function tests, with measurement of thyroid-stimulating hormone and thyroid hormone (free thyroxine (T_4)) will out rule secondary hypothyroidism, which is manifest by a low serum free T_4 in the presence of an inappropriately normal or low thyroid-stimulating

hormone. Gonadotropins (follicle-stimulating and luteinizing hormone) and sex steroid concentrations (menstrual history in pre-menopausal women) should be checked in all patients undergoing screening. The presence of oligo- or amenorrhea in women without an elevation in gonadotropin levels is in keeping with hypothalamic-pituitary disease. Similarly, in men with low libido and/or erectile dysfunction, the presence of a low serum testosterone in the absence of elevated gonadotropins is suggestive of hypothalamic/pituitary damage.

Assessment of GH and ACTH reserve generally requires a dynamic stimulation test. Hypoglycemia is a potent stimulus of both GH and ACTH. The insulin tolerance test measures GH and ACTH reserve by inducing hypoglycemia with a bolus of intravenous insulin (0.15 units/kg). GH and cortisol levels are measured every 15–30 minutes for two hours. It can be safely conducted in an experienced center, but is contraindicated in patients with a history of seizures or heart disease. Also, it is unpleasant for the patient, and requires hospital admission and close medical supervision. The glucagon stimulation test is a suitable alternative when the insulin tolerance test is contraindicated.

GH replacement requires a daily subcutaneous injection and is generally not prescribed to those over the age of 70. In addition, its prescription is restricted to those with severely impaired quality of life in some jurisdictions. GH reserve should, therefore, only be tested in those who are being considered for a trial of replacement. If assessment of GH status is not required then the short corticotropin (ACTH) test provides a practical alternative for the assessment of adrenal reserve, due to its simplicity and usefulness in excluding clinically significant adrenal insufficiency [100]. This test relies on the assumption that long-standing ACTH deficiency results in adrenal gland atrophy. A large dose of synthetic ACTH (250 µg cosyntropin) is injected intramuscularly and the adrenal cortisol response is measured after 30 minutes. A subnormal cortisol response, in the context of potential pituitary injury and symptoms of hypopituitarism, is taken as surrogate evidence of ACTH deficiency. Alternatively, an early-morning (9 a.m.) serum cortisol of greater than 18 µg/dL (500 nmol/L) provides reassuring evidence of normal ACTH reserve.

Following normal pituitary function tests in patients with persistent or late-onset post-concussive symptoms, repeat testing is not usually required unless new symptoms emerge or they have been exposed to further episodes of CBI.

Hormone Replacement

Pituitary hormone replacement is complex and requires specialist supervision by an endocrinologist. Close patient monitoring and careful attention to the potential interaction between different hormones are required.

ACTH and resultant cortisol deficiency following brain injury is potentially life threatening and steroid replacement should be instituted prior to any other hormone replacement. Oral glucocorticoids such as hydrocortisone, at 10–20 mg/day in divided doses, provide adequate replacement. Cortisone acetate, dexamethasone, and prednisolone, at equivalent doses, are suitable alternatives. Dosing in children is based on body surface area and should be monitored by a pediatric endocrinologist. Patients should be carefully counseled about the need to double or treble the dose of glucocorticoids in the event of intercurrent illness to avoid a life-threatening adrenal crisis. In addition, they should be given advice to seek medical attention for parenteral glucocorticoids if they suffer from a vomiting illness, when absorption of oral medication is unreliable.

Thyroid-stimulating hormone deficiency can be easily treated with once-daily oral thyroxine replacement. This should only be commenced once glucocorticoid replacement has been established in those with concomitant ACTH/cortisol deficiency. Once the patient has been established on a stable dose of thyroxine, an annual measurement of serum free T_4 will typically suffice to monitor replacement. In contrast to primary hypothyroidism, thyroid-stimulating hormone cannot be used as a guide to judge thyroxine replacement in central hypothyroidism. The aim of treatment should be to maintain serum free T_4 levels in the mid-normal range.

Estrogen replacement is advised for pre-menopausal women with hypogonadotropic hypogonadism following head trauma. Both oral and transdermal preparations are available. The aim of treatment is to alleviate symptoms of estrogen deficiency, including hot flashes, mood disturbance, and vaginal dryness. Estrogen supplementation will also prevent premature osteoporosis and may reduce cardiovascular risk in young hypogonadal women. Patients with an intact uterus should also receive cyclical progesterone to induce a regular withdrawal bleed and prevent endometrial hyperplasia.

Testosterone replacement can improve many of the symptoms of sex steroid deficiency in men. Transdermal preparations must be applied daily. Care must be taken to wash hands carefully after application in order to avoid transfer to close contacts. Many patients find intramuscular preparations, which are available as monthly or three-monthly injections, more convenient. Serum testosterone levels should be maintained in the mid-normal range. Excess replacement can lead to hemoconcentration and elevation of the hematocrit. Also, testosterone replacement should be avoided in men with concomitant prostate cancer, which is increasingly common in aging men. For these reasons, monitoring of treatment should include a complete blood count and prostate-specific antigen level in conjunction with the serum testosterone.

GH is a potent mitogenic hormone which should be replaced in deficient children and adolescents until final height is achieved. Current preparations must be administered daily by sub-cutaneous injection. The dose is titrated to achieve satisfactory linear growth. Serum IGF-1, a liver-derived protein which mediates most of the actions of GH, can also be monitored to ensure adequate dosing. GH is licensed for the syndrome of adult GHD which has considerable cross-over with persistent or late-onset post-concussive symptoms. Serum IGF-1 levels are used to titrate the dose in adulthood.

Many clinicians also use the response to the disease-generated Quality of Life Assessment of Growth Hormone Deficiency in Adulthood (QoL-AGHDA) questionnaire to assess response to treatment [101]. This 25-point questionnaire was designed to assess health-related quality in GH-deficient subjects. Higher scores are indicative of a poorer quality of life. Replacement is generally not continued beyond the age of 70 years to take account of the natural age-related decline in GH levels.

Conclusion

Anterior hypopituitarism is a relatively common consequence of closed head injury. It was formerly considered to be a common complication of moderate to severe TBI. It has become apparent more recently that this problem is common among survivors of repetitive CBIs, and that even a single typical concussion may trigger persistent and clinically significant hypopituitarism. There is considerable overlap between symptoms of chronic pituitary hormone deficiency and persistent post-concussive symptoms – although further research is required to determine the degree to which the neurobehavioral problems that occur in roughly 36% of concussion victims are actually signs of a treatable hormone deficiency. Future prospective, longitudinal studies may clarify the risk factors for development of hypopituitarism following single and repetitive concussions and the natural history of this disorder. Based on currently available evidence, high-risk individuals should be offered screening under specialist supervision. The potential role of appropriate hormone replacement in attenuating the features of chronic traumatic encephalopathy is an exciting area of future research.

References

1. Cyran E. Hypophysenschädigung durch Schädelbasisfraktur. *Dtsch Med Wschr* 1918; 44: 1261.
2. Escamilla RF, Lisser H. Simmonds' disease. A clinical study with review of the literature; differentiation from anorexia nervosa by statistical analysis of 595 cases, 101 of which were proved pathologically. *J Clin Endocrinol Metab* 1942; 2: 65–96.
3. Daniel PM, Prichard MM, Treip CS. Traumatic infarction of the anterior lobe of the pituitary gland. *Lancet* 1959; 2: 927–931.
4. Harper CG, Doyle D, Adams JH, Graham DI. Analysis of abnormalities in pituitary gland in non-missile head injury: Study of 100 consecutive cases. *J Clin Pathol* 1986; 39: 769–773.
5. Schneider HJ, Kreitschmann-Andermahr I, Ghigo E, Stalla GK, Agha A. Hypothalamopituitary dysfunction following traumatic brain injury and aneurysmal subarachnoid hemorrhage: A systematic review. *JAMA* 2007; 298: 1429–1438.
6. Tanriverdi F, Unluhizarci K, Kelestimur F. Pituitary function in subjects with mild traumatic brain injury: A review of literature and proposal of a screening strategy. *Pituitary* 2010; 13: 146–153.
7. Tanriverdi F, De Bellis A, Bizzarro A, Sinisi AA, Bellastella G, Pane E, Bellastella A, et al. Antipituitary antibodies after traumatic brain injury: Is head trauma-induced pituitary dysfunction associated with autoimmunity? *Eur J Endocrinol* 2008; 159: 7–13.
8. Salehi F, Kovacs K, Scheithauer BW, Pfeifer EA, Cusimano M. Histologic study of the human pituitary gland in acute traumatic brain injury. *Brain Inj* 2007; 21: 651–656.
9. Crompton MR. Hypothalamic lesions following closed head injury. *Brain* 1971; 94: 165–172.
10. Tanriverdi F, Unluhizarci K, Kocyigit I, Tuna IS, Karaca Z, Durak AC, et al. Brief communication: Pituitary volume and function

in competing and retired male boxers. *Ann Intern Med* 2008; 148: 827–831.

11. Aimaretti G, Ambrosio MR, Benvenga S, Borretta G, De Marinis L, De Menis E, Di Somma C., et al. Hypopituitarism and growth hormone deficiency (GHD) after traumatic brain injury (TBI). *Growth Horm IGF Res* 2004; 14: S114–S117.

12. Masel BE. Rehabilitation and hypopituitarism after traumatic brain injury. *Growth Horm IGF Res* 2004; 14: S108–S113.

13. Aimaretti G, Ghigo E. Traumatic brain injury and hypopituitarism. *Sci World J* 2005; 5: 777–781.

14. Bondanelli M, Ambrosio MR, Zatelli MC, De Marinis L, degli Uberti EC. Hypopituitarism after traumatic brain injury. *Eur J Endocrinol* 2005; 152: 679–691.

15. Dogru O, Koken R, Bukulmez A, Melek H, Ovali F, Albayrak R. Delay in diagnosis of hypopituitarism after traumatic head injury: A case report and review of the literature *Neuroendocrinol Lett* 2005; 26: 311–313.

16. Popovic V. GH deficiency as the most common pituitary defect after TBI: Clinical implications. *Pituitary* 2005; 8: 239–243.

17. Popovic V, Aimaretti G, Casanueva FF, Ghigo E. Hypopituitarism following traumatic brain injury. *Growth Horm IGF Res* 2005; 15: 177–184.

18. Samadani U, Reyes-Moreno I, Buchfelder M. Endocrine dysfunction following traumatic brain injury: Mechanisms, pathophysiology and clinical correlations. *Acta Neurochir* 2005 [Suppl] 93: 121–125.

19. Powner DJ, Boccalandro C, Alp MS, Vollmer DG. Endocrine failure after traumatic brain injury in adults. *Neurocrit Care* 2006; 5: 61–70.

20. Urban RJ. Hypopituitarism after acute brain injury. *Growth Horm IGF Res* 2006; 16: S25–S29.

21. Behan LA, Agha A. Endocrine consequences of adult traumatic brain injury. *Horm Res Paediatr* 2007; 68: 18–21.

22. Einaudi S, Bondone C. The effects of head trauma on hypothalamic–pituitary function in children and adolescents. *Curr Opin Pediatr* 2007; 19: 465–470.

23. Medic-Stojanoska M, Pekic S, Curic N, Djilas-Ivanovic D, Popovic V. Evolving hypopituitarism as a consequence of traumatic brain injury (TBI) in childhood – Call for attention. *Endocr* 2007; 31: 268–271.

24. Rothman MS, Arciniegas DB, Filley CM, Wierman ME. The neuroendocrine effects of traumatic brain injury. *J Neuropsychiatry Clin Neurosci* 2007; 19: 363–372.

25. Acerini CL, Tasker RC. Neuroendocrine consequences of traumatic brain injury. *J Pediatr Endocrinol Metab* 2008; 21: 611–619.

26. Behan LA, Phillips J, Thompson CJ, Agha A. Neuroendocrine disorders after traumatic brain injury. *J Neurol Neurosurg Psychiatry* 2008; 79: 753–759.

27. Klose M, Feldt-Rasmussen U. Does the type and severity of brain injury predict hypothalamo–pituitary dysfunction? Does posttraumatic hypopituitarism predict worse outcome? *Pituitary* 2008; 11: 255–261.

28. Powner DJ, Boccalandro C. Adrenal insufficiency following traumatic brain injury in adults. *Curr Opin Crit Care* 2008; 14: 163–166.

29. Kelestimur F. Growth hormone deficiency after traumatic brain injury in adults: When to test and how to treat? *Pediatr Endocrinol Rev* 2009; 6: 534–539.

30. Blair JC. Prevalence, natural history and consequences of post-traumatic hypopituitarism: A case for endocrine surveillance. *Br J Neurosurg* 2010; 24: 10–17.

31. Guerrero AF, Alfonso A. Traumatic brain injury-related hypopituitarism: A review and recommendations for screening combat veterans. *Milit Med* 2010; 175: 574–580.

32. Guttikonda S, Ahmadi S, Urban RJ. Pituitary dysfunction after traumatic brain injury: Screening and hormone replacement. *Exp Rev Endocrinol Metab* 2011; 6: 697–703.

33. Sundaram NK, Geer EB, Greenwald BD. The impact of traumatic brain injury on pituitary function. *Endocrinol Metab Clin N Am* 2013; 42: 565–583.

34. Richmond E, Rogol AD. Traumatic brain injury: Endocrine consequences in children and adults. *Endocrine* 2014; 45: 3–8.

35. Fernandez-Rodriguez E, Bernabeu I, Castro AI, Casanueva FF. Hypopituitarism after traumatic brain injury. *Endocrinol Metab Clin N Am* 2015; 44: 151–159.

36. Masel BE, Urban RJ. Chronic endocrinopathies in traumatic brain injury disease. *Neurotrauma* 2015; 32: 1902–1910.

37. Paterniti I, Cordaro M, Navarra M, Esposito E, Cuzzocrea S. Emerging pharmacotherapy for treatment of traumatic brain injury: Targeting hypopituitarism and inflammation. *Exp Opin Emerg Drugs* 2015; 20: 583–596.

38. Reifschneider K, Auble B, Rose S. Update of endocrine dysfunction following pediatric traumatic brain injury. *J Clin Med* 2015; 4: 1536–1560.

39. Tanriverdi F, Schneider HJ, Aimaretti G, Masel BE, Casanueva FF, Kelestimur F. Pituitary dysfunction after traumatic brain injury: A clinical and pathophysiological approach. *Endocrinol Rev* 2015; 36: 305–342.

40. Renner C. Interrelation between neuroendocrine disturbances and medical complications encountered during rehabilitation after TBI. *J Clin Med* 2015; 22: 1815–1840.

41. Tanriverdi F, Kelestimur F. Pituitary dysfunction following traumatic brain injury: Clinical perspectives. *Neuropsychiatr Dis Treat* 2015; 11: 1835–1843.

42. Tritos NA, Yuen KC, Kelly DF, AACE Neuroendocrine and Pituitary Scientific Committee. American Association of Clinical Endocrinologists and American College of Endocrinology disease state clinical review: A neuroendocrine approach to patients with traumatic brain injury. *Endocrinol Pract* 2015; 21: 823–831.

43. Karaca Z, Tanriverdi F, Unluhizarci K, Kelestimur F. GH and pituitary hormone alterations after traumatic brain injury. *Prog Mol Biol Translat Sci* 2016; 138: 167–191.

44. Aimaretti G, Ambrosio MR, Di Somma C, Fusco A, Cannavò S, Gasperi M, Scaroni C, et al. Traumatic brain injury and subarachnoid haemorrhage are conditions at high risk for hypopituitarism: Screening study at 3 months after the brain injury. *Clin Endocrinol* 2004; 61: 320–326.

45. Aimaretti G, Ambrosio MR, Di Somma C, Gasperi M, Cannavo' S, Scaroni C, Fusco A, et al. Residual pituitary function after brain injury-induced hypopituitarism: A prospective 12-month study. *J Clin Endocrinol Metab* 2005; 90: 6085–6092.

46. Tanriverdi F, Senyurek H, Unluhizarci K, Selcuklu A, Casanueva FF, Kelestimur F. High risk of hypopituitarism after traumatic brain injury: A prospective investigation of anterior pituitary function in the acute phase and 12 months after trauma. *J Clin Endocrinol Metab* 2006; 91: 2105–2111.

47. Englander J, Bushnik T, Oggins J, Katznelson L. Fatigue after traumatic brain injury: Association with neuroendocrine, sleep, depression and other factors. *Brain Inj* 2010; 24: 1379–1388.

48. Kokshoorn NE, Smit JWA, Nieuwlaat WA, Tiemensma J, Bisschop PH, Veldman RG, Roelfsema F, et al. Low prevalence of hypopituitarism after traumatic brain injury: A multicenter study. *Eur J Endocrinol* 2011; 165: 225–231.

49. Moreau OK, Yollin E, Merlen E, Daveluy W, Marc Rousseaux M. Lasting pituitary hormone deficiency after traumatic brain injury. *J Neurotrauma* 2012; 29: 81–89.

50. Klose M, Stochholm K, Janukonyt J, Christensen LL, Frystyk J, Andersen M, Laurberg P. et al. Prevalence of posttraumatic growth hormone deficiency is highly dependent on the diagnostic

set-up: Results from the Danish National Study on Posttraumatic Hypopituitarism. *J Clin Endocrinol Metab* 2014; 99: 101–110.

51. Lieberman SA, Oberoi AL, Gilkison CR, Masel BE, Urban RJ. Prevalence of neuroendocrine dysfunction in patients recovering from traumatic brain injury. *J Clin Endocrinol Metab* 2001; 86: 2752–2756.

52. Giordano G, Aimaretti G, Ghigo E. Variations of pituitary function over time after brain injuries: The lesson from a prospective study. *Pituitary* 2005; 8: 227–231.

53. Kelly DF, McArthur DL, Levin H, Swimmer S, Dusick JR, Cohan P, Wang C, et al. Neurobehavioral and quality of life changes associated with growth hormone insufficiency after complicated mild, moderate, or severe traumatic brain injury. *J Neurotrauma* 2006; 23: 928–942.

54. Bushnik T, Englander J, Laurence Katznelson L. Fatigue after TBI: Association with neuroendocrine abnormalities. *Brain Inj* 2007; 21(6); 559–566,

55. Schneider HJ, Saånmann PG, Schneider M, Croce CG, Corneli G, Sievers C, Ghigo E, et al. Pituitary imaging abnormalities in patients with and without hypopituitarism after traumatic brain injury. *J Endocrinol Invest* 2007; 30: RC9-RC12.

56. Bavisetty S, Bavisetty S, McArthur DL, Dusick JR, Wang C, Pejman C, Boscardin WJ, et al. Chronic hypopituitarism after traumatic brain injury: Risk assessment and relationship to outcome. *Neurosurg* 2008; 62: 1080–1094.

57. Kreitschmann-Andermahr I, Hartmann Y, Poll E, Schneider HJ, Buchfelder M, Stalla GK. The German database on hypopituitarism after traumatic brain injury and aneurysmal subarachnoid hemorrhage – Description, objectives and design. *Exp Clin Endocrinol Diab* 2011; 119: 15–20.

58. Rosario ER, Aqeel R, Brown MA, Sanchez G, Moore C, Patterson D. Hypothalamic–pituitary dysfunction following traumatic brain injury affects functional improvement during acute inpatient rehabilitation. *J Head Trauma Rehabil* 2008; 28: 390–396.

59. Alavi SA, Tan CL, Menon DK, Simpson HL, Hutchinson PJ. Incidence of pituitary dysfunction following traumatic brain injury: A prospective study from a regional neurosurgical centre. *Br J Neurosurg* 2016; 30: 302–306.

60. Kopczak A, Krewer C, Schneider M, Kreitschmann-Andermahr I, Schneider HJ, Stalla GK. The development of neuroendocrine disturbances over time: Longitudinal findings in patients after traumatic brain injury and subarachnoid haemorrhage. *Int J Mol Sci* 2016; 17: 1–12.

61. Kelly DF, Chaloner C, Evans D, Mathews A, Cohan P, Wang C, Swerdloff R, et al. Metabolic syndrome, and impaired quality of life in retired professional football players: A prospective study. *J Neurotrauma* 2014; 31: 1161–1171.

62. Nourollahi S, Wille J, Weiß V, Wedekind C, Lippert-Grüner M. Quality-of-life in patients with post-traumatic hypopituitarism. *Brain Inj* 2014; 28: 1425–1429.

63. Aimaretti G, Corneli G, Di Somma C, Baldelli R, Gasco V, Rovere S, Migliaretti G, et al. Different degrees of GH deficiency evidenced by GHRH+arginine test and IGF-I levels in adults with pituitary disease. *J Endocrinol Invest* 2005; 28: 247–252.

64. Bondanelli M, De Marinis L, Ambrosio MR, Monesi M, Valle D, Zatelli MC, et al. Occurrence of pituitary dysfunction following traumatic brain injury. *J Neurotrauma* 2004; 21: 685–696.

65. Kelly DF, Gonzalo IT, Cohan P, Berman N, Swerdloff R, Wang C. Hypopituitarism following traumatic brain injury and aneurysmal subarachnoid hemorrhage: A preliminary report. *J Neurosurg* 2000; 93: 743–752.

66. Klose M, Juul A, Poulsgaard L, Kosteljanetz M, Brennum J, Feldt-Rasmussen U. Prevalence and predictive factors of post-traumatic hypopituitarism. *Clin Endocrinol* 2007; 67: 193–201.

67. Klose M, Juul A, Struck J, Morgenthaler NG, Kosteljanetz M, Feldt-Rasmussen U. Acute and long-term pituitary insufficiency in traumatic brain injury: A prospective single-centre study. *Clin Endocrinol* 2007; 67: 598–606.

68. Krewer C, Schneider M, Schneider HJ, Kreitschmann-Andermahr I, Buchfelder M, Faust M, Berg C, et al. Neuroendocrine disturbances one to five or more years after traumatic brain injury and aneurysmal subarachnoid hemorrhage: Data from the German database on hypopituitarism. *J Neurotrauma* 2016; 33: 1544–1553.

69. Silva PPB, Bhatnagar S, Herman SD, Zafonte R, Klibanski A, Miller KK, Tritos NA. Predictors of hypopituitarism in patients with traumatic brain injury. *J Neurotrauma* 2015; 32: 1789–1795.

70. Tanriverdi F, Ulutabanca A, Kursad Unluhizarci K, Selcuklu A, Casanueva FF, Kelestimur F. Three years prospective investigation of anterior pituitary function after traumatic brain injury: A pilot study. *Clin Endocrinol* 2008; 68: 573–579.

71. Tanriverdi F, De Bellis A, Ulutabanca H, Bizzarro A, Sinisi AA, Bellastella G, Paglionico VA, et al. A five year prospective investigation of anterior pituitary function after traumatic brain injury: Is hypopituitarism long-term after head trauma associated with autoimmunity? *J Neurotrauma* 2013; 30: 1426–1433.

72. Wachter D, Gündling K, Oertel MF, Stracke H, Karsten Böker D-K. Pituitary insufficiency after traumatic brain injury. *J Clin Neurosci* 2009; 16: 202–208.

73. Wilkinson CW, Pagulayan KF, Petrie EC, Mayer CL, Colasurdo EA, Shofer JB, Hart KL, et al. High prevalence of chronic pituitary and target-organ hormone abnormalities after blast-related mild traumatic brain injury. *Front Neurol* 2012; 3: 1–12.

74. Dimopoulou I, Tsagarakis S, Theodorakopoulou M, Douka E, Zervou M, Kouyialis AT, Thalassinos N, et al. Endocrine abnormalities in critical care patients with moderate-to-severe head trauma: Incidence, pattern and predisposing factors. *Intens Care Med* 2004; 30: 1051–1057.

75. Renner C, Hummelsheim H, Kopczak A, Steube D, Schneider HJ, Schneider M, Kreitschmann-Andermahr I, et al. The influence of gender on the injury severity, course and outcome of traumatic brain injury. *Brain Inj* 2012; 26: 1360–1371.

76. Lauzier F, Turgeon AF, Boutin A, Shemilt M, Cote I, Lachance O, Archambault PM, et al. Clinical outcomes, predictors, and prevalence of anterior pituitary disorders following traumatic brain injury: A systematic review. *Crit Care Med* 2014; 42: 712–721.

77. GH Research Society. Consensus guidelines for the diagnosis and treatment of growth hormone (GH) deficiency in childhood and adolescence: Summary statement of the GH Research Society. *J Clin Endocrinol Metab* 2000; 85: 3990–3993.

78. Hoeck HC, Vestergaard P, Jakobsen PE, Laurberg P. Test of growth hormone secretion in adults: Poor reproducibility of the insulin tolerance test. *Eur J Endocrinol* 1995; 133: 305–312.

79. Riedy G, Senseney JS, Liu W, Ollinger J, Sham E, Krapiva P, Patel JB, et al. Findings from structural MR imaging in military traumatic brain injury. *Radiology* 2016; 279: 207–215.

80. Baxter D, Sharp DJ, Feeney C, Papadopoulou D, Ham TE, Jilka S, Hellyer PJ, et al. Pituitary dysfunction after blast traumatic brain injury: The UK BIOSAP study. *Ann Neurol* 2013; 74(4): 527–536.

81. Tanriverdi F, Taheri S, Ulutabanca H, Caglayan AO, Ozkul Y, Dundar M, Selcuklu A, et al. Apolipoprotein E3/E3 genotype decreases the risk of pituitary dysfunction after traumatic brain injury due to various causes: Preliminary data. *J Neurotrauma* 2008; 25: 1071–1077.

82. Tanriverdi F, Unluhizarci K, Kocyigit I, Tuna IS, Karaca Z, Durak AC, et al. Brief communication: Pituitary volume and function in competing and retired male boxers. *Ann Intern Med* 2008; 148: 827–831.

83. Tanriverdi F, Unluhizarci K, Coksevim B, Selcuklu A, Casanueva FF, Kelestimur F. Kickboxing sport as a new cause of traumatic brain injury-mediated hypopituitarism. *Clin Endocrinol* 2007; 66: 360–366.

84. Kelestimur F, Tanriverdi F, Atmaca H, Unluhizarci K, Selcuklu A, Casanueva FF. Boxing as a sport activity associated with isolated GH deficiency. *J Endocrinol Invest* 2004; 27: RC28–RC32.

85. Heather NL, Jefferies C, Hofman PL, Derraik JG, Brennan C, Kelly P, et al. Permanent hypopituitarism is rare after structural traumatic brain injury in early childhood. *J Clin Endocrinol Metab* 2012; 97: 599–604.

86. Pickles W. Disturbances of metabolism associated with head injuries. *NEJM* 1947; 236: 858–862.

87. Agha A, Thornton E, O'Kelly P, Tormey W, Phillips J, Thompson CJ. Posterior pituitary dysfunction after traumatic brain injury. *J Clin Endocrinol Metab* 2004; 89: 5987–5992.

88. Hannon MJ, Finucane FM, Sherlock M, Agha A, Thompson CJ. Disorders of water homeostasis in neurosurgical patients. *J Clin Endocrinol Metab* 2012; 97: 1423–1433.

89. Foley CM, Wang DH. Central diabetes insipidus following a sports-related concussion: A case report. *Sports Health* 2012; 4: 139–141.

90. Jang SH, Yi JH, Kim SH, Kwon HG. Relation between injury of the hypothalamus and subjective excessive daytime sleepiness in patients with mild traumatic brain injury. *J Neurol Neurosurg Psychiatry* 2016; 87: 1260–1261.

91. Zhou Y. Abnormal structural and functional hypothalamic connectivity in mild traumatic brain injury. *J Magn Reson Imaging* 2017; 45: 1105–1112.

92. McKee AC, Daneshvar DH. The neuropathology of traumatic brain injury. *Handb Clin Neurol* 2015; 127: 45–66.

93. Agha A, Phillips J, O'Kelly P, Tormey W, Thompson CJ. The natural history of post-traumatic hypopituitarism: Implications for assessment and treatment. *Am J Med* 2005; 118: 1416.

94. Tanriverdi F, De Bellis A, Bizzarro A, Sinisi AA, Bellastella G, Pane E, et al. Antipituitary antibodies after traumatic brain injury: Is head trauma-induced pituitary dysfunction associated with autoimmunity? *Eur J Endocrinol* 2008; 159: 7–13.

95. Ives JC, Alderman M, Stred SE. Hypopituitarism after multiple concussions: A retrospective case study in an adolescent male. *J Athl Train* 2007; 42: 431–439.

96. Thomas JD, Monson JP. Adult GH deficiency throughout lifetime. *Eur J Endocrinol* 2009; 161(Suppl 1): S97-S106.

97. Tanriverdi F, Suer C, Yapislar H, Kocyigit I, Selcuklu A, Unluhizarci K, et al. Growth hormone deficiency due to sports-related head trauma is associated with impaired cognitive performance in amateur boxers and kickboxers as revealed by P300 auditory event-related potentials. *Clin Endocrinol* 2013; 78: 730–737.

98. Abs R, Mattsson AF, Bengtsson BA, Feldt-Rasmussen U, Góth MI, Koltowska-Häggström M, et al. Isolated growth hormone (GH) deficiency in adult patients: Baseline clinical characteristics and responses to GH replacement in comparison with hypopituitary patients. A sub-analysis of the KIMS database. *Growth Horm IGF Res* 2005; 15: 349–359.

99. Alexander GM, Swerdloff RS, Wang C, Davidson T, McDonald V, Steiner B, et al. Androgen–behavior correlations in hypogonadal men and eugonadal men. II. Cognitive abilities. *Horm Behav* 1998; 33: 85–94.

100. Agha A, Tomlinson JW, Clark PM, Holder G, Stewart PM. The long-term predictive accuracy of the short synacthen (corticotropin) stimulation test for assessment of the hypothalamic–pituitary–adrenal axis. *J Clin Endocrinol Metab* 2006; 91: 43–47.

101. McKenna SP, Doward LC, Alonso J, Kohlmann T, Niero M, Prieto M, Wiren L. The QoL-AGHDA: An instrument for the assessment of quality of life in adults with growth hormone deficiency. *Qual Life Res* 1999; 8: 373–383.

Chapter

27

Evidence-Based Rehabilitation in Typical Concussive Brain Injury: Results of a Systematic Review

Jon Pertab

In concussion of the brain, as soon as the blow which strikes the skull has caused the symptoms of concussion, the physical disturbance of the brain, whatever it may be, has been produced ... Such a disturbed brain ... soon becomes fatigued from use; and if claims are made upon it too soon after the injury – that is, before the structural and physiological integrity is reacquired – the patient is very likely to suffer from serious disease of the brain. Cerebral exercise or mental occupation should always in such cases be short of fatigue.

John Hilton, 1867 [1]

Introduction

Clinicians tasked with intervening in cases of concussion to the brain have been considering appropriate interventions for hundreds, if not thousands, of years [2]. While subjective symptoms tend to abate without treatment in many concussed patients, some experience lingering symptoms and present for treatment at clinics and hospitals. Others may feel well yet harbor persistent deleterious brain change (for instance, maintaining performance only at the expense of increased cerebral energy consumption). Currently, many published consensus statements and practice recommendations exist but sparse evidence demonstrates the efficacy of the recommended interventions to mitigate lingering symptoms after concussion. A major reason for that problem is that neurology has yet to identify biologically homogeneous subtypes of CBI – a first step toward determining whether specific therapies address specific disorders. The good news is that the concept of subtypes is rapidly gaining acceptance and beginning to inform clinical trials. That is, it is increasingly clear that different problems dominate at different stages post concussion, and that different symptoms at each stage require different interventions. The present chapter qualitatively evaluates available data on post-acute concussion treatment, determines if the quality warrants research-based rehabilitation recommendations, identifies opportunities for future research, and discusses implications for clinicians.

"Mild Traumatic Brain Injury" as a Diagnostic Construct

Research focused on rehabilitation in "mild traumatic brain injury"(mTBI) faces a number of challenges. Among the most prominent is the fact that in "mTBI" *mild* has no neurological meaning. As a result, "mTBI" is a clinical construct for which a number of committees have generated competing operational definitions, criteria, and guidelines. Although a variety of biomarkers related to "mTBI" are being explored [3, 4], currently the diagnosis continues to rely on subjective symptoms, observed signs, and arbitrary cut-offs. Even those systems employed most frequently in research are structured so that a wide range of presentations meet criteria for diagnosis [5, 6]. For example, one of the most commonly used definitions used in "mTBI" research was developed by the American Congress of Rehabilitation Medicine in 1993 [5], and is summarized in Table 27.1.

Unfortunately, the American College of Rehabilitation Medicine definition, like others used in rehabilitation research, has no biological specificity. It does not refer to a particular neurological disorder, but instead to a broadly characterized subset of head injuries that vary in terms of mechanism of injury, symptoms, signs, and clinical course – guaranteeing that cohorts identified using these criteria will exhibit biological heterogeneity. For example, the athlete who feels dazed for a few moments after a collision and experiences no subsequent symptoms meets criteria for diagnosis of "mTBI." So does the concussion survivor who was rendered unconscious for 20 minutes in a motor vehicle accident, subsequently suffering with permanent symptoms and lifelong disability.

The subjectivity and heterogeneity associated with the use of *mild* muddy scientific enquiry into the condition from the outset. The unique features specific to any individual patient may require a very different treatment approach compared with any other person in the concussed population. Despite the limitations in the construct, due to both the high incidence of concussive brain injury (CBI) and the newly discovered

Table 27.1 American Congress of Rehabilitation Medicine definition of mild traumatic brain injury [5]

Definition

A patient with mild traumatic brain injury is a person who has had a traumatically induced physiological disruption of brain function, as manifested by at least one of the following:

1. any period of loss of consciousness
2. any loss of memory for events immediately before or after the accident
3. any alteration in mental state at the time of the accident (e.g., feeling dazed, disoriented, or confused); and
4. focal neurological deficit(s) that may or may not be transient;

but where the severity of the injury does not exceed the following:

- loss of consciousness of approximately 30 minutes or less
- after 30 minutes and initial Glasgow Coma Scale of 13–15
- posttraumatic amnesia not greater than 24 h

Comments

This definition includes:

1. the head being struck
2. the head striking an object
3. the brain undergoing an acceleration / deceleration movement (i.e., whiplash) without direct external trauma to the head

potential for lasting sequelae, there is widespread acceptance that "mTBI" is a worthy target for health research and intervention [7].

Post-Concussive Symptoms

Another research challenge relates to the nature of the symptoms associated with concussion. Symptoms that typically linger in the days, weeks, and months following mTBI are typically referred to as post-concussive symptoms (PCS) and include sleep disruption, cognitive complaints, emotional disturbance, and physical symptoms such as fatigue and headache [8–11]. As pointed out in the introductory chapter by Victoroff, it is important to note that the symptoms popularly associated with so-called "mTBI" are not unique to concussion and occur both in general population samples and in multiple clinical groups, including general trauma controls, patients with a variety of psychiatric diagnoses, and chronic pain patients [12–24]. These observations have stirred debate regarding the etiology of PCS [25–30]. As discussed earlier in this volume and illustrated with a modified Haddon matrix, multi-symptomatic human neurobehavioral problems of uncertain (or diverse) pathophysiology do not lend themselves to facile causal classification. They are virtually always the product of interactions between unique individual pre-exposure traits (i.e., genetic, epigenetic, and environmental factors and their interplay), injury traits, response-to-injury traits, and the recovery environment. For the purposes of this chapter the causality debate is not considered further. Rather,

the chapter evaluates potential interventions for symptoms that manifest after a typical CBI.[1]

Treatment-Seeking CBI Patients

Given the diversity of the CBI population, it is not surprising that there is a wide range in prevalence estimates for persistent PCS. While the prevalence of PCS in the entire CBI population (treatment-seeking and non-treatment-seeking) may be relatively low [25], there are much higher rates in the subsample of patients (approximately 35% of the CBI population at large [31]) who present for evaluation and treatment at an emergency department (ED). Multiple cohort studies from around the globe confirm that many ED CBI patients report symptoms and functional impairment months, and even years, post injury [32–36]. Although interpretation of findings should be made cautiously due to methodological limitations (varying criteria used for diagnosis, varying methods of symptom sampling, co-occurring injuries, pre-existing pathologies), the overall picture points to lingering complaints in both litigating and non-litigating samples. In the ED CBI population, it is not uncommon for prevalence estimates of PCS complaints lingering beyond three months to be in the range of 30–50%, and roughly 36.5% remain symptomatic for one year or longer. With an estimated prevalence of 600 concussions for every 100,000 adults per year [37], the number of affected individuals represents a significant global health problem. For the subset of CBI patients who present at an ED, a substantial proportion will have a protracted recovery pattern and seek treatment for lingering concerns.

The previous discussion illustrates that: (1) whether one employs the new paradigm encouraged in this volume that CBI is a biological problem (deleterious effects of brain rattling) or the 20th-century notion of mTBI (referring to one of many committee-generated symptom clusters), the construct under discussion comprises a wide range of brain pathology and patient characteristics – a fact that will delay progress until biomarkers permit rational classification; (2) symptoms that correlate with CBI have substantial overlap with other conditions and are also present in the general population; and (3) despite the limitations in our basic understanding of the CBI construct and the causation of lingering problems, a significant proportion of the CBI population present for treatment of lingering difficulties.

Chapter Focus

For decades, authors have advocated for systematic research to inform evidence-based CBI rehabilitation [38]. This chapter presents the results of a systematic review of CBI treatment research to date. The review is limited to a specific focus – interventions that might typically fall under the broad umbrella of the following rehabilitation professionals – psychology /

---

[1] "Typical CBI" refers to the overwhelming majority of CBIs presenting for medical attention. For practical purposes, one might characterize such traumas as brain injuries due to abrupt external force to the head without brain penetration, prolonged coma, or gross intracranial hemorrhage. Pending discovery of a biomarker that permits a more scientific classification of CBIs, further specification is left to future study.

neuropsychology, occupational therapy, speech therapy, and physical therapy / physiotherapy. Interventions that typically fall outside of the purview of these members of the rehabilitation team are not included in the review (medications, hyperbaric therapy, dietary supplementation, acupuncture, chiropractic interventions, naturopathic intervention).

Methods

The 2011 American Academy of Neurology (AAN) *Clinical Practice Guideline Process Manual* informed the methodology for the systematic review strategy. Results interpretation was supplemented by considerations in the *Cochrane Handbook for Systematic Reviews of Interventions* [39, 40].

The Clinical Question (Population, Intervention, Co-intervention, Outcome / PICO Format)

One might characterize the current state of the literature as transitional. That is, although it is universally known that "mild" does not refer to a specific brain condition or neurobiological phenomenon, the phrase "mild traumatic brain injury" has dominated empirical CBI literature for about two decades. Hence, a systematic review attempting to compile data pertinent to CBI is obliged to employ the older terminology in its searches. One must candidly acknowledge that the resulting conclusions are derived from studies of heterogeneous cohorts. For patients who have been diagnosed with "mTBI" and experience PCS symptoms (*population*), are rehabilitation therapies that are typically delivered by psychology/neuropsychology, physical therapy, speech therapy, or occupational therapy (*intervention*) more effective than non-specific support and attention – placebo therapeutic conditions (*co-intervention*) in reducing either PCS or associated functional impairments (*outcome*) (PICO)?

Search Strategy

The literature search was performed in six electronic databases: Embase, PubMED (MEDLINE), PsycINFO, CINAHL, and the Cochrane Register of Controlled Trials. A Boolean search strategy comprising (population of interest) AND (treatments of interest) was employed which utilized the following initial structure: (mild traumatic brain injury OR concussion OR mild head injury OR postconcussion syndrome) AND (treatment OR intervention OR therapy OR rehabilitation).

This initial structure was adapted for each electronic database. To capture the population of interest, medical subheadings (or their equivalent) were consulted and these were added to the search algorithm. Terms in the initial structure were also added as keywords in singular and duplicate (e.g., ("head injury" AND mild) OR ("head injuries" AND mild)). Medical subheadings were also consulted to ensure a wide net was cast for the treatments of interest, with the following terms incorporated into the search: physical therapy, physiotherapy,

cognitive rehabilitation, occupational therapy, speech therapy, recreation therapy, exercise therapy, sleep therapy, cognitive therapy, behavior therapy, psychotherapy. Where the broad terms treatment, therapy, intervention, or rehabilitation did not subsume the treatments of interest listed above they were entered into the model individually as keywords. This resulted in a final Boolean search that was unique to each database.

The search results were exported and combined in Endnote referencing software and duplicates were exported to a separate library. As a check of the validity of the search strategy, a previous systematic review was identified that had a similar breadth to the present chapter. Comper et al. conducted a systematic review of treatments for mTBI which was published in 2005 [41]. The search strategy employed in the present chapter captured 18 of the 21 articles included in Comper's final analysis. As initial literature searches typically only identify 30–80% of relevant trials [40], the search strategy was validated and not modified further.

Additional articles were identified from the personal collection of the author, the reference lists of articles that met criteria for inclusion in the study, and the reference lists of recent review articles, clinical guidelines, and systematic reviews.

The initial search was conducted in mid-December 2013 with automated alerts for any additions to the databases tracked through the end of December 2013. The number of references identified in each search engine was: Embase (3965), PubMED (2012), PsycINFO (1024), CINAHL (1244), and Cochrane (169). Removing duplicates resulted in 6171 total references published between 1967 and 2013. Titles and abstracts were reviewed and 6067 discarded as irrelevant – leaving 107 potentially relevant articles. These were combined with 22 articles identified from reference lists and the personal collection of the author, resulting in a final sample of 129 articles for full text review. Subsequent to that systematic search, in the interval prior to publication, further searches were conducted in PubMED and OVID – in addition to hand searches of newly identified bibliographies – with the goal of capturing and incorporating the most current developments into this chapter as of early 2017.

Inclusion / Exclusion Criteria

Articles for full text review were entered into a spreadsheet for analysis if they met the following criteria:

1. presents data targeted at evaluating a rehabilitation intervention for an mTBI population that can be broadly construed as applicable to the following disciplines: neuropsychology / psychology, speech therapy, physical therapy / physiotherapy, or occupational therapy

2. where non-mTBI participants are included in the study, results for an mTBI-like subgroup were reported separately. American Congress of Rehabilitation Medicine mTBI diagnostic criteria were used to determine categorization where the article included multiple groups (such as those based on amnesia duration) [5]

3. employed at a minimum some type of control condition (not necessarily randomized)

4. were written in English or a translation was available.

Studies were not excluded based on the target (symptoms) of the intervention. Nor were treatments of co-morbid conditions (such as post-traumatic stress disorder (PTSD)) excluded due to the prominent overlap of the symptoms of co-morbid conditions with PCS. Studies were not excluded based on age, demographics of participants, or mechanism of injury (sports, blast, blunt trauma, military, civilian). Studies were not excluded based on publication status (thus including dissertations and other non-peer-reviewed material) – where there was accessible information it was systematically evaluated.

Each study that met these criteria was entered into a spreadsheet which collated information regarding demographics of the population and sample, the type of intervention (cognitive rehabilitation, exercise), the method of group assignment, the specifics associated with the intervention and control conditions, outcome measures, and a section related to risk of bias based on criteria published by the AAN classification system for study quality [39].

Method for Evaluating Study Quality and Determining Practice Recommendations

Each study that met inclusion criteria was evaluated for quality and risk of bias using the classification criteria of the AAN – those criteria relevant to the sample of studies identified are listed in the headings of Table 27.2.

Once the quality of individual studies has been evaluated, the AAN presents specific guidelines for making practice recommendations based on the quality of evidence addressing a specific problem with a specific intervention [39]:

- multiple class I studies demonstrating positive effects lead to the treatment being described as: "highly likely to be effective"
- multiple class II studies or a single class I study: "likely effective"
- multiple class III studies or a single class II study: "possibly effective"
- multiple class IV studies or a single class III study: "insufficient evidence to support or refute the effectiveness."

The guidelines also provide direction on when to apply further statistical or meta-analysis techniques. In general this is when the methodological similarity in population, treatment, and outcome warrants the combining of study results and not otherwise. "Meta-analysis is a technique that reduces random error but not systematic error" [39].

Results from applying the AAN guidelines to the PICO question regarding mTBI interventions are presented below.

Results

Of the 128 articles that were reviewed in full text, 34 met inclusion criteria for the analysis. The methodological quality of these studies as a whole is summarized in Table 27.2. Studies are divided into six rationally based rehabilitation umbrellas which form the sections of this results section. Within each area the details of the studies were evaluated to determine if

any specific practice recommendations or meta-analytic combination of results was warranted.

Cognitive Rehabilitation

The initial search identified four studies that investigated treatments falling under the broad umbrella of cognitive rehabilitation. These comprised one class 2 study, one class 3 study and two class 4 studies.

The treatments investigated were diverse. Cicerone [42] compared four mTBI patients who completed weekly attention remediation tasks (11–27 weeks) to mTBI patients in a waitlist control in a total sample of eight patients. Actively treated subjects reportedly exhibited better working memory. Nelson et al. [43] compared the addition of "interactive metronome therapy" (a biofeedback conditioning technology in which subjects perform movements in time to a metronome, allegedly enhancing neuroplasticity under cognitive stress) to standard multidisciplinary rehabilitation in a total sample of 46 patients. The biofeedback group reportedly exhibited greater improvements on multiple neuropsychological measures.

Riegler et al. [44] compared a web and telephone coping strategy education intervention to a clinic delivered intervention that "loosely mirrored" the web/telephone group in a total sample of 12 mTBI patients. The study found equivalent benefits to memory and learning under both conditions – in essence reporting that two cognitive rehabilitation methods both helped without having compared either one with an alternative treatment.

Tiersky et al. [45] compared attention process training combined with cognitive behavioral therapy to a minimal-support (waitlist) control condition in a total sample of 29 mTBI patients. This study is notable for its combination of psychotherapy with cognitive rehabilitation. Actively treated subjects reportedly had both improved emotional status and better performance on an attention task.

The author's follow-on review identified several more recent reports from the civilian and military literature. For instance, Cantor et al. [76] studied 98 subjects with TBI and persistent executive dysfunction. Fifty percent of the cohort had "mild" injuries. An average of 10.7 years had elapsed since injury in the active treatment group. The treatments included training in problem solving, emotional regulation, and attention as well as the use of cognitive supports. Twelve weeks of training (nine hours per week) were associated with significant improvement in some executive function measures. Results were not stratified by severity, but secondary analysis suggested that severity did not alter the findings. There was no evidence of benefits on other measures of neuropsychological function and no significant improvements in emotional regulation, self-awareness, affective distress, self-efficacy, participation, or quality of life. It is nonetheless intriguing that concussion survivors more than a decade post injury apparently derived some benefit.

In the military domain, Twamley et al. [77] reported a 12-week pilot project with 34 veterans who had survived mostly "mild" TBIs. Half the group received supported employment; half also received psychoeducation and advice on managing sleep,

Table 27.2 Methodological quality of included studies – American Academy of Neurology (AAN) (2011) rating criteria [39]

Area / Author (year)	Class 1 requirements								Downgrades			AAN class
	Concurrent controls with randomized allocation	Representative population	Baseline features equivalent/statistical adjustment	Masked/objective outcome assessment[a]	(a) Concealed allocation	(b) Primary outcomes clearly defined and relevant	(c) Exclusion/inclusion criteria clearly defined	(d) <20% attrition or statistical adjustment	Meets class 2 criteria[b]	Unmasked/subjective outcome assessment (class 3)[c]	Study conditions lacking precision (class 4)[d]	
Cognitive rehabilitation												
Cicerone (2002) [42]	No	Yes	No	Yes	No	Yes	Yes	N/A	No	No	Yes	4
Nelson et al. (2013) [43]	Yes	Yes	Yes	Yes	Yes	Yes	Yes	No	Yes	No	No	2
Riegler et al. (2013) [44]	No	No	Yes	Yes	No	Yes	Yes	N/A	No	Yes	Yes	4
Tiersky et al. (2005) [45]	Yes	Yes	Yes	No	Yes	Yes	Yes	No	No	Yes	No	3
Psychotherapy												
Bryant et al. (2003) [46]	Yes	Yes	Yes	Yes	Yes	Yes	Yes	Yes	N/A	No	No	1
Leonard (2002) [47]e	Yes	Yes	Yes	Yes	Yes	Yes	Yes	Yes	No	Yes	No	3
Silverberg et al. (2013) [48]	Yes	Yes	Yes	No	Yes	Yes	Yes	Yes	No	Yes	No	3
Exercise-based interventions												
Baker et al. (2012) [49]	No	No	No	No	N/A	Yes	No	No	No	No	Yes	4
Leddy et al. (2013) [50]	Yes	No	No	Yes	No	Yes	Yes	Yes	No	Yes	No	3
Physical therapy interventions												
Jensen et al. (1990) [51]	Yes	Yes	Yes	No	Yes	Yes	Yes	Yes	No	Yes	No	3
Schneider et al. (2014) [52]f	Yes	Yes	Unclear	Yes	Unclear	Yes	Unclear	Yes	Unclear	No	Yes	4
Mixed multidisciplinary interventions												
Andersson et al. (2007, 2011) [53, 54]	Yes	Yes	Yes	No	Yes	Yes	Yes	Yes	No	Yes	Yes	4

Study										
Ghaffar et al. (2006) [55]	Yes	Yes	Unclear	Yes	Yes	Yes	No	No	Yes	4
Goranson et al. (2003) [56]	No	No	N/A	Yes	Yes	N/A	No	Yes	Yes	4
Matuseviciene et al. (2013) [57]	Yes	Unstated	Unstated	Yes	Yes	Yes	No	Yes	Yes	4
Wade et al. (1997) [58]	Yes	Yes	Yes	Yes	Yes	No	No	Yes	Yes	4
Wade et al. (1998) [59]	Yes	Yes	Yes	Yes	Yes	No	No	Yes	Yes	4
Early single-session interventions										
Lowdon et al. (1989) [60]	Yes	Yes	Unstated	Yes	Yes	No	No	Yes	No	4
Mittenberg et al. (1996) [61]	Yes	Yes	Unclear	Yes	Yes	No	No	Yes	Yes	4
Ponsford et al. (2001) [62]	Yes	Yes	No	Yes	Yes	Yes	Yes	No	No	2
Ponsford et al. (2002) [63]	Yes	Yes	No	Yes	Yes	No	Yes	No	No	2
Wrightson and Gronwall (1981) [64]	Yes	Unclear	Unclear	Yes	Unclear	Yes	No	Yes	Yes	4
Early brief interventions										
Alves et al. (1993) [65]	Unclear	No	Unstated	No	Yes	No	No	Yes	Yes	4
Bell et al. (2008) [66]	Yes	Yes	Yes	Yes	Yes	Yes	No	Yes	No	3
de Kruijk et al. (2002) [67]	Yes	Yes	Unstated	Yes	Yes	Yes	No	Yes	No	3
Gronwall (1986) [68]	No	No	N/A	Yes	Yes	Unstated	No	No	Yes	4
Hekstad et al. (2010) [69]	Yes	Unstated	No	Yes	No	No	No	Yes	Yes	4
Hinkle et al. (1986) [70]	Yes	Unstated	No	Yes	Yes	No	No	No	Yes	4
Minderhoud et al. (1980) [71]	No	No	Unstated	Yes	Yes	No	No	Yes	Yes	4

(continued)

Table 27.2 (*Cont.*)

Area Author (year)	Class 1 requirements								Downgrades			AAN class
	Concurrent controls with randomized allocation	Represent-ative population	Baseline features equivalent/ statistical adjustment	Masked / objective outcome assessment[a]	(a) Concealed allocation	(b) Primary outcomes clearly defined and relevant	(c) Exclusion/ inclusion criteria clearly defined	(d) < 20% attrition or statistical adjustment	Meets class 2 criteria[b]	Unmasked/ subjective outcome assessment (class 3)[c]	Study conditions lacking precision (class 4)[d]	
Paniak et al. (1988, 2000) [72, 73]	Yes	Yes	Yes	No	Unclear	Yes	Yes	Yes	No	Yes	Yes	4
Relander et al. (1972) [74]	Yes	Yes	Yes	Yes	Unstated	Yes	Yes	Yes	No	No	Yes	4
Suffoletto et al. (2013) [75]	Yes	Yes	Yes	No	Yes	Yes	Yes	Yes	No	Yes	No	3

[a] Required for class 1 or class 2, for purpose of this chapter cognitive or neuropsychological assessment measures considered objective, days to return to work considered objective, where objective *and* subjective measures (e.g., patient questionnaire) both used as primary measures, the study is rated as meeting objectivity criteria.

[b] Either cohort / matched design that meets a–d or randomized controlled trial lacking one or two of b–d, must have objective or masked outcome assessment, consideration prior to class 3 and 4 downgrades.

[c] Includes subjective self-report of participant (questionnaires, checklists, etc.).

[d] For the purpose of this chapter defined as inadequate information to allow a reasonable approximation for a replication study – includes intervention protocol, protocol for control group, and measures used. If intervention was manualized, described in detail, or similarly structured this condition was considered met.

[e] Dissertation.

[f] Poster abstract.

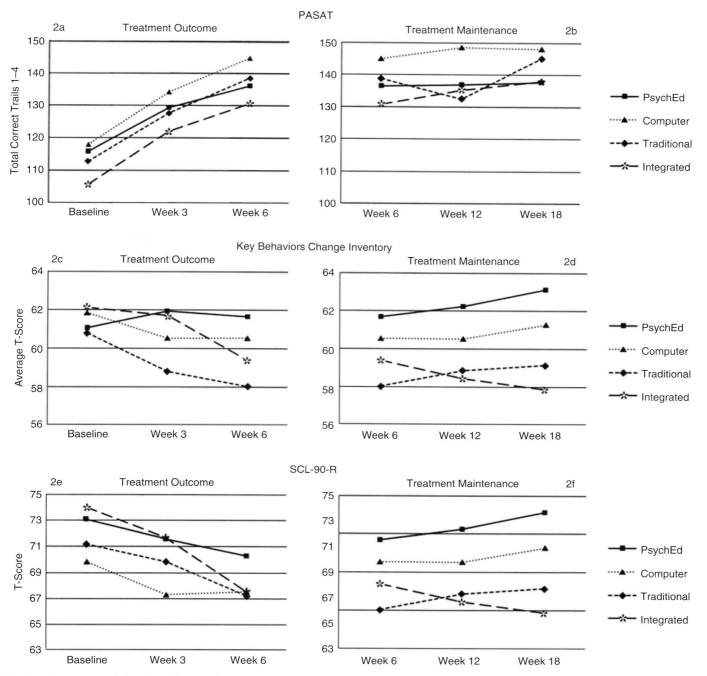

Fig. 27.1 Cognitive, psychological, and functional treatment outcomes and treatment maintenance, comparing four six-week treatments. PASAT: Paced Auditory Serial Addition Test [80]; SCL-90-R: Symptom Checklist-90-R [81].

Source: Cooper et al., 2017 [78] with permission from Lippincott Williams & Wilkins, Inc./Wolters Kluwer

headaches, and fatigue, plus compensatory cognitive strategies (a program the authors called CogSMART). The second group reported significantly reduced PCS but, again, did not differ in neuropsychological performance.

One recent study is noteworthy for focusing exclusively on mTBI survivors with persistent cognitive symptoms and earnestly attempting to control for non-specific treatment effects. Cooper et al. [78] randomized 126 service members to one of four treatments: psychoeducation alone, computer-based cognitive rehabilitation, therapist-directed cognitive rehabilitation,

or the latter combined with cognitive behavior therapy. The outcome measures included: (1) a test of cognition (the challenging Paced Auditory Serial Addition Test); (2) a measure of subjective symptoms (the Symptom Checklist–90 Revised); and (3) the Key Behaviors Change Inventory (a family/observer-rated scale of behaviors [79]. Interestingly, all four treatment groups showed significant improvement on all three measures, and both therapist-directed groups had better outcome than the psychoeducational group. Figure 27.1 illustrates those findings, as well as the observation that benefits persisted on 18-week follow-up.

How should one interpret such data? It is not possible to isolate the cognitive rehabilitation element from other potentially beneficial factors, which leaves open the question of cognitive rehabilitation's efficacy. The baselines were different. The computer treatment group reportedly had lower education. Yet it stands out that psychoeducation alone had the least lasting benefit, and that therapist contact seems to have been especially helpful.

A major barrier to interpreting these cognitive rehabilitation studies is the failure to control for the impact of recruitment, enrollment, solicitous attention, and the benefit of the control condition. As Cooper et al. put it, "A challenge in this area of research is the difficulty of isolating the effect of cognitive rehabilitation interventions, which are often provided in addition to standard care" ([82], p. 415). Thus, while multiple studies reported positive findings for the treatment condition [42, 44, 45, 76–78], none included a genuine placebo condition (such as sham treatment) to control for the increased non-specific support and attention the patients in the treatment conditions received. Moreover, simultaneous administration of more than one treatment element frustrates an attempt to isolate a possible benefit from cognitive rehabilitation. Investigators often compared multi-component treatments with one another (e.g., [78]) or compared multi-component treatments with "usual care." Janak et al. [83], for example, reported benefits from cognitive rehabilitation plus vestibular interventions plus headache management plus integrated behavioral health care in a cohort of 257 active duty military concussion survivors.

Given concerns about denying care that might ameliorate PCS, it may no longer be realistic to expect clinical trials to administer a single treatment element. Nor is there an easy way to control for the salubrious effects of therapist contact. Thus, although promising evidence suggesting efficacy has emerged, a survey of the field confirms that methodological limitations continue to hamper certainty regarding what form of cognitive rehabilitation, administered by whom, to which concussion survivors, at what stage of recovery might be effective.

In the light of that observation, the following conclusion is made based on AAN guidelines:

> For patients who have been diagnosed with "mTBI" and experience PCS, there is insufficient evidence to support or refute a contention that any cognitive rehabilitation intervention is more effective than non-specific support and attention in reducing either PCS or associated functional impairments.

That having been said, the author acknowledges that this may not be the most pressing question. Our goal is to determine what works. Although there may be no practical way to evaluate whether cognitive rehabilitation works as a stand-alone treatment, some evidence supports the conclusion that combined therapies that include cognitive rehabilitation may be superior to those that do not.

Psychotherapy

An example of consensus advice, in this case from the "Updated clinical practice guidelines for concussion/mild traumatic brain injury and persistent symptoms" published in 2015 by the mTBI Expert Consensus Group [84], reads: "Cognitive-Behavioural Therapy (CBT) has well-established efficacy for treatment of primary mood and anxiety disorders; as such, it may be appropriate in the treatment of mood and anxiety symptoms following mTBI" (p. 695). Clinicians cannot put faith in the reasoning that, since a treatment works for an idiopathic primary psychiatric symptom, it will surely work for that symptom regardless of etiology. One hopes for more authentic scientific support. The review identified three studies of interventions that fall under the broad umbrella of psychotherapy.[2] These comprised one class 1 study (that could be argued as a class 2), and two class 3 studies.

Two of these studies included a placebo control condition that accounted for the increased non-specific support and attention the patients in the treatment conditions received: Bryant et al. designed a study to determine if brief, manualized, cognitive behavioral therapy reduces symptoms associated with acute stress disorder in mTBI; and prevents progression of symptoms to PTSD [47]. A control condition with an equal number of supportive counseling sessions was employed. While the focus of the intervention may be seen as diverging from the purpose of the present evaluation (mTBI rehabilitation), it was included based on the observation that it has not yet been possible to disentangle symptoms of PTSD and PCS [85, 86]. Clinically significant benefits favoring the intervention group were noted on semi-structured symptom interviews (blinded). It is noted that the sample size in each group was small ($n = 12$ in each condition), which could arguably downgrade this research to class 2.

The dissertation of Leonard describes a three-condition intervention comparing four-session group cognitive behavior therapy, four-session group education and support, and waitlist control [47]. The target was PCS. There were no significant differences between the two group therapy conditions, but both conditions demonstrated fewer symptoms at three-month follow-up than the waitlist control condition. Thus, while well controlled, this study does not provide evidence of any specific psychotherapy techniques that have benefits over and above non-specific support and attention.

The third study in this area by Silverberg et al. compared usual treatment (education and reassurance from an occupational therapist) versus that treatment plus six sessions of cognitive behavioral therapy in a randomized, open trial. These mTBI subjects were pre-selected on the basis of a judgment that they were "at risk" for "post-concussive syndrome" [48]. The addition of CBT was associated with reduced rates of "post-concussive syndrome." Again, there was no control for the possible effects of the extra attention provided to the CBT subjects.

---

[2] As previously described, Tiersky et al. [45] combined psychotherapy (cognitive behavioral therapy) with cognitive remediation and should be considered part of this list.

Cerebral blood flow response to increasing exercise intensity and the engagement and role of the three mechanisms that control it

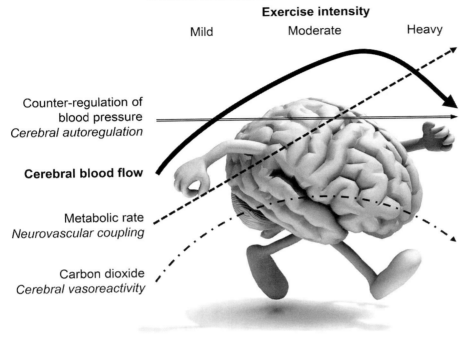

Fig. 27.2

Blood pressure increases proportionally to exercise intensity, engaging autoregulation that serves to maintain constant flow. However, at mild and moderate intensities, both metabolic rate and carbon dioxide increase, hence both neurovascular coupling and cerebrovascular reactivity result in increased cerebral blood flow. With heavy exercise intensities, there is a pronounced hypocapnia, and so the net result of the three controlling mechanisms is a decrease in cerebral blood flow.

Source: Tan et al. (2014) [88] (p. 1669) with permission from American Academy of Neurology; Wolters Kluwer

For the area of psychotherapy for PCS after CBI, the evidence supports the following conclusion:

For patients who have been diagnosed with "mTBI" and experience acute stress disorder symptoms, brief cognitive behavioral therapy (as per the Bryant manual) is likely effective in reducing acute stress disorder symptoms when compared to the effects of non-specific support and attention. There is insufficient evidence to support or refute a contention that any other psychotherapy intervention is more effective than non-specific support and attention.

Exercise-Based Interventions

As noted in the introduction to this chapter, it is clear that different problems dominate during different stages post CBI; hence, the focus of therapies needs to shift in an agile way as the concussion survivor's brain changes. Timing is especially important in considering exercise-based interventions. Many reviewers agree that, in the acute phase, concussion survivors are more likely to benefit from rest than from exercise, whereas in the post-acute phase patients might benefit from symptom-limited exercise (especially aerobic) and cognitive activity [82, 87–93]. This may be explained, at least in part, by a series of important rodent experiments published over a decade by Griesbach et al. [94], strongly suggesting that both the timing and circumstances of post-concussive exercise influence its neurobiological effects: immediate post-concussive exercise was found to both provoke autonomic dysfunction and to interfere with the usual up-regulation of neuroplasticity factors, including phosphorylated cyclic AMP response element-binding protein, phosphorylated synapsin I, and

mitogen-activated protein kinase. In contrast, voluntary exercise that was delayed for two weeks post injury was associated with increased production of brain-derived neurotrophic factor in the hippocampus [95, 96]. Such peptide production, in turn, was shown to correlate with cognitive improvement [97]. Of interest, *involuntary* delayed exercise was *not* found to elevate brain-derived neurotrophic factor levels in mildly concussed rats – a difference attributed by the authors to stress [98, 99]. Collectively, these findings suggest that a therapeutic window exists after concussion during which voluntary, submaximal aerobic exercise enhances recovery.

Although the ideal post-concussive exercise prescription remains to be discovered, evidence suggests that humans also benefit from light (typically symptom-limited) aerobic exercise. As illustrated in Figure 27.2, mild or moderate exercise is theoretically better than strenuous exercise because it optimizes cerebral blood flow. Moreover, since adults tend to have more room for improvement in maximal exercise capacity, they are theoretically more likely than adolescents to exhibit benefits from such training [88].

Theory and observational studies aside, little empirical evidence from controlled investigations is available to recommend the best kind and amount of exercise at the best time post injury. The initial review identified just two studies that tested the efficacy of exercise rehabilitation. These comprised one class 3 study, and one class 4 study.

The Baker et al. study was designed to determine if there is a differential response to exercise in mTBI participants who had exercise-related exacerbation of PCS, versus those who could exercise to their maximum heart rate without exacerbation of PCS [49]. There were no differences between these groups on PCS response to treatment and thus this study is not informative to the research question of this chapter (post hoc evaluation of completers vs. non-completers is also of limited utility).

The study by Leddy et al. was a pilot of exercise treatment for PCS with randomized allocation (unconcealed) to the exercise group or a stretching control condition [50]. The sample size was very small, with $n = 4$ in each group; differences in baseline characteristics are noted. The study found large effect sizes on both exercise capacity and PCS; functional magnetic resonance imaging (fMRI) differences between groups were also noted. This pilot had many positive design features and strong effects; however, the small sample size (pilot study), non-equivalent groups, and different duration of the intervention and control conditions limit the ability to draw conclusions related to the present research question.

The author's follow-on review identified little additional evidence. Kurowski et al. [100] randomized 30 adolescents with one to four months of persistent symptoms to either subsymptomatic aerobic exercise or full-body stretching. At six weeks the aerobic exercise group reported significantly fewer PCS. However, the study did not systematically assess lasting benefits. Perhaps importantly, the subjects had not been selected for exercise intolerance. As discussed later in this chapter, some evidence suggests that a biologically distinct subset of concussion survivors can be diagnosed based on response to exercise and these patients may be significantly more likely to benefit from an exercise prescription.

While the results of these studies are encouraging and present strong support for further research in this area, in terms of PICO question for this chapter, the following conclusion is drawn:

> For patients who have been diagnosed with "mTBI" and experience PCS, there is insufficient evidence to support or refute a contention that any exercise-based intervention is more effective than non-specific support and attention in reducing either PCS or associated functional impairments.

Physical Therapy Interventions

Two studies examined interventions that fall under the umbrella of physical therapy rehabilitation. These comprised one class 3 study, and one class 4 study.

Jensen et al. report a study exploring if two-session manual spine therapy is more effective in reducing post-traumatic headache vs. a cold-pack control group in a sample of 19 patients [51]. Large effects were found post treatment on subjective self-report measures but these were not maintained in follow-up.

A poster abstract regarding a physical therapy intervention to speed clearance to return to sport was identified that had limited information about the specifics of the study [52]. The abstract by Schneider et al. describes an eight-session multimodal physical therapy treatment contrasted with eight sessions with a physical therapist focused on gradual exertion – improvements were more prominent in the multimodal group (total sample 31 patients). Based on only the details of

the abstract, this study meets class 4 criteria but if a full publication becomes available the design features reported would lend themselves to a higher rating.

At this stage, the results of these two studies present compelling support for further research in this area, but in terms of the PICO question for this chapter, the following conclusion is drawn:

> For patients who have been diagnosed with"mTBI" and experience PCS, there is insufficient evidence to support or refute a contention that any physical therapy-based intervention is more effective than non-specific support and attention in reducing either PCS or associated functional impairments.

Mixed, Multidisciplinary Interventions

In addition to the previously mentioned studies that involved more than one treatment component, six studies examined interventions that fall under the broad umbrella of mixed multidisciplinary rehabilitation. Several included physician involvement but these were not excluded as they also included interventions relevant to the professions examined in the present chapter.

All of the studies in this section were classified as class 4 – in general because the interventions and / or control conditions were poorly defined, which results in an automatic downgrade to class 4 under the AAN grading system. For example, the most recently published study in this area [57] described the intervention as a follow-up visit with a physician 14–21 days post injury, which is described in some detail, but the description also included the statement, "Interventions for identified problems related to the MTBI or to comorbidities were provided as needed, such as prescription of drugs for pain, anxiety or depression or referral to other specialists or teams." How these treatment and referral decisions were made and what interventions were actually delivered in this condition was not further described. The control condition is also loosely described as: "TAU [treatment as usual] was provided according to local routines for all patients and could comprise contact with a general practitioner at the patient's discretion but no routine follow-up."

In general, most studies in this area reflected the same pattern – the group conditions were poorly defined and ability to gain even a rough idea of what actually occurred in the treatment and/or control groups was poor. Even when significant effects were found (one study [56]) the lack of specificity about the conditions was not conducive to determining the likely cause of these effects. On the one hand, it would be no surprise if it were eventually determined that an individualized combination of treatments selected with care and targeting a patient's particular symptoms yielded greater average benefits than did either a single treatment or the administration of a multi-component program without regard to symptom profile. On the other hand, the existing literature is essentially uninterpretable. Not only were the descriptions of multi-component programs too imprecise to meaningfully communicate the method, but also no studies assigned patients with particular symptoms to targeted interventions.

With regard to the research question of this chapter, the following conclusion is made:

For patients who have been diagnosed with "mTBI" and experience PCS, there is insufficient evidence to support or refute a contention that mixed multimodal rehabilitation intervention (however this might be loosely defined in the studies available thus far) is more effective than non-specific support and attention in reducing either PCS or associated functional impairments.

Early Single-Session Interventions and Early Brief Interventions

Fifteen studies fell under the umbrella of early single-session intervention or early brief interventions. Most targeted PCS, evaluating the effects of information, reassurance, bed rest, and psychotherapy techniques to reduce persistence of PCS.

The vast majority, ten of 15, had similar limitations to studies in the previous section – poorly defined intervention and / or control conditions (Table 27.2). These are non-instructive to the current chapter and are not considered further in the results section.

In the remainder of the single-session interventions, only two class 2 studies were identified. Ponsford et al. evaluated the effects of an information booklet on both neuropsychological test scores and self-reported symptoms [62, 63]. The study in the adult population did not control for the extra attention associated with an initial assessment, but in the child study the assessment conditions were equivalent. No differences in objective test scores were identified at three months post injury but modest benefits of the brief interventions were noted on subjective PCS in both studies. Although the studies are rated as class 2 and have some objective outcome assessment measures, the significant findings were found only on the subjective measures (class 3 evidence). This results in the following conclusion in the subsection of single-session interventions:

For patients who have been diagnosed with "mTBI" and experience PCS, there is insufficient evidence to support or refute a contention that early single-session interventions are more effective than non-specific support and attention in reducing either PCS or associated functional impairments.

In the non-class 4 studies evaluating early brief interventions (three studies out of ten total), one evaluated differential prescription of bed rest, one evaluated the benefits of text messaging advice, and one evaluated the impact of telephone call advice [66, 67, 75]. In general, these were well-designed randomized controlled trials but effects were modest and suffered from the lack of an outcome measure not based on self-report, resulting in automatic downgrade to class 3 per AAN criteria. With regard to the research question of this chapter, the following conclusion is made:

For patients who have been diagnosed with "mTBI" and experience PCS, there is insufficient evidence to support or refute a contention that early brief intervention (in any of its varieties) is more effective than non-specific support and attention in reducing either PCS or associated functional impairments.

Discussion

Evidence refers to information from studies of clinically important outcomes, in patients with specific conditions undergoing specific interventions. American Academy of Neurology (2011).

[39]

The purpose of the present chapter is to systematically identify and evaluate evidence that has the potential to inform rehabilitation in CBI under the scope of the following professions – psychology / neuropsychology, physical therapy / physiotherapy, speech therapy, or occupational therapy. The method was designed to identify all controlled studies of rehabilitation interventions applied in the "mTBI" population through the end of December 2013. The methodology of the 34 studies initially identified was evaluated using the process advocated by the AAN with a view to providing clinical practice guidelines if warranted by the evidence. A follow-on search of PubMed/OVID updated the search to the beginning of 2017.

Note that the AAN's definition of *evidence* refers to "specific conditions." At this transition stage of CBI studies, one must temper any conclusions with the admonition that "mTBI" is not a specific condition. It is one of dozens of consensus-derived operational definitions that facilitate the selection of subjects for study, even though the subjects' degree of biological similarity is unknown. One must exercise caution in assuming that findings from "mTBI" research are relevant to typical CBI.

Perhaps even more importantly, many empirical investigations treated subjects as if they were comparable, and cohorts as if they were homogeneous, and outcomes as if they could be measured by a single score. For progress to occur, it is critical to abandon the 20th-century paradigm of a "post-concussive syndrome." Evidence strongly suggests not only that: (1) the symptoms that are most likely to dominate the clinical presentation at the acute, post-acute, and chronic stages are different; and that (2) innumerable individual factors guarantee that no two concussion survivors will ever exhibit the same symptoms and course; and yet that (3) biologically differentiable subtypes of the post-concussive condition possibly follow somewhat distinct trajectories and, if so, probably respond to different treatments.

For instance, despite the likelihood that all CBIs share common neurobiological elements – i.e., brain rattling, axonal stretching, and threatened shortfall of cellular energy – it seems legitimate to consider the possibility that lower-speed sports-related concussion is systematically different from higher-speed motor vehicle-related concussion. It is also virtually certain that genetic variation in cerebral response to abrupt force influences the spectrum of changes in the post-concussive state.

On another front, several authorities have specifically urged that a distinction be made between concussion survivors with a physiological problem of persistent global metabolic dysfunction versus survivors in whom isolated neurobiological factors such as vestibulo-ocular or cervicogenic dysfunction are dominant. Ellis et al. [90] referred to the first problem as "physiological post-concussion disorder." Members of this subgroup are posited to suffer from altered cerebrovascular reactivity, CO_2 sensitivity, neurovascular regulation, and autonomic dysfunction that represents, in part, a longer-than usual neurometabolic cascade with insufficient provision of energy to fulfill neural demands. Such patients can reportedly be distinguished from patients with other underlying post-concussive problems because they exhibit a marked, diagnostically meaningful exacerbation of symptoms on exposure to aerobic stress. For example, the Buffalo Concussion Treadmill Test is a graded exercise method, recommended for assessment of sports-related concussion, in which the athlete performs progressively more strenuous exercise (incline and speed) while being monitored for clinical symptoms and cardiovascular response [91, 101, 102]. Patients with "physiological" PCS reportedly complain of test-induced exacerbation of headache, dizziness, fatigue, and light sensitivity. They are proposed to benefit from submaximal aerobic exercise. Patients from the other subgroups reportedly show no such symptom exacerbation and are less likely to benefit from an exercise prescription [90].

Another fragment of evidence possibly supports the notion that the benefits of aerobic exercise are associated with cerebral blood flow: Leddy et al. conducted a pilot study comparing fMRI response to a mathematical task among concussed persons who had undergone aerobic training versus those who stretched. The pattern of activation only normalized in the aerobic exercise group [50].

Should the theory of a subgroup with prolonged metabolic/vascular dysfunction gain support from further research, exercise intolerance would permit biomarker-based classification of patients with persistent symptoms. More importantly, valid and reliable diagnosis of a neurobiologically distinct subgroup would enable rational design of interventions and clinical trials targeting specific metabolic/vascular/autonomic problems in a homogeneous cohort. That is, whether or not this particular theory is proven, the concept is vital: rehabilitation of persistent PCS is unlikely to progress until biological subgroups are identified and treatments can be tailored to etiologies.

Unfortunately, despite all of the pre-clinical and clinical evidence suggesting the benefit of post-acute submaximal symptom-limited aerobic exercise, that intervention has yet to be studied in a rigorous and systematic way employing large enough cohorts of demonstrably physiologically similar patients with appropriate controls and adequate follow-up to judge efficacy. Hence, with the exception that early brief cognitive behavioral therapy is likely effective in reducing symptoms of acute stress disorder in the adult "mTBI" population, the following conclusion is reached:

> For patients who have been diagnosed with "mTBI" and experience PCS, there is insufficient evidence to support or refute a contention that any rehabilitation intervention is more effective than non-specific support and attention in reducing either PCS or associated functional impairments.

The research to date has not provided robust information regarding the efficacy of rehabilitation interventions in "mTBI" (or CBI). The findings of this chapter highlight that non-equivalent or waitlist control conditions, case studies, and quasi-experimental pre–post designs may be instructive in generating hypotheses, but they are inadequate to inform evidence-based treatment recommendations by applying current guidelines. Many hypotheses have been developed in the past few decades of CBI research and well-designed, controlled treatment trials are needed to inform clinical practice and enhance patient outcomes. Several salient research opportunities and design considerations became apparent during the construction of this chapter and the most prominent are discussed in subsequent sections.

Outcome Measures

Many studies reviewed in this chapter targeted PCS as an outcome measure. Even well-designed trials (e.g., [48, 66, 75]) suffered from lack of an available primary outcome measure for PCS that is not based on a subjective, self-report symptom checklist. By AAN criteria, using subjective patient ratings on checklists results in an automatic downgrade to a class 3 study where otherwise the design would have warranted a class 1 or class 2 grading. There appears to be some weight to the argument that self-report questionnaires may provide divergent results to measures based on more robust forms of symptom enquiry such as semi-structured interview [103, 104].

It would be worthwhile fostering research resulting in a reliable, validated, semi-structured interview assessment for PCS. This process might reasonably be modeled on the development of the Clinician Administered Posttraumatic Stress Disorder Scale [105] or other such similar measures. Due to the broad overlap of PCS with the effects of chronic pain, chronic fatigue, and orthopedic trauma, such a scale might not necessarily be solely targeted at CBI but have broad applicability to a variety of overlapping conditions in the general rehabilitation field, thus avoiding the problems associated with identifying symptoms that discriminate CBI sequelae from other conditions, or having to revamp the scale every time a new diagnostic system for PCS became prominent. Incorporating validity items into such a measure is indicated. A brief self-report version (while subjective) would also be a useful adjunct for session-by-session or daily symptom tracking.

Using Sensitive Measures

While not explored in this chapter, there is a growing awareness in neuropsychological literature that traditional assessment measures (standardized paper-and-pencil tests) developed in more severely impaired populations with diverse diagnoses are only sensitive to the earliest neurobiological effects of CBI, and largely blind to persistent and subtle deficits of cognitive or non-cognitive behavior. Furthermore, there is evidence that measurable neuropathology persists in patients even if they are asymptomatic and not impaired on traditional cognitive measures [106, 107]. Studies are beginning to emerge that use mixed methodologies for outcome assessment, combining traditional neuropsychological outcome measures with experimental cognitive measures, neurophysiological measurements such as electroencephalogram or evoked potentials, or advanced neuroimaging methods such as fMRI and diffusion tensor imaging [50, 108–110]. Such combined methodologies will increase the sensitivity of studies.

The caveat for rehabilitation research is that pragmatic measurements that are relevant to the targets of treatment (such as functioning in activities of daily living, time to return to work, sports, school) should not be abandoned. There is the risk that we may gain a fantastic appreciation of functional brain-scanning changes in response to treatment or during the natural course of recovery, but lose the outcomes that are most important to our patients – how neurologic changes correlate with subjective experience and daily functioning.

Sampling Subpopulations

It is promising that many of the studies evaluated in the present chapter have recognized the heterogeneity of the "mTBI" population and have restricted sampling to specific subpopulations – for example, concussed patients meeting criteria for acute stress disorder [46], concussed patients with risk factors for lingering PCS [48, 57], and concussed patients with exercise-induced symptom exacerbation [49, 50]. In rare cases, there may be some rehabilitation intervention that may have broad applicability to the CBI population as a whole. More commonly, a specific sub-sample will be more appropriate.

For example, if one were interested in designing a study targeting intervention for sleep disturbance after CBI, it would be more instructive (and likely increase study power) to target a well-defined age group (20–45 years, for example), at a specific duration since injury (three to four months post injury), with a specific sleep problem (delayed sleep onset >1 h), rather than attempt such a study in a more general population.

Clarifying the Construct

The growing body of literature in the field of animal and human neuroscience provides hope regarding two current limitations in CBI intervention research: (1) the lack of a biologically based diagnostic system; and (2) confusion regarding the etiology of persisting PCS. Developments in neuroscience research show promise of remedying these limitations that have led to the stuttering nature of CBI rehabilitation research to date.

There has been an explosion in concussion research in neuroscience – leading to a slow-growing understanding of the neurobiological changes associated with lingering sequelae. Since death shortly after CBI is exceedingly rare, human CBI research will forever face the special challenge that prompt post-mortem brain study is almost impossible. Yet advances in non-invasive *in vivo* assessment technologies (e.g., advanced neuroimaging) have hugely accelerated progress. It is important for rehabilitation professionals to become more involved in this global research endeavor, and move beyond observational research designs. Many compelling hypotheses have been raised by previous research. Future investigations employing rigorous, equivalent control research designs are needed to evaluate these hypotheses and ground CBI rehabilitation in evidence-based practice.

Guiding Principles for Clinical Practice

For many rehabilitation providers, the finding that treatment literature is largely barren of robust controlled trials to inform treatment for CBI patients may be sobering. It is important to recognize that the sample of research considered by this chapter is a small subsample of the wider research in the concussion field. Specific research evidence (in the form of controlled trials) is not the only information clinicians recruit to make treatment decisions. This concept is highlighted in the AAN guidelines that informed the method for this chapter: "Evidence is only one source of knowledge clinicians use to make decisions. Other sources include established principles and judgment" [39]. In the course of developing this chapter, over 6000 abstracts related to "mTBI" intervention were reviewed. While the research is not sufficiently developed to inform evidence-based practice guidelines (by AAN criteria), it is adequate to identify guiding philosophies that can be employed in clinical practice.

Some of the most compelling developments in the field relate to research and commentaries that encourage clinicians to look beyond a simplistic "concussion causes PCS" framework and understand PCS from the perspective of a complex interface between: (1) the individual's pre-morbid genetic traits, experiences, and temperament; (2) the neurobiological stresses associated with abrupt external force rattling the brain; and (3) the biopsychosocial factors associated with acute/chronic stress, sleep disorder, autonomic dysregulation, sensory and vestibular anomalies, pituitary dysfunction, and chronic pain [23, 111–118]. The neurobiological changes associated with these interacting clinical features have not been fully elucidated, but even at this stage, the broader framework can alert clinicians to intervention opportunities that would otherwise have been missed under a more simplistic model.

Acute and Sub-Acute Management

If the patient is presenting acutely (within the first two days) or sub-acutely (for instance, within the first two weeks), the first step is to ensure that the possibility of complications such as intracranial bleeding has been excluded by appropriate medical providers. It is also important to stress that patients ought to avoid situations that place them at risk for a second concussion until their symptoms resolve. In many cases where symptoms seem to be following a rapidly improving course, simple education regarding neurophysiology and behavioral principles that will promote or hinder recovery may be sufficient. That information could be summarized in a handout.

Fortunately, the majority of survivors of typical concussions tend to have an uncomplicated resolution of symptoms without further or ongoing intervention. Unfortunately, evidence is growing that a substantial proportion of patients probably suffer from cerebral dysfunction, of which they may or may not be aware – and which may or may not produce late effects. Patients should be advised to seek early and active follow-up if the trajectory of their recovery falters within the first few weeks and be given information about appropriate clinical resources. Despite the poverty of empirical evidence, as summarized in this chapter, various professional groups will surely continue to publish guidelines regarding appropriate management, especially in the case of sports-related concussion [119]. Specific applications of rehabilitation principles to veteran populations are discussed in other chapters of this volume. One hopes that prudence and progress will eventually improve the average treatment of CBI survivors who present for medical attention.

Post-Acute Assessment

For patients who present with persistent complaints beyond a month, a more active rehabilitation approach is indicated. Given our awareness that many conditions mimic, overlap, or interact with post-concussive complaints (sleep deprivation, anxiety, depression, chronic pain, general physical trauma), an initial assessment to consider the relevance of a concussion history to current presentation is the first step.

If an individual sustained a well-documented concussion but had minimal initial disruption to his or her life in terms of symptoms or functional difficulties in the first few weeks, clinicians sometimes assume that emotional symptoms with onset three to nine months post-concussion are unrelated, or "psychological" complications, or influenced by litigation. In fact, evidence suggests that delayed-onset depression is more the rule than the exception. Although the underlying neurobiology of delayed or late-onset PCS has yet to be elucidated, it is appropriate to consider a variety of potentially modifiable factors beyond pre-morbid vulnerabilities and direct effects of cerebral damage, such as chronic pain, sleep disturbance, stress, undetected endocrine dysfunction, and multi-determined psychiatric symptoms.

For patients with clear concussion-related symptoms, traditional neuropsychological assessment with extensive cognitive testing is rarely informative to treatment planning in the early stages over and above data gathered in a clinical interview (limited incremental validity). Moreover, such testing was not designed for, and is usually not sensitive to, the effects of CBI after the acute stage. Yet selective testing may help inform decisions related to return to work and school as the patient stabilizes or plateaus, and may help to monitor treatment response.

The subjectivity and heterogeneity associated with the "mTBI" diagnosis result in a wide array of presentations falling under that rhetorical umbrella. As previously mentioned, the unique features specific to each individual concussion survivor may require a very different treatment approach to any other person in the CBI population. It is beyond the scope of this chapter to discuss in detail the wide range of research information that can inform CBI rehabilitation; however, some of the most salient factors that can contribute to a treatment heuristic are discussed below.

Neurobiology as a Guiding Principle

We have a growing understanding of the neurobiology associated with concussion and these findings will gradually inform clinical practice. One of the most widely cited summaries of research into the biology of concussion was produced by the UCLA research group in 2001 [120]. The authors describe the "neurometabolic cascade of concussion" triggered by traumatic insult to the brain, and the resultant "cellular energy crisis." Applying this research to clinical practice results in the following rehabilitation principle:

> Concussed patients are faced with reduced neural resources which contribute to post-concussive complaints. Temporarily reducing neural demands has the potential to speed recovery, as resources which would otherwise be depleted by these demands can be applied to restoring neurochemical homeostasis.

There are a number of factors that research has identified when considering which "neural demands" clinicians can target to free resources for brain-healing processes and these are considered in subsequent sections.

Although the "neurometabolic cascade" is an inaccurate metaphor for the actual pathophysiology of CBI, it can be a valuable educational tool to share with patients in a simplified form. It provides an easy-to-communicate rationale for treatment structure and targets. When patients grasp the physiology behind their symptoms, they may be more compliant with treatment recommendations. For patients in the post-acute phase, the present author reviews with them a booklet with a simplified, plain-language explanation of the "neurometabolic cascade" as the first stage of developing a treatment plan. Most patients have never had the neurobiology associated with their symptoms explained to them and are generally relieved when they realize that they can be active participants in their rehabilitation and recovery and work toward creating the most ideal conditions for their brain chemistry to normalize.

Again, the so-called "neurometabolic cascade" is only one aspect of a very large variety of neurobiological changes associated with concussion. Other factors, such as axonal stretch, axolemmal disruption, micro-hemorrhage, neuro-inflammation, immunomodulatory changes, and gene expression changes, may also be at play in the individual patient [24, 121–124]. Moreover, the "cascade" analogy fails to consider the simultaneous occurrence of multiple neuroprotective and regenerative phenomena in what amounts to a battle for the health of the brain that perhaps persists for months or years. Still, the author has not found it useful to overwhelm the patient with a comprehensive 21st-century understanding of CBI. The simplified UCLA model may be sufficient for preliminary education in most cases.

Balancing Rest vs. Activity / Fatigue Management

Post-concussive fatigue is addressed in depth elsewhere in this volume (Chapter 24). This section focuses on rehabilitation interventions. The goal of fatigue management is to encourage initial reduction in intensity and duration of demanding activities to a level that is sustainable (not leading to periods of symptom exacerbation) and then gradually increase functional activity over time, as tolerated by the patient. In the author's experience, an essential component to fatigue management is a system to track activities on a daily basis, rate level of fatigue at regular intervals during the day, and track other idiosyncratic symptoms that indicate the patient has "overdone it" (often headaches or dizziness). By reviewing such data from a tracking sheet the practitioner can be alerted to patterns of behavior that lead to exacerbation in symptoms and address these in the treatment session.

Typically, exposure to high-stimulus environments (busy shopping malls, dance clubs) is to be minimized, and environmental manipulations to reduce over-stimulation and promote functioning are to be encouraged (such as clearing clutter from a workspace or reducing multitasking and environmental noise). It is important to note that what triggers symptoms for one concussion survivor may be relaxing and restorative for another. Tracking sheets produce the data needed to make effective recommendations – for some patients reading, computer games, light exercise, and social activity will be problematic, but for other patients they will not.

Traditionally, rest has been the primary prescribed recommendation for CBI patients. The historical recommendation for "no activity until asymptomatic" appears to have been promoted by consensus recommendations for acute sports concussion management [125]. However, it should be highlighted that the universal application of this recommendation in the post-acute phase can be iatrogenic and expose the patient to the risks associated with inactivity and deconditioning [126]. Furthermore, there is currently no controlled research to support the contention that striving for no activity is helpful at any stage of the rehabilitation process in sports populations or otherwise. Rather, the research that is available supports the approach of encouraging moderate gradual increases in levels of physical activity and cognitive challenge, but not to the extent that the neural energy reserves are depleted via overexertion. Schneider et al. provide a review of this issue relating to sports populations [127]. Silverberg and Iverson's 2013 review addresses the same issue from a general population perspective [126] and provides research-based principles to guide activity resumption recommendations in clinical practice.

Prioritizing and Treating Co-Morbidities

The clinician must also be attuned to, and provide access to, interventions for co-morbid conditions that have the potential to interact with, and hamper, recovery from concussion. The most prominent co-morbid factors identified in the research regarding "mTBI" rehabilitation are sleep disruption, chronic pain, and post-traumatic anxiety symptoms [128–132]. Research regarding these conditions in general suggests that they can independently impair functioning, produce symptoms similar to and overlapping with PCS, and compete with neural resources that could otherwise be applied to brain recovery. Where these co-morbidities are apparent, early targeted intervention is indicated.

Multidisciplinary intervention targeted at reducing disability by addressing sleep, pain, and anxiety tends to have positive benefits on both target symptoms and post-concussive complaints [133]. In the author's clinical experience, sleep stabilization is so important to the progress of most concussion survivors that other areas of intervention are typically not prioritized until the patient's sleep is effectively treated with cognitive behavioral interventions for sleep disruption (sleep restriction, stimulus control, cognitive restructuring, relaxation protocols), augmented as needed by medications.

Tailoring Subsequent Treatment to the Individual

It should be clear to the reader that each concussion survivor presents with a unique variety of clinical needs. Pending progress in precision medicine tailored to each genome and epigenome, and progress in detecting the specific modifiable etiologies of each symptom in each patient, the clinician's capacity to individualize CBI care is limited. It is also clear that access to health care varies tremendously, and that too few patients will receive anything approaching an ideal, personalized rehabilitation program. Still, several rough rules of the road may help guide the provision of appropriate therapies. For instance, practitioners should be cautious about over-prescribing multiple interventions in the context of a patient prone to fatigue and often struggling with demands of reduced capacity for work or school, limited financial resources, and compounding daily demands. Ideally, CBI patients would benefit from initial consultation with a physician and rehabilitation psychologist who specialize in concussion. These providers can typically manage the core treatment functions previously described – education, fatigue management, sleep stabilization, brief cognitive behavioral anxiety interventions, and referral to physical therapy for treatment of pain (physical therapists can also be consulted regarding graduated exercise programs if indicated). Given these services, most patients progress toward their typical level of functioning. The clinical team can work with employers, school personnel, and families to minimize the stresses associated with temporarily impaired functioning on employment, educational progress, and family functioning. High levels of stress impact neurochemistry and will likely impair recovery.

By applying the principles above, specific PCS (such as headaches, dizziness, and memory difficulties) tend to resolve without targeting these symptoms directly. In addition to daily activity and symptom tracking, the author's clinic also gathers symptom data at each appointment (from a checklist) and graphs this data at the beginning of the appointment to determine if the treatment plan is effective or requires revision. For some patients, persistent residual symptoms are apparent and a secondary referral for endocrine assessment, vestibular rehabilitation, neuro-optometry intervention, and formal cognitive rehabilitation should be considered as progress plateaus or if the symptom profile suggests that specific difficulties are impairing the rate of progress.

While research progress is encouraging, it is still the case that there is very limited controlled research that clinicians can draw on to inform their practice. It is important for rehabilitation professionals to be embedded in CBI research programs to design studies that are targeted at improving outcomes in the large number of patients who present with persistent PCS. The lack of evidence highlights the importance of being responsive and not rigid in our notions of what is useful and not useful in CBI rehabilitation. This applies both on individual patient level and systems level considerations.

As noted above, this volume appears at a time of transition. It is clear that the 20th-century paradigm of "mTBI" lacks biological meaning, but neuroscience has yet to discover a valid and reliable way to distinguish neurobiologically homogeneous subsets of the concussed population. As with other neurological disorders, breakthroughs in clinical management will only accelerate after clinicians have practical markers that reveal specific, hopefully modifiable, cerebral changes. Nonetheless, current knowledge informs guiding philosophies that can already be employed in clinical practice. Close monitoring of patient response to interventions that are employed will facilitate changes to the treatment plan if they prove unfruitful. Health care systems need to accommodate the newly apparent significance of concussion. Although this raises the specter of escalating cost, society will perhaps discover that early, expert, multidisciplinary management more than pays off in long-term benefits. And rehabilitation teams must be open to revising practice algorithms as more information about effective interventions for CBI come to light.

References

1.   Hilton J. *On rest and pain: A course of lectures on the influence of mechanical and physiological rest in the treatment of accidents and surgical diseases and the diagnostic value of pain,* second edition. New York: William Wood, 1867.

2.   Halstead ME. Historical perspectives on concussion. In: Niskala J, Walter KD, editors. *Pediatric and adolescent concussion: Diagnosis, management, and outcomes.* New York: Springer Science, 2012, pp. 3–8.

3.   Siman R, Giovannone N, Hanten G, Wilde EA, McCauley SR, Hunter JV, et al. Evidence that the blood biomarker SNTF predicts brain imaging changes and persistent cognitive dysfunction in mild TBI patients. *Front Neurol* 2013; 4: 190.

4.   Zetterberg H, Smith DH, Blennow K. Biomarkers of mild traumatic brain injury in cerebrospinal fluid and blood. *Nat Rev Neurol* 2013; 9: 201–210.

5.   American Congress of Rehabilitation Medicine. Definition of mild traumatic brain injury. *J Head Trauma Rehabil* 1993; 8: 86–87.

6.   Carroll LJ, Cassidy JD, Holm L, Kraus J, Coronado VG, WHO Collaborating Centre Task Force on Mild Traumatic Brain Injury. Methodological issues and research recommendations for mild traumatic brain injury: The WHO Collaborating Centre Task Force on Mild Traumatic Brain Injury. *J Rehabil Med* 2004; 43 (Suppl): 113–125.

7.   Centers for Disease Control and Injury Prevention. *Report to U.S. Congress on mild traumatic brain injury: Steps to prevent a serious public health problem.* Atlanta, GA: National Center for Injury Prevention and Control, 2003.

8.   Lovell MR, Collins MW. Neuropsychological assessment of the college football player. *J Head Trauma Rehabil* 1998; 13: 9–26.

9.   Lovell MR, Iverson GL, Collins MW, Podell K, Johnston KM, Pardini D, et al. Measurement of symptoms following sports-related concussion: Reliability and normative data for the post-concussion scale. *Appl Neuropsychol* 2006; 13: 166–174.

10. King NS, Crawford S, Wenden FJ, Moss NE, Wade DT. The Rivermead Post Concussion Symptoms Questionnaire: A measure of symptoms commonly experienced after head injury and its reliability. *J Neurol* 1995; 242: 587–592.

11. Kontos AP, Elbin RJ, Schatz P, Covassin T, Henry L, Pardini J, Collins MW. A revised factor structure for the post-concussion symptom scale: Baseline and postconcussion factors. *Am J Sports Med* 2012; 40: 2375–2384.

12. Iverson GL, Lange RT. Examination of 'postconcussion-like' symptoms in a healthy sample. *Appl Neuropsychol* 2003; 10: 137–144.

13. Mickeviciene D, Schrader H, Obelieniene D, Surkiene D, Kunickas R, Stovner LJ, Sand T. A controlled prospective inception cohort study on the post-concussion syndrome outside the medicolegal context. *Eur J Neurol* 2004; 11: 411–419.

14. Tiersky LA, Cicerone KD, Natelson BH, DeLuca J. Neuropsychological functioning in chronic fatigue syndrome and mild traumatic brain injury: A comparison. *Clin Neuropsychol* 1998; 12: 503–512.

15. Landre N, Poppe CJ, Davis N, Schmaus B, Hobbs SE. Cognitive functioning and postconcussive symptoms in trauma patients with and without mild TBI. *Arch Clin Neuropsychol* 2006; 21: 255–273.

16. Trahan DE, Ross CE, Trahan SL. Relationships among postconcussional-type symptoms, depression, and anxiety in neurologically normal young adults and victims of mild brain injury. *Arch Clin Neuropsychol* 2001; 16: 435–445.

17. Wong JL, Regennitter RP, Barrios F. Base rate and simulated symptoms of mild head injury among normals. *Arch Clin Neuropsychol* 1994; 9: 411–425.

18. Machulda MM, Bergquist TF, Ito V, Chew S. Relationship between stress, coping, and postconcussion symptoms in a healthy adult population. *Arch Clin Neuropsychol* 1998; 13: 415–424.

19. Garden N, Sullivan KA, Lange RT. The relationship between personality characteristics and postconcussion symptoms in a non-clinical sample. *Neuropsychol* 2010; 24: 168–175.

20. Donnell AJ, Kim MS, Silva MA, Vanderploeg RD. Incidence of postconcussion symptoms in psychiatric diagnostic groups, mild traumatic brain injury, and comorbid conditions. *Clin Neuropsychol* 2012; 26: 1092–1101.

21. Smith-Seemiller, L., Fow NR, Kant R, Franzen MD. Presence of post-concussion syndrome symptoms in patients with chronic pain vs mild traumatic brain injury. *Brain Inj* 2003; 17: 199–206.

22. Laborey, M., Masson F, Ribereau-Gayon R, Zongo D, Salmi LR, Lagarde E. Specificity of postconcussion symptoms at 3 months after mild traumatic brain injury: Results from a comparative cohort study. *J Head Trauma Rehabil* 2014; 29: E28–E36.

23. Lagarde E, Salmi LR, Holm LW, Contrand B, Masson F, Ribéreau-Gayon R, Laborey M, Cassidy JD. Association of symptoms following mild traumatic brain injury with posttraumatic stress disorder vs postconcussion syndrome. *JAMA Psychiatry* 2014; 71: 1032–1040.

24. Iverson GL. Outcome from mild traumatic brain injury. *Curr Opin Psychiatry* 2005; 18: 301–317.

25. Davies R, McMillan TM. Opinion about post-concussion syndrome in health professionals. *Brain Inj* 2005; 19: 941–947.

26. Silverberg ND, Iverson GL. Etiology of the post-concussion syndrome: Physiogenesis and psychogenesis revisited. *NeuroRehabil* 2011; 29: 317–329.

27. Prigatano GP, Gale SD. The current status of postconcussion syndrome. *Curr Opin Psychiatry* 2011; 24: 243–250.

28. Macleod SAD. Post concussion syndrome: The attraction of the psychological by the organic. *Med Hypotheses* 2010; 74: 1033–1055.

29. King NS. Post-concussion syndrome: Clarity amid the controversy? *Br J Psychiatry* 2003; 183: 276–278.
30. Ruff RM. Mild traumatic brain injury and neural recovery: Rethinking the debate. *Neurorehabil* 2011; 28: 167–180.
31. Sosin DM, Sniezek JE, Thurman DJ. Incidence of mild and moderate brain injury in the United States, 1991. *Brain Inj* 1996; 10: 47–54.
32. Lannsjö M, af Geijerstam JL, Johansson U, Bring J, Borg J. Prevalence and structure of symptoms at 3 months after mild traumatic brain injury in a national cohort. *Brain Inj* 2009; 23: 213–219.
33. Fourtassi M, Hajjioui A, Ouahabi AE, Benmassaoud H, Hajjaj-Hassouni N, Khamlichi AE. Long term outcome following mild traumatic brain injury in Moroccan patients. *Clin Neurol Neurosurg* 2011; 113: 716–720.
34. Thornhill S, Teasdale GM, Murray GD, McEwen J, Roy CW, Penny KI. Disability in young people and adults one year after head injury: Prospective cohort study. *BMJ* 2000; 320: 1631–1635.
35. Jakola AS, Muller K, Larsen M, Waterloo K, Romner B, Ingebrigtsen T. Five-year outcome after mild head injury: A prospective controlled study. *Acta Neurol Scand* 2007; 115: 398–402.
36. Chan HF, Chor CM, Ling WY, Wong GKC, Ng SCP, Poon WS. Long-term disability in the local population 2 years after mild head injury: Prospective cohort study. *Surg Practi* 2005; 9: 8–11.
37. Cassidy JD, Carroll LJ, Peloso PM, Borg J, von Holst H, Holm L, et al. Incidence, risk factors and prevention of mild traumatic brain injury: Results of the WHO Collaborating Centre Task Force on Mild Traumatic Brain Injury. *J Rehabil Med* 2004; 43 (Suppl): 28–60.
38. Ryan TV, Ruff RL. The efficacy of structured memory retraining in a group comparison of head trauma patients. *Arch Clin Neuropsychol* 1988; 3: 165–179.
39. American Academy of Neurology. *Clinical practice guideline process manual.* St. Paul, MN: American Academy of Neurology, 2011.
40. Higgins J, Green S, editors. *Cochrane handbook for systematic reviews of interventions.* West Sussex, UK: Wiley-Blackwell, 2008.
41. Comper P, Bisschop SM, Carnide N, Tricco A. A systematic review of treatments for mild traumatic brain injury. *Brain Inj* 2005; 19: 863–880.
42. Cicerone KD. Remediation of 'working attention' in mild traumatic brain injury. *Brain Inj* 2002; 16: 185–195.
43. Nelson LA, Macdonald M, Stall C, Pazdan R. Effects of interactive metronome therapy on cognitive functioning after blast-related brain injury: A randomized controlled pilot trial. *Neuropsychol* 2013; 27: 666–679.
44. Riegler LJ, Neils-Strunjas J, Boyce S, Wade SL, Scheifele PM. Cognitive intervention results in web-based videophone treatment adherence and improved cognitive scores. *Med Sci Monit* 2013; 19: 269–275.
45. Tiersky LA, Anselmi V, Johnston MV, Kurtyka J, Roosen E, Schwartz T, Deluca J. A trial of neuropsychologic rehabilitation in mild-spectrum traumatic brain injury. *Arch Phys Med Rehabil* 2005; 86: 1565–1574.
46. Bryant RA, Moulds M, Guthrie R, Nixon RD. Treating acute stress disorder following mild traumatic brain injury. *Am J Psychiatry* 2003; 160: 585–587.
47. Leonard KN. Cognitive-behavioral intervention in persistent postconcussion syndrome: A controlled treatment outcome study. Thesis. Texas Scholar Works; University of Texas at Austin. 2002. Available at https://repositories.lib.utexas.edu/handle/2152/11143
48. Silverberg ND, Hallam BJ, Rose A, Underwood H, Whitfield K, Thornton AE, Whittal ML. Cognitive-behavioral prevention of postconcussion syndrome in at-risk patients: A pilot randomized controlled trial. *J Head Trauma Rehabil* 2013; 28: 313–322.
49. Baker JG, Freitas MS, Leddy JJ, Kozlowski KF, Willer BS. Return to full functioning after graded exercise assessment and progressive exercise treatment of postconcussion syndrome. *Rehabil Res Pract* 2012; 2012: 705309.
50. Leddy JJ, Cox JL, Baker JG, Wack DS, Pendergast DR, Zivadinov DR, Willer B. Exercise treatment for postconcussion syndrome: A pilot study of changes in functional magnetic resonance imaging activation, physiology, and symptoms. *J Head Trauma Rehabil* 2013; 28: 241–249.
51. Jensen OK, Nielsen FF, Vosmar L. An open study comparing manual therapy with the use of cold packs in the treatment of post-traumatic headache. *Cephalalgia* 1990; 10: 241–250.
52. Schneider K, Meuwisse WH, Nettel-Aguirre A, Barlow K, Boyd L, Kang J, Emery CA. Cervicovestibular rehabilitation in sport-related concussion: A randomised controlled trial. *Br J Sports Med* 2014; 48: 1294–1298.
53. Andersson EE, Bedics BK, Falkmer T. Mild traumatic brain injuries: A 10-year follow-up. *J Rehabil Med* 2011; 43: 323–329.
54. Andersson EE, Emanuelson I, Bjorklund R, Stalhammar DA. Mild traumatic brain injuries: The impact of early intervention on late sequelae. A randomized controlled trial. *Acta Neurochir* 2007; 149: 151–160.
55. Ghaffar O, McCullagh S, Ouchterlony D, Feinstein A. Randomized treatment trial in mild traumatic brain injury. *J Psychosom Res* 2006; 61: 153–160.
56. Goranson TE, Graves RE, Allison D, La Freniere R. Community integration following multidisciplinary rehabilitation for traumatic brain injury. *Brain Inj* 2003; 17: 759–774.
57. Matuseviciene G, Borg J, Stålnacke BM, Ulfarsson T, de Boussard C. Early intervention for patients at risk for persisting disability after mild traumatic brain injury: A randomized, controlled study. *Brain Inj* 2013; 27: 318–324.
58. Wade DT, Crawford S, Wenden FJ, King NS, Moss NE. Does routine follow up after head injury help? A randomised controlled trial. *J Neurol Neurosurg Psychiatry* 1997; 62: 478–484.
59. Wade DT, King NS, Wenden FJ, Crawford S, Caldwell FE. Routine follow up after head injury: A second randomised controlled trial. *J Neurol Neurosurg Psychiatry* 1998; 65: 177–183.
60. Lowdon IM, Briggs M, Cockin J. Post-concussional symptoms following minor head injury. *Injury* 1989; 20: 193–194.
61. Mittenberg W, Tremont G, Zielinski RE, Fichera S, Rayls KR. Cognitive-behavioral prevention of postconcussion syndrome. *Arch Clin Neuropsychol* 1996; 11: 139–145.
62. Ponsford J, Willmott C, Rothwell A, Cameron P, Ayton G, Nelms R, Curran C, Ng K. Impact of early intervention on outcome after mild traumatic brain injury in children. *Pediatrics* 2001; 108: 1297–1303.
63. Ponsford J, Willmott C, Rothwell A, Cameron P, Kelly AM, Nelms R, Curran C. Impact of early intervention on outcome following mild head injury in adults. *J Neurol Neurosurg Psychiatry* 2002; 73: 330–332.
64. Wrightson P, Gronwall D. Time off work and symptoms after minor head injury. *Injury* 1981; 12: 445–454.
65. Alves W, Macciocchi SN, Barth JT. Postconcussive symptoms after uncomplicated mild head injury. *J Head Trauma Rehabil* 1993; 8: 48–59.
66. Bell KR, Hoffman JM, Temkin NR, Powell JM, Fraser RT, Esselman PC, Barber JK, Dikmen S. The effect of telephone counselling on reducing posttraumatic symptoms after mild traumatic brain injury: A randomised trial. *J Neurol Neurosurg Psychiatry* 2008; 79: 1275–1281.
67. de Kruijk JR, Leffers P, Meerhoff S, Rutten J, Twijnstra A. Effectiveness of bed rest after mild traumatic brain injury: A

randomised trial of no versus six days of bed rest. *J Neurol Neurosurg Psychiatry* 2002; 73: 167–172.

68. Gronwall D. Rehabilitation programs for patients with mild head injury: Components, problems, and evaluation. *J Head Trauma Rehabil* 1986; 1: 53–62.

69. Heskestad B, Waterloo K, Baardsen R, Helseth E, Romner B, Ingebrigtsen T. No impact of early intervention on late outcome after minimal, mild and moderate head injury. *Scand J Trauma Resusc Emerg Med* 2010; 18: 1–5.

70. Hinkle JL, Alves WM, Rimell RW, Jane JA. Restoring social competence in minor head-injury patients. *J Neurosci Nurs* 1986; 18: 268–271.

71. Minderhoud JM, Boelens ME, Huizenga J, Saan RJ. Treatment of minor head injuries. *Clin Neurol Neurosurg* 1980; 82: 127–140.

72. Paniak C, Toller-Lobe G, Durand A, Nagy J. A randomized trial of two treatments for mild traumatic brain injury. *Brain Inj* 1998; 12: 1011–1023.

73. Paniak C, Toller-Lobe G, Reynolds S, Melnyk A, Nagy J. A randomized trial of two treatments for mild traumatic brain injury: 1 year follow-up. *Brain Inj* 2000; 14: 219–226.

74. Relander M, Troupp H, Af Bjorkesten G. Controlled trial of treatment for cerebral concussion. *Br Med J* 1972; 4: 777–779.

75. Suffoletto B, Callaway CW, Kristan J, Monti P, Clark DB. Mobile phone text messaging to assess symptoms after mild traumatic brain injury and provide self-care support: A pilot study. *J Head Trauma Rehabil* 2013; 28: 302–312.

76. Cantor J, Ashman T, Dams-O'Connor K, Dijkers MP, Gordon W, Spielman L, et al. Evaluation of the short-term executive plus intervention for executive dysfunction after traumatic brain injury: A randomized controlled trial with minimization. *Arch Phys Med Rehabil* 2014; 95: 1–9.

77. Twamley EW, Jak AJ, Delis DC, Bondi MW, Lohr JB. Cognitive Symptom Management and Rehabilitation Therapy (CogSMART) for veterans with traumatic brain injury: Pilot randomized controlled trial. *J Rehabil Res Develop* 2014; 51: 59–70.

78. Cooper DB, Bowles AO, Kennedy JE, Curtiss G, French LM, Tate DF, Vanderploeg RD. Cognitive rehabilitation for military service members with mild traumatic brain injury: A randomized clinical trial. *J Head Trauma Rehabil* 2017; 32: E1–E15.

79. Belanger HG, Brown KM, Crowell TA, Vanderploeg RD, Curtiss G. The key behaviors change inventory and executive functioning in an elderly clinic sample. *Clin Neuropsychol* 2002; 16: 251–257.

80. Gronwall DMA. Paced auditory serial-addition task: A measure of recovery from concussion. *Percep Motor Skills* 1977; 44: 367–373.

81. Derogatis LR. *SCL-90-R. Symptom Checklist-90-R: Administration, scoring, and procedures manual.* Minneapolis, MN: National Computer Systems, 1994.

82. Cooper DB, Bunner AE, Kennedy JE, Balldin V, Tate DF, Eapen BC, Jaramillo CA. Treatment of persistent post-concussive symptoms after mild traumatic brain injury: A systematic review of cognitive rehabilitation and behavioral health interventions in military service members and veterans. *Brain Imaging Behav* 2015; 9: 403–420.

83. Janak JC, Cooper DB, Bowles AO, Alamgir AH, Cooper SP, Gabriel KP, Perez A, Orman JA. Completion of multidisciplinary treatment for persistent postconcussive symptoms is associated with reduced symptom burden. *J Head Trauma Rehabil* 2017; 32: 1–15.

84. Marshall S, Bayley M, McCullagh S, Velikonia D, Berrigan L, Ouchterlony D. Weegar K, mTBI Expert Consensus Group. Updated clinical practice guidelines for concussion/mild traumatic brain injury and persistent symptoms. *Brain Inj* 2015; 29: 688–700.

85. Morissette SB, Woodward M, Kimbrel NA, Meyer EC, Kruse MI, Dolan S, Gulliver SB. Deployment-related TBI, persistent postconcussive symptoms, PTSD, and depression in OEF/OIF veterans: Separating deployment-related traumatic brain injury and posttraumatic stress disorder in veterans: Preliminary findings from the Veterans Affairs traumatic brain injury screening program. *Rehabil Psychol* 2011; 56: 340–350.

86. Hill JJ, Mobo BH Jr, Cullen MR. Separating deployment-related traumatic brain injury and posttraumatic stress disorder in veterans: Preliminary findings from the Veterans Affairs traumatic brain injury screening program. *Am J Phys Med Rehabil* 2009; 88: 605–614.

87. Elbin RJ, Schatz P, Lowder HB, Kontos AP. An empirical review of treatment and rehabilitation approaches used in the acute, sub-acute, and chronic phases of recovery following sports-related concussion. *Curr Treat Options Neurol* 2014; 16: 320.

88. Tan CO, Meehan WP 3rd, Iverson GL, Taylor JA. Cerebrovascular regulation, exercise, and mild traumatic brain injury. *Neurology* 2014; 83: 1665–1672.

89. Broglio SP, Collins MW, Williams RM, Mucha A, Kontos AP. Current and emerging rehabilitation for concussion: A review of the evidence. *Clin Sports Med* 2015; 34: 213–231.

90. Ellis MJ, Leddy J, Willer B. Multi-disciplinary management of athletes with post-concussion syndrome: An evolving pathophysiological approach. *Front Neurol* 2016; 7: 136.

91. Leddy JJ, Baker JG, Willer B. Active rehabilitation of concussion and post-concussion syndrome. *Phys Med Rehabil Clin N Am* 2016; 27: 437–454.

92. Miller Phillips M, Reddy CC. Managing patients with prolonged recovery following concussion. *Phys Med Rehabil Clin N Am* 2016; 27: 455–474.

93. Sawyer Q, Vesci B, McLeod TC. Physical activity and intermittent postconcussion symptoms after a period of symptom-limited physical and cognitive rest. *J Athl Train* 2016; 51: 739–742.

94. Griesbach GS, Gomez-Pinilla F, Hovda DA. The upregulation of plasticity-related proteins following TBI is disrupted with acute voluntary exercise. *Brain Res* 2004; 1016: 154–162.

95. Griesbach GS, Hovda DA, Molteni R, Wu A, Gomez-Pinilla F. Voluntary exercise following traumatic brain injury: Brain-derived neurotrophic factor upregulation and recovery of function. *Neurosci* 2004; 125: 129–139.

96. Griesbach GS, Gómez-Pinilla F, Hovda DA. Time window for voluntary exercise-induced increases in hippocampal neuroplasticity molecules after traumatic brain injury is severity dependent. *J Neurotrauma* 2007; 24: 1161–1171.

97. Griesbach GS, Hovda DA, Gomez-Pinilla F. Exercise-induced improvement in cognitive performance after traumatic brain injury in rats is dependent on BDNF activation. *Brain Res* 2009; 1288: 105–115.

98. Griesbach GS, Tio DL, Vincelli J, McArthur DL, Taylor AN. Differential effects of voluntary and forced exercise on stress responses after traumatic brain injury. *J Neurotrauma* 2012; 29: 1426–1433.

99. Griesbach GS, Tio DL, Shyama N, Hovda DA. Recovery of stress response coincides with responsiveness to voluntary exercise after traumatic brain injury. *J Neurotrauma* 2014; 31: 674–682.

100. Kurowski BG, Hugentobler J, Quatman-Yates C, Taylor J, Gubanich PJ, Altaye M, Wade SL. Aerobic exercise for adolescents with prolonged symptoms after mild traumatic brain injury: An exploratory randomized clinical trial. *J Head Trauma Rehabil* 2017; 32: 79–81.

101. Leddy JJ, Kozlowski K, Donnelly JP, Pendergast DR, Epstein LH, Willer B. A preliminary study of subsymptom threshold exercise training for refractory postconcussion syndrome. *Clin J Sport Med* 2010; 20: 21–27.

102. Leddy JJ, Baker JG, Kozlowski K, Bisson L, Willer B. Reliability of a graded exercise test for assessing recovery from concussion. *Clin J Sport Med* 2011; 21: 89–94.

103. Iverson GL, Brooks BL, Ashton VL, Lange RT. Interview versus questionnaire symptom reporting in people with the postconcussion syndrome. *J Head Trauma Rehabili* 2010; 25: 23–30.

104. Nolin P, Villemure R, Heroux L. Determining long-term symptoms following mild traumatic brain injury: Method of interview affects self-report. *Brain Inj* 2006; 20: 1147–1154.

105. Blake DD, Weathers FW, Nagy LM, Kaloupek DG, Gusman FD, Charney DS, Keane TM. The development of a clinician-administered PTSD scale. *J Trauma Stress* 1995; 8: 75–90.

106. Hammeke TA, McCrea M, Coats SM, Verber MD, Durgerian S, Flora K, et al. Acute and subacute changes in neural activation during the recovery from sport-related concussion. *J Int Neuropsychol Soc* 2013; 19: 863–872.

107. Teel EF, Ray WJ, Geronimo AM, Slobounov SM. Residual alterations of brain electrical activity in clinically asymptomatic concussed individuals: An EEG study. *Clin Neurophysiol* 2014; 125: 703–707.

108. Chen AJ, Novakovic-Agopian T, Nycum TJ, Song S, Turner GR, Hills NK, et al. Training of goal-directed attention regulation enhances control over neural processing for individuals with brain injury. *Brain* 2011; 134: 1541–1554.

109. Strangman GE, O'Neil-Pirozzi TM, Goldstein R, Kelkar K, Katz DI, Burke D, et al. Prediction of memory rehabilitation outcomes in traumatic brain injury by using functional magnetic resonance imaging. *Arch Phys Med Rehabil* 2008; 89: 974–981.

110. Baillargeon A, Lassonde M, Leclerc S, Ellemberg D. Neuropsychological and neurophysiological assessment of sport concussion in children, adolescents and adults. *Brain Inj* 2012; 26: 211–220.

111. Bryant R. Post-traumatic stress disorder vs traumatic brain injury. *Dial Clin Neurosci* 2011; 13: 251–262.

112. Leddy JJ, Willer B. Use of graded exercise testing in concussion and return-to-activity management. *Curr Sports Med Rep* 2013; 12: 370–376.

113. Leddy JJ, Sandhu H, Sodhi V, Baker JG, Willer B. Rehabilitation of concussion and post-concussion syndrome. *Sports Health* 2012; 4: 147–154.

114. Khoury S, Chouchou F, Amzica F, Giguère JF, Denis R, Rouleau GA, Lavigne GJ. Rapid EEG activity during sleep dominates in mild traumatic brain injury patients with acute pain. *J Neurotrauma* 2013; 30: 633–641.

115. Ruff RL, Riechers RG 2nd, Wang XF, Piero T, Ruff SS. For veterans with mild traumatic brain injury, improved posttraumatic stress disorder severity and sleep correlated with symptomatic improvement. *J Rehabil Res Dev* 2012; 49: 1305–1320.

116. Tanriverdi F, Unluhizarci K, Kelestimur F. Pituitary function in subjects with mild traumatic brain injury: A review of literature and proposal of a screening strategy. *Pituitary* 2010; 13: 146–153.

117. Pogoda TK, Hendricks AM, Iverson KM, Stolzmann KL, Krengel MH, Baker E, et al. Multisensory impairment reported by veterans with and without mild traumatic brain injury history. *J Rehabil Res Dev* 2012; 49: 971–984.

118. Reger ML, Poulos AM, Buen F, Giza CC, Hovda DA, Fanselow MS. Concussive brain injury enhances fear learning and excitatory processes in the amygdala. *Biol Psychiatry* 2012; 71: 335–343.

119. Putukian M, Kutcher J. Current concepts in the treatment of sports concussions. *Neurosurg* 2014; 75 (Suppl 4): S64–S70.

120. Giza CC, Hovda DA. The neurometabolic cascade of concussion. *J Athl Train* 2001; 36: 228–235.

121. Patterson ZR, Holahan MR. Understanding the neuro-inflammatory response following concussion to develop treatment strategies. *Front Cell Neurosci* 2012; 6: 58.

122. Bigler ED. Neuropsychology and clinical neuroscience of persistent post-concussive syndrome. *J Int Neuropsychol Soc* 2008; 14: 1–22.

123. Barkhoudarian G, Hovda DA, Giza CC. The molecular pathophysiology of concussive brain injury. *Clin Sports Med* 2011; 30: 33–48.

124. Niogi SN, Mukherjee P, Ghajar J, Johnson C, Kolster RA, Sarkar R, et al. Extent of microstructural white matter injury in postconcussive syndrome correlates with impaired cognitive reaction time: A 3T diffusion tensor imaging study of mild traumatic brain injury. *AJNR Am J Neuroradiol* 2008; 29: 967–973.

125. McCrory P, Meeuwisse WH, Aubry M, Cantu RC, Dvořák J, Echemendia RJ, et al. Consensus statement on concussion in sport: The 4th International Conference on Concussion in Sport held in Zurich, November 2012. *J Athl Train* 2013; J48: 554–575.

126. Silverberg ND. Iverson GL. Is rest after concussion "the best medicine?": Recommendations for activity resumption following concussion in athletes, civilians, and military service members. *J Head Trauma Rehabil* 2013; 28: 250–259.

127. Schneider KJ, Iverson GL, Emery CA, McCrory P, Herring SA, Meeuwisse WH. The effects of rest and treatment following sport-related concussion: A systematic review of the literature. *Br J Sports Med* 2013; 47: 304–307.

128. Wood RL, O'Hagan G, Williams C, McCabe M, Chadwick N. Anxiety sensitivity and alexithymia as mediators of postconcussion syndrome following mild traumatic brain injury. *J Head Trauma Rehabil* 2014; 29: E9–E17.

129. Chaput G, Giguère JF, Chauny JM, Denis R, Lavigne G. Relationship among subjective sleep complaints, headaches, and mood alterations following a mild traumatic brain injury. *Sleep Med* 2009; 10: 713–716.

130. Schreiber S, Barkai G, Gur-Hartman T, Peles E, Tov N, Dolberg OT, Pick CG. Long-lasting sleep patterns of adult patients with minor traumatic brain injury (mTBI) and non-mTBI subjects. *Sleep Med* 2008; 9: 481–487.

131. Weyer Jamora C, Schroeder SC, Ruff RM. Pain and mild traumatic brain injury: The implications of pain severity on emotional and cognitive functioning. *Brain Inj* 2013; 27: 1134–1140.

132. Hou L, Han X, Sheng P, Tong W, Li Z, Xu D, et al. Risk factors associated with sleep disturbance following traumatic brain injury: Clinical findings and questionnaire based study. *PLoS One* 2013; 8: e76087.

133. Richter KJ, Cowan DM, Kaschalk SM. A protocol for managing pain, sleep disorders, and associated psychological sequelae of presumed mild head injury. *J Head Trauma Rehabil* 1995; 10: 7–15.

Chapter 28

A Modest Plea

Jeff Victoroff

破釜沉舟

Break the kettles and sink the boats.

Xiang Yu, 207 B C E

- On September 9, 2010 the author asked the current Director of the National Institute of Neurologic Disorders and Stroke (NINDS), Walter Koroshetz, "Why has NINDS never funded a single prospective longitudinal study of the late effects of concussion?" Walter mumbled an excuse, turned his back, and walked away.
- On September 9, 2016 the author sent a nine-page letter to the former Director of NINDS, Story Landis, asking, "Why has NINDS never funded a single prospective longitudinal study of the late effects of concussion?" Story never responded.
- To the best of the author's limited knowledge, there was at least one person affiliated with the National Institutes of Health (NIH) who had the authority, the intellectual wherewithal, and the vision to act for the good of concussed persons. That was Tom Insel, long-time Director of the National Institute of Mental Health. Tom retired to work for a multinational corporation.
- A research project exists called Late Effects of Traumatic Brain Injury (ID number 13–0751) [1]. The Late Effects of Traumatic Brain Injury Brain Donor Program is a four-year, $6 million project funded by the Foundation for the NIH and NINDS. It may be worthwhile reviewing that project's somewhat cringe-inducing self-promotional materials:

The Late Effects of Traumatic Brain Injury (LE-TBI) Project aims to learn more about the long-term effects of TBI in the general population … There is no brain bank in the United States that focuses on collecting brain tissue from individuals who survived a TBI. When brain tissue from TBI survivors becomes available, in most cases very little is known about the person before they died. The LE-TBI Project will address this problem by enrolling living TBI survivors into the LE-TBI Brain Donor Program. All participants involved in the LE-TBI Brain Donor Program at Mount Sinai will participate in an assessment of their cognitive, emotional, and behavioral functioning, an MRI [magnetic resonance imaging] scan, and genomic analysis. Those individuals who die during the course of the study and who consent to brain donation will undergo additional neuroimaging and an extensive neuropathological exam using techniques designed to identify the specific proteins involved in TBI. To date, this project represents the most systematic and scientifically rigorous effort to develop a more complete understanding of the long-term outcomes of single and multiple TBI. This study is unique in that it involves brain banking – traumatic brain injury has never been studied in the general population with brain autopsy as a major focus.

[1]

The methodological limitations of this project are obvious and fatal. It is entirely retrospective. No valid or reliable assessments will be made of pre-injury brain function or behavior. No valid or reliable assessments will be available regarding any TBI. No valid or reliable data will track the trajectory of brain or behavior change after injury. No properly selected controls (monozygotic twins discordant for injury) will be studied. As a result (and setting aside the principal investigator's apparent allegiance to a benighted nosology), the best possible outcome of this costly boondoggle will be to catalog a few case reports without knowing whether they are representative or what happened to the subjects. It would be generous to say that the findings will be hard to interpret.

And better research is in jeopardy. Functional neuroimaging is a work in progress. As explained earlier in this text, its findings and conclusions are inconsistent and not yet credible. Yet both editors of this volume predict that advances over the coming decades are likely to improve spatial and temporal resolution and biological validity. Once we can non-invasively video proteins folding and mitochondria respiring, we can better search for biomarkers of concussive brain injury (CBIs). That work is likely to reveal the secrets of concussion half a century before longitudinal studies are done. That work depends, of course, on knowing what's normal.

On August 11, 2017 the NIH announced that functional neuroimaging studies of normal people will be reclassified as "clinical trials." Throughout this text, the editors have championed the necessity of using words meaningfully. A *clinical trial* involves an intervention. The effect of that intervention on the health status of experimental subjects is compared with the effect of not intervening (or intervening differently) on control subjects. Typically, a clinical trial involves doing something to people with knives or chemicals. Non-invasive functional brain imaging of healthy people is not, in any honest world, a clinical trial. "Researchers say the new requirements … are unnecessary, and they will confuse the public and stifle basic cognitive studies" [2].

The present author agrees that protection of human subjects takes priority over all other clinical research considerations. He would merely inquire whether, in this case, the baby is being tossed with the bath water.

Neurology's Psychology: A Speculation

Neurology is a fascinating discipline with great potential. It has failed to live up to that potential. For more than 100 years, the field has been hamstrung by its resistance to logical nosology. As a result, it has underserved the interests of global public health. To help the suffering, one must figure out what's wrong and what works to mitigate that wrongness. Rigid loyalty to scientifically indefensible classifications of human distress derived from antiquated and ill-conceived paradigms is a dangerous drag on progress. The irrational assignment of artificial categorical distinctions across the continuum of TBI – for instance, the misleading persistence of the term "mild," contrary to the evidence of infinite continuity – has undermined generations of empirical work.

Why has neurology failed in this way? Absent concentrated, rigorous, objective study, one must remain humble about proposing a given chain of causality. The present author merely speculates and would instantly defer to any better-investigated explanation. That caveat confessed, one possibility comes to mind.

The author predicts that medical students and non-neurologist physicians, surveyed, would probably agree with the statement, "Neurologists are different." Respondents might not wrangle sufficient psychologizing rhetoric to better characterize their instinctive observation. For the sake of argument, what would respondents mean by "different"? One trait that is probably attributed to neurologists is relative emotional ease with neuroanatomy – a subject that often provokes dis-ease among students. Comfort with neuroanatomy seems to be dependent, at least in part, on three-dimensional visualization and mental rotation. Mental rotation is almost unique among cognitive constructs in the degree to which expertise depends on sex. Although sexual differences in human cognition are mostly subtle, mental rotation is the prototypical exception.

How might that cognitive trait pertain to neurologists' rigid defense of an indefensible nosology? Baron-Cohen [3] has theorized that autism spectrum mental disorders can be regarded as extreme maleness – an excessive concentration of XYness to the point of cerebral toxicity. In his view, the prototypical characteristic of XYness is systematization. That is, a tendency perhaps exists for XY humans to be biased in favor of systematizing their observations of perceived phenomena, while XXness is perhaps a little more strongly associated with a tendency toward empathy. These are obviously neither categorical associations – the overlap in the distribution curves is much more impressive than the separation of the modes – nor reliable ones. They are just barely detectable trends of yet-to-be-measured significance. So-called *systematizers* purportedly exhibit several other traits. These people tend to be socially awkward and insensitive to others' feelings. Their decisions tend to be final, even in the light of new evidence. They may be deficient in theory of mind; perhaps they're a bit short on mirror neurons? And they tend to be enthusiasts of authoritarian dogma who are intolerant of ambiguity.

In fact, the vast majority of humans are blessed with complex mixtures of traits that are sometimes labeled "male" or "female" to satisfy a desperation for irrationally simplistic order in the universe. Thus, one may credit the Baron-Cohen school for detecting important human behavioral traits and their tendency to cluster, but that legitimate observation deserves a better conceptual framework than "extreme male." As always, inventing a dichotomy is a pitiful way to describe nature's continuum. There are not warring tribes of male systematizers and female empaths. Everyone has some degree of both traits.

That caveat in mind, one admits that these traits exist, and one suspects that different occupational identities might attract those with more of one trait and less of another. Medical students run the personality gamut. A tiny minority choose to become neurologists. Conceivable, self-selection favors that choice among those who are especially attracted to the concrete comforts of three-dimensional mechanics and ill at ease in a vacuum of labels. That would help to explain the Swiss Watch Fallacy of the localizationists – the unseemly eagerness, directly evolved from Gall and Spurzheim's phrenology [4], to assign specific functions to bits of cortex as if it were a timepiece. (Perhaps the same desire for black-and-white certainty helps explain why a small subset of neuropsychologists cling to the claims that paper-and-pencil tests validly and reliably detect brain damage and that neuropsychological tests find the focus of harm.) Intolerance of ambiguity would also bias those bearing this phenotypic trait toward embracing arbitrary, artificially certain classifications to soothe their dread of uncertainty. "Hey, better to use the phrase 'Alzheimer's disease' without having demonstrated any specific biological meaning than to suffer the indignity of saying, 'We have yet to conceptualize the boundaries of normal aging.'"

If this type of cognitive bias is commonplace among neurologists it would favor the perpetuation of resistance to acknowledging new empirical data that threaten their fortress of dogma. Moreover, if neurologists who most assertively display resistance to rational classification are judged to be prototypical among their peers, social psychology predicts those will become our leaders. As a result, one might be concerned that the innate conservatism of neurology has assisted close-minded persons to become chairpersons of departments, chairs of study sections, and journal editors. The demagoguery of systematizers, in consequence, may represent a structural barrier to the promotion of open minded assistant professors and to progress in medical discovery.

The need for cognitive closure and intolerance of ambiguity are by no means unique to neurologists. Neither physicians (of any variety) nor patients can function comfortably without faith in some system. For that reason, disease naming is a necessary evil – even if it is premature, misguided, and risks causing harm and death due to stiff-necked loyalty to biologically bankrupt diagnoses. One can bemoan this pre-Enlightenment tradition in neurology, but only with fair-minded acknowledgment of its inevitability and comforting powers. Unless and until science advances to the point that empiricism supports more logical and rational classification and the weight of evidence grows sufficiently to squash the daemons of dogmatic conservatism, who can fault medicine's popular faith in cupping, bleeding, clysters, and "Alzheimer's disease"?

What Might Help?

It is traditional, to the point of being boilerplate, to end a scientific document with a plea. Most often, that plea is for money. Too often, that plea is preceded by a rather egregious deviation from scientific expression. "Having honestly reported our materials, methods, results, and conclusions – having acknowledged the limitations inherent in our approach and dressed our opinions in the piebald motley of false humility – we now abandon all restraint to nakedly declare that we have no idea how to interpret our results but our lab's pizza budget and the future well-being of humanity are dependent on the research dollars we personally scare up with this sentence."

Periodically, in this collaborative book, authors have noted limitations that have delayed progress in understanding concussive brain injury. In many cases, those limitations have more to do with failures of imagination and rigorous thought than of adequate funding. In some cases – such as the limits of certainty due to inordinate reliance on cross-sectional rather than longitudinal research and numbers far too small to permit stratification by more than a couple of the large number of obvious confounding variables – funding is indeed a rate-limited factor. For example, the renowned U.S. neuropathologist, Ann McKee, recently and eloquently crystallized how money could revolutionize knowledge in the domain of sports-related CBI:

We need a very well-constructed longitudinal study looking at young individuals playing these sports. We need to follow them for decades. We need to take measurements throughout their lives and playing careers so we can begin to detect when things start to go wrong. If we can detect early changes, that's when we could really make a difference.
[5]

The present author heartily agrees. He will, however, make a less traditional plea.

Among the uncertainties surrounding our subject, one of the most compelling is the uncertainty regarding how much our subject matters. If typical, clinically attended CBIs are as common as estimated in Chapter 2, and if symptomatic

persistent traumatic encephalopathy is as common as reported in Chapter 5, and if both symptomatic and asymptomatic persistent encephalopathy predispose concussion survivors to acceleration of time-passing-related brain changes, then about ten million new concussion survivors are created in the United States each year, of whom about 3.6 million are lastingly impaired in a grossly apparent way and as many as ten million will be harmed in a way that might multiply the risk of that person becoming a long-term burden to his or her family and society. The magnitude of the health impact on the population is dynamic, since new brain-impaired people replace those with apparent recovery or death. Yet we may be on the cusp of a crisis, since traumatic brain change is spreading with the aging (and falling) of the global population.

Violating our own recommendation and dichotomizing a continuum, there are two possibilities:

1. CBI is a major global public health problem.
2. CBI is not a major global public health problem.

But we don't know! Unlike some public health problems, the dimensions of this threat are hard to nail down.

If number 1 is true, then, like man-made global warming, due to more accurate interpretation of existing data, new data, and the paradigm shifts outlined in this volume, the current generation has just discovered a massive threat to humanity and must take immediate action. A gigantic escalation in funding for translatable research is justified and would perhaps be highly cost-efficient. If number 2 is true, then not so much. The truth is inaccessible at the time of this writing.

How soon will we know the answer? Progress is finally under way. As discussed in the Introduction, at least three recently funded large-scale projects will follow concussion survivors longitudinally: (1) the National Study on the Effects of Concussion in Collegiate Athletes and U.S. Military Service Academy Members (CARE consortium) [6]; (2) the Transforming Research and Clinical Knowledge in Traumatic Brain Injury (TRACK-TBI) study [7]; and (3) the Chronic Effects of Neurotrauma Consortium (CENC) multicenter observational study [8]. Unfortunately, none actualizes the vision of a long-term population–based prospective cohort study in the vein of Framingham. Therefore, none will tell us the magnitude of the human threat. Still, simply knowing the spectrum of long-term clinical courses among thousands of similarly assessed CBI survivors will be a tremendous advance. Within 50 years we be better able to estimate the proportion of such patients likely to exhibit lasting harm.

Therefore, rather than begging for more money to study CBI, the present author will focus a plea on two inextricably intertwined issues.

One: it would be good to know whether number 1 or 2 is true. Setting aside the myriad domains of TBI inquiry deserving our sustained attention, perhaps the highest-priority question society should try to answer is, "How much does it matter whether we understand – and learn to mitigate the effects of – CBI?" That is, *some* escalation of research funding is already justified by the *possibility* that a gigantic escalation is required and our urgent need to determine whether that is in fact the case. Funding *must* be found to support big, sophisticated studies just to answer our preliminary question: how common are disabling late effects (including an increased risk of neurobehavioral troubles five to 75 years post injury)?

Two: in order for the universe of interested parties to work collectively and collaboratively toward finding the correct answer to that preliminary question, a sufficient number of individual scholars must assert their freedom from cant. Sometimes, Dr. Bigler and I dream that this brief introductory textbook might encourage a quiet intellectual renaissance and incite an academic revolution. Vividly aware of our own limitations, and of the innate conservatism of neurology, we cannot expect that. Yet the tyranny of terms of art must be defeated. The fallacy of illogical nosologies must be exposed. The cycle of slavish replication of bad hypothesis testing in the hopes of publications and grants must be broken. If we have supported a baby step in the direction of truth, we will die content.

Thus we complete the circle, closing in on a concept introduced in this book's Introduction: the political psychology of concussion research.

An Invitation to Young Thinkers

Medicine has become an anti-intellectual guild. Need proof? Ask your primary care provider to define "disease." Out of compassion, when you hear what next comes from his or her mouth, restrain your guffaw.

At the time of this writing (21st-century CE) moral intellectual children both self-select and are bureaucratically selected away from medical careers.[1] Still, although medicine is unfriendly to moral thinkers, it desperately needs them. Young readers who may happen to stumble upon this prose are invited to weigh the risks and benefits: in its favor, medicine is a milieu with a higher proportion of well-intentioned practitioners than politics, street gangs, or investment banking. Pursued with realistic expectations, well-being can occasionally be found in some medical careers. If you are one of those who slip through the cracks and, against all odds, find yourself with an MD, have fun! Frustration at medicine's systematic resistance to serious thought is distracting. Resentment is self-indulgent. Just brace yourself for a decade of inequitable assignment to the Dalit stratum of a primitive caste system, keep your eyes wide open, and do your best for patients.

Thoughtful readers may be outraged at the current state of medical care – especially in the United States. Human misery is unnecessarily magnified and prolonged by willful ignorance – in medicine as in politics and interpersonal relations. That, however, is the way of the world. Outrage is justifiable. Surprise is not. A revolution would have to occur for neurology to think through its miserable nosology and correct it. A revolution would have to occur for medical schools to attract and select youth who are moral and intellectual. Come the revolution, the

editors of this book will be dead. We have a strategy, however, to stay in touch with readers: new evidence shows that some of you will be built from quarks that once built us! We will try to pass on the good ones.

Concussive Brain Injury Meets the Law

The present author feels compelled to make one additional plea. It is a less important, lower-priority plea than understanding concussion. Yet the quality of perhaps thousands of lives and the redistribution of perhaps hundreds of millions of dollars are at stake every year. Sometimes a CBI results in a legal action. Under those trying circumstances, one wishes for polices that encourage virtue.

Both editors of this text occasionally try to understand cases under litigation. The experience is strange and often disheartening. Medical training isolates one in the bubble of Hippocrates. The goal of one's existence becomes to figure out the truth and use that to help dis-eased people. Many who join the clergy perhaps have a similar goal. Teachers, military volunteers, public safety officers, journalists, and (in very rare cases) political activists possibly share a similar vulnerability to the allure of altruism. Lawyers who focus on injury claims? Western law banished morality as an attorney's guiding star about 2000 years ago. Expert witnesses? In the United Kingdom, expert witnesses are free from pressures to tilt their testimony. They serve the court, not the attorney. In the United States, experts are pressured to act badly. Too often, they do.

Where did Expert Witnesses Come From?

Few readers will have met John Smeaton. More will know of the sunny morning in 1763 when he introduced the use of hydraulic lime in concrete. Even those readers may have forgotten Smeaton's other claim to notoriety. Silting threatened to make Well's Harbour, Norfolk, unnavigable. A solution was needed, but it would be costly for someone. In 1782, an English judge invited the greatest civil engineer of the time (Mr. Smeaton) to provide expert testimony. Since then, and increasingly so since the mid 20th century, the United Kingdom has turned to experts to teach and explain technical matters.

One could trace the employment of expert witnesses back even further, perhaps to the days when Roman Emperor Claudius ill-advisedly invented lawyers. That is, unlike the Greeks who prohibited advocates from taking money, Claudius for the first time approved a profession of men who sought payment (as much as 10,000 sesterces) to attend court and advocate on behalf of others.

The predictable result? While medical schools inculcate a value – do good – law schools don't. Justice is mentioned in passing, like a celebrity's driveway on a Hollywood tour. The law student is often educated by mentors who set aside concerns about truth and right, justice and virtue, and instead

---

[1] The author was once asked to better specify his call for moral selectivity in medical school admissions. The best he could come up with on the fly: "A senior medical school student who has yet to publicly criticize a full professor for insensitivity to patients probably does not deserve to have gained admission." As the old saying (which the author just invented) goes: the trembling hare does nothing for the husk.

demonstrate how to seek money by persuading judges and juries with articulate guile. It is testimony to the courage of a laudable minority that they escape from law school with ideals.[2]

In the Middle Ages, inquisitions were widely employed instead of trials. In an inquisition, the jury is composed of people brought in by the court due to their special knowledge of the matter at hand. Inquisitions, in effect, sought justice by empaneling a jury of experts. Medieval experts were granted a fair amount of leeway and became creative in the application of truth extraction methods, although recent evidence suggests that truth is not the most common result of torture. But a Renaissance transition occurred in Britain. In a dramatic turnabout from the inquisitional system, jurors were selected based on their *lack* of knowledge of the case [9, 10]. That is why today jurors are routinely disqualified if they possess special knowledge relevant to the case. This transition required that verdicts be rendered entirely on the basis of direct witness knowledge, e.g. "I jumped off my wombat, grabbed my longbow, and there she was."

The predictable result? Whenever lay or "common" knowledge was insufficient to analyze a witnessed fact, the British court might solicit the help of a teacher and explainer. One interesting consequence: expert witnesses in the British system play a role that is virtually the opposite of that played by all other witnesses. As Coke clarified in 1622: "tis no satisfaction for a witness to say that he 'thinketh' or 'persuadeth himself'" [11]. In other words, for almost every witness, opinion is not testimony. For experts, in contrast, opinion is *exactly* what is sought. Experts are expected to rely on their own informed knowledge and conclusions about a subject. Baker (1992) explained:

> Although witnesses are generally governed by the opinion rule, expert witnesses have never been subject to the rule. The opinion rule and the use of expert testimony developed to fill a need for information resulting from the transformation to the adversarial trial system.
>
> ([11], p. 326)

Consider the incentives of the adversaries in a species that still lacks accurate lie detection. Plaintiffs and defendants, of course, seek their own self-interests. As much as one hopes for honesty, the system rewards duplicity. Advocates (lawyers) for plaintiffs and defendants are animated by the same drivers. To maximize their incomes, the Western system obliges attorneys to prioritize winning over truth or justice. Judges and jurors, if they truly have no special knowledge or stake in the outcome, are thankfully free from that pressure to dissimulate – although

they invariably bring to the bench a lifetime of cognitive biases, gaps in knowledge, and emotional confounders. Expert witnesses, under the British system, are similarly, gloriously, free from perverse incentives. They may have biases particular to their guild or personal pride, but hopefully not particular to the plaintiff or defendant. The British expert's duty is to the court. As stated by the U.K. Ministry of Justice's Rules and Practice Directions under its Procedural Rules for the Civil Courts pertaining to Experts and Assessors, Part 35, Rule 35.3 [12]:

1. It is the duty of experts to help the court on matters within their expertise.
2. This duty overrides any obligation to the person from whom experts have received instructions or by whom they are paid.

U.S. Deviance

Things are different in the United States. Exceptionalism, in this case, is unworthy of a boast. As Timmerbeil put it [13]: "The U.S. civil trial system seems to be basically a battle of the parties in which the lawyers are protagonists and warlords."

Although every state has its own Code of Civil Procedures, many are direct descendants of the U.S. Federal Code. The most relevant five Federal Rules of Evidence (FREs):

1. FRE 702: Testimony by Expert Witnesses
2. FRE 703: Bases of an Expert
3. FRE 704: Opinion on an Ultimate Issue
4. FRE 705: Disclosing the Facts or Data Underlying an Expert
5. FRE 706: Court-Appointed Expert Witnesses.

Each makes good reading. Yet the idiosyncratic nature of U.S. civil jurisprudence is instantly apparent. The U.K. Ministry for Justice requires that experts work for the court – that is, for justice. The U.S. code begins with lip service to that goal: One of the four desirable qualifications for an expert under FRE 702 is that "the expert's scientific, technical, or other specialized knowledge will help the trier of fact to understand the evidence or to determine a fact in issue" [14]. That defines a *capacity* to help. *Yet nothing in the code requires the expert to actually provide that help!*

The FRE does not formally define the duties of an expert witness nor does it contain any specific written obligation for the expert to be independent. This distinction between the UK and US jurisdictions has prompted views of greater expert partisanship in the US. Nevertheless, there

---

[2] One is gratified to encounter many exceptional attorneys, typically active in altruistic by-ways such as legal aid, public defense, environmental defense, and non-governmental organizations (e.g., Human Rights Watch). Consider for a moment a revolutionary idea: what if, as medical schools idealize the selfless provision of health care, law schools idealized the selfless provision of justice? What if America thumbed its nose at Emperor Claudius, entombed his adversarial system in a distant asteroid, and reinvented the purpose of lawyers? Can the reader imagine a world in which that entire profession was devoted to doing the right thing? Lawyers would be an astonishing boon to civil life. That seems implausible, yet there are already judges and mediators. In the present author's admittedly untutored opinion, America would profit if society devised some way to distinguish between justice-seeking attorneys and the others. Since they serve different muses, they deserve different titles. Justice seekers might be celebrated like firemen, and awarded the honorific *Juris Doctor and Prince of Peace*. The others? Perhaps *Dog Food with a Degree*.

appears to be little enthusiasm for any change in the FRE to deal with this and the US appears to be content with the current governance of experts.

(Huyghe & Chan, 2013 [15], p. 16)

What do the other rules say? FRE 703 only discusses the source of opinions. FRE 704 allows the expert to opine regarding ultimate issues. FRE 705 frees the expert to announce his or her opinion without discussing the relevant facts. Timmerbeil again [13]:

In U.S. civil litigation … The party has the choice which expert it hires. This so-called "expert shopping" gives the party the opportunity to hire an expert who best supports the party's view. The parties are not interested "in finding the best scientist, but the best witness" … However, this is not the end. It is likely that the defendant will also hire an expert. Of course, the defendant will select an expert who supports the defendant's view.

One could argue that Western justice took one hit in ancient Rome, when Claudius legalized paid advocates, and a second hit across the pond, when U.S. authorities legalized expert shopping.

However: a flicker of light appears at the end of the tunnel. There is FRE 706. FRE 706 states: "The court may appoint any expert that the parties agree on and any of its own choosing." That means judges need not plug their ears with sealing wax and doze through the biased rants of paid experts. If they really want the truth, they can hire an impartial expert.

Many readers may have blinked with surprise. "Huh? When did this happen? I never heard of such a thing! That's a great idea! Why don't they do it all the time?"

Good question. Here is a good answer:

Court-appointed experts are rarely used in U.S. civil litigation. A survey of federal judges revealed that 81% had never appointed an expert under FRE 706, and only 8% had appointed a court expert more than one time. The court does not often appoint its own expert because of the adversarial tradition and the problem of compensation, despite FRE 706. Moreover, many judges and lawyers may be unaware of the possibility to appoint a court expert.

(Timmerbeil, 2003 [13], p. 168)

That last sentence, to the present author, is astounding. Since expert shopping is a glaring fault of U.S. jurisprudence and FRE 706 is ready at hand to enhance the odds of justice, how does it happen that American judges are unaware?

By the way, the United Kingdom is not the only place where the expert's duty is to help the court. German rules of evidence regarding expert testimony (*Sachverständigenbeweis*) are equally well crafted to facilitate the quest for truth:

Contrary to U.S. practice, the parties do not nominate their own expert witnesses but designate the factual allegations to be submitted to an expert. The selection and appointment of the expert is the responsibility of the court.

(Bastuck & Gopfert, 1994 [16], p. 616)

The present author has almost no knowledge of law. Others are far better suited to addressing these weighty issues. Nonetheless, after more than 25 years of expert testimony, he cannot help but have formed an opinion. In his opinion, civil litigation regarding TBI in the United States is deeply flawed, often denies jurors truths about brains, and routinely heartless. Built-in incentives to lie and cheat infest the process from top to bottom. Add to that the rarity of authentic TBI expertise and the legitimate confusion about the nature of brain injury, and one has written the recipe to bake injustice. In this respect – as in the delivery of health care – the United States stands ashamed before the rest of the modern world.

Where Lies Hope?

The present author sees two promptly accessible balms for this socio-political disease. The problem, in each case, is the need for virtue.

One has already been mentioned: FRE 706. Speaking with almost a dozen judges in recent years, the author has asked the same question: "How come federal judges almost never retain experts – almost never take advantage of this brilliant stratagem for enhancing justice?" In every case but one (the last judge did not know she could retain experts), the answer was the same: inadequate funding. The courts are overburdened. The judges are close to being overwhelmed. And who wants to pay for scientific truth, when the attorneys will gladly hire biased explainers on their own dimes?

The answer to finding the money to liberate America from biased experts is so far afield from the author's limited domains of study as to rival alien mathematics. He cannot even begin to mull the socio-economic–legal–public policy steps that could actualize FRE 706's potential in the U.S. federal, state, and municipal court systems. Yet if other modern nations can do it, he must ask those with better vision: "Why can't we?"

The Duty Clause

The second mitigator that comes to mind is perhaps even more far-fetched than asking judges to follow federal law. It involves asking experts to do the right thing.

The present author has no way of predicting whether this book will be read. If it is read, there is no way to predict its influence. In candor, one cannot expect much. The ingrained incentives of U.S. tradition present a virtually impermeable barrier to the diffusion of justice into civil torts. Trial lawyers will surely remain wealthy so long as they fight to maintain the perverse status quo. Congress will not act without pressure from constituents, few of whom read Holdsworth for pleasure. Experts are completely disorganized and many seem to slaver over the lucre they get by misrepresenting science in court. And the only way this issue might come before the Supreme Court is if some day an ideal case arises that exposes the question: "Does paying scientists to advocate, an obviously bad idea, comport with the Constitution?"

There is, however, a simple solution. A voluntary duty clause.

The present author has struggled for decades to optimize the terms of contracts that will fairly alert attorneys to his atypical position: he is occasionally willing to evaluate a forensic neurobehavioral matter. He may even accept dollars from attorneys if they regard truth as a good investment. He will never work for an attorney. His duty is solely to the court and to the triers of fact. The amount of money that would sway his opinion does not exist on Earth.

Three factors undermine his policy. First, preliminary evidence suggests that he is human.[3] Second, few attorneys believe him until it is too late. Third, his region is overrun with doctors claiming TBI expertise. Attorneys can effortlessly find a paragon of moral laxity.

Awareness of the U.K.'s Rule 35.3 has been handy. The author now includes a brief clause in his contracts to harmonize with that language:

> The expert agrees to retention on the condition that the retaining attorney knows and accepts the expert's duty. The expert's duty is to the court. The expert will make a concerted and impartial effort to understand a case scientifically. The expert will make a concerted and impartial effort to teach and explain that science to the judge and triers of fact.

The inclusion of this duty clause in his every contract might possibly increase the likelihood of communicating to the attorney that the expert rejects the U.S. tradition of expert mendacity. It possibly pre-empts some later expressions of shock when he tells the truth. It does nothing, however, to defeat the damage done by the hoards of dishonest experts. That would require cooperation.

Collective Bargaining

Let's start small. How about California? The author hereby proposes a collective initiative – and a challenge. He pleads: if every neurologist and neuropsychologist licensed in California includes the duty clause in his or her forensic contracts, dishonest Southwestern attorneys will find it more difficult to conspire with a doctor to defraud a judge and jury. Of course, they can shop elsewhere. Globalization has made that clear. But collective bargaining, in which a guild or union insists on minimum basic standards, has somewhat revolutionized some human enterprises. Doctors are not joiners. Many are cowboys at heart. But only a cooperative effort of this kind could turn the tide. Unless and until U.S. jurisprudence matures to meet the ethical standards of Western democracies, such grassroots initiatives may be one of the few methods we can employ to fight for that which is right and good.

Conclusion

Dr. Bigler and I hope that this brief introductory textbook on CBI will excite a scholarly renaissance and incite an academic revolution, all to the benefit of the patient. Vividly aware of our own limitations, and of the innate conservatism of neurology, we must not count on that. Yet the tyranny of terms of art must be defeated. The fallacy of illogical nosologies must be exposed. The cycle of slavish replication of bad hypothesis testing in the hopes of publications and grants must be broken. If we have supported a baby step in the direction of truth, we will die content.

A book is inanimate. A thought? Not so clear. But one thing is clear: without a thoughtful reader, this book has all the precious value of a pail of sand. Dr. Bigler and I realize who is really most worthy of acknowledgment: only you can bring these words to life.

References

1. Late effects of traumatic brain injury. ID number 13–0751. Icahn School of Medicine at Mt. Sinai. Available at: http://icahn.mssm.edu/research/clinical-trials/health-topics/aging/13–0751.
2. Anonymous. Clinical trial definition expands. *Science* 2017;357:736.
3. Baron-Cohen S. The evolution of empathizing and systematizing: Assortative mating of two strong systematizers and the cause of autism. In: Dunbar R, Barrett L, editors. *Oxford handbook of evolutionary psychology*. Oxford, UK: Oxford University Press, 2009.
4. Gall FJ, Spurzheim JC. *Anatomie et physiologie du système nerveux en général, et du cerveau en particulier*. Paris: Schoell, 1810.
5. McKee A. Interview by Tom Goldman T. National Public Radio; All things considered, July 25th 2017. Available at www.npr.org/2017/07/25/539198429/study-cte-found-in-nearly-all-donated-nfl-player-brains.
6. Broglio SP, McCrea M, McAllister T, Harezlak J, Katz B, Hack D, et al. A national study on the effects of concussion in collegiate athletes and US Military Service Academy members: The NCAA–DoD Concussion Assessment, Research and Education (CARE) Consortium structure and methods. *Sports Med* 2017;47:1437–1451.
7. Track-TBI. Transforming Research and Clinical Knowledge in Traumatic Brain Injury. International Traumatic Brain Injury Research Initiative. Available at https://tracktbi.ucsf.edu/.
8. Walker WC, Carne W, Franke LM, Nolen T, Dikmen SD, Cifu DX, et al. The Chronic Effects of Neurotrauma Consortium (CENC) multi-centre observational study: Description of study and characteristics of early participants. *Brain Injury* 2016; 30:1469–1480.
9. Holdsworth WS. *A history of English law*. New York: Little Brown, 1924.
10. Pollock F, Maitland FW. *The history of English law*, vol. 1: *Before the time of Edward I*, 2nd edition. Cambridge, UK: Cambridge University Press, 1968.

---

[3] One earnestly attempts to be utterly impartial. Ideally, by bravely seeking insight and facing our own embarrassing limits we can become alert to our prejudices and then nimbly dodge the errors of unconscious bias. But (as Freud perhaps discovered on his death bed), true insight is not available in this life. In a valuable recent book, Mercier and Sperber discuss human reason. They eloquently expose the hogwash of rationality among those who sport human brains. Bias is an evolutionary treat [17]. Zebrafish brains? The evidence regarding prejudice is mixed. Human brains? Biased. The author, therefore, is duty-bound to confess that, best intentions notwithstanding, if he has a human brain he is biased.

11. Baker TE. The impropriety of expert witness testimony on the law. 40 *U Kan L Rev* 1992; 325–364. Available at: http://ecollections.law.fiu.edu/faculty_publications/180.

12. U.K. Ministry of Justice. Courts. Procedure rules; civil; Rules & practice directions, Part 35: Experts and assessors. Available at: www.justice.gov.uk/courts/procedurerules/civil/rules/part35#IDASLICC.

13. Timmerbeil S. The role of expert witnesses in German and U.S. civil litigation. *Ann Survey Int Compar Law* 2003;9:Article 8. Available at: http://digitalcommons.law.ggu.edu/annlsurvey/vol9/iss1/8.

14. Federal Rules of Evidence. Washington, DC: U.S. Government Printing Office, 2014. Available at www.uscourts.gov/sites/default/files/Rules%20of%20Evidence.

15. Huyghe S, Chan A. The evolution of expert witness law under UK and US jurisdictions. *Construction Law Int* 2013;8:14–18.

16. Bastuck B, Gopfert B. Admission and presentation of evidence in Germany; 16. *Loyola LA Int Comp Law Rev* 1994;16:609–627. Available at: http://digitalcommons.lmu.edu/ilr/vol16/iss3/1.

17. Mercier H, Sperber D. *The enigma of reason*. Cambridge, MA: Harvard University Press, 2017.

Index

second impact syndrome, 103, 113
Sensory Organization Test (SOT), 676
sex differences in outcomes in pediatric patients, 652
sex differences in risk, 112–13
sideline tools, 672–75
skateboarding, 126
skiing, 126
snowboarding, 126
soccer, 126–28
Sport Concussion Assessment Tool - 3rd edition (SCAT-3), 675
sports participation rates, 110–11
Standardized Assessment of Concussion (SAC), 673
summary of assessment tools, 679–80
symptom checklists, 672–73
taekwondo, 124
virtual reality (VR) testing environment, 676–77
why prevalence of brain injury may never be known, 128–29
wrestling, 127
Sports Concussion Assessment Tool (SCAT), 647–48, 657
sports neuropsychology, 411–12
Sports Neuropsychology Society, 411
Standardized Assessment of Concussion (SAC), 653, 657, 673
straw man issue of mind/body dualism, 328
stress granules (SGs), 171
Stress Inoculation Training (SIT), 449, 469
stress vulnerability genes, 312–13
Stressful Life Events Screening Questionnaire, 459
stretch or strain forces in CBI, 139
striatum, 388, 389
Strich, Sabrina, 50, 60–61, 262
structural MRI, 263–75
range of techniques, 264
structural neuroimaging, 263
future technologies, 633–35
near-future technologies, 632–33
persistent or delayed-onset encephalopathy following repeated CBI, 630–31
potential contributions to TBI management, 635
present technologies, 631–32
Structured Interview for TBI Diagnosis, 687, 689
Stuss, DT, 406
subconcussions, 65, 528
functional neuroimaging, 564–65

neuroimaging of repeated subconcussive trauma, 567
pediatric patients, 664–65
substance use in TBI patients, 751
Suicidal Behaviors Questionnaire–Revised, 436
Suicide Ideation Questionnaire, 436
suprachiasmatic nucleus (SCN), 757
suvorexant, 764
SWI (susceptibility weighted imaging), 264t6.1
Swiss Watch Theory of Behavioral Neurology, 22, 292–93, 296, 402
Symbol Digit Modalities Task (mSDMT), 746
Symonds, Charles, 55, 56, 154, 212, 249, 328
symptom checklists, 672–73
symptoms
assessment of pediatric patients, 657
denial, 346
imaginary/intentional dichotomy, 13–14
misplaced faith in a dated trichotomy, 11–14
organic/psychological dichotomy, 12–13
pressures on athletes not to report, 25–26
under-reporting, 353
syndrome of inappropriate antidiuresis (SIAD), 773

T-maze, 166
T-tau biomarker, 640
taekwondo
concussion risk, 124
tau
disruption by axonal stretch in TBI, 332–34
hyperphosphorylation and aggregation, 639
pathology after TBI, 576–78
role in neurodegeneration, 168–71
as a serum biomarker, 642
tau oligomers
efforts to mitigate late effects in CBI, 543–44
role in late effects of CBI, 543–44
tauopathy
in CTE, 527
inflammatory hypothesis of development, 536
relationship to repeated CBI, 534
risk in persons exposed to repeated concussions, 534–35
role in CTE, 530–32

seeding hypothesis of development, 536
vascular hypothesis of development, 536
TBI Identification Clinical Interview, 687
TBI Quality of Life (TBI-QOL) Fatigue Short Form, 748t24.2
TDP-43 biomarker, 642
TDP-43 proteinopathies, 537–38
Tedeschi, C.G., 59–60
Tef gene, 762
temporomandibular joint dysfunction (TMJD) headache caused by, 731
tension-type headache, 732–33
testosterone replacement therapy, 776
Teuber, Hans-Lucas, 3
thalamus, 179, 388
Thematic Apperception Test (TAT), 403
third occipital nerve headache, 732
threat response
abnormal response following TBI, 447–48
three-month myth, 210–12
thyroid stimulating hormone (TSH), 767
deficiency symptoms, 768t26.1
deficiency treatment, 776
time after impact of CBI
outcome variance related to, 302–5
Trail Making tests, 405
transcriptomics, 305–10
Transforming Research and Clinical Knowledge in TBI (TRACK-TBI), 710
trauma-triggered migraine, 734–35
traumatic brain injury (TBI)
distinguishing mild TBI from PTSD, 390
overlap of symptoms with PTSD, 390
structural brain changes overlap with PTSD, 392–93
Traumatic Brain Injury Act, 6, 7
traumatic encephalopathy
classification of TBI-induced neurodegenerative disorders, 578–79
etiologies, 582
features of, 582
lack of clinical diagnostic criteria, 582
neuropathology, 582
origin of the term, 582
original meaning of the term, 526–27
terms used to describe, 582
traumatic encephalopathy review
approach to review of published cases, 582

challenges to discovery of diagnostic criteria, 585–91
lack of clinical diagnostic criteria, 582
limitations of the review process, 585–91
method, 583
provisional research diagnostic criteria, 585
results, 583–85
Traumatic Life Events Questionnaire, 687
treatment after mTBI
appropriate interventions, 780
mTBI as a diagnostic construct, 780–81
post-concussive symptoms, 781
treatment-seeking CBI patients, 781
treatment of CBI
acute and sub-acute management, 793–94
balancing rest versus activity, 794–95
fatigue management, 794–95
guiding principles for clinical practice, 793–96
neurobiology as a guiding principle, 794
post-acute assessment, 794
prioritizing and treating comorbidities, 795
tailoring subsequent treatment to the individual, 795–96
treatment research systematic review, 781–82
challenge to define evidence-based rehabilitation interventions, 791–93
clarifying the construct, 793
clinical question, 782
cognitive rehabilitation, 783–88
determination of practice recommendations, 783
discussion, 791–93
early brief interventions, 791
early single session interventions, 791
exercise interventions, 789–90
guiding principles for clinical practice, 793–96
heterogeneity of the CBI population, 793
inclusion/exclusion criteria, 782–83
lack of consistent outcome measures, 792
methodology, 782
mixed, multidisciplinary interventions, 790–91